Clinical
Ocular
Pharmacology

Clinical Ocular Pharmacology

Third Edition

Edited by

Jimmy D. Bartlett, O.D., D.O.S.
Professor of Optometry, University of Alabama at Birmingham, School of Optometry;
Professor of Pharmacology, Department of Pharmacology and Toxicology, University
of Alabama, School of Medicine, Birmingham

Siret D. Jaanus, Ph.D.
Professor of Pharmacology, Department of Biological Sciences, State University of
New York, State College of Optometry, New York; Professor Emeritus, Southern
California College of Optometry, Fullerton

Butterworth–Heinemann
Boston   Oxford   Melbourne   Singapore   Toronto   Munich   New Delhi   Tokyo

Library of Congress Cataloging-in-Publication Data

Clinical ocular pharmacology / edited by Jimmy D. Bartlett, Siret D. Jaanus. — 3rd ed.
        p.   cm.
    Includes bibliographical references and index.
    ISBN 0-7506-9448-3 (hc)
    1. Ocular pharmacology.   I. Bartlett, Jimmy D.   II. Jaanus, Siret D.
    [DNLM: 1. Eye Diseases—drug therapy.   2. Eye—drug effects.   WW 166 C641 1995]
    RE994.C55   1995
    617.7'061—dc20
    DNLM/DLC
    for Library of Congress   95-19146
                                                                           CIP

British Library Cataloguing-in-Publication Data
A catalogue record for this book is available from the British Library.

The publisher offers discounts on bulk orders of this book.
For information, please write:

Manager of Special Sales
Butterworth–Heinemann
313 Washington Street
Newton, MA 02158–1626

10 9 8 7 6 5 4 3 2

Printed in the United States of America

*Dedicated to the profession of optometry
and to those individuals who have inspired and guided
our professional lives.*

Contents

Contributing Authors

Larry J. Alexander, O.D.
Adjunct Professor of Optometry, University of
Alabama at Birmingham, School of Optometry,
Birmingham; Director, Department of Comprehensive
Consultative Optometry, Retina Associates Public
Service Corporation, Louisville
  *23. Neuro-Ophthalmic Disorders; 32. Diseases of
  the Retina*

David M. Amos, O.D.
Private Practice, Overland Park; Consultant, Kansas
City Veterans Administration Medical Center, Kansas
City, Missouri; formerly, Associate Professor of
Ophthalmology, Department of Ophthalmology,
University of Kansas Medical Center, Kansas City
  *22. Cycloplegic Refraction; 34.Pharmacologic
  Management of Strabismus*

John F. Amos, O.D., M.S.
Professor and Chair, Department of Optometry and
Director of the Professional Program, University of
Alabama at Birmingham, School of Optometry,
Birmingham
  22. Cycloplegic Refraction

Jimmy D. Bartlett, O.D., D.O.S.
Professor of Optometry, University of Alabama at
Birmingham, School of Optometry; Professor of
Pharmacology, Department of Pharmacology and
Toxicology, University of Alabama, School of
Medicine, Birmingham
  *1. Pharmacotherapy of the Ophthalmic Patient;
  3. Ophthalmic Drug Delivery; 6. Local Anesthetics;
  7. Analgesics for Treatment of Acute Ocular Pain;
  10. Antiglaucoma Drugs; 20. Topical and Regional
  Anesthesia; 21. Dilation of the Pupil; 23. Neuro-
  Ophthalmic Disorders; 24. Diseases of the Eyelids;
  35. Medical Management of the Glaucomas;
  37. Ocular Effects of Systemic Drugs*

Debra J. Bezan, M.Ed., O.D.
Professor of Optometry, Northeastern State University,
College of Optometry; Clinic Director, Department of
Optometry, W.W. Hastings Indian Health Service
Hospital, Tahlequah, Oklahoma
  31. Postoperative Care of the Cataract Patient

Kari E. Blaho, Ph.D.
Research Director, Department of Emergency Medicine
and Clinical Toxicology, University of Tennessee,
College of Medicine, Memphis
  19. Adjunctive Agents

Neal L. Burstein, Ph.D.
Director, The Rabbi Mordecai M. Burstein Library of
Vision, Boulder
  2. Ophthalmic Drug Formulations

John H. Carter, O.D., Ph.D. (deceased)
Professor of Bioscience, The New England College of
Optometry, Boston
  9. Cycloplegics

Linda Casser, O.D.
Associate Professor of Optometry, Indiana University,
School of Optometry, Bloomington; Director,
Indianapolis Eye Care Center, Indiana University,
Indianapolis
  27. Diseases of the Cornea

John G. Classé, O.D., J.D.
Professor of Optometry, University of Alabama at
Birmingham, School of Optometry, Birmingham;
Member of the Bar of Alabama
  5. Legal Aspects of Drug Utilization

Richard J. Clompus, O.D.
Adjunct Faculty, Pennsylvania College of Optometry, Philadelphia; Consultant, Bryn Mawr Rehabilitation Hospital, Malvern, Pennsylvania
> 25. *Diseases of the Lacrimal System*

Timothy R. Covington, Pharm.D.
Bruno Professor of Pharmacy and Director, Managed Care Institute, Samford University, School of Pharmacy, Birmingham
> 4. *Pharmaceutical and Regulatory Aspects of Ocular Drug Administration*

Murray Fingeret, O.D.
Associate Clinical Professor of Optometry, State University of New York, State College of Optometry, New York; Chief, Optometry Section, Brooklyn/Saint Albans Veterans Administration Medical Center, Brooklyn
> 30. *Uveitis;* 35. *Medical Management of the Glaucomas*

Felicia A. Fodera, O.D.
Adjunct Assistant Clinical Professor of Clinical Sciences, State University of New York, State College of Optometry, New York; Supervisor of Externs, Optometry Service, F.D.R. Veterans Administration Hospital, Montrose, New York
> 30. *Uveitis*

Eduardo Gaitan, M.D.
Professor of Medicine and Attending Physician, University of Mississippi, School of Medicine; Chief, Endocrinology Section and Attending Physician, Medical Service, Veterans Affairs Medical Center and Veterans Affairs Memorial Hospital, Jackson
> 33. *Thyroid-Related Eye Disease*

Sally L. Hegeman, Ph.D.
Associate Professor of Optometry, Indiana University, School of Optometry, Bloomington; Adjunct Associate Professor of Pharmacology, Indiana University, School of Medicine, Bloomington
> 13. *Antiallergy Drugs and Decongestants*

Jeffrey A. Hiett, O.D., M.S.
Adjunct Associate Professor of Optometry, The Pacific University, College of Optometry, Forest Grove, Oregon; Chief, Optometry Program, Department of Ambulatory Care, American Lake Veterans Administration Medical Center, Tacoma, Washington
> 10. *Antiglaucoma Drugs;* 37. *Ocular Effects of Systemic Drugs*

Nicky R. Holdeman, O.D., M.D.
Chief, Department of Medical Services and Director, The University Eye Institute, University of Houston, College of Optometry, Houston
> 7. *Analgesics for Treatment of Acute Ocular Pain*

Gary A. Holt, M.Ed., Ph.D., R.Ph.
Associate Professor of Pharmacy and Health Administration, Northeast Louisiana University, School of Pharmacy, Monroe
> 4. *Pharmaceutical and Regulatory Aspects of Ocular Drug Administration*

Siret D. Jaanus, Ph.D.
Professor of Pharmacology, Department of Biological Sciences, State University of New York, State College of Optometry, New York, New York; Professor Emeritus, Southern California College of Optometry, Fullerton
> 6. *Local Anesthetics;* 8. *Mydriatics and Mydriolytics;* 9. *Cycloplegics;* 10. *Antiglaucoma Drugs;* 12. *Anti-Inflammatory Drugs;* 13. *Antiallergy Drugs and Decongestants;* 14. *Lubricants and Other Preparations for Ocular Surface Disease;* 15. *Anti-Edema Drugs;* 37. *Ocular Effects of Systemic Drugs*

William L. Jones, O.D.
Optometry Section, Veterans Affairs Medical Center, Albuquerque, New Mexico
> 29. *Diseases of the Sclera*

Gary A. Lesher, Ph.D.
Professor of Pharmacology and Toxicology, Department of Basic and Health Sciences, Illinois College of Optometry, Chicago
> 12. *Anti-Inflammatory Drugs*

Nada J. Lingel, O.D., M.S.
Associate Professor of Optometry and Assistant Dean for Clinical Affairs, The Pacific University, College of Optometry, Forest Grove, Oregon
> 27. *Diseases of the Cornea*

Gerald E. Lowther, O.D., Ph.D.
Professor of Optometry, Indiana University, School of Optometry, Bloomington
> 18. *Contact Lens Solutions and Care Systems*

Gerald G. Melore, O.D., M.P.H.
Assistant Clinical Professor of Optometry, The Pacific University, College of Optometry, Forest Grove, Oregon; Chief, Optometry Service, Veterans Administration Medical Center, Portland, Oregon
> 24. *Diseases of the Eyelids*

John H. Nishimoto, O.D.
Assistant Professor of Optometry and Director of
Residencies, Southern California College of
Optometry, Fullerton
  28. Allergic Eye Disease

Gary D. Novack, Ph.D.
President, PharmaLogic Development, Incorporated,
Irvine, California
  10. Antiglaucoma Drugs

Neal Nyman, O.D.
Associate Professor of Optometry, Department of
Clinical Sciences, Pennsylvania College of Optometry,
Philadelphia; Chief, Primary Care Service Module 4,
The Eye Institute of the Pennsylvania College of
Optometry, Philadelphia
  8. Mydriatics and Mydriolytics

Gary E. Oliver, O.D.
Chief, Ocular Disease and Special Testing Service,
Department of Clinical Sciences, State University of
New York, State College of Optometry, New York
  26. Diseases of the Conjunctiva

Paul L. Owens, O.D., M.D., Sc.D.
Assistant Clinical Professor of Ophthalmology,
Department of Clinical Sciences, State University of
New York, State College of Optometry; Associate
Attending Surgeon, Department of Ophthalmology,
Manhattan Eye, Ear, Nose and Throat Hospital,
New York
  34. Pharmacologic Management of Strabismus

Marlon L. Priest, M.D.
Associate Professor of Surgery, University of Alabama,
School of Medicine, Birmingham
  38. Life-Threatening Systemic Emergencies

Christopher J. Quinn, O.D.
Center Director, OMNI Eye Services, Iselin,
New Jersey
  26. Diseases of the Conjunctiva

Cristina M. Schnider, O.D., M.S.
Associate Professor of Optometry and Chief, Contact
Lens Services, The Pacific University, College of
Optometry, Forest Grove, Oregon
  17. Dyes

Leo P. Semes, O.D.
Associate Professor of Optometry, University of
Alabama at Birmingham, School of Optometry,
Birmingham; Consultant, Department of Optometry,
Birmingham Veterans Administration Medical Center,
Birmingham
  25. Diseases of the Lacrimal System

David P. Sendrowski, O.D.
Chief, Ocular Disease and Special Testing Service,
Southern California College of Optometry, Fullerton;
Director, Department of Optometric Services, North
Orange County Community Clinic, Anaheim
  33. Thyroid-Related Eye Disease

Mordechai Sharir, M.D., Ph.D.
Assistant Professor of Ophthalmology, Tel-Aviv
University, Sackler School of Medicine, Tel-Aviv;
Head of Glaucoma Service, Department of
Ophthalmology, The Edith Wolfson Hospital,
Holon, Israel
  10. Antiglaucoma Drugs

Leonid Skorin, Jr., O.D., D.O.
Adjunct Assistant Professor of Ophthalmology,
Chicago College of Osteopathic Medicine, Chicago;
Clinical Assistant Professor of Ophthalmology and
Visual Sciences, University of Illinois Eye and Ear
Infirmary, Chicago; Clinical Instructor of
Ophthalmology, Department of Osteopathic Medicine,
Division of Ophthalmology, Michigan State University,
College of Human Medicine, East Lansing
  23. Neuro-Ophthalmic Disorders

Mark W. Swanson, O.D.
Assistant Professor of Optometry, University of
Alabama at Birmingham, School of Optometry,
Birmingham; Consulting Staff, Department of
Medicine, University Hospital, Birmingham
  13. Antiallergy Drugs and Decongestants

David K. Talley, O.D.
Assistant Professor and Director of Continuing
Education, Northeastern State University, College of
Optometry, Tahlequah; Staff Optometrist, Department
of Optometry, W.W. Hastings Indian Health Service
Hospital, Tahlequah, Oklahoma
  20. Topical and Regional Anesthesia

David S. Tatro, Pharm.D.
Drug Information Consultant, San Carlos, California
  36. Drug Interactions

J. James Thimons, O.D.
Associate Professor of Optometry and Chairman,
Department of Clinical Sciences, State University of
New York, State College of Optometry, New York
   26. Diseases of the Conjunctiva

David R. Whikehart, Ph.D.
Professor of Physiological Optics, Vision Science
Research Center, University of Alabama at
Birmingham, School of Optometry, Birmingham
   16. Irrigating Solutions

Diane P. Yolton, Ph.D., O.D.
Professor of Optometry, The Pacific University,
College of Optometry, Forest Grove, Oregon
   11. Anti-Infective Drugs

John R. Yuen, Pharm.D.
Consultant in Pharmacology, University of Southern
California, School of Pharmacy, Los Angeles; Clinical
Pharmacist, Department of Pharmacy Services, Estelle
Doheny Eye Hospital/Doheny Eye Institute,
Los Angeles
   1. Pharmacotherapy of the Ophthalmic Patient

Preface

The third edition of *Clinical Ocular Pharmacology* was written during a time in which the organization of health care delivery in the United States and its payment mechanisms were receiving considerable attention and undergoing radical changes. The delivery of comprehensive eye care services, involving networks of optometrists and ophthalmologists, is increasingly delegating to the optometrist the responsibility for primary care. It is clear that as health care reform continues, optometry and ophthalmology must finally come to grips with providing high-quality eye care in an efficient and cooperative environment that encourages each provider to function at his or her highest level of expertise and training. To that end, our purpose with this edition remains much the same as its predecessors—to give both the student and practitioner clinically relevant information based on sound scientific principles that will enhance care of the ophthalmic patient. Our purpose is not solely to provide insight into pharmacologic mechanisms of ocular drugs, but rather to take the reader from the classroom to the clinic by emphasizing practical uses of drugs in the primary care of eye patients.

In this edition we have reorganized large portions of the text. By reordering several chapters, we believe the material has a more logical presentation. A key feature of this reorganization is the use of therapeutic rather than the classic pharmacologic drug classifications for the chapters in Part II. We believe this philosophical change in presentation will be welcomed by clinicians and clinicians-in-training, whose primary interest is the clinical uses of ocular drugs rather than their pharmacologic mechanisms. For example, all antiglaucoma drugs are now discussed in a single chapter rather than in three chapters as in the previous editions. As a part of this reorganization, we have added important new chapters that properly reflect the current scope of primary eye care practice. Unfortunately, the extent of the reorganization and additional material precluded our continued use of the color plates from the second edition.

Since the second edition was prepared, there has been a veritable explosion of scientific literature in ophthalmic pharmacology and ocular disease. Although we have attempted to consolidate this literature and to provide meaningful references for each chapter, we were often forced to choose among key references for the sake of brevity, and in these instances, we often selected among the most recent citations and important review articles. In this way, the scientific foundations of the various discussions have been preserved while limiting the number of cited references. In other instances, however, it was extremely difficult to eliminate classic or important new citations, and these references have remained for the use of our readers who want more information. In the area of glaucoma alone, we have over 1000 references regarding antiglaucoma medications and the diagnosis and clinical management of glaucoma.

We are deeply grateful for our contributing authors, both those who are new to this edition and those who have contributed to previous editions. Without their enthusiasm, commitment, and expert contributions, the preparation of this book would have been impossible. The helpful suggestions from our colleagues, and the expert advice from peer referees who offered insightful and useful comments regarding each new and revised chapter, have improved both the presentation and accuracy of the text. This has resulted, we believe, in a text that more appropriately reflects contemporary thought and practice in the clinical uses of ophthalmic drugs in primary eye care. Our secretaries Brenda McKenzie and Lucille Rose are commended for their continuing patience and perseverance as well as expert technical skills in word processing. Robert Hollingsworth spent uncountable hours retrieving scientific literature, and we especially appreciate the unique skills of our medical librarians Caren Hughes, Carolyn McLean, Patricia Carlson, and Claudia Perry. We are also grateful for the invaluable technical assistance of Ann DeLaney, Pat Humpres, Char Brazil, Robin Fogel, Bonnie Gauer, Fran Tabor, and Laurel Gregory. A special mention must be made of the superb medical illustrations provided by Ken Norris. His exceptional artistic skills, together with his keen interpretative abilities, have combined to elevate the quality of this book to new heights.

We also thank our readers, who have continually given us positive feedback regarding the usefulness of this book in both the learning of ocular pharmacology and in the "real world" of day-to-day patient care.

Most of all, we must thank our families, whose endurance and sacrifice on behalf of this project often reached the limits of understanding. We mourn the enumerable hours lost from our time with Jaak, Cindy, Andrew, Kenton, and Harrison.

J.D.B.
S.D.J.

PART I

Fundamental Concepts in Ocular Pharmacology

There is no great danger in our mistaking the height of the sun, or the fraction of some astronomical computation; but here where our whole being is concerned, 'tis not wisdom to abandon ourselves to the mercy of the agitation of so many contrary winds.

—Hippocrates

Pharmacotherapy of the Ophthalmic Patient

John R. Yuen
Jimmy D. Bartlett

As its title implies, this book is about clinical ocular pharmacology and patient care. Its goal is to give both the student and the practitioner clinically relevant information based on sound scientific principles that will enhance care of the ophthalmic patient. *Clinical Ocular Pharmacology* is perhaps unique among pharmacology texts in this regard. Its ultimate purpose is not solely to provide information about pharmacologic mechanisms of ocular drugs, but rather, to take the reader from the classroom to the clinic by emphasizing practical applications of drug use in the primary care of ophthalmic patients. This book concerns the use of ocular drugs in patients with either acute or chronic ocular diseases for which drug therapy is indicated, as well as in asymptomatic patients who need only routine care.

In this chapter the term *pharmacotherapy* refers to the use of drugs for the examination, diagnosis, or treatment of patients with eye or vision problems, or for asymptomatic patients who are undergoing comprehensive eye examinations. This chapter addresses ophthalmic patients as individuals. It emphasizes that people with eye problems are no different from people with conditions such as the common cold, asthma, rheumatoid arthritis, or diabetes. From a health care perspective, all these individuals have medical histories, may be taking certain medications that could interact with administered or prescribed ocular drugs, may have certain socioeconomic positions or illnesses that make prescribed medications unaffordable, and have the desire or need to overcome health problems. Thus, the treatment of eye problems involves many of the same things as the treatment of general medical illnesses. This chapter discusses some of the fundamental issues that must be ad-

dressed if ophthalmic patients are to benefit fully from drug use. The clinical applications of these pharmacotherapeutic principles are stressed throughout this book.

Initiating and Monitoring Ocular Pharmacotherapy

The decision of whether to use drugs for diagnosis or treatment is often straightforward. Topical anesthetics are needed for accurate tonometry, and mydriatics are required for adequate ophthalmoscopic examinations. Pharmacologic intervention is clearly needed for patients who have glaucoma with the diagnostic triad of elevated intraocular pressure (IOP), optic disc damage, and visual field loss. Less clear-cut, however, are patients with mild, almost asymptomatic blepharitis, who may or may not need eyelid scrubs. Patients with dry eyes with only intermittent symptoms and no ocular surface abnormality may not require pharmacotherapeutic intervention using artificial tears or lubricants. In some cases, treatment may entail drugs, physical therapeutic measures (e.g., hot compresses), or sometimes both. Simple reassurance therapy can be sometimes entirely sufficient, and the disease process may run its natural course.[1] A subconjunctival hemorrhage, for example, generally requires only patient reassurance. In general, the decision to intervene with diagnostic or therapeutic pharmaceutical agents should be based on patients' symptoms, ocular signs, knowledge of the natural history of the disease process, and identification of any underlying ocular or general medical contraindications.

One of the factors often overlooked in prescribing for ophthalmic patients is the affordability of ordered medications. Because of limitations of Medicare and private health care insurance, much of the expense incurred for eye care for elderly patients is paid out-of-pocket.[2] Medications that are not purchased are not used. This explains why patients at lower socioeconomic levels have chronic eye conditions such as glaucoma that often deteriorate. To control medication costs and thus enhance compliance with drug usage, patients should be encouraged to comparison-shop. This is especially important for medications that are used on a chronic basis. Several studies[3–5] have documented that prescription drug prices vary considerably among pharmacies. Patients may need to receive guidance in choosing community pharmacies that combine reasonable prices with necessary services. Moreover, prescribing generic drugs when feasible may help to control the costs of therapy, especially for chronic diseases such as glaucoma.[3] The long-term control of chronic eye conditions depends in large measure on good patient compliance, patient understanding of the ocular condition, and a budgeted medical care plan. Clinicians' best intentions and efforts toward patient education are unsuccessful if the medical and pharmacotherapeutic plan is not practicable.

Patient education can also have a substantial impact on the ability or willingness of patients to use prescribed medications. If patients are not educated and counseled in the simplest, most direct manner possible, they often misunderstand instructions and consequently fail to use medications correctly. In addition to verbal communication, practitioners should incorporate written and visual aids to counsel patients on proper medication use. Written dosage schedules should be tailored for each patient as a reminder of when and how to use topical medications such as eyedrops or ointments.[6] Written dosage schedules help teach and reinforce proper medication use, avoid confusion, and enhance compliance. This is especially important for patients who require chronic therapy for conditions such as primary open-angle glaucoma and dry eye syndrome. When patients are fully informed about their disease or condition and the need to adhere to prescribed dosage schedules, compliance with drug therapy is personalized, thus speeding recovery and reducing ocular morbidity.

One of the most important decisions to make when instituting ocular pharmacotherapy is the route of drug administration. In most cases this is straightforward. Patients undergoing tonometry or pupillary dilation are given the diagnostic agent as eyedrops, which are formulated for ophthalmic use only as topical preparations. Patients with infectious or inflammatory disease, however, can be given therapeutic agents in a variety of forms. Most infections of the ocular surface, such as blepharitis or conjunctivitis, are best treated using topical antibiotic eyedrops or ointments, but some infections of the adnexa are treated more effectively with orally administered antibiotics. Two examples are internal hordeolum and preseptal cellulitis, which respond more quickly to oral than to topical pharmacotherapy. When topical therapy is used, practitioners must choose the proper drug formulation from among a vast array of available products.

Most patients require traditional topical ophthalmic formulations (e.g., solutions, suspensions, ointments). Some clinical situations, however, warrant specialized drug delivery methods such as sprays, eyelid scrubs, gels, soft contact lenses, collagen shields, or cotton pledgets[7] (see Chapter 3). Less commonly, patients need injections into or around the eye. Such periocular, intracameral, and intravitreal injections are discussed in Chapter 3. These methods of drug administration are used more often in surgery or for the treatment of complicated inflammatory or infectious diseases that respond poorly to topical therapy alone.

Determining Contraindications to Drug Use

Successful diagnosis and management of ocular disease requires rational drug selection and administration. Poorly chosen and contraindicated drug regimens can contribute to iatrogenic ocular or systemic disease with potentially adverse medicolegal consequences. To avoid using drugs that may be contraindicated in certain patients, pharmacotherapy should follow guidelines recommended by the Food and Drug Administration (FDA), and pharmacists or other qualified drug experts should be consulted when necessary. A careful patient history and clinical examination should precede the initiation of drug therapy.

Patient History

A systematic history (Table 1.1) is essential before any drug is administered or prescribed. A careful history alerts practitioners to possible adverse drug reactions and assists in deciding the best pharmacotherapy for the patient.

OCULAR HISTORY

A careful and complete ocular history is vitally important because the eye is the primary focus of ophthalmic practitioners. Clinicians should ask about past as well as current eye disease. Abnormalities such as narrow anterior chamber angles or frank angle-closure glaucoma can contraindicate the use of mydriatics for diagnostic examination. Past ocular trauma can be important because patients with traumatic ectropion may not be able to tolerate or retain ocular inserts such as the collagen shield or Ocusert. The presence of strabismus or amblyopia may contraindicate the use of pressure patching in patients with corneal trauma. Patching one eye can severely limit mobility in patients with reduced

TABLE 1.1
Essential Elements of the Patient History

Ocular history
    Past or current eye disease
    Trauma
    Strabismus or amblyopia
    Contact lens wear
    Current ocular medications
    Eye surgery
Medical history
    Cardiovascular disease
    Pulmonary disorders
    Thyroid disease
    Diabetes
    Seizure disorders
    Affective and mental disorders
    Pregnancy
    Myasthenia gravis
    Erythema multiforme
    Blood dyscrasias
    Immune status
Medication history
    Dopamine or dobutamine
    Bronchodilators
    Tricyclic antidepressants
    Over-the-counter antihistamines, decongestants
    Allergies (preservatives, penicillins, sulfonamides, neomycin,
      opioids)
Family history
    Open-angle glaucoma
Social/Cognitive history
    Drug abuse
    Mental abuse
Occupational history

visual acuity in the fellow eye. Because many topically applied medications can cause corneal complications when used in the presence of soft contact lenses,[8] practitioners should also inquire about a history of contact lens wear. A history of current ocular medications is essential, because if their continued use is necessary, the old and new medications need to be spaced properly if maximum benefit is to be achieved from both. A history of ocular surgery is also important. For example, topically applied epinephrine for treatment of glaucoma can cause a high incidence of cystoid macular edema in aphakic patients.[9]

MEDICAL HISTORY

A careful medical history, including review of systems, is essential to identify drugs that may be contraindicated on the basis of systemic disease. Topically applied ocular medications such as β blockers readily enter the systemic circulation and have high bioavailability throughout the body.[10,11]

Cardiovascular Disease.   Patients with systemic hypertension, arteriosclerosis, and other cardiovascular diseases may be at risk when high concentrations of topically administered adrenergic agonists such as phenylephrine are used. Repeated topical doses or soaked cotton pledgets placed in the conjunctival sac have been associated with adverse cardiovascular effects.[12] Likewise, β blockers should be avoided or used with caution in patients with congestive heart disease, severe bradycardia, and high-grade AV block.[13] Topical β blockers may, however, be used safely in patients with cardiac pacemakers.[13]

Respiratory Disorders.   Because topically applied β blockers can induce asthma or dyspnea in patients with preexisting chronic obstructive pulmonary disease (COPD),[13–16] clinicians should inquire about a history of pulmonary disorders before initiating glaucoma treatment with β blockers.

Thyroid Disease.   Elevated blood pressure or other adverse cardiovascular effects can sometimes result when patients with Graves' disease receive adrenergic agonists.[17] This occurs because of the increased catecholamine activity associated with hyperthyroidism. Agents to be avoided or used cautiously include topically applied phenylephrine for routine pupillary dilation or topical epinephrine for treatment of glaucoma.

Diabetes Mellitus.   Systemic administration of hyperosmotic agents can cause clinically significant hyperglycemia in patients with diabetes. This is of particular concern in ophthalmic practice when oral glycerin is given for treatment of acute angle-closure glaucoma. Systemic corticosteroid therapy may also represent a significant risk in patients with diabetes because of drug-induced hyperglycemia. Furthermore, it is often more difficult to achieve adequate dilation of the pupils in patients with diabetes when using topically administered mydriatics. Practitioners may exceed the usual mydriatic dosage and subject patients to potential adverse systemic side effects.

Seizure Disorders.   Clinicians should be cautious when using topically applied central nervous system (CNS) stimulants such as cyclopentolate. High concentrations of these drugs in normal children, and occasionally in adults, have resulted in transient CNS effects. The risk may be greater in patients with documented seizure disorders who are not under medication or not taking their prescribed drug regimens.[18,19]

Affective and Mental Disorders.   Anxiety and emotional instability can be associated with psychogenic reactions that may appear drug related, including vasovagal syncope. Attention to patients' systemic medications and various innuendos during the initial patient interview may alert clinicians to such a possibility. Treatment of these disorders, moreover, may potentiate the activity of ophthalmic medications. For example, use of monoamine oxidase (MAO) inhibitors or tricyclic antidepressants (TCAs) can enhance the systemic effects of topically applied phenylephrine.[20]

Pregnancy.   Systemic drugs should not be administered to pregnant women unless absolutely essential for the well-being of either the expectant mothers or the fetus. Most topically administered medications, however, are permissible if given in relatively low concentrations for brief periods.[21] Pharmacotherapy of pregnant ophthalmic patients is discussed later in this chapter.

Other Medical Conditions.   Other systemic disorders can be affected by or contraindicate topically applied medications. Examples include myasthenia gravis, which can be worsened with topical timolol,[22] and erythema multiforme (Stevens-Johnson syndrome), which can be caused or exacerbated by topical ocular sulfonamides.[23,24]

MEDICATION HISTORY

A thorough medication history should be taken. Patients may be taking systemic drugs that have a high potential for adverse interactions with ocular pharmacotherapeutic agents. Such interactions can play a significant role in enhancing drug effects and may exacerbate adverse reactions. Several drug-drug interactions between ocular antiglaucoma and systemic medications have been well documented (Table 1.2).[11] For example, β blockers are contraindicated in patients with cardiac failure, bradycardia, and second- or third-degree AV block. Patients with cardiac disease who are being treated with potent inotropic agents such as dopamine or dobutamine should not be given topical ocular β blockers.[11] Likewise, nonselective β blockers are contraindicated in patients with chronic obstructive pulmonary disease (COPD). These drugs block exogenous stimulation of β_2-receptors by medications such as isoproterenol, metaproterenol, and albuterol.[11] Use of nonselective β blockers in patients with COPD can induce bronchospasm, so cardioselective β blockers such as betaxolol are preferred as long as respiratory function is closely monitored. Phenylephrine should be used with caution for pupillary dilation in patients taking TCAs and MAO inhibitors because the risk of adverse cardiovascular effects is increased.[20]

It is important for clinicians to be aware of all over-the-counter (OTC) medications and folk medicines (i.e., home remedies) that patients may be using. Many patients may not consider OTC agents, especially antihistamines and decongestants for hay fever and colds, as "drugs" that can affect the autonomic nervous system (ANS). OTC preparations can potentially interact with ocular drugs such as homatropine and phenylephrine that also influence autonomic func-

TABLE 1.2
Adverse Interactions Between Antiglaucoma and Systemic Medications

Systemic Drug	Ocular Drug	Adverse Effect
Cardiac glycosides	β blockers	Cardiac depression
Quinidine	β blockers	Cardiac depression
Xanthines	β blockers	Bronchospasm
β-adrenergic agonists	β blockers	Cardiac depression Bronchospasm
Succinylcholine	Cholinesterase inhibitors	Prolonged respiratory paralysis (apnea)

tions. The prevention, identification, and management of potential drug interactions are discussed in Chapter 36.

Although the risk of anaphylactic reactions associated with topically administered drugs is extremely remote, inquiry regarding drug allergies is essential. Hypersensitivity to thimerosal is not uncommon among contact lens patients,[25] and knowledge of allergy to topically and systemically administered antibiotics is helpful when initiating antimicrobial therapy. For example, penicillin-allergic patients should not be given penicillins or cephalosporins, and sulfonamide-allergic patients should not be given topical ocular sodium sulfacetamide or carbonic anhydrase inhibitors. Narcotic analgesics should be avoided in patients allergic to opioids. Cross-sensitivity of proparacaine with other local anesthetics is rare and usually not an important clinical consideration (see Chapter 6). A history of hypersensitivity to specific local anesthetics should nevertheless be noted.

FAMILY HISTORY

A history of familial eye disease can be helpful in identifying contraindications to drug use. For example, it has been demonstrated that about 70% of the first-degree offspring of individuals with primary open-angle glaucoma have clinically significant elevations of IOP when given long-term topical steroids.[26] Thus, when topical steroid therapy is contemplated in close relatives of individuals with glaucoma, steroids with less propensity to elevate IOP should be chosen. In addition, the IOP should be monitored carefully.

SOCIAL/COGNITIVE HISTORY

Questions regarding the social history may uncover important patient attributes that can either enhance or preclude successful pharmacotherapy. For example, a history of drug abuse may indicate personal instability and thus may suggest noncompliance with the intended drug therapy. Observation of patients' mental status is often helpful in designing a suitable pharmacotherapeutic program with which patients are likely to comply. Simple, straightforward, inexpensive drug regimens should be stressed, especially for patients who may have difficulty understanding more sophisticated treatments.

Clinical Examination

PHYSICAL LIMITATIONS AFFECTING COMPLIANCE

Unlike oral drug therapy, in which the usual dosage unit is a tablet or capsule that is simply swallowed, ocular pharmacotherapy requires some degree of manual dexterity if the topical solutions or ointments are to be instilled successfully. Clinicians should examine patients' hands and fingers for limitations that might affect the proper use of ocular solutions or ointments. For example, elderly patients with arthritis may have exceptional difficulty manipulating bottle caps or tubes of ocular medications. If the physical maneuver of instilling eyedrops or ointments cannot be mastered, even the best planned drug therapy cannot possibly be beneficial despite patients' best intentions. When patients cannot successfully learn to instill ocular medications, alternative approaches include orally administered drugs or drug administration by family members or attendants.

COMPREHENSIVE EYE EXAMINATION

A complete eye examination is essential to establish the definitive diagnosis and to identify possible contraindications to the intended pharmacotherapy. Some portions of this evaluation should be performed before drug use because various clinical procedures can be influenced by previously administered drugs. This practice not only legally protects clinicians but also provides certain baseline clinical information that may be unobtainable following drug administration. These procedures include the following.[27]

Visual Acuity.   Corrected visual acuity should be the initial clinical test performed at every patient visit. This "entrance" acuity measurement legally protects clinicians and provides baseline information when patients are monitored on successive visits. For example, topically applied ointments often have a transient detrimental effect on visual acuity.

Pupil Examination.   A meaningful evaluation of pupils following drug-induced mydriasis or miosis is impossible. Thus, pupillary examination, including pupil size and responsiveness, should be recorded before instilling mydriatics or miotics. The presence and nature of the direct reflexes, as well as the presence or absence of an afferent pupillary defect, should be recorded.

Manifest Refraction.   Because topically applied cycloplegics often affect the manifest (subjective) refractive error, refraction influenced by drugs is undesirable. When indicated, cycloplegic refraction may be performed following the initial manifest refraction or as the initial refractive procedure in children (see Chapter 22).

Amplitude of Accommodation.   Because of the cycloplegic and mydriatic effects of anticholinergic drugs, amplitude of accommodation should be measured before administering these agents.

Tests of Binocularity.   Binocular vision, including accommodation-convergence relationships, should be evaluated before administering cycloplegics. In many cases these drugs produce dramatic alterations in the observed heterophoria or heterotropia measurements. For example, esophoria or esotropia associated with uncorrected latent or manifest hyperopia often worsens with cycloplegics.

Biomicroscopy.   It is important to evaluate the cornea and other anterior segment structures before instilling any drug, including dyes. Any topically applied drugs, especially anesthetics, or procedures such as applanation tonometry and gonioscopy may possibly compromise the corneal epithelium. The indiscrete application of a sodium fluorescein-impregnated filter paper strip may result in corneal staining patterns associated with the iatrogenic foreign body abrasion. Because certain mydriatics, such as phenylephrine, can produce nonpathologic (pigmented) cells in the anterior chamber, it is of diagnostic importance to know whether such cells are iatrogenic. Thus, careful evaluation of the aqueous using a short or conical slit lamp beam is essential before pupillary dilation. Furthermore, examination of the anterior chamber angle is of value before administering mydriatics to dilate the pupil (see Chapter 21). In other instances, certain drugs should precede others so that the corneal epithelium and precorneal tear film are not disturbed. For example, sodium fluorescein should be instilled for determining the tear breakup time (BUT) before a topical anesthetic is administered for tonometry. The anesthetic can adversely affect the BUT measurement.

Tonometry.   In eyes with narrow anterior chamber angles, it is important to record the IOP before dilating the pupil with mydriatics. Although cycloplegics can cause slight increases of pressure even in eyes with open angles,[28,29] acute and dangerous pressure elevation is common in eyes that are undergoing attacks of angle-closure glaucoma induced by mydriatics. Thus, baseline tonometry is essential before dilating pupils in eyes with narrow angles.

Tests of Cardiovascular Status.   It is of value to note pulse strength, regularity, and rate during routine sphygmomanometry, because some topically administered ocular drugs such as atropine and β blockers can affect systemic blood pressure and cardiac activity. This is especially important prior to and during chronic treatment of patients with glaucoma, who routinely use β blockers that can have adverse cardiovascular effects.

Minimizing Drug Toxicity and Other Adverse Reactions

Side effects associated with ocular drugs are not uncommon, but serious reactions are extremely rare. In most instances these adverse reactions are manifestations of drug hypersensitivity (allergy) or toxicity. The allergic or toxic reaction usually occurs in the eye itself, but occasionally, as in erythema multiforme potentiated by sulfonamide agents, it can manifest as a systemic response.

Ocular Effects of Locally Administered Drugs

Numerous adverse ocular effects from topically administered drugs have been observed[30] (Table 1.3). Topical ophthalmic medications can produce adverse ocular events through a variety of mechanisms,[31] and the ocular tissues respond by manifesting cutaneous changes, conjunctivitis, keratitis, hyperpigmentation or hypopigmentation, or infectious complications.[32] Clinicians who administer or prescribe ocular drugs must be aware of these potential complications.

In general, any topically applied drug or its inactive ingredients can elicit a hypersensitivity response. Such local allergic reactions are especially common with neomycin and with thimerosal[25] or chlorhexidine used as preservatives in some older contact lens solutions. Practitioners should diminish the risk of allergic responses by carefully questioning patients about any previous drug reactions. If an allergic profile is identified by history or examination, this fact should be recorded on the chart and alternative drug regimens should be selected. Clinicians should inform patients about expected side effects of drugs as well as allergic and other adverse drug reactions. Patients may incorrectly identify the transient burning and stinging of certain eyedrops as an allergic response. Topical ophthalmic agents that are commonly misinterpreted as causing allergic reactions include the mydriatic/cycloplegic agents, β-adrenergic blockers, adrenergic agonists, and some anti-infective agents. Management of the mild hypersensitive reactions that occasionally occur from topical application of ocular drugs is considered in later chapters.

Although iatrogenic infection is possible with locally

TABLE 1.3
Adverse Ocular Effects from Topically Administered Drugs

Eyelids
   Urticaria and angioedema
   Allergic contact dermatoconjunctivitis
   Allergic contact dermatitis
   Photoallergic contact dermatitis
   Irritative or toxic contact dermatitis
   Phototoxic dermatitis
   Cumulative deposition
   Melanotic hyperpigmentation or hypopigmentation
   Microbial imbalance

Conjunctiva
   Anaphylactoid conjunctivitis
   Allergic contact (dermato) conjunctivitis
   Cicatrizing allergic conjunctivitis
   Nonspecific (papillary) irritative or toxic conjunctivitis
   Follicular irritative or toxic conjunctivitis
   Cicatrizing and keratinizing irritative or toxic conjunctivitis
      (including pseudotrachoma)
   Cumulative deposition
   Microbial imbalance

Cornea
   Anaphylactoid keratitis
   Allergic contact keratitis
   Irritative or toxic keratitis
   Phototoxic keratitis
   Toxic calcific band keratopathy
   Pseudotrachoma
   Cumulative deposition
   Microbial imbalance

Intraocular pressure
   Elevation (glaucoma)
   Reduction (hypotony)

Uvea
   Hypertrophy of pupillary frill (iris "cyst")
   Iridocyclitis
   Iris sphincter atrophy

Crystalline lens
   Anterior subcapsular opacification
   Posterior subcapsular opacification

Retina
   Detachment
   Cystic or hemorrhagic toxic maculopathy

Modified from Wilson FM. Adverse external ocular effects of topical ophthalmic medications. Surv Ophthalmol 1979;24(2):57–88.

applied drugs, it can usually be avoided by handling medications carefully. Airborne contamination is usually of little significance.[33] The main source of pathogens is the dropper tip that has been allowed to come in contact either with practitioners' fingers or with the nonsterile surface of patients' lids, lashes, or face.[34–36] Care must therefore be exercised when instilling topical medications. In addition, labeled expiration dates should be respected, and old or contaminated solutions should be discarded. Prescription directions for eyedrops should include special medication expiration dates that do not exceed 90 days following opening of the safety seal. This ensures that the volume of drops dispensed is used within a reasonable and expected period. Furthermore, patients, practitioners, and drug manufacturers are protected against untoward and potential idiosyncratic effects of expired or contaminated ophthalmic solutions.

The use of topical steroids in patients with infectious external disease is controversial.[37] When the inflammatory response is suppressed by steroids in the absence of an effective antimicrobial agent, microorganisms can reach higher tissue concentrations and spread to adjacent tissue, thereby worsening the infectious process.[38] Topical steroids can be used selectively for certain ocular infections but only if specific guidelines are carefully followed (see subsequent chapters).

Mydriatics should be used with caution in patients with extremely narrow anterior chamber angles. These drugs may precipitate an attack of acute angle-closure glaucoma. Furthermore, topically administered steroids can raise IOP to dangerous levels, especially in patients who already have open-angle glaucoma or in these patients' first-degree offspring.[26]

In recent years considerable attention has been devoted to developing artificial tears and lubricants without preservatives, because the long-term use of agents with preservatives can damage the ocular surface. This toxicity can manifest itself clinically as superficial punctate keratitis accompanied by irritation, burning, or stinging. Preservative-free artificial tear preparations can generally be used at frequent dosage intervals for long periods without compromising the ocular surface.[39]

The long-term use of topical antiglaucoma medications can also induce local metaplastic changes in the conjunctiva, related either to the active medications themselves, their preservatives, or to the duration of topical treatment.[83] Conjunctival shrinkage with foreshortening of the inferior conjunctival fornix is a possible consequence.[84]

Some topically administered ocular preparations affect visual acuity. Notable examples are the lubricating ointments for dry eye and the antimicrobial ointments for ocular infections. Although acuity is only slightly reduced, this effect can be annoying to patients and may lead to noncompliance. The precipitous reduction of acuity associated with retrobulbar anesthetics, however, is more serious. Contralateral amaurosis has been reported following injection of these anesthetics.[40,41]

The abuse of topically administered drugs by either practitioners or patients can cause significant ocular toxicity. Infiltrative keratitis has occurred from the chronic use of anesthetic eyedrops for relief of pain associated with corneal abrasions.[42] Bilateral posterior subcapsular cataracts have developed in a 24-year-old patient following the topical administration of prednisolone acetate 0.12% twice daily for four years.[43] Practitioners should carefully monitor patients treated with drugs known to have potentially significant ocular or systemic side effects.

Systemic Effects of Topically Administered Drugs

As mentioned previously, topically applied ocular drugs can have systemic effects. Drugs are absorbed from the conjunctival sac into the systemic circulation through the conjunctival capillaries, from the nasal mucosa after passage through the lacrimal drainage system, or, after swallowing, from the pharynx or the gastrointestinal tract.[44] Because topically applied drugs avoid the first-pass metabolic inactivation that normally occurs in the liver, these drugs can exert the same substantial pharmacologic effect as a similar parenteral dose. Each 50 μl-drop of a 1.0% solution contains 0.5 mg of drug, which means that solutions applied topically to the eye may exceed the minimum toxic systemic dose. Table 1.4 summarizes some of the clinically important systemic effects caused by topical ocular medications.[10,11,13,44–47]

The prevention of systemic effects associated with topically applied ocular drugs is largely a matter of a very careful patient interview and examination before administering or prescribing any medication. In addition, adherence to the following general guidelines may reduce the risk of adverse reactions.

- Advise patients to store all medications out of children's reach. As few as 20 drops of 1% atropine can be fatal if swallowed.[48]
- Instruct patients to wipe excessive solution or ointment from the lids and lashes after instillation.
- Use the lowest concentration and minimal dosage frequency consistent with a drug's clinical purpose. Avoid overdosage.
- Confirm the dosage of infrequently used drugs before prescribing or administering them.
- Consider the potential adverse effects of a drug relative to its potential diagnostic or therapeutic benefit to patients before prescribing or administering them.
- Consult with each patient's primary physician before prescribing β blockers for patients with cardiac or pulmonary contraindications.
- Recognize adverse drug reactions. Practitioners often fail to recognize the clinical signs of drug toxicity or allergy, which can occur only a few seconds or minutes after drug administration or months or years later.
- Consider the use of manual nasolacrimal occlusion in the office or recommend it for home use, particularly in patients who are at high risk for systemic complications

TABLE 1.4
Clinically Significant Systemic Effects Caused by Ocular Medications

Ocular Drug	Clinical Circumstance Under Which Adverse Effect Occurs	Systemic Effect
β blockers	Treatment of open-angle glaucoma	Decreased cardiac rate, syncope, exercise intolerance, bronchospasm, emotional or psychiatric disorders
Echothiophate	Treatment of open-angle glaucoma when succinylcholine is used as skeletal muscle relaxant during surgery requiring general anesthesia	Prolonged apnea
Pilocarpine	Overdosage of acute angle-closure glaucoma	Nausea, vomiting, sweating, tremor, bradycardia
Cyclopentolate	Overdosage for cycloplegic refraction	Hallucinatory behavior
Chloramphenicol	Treatment of ocular infections	Bone marrow depression, fatal aplastic anemia

associated with certain topically applied drugs (e.g., use of β blockers in patients with COPD). This procedure can reduce systemic drug absorption.[49]

Ocular Effects of Systemically Administered Drugs

Practitioners must be aware of toxic ocular changes caused by systemic medications used for nonocular reasons even though these effects do not relate directly to ocular pharmacotherapy. These medications can have many ocular or visual effects that must be considered when evaluating the ocular health of patients. Many of these drug-induced changes, such as mild symptoms of dry eye associated with anticholinergic drugs, are common but benign. In other instances they can be serious enough to threaten permanent loss of vision, such as ethambutol-induced optic neuropathy.[50,51] Knowledge of the systemic medications taken by individual patients can reduce potential ocular morbidity associated with drug use.

Almost half of the more than 1.5 billion prescriptions dispensed annually from retail pharmacies are for cardiovascular, anti-infective, psychotherapeutic, and diuretic agents.[52] Use of cardiovascular drugs and diuretics has increased substantially in recent years, probably as a result of the increasing proportion of elderly in the population.[52] *Polypharmacy*, the prescription or use of more medications than are clinically necessary, is especially common in patients over the age of 65 years.[53,54] Such use of multiple medications increases the risk of adverse drug interactions and other toxic effects. In the general optometric population, 75% to 90% of the elderly use at least one prescription or nonprescription drug,[55,56] and the average person over age 65 takes two or three prescription medications.[57] The trend toward drug use in individuals over age 80 is even higher.[54]

Therefore, many patients may experience adverse ocular effects associated with systemic medications. The mechanisms underlying these adverse effects are diverse and complex. The diagnosis and clinical management of these conditions are discussed in Chapter 37.

Managing Special Patient Populations

Practitioners who use ophthalmic medications must be knowledgeable about the unique needs of certain patients to enhance the effectiveness of drugs and avoid or minimize side effects. Optometrists and ophthalmologists are particularly interested in certain groups of patients.

Pregnant or Lactating Women

Mothers are the principal targets for drugs administered during pregnancy. In reality, however, their fetuses become inadvertent drug recipients. Some effects on fetuses can be expected throughout pregnancy, the intrapartum period, and even into early neonatal life as drugs are delivered to infants through breast milk.

SPECIAL PRECAUTIONS

Practitioners should pay special attention to the phase of pregnancy when making decisions about medication use and dose. The highest risk of fetal dysmorphosis occurs during early pregnancy, usually the first 6 weeks' postconception or the first 8 weeks after the start of the last menstrual period.[58]

Medications should be avoided during pregnancy and lactation. Chronic diseases, however, such as diabetes, thyroid conditions, rheumatoid arthritis, seizure disorders, and psychological conditions, warrant the continuation of medications with close monitoring to ensure maternal well-being while minimizing potential hazards to the fetus.[59]

DOSAGE CONSIDERATIONS

Medications used in pregnancy must be given with extreme caution and responsibility. Most drugs administered to mothers pass to fetuses to at least some degree and may have *in utero* or postpartum effects.[58] Whenever possible, nonpharmacologic intervention should be employed. If drugs are used, doses should be low yet effective, and the duration of treatment should be as short as possible. Teratogenic and neonatal effects of drugs used during pregnancy and lactation are minimal, and most of the applicable information comes from isolated case reports.[58] Animal studies are performed extensively in the drug development and approval process, although the degree of cross-species relevance is variable.[59]

PRACTICAL CONSIDERATIONS

When oral pharmacotherapy is necessary for treatment of an ocular condition, morning sickness or other pregnancy-related nausea, vomiting, and gastrointestinal upset may preclude successful treatment. Patients should be advised to consume smaller but more frequent meals consisting of foods known to be agreeable. They should avoid foods, liquids, fragrances, and other stimuli that may provoke nausea and vomiting. All other drug therapy should also be avoided, if possible. If necessary, OTC antinauseants can be used. For persistent nausea and vomiting, mild antihistamines may be used in consultation with patients' primary physicians. The use of OTC antacids may be of benefit for gastrointestinal upset when changes in dietary selection and schedules are unsuccessful.

Consumption of caffeine-containing products, including analgesics, as well as alcohol and tobacco should be stopped for the duration of the pregnancy and breastfeeding period as soon as women know they are pregnant. Caffeine and alcohol are readily transferred to young infants through breast milk. Eliminating these products minimizes the risk of unplanned abortions, premature births, low birth weights, and developmental disorders.

When topical ophthalmic drugs must be administered to pregnant patients, they should be administered at minimally effective doses and for as short a time as possible. The use of nasolacrimal occlusion following the instillation of eye medications minimizes systemic drug absorption and should always be recommended.[60] Patients who take medications should also be advised about the potential risks to newborns during breastfeeding. Table 1.5 summarizes current recommendations for use of ophthalmic medications during pregnancy and breastfeeding.[61]

Pediatric Patients

Eye injuries account for the majority of eye problems in older children. Each year over 70,000 children under 15 years of age are treated for eye injuries.[62] Other conditions commonly seen during childhood include hordeolum, blepharitis, conjunctivitis, dacryocystitis, and strabismus. Pharmacotherapeutic intervention is commonly employed for most of these disorders, and both topical and systemic routes of administration are used. Special considerations for drug therapy for pediatric patients are also discussed in Chapters 21, 22, and 34.

DOSAGE CONSIDERATIONS

Pediatric dosage calculations for systemic drugs are not simply fractionated equivalencies based on average adult body weights and recommended adult dosages. A more complete determination of pediatric dosing requires knowledge of the individual patient, the disease group, the age group, the drugs to be administered, pharmacokinetic data for children, and sometimes an understanding of the dose-response relationship of specific drug receptors in growth and development.[63] Acquiring this knowledge, however, can be extremely difficult, and pediatric dosing is often fraught with error by unintentional carelessness on the part of clinicians.

Three objective parameters are traditionally used to calculate systemic dosages: age, weight, and body surface area. Children's doses determined by percentage of adult doses based on body weight and surface area can vary widely. Many dosage guidelines based on age and weight inadequately reflect the complexities of physiologic growth, human development, and our increasing knowledge of drugs.[63] Examples of age and weight calculations include Young's Rule and Clark's Rule, respectively. Clinicians should note that dosage determinations based on age and weight are conservative and may actually underestimate the required dose.[64]

Young's Rule (using age):

$$\text{pediatric dose} = \text{adult dose} \times \frac{\text{age (years)}}{\text{age} + 12}$$

Clark's Rule (using weight):

$$\text{pediatric dose} = \text{adult dose} \times \frac{\text{weight (kg)}}{70} \text{ or}$$

$$\text{pediatric dose} = \text{adult dose} \times \frac{\text{weight (lb)}}{150}$$

Dosage determinations based on body surface area may be the most sensitive approach to approximating age-dependent variations in drug disposition.[63-65] Several body surface area

TABLE 1.5
Recommended Use of Ophthalmic Drugs During Pregnancy or Lactation

Drug	Toxicity During Pregnancy	Recommendation	Toxicity During Lactation	Recommendation
β Blockers				
Betaxolol	Neonatal hypoglycemia	Use caution	β blockade (?)	Avoid
Levobunolol	Neonatal bradycardia	Use caution	β blockade (?)	Avoid
Timolol	Neonatal depression	Use caution	β blockade (?)	Avoid
Carbonic Anhydrase Inhibitors (Oral)				
Acetazolamide	Teratoma, renal and limb deformities (animals)	Use caution	Renal and metabolic effects (?)	Avoid
Methazolamide	No data available	Use caution	Renal and metabolic effects (?)	Avoid
Miotics				
Pilocarpine	Neonatal hyperthermia, restlessness, seizures, diaphoresis	Use caution	No data available	Use caution
Mydriatics/Cycloplegics				
Atropine	Minor fetal malformations	Use caution	Anticholinergic effect (?)	Avoid
Cyclopentolate	No data available	Use caution	Anticholinergic effect (?)	Avoid
Dipivefrin	No data available	Use caution	No data available	Use caution
Epinephrine	Fetal hypoxia, inguinal hernia, cataracts (animals)	Avoid	No data available	Use caution
Homatropine	Minor fetal malformations	Use caution	Anticholinergic effect (?)	Avoid
Phenyleprine	Fetal hypoxia, inguinal hernia, clubfoot	Avoid	Hypertension	Avoid
Scopolamine	Minor fetal malformations, neonatal tachycardia, decreased heart rate variability	Use caution	Anticholinergic effect (?)	Avoid
Tropicamide	No data available	Use caution	Anticholinergic effect (?)	Avoid
Corticosteroids				
Prednisolone, dexamethasone, medrysone	Fetal hypoadrenalism, stillbirth, growth or mental development suppression, cataracts, cleft lip and palate (animals)	Use caution	Growth suppression, interferes with endogenous corticosteroid production	Avoid
Antibacterials				
Erythromycin	No data available	Probably safe	No adverse effects reported	Use caution
Gentamicin	Ototoxicity (?)	Use caution	Ototoxicity (?)	Avoid
Neomycin	Ototoxicity (?)	Use caution	Ototoxicity (?)	Avoid
Polymyxin B	No data available	Probably safe	No data available	Probably safe
Penicillins	No data available	Use caution	Diarrhea or allergy	Avoid
Cephalosporins	Safety not established	Use caution	Alteration of bowel flora	Avoid
Sulfonamides	Hemolysis in glucose-6-phosphate deficiency, kernicterus, skeletal malformations (animals)	Use caution	Diarrhea, rash	Probably safe[a]
Tetracycline	Growth suppression, dental staining	Avoid	Growth suppression, dental staining	Avoid
Tobramycin	Ototoxicity (?)	Use caution	Ototoxicity (?)	Avoid
Antivirals				
Acyclovir	No data available	Use caution	No data available	Avoid
Trifluridine	Teratogenic (animals)	Use caution	No data available	Avoid
Vidarabine	Teratogenic (animals)	Use caution	No data available	Avoid

TABLE 1.5
Recommended Use of Ophthalmic Drugs During Pregnancy or Lactation (continued)

Drug	Toxicity During Pregnancy	Recommendation	Toxicity During Lactation	Recommendation
Fluorescein (Intravenous)	Little data available	Use caution	Little data available	Use caution
Analgesics				
Aspirin	Hemorrhage, prolonged labor, adverse fetal effects such as low birth weight and intracranial hemorrhage	Avoid	Excreted in low concentrations	Avoid
Acetaminophen	Not teratogenic	Safe for short-term use	Excreted in low concentrations	Safe
Ibuprofen	Safety not established	Avoid	Possible cardiovascular effects	Avoid
Narcotic analgesics	Teratogenic, withdrawal symptoms	Avoid	Excreted, but effects may not be significant	Use caution
Antihistamines				
Chlorpheniramine, diphenhydramine, astemizole, terfenadine, loratadine	Safety not established	Avoid during third trimester	No data available	Avoid

^aContraindicated in premature, hyperbilirubinemic, or glucose-6-phosphate-deficient infants.
Adapted from Samples JR, Meyer SM. Use of ophthalmic medications in pregnant and nursing women. Am J Ophthalmol 1988;106:616–623.

dosing nomograms are available in chart and slide-rule formats.[65,66] Clinicians should note, however, that body surface area dosing guidelines are not clearly established for most drugs. The use of body surface area formulas allows drug dosing to be more closely related to blood volume, cardiac output, renal blood flow, glomerular filtration, and caloric and fluid requirements.[63]

Most pharmacokinetic pediatric dosing focuses on the measurement of drug concentrations within body fluids.[65] For drugs with a narrow therapeutic index, such as systemic aminoglycoside antibiotics and theophylline, pharmacokinetic evaluations of blood serum concentration and renal function have proven effective as parameters for monitoring drug therapy.

Most drugs approved for systemic use in children have dosage recommendations stated in milligrams of medication per kilogram body weight. However, the safety, efficacy, and dosage guidelines for many ophthalmic drugs have not been established for children. In general, it is prudent to follow manufacturer's guidelines when they are available, and pediatric doses should not exceed maximum recommended adult doses. Unlike systemic drug dosages, however, topical ocular doses are generally not reduced in children.

PRACTICAL CONSIDERATIONS

Children and their parents or caregivers should be present for drug counseling, and they should be given the opportunity to ask questions about the prescribed medications. Children, like adults, tolerate eyedrop formulations better than eye ointments because the visual and sensory effects are more transient with drops. Pediatric patients with glaucoma who use chronic ocular hypotensive medications and patients who require immunosuppressive therapy with corticosteroids are exceptions. Ointments applied at bedtime have proved effective and easy to use in such patients.

The variable absorption of ophthalmic drops is least predictable in crying, intolerant infants. These patients have minimal corneal absorption as a result of the dilutional and washing effect of the tears. Thus, special care must be given to the quantity and absorption of topical ophthalmic solutions and ointments in children. Children may receive systemic doses from topical ophthalmic medications sufficient to cause undue harm. When appropriate, the oral route of drug administration may be preferred for some pediatric patients. For example, this may be feasible when treating infections of the lacrimal drainage system, such as dacryocystitis, and in cases of orbital or preseptal cellulitis. Young patients are able to swallow liquid suspensions and solutions easier than oral solids (e.g., tablets or capsules). Because oral medications are the most reliable form of dosing and delivery, they continue to be a mainstay in pediatric drug therapy.

Family members and children's teachers are the best resources to assist with compliance with regimented ophthalmic pharmacotherapy. These individuals should be encouraged to inform the prescribing optometrist or ophthalmologist of any apparent or suspected problems with the drug therapy.

Geriatric Patients

The management of many eye conditions requires treatment procedures that are inherently difficult for elderly patients. For example, these patients may need short-term prophylactic or suppressive therapy following cataract extraction. Chronic conditions treated in the elderly, such as glaucoma and keratoconjunctivitis sicca (dry eye syndrome), require continuous, repetitive, and sometimes complex pharmacotherapeutic regimens. In addition, the need for multiple drug therapy promotes patient noncompliance.

SPECIAL PRECAUTIONS

Due to systemic disease and multiple drug therapy, geriatric patients may experience more adverse drug reactions.[67,68] Systemic absorption of topically applied drugs may cause adverse drug effects. On the other hand, weakened lid turgor, as occurs in age-related ectropion, may increase the retention time of ophthalmic drugs in the conjunctival sac, thus exacerbating the local drug effect or ocular toxicity.[69]

Poor compliance with eyedrop dosage schedules is common in the geriatric population.[70] Cognitive difficulties in following directions for drug administration must be evaluated. Not only can preexisting conditions such as stroke and Alzheimer's disease impair cognitive function, but the use of ophthalmic medications such as β blockers and carbonic anhydrase inhibitors may also contribute to patient confusion and cognitive impairment.

Arthritis, tremors, and other conditions may impair fine motor skills and thus preclude proper self-administration of topical ophthalmic formulations. Some elderly patients find the construction of ophthalmic bottles too rigid to enable drops to be easily squeezed out.

Clinicians must be aware of systemic conditions that may affect ocular pharmacotherapy and require continued management. Special attention should be given to the combined ophthalmic and systemic use of β blockers and steroids. Certain cardiac agents, psychotropic drugs, antidepressants, and antiarthritic agents may have adverse ocular effects (see Chapter 37), and practitioners must detect evidence of ocular toxicity before significant damage occurs.

Topically applied epinephrine may have deeper intraocular penetration in aphakic patients. Clinicians must be aware of drug-related retinal effects, such as cystoid macular edema, in such patients. Polypharmacy may prevent elderly patients from receiving adequate ocular and systemic drug therapy. Patients may have contraindicated drug combinations, redundant medications prescribed by several clinicians, erroneous duplications of drugs or categories of drugs, interactions from prescription and OTC medications, and outdated drugs or dosage schedules. Inappropriate drug prescribing for elderly patients is a growing problem requiring greater community-based educational and perhaps regulatory efforts.[85]

DOSAGE CONSIDERATIONS

Therapeutic dosages for systemic medications in geriatric patients are generally lower than the "normal adult dosage" cited in the drug manufacturer's product information. It is not uncommon for the appropriate dose to be 25–50% of the average adult dose. Systemic drug therapy should be started with doses at the lower end of the recommended adult dosage range. Doses can then be slowly titrated at a minimum time interval of three geriatric half-lives between each increase in dose.[71] However, topical dosages of ophthalmic medications are not adjusted.

Renal function is the most important factor in determining dosage regimens in elderly patients. Geriatric dosing usually makes allowances for reduced renal clearance. An age-related decline in creatinine clearance occurs in approximately two-thirds of the population as a function of renal elimination.[71] Because the kidney serves as the principal organ for drug elimination from the body, elderly patients are prone to potentially toxic accumulations of drugs and their metabolites.

Drug characteristics such as protein-binding, hepatic metabolites, and lipophilicity affect drug distribution.[68] Clinical pharmacokinetic evaluations provide quantitative analyses of renally eliminated drugs. Such analyses consider variables such as the linear relationship of creatinine clearance, volume of distribution, and the unique elimination constant of a drug, which is a measure of its half-life. This information can be useful for agents that have a narrow therapeutic index, such as the therapy of serious ocular infections with systemic aminoglycosides.

Independent of the dosing guidelines selected, clinical judgement and common sense must remain sovereign over simple dosage calculation. Because elderly patients are more sensitive to the therapeutic as well as the nontherapeutic effects of drugs, the best individualized drug regimen must be determined to preserve the vitality and independence of geriatric living. Elderly patients with glaucoma who use long-term topical β-blocker therapy are an example of balancing the risk-benefit dichotomy. An adequate degree of IOP control must be maintained without precipitating adverse events such as confusion, syncope, falls, and sexual dysfunction, which can occur with these agents.

PRACTICAL CONSIDERATIONS

Understanding and compliance are two goals of patient education. Clinicians should keep dosage directions clear, simple, and achievable. Elderly patients appreciate handwritten dosing charts, large numerals written on bottles to signify dosage frequency, and color codes for drug identification. Dosage schedules should be established to fit patients' life-styles (e.g., four-times-a-day dosing should be done at wake-up, lunch, dinner, and bedtime). Patients should be asked to repeat the identification of prescribed medications and the dosing schedules. In addition, they should be able to find telephone numbers of their prescribers and dispensing pharmacy readily.

Patient education should be confirmed by all allied health professionals. At a minimum, medication counseling should be provided by prescribing clinicians and issuing pharmacists. Some third-party reimbursement programs and most state boards of pharmacy now require that a registered pharmacist counsel patients about their medications. Nurses, technicians, and other ophthalmic personnel should also be trained in practical aspects of ocular pharmacology to assist in patient counseling.

Attention should also be directed toward both the ophthalmic and systemic medication schedules of geriatric patients. Patients who receive ophthalmic medications may stop or become confused about continuing their systemic medications. When several ophthalmic and systemic medications are prescribed, patients should be referred to a community pharmacy. Their prescriptions should be processed, evaluated, and managed for appropriateness, allergies, contraindications, pricing, polypharmacy abuse, prescription redundancy, and medication record keeping among multiple prescribers. Medication management through a single pharmacy is advantageous because a complete medication history results and patients who need to have their dosage regimen simplified benefit.

Practitioners should develop provisions for additional health care needs and continuity of care for elderly patients. Family members or close friends may accept responsibility for assisting or overseeing drug scheduling and administration. These individuals should be included in the drug counseling process. Community geriatric assistance is available through third-party insurance carriers, skilled nursing facilities, and independent agencies. Health maintenance organizations (HMOs) are incorporating innovative alternatives for managing high-risk geriatric patients by providing comprehensive health care that does not require restrictive fee-for-service reimbursements.[72]

Visually Impaired Patients

Over ten million people in the United States have irreversible vision loss.[73] Visually impaired patients may find complying with prescribed drug regimens inherently difficult, and their problems can extend beyond the scope of visual compromise. The low-vision specialist can serve a key role in helping visually impaired patients maintain good health by maximizing adherence to medication activities requiring visual capabilities.

SPECIAL PRECAUTIONS

Vision loss can have deleterious effects on people's ability to perform basic activities of daily living such as eating, walking, dressing, and performing personal hygiene. It can also limit the proper use of topical or systemic medications, especially when multiple drug therapies require differentiation of one medication from another.

Age-related ocular conditions such as cataracts, glaucoma, and macular degeneration make elderly patients especially prone to low-vision life-style changes. Two chronic conditions, diabetes and glaucoma, have major visual implications for patients who cannot take their medications appropriately because drug therapy is the primary mode of treatment for most patients afflicted with these conditions.

DOSAGE CONSIDERATIONS

Dosage considerations for visually impaired patients are directed toward compliance and the ability of patients to fully carry out directions for use of prescribed medications.

PRACTICAL CONSIDERATIONS

Many visually impaired patients are capable of recognizing their topical ophthalmic medications but find it difficult to be sure that an administered drop has reached the intended eye. Solutions or suspensions that are stored in the refrigerator can provide enough cold temperature sensation for patients to feel the drop when instilled into the eye.[74]

As with geriatric patients, individuals with low vision appreciate handwritten dosing charts using large print, large numerals displayed on bottles to signify dosage frequency (Fig. 1.1), and color codings for drug identification.

It is imperative that visually impaired patients be able to identify their medications and the dosing schedules for each drug. In addition, these patients should be able to use the telephone to contact their prescriber and dispensing pharmacy. Magnifiers, large-print telephone dials, or other visual or nonoptical aids may be required and should be recommended when needed.

Patients with Low Cognitive Function

Rarely does formal clinical training fully prepare ophthalmic clinicians for the challenges presented by patients with low cognitive function. These patients often have complex ocular problems that require outpatient therapy with multiple drugs. Both delirium and dementia are characterized by a clouded state of consciousness and some degree of disorientation and memory loss. Depression can coexist with these conditions and cause further complications for patients with low cognitive function.[75]

Drug therapy, in particular, can directly affect cognition. Adverse drug reactions, which account for 3% to 10% of all hospitalizations among elderly patients, can contribute to cognitive impairment.[72,76] Elderly patients over 65 years of age are more often afflicted with low cognition. These conditions are much easier to recognize clinically than to define etiologically. Medications, sys-

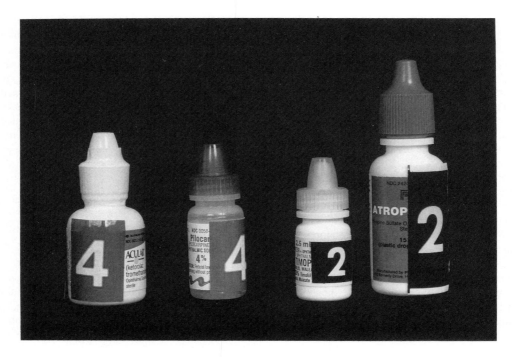

FIGURE 1.1   **Large, stick-on numerals, such as those used on office charts, can indicate dosage frequency for medications used by visually impaired patients.**

temic illnesses, and organic factors must be considered in the definitive diagnosis and differentiation of cognitive impairment.

SPECIAL PRECAUTIONS

Evaluating patients' mental status is a quick way to assess cognitive function.[77,78] Elaborate, graded examinations with neurologic components are not necessary for ophthalmic clinicians. Basic assessments of orientation, short-term memory, and performance of simple cognitive tasks may be completed in a matter of minutes using the Mini-Mental State Examination (MMSE) or shortened versions of this test.[77,78] Based on these assessments, clinicians should be able to determine whether patient education efforts will be successful, whether self-administration of ophthalmic medications is feasible, and if ancillary medical assistance by family, friends, or professionals will be necessary.

Clinicians should take a careful drug history of all prescription and OTC medications, including both systemic and ophthalmic drugs. Antianxiety agents, sedatives, antidepressants, and anticholinergic psychotropic medications may lower cognitive function. If low cognition is suspected for the first time, referral to a neurologist is warranted. It is important to rule out depression, delirium, dementia, and drug-related adverse reactions.

DOSAGE CONSIDERATIONS

Dosages for patients with low cognitive function cannot be formally calculated. Treatment must be individualized to meet the needs of patients and to enhance compliance with drug therapy. For example, it is not uncommon to prescribe multiple ophthalmic steroids (e.g., a steroid suspension and a combination steroid-antibiotic suspension) to patients with low cognitive functioning who are receiving short-term treatment following cataract extraction or glaucoma filtering procedures. If steroid therapy is warranted, a dosing regimen that carries a high likelihood of some steroid administration is necessary in patients who are unlikely to fully carry out the prescribed directions for drug use. Careful evaluation and monitoring is necessary, because these patients may also overmedicate themselves.

PRACTICAL CONSIDERATIONS

In addition to required prescription label information for each medication, simplified directions and color- or number-coded labels may be necessary. Clinicians should expect to spend four to five times the usual drug counseling time with patients with low cognitive functioning. Patients must be taught to identify and administer the prescribed medications, and they should recite this information. Practitioners should note that relatively complex techniques of ophthalmic drug administration such as nasolacrimal occlusion may exceed the abilities of patients with low cognitive functioning. Persistent encouragement to learn these procedures may only aggravate patient confusion and result in further compliance problems.

Supportive care systems are the best short-term solution to treating patients with low cognitive functioning. Family members, close friends, and reliable neighbors may serve as sufficient lay support in the scheduling, supervision, and proper administration of medications. These individuals also serve as excellent sources of feedback concerning the therapeutic improvement of patients. The person or persons who assist patients should be given thorough drug education counseling, because they provide an important link in the total pharmacotherapeutic program. Although formal health care programs for patients with low cognitive functioning are variable and costly, they may be the only viable option for the short-term or long-term well-being of some patients. Access to referral information for established medical assistance agencies is necessary for management of patients with low cognitive functioning, especially if they have no outside support systems.

Patients with Acquired Immunodeficiency Syndrome

Acquired immunodeficiency syndrome (AIDS) has had a staggering effect on the health and vitality of the world. By the mid-1990s, over 300,000 patients had been diagnosed with AIDS in the United States, and over 800,000 worldwide.[79] The most serious vision-threatening manifestation of AIDS is cytomegalovirus (CMV) retinitis.[80] Other ophthalmic disorders include ocular toxoplasmosis, *Pneumocystis carinii* choroiditis, optic neuritis, *Candida* uveitis, herpetic retinal necrosis, herpes zoster ophthalmicus, and keratoconjunctivitis.[81]

SPECIAL PRECAUTIONS

Drug therapy for patients with AIDS can be complex and expensive. It is not uncommon for ambulatory patients to have over 15 different prescriptions for drugs, which are given orally, subcutaneously, intravenously, intramuscularly, or topically to the skin or eye. Many of these regimens involve prophylactic coverage against the great variety of opportunistic infections that commonly occur in AIDS. Patients with AIDS may also be using several investigational medications.

Attention must be given to the economic aspects of AIDS treatment. Health care expenses for patients with AIDS are financially devastating. In 1992 the annual costs for treatment of an individual patient exceeded $30,000. This figure can easily double or triple for patients who use ganciclovir or foscarnet for treatment of CMV retinitis.[82]

Ophthalmic medications for patients with AIDS can be difficult to manage. These patients are more susceptible to

bacterial and fungal conjunctivitis and keratitis. Treatment for these infections may require fortified topical ophthalmic solutions that are specially prepared by pharmacies that are capable of extemporaneously preparing ophthalmic drugs under aseptic conditions (see Chapter 4). Fortified ophthalmic solutions are concentrated preparations that may be five times more potent than commercially available formulations. When stored under refrigeration, the average expiration date for fortified ophthalmic solutions is 7 to 10 days after preparation. Patients can be advised that the cost for these extemporaneously prepared medications may be as much as 3 to 6 times greater than that of the less potent, commercially available products.

Patients with AIDS are also more susceptible to the side effects of medications. Many of the systemic antimicrobial agents cause severe gastric upset, dermatologic manifestations, and CNS effects at higher dosages. Because these patients must often take TCAs, narcotic analgesics, and other federally controlled substances, the risk of CNS disturbances is greater.

DOSAGE CONSIDERATIONS

Dosage regimens for patients with AIDS are far from established. In light of new clinical manifestations of the AIDS complex, clinicians are continually redefining the limits of dosage regimens for the pharmacotherapy of infectious diseases.

PRACTICAL CONSIDERATIONS

Medication regimens should be as consistent and simple as possible because patients are burdened by great physical, mental, emotional, and financial distress. It helps patients with AIDS if refills are regularly updated and necessary triplicate prescriptions for controlled medications are available when warranted. Special attention should be given to medication counseling, drug compliance, and the identification and management of medication side effects. The pharmacy department or community pharmacy that dispenses patients' medications should have complete historical records available, including all medications, dosages, refills, dates, prescribers, and costs of drugs issued.

Patients with AIDS may need assistance in establishing medical and personal support during therapy. Community-based assistance for medical, social, emotional, and financial needs should be made available.

References

1. Blume AJ. Reassurance therapy. In: Amos JF, ed. Diagnosis and management in vision care. Boston: Butterworth, 1987:715–718.
2. McPhillips R. Can the elderly afford eye care? Can we afford eye care for the elderly? Ophthalmology 1987;94:1199–1204.

3. Kass MA, Gordon M. The effect of a generic drug law on the retail cost of antiglaucoma medications. Am J Ophthalmol 1981;92:273–278.

4. Ball SF, Schneider E. Cost of β-adrenergic receptor blocking agents for ocular hypertension. Arch Ophthalmol 1992;110:654–657.

5. Gelvin JB, Goen TM. Dosage cost analysis in glaucoma management. J Am Optom Assoc 1989;60:768–770.

6. Fingeret M, Schuettenberg SP. Patient drug schedules and compliance. J Am Optom Assoc 1991;62:478–480.

7. Chiou GCY, Watanabe K. Drug delivery to the eye. Pharmacol Ther 1982;17:269–278.

8. Bartlett JD. Medications and contact lens wear. In: Silbert J, ed. Anterior segment complications of contact lens wear. New York: Churchill Livingstone, 1994:473–485.

9. MacKool RJ, Muldoon T, Fortier A, Nelson D. Epinephrine induced cystoid macular edema in aphakic eyes. Arch Ophthalmol 1977;95:791–793.

10. Hugues FC, LeJeunne C, Munera Y. Systemic effects of topical antiglaucomatous drugs. Glaucoma 1992;14:100–104.

11. Gerber SL, Cantor LB, Brater DC. Systemic drug interactions with topical glaucoma medications. Surv Ophthalmol 1990;35:205–218.

12. Fraunfelder FT, Scafidi AF. Possible adverse effects from topical ocular 10% phenylephrine. Am J Ophthalmol 1978;85:447–453.

13. Collignon P. Cardiovascular and pulmonary effects of β-blocking agents: Implications for their use in ophthalmology. Surv Ophthalmol 1989;33 (suppl):455–456.

14. Van Buskirk EM. Adverse reactions from timolol administration. Ophthalmology 1980;87:447–450.

15. Fraunfelder FT. Ocular β-blockers and systemic effects. Arch Intern Med 1986;146:1073–1074.

16. Roholt PC. Betaxolol and restrictive airway disease. Arch Ophthalmol 1987;105:1172.

17. Zimmerman TJ. Agents for glaucoma. In: Bartlett JD, Ghormley NR, Jaanus SD, et al, eds. Ophthalmic drug facts. St. Louis: Facts and Comparisons, 1995:157–202.

18. Kennerdell JS, Wucher FP. Cyclopentolate associated with two cases of grand mal seizure. Arch Ophthalmol 1972;87:634–635.

19. Awan KJ. Adverse systemic reactions to topical cyclopentolate hydrochloride. Ann Ophthalmol 1976;8:695–698.

20. Meyer SM, Fraunfelder FT. Phenylephrine hydrochloride. Ophthalmology 1980;87:1177–1180.

21. Fraunfelder FT, Samples JR. Ophthalmic medications during pregnancy. JAMA 1988;259:2021–2022.

22. Verkijik A. Worsening of myasthenia gravis with timolol maleate eyedrops. Ann Neurol 1985;199:211–212.

23. Gottschalk HR, Stone OJ. Stevens-Johnson syndrome from ophthalmic sulfonamide. Arch Dermatol 1976;112:513–514.

24. Jenvert GI, Cohen EJ, Donnenfeld ED, et al. Erythema multiforme after use of topical sulfacetamide. Am J Ophthalmol 1985;99:465–468.

25. Tosti A, Tosti G. Thimerosal: A hidden allergen in ophthalmology. Contact Dermatitis 1988;18:268–273.

26. Bartlett JD, Woolley TW, Adams CM. Identification of high intraocular pressure responders to topical ophthalmic corticosteroids. J Ocular Pharmacol 1993;9:35–45.

27. Eskridge JB, Amos JF, Bartlett JD, eds. Clinical procedures in optometry. Philadelphia: J.B. Lippincott, 1991.

28. Harris LS. Cycloplegic-induced intraocular pressure elevations. A study of normal and open-angle glaucomatous eyes. Arch Ophthalmol 1968;79:242–246.

29. Portney GL, Purcell TW. The influence of tropicamide on intraocular pressure. Ann Ophthalmol 1975;7:31–34.

30. Wilson FM. Adverse external ocular effects of topical ophthalmic therapy. An epidemiologic, laboratory, and clinical study. Trans Am Ophthalmol Soc 1983;81:854.

31. Wilson FM. Adverse external ocular effects of topical ophthalmic medications. Surv Ophthalmol 1979;24:57–88.

32. Fiore PM, Jacobs IH, Goldberg DB. Drug-induced pemphigoid. A spectrum of diseases. Arch Ophthalmol 1987;105:1650–1663.

33. Lyle WM, Hopkins GA. The unwanted ocular effects from topical ophthalmic drugs. Their occurrence, avoidance and reversal. J Am Optom Assoc 1977;48:1519–1523.

34. Coad CT, Osato MS, Wilhelmus KR. Bacterial contamination of eyedrop dispensers. Am J Ophthalmol 1984;98:548.

35. Schein OD, Wasson PJ, Boruchoff SA, et al. Microbial keratitis associated with contaminated ocular medications. Am J Ophthalmol 1988;105:361–365.

36. Schein OD, Hibberd PL, Starck T, et al. Microbial contamination of in-use ocular medications. Arch Ophthalmol 1992;110:82–85.

37. O'Day DM. Corticosteroids: An unresolved debate. Ophthalmology 1991;98:845–846.

38. Stern GA, Buttross M. Use of corticosteroids in combination with antimicrobial drugs in the treatment of infectious corneal disease. Ophthalmology 1991;98:847–853.

39. Berdy GJ, Abelson MB, Smith LM, George MA. Perservative-free artificial tear preparations: Assessment of corneal epithelial toxic effects. Arch Ophthalmol 1992;110:528–532.

40. Nicoll JMV, Acharya PA, Ahlen K, et al. Central nervous system complications after 6000 retrobulbar blocks. Anesth Analg 1987;66:1298–1302.

41. Friedberg HL, Kline OR. Contralateral amaurosis after retrobulbar injection. Am J Ophthalmol 1986;101:688–690.

42. Michaels RH, Wilson FM, Grayson M. Infiltrative keratitis from abuse of anesthetic eyedrops. J Indiana State Med Assoc 1979;72:51–54.

43. Gasset AR, Bellows RT. Posterior subcapsular cataracts after topical corticosteroid therapy. Ann Ophthalmol 1974;6:1263–1265.

44. Urtti A, Salminen L. Minimizing systemic absorption of topically administered ophthalmic drugs. Surv Ophthalmol 1993;37:435–456.

45. Fraunfelder FT, Morgan RL, Yunis AA. Blood dyscrasias and topical ophthalmic chloramphenicol. Am J Ophthalmol 1993;115:812–813.

46. Everitt DE, Avon J. Systemic effects of medications used to treat glaucoma. Ann Intern Med 1990;112:120–125.

47. Fraunfelder FT, Meyer SM. Systemic adverse reactions to glaucoma medications. Int Ophthalmol Clin 1989;29:143–146.

48. Havener WH. Ocular pharmacology. St. Louis: C.V. Mosby Co, 1983;5:261–417.

49. Zimmerman TJ, Sharir M, Nardin GF, Fuqua M. Therapeutic index of pilocarpine, carbachol, and timolol with nasolacrimal occlusion. Am J Ophthalmol 1992;114:1–7.

50. Bartlett JD. Ophthalmic toxicity by systemic drugs. In: Chiou GCY, ed. Ophthalmic toxicology. New York: Raven Press, 1992:167–217.

51. Jaanus SD. Ocular side effects of selected systemic drugs. Optom Clin 1992;2:73–96.

52. Baum C, Kennedy DL, Knapp DE, et al. Prescription drug use in 1984 and changes over time. Medical Care 1988;26:105–114.

53. Montamat SC, Cusack B. Overcoming problems with polypharmacy and drug misuse in the elderly. Clin Geriatr Med 1992;8:143–158.

54. LeSage J. Polypharmacy in geriatric patients. Nurs Clin North Am 1991;26:273–290.

55. Health care financing administration: Medicare and Medicaid. Requirements for long-term care facilities. Federal Register 1989;54:5316.

56. Wilcox TK, Bartlett JD. Systemic drug profiles in adult optometric outpatients. J Am Optom Assoc 1988;59:122–126.

57. Nolan L. Prescribing for the elderly. II. Prescribing patterns: Differences due to age. J Am Geriatr Soc 1988;36:245.

58. Biggs JSG, Allan JA. Medication and pregnancy. Drugs 1981;21:69–75.

59. Hill RM, Stern L. Drugs in pregnancy: Effects on the fetus and newborn. Drugs 1979;17:182–197.

60. Kooner KS, Zimmerman TJ. Clinical ocular pharmacology: Some overlooked features. Ophthalmol Clin North Am 1989;2:2–14.

61. Samples JR, Meyer SM. Use of ophthalmic medications in pregnant and nursing women. Am J Ophthalmol 1988;106:616–623.

62. American Association for Pediatric Ophthalmology and Strabismus Committee. Eye care for the children of America. J Pediatr Ophthalmol Strabismus 1991;28:64–67.

63. Milsap R, Szefler SJ. Special pharmacokinetic considerations in children. In: Evans WE, Schentag JJ, Jusko WJ, Harrison H, eds. Applied pharmacokinetics: Principles of therapeutic drug monitoring, ed. 2. Spokane, WA: Applied Therapeutics, Inc., 1986:294–330.

64. Cohen MS. Special aspects of perinatal and pediatric pharmacology. In: Katzung BG, ed. Basic and clinical pharmacology. Norwalk, CT: Appleton & Lange, 1992:860.

65. Maxwell GM. Pediatric drug dosing: Body weight versus surface area. Drugs 1989;37:113–115.

66. Carpenter TM. Tables, factors and formulas for computing respiratory exchange and biological transformations of energy. Publication 303C, ed. 4. Washington DC: Carnegie Institute, 1948:107–108.

67. Vestal RE, Cusack BJ. Pharmacology and aging. In: Schneider EL, Rowe JW, eds. Handbook of the biology of aging, ed. 3. New York: Academic Press, 1990:349–383.

68. Jaanus SD. Pharmacologic aspects of aging. In: Rosenbloom A, Morgan M, eds. Vision and aging, ed. 2. Boston: Butterworth, 1993:160–177.

69. Fraunfelder FT, Meyer SM. Safe use of ocular drugs in the elderly. Geriatrics 1984;39:97–102.

70. Rumsey KE. Pharmacological considerations in older adults. J Am Optom Assoc 1989;60:520–530.

71. Katzung BG. Special aspects of geriatic pharmacology. In: Katzung BG, ed. Basic and clinical pharmacology. Norwalk, CT: Appleton & Lange, 1992:863–869.

72. Kramer AM, Fox PD, Morgenstern N. Geriatric care approaches in health maintenance organizations. J Am Geriatr Soc 1992;40:1055–1067.

73. Hood CM, Siedman KR. Setting up a low vision practice. Probl Optom 1992;4:107–116.

74. Mansour AM. Tolerance to topical preparations: Cold or warm? Ann Ophthalmol 1991;23:21–22.

75. Francis J. Delirium in older patients. J Am Geriatr Soc 1992;40:829–838.

76. Cole HC, Shapiro AP. Drug-induced illness as a cause for admission to a community hospital. J Am Geriatr Soc 1989;37:323–326.

77. Braekhus A, Laake K, Engedal K. The mini-mental state examination: Identifying the most efficient variables for detecting cognitive impairment in the elderly. J Am Geriatr Soc 1992;40:1139–1145.

78. Zisok S, Braff DL. Delirium: Recognition and management in the older patient. Geriatrics 1986;41:67–78.

79. Anonymous. Acquired immunodeficiency syndrome (AIDS)—data as at 31 December 1993. Weekly Epidemiol Rec 1994; 69(2):5–6.

80. Anonymous. National Eye Institute issues clinical alert about CMV retinitis in AIDS. JAMA 1991;266:2665.

81. Friedman WR, Helm M. Retinal and ophthalmologic manifestations of AIDS. In: Ryan SJ, ed. Retina. St. Louis: C.V. Mosby Co, 1989:597–616.

82. Holland GN. Acquired immunodeficiency syndrome and ophthalmology: The first decade. Am J Ophthalmol 1992;114:86–95.

83. Brandt JD, Wittpenn JR, Katz LJ, et al. Conjunctival impression cytology in patients with glaucoma using long-term topical medication. Am J Ophthalmol 1991;112:297–301.

84. Schwab IR, Linberg JV, Gioia VM, et al. Foreshortening of the inferior conjunctival fornix associated with chronic glaucoma medications. Ophthalmology 1992;99:197–202.

85. Willcox SM, Himmelstein DU, Woolhandler S. Inappropriate drug prescribing for the community-dwelling elderly. JAMA 1994;272:292–296.

CHAPTER 2

Ophthalmic Drug Formulations

Neal L. Burstein

Drugs affect ocular tissues based on the special pharmacokinetic properties of the eye. *Pharmacokinetics* is the study of the time course of absorption, distribution, metabolism, and elimination of an administered drug.[1] Drug absorption depends on the molecular properties of the drug, the viscosity of its vehicle, and the functional status of the tissue forming the barrier to penetration.[2] Drug distribution over time and bioavailability at the desired site of action can usually be predicted by the interrelationships of the compartments and barriers of the eye.[3] Metabolism plays an important part in eliminating drugs and their sometimes toxic by-products from the eye and from the body.[4] Metabolic enzymes have recently been studied to assist in the design of *prodrugs*, which are molecules that are converted to an active form after tissue penetration has occurred.[5]

This chapter considers the unique structural aspects of ocular tissues as they relate to pharmacokinetics. Examples of how ocular drugs are designed and formulated to enhance bioavailability will also be considered.

Physicochemical Factors Affecting Drug Bioavailability

Medicinal chemistry involves the study of existing drugs and the design and synthesis of molecules with improved activity, bioavailability, toxicity, and other characteristics. An understanding of the action of any drug is based on analysis of its quantitative structure-activity relationships, which are unique to each molecular structure. Computer analysis of these relationships and of three-dimensional molecular conformations has contributed to rapid development in this field. Some of the quantifiable properties used in evaluating molecular drugs for therapeutic consideration are described below.

Solubility and Partition Coefficient

Molecular diffusion through cell membranes can occur by two major pathways.[6] The first is entry through the lipid portion of the membrane by lipophilic ("fat-loving") compounds. The second is diffusion through "water pores" in the membrane by hydrophilic ("water-loving") compounds. Because the cell membrane is largely composed of lipids, there are few restrictions on the penetration of lipophilic compounds, even considering molecular size. Hydrophilic compounds, in contrast, are more limited in diffusion except where an extracellular fluid pathway exists for transport.[7] The hydrophilic versus lipophilic migrational tendencies of a compound, as well as its absolute solubilities in each phase, greatly affect its pharmacokinetics.[8]

A useful expression for the relative lipophilic versus hydrophilic nature of a molecule is the octanol-water partition coefficient. In a simple test, a molecular species is suspended and well stirred in a flask containing equal portions of buffered water and octanol. Organic solutes such as hexane are sometimes substituted for octanol as the lipid phase. The pH of the buffer is important because it affects the partitioning of a weak acid or base. After equilibrium occurs, the two phases are each analyzed for concentration of the test species. The result is expressed as the log of concentration ratios between octanol and water. A wide range of solubilities in aqueous and lipid phases can be expressed by the coefficient derived from this method.[8,9]

Molecular Size and Shape

Molecular size is often less important than the molecular charge and partitioning characteristics in determining ocular drug penetration.[9] However, very large molecules are sterically hindered by their bulk, which impedes their diffusion through narrow spaces.[3] The size of a globular molecule increases as the cube root of the molecular weight, which is usually expressed in daltons (d). The water of solvation surrounding a charged molecule must be considered in determining the total size for diffusion calculations. The diffusion coefficient decreases with increasing molecular size. The molecular configuration becomes important for proteins and other macromolecules, where the shape can vary from a folded globular form to an elongate helix.

In ophthalmic medications, the concentration of the active drug is usually expressed as a percentage. However, a high molecular weight compound is present at a lower molarity than a smaller molecule when both are supplied at the same percentage. Some commercially available compounds with similar active sites but different groups substituted in the inactive portions of the molecule are supplied at concentrations that appear to be the same on a weight basis. However, they vary considerably in molarity due to the difference in molecular size or the size of the inactive ion.

Dissociation Constant

Any drug that is at least partially water soluble ionizes to a degree dependent on the ionizable groups of the molecule and the pH of the solute. Many ophthalmic drugs with charged groups act as weak bases. For example, pilocarpine hydrochloride undergoes hydrolysis to an equilibrium dependent on the hydrogen ion concentration, as follows:[10]

$$C_{11}H_{16}N_2O_2HCl \rightarrow C_{11}H_{16}N_2O_2H^+$$
Pilocarpine HCl   Pilocarpine ion

$$+ Cl^-$$
Chloride ion   (2.1)

$$C_{11}H_{16}N_2O_2H^+ + HOH \rightarrow C_{11}H_{16}N_2O_2HOH$$
Pilocarpine ion   Pilocarpine base

$$+ H^+$$
Hydrogen ion   (2.2)

The pK_b of a base is the pH at which 50% of the molecule is dissociated. Table 2.1 shows the pK_b for several ophthalmic drugs. At a pH lower than the pK_b, more than half the weak base is dissociated. Figure 2.1 shows the ion-base equilibrium of these drugs. Drugs such as pilocarpine, which are present in both base and ionic forms at ocular pH, penetrate most ocular barriers readily. When a drug is biologically active but has difficulty reaching its site of action, adjusting the dissociation constant by modifying ionizable groups can markedly alter drug penetration.[10] However, it is not practical in clinical use to make the pH of formulations lower than 4 or higher than 10. The effects of pH on the storage properties and comfort of ophthalmic formulations are discussed later in this chapter.

Ocular Tissue Structure and Pharmacokinetics

The eye is composed of numerous tissues, each of distinct developmental origin, and each with a specific role in the functioning visual system. These tissues include the smooth and striate musculature, a variety of simple and mucoid epithelia, connective tissues, sympathetic and parasympathetic nerves, and the retina. The retina is often considered a direct extension of the brain because it and the optic nerve are formed together from an outfolding of the embryonic neural tube.

The organization of the eye must provide a path for light through the clear tissues that form the optical imaging system, while providing for the nutrition of those same tissues in the absence of a blood supply. This avascularity allows a direct route for ocular drug penetration without absorption by the systemic circulation.

In this section, some special properties of each of the

TABLE 2.1
Percentage of Free Base in Equilibrium with Salts of Alkaloids

Drug	pK_b	pH 4.0	pH 7.4	pH 9.0
Atropine	4.35	0.0002	0.6	18.3
Ephedrine	4.64	0.0004	1.1	30.4
Procaine	5.15	0.001	3.4	58.5
Cocaine	5.59	0.004	8.9	79.6
Pilocarpine	7.15	0.141	78.1	99.3

From Hind HW, Goyan FM. A new concept of the role of hydrogen ion concentration and buffer systems in the preparation of ophthalmic solutions. J Am Pharm Assoc 1947;36:33–41.

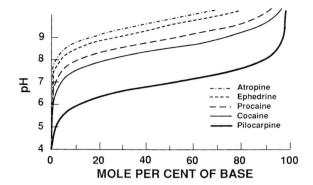

FIGURE 2.1 **The ion-base equilibrium of drugs that are weak bases is plotted as a function of pH. The pK$_b$ is the pH at which 50% of the drug is ionized (see Table 2.1 for numerical values). (Modified from Hind HW, Goyan FM. A new concept of the role of hydrogen ion concentration and buffer systems in the preparation of ophthalmic solutions. J Am Pharm Assoc 1947;36:33–41.)**

clear axial components of the eye, together with their nutritional and metabolite exchange through the adjoining vascular tissues, are discussed. A model is then developed wherein the ocular tissues and fluids function as barriers and depots. Such a model can be useful in predicting ocular distribution of drugs over time.

Tear Structure and Chemical Properties

The tear film covering the cornea and defining the major optical surface of the eye is composed of three layers[11,12] (see Figure 14.1). The outermost, oily layer is usually considered to be a lipid monolayer and is produced primarily by the meibomian glands located in the eyelids. The primary function of the oily layer is to stabilize the surface of the underlying aqueous fluid layer and retard evaporation. Tear surface lipids are readily washed away if the eye is flushed with saline or medication, resulting in a tear evaporation increase of more than tenfold.[13] Minor infections of the meibomian glands, particularly with *Staphylococcus*, can also decrease tear film stability. This is due to an alteration of the chemical nature of meibum, the secretion product of the gland.

The aqueous phase of the tears comprises more than 95% of the total volume and covers the cornea with a layer that averages about 7 μm thick. This layer is inherently unstable, however, and begins to thin centrally at the end of each blink. The tear film in healthy subjects has a breakup time (BUT) that averages between 25 and 30 seconds.[14]

The inner, or basal, layer of the tears is composed of glycoproteins and is secreted by goblet cells in the conjunc-

tiva. This mucinous layer is present both as a thin hydrophilic coating covering the cornea and conjunctiva and as thick rolls and strands that cleanse the tears of particulate debris at each blink (Fig. 2.2).[15]

The pH of the tears is about 7.4,[16] and the tear layer contains small amounts of protein including lysozymes, lactoferrins, gamma globulins, and other immune factors. The tears are primarily responsible for supplying the oxygen requirements of the corneal epithelium.

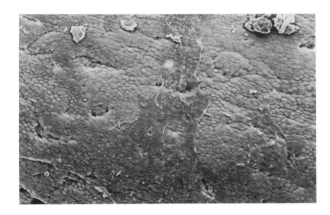

A

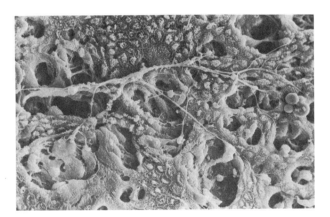

B

FIGURE 2.2 **The conjunctiva of a rabbit is shown by scanning electron microscopy with surface mucins intact. Note the sheets and folds that allow the mucins to entrap particles and remove them from the tears. The tears form a reservoir for drug compounds, including those that are delivered as particulate suspensions. (From Burstein NL. The effects of topical drugs and preservatives on the tears and corneal epithelium in dry eye. Trans Ophthalmol Soc UK 1985;104:402–409.)**

Tear Volume

The normal volume of the tear layer is 8 to 10 µl, including the fluid trapped in the folds of the conjunctiva.[17] A total volume of perhaps 30 µl can be held for a brief time if the eyelids are not squeezed after dosing. When a single drop of medication of 50 µl (1/20 ml) is applied, the nasolacrimal duct rapidly drains the excess. Increasing drop size, therefore, does not result in more medication penetrating the cornea.[18] However, the systemic load is increased linearly with drop size, because after drainage through the nasolacrimal duct the drug is usually absorbed through the nasal mucosa or swallowed. For drugs with major systemic side effects, such as β blockers, efforts have been made to limit drop size.[19] A metering dispenser delivering small drops (25 µl) has been introduced to decrease the ratio of systemic to ocular effect. Such a device, however, cannot take the place of careful supervision during initial dosing and monitoring of patient compliance.[20]

It is difficult to limit the volume of a drop dispensed by gravity from a dropper tip below about 25 µl, three times the normal tear reservoir. Chrai and associates[21] have proposed that the theoretical optimum volume of drug solution to deliver is zero volume, because increasing the instilled volume increases the volume lost and the percentage of drug lost. Although this theoretical extreme is impossible to achieve, it is practical to dispense accurately measured drops as small as 2 to 5 µl by reducing the bore size of commercial dropper dispensers.[22] Small drop volumes can also be dispensed from a micrometer syringe by touching a flexible polyethylene tip to the conjunctiva. For investigational purposes this allows instillation of drugs without greatly affecting size of the tear reservoir.

Tear Flow

The normal rate of basal (unstimulated) tear flow in humans is about 0.5 to 2.2 µl/min and decreases with age.[17,23] Tear flow rate is stimulated by the ocular irritation resulting from many topical medications. The concentration of drug available in the tears for transcorneal absorption is inversely proportional to the tear flow, due to the drug's dilution and removal by the nasolacrimal duct and by lid spillover. Therefore, both the flow rate and tear volume influence drug absorption by the anterior segment of the eye.[23]

To enhance corneal drug absorption, the tear film concentration can be prolonged by manually blocking the nasolacrimal ducts or by tilting the head back to reduce drainage[24] (see Chapter 3). Another effective technique to increase corneal penetration is to give a series of drops at intervals of about 10 minutes.[18] It has been determined, however, that when different drug formulations are given as drops in rapid succession, the medications first applied are diluted and do not achieve full therapeutic potential.[21]

Patients with a flow rate near the lower limit of 0.5 µl/min, often due to aging or atrophy of the lacrimal ducts and glands, are usually considered to have dry eye (keratoconjunctivitis sicca).[25] This group includes many elderly patients, individuals with rheumatoid arthritis, some postmenopausal women, and persons with exposure keratitis associated with dry climate or dusty work conditions.[15] Several factors contribute to greatly increased drug absorption in these individuals. Their total tear volume is less than normal, so that a drop of medication is not diluted as much as usual. Because lacrimation is reduced, the drug is not rapidly diluted by tears and has a prolonged residence time next to the corneal surface, where the majority of absorption occurs. Since epithelial surface damage is usually present in patients with dry eye, the final result is greatly increased ocular absorption.

Drugs (e.g., pilocarpine) that cause rapid lacrimation by stinging or by stimulation of lacrimal glands in normal individuals are formulated at high concentration to offset the dilution and washout that occur from tear flow. Patients with dry eyes that do not tear readily can absorb greatly exaggerated doses of topically applied medications. In children, who cry and lacrimate more easily than adults, rapid drug washout can prevent adequate absorption of topically applied medications.

Cornea and Sclera

The cornea is a five-layered, avascular structure[26] (Fig. 2.3). It comprises the major functional barrier to ocular penetration, and it is also the major site of absorption for topically applied drugs. The epithelium and stroma have a major influence on pharmacodynamics, since they constitute depots or reservoirs for lipophilic and hydrophilic drugs, respectively.

The sclera is an opaque, vascular structure continuous with the cornea at the limbus. The loose connective tissue overlying the sclera, the conjunctiva, is also vascularized. The conjunctiva and sclera, as routes of drug penetration, are responsible for less than one-fifth of all drug absorption to the iris and ciliary body. This limited absorption is due to the extensive vascularization of these tissues, which results in removal of most drugs.[27,28] An elegant visualization of the route of scleral penetration was achieved by Bienfang,[29] who applied a piece of filter paper moistened with epinephrine to the white of the eye in a human subject. He was able to obtain mydriasis in an isolated sector of iris adjacent to the site of scleral application.

The conjunctival sac forms a large area, about 32 cm² for both eyes. Its surface functions as a major depot for some drugs that are superficially absorbed, then re-released to the tears. Trapped particles from a suspension may allow active drug to dissolve slowly from the conjunctival sac and saturate tear drug levels.[30]

CORNEAL EPITHELIUM

The corneal epithelium is 5 to 6 cell-layers thick centrally and 8 to 10 cell-layers thick at the periphery. It is composed of a basal germinative layer, intermediate wing cells, and a surface squamous layer that possesses structures known as *zonula occludens,* or tight junctions. These junctions comprise a continuing border between epithelial cells formed by the fusion of the outer plasma membrane.[31] Mucopolysaccharides bound to the outer plasma membrane, shown in Figure 2.4A, stabilize the tears. The cornea relies on diffusion of nutrients from the aqueous humor to supply its metabolic needs.[16]

Over half the total corneal electrical resistance is contained in the uppermost squamous cell layer.[32] Because the healthy epithelium presents a continuous layer of plasma membrane to the tear film (Fig. 2.4B), it largely resists the penetration of hydrophilic drugs.[33] The anionic diagnostic agent sodium fluorescein is a good example of such a hydrophilic agent. The amount of fluorescein penetrating the intact epithelium is small. If a slight break in the outer cellular layer occurs, then fluorescein can penetrate easily and is visible as a green stain for several minutes in the beam of a blue excitation filter. Epithelial erosion or the action of cationic preservatives can greatly increase the penetration of hydrophilic drugs in the same manner.

The interstices between the epithelial cell layers communicate directly by an aqueous pathway with the stroma and aqueous humor. This has been demonstrated by Tonjum,[34] who injected horseradish peroxidase, an enzyme used experimentally as a molecular tracer, into aqueous humor. It diffused readily across the entire cornea and accumulated adjacent to the epithelial tight junctional complex, where it was blocked from passage to the tear side. When applied to the tears, however, it did not penetrate the outer corneal layer.

Lipophilic drugs can readily enter the epithelium, because its barrier is composed of phospholipid membranes.[35] Since the epithelium contains more than two-thirds of the plasma membrane mass of the cornea, it is the most significant storage depot for agents that readily partition into lipid media. The release rate of drugs from the epithelium depends on their tendency to reenter an aqueous phase. Thus, agents that are very lipophilic have a very long half-life once in the epithelium. For example, cyclosporins have a half-life of about 24 hours in epithelium. They are effective when administered topically every 48 hours, because they have sufficient biologic activity to remain effective at the very low levels released from the cornea.[36]

To penetrate the cornea effectively, a drug must possess a balance of hydrophilic and lipophilic properties and must be able to partition between both media. This phenomenon is well known through the study of series of compounds of similar properties, such as β blockers.[37] A plot of partition coefficient versus corneal permeability usually results in the

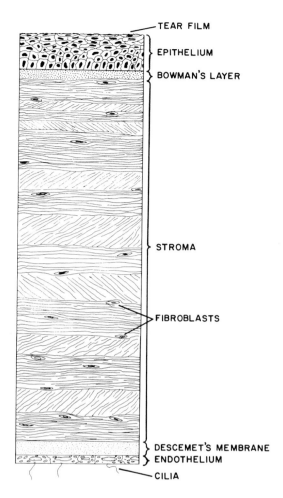

FIGURE 2.3   **Cross-sectional diagram of the cornea. Note the epithelium is only about one-tenth the total corneal mass. Nevertheless, it can be considered a separate storage depot for certain lipophilic drugs.**

formation of a parabola.[8] An example is shown in Figure 2.5. Molecular species with the appropriate partition coefficient at or near the peak are thus readily transferred through the cornea. Those with too low a coefficient do not penetrate well through the outer epithelial barrier. Those with too high a partition coefficient tend to remain in the epithelium and partition into the anterior chamber slowly, resulting in low but prolonged aqueous humor levels.[8]

CORNEAL STROMA

Bowman's layer is the modified anterior border of stroma in humans. This layer is 8 to 14 μm thick and is composed of clear, randomly oriented collagen fibrils surrounded by mucoprotein ground substance.[26,38] Numerous pores in the

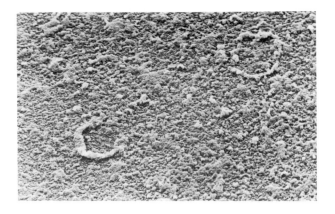

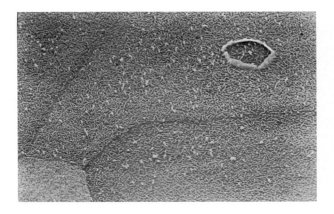

A   B

FIGURE 2.4   Scanning electron micrographs of the corneal epithelium of a rabbit. *(A)* Mucins are fixed in place as they are normally, to stabilize the tear film. The pits seen in the photograph are normal for rabbits and are not present in humans. *(B)* The mucins are washed away by acetylcysteine to reveal the underlying pattern of microvilli and microplicae visible on the cell surface. (From Burstein NL. The effects of topical drugs and preservatives on the tears and corneal epithelium in dry eye. Trans Ophthalmol Soc UK 1985;104:402–409.)

inner structure allow the passage of terminal branches of corneal nerves from the stroma into epithelium. The surface of Bowman's layer adjoins the structurally distinct epithelial basal lamina. The drug penetration characteristics of Bowman's layer are probably similar to those of the stroma.

The stroma occupies 90% of the corneal thickness and contains about one-third of the cells of the cornea in the form of keratocytes. The connective tissue of the stroma is composed of multiple layers of closely knit collagen bundles, or lamellae, arranged to distribute evenly the stress of the intraocular pressure (IOP) to the limbus, the thickened zone that joins the cornea and sclera. The collagen bundles are hexagonally packed and more ordered in the cornea than in the sclera. Their organization, together with the interspersed proteoglycans, is largely responsible for the clarity of the cornea.[39]

The collagen fibrils occupy space and also increase the path of diffusion, with the net effect of impeding diffusion by the equivalent of a fluid layer several times the actual stromal thickness. Nevertheless, the stroma is transparent to molecular species below about 500,000 d.[3] The stroma serves as the major ocular depot for topically applied hydrophilic drugs, and the keratocytes presumably provide a reservoir for lipophilic compounds as well.

The posterior border of the stroma is the endothelial basal lamina, termed Descemet's layer. Approximately 3 to 4 μm thick at birth, it becomes about 10 to 12 μm thick by 50 years of age. It is highly elastic and is formed of prenatal banded collagen and unbanded collagen secreted after birth by the endothelium. Descemet's layer stains distinctly periodic acid–Schiff (PAS) positive because of the presence of carbohydrate not found in stroma and has a structural pattern

evident in cross-section that is not present in any other known tissue.[26,40] Descemet's layer appears to pass molecular species as readily as the stroma and is not known to act as a separate drug depot.

CORNEAL ENDOTHELIUM

The corneal endothelium, a monolayer of polygonal cells about 3 μm thick,[41] has a structure and properties unique in the body. It should not be confused with the blood vessel endothelium, which is of different developmental origin and has different characteristics. The nonregenerative property of the corneal endothelium requires that existing cells stretch to cover the space of any neighbors that are destroyed by physical damage or senescence. The endothelial cell layer has the remarkable ability to pump its own weight in fluid from the stromal side into the anterior chamber in five minutes. The intercellular borders form a junction that is open along its full length and allows a rapid leakage of water and solutes in the reverse direction to the fluid pump.[40,42]

The fluid pump is probably a bicarbonate-based ion transport, which may be coupled to Na^+–K^+ ATPase by an unknown mechanism.[43,44] The leak is composed of a channel that is 12 μm long and 20 nm wide, narrowing to 5.0 nm at the edge facing the anterior chamber.[45] This space is large enough to conduct large molecules, such as 3.5 nm diameter colloidal gold and colloidal lanthanum particles (Fig. 2.6). The ultrastructure and ability to pass large molecules make the endothelial border a special type of leaky junction, rather than a tight junction *(zonula occludens)* as sometimes stated. Globular proteins above 1,000,000 d cannot pass readily, but smaller molecules are not hindered. Pinocytosis does occur in the endothelium and allows the transport of high molecular weight proteins. Because of the thinness and small volume of the endothelial layer, it is not considered a major reservoir for drugs.[3]

The cornea can concentrate certain substances from the aqueous, allowing the corneal stroma to hold more drug than would be expected from its fluid mass. This may result from the constant inward leakage of whole aqueous from the anterior chamber to the stroma, offset by the return of osmotic water by the fluid pump. Fluorescein given by mouth or vein thus accumulates rapidly in the corneal stroma from the aqueous. An alternative explanation for this accumulation is the ionic binding of substances by negative charges in stroma, reducing the diffusible pool of solute. Because fluorescein is itself an anion, however, this explanation is not fully satisfactory.[3]

Iris

The iris functions primarily to adjust the amount of light reaching the retina, simultaneously altering the visual depth of focus without changing the field of vision. It does this by controlling the total area of the visual pathway between the two major refractive components of the eye—the cornea and lens. It therefore contains pigment to absorb light. To accomplish this function, two groups of muscles, the sphincter and the dilator, work in opposition. These are supplied by cholinergic and adrenergic innervation, respectively. Miosis (pupillary constriction) can be accomplished by endogenous or exogenous acetylcholine or by cholinergic stimulation. Mydriasis (dilation) can be accomplished by an adrenergic stimulant such as epinephrine, which acts on the dilator musculature, or by an antagonist to acetylcholine, which allows relaxation of the sphincter. The readily observed behavior of the iris has made its action an excellent model for the study of drug penetration in the human eye.[2]

The pigment granules of the iris epithelium absorb light and can also absorb lipophilic drugs. This type of binding is characteristically reversible, allowing release of drug over time. It is usually termed nonspecific or low-affinity binding, indicating that a specific high-affinity drug receptor is not involved. As a result, the iris can serve as a depot or reservoir for some drugs, concentrating and then releasing them for longer than otherwise expected.

Nonspecific binding can prevent or delay a single dose of a lipophilic drug from reaching an effective level within the eye. On multiple dosing, however, a saturation equilibrium is reached when the amount of drug being bound is the same as that being released from the reservoir. Once this occurs, effective dosing is achieved. Individual iris pigmentation varies widely, and some drugs show a far greater response after the first dose in blue-eyed individuals than in patients

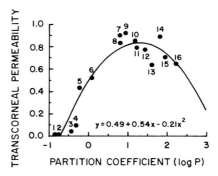

FIGURE 2.5 **Parabolic curve of corneal penetration versus octanol-water partition coefficient. As the drug becomes too lipophilic or too hydrophilic, penetration through the cornea is diminished. Numbers refer to reagents. (Adapted from Kishida K, Otori T. Quantitative study on the relationship between transcorneal permeability of drugs and their hydrophobicity. Jpn J Ophthalmol 1980;24:251–259.)**

with dark irides. Shell[1] demonstrated constriction of the pupil (miosis) after a single dose of pilocarpine continuing for 4.7 hours in darkly pigmented subjects compared with only two hours in subjects with blue eyes.

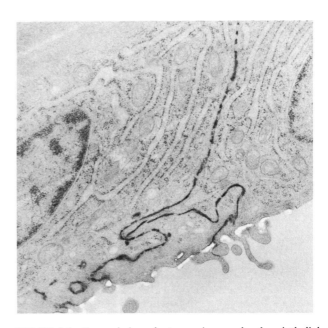

FIGURE 2.6 **Transmission electron micrograph of endothelial cells showing a border between two cells. The dense material is lanthanum, which was added one minute before the tissue was fixed by rapid freezing. The area of cytoplasm bordering cells at bottom center is probably an interdigitation from one of the two cells.**

Aqueous Humor

Aqueous humor is formed by the ciliary body and occupies the posterior and anterior chambers, a compartment measuring about 0.2 ml, although the total volume decreases with age as the lens grows. The fluid is constantly generated by the pigmented and nonpigmented epithelium of the ciliary body, which is supplied by a rich bed of capillaries. It flows from the posterior chamber through the pupil and then slowly circles in the anterior chamber, circulated by the thermal differential between the cornea and the deeper ocular tissues.[46] The aqueous exits at the angle between the cornea and iris through the sieve-like trabecular meshwork. It then enters the canal of Schlemm, which leads directly into low-pressure episcleral veins and finally into the general circulation. Drugs absorbed through the cornea can leave the aqueous through this so-called conventional route or through the walls of the iris or other tissues comprising the margins of the anterior chamber, the "uveoscleral route" of aqueous humor outflow.

Ciliary Body

The major function of the ciliary body is aqueous humor production. Aqueous is composed of a clear ultrafiltrate of blood plasma devoid of large proteins, together with some substances actively transported across the blood-aqueous barrier.

The capillaries of the ciliary body are many and possess no tight junctions to limit the diffusion of drugs or proteins. However, drugs are usually limited by the apically tight junctions of the nonpigmented cells at the paired layers making up the ciliary epithelium.[47] Systemic drugs enter the anterior and posterior chambers largely by passing through the ciliary body vasculature and then diffusing into the iris where they can enter the aqueous humor.

The ciliary body is the major ocular source of drug-metabolizing enzymes responsible for the two major phases of reactions that begin the process of drug detoxification and removal from the eye. The localization of these enzymes together in a single tissue is important, because the oxidative and reductive products from phase I reactions of the cytochrome P-450 system are highly reactive and potentially more toxic than the parent compounds.[4] Conjugation by glucuronidation, sulfonation, acetylation, methylation, or with amino acids or glutathione in phase II reactions can then be accomplished by detoxifying enzymes. The uveal circulation provides up to 88% of the total blood flow and can rapidly remove these conjugated products from the eye.[48] Melanin granules of the pigmented ciliary epithelium adsorb polycyclic compounds such as chloroquine, storing them for metabolism and removal.[49]

Crystalline Lens

The normal human lens originates from a double layer of epithelium. Its thickened outer basal lamina (the capsule) is analogous to Descemet's layer. The lens grows to become a thick, flexible tissue composed of cells densely packed with clear proteins known as crystallins. By the age of 50 years, flexibility is reduced, thus diminishing accommodation.[50] The capsule reaches a thickness of several microns anteriorly and is ten times thinner posteriorly. The anterior lens epithelium is the most active region metabolically, conducting cation transport and cell division. This region is also the most prone to damage from drugs or toxic substances.[51]

Hydrophilic drugs of high molecular weight cannot be absorbed by the lens from the aqueous humor, because the lens epithelium is a major barrier to entry.[52] The capsule prevents the entry of large proteins. Lipid-soluble drugs, however, can pass slowly into and through the lens cortex.[51] Fluorescein, a hydrophilic molecule, can penetrate the capsule and reach the nucleus in a few weeks.[46] The lens can be viewed primarily as a barrier to rapid penetration of drugs from aqueous to vitreous humor.

The lens grows with age, and colorations or opacities may develop and interfere with vision. Cataract formation may be enhanced by some miotics, steroids, and phenothiazines.[51] Aldose reductase inhibitors, which prevent the conversion of sugars to polyols, appear to prevent or delay diabetic cataract.[53] Levels of glutathione and other compounds drop during the formation of some types of cataract.[54] The pharmacokinetics of delivery and penetration of such compounds into the crystalline lens is currently of great interest.

When cataracts necessitate lens removal to restore vision, the kinetics between aqueous and vitreous humor change. A major barrier to molecular transport is removed, and more rapid exchange can occur between aqueous and vitreous contents and various ocular components. In one experimental study,[55] the concentration of a topically applied anti-inflammatory agent, flurbiprofen, was increased in retinal tissues, vitreous humor, and choroid after lens removal.

Vitreous Humor

The vitreous humor is a viscoelastic connective tissue composed of small amounts of glycosaminoglycans, including hyaluronic acid, and proteins such as collagen. The collagen fibrils are anchored directly to the basal lamina, which forms the boundaries of the lens, the ciliary body epithelium, and the neuroglial cells of the retina.[56] Although the anterior vitreous is cell-free, the posterior vitreous contains a few phagocytic cells called hyalocytes and is sometimes termed the cortical tissue layer.[57]

At birth, the material of the vitreous is gel-like in humans and primates. A central remnant of the hyaloid artery, Cloquet's canal, which is free of collagen fibrils, runs from the posterior lens capsule to the optic disc. Because the total volume of the vitreous expands with age while the amount of hyaluronate remains constant, the gel-like material develops a central viscous fluid lake completely surrounded by the gel vitreous. These events can cause condensation and tearing of the sheath of Cloquet's canal, forming structures termed floaters, which can interfere with vision.[58,59]

The vitreous comprises approximately 80% of the ocular mass. It may be considered an unstirred fluid with free diffusion for small molecules.[60] Some molecular species can diffuse between the posterior chamber and the vitreous. However, very high molecular weight substances, such as hyaluronate, are held in place by the zonules and lens capsule and diffuse out of the vitreous only after intracapsular lens extraction.[61–64] From this discussion it is apparent that the vitreous can serve as a major reservoir for drugs as well as a temporary storage depot for metabolites. For low molecular weight substances, a free path of diffusion exists from the ciliary body through the posterior aqueous humor.

Hydrophilic drugs such as gentamicin, which do not cross the blood-retinal barrier readily, have a prolonged half-life of 24 hours or more in the vitreous humor.[3] Their major route of exit is across the lens zonules and into the aqueous humor and then through the aqueous outflow pathways. For the vitreous to act as a depot for these drugs, they must be injected or introduced by iontophoresis.[63,65]

Retina and Optic Nerve

Tight junctional complexes, *zonula occludens,* in the retinal pigment epithelium (RPE) prevent the ready movement of antibiotics and other drugs from the blood to the retina and vitreous. The retina is a developmental derivative of the neutral tube wall and can be viewed as a direct extension of the brain, and it is not surprising that the blood-retinal barrier somewhat resembles the blood-brain barrier in form and function. Experimental evidence for this similarity comes from the work of Cunha-Vaz,[66,67] who showed that histamine does not alter the vascular permeability of the retina but does affect that of all other ocular tissues. The retina closely resembles the brain with respect to this trait.

The capillaries of the retina are lined by continuous, close-walled endothelial cells, which are the primary determinant of the molecular selectivity that is the major function of the blood-retinal barrier.[68,69] Bruch's membrane is a prominent structure associated with the retinal-vitreous barrier, yet it contributes relatively little to the barrier's filtration properties.

The barrier protects against the entry of a wide variety of metabolites and toxins and is effective against most hydrophilic drugs, which do not cross the plasma membrane. Glucose, however, can cross much more easily than would be expected from its molecular structure. This diffusion is probably facilitated by an active transport system involving a transmembrane carrier molecule. Lipophilic drugs cross the barrier easily in either direction due to their membrane fluidity. A number of agents, including topical epinephrine, systemic agents such as digitalis, phenothiazines, quinine, methyl alcohol and quinoline derivatives, can cause retinal toxicity.[70,71] A growing number of substances have been shown to be transported from the vitreous and retina into the blood plasma, including ions, drugs, and the prostaglandins associated with ocular inflammation.[72–74]

The optic nerve is of interest here because some drugs are toxic to this tissue.[71,75] The antibiotics chloramphenicol, ethambutol, streptomycin, and sulfonamides can cause optic neuritis. Vitamin A, especially in large doses, can result in papilledema. Digitalis can cause retrobulbar neuritis (see Chapter 37).

Blood Supply and Removal of Drugs and Metabolites

The parenteral route of administration is effective only for drugs of low systemic toxicity that can be introduced into the eye at therapeutic concentrations. An important example of systemic dosing is the case of internal ocular infections, such as endophthalmitis, where a high concentration of antibiotic must be maintained. The systemic dose can also be augmented by topical drug applications to the eye.[76]

Drugs that are unacceptable as systemic medications due to toxicity to certain organs such as liver or kidney can be especially useful for topical ocular dosing. Certain drugs are also well suited for topical use in the eye or for injection, because they are rapidly diluted by the bloodstream to levels that are nontoxic.

The bloodstream is responsible for removing drugs and drug metabolites from ocular tissues. The two circulatory pathways in the eye, the retinal vessels and the uveal vessels, are quite different. The retinal vessels can remove many drugs, metabolites, and such agents as prostaglandins from the vitreous humor and retina, apparently by active transport.[69] The uveal vessels remove drugs by bulk transport from the iris and ciliary body. The direct outflow pathway from aqueous humor through trabecular meshwork and canal of Schlemm into the episcleral vessels is another major source of drug removal from the eye.

Compartment Theory and Drug Kinetics

The eye is a unique structure, because several of its fluids and tissues—the tear film, cornea, aqueous humor, lens, and vitreous humor—are almost completely transparent. These

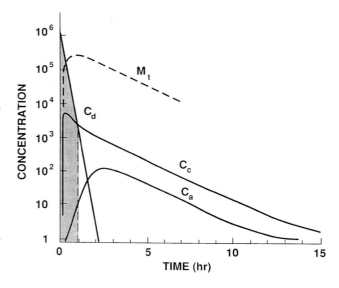

FIGURE 2.7 **Pharmacokinetics of sodium fluorescein in tears, cornea, and aqueous humor after instillation. The concentration of fluorescein in each compartment is plotted as a function of time. The tear concentration (C_d) falls rapidly, and significant drug is transferred to the cornea only while the tear concentration remains higher than the corneal concentration (C_c). The cornea then functions as a storage depot for the aqueous humor, whose concentration (C_a) parallels that of the cornea for many hours. The dotted line M_t represents the total mass of the drug in all tissues. This curve can be experimentally verified in the living human eye by fluorophotometry. (Modified from Maurice DM, Mishima S. Ocular pharmacokinetics. In: Sears ML, ed. Pharmacology of the eye. Handbook of experimental pharmacology. Berlin: Springer-Verlag, 1984;69:19–116.)**

components of the ocular system have no direct blood supply in the healthy state. Each can be considered a separate chamber or compartment. A compartment is defined here as a region of tissue or fluid through which a drug can diffuse and equilibrate with relative freedom. Each compartment is generally separated by a barrier from other compartments, so that flow between adjacent compartments takes more time than diffusion within each compartment.

The tears are an example of a compartment with constant turnover, since the inflow of lacrimal fluid is constant and equal to the outflow through the puncta. Consider the fate of sodium fluorescein, a diagnostic tracer representative of a highly hydrophilic drug. Once instilled, it mixes rapidly with the tears, and the tear flow carries away a portion per unit time dependent on the drug concentration present.

Approximately 99% of fluorescein or of a hydrophilic drug exits the tears by lacrimal drainage, yet a very small amount penetrates the corneal epithelial barrier and enters the stroma. A barrier is a region of lower permeability or restricted diffusion that exists between compartments. If the epithelium is considered to be a barrier to drug penetration from the tears and the bulk of the cornea a compartment, a two-compartment model can be described. In the absence of an active transport mechanism, drugs diffuse across barriers according to the laws of thermodynamics, from a region of higher to one of lower concentration. Fick's first law of diffusion states that the rate of diffusion across a barrier is proportional to the concentration gradient between the compartments on either side of the barrier.

From Fick's law, the rate of diffusion of a drug across a barrier is linearly dependent on the concentration difference between the compartments on either side of the barrier. As soon as the concentration of drug in the cornea equals that of the tears, drug no longer penetrates inward. Therefore, cor-

neal absorption depends on the integral, or "area under the curve," of tear film concentration during the first 10 to 20 minutes after instillation of drug, as indicated by the shaded area in Figure 2.7. Absorption is subject to modification by many factors, including other drugs, preservatives, infection, inflammation, or neuronal control, which can greatly affect drug bioavailability at the desired site of action.

The diffusion of drug from the cornea to the aqueous humor is similar to that from tears to cornea, except that for the corneal depot, the aqueous humor receives the major proportion of drug. Both lateral diffusion across the limbus and diffusion back across the epithelium contribute relatively little to the total diffusion.

The majority of the corneal drug depot eventually enters the aqueous humor, and the aqueous level rises to a maximum over about three hours. After this time, the concentration of drug in the cornea and in the aqueous humor drop in parallel as the aqueous humor level decays logarithmically, as shown in Figure 2.7.

The compartment model just described can estimate the concentrations of drugs within various ocular tissues. A more complex compartment model, which includes drug movement through the posterior aqueous, vitreous, and retina, is shown in Figure 2.8. This model becomes useful when a drug is introduced directly into the vitreous or systemic circulation, or when the very slight amount of a topically applied drug reaching the lens, vitreous, or retina must be considered.

The molecular properties of drugs influence which tissues act as reservoirs for them and which act as barriers. Modeling parameters vary considerably for drugs with different penetration and partitioning properties. For example, the distribution and elimination of a lipophilic drug that is also water-soluble and penetrates the corneal epithelium readily

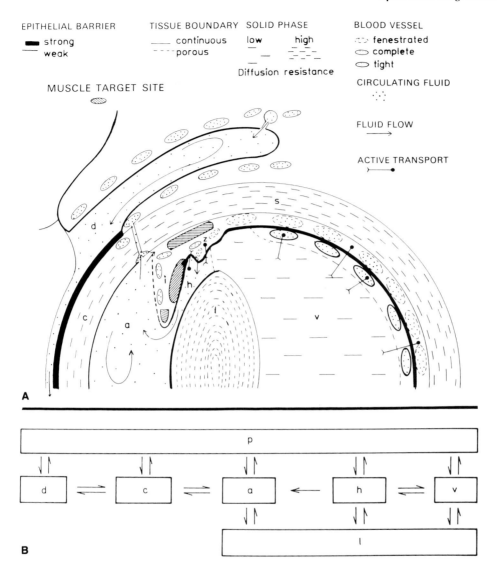

FIGURE 2.8 **Pharmacokinetic model of the eye.** *(A)* Physical relationships, including the major barriers and active pumping mechanisms. *(B)* Compartment model. p, plasma; d, tear reservoir; c, cornea; a, anterior chamber aqueous; h, posterior chamber aqueous; l, lens; i, iris; z, ciliary body; s, sclera; v, vitreous humor. (From Maurice DM, Mishima S. Ocular pharmacokinetics. In: Sears ML, ed. Pharmacology of the eye. Handbook of experimental pharmacology, Berlin: Springer-Verlag, 1984;69:19–116.)

occurs more rapidly than the example of fluorescein illustrated in Figure 2.7.

Active Transport and Diffusion Kinetics

Drug distribution usually depends on the rate of passive diffusion within and between compartments. It is governed by the barrier resistance between any two compartments where the distribution is unequal at a given time. In some cases, however, molecules accumulate against a concentration gradient on one side of a barrier.[6] Either of two phenomena is responsible for such an observation. One, coupled pumping mechanisms in the cell may provide the energy necessary for active transport.[7] Two, nonspecific binding due to ionic or other forces may cause an apparent accumulation of molecules against a concentration gradient.[3]

The properties of passive drug release from a tissue or from an artificial device can vary under certain circumstances. One example is *zero-order kinetics*, a term used when the release of a drug is constant over time. Zero-order kinetic conditions are satisfied when the concentration of a drug released over time is independent of concentration. Drugs usually obey zero-order kinetics when there is a rate-limiting barrier, as when a carrier system is saturated by an excess of drug. The Ocusert, which is a small membrane-bound delivery system designed for insertion in the conjunctival sac, is an example of drug dosing by zero-order kinetics (see Fig. 3.25). A reservoir of pilocarpine is released at a nearly constant rate over a one-week period for treatment of glaucoma.[1]

First-order kinetics is most commonly encountered in ocular drug movement (Fig. 2.9). Here the rate of movement is directly proportional to the concentration difference across the barrier, and the rate changes with time as the concentration differential across the barrier changes. The passive diffusion of molecules across a nonsaturated barrier generally adheres to first-order kinetics.[6]

Prodrugs

When the metabolite of a drug is more active at the receptor site than the parent form, the drug is often termed a *prodrug*. To be therapeutically useful, a prodrug must metabolize predictably to the effective drug form before it reaches the receptor site. The greatest advantage of prodrugs is the potential to add groups that mask features of the drug molecule that prevent penetration or have other undesirable

effects. Prodrug design can be a useful way of increasing penetration of a therapeutic agent through corneal or other barriers.

Dipivalyl epinephrine is the first successful example of the ophthalmic prodrug concept. A pair of pivalyl groups is attached to the two charged groups on epinephrine. The epithelial penetration is increased 10-fold by this diesterification because of the lipophilic nature of the modified prodrug.[1] The pivalyl groups are removed by esterases in the cornea, leaving epinephrine to act at the receptor site. Thus, a topically applied dipivalyl derivative need only be one-tenth the concentration of epinephrine to achieve bioavailability equivalent to epinephrine.[5] Systemic absorption of the drug is thereby greatly reduced. Since its introduction, dipivalyl epinephrine has achieved wide acceptance for intraocular pressure control in the treatment of glaucoma.

A prodrug that can cross the blood-vitreous barrier into the vitreous humor by virtue of lipophilicity may then be metabolized into a drug that has a greater ionic charge. As a charged compound, it cannot readily recross the barrier. An anti-inflammatory drug or antibiotic of low systemic toxicity could thus be introduced by the systemic route into the eye at relatively infrequent intervals and become trapped by metabolic alteration. It could then supply the aqueous and corneal tissues with a near-zero-order supply of drug over a prolonged period. The vitreous could thus become a drug reservoir of major consequence.

The future design and use of prodrugs holds much promise in ocular drug delivery, particularly where lipophilic prodrugs can be induced to penetrate the blood-vitreous barrier readily and then metabolized to a form that is trapped in the vitreous compartment. Because of their selective permeability, drugs could reach an effective concentration in the eye by entrapment within the vitreous compartment. A major problem with this approach is that the brain may sequester drug in the same manner as the vitreous humor. This could potentially be avoided by identifying a suitable enzyme that is present in vitreous humor and not in the brain.

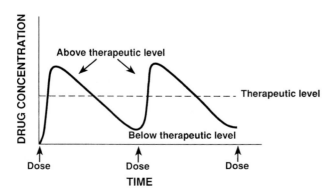

FIGURE 2.9   **First-order kinetics of ocular drugs in solution or ointment. This results in periods of overdosage and underdosage. (Modified with permission from Place V, Benson H. Local effects of topically applied steroids. J Steroid Biochem 1975;6:717–722, copyright 1975, Pergamon Press, Ltd.)**

Receptors

Endogenous hormones and neurotransmitters are internally secreted substances that change tissue responses by binding at sites of action known as *receptors*. Exogenous drugs, with a few notable exceptions, are administered compounds that mimic, block, or change the response of tissue receptors to endogenous molecules. The response of each tissue to a given drug depends on the type and number of receptors it contains. This in turn depends on the recent history of stimulation, which affects the size of the receptor population.

In recent years the isolation of well-defined membrane molecules, some of which have been successfully isolated,

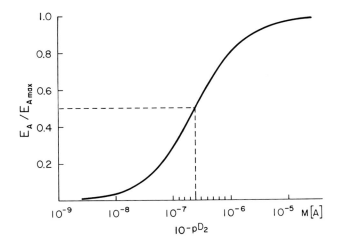

FIGURE 2.10 **Classic dose-response curve for a drug agonist, A. The sigmoid curve defines the theoretical effect on a specific receptor for varying concentrations of the agonist. The value labeled pD_2 is the negative log of the molar concentration of agonist producing 50% of maximal receptor effect, the ED_{50}. (From Van Den Brink FG. General theory of drug-receptor interactions. In: Van Rossem JM, ed. Kinetics of drug action. Handbook of experimental pharmacology, Berlin: Springer-Verlag, 1977;47.)**

purified, and reconstituted by modern techniques, has led to new knowledge of receptor function.[77] A receptor is viewed as a molecule or molecular complex residing in the membrane of a cell that binds a ligand and initiates or redirects cellular activity. A ligand is an endogenous hormone, neurotransmitter, or exogenous drug or substance with high affinity and high specificity for receptor binding. The ligand binding to the receptor may be by weak van der Waals forces, attraction of oppositely charged ionic pairs, covalent bonding, or a combination of these.[78] The specific effect of a ligand is presumed to be caused by the interaction with its receptor, which is viewed as a reversible, biomolecular interaction.[79] The mammalian receptor model is not valid for the effects of membrane-active anesthetic agents.

Agonists and Antagonists

A dose-response curve can be generated to show the effects of increasing drug levels. Usually this reaches a plateau beyond which no further increase in cell activity can be elicited by increasing the drug level, as shown in Figure 2.10. The proportion of maximal activity, $E_A/E_{A max}$, is a function of the molar concentration of the agonist, A. Over the central range of the drug-receptor interaction, a nearly linear dose-response function is generated. The concentration of drug that yields half-maximal effect is used to calculate the receptor affinity of the drug and is often expressed as the negative logarithm of molar concentration, pD_2.[79]

A partial agonist binds to a receptor without producing the maximal response. No direct relationship exists between the binding affinity of a ligand and its ability to stimulate the receptor. These two independent properties together determine drug activity. For example, a drug that binds strongly yet does not cause maximal response can act both as a partial

agonist and as an antagonist simultaneously because it blocks other ligands from binding and eliciting the maximal or normal response.

An antagonist blocks stimulation of a drug receptor by binding at a site, interfering with ligand binding, or by altering the molecular conformation of the binding site. Antagonists can be classified as competitive or noncompetitive inhibitors depending on whether they compete for the same molecular binding site as the ligand. Since antagonists often bind strongly, remaining in position on the receptor without internalization or destruction, they can exert their effects at very low concentrations and act as powerful drug substances. Antagonists may have an intrinsic partial agonist activity of their own. Graded transitions between agonist and antagonist activity are a common feature of molecular structure-activity relationships.[80]

Down Regulation of Receptors

The eye can adjust its sensitivity to naturally released transmitter substances. If an endogenous neurotransmitter is present at abnormally high levels, the number of receptors for that drug may be reduced proportionately to compensate and allow normal physiologic function. This can also occur when a drug is administered at frequent intervals; it is termed *down regulation*.[81] Adrenergic agonists typically produce a strong response on initial application and then have reduced effect when dosing is continued at frequent intervals. Adrenergic receptors have been shown to be regulated experimentally in corneal tissue in response to epinephrine.[82] When drug use is discontinued, normal sensitivity returns in a few days. Antagonist drugs generally cause less down regulation than agonists, or none at all, since they do not stimulate maximal receptor response.

Properties of Drug Formulations Affecting Bioavailability

Biopharmaceutics involves the development of optimum dosage forms for the delivery of a given drug.[1] For example, preservatives that compromise the health of corneal epithelial cells have been eliminated from unit-dose medications intended for dry eye sufferers and other sensitive individuals. Major advances are also taking place in the development of vehicles and specific formulations to enhance ocular bioavailability and decrease systemic absorption of drugs.[83] In this section some of the properties of ocular formulations are considered in terms of their effects on drug bioavailability. Side effects of drugs and preservatives are also discussed.

Bioavailability

Bioavailability describes the amount of drug present at the desired receptor site. The dose level producing a response that is 50% of maximum is termed the ED_{50} (see Fig. 2.10). An effective dose level must be present for a time sufficient to produce the desired action. The requirements for concentration and time to achieve ED_{50} differ widely depending on the mechanism of action of the drug and the desired response. Two challenging examples of drug bioavailability problems have been selected to illustrate markedly different requirements for effective therapeutic dosing.

A bicarbonate pump located in the membrane of the ciliary body is important in the production of aqueous humor. Inhibition of the enzyme carbonic anhydrase (CA) reduces the ciliary body fluid output by as much as one-third.[84] Such inhibition is desirable in treating glaucoma because it lowers IOP. The CA enzyme must be almost completely inhibited to produce the desired reduction of fluid transport. This can easily be achieved in a tissue bath where a sufficiently high concentration of a carbonic anhydrase inhibitor (CAI) such as acetazolamide can be maintained. However, orally administered CAIs of sufficient dosage to allow therapeutic ocular effects can also cause acidosis and gastric upset. Topical application of CAIs has only recently achieved clinical success due to the problem of insufficient corneal penetration and bioavailability (see Chapter 10).

Epidermal growth factors (EGF), derived originally from mouse salivary glands, are of interest in corneal epithelial wound healing and potentially in stimulating endothelial cell division as well. They are medium-length peptides that can stimulate DNA synthesis and reproduction in epithelial and certain other cells. A single dose of EGF, internalized through the cell receptors, can cause events leading to mitosis. Great success has been achieved in obtaining cell growth in culture. However, prolonged contact for at least 20 minutes with the cell membrane is required to stimulate binding

and internalization. A complicating factor is that EGF actually inhibits cell reproduction in high concentrations. Moreover, it is not easy to demonstrate efficacy using topically applied EGF because of the rapidly changing concentration in the tear film, which is initially so high that it is inhibitory and then becomes so low that it is ineffectual in minutes.[85] Research is now directed at methods of altering cells at secondary receptor sites to render them more receptive to rapid binding and incorporation of EGF.

These two examples illustrate the bioavailability considerations that must be taken into account in the practical design of drugs that are to be therapeutically useful in humans once a mechanism of action is characterized.

Active Ingredients

Therapeutic and diagnostic drugs given topically or systemically can have major effects on uptake of other drugs as a result of their own actions on tissue permeability, blood flow, and fluid secretion. Preservatives, buffers, and vehicles also can have significant effects on drug absorption.[86] Table 2.2 categorizes some topical medications and preservatives and their effects on the corneal epithelium, as evaluated by scanning electron microscopy.[87]

Many drugs used to treat glaucoma decrease aqueous humor formation and thereby slow their own kinetics of removal and removal of other drugs by the aqueous route. In a like manner, anti-inflammatory agents compensate for the increased permeability of the blood-aqueous barrier and help to bring it back within normal limits, thus altering the kinetics of drugs within the eye. Many similar examples of drug modification of pharmacokinetics can be found (e.g., the inhibition of tear flow by systemically administered anticholinergic agents).

Stability

No complex drug molecule is indefinitely stable in solution. The determination of drug stability is of major concern to the pharmaceutical industry. In the United States, a manufacturer must demonstrate that at least 90% of the labeled concentration of a drug is present in the active form after storage at room temperature for the shelf life requested. In many cases, a manufactured drug may contain 110% of the labeled amount of medication, so that 18% of the drug can degrade before the minimum acceptable level is reached. A shelf life of less than 18 months usually makes warehousing and distribution of a drug economically impractical, unless the drug is in very high demand.

Once a sealed bottle is opened, the contents are subject to the risk of excessive oxidation and microbial contamination. The bottle may be subject to heating if left on a table, in a car, or in a pocket. These conditions all contribute to acceler-

TABLE 2.2
Effects of Topical Ocular Drugs, Vehicles, and Preservatives on the Corneal Epithelium of the Rabbit Eye

	Topical Preparation		*SEM[a] Evaluation of Effects on Corneal Epithelium*
Preparations causing no epithelial damage		%	
Drugs	Atropine	1.0	Surface epithelial microvilli normal in size, shape, and
	Chloromycetin	0.5	distribution
	Epinephryl borate	1.0	No denuded cells
	Gentamicin	0.3	Cell junctions intact
	Proparacaine	0.5	Plasma membranes not wrinkled
	Tetracaine	0.5	Usual number of epithelial "holes"
Vehicles	Boric acid in petrolatum-mineral oil	5.0	
	Methylcellulose	0.5	
	Polyvinyl alcohol	1.6	
	Saline	0.9	
Preservatives	Chlorobutanol	0.5	
	Disodium edetate	0.1	
	Thimerosal	0.01	
Preparations causing moderate epithelial damage		%	
Drugs	Echothiophate iodide	0.25	Most cells normal
	Pilocarpine	2.0	Some cells showed loss of microvilli and wrinkling of
	Fluorescein	2.0	plasma membranes
	Fluor-I-Strip (wet with 1 drop 0.9% saline)		A small number of cells showed disruption of plasma membrane with premature cellular desquamation
Preparations causing important epithelial damage		%	
Drugs	Cocaine	4.0	Complete loss of microvilli
	Neopolycin	(no BAK)	Wrinkling of plasma membranes
			Premature desquamation of top layer of cells
Preservatives	Benzalkonium chloride	0.01	Severe epithelial microvillous loss
Drug + preservative	Pilocarpine	2.0	Severe membrane disruption
	Gentamicin	0.3	Death and desquamation of two superficial layers of
	Benzalkonium chloride	0.01	cells over 3-hour period

[a]Scanning electron microscope.
Adapted from Pfister RR, Burstein NL. The effects of ophthalmic drugs, vehicles, and preservatives on corneal epithelium: A scanning electron microscope study. Invest Ophthalmol 1976;15:246–259.

ated drug degradation. Diagnostic agents must be replaced on a routine basis to prevent their use too long after opening. This is particularly true for topical anesthetics, which can rapidly deteriorate once opened. Any drug formulation that has a brownish discoloration or that stings more than usual should be suspect, even if still apparently in date.

Drugs formulated in an acid solution are sometimes more stable than those at neutral or alkaline pH, particularly when the drug is a weak base.[10] Often such a drug must be stored at an acid pH to increase protonation and prevent rapid degradation. Polypeptides such as growth factors, which are now of interest in ophthalmic formulations, may require alkaline storage. In the eye, the normal pH is approximately 7.4.[16]

Tear pH can remain altered for over 30 minutes after addition of a strongly buffered solution. A change of tear pH can cause such irritation and stimulation of lacrimation that drug penetration is decreased. The use of a low concentration of buffer in the drug vehicle can allow the natural ocular buffering system to reestablish normal tear film pH rapidly after drug instillation.

Certain drug formulations are not stable in solution. As an example, an antioxidant such as sodium metabisulfite must be added to the formulation of adrenergic drugs such as epinephrine to prevent the rapid formation of an irritating brownish degradation product. An extreme stability problem is posed by acetylcholine, a very useful drug in rapidly and reversibly constricting the pupil in some surgical procedures such as cataract extraction. This agent degrades within minutes in solution. Therefore, a system for packaging has been developed using a sterile aqueous solution in one compartment and lyophilized (freeze-dried) drug in the other. A plunger displaces a stopper between chambers, allowing mixing just before use.

Osmolarity

The combination of active drug, preservative, and vehicle together usually result in a hypotonic formulation (less than 290 milliOsmoles [mOsm]). Simple or complex salts, buffering agents, or certain sugars are often added to adjust osmolarity of the solution to the desired value. An osmolarity of 290 mOsm is equivalent to 0.9% saline, and this is the value sought for most ophthalmic as well as intravenous medications. The ocular tear film has a wide tolerance for variation in osmotic pressure. However, increasing tonicity above that of the tears causes immediate dilution by osmotic water movement from the lids and eye.[88] Hypotonic solutions are sometimes used to treat dry eye conditions and reduce tear osmolarity from abnormally high values.[89]

Preservatives

The formulation of ocular medications has included antimicrobial preservatives since the historic problem of fluorescein contamination in the 1940s. *Pseudomonas,* a soil bacterium that can cause corneal ulceration, uses the fluorescein molecule as an energy source for metabolism. Many years ago this bacterium caused serious consequences for practitioners who kept unpreserved solutions of fluorescein in the office to assist in the diagnosis of corneal abrasions. As a result of several tragic infections, two actions have been taken by manufacturers. One, fluorescein is now most commonly supplied as a dried preparation on filter paper, which prevents the growth of pathogens.[86] Two, as a precautionary measure, all ophthalmic solutions designed for nonsurgical, multiple use after opening now contain preservatives. However, as noted by Lemp and associates,[90] preservatives employed at high concentrations can irritate and damage the ocular surface.

Two distinct types of preservatives are currently available for commercial use. One group, the surfactants, are ionically charged molecules that disrupt the plasma membrane and are usually bactericidal. The other group of chemical toxins includes mercury and iodine and their derivatives as well as alcohols. These compounds block the normal metabolic processes of the cell. They are considered bacteriostatic if they only inhibit growth, or bactericidal if they destroy the ability of bacteria to reproduce. In contrast to antibiotics, which selectively destroy or immobilize a specific group of organisms, the preservatives act nonselectively against all cells.

BENZALKONIUM CHLORIDE AND OTHER SURFACTANTS

The quaternary surfactants benzalkonium chloride and benzethonium chloride are preferred by many manufacturers because of their stability, excellent antimicrobial properties in acid formulation, and long shelf life. They exhibit toxic effects on both the tear film and the corneal epithelium and have long been known to increase drug penetration.[91,92] The toxicity of these compounds is increased by the degree of acidity of the formulation.[93]

A single drop of 0.01% benzalkonium chloride can break the superficial lipid layer of the tear film into numerous oil droplets[12] because it can interface with the lipid monolayer of the tear surface and disrupt it by detergent action. Benzalkonium chloride reduces the BUT of the tear film by one-half.[94] Repeated blinking does not restore the lipid layer for some time. The inclusion of benzalkonium chloride in artificial tear formulations is questionable. It neither protects the corneal epithelium nor promotes a stable, oily tear surface.

Patients who receive anti-inflammatory agents are at particularly high risk of experiencing tear film breakup and corneal erosion due to the benzalkonium chloride present as a preservative. The repeated application of these drops can further compromise an eye in which the tear film or cornea may already be damaged.[95] It may be necessary in superficial inflammation or corneal erosion to eliminate all medications. This alone may allow healing. In many cases of superficial inflammation, a lubricating eyedrop without preservatives may be the best course of treatment.[96]

The ability of surfactants to disrupt membranes or to alter their permeability is related to their charge and to the size of their hydrophobic (lipophilic) group. These agents are usually cationic. Marsh and Maurice[97] studied the ability of cationic surfactants to alter corneal permeability. They observed a significant increase in permeability that, however, was coupled with objectionable irritation. Cadwallader and Ansel[98] studied the effects of benzalkonium chloride of varying molecular chain lengths and found that the C_{14} length was the most toxic. This length most easily fits into the bilaminar model of the plasma membrane first proposed by Davson and Danielli[6,99] (Fig. 2.11).

CHLORHEXIDINE

Chlorhexidine is a diguanide that contains two charges arranged so that it does not intercalate readily into the phospholipid membrane. It is useful as an antimicrobial agent in the same range of concentrations as is benzalkonium chloride, yet it is used at lower concentrations in marketed formulations. It does not alter corneal permeability to the same degree as does benzalkonium chloride[99] for perhaps two major reasons. One, the structure of chlorhexi-

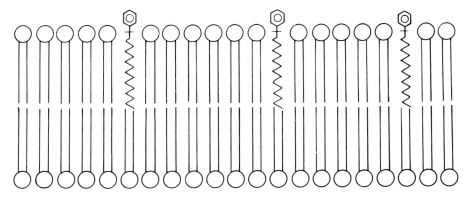

FIGURE 2.11   **Comparison of the structures of benzalkonium chloride (BAC) and chlorhexidine (CDG). Benzalkonium chloride can intercalate readily into a plasma membrane, as seen below. Chain length affects binding ability. Chlorhexidine cannot bind effectively into the membrane and causes far less surface disruption. (From Burstein NL. Preservative alteration of corneal permeability in humans and rabbits. Invest Ophthalmol Vis Sci 1984;25:1453–1457.)**

dine is such that it has two positive charges separated by a long carbon backbone, and it cannot intercalate into a lipid layer in the same manner as does benzalkonium chloride. Two, Green and associates[100] have shown that proteins neutralize the toxicity of chlorhexidine, and this may occur in the tear film.

MERCURIALS

Of the mercurial preservatives, thimerosal is less subject to degradation into toxic mercury than either phenylmercuric acetate or phenylmercuric nitrate. Thimerosal is most effective in weakly acidic solutions. Some patients, however, develop a contact sensitivity and must discontinue use after several weeks or months of exposure.[101] Because thimerosal affects internal cell respiration and must be present at high continuous concentrations to have biologic effects, its dilution by the tear film prevents short-term epithelial toxicity on single application.[102] It has no known effects on tear film stability. A concentration of 1% thimerosal is required to equal the effects on corneal oxygen consumption of 0.025% benzalkonium chloride.[103]

CHLOROBUTANOL

Chlorobutanol is less effective than benzalkonium chloride as an antimicrobial and tends to disappear from bottles during prolonged storage.[104] No allergic reactions are apparently associated with prolonged use. Scanning electron microscopy of rabbit corneal epithelial cells also indicates that twice-daily administration of a chlorobutanol-preserved artificial tear results in only modest exfoliation of corneal epithelial cells.[144] Chlorobutanol is not a highly effective preservative when used alone and therefore is often combined with EDTA in ophthalmic drug formulations.[88,105]

MISCELLANEOUS PRESERVATIVES

Methylparaben and propylparaben have been introduced into some medications in recent years, especially artificial tears and nonmedicated ointments. They can cause allergic reactions and are unstable at high pH.[105]

Disodium ethylenediaminetetra-acetic acid (EDTA) is a special type of molecule known as a chelating agent. EDTA can preferentially bind and sequester divalent cations in the increasing order: Ca^{++}, Mg^{++}, Zn^{++}, Pb^{++}. Its role in preservation is to assist the action of thimerosal, benzalkonium chloride, and other agents. By itself, EDTA does not have a highly toxic effect on cells, even in culture.[106] Contact dermatitis is known to occur from EDTA.[105]

When instilled topically in the eye, mercurial and alcoholic preservatives are rapidly diluted below the toxic threshold by tears. However, surfactant preservatives rapidly bind by intercalating into the plasma membrane and can increase corneal permeability before dilution can occur. The changed barrier property of the cornea can allow large hydrophilic molecules to penetrate the cornea far more readily.

Vehicles

An ophthalmic vehicle is an agent other than the active drug or preservative added to a formulation to provide proper tonicity, buffering, and viscosity to complement drug action[104,107] (Table 2.3). The use of one or more high molecular weight polymers increases the viscosity of the formulation, delaying washout from the tear film and increasing bioavailability of drugs. Polyionic molecules can bind at the corneal surface and increase drug retention as well as stabilize the tear film. Petrolatum or oil-based ointments provide even longer retention of drugs at the corneal surface and provide a temporary lipid depot. In artificial tears, the vehicles themselves may be the therapeutically active ingredients that moisturize and lubricate the cornea and conjunctiva and augment the tear film, preventing desiccation of epithelial cells.

The therapeutic index of drugs, particularly those that are systemically absorbed, can be maximized in many ways, including modifying the vehicle used for drug delivery. The β blockers are an example of such a group. Increased viscosity and controlled-depot drug release are vehicular strategies that can contribute to increased specificity of these drugs.[108]

The monomer unit structure of the vehicle and its molecular weight and viscosity control the behavior of the vehicle. In the manufacture and purification of polymers, a range of molecular sizes is usually present in the final product.[109]

Molecular viscosity, which is measured in centistokes, is a nonlinear function of molecular weight and of concentra-

TABLE 2.3
Excipients Used in Ophthalmic Formulations

Classification	*Representative Products*
Viscous Agents	Methylcellulose
	Polyvinyl alcohol
	Polyvinylpyrrolidone (povidone)
	Propylene glycol
	Polyethylene glycol
	Polysorbate 80
	Dextran
	Gelatin
Antioxidants	Sodium sulfites
	EDTA
Wetting Agents	Polysorbate
	Poloxamer
	Tyloxapol
Buffers	Acetic, boric, and hydrochloric acids
	Potassium and sodium bicarbonate
	Potassium and sodium borate
	Potassium and sodium phosphate
	Potassium and sodium citrate
Tonicity Agents	Buffers
	Dextrans
	Dextrose
	Glycerin
	Propylene glycol
	Potassium and sodium chloride

Adapted from Bartlett JD, Ghormley NR, Jaanus SD, et al., eds. Ophthalmic Drug Facts. St. Louis: Facts and Comparisons, 1995.

tion. Thus, a 2% solution of polymer in water usually does not have twice the viscosity of a 1% solution. Each batch of a commercial polymer must therefore be measured for viscosity at the appropriate concentration. The addition of salts can affect the final viscosity of some polymers. Divalent anions and cations can have a major effect on the conformation of polymers in solution, occasionally causing incompatibilities when formulations are mixed together in the eye.

POLYVINYLPYRROLIDONE

Polyvinylpyrrolidone (PVP) (U.S. Pharmacopeia name: povidone) is the homopolymer of N-vinyl-2-pyrrolidone, which was used as a blood plasma substitute during World War II. Although PVP is considered to be a nonionic polymer, it has specific binding and detoxification properties that are of great interest in health care. For example, it complexes iodine, reducing its toxicity 10-fold, while still allowing bactericidal action to occur. This occurs through the formation of iodide ions by reducing agents in the polymer, which then complex with molecular iodine to give tri-iodide ions.[109] Povidone can also complex with mercury, nicotine, cyanide, and other toxic materials to reduce their damaging effects.[110]

The pharmacokinetics of povidone are well understood as a result of its experimental use to determine the properties of pores in biological membranes. Povidone molecules can readily penetrate hydrophilic pores in membranes if they are small enough, and they are also taken up by pinocytotic vesicles. Apparently povidone is not detectably bound to membrane surfaces and hence does not provide long-lasting viscosity enhancement beyond the normal residence time in the tears.

Povidone has very low systemic toxicity, shows no immune rejection characteristics, and is easily excreted by the kidneys at molecular weights up to 100,000 d.[111] The pK_a of the conjugate acid (PVP · H$^+$) is between 0 and 1, and the viscosity of povidone does not change until near pH 1, when it doubles. Therefore, the ionic character of the PVP chain should not be appreciable at pharmaceutical or physiologic pH values. However, with ionic cosolutes, anions are bound much more readily than cations by povidone. Cosolute binding can cause a change in the size of the polymer coil, influencing the viscosity and other properties of the solution.

POLYVINYL ALCOHOL

Introduced into ophthalmic practice in 1942, polyvinyl alcohol (PVA) is a water-soluble viscosity enhancer with both hydrophilic and hydrophobic sites.[107] A common concentration used in ophthalmic preparations is 1.4%.[104] PVA is useful in the treatment of corneal epithelial erosion and dry eye syndromes because it is nonirritating to the eye and actually appears to facilitate healing of abraded epithelium.[112] It is also used to increase the residence time of drugs in the tears, aiding ocular absorption.[113]

HYDROXYPROPYL METHYLCELLULOSE

Like polyvinyl alcohol, the viscosity enhancer hydroxypropyl methylcellulose (HPMC) is available in a variety of molecular weights and in formulations with different group substitutions. It has been shown to prolong tear film wetting time and to increase the ability of fluorescein and dexamethasone to penetrate the cornea. HPMC 0.5% has been shown to exhibit twice the ocular retention time of 1.4% PVA.[114,115]

CARBOXYMETHYLCELLULOSE

Carboxymethylcellulose is a vehicle whose properties in solution resemble another cellulose ether, hydroxymethylcellulose. However, the carboxylic and hydroxylic groups provide anionic charge, which may be valuable in promoting mucoadhesion and increasing tear retention time.[116,117] Tensiometric testing has shown that carboxymethylcellulose has a greater adhesion to mucins than do other viscous vehicles currently used in ocular formulations.[118] Grene and associates[119] demonstrated the efficacy of unpreserved artificial tears containing carboxymethylcellulose over a preserved formulation of hydroxypropyl methylcellulose. Direct comparison of the two agents in similar, unpreserved formulations has yet to be demonstrated.

SODIUM HYALURONATE

High molecular weight polymers, including mucin, collagen, and sodium hyaluronate (SH), have a viscosity that rises more rapidly than would be expected from increased concentration alone. When these substances are exposed to shear (e.g., with the motion of blinking), the viscosity decreases as the molecules orient themselves along the shear forces. This non-Newtonian property is termed "shear thinning." An advantage of shear-thinning polymers is that they have a high viscosity in the open eye, stabilizing the tear film.[120] When blinking occurs they thin, preventing the feeling of irritation that would occur with a high-viscosity Newtonian fluid.

Several studies have demonstrated that SH remains in contact with the cornea for a longer time than isotonic saline. Gamma scintigraphy has also shown that a solution of 0.25% has a longer residence time in the precorneal area of humans than does phosphate buffer solution (PBS).[121–123] In addition, when 0.25% SH is combined with certain agents, it can enhance their ocular bioavailability.[124,125] Compared with PBS solution, 0.25% SH significantly increases tear concentrations of topically applied gentamicin sulfate at 5 and 10 minutes following instillation.[125] More studies are necessary to establish the safety of SH and its ability to maintain efficient drug levels in the precorneal area.

GEL-FORMING SYSTEMS

A newer development in ocular drug delivery systems is the use of large molecules that exhibit reversible phase transitions whereby an aqueous drop delivered to the eye will reversibly gel upon contact with the precorneal tear film.[126,143] Such changes in viscous properties can be induced by alterations in temperature, pH, and electrolyte composition.[83] Gelrite, a polysaccharide, low-acetyl gellan gum, forms clear gels in the presence of mono- or divalent cations typically found in tear fluid.[126] It enhances the penetration and prolongs the action of topically applied ocular drugs[127–131] (Fig. 2.12). Comparison of timolol in the gel formulation (Timoptic-XE) to a standard solution has shown that a single daily dose of the gel is similarly effective in lowering IOP in patients with open-angle glaucoma as twice-daily instillation of the solution.[130] Evidence also indicates that the Gelrite vehicle may slightly prolong the action of topical ocular CAIs.[131]

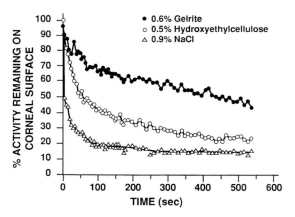

FIGURE 2.12 **The corneal residence of three ophthalmic vehicles in humans (mean data, n = 8). The ocular retention time of Gelrite is longer than that of hydroxyethylcellulose or saline. SEM within 10% of the mean. (Modified from Greaves JL, Wilson CG, Rozier A, et al. Scintigraphic assessment of an ophthalmic gelling vehicle in man and rabbit. Curr Eye Res 1990;9:415–420.)**

POLYIONIC VEHICLES

Recent advances in chemical synthesis and in an understanding of the tear film of the eye have resulted in the development of compounds with two or more regions that vary in both their lipophilic nature and binding. The first of these to be tested in the eye was poloxamer 407, a polyionic vehicle with a hydrophobic nucleus of polyoxypropylene, and hydrophilic end groups of polyoxyethylene.[132] The conceptual function of this vehicle in the tear film is shown in Figure 2.13.

One advantage of poloxamers is their ability to produce an artificial microenvironment in the tear film, which can greatly enhance the bioavailability of lipophilic drugs such as steroids. In one series of experiments in rabbits[a], a 10-fold increase in penetration of progesterone was achieved with a poloxamer vehicle.

CATION EXCHANGE RESIN (AMBERLITE)

Emulsions are biphasic lipid-water or water-lipid combinations that can dissolve and deliver both hydrophilic and lipophilic compounds. A binding agent, such as the polyacrylic acid polymer carbopol 934P, is added to the mixture to enhance physical stability and ease of resuspendability of the product.[133] This system has been used with the topical antiglaucoma drugs betaxolol, timolol, and pilocarpine.[133] Betaxolol, for example, is first combined with a cation exchange resin to which it binds. This binding reduces the

amount of free drug in solution and enhances ocular comfort following topical application (Fig. 2.14). The drug-resin particles are then incorporated into a vehicle containing the carbopol 934P, which increases viscosity of the formulation and prolongs ocular contact time of the drug.[133] Both animal models and human clinical trials have shown that the ocular bioavailability of 0.25% betaxolol suspension (Betoptic-S) is equivalent to that of 0.5% betaxolol solution.[133] The uniqueness of this suspension is demonstrated by its ability to provide uniform dosing of betaxolol for up to four weeks without resuspending the product.[133]

SUBMICRON EMULSIONS

A submicron emulsion (SME) vehicle has also been developed to enhance ocular bioavailability of topically applied drugs.[134,135] This emulsion offers a biphasic medium (lipid-water) that may dissolve and deliver both lipophilic and hydrophilic compounds. When used to deliver pilocarpine, SME vehicle permits a 12-hour duration of action and may thus reduce the dosing frequency of this antiglaucoma medication.[135]

OINTMENTS

Ointments are commonly used for topical application of drugs to the eye. These vehicles are primarily mixtures of white petrolatum and liquid mineral oil with or without a water-miscible agent such as lanolin.[136] The mineral oil is added to the petrolatum to allow the vehicle to melt at body temperature, and the lanolin is added to the nonemulsive ointment base to absorb water. This allows for water and

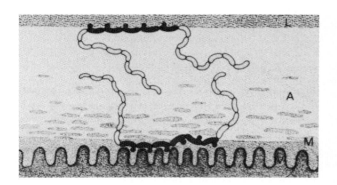

FIGURE 2.13 **Poloxamer 407, represented schematically in the tear film. The lipophilic center of the molecule tends to bind at the corneal surface, while the hydrophilic end chains stabilize the tears. Such polyionic vehicles may provide improved drug delivery in the future. L, lipid layer; A, aqueous layer; M, mucin layer. (From Waring GO, Harris RR. Double-masked evaluation of a poloxamer artificial tear in keratoconjunctivitis sicca. In: Leopold IH, Burns RP, eds. Symposium on ocular therapy. New York: John Wiley & Sons, 1979;11:127–139. Reprinted by permission of John Wiley & Sons, Inc.)**

---

[a]Krezanoski JZ, Weinreb R, Polanski J, Burstein NL, unpublished data, 1981.

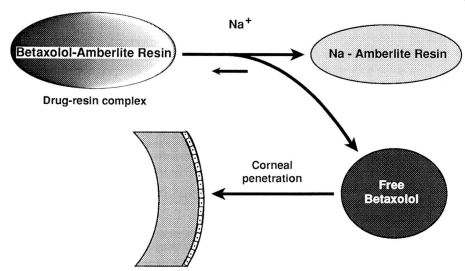

FIGURE 2.14 **Diagram showing how Amberlite resin and betaxolol work. Betaxolol binds to the resin, reducing the concentration of free betaxolol. In the presence of Na+ or K+ in the tear fluid, the resin binds to the cation, thus releasing free betaxolol, which becomes available for corneal penetration. (Adapted from Jani R, Gan O, Ali Y, et al. Ion exchange resins for ophthalmic delivery. J Ocular Pharmacol 1994;10:57–67.)**

water-soluble drugs to be retained in the delivery system. Commercial ophthalmic ointments are derivatives of a hydrocarbon mixture of 60% petrolatum USP and 40% mineral oil USP, forming a molecular complex that is semisolid but that melts at body temperature.[137] In general, ointments are well tolerated by the ocular tissues, and when antibiotics are incorporated, they are usually more stable in ointment than in solution.[138]

The primary clinical purpose for an ointment vehicle is to increase the ocular contact time of the applied drugs. The ocular contact time is about twice as long in the blinking eye and four times longer in the nonblinking (patched) eye compared with a saline vehicle.[136] Ointments are retained longer in the conjunctival sac because the large molecules of the ointment are not easily removed into the lacrimal drainage system by blinking. A nonpolar oil is a component of tears, and this is another factor in the prolonged retention. Because ointments are nonpolar oil bases, they are readily absorbed by the precorneal and conjunctival tear films.[139] Ointments are used to increase drug absorption for nighttime therapy or for conditions in which antibiotics are delivered to a patched eye, such as corneal abrasions, because they markedly increase contact time. They are also useful in children, since they do not wash out readily with tearing.

Ointments have several disadvantages. They may be difficult to self-administer, particularly by partially sighted patients who may occasionally traumatize the ocular surface with the applicator tip. In addition, dosing is imprecise. Furthermore, many patients report transient blurred vision with the use of ophthalmic ointments. Because ointments cause blurred vision, they are not often used for daytime therapy except where necessitated by postsurgical, infectious, or other special circumstances. Some patients incur contact dermatitis from ophthalmic ointments, espe-cially atropine ointment and formulations containing neomycin.

DRUG RELEASE SYSTEMS

Soft contact lenses and collagen shields absorb drugs from solution and then slowly release them when placed on the eye. This form of drug therapy can be valuable when continuous treatment is desired (see Chapter 3).[83,140–142]

Two major types of advanced drug release systems have been designed based on the insertion of a solid device in the eye. The first is a device of low permeability filled with drug, and the second is a polymer that is completely soluble in lacrimal fluid, formulated with drug in its matrix.[141] Both of these systems can be made to approach zero-order kinetics.[1]

The advantages of these systems are significant for the treatment of certain conditions, including glaucoma. Inserts may also increase the noncorneal route of drug absorption across the sclera.[83] To date, the expense of the slow-release inserts compared with the economy of eyedrops has hindered their acceptance. However, both theory and clinical experience support the rationality of this approach to ocular dosing. Future improvements in technology and reduced cost would allow increased use of this dosage form.

Ocular Drug Development and the Patient

Many steps are involved in the successful design of an ocular drug formulation. The first is selection of an appropriate drug molecule that maximizes therapeutic benefit and bioavailability while minimizing toxicity. A formulation must then be developed to include a vehicle, a preservative, and a buffer. Stability, toxicity, and efficacy must then be evaluated for the complete formulation. An effective dosing regimen must also be developed before beginning clinical trials on a wide scale. The Food and Drug Administration (FDA) is involved in evaluating these steps to provide formulations that are efficacious and safe (see Chapter 4).

Of the numerous factors that influence ocular drug efficacy and safety, one of the most important remains that of patient compliance. Determining the proper dosage regimen and getting the patient to administer the medication is a primary responsibility of the practitioner. These factors are considered in Chapters 1 and 4.

References

1. Shell JW. Pharmacokinetics of topically applied ophthalmic drugs. Surv Ophthalmol 1982;26:207–218.
2. Burstein NL, Anderson JA. Review: Corneal penetration and ocular bioavailability of drugs. J Ocular Pharmacol 1985;1:309–326.
3. Maurice DM, Mishima S. Ocular pharmacokinetics. In: Sears ML, ed. Pharmacology of the eye, Handbook of experimental pharmacology. Berlin: Springer-Verlag, 1984;69:19–116.
4. Shichi H. Biotransformation and drug metabolism. In: Sears ML, ed. Pharmacology of the eye, Handbook of experimental pharmacology. Berlin: Springer-Verlag, 1984;69:117–148.
5. Anderson JA, Davis WL, Wei CP. Site of ocular hydrolysis of a prodrug, dipivifrin, and a comparison of its ocular metabolism with that of the parent compound, epinephrine. Invest Ophthalmol Vis Sci 1980;19:817–823.
6. Davson H, Danielli JF. The permeability of natural membranes. Cambridge: University Press, 1943.
7. Ussing HH. Transport of electrolytes and water across epithelia. Harvey Lectures, Series 59, 1965.
8. Hansch C, Clayton JM. Lipophilic character and biological activity of drugs. II. The parabolic case. J Pharm Sci 1973;62:1–21.
9. Kishida K, Otori T. Quantitative study on the relationship between transcorneal permeability of drugs and their hydrophobicity. Jpn J Ophthalmol 1980;24:251–259.
10. Hind HW, Goyan FM. A new concept of the role of hydrogen ion concentration and buffer system in the preparation of ophthalmic solutions. J Am Pharm Assoc 1947;36:33–41.
11. Holly FJ. Formation and stability of the tear film. Int Ophthalmol Clin 1973;13:73–96.
12. Holly FJ. Tear film formation and rupture. In: Holly FJ, ed. The precorneal tear film. Dry Eye Institute, 1986.
13. Mishima S, Maurice DM. Oily layer of tear film and evaporation from corneal surface. Exp Eye Res 1961;1:39–45.
14. Norn MS. Desiccation of the precorneal tear film. I. Corneal wetting-time. Acta Ophthalmol 1969;47:865–880.
15. Burstein NL. The effects of topical drugs and preservatives on the tears and corneal epithelium in dry eye. Trans Ophthalmol Soc UK 1985;104:402–409.
16. Hind HW, Goyan FM. The hydrogen ion concentration and osmotic properties of lacrimal fluid. J Am Pharm Assoc 1949;38:477–479.
17. Mishima S, Gasset A, Klyce SD Jr, Baum JL. Determination of tear volume and tear flow. Invest Ophthalmol 1966;5:264–276.
18. Chrai SS, Makoid MC, Eriksen SP, Robinson JR. Drop size and initial dosing frequency problems of topically applied ophthalmic drugs. J Pharm Sci 1974;63:333–338.
19. Patton TF, Francoeur M. Ocular bioavailability and systemic loss of topically applied ophthalmic drugs. Am J Ophthalmol 1978;85:225–229.
20. Kaila T, Salminen L, Huupponen R. Systemic absorption of topically applied ocular timolol. J Ocular Pharmacol 1985;1:79–83.
21. Chrai SS, Patton TF, Mehta A, Robinson JR. Lacrimal and instilled fluid dynamics in rabbit eyes. J Pharm Sci 1973;62:1112–1121.
22. Gray RH, Franklin SJ, Reeves BC. Visual recovery using small dilating drops. J Pharm Pharmacol 1992;44:682–684.
23. Mishima S. Clinical pharmacokinetics of the eye. Invest Ophthalmol Vis Sci 1981;21:504–541.
24. Fraunfelder FT. Extraocular fluid dynamics: How best to apply topical ocular medications. Trans Am Ophthalmol Soc 1976;74:457–487.
25. Roen JL, Stasior OG, Jakobiec FA. Aging changes in the human lacrimal gland: Role of the ducts. CLAO J 1985;11:237–242.
26. Spencer WH, ed. Ophthalmic pathology: An atlas and textbook, 3 vols., ed. 3. Philadelphia: W.B. Saunders Co, 1985.
27. Ahmed I, Patton TF. Importance of the noncorneal absorption route in topical ophthalmic drug delivery. Invest Ophthalmol Vis Sci 1985;26:584–587.
28. Doane MG, Jensen AD, Dohlman CH. Penetration routes of topically applied eye medications. Am J Ophthalmol 1978;85:383–386.
29. Bienfang DC. Sector pupillary dilatation with an epinephrine strip. Am J Ophthalmol 1973;75:883–884.
30. Ehlers N. On the size of the conjunctival sac. Acta Ophthalmol 1965;43:205–210.
31. Porter KR, Bonneville MA. Fine structure of cells and tissues, ed. 3. Philadelphia: Lea & Febiger, 1968.
32. Klyce SD. Electrical profiles in the corneal epithelium. J Physiol 1972;226:407–429.
33. Maurice DM. Review: The permeability of the cornea. Ophthal Lit 1953;7:1–26.
34. Tonjum AM. Permeability of rabbit corneal epithelium to horseradish peroxidase after the influence of benzalkonium chloride. Acta Ophthalmol 1975;53:335–347.
35. Swan KC, White NG. Corneal permeability. I. Factors affecting penetration of drugs into the cornea. Am J Ophthalmol 1942;25:1043–1057.
36. Wiederholt M, Kössendrup D, Schulz W, Hoffmann F. Pharmacokinetics of topical cyclosporin A in the rabbit eye. Invest Ophthalmol Vis Sci 1986;27:519–524.
37. Huang HS, Schoenwald RD, Lach JL. Corneal penetration behavior of beta blocking agents. II. Assessment of barrier contributions. J Pharm Sci 1983;72:1272–1279.
38. Hogan MJ, Alvarado JA, Weddell JE. Histology of the human eye. Philadelphia: W.B. Saunders Co, 1971.
39. Maurice DM. The chemical and physical basis of corneal transparency. Biochemistry of the eye, Symp. Tutzing Castle, August 1966:51–61.
40. Davson H. Physiology of the eye. New York: Academic Press, 1980.

41. Johnston MC, Noden DM, Hazelton RD, et al. Origins of avian ocular and periocular tissues. Exp Eye Res 1979;29:27–43.
42. Maurice DM. The cornea and sclera. In: Davson H, ed. The eye. New York: Academic Press, 1984;1b.
43. Hodson S, Miller F. The bicarbonate ion pump in the endothelium which regulates the hydration of rabbit cornea. J Physiol 1976;263:563–577.
44. Whigham C, Hodson S. The movement of sodium across short-circuited rabbit corneal endothelium. Curr Eye Res 1985;4:1241–1245.
45. Burstein NL, Maurice DM. Cryofixation of tissue surfaces by a propane jet for electron microscopy. Micron 1978;9:191–198.
46. Maurice DM. The use of fluorescein in ophthalmological research. The Friedenwald Memorial Lecture. Invest Ophthalmol 1967;6:464–477.
47. Burstein NL, Fischbarg J, Liebovitch L. Electrical potential, resistance, and fluid secretion across isolated ciliary body. Exp Eye Res 1984;39:771–779.
48. Friedman E, Kopald HH, Smith TR, Mimura S. Retinal and choroidal blood flow determined with krypton-85 anesthetized animals. Invest Ophthalmol 1964;3:539–547.
49. Yamashita H, Uyama M, Sears ML. Comparative study by electron microscopy of response to urea between ciliary epithelia of albino and pigmented rabbits. A function of the ciliary pigmented epithelium. Jpn J Ophthalmol 1981;25:313–320.
50. Fisher RF, Hayes BP. Thickness and volume constants and ultrastructural organization of basement membrane (lens capsule). J Physiol 1979;293:229–245.
51. Paterson CA. Effects of drugs on the lens. In: Ellis PP, ed. Side effects of drugs in ophthalmology. Int Ophthalmol Clin 1971;11:63–98.
52. Kaiser RJ, Maurice DM. The diffusion of fluorescein in the lens. Exp Eye Res 1964;3:156–165.
53. Kinoshita JH. Mechanisms of cataract formation. Invest Ophthalmol 1974;13:713–724.
54. Reddy VN. Metabolism of glutathione in the lens. Exp Eye Res 1971;11:310–328.
55. Anderson JA, Chen CC, Vita JB, Shackleton M. Disposition of topical flurbiprofen in normal and aphakic rabbit eyes. Arch Ophthalmol 1982;100:642–645.
56. Balazs EA. Physiology of the vitreous body in retinal surgery with special emphasis on reoperations. In: Schepens CL, ed. Proceedings of the II Conference of the Retina Foundation, Ipswich, May 30–31, 1958. St. Louis: C.V. Mosby Co, 1960.
57. Balazs EA. Molecular morphology of the vitreous body. In: Smelser GK, ed. The structure of the eye. New York: Academic Press, 1961;293–310.
58. Balazs EA, Flood MT. Age-related changes in the physical and chemical structure of human vitreous (abstr.). Third International Congress for Eye Research, Osaka, Japan, 1978.
59. Balazs EA, Denlinger JL. The vitreous. In: Davson H, ed. The eye, ed. 3. New York: Academic Press, 1984;1a:533–589.
60. Maurice DM. The exchange of sodium between the vitreous body and the blood and aqueous humour. J Physiol 1957;137:110–125.
61. Osterlin S. On the molecular biology of the vitreous in the aphakic eye. Acta Ophthalmol 1977;55:353–361.
62. Osterlin S. Vitreous changes after cataract extraction. In: Freeman HM, Hirose T, Schepens CL, eds. Vitreous surgery and fundus diagnosis and treatment. New York: Appleton-Century-Crofts, 1977.
63. Maurice DM. Injection of drugs into the vitreous body. In: Leopold IH, Burns RP, eds. Symposium on ocular therapy. New York: John Wiley & Sons, 1976;9:59–71.
64. Balazs EA, Denlinger JL. The pharmacology of the vitreous. In: Dikstein S, ed. Drugs and ocular tissues. Basel: S. Karger, 1977:524–538.
65. Burstein NL, Bernacchi D, Leopold IH. Gentamicin iontophoresis into vitreous humor. J Ocular Pharmacol 1985;1:63–368.
66. Cunha-Vaz J. The blood-ocular barriers. Surv Ophthalmol 1979;23:279–96.
67. Henkind P. Ocular circulation. In: Records RE, ed. Physiology of the eye and visual system, Hagerstown, MD: Harper & Row, 1975;5:98–155.
68. Bill A. The blood-aqueous barrier. Trans Ophthalmol Soc UK 1986;105:149–155.
69. Alm A, Bill A. Ocular circulation. In: Moses R, ed. Adler's physiology of the eye: Clinical applications, ed. 8. St. Louis: C. V. Mosby Co, 1987.
70. Cerasoli JR. Effects of drugs on the retina. In: Ellis PP, ed. Side effects of drugs in ophthalmology. Int Ophthalmol Clin 1971;11:121–136.
71. Leopold IH. Ocular complications of drugs: Visual changes. JAMA 1968;205:631.
72. Bito LZ, Davson H, Levin E, et al. The relationship between the concentration of amino acids in the ocular fluids and the blood plasma of dogs. Exp Eye Res 1965;4:374–380.
73. Bito LZ. Absorptive transport of prostaglandins from intraocular fluids to blood: A review of recent findings. Exp Eye Res 1973;16:299–306.
74. Bito LZ, DeRousseau CJ. Transport functions of the blood-retinal barrier system of the micro environment of the retina. In: Cunha-Vaz J, ed. Blood-retinal barriers. 1980:133–163.
75. Leibold JE. Drugs having a toxic effect on the optic nerve. In: Ellis PP, ed. Side effects of drugs in ophthalmology. Int Ophthalmol Clin 1971;11:137–158.
76. Leopold IH. Anti-infective agents. In: Sears ML, ed. Pharmacology of the eye, Handbook of experimental pharmacology. Berlin: Springer-Verlag, 1984;69:385–458.
77. Levitzki A. Reconstitution of membrane receptor systems. Biochim Biophys Acta 1985;822:127–153.
78. Goldstein A, Aronow L, Kalman SM. Principles of drug action. New York: Harper & Row, 1974.
79. Van den Brink FG. General theory of drug-receptor interactions. In: Van Rossum JM, ed. Kinetics of drug action. Berlin: Springer-Verlag, 1977.
80. Triggle DJ. Receptor theory. In: Smythies JR. Receptors in pharmacology. New York: Marcel Dekker, 1978:1–66.
81. Gavin JR, Roth J, Neville DM, et al. Insulin-dependent regulation of insulin receptor concentrations: A direct demonstration in cell culture. Proc Natl Acad Sci USA 1974;71:84–88.
82. Candia OA, Neufeld AH. Topical epinephrine causes a decrease in density of beta-adrenergic receptors and catecholamine-stimulated chloride transport in the rabbit cornea. Biochim Biophys Acta 1978;543:403–408.
83. Lee VHL. Review: New directions in the optimization of ocular drug delivery. J Ocular Pharmacol 1990;6:157–164.
84. Becker B. Decrease in intraocular pressure in man by a carbonic anhydrase inhibitor, Diamox. Am J Ophthalmol 1954;37:13–15.
85. Burstein NL. Review: Growth factor effects on corneal wound healing. J Ocular Pharmacol 1987;3:263–277.

86. Burstein NL. Corneal cytotoxicity of topically applied drugs, vehicles, and preservatives. Surv Ophthalmol 1980;25:15–30.

87. Pfister RR, Burstein NL. The effects of ophthalmic drugs, vehicles, and preservatives on corneal epithelium: A scanning electron microscope study. Invest Ophthalmol 1976;15:246–259.

88. Maurice DM. The tonicity of an eye drop and its dilution by tears. Exp Eye Res 1971;11:30–33.

89. Gilbard JP, Kenyon KR. Tear diluents in the treatment of kerato-conjunctivitis sicca. Ophthalmology 1985;92:646–650.

90. Lemp MA, Goldberg M, Roddy MR. The effect of tear substitutes on tear film breakup time. Invest Ophthalmol 1975; 14:255–258.

91. Burstein NL. Preservative cytotoxic threshold for benzalkonium chloride and chlorhexidine digluconate in cat and rabbit corneas. Invest Ophthalmol Vis Sci 1980;19:308–313.

92. Leopold IH. Local toxic effect of detergents on ocular structures. Arch Ophthalmol 1945;34:99–102.

93. Keller N, Moore D, Carper D, Longwell A. Increased corneal permeability by the dual effects of transient tear film acidification and exposure to benzalkonium chloride. Exp Eye Res 1980;30:203–210.

94. Wilson WS, Duncan AJ, Jay JL. Effect of benzalkonium chloride on the stability of the precorneal tear film in rabbit and man. Br J Ophthalmol 1975;59:667–669.

95. Olson RJ. Anti-inflammatory drugs. In: Ellis PP, ed. Current topics in ocular inflammation. Littleton, CO: Postgraduate Institute for Medicine, 1993:47–53.

96. Friedlaender M. External disease and allergy. In: Ellis PP, ed. Current topics in ocular inflammation. Littleton, CO: Postgraduate Institute for Medicine, 1993:29–34.

97. Marsh RJ, Maurice DM. The influence of nonionic detergents and other surfactants on human corneal permeability. Exp Eye Res 1971;11:43–48.

98. Cadwallader DE, Ansel HC. Hemolysis of erythrocytes by antibacterial preservatives. II. Quaternary ammonium salts. J Pharm Sci 1965;54:1010–1012.

99. Burstein NL. Preservative alteration of corneal permeability in humans and rabbits. Invest Ophthalmol Vis Sci 1984;25:1453–1457.

100. Green K, Livingston V, Bowman K. Chlorhexidine effects on corneal epithelium and endothelium. Arch Ophthalmol 1980;98:1273–1278.

101. Abrams JD, Davies TG, Klein M. Mercurial preservatives in eyedrops. Br J Ophthalmol 1965;49:146–147.

102. Burstein NL, Klyce SD. Electrophysiologic and morphologic effects of ophthalmic preparations on rabbit corneal epithelium. Invest Ophthalmol Vis Sci 1977;16:899–911.

103. Burton GD, Hill RM. Aerobic responses of the cornea to ophthalmic preservatives, measured *in vivo*. Invest Ophthalmol Vis Sci 1981;21:842–845.

104. Mullen W, Shepherd W, Leibowitz J. Ophthalmic preservatives and vehicles. Surv Ophthalmol 1973;17:469–483.

105. Mondino BJ, Salamon SM, Zaidman GW. Allergic and toxic reactions in soft contact lens wearers. Surv Ophthalmol 1982;26:337–344.

106. Adams J, Wilcox MJ, Trousdale MD, et al. Morphologic and physiologic effects of artificial tear formulations on corneal epithelium derived cells. Cornea 1992;11:234–241.

107. Hind HW. Aspects of contact lens solutions. The Optician, May 2, 1975.

108. Urtti A, Salminen L. Minimizing systemic absorption of topically administered ophthalmic drugs. Surv Ophthalmol 1993;37:435–456.

109. Molyneux P. The physical chemistry and pharmaceutical applications of polyvinylpyrrolidone. In: Digenis GA, Ansell J, eds. Proceedings of the International Symposium on Povidone. Louisville: University of Kentucky College of Pharmacy, 1983.

110. Shelanski HA, Shelanski MV, Cantor A. Polyvinyl pyrrolidone (PVP)—a useful adjunct in cosmetics. J Soc Cos Chem 1954;5:129–132.

111. Schwartz FL. Evaluation of the safety of povidone and crospovidone. Yakuzaigaku 1981;41:205–217.

112. Sabiston DW. The dry eye. Trans Ophthalmol Soc NZ 1969;21:96–100.

113. Krishna N, Mitchell B. Polyvinyl alcohol as an ophthalmic vehicle: Effect on ocular structures. Am J Ophthalmol 1965;59:860–864.

114. Linn ML, Jones LT. Rate of lacrimal excretion of ophthalmic vehicles. Am J Ophthalmol 1968;65:76–78.

115. Trueblood JH, Rossomondo RM, Carlton WH, Wilson LA. Corneal contact times of ophthalmic vehicles. Arch Ophthalmol 1975;93:127–130.

116. Holly FJ. Aqueous tear substitutes. In: Lamberts DW, Potter DE, eds. Clinical ophthalmic pharmacology. Boston: Little, Brown, 1987:497–518.

117. Peppas NA, Buri PA. Surface, interfacial and molecular aspects of polymer bioadhesion of soft tissues. J Controlled Release 1985;2:257–275.

118. Hunt G, Kearney P, Kellaway IW. Mucoadhesive polymers in drug delivery systems. In: Jensen P, Lloyd-Jones TG, eds. Drug delivery systems fundamentals and techniques. Weinham, Germany. VCH 180–199, 1987.

119. Grene RB, Lankston P, Mordaunt J, et al. Unpreserved carboxymethylcellulose artificial tears evaluated in patients with keratoconjunctivitis sicca. Cornea 1992;11:294–301.

120. Snibson GR, Greaves JL, Soper NDW, et al. Ocular surface residence times of artificial tear solutions. Cornea 1992;11:288–293.

121. Snibson GR, Greaves JL, Soper NDW, et al. Precorneal residence times of sodium hyaluronate solutions studied by gamma scintigraphy. Eye 1990;4:594–602.

122. Gurny R, Ryser JE, Tabatabay CC, et al. Precorneal residence time in humans of sodium hyaluronate as measured by gamma scintigraphy. Graefe's Arch Clin Exp Ophthalmol 1990;228:510–512.

123. Ludwig A, Van Ooteghem M. Evaluation of sodium hyaluronate as viscous vehicle for eye drops. J Pharm Belg 1989;44:391–397.

124. Moreira CA, Armstrong AT, Jelliffe RW,et al. Sodium hyaluronate as a carrier for intraocular gentamicin. Acta Ophthalmol 1991;69:45–49.

125. Bernatchetz SF, Tabatabay C, Gurny R. Sodium hyaluronate 0.25% used as a vehicle increases the bioavailability of topically administered gentamicin. Graefe's Arch Clin Exp Ophthalmol 1993;231:157–171.

126. Rozier A, Mazuel C, Grove J, et al. Gelrite: A novel ion-activated, in-situ gelling polymer for ophthalmic vehicles. Effect on bioavailability of timolol. Int J Pharmacol 1989;57:163–168.

127. Greaves JL, Wilson CG, Rozier A, et al. Scintigraphic assessment of an ophthalmic gelling vehicle in man and rabbit. Curr Eye Res 1990;9:415–420.

128. Maurice DM, Srinivas SP. Use of fluorometry in assessing the efficacy of a cation-sensitive gel as an ophthalmic vehicle: Comparison with scintigraphy. J Pharm Sci 1992;7:615–619.

129. Vogel R, Kulaga SF, Laurence JK, et al. The effect of Gelrite vehicle on the efficacy of low concentrations of timolol. Invest Ophthalmol Vis Sci 1990;31(suppl):404.

130. Shedden AH, Laibovitz RA, Repass R, et al. 24 hour diurnal evaluation of IOP following administration of Timoptic-XE (TXE) QD as compared to Timoptic (TS) BID. Invest Ophthalmol Vis Sci 1993;34(suppl):235.

131. Gunning FB, Greve EL, Bron AM, et al. Two topical carbonic anhydrase inhibitors sezolamide and dorzolamide in Gelrite vehicle: A multiple-dose efficacy study. Graefe's Arch Clin Exp Ophthalmol 1993;231:384–388.

132. Waring GO, Harris RR. Double-masked evaluation of a poloxamer artificial tear in keratoconjunctivitis sicca. In: Leopold IH, Burns RP, eds. Symposium on ocular therapy. New York: John Wiley & Sons 1979;11:127–139.

133. Jani R, Gan O, Ali Y, et al. Ion Exchange resins for ophthalmic delivery. J Ocular Pharmacol 1994;10:57–67.

134. Bar-Ilan A, Aviv H, Friedman D, et al. Improved performance of ocular drugs formulated in submicron emulsions. Invest Ophthalmol Vis Sci 1993;34(suppl):1488.

135. Melamed S, Kurtz S, Greenbaum A, et al. Effect of pilocarpine in submicron emulsion on IOP in healthy volunteers. Invest Ophthalmol Vis Sci 1993;34(suppl);926.

136. Fraunfelder FT, Hanna C. Ophthalmic drug delivery systems. Surv Ophthalmol 1974;18:292–298.

137. Scruggs J, Wallace T, Hanna C. Route of absorption of drug and ointment after application to the eye. Ann Ophthalmol 1978;10:267–271.

138. Mackeen DL. Aqueous formulations and ointments. Int Ophthalmol Clin 1980;20:79–92.

139. Hardberger R, Hanna C, Boyd CM. Effects of drug vehicles on ocular contact time. Arch Ophthalmol 1975;93:42–45.

140. Kaufman HE, Uotila MH, Gasset AR, et al. The medical uses of soft contact lenses. Trans Am Acad Ophthalmol Otolaryngol 1971;75:361–373.

141. Chiou GCY, Watanabe K. Drug delivery to the eye. Pharmacol Ther 1982;17:269–278.

142. Milani JK, Verbukh I, Pleyer U, et al. Collagen shields impregnated with gentamicin-dexamethasone as a potential drug delivery device. Am J Ophthalmol 1993;116:622–627.

143. Kumar S, Haglund BO, Himmelstein KS. In situ-forming gels for ophthalmic drug delivery. J Ocular Pharmacol 1994;10:47–56.

144. Doughty MJ. Acute effects of chlorobutanol- or benzalkonium chloride-containing artificial tears on the surface features of rabbit corneal epithelial cells. Optom Vis Sci 1994;71:562–572.

CHAPTER 3

Ophthalmic Drug Delivery

Jimmy D. Bartlett

The pharmacotherapy of eye disease generally requires high local concentrations of drug at the ocular tissues. Treatment of ocular surface infections or inflammations necessitates effective drug delivery to the eyelids, conjunctiva, or cornea. In contrast, treatment of uveitis, glaucoma, or retinitis involves therapeutic drug levels at appropriate target sites deep within the globe. Although many systems have been developed specifically for drug delivery to the eye, most of them suffer from lack of precision, and those associated with intraocular drug delivery can lead to unacceptable toxicity. This chapter discusses the most clinically useful drug delivery systems developed for ocular pharmacotherapy, with emphasis on those used in primary eye care.

Topical Administration

Topical application, the most common route of administration for ophthalmic drugs, is convenient, simple, and noninvasive, and patients can self-administer the medication. The primary source of drug loss in topical administration is diffusion into the circulating blood.[1] Diffusion into the blood takes place through blood vessels of the conjunctiva, episclera, intraocular vessels, and vessels of the nasal mucosa and oral pharynx after drainage through the nasolacrimal system. Because of these blood losses of drug, topically administered medications do not typically penetrate in useful concentrations to the posterior ocular structures and therefore are of no therapeutic benefit for diseases of the posterior segment. The occurrence of systemic side effects sometimes associated with the topical application of ocular drugs has created much interest in devising various drug delivery systems to minimize the risk of systemic toxicity.

The following discussion considers these and other forms of topical drug delivery systems.

Solutions and Suspensions

Solutions are the most commonly used mode of delivery for topical ocular medications. Solutions or suspensions are usually preferred over ointments, because the former are more easily instilled, interfere less with vision, and have fewer potential complications.[2] Disadvantages of topically applied solutions include short ocular contact time,[2] imprecise and inconsistent delivery of drug, frequent contamination,[3] and the possibility of ocular injury with the dropper tip.[4,5] Furthermore, aqueous suspensions have the problem of precipitation. Suspensions must be resuspended by shaking to provide an accurate dosage of drug, and the degree of resuspension varies considerably among preparations and among patients. The best corticosteroid formulations, for example, are not always adequately resuspended even by the most compliant and carefully instructed patients.[6]

PACKAGING

Most eyedrop containers consist of two parts, an eyedropper tip and a bottle containing the solution or suspension.[7] The eyedropper tip for many ophthalmic medications is constructed with an inner chamber and an outer chamber separated by a narrow aperture[7,8] (Fig. 3.1). This design increases the resistance to fluid flow so that squeezing the bottle produces a single drop rather than multiple drops or a stream of medication. The outer surface dimensions of the tip affect drop size. Eyedrops of different sizes are produced by

47

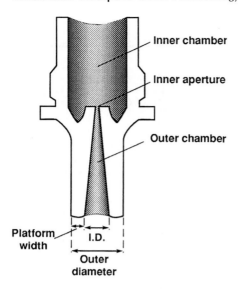

FIGURE 3.1 **Cross section of an eyedropper tip. An inner chamber is separated from an outer chamber by an inner aperture. The outer diameter, platform width, and inner diameter (I.D.) are critical dimensions in determining the eyedrop's size. (From Brown RH, Hotchkiss ML, Davis EB. Creating smaller eyedrops by reducing eyedropper tip dimensions. Am J Ophthalmol 1985;99:460–464.)**

changing the outer diameter and platform width (see Fig. 3.1).[7,8]

Because it is advantageous to administer small volumes of medication to minimize systemic absorption of topically applied solutions or suspensions, some manufacturers have attempted to reduce eyedrop volume by modifying or redesigning dropper tips.[8] Traditionally, commercial eyedrops have ranged in size from 50 to 70 μl.[9] The typical volumes now delivered by commercial glaucoma medications are in the range of 25 to 56 μl.[10]

To help reduce confusion in labeling and identification among various topical ocular medications, drug packaging standards have also been proposed.[11] When fully implemented by the ophthalmic drug industry, the standard colors for drug labeling and bottle caps will be yellow, blue, or both for β blockers, red for mydriatics and cycloplegics, green for miotics, gray for nonsteroidal anti-inflammatory drugs, and brown or tan for anti-infective agents.

STORAGE

Solutions of drugs should be stored in the examination room in a manner allowing easy identification of labels (Fig. 3.2). Containers of solutions often differ little in size, shape, or labeling, and numerous cases of bottle confusion between drugs with similar packaging have been reported.[12,13] The drug name should be confirmed by inspection each and every time a medication is used.

Although refrigeration of solutions may help to prolong

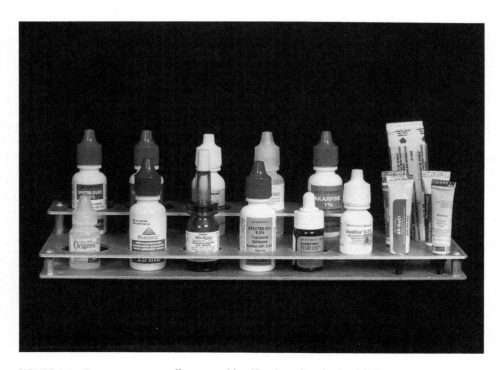

FIGURE 3.2 **Drug storage tray allows easy identification of packaging labels.**

shelf life, there appears to be little difference in local ocular irritation caused by eyedrops stored in the refrigerator or at room temperature.[14] Cold drops, however, can serve to reinforce proper eyedrop self-administration technique for patients who have difficulty ascertaining when the drops have been properly instilled.

Many practitioners have been annoyed by the bubbles contained in even the more viscous gonioscopic or fundus contact lens solutions. These troublesome bubbles can be minimized or eliminated by simply storing the solution inverted in the plastic vial in which many topical ophthalmic preparations are commercially packaged (Fig. 3.3). In this way the bubbles float to the top of the solution during storage and do not subsequently interfere with the clinical procedure.

Expiration dates of solutions should be respected. Practitioners should periodically survey ophthalmic preparations in the office and discard solutions that have reached the expiration date. The use of old solutions can increase liability as well as introduce the risk of potential drug toxicity or iatrogenic infection.[15] Some commonly used ophthalmic solutions, such as proparacaine, may change color, indicating deterioration (Fig. 3.4). Others, however, show no visible signs of deterioration.

TECHNIQUES OF INSTILLATION

Two methods are commonly used to instill topical ocular solutions.

1. With the patient looking down and the upper lid retracted, one or two drops of solution are applied to the superiorly exposed bulbar conjunctiva.
2. With the patient's head inclined backward so that the optical axis is as nearly vertical as possible, the lower lid should be retracted and the upper lid stabilized. The patient should be instructed to elevate the globe to move the cornea away from the instillation site to minimize the blink reflex. The solution should be instilled, and the dropper tip should be kept at least 2 cm from the globe to avoid contact contamination[15] (Fig. 3.5). After the lids are gently closed, the patient should be cautioned to avoid lid squeezing. Pressure should be applied with the fingertips over the puncta and canaliculi to minimize nasolacrimal drainage[16] (Fig. 3.6). This position should be maintained for 2 to 3 minutes.[17]

Several investigators[1,16–18] have shown that simple eyelid closure alone significantly retards medication drainage and thereby minimizes potential side effects associated with systemic drug absorption. Moreover, Zimmerman and associates[19,20] have demonstrated that when nasolacrimal occlusion is used in conjunction with eyelid closure, intraocular drug absorption may be enhanced. The same maximal drug effect can be achieved with many antiglaucoma drugs at

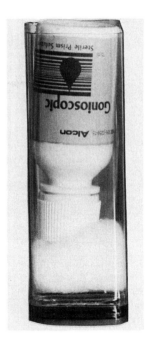

FIGURE 3.3 **Inverted storage of gonioscopic solution minimizes interference by bubbles.**

lower concentrations and with lower dosage frequencies than those generally recommended. This is true for use of pilocarpine, carbachol, and timolol[19] but not for epinephrine or dipivefrin.[20]

Various modifications of the latter technique have resulted in increased ocular contact time for the applied solution.

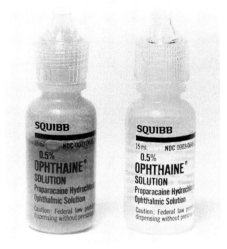

FIGURE 3.4 **Change in color of proparacaine solution (left) indicates deterioration of the preparation.**

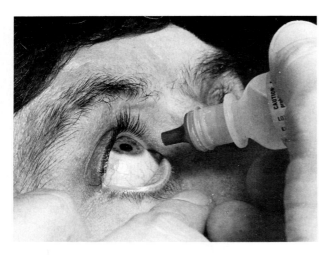

FIGURE 3.5 **Traditional technique for instillation of topical ocular solutions. The patient's head is inclined backward, the lower lid is retracted, the globe is elevated, and the dropper tip is kept at least 2 cm from the globe.**

Fraunfelder[21] modified the procedure by gently pulling the lid away from the globe at right angles to the plane of the head and placing the drop in the inferior conjunctival sac without touching ocular tissues or lashes. After waiting to allow gravity to deliver the drop to the most dependent area of the

fornix, he moved the lid parallel to the plane of the head until it came in contact with the globe (Figs. 3.7 and 3.8). This "pouch" method thus allows the topically applied solution to act as a "depot" deposit. Even with the patient's head vertical and with a normal blink rate or with the lids closed, 80% or 96% of the drop, respectively, remains in the ocular area for five minutes.[21] This method increases the ocular retention rate of a 13 μl drop twice as much over simply applying drops to the superior bulbar conjunctiva. The effect is even more striking with the more flaccid lids commonly encountered in older age groups.[21] Regardless of the method of initial drop instillation, closure of the lids following drop instillation markedly increases the contact time of the drug with the ocular tissues.[21] Tables 3.1 and 3.2 summarize the recommended procedures for drop instillation.

Administering topical solutions to uncooperative children is often disconcerting. Several techniques may be used to facilitate drug administration to these patients.[22] The hand can be placed on the forehead, which proprioceptively reinforces upward gaze. In addition, the palpebral aperture can be widened for drop instillation by telling children to open their mouths. A spread of the neural impulse from the mesencephalic root of the fifth cranial nerve to the nucleus of the levator may explain the effectiveness of this maneuver.[22] Another useful method of administering drops to uncooperative pediatric patients is to instruct them to close

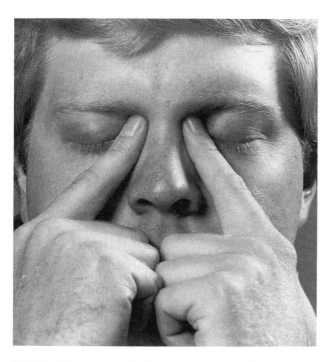

FIGURE 3.6 **Nasolacrimal drainage of solutions may be minimized by applying pressure over the puncta and canaliculi.**

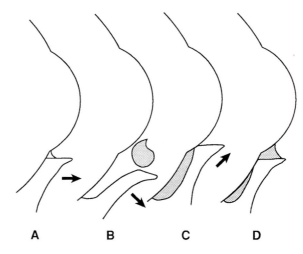

A   B   C   D

FIGURE 3.7 **Schematic representation of technique described by Fraunfelder[21] to administer topical solutions to the eye. *(A)* The lid is gently pulled away at right angles to the plane of the head. *(B)* The drop is placed in the inferior conjunctival sac without touching ocular tissues or lashes. *(C)* After waiting a moment to allow gravity to deliver the drop to the most dependent area of the fornix, the lid is then moved parallel to the plane of the head until it comes in contact with the globe. *(D)* A portion of the drop is entrapped under the eyelid. (From Fraunfelder FT. Extraocular fluid dynamics: How best to apply topical ocular medication. Trans Am Ophthalmol Soc 1976;74:457–487, with permission of the author and publisher.)**

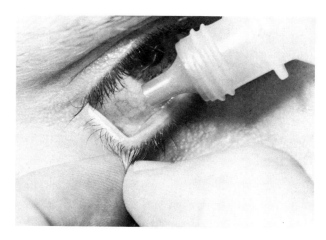

FIGURE 3.8   **Technique described by Fraunfelder[21] to administer topical solutions to the eye. The drop is placed in a "pouch" created by gently pulling the lower lid away at right angles to the plane of the head.**

their eyes. They usually will not resist and are unable to see the approach of the dropper bottle. By gently retracting the lower lid, a small opening through the lashes into the conjunctival sac is created, and the drop can be instilled. The simple placement of the drop on the eyelashes of the closed eyelids has also been shown to achieve effective mydriasis and cycloplegia in the pediatric population.[23,24]

The self-administration of topical solutions by elderly patients can sometimes be difficult because of arthritis, tremors, or other physically debilitating diseases. Burns and Mulley[25] have shown that, indeed, most patients over the age of 75 years have difficulty applying their eyedrops. Although some patients recognize the problem, many are observed to have difficulty but do not acknowledge their inadequacies at eyedrop installation. Thus, simply asking patients about their eyedrop technique is not likely to reveal

TABLE 3.1
Recommended Procedure for Instilling Topical Ocular Solutions

1. Tilt patient's head backward.
2. Instruct patient to direct gaze toward ceiling.
3. Gently grasp lower outer eyelid below lashes and pull eyelid away from globe.
4. Without touching lashes or eyelids, instill one drop of solution into conjunctival sac.
5. Continue to hold eyelid in this position for a few seconds to allow solution to gravitate into deepest portion of lower fornix.
6. Instruct patient to gaze downward while lifting the eyelid upward until it contacts the globe.
7. Instruct patient to gently close eyes.
8. Patient should keep eyes closed for 1–2 minutes.

TABLE 3.2
Instructions to Patients for Self-Administration of Solutions or Suspensions

1. Tilt head backward.
2. With clean hands, gently grasp lower outer eyelid below lashes and pull eyelid away from the eye.
3. Place dropper over eye by looking directly at it.
4. Just before applying a drop, look upward.
5. After applying the drop, look downward for a few seconds.
6. Lift eyelid upward until it contacts the eye.
7. Gently close eyes for 1–2 minutes.

patients in need of instruction.[25] A better approach is to actually observe eyedrop instillation technique and to make sure that it is taught to all patients or their caregivers before patients leave the office.[26] The instillation of ocular drugs may be facilitated in these patients by using a pair of spectacle lenses into which a hole has been drilled through the center of each lens.[27] The patient inserts the dropper tip into the hole, gazes superiorly, and squeezes the bottle (Fig. 3.9). Only polycarbonate lenses should be used, because the risk associated with drilling into a conventional glass or plastic lens is considerable. Various commercial devices are also available (Fig. 3.10).[28]

Solutions characterized by significant local toxicity or staining potential (e.g., silver nitrate, rose bengal) can be instilled using a cotton swab as applicator. This technique serves essentially to minimize drop size and subsequent overflow onto the patient's cheek or clothing.

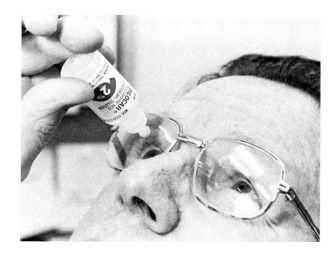

FIGURE 3.9   **Modification of polycarbonate spectacle lenses to facilitate drop instillation. After a hole is drilled through the center of each lens, the patient inserts the dropper tip into the hole, gazes superiorly, and squeezes the bottle.**

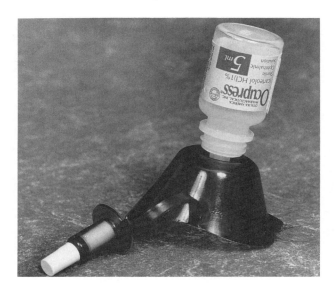

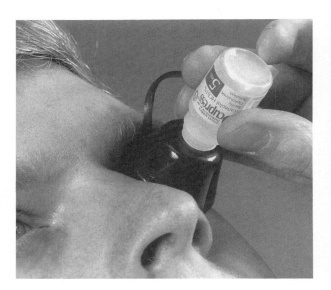

A   B

FIGURE 3.10   **Commercial eyedrop assistance device. *(A)* Insertion of dropper bottle into device. *(B)* Device in use.**

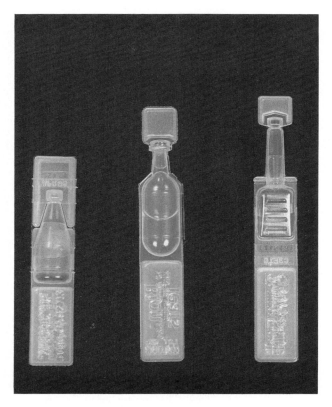

FIGURE 3.11   **Unit-dose dispensers.**

UNIT-DOSE DISPENSERS

Recognizing that chronic therapy with frequently applied, preserved solutions can be toxic to the ocular surface, several manufacturers have formulated some ophthalmic solutions in unit-dose dispensers without preservatives (Fig. 3.11). Unpreserved artificial tears are available in this form, as are timolol, phenylephrine, and apraclonidine.[29]

Most unit-dose dispensers accommodate solution volumes ranging from 0.1 to 0.6 ml. Because these solutions are unpreserved, they are designed for short-term use (not exceeding 12 hours), after which the unit is discarded.

It is important for patients to fully understand how these dispensers should be used. The plastic top should be twisted completely off before use; if the cap is only partially twisted or pulled off, a small "barb" can remain (Fig. 3.12), which has the potential to cause ocular injury in the form of traumatic conjunctivitis[30] or corneal abrasion.[31]

SPRAYS

The topical administration of solutions to the eye is often an unpleasant procedure associated with significant burning, stinging, lacrimation, and emotional ambivalence, especially in children. Topical sprays represent an alternative method of administering ophthalmic solutions that may be less irritating and less objectionable. Pilocarpine, epinephrine, and other agents were once commercially available in mist-dispensing bottles, but these are no longer manufactured. Combinations of mydriatics and cycloplegics such as phenylephrine-tropicamide or phenylephrine-tropicamide-cyclopentolate can be used as sprays for routine mydriasis in adults or for cycloplegia in children.[23,24] The spray can be produced by using a refillable perfume atomizer (Fig. 3.13) or plastic spray bottle that has first been sterilized with ethylene oxide gas or hydrogen peroxide before filling with the appropriate mydriatic or cycloplegic combination (see Chapter 21). The unit is held 5 to 10 cm from the eye before activating the spray.

One advantage of a spray is that the drug can be applied to closed eyelids. Following drug application, patients should be instructed to blink. If the medication reaches the precorneal tear film, mild stinging is expected. After blinking several times, patients should wipe off the excess solution. If no mild burning or stinging occurs after the eye has been sprayed, it is likely that none of the drug reached the precorneal tear film from the lid margin, and another application is necessary. This may occur in patients who have tightly closed lids in which redundancy of the skin shields the lid margins from the spray.

Several investigators[23,24] have compared the efficacy of sprays to topically applied eyedrops and found sprays to provide both mydriasis and cycloplegia comparable to those obtained with eyedrops (Fig. 3.14). This occurs even when sprays are applied to the closed eyelids. The effectiveness of sprays under "closed eye" conditions is probably explained by the minimal quantities of drug in the tear film actually required for maximum mydriasis and cycloplegia.[32]

The use of sprays is a rapid and effective method for drug delivery. Patient resistance is less when the spray is directed to the closed eye.[23,24] The clinical use of mydriatic and cycloplegic sprays has been well tolerated by patients and is particularly well received by children, because the patients do not need to assume an awkward position to receive the spray.

Ointments

Although solutions are the most commonly used vehicles for topical ocular medications, ointments are also frequently used for application to the eye. When applied to the inferior conjunctival sac, ophthalmic ointments melt quickly, and the excess spreads out onto the lid margins, lashes, and skin of the lids, depending on the amount instilled and on the extent of lacrimation induced by any irritation. The ointment at the lid margins acts as a reservoir and enhances drug contact time.[33]

TECHNIQUES OF APPLICATION

Patients are instructed to elevate the gaze, and with the lower lid retracted, the ointment is instilled into the inferior conjunctival sac in a sweeping fashion from canthus to canthus (Fig. 3.15). A pressure patch can then be applied. The daytime use of ointments frequently leads to complaints of blurred vision. For bedtime use at least 1 cm of ointment is

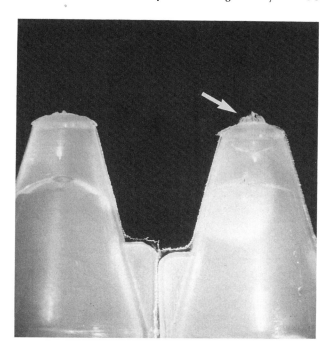

FIGURE 3.12   "Barb" (arrow) on unit-dose dispenser created by abrupt and incomplete twisting of the cap.

generally applied. If the ointment is not to be applied at bedtime or used under a pressure patch, smaller volumes of ointment should be instilled.

An alternative method of application involves placing the ointment on a cotton-tipped applicator and applying it to the upper lid margin and lashes as well as the medial and lateral canthi.[34] In this way the ointment causes minimal blurring of

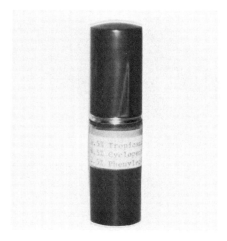

FIGURE 3.13   Refillable perfume atomizer can be used to deliver solutions in the form of a spray.

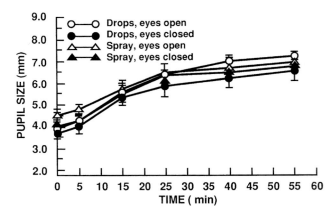

FIGURE 3.14 **Mydriatic effect of ophthalmic spray applied to closed eyes is comparable to that of eyedrops applied to open eyes.** (From Wesson MD, Bartlett JD, Swiatocha J, et al. Mydriatic efficacy of a cycloplegic spray in the pediatric population. J Am Optom Assoc 1993;64:637–640.)

vision, and drug irritation is minimized. In addition, the ointment acts as a drug reservoir and has a therapeutic effect for approximately 6 hours. This method of application may be of practical value in the treatment of ocular infections in all patients, but especially those in the pediatric and geriatric age groups.

Once the ointment has been instilled, the bioavailability of subsequently instilled solutions may be altered because the solution is blocked from contact with the ocular surface.[35] Whenever both solution and ointment formulations are used in therapy, the solution should be instilled before the ointment is applied.

COMPLICATIONS

Contact dermatitis of the lids sometimes occurs during use of ointments containing sensitizing agents such as atropine

or neomycin, because ointments are characterized by prolonged ocular contact time. Hypersensitivity to the incorporated preservatives may also occur.

Blurred vision is one of the most frequent adverse effects from ophthalmic ointments. This problem can often be alleviated or minimized by simply reducing the volume of ointment instilled during the daytime. Another option involves instructing patients to apply the ointment to each eye on an alternating schedule.[36] This allows patients to have acceptable vision with at least one eye at all times during the waking hours.

The effect of ophthalmic ointments on the healing of corneal wounds has received considerable attention. Early formulations of ophthalmic ointments contained waxy grades of petrolatum or unwashed lanolin, which interfered with corneal wound healing.[37,38] Contemporary ophthalmic ointments, however, are nonemulsive and do not contain the

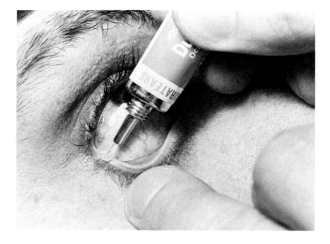

A

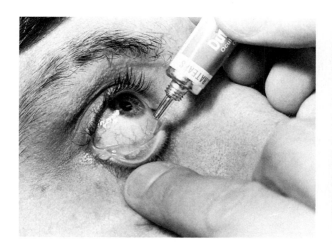

B

FIGURE 3.15 **Technique of ointment instillation. With the globe elevated and the lower lid retracted, ointment is instilled into the inferior conjunctival sac in a sweeping fashion from lateral canthus (A) to medial canthus (B).**

coarse grade of white petrolatum.[37] Ophthalmic ointments contain the less viscous petrolatum or are made even less viscous by the addition of liquid mineral oil. Because highly purified lanolin has little or no inhibitory effect on the healing of epithelial wounds,[38] purified lanolin is occasionally added to the white petrolatum-mineral oil nonemulsive base. This allows water and many water-soluble drugs to be retained in the nonemulsive ointment preparation. These ointments cause no significant inhibition of corneal wound healing, even when maximum dosage frequencies of every 30 minutes are employed.[37]

Ointments rarely become entrapped within the cornea.[35,39,40] The inability to trap ophthalmic ointments during corneal wound healing appears to be related to the rapid melting of these preparations. Almost all commercial ophthalmic ointments melt below body temperature and become an oil within minutes. This rapid melting allows the ointment to float above the precorneal tear film and permits migration and mitosis of the underlying epithelial cells without interference. Entrapment of ointment occurs only after direct injection into the stroma or, rarely, in corneal wounds in which stroma-to-stroma contact occurs anterior to the ointment. However, "pseudoentrapment" of ointment in the cornea sometimes occurs in corneal lesions with stromal loss or distortion of the normal stromal architecture that have been administered ointments and pressure patched. This situation allows ointment globules to lie below the corneal surface.[39] Although the clinical picture is that of a cluster of large ointment globules lodged within the corneal defect, the ointment is actually trapped only within the wound exudates below the plane of the corneal surface (Fig. 3.16). No treatment is necessary, because the ointment usually extrudes spontaneously within 24 to 48 hours even if the pressure dressing is continued. No complications are associated with this condition.

It has been generally assumed that ointments are not eliminated through the nasolacrimal drainage system.[33,41] Scruggs and associates[33] have shown that topically applied ophthalmic ointments travel through the lacrimal drainage system, although more slowly than do solutions. These investigators demonstrated that the total amount of drug absorbed systemically is similar regardless of whether solution or ointment is used. The slower drainage of ointments through the nasolacrimal system and the resulting slower systemic absorption may explain why systemic drug toxicity is much less common with topical ointments than with solutions. An ointment delivers a much smaller total amount of drug compared to the "bolus" effect of drop therapy,[35] which is another important factor that contributes to the reduced systemic toxicity of ointment preparations. Serious side effects can indeed occur with ointment therapy, however. Death has occurred following the administration of topical atropine ointment.[42,43]

The following guidelines are suggested for the clinical utilization of ophthalmic ointments.[44]

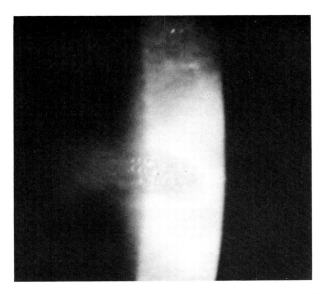

FIGURE 3.16 **Pseudoentrapment of ointment in cornea in case of recurrent corneal erosion. The photograph was taken three hours after removal of firm pressure dressing. (From Fraunfelder FT, Hanna C, Woods AH. Pseudoentrapment of ointment in the cornea. Arch Ophthalmol 1975;93:331–334. Copyright 1975, American Medical Association.)**

- Ointments may be used immediately after intraocular surgery under a conjunctival flap or in corneal incisions with excellent wound approximation, because the risk of entrapment of ointment is minimal. Ointments should not be used, however, in any surgical wound in which there is a question of wound integrity, such as when difficulty is experienced maintaining the anterior chamber at surgery. In such cases, ointment application should be delayed for several days until after the first dressing change. Ointments should be used with caution in jagged or flaplike corneal lacerations, in eyes with impending corneal perforation, and in open conjunctival lacerations.
- Ointments can be used routinely for superficial corneal abrasions. However, any abrasion involving corneal tissues deeper than the epithelium should be managed on an individual basis depending on the configuration of the wound edges.
- Ointments may be applied to corneal ulcers with little risk of entrapment or inhibition of wound healing. However, they should be used with caution in ulcers with an impending perforation or large overhanging margins because there is a risk of ointment entrapment under a flap.

Lid Scrubs

Application of solutions or ointments directly to the lid margin is especially helpful in treating seborrheic or infec-

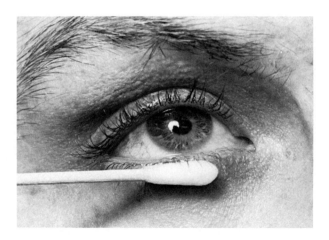

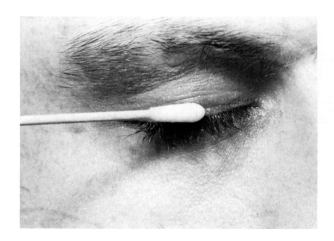

A   B

FIGURE 3.17   **Technique of lid scrub. Drug application to the lid margin is accomplished with a cotton-tipped applicator applied to the opened *(A)* or closed *(B)* eyelids.**

tious blepharitis. This direct application is probably more effective therapeutically than is the simple instillation of topical solutions or ointments into the conjunctival sac. After several drops of the antibiotic solution or detergent, such as baby shampoo, are placed on the end of a cotton-tipped applicator, the solution is applied to the lash line of the lid margin with the eyelids either opened or closed (Fig. 3.17). Antibiotic ointments are applied in the same way.

Although baby shampoo is frequently used for cleaning the eyelid margin, commercially available eyelid cleansers are effective, with potentially less ocular stinging, burning, or toxicity.[45–47] Commercial lid scrub products are designed to aid in removal of oils, debris, or desquamated skin associated with the inflamed eyelid. The lid scrubs can also be used for hygienic eyelid cleansing in contact lens wearers. Although these solutions are designed to be used full strength on eyelid tissues, they must not be instilled directly into the eyes. Some of the products (Table 3.3) are packaged with presoaked gauze or cotton pads (Fig. 3.18), which provide an abrasive action to augment the cleansing properties of the detergent.[29]

Gels

Pilocarpine is commercially available in a carbomer gel vehicle.[29,48,49] The ocular hypotensive and miotic effects of this formulation have been compared with traditional drop instillation. The 4% pilocarpine gel is packaged in a 3.5-g tube similar to that in which ophthalmic ointments are packaged. A practical advantage of this sustained pulse delivery system is the once-daily dosage regimen, usually administered at bedtime. Other advantages include im-

proved patient compliance as well as a reduction in ocular side effects such as drug-induced myopia during the waking hours.[50] The major disadvantage of pilocarpine gel is its significant loss of ocular hypotensive effect during the hours before the next bedtime dose.[51,52] Minor side effects include superficial corneal haze, which may occur after long-term use (> 8 weeks)[48] and superficial punctate keratitis, which can affect almost one-half the treated patients but usually resolves spontaneously.[52]

Solid Delivery Devices

One of the significant problems with the delivery of drugs in solution is that drug administration is pulsed, with an initial period of overdosage followed by a period of relative underdosage (see Fig. 2.9). The development of solid drug delivery devices has been an attempt to overcome this disadvantage.

HYDROGEL CONTACT LENSES

The effect of topically applied ophthalmic drugs can be enhanced by several methods. "Lamellae," described as early as 1948, were atropine-containing gelatin wafers intended for placement in the conjunctival sac. A Russian study in 1966[53] reported use of pilocarpine-impregnated disks of polyvinyl alcohol that were designed to provide sustained miosis and reduce intraocular pressure (IOP). The use of soft contact lenses as a vehicle for the delivery of pilocarpine was first suggested by Sedlacek, a Czechoslovakian ophthalmologist, in 1965.[54] In the United States the use of hydrogel contact lenses for drug delivery was initially

TABLE 3.3
Eyelid Scrub Products

Trade Name (Manufacturer)	Ingredients	Formulation
Lids & Lashes (Allergan)	Cocoamphodiacetate, sodium trideceth sulfate, hexylene glycol, PPG-10 methyl glucose ether, PEG-20 methyl glucose sesquistearate, boric acid, quaternium-15, purified water USP	Premoistened pads
Eye-Scrub (Ciba Vision)	PEG-200 glyceryl monotallowate, disodium laureth sulfosuccinate, cocoamido propyl amine oxide, PEG-78 glyceryl monococoate, benzyl alcohol, EDTA	Solution and premoistened pads
OcuClenz (Storz/Lederle)	Disodium oleamido PEG-2 sulfosuccinate, cocoamphodiacetate, poloxamer 185, poloxamer 188, methylparaben, propylparaben, citric acid, EDTA	Solution
Lid Wipes SPF (Akorn)	PEG-200 glyceryl monotallowate, PEG-80 glyceryl monococate, laureth-23, cocoamido propylamine oxide, NaCl, glycerin, sodium dihydrogen phosphate, sodium hydroxide	Premoistened pads
OCuSOFT (Cynacon/OCuSOFT)	PEG-80 sorbitan laurate, sodium trideceth sulfate, PEG-150 distearate, cocamido propyl hydroxysultaine, lauroamphocarboxyglycinate, sodium laureth-13 carboxylate, PEG-15 tallow polyamine, quaternium-15	Solution and premoistened pads
Prescribed Care (Almay)	Water, poloxamer 184, butylene glycol, disodium lauroamphodiacetate, sodium trideceth sulfate, hexylene glycol, phenoxyethanol, citric acid, benzyl alcohol	Premoistened pads

Adapted from Bartlett JD, Ghormley NJ, Jaanus, SD, et al., eds. Ophthalmic drug facts. St. Louis: Facts and Comparisons, 1995.

proposed by Waltman and Kaufman in 1970.[55] The use of hydrogel lenses to prolong drug contact with the eye seems to be effective at least for some of the medications studied.

Drugs penetrate soft contact lenses at a rate that depends on the pore size between the cross-linkages of the three-dimensional lattice structure of the lens, the concentration of drug in the soaking solution, the soaking time, the water content of the lens, and the molecular size of the drug. Lenses with higher water contents absorb more water-soluble drug for later release into the precorneal tear film.[2,56-58]

The degree of permeability is also related to lens thickness. A thinner lens allows a greater amount of topically applied drug to pass into the lens-cornea interface, whereas a

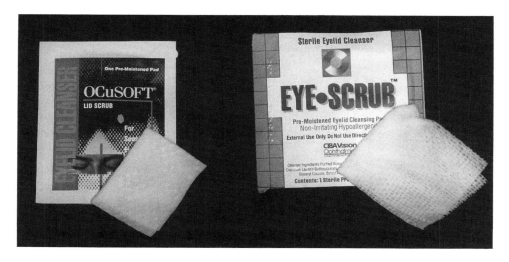

FIGURE 3.18 **Commercial eyelid scrub products.**

thicker lens stores a greater amount of the drug without releasing it to the cornea.[58]

Maximum drug delivery is obtained by presoaking the lens.[55,59–62] This produces a more sustained high yield of drug.[59] In addition, a prolonged soaking to a state of equilibrium before clinical use produces a more standardized form of presoaked lens.

In addition to pilocarpine,[57,59,60,63] many other drugs have been used in hydrogel contact lens delivery systems. The release rates of antibiotics, including chloramphenicol, tetracycline, bacitracin, gentamicin, tobramycin, and polymyxin B, have been studied.[64–66] Other drugs have been delivered with these lenses, including ethylenediaminetetra-acetic acid (EDTA) for alkali burns,[64] cystein hydrochloride,[64] acetylcysteine,[67] lubricating solutions,[68] normal saline solution,[69] idoxuridine,[69] corticosteroids,[69] and hypertonic solutions.[2]

Jain[70] compared soft contact lens with subconjunctival delivery of chloramphenicol, gentamicin, and carbenicillin. Soft contact lenses provided significantly higher aqueous drug levels than did subconjunctival injection (Fig. 3.19).

Early in the use of soft contact lenses as a drug delivery system, it was suggested never to soak lenses in solutions containing preservatives because the prolonged delivery of relatively high concentrations of preservatives might be toxic to the eye. Ocular irritation as well as superficial punctate erosions of the cornea could result.[71] However, Lemp[68] found no evidence of benzalkonium chloride in hydrogel contact lenses used as drug delivery devices. He also failed to find clinical evidence of corneal toxicity associated with the preservative. Thus, the use of ophthalmic medications containing benzalkonium chloride as a preservative in conjunction with hydrogel contact lenses is probably a clinically acceptable procedure.[72] Further studies, however, are needed to clarify the safety of other preservatives used in conjunction with this drug delivery system.

Currently, disposable soft contact lenses[73] are used for drug delivery and appear to be of greatest clinical value in the treatment of bullous keratopathy, dry eye syndromes, and corneal conditions requiring protection.[2] The most significant disadvantage of this mode of therapy, however, is the rapid loss of most drugs from the lens. Drug-impregnated hydrogel lenses are characterized by first-order kinetics,[70] so they only occasionally offer any significant advantage over topically applied solutions or ointments.

COLLAGEN SHIELDS

Shaped like contact lenses, collagen shields are thin membranes of porcine or bovine scleral collagen that conform to the cornea when placed on the eye. They are packaged in a dehydrated state and require rehydration before application (Fig. 3.20). When a shield is rehydrated in a solution containing a water-soluble drug, the drug becomes trapped in the collagen matrix.[74] Collagen shields have been studied extensively for their potential usefulness as drug delivery devices, because the drug is released as the shield dissolves. They have been evaluated for the delivery of antibacterial, antifungal, antiviral, anti-inflammatory, and immunosuppressive drugs, as well as anticoagulants.[75]

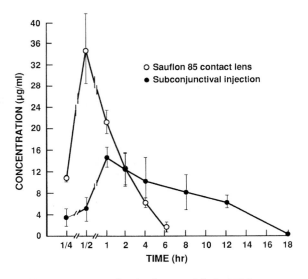

FIGURE 3.19 **Aqueous levels of gentamicin in 150 human eyes. The gentamicin was delivered subconjunctivally or with a Sauflon 85 soft contact lens. (From Jain MR. Drug delivery through soft contact lenses. Br J Ophthalmol 1988;72:150–154.)**

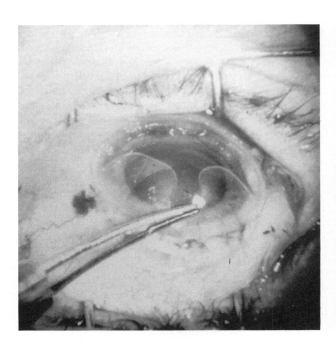

FIGURE 3.20 **Rehydrated collagen shield on eye. (Courtesy of Bausch & Lomb, Inc.)**

TABLE 3.4
Commercially Available Collagen Shields

Trade Name	Manufacturer	Collagen Source	Diameter (mm)	Base Curve (mm)	Water Content (%)	Duration (hrs)
Bio-Cor	Bausch & Lomb	Porcine sclera	14.5	9.0	63.0	12, 24, 72
MediLens	Chiron	Bovine corium	16.0	8.8	83.0	24
Collagen Shield	Chiron	Bovine corium	14.0	9.1	80.0	24
Soft Shield	Oasis	Bovine collagen	14.5	9.0	80–85	12, 24, 72
Proshield	Alcon	Bovine collagen	14.6	8.8	—	12
			16.0	8.8	—	24

Currently available collagen shields are listed in Table 3.4. The Bio-Cor (Bausch & Lomb) shield has a variable dissolution rate of 12, 24, or 72 hours depending on the amount of collagen cross-linking induced by ultraviolet radiation during the manufacturing process.[76] Shields dissolve as a result of proteolytic degradation by the tear film.[77,78] The oxygen permeability is comparable to that of a hydroxyethyl-methacrylate (HEMA) lens of similar water content.[79] Before insertion, the shields must be rehydrated for at least three minutes in saline, lubricating solution, antibiotic or steroid. Because the shields are floppy when hydrated, use of a topical anesthetic may be required.[74]

The results of numerous animal studies,[75,77,80–85] primarily using the rabbit model, that involved the use of collagen shields as drug delivery devices have generally been favorable. However, extrapolation of conclusions from animal experiments to clinical practice can be difficult or even erroneous. Phinney and associates[80] demonstrated *in vitro* that presoaked shields release most of the gentamicin within the first 30 minutes, whereas vancomycin was released gradually over 6 hours. After soaking in gentamicin, vancomycin, or a combination of the two, the shields produced tear, cornea, and aqueous levels in rabbits that were comparable to or higher than those achieved by frequent application of eyedrops (Fig. 3.21). Several investigators[75,81,85] have studied the use of collagen shields to deliver aminoglycosides for treatment of experimental *Pseudomonas* keratitis in rabbits. Although the results have shown that shields rehydrated in a water-soluble antibiotic such as gentamicin or tobramycin may be an effective and convenient mode of therapy for this condition, they should not entirely replace traditional antibiotic eyedrop therapy. Instead, they may be more effective with topical eyedrop supplementation to increase the amount of drug available during therapy. Delivery of other antibiotics has also been investigated. Schwartz and associates[83] found that amphotericin B delivered to the cornea by collagen shields is comparable to frequent eyedrop application. Polypeptides such as tissue plasminogen activator (tPA), which cannot normally penetrate the cornea in

significant amounts when given as eyedrops, have been delivered efficiently to the eye using shields rehydrated for 20 minutes in a solution containing tPA.[82] This may suggest that tPA could be administered by collagen shields to lyse fibrin clots in the anterior chamber, thus avoiding intraocular injections.

Although the animal data are sound and have positive implications for clinical practice, relatively few studies demonstrate the utility or efficacy of collagen shields in patients with eye disease. Colin and associates[86] treated 18 patients with typical herpes simplex virus epithelial keratitis. Collagen shields were used after rehydrating with trifluridine for 15 minutes. In addition, trifluridine eyedrops were given five times daily. The average healing time was 2.9 days (range: 1 to 7 days). No allergic reactions occurred, but punctate keratitis was observed in three eyes. The investigators concluded that collagen shields used in conjunction with topical trifluridine therapy can shorten the average epithelial healing time compared with traditional antiviral eyedrop therapy. These results, which confirm those of other researchers,[78] suggest that shields may be superior to topical eyedrops or soft contact lenses in delivering water-soluble drugs to the human cornea.

Clinical experience indicates that the collagen shield is relatively safe when used as a drug delivery device. Pflugfelder and Murchison[87] reported a patient, however, who had persistent corneal edema when treated with a 12-hour shield soaked in tobramycin (40 mg/ml), vancomycin (50 mg/ml), and dexamethasone sodium phosphate (4 mg/ml). It is recommended that antibiotic/steroid-soaked shields used for prophylaxis of postoperative endophthalmitis should be used with caution or avoided in patients with reduced corneal endothelial cell counts or poor tear clearance. Moreover, Wentworth and associates[84] have recently shown that collagen shield treatment of alkali corneal injuries may actually accelerate corneal ulceration and perforation. This may result from trapping of activated polymorphonuclear leukocytes (PMNs) in the collagen shields, causing a locally high concentration of metalloproteinases. Alternatively,

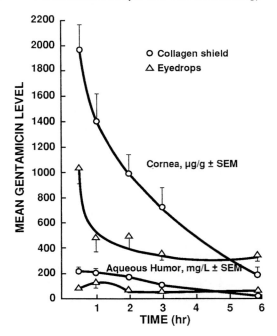

FIGURE 3.21 **Gentamicin delivered by eyedrops or collagen shield. Mean corneal and aqueous gentamicin levels were measured in collagen shield-treated and eyedrop-treated eyes of rabbits for 6 hours. Collagen shields were soaked for 2 hours in gentamicin (40 mg/ml) prior to application. A five-drop loading dose of gentamicin (15 mg/ml) eyedrops was followed by hourly application. Vertical bars indicate SEM. (From Phinney RB, Schwartz SD, Lee DA, et al. Collagen-shield delivery of gentamicin and vancomycin. Arch Ophthalmol 1988;106:1599–1604. Copyright 1988, American Medical Association.)**

breakdown of the collagen shield may generate collagen-derived peptides chemotactic for PMNs, enhancing the influx of PMNs and the release of destructive enzymes. Thus, use of collagen shields should probably be avoided in patients with significant chemical injury.

Collagen shields appear to have numerous advantages compared with contact lenses, subconjunctival injections, or frequent topical eyedrop therapy. Frequent topical application of eyedrops can be labor-intensive and irritating, thus contributing to poor compliance. Subconjunctival injections can be painful and even dangerous. Drug delivery using impregnated collagen shields is potentially more comfortable and reliable than frequent applications of eyedrops or daily subconjunctival injections.[80] The available data seem to suggest that collagen shields provide drug delivery comparable or superior to that achieved with topical eyedrops, subconjunctival injection, or soft contact lenses.[74–76]

Collagen shields have some potential complications that may limit their usefulness. In addition to high cost, shields are available in a limited number of base curves and diame-

ters and thus may not fit properly to maintain position over the cornea and limbus. They can fit too tightly, inducing corneal hypoxia associated with tight lens syndrome. Furthermore, although the shields degrade over a short time, sharp edges or tears can cause foreign body irritation or corneal compromise. Allergic reactions can also occur.[88] Another potential problem can result when the shields are used to deliver drug combinations. Two antibiotics are usually employed for the initial treatment of infectious corneal ulcers. The combination of gentamicin and cefazolin can result in precipitation, which precludes incorporation of this combination into a collagen shield.[80] Practitioners must use only drugs that are compatible pharmacologically, and they should be especially careful when using combinations of drugs to be sure that the combination does not cause precipitation.[74]

FILTER PAPER STRIPS

Two staining agents, sodium fluorescein and rose bengal, are commercially available as drug-impregnated filter paper strips (Fig. 3.22). This form of drug delivery allows these agents to be more easily administered to the eye in dosage amounts adequate for their intended clinical purpose. Administration of excessive drug is eliminated, thus avoiding unintentional staining of lid tissues or patients' clothing. Furthermore, the availability of fluorescein-impregnated paper strips eliminates the risk of solution contamination with *Pseudomonas aeruginosa*.

For administration, the drug-impregnated paper strip is moistened with a drop of normal saline or extraocular irrigating solution, and the applicator is gently touched to the superior or inferior bulbar conjunctiva or to the inferior conjunctival sac. Some practitioners prefer to moisten the fluorescein-impregnated strip with a drop of rose bengal solution before application, allowing for the simultaneous administration of both the sodium fluorescein and rose bengal. To avoid the risk of cross-contamination between eyes, practitioners should use separate applicators for dye delivery to eyes with suspected infection.

COTTON PLEDGETS

Cotton pledgets saturated with ophthalmic solutions are of value in several clinical situations. These devices allow prolonged ocular contact time with solutions that are normally topically instilled into the eye. A pledget is constructed by simply teasing the cotton tip of an applicator to form a small (approximately 5 mm), elongated body of cotton. After placing one or two drops of the ophthalmic solution on the pledget, the device is placed into the inferior conjunctival fornix (Fig. 3.23).

The clinical use of pledgets is usually reserved for administration of mydriatic solutions such as cocaine, phenylephrine, or hydroxyamphetamine. This method of drug delivery allows maximum mydriasis in attempts to break posterior

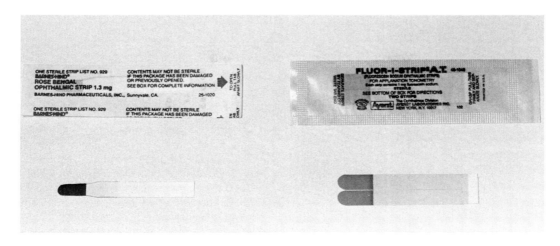

FIGURE 3.22   **Drug-impregnated filter paper strips. Rose bengal (left) and sodium fluorescein (right).**

synechiae or dilate sluggish pupils. Mydriasis of the inferior pupillary quadrant for intentional sector dilation of the pupil can also be achieved (see Chapter 21).

ARTIFICIAL TEAR INSERTS

In 1977 Katz and Blackman[89] first described a soluble ophthalmic drug delivery insert developed in the United States for treating dry eye syndromes (Lacrisert). The Lacrisert consists of a rod-shaped pellet of hydroxypropyl cellulose without preservative. In its dehydrated state, each dosage unit measures approximately 1 mm in diameter and 4 mm in length, and it contains 5 mg of the synthetic polymer. Lacrisert is supplied to patients in hermetically sealed blister packs. Each dosage unit is inserted into the inferior conjunctival fornix with a specially designed applicator (Fig. 3.24). Following placement into the conjunctival sac, its hypertonicity causes it to absorb basal tear production and fluid from the capillaries of the conjunctiva, and it consequently swells, becoming a gelatinous mass. During the following several hours the insert dissolves and releases the polymer into the tear film.

This device is useful for patients with moderate to severe dry eye syndromes for whom conventional therapies have failed or are inconvenient. Although the device may be reasonably well tolerated and generally does not migrate or become displaced, the most annoying side effect, associated with the intense release of polymer, is blurring of vision after 4 to 6 hours.[90,91] Many patients are able to minimize or eliminate the blurred vision by removing the insert after 3 to 4 hours and inserting a second device several hours later or by inserting the device at bedtime. Because transient blurring of vision is common, patients should be instructed to be cautious when operating hazardous machinery or driving a motor vehicle.[92]

Local discomfort is another significant problem. Most patients seem to experience at least some foreign body discomfort.[93] In patients with insufficient remaining basal tear secretion, the inserts do not imbibe fluid, dissolve, or release polymer to the eye. Thus, the absence of measurable tear secretion, as demonstrated by a very low Schirmer test value, may predict treatment failure with this device.[93,94]

The continuous delivery of a tearlike substance may be more similar to the natural physiologic condition than is the intermittent instillation of artificial tears and lubricants, and patients with chronic severe dry eye syndromes may more satisfactorily alleviate both objective corneal findings as well as subjective symptoms.[90] In most patients, the duration

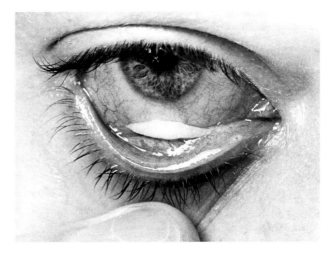

FIGURE 3.23   **Cotton pledget positioned in inferior conjunctival fornix.**

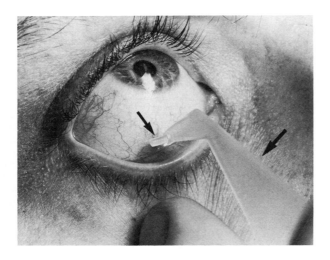

FIGURE 3.24   **Insertion of artificial tear insert (small arrow) into inferior conjunctival fornix with specially designed applicator (large arrow).**

of action of the insert is about 24 hours, and once-daily application is usually sufficient to relieve symptoms. Some patients, however, may require twice-daily application.

MEMBRANE-BOUND INSERTS

Thin, multilayered, drug-impregnated, copolymeric plastic devices placed into the conjunctival sac have been designed to release a specified amount of drug over an extended period. The only such device marketed in the United States became commercially available in 1974 (Ocusert, Alza). The device consists of a two-membrane sandwich of ethylene vinylacetate with a pilocarpine reservoir in the center. A white titanium dioxide ring incorporated between the copolymeric membranes aids in visualizing and handling the insert (Fig. 3.25). This elliptical device contains one of two commercially available quantities of pilocarpine. The pilocarpine is bound to alginic acid and is present as a free base, partly in an ionized (water-soluble) and partly in an unionized (lipid-soluble) form.[62] The device is sterile and contains no preservatives. The physical and drug release characteristics of the Ocusert are listed in Table 3.5.[4,95]

Membrane-controlled drug devices such as the Ocusert are characterized by zero-order drug delivery, in which the drug is released into the tear film at a constant rate over almost the entire lifetime of the device.[62,90] Drug release terminates when the reservoir is exhausted. The controlled rate of drug delivery is provided by interaction between the polymeric membrane molecules and the molecules of the drug contained in the reservoir. The driving force of the concentration gradient maintained by the saturated concentration of drug within the reservoir is a major factor in the rate of drug release. As long as this gradient exists, there is zero-order drug delivery through the membrane.[90] The concentration of drug outside the membrane is another factor in the rate of drug release. Released drug must be removed or the driving force (gradient) is diminished. The eye provides an excellent environment for such a drug delivery system because tear flow prevents the buildup of a stagnant layer of drug around the device. During the initial 6 to 8 hours following insertion of the device, the pulse release of pilocarpine from the device is higher as a result of the amount of drug previously equilibrated into the barrier membranes.[90] During this period the Ocusert releases 3 to 4 times the amount of pilocarpine it does at later times.[96] Following this initial period, the pilocarpine is released at a constant rate of 20 μg/hr (Ocusert Pilo-20) or 40 μg/hr (Ocusert Pilo-40) for approximately 7 days. Figure 3.26 illustrates the time course of pilocarpine release from the Ocusert Pilo-20 system.

Because of individual differences, direct comparisons between the Ocusert systems and various concentrations of pilocarpine drops cannot be made. However, a majority of glaucoma patients controlled with pilocarpine 0.5% and 1% drops can usually be controlled with the Ocusert Pilo-20.[96] Most patients who require 2% or 4% solutions of pilocarpine require the Ocusert Pilo-40.

The clinical advantages of the pilocarpine Ocusert over pilocarpine drops are numerous. One of the distinct advantages of the Ocusert is the substantially less total drug delivered to the eye for adequate control of IOP. Such reservoir membrane delivery systems are capable of only a very low drug release rate, but because these systems are characterized by zero-order drug delivery, the therapeutic effect can be achieved with much smaller amounts of drug. The Ocusert Pilo-20 releases 3.4 mg of drug over a 7-day period, whereas the Ocusert Pilo-40 contains twice the amount of pilocarpine and releases it at twice the rate. By comparison, administration of one drop (0.05 ml) of 2% pilocarpine solution four times daily delivers 28 mg of drug per eye over a 7-day period, four or eight times the amount released from an Ocusert over the same period.[97] Because the total dose of pilocarpine delivered by the Ocusert is considerably less than that delivered by pilocarpine drop instillation, the risk of ocular or systemic pilocarpine toxicity is reduced. In patients with open but narrow anterior chamber angles, pilocarpine can precipitate angle closure by inducing pupillary block and forward movement of the lens-iris diaphragm.[98] Although both the Pilo-20 and Pilo-40 Ocusert systems produce shallowing of the anterior chamber, the shallowing produced by the Ocusert (0.08 mm with Pilo-20) is less than that produced by 2% pilocarpine drops (0.265 mm).[98,99] Despite this advantage, however, retinal detachment has been reported with Ocusert use.[100,101]

In addition, visual disturbances associated with drug-induced miosis or myopia do not occur to the same extent with the Ocusert systems as they do with pilocarpine solu-

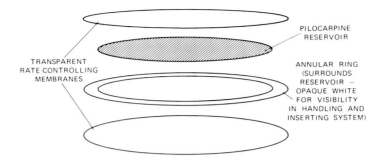

TRANSPARENT
RATE-CONTROLLING
MEMBRANES

PILOCARPINE
RESERVOIR

ANNULAR RING
(SURROUNDS
RESERVOIR —
OPAQUE WHITE
FOR VISIBILITY
IN HANDLING AND
INSERTING SYSTEM)

A

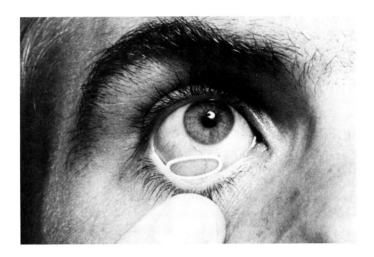

B

FIGURE 3.25   *(A)* **Schematic diagram of pilocarpine Ocusert.** *(B)*
Ocusert in situ.

tions (Fig. 3.27). In one study,[99] average pupil size after the instillation of 2% pilocarpine solution was 1.35 mm; after insertion of the Ocusert Pilo-20 it was 3.0 mm. The mean accommodative myopia was significant for the solution-treated group (3.10 D) but was negligible for the Ocusert-treated group (0.45 D). In the younger age group, the changes were more pronounced. There was a mean accommodative myopia of 5.84 D in the solution-treated group between the ages of 20 and 40 years, and the maximum accommodative myopia was 11.0 D. In the age group between 40 and 60, the maximum accommodative myopia was 5 D after instillation of one drop of 2% pilocarpine. After

age 60 years, however, accommodative myopia was usually insignificant, reaching a maximum of only 1.25 D in the Ocusert-treated group.

Since the device is inserted only once per week, drug application is convenient, and good patient compliance results. The Ocusert also enjoys a distinct advantage for patients such as the elderly who must rely on others for treatment.

Despite these advantages, this membrane-bound insert is rarely used in clinical practice. The major problems preventing satisfactory use of the Ocusert in practice are foreign body sensation, especially when it becomes folded, and

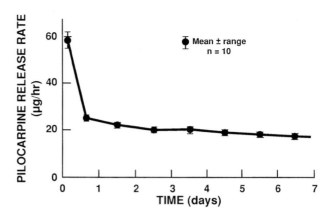

FIGURE 3.26   **Time course of pilocarpine release from the Ocusert Pilo-20 system. (Modified from Shell JW, Baker RW. Diffusional systems for controlled release of drugs to the eye. Ann Ophthalmol 1974;6:1037–1045.)**

difficulty with retention of the device.[95] When the Ocusert becomes folded, it must be replaced with a fresh one because it usually cannot be straightened to its original smooth shape. Retention problems may be solved in some cases by instructing patients to wear the device in the upper fornix, especially while sleeping. Other significant disadvantages associated with the device include the need for detailed instruction and encouragement of patients, and significantly higher cost compared with other antiglaucoma medications.

Continuous Flow Devices

When relatively small amounts of drug are required for delivery to the eye, the use of solutions, ointments, or inserts is usually satisfactory. However, when large volumes of fluids are required, such as in the treatment of acute chemical burns, other drug delivery systems are necessary. Various methods for delivering large volumes of fluids continuously to the eye have been developed.

TABLE 3.5
Characteristics of the Pilocarpine Ocusert

Characteristics	Pilo-20	Pilo-40
Long axis (mm)	13.4	13.0
Short axis (mm)	5.7	5.5
Thickness (mm)	0.3	0.5
Weight of device (mg)	19.0	29.0
Weight of drug (mg)	5.0	11.0
Pilocarpine release rate (μg/hr)	20	40
Therapeutic lifetime (days)	7	7
Total pilocarpine released (mg)	3.4	6.7

Modified from Novak S, Stewart RH. The Ocusert system in the management of glaucoma. Tex Med 1975;71(12):63–65, with permission of the authors and publisher.

CONVENTIONAL IRRIGATING SYSTEMS

Extraocular irrigation is often employed in the initial treatment of ocular foreign bodies or chemical burns in an effort to dislodge foreign material. It is also used to remove excessive drug from the eye after fluorescein or rose bengal staining or following gonioscopic or fundus contact lens procedures in which viscous lens-bonding solutions have been used. The conventional delivery system for irrigation fluids consists simply of the container of irrigating solution and a means—usually a tissue, towel, or emesis basin—with

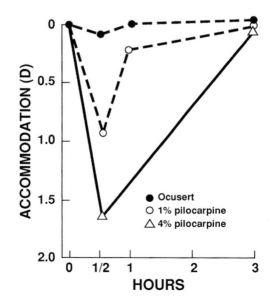

FIGURE 3.27   **Accommodative spasm resulting from one drop of 4% pilocarpine, one drop of 1% pilocarpine, or pilocarpine Ocusert. (Modified from Brown HS, Meltzer G, Merrill RC, et al. Visual effects of pilocarpine in glaucoma. Arch Ophthalmol 1976;94:1716–1719. Copyright 1976, American Medical Association.)**

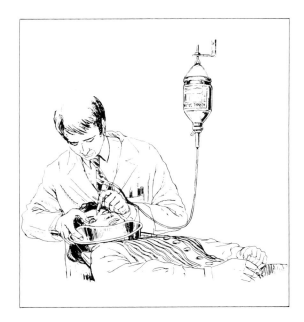

FIGURE 3.29 **Ocular irrigation unit consisting of a standard 1000 ml bottle of sterile normal saline, intravenous tubing with stopcock (needle removed), and a hanger. (From Flora MR. How to make a simple ocular irrigation unit. Rev Optom 1980;117:59, with permission of the author and publisher.)**

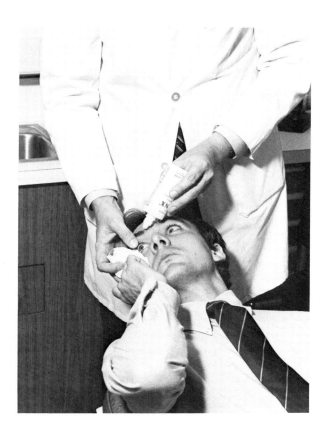

FIGURE 3.28 **Conventional irrigation system. The head is tilted toward the side to be irrigated, and the irrigation solution is collected in a tissue or towel after it has bathed the extraocular tissues.**

which to collect the fluid after bathing the eye. Patients should be in a supine position with head tilted toward the side to be irrigated (Fig. 3.28). The irrigating solution should be at room temperature to minimize patient discomfort during the procedure. With the upper and lower lids retracted, clinicians gently bathe the extraocular surfaces with the solution, taking care to collect the fluid in the tissue, towel, or emesis basin and to avoid staining patients' clothing. In most cases no topical anesthesia is required, except if patients, because of severe pain or ocular involvement, are unable to open the eye.

A simple, inexpensive, yet effective ocular irrigation unit can be assembled by using a standard 500 or 1000 ml bottle or bag of sterile normal saline commonly used for intravenous infusion, intravenous tubing with stopcock (needle removed), and a hanger made from a metal bracket and threaded ring (Fig. 3.29).[102,103] The bag and tubing can be hung from a wall or mobile stand. A mobile stand allows the unit to be moved to any treatment room. Such a unit permits

irrigation at rates varying from the standard intravenous drip to a maximum of 200 ml/min. Excess irrigating solution is collected in an emesis basin.

The obvious limitation of these conventional irrigating systems is the need to have an attendant administer the fluid, but the advantage is the ease and simplicity with which the solution can be administered. In addition, conventional irrigating systems represent the most cost-effective means of administering fluids continuously to the eye.

CONTINUOUS IRRIGATING SYSTEMS

To circumvent the need for an attendant to administer the irrigating fluid or drug, various methods have been developed that enable the continuous delivery of fluid on a long-term basis. Most methods that have been devised for continuous ocular irrigation are suitable for relatively short periods in nonambulatory patients. Polyethylene tubing is sometimes simply passed with a minor surgical procedure through the lid and into the conjunctival fornix, and the fluid or drug to be perfused is supplied from an overhead infusion bottle. The tubing is anchored to the skin with sutures at the zygoma and forehead and may also be secured by tape. An adaptor may be attached to the tubing and to the intravenous infusion apparatus, which allows the system to be disconnected for ambulation. Many patients tolerate this apparatus well, with no apparent discomfort. In cases in which it is undesirable to penetrate the lids surgically, various configurations of tubing, loops, rings, and haptic contact lens shells have been successfully employed.[104,105]

Periocular Administration

When higher concentrations of drugs, particularly corticosteroids and antibiotics, are required in the eye than can be delivered by topical, oral, or parenteral administration, local injections into the periocular tissues can be considered. Periocular drug delivery includes subconjunctival, sub-Tenon's, retrobulbar, and peribulbar administration.

Subconjunctival Injection

Although repeated topical applications of most ocular drugs results in intraocular drug levels comparable to those achieved with subconjunctival injections, subconjunctival injections offer an advantage in the administration of drugs, such as antibiotics, with poor intraocular penetration. Although the value of subconjunctival injections as a useful route of drug administration is still questionable in many clinical circumstances, this mode of drug delivery appears to offer the following advantages:[2]

- High local concentrations of drug can be obtained with the use of small quantities of medication, thereby avoiding adverse systemic effects.
- High tissue concentrations can be obtained with drugs that poorly penetrate the epithelial layer of the cornea or conjunctiva. This method is useful in patients who do not reliably use topical medication.
- Drugs can be injected at the conclusion of surgery to avoid the necessity of topical or systemic drug therapy.

Subconjunctival injection involves passing the needle between the anterior conjunctiva and Tenon's capsule (Fig. 3.30). This can be performed through the lid, as illustrated in Figure 3.30, or directly into the subconjunctival space. Although the injection can be placed in any quadrant, the superotemporal quadrant is preferred because this is the only quadrant between two rectus muscles that is not traversed by a portion of an oblique muscle or a tendon. In some cases, however, an injection site adjacent to the intraocular inflammation may be desirable. Tenon's capsule lies between the injected drug and the globe, so the amount of drug absorbed across the sclera is minimized. In fact, the mechanism of drug absorption following subconjunctival injection may relate to simple leakage of drug through the needle puncture site with subsequent absorption through the cornea.[106] McCartney and associates,[107] however, have shown that, at least for corticosteroids, a subconjunctivally administered drug does penetrate the underlying sclera, suggesting

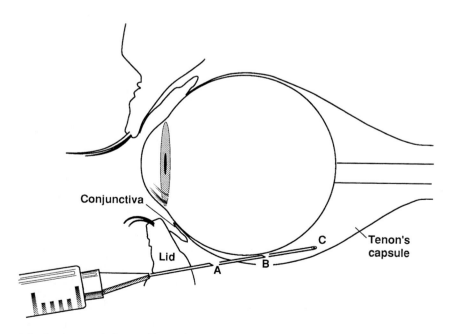

FIGURE 3.30   **Relative positions of periocular injections.** *(A)* **Subconjunctival.** *(B)* **Sub-Tenon's.** *(C)* **Retrobulbar.**

a rationale for placing the drug directly adjacent to the site of inflammation rather than injecting it randomly.

The specific technique of drug administration used by most practitioners is relatively simple.[108] After the eye is anesthetized with a drop of local anesthetic, such as proparacaine instilled five times at one-minute intervals, patients are instructed to look down while the upper eyelid is retracted. The conjunctiva is grasped with fine-toothed forceps between the superior and lateral rectus muscles and midway between the limbus and equator of the eye, and the drug is injected with a 25- or 27-gauge hypodermic needle. Following injection, the puncture site is firmly grasped with forceps for a few minutes to prevent leakage of drug after the needle has been withdrawn. An eye pad is applied for several hours. Although most patients often feel minor discomfort for 24 to 36 hours, they are usually able to continue with their daily activities.

Probably the greatest clinical benefit associated with the subconjunctival route of drug administration is in the treatment of severe corneal disease such as bacterial ulcers. Much higher concentrations of antibiotics can be achieved in the affected corneal tissues with subconjunctival injection than can be obtained by systemic drug administration.[109] Subconjunctival antibiotic administration is also useful as an initial supplement to the systemic or intravitreal antibiotic treatment of bacterial endophthalmitis.[110] A variety of ocular diseases are treated with subconjunctival corticosteroids. Subconjunctival injection of 5-fluorouracil, an antifibroblast agent, is commonly used following high-risk trabeculectomy surgeries for glaucoma.[111,112]

Anterior Sub-Tenon's Injection

Although the terms *subconjunctival* and *anterior sub-Tenon's* are often used interchangeably, they are technically different forms of drug administration. Either one of two techniques may be used:[113] one involves injection through the eyelid, and the other involves injection directly under Tenon's capsule.

Sub-Tenon's injection offers no significant advantages over subconjunctival drug administration. In fact, sub-Tenon's injection delivers lower quantities of drug to the eye and is associated with a greater risk of perforating the globe.[109] Despite these disadvantages, however, sub-Tenon's injections are occasionally used in the treatment of severe uveitis.

Posterior Sub-Tenon's Injection

As with the subconjunctival and anterior sub-Tenon's routes of administration, posterior sub-Tenon's injections can be administered through two routes, conjunctival or skin. To minimize the risk of perforating the globe, the tip of the needle may be moved from side to side as it is passed posteriorly following the curvature of the globe. Because neither the injected drug nor the tip of the needle is visible during the injection procedure, the precise location of the inoculation site is unknown. However, the posterior portion of Tenon's space is the desired target.

Posterior sub-Tenon's injection of corticosteroids is most often used in the treatment of chronic equatorial and midzone posterior uveitis, including inflammation of the macular region.[114] Cystoid macular edema following cataract extraction is also treated occasionally with sub-Tenon's repository steroids.[115] In the treatment of macular disease, however, there may be little difference in clinical effectiveness between a posterior sub-Tenon's injection and a retrobulbar injection because these tissue spaces freely intercommunicate.[116]

Retrobulbar Injection

Drugs have been administered by retrobulbar injection for over 75 years.[117,118] The procedure was originally developed to anesthetize the globe for cataract extraction and other intraocular surgeries, and this remains its principal clinical use. However, antibiotics, vasodilators, corticosteroids, and alcohol have also been administered through this route. Currently, retrobulbar anesthetics are used routinely, retrobulbar corticosteroids are used occasionally (although their clinical value remains controversial and unproved), and retrobulbar alcohol is rarely administered.

The specific technique usually involves injection through the skin of the lower lid with a 23- or 25-gauge needle inserted immediately above the inferotemporal orbital rim and directed toward the orbital apex[119,120] (see Fig. 3.30). Retrobulbar injections may also be administered inside the lower eyelid through the conjunctival fornix. In general, 35 mm (1⅜-inch) needles are usually adequate to deliver the drug within the muscle cone, although 50 mm (2-inch) needles can be used to produce a deeper anesthetic injection to ensure a more complete motor block. Blunted needles may reduce the likelihood of retrobulbar hemorrhage and penetration of the globe.[121,122]

Regardless of the drug to be injected, it is advisable to attempt aspiration of blood before injecting any significant amount of medication to ensure that the tip of the needle is not within a blood vessel. It has also been suggested that injecting small amounts of the drug as the needle is gently inserted may tend to push away tissues from the needle tip. Supplemental measures following injection include massage after anesthetic injections to increase diffusion of the drug. Following alcohol injection, ice compresses are often applied to reduce lid and conjunctival swelling.[123]

Retrobulbar injections have been used for a variety of ocular diseases. Dramatic relief of pain has often been

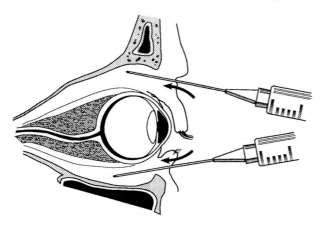

FIGURE 3.31   Peribulbar injection technique, in which the needle avoids the intraconal space. (Adapted from Fry RA, Henderson J. Local anaesthesia for eye surgery. The periocular technique. Anaesthesia 1989;45:14–17.)

achieved with retrobulbar injection of alcohol (95% ethanol). In most cases, this therapy has been reserved for patients with blind eyes, such as in absolute glaucoma, but it has also been used in patients who are partially sighted.[124,125] Duration of relief of pain may be for several months or as long as a year or more. Retrobulbar injection of 6.7% aqueous phenol has been reported to give pain relief lasting 4.5 to 48 months. Retrobulbar phenol may be preferable to alcohol because the former causes less pain during injection.[126] Although retrobulbar injections of alcohol or phenol may offer an alternative to enucleation of blind and painful eyes, they should not be used if the internal structures of the eye cannot be examined. The incidence of unsuspected melanomas in such eyes is alarmingly high, and misdiagnosis or mismanagement can result if retrobulbar alcohol or phenol therapy is used.[125]

Although the use of retrobulbar steroids is controversial, this therapeutic modality has been advocated and continues to be used in the treatment of Graves' ophthalmopathy and inflammatory diseases of the posterior segment, including the macula. In some instances retrobulbar steroid therapy has been successful when high doses of oral steroids have failed to produce a satisfactory clinical response. The singular advantage of retrobulbar steroid therapy is that higher local drug concentrations can be obtained with less systemic toxicity than is possible with high doses of systemic steroids.[127]

Peribulbar Injection

More than one million retrobulbar anesthetic injections are performed annually in the United States. Because of the

risks associated with this procedure, the peribulbar technique was introduced during the mid-1980s.[128,129] The procedure consists of placing one or more injections of local anesthetic around the globe but not directly into the muscle cone (Fig. 3.31).[120,128–132] Because the fascial connections of the extraocular muscles are incomplete, the anesthetic injected around the globe eventually infiltrates the muscle cone to provide anesthesia and akinesia.[120] Although both retrobulbar and peribulbar procedures do not allow visualization of the injection site, the retrobulbar technique intentionally aims for the muscle cone, which contains vital structures. This can be accomplished only by placing the needle extremely close to the globe. In contrast, the peribulbar procedure intentionally avoids the globe and the muscle cone, making it safer.[130]

When compared with the retrobulbar technique, peribulbar anesthesia provides similar anesthesia and akinesia,[132–135] but some patients may have inadequate akinesia and require additional injections.[132] In addition, the onset time of blockade is not as rapid as with retrobulbar injection.[134] Nevertheless, the overwhelming advantage of the peribulbar technique relates to deposition of the anesthetic outside the muscle cone. This reduces the potential for inadvertent globe penetration, retrobulbar hemorrhage, and direct optic nerve injury.[128,129,134,135]

Complications of Periocular Injection

Because of the disadvantages and complications associated with periocular drug administration, this form of drug delivery should generally be reserved for ocular disorders that fail to respond adequately to topical drug therapy. A major disadvantage of subconjunctival injections is the very low tissue drug concentrations during the intervals between injections.[109] In addition, local effects include massive subconjunctival hemorrhage, markedly irritated eyes, dellen formation, chemosis, pain, and retained subconjunctival drug deposits.[2] Periocular drug administration involves injection directly into the ocular tissues, and patient apprehension is a significant limiting factor.

Although serious complications with retrobulbar and peribulbar injections are uncommon, numerous complications have been reported[128,136–138] (Table 3.6). Some unique problems have been associated with the periocular administration of corticosteroids. Glaucoma has resulted from the periocular injection of such drugs. Surgical excision is the only means of removing the steroid once it is deposited.[116,139] Diplopia and limited elevation of the involved eye have followed the periocular injection of steroids into the region of the superior fornix.[140] Cataract has also been reported as a complication of periocular steroids.[141] In one study a patient developed numerous complications following a series of 20 retrobulbar injections of steroid administered weekly for the treatment of presumptive toxoplasmic retinitis.[141] These

TABLE 3.6
Complications of Retrobulbar or Peribulbar Injections

- Retrobulbar hemorrhage
- Conjunctival and eyelid ecchymosis
- Proptosis
- Exposure keratopathy
- Elevated intraocular pressure
- Contralateral amaurosis
- Respiratory arrest
- Bradycardia
- Central retinal artery/vein occlusion
- Optic atrophy
- Transient reduction in visual acuity
- Extraocular muscle palsies
- Ptosis
- Pupillary abnormalities
- Chemosis
- Eyelid swelling
- Pain
- Cardiovascular or central nervous system drug toxicity
- Accidental perforation of the globe

complications included pseudoptosis, proptosis, Cushing's syndrome, systemic hypertension, increased susceptibility to bruises, and weight loss. Intralesional periocular injection of steroids has resulted in both retinal and choroidal vascular occlusion.[142,143]

One of the most significant and serious complications associated with periocular injections is accidental perforation of the globe.[121,128,144,145] Steroid preparations have been accidentally injected into the choroidal vasculature, retina, and the intraocular compartment.[144] The globe can be perforated so easily, and without noticeable resistance, that practitioners may not realize that the globe has been penetrated.[146] In some cases perforation may go undetected for several weeks. The immediate effects associated with perforation of the globe during periocular steroid administration may include pain, reduced vision, ocular hypertension, ocular hypotony, an obvious white mass in the vitreous cavity, visible subretinal material, and intraocular hemorrhage. Delayed effects have included pseudohypopyon in aphakia from prolapse of drug from the vitreous cavity, vitreoretinal traction bands, preretinal membrane formation, retinal detachment, toxic pigmentary atrophy, and optic atrophy.[128,144] The injected intraocular steroid material may require 6 to 8 weeks to disappear, which is followed by either complete recovery of vision or permanent vision loss of varying degrees.[128,144,145] Emergency vitrectomy may also be required.[144]

The use of periocular injections less than 4 to 6 weeks following cataract extraction is contraindicated.[113] The tendency for patients receiving periocular injections to squint or squeeze the lids during the procedure mandates that the

procedure be delayed until the surgical wound has adequately healed.

Intracameral Administration

Intracameral administration involves injecting a drug directly into the anterior chamber of the eye. The most common clinical application is the injection of viscoelastic substances into the anterior chamber during cataract extraction and glaucoma filtering surgeries to protect against corneal endothelial cell loss and flat anterior chamber.[147] Ethacrynic acid[148] and tPA[149] have also been administered intracamerally.

When antibiotics are used, however, this procedure is associated with a significant risk of drug toxicity but has the advantage of rapidly achieving high intraocular concentrations of drug. Intracameral antibiotic administration may be particularly valuable in the treatment of nonsterile conditions requiring surgery such as closure of a ruptured operative wound or repair of a laceration. Only very minute quantities of antibiotics are tolerated in the anterior chamber. Irrigation of the anterior chamber with excessive amounts of antibiotics often causes destruction of the corneal endothelium, dense corneal opacification, anterior uveitis with neovascularization, or cataract.

Intravitreal Administration

Many drugs have been injected directly into the vitreous. These include antibacterial and antifungal agents for treatment of bacterial and fungal endophthalmitis, respectively, and antivirals for treatment of viral retinitis. The treatment of many intraocular diseases using systemically administered drugs is hampered because of poor drug penetration into the eye. The tight junctional complexes of the retinal pigment epithelium and retinal capillaries serve as the blood-ocular barrier, which inhibits penetration of antibiotics into the vitreous.[150] Reports[110] have demonstrated that patients with endophthalmitis can be successfully treated using intravitreal and subconjunctival rather than systemically administered antibiotics. Although systemic antibiotics are often used to treat bacterial endophthalmitis, the systemic route of administration has limited efficacy as well as potential side effects that limit therapeutic success. Thus, the role of systemic antibiotics in the treatment of endophthalmitis is uncertain.[151]

Intravitreal antineoplastic agents have also been evaluated for the prevention of cellular proliferation in the vitreous cavity following retinal reattachment surgery, which can lead to proliferative vitreoretinopathy.[150] Many of these patients undergo vitrectomy, and drug penetration throughout

TABLE 3.7
Maximum Nontoxic Intravitreal Doses of Antibacterial, Antifungal, and Antiviral Agents

Agent	Maximum Nontoxic Dose (μg/ml)
Single	
Chloramphenicol	10
Clindamycin	9
Amikacin	10
Tobramycin	10
Gentamicin	8
Methicillin	20
Lincomycin	10
Oxacillin	10
Penicillin	80
Amphotericin B methyl ester	75[a]
Ganciclovir	4000[b]
Foscarnet	10000[b]
Combination	
1. Gentamicin	8
Oxacillin	10
2. Clindamycin	9
Gentamicin	8
3. Methicillin	20
Gentamicin	8
4. Penicillin	80
Gentamicin	8

[a]Recommended dose is 10 μg/ml.
[b]Intact vitreous.
Adapted from Peyman GA, Schulman JA. Intravitreal drug therapy. Jpn J Ophthalmol 1989;33:392–404.

the intraocular cavity can be enhanced. Intravitreally injected drugs may have the potential for increased retinal toxicity. Peyman and Schulman[150] have delineated drug concentrations that would be nontoxic when administered intravitreally in vitrectomized eyes (Table 3.7).

Antiviral agents are sometimes injected intravitreally for treatment of cytomegalovirus (CMV) retinitis in patients with acquired immunodeficiency syndrome (AIDS).[152–154] Intravitreal ganciclovir may be an effective alternative to systemic ganciclovir in patients with severe neutropenia as well as in patients who desire to remain on systemic zidovudine.[153] High doses of intravitreal ganciclovir can effectively suppress CMV retinitis and preserve vision without adverse systemic effects.[154] An intraocular sustained-release ganciclovir implant has recently been shown to be effective for treatment of newly diagnosed CMV retinitis in patients with AIDS. The device delivers ganciclovir at a rate of 1 μg/h.[155]

Silicone oil has also been injected intravitreally for treatment of complicated retinal detachments.[156–158]

Iontophoresis

In the early part of this century iontophoresis was commonly used in the treatment of ocular infections, but this procedure is almost never used today.[109,159] The technique involved applying a cup containing a solution of antibiotic to the eye. An electrode was attached to the bottom of the cup, and another electrode was usually held by patients to complete the circuit. Electric current was passed through this circuit in a direction appropriate to the net charge of the active portion of the antibiotic molecule. This technique was used to enhance the corneal penetration of water-soluble antibiotics. The crystalline lens-iris barrier can be bypassed by applying the current through the pars plana to produce high vitreal drug concentrations.[76] Using a rabbit model, Sarraf and associates[160] have shown that such transscleral iontophoresis of foscarnet may prove to be an effective and safe technique for antiviral treatment of CMV retinitis in patients with AIDS.

References

1. Urtti A, Salminen L. Minimizing systemic absorption of topically administered ophthalmic drugs. Surv Ophthalmol 1993;37:435–456.

2. Fraunfelder FT, Hanna C. Ophthalmic drug delivery systems. Surv Ophthalmol 1974;18(4):292–298.

3. Templeton WC, Eiferman RA, Snyder JW, et al. *Serratia* keratitis by contaminated eyedroppers. Am J Ophthalmol 1982;93:723–726.

4. Halberg GP, Kelly SE, Morrone M. Drug delivery systems for topical ophthalmic medication. Ann Ophthalmol 1975;7(9):1199–1209.

5. Nelson JD. Hazards of unit dose artificial tears. Arch Ophthalmol 1991;109:173–174.

6. MacKeen DL. Aqueous formulations and ointments. Int Ophthalmol Clin 1980;20(3):79–92.

7. Brown RH, Hotchkiss ML, Davis BB. Creating smaller eyedrops by reducing eyedropper tip dimension. Am J Ophthalmol 1985;99:460–464.

8. Brown RH, Lynch MG. Design of eyedropper tips for topical beta-blocking agents. Am J Ophthalmol 1986;102:123–124.

9. Shell JW. Pharmacokinetics of topically applied ophthalmic drugs. Surv Ophthalmol 1982;26:207–218.

10. Lederer CM, Harold RE. Drop size of commercial glaucoma medications. Am J Ophthalmol 1986;101:691–694.

11. Fraunfelder FT. Drug-packaging standards for eye drop medications. Arch Ophthalmol 1988;106:1029.

12. Frenkel REP, Hong YJ, Shin DH. Misuse of eyedrops due to interchanged caps. Arch Ophthalmol 1988;106:17.

13. Lyons C, Stevens J, Bloom J. Superglue inadvertently used as eyedrops. BMJ 1990;300:328.

14. Mansour AM. Tolerance to topical preparations: Cold or warm? Ann Ophthalmol 1991;23:21–22.

15. Schein OD, Hibbert PL, Starck T, et al. Microbial contamination of in-use ocular medications. Arch Ophthalmol 1992;110:82–85.

16. Zimmerman TJ, Kooner KS, Kandarakis AS, et al. Improving the therapeutic index of topically applied ocular drugs. Arch Ophthalmol 1984;102(4):551–552.

17. White WL, Glover AT, Buckner AB. Effect of blinking on tear elimination as evaluated by dacryoscintigraphy. Ophthalmology 1991;98:367–369.

18. Whitson JT, Love R, Brown RH, et al. The effect of reduced eyedrop size and eyelid closure on the therapeutic index of phenylephrine. Am J Ophthalmol 1993;115:357–359.

19. Zimmerman TJ, Sharir M, Nardin GF, Fuqua M. Therapeutic index of pilocarpine, carbachol, and timolol with nasolacrimal occlusion. Am J Ophthalmol 1992;114:1–7.

20. Zimmerman TJ, Sharir M, Nardin GF, Fuqua M. Therapeutic index of epinephrine and dipivefrin with nasolacrimal occlusion. Am J Ophthalmol 1992;114:8–13.

21. Fraunfelder FT. Extraocular fluid dynamics: How best to apply topical ocular medications. Trans Am Ophthalmol Soc 1976;74:457–487.

22. Gray LG. Avoiding adverse effects of cycloplegics in infants and children. J Am Optom Assoc 1979;50(4):465–470.

23. Wesson MD, Bartlett JD, Swiatocha J, Woolley T. Mydriatic efficacy of a cycloplegic spray in the pediatric population. J Am Optom Assoc 1993;64:637–640.

24. Bartlett JD, Wesson MD, Swiatocha J, Woolley T. Efficacy of a pediatric cycloplegic administered as a spray. J Am Optom Assoc 1993;64:617–621.

25. Burns E, Mulley GP. Practical problems with eye-drops among elderly ophthalmology outpatients. Age and Aging 1992;21:168–170.

26. Donnelly D. Instilling eyedrops: Difficulties experienced by patients following cataract surgery. J Adv Nursing 1987;12:235–243.

27. Tennant JS. Instillation of eye drops (letter). Am J Ophthalmol 1979;87(1):104–105.

28. Sheldon GM. Self-administration of eyedrops. Ophthalmic Surg 1987;18:393–394.

29. Bartlett JD, Ghormley NR, Jaanus SD, et al. Ophthalmic drug facts. St. Louis: Facts and Comparisons, 1995.

30. Loeffler M, Hornblass A. Hazards of unit dose artificial tear preparations. Arch Ophthalmol 1990;108:639–640.

31. Nelson JD. Corneal abrasions resulting from a unit dose artificial tear dispenser. Am J Ophthalmol 1987;103:333–334.

32. Loewenstein A, Bolocinic S, Goldstein M, Lazar M. Application of eye drops to the medial canthus. Graefe's Arch Clin Exp Ophthalmol 1994;232:680–682.

33. Scruggs J, Wallace T, Hanna C. Route of absorption of drug and ointment after application to the eye. Ann Ophthalmol 1978;10(3):267–271.

34. Wallace T, Hanna C, Boozman F, et al. New application of ophthalmic ointments (letter). JAMA 1975;233(5):418.

35. Robin JS, Ellis PP. Ophthalmic ointments. Surv Ophthalmol 1978;22(5):335–340.

36. Putterman AM. Instilling ocular ointments without blurred vision. Arch Ophthalmol 1985;103:1276.

37. Hanna C, Fraunfelder FT, Cable M, et al. The effect of ophthalmic ointments on corneal wound healing. Am J Ophthalmol 1973;76(2):193–200.

38. Heerema JC, Friedenwald JS. Retardation of wound healing in the corneal epithelium by lanolin. Am J Ophthalmol 1950;33(9):1421–1427.

39. Fraunfelder FT, Hanna C, Woods AH. Pseudoentrapment of ointment in the cornea. Arch Ophthalmol 1975;93(5):331–334.

40. Fraunfelder FT, Hanna C, Cable M, et al. Entrapment of ophthalmic ointment in the cornea. Am J Ophthalmol 1973;76(4):475–484.

41. Norn MS. Role of the vehicle in local treatment of the eye. Acta Ophthalmol 1964;42(4):727–734.

42. Heath WE. Death from atropine poisoning. BMJ 1950;2:608.

43. Hughes CA. Poisoning from use of atropine ointment. Trans Ophthalmol Soc UK 1938;58:444–446.

44. Fraunfelder FT, Hanna C. Ophthalmic ointment. Trans Am Acad Ophthalmol Otolaryngol 1973;77:467–475.

45. Avisar R, Savir H, Deutsch D, Teller J. Effect of I-Scrub on signs and symptoms of chronic blepharitis. DICP Ann Pharmacother 1991;25:359–360.

46. Polack FM, Goodman DF. Experience with a new detergent lid scrub in the management of chronic blepharitis. Arch Ophthalmol 1988;106:719–720.

47. Leibowitz HM, Capino D. Treatment of chronic blepharitis. Arch Ophthalmol 1988;106:720.

48. Johnson DH, Kenyon KR, Epstein DL, et al. Corneal changes during pilocarpine gel therapy. Am J Ophthalmol 1986; 101(1):13–15.

49. Johnson DH, Epstein DL, Allen RC, et al. A one-year multicenter clinical trial of pilocarpine gel. Am J Ophthalmol 1984;97(6): 723–729.

50. Mandell AI, Bruce LA, Chalifa MA. Reduced cyclic myopia with pilocarpine gel. Ann Ophthalmol 1988;20:133–135.

51. Maas S, Ros FE, DeHeer LJ, et al. Efficacy and safety of the combination therapy pilogel/β-blocker: Interim results. Doc Ophthalmol 1989;72:391–398.

52. Maas S, Ros FE, DeHeer LJ, et al. Long-term treatment with Pilogel/β-blocker in glaucoma patients. Int Ophthalmol 1991;15:281–284.

53. Yakovlev AA, Lenkevich MM. Use of pilocarpine- impregnated alcohol films in the treatment of glaucomatous patients. Vestn Oftalmal 1966;79(6):40–42.

54. Sedlacek J. Possibility of the application of ophthalmic drugs with the use of gel contact lenses. Cesk Oftalmal 1965;21:509–512.

55. Waltman SR, Kaufman HE. Use of hydrophilic contact lenses to increase ocular penetration of topical drugs. Invest Ophthalmol Vis Sci 1970;9(4):250–255.

56. Scullica L, Squeri CA, Ferreri G. "Minor" applications of soft contact lenses. Trans Ophthalmol Soc UK 1977;97(1):159–161.

57. Ruben M, Watkins R. Pilocarpine dispensation for the soft hydrophilic contact lens. Br J Ophthalmol 1975;59(8):455–458.

58. Aquavella JV. New aspects of contact lenses in ophthalmology. Adv Ophthalmol 1976;32:2–34.

59. Hillman JS. Management of acute glaucoma with pilocarpine-soaked hydrophilic lens. Br J Ophthalmol 1974;58(7):674–679.

60. Podos SM, Becker B, Asseff C, et al. Pilocarpine therapy with soft contact lenses. Am J Ophthalmol 1972;73(3):336–341.

61. Maddox YT, Bernstein HN. An evaluation of the Bionite hydrophilic contact lens for use in a drug delivery system. Ann Ophthalmol 1972;4(9):789–802.

62. Lamberts DW. Solid delivery devices. Int Ophthalmol Clin 1980;20(3):63–77.

63. Hillman JS, Marsters JB, Broad A. Pilocarpine delivery by hydrophilic lens in the management of acute glaucoma. Trans Ophthalmol Soc UK 1975;68(1):79–84.

64. Krejci L, Brettschneider I, Praus R. Hydrophilic gel contact lenses as a new drug delivery system in ophthalmology and as a therapeutic bandage lenses. Acta Univ Carol [Med] (Praha) 1975; 21(5/6):387–396.

65. Praus R, Krejci L. Elution and intraocular penetration of the ophthalmic drugs of different molecular weights from the hydrophilic contact lenses through the intact and injured cornea. Acta Univ Carol [Med] (Praha) 1977;23:3–10.

66. Matoba AY, McCulley JP. The effect of therapeutic soft contact lenses on antibiotic delivery to the cornea. Ophthalmology 1985;92:97–99.

67. Shaw EL, Gasset AR. Management of an unusual case of keratitis mucosa with hydrophilic contact lenses and acetylcysteine. Ann Ophthalmol 1974;6(10):1054–1056.

68. Lemp MA. Bandage lenses and the use of topical solution containing preservatives. Ann Ophthalmol 1978;10(10):1319–1321.

69. Wilson M, Leigh E. Therapeutic use of soft contact lenses. Proc R Soc Med 1975;68(1):55–56.

70. Jain MR. Drug delivery through soft contact lenses. Br J Ophthalmol 1988;72:150–154.

71. Kaufman HE, Uotila MH, Gasset AR, et al. The medical uses of soft contact lenses. Trans Am Acad Ophthalmol Otolaryngol 1971;75:361–373.

72. Iwasaki W, Kosaka Y, Momose T, et al. Absorption of topical disodium cromoglycate and its preservatives by soft contact lens. CLAO J 1988;14:155–158.

73. Sulewski ME, Kracher GP, Gottsch JD, Stark WJ. Use of the disposable contact lens as a bandage contact lens. Arch Ophthalmol 1991;109:318.

74. Mondino BJ. Collagen shields. Am J Ophthalmol 1991;112:587–590.

75. Silbiger J, Stern GA. Evaluation of corneal collagen shields as a drug delivery device for the treatment of experimental Pseudomonas keratitis. Ophthalmology 1992;99:889–892.

76. Friedberg ML, Pleyer U, Mondino J. Device drug delivery to the eye. Collagen shields, iontophoresis and pumps. Ophthalmology 1991;98:725–732.

77. Finkelstein I, Trope GE, Heathcote JG, et al. Further evaluation of collagen shields as a delivery system for 5-fluorouracil: Histopathological observations. Can J Ophthalmol 1991;26:129–132.

78. Reidy JJ, Limberg M, Kaufman HE. Delivery of fluorescein to the anterior chamber using the corneal collagen shield. Ophthalmology 1990;97:1201–1203.

79. Weissman BA, Brennan NA, Lee DA, Fatt I. Oxygen permeability of collagen shields. Invest Ophthalmol Vis Sci 1990;31:334–338.

80. Phinney RB, Schwartz SD, Lee DA, Mondino BJ. Collagen-shield delivery of gentamicin and vancomycin. Arch Ophthalmol 1988;106:1599–1604.

81. Brockman EB, Tarantino PA, Hobden JA, et al. Keratotomy model of Pseudomonas keratitis: Gentamicin chemotherapy. Refract Corneal Surg 1992;8:39–43.

82. Murray TG, Jaffe GJ, McKay BS, et al. Collagen shield delivery of tissue plasminogen activator. Functional and pharmacokinetic studies of anterior segment delivery. Refract Corneal Surg 1992;8:44–48.

83. Schwartz SD, Harrison SA, Engstrom RE, et. al. Collagen shield delivery of amphotericin B. Am J Ophthalmol 1990;109:701–704.

84. Wentworth JS, Paterson CA, Wells JT, et. al. Collagen shields exacerbate ulceration of alkali-burn rabbit corneas. Arch Ophthalmol 1993;111:389–392.

85. Hobden JA, Reidy JJ, O'Callaghan RJ, et al. Treatment of experimental Pseudomonas keratitis using collagen shields containing tobramycin. Arch Ophthalmol 1988;106:1605–1607.

86. Colin J, Malet F, Chastel C, Richard MC. Use of collagen shields in the treatment of herpetic keratitis. Curr Eye Res 1991;10:189–191.

87. Pflugfelder SC, Murchison JF. Corneal toxicity with an antibiotic/steroid soaked collagen shield. Arch Ophthalmol 1992;110:20.

88. Keats RH, Shriver PA, Martines E. Complications of collagen corneal shields. CLAO J 1992;18:14–15.

89. Katz IM, Blackman WM. A soluble sustained-release ophthalmic delivery unit. Am J Ophthalmol 1977;83:728–734.

90. Zimmerman TJ, Leader B, Kaufman HE. Advances in ocular pharmacology. Ann Rev Pharmacol Toxicol 1980;20:415–428.

91. LaMotte J, Grossman E, Hersch J. The efficacy of cellulosic-ophthalmic inserts for treatment of dry eye. J Am Optom Assoc 1985;56(4):298–302.

92. Lacrisert Product Information, Merck and Co. Inc., West Point, Pennsylvania, 1981.

93. Lindahl G, Calissendorff B, Carle B. Clinical trial of sustained-release artificial tears in keratoconjunctivitis sicca and Sjögren's syndrome. Acta Ophthalmol 1988;66:9–14.

94. Prause JU. Treatment of keratoconjunctivitis sicca with Lacrisert. Scand J Rheumatol 1986;61:261–263.

95. Novak S, Stewart RH. The Ocusert system in the management of glaucoma. Tex Med 1975;71(12):63–65.

96. Quigley HA, Pollack IP, Harbin TS. Pilocarpine Ocuserts. Long-term clinical trials and selected pharmacodynamics. Arch Ophthalmol 1975;93(9):771–775.

97. Hitchings, RA, Smith RJH. Experience with pilocarpine Ocuserts. Trans Ophthalmol Soc UK 1977;97(1):202–205.

98. Drance SM, Mitchell DWA, Schulzer M. The effects of Ocusert pilocarpine on anterior chamber depth, visual acuity, and intraocular pressure in man. Can J Ophthalmol 1977;12(1):24–28.

99. Francois J, Goes F, Zagorski Z. Comparative ultrasonographic study of the effect of pilocarpine 2% and Ocusert P 20 on the eye components. Am J Ophthalmol 1978;86(2):233–238.

100. Puustjarvi T. Retinal detachment during glaucoma therapy. Review. A case report of an occurence of retinal detachment after using membranous pilocarpine delivery system. Ophthalmologica 1985;190:40–44.

101. Wesley P, Liebmann, J, Ritch R. Rhegmatogenous retinal detachment after initiation of Ocusert therapy. Am J Ophthalmol 1991;112:458–59.

102. Flora MR. How to make a simple ocular irrigation unit. Rev Optom 1980;117(1):59.

103. Herr RD, White GL, Bbrnhisel K, et al. Clinical comparison of ocular irrigation fluids following chemical injury. Am J Emerg Med 1991;9:228–231.

104. Doane MG. Methods of ophthalmic fluid delivery. Int Ophthalmol Clin 1980;20(3):93–101.

105. Yamabayashi S, Furuya T, Gohd T, et al. Newly designed continuous corneal irrigation system for chemical burns. Ophthalmologica 1990;201:174–179.

106. Wine NA, Gornall AG, Basu PK. The ocular uptake of subconjunctivally injected C^{14} hydrocortisone. I. Time and major route of penetration in a normal eye. Am J Ophthalmol 1964;58(3):362–366.

107. McCartney HJ, Drysdale IO, Gornall AG, et al. An autoradiographic study of the penetration of subconjunctivally injected hydrocortisone into the normal and inflamed rabbit eye. Invest Ophthalmol 1965;4(3):297–302.

108. Garber MI. Methylprednisolone in the treatment of exophthalmos. Lancet 1966;1(7444):958–960.

109. Baum JL, Barza M, Weinstein L. Preferred routes of antibiotic administration in treatment of bacterial ulcers of the cornea. Int Ophthalmol Clin 1973;13(4):31–37.

110. Pavan PR, Brinser JH. Exogenous bacterial endophthalmitis treated without systemic antibiotics. Am J Ophthalmol 1987;104:121–126.

111. Ophir A, Ticho U. A randomized study of trabeculectomy and subconjunctival administration of fluorouracil in primary glaucomas. Arch Ophthalmol 1992;110:1072–1075.

112. Zalish M, Leiba H, Oliver M. Subconjunctival injection of 5-fluorouracil following trabeculectomy for congenital and infantile glaucoma. Ophthalmic Surg 1992;23:203–205.

113. Giles CL. Bulbar perforation during periocular injection of corticosteroids. Am J Ophthalmol 1974;77(4):438–441.

114. Leon CR, Lloyd WC. Treatment protocol for orbital inflammatory disease. Ophthalmology 1985;92:1325.

115. Suckling RD, Maslin KF. Pseudophakic cystoid macular oedema and its treatment with local steroids. Aust NZ J Ophthalmol 1988;16:353–359.

116. Havener WH. Ocular pharmacology. St. Louis: C.V. Mosby Co, 1983;5:18–43.

117. Ellis PP. Retrobulbar injections. Surv Ophthalmol 1974;18(6):425–430.

118. Feibel RM. Current concepts in retrobulbar anesthesia. Surv Ophthalmol 1985;30(2):102–110.

119. Davison JA. Features of a modern retrobulbar anesthetic injection for cataract surgery. J Cataract Refract Surg 1993;19:284–289.

120. Simonson D. Retrobulbar block: A review for the clinician. JAANA 1990;58:456–461.

121. Grizzard WS, Kirk NM, Pavan PR, et al. Perforating ocular injuries caused by anesthesia personnel. Ophthalmology 1991;98:1011–1016.

122. Waller SG, Taboada J, O'Connor P. Retrobulbar anesthesia risk. Do sharp needles really perforate the eye more easily than blunt needles? Ophthalmology 1993;100:506–510.

123. May DR, May WN. Decreasing discomfort caused by retrobulbar alcohol injection. Am J Ophthalmol 1981;95(2):262–263.

124. Maza CE. A safer technique for retrobulbar alcohol injections. Ophthalmic Surg 1989;20:823.

125. Al-Faran MF, Al-Omar OM. Retrobulbar alcohol injection in blind painful eyes. Ann Ophthalmol 1990;22:460–462.

126. Birch M, Strong N, Brittain P, et. al. Retrobulbar phenol injection in blind painful eyes. Ann Ophthalmol 1993;25:267–270.

127. Freeman WR, Green RL, Smith RE. Echographic localization of cortiosteroids after periocular injection. Am J Ophthalmol 1987;104(3):281–288.

128. Duker JS, Belmont JB, Benson WE, et. al. Inadvertent globe perforation during retrobulbar and peribulbar anesthesia. Patient characteristics, surgical management, and visual outcome. Ophthalmology 1991;98:519–526.

129. Davis DB, Mandel MR. Posterior peribulbar anesthesia: An alternative to retrobulbar anesthesia. J Cataract Refract Surg 1986;12:182–184.

130. Pannu JS. Retrobulbar vs. peribulbar. Ophthalmic Surg 1988;19:828.

131. Ahmad S, Ahmad A, Benzon HT. Clinical experience wth the peribulbar block for ophthalmologic surgery. Regional Anesth 1993;18:184–188.

132. Apel A, Woodward R. Single-injection peribulbar local anaesthesia—a study of fifty consecutive cases. Aust NZ J Ophthalmol 1991;19:149–153.

133. Ropo A, Nikki P, Ruusuvaara P, et. al. Comparison of retrobulbar and periocular injections of lignocaine by computerized tomography. Br J Ophthalmol 1991;75:417–420.

134. Fry RA, Henderson J. Local anaesthesia for eye surgery. The periocular technique. Anaesthesia 1989;45:14–17.

135. Whitsett JC, Balyeat HD, McClure B. Comparison of one-injection-site peribulbar anesthesia and retrobulbar anesthesia. J Cataract Refract Surg 1990;16:243–245.

136. Nicoll JMV, Acharya PA, Ahlen K, et al. Central nervous system complications after 6,000 retrobulbar blocks. Anesth Analg 1987;66:1298–1302.

137. Cohen SM, Sousa FJ, Kelly NE, et. al. Respiratory arrest and new retinal hemorrhages after retrobulbar anesthesia. Am J Ophthalmol 1992;113:209–211.

138. Edge KR, Nicoll JMV. Retrobulbar hemorrhage after 12,500 retrobulbar blocks. Anesth Analg 1993;76:1019–1022.

139. Mills DW, Siebert LF, Climehaga DB. Depot triamcinolone-induced glaucoma. Can J Ophthalmol 1986;21(4):150–152.

140. Raab EL. Limitation of motility after periocular corticosteroid injection. Am J Ophthalmol 1974;78(6):996–998.

141. Nozik RA. Periocular injection of steroids. Trans Am Acad Ophthalmol Otolaryngol 1972;76(3):695–705.

142. Shorr N, Seiff S. Central retinal artery occlusion associated with periocular corticosteroid injection for juvenile hemangioma. Ophthalmic Surg 1986;17(4):229–231.

143. Thomas EL, Laborde RP. Retinal and choroidal vascular occlusion following intralesional corticosteroid injection of a chalazion. Ophthalmology 1986;93(3):405–407.

144. Wilson DR, Kimble JA, Witherspoon CD, Morris R. Retinal toxicity from accidental intraocular injection of a depot corticosteroid: A case report. Ann Ophthalmol–Glaucoma 1994;26:126–130.

145. Hay A, Flynn HW, Hoffman JI, et. al. Needle penetration of the globe during retrobulbar and peribulbar injections. Ophthalmology 1991;98:1017–1024.

146. Schlaegel TF, Wilson FM. Accidental intraocular injection of depot corticosteroids. Trans Am Acad Ophthalmol Otolaryngol 1974;78(6):847–855.

147. Barak A, Alhalel A, Kotas R, et al. The protective effect of early intraoperative injection of viscoelastic material in trabeculectomy. Ophthalmic Surg 1992;23:206–209.

148. Melamed S, Kotas-Neumann R, Barak A, et al. The effect of intracamerally injected ethacrynic acid on intraocular pressure in patients with glaucoma. Am J Ophthalmol 1992;113:508–512.

149. Snyder RW, Sherman MD, Allinson RW. Intracameral tissue plasminogen activator for treatment of excessive fibrin response after penetrating keratoplasty. Am J Ophthalmol 1990;109:483–484.

150. Peyman GA, Schulman JA. Intravitreal drug therapy. Jpn J Ophthalmol 1989;33:392–404.

151. Doft BH. The endophthalmitis vitrectomy study. Arch Ophthalmol 1991;109:487–489.

152. Diaz-Llopis M, Chipont E, Sanchez S, et. al. Intravitreal foscarnet for cytomegalovirus retinitis in a patient with acquired immunodeficiency syndrome. Am J Ophthalmol 1992;114:742–747.

153. Cantrill HL, Henry K, Melroe NH, et. al. Treatment of cytomegalovirus retinitis with intravitreal ganciclovir. Long-term results. Ophthalmology 1989;96:367–374.

154. Young SH, Morlet N, Heery S, et. al. High-dose intravitreal ganciclovir in the treatment of cytomegalovirus. Med J Aust 1992;157:370–373.

155. Martin DF, Parks DJ, Mellow SD, et al. Treatment of cytomegalovirus retinitis with an intraocular sustained-release ganciclovir implant. A randomized controlled clinical trial. Arch Ophthalmol 1994;112:1531–1539.

156. Nguyen QH, Lloyd MA, Heuer DK, et. al. Incidence and management of glaucoma after intravitreal silicone oil injection for complicated retinal detachments. Ophthalmology 1992;99:1520–1526.

157. Chan C, Okun E. The question of ocular tolerance to intravitreal liquid silicone. A long-term analysis. Ophthalmology 1986;93(5):651–660.

158. Grisolano J, Peyman GA. Special short needles to inject and aspirate high-viscosity silicone oil. Arch Ophthalmol 1986;104(4):608.

159. Hughes L, Maurice DM. A fresh look at iontophoresis. Arch Ophthalmol 1984;102(12):1825–1829.

160. Sarraf D, Lee DA. The role of iontophoresis in ocular drug delivery. J Ocular Pharmacol 1994;10:69–81.

Pharmaceutical and Regulatory Aspects of Ocular Drug Administration

Timothy R. Covington
Gary A. Holt

Drugs and the drug-benefit component of managed health care plans remain among the "best buys" in American health care. Clinicians, health care economists, and fiscal managers are beginning to realize that 85% to 90% of all acute and chronic illnesses are cured or symptomatically relieved by drug therapy. All health care providers should work more deliberately to:

- Promote the safe, appropriate, effective, and economical use of both prescription and nonprescription drugs.
- Assist in producing optimal therapeutic outcomes by fostering precision in drug therapy management.
- Foster the evolution of highly cognitive, outcome-oriented pharmaceutical care by maximizing the benefits of drug therapy and identifying, resolving, and preventing drug-related problems and therapeutic misadventures.

Efforts that lead to proper drug and dosage selection, fewer adverse drug reactions, fewer drug-drug interactions, and better patient compliance produce significant dividends in quality and cost of care.

Quality of Care Considerations

All payers of health care bills in the United States are strongly focused on issues of quality and value. Accrediting agencies are following a similar strategy as they look for positive health outcome indicators. A cost-benefit disparity appears to exist in many health care encounters. The ultimate payer is moving health care providers into an era of assessment and accountability since too little objective evidence exists supporting a positive correlation between rising costs, quality of care, and optimal health outcomes.

The United States leads the world in health care costs. Despite expenditures, however, evidence that drug therapy management is far less than optimal is abundant and growing. Evidence of improper drug selection and use and "therapeutic misadventuring" is manifest in the following facts:[1]

- Approximately 30% to 50% of the 1.8 billion prescriptions dispensed annually are taken or used incorrectly by patients.
- The overall cost of failure to use drugs properly exceeds $30 billion per year in outpatient care, hospitalization, time off work, lost productivity, and other factors.
- Approximately 7% of patients never get their original prescription filled.
- Approximately 15% of patients do not take the full course of their prescribed medication.
- Approximately 32% of patients do not have their prescriptions refilled, even though they need to do so.
- Between 24% and 66% of hospital antibiotic use is unnecessary or otherwise inappropriate, as judged by expert panels.

- Approximately 8% to 11% of all hospital admissions are related to failure to take drugs properly.
- Approximately 3% to 5% of all hospital admissions are directly attributable to drug-induced toxicity, much of which is preventable.
- Approximately 16% of all hospital admissions of patients ≥70 years of age result from adverse drug reactions.
- Noncompliance with drug therapy results in the loss of over 20 million workdays per year.
- Approximately 23% of nursing home admissions result from the inability to manage medication use in the home environment.
- Approximately 125,000 Americans die annually from failure to take drugs properly.

Cost of Care Considerations

Payers of health care bills in the United States are experiencing "sticker shock." The $939 billion US health care expenditure of 1993 is projected to grow to $1.5 trillion by the year 2000. Annual health care costs were $204 per person in 1965, $3160 per person in 1992, and are projected to be about $5500 per person by the year 2000. A past president of the American Medical Association has declared that the United States is heading for a health care "meltdown" if spiraling costs are not brought under control.

The current shift in the health care paradigm is toward "applying the brake" to health care expenditures without adversely impacting quality of care. Cost and quality issues suggest that great emphasis be placed on optimal drug use. This chapter presents some of the most fundamental yet vital components of ophthalmic drug use.

Guidelines for Prescription Writing

The Prescription

A prescription is defined as a verbal or written order for a drug issued by a properly licensed and authorized health care practitioner. Prescriptions are a vital element of the prescriber-patient-pharmacist relationship. The prescription generally completes the initial prescriber-patient encounter but initiates a series of actions on the part of pharmacists that are designed to ensure that the health outcome of patients is optimal.

In the United States drugs can be legally classified into two groups. Drugs that can be obtained only by prescription have a somewhat lower safety profile than the other class of drugs, referred to as nonprescription or over-the-counter (OTC) drugs. Prescription drugs are also known as *legend* drugs. A legend drug is one that reflects the classification on the manufacturer's label, which states, "Caution: Federal Law Prohibits Dispensing Without Prescription."

The mechanical act by pharmacists of filling prescriptions is designed to ensure that patients receive the proper drug in the correct dosage and that the drug is used as prescribed, consistent with the manufacturer's labeling. In addition, they provide numerous cognitive services. Pharmacists typically screen for potential drug-related complications before patients receive a particular drug. This activity is known as the drug-use-evaluation (DUE) process, which is designed to optimize drug therapy management by attempting to identify, resolve, and prevent drug-related problems. This process does much to positively impact quality of drug use and clinical outcomes. Well-designed DUE activity focuses on assessing (1) appropriateness of drug use; and (2) drug overutilization or underutilization. Table 4.1 lists the elements of a comprehensive DUE activity.

Pharmacists then deliver prescribed drugs to patients, or patients' designees, and provide counseling on proper drug use. Elements of patient education and counseling on proper drug use usually address or should address the following:[2]

- For whom the drug is intended
- Use of the drug and what to expect
- When to take or use the drug
- What special preparation, if any, is required for use
- Precautions to be observed while taking the drug
- Side effects that commonly occur
- Steps to take to avoid or minimize side effects
- What to do if side effects occur
- How to properly store the drug
- Conditions or situations to avoid while taking or using the drug
- Other drugs or foods to avoid or to consume with caution while taking the drug
- Refill information
- Action to take if one or more doses are missed
- Any other information regarding drug use appropriate to the situation

TABLE 4.1
Elements of a Comprehensive Drug-Use-Evaluation (DUE)

I. Appropriateness of drug use
  A. Indications
  B. Contraindications
  C. Risk factors
  D. Age
  E. Gender
  F. Concurrent drug use (drug interactions)
II. Overutilization/underutilization
  A. Dosage
  B. Quantity dispensed
  C. Frequency of dose
  D. Interval between prescriptions
  E. Duration of therapy

Pharmacists and prescribers should be highly cooperative in discussing patients' drug regimens. This collegiality is vital to patients' best health care interests and often results in excellent refinements in the drug use process. The spirit of trust and commitment to high ethical and professional standards with regard to confidentiality of patient information is, of course, essential in the prescriber-pharmacist relationship.

Anatomy of the Prescription

Prescriptions are usually written on preprinted forms provided in the form of a pad of blank prescriptions. These preprinted forms are called prescription blanks. Examples of the format are shown in Figure 4.1. It is recommended that the prescriber's name, office address, telephone number and other pertinent information (e.g., facsimile [FAX] number) be printed at the top. Although use of specially printed prescription blanks is encouraged, prescription blanks for routine drug orders are not required. Prescribers may write a routine prescription on any paper or writing material. However, prescriptions for certain controlled substances may require special prescription blanks.

The fundamental elements of a prescription include the following:[3,4]

- Patient's name and current address
- Date the prescription was written
- Rx symbol (superscription)
- Medication prescribed (inscription)
- Dispensing directions to pharmacist (subscription)
- Directions for patient use (signa or signatura)
- Refill, special labeling, or other instructions
- Prescriber's signature, address and other appropriate information (e.g., telephone, FAX, pager numbers)

Patient information is essential for identification purposes. Although prescription forgeries and fraud in the drug acquisition process are not common, they are a reality. As with any part of the prescription, legibility is strongly encouraged. Sloppy, unclear, or barely legible prescription information substantially increases the risk of medication error. Many prescribers go beyond the name and address in providing patient information. Some prescribers provide the pharmacist with the diagnosis on the prescription. This helps tremendously in the DUE process, particularly if a drug has multiple Food and Drug Administration (FDA)-approved indications for use. Some prescribers provide height, weight, and age information for pediatric patients.

The date the prescription was written is critical. A significant lapse of time between the date the prescription was written and when it is presented for dispensing can have negative health implications. A delay in presenting the prescription to a pharmacy may warrant a call from the pharma-

cist to the clinician to determine whether the intent of the prescriber and needs of the patient can still be met. This matter is more crucial in the management of acute rather than chronic illnesses and in the dispensing and sale of controlled substances.

The Rx symbol, or superscription, is an ancient symbol associated with healing.[4] The current Rx symbol is actually a distortion or contraction of the Latin verb recipe, meaning "take thou" or "you take."

The medication prescribed, or inscription, is the primary portion of a prescription.[4] This portion of the prescription contains the name of the drug to be dispensed, its concentra-

JOHN A. SMITH, O. D.
Optometry

1234 Hospital Drive   Telephone (100) 123-2020
Anytown, U.S.A. 12345   DEA No. AH6650431

NAME _____ Frank Q. Smith _____ AGE __ 65 __
ADDRESS __ 123 Main St. __ DATE 2/14/95

℞   Pred-G ophthalmic susp.

#5 ml.

Sig.: ˙T gt. O. D. q.i.d. X

1 week for eye inflammation

☒ Label
☒ No Refill   _John A. Smith_ ,O. D. _____ ,O. D.
☐ Refill X ___ Dispense as Written   Product Selection Permitted

A

JOHN A. SMITH, O. D.
Optometry

1234 Hospital Drive   Telephone (100) 123-2020
Anytown, U.S.A. 12345   DEA No. AH6650431

NAME _____ Donald Q. Doe _____ AGE __ 13 __
ADDRESS __ 456 Peach Ave. __ DATE 2/14/95

℞   Erythromycin ophthalmic ung.
#3.5 g.
Sig.: scrub eyelids using
cotton-tipped applicator
b.i.d.

☒ Label
☐ No Refill   _____ ,O. D. _John A. Smith_ ,O. D.
☒ Refill X _2_ Dispense as Written   Product Selection Permitted

B

FIGURE 4.1   **Typical prescription format.** *(A)* Ophthalmic suspension. *(B)* Ophthalmic ointment.

tion or dosage units, and its formulation (e.g., solution, ointment, capsule). Prescribers may refer to it by generic or brand name. Most prescriptions are dispensed in premanufactured dosage forms. Compounded prescriptions are those in which various ordered ingredients are formulated by pharmacists. Compounded prescriptions are increasing in numbers so that prescribers may meet special needs of their patients.

Dispensing directions to pharmacists (subscription) are usually brief.[4] If the product is premanufactured, the subscription usually consists of the number of dosage units preceded by a "#" sign. If the subscription is for a compounded prescription, dispensing directions are much more complex.

The specific directions to patients on how to properly use the prescription comprise the signatura (Sig.) of the prescription.[4] The Latin translation of signatura is "mark thou." The directions for use are commonly written using abbreviated forms of both English and Latin terms. These directions are translated by pharmacists and placed on the label of the prescription container. Pharmacists often verbally expand these directions. Written patient information leaflets designed to foster safe and appropriate drug use may also be dispensed with the prescription by pharmacists. In a few instances, such as with estrogens, federal law dictates that manufacturers provide FDA-approved patient package inserts (PPIs).

Additional instructions to patients or to pharmacists may be included on the prescription. Some prescribers want patients to know the name and strength of the prescription drug. This is accomplished by writing or checking "label" on the prescription. This fosters communication among pharmacists, prescribers, and patients and allows rapid identification in emergencies and cases of accidental or intentional overdosage. The manufacturer's expiration date may also be requested. The number of authorized refills should be indicated on every prescription. If no refill information is provided, it is understood that no refills are authorized. Because of potential abuse and other safety considerations, refills are never authorized for any schedule II controlled substance.

Pharmacists frequently make additional notations on prescriptions. This typically includes the dispensing pharmacist's initials, the retail price of the drug, the brand name or generic product dispensed, and any other appropriate notations. Prescriptions become part of a master prescription file, and such records are usually kept for many years. Prescription information is also typically entered into a computer to develop an electronic file of each patient's medication history.

Language of the Prescription

Elements of prescription nomenclature have their roots in antiquity. Many of the root words are derived from Latin,

TABLE 4.2
Selected Prescription Abbreviations and Their Meaning

Abbreviation	English Meaning
a.c.	before meals
b.i.d.	twice a day
$\bar{c}$	with
caps.	capsule
d.	day
gt(t)	drop(s)
h.	hour
h.s.	at bedtime
o.d.	right eye
o.h.	every hour
o.s.	left eye
o.u.	each eye
p.c.	after meals
p.o.	by mouth
p.r.n.	as needed
q.	each, every
q.h.	every hour
q.i.d.	four times a day
q.o.d.	every other day
$\bar{s}$	without
sig.	label
sol.	solution
susp.	suspension
tab.	tablet
tbsp.	tablespoonful
t.i.d.	three times a day
tsp.	teaspoonful
ung.	ointment
ut dict.	as directed

and most are abbreviated. The translations of commonly employed prescription abbreviations are listed in Table 4.2.[4]

Prescribers use numerous other colloquial shorthand abbreviations for drugs and conditions. The use of some of these is so widespread that they are accepted as standard abbreviations. For example, ASA is commonly written for aspirin and CPM for chlorpheniramine maleate. Frequently used abbreviations for disease conditions include CHF for congestive heart failure, UTI for urinary tract infection, DM for diabetes mellitus, HBP or Htx for hypertension, and URI for upper respiratory infection.

The system of measurement employed in prescription writing has shifted from the avoirdupois and apothecary system to the metric system, although the apothecary system is still occasionally employed. The metric system is the preferred system and its use is encouraged.

Ophthalmic practitioners are encouraged to recommend auxiliary labeling on prescription labels whenever appropriate. Such auxiliary labeling can be efficient in fostering

TABLE 4.3

Commonly Employed Auxiliary Information for Use on Prescription Labels or Containers

Shake well
For external use only
For the eye
Keep in refrigerator. Do not freeze
Keep out of the reach of children
No refills
____ refills available
Take until gone
Store in a cool, dry place
Take with food
Avoid alcohol
May cause drowsiness
Take on an empty stomach
Take 30 minutes to 60 minutes before bedtime
Take every ____ hours around the clock

compliance and ensuring the safe, appropriate, and effective use of the prescription. Common auxiliary language that may be included as appropriate on prescription labels includes phrases listed in Table 4.3.[4]

Types of Prescriptions

Prescriptions may be transmitted via written prescription, telephone, or FAX. The majority of prescriptions are written on preprinted forms. Although the telephone has been used for over 100 years, it is a bit depersonalizing, and basic rules of telephone etiquette are often ignored or not properly applied. Optimal telephonic interaction requires a friendly voice; courtesy; an unhurried caller (prescriber); good listening skills; alertness; clearly spoken, carefully chosen words; accurate information; and an opportunity for questions and dialogue. Telephone calls should be logged or otherwise documented.

Prescribers should identify themselves before a prescription order is placed over the telephone. Ophthalmic practitioners should verify that the prescription was received and transcribed accurately. They should remember that it is patients who suffer the consequences of inappropriate translations and transcriptions. Relationships with pharmacists should be collegial, with the best interest of patients taking precedence over all other considerations. Prescribers should not be oversensitive to pharmacists who telephone them to verify prescriptions apparently called in by office personnel or nurses. Prescription drug fraud is committed by nonmedical individuals periodically. In fact, it is far preferable for prescribers not to delegate the function of calling prescriptions in to pharmacies.

FAX transmission of prescriptions lends itself to prescription fraud and drug diversion. It is difficult to ascertain the origin of the FAX, and FAX prescriptions could be forgeries. Since a FAX prescription order is only a copy, the original prescription could be available to patients, who may then take it to a second pharmacy for dispensing. The checks and balances on FAX transmission are inadequate, and such practices should be avoided or minimized.

Many states have ruled that a prescription transmitted by FAX is not valid for dispensing purposes. Some states allow FAX transmission of prescriptions only within a single hospital or between hospitals and nursing homes. Other states permit prescription transmission by FAX but require verification.

Steps for Effective Prescription Writing

Ineffective or inefficient prescription writing may limit optimal therapeutic outcomes. A properly written prescription is fundamental to compliance and the safe, appropriate, and effective use of drugs. The prescription is a vital communication tool. Casual prescribing practices contribute to therapeutic misadventures in which patients bear the consequences, both economically and medically.

Legibility is fundamental to good prescription writing. Illegibility increases the risk of patient-sustained medication errors. The use of potentially confusing abbreviations such as q.d., q.i.d., or q.o.d. should be avoided. Bold periods and sloppy lettering have resulted in q.o.d. (every other day) being translated to q.i.d. (four times daily). This results in an eightfold (800%) increase in the intended dosage. A recent malpractice case involved a misinterpretation of q.d. and q.i.d. Rather than a thyroid supplement being consumed once per day, it was consumed four times daily and iatrogenic hyperthyroidism resulted. OD can be interpreted as once daily or right eye. Abbreviations of drug names are discouraged. For example, zidovudine is often expressed as AZT, but this abbreviation has also been interpreted to be azathioprine or aztreonam.

Decimals should be avoided whenever possible, since decimal designations are difficult to comprehend.[4] Therefore, a 500-mg designation is preferable to a 0.5-g designation. "Naked" decimals should also be avoided. For example, 0.25 ml is preferable to .25 ml. If a decimal point is not seen, tremendously large multiples of the intended dose occur. The health consequences of such errors can produce profound morbidity and even mortality.

When appropriate, practitioners should indicate on the prescription exactly when during the day the prescribed drug should be administered. For example, rather than prescribing a drug four times daily, the exact times should be stated (e.g., 9:00 a.m., 1:00 p.m., 5:00 p.m. and 9:00 p.m.). If a drug should be dosed around the clock, the specific hours should be stated. Otherwise, patients tend to take medication only during the waking hours.

Prescribers are encouraged to include on the prescription why the drug is prescribed. For example, "instill one drop in each eye at 7:00 a.m. and 7:00 p.m. for glaucoma"; "take one capsule before bedtime for eye infection"; "take one teaspoonful at 8:00 a.m., 2:00 p.m., 8:00 p.m., and 2:00 a.m. for eye infection"; and "instill one drop in each eye at 9:00 a.m., 3:00 p.m., and 9:00 p.m. to treat eye inflammation."

Vague instructions such as "take as necessary," "take as needed," "use as directed," or "take as directed" are strongly discouraged.[5] "Take as needed" gives patients license to self-assess and self-treat. This introduces subjectivity into the drug use process and invites over- or underutilization, both of which have the potential to produce adverse health consequences. Underutilization predisposes to therapeutic failure and all its attendant complications. Overutilization predisposes to drug-induced toxicity and adverse effects. "Take as directed" or "use as directed" also invites patient subjectivity. Furthermore, it presumes that patients will remember in full the verbal directions provided by prescribers or pharmacists. It is a dangerous practice to assume that the patient population, which is highly stratified intellectually, to remember what was intended by prescribers.

Ophthalmic practitioners should request that the name and strength or concentration of the prescribed medication be placed on the prescription label. Because this information is in the public health interest, most pharmacists routinely provide this information unless directed otherwise by prescribers. In expressing strengths of medication and any other weight or measure, the metric system should be used whenever possible.

The prescription should indicate the number of authorized refills. Medication prescribed for acute ocular diseases should have few, if any, refills. This is particularly true when prescribing corticosteroids. If a course of therapy for an acute infection or inflammation does not produce the desired clinical result, prescribers may need to see patients again, reevaluate their condition, and refine the drug therapy. Multiple refills, however, are often appropriate for managing chronic diseases such as open-angle glaucoma. Instructions to pharmacists such as "refill prn" or "refill ad lib" are generally inappropriate. Such a practice may discourage appropriate medical follow-up.

Legal and Regulatory Considerations

PRESCRIPTIVE AUTHORITY

The authority to prescribe is a privilege conferred on various health professionals by legislative and regulatory actions of both federal and state governments. Federal law states that legal drugs may be prescribed by practitioners licensed by law to perform such acts. Since most states license health practitioners, prescriptive authority falls largely under the purview of individual state regulatory agencies and licensing boards. Even the Controlled Substances Act does not establish specific criteria regarding who may do the prescribing. Rather, it requires that the prescriber be licensed to prescribe under state law and be registered with the Drug Enforcement Administration (DEA).

Physicians, including osteopaths, have the widest latitude with respect to prescription-writing activity. All medical specialties and subspecialties fall under the general category of physician and have broad prescription-writing privileges. Numerous states have extended prescriptive authority to nonphysician health practitioners with some limitations. Veterinarians may prescribe drugs for animals, podiatrists for medical disorders associated with the foot, dentists for disorders associated with the oral cavity, and optometrists for disorders of the eye. Prescriptive authority has also been granted to physician's assistants, nurse practitioners, pharmacists, and others, although this authority is neither consistent nor universal among the states.

CONTROLLED SUBSTANCES

The Comprehensive Drug Abuse Prevention and Control Act of 1970, most commonly known as the Controlled Substances Act,[6] is enforced by the US Department of Justice. The Controlled Substances Act regulates use of drugs acting on the central nervous system that possess significant abuse potential and potential to produce psychological and physical dependency. All practitioners authorized to prescribe a drug regulated by the DEA must register with the DEA and be assigned a DEA number, which should not be preprinted on prescription blanks and pads. The DEA number should be handwritten in ink on prescriptions for drugs covered under the Controlled Substances Act. Widespread dissemination of a DEA number on routine prescriptions containing this number fosters fraud, forgeries, drug diversion and illegal drug use. Furthermore, prescription pads should be held under relatively tight security because they can be valuable in the hands of persons with illegal motives. Prescribers should never presign prescriptions because such prescriptions represent "blank checks" for illegal acquisition of prescription drugs of all types. Prescriptions issued for (1) the purpose of abetting the habit of addicts or for continuing addicts' drug dependence, (2) a fictitious person or person other than the one named on the prescription, (3) prescribers' office use, or (4) use outside the normal course of prescribers' professional practice are invalid and should not be dispensed by pharmacists.

Controlled substances are divided into five schedules or classes.[6] Schedule I substances have no accepted and approved medical use in the United States, possess significant potential for abuse and dependency, and lack adequate evidence of safety. Agents such as heroin, lysergic acid diethyl-amide (LSD), marijuana, mescaline, peyote, and psilocybin are schedule I drugs. Placement of drugs in schedule I does not mean some of these agents do not have medical potential. Drugs with medical potential can be evaluated as investigational under appropriate protocols and FDA oversight.

Schedule II drugs are accepted for medical use, but limitations on their use are strict because of their high abuse and dependency potential. Prescriptions for schedule II drugs must be in ink, personally signed by prescribers, and cannot be refilled. They should be limited to the smallest quantity possible to treat the medical condition effectively. Prescriptions for chronic use of all scheduled medications warrant suspicion, and calls from pharmacists to explore the medical circumstances requiring chronic use should be expected. Examples of schedule II drugs are morphine, hydromorphone, codeine (larger doses), meperidine, oxycodone, methadone, amphetamines, cocaine, barbiturates, and methylphenidate.

Schedule III agents possess significant but less potential for abuse and dependency than do schedule I and II agents. Schedule III agents may contain limited quantities of certain narcotics (e.g., codeine, hydrocodone), barbiturates, and selected antianxiety agents and sleep aids.

Schedule IV drugs have relatively low abuse potential and limited dependency potential. Whereas prescriptions for schedule II drugs must be written, prescriptions for schedule III and IV drugs may be verbal. Unlike schedule II drugs, which cannot be refilled, schedule III and IV drugs can be refilled up to five times in 6 months if authorized by prescribers. Examples of schedule IV drugs are some of the benzodiazepine tranquilizers, nonbenzodiazepine tranquilizers, propoxyphene, and some amphetamine-like stimulants.

Schedule V agents have low abuse potential. Many of the products are used to suppress cough and treat diarrhea. None of these agents is commonly used for ophthalmic purposes. Some states require prescriptions, whereas others allow OTC sale by pharmacists.

Federal regulations concerning controlled substances may be superseded by stricter state regulations. Prescribers must recognize that if scheduled medication is inventoried in the office practice, an additional registration must be filed with the DEA, accurate records must be kept on receipt and disbursement of scheduled drugs, and practitioners must submit to DEA inspections. Controlled substances commonly used in outpatient ophthalmic practice are listed in Table 4.4. The clinical uses of cocaine are described in Chapters 20 and 23, and the uses of opioid analgesics are discussed in Chapter 7.

UNLABELED USE

When a drug receives FDA approval for marketing, the drug also receives approval of the official labeling. Labeling includes information that appears on the label of the drug's

TABLE 4.4
Controlled Substances Commonly Used in Outpatient Ophthalmic Practice

Schedule	Drug(s)
I	Not commercially available
II	Cocaine, oxycodone
III	Aspirin with codeine, acetaminophen with codeine, acetaminophen with hydrocodone
IV	Propoxyphene
V	None commonly used

container and in the package insert. This includes information on indications, contraindications, warnings, precautions, adverse effects, drug interactions, and administration and dosage guidelines. The FDA requires that all statements submitted by the manufacturer and contained in the labeling be supported by documentation on file with the FDA. Thus, FDA-approved labeling determines which uses (indications) of the drug are supported by experience and data. The FDA limits claims that may appear in advertisements and promotional material.

Official labeling, the package insert, and the FDA-approved indications do not necessarily constrain prescribers in ophthalmic practice. The FDA has no statutory or regulatory authority over the professional practice of health care personnel. Therefore, "off-label" or "unlabeled" use of a drug for indications or dosages other than those listed in FDA-approved labeling can occur under appropriate conditions.[7]

However, indiscrete, uninformed prescribing for an "off-label" use unsupported by clinical studies is discouraged. Unlabeled indications or dosages supported by clinical studies, the published peer-reviewed literature, and a consensus among prescribers is usually adequate to support drug use for a non-FDA approved indication or dosage. Unlabeled uses are typically supported by further investigation and a significant body of clinical documentation. Moreover, the pharmaceutical manufacturer, at some point in the evolution of "off-label" use, generally applies to the FDA for the new indication or dosage. Unfortunately, the time period between the application and FDA approval for new indications is often lengthy.

Prescribing of an FDA-approved drug for an "off-label" use does not require prior consent of patients, is not considered research, and does not require special consideration or approval by an Institutional Review Board or other body concerned with the protection of human subjects. Prescribers have considerable freedom to prescribe for "off-label" uses but are vulnerable if such uses are not supported by safety and efficacy data. Thus, it is best to obtain patients'

TABLE 4.5
Drugs with Unlabeled Ophthalmic Uses

Generic (Trade)	Labeled Indication	Unlabeled Ophthalmic Use
Acetylcysteine (*Mucomyst*)	Mucolytic agent in bronchopulmonary conditions	Topical mucolytic treatment of vernal conjunctivitis, giant papillary conjunctivitis, filamentary keratitis
Acyclovir (*Zovirax*)	Treatment of varicella-zoster and genital herpes simplex	Treatment of epithelial herpes simplex keratitis
Aminocaproic acid (*Amicar*)	Antifibrinolytic agent for the treatment of excessive bleeding	Oral treatment of traumatic hyphema
Aspirin (e.g., *Bayer*)	Anti-inflammatory, analgesic, antipyretic agent	Oral treatment of vernal conjunctivitis
Diclofenac sodium (*Voltaren*)	Treatment of postoperative cataract inflammation	Anti-inflammatory treatment following argon laser trabeculoplasty; treatment of seasonal allergic conjunctivitis; and pain associated with radial keratotomy and photorefractive keratectomy
Fluorescein sodium (e.g., *Fluorescite*)	Topical or intravenous diagnostic ophthalmic dye	Oral fluorography for diagnosis of retinal vascular diseases
Polyhexamethylene biguanide	Swimming pool and contact lens disinfectant	Treatment of *Acanthamoeba* keratitis
Sodium hyaluronate (*Amvisc*) Chondroitin sulfate (*Viscoat*)	Viscoelastic agents in intraocular surgery	Topical treatment of severe dry eye disorders
Suprofen (*Profenal*)	Prevention of intraoperative miosis during cataract extraction	Topical treatment of contact lens-associated giant papillary conjunctivitis

Adapted from Bartlett JD, Ghormley NR, Jaanus SD, et al, eds. Ophthalmic Drug Facts. St. Louis: Facts and Comparisons, 1995: 273–280.

informed consent before using or prescribing any drug for an unlabeled purpose (see Chapter 5).

Prescribers should exercise sound judgment when deviating from FDA-approved indications and dosages. In the event of litigation, the burden of proof for demonstrating that prescribing and dispensing of a drug for an unlabeled indication was within the limits of good medical practice rests primarily with prescribers. Departure from FDA-approved labeling may be considered *prima facie* evidence of negligence in the absence of sound professional judgment and clinical and scientific literature that supports the particular "off-label" use, especially if the drug has been used in an irrational, unsafe, and unreasonable manner. Drugs that have well-documented "unlabeled" ophthalmic uses are listed in Table 4.5.

Guarding Against Prescription Forgery

Prescribers can do much to minimize prescription forgeries. Security of prescription pads is crucial. Preprinted prescription forms are "blank checks" for drugs, and prescription blanks with preprinted DEA numbers are an invitation to forgeries for scheduled medication with moderate to high abuse and dependency potential. Moreover, use of this number may allow others to place the DEA number on additional forged prescriptions.

Prescription forgeries are a substantial problem. Prescribers and pharmacists seem to develop a "sixth sense" about patients who are prone to drug abuse and forgeries. Ophthalmic practitioners and pharmacists are encouraged to collaborate thoroughly in the prescription verification process. Figure 4.2 illustrates a prescription for a controlled substance in which the number of dosage units to be dispensed is specified parenthetically to prevent alteration of the dosage units.

Generic Versus Brand Name Drugs

The generic drug industry is a vigorous and dynamic component of the health care complex. Generic drug utilization has increased dramatically since 1975, when 9.5% of all prescriptions were generic versions. Currently over 40% of all drugs prescribed are generic versions of an innovator's product that has lost its patent exclusivity. Interestingly, several large brand-name pharmaceutical companies have purchased generic drug companies, formed their own generic drug divisions, or begun to distribute products manufactured for them by generic drug firms under the brand name label. Thus, the large brand name firms control a large portion of the generic drug market either directly or indirectly.

Recent and impending patent expirations are expected to contribute even more significantly to a trend of increasing generic drug utilization. From 1991–1994 patent expirations have allowed generic versions of drugs that had cumulative sales of $8.1 billion in 1989. By 1999, 45% of the current top 50 brand-name drugs will be "off patent."

A major event in 1984 has led to a significant upward spiral in generic drug use. This event, passage of the Drug Price Competition and Patent Term Restoration Act (Waxman-Hatch Act), permits the FDA to employ an expedited review process for approval of generic versions of brand name drugs already found to be safe and effective for clinical use but no longer protected by a patent. The expedited review process is known as an abbreviated new drug application (ANDA).

The Waxman-Hatch Act of 1984 was motivated to a significant degree by cost considerations, but quality issues concerning bioequivalency and therapeutic equivalency were addressed as well. The FDA evaluates and considers as therapeutically equivalent those drugs that satisfy approval criteria within the following three categories:[8] (1) product characteristics and labeling, (2) manufacturing and quality control, and (3) bioequivalency.

All FDA-approved drugs (pioneer brand name and generic versions) are required to meet the same FDA standards of quality. Generic versions must be bioequivalent to the innovator's product, within predetermined limits, to ensure therapeutic equivalency and no greater risk for drug-induced toxicity.

The Waxman-Hatch Act does not require a generic manufacturer to repeat clinical trials and redemonstrate drug safety and efficacy. Under the ANDA process, generic manufacturers must provide evidence that the generic version:[8]

1. Contains the same active ingredient as the brand name drug.
2. Is of similar bioequivalency/bioavailability.
3. Produces the same pharmacologic and therapeutic activity in the body (*in vivo*) as the brand name product.
4. Is manufactured according to stringent and universally applied FDA requirements.
5. Meets FDA requirements for stability, purity, strength, and quality.
6. Is labeled with the same claims, warnings, and other information as the innovator's product.

FDA approval of generic drugs is based, to a significant extent, on evidence of comparable *in vivo* bioavailability. Bioequivalent drug products are defined as those pharmaceutically equivalent products (i.e., drug products that contain the same active ingredient in the same concentration and dosage form and administered by the same route of administration) that display comparable bioavailability (i.e., comparable rate and extent to which the active or therapeutic ingredient is absorbed from a drug product and becomes available at the site of drug action when studied under similar experimental conditions).[8]

The graphic representation of bioavailability for systemic medications is generally represented by a serum concentration/time curve that plots serum drug concentration against time.[8] The variables evaluated are the area under the curve (AUC), maximal serum concentration (C_{max}), and the time to reach the maximal concentration (T_{max}). Total drug absorption is reflected by AUC. C_{max} and T_{max} are also important because the pharmacologic effect of several drugs depends on their rate of absorption. When comparing generic formulations with the innovator's product, the more superimposable the concentration/time curves, the more likely the two products are to be bioequivalent and therapeutically equivalent.

Statistical questions remain concerning how much the bioavailability values obtained from the innovator's product and generic versions should be allowed to vary. Although different standards are set for different classes or types of drugs, the general bioavailability standard is an upward or downward variation of no more than 20% between the innovator's product and the generic drug's AUC and the average maximum and minimum concentrations. In addition, the time to reach T_{max} should not differ significantly. Most generic versions tested to date have demonstrated plasma levels within 3% to 5% of the innovator drug. Sentiment seems to be growing for what appears to be an achievable ±10% bioavailability criterion.[8]

The FDA "Orange Book," officially titled *Approved Drug Products With Therapeutic Equivalency Evaluations*, provides a list of all drugs fully reviewed by the FDA for

JOHN A. SMITH, O. D.
Optometry

1234 Hospital Drive — **Telephone (100) 123-2020**
Anytown, U.S.A. 12345 — **DEA No. AH6650431**

NAME Jane R. Jones **AGE** 42
ADDRESS 123 Oak St. **DATE** 2/14/95

℞ Tylenol w/codeine no. 3
#12 (twelve)
Sig.: i tab. p.o. q. 4 h.
p.r.n. pain

☒ Label
☒ No Refill
☐ Refill X ___ ______ ,O. D. Dispense as Written — John A. Smith ,O. D. Product Selection Permitted

FIGURE 4.2 **Prescription for a controlled substance.**

both safety and efficacy and for which new drug applications (NDAs) and abbreviated new drug applications (ANDAs) have been approved.[8] Equivalence evaluations are provided for generic drugs that are pharmaceutical and therapeutic equivalents of brand name drugs when administered according to the labeling. Products not included are generally those marketed before 1938 or those brought to market between 1938 and 1962 that the FDA has certified as safe but has not yet approved as effective.

Of the over 10,000 drugs in the "Orange Book," approximately 80% are generic versions.[8] Of the approximately 8,000 multisource generic drugs, over 90% are considered therapeutically equivalent to the innovator's product.[8]

All products with a two-letter code beginning with an "A" are considered therapeutically equivalent to the innovator's product. "A" rated products for which there are no known or suspected bioequivalency problems are further designated, largely by dosage form, with a second letter (Table 4.6).[8] Products with a two-letter code beginning with a "B" are products not considered therapeutically equivalent to "A"-rated products and have actual or potential bioequivalence problems that have not been resolved by appropriate testing.[8] "B"-rated products are further classified with a second letter (see Table 4.6). The "Orange Book" is updated monthly to reflect new scientific information that justifies a change in drug ratings.

Ophthalmic practitioners may wish to collaborate with pharmacists in selecting generic versions of drugs. Pharmacists are particularly knowledgeable regarding bioequivalency of generic drugs, product quality, and manufacturer reliability relative to service and source of supply. Prescribers are encouraged to abide by the following guidelines in prescribing generic drugs:[8]

1. Seek bioequivalency information. Only "A"-rated multisource products should be prescribed.
2. Realize that several companies with large generic drug lines are distributors only. They repackage drugs manufactured by other companies. The manufacturer's reputation and history of producing high-quality generics is paramount. Prescribers may want to specify on the prescription the manufacturer of generic versions.
3. Do not assume that different dosage forms of the same drug and strength are equivalent.
4. If a bioequivalent generic product is selected, discourage a change in source of supply. Patients become confused when they receive generically equivalent drugs upon refill that are a different color or shape than the medication originally dispensed.
5. Assess patient status. Medically fragile patients should avoid changing source of supply.
6. Prescribe with great care drugs or drug classes with known bioavailability problems or a narrow therapeutic range.
7. Reassure patients that high-quality generic drugs exist in abundance.

TABLE 4.6
FDA Rating System for Designation of Equivalence

Principal Categories

A—Drug products that are considered to be therapeutically equivalent to other pharmaceutically equivalent products.

B—Drug products not considered at this time to be therapeutically equivalent to other pharmaceutically equivalent products.

Subgroups of "A"-rated products (considered to be therapeutically equivalent)

AA—Products in conventional dosage forms not presenting bioequivalence problems.

AB—Products meeting necessary bioequivalence requirements.

AN—Bioequivalent solutions and powders for aerosolization.

AO—Bioequivalent injectable oil solutions.

AP—Bioequivalent injectable aqueous solutions.

AT—Bioequivalent topical products.

Subgroups of "B"-rated products (considered not to be therapeutically equivalent)

BC—Extended-release dosage forms (tablets, capsules, injectables).

BD—Documented bioequivalence problems with active ingredients and dosage forms.

BE—Delayed release oral dosage forms.

BN—Products in aerosol-nebulizer delivery system.

BP—Potential bioequivalence problems with active ingredients and dosage forms.

BR—Suppositories or enemas that deliver drugs for systemic absorption.

BS—Products having drug-standard deficiencies.

BT—Topical products with bioequivalence issues.

BX—Drug products for which the data are insufficient to determine therapeutic equivalence.

Generic drugs represent a low-cost alternative to more expensive brand name products. The place of generic drugs in contemporary health care is secure and growing. Prescribers should appreciate marketplace realities and take appropriate steps to ensure the prudent use of generic drugs.

Extemporaneous Compounding

The large-scale process of manufacturing must be differentiated from compounding in the context of prescription drug therapy. *Manufacturing* involves production, preparation, propagation, conversion, and processing of a drug or device, whether directly or indirectly by extraction from substances of natural origin or independently by means of chemical or biological synthesis.[9] It includes any packaging or repackaging of the substances, labeling or relabeling of the containers, and promotions and marketing of such drugs or devices. Manufactured products are commercially available for resale.

Compounding is defined as the preparation, mixing, assembling, packaging, and labeling of a drug or device pursuant to the receipt of a prescription or for purposes of teaching, research, or chemical analysis.[9] Pharmacists typically compound drugs extemporaneously upon receipt of a valid prescription. Bulk or batch compounding in anticipation of several prescriptions may occur.

Compounding is a traditional pharmacy function, and the art and science of compounding has enjoyed a resurgence over the past several years. Although pharmaceutical manufacturers essentially usurped pharmacists' traditional compounding function by providing premanufactured products in the post-World War II era, the last decade has seen an increased demand for specialty dosage forms that are not commercially available.

The FDA protects traditional compounding by pharmacists but expressly prohibits health professionals from independent, large-scale manufacturing conducted under the guise of compounding. The FDA prohibits the following:[9]

- Compounding large quantities of drug products that are commercially available
- Receipt, storage, and use of drug substances from sources that are not FDA-approved
- Receipt, storage, and use of drug components that do not meet compendial requirements (e.g., purity, stability, clarity, bioavailability, sterility)
- Compounding using commercial scale manufacturing or testing equipment
- Compounding amounts of drug products in excess of what is needed for valid prescription orders
- Solicitation of business to compound specific drug products or product classes

Organized medicine is opposed to compounding by prescribers. This opposition is based primarily on grounds of conflict of interest, but medicolegal considerations are also important. Most prescribers and many pharmacists are unaware of the Good Manufacturing Practices (GMP) standards of the FDA. Compounding of elegant, stable, therapeutically effective dosage forms requires special knowledge. Knowledge and techniques that ensure purity, sterility, clarity, bioavailability, predictable pharmacokinetics, stability, potency, and the expected therapeutic response necessitate a high level of professional sophistication and appropriate compounding and analytical equipment. Prescribers should write sparingly for dosage forms and delivery systems that require manipulation and compounding, and only when they are reasonably certain that pharmacists are particularly qualified and equipped to meet prescribers' objectives and patients' therapeutic needs. Product safety and efficacy are of paramount importance.

Compliance with Prescribed Drug Regimen

The fundamental, ubiquitous problem of patient noncompliance continues to be significant in the management of ocular disease in ambulatory outpatients. Much time, effort, and expense are directed at diagnosis and the subsequent selection of drug therapy, but what occurs beyond that point is often left to chance and its potential associated complications.

Some clinicians consider therapeutic noncompliance to be one of the most significant dilemmas facing medical practice today. It is discouraging that in an era when efficacious therapies exist, only about 50% to 75% of patients for whom appropriate therapy is prescribed derive full benefit from that therapy through strict adherence.

Clinicians tend to transfer to patients the blame for failure to comply with a prescribed drug regimen. Although this blame may be appropriately placed in some instances, prescribers and dispensers of medication have a large responsibility for ensuring that patients use their drugs properly. Greater appreciation of the incidence, causes, and clinical implications of therapeutic noncompliance allows a higher degree of role clarification, proper perspective, and, it is hoped, more vigorous and meaningful efforts to optimize therapeutic compliance and ocular health outcomes.

Incidence of Noncompliance

In an ambulatory population-at-large, a typical range of noncompliance is approximately 25% to 50%.[10] The range of noncompliance in a review of 50 compliance studies varied from 11% to 92%. Patients reportedly take only about 75% of prescribed doses of pilocarpine drops; 15% take less than one-half of the doses, and 6% take less than one-fourth the doses.[11] Unfortunately, no simple screening device helps practitioners identify the unreliable patient or accurately predicts the potential for patient noncompliance at the time of initial diagnosis.[12]

The failure to use medication properly takes many forms. Compliance errors involve skipping doses; taking medication for the wrong purpose, in the wrong dose, or at the wrong time; using outdated medication; using improper administration techniques; or prematurely discontinuing a prescription for an acute illness. The ultimate error in noncompliance is failing to get the prescription filled. Approximately 7% (126 million) of the 1.8 billion prescriptions written each year are never purchased. Compliance errors tend to result in overutilization or underutilization of one or more drugs.

Clinical Implications of Noncompliance

Noncompliance with a prescribed regimen frequently produces adverse sequelae. The nature of the consequences depends on the type of error. The most common errors of compliance are overutilization, underutilization, and administration of medications at inappropriate time intervals. The implications of underutilization are obvious. A large number of therapeutic failures result. In some cases noncompliant patients have been judged refractory to the prescribed treatment, and a more aggressive approach to treatment with a higher degree of side effect potential has been instituted.

Noncompliance that results in overutilization predisposes to drug-induced adverse effects. Some overzealous patients believe that if one dose is good, an extra one or two doses per day will be better and will hasten a cure or relief of symptoms. To compensate for missed doses, many patients, unaware of the biopharmaceutics, pharmacokinetics, and side effect profile of a particular drug, may double or triple doses at the next dosing interval.

Other compliance errors, including improper technique of administration, using medication for the wrong purpose, or using outdated medication, also have clinical implications. To optimize absorption, it is essential that appropriate techniques of administration be employed. This is particularly critical with routine ophthalmic solutions, suspensions, and ointments, special ophthalmic devices such as sustained-release inserts (e.g., Lacrisert, Ocusert), and unique packaging features such as the C-Cap Compliance caps available on several antiglaucoma medications (see Chapter 35). In addition, many patients may self-diagnose and use stored "left over" prescription medication to treat symptoms perceived to be similar to those for which the prescription was originally issued. If a drug is used to treat similar symptoms at a later date, the drug could have aged or otherwise deteriorated due to excessive extremes of heat and moisture to subpotent, inactive or toxic constituents.

Reasons for Noncompliance

The correlation between noncompliance and several variables has been tested. Significant relationships appear to exist between noncompliance and the factors listed in Table 4.7.[13] The most important reasons for therapeutic noncompliance appear to relate most often to (1) complexity of the drug regimen, (2) lack of understanding of the nature of the illness and the importance of drug therapy, and (3) failure to thoroughly understand the instructions for proper use. Frequency of interpretive errors of instructions on prescription labels ranges between 9% and 64%. For example, a label instructing patients taking the diuretic furosemide to "take one tablet as needed for fluid retention" led one patient to believe the drug would cause fluid retention. The instruction to "force fluids" on a prescription for a sulfonamide-containing prescription was interpreted to mean "strain during urination."

It is a mistake for ophthalmic practitioners to assume that the drug-consuming public is knowledgeable and understanding. The public's knowledge level and ability to comprehend is highly stratified. Health professionals tend to overestimate intellectual sophistication of patients, who generally make no request for clarification or additional information. Documented research shows that it may not

TABLE 4.7
Factors Associated with Noncompliance

Advancing age
Duration of therapy
Number of drugs in the regimen
Frequency of administration
Drug-induced adverse effects
Asymptomatic disease or relief of symptoms
Fear of drug dependence or addiction
Interference with daily routine
Poor palatability of drug
Absence of a viable patient-prescriber relationship
Excessive waiting to see the prescriber or pharmacist
Distrust of the health care system
Lack of continuity of care
Nature of the illness
Cost of the medication

even be enough to supplement written words with verbal instructions. Practitioners should make sure that patients truly comprehend the essence of the message by asking them questions or by encouraging them to ask questions. This validation is frequently missing in practitioner-patient encounters.

To some degree, maximizing compliance must be an individualized process. Good communication skills are essential. Warm, empathetic, sincere prescribers generate confidence and trust. Patients cannot be frightened, coerced, or threatened into compliance. Instead, they should be educated, advised, and encouraged. Patient education and understanding are cornerstones in achieving high levels of pharmacotherapeutic compliance.

Patient Education and Counseling Considerations

Recognition by both health care providers and patients that medication can be of maximal benefit only if used properly is still not sufficiently reflected in patient compliance and drug consumption patterns. Some have suggested that far better instructions are provided on the use and maintenance of automobiles, cameras, television sets, and kitchen appliances than potent drugs. These medications have the potential not only to do great good but also to produce morbidity and even mortality if not used properly.

Many factors contribute to effective patient education and counseling, including the verbal communication skills of prescribers and pharmacists, the counseling atmosphere and environment, and the receptivity of patients. The education and counseling of patients about their ocular disease and drug therapy involves the following fundamentals:[14]

1. Name of the person for whom the medication is intended. Make patients aware that prescription medication is to be used only by the individual whose name appears on the label. Potent prescription drugs are never to be used for what are perceived to be similar symptoms in other individuals. Lay people are simply not qualified to make an objective, informed differential diagnosis of others and then prescribe medication for them. Such practices have led to serious adverse health consequences.

2. Purpose of the medication. With few exceptions, patients should know what the prescribed medication is intended to treat. General terms understood by lay people are preferred (e.g., "pink eye," glaucoma, granulated eyelids, stye).

3. Name of the medication. A prescription label should contain the generic name of the drug (and brand name if applicable). Exceptions to this routine practice rarely exist. This information can be valuable for discussions of drug therapy with health care providers and dispensing pharmacists. This practice also allows easier and more positive identification of the drug if overdose occurs.

4. Directions for using the medication. It is dangerous to assume that most patients use all medication properly. Prescription labels and any instructional "how to use" information contained in the package may be difficult to understand or may be subject to multiple interpretations. Furthermore, the various precautions and warnings that exist for all drugs must be observed if therapy is to be optimal. Patients themselves bear considerable responsibility for the achievement of the best possible therapeutic outcome, but they can fulfill their responsibility only if health care providers supply effective "how to use" information. Particular attention should be given to counseling patients who use drugs other than in oral forms. Most ophthalmic pharmacotherapy involves topical preparations, and special attention should be given to careful instruction in the use of eyedrops and ointments.

5. Schedule for medication administration. Patients must be made aware of appropriate time intervals between drug doses. Timing of administration may affect absorption and blood or ocular levels of the drug. Clinicians should provide verbal definition of label instructions (e.g., before meals, after meals, at bedtime; 2, 3, or 4 times daily; every 4, 6, or 12 hours; on an empty stomach). "As directed" is considered an inappropriate form of patient instruction.

6. Duration of treatment. Patients should be encouraged to take a full course of therapy for an acute condition unless untoward events occur. This is particularly critical with antibiotics and other anti-infectives, where failure to take the full course of therapy may lead to a therapeutic failure and reinfection. Patients on chronic maintenance therapy should be counseled about the importance of acquiring refills on time, continuous therapy, and potential risk associated with abrupt discontinuation of certain drugs such as corticosteroids.

7. Maximum daily dose. The dose recommended on the prescription label is considered the maximum daily dose and should not be exceeded unless authorized. This is particularly critical with drugs having a narrow therapeutic index or high abuse potential. Clinicians should note that almost all drug-induced adverse events are dose-related. Increasing doses beyond those prescribed seldom results in additional therapeutic benefits but may markedly increase the risk of experiencing one or more serious adverse drug effects.

8. Side effects. All drugs have the potential to produce side effects. Patients should be warned about those most likely to occur and told when they should report these untoward events. In many instances, precautions may be taken to minimize risk. Slight decreases in drug doses sometimes diminish substantially the intensity of one or more side effects without compromising the therapeutic benefit.

9. Drug interactions. Many prescription and nonprescription drugs may interact adversely with one another, and certain drugs may also interact with components of some foods (see Chapter 36). Drugs may also alter the results of some laboratory tests. Many drug interactions are of little or no clinical significance, and some drugs or foods may be given together if the potential value of the drug combination outweighs the potential risk. Some interactions lead to such significant problems, however, that some drug combinations are absolutely contraindicated. Prescribers have the clinical ability to differentiate levels of significance and act accordingly on the behalf of patients.

10. Storage. Special requirements for storage of certain drugs are frequently underappreciated or overlooked. Proper storage is required for drug stability and maintenance of potency. Patients must understand the importance of proper storage (e.g., refrigeration, protection from sunlight, protection from moisture, avoidance of extreme heat). Practitioners should repeat the importance of keeping all medication out of children's reach.

11. Miscellaneous considerations. A variety of specific instructions unique to a particular drug regimen or a specific patient may be required. For example, patients may require special directions for preparation or administration of drugs, reviews of precautions to be observed during therapy, techniques for self-monitoring therapy, prescription refill information, or action to take in the event of a missed dose. Providing this information requires professional judgement and communication skills. Both ophthalmic practitioners and dispensing pharmacists are responsible for tailoring drug information to meet specific therapeutic goals and needs of patients in a manner conducive to their understanding.

Professional practice standards for patient education and counseling are rapidly becoming legal and regulatory mandates. Overreliance on prescription labels to communicate the essential message is not in the public interest, primarily because of the size limitations of prescription labels. The synergistic combination of a complete prescription label and appropriate verbal counseling appears to be effective in patients' ability to recall critical information. Supplemental instructional leaflets, brochures, or information sheets make an optimal therapeutic outcome even more probable.

Practitioners, however, must recognize the great difference between "providing information" and "educating." Validation of understanding is critical. Patients should be encouraged to comment and ask questions. Further initiatives in the realm of patient education and counseling relative to proper drug use are needed.

The Drug Development and Approval Process

The US drug development and approval process is complex and laborious but brings new drugs to the marketplace with a high assurance of both safety and efficacy.[15-17] The United States remains the global leader in pharmaceutical development, and over $200 million in research and development costs is required to bring a single new drug to the market. The FDA interprets, enforces, and manages the reasonably well-defined new drug approval process, which has its foundation in the Food, Drug and Cosmetic Act of 1938 and numerous subsequent amendments. The new drug approval process has been given further definition and structure in numerous additional federal regulations, legislation, and guidelines. The new drug approval process has three principal elements.[17]

- Testing for safety and efficacy through nonclinical and clinical studies
- Preparing and submitting drug and drug-related data and information to the FDA through investigational new drug applications (INDs) and new drug applications (NDAs)
- FDA review of IND and NDA submissions

These elements are detailed further in the following steps.[17]

Discovery

Discovery begins in the laboratory where various scientific applications converge. People tend to think of this phase as the stage of drug development where new molecular entities and "breakthrough" drugs are discovered, but in fact, drugs may meet criteria for qualification as a "new" drug in many ways. New drugs may be new, novel molecular entities never before used as drugs, chemicals known for some time but never used as medicines in the United States (e.g., naturally occurring substances, chemicals marketed as drugs in other countries), or drugs previously approved by the FDA for which new uses, dosage forms, routes of administration, or other clinically significant applications are requested.

Preclinical Testing

Preclinical screening and testing in laboratory and animal studies is performed to obtain basic toxicologic and pharmacologic information and to assess primary safety and biologic activity. Toxicity testing may evaluate acute, subacute, and chronic toxicity; carcinogenicity; mutagenicity; and teratogenic potential. Preclinical studies in laboratory and animal models are imperfect predictors of clinical response, but they remain the best practical screening methodology for assessing dose-response characteristics, adverse effects, pharmacokinetic characteristics, mechanisms, and sites and durations of drug action for potential use in humans. Preclinical testing requires an average of 3.5 years for compounds that show promise. Only about one in five potential therapies progresses past animal testing, and only about one of every 1,000 compounds originally tested in preclinical studies becomes commercially available.

Investigational New Drug Application (IND)

If a drug shows promise in preclinical testing, the drug sponsor files an IND with the FDA seeking permission to begin drug testing in humans. The FDA generally requires that the IND contain a pharmacologic profile, acute toxicity data in several species of animals using the route of administration proposed for clinical use, and short-term toxicity studies (2 weeks to 3 months). The drug sponsor submits prescribed information in four specific areas: animal toxicology, manufacturing information, clinical protocols for proposed human testing, and investigator qualifications. The FDA requires that the holders of INDs continually update their IND with information that periodically allows the FDA to reassess the safety of ongoing and proposed clinical trials as well as to inspect investigator qualifications. The IND allows for interstate shipment of unapproved drugs to investigators. The IND becomes effective if the FDA does not disapprove it within 30 days of submission.

As the drug progresses to clinical testing, the FDA sets standards for clinical evaluation to ensure that data derived from trials are accurate. It also attempts to protect human subjects involved in testing. FDA guidelines known as Good Clinical Practice (GCP) standards and General Considerations for the Clinical Evaluation of Drugs and other guidelines assist sponsors, investigators, monitors, Institutional Review Boards, and others relative to appropriate clinical testing standards and expectations. Sponsors are required to report data to the FDA after the completion of each phase of clinical testing.

Phase I Clinical Trials

Phase I studies represent the first use of a new drug in humans. The focus of this highly exploratory phase of testing is determination of the safety profile and safe dosage range of the drug. The drug's pharmacokinetics and pharmacodynamics are assessed, and data are obtained concerning such parameters as onset and duration of action. Whether single-dose or short-term multiple dose studies, they should be placebo-controlled. Between 20 and 100 subjects, who should be healthy volunteers free from abnormalities that might complicate interpretation of results, are usually involved. Historically, a gender bias toward males has existed. Phase I clinical testing usually requires 6 months to 1 year to complete, and approximately 30% of drugs studied are not tested further.

Phase II Clinical Trials

Phase II trials shift the focus from safety to efficacy. Patients who suffer from the disease or condition the drug is intended to treat are used as subjects. Because adverse effects or drug toxicity are still a concern, 100 to 500 fairly homogeneous volunteers make up the study population. Relatively short, closely monitored, placebo-controlled or dose-comparison, double-masked, randomized studies are used to assess efficacy, optimal dose, and adverse effects. Phase II trials may take 2 to 5 years. Approximately 35% of drugs studied are not tested further.

Phase III Clinical Trials

Phase III ("pivotal") testing involves drug evaluation under conditions more closely resembling those under which the drug would be used if approved for marketing. The total study population usually ranges between 1,000 and 3,000 patients. To ensure a more representative population, volunteers are more heterogeneous than those selected for phase II studies. Phase III studies tend to be multicenter, double-masked, placebo-controlled, multiple end-point and long-term with a continuing focus on safety, efficacy, and optimal dosing. Testing may take 2 to 4 years. Approximately 5% of drugs in phase III trials are not studied further.

New Drug Application (NDA)

The NDA is the vehicle through which a sponsor formally requests FDA approval to market a new drug in the United States. After all three phases of clinical testing are completed, thousands of pages of data and information supporting the safety and efficacy of the drug for its proposed use are submitted to the FDA for review. Explicit NDA content and formatting requirements have recently been revised and restructured to expedite FDA review. The NDA assesses the drug's chemistry, processes of manufacturing and control, preclinical pharmacology and toxicology, human pharmacokinetics and bioavailability, and microbiology (if applicable). Clinical data, statistical evaluations, proposed labeling and packaging, case report tabulations (if necessary), case report forms, and publications are also evaluated.

If a drug has been previously approved and the sponsor wishes to change the manufacturing process or specific sections of the labeling, a less rigorous submission process is available through a Supplemental New Drug Application (SNDA). Changes in indications, labeling (package insert), manufacturing and quality control methods, route of administration, dosage form, dosage schedule, strength, formulation, and container or closure system require an SNDA.

Food and Drug Administration Review of New Drug Applications

Voluminous and complex NDAs, once received by the FDA, are assigned to one of nine review divisions of the FDA Center of Drug Evaluation and Research (CDER). Major steps in the FDA review of a submitted NDA are acknowledgement of receipt; designation of sponsor's contact person at FDA; determination of suitability for filing, which must occur within 60 days of receipt; setting of review priority; simultaneous review by FDA review teams; sponsor-FDA dialogue; provision of safety updates and additional data by sponsor; and issuance of FDA action letter (approvable, approval, or nonapprovable). Once approved, the drug may be released to the market.

According to federal law, the FDA must send the action letter to the sponsor within 180 days of receipt. The 180-day FDA review may be extended only when major amendments are submitted to the NDA. However, the average FDA review requires 24 to 30 months. Several factors contribute to this delay, including insufficient FDA funding and staffing, highly error-intolerant US Congress and public, backlog of submissions, priority for breakthrough drugs, increasing complexity of submissions, and accountability of sponsors and reviewers.

Phase IV Clinical Trials

Phase IV testing, which may continue after FDA approval of an NDA, is a component of postmarketing surveillance activity. This testing represents an excellent method of gathering more data on safety and efficacy or identifying some competitive health outcome, quality of life, cost-benefit, or cost-effectiveness advantage for a product.

Phase IV studies may be FDA-requested or sponsor-initiated. The FDA, however, does not have the legal or regulatory authority necessary to require phase IV testing. Between 1986 and 1988 the FDA requested phase IV testing in 22% of cases, and voluntary compliance by drug sponsors to postmarketing data requests by the FDA is high.

The FDA drug review and approval process has been refined substantially over time, particularly since the early 1990s. Several relatively new developments and potential changes in the FDA new drug review and approval process appear to be in the public's best health interests. These include attention to expedited clinical testing and accelerated approval for drugs that show significant promise against serious, life-threatening diseases such as cancer and acquired immunodeficiency syndrome (AIDS); parallel tracks allowing use of experimental therapies in AIDS patients as soon as possible in the drug development process; compassionate-use protocols in patients with severe or life-threatening conditions under a treatment IND; and safety testing harmonization that would sanction recognition by the FDA of safety data obtained in foreign countries in the US equivalent of phase I testing. External review committees, expanded use of advisory committees, users' fees, and electronic NDA submissions have also refined the drug approval process.

References

1. Olin BR (ed). The Professionals Guide to Patient Drug Facts. St. Louis: Facts and Comparisons. 1994, IX–X.
2. Anon. Practice Standards of ASHP. Bethesda: American Society of Hospital Pharmacists. 1991–92. 24.
3. Ansel HC. The Prescription. In: Remington's Practice of Pharmacy. Philadelphia: Mack Publishing. 1990;1828–41.
4. Holt GA, Parker R. Introduction to Pharmacy Practice. Birmingham: Holt Publishing, 1993;65.
5. Covington TR. Patient Education and Compliance. In: Brown TR, Smith MC. Handbook of Institutional Pharmacy Practice, ed. 2. Chapter 57. Baltimore: Williams & Wilkins. 1986.
6. Holt GA, Parker R. Introduction to Pharmacy Practice. Birmingham: Holt Publishing, 1993;100.
7. Tatro DS. Unlabeled Use of FDA-Approved Drugs. Facts and Comparisons Drug Newsletter. 1990;9:49–50.
8. Covington TR. Generic Drug Utilization: Overview and Guidelines for Prudent Use. American Druggist. 1991 (Suppl).
9. Holt GA, Parker R. Introduction to Pharmacy Practice. Birmingham: Holt Publishing, 1993;196.
10. Knowles MR. Improving Patient Compliance. Proceedings of a Symposium. Washington, DC. National Pharmaceutical Council. 1985.
11. Kass MA, Meltzer DW, Gordon M, et al. Compliance with topical pilocarpine treatment. Am J Ophthalmol 1986;101:515–23.
12. Kass MA, Gordon M, Meltzer DW. Can ophthalmologists correctly identify patients defaulting from pilocarpine therapy? Am J Ophthalmol 1986;101:524–30.
13. Bond WS. Medication noncompliance. Facts and Comparisons Drug Newsletter. 1990;9:33–35.
14. Covington TR. Talk About Prescriptions. Facts and Comparisons Drug Newsletter. 1990;9:76–77.
15. Novack GD. The development of new drugs for ophthalmology. Am J Ophthalmol 1992;114:357–64.
16. Young FE. From test tube to patient: New drug development in the United Sates. Washington, DC: Food and Drug Administration Special Report. 1988.
17. Covington TR. Birth of a Drug: The U.S. Drug Development and Approval Process. Facts and Comparisons Drug Newsletter. 1992;11:73–75.

CHAPTER 5

Legal Aspects of Drug Utilization

John G. Classé

Numerous legal issues are involved in the use or prescription of pharmaceutical agents by optometrists. Legislation permitting ophthalmic drug use is the most significant legal event affecting optometry in the past 25 years. Issues such as certification, registration, and comanagement are contemporary offshoots of the regulatory process. Responsibility for care is another important legal issue, requiring optometrists to understand and comply with the demands of informed consent, negligence law, and product liability law. Each of these legal concepts has a unique influence on the clinical practice of optometry and the use of ophthalmic drugs. In the following sections, these issues and their relevance for practitioners of optometry are described, beginning with the most fundamental consideration of all, the legal authority by which clinicians are permitted to use pharmaceutical agents.

Legal Basis for Drug Use in Optometry

The use of drugs while rendering professional services has not traditionally been included within the clinical scope of optometry. The reason lies in the historical basis for the licensure of optometrists. The clinical practice of optometry began as an extension of the science of optics, in a lineage that can be traced back for centuries.[1] This development occurred quite independently of medicine, which eschewed refractive services in favor of the use of drugs and surgery to treat disorders of the eye. In America, the two callings continued to evolve separately, although the clinical distinction between them lessened when physicians began practicing refraction as a "medical" function. The situation was further complicated by the emergence of two types of opticians: dispensing opticians, who performed no refractive services and whose sole function was to dispense ophthalmic materials on a physician's prescription; and refracting opticians (the forerunners of optometrists), who performed refractions, detected disease, and dispensed their own ophthalmic materials. In performing these services the refracting opticians were in direct competition with physicians who offered eyecare.[a] By the late 1800s physicians began to regard these services as "infringing" on the practice of medicine because of the licensure laws passed by the states to regulate medicine.

The practice of medicine was largely unregulated during the first half of the 19th century, and legitimate physicians dispaired over their inability to prevent quackery and to stem the proliferation of cult practitioners and unsound practices.[2] Their major problem was the lack of regulatory standards for medical schools, which produced graduates of widely varying levels of knowledge, skill, and experience. A solution was found in licensure: medical school graduates would be required to pass an examination and receive a license before they would be legally entitled to practice their profession within a state. Beginning in the 1870s the "modern" medical practice acts were passed to achieve this end, and they succeeded in elevating both the competence and the esteem of physicians nationwide.[2] However, out of necessity the laws incorporated a definition of medicine that was suffi-

---

[a]Physicians were themselves divided into different camps: ophthalmologists, who were physicians who had undergone a residency in medical and surgical management of the eye and had restricted their practice to the eye; and oculists, who were physicians who had learned eyecare through experience (without the benefit of formal training) and who specialized in treatment of the eye. In addition, general practitioners treated eye problems, including refractive errors, as part of the general practice of medicine.

ciently broad to regulate any form of medical practice, including refraction. Refracting opticians, themselves unlicensed, found that their historical right to practice their calling was subservient to the legal right of the states to prevent them from doing so (under the guise of illegally practicing medicine). It was a situation ripe for conflict between the refracting opticians and their physician rivals, the ophthalmologists.

Legislative Authorization

The "legalization" of optometry began with the efforts of Charles Prentice of New York City, whose Optical Society for the State of New York drafted the first bill intended to regulate the practice of "optometry."[3] Introduced in the New York legislature in 1897, the law required licensure of any individual—whether optician or physician—seeking to practice refraction and related services. Regulation was to be achieved through a four-member Board of Optometry. Prentice and his colleagues, realizing that compromise was necessary to have the bill passed, agreed to an all-physician board as demanded by the opposing ophthalmologists. Despite this concession, physicians killed the bill, thereby ending the best opportunity they were to have to prevent the licensure of optometrists.[4] But Prentice's idea caught the imagination of refracting opticians across the country, and in 1901 the state of Minnesota enacted the first optometry practice act.[1] This law recognized the practice of optometry, provided for examination and licensure, and established an all-optician board for regulatory purposes. Physicians were expressly exempted from the provisions of the law. In states throughout the nation similar laws were introduced, but to secure their passage the legislatures had to be convinced that the practice of optometry was not an aspect of medicine. Prentice and others devised strategies to impress this point on legislators, inventing slogans such as "a lens is not a pill" and "a lens treats light" to illustrate the difference between the two professions. A widely discussed lawsuit, brought at the urging of Albert Fitch of Philadelphia,[5] resulted in a ruling that optometry was not a branch of medicine and thus could not be regulated by physicians.[6] The distinction was further emphasized by the actual bills being introduced in the legislatures, which expressly or implicitly prohibited the use of drugs and surgery because these were "medical" functions. This strategy was successful; by 1924 all states and the District of Columbia had passed optometry laws. But the result was a drugless profession.

Judicial Regulation

By the late 1960s optometrists found the restrictive nature of these laws to be incompatible with their newly assumed role as health care providers. The ophthalmoscope was routinely used to detect abnormalities; the tonometer and the contact lens required physical contact with the eye; and participation in Medicare, Medicaid, and other health insurance plans obligated the optometrist to make "medical" diagnoses. As a result, optometry became recognized as an aspect of health care, serving as an entry point into the system for persons with eye disease or ocular manifestations of systemic disease. Clinicians were frustrated because they were prevented from using some ophthalmic equipment and instrumentation by the statutory prohibitions against use of pharmaceutical agents in state optometry laws. Thus began a movement that has not yet run its course, the effort to amend the original optometry practice acts to permit optometrists to use pharmaceutical agents.

The first state law expressly authorizing the use of ophthalmic drugs was enacted in 1971 by the Rhode Island legislature, after three years of effort. This law, which allowed Rhode Island optometrists to use drugs for diagnostic purposes, was the beginning of a new era in optometry. It was also the cause of a lawsuit, testing the right of state legislatures to pass such laws.[7]

Although the right to enact laws is strictly a legislative function, it is the duty of the courts, when presented with a case or controversy, to examine laws to ensure that they do not conflict with the constitution. Therefore, although a law may be duly enacted, it is void if the courts rule it is unconstitutional. Such was the purpose of the Rhode Island case. The lawsuit was brought by the Rhode Island Ophthalmological Society, which maintained that the legislature had endangered the public health by permitting optometrists to use ophthalmic drugs for diagnosis. The ophthalmologists argued that the law was an unconstitutional exercise of legislative power and that it would cause them economic injury. Both the trial court and the Rhode Island Supreme Court rejected the ophthalmologists' arguments, and the law was not subjected to further challenge.[8] A similar fate awaited the first law authorizing optometric use of drugs for therapeutic purposes, passed by the West Virginia legislature in 1976. The law was immediately subjected to legal attack by ophthalmologists, who argued that it was an unconstitutional application of the legislature's duty to protect the public from injury.[8,9] But again this argument was rejected, with the courts observing that the scope of optometric services was a legislative matter and that if the legislature conferred on optometrists the authority to use drugs for therapeutic purposes, such an exercise of legislative power was constitutional.[9]

Further changes in the scope of optometry practice acts may bring additional litigation. It should be noted, however, that no power ever granted to optometrists by the legislatures has been ruled unconstitutional by the courts, and it seems reasonable to assume that subsequent amendments of state optometry laws permitting an expanded scope of practice will meet a similar judicial response if challenged.

Administrative Regulation

Although the right to use ophthalmic drugs may be authorized by a jurisdiction's optometry statutes, various legal requirements may have to be satisfied to exercise this right. Two common requirements are certification and registration.

CERTIFICATION

To use pharmaceutical agents, optometrists must have been granted this right at licensure[b] or must be certified by the board of optometry as qualified to exercise it. Certification—a process of education and examination—is necessary to ensure that ophthalmic drugs are used only by qualified practitioners. Optometrists who have satisfied the educational requirements and have passed the examination are given a certificate, which usually must be displayed with the optometrist's license. Certification confers legal standing on practitioners to use the permitted pharmaceutical agents within the bounds of state law. If optometrists act outside the scope of certification, however, such actions may subject them to discipline by the state board of optometry. Similarly, if optometrists use drugs in the course of patient care without first obtaining the necessary certification, they may be disciplined by the board, even though state law authorizes use of the drug by optometrists.[10] Certification is a legal prerequisite to drug use in these circumstances, and failure to satisfy certification requirements violates the optometry practice act.

REGISTRATION

Even if optometrists have complied with licensure and certification requirements, certain federal regulations must be observed if they wish to use controlled substances. The dispensing of central nervous system drugs with significant potential for abuse is regulated by federal law,[11,12] and enforcement is the responsibility of the Drug Enforcement Administration (DEA). If a state optometry practice act (or board ruling) authorizes the use of controlled substances, optometrists must register with the DEA and obtain a registration number before using these drugs clinically. The DEA number must also be written on any prescription for controlled substances given to patients. Failure to observe these requirements violates federal law (see Chapter 4). An addi-

tional administrative matter concerns the dispensing of drugs to patients by optometrists. Although state pharmacy acts regulate the sale of pharmaceutical products to consumers, direct sale by licensed health care practitioners to patients is usually excluded from the provisions of these laws. Therefore, unless prohibited by the optometry practice act, optometrists may dispense pharmaceutical agents to patients directly. If controlled substances are among the drugs provided to patients, optometrists must be certain to comply with all record-keeping requirements.

COMANAGEMENT

Under certain circumstances optometrists may, in conjunction with physicians, participate in the prescribing or dispensing of pharmaceutical agents under the physicians' authority. These circumstances most commonly arise in multidisciplinary settings and in practices in which optometrists and physicians work together. Practitioners in separate offices may also find cooperation necessary under certain types of circumstances, such as postoperative care or long-term management of disease. The physician and optometrist comanage patients' care through a delegation of responsibility to the optometrist, who acts in place of the physician to examine patients and monitor treatment. The optometrist's role is described in a comanagement protocol that is specifically written for the individual optometrist and that carefully delineates the conditions for which cooperative care may be undertaken.[13] The mode of treatment (tests to be performed, drug dosages, scheduled patient follow-up) are also specified in the document (Fig. 5.1). The optometrist, while following the comanagement protocol, is acting as the agent of the physician, who remains primarily responsible for the patient's well-being. Communication between practitioners is an essential feature of this type of care. The optometrist should confer with the physician within a reasonable period after examination concerning patient findings, and the physician should receive a written copy of the optometrist's records (by mail or facsimile transmission) following the examination. These formalities are necessary to ensure that the comanagement protocol is being properly followed.

Should the optometrist be negligent while acting within the scope of the comanagement protocol, both the physician and optometrist share legal responsibility for any injury suffered by patients.[14] If the optometrist acts outside the limits of delegated authority, or in contravention to them, the optometrist is solely liable for any negligence. For this reason the physician must place great confidence in the optometrist's knowledge and skill before entering into a comanagement arrangement. To limit the potential for liability problems, legal and insurance counsel should be consulted before initiating a comanagement relationship. Under a comanagement protocol, the prescribing of drugs for treatment remains the responsibility of the physician. An optom-

---

[b]A license confers upon the licensee all rights that may be exercised in the jurisdiction. Therefore, optometrists who qualify for licensure within a state receive a license that enables them to employ all the techniques and methods available to optometrists within that state. For example, if the state allows the use of therapeutic pharmaceutical agents by optometrists, successful passage of the licensing examination confers on optometrists the right to use these agents. Optometrists who are already licensed at the time the definition of optometry is changed will have to be certified before they can use this new right. Thus, certification inevitably occurs after licensure.

All glaucoma patients will receive follow-up care according to the following criteria:

Primary Open-angle Glaucoma

1. All glaucoma suspects should be worked up on the attached form—Initial Glaucoma Workup form.
2. Gonioscopy should be performed only with Cell-U-Visc to minimize corneal trauma prior to visual field test performance.
3. The attending physician must be consulted prior to the visual field test to determine which field is to be performed.
4. Perform the visual field test with the appropriate correcting lens in place for 33 cm and always enter the patient's birthdate.
5. A consultation must be scheduled on Glaucoma Day or Family Practice Day prior to initiation of therapy except in the instance of emergencies.
6. All diagnosed and treated glaucoma patients must have a Glaucoma Control Flow Chart attached to the outside of their progress note cover.
7. All glaucoma progress checks must be entered on the Glaucoma Follow-up form and are to be faxed to the prescribing physician the day of the visit.
8. All patients must receive a schedule of when to use the medications on the Med Use form as well as a patient information sheet.
9. Glaucoma patients should be scheduled every 3 months and must be seen once a year by the prescribing ophthalmologist. The appointment should be made prior to leaving the clinic.
10. Patients requiring a refill or medication change necessitate a phone call to the prescribing physician, with the record faxed to the physician's office that day. The physician needs the name and phone number of the pharmacy when the phone call is placed.
11. Visual field tests are to be repeated on at least a yearly basis.

Argon Laser Trabeculoplasty

1. A referral letter must be sent to the ophthalmologist at the time the appointment is made for argon laser trabeculoplasty.
2. The patient is usually returned 1 week post-op using a topical steroid.
3. The patient is to be billed at 10% of the surgical fee for post-op care.
4. If pressure spiked above pre-op level, call the surgeon. If IOP is reduced below or at pre-op level, taper the steroid.
5. Reschedule for continuing follow-up visits according to the guidance of the attending physician, maximum 1 month later.

FIGURE 5.1   Example protocol for the management of patients with open-angle glaucoma. (Courtesy of the School of Optometry, University of Alabama at Birmingham.)

etrist who uses a pharmaceutical agent that is outside the scope of practice commits an act for which discipline may be imposed by the appropriate state regulatory agency.[c] Even an averral that the circumstances constituted an "emergency" cannot provide legal justification for such an act, for Good Samaritan statutes do not provide legal immunity for in-office procedures even if the condition threatens vision.[d]

---

[c]Optometrists who commit an act that is outside the scope of licensure are subject to discipline by the state board of optometry. Disciplinary measures that the board may use include reprimand, suspension of licensure, and revocation of licensure. Boards may also seek injunctions against continuation of the prohibited activity or may enter into consent agreements in which the defendant optometrist agrees not to continue the proscribed conduct. See Classé JG. Legal aspects of optometry. Boston: Butterworth, 1989;152–180.

[d]Good Samaritan statutes in most states do not include optometrists as a covered party. Furthermore, these statutes do not provide legal protection for in-office treatment of routine ocular urgencies or emergencies. See Classé JG. Legal aspects of optometry. Boston: Butterworth, 1989;201–206.

Optometrists must understand the proscriptions of state optometry laws with regard to the use of ophthalmic drugs and must observe these limitations. Although comanagement allows an optometrist to participate in the medical management of certain types of patients (e.g., patients with glaucoma, individuals needing postoperative care for cataract), the role of the optometrist is to monitor care under the physician-initiated treatment plan. It does not provide legal justification for acts outside the scope of licensure.

The right to use drugs entails certain legal obligations, which are intended to protect patients from the risk of injury. These obligations include the doctrine of informed consent, which in some circumstances requires optometrists to inform patients of the side effects and risks of drug use; the duty to conform to the standard of care, the breach of which may subject optometrists to an action for negligence; and product liability law, under which optometrists can be drawn into the legal dispute created by a drug that is unreasonably dangerous and injures patients. These matters are discussed in the following sections.

Informed Consent

An important legal duty that must be observed by health care practitioners is the duty of affirmative disclosure, which obliges practitioners to communicate warnings, findings, and other pertinent information to patients. The reason for this obligation lies in the legal status that doctors occupy as *fiduciaries*, persons who occupy a special position of trust and confidence with those they serve.[15] The function of this duty of disclosure is to enable the less knowledgeable patient to understand the treatment recommended by the doctor. It has long been a precept of American law that no treatment may be undertaken without the consent of the patient, a philosophy succinctly stated by Judge Benjamin Cardozo[16]: "Any human being of adult years and sound mind has a right to determine what shall be done with his own body; and a surgeon who performs an operation without his patient's consent commits an assault, for which he is liable for damages."

Cardozo's opinion concerned a case in which surgery was performed without the patient's consent, but the principle he expressed can be applied to any procedure that contains some risk of patient harm. Treatment may not be instituted without the patient's consent, and this consent cannot be legally secured without the patient's being informed of the hazards, the possible complications, and both the expected and the unexpected results of treatment. In addition, practitioners must not make any misrepresentations, either by misstating known facts or by withholding pertinent information. This requirement forms the basis for the doctrine of informed consent.

Requirements for informed consent can arise in many areas of optometry: in the diagnosis of disease,[17] in contact lens practice,[18] when recommending binocular vision therapy,[19] or when ophthalmic drugs are used.[20] The latter category is one that has grown in importance as optometric drug utilization has increased. Optometrists must understand their legal obligation to discuss the risks of pharmaceutical use and must comply with the doctrine of informed consent when doing so. This legal duty has two aspects: (1) recognizing when the duty arises, and (2) determining the amount of information that must be divulged.

Disclosure Requirements

Generally speaking, optometrists must disclose to patients information sufficient to engender informed consent. But the legal test of how much information must be divulged to satisfy this duty varies among the states. In fact, conflicting opinions have been expressed by the courts and have proved to be a source of consternation for health care practitioners.[21] Even so, these opinions must be understood and complied with, since informed consent issues routinely arise in clinical practice.[22]

Two standards may be applied to determine if practitioners have met disclosure requirements: a "professional community" standard and a "reasonable patient" standard.

THE "PROFESSIONAL COMMUNITY" STANDARD

The first court decisions applied the same legal test to informed consent cases as was applied to negligence cases: the practitioner was held to the standard of the reasonable person.[23] Liability was imposed if the practitioner was found to have breached the duty to act as a reasonable practitioner would have acted under the same or similar circumstances. In determining the standard of care expected of the practitioner, the courts allowed other practitioners to testify concerning the warnings or disclosures that were necessary. Hence, the standard was a profession-set one, based on expert testimony and determined by the conduct of other practitioners. If the defendant practitioner divulged that amount of information deemed to be reasonable by other practitioners, then a breach of duty did not occur.

A sample case may be used to illustrate the application of the "professional community" rule.[24] A patient with a corneal foreign body was examined by an ophthalmologist, who removed the metallic foreign body and attempted to debride the rust ring that had formed around it. The procedure resulted in permanent corneal scarring. The patient sued the ophthalmologist, alleging that the risk of scarring had not been described and that the attempt to remove the rust ring had been undertaken without the patient's consent. In determining that the ophthalmologist was not liable, the court held that the scope of the physician's disclosure should be measured by the disclosures that would be made by an ophthalmologist in the community acting under the same or

TABLE 5.1
States Applying the "Professional Community" Standard

Arizona	Illinois	Nevada
Arkansas	Indiana	New Hampshire
Colorado	Kansas	North Carolina
Delaware	Maine	North Dakota
Florida	Massachusetts	South Carolina
Georgia	Michigan	South Dakota
Hawaii	Missouri	Virginia
Idaho	Montana	Wyoming

Adapted from "Modern status of views as to general measure of physician's duty to inform patient of risks of proposed treatment," 88 ALR 3d 1008.

similar circumstances. The defendant was found to have met this requirement.

The "professional community" rule was adopted in a number of states (Table 5.1), but it was soon rivaled by another rule, which is found today in a majority of jurisdictions.

THE "REASONABLE PATIENT" STANDARD

This standard is based on what a reasonable patient must know rather than on what a reasonable practitioner must divulge.[25] Evidence is offered to establish what a prudent person in the patient's position would have done if adequately informed of all significant risks. Patients no longer must obtain expert testimony, because the issue concerns what they need to know rather than what practitioners are reasonably expected to divulge.

The standard may be illustrated by a sample case.[26] A patient with an eye laceration was treated by an ophthalmologist, who repaired the laceration but did not attempt to remove a metallic corneal foreign body. By the next day an infection developed, and the patient was referred by the ophthalmologist to another physician. Although treatment was instituted and the foreign body removed, the infection ultimately resulted in enucleation. The patient sued the ophthalmologist, arguing that the doctrine of informed consent required the ophthalmologist to inform the patient of the risk of delay in removing the foreign body. The court held that the ophthalmologist had a duty to disclose the risks or hazards that a reasonable person would need to know in order to make an informed decision concerning a medical or surgical procedure. Failure to make this disclosure, if it would have caused the patient to proceed differently, constituted a breach of the doctrine of informed consent. The "reasonable patient" standard has become the subject of much discussion in the medical profession, although studies of professional liability cases have shown that physicians are rarely subjected to informed consent claims.[27] Jurisdictions that have adopted this objective standard are listed in Table 5.2.[28]

TABLE 5.2
States Applying the "Reasonable Patient" Standard

Alabama	Minnesota	Pennsylvania
Alaska	Mississippi	Rhode Island
California	Nebraska	Tennessee
Connecticut	New Jersey	Texas
District of Columbia	New Mexico	Utah
Iowa	New York	Vermont
Kentucky	Ohio	Washington
Louisiana	Oklahoma	West Virginia
Maryland	Oregon	Wisconsin

Adapted from "Modern status of views as to general measure of physician's duty to inform patient of risks of proposed treatment," 88 ALR 3d 1008.

The Duty to Disclose Risks of Proposed Treatment

Under certain circumstances practitioners may incur a duty to warn patients of the risks of ophthalmic drug use, both for drugs used diagnostically and for those used therapeutically. Of the two classes, the greater obligation arises when therapeutic agents are employed. Occasions may also arise when patients should be warned of the potential risks of refusing to allow a drug to be administered.

DIAGNOSTIC AGENTS

The common diagnostic drugs used by optometrists are anesthetics, mydriatics, cycloplegics, and dyes. Routine use of these drugs creates a risk of injury only in very unusual circumstances. Therefore, informed consent is rarely a legal issue when they are employed.

The use of topical anesthetics creates a small risk that patients will experience a toxic response resulting in the disruption or desquamation of the corneal epithelium. Because this is an idiosyncratic response and cannot be predicted, it does not create the kind of risk for which informed consent is necessary. Even if a toxic reaction does occur, the effect is transient and limited. Thus, informed consent should not prevent prudent practitioners from administering these drugs when clinically appropriate.

Dilation of the pupil is a diagnostic procedure with potentially serious side effects (i.e., angle-closure or pupillary-block glaucoma), but the risk of injury must be communicated only to patients for whom it is significant. Studies have determined that only 2% to 6% of the general population have angles anatomically narrow enough to close,[29] and that for the patient population most at risk—those over 30 years of age—the chance of precipitating an angle-closure glaucoma is 1 in 45,000.[30] These statistics indicate that for the great majority of patients the risk is minimal or nonexistent. Thus, when performing routine dilation, clinicians have no duty to discuss the potential complications of mydriasis.

For that small percentage of the population with anterior chamber angles narrow enough to be closed by pupillary dilation, however, the decision to dilate should be made jointly with patients after they have been informed of the benefits of dilation and of the risks and implications of angle closure. The determination of whether to employ dilation should be made in light of the need for it (e.g., if ophthalmoscopy of the retinal periphery is deemed necessary) and after the risk of angle closure has been reasonably determined (e.g., through the use of gonioscopy). The patient's decision should be documented and retained in the record. Figure 5.2 shows a form ideally suited for this purpose.[31]

Cycloplegia is reserved for a limited number of conditions (e.g., suspected latent hyperopia or accommodative esotropia). Hyperopic patients may have shallow anterior chamber angles that require assessment before instilling the cycloplegic. Because this technique is most often needed for young patients, careful attention must be given to the concentration and dosage of the cycloplegic used, so that the risk of toxic effects can be minimized. Assuming that the angle is open and that the appropriate drug is selected for use, the risk of angle closure is no different than in patients undergoing routine mydriasis. Consequently, clinicians do not have to obtain informed consent. If risk factors are present and clinical complications are a consideration, practitioners should discuss these factors with patients (or, if children, with parents or guardians) and obtain the necessary consent to administer the drug. The administration of atropine to infants before performing a cycloplegic examination may also necessitate communication. The use of atropine is probably justified clinically only in patients 4 years of age or younger who are suspected of having accommodative esotropia,[20] and it should be used conservatively in terms of concentration and dosage. The signs and symptoms of atropine toxicity may be explained to parents in these cases to minimize the risk of an overlooked toxic drug reaction.

Although sodium fluorescein and rose bengal are routinely administered topically to the eye as indicator dyes, sodium fluorescein can also be administered orally to evaluate retinal and choroidal lesions. Such oral fluorography (or angioscopy) has been documented to be safe and effective for some clinical conditions,[32] but the oral administration of sodium fluorescein is not yet approved by the Food and Drug Administration (FDA). In these circumstances it is permissible for practitioners to use the oral route of administration, but informed consent should be obtained and documented (Table 5.3).

The preceding circumstances are not the only ones in which risks may have to be communicated to patients. Occasionally, patients refuse to allow a drug to be administered for diagnostic purposes. The usual circumstances involve mydriatics for dilation and topical anesthetics for tonometry.[33] Patients have the right to refuse any test, and clinicians cannot obtain a lawful consent by coercion to legally perform a test against the patient's will. Clinicians,

What You Need to Know About Dilation of the Pupil

Dilation of the pupil is a common diagnostic procedure used by optometrists to better examine the interior of the eye. It allows a more thorough examination by making the field of view wider and by permitting the doctor to see more of the inside of the eye. Being able to examine the inside of the eye is essential to determining that your eye is healthy.

To dilate the pupil, eye drops must be administered. They require roughly half an hour to take effect. Once your pupils are dilated, it is common to be sensitive to light, a symptom that is usually alleviated by sunglasses. If you do not have any sunglasses, a disposable pair will be provided for you. Another common symptom is blurred vision, especially at near. It will require about 4 to 6 hours for your vision to return to normal. During this time you must exercise caution when walking down steps, driving a vehicle, operating dangerous machinery, or performing other tasks that may present a risk of injury. If you have any special transportation needs, please let us know so that they can be arranged prior to dilation.

In about 2% of people there is a possible complication of dilation of the pupil; it has been determined that you fall into this category. You must understand this complication before you give your consent to have this procedure performed.

The doctor's examination has revealed that there is a possibility of elevating the pressure inside your eye when dilation is performed. The medical term for this eventuality is "angle closure glaucoma". Because of this possibility, once your pupil is dilated and the interior of the eye has been examined, the pressure will be checked again. Should it become elevated, it will be necessary to lower the pressure by administering eyedrops and oral medication. Afterwards, it may be necessary to refer you to an eye surgeon for treatment with a laser to prevent further occurrences of this kind.

Because of the structure of your eyes, it is possible for an angle closure to occur at some other time, when the symptoms may not be recognized and treatment may not be immediately provided. Such an eventuality could seriously affect your vision. Therefore, there is a benefit to you in having dilation perfomed today and in allowing this complication, if it occurs, to be diagnosed and treated immediately.

The decision to undergo dilation is yours. You may choose not to have dilation performed, but because of your history, symptoms, or examination findings, the doctor recommends that dilation of the pupil be used today to examine your eye for disease. If you have any questions concerning the procedure, please ask them so that we may answer them. Then please sign your name in the appropriate place below to signify your decision.

[] I understand the risks and benefits of pupillary dilation and I consent to have the procedure performed.

[] The risks and benefits of pupillary dilation have been adequately explained to me and I understand them, but I do not wish to undergo the procedure.

_____   _____
Date   Signature of Patient

_____
Attest (initials)

© 1991 John G. Classé

FIGURE 5.2 **Example of informed consent document for dilation of the pupil when the patient has a narrow anterior chamber angle.**

however, are obliged to ensure that patients understand the potential ramifications of refusal. For example, elderly patients with visual field loss and optic disc cupping should be warned of the need for tonometry, and patients with reduced visual acuity who complain of floaters and flashes have an obvious need for ophthalmoscopy through a dilated pupil. Practitioners must weigh the need for the test in light of the clinical situation and must advise patients accordingly. Re-

TABLE 5.3
Informed Consent for Oral Fluorography

I, _____, hereby consent to photography of my eyes or associated areas for the documentation and/or diagnosis of certain retinal conditions or diseases that may be present.

I also understand that the photographs may be used to document my ocular status as well as for future use in publications, video tapes, or other educational presentations that may or may not benefit me.

I understand that the medication, sodium fluorescein, is not yet approved by the Food and Drug Administration for oral use, although it has been documented to be effective in revealing certain abnormalities of the retina when taken orally. I also understand that no side effects have been reported from the use of oral fluorescein with the occasional exception of slight discoloration of the skin or urine lasting up to 24 hours. Possible side effects include nausea, vomiting, and allergic reactions such as hives or anaphylactic shock (breathing, heart, and blood pressure problems).

Signed:	_____
Witness:	_____
Dated:	_____

Used with permission from the School of Optometry, University of Alabama at Birmingham.

fusals should always be documented in the patient record (Fig. 5.3).[31] Some practitioners use forms that are signed by patients and retained in the patient record, and these are a satisfactory means of documenting patients' decisions. If a patient refuses to undergo a procedure, the potential adverse consequences of that decision must be explained to the patient (e.g., the symptoms of retinal detachment for a patient reporting the acute onset of flashes and floaters).

THERAPEUTIC AGENTS

The duty to inform patients of the potential toxic effects of drug therapy is greatest when therapeutic agents are prescribed.[20] The reason for this is due, in part, to clinicians' lack of control over drug administration. Whereas the use of drugs for diagnostic purposes is carefully controlled by practitioners and is usually an in-office procedure, the prescribing of therapeutic agents results in extended drug use that is entirely within patients' control. Abuse of therapeutic agents has been documented in the ophthalmologic patient population,[34,35] and optometrists should be aware of this potential problem, especially when using therapeutic agents such as steroids and antiglaucoma medications.

Patients should be warned of the side effects of extended use of therapeutic agents and should be required to consult

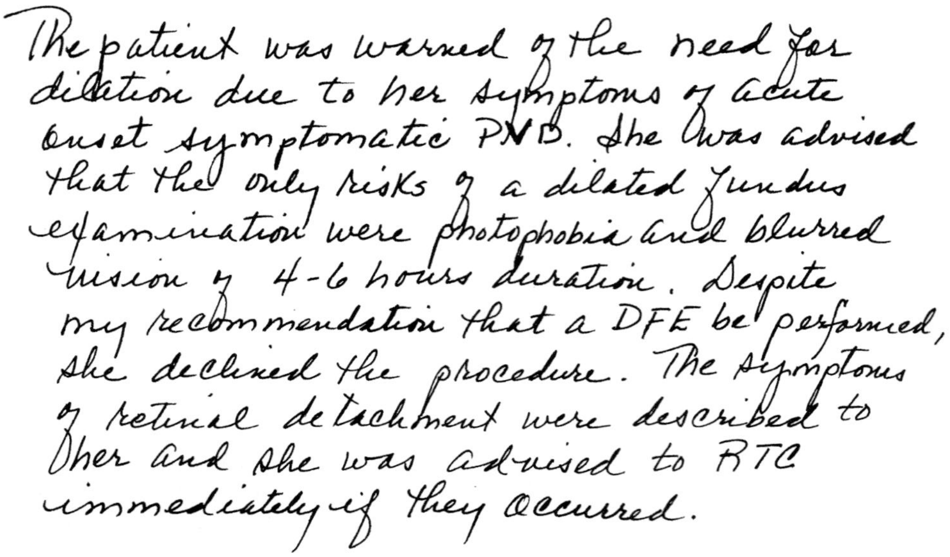

FIGURE 5.3 **Example of handwritten record entry to document informed consent when a patient refuses pupillary dilation.**

The patient was warned of the need for dilation due to her symptoms of acute onset symptomatic PVD. She was advised that the only risks of a dilated fundus examination were photophobia and blurred vision of 4–6 hours duration. Despite my recommendation that a DFE be performed, she declined the procedure. The symptoms of retinal detachment were described to her and she was advised to RTC immediately if they occurred.

the prescribing clinician if additional prescription renewals are needed. As with diagnostic agents, the need to communicate with patients depends on the clinician's assessment of risk. If a drug is used for only a brief time, the risk is far less than if an extended period of treatment is anticipated. Likewise, greater dosages create larger risks and greater necessity for disclosure. Optometrists must be familiar with the allergic and toxic effects of the therapeutic drugs they prescribe and should inform patients of potential risks under the appropriate circumstances.

Of the commonly used therapeutic drugs, the greatest risks are encountered when clinicians prescribe topical steroids (for extended periods), systemic steroids, β blockers, miotic antiglaucoma agents, and oral carbonic anhydrase inhibitors (CAIs).[16] Optometrists should be aware of the toxic effects that attend the use of these drugs and should warn patients accordingly. Disclosures should be documented in the patient record.

The doctrine of informed consent may also be applied to situations in which optometrists fail to disclose alternatives to therapy. This issue can occasionally arise when optometrists use drugs for therapy.

Alternatives to Therapy

Disclosure requirements obligate clinicians not only to warn of the risks of treatment but also to describe alternatives to therapy.[36] This duty may arise in various ways when drug use is contemplated. For example, if echothiophate therapy is recommended for the treatment of accommodative esotropia in a young child, alternative treatment—such as lens therapy—should be discussed as well. Another example involves glaucoma suspects. Patients with elevated intraocular pressure (IOP) and no optic disc damage or visual field loss should be appraised of the clinical alternatives: receive medical therapy or be monitored by the optometrist until disc damage or measurable field loss occurs. In these and analogous situations, clinicians should avoid dictating the mode of treatment and should ensure that the course of therapy is obtained with patient consent.

In clinical situations in which there are alternatives to treatment, optometrists should note in the patient record that the alternatives were discussed and that the treatment chosen was obtained with the patient's consent.

Disclosure of Abnormalities

Not infrequently, diagnostic drug use discloses an ambiguous or suspicious finding. Clinicians must explain these findings so that patients can determine if they wish to undergo further testing.[36] A sample case illustrates how informed consent can be applied to such a situation.[37]

A 58-year-old woman complaining of poor focus and of gaps in her vision was examined by an ophthalmologist. The cause of these complaints was attributed to her contact lenses, but during the course of the examination Schiotz tonometry was performed, with readings of 23.8 mm Hg obtained in each eye. Despite this result, no dilated fundus examination or visual field assessment was performed, and the potential significance of the IOP findings was not discussed with the patient. During the next 2 years the patient was seen a dozen times, but it was not until the end of this period that she was diagnosed as having open-angle glaucoma. Despite medical and surgical therapy, her visual acuity decreased to 20/200 and she suffered a profound visual field loss. She sued the ophthalmologist, alleging that he was negligent for failing to diagnose the disease and to warn of the elevated IOPs. Although a judgment in favor of the physician was rendered after trial, the woman filed an appeal. The state supreme court reversed the decision of the trial court, ruling that under the doctrine of informed consent the ophthalmologist was under a duty to inform the woman of any abnormal findings and to advise her of any diagnostic procedures that could be undertaken to determine the significance of the findings.

Optometrists have a similar duty to discuss the results of diagnostic tests with patients and to advise patients of the availability of further testing to rule out the presence of disease.[17] Ambiguous or suspicious findings should be resolved, and if patients do not return for recall appointments or do not wish to undergo further evaluation, these facts should be documented in the patient record.

Documentation of Warnings

Communications with patients required by the doctrine of informed consent should be documented in the patient record. Either a handwritten entry or a form signed by the patient is adequate for legal purposes. Failure to record communications or inadequate entries concerning such communications may result in a successful legal claim against the practitioner.

In a case involving a military optometrist,[38] a middle-aged military retiree complained of the acute onset of "black spots" in one eye. The optometrist found the patient's best corrected acuity was 20/30 and 20/40, which was due to cataracts. The optometrist performed a dilated fundus examination with a binocular indirect ophthalmoscope and diagnosed the patient's condition as posterior vitreous detachment. The patient returned home, but 4 weeks later, while climbing a ladder he experienced a bright flash of light in the affected eye. The man called the eye clinic and obtained an appointment for 6 days later. At that examination his visual acuity was 20/200, because of a large retinal detachment that involved the macula. Despite surgery, vision in the eye remained greatly reduced. He sued the optometrist, alleging that the practitioner was negligent in failing to detect the retinal detachment and that he had breached the doctrine of informed consent by failing to warn the patient of the symptoms of retinal detachment.

At the trial the surgeon who repaired the eye testified that the retinal detachment could not have been present at the time of the optometrist's examination, thereby exonerating the optometrist of the negligence claim. The key evidence concerning the informed consent claim came from the optometrist's record. Although the optometrist testified that he had warned the patient of the symptoms of detachment, his record stated: "PVD. Reassure. RTC PRN." The court found this terse entry to be inadequate to support the optometrist's contention that a warning had been given and awarded a judgment in favor of the patient.

Negligence

Although the doctrine of informed consent is an important legal consideration when ophthalmic drugs are employed, the most likely source of a professional liability claim against an optometrist is negligence. As various reports have demonstrated,[39,40] large liability claims against optometrists typically allege misdiagnosis, and the need for topical anesthesia and mydriasis is common to these claims. In the majority of instances the misdiagnosis is due to failure to use the appropriate pharmaceutical agent rather than toxic or allergic drug reactions.[40] Consequently, it may be argued that the likelihood of a negligence claim is highest when optometrists fail to use an ophthalmic drug that, when employed appropriately, would permit a proper diagnosis. Claims most commonly allege failure to diagnose open-angle glaucoma,[41] tumors affecting the visual system,[42] or retinal detachment.[43]

Misdiagnosis is also an important aspect of claims involving the use of therapeutic ophthalmic agents. Although the toxic effects of these drugs have been a common cause of liability claims against ophthalmologists,[34,35] failure to make the correct diagnosis, followed by institution of an inappropriate therapeutic regimen, has become the major concern of optometrists.[20,40] Because of the restricted nature of most optometry practice acts, which usually limit therapy to the anterior segment of the eye, claims against optometrists most frequently allege mismanagement of corneal problems.

Although negligence represents the most important legal complication of clinical practice, the exposure of optometrists to malpractice claims remains at a relatively low level, far below that of physicians.[44–46] Within optometry there is no difference between diagnostic and therapeutic drug use with regard to the risk of malpractice, since professional liability insurance premiums do not vary on this basis.[e] However, as optometry laws continue to be amended to enable optometrists to serve as primary providers of eyecare, this increased clinical responsibility inevitably will result in increased litigation. Because the use of pharmaceutical agents is an integral part of these responsibilities, optometrists must be familiar with the concept of negligence and must understand how negligence may arise in clinical practice.

Proof of Negligence

The law holds every individual to a reasonable standard of conduct, and failure to exercise reasonable care creates liability if it results in harm to others. Accordingly, negligence may be defined as "the omission to do something which a reasonable man, guided by those ordinary considerations which ordinarily regulate human affairs, would do, or the doing of something which a reasonable and prudent man would not do."[47]

Optometrists have an obligation to adhere to a reasonable standard of care when rendering services to patients. This standard may be summarized by the question, "What would a reasonable optometrist do under the same or similar circumstances?" From this question it is apparent that the defendant optometrist's conduct is to be compared with the conduct expected of a hypothetical "reasonable optometrist."[48] If the defendant optometrist's conduct fails to measure up to the conduct expected of this reasonable practitioner, a breach of the standard of care occurs. However, proof of negligence entails more than a demonstration that the defendant optometrist has violated the standard of care. There are, in fact, four elements to this tort,[f] and to state a cause of action in a court of law the plaintiff-patient must offer evidence in support of each.[48] These four elements are:

1. A duty on the part of the practitioner to adhere to a reasonable standard of care, which is intended to minimize the risk of injury to the patient.

---

[e]The nation's largest carrier of malpractice coverage for optometrists has monitored drug-related claims over the past two decades and has reported no significant liability risk associated with therapeutic drug use by optometrists. For a discussion, see Classé JG. Liability for the treatment of anterior segment eye disease. Optom Clin 1991;1(4):1–16.

[f]A tort is a "breach of duty (other than a contractual or quasicontractual duty) which gives rise to an action for damages." (Prosser WL. Law of torts, ed. 4. St. Paul, MN: West, 1971;1.) This rather unsatisfactory definition leaves one with more of an indication of what a tort is not; it is not a crime, it is not based on contract, and it does not result in loss of liberty. It is a civil action, brought for the purpose of receiving monetary compensation for damages, and is based on a breach of duty.

2. Breach of this standard of care by the practitioner.
3. Actual, physical injury suffered by the patient.
4. A proximate relationship between the patient's injury and the practitioner's actions (or failure to act).

DUTY

The duty to adhere to a reasonable standard of care is established by the doctor-patient relationship. Proof of the duty is rarely a problem for plaintiff-patients, since in the great majority of cases patients are examined by optometrists in an office or under circumstances that make the relationship apparent. The lack of formal surroundings, or even failure of the optometrist to charge for services, does not defeat the duty if a doctor-patient relationship has been formed. Once an optometrist has created the relationship, the optometrist is legally obligated to adhere to the standard of care expected of a reasonable practitioner acting under the same or similar circumstances. Since proof of this standard can be offered only by individuals actually familiar with it, expert testimony is required.

BREACH OF THE STANDARD OF CARE

Expert witnesses, unlike other witnesses, are not limited to reporting the perceptions of their senses but may offer opinions. Such witnesses first must be qualified, which is a process intended to convince the trial judge that the individual being offered as an expert is competent to testify about the matter at issue. Traditionally, only practitioners of the same "school" have been considered competent to testify about the standard of care expected of defendant practitioners.[49] However, the growing liberality of rules of evidence and the lessening distinction clinically between optometrists and ophthalmologists have combined to change this traditional pattern, and ophthalmologists are frequently deemed competent to testify concerning the standard of care expected of optometrists. This development has led to the imposition of a medical standard of care for optometrists in cases involving misdiagnosis or mismanagement of ocular disease.[50]

The likelihood of testimony by physicians—and the imposition of a medical standard of care—is greatest in cases involving ophthalmic drugs because of the use of these agents to diagnose or treat disease. Of course, expert testimony on behalf of a defendant optometrist may allege that the optometrist acted in conformance with the standard of care. It is then left to the jury to determine liability. This element of proof is usually the most difficult for plaintiffs to establish and is frequently the most contentious aspect of a malpractice trial.

INJURY

Assessment of patients' injuries is also a matter requiring an expert's opinion, and either optometrists or ophthalmolo-gists may provide this testimony. Visual impairment is usually evaluated as loss of visual acuity, loss of visual field, restriction of ocular motility, or a combination of these three factors.[51] Other ocular disturbances that result in loss of functions such as color vision, accommodation, and binocular vision may also be evaluated, as may deformities or disfigurements of the orbit or face.[51] Optometrists who testify concerning the degree of injury suffered by patients should be familiar with the accepted standards used in legal proceedings.[g]

PROXIMATE CAUSE

The fourth element of negligence is proximate cause, sometimes referred to as legal cause, which serves to tie together the negligent act (or failure to act) and the resulting injury.[48] For example, failure to employ a mydriatic drug for an ophthalmoscopic examination may be the proximate cause of a clinician's failure to detect an intraocular disease. Expert testimony is necessary to link together what the practitioner did (or did not do) and the injury.

Plaintiff-patients must prove each of these four elements by a preponderance of the evidence. As the preceding discussion has demonstrated, expert testimony is crucial to the presentation of this evidence, and it is equally important to defendant optometrists, since they seek to refute plaintiffs' allegations. The focus of a malpractice case is usually the standard of care, which has particular requirements when applied to the use of ophthalmic drugs.

Standard of Care

Optometrists are expected to display that degree of skill and learning that is commonly possessed by members of the profession who are in good standing and to exercise what is referred to as "due care."[h] This obligation has broad implications whenever optometrists use ophthalmic drugs, since the standard of care requires that optometrists:

1. Understand the allergic and toxic side effects of all drugs administered or prescribed.
2. Take an adequate history to determine if there has been any previous allergic or toxic response to a drug, especially an ophthalmic agent.
3. Select the appropriate drug for patients' needs or conditions.

---

[g]The assessment of visual impairment is described in *Guides to the Evaluation of Permanent Impairment,* ed. 2. Chicago: American Medical Association, 1984;141–151. *The Physician's Desk Reference for Ophthalmology* contains a reprint of this information.

[h]Due care may be defined as "that care which an ordinarily prudent person would have exercised under the circumstances." (Black's Law Dictionary, rev. ed. 4. St. Paul, MN: West, 1968.)

4. Warn patients of side effects of drug use that may create a risk of injury.
5. Monitor patients while they are under the influence of the diagnostic or therapeutic agent so that complications can be managed in a timely manner.

To conform to these due care requirements, an optometrist is expected to act in the same manner as a reasonable practitioner by observing the following clinical and legal guidelines.

KNOWLEDGE

Practitioners are under a legal duty to keep abreast of new developments, especially information that affects patient care, such as reports of drug toxicity.[52] Therefore, practitioners not only must understand the properties of any drugs that are used for patient care, but also must remain knowledgeable concerning more efficacious drugs or reports of adverse events. Failure to stay abreast of these developments has resulted in successful claims against physicians[53] and could also serve as a cause of action against optometrists.

HISTORY

The standard of care requires that an adequate drug history be taken, including:

- The patient's history of past drug use
- Drugs currently being taken
- Any allergic or toxic reactions to drugs, past or present
- History of ophthalmic drug use, including a determination of whether anesthesia and mydriasis have been employed at a previous examination

Failure to take an adequate history that results in an allergic or toxic response to a drug may render practitioners liable for this otherwise preventable injury.[54]

USE OF THE APPROPRIATE AGENT

Adherence to the standard of care is necessary to minimize the risk of injury to patients. An optometrist is obligated to choose the pharmaceutical agent that fulfills this requirement and, in so doing, is expected to exercise that degree of skill and learning that is commonly possessed by like practitioners. The drug that is most appropriate for the patient's condition and its most appropriate route of administration must be determined to minimize the risk of adverse effects. If an optometrist uses an inappropriate agent—such as a topical β blocker for a glaucoma patient who has chronic obstructive pulmonary disease, thereby precipitating an otherwise preventable injury—the optometrist has failed to meet this duty and is legally responsible for both transient and permanent effects of the drug's use. The same would be true if an optometrist attempted to treat an anterior uveitis

with a systemic steroid without first establishing that a topical route of administration was inadequate or inappropriate.[34,35] In each instance the optometrist's conduct must measure up to that of a reasonable optometrist or liability may result.

WARNINGS

Because of the doctrine of informed consent, under some circumstances optometrists must discuss the risks and possible side effects of drug use with patients. For example, if a patient were to undergo prolonged treatment with topical steroids, the optometrist would be obligated to warn the patient of potential side effects, including glaucoma, ocular infection, and cataract. Although the amount of information that must be communicated to patients varies among states due to different evidentiary requirements, the circumstances under which warnings are necessary generally do not vary. For example, all patients receiving a dilated fundus examination should be warned of the potential photophobia, discomfort, and blur caused by pupillary dilation. Warnings are an essential aspect of drug use and should not be overlooked or ignored.

MANAGEMENT OF SIDE EFFECTS

If patients experience a drug-related allergic or toxic effect, clinicians must meet reasonable standards of detection and management. For example, a postdilation telephone call from a patient complaining of severe headache and blurred vision requires an examination instead of the proverbial "take an aspirin and call me in the morning." Likewise, a patient who is being treated with topical steroids must be recalled with sufficient regularity to detect adverse events before they have significantly affected the patient's vision.

For each of these due care requirements, optometrists must satisfy reasonable standards of conduct, and because the use of ophthalmic drugs is essentially a medical act, ophthalmologists may be competent to state the standard of care expected of optometrists under these circumstances.[50]

Another aspect of the standard of care involves optometrists who decide, for personal or professional reasons, not to employ pharmaceutical agents. No optometrist is under a legal duty to use these agents, but individuals who choose not to use ophthalmic drugs face some formidable standard of care issues, particularly with regard to the use of drugs for diagnostic purposes. If a patient seeks an optometrist's care, and if during the course of the examination a reasonable optometrist would have recognized that the use of an ophthalmic drug was necessary to make the appropriate diagnosis of the patient's condition, then a legal duty arises either to use the ophthalmic agent or to refer the patient to another practitioner for the necessary examination. The most common drugs that create this situation are mydriatics.

A hypothetical example illustrates how the standard of care can be applied to practitioners who do not use drugs for diagnostic purposes. If a patient has received a blow to the eye from a fist, ball, or other blunt object, the optometrist must rule out the possibility of a retinal break.[55] To perform a reasonable examination—one that conforms to the expected standard of care—dilation of the pupil is necessary.[33,56] In fact, it may be argued that examination of the retinal periphery with a binocular indirect ophthalmoscope is required under these circumstances. If the optometrist does not dilate the pupil, any ophthalmic examination is below the standard of care. The only recourse available to the optometrist is to refer the patient to another clinician so that the patient can receive the appropriate evaluation. Optometrists who choose not to use drugs are subject to the same standard as clinicians who do. For a patient suffering blunt ocular trauma, a reasonable practitioner would realize that a dilated fundus examination is necessary to rule out the presence of peripheral retinal disease. Optometrists who do not measure up to this standard are liable for any injury patients suffer due to failure to receive a timely diagnosis.

Misdiagnosis

Misdiagnosis of open-angle glaucoma, tumors affecting the visual system, and retinal detachment is the leading cause of large malpractice claims against optometrists.[40] In the great majority of cases, failure to make the appropriate diagnosis is linked to failure to perform a key diagnostic test (e.g., tonometry, or ophthalmoscopy through a dilated pupil). Therefore, the legal problem most likely to be encountered by a clinician is failure to use an ophthalmic agent. Example cases may be used to illustrate how claims of misdiagnosis can arise when these three important disorders are encountered.

OPEN-ANGLE GLAUCOMA

The standard of care for the detection of open-angle glaucoma has been established by a series of cases involving ophthalmologists.[37,57,58] The leading case[57] involved a 22-year-old woman who was fitted for contact lenses and examined intermittently over the course of 10 years before the ophthalmologists discovered that she had open-angle glaucoma and that her visual field was reduced to less than 10 degrees. She sued the ophthalmologists for negligence, and at trial tonometry became the key issue. She alleged that the physicians had a duty to perform the test while she was a contact lens patient; they defended the claim on the basis that tonometry was not a routine test for patients under 40 years of age.

Although the ophthalmologists won the trial, the case was reversed on appeal, a decision that evoked a storm of commentary.[59] Ironically, the court's opinion proved to be a legal dead end, but the intense publicity surrounding the case succeeded in changing the standard of care in both ophthalmology and optometry.[60]

Cases brought today against optometrists for failure to diagnose open-angle glaucoma almost uniformly allege failure to perform tonometry. Just as uniformly, defendant optometrists resort to procedural defenses that seek to avoid this issue.[61–64] The result has been a standard of care that requires routine use of tonometry regardless of patient age. For this reason, topical anesthesia is an important procedure. Dilation of the pupil for ophthalmoscopy, visual field assessment, and other appropriate tests for glaucoma may be necessary as well.

TUMORS AFFECTING THE VISUAL SYSTEM

Tumors may be external, such as squamous cell carcinomas, or intraocular, such as malignant melanomas, or intracranial, such as pituitary adenomas. All three types of tumors may be considered "ocular," and all pose unique clinical challenges. The detection of intraocular tumors presents one of the most difficult diagnostic dilemmas encountered by optometrists. To make the diagnosis, a dilated fundus examination is needed, but patients with "silent" tumors may not evince symptoms that would lead a reasonable practitioner to determine that dilation is required. Practitioners are not legally obligated to discover all that may be wrong with patients but rather to perform an examination that is in keeping with the standard of care.[65] Therefore, failure to detect a "silent" tumor because dilation is not demanded by the patient's complaint or history may not be construed as negligence. A recent case challenges this assumption, however, and imposes a medical standard of care for the use of pupillary dilation.[66]

A 4½-year-old child with accommodative esotropia was examined by a military optometrist, who found 20/30 acuity in each eye and good eye alignment with spectacles. Direct ophthalmoscopy performed through an undilated pupil revealed no evidence of posterior pole disease. The optometrist saw the patient on two other occasions over the next seven months, but no pathology was observed. About 13 months after the initial examination the child was found to have leukocoria in the deviating eye. A dilated fundus examination by a base ophthalmologist revealed a 15 DD retinoblastoma located at the equator of the eye and spreading anteriorly. The child was referred to a specialist for treatment, and irradiation was used successfully to destroy the tumor. The irradiation caused cataract, however, and the tumor caused retinal detachment, resulting in a best corrected acuity in the eye of 20/300. A suit was brought against the optometrist, alleging that he was negligent for failing to perform a dilated fundus examination with a binocular indirect ophthalmoscope at the initial examination and periodically thereafter. After a trial found in favor of the optometrist, the case was appealed to a federal appellate court, which ruled that the optometrist had breached the standard of care in failing to perform a dilated fundus examination. The court relied exclusively on medical testimony in reaching its opinion, thereby imposing a medical standard of care on the defendant optometrist.[67] Although the optometrist was ultimately found not liable, the court's opinion established a precedent for the use of pupillary dilation in patients with "silent" tumors.[68]

The use of pupillary dilation is required for symptomatic patients, as illustrated by the following case.[69] An optometrist employed by a multidisciplinary clinic examined a middle-aged woman who complained of reduced vision and found her best-corrected visual acuity to be 20/25 and 20/40. The optometrist attributed this to cataracts. Although refraction, tonometry, and ophthalmoscopy were performed, the optometrist did not dilate the patient's pupils. After discussing his findings with the patient he dismissed her. Two months later she realized that the vision in one eye was markedly reduced, and she returned to the clinic, where the diagnosis of retinal detachment secondary to a von Hippel-Lindau tumor was made. Despite surgery, the patient was left with a permanent loss of acuity. She sued the optometrist, alleging that he was negligent for failing to make the diagnosis in a timely manner. Although the optometrist prevailed at the trial, the patient was awarded damages on appeal, with the court stating that, "the evidence is overwhelming that the (plaintiff's) eye should have been dilated" and that the optometrist should be held to "the same rules relating to the duty of care and liability as ophthalmologists."[70]

The rationale for the court's opinion was that the diagnosis of cataract (a "disease") required dilation of the pupil and that had dilation been performed at the time of the optometrist's examination, the possibility of a retinal detachment could have been ruled out. In finding the optometrist liable, the court imposed a medical standard of care. Therefore, a dilated fundus examination should be employed whenever best-corrected visual acuity is reduced, and coexisting disease should be considered a possibility until an examination determines otherwise. Optometrists may be held responsible for the diagnosis of intraocular tumors—even those as rare as malignant melanoma—in symptomatic patients.[42]

RETINAL DETACHMENT

The necessity for dilation of the pupil is probably most evident in cases where retinal detachment is, or should be, suspected. Many patients are at risk for retinal detachment, and it can be argued that pupillary dilation is necessary whenever patients are found to have any of the following[43,56]:

- Significant myopia
- Aphakia or pseudophakia
- Recent YAG capsulotomy
- Glaucoma therapy with miotics

- Lattice degeneration
- Blunt trauma to the eye
- History of retinal detachment in the fellow eye
- Proliferative retinopathy (e.g., proliferative stage of sickle cell, diabetes, branch retinal vein occlusion)

Another important precursor of retinal detachment is acute onset, symptomatic, posterior vitreous detachment (PVD). It has been reported that 7% to 15% of patients with acute, symptomatic PVD have a retinal tear.[71,72] About one-third of these tears progress to retinal detachment.[73] If patients complain of spots, specks, floaters, or other entoptic phenomena that indicate the possibility of PVD, optometrists must conduct a dilated fundus examination to rule out the presence of a tear. Although failure to detect the detachment may not be below the standard of care, failure to examine patients under conditions of dilation may be so construed.[34,35]

Symptoms of reduced visual acuity also require careful assessment of the interior of the eye. In a case involving a diabetic patient who complained of blurred vision,[74] the defendant optometrist performed a refraction and prescribed spectacles that he assured the patient would relieve her symptoms. Because of the patient's history of diabetes and the complaint of reduced acuity, the standard of care required a dilated fundus examination. The optometrist did not perform this evaluation, however, and after dispensing spectacles to the patient did not undertake any further treatment. Six months later the patient consulted an ophthalmologist, who found that the patient had proliferative retinopathy due to diabetes and had suffered a retinal detachment in one eye and unmanageable complications in the other. A lawsuit was instituted against the optometrist for negligence in failing to make the diagnosis and to refer the patient for treatment. It is important to note that diabetic patients constitute an important and challenging clinical problem for optometrists because of the number of affected individuals, the frequency of ocular complications, and the long-term management required.[75,76]

Although other causes of misdiagnosis have been alleged against optometrists,[40,44,77–80] these three types of claims are the most frequent and represent the most significant clinical and legal challenges to diagnostic skill. Failure to diagnose these conditions poses the greatest risk of litigation for optometrists.

Complications of Diagnostic Drug Use

Optometrists must be familiar with the allergic and toxic effects of any ophthalmic drugs used for diagnostic purposes and must be prepared to manage these complications when they occur.[20] This obligation is frequently encountered when using the common diagnostic agents: anesthetics, mydriatics, and cycloplegics.

ANESTHETICS

Topical anesthesia is necessary for applanation tonometry and gonioscopy. Proparacaine and benoxinate are the agents most commonly employed. Because use of these agents may cause an allergic or toxic response, optometrists should determine if patients have experienced a previous adverse reaction before using the drug. If optometrists observe such a reaction, this fact should be noted conspicuously in the patient record to prevent a second episode at a subsequent examination. Of course, optometrists may choose an alternative drug in this event, since proparacaine and benoxinate are structurally dissimilar and an allergic reaction to one drug does not mean that patients are also allergic to the other (see Chapter 6). If a patient experiences an adverse reaction, the worst result—desquamation of the corneal epithelium—is transient and the discomfort is not severe.[81] Most episodes resolve within 24 to 48 hours, with no permanent effect on vision. There is little opportunity for negligence or for substantial damages.

Injury may be permanent, however, if a topical anesthetic is applied copiously to a compromised cornea.[82] Anesthetics should never be dispensed to patients for use at home, and if other practitioners have dispensed anesthetics to patients for use on an ''as needed'' basis, these patients should be counseled concerning this ill-advised use of topical anesthesia.

MYDRIATICS

These drugs constitute the most important class of diagnostic agents because of their use for dilating the pupil for ophthalmoscopy. A history must be taken to ensure that patients have not experienced angle closure after dilation by previous examiners, and the anterior chamber angle should be examined to determine the risk of precipitating an angle-closure attack. It has been estimated that only 2% to 6% of the population has angles that are sufficiently narrow to close,[29] and that for the general population, the risk of angle closure following pupillary dilation is 1 in 180,000.[30]

Therefore, for 94% to 98% of individuals—those whose angles cannot be closed—there is no requirement under the doctrine of informed consent to warn them of this risk. Only those rare individuals whose histories or anterior chamber angles indicate a risk must be informed of the possibility of angle closure, so that their consent can be obtained before performing the procedure. Clinicians should document that the warning was given and that patients' consent was received (see Fig. 5.2). The use of prophylactic laser peripheral iridotomy in lieu of pupillary dilation should also be considered and discussed with patients if management of angle closure would be inappropriate. A clinical and legal issue of some importance is posed by the necessity for pupillary dilation. If there is litigation, the use of expert testimony is required to determine if dilation was needed to conform to the standard of care in a specific instance. If a reasonable practitioner would have realized that a dilated fundus examination was necessary under the circumstances, then the patient must receive that evaluation or be referred to another practitioner so that it can be performed. There are numerous circumstances under which the obligation to use pupillary dilation seems to arise (see Chapter 21).

Because patients who have undergone mydriasis typically experience photophobia, discomfort, and loss of accommodation (if tropicamide is used), optometrists should be certain to safeguard them from injury while they are in the office and on the premises. Elderly[83] and handicapped[84] patients are particularly susceptible to injury from falls or similar mishaps and may successfully claim damages if it can be shown that optometrists did not take reasonable steps to protect them. Clinical and office staff should be prepared to assist patients who are on the premises. An example case illustrates the potential for injury.[83]

An elderly patient who was to be examined by an ophthalmologist received drops of tropicamide from a nurse and then was seated in the waiting room without being informed of the drug's effects. When she was called for examination, the patient's blurred vision caused her to fall as she attempted to get up from the chair and cross the room. Despite her complaints of pain, the physician persisted in performing the examination, and after she insisted she could not walk to leave the office, an ambulance was called and she was taken to the hospital. She was found to have fractured her hip and spent considerable time recovering from complications. She sued the ophthalmologist for negligence, and the trial court awarded her both compensatory and punitive damages.

Because patients whose pupils have been dilated usually leave the premises with their vision impaired, the optometrist's obligation is extended to include a warning of the effects of mydriasis on such tasks as driving a motor vehicle, operating machinery, or other foreseeable activities for which there is a risk of injury.[85] In some cases, it may be necessary to administer an α-adrenergic blocking agent (e.g., dapiprazole) to speed the return of acuity.[86] If it is known in advance that patients will undergo a dilated fundus examination, they should be advised when making the appointment so that appropriate arrangements for transportation can be made. If the risk of injury to the patient is deemed significant, a reschedule examination may be arranged (e.g., at the same time ophthalmic materials are to be dispensed) so that the patient can make provisions for transportation. In all cases it is wise to ensure that the patient has sunglasses to protect against glare or to provide the patient with disposable mydriatic sunglasses designed for this purpose (see Chapter 21).

Failure to warn patients not only subjects optometrists to claims for injuries suffered by patients, but also can widen liability to include third parties who may be injured by patients (e.g., in an automobile accident).[87,88] Optometrists should routinely document the warnings given to patients rather than relying on the patient's memory after the fact.[i]

Another important matter that should be documented is a patient's refusal to undergo dilation of the pupil. Optometrists are obligated to explain the importance of a dilated fundus examination to patients in terms that engender understanding. If despite the warning, a patient refuses to undergo the procedure, an entry should be made in the patient record (see Fig. 5.3), or the patient can be asked to sign a form that asserts the patient has rejected the optometrist's advice and understands the significance of the refusal. In rare cases, the matter may be of such importance that a certified letter, return receipt requested, should be sent to the patient, with a copy retained in the patient record. By whatever means selected, optometrists should not overlook the necessity for documentation in these cases.

CYCLOPLEGICS

Among the cycloplegics most frequently used are cyclopentolate and atropine. Because of their potential side effects, a careful history and assessment of the anterior chamber angle are necessary before use. Selection of the appropriate agent is also important (see Chapter 22). If there is a risk of angle closure, this risk must be communicated to patients, and informed consent should be obtained before the drug is administered.

If atropine is used, clinicians must be aware of the signs and symptoms of atropine toxicity. A similar concern exists when 2% cyclopentolate is used in infants or children.[89] If patients experience side effects, optometrists should be prepared to manage them either through direct intervention or referral to other practitioners.

Patients may be affected by photophobia and loss of accommodation, as they are with mydriatics. Therefore, patients must be monitored while in the office and on the premises and must be warned of the drug's effects while operating a vehicle or performing other tasks that pose a risk of injury to patients or others. Documentation of this warning should be included in the patient record.

Interestingly, failure to employ cycloplegia for the purpose of prescribing spectacles for a young patient with latent hyperopia has resulted in a claim of negligence against an optometrist.[90] However, the opportunity for a "slip and fall" injury or an automobile accident poses the greatest legal risks if no warning is given or no protection against glare is provided.

Although the toxic and allergic side effects of diagnostic pharmaceutical agents can be the cause of a malpractice claim, the side effects of therapeutic drugs are potentially a more likely source of litigation.

Complications of Therapeutic Drug Use

The complications of therapeutic drug use are a leading cause of malpractice claims against ophthalmologists[34,35] and potentially pose a significant malpractice risk for optometrists.[20,40] Because drug use occurs outside practitioners' offices and may involve use for an extended period of time, the opportunity for complications to arise, particularly those related to drug toxicity, is greater. If patient follow-up is not timely, the complications may go undetected, thus compounding the injury. Worst of all, if practitioners fail to make the correct diagnosis, the treatment not only fails to remedy patients' problems but also delays institution of the correct therapy. For these reasons optometrists using therapeutic agents face malpractice risks that differ from those encountered with diagnostic agents.

Negligence claims against ophthalmologists involving the use of therapeutic agents may be grouped into three categories: (1) misuse of steroids, (2) complications of antiglaucoma agents, and (3) misdiagnosis, followed by institution of an inappropriate therapeutic regimen.[34,35] Each of these problems has important legal implications for optometrists.

STEROIDS

The leading cause of drug-related claims against ophthalmologists is misuse of steroids, particularly the topically applied agents.[34,35] The usual situation is one in which patients use the drug for prolonged therapy, resulting in cataracts, open-angle glaucoma, or both.[91] Two legal issues are present in these cases. The first involves a practitioner's obligation to warn patients of side effects as required by the doctrine of informed consent. Failure to satisfy this duty can result in successful liability claims against the practitioner.[92] Prudent practitioners also ensure that this warning is documented in the patient record. The second issue concerns patients' ability to obtain prescription refills, which is often a complex web of entanglements among prescribing practitioners, practitioners' staff, patients, and pharmacists who fill the prescription. To reduce the opportunity for misunderstanding or mistake, the prescription should specify the drug quantity and the number of refills and should include a statement that these orders may not be changed. Practitioners should always retain a copy of the prescription given to patients (see Chapter 4).

Systemic steroids are also the cause of numerous negligence claims. These drugs have side effects that can result in serious injury, even death, and consequently must be used

---

[i]The ability of patients to recall warnings is highly suspect. Several studies have revealed that patients in fact remember very little. See Robinson G, Merav A. Informed consent: Recall by patients tested postoperatively. Ann Thorac Surg 1976;22:209–212; Priluck IA, Robertson DM, Buettner H. What patients recall of the preoperative discussion after retinal detachment surgery. Am J Ophthalmol 1979;87:620–623; and Morgan LW, Schwab IR. Informed consent in senile cataract extraction. Arch Ophthalmol 1986;104:42–45.

conservatively. Systemically administered drugs, with their risk of systemic complications, should not be used if a topical route of administration suffices, and practitioners must be prepared to justify the selection of a systemic route of administration when complications result and a topical route of administration was not used first.[34,35] Whenever systemic steroids are prescribed, practitioners must warn patients of side effects, monitor patients adequately so that preventable injuries can be detected, and document the care rendered.

ANTIGLAUCOMA AGENTS

Legal claims arising from glaucoma therapy may be divided into three categories: (1) adverse effects of β blockers, (2) retinal detachments following initiation of miotic therapy, and (3) complications resulting from use of CAIs.

Beta blockers are often the drug of choice for the initial treatment of primary open-angle glaucoma, but these drugs are contraindicated for use in persons with chronic obstructive pulmonary disease and heart block (see Chapter 10). A careful history should be taken prior to initiating therapy to avoid potentially fatal ramifications. It is advisable to monitor patients who are taking β blockers (e.g., pulse, blood pressure) and to inquire about side effects at periodic follow-up examinations.

In a sample case,[93] a 68-year-old woman with cataracts underwent uneventful extracapsular cataract extraction. On the first postsurgical day the ophthalmologist dispensed timolol to control elevated IOP. The patient had a long history of asthma and was taking medications for the condition, including prednisone, but the physician had not taken note of them. After the first administration of the timolol, the woman experienced severe bronchospasm, collapsed, and died. The use of miotics in myopic patients has been the cause of negligence claims when therapy has resulted in retinal detachment.[94] Patients who are at risk for detachment should be treated with nonmiotic agents initially. To comply with the doctrine of informed consent, the use of miotics should be preceded by a discussion with patients of the risks and benefits of the drug chosen. When miotics are the drug of choice for treatment, patients should be examined carefully to rule out the presence of risk factors (e.g., lattice degeneration) that may increase the likelihood of a retinal detachment.

CAIs such as acetazolamide have well-known side effects (e.g., renal calculi) that require an assessment of the benefits and risks of the use of these drugs before initiating therapy. If a practitioner cannot demonstrate that topically applied drugs are inadequate to control a patient's glaucoma, the choice of an oral CAI may be difficult to justify.[34,35] The risks of a systemic route of administration obligate practitioners to discuss potential complications and to obtain informed consent from patients. Because of the prolonged nature of glaucoma therapy, patients must be examined periodically both to assess the effectiveness of treatment and to rule out the presence of drug-related complications. An extremely rare complication, aplastic anemia, has been the subject of unsuccessful legal claims alleging that the treating practitioner had a legal duty to warn of this side effect and to monitor patients for signs of its occurrence.[34,35]

MISDIAGNOSIS

Unlike claims of misdiagnosis involving diagnostic agents, which usually concern intraocular disorders, allegations involving therapeutic agents usually concern the cornea and the anterior segment.[20,40] Optometrists who undertake to treat diseases of the cornea and the external adnexa may be held to a medical standard of care and must be prepared to justify the treatment rendered accordingly. This area of therapeutic drug use is probably the one in which optometrists are most vulnerable to legal claims.

Litigation can arise out of misdiagnosis of corneal complications associated with herpes simplex,[95] *Pseudomonas* ulcers,[96] fungal infections,[34] and corneal abrasions occurring in the contact lens population, particularly among patients fitted with extended wear lenses.[97] Optometrists must be certain to conform to the standard of care in making diagnoses, scheduling patient follow-up visits, and arranging consultations and referrals. Because complications can rapidly lead to permanent injuries and loss of visual acuity, optometrists must be vigilant when diagnosing and managing corneal and external disease. The treatment rendered should be documented with the same meticulous concern.

Documentation

The patient record is vital in any litigation in which optometrists are charged with negligence. A properly maintained record may offer an irrefutable defense, and an inadequate record may make the optometrist's position indefensible. Recordkeeping is an important task that should not be neglected.[98-100] Although there are no legally established requirements for organizing or maintaining records, because of the episodic nature of much of the care rendered by optometrists (particularly when using therapeutic pharmaceutical agents), the problem-oriented recordkeeping system is preferable.[101]

Optometrists should record each patient's drug history, the drugs used for diagnosis or treatment, any appropriate warnings, and the outcome of the case if there are complications (Table 5.4). For clinical and legal reasons, optometrists should be certain to document recalls and referrals.

RECALLS

If patients require follow-up care, a recall appointment is necessary. Recalls should be scheduled for a specific date and time before patients leave the office, even if the date of

TABLE 5.4
Documentation of Drug Use

Documentation should include:

1. All drugs the patient is taking, including any drugs taken for prolonged periods that may have adverse effects on the eyes or vision
2. Previous allergic or toxic responses to any drugs, including ophthalmic drugs
3. Drugs employed by the optometrist for diagnostic or therapeutic purposes, including concentration and dosage. If therapeutic drugs are prescribed, a copy of the prescription should be retained in the patient's record
4. Allergic or toxic responses to any drugs administered, which should be conspicuously noted
5. Warnings concerning the risks of drug use that are communicated to the patient
6. Treatment or disposition of the patient if an adverse event is experienced
7. Recalls and referrals or consultations

the appointment is weeks or months away. Optometrists should note the reason for the recall on the patient's record and should be certain that the recall examination addresses the problem for which the patient is required to return. To minimize "no show" appointments, it is best to contact patients before the scheduled date to confirm the day and time of the appointment. In some instances, "no show" patients may need to be contacted to determine why they failed to keep the appointment.[j]

REFERRALS

The preferable means of making a referral is to choose the practitioner and arrange the appointment before the patient has left the office. This information, along with any other pertinent data relative to the referral, should be noted in the patient's record. If a referral letter is written, a copy of the letter should also be retained in the record. Because of the importance of documenting referrals,[102] clinicians should establish a "fail-safe" system of review that ensures that appropriate entries have been made. The omission of this information, if litigation should ensue, unalterably weakens the optometrist's defense.[102]

CONSULTATIONS

Consultations with other practitioners should be scheduled and documented in the same manner as referrals. Consultation creates a joint venture in which liability for negligence may be shared. For this reason, consultants should be selected with due care. Patients' records should contain any correspondence to consultants, the consultants' written rec-

ommendations, and accounts of the action taken based on consultants' findings.

Product Liability

Drug-related product liability claims involving clinicians are rare. Because drugs are customarily sold to patients by pharmacists on the prescription of a duly licensed practitioner, it is the manufacturer or seller of the drug who is held liable if patients suffer an injury because the drug is "defective." However, clinicians may become defendants because the drug was inappropriately or improperly prescribed or because of insufficient patient follow-up while patients were taking the drug. Clinicians may also be charged with failing to comply with the doctrine of informed consent by inadequately warning patients of drug-related side effects.[103] Therefore, optometrists, as clinicians who prescribe and dispense drugs, should be familiar with the requirements of product liability law, because the adverse effects of a drug may precipitate a legal dispute among patients, pharmacists, and drug manufacturers, to which optometrists are a party.

A sample case can be used to illustrate a typical product liability claim.[104] A man who was severely allergic to a variety of substances was treated by a physician who prescribed an extensive course of therapy, including steroids taken topically, orally, and by injection. After more than 20 years of treatment, the patient developed osteoporosis and bilateral cataracts, which were removed surgically. He subsequently sued the manufacturer of the steroids, alleging that the drug was a defective product because the package inserts did not warn specifically enough of its dangerous side effects. He also sued the physician for negligence, alleging that the physician had failed to warn him of the risks associated with the use of steroids and had inadequately monitored the effects of treatment.

Because drug-related side effects may provide the motivation for a lawsuit, optometrists should be familiar with the ophthalmic drugs that have been the subject of product

---

[j]Although practitioners are under no legal duty to contact patients who fail to keep appointments, there are circumstances under which follow-up may be wise. For example, a patient who is undergoing treatment with therapeutic agents and who is in need of further evaluation faces a much higher risk of complication than a daily wear contact lens patient who fails to keep a 6-month recall appointment. Follow-up in the former case may prevent an injury—and a lawsuit.

liability claims. This section describes these medications, the theory of product liability, and how together they may be applied to the practice of optometry.

Basis for Product Liability

Product liability law is an attempt to reduce the economic impact of product-caused injuries on consumers. The underlying social theory is that the designer, manufacturer, and seller of a product are better able to absorb the economic loss through the purchase of liability insurance, which becomes part of the cost of the product, than is the injured consumer, who suffers lost time from work and the cost of medical and hospital bills as well as the possibility of impairment. Product liability claims allow the consumer to recover these costs and to receive compensation for both temporary and permanent injuries.

If a product is being used for its customary and intended purpose, without having undergone substantial change in the condition in which it was sold, and the product injures a consumer as a result of defective design or manufacture, then the designer, manufacturer, and seller bear the legal responsibility for the consumer's injury as a matter of law.[105] This rule applies even though the designer, manufacturer, and seller have exercised all possible care in the preparation and sale of the product. The distinction between product liability law and negligence is made most apparent by the "strict liability" of the former. The standard of care is no longer the legal measure; rather, it is the "defective" character of the product that establishes the defendant's liability.

Proof that a drug is "defective" requires evidence that it is unreasonably dangerous for the purpose sold or, alternatively, that it does not meet the expectations of an ordinary consumer as to its safety. Injury caused by the side effects of a drug, however, does not create an action for which damages may be awarded if the manufacturer has adequately issued a warning of the known side effects. In a representative case,[106] a woman who received chloroquine over an 8-year period for the treatment of systemic lupus erythematosus developed retinopathy and ultimately became almost totally blind. She sued the drug manufacturer for failure to warn, and the company defended the claim by producing evidence that warnings had been issued after investigators had established a scientific basis for attributing the retinal changes to the drug. These warnings were not issued, however, until years after publication of the first case reports that linked the drug to ocular side effects. The trial court found in favor of the manufacturer, but the decision was reversed on appeal, with the apellate court holding that the manufacturer failed to issue a timely warning. A similar conclusion has been reached in other cases.[107,108]

The manufacturer's duty to warn extends to the prescriber of the drug and not to the patient.[109] For example, a woman who had taken thioridazine (Mellaril) for a psychiatric disorder experienced a pigmentary retinopathy so severe that she became legally blind.[110] She sued the manufacturer, alleging that the warning of drug side effects was inadequate. The manufacturer's defense was that the risk of pigmentary retinopathy was well known, that this risk had been communicated to physicians for more than 20 years, and that the warning on the package insert was sufficient. The jury found in favor of the manufacturer and the patient appealed, but the appellate court upheld the decision, noting that the drug manufacturer's duty was to provide an adequate warning to the physician and not to her.[110]

Because clinicians must communicate such a warning to patients, as required by the doctrine of informed consent, optometrists are legally obligated to understand the side effects of any drugs that are prescribed.[111] Optometrists must stay abreast of reports in the literature and warnings from drug manufacturers and must explain these risks to patients before initiating treatment. The duty to warn also extends to the side effects of drugs administered systemically. A series of cases has delineated the obligation to warn patients of drugs that will impair operation of a motor vehicle and has resulted in the imposition of liability against practitioners for failing to fulfill this obligation, including cases in which patients injure a third party.[87,88,112] For example, a bus driver who was given a prescription for the antihistamine, tripelennamine, became groggy and drowsy after taking a tablet before work and "blacked out or went to sleep" while driving, causing the bus to strike a telephone pole and injure a passenger.[113] In the resulting lawsuit, the passenger alleged that the prescribing physician was negligent for failing to warn the driver of the effects of the drug. Although the claim was dismissed by the trial court, it was upheld on appeal. The appellate court ruled that even if a jury found the driver to be negligent, the physician could also be held liable if the jury found he had failed to warn of the side effects of the drug.

A common source of information concerning the risks of drug use is the package insert that accompanies the drug. The package insert also describes the recommended dosage and treatment regimen for the drug. Optometrists should be familiar with this information and should be prepared to justify any deviation from these recommendations. The risk of side effects and the expected benefit must be discussed with patients before informed consent that meets legal requirements can be secured. Because the treatment of eye disease raises the possibility that a court will impose a medical standard of care on a defendant optometrist, deviation from a recommended treatment regimen described in the package insert should be undertaken only with clear clinical justification (see Chapter 4).

Another aspect of this obligation concerns the management of adverse reactions. Practitioners are fiduciaries and owe patients a duty of affirmative disclosure, which means that not only misleading statements but also silence may constitute a breach of the practitioner's obligations.[114] A sample case[115] illustrates this principle. A man who complained of chronic eyelid problems that caused numerous hordeola was treated by an ophthalmologist with Inflamase ⅛%. The treatment was successful, but 2 years after therapy began a pharmacist mistakenly refilled the prescription with Inflamase 1%, which caused blurred vision and pain due to disruption of the corneal epithelium. Afterwards the ophthalmologist avoided the patient's inquiries about the effects of the medication on his vision. Ultimately the patient sued the drug manufacturer, alleging that the product was defective, and the ophthalmologist, claiming that the physician was negligent and that his conduct constituted fraud. Although the trial court found that the statute of limitations barred the claim, the decision was reversed on appeal, with the appellate court ruling that the ophthalmologist's conduct in avoiding the patient's questions could not be used as a basis on which to defeat the patient's claim as a matter of law.

The nexus among drug side effects, the duty to warn, and the torts of product liability and negligence make it necessary for clinicians to recognize those drugs that have been the cause of legal claims in order to take the steps necessary to minimize the risk of injury and possible litigation.

Ophthalmic Drugs and Liability Claims

The ophthalmic drugs that have been the most frequent causes of product liability and negligence claims are (1) acetazolamide, (2) echothiophate iodide, (3) hydrocortisone, (4) neomycin sulfate with dexamethasone sodium phosphate, and (5) prednisolone acetate with phenylephrine hydrochloride. Cases are used to illustrate the basis for legal claims involving these drugs.

ACETAZOLAMIDE

This CAI is used in the treatment of glaucoma (see Chapters 10 and 35). A known side effect of prolonged use is the formation of kidney stones.

A woman with glaucoma who had been using acetazolamide (Diamox) for many years was hospitalized twice within 2 years for kidney stones.[116] After the second hospitalization another drug was substituted for the acetazolamide, and the patient's IOP was well controlled without further complications. The patient then sued the physician who had prescribed the Diamox, alleging that the physician was negligent, and this claim was eventually settled for an undisclosed sum. She also sued the drug manufacturer, alleging that there was a failure to warn users of the drug of its potential side effects. The manufacturer, however, was held not to be liable; the court found that the manufacturer had satisfied the legal duty to warn the physician and that there was no legal duty to warn the patient.

ECHOTHIOPHATE IODIDE

This strong miotic may be used in the treatment of open-angle glaucoma when the disease does not respond to more conventional forms of therapy (see Chapters 10 and 35). A suspected side effect of treatment is retinal detachment, particularly in "at risk" patients, such as those with high myopia.

A man who had received glaucoma therapy for 8 years was changed to Phospholine Iodide.[94] Three weeks later he began seeing "spots" before his eyes, and 4 days later he suffered an acute loss of vision. Because the physicians he consulted were unable to see him immediately, the diagnosis of retinal detachment was delayed for one week. Surgery was unsuccessful, and the patient filed suit against the manufacturer of the drug and the physicians who had prescribed it. Although the drug manufacturer denied the existence of a causal relationship between the use of echothiophate and the detachment, the patient's product liability claim was settled before trial. After a jury trial, a substantial judgment was awarded to the patient for the negligence claim.

HYDROCORTISONE

This anti-inflammatory agent is found in a number of antibacterial-steroid combinations and is a well-documented cause of open-angle glaucoma when used for an extended period of time. A 10-year-old boy was given Cortisporin by an ophthalmologist to treat a rash that affected the patient's eyelids.[117] The child's mother administered the drug for 15 months before doctors discovered that her son had bilateral open-angle glaucoma that caused loss of vision in one eye and severe visual impairment in the other. A lawsuit was filed against the prescribing physician and the pharmacy that had supplied the drug, and the case was settled before trial for a substantial amount.

NEOMYCIN SULFATE WITH DEXAMETHASONE SODIUM PHOSPHATE

This antibiotic-steroid combination is applied topically for numerous ocular disorders. Known side effects of prolonged use include cataracts and open-angle glaucoma.

A pediatrician prescribed NeoDecadron for a young girl who had conjunctivitis, and the child's mother used the ointment intermittently for 2 years, during which time the prescription was refilled 6 times.[118] By the end of this period the girl had developed bilateral open-angle glaucoma that caused loss of vision. The physician did not monitor her IOP during the time she was receiving treatment. A sizable judgment was awarded the child by the trial court.

PREDNISOLONE ACETATE WITH PHENYLEPHRINE HYDROCHLORIDE

This steroid-vasoconstrictor combination has been applied topically to treat various ocular inflammations. Long-term use of the drug is known to cause open-angle glaucoma.

An ophthalmologist prescribed Prednefrin ⅛% solution for a woman with conjunctivitis, and one month later the patient's pharmacist called the physician to ask if she could refill the prescription in two bottles (she requested one for work and one for home).[92] The ophthalmologist gave permission but offered no advice concerning future refills. The pharmacist continued to refill the prescription over 5 months. At an examination 1 year later the patient was found to have elevated IOP. Eventually the patient was diagnosed as having open-angle glaucoma and cataracts, and she filed suit against the ophthalmologist, the pharmacist, and the drug manufacturer. During the trial she settled her claims against the ophthalmologist and the pharmacist, but the jury found in favor of the drug manufacturer, holding that the patient had misused the drug.

Documentation

Documentation of patient care is essential to the defense of legal claims. If pharmaceutical agents are used, clinicians should ensure that the patient record includes an adequate history, a description of drugs used, any warnings communicated to the patient, required recall appointments (including "no show" appointments), and an explanation of the treatment rendered if patients experience allergic or toxic side effects.

If this information is recorded, clinicians are able to substantiate the treatment rendered, and as long as that treatment has been in compliance with the standard of care, clinicians will defeat an action for damages. Inadequate documentation, however, may produce the opposite result. Clinicians should take the time to maintain accurate, thorough, contemporaneous records that reflect the care and attention given to each patient.

References

1. Hirsch M, Wick R. The optometric profession. Philadelphia: Chilton, 1968.
2. Shyrock RH. Medical licensing in America, 1650–1965. Baltimore: Johns Hopkins University Press, 1967.
3. Prentice C. Legalized optometry and memoirs. Seattle: Casperin Fletcher Press, 1926;128–133.
4. Stevens R. American medicine and the public interest. New Haven: Yale University Press, 1977;103–109.
5. Fitch A. My fifty years in optometry. Philadelphia: Press of the Pennsylvania State College of Optometry, 1955;7–8.
6. *Martin v. Baldi,* 249 Pa. 253, 94 A. 1091 (1915).
7. *Rhode Island Ophthalmological Society v. Cannon,* 317 A. 2d 124 (1974).
8. Classé J. The right to practice primary care. J Am Optom Assoc 1986;57:549–553.
9. *Esposito v. Shapero,* Civil Action 76-1214, West Virginia Circuit Court, Cabell County, December 16, 1976 (cert. denied June 6, 1977).
10. *Molina v. McQuinn,* 758 P. 2d 798 (New Mex. 1988).
11. Comprehensive Drug Abuse Prevention and Control Act of 1970. In: Physician's manual: An information outline of the Controlled Substances Act of 1970. Washington, DC: U.S. Department of Justice, 1978.
12. Bartlett JD, Wood JW. Optometry and the Drug Enforcement Administration. J Am Optom Assoc 1981;52:495–498.
13. Adams CM, Alexander LJ, Bartlett JD, Classé JG. Comanagement of patients with glaucoma. Optom Clin 1992;2(4):143–156.
14. Holder A. Medical malpractice law. New York: John Wiley & Sons, 1975;200–204.
15. *Black's Law Dictionary,* rev. ed. 4. St. Paul, MN: West, 1968.
16. *Schloendorff v. Society of New York Hospital,* 211 N.Y. 125, 105 N.E. 92 (1914).
17. Thal LS. *Gates v. Jensen:* Another precedent for glaucoma testing. J Am Optom Assoc 1981;52:349–353.
18. Harris MG, Dister RE. Informed consent in contact lens practice. J Am Optom Assoc 1987;58:230–236.
19. Luttjohann L. Informed consent and release of patient records. Kansas Optom J 1984;51:6–7.
20. Classé J. Liability and ophthalmic drug use. Optom Clin 1992;2(4):121–134.
21. Kraushar MF, Steinberg JA. Informed consent: Surrender or salvation? Arch Ophthalmol 1986;104:352–355.
22. Gold JA. Informed consent. Arch Ophthalmol 1993;111:321–323.
23. *Natanson v. Cline,* 187 Kan. 186, 354 P. 2d 670 (1960).
24. *Welch v. Whitaker,* 317 S.E. 2d 758 (S.C. App. 1984).
25. *Woods v. Brumlop,* 1 N.M. 2d 221, 377 P. 2d 520 (1962); *Canterbury v. Spence,* 464 F. 2d 772 (D.C. Cir. 1972); and *Cobbs v. Grant,* 8 Cal. 3d 229, 502 P. 2d 1 (1972).
26. *Ford v. Ireland,* 699 S.W. 2d 587 (Tex. App. 1985).
27. Curran WJ. Malpractice claims: New data and new trends. N Engl J Med 1979;300:26.
28. Modern status of views as to general measure of physician's duty to inform patient of risks of proposed treatment, 88 ALR 3d 1008.
29. Cockburn DM. Prevalence and significance of narrow anterior chamber angles in optometric practice. Am J Optom Physiol Opt 1981;58:171–175.
30. Keller JT. The risk of angle closure from the use of mydriatics. J Am Optom Assoc 1975;46:19–21.
31. Classé J. Pupillary dilation: an eye-opening problem. J Am Optom Assoc 1992;63:733–740.
32. Potter JW, Bartlett JD, Alexander LJ, et al. Oral fluorography. J Am Optom Assoc 1985;56:784–792.
33. Alexander LJ, Scholles J. Clinical and legal aspects of pupillary dilation. J Am Optom Assoc 1987;58:432–437.
34. Bettman JW. A review of 412 claims in ophthalmology. Int Ophthalmol Clin 1980;20(4):131–142.
35. Bettman JW. Seven hundred medicolegal cases in ophthalmology. Ophthalmology 1990;97:1379–1384.
36. Classé JG. Legal aspects of optometry. Boston: Butterworth, 1989;295–301.
37. *Gates v. Jensen,* 92 Wash. 2d 246, 595 P. 2d 919 (1979).
38. *Koenig v. United States,* case 86-CV-10269-BC, U.S. District Court, Eastern District of Michigan (Jan. 20, 1989).
39. Scholles J. A review of professional liability claims in optometry. J Am Optom Assoc 1986;57:764–766.

40. Classé JG. A review of 50 malpractice claims. J Am Optom Assoc 1989;60:694–706.
41. Classé JG. Optometrist's duty to test for glaucoma. South J Optom 1984;2:6–10.
42. Classé JG. Optometrist's duty to detect ocular tumors. South J Optom 1985;3:26–32.
43. Classé JG. Optometrist's duty to detect retinal detachment. South J Optom 1985;3:7–13.
44. Classé JG. Liability for the treatment of anterior segment eye disease. Optom Clin 1991;1(4):1–16.
45. National Association of Insurance Commissioners. Malpractice Claims, vol. 2, no. 2. Madison, Wis: National Association of Insurance Commissioners, 1980.
46. Elmstrom G. Malpractice: What can ODs expect? Opt J Rev Optom 1977;114:42–45.
47. Black's Law Dictionary, rev. ed. 4. St. Paul, MN: West, 1968.
48. Prosser WL. Law of torts, ed. 4. St. Paul, MN: West, 1971;139–235.
49. Prosser WL. Law of torts, ed. 4. St. Paul, MN: West, 1971;162–163.
50. Classé J. Liability and the primary care optometrist. J Am Optom Assoc 1986;57:926–929.
51. Guides to the evaluation of permanent impairment, ed. 2. Chicago: American Medical Association, 1984;141–151.
52. Reed v. Church, 8 S.E. 2d 285 (Va. 1940).
53. Trogun v. Fruchtman, 209 N.W. 2d 297 (Wis. 1973).
54. Yorston v. Pennell, 153 A. 2d 255 (Pa. 1959).
55. Cox MS, Schepens CL, Freeman HM. Retinal detachment due to ocular contusion. Arch Ophthalmol 1966;76:678–685.
56. Classé JG. Clinicolegal aspects of vitreous and retinal detachment. Optom Clin 1992;2(3):113–125.
57. Helling v. Carey, 83 Wash. 2d 514, 519 P. 2d 981 (Wash. 1974).
58. Harris v. Groth, 90 Wash. 2d 438, 663 P. 2d 113 (Wash. 1983).
59. Wechsler S, Classé JG. Helling v. Carey: Caveat medicus (let the doctor beware). J Am Optom Assoc 1977;48:1526–1529.
60. Classé JG. Helling revisited: How the "tale" wagged the dog. J Am Optom Assoc 1987;58:343–345.
61. McMahon v. Glixman, 393 N.E. 2d 875 (Mass. 1979).
62. Collins v. American Optometric Association, 693 F. 2d 636 (7th Cir. 1982).
63. Holmes v. Iwasa, 104 Ida. 179, 657 P. 2d 476 (1983).
64. Feharne v. Dunlap, 565 N.Y.S. 2d 664 (1991).
65. Semes L, Gold A. Clinical and legal considerations in the diagnosis and management of ocular tumors. J Am Optom Assoc 1987;58:134–139.
66. Classé JG. The eye opening case of Keir v. United States. J Am Optom Assoc 1989;60:471–476.
67. Keir v. United States, 853 F. 2d 398 (6th Cir. 1988).
68. Classé JG. A dark victory. Optom Economics 1991;1(2):44–45.
69. Fairchild v. Brian, 354 So. 2d 675 (La. App. 1977).
70. 354 So. 2d at 679.
71. Byer NE. Natural history of posterior vitreous detachment with early management as the premier line of defense against retinal detachment. Ophthalmology 1994;101:1503–1514.
72. Tasman WS. Posterior vitreous detachment and peripheral breaks. Trans Am Acad Ophthalmol Otolaryngol 1968;72:217–224.
73. Davis MD. Natural history of retinal breaks without detachment. Arch Ophthalmol 1974;92:183–194.
74. Whitt v. Columbus Cooperative Enterprises, 64 Ohio St. 355, 415 N.E. 2d 985 (1980).
75. Alexander LJ. Vision care for the patient with diabetes (editorial). J Am Optom Assoc 1987;58:872–873.
76. Lipson LG, ed. Diabetes mellitus in the elderly. Am J Med 1986;80:1–56.
77. Steele v. United States, 463 F. Supp. 321 (D.C. Alaska 1978).
78. Tempchin v. Sampson, 262 Md. 156, 277 A. 2d 67 (Md. 1971).
79. Kime v. Aetna, 66 Ohio App. 277, 33 N.E. 2d 1008 (Ohio App. 1940).
80. Wills v. Klingenbeck, 455 So. 2d 806 (Ala. 1984).
81. Norden LC. Adverse reactions to topical ocular anesthetics. J Am Optom Assoc 1976;47:730–733.
82. Burns RP, Forster RK, Laibson P, Gibson IK. Chronic toxicity of local anesthetics on the cornea. In: Leopold IH, Burns RP, eds. Symposium on ocular therapy. New York: John Wiley & Sons, 1977;10:31–44.
83. Graham v. Whitaker, 321 S.E. 2d 40 (S.C. 1984).
84. Truxillo v. Gentilly Medical Building, Inc., 225 So. 2d 488 (La. 1969).
85. Welke v. Kuzilla, 144 Mich. App. 245, 375 N.W. 2d 403 (Mich. App. 1985).
86. Bartlett JD, Classé JG. Dapiprazole: Will it affect the standard of care for pupillary dilation? Optom Clin 1992;2(4):113–120.
87. Gold AR. Failure to warn. J Am Optom Assoc 1986;57:317–319.
88. Classé JG. Optometrist's duty to warn of vision impairment. South J Optom 1986;4:66–69.
89. Gray LG. Avoiding adverse effects of cycloplegics in infants and children. J Am Optom Assoc 1979;50:465–470.
90. Kahn v. Shaw, 65 Ga. App. 563, 16 S.E. 2d 99 (Ga. App. 1941).
91. Lorentzon v. Rowell, 321 S.E. 2d 341 (Ga. App. 1984).
92. Ortiz v. Allergan Pharmaceuticals, 489 S.W. 2d 135 (Tex. Civ. App. 1972).
93. Westmoreland v. Doe, case no. CL92–423, City of Petersburg Circuit Court, Petersburg, Va. Reported in Medical Malpractice: Verdicts, Settlements, and Experts 1992;9(2):11.
94. Fykes v. Chatow, docket no. 976896, Superior Court, Los Angeles County, Cal., 1974. Reported in The Citation, 1975;30:120.
95. Classé JG, Harris MG. Liability and extended wear contact lenses. J Am Optom Assoc 1987;58:848–854.
96. Classé JG. Optometrist's liability for contact lenses. South J Optom 1986;4:52–57.
97. Beaman v. Schwartz, 738 S.W. 2d 632 (Tenn. App. 1986).
98. Scholles J. Documentation and record-keeping in clinical practice. J Am Optom Assoc 1986;57:141–143.
99. Miller PJ. Documentation as a defense to legal claims. J Am Optom Assoc 1986;57:144–145.
100. Classé JG. Record-keeping and documentation in clinical practice. South J Optom 1987;5:11–25.
101. Scope of practice: Patient care and management manual. St. Louis: American Optometric Association, 1986.
102. Gerber P. How to blow your own malpractice defense. Optom Man 1981;17:19–25.
103. McMickens v. Callahan, 533 So. 2d 589 (Ala. 1988).
104. Hill v. Squibb and Sons, 592 P. 2d 1383 (Mont. 1979).
105. Section 402A of the Restatement of Torts, 2nd. (May not be applicable in all jurisdictions.)
106. Basko v. Sterling Drug, Inc., 416 F. 2d 417 (D.C. Conn 1969).
107. Krug v. Sterling Drug, Inc., 416 S.W. 2d 143 (Mo. 1967).
108. Kershaw v. Sterling Drug, Inc., 415 F. 2d 1005 (5th Cir. 1969).
109. Dixon MG. Drug product liability. New York: Matthew Bender, 1974:§9.01–9.09.

110. *Hatfield v. Sandoz-Wander, Inc.,* 464 N.E. 2d 1105 (Ill. App. 1984).

111. Dixon MG. Drug product liability. New York: Matthew Bender, 1974:§7.01–7.26.

112. *Wilschinsky v. Medina,* 775 P. 2d 713 (New Mex. 1989).

113. *Kaiser v. Suburban Transportation System,* 65 Wash. 2d 461, 398 P. 2d 14, modified 401 P. 2d 350 (Wash. 1965).

114. Holder AR: Medical malpractice law. New York: John Wiley & Sons, 1975;225.

115. *Lorentzon v. Rowell,* 321 S.E. 2d 341 (Ga. App. 1984).

116. *Bacardi v. Holzman,* 182 N.J. Super. 422, 442 A. 2d 617 (N.J. 1981).

117. *Kong v. Clay-Grant Pharmacy,* docket no. 619350, Superior Court, San Francisco County, Cal., 1972. Reported in The Citation 1973;26:122.

118. *Aetna Casualty and Surety Co. of Illinois v. Medical Protective Co. of Ft. Wayne, Indiana,* 575 F. Supp. 901 (Ill. D.C. 1983).

PART II

Pharmacology of Ocular Drugs

Drug therapy must be based upon correlation of effects of drugs with physiologic, biochemical and microbiologic kinetic aspects of diseases. Only through basic knowledge can we understand toxicology and limitations of drugs and how these can be overcome.

—I.H. Leopold

CHAPTER 6

Local Anesthetics

Jimmy D. Bartlett
Siret D. Jaanus

Local anesthetics are drugs that block nerve conduction when applied locally to nerve tissue in appropriate concentrations.[1] Although a variety of factors can interfere with nerve conduction, including hypothermia, anoxia, and various chemical substances, the clinical advantage of local anesthetics is that their action is reversible. Nerve function recovers completely, with no evidence of structural damage to nerve fibers or cells. Another prominent clinical feature of local anesthesia is that loss of sensation occurs without loss of consciousness.[1,2] This chapter considers the pharmacologic properties of anesthetics currently used for ophthalmic procedures.

Historical Perspective

The first documented use of local anesthesia was in approximately 800 AD, when cocaine-filled saliva, obtained by chewing the leaves of the shrub *Erythroxylon coca,* was placed on the skull for trephining operations.[3] In 1860 Albert Niemann isolated the active alkaloid from the coca plant and named it cocaine.[4] It remained, however, for Karl Koller to complete the discovery of local anesthesia. In 1884 he instilled a drop of cocaine solution into the eye of a frog. Within one minute the frog permitted its cornea to be touched. Koller subsequently tested the drug in his own eye. He observed that his cornea was devoid of sensation when touched with a pin. He also noted that the local anesthetic effect of cocaine was accompanied by a widening of the palpebral fissure, pupillary dilation, and a slight paresis of accommodation.[4] Within one year of Koller's discovery, cocaine was widely used in ophthalmic practice.

The initial clinical success of cocaine anesthesia was soon dampened by reports of both acute and chronic adverse effects due to local and systemic toxicity and to cocaine's addicting properties.[2] As a result, an intense effort was made to develop local anesthetics with a more favorable therapeutic index. The chemical identification of cocaine as a benzoic acid ester led to the synthesis of procaine in 1905. Numerous similar compounds were developed, including tetracaine and other anesthetics used today in ophthalmic practice.[2,5]

Pharmacologic Properties

Structural Features

Local anesthetics, except for cocaine, are synthetic, aromatic, or heterocyclic compounds. Nearly all local anesthetics in current clinical use are weakly basic tertiary amines. Their general configuration is shown in Figure 6.1. The structural components consist of an aromatic lipophilic portion, an intermediate alkyl chain, and a hydrophilic hydrocarbon group that is usually a tertiary amine but may also be a secondary amine. The lipophilic portion is usually an unsaturated aromatic ring and is essential for anesthetic activity. The lipophilic section determines potency, duration of action, and potential toxicity of the anesthetic. Changes in either the aromatic or amine portions can alter the lipid solubility of a local anesthetic and thereby alter its anesthetic potency. In general, highly lipid-soluble anesthetics are the most potent, with the longest durations of action.[1,5] The intermediate chain, usually of four to five carbons, is linked to the aromatic group by either an ester (–CO–) or amide (–NHC–) linkage, the nature of which determines certain pharmacologic properties of the molecule, including its me-

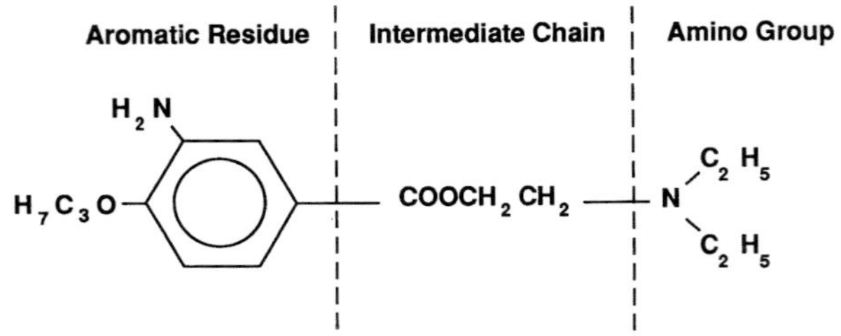

FIGURE 6.1   **Molecular structure of proparacaine, consisting of a lipophilic aromatic residue, an intermediate alkyl chain, and a hydrophilic amino group.**

tabolism.[1,5,6] All commonly used topical anesthetics are of the ester type, whereas most injectable anesthetics have an amide linkage (Table 6.1).

Physiochemical Characteristics

All local anesthetics exist in solution as the uncharged amine or as the positively charged substituted ammonium cation. In the amine form they tend to be only slightly soluble in water and are therefore usually formulated in solution in the form of acidic hydrochloride salts, which are water soluble[1,5,7] and contribute to stability of the anesthetic in solution. The degree of ionization is also important in the distribution of the anesthetic to its site of action, because only the nonionized form readily crosses cell membranes. Since the local anesthetics are weak bases, with a pK_a between 8.0 and 9.0, they tend to ionize in acidic solutions, thus enhancing both stability and shelf life.[1,5,7] On contact with neutral or alkaline environments, such as tears, the uncharged form predominates. If a local anesthetic is ap-

TABLE 6.1
Classification of Local Anesthetics

Ester linkage
  Esters of benzoic acid
    Cocaine
  Esters of meta-aminobenzoic acid
    Proparacaine
  Esters of para-aminobenzoic acid
    Procaine
    Chloroprocaine
    Tetracaine
    Benoxinate
Amide linkage (Amides of benzoic acid)
  Lidocaine
  Mepivacaine
  Bupivacaine
  Etidocaine

plied or injected into an acidic environment, such as in the presence of infection, the ionized fraction of the drug increases.[1,5]

Mechanism of Action

Local anesthetics prevent both the generation and conduction of nerve impulses. Their main site of action appears to be the cell membrane, where they block the transient increase in membrane permeability to sodium ions.[1,5,7] Blockade of the sodium channel is thought to occur by interaction of the local anesthetic with a specific binding site associated with the sodium channel.[1] Following application, anesthetics cross the cell membrane in the uncharged (lipid-soluble) form, but at the site of action, the charged form binds to the receptor.[1]

The duration of action of local anesthetics is proportional to the time they are in contact with the nerve tissue.[1] Consequently, any agent or procedure that keeps anesthetics at their site of action prolongs the period of anesthesia. In clinical practice, formulation of anesthetics with vasoconstrictors helps localize the anesthetic at the desired site. Local vasoconstriction may also offer the advantage of slowing absorption into the systemic circulation, which reduces the potential for systemic anesthetic toxicity.

In addition, the intrinsic vasodilator activity and degree of plasma protein binding of anesthetics can influence their clinical potency and duration of action. Compared to mepivacaine, lidocaine exhibits enhanced vasodilator action, which results in a clinically shorter duration of action.[5] Although protein binding generally reduces the amount of free drug available for receptor interaction, it can provide a drug depot for maintenance of anesthetic effect. This may partly explain the prolonged duration of action of highly protein-bound anesthetics such as bupivacaine and etidocaine.[8]

Anesthetics in current clinical use have relatively low systemic and ocular toxicity. Compared with cocaine, they do not alter pupil size or affect accommodation. Their sufficiently long duration of action, low cost, stability in solution, and general lack of interference with actions of other drugs make them useful agents for such ocular procedures as tonometry, foreign body and suture removal, gonioscopy, nasolacrimal duct irrigation and probing, and minor eyelid surgery.

Injectable Anesthetics

A wide variety of ocular diagnostic and surgical procedures may be performed under local anesthesia. Many procedures, such as suture removal, removal of superficial foreign bodies in the cornea, nasolacrimal irrigation, and tonometry

TABLE 6.2
Local Anesthetics for Regional Infiltration and Peripheral Nerve Block

Anesthetic (Trade Name)	Formulation (% solution)[a]	Onset of Action (min)	Duration of Action (hr)	Maximum Dose (mg)[b]
Procaine (Novocain)	1, 2, 10	7–8	½–¾	600 (10.0 mg/kg)
Lidocaine (Xylocaine)	0.5, 1, 1.5 2, 4	4–6	⅔–1 (1–2 with epinephrine)	300 (4.5 mg/kg) 500 (7.0 mg/kg with epinephrine)
Mepivacaine (Carbocaine)	1, 1.5, 2	3–5	2–3	400
Bupivacaine (Marcaine, Sensorcaine)	0.25, 0.50 0.75	5–10	4–12	175
Etidocaine (Duranest)	1, 1.5	3–5	5–10	400 (8.0 mg/kg)

[a]1% solution = 10 mg/ml. Some concentrations are commercially available with epinephrine. Hyaluronidase may be added to the retrobulbar or peribulbar injection to increase diffusion of anesthetic.
[b]For healthy adults. Use lowest dosage that provides effective anesthesia.

Adapted from Raj PP. Handbook of regional anesthesia. New York: Churchill Livingstone, 1985; Bartlett JD, Ghormley NR, Jaanus SD, et al., eds. Ophthalmic Drug Facts, St. Louis: Facts and Comparisons, 1995; Crandali DG. Pharmacology of ocular anesthetics. In: Duane TD, Jaeger EA, eds. Biomedical foundations of ophthalmology. Philadelphia: JB Lippincott, 1994; and Sobol WM, McCrary JA. Ocular anesthetic properties and adverse reactions. Int Ophthalmol Clin 1989;29:195–199.

require only topical administration of surface active anesthetics. However, when more extensive procedures are to be undertaken, administration of anesthetics by injection is necessary (Table 6.2). Facial nerve block, retrobulbar injection, or tissue infiltration are widely used, and discomfort associated with these procedures may be reduced by preheating anesthetics before injection.[9]

The required duration of a complete nerve block for a procedure is of great importance to the clinician in selecting a suitable local anesthetic. The duration of the anesthetic effect is determined by the length of time the drug stays bound to the nerve protein. This is dictated by the chemical structure of the drug, the concentration and amount administered, and the rate of removal by diffusion and circulation.

The most commonly used anesthetics for retrobulbar or peribulbar anesthesia are lidocaine and bupivacaine.[10,11] Lidocaine provides a rapid onset of anesthesia and akinesia, and bupivacaine has the advantage of offering prolonged postoperative pain relief.[12] These properties of the individual agents provide justification for using combinations of these anesthetics to achieve both rapid onset and prolonged duration of anesthesia and akinesia produced by retrobulbar or peribulbar injections.[11,13] Combinations, however, are not usually used for tissue infiltration procedures involving the eyelids. Instead, individual anesthetics, usually lidocaine, are used alone.

The addition of epinephrine, a vasoconstrictor, to an injectable anesthetic prolongs the duration of anesthesia and decreases the rate of systemic absorption, thereby decreasing the risk of systemic toxicity. The duration of bupivacaine, however, an already long-acting anesthetic, cannot be significantly extended by adding epinephrine.[12] The epinephrine also decreases local bleeding. Effective vasoconstriction is obtained with a concentration of 1:100,000 or even 1:200,000. The usual concentrations of epinephrine used for ophthalmic procedures range from 1:50,000 to 1:200,000. Recently, however, the rationale for the use of epinephrine has been questioned on the basis of the relative safety of anesthetics used for retrobulbar or peribulbar anesthesia, the risk of epinephrine side effects such as cardiac arrhythmia following accidental intravascular injection, and lack of enhanced anesthetic effect.[10]

When epinephrine is subjected to heat, its potency is destroyed. Consequently, solutions containing epinephrine should not be subjected to heat sterilization. Although epinephrine is widely used as an adjunctive agent in local anesthetics, undesirable effects on local tissue can occur. Epinephrine may delay wound healing and cause occasional necrosis and intense vasoconstriction. It may also produce adverse systemic reactions such as apprehension, anxiety, restlessness, tremor, pallor, tachycardia, dyspnea, hypertension, palpitation, headaches, and precordial distress. When subjective palpitation occurs with or without a throbbing

TABLE 6.3
Topical Anesthetics

Anesthetic	Trade Name (Manufacturer)	Formulation
Cocaine hydrochloride	Schedule II controlled substance	1–10% solution prepared from the bulk powder[a]
Tetracaine hydrochloride	Pontocaine (Sanofi Winthrop)	0.5% solution and ointment
Benoxinate hydrochloride with sodium fluorescein	Fluress (Pilkington/Barnes-Hind)	0.4% solution, combined with 0.25% sodium fluorescein
Proparacaine hydrochloride	AK-Taine (Akorn) Alcaine (Alcon) Ophthaine (Apothecon) Ophthetic (Allergan)	0.5% solution; also available as preservative-free 1 ml unit-dose
Proparacaine hydrochloride with sodium fluorescein	Fluoracaine (Akorn) Fluorocaine (Medical Ophthalmics)	0.5% solution, combined with 0.25% sodium fluorescein

[a]Fiscella RG, Lam J, Schell J, Siegel FP. Cocaine hydrochloride topical solution prepared for ophthalmic use. Am J Hosp Pharm 1993;50:1572.

headache, tachycardia, and hypertension, a diagnosis of reaction to epinephrine rather than to the local anesthetic is indicated. Although these reactions are temporary, patients with cardiovascular disease may suffer cardiac arrhythmias, angina attacks, or cerebral ischemia.

Hyaluronidase (Wydase), an aqueous testicular extract, is often added to anesthetics for retrobulbar or peribulbar injection to enhance spread of anesthetics through the retrobulbar tissues.[10] This enzyme depolymerizes hyaluronic acid, which acts as tissue cement, thus causing the anesthetic to diffuse more rapidly through local tissues.[14] A more effective akinesia of the orbicularis and extraocular muscles is generally achieved with the concomitant use of hyaluronidase in retrobulbar and peribulbar injections of anesthetics. A dose of 75 units (0.5 ml) per 10 ml anesthetic solution is usually sufficient to produce enhanced anesthesia and akinesia.[11]

Topical Anesthetics

The efficacy of topical anesthetics is usually determined by their ability to suppress corneal sensitivity. When a dose-response relationship is determined for various anesthetics, a concentration for each drug is obtained beyond which no further increase in activity occurs. The concentration at which this maximum efficacy occurs is termed the *maximum effective concentration*. Thus, increasing the concentration of the anesthetic beyond the maximum effective concentra-

tion serves no useful purpose but increases the risk of local and systemic toxicity.

The maximum effective concentrations of proparacaine, tetracaine, and cocaine are 0.5%, 1%, and 20%, respectively. However, in clinical practice, the optimum effective concentration of the drug may be less than the maximum effective concentration. For instance, 0.5% tetracaine is less irritating to the eye than the maximum effective concentration of 1% and thus is better suited for clinical use. The topical application of a combination of two or more local anesthetics does not produce an additive effect, yet increases the risk of side effects. The use of combinations of anesthetics is therefore contraindicated. The commonly used topical anesthetics are listed in Table 6.3.

Cocaine

Cocaine is unique among local anesthetics because it exhibits both anesthetic and adrenergic agonist activity. It is not commercially available in an ophthalmic solution. For clinical use the salt form of cocaine, cocaine hydrochloride, must be specially formulated in aqueous solution. Although not approved by the Food and Drug Administration (FDA) for ophthalmic use, solutions of cocaine (4%, 10%, Roxane) intended for otolaryngological purposes are commercially available. Clinical experience indicates that these are apparently effective and safe for ocular use. The usual concentration for topical ocular use is 1% to 4%,[15] but the 10% solution is often used, due to its adrenergic stimulatory effects, for the diagnosis of Horner's syndrome. One drop of a 2% solution produces excellent corneal anesthesia within 5 to 10 minutes.[16] Complete anesthesia lasts about 20 minutes, with incomplete surface anesthesia lasting for approximately 1 to 2 hours.[16] Anesthesia of the conjunctiva and insertions of the rectus muscles is sufficiently complete to permit painless grasping of the eye with forceps (in forced duction testing) for about 10 minutes.[17] Incomplete conjunctival anesthesia lasts for an additional 5 to 10 minutes.[17]

In addition, cocaine is used as a nasal spray or in a nasal pack during dacryocystorhinostomy (DCR). When applied to the nasal mucosa in a gauze pack, cocaine anesthetizes the contact area for an hour or longer.[18] Cocaine, due to its adrenergic effects, causes vasoconstriction, thus retarding its own absorption. Hence, cocaine constricts the conjunctival and nasal vasculatures when applied topically to these mucous membranes. Because of this vasoconstrictor action, use of epinephrine with cocaine is not only unnecessary but may be harmful, since cocaine causes sensitization to exogenous epinephrine.[18] Although cocaine has not been compared with other topical anesthetics in well-controlled clinical studies, there is a strong clinical impression that use of cocaine as a topical anesthetic has several potential advantages[19]: (1) cocaine is considerably more effective and longer acting than the other available topical anesthetics for achieving anesthesia of the conjunctiva; (2) cocaine has a more prolonged action than the other topical anesthetics in anesthetizing the cornea, but the intensity of anesthesia is not greater; and (3) cocaine may loosen the corneal epithelium to a greater extent than other topically applied anesthetics, thus facilitating debridement of the corneal epithelium.

Because cocaine blocks reuptake of norepinephrine and has an adrenergic potentiating effect, its use is contraindicated in patients with systemic hypertension or patients taking adrenergic agonists.[18] The interaction between cocaine and catecholamines contraindicates the use of cocaine in patients taking drugs that modify adrenergic neuronal activity, such as guanethidine, reserpine, tricyclic antidepressants, methyldopa, or monoamine oxidase (MAO) inhibitors.[15,18] Conversely, drugs that act directly on adrenergic receptors, such as phenylephrine, are contraindicated with use of cocaine.[18] Systemic toxicity can be prevented by anticipating potential drug interactions or hypertensive crises. Furthermore, since cocaine has a mydriatic effect, it is contraindicated in patients predisposed to angle-closure glaucoma.

The major side effect of cocaine is significant corneal epithelial toxicity. Grossly visible grayish pits and irregularities are readily produced by this drug.[15] These are followed by loosening of the corneal epithelium, which may result in large erosions. Although this characteristic is generally considered to be an adverse effect, it is clinically useful in cases requiring corneal epithelial debridement, as in treatment of herpetic ulcers. However, the corneal epithelial effects of cocaine contraindicate its use in any procedure requiring good visualization through the cornea, such as in retinal detachment surgery or in routine ophthalmoscopy or gonioscopy.

Acute systemic cocaine toxicity may result from as little as 20 mg (10 drops of a 4% solution) of drug.[17] Systemic side effects can potentially occur from the excessive topical application of the drug to the eye. Therefore, the total dose of cocaine should not exceed 3 mg/kg body weight. Typical manifestations of systemic toxicity include excitement, restlessness, headache, rapid and irregular pulse, dilated pupils, nausea, vomiting, abdominal pain, delirium, and convulsions.[20] The usual fatal dose is 1.2 g,[1] and death commonly results from respiratory failure.[21] Propranolol, a β-adrenergic blocking drug, has been reported to be an effective antagonist to the toxic cardiovascular effects of cocaine.[18]

Because of its potential ocular and systemic toxicity, cocaine has generally been replaced by the safer, synthetic local anesthetics. Nevertheless, it remains a drug of choice for topical anesthesia preceding corneal epithelial debridement and forced duction testing. Its only nonanesthetic ophthalmic use is in the pharmacologic diagnosis of suspected Horner's syndrome (see Chapter 23). Because of the strong abuse potential of cocaine, its distribution and clinical use are subject to federal and state controlled substance regulations under supervision of the Drug Enforcement Administration (DEA).[22]

Tetracaine

Tetracaine, an ester of para-aminobenzoic acid, has been widely used for topical anesthesia of the eye. It is currently available in a 0.5% solution and a 0.5% ointment. Its onset, intensity, and duration of anesthesia are comparable to those of proparacaine and benoxinate (Fig. 6.2). Onset of anesthesia sufficient to permit tonometry or other minor procedures involving the superficial cornea and conjunctiva is 10 to 20 seconds, and duration of anesthesia is 10 to 20 minutes. It has been reported, however, that the 1% solution produces anesthesia lasting nearly an hour.[23]

Tetracaine causes rapid surface anesthesia, but even repeated applications to the conjunctival surface may fail to achieve effective scleral anesthesia.[17] For ocular use as a local anesthetic, tetracaine should never be injected.[17] Moreover, since the 0.5% ointment produces prolonged anesthesia, this formulation is preferred for long-term topical anesthesia, which may be occasionally necessary for procedures such as electroretinography (ERG), where reinstillation of the topical anesthetic solution during the procedure is impractical. The ointment formulation may be used following removal of corneal foreign bodies to allow prolonged comfort of the patched eye. Tetracaine ointment is also helpful following cauterization of corneal or conjuncti-

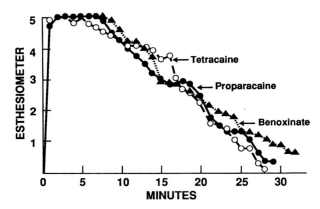

FIGURE 6.2 **Comparison of onset, intensity, and duration of anesthesia obtained with tetracaine 0.5%, proparacaine 0.5%, and benoxinate 0.4%. (Reprinted with permission from The American Journal of Ophthalmology 1955;40:697–704. Copyright, The Ophthalmic Publishing Company.)**

val lesions requiring that the eye be pressure-patched. It is important to note, however, that the patient should *never* be allowed to self-administer this or any other topical anesthetic. Serious corneal complications may result (see Contraindications).

Practitioners are cautioned to consider tetracaine a potent and potentially toxic local anesthetic. Dangerous overdoses may occur if it is administered in doses higher than 1.5 mg/kg body weight.[15]

A variety of side effects often accompany the use of topical tetracaine. Tetracaine appears to produce greater corneal compromise than proparacaine.[17,24,68] Perhaps the greatest objection, however, to the use of tetracaine is the moderate stinging or burning sensation that almost always occurs immediately following its topical instillation. This typically lasts 20 to 30 seconds following drug application. Another problem associated with use of tetracaine is allergic reactions. Local allergy to tetracaine may develop because of repeated use (e.g., in tonometry of glaucoma patients), but this is uncommon. Tetracaine exhibits no cross-sensitivity with proparacaine.[20]

Benoxinate

Benoxinate is commercially available only in combination with sodium fluorescein 0.25% (Fluress). Benoxinate 0.4%, an ester of para-aminobenzoic acid (PABA), has an onset, intensity, and duration of anesthesia similar to those of tetracaine 0.5% and proparacaine 0.5% (see Fig. 6.2).[15,16,25] Because benoxinate is available only in combination with sodium fluorescein, its primary clinical use is for applanation tonometry.[26] Although solutions of fluorescein serve as

good culture media for *Pseudomonas aeruginosa*,[27] the benoxinate-sodium fluorescein combination has been shown to have substantial bactericidal properties.[16,28] Thus, the benoxinate-sodium fluorescein combination is ideal for use in applanation tonometry, since it does not have the same risk for *Pseudomonas* contamination characteristic of sodium fluorescein solutions.

When the anesthetic effect of low concentrations (0.1% and 0.2%) of benoxinate is compared with the commercially available 0.4% solution, the maximum increase in sensitivity threshold that can be measured following instillation of 50 μl of each concentration is 200 mg/mm^2.[29] All three anesthetic solutions produce this amount of decreased corneal sensitivity, although the lower concentrations have the shortest duration of anesthetic effect. Thus, lower concentrations of benoxinate than are commercially available may be sufficient for routine applanation tonometry and other procedures requiring only minimal superficial anesthesia.[29]

Relatively few side effects are associated with the clinical use of benoxinate as an ocular anesthetic. Topical instillation typically produces a sensation of stinging or burning that is greater than that produced by the instillation of proparacaine but less than that produced by tetracaine.[15,30] In addition, benoxinate appears to cause less corneal epithelial desquamation than proparacaine, but this has not been substantiated by controlled clinical studies. Local allergic reactions to benoxinate are rare.[23] Benoxinate may be safely administered to some patients who are allergic to tetracaine, another ester of PABA, without allergic reactions, suggesting that the allergenic potential of benoxinate is extremely low.[31] There is no apparent cross-sensitivity between this agent and proparacaine.[20]

Proparacaine

Proparacaine is commercially available in a 0.5% solution, both with and without sodium fluorescein 0.25% (see Table 6.3). The onset, intensity, and duration of anesthesia from these preparations are similar to those of tetracaine 0.5% and benoxinate 0.4% (see Fig. 6.2).[15,25] Proparacaine, however, does not appear to penetrate into the cornea or conjunctiva as well as does tetracaine.[32]

When used without sodium fluorescein, proparacaine is widely employed as a general-purpose topical anesthetic. It produces little or no discomfort or irritation on instillation and is therefore readily accepted by most patients. Unopened bottles may be stored at room temperature, but once opened the bottles should be tightly capped and, ideally, refrigerated to retard discoloration.[16] Discolored solutions of proparacaine should be discarded (see Fig. 3.4).

Several investigators[29,30] have studied the anesthetic effects from low concentrations of proparacaine and found that 0.25% proparacaine is an effective anesthetic in all patients and that 0.125% proparacaine is effective in patients over age 40 years. Thus, as with benoxinate, lower concentrations of proparacaine than are commercially available may be sufficient for procedures requiring only minimal superficial anesthesia.

Proparacaine has few side effects. Although localized hypersensitivity reactions may develop, these are rare and occur less frequently with proparacaine than with tetracaine.[23] Allergic reactions may be characterized by conjunctival hyperemia and edema, edematous eyelids, and lacrimation.[24] Following topical ocular instillation in recommended doses, allergic systemic manifestations are extremely rare. Topically instilled proparacaine has been reported to have had a possible role in the development of a hypersensitivity reaction resulting in exacerbation of Stevens-Johnson syndrome.[33]

Proparacaine does not exhibit cross-sensitivity with tetracaine.[17] However, since proparacaine and tetracaine both contain an ester linkage, it is theoretically possible for them to exhibit cross-sensitivity.[15] Wilson and Fullard[34,35] have studied the effects of commercially prepared 0.5% proparacaine (Ophthaine) on the rate of corneal epithelial desquamation and observed that the drug initially reduces the rate of normal cell sloughing. Then increased epithelial cell desquamation is apparent for at least 6 hours (Fig. 6.3). These investigators proposed that the proparacaine solution may cause desquamation by interfering with normal epithelial cell-membrane activity or by inhibiting a factor, released by functioning nerves, that mediates cell desquamation.

Bupivacaine

Many painful ocular conditions could potentially benefit from the long-term local application of a nontoxic anesthetic.[36] Examples include mechanical, chemical, and thermal injuries, infectious corneal ulcers, and following keratoplasty, radial keratotomy or excimer laser procedures. Bupivacaine, a long-acting injectable anesthetic, is not commercially available as a topical ocular anesthetic. However, it has been studied in rabbits for potential efficacy as a long-acting topical anesthetic.[37] Bupivacaine 0.75% was found to be less toxic than 0.5% proparacaine to the corneal epithelium, but not significantly different from proparacaine in onset or duration of anesthetic activity. Modification of the bupivacaine molecule or formulation may be necessary to extend the anesthetic's duration of action when topically applied.

Side Effects

When used in recommended dosages, severe local reactions to topically applied anesthetics are exceedingly rare, and systemic reactions are even more uncommon. Al-

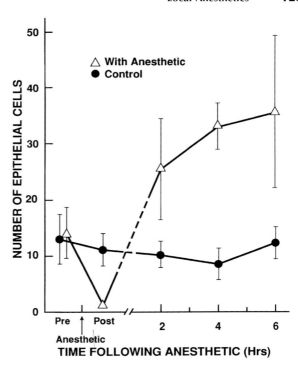

FIGURE 6.3 **Number of epithelial cells (mean ± SE) irrigated from precorneal tear film at different times. In the 2 to 6-hour period after instillation of 0.5% proparacaine, the number of cells was significantly greater with the anesthetic than with the control ($P < 0.001$, paired *t*-test). (From Wilson GS, Fullard RJ. Proparacaine sloughs cells. J Am Optom Assoc 1988;59:701–702.)**

though side effects can occur following use of topical anesthetics, adverse reactions are much more likely to occur with use of local anesthetics injected for infiltration or regional nerve block. Any use of local, including topically applied, anesthetics can cause systemic toxicity, but the vast majority of such systemic reactions occur as a result of overdosage of drug rather than true allergic hypersensitivity.[38] In general, patients who are particularly susceptible to the development of adverse reactions include those with known drug allergies, asthma, cardiovascular disease, liver disease, and hyperthyroidism.[39] Elderly patients, debilitated patients, and infants are also more vulnerable.

Local reactions include relatively minor allergic or toxic involvement of the cornea, conjunctiva, or lids. Although the small amounts of anesthetic normally used in topical ocular applications are usually insufficient to cause toxic systemic effects,[40] systemic toxicity can potentially occur in any patient if the topical anesthetic is applied in dosages exceeding those normally recommended. There has been only one report of a severe systemic reaction to a topically applied ocular anesthetic. Cohn and Jocson[31] reported a case

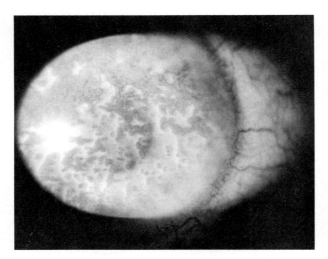

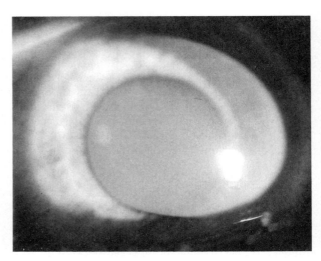

A

B

FIGURE 6.4 *(A)* Severe toxic corneal epithelial desquamation following instillation of proparacaine 0.5%. *(B)* Same cornea 24 hours later, demonstrating the rapidity with which healing occurs.

of grand mal seizures occurring in a 28-year-old patient following administration of a benoxinate-sodium fluorescein solution. These authors acknowledged that the anesthetic component, benoxinate, may not necessarily have been implicated, since the combination solution also contained sodium fluorescein as an indicator dye, polyvinylpyrrolidone as a vehicle, and chlorobutanol as a preservative. Furthermore, appropriate testing for a possible immune mechanism could not be performed. Because of the speed and severity of the reaction, the authors preferred to characterize the reaction as idiosyncrasy rather than as an immune response. There have been no other reports of severe systemic toxic or allergic reactions to topically applied ocular anesthetics.[23,39] In general, all serious ocular or systemic side effects from local anesthetics have been associated with the use of cocaine or anesthetics for infiltration or regional nerve block, or have developed as a result of prolonged use by self-administration.[39]

Toxicity

OCULAR

It is not uncommon for topically applied anesthetics, especially benoxinate and tetracaine, to cause mild local stinging or burning following instillation. As discussed previously, however, this lasts only momentarily and requires no specific treatment other than patient reassurance.

In some patients, especially those over age 50 years, a localized or diffuse desquamation of corneal epithelium becomes evident. This epithelial reaction usually consists of superficial punctate keratitis and probably results from exposure and tear film instability associated with decreased reflex tearing, infrequent blinking, and increased tear evaporation.[41] The punctate keratopathy is frequently absent immediately following anesthetic instillation but may appear 5–30 minutes later. Although it is usually mild and of no clinical significance, occasionally it can be extensive enough to reduce vision to 20/80 (6/24) to 20/200 (6/60) (Fig. 6.4). In its most severe form, it may be characterized by a diffuse, necrotizing, epithelial keratitis with filament formation and corneal edema, but this has been reported to occur in only 1 of every 1,000 patients receiving a topical ocular anesthetic.[39] The cornea can appear gray because of the epithelial and stromal edema, and folds may develop in Descemet's membrane.[39] The conjunctiva can be hyperemic, and the patient may complain of blurred vision or photophobia. There may be lacrimation and mild to intense ocular pain, but there tends to be little pain initially because of the corneal anesthesia. Treatment other than reassurance or ocular lubricating agents is usually not required because the corneal epithelium begins to spontaneously regenerate almost immediately (see Fig. 6.4)[23,39] In moderate to severe cases the episode should be treated as a superficial corneal abrasion, using a cycloplegic, antibacterial ointment, and pressure-patching (see Chapter 27). Systemic analgesics such as acetaminophen or ibuprofen should be administered (see Chapter 7), and the patient should be advised to use cold compresses for additional relief of local discomfort. Toxic reactions should be recorded in the patient's chart, and a different topical anesthetic should be used on subsequent patient visits.

The repeated administration of topical ocular anesthetics should be avoided because it may significantly retard healing of corneal epithelial wounds. Topical anesthetics are particularly dangerous when given to patients for self-administration. The diagnosis and treatment of severe corneal toxicity associated with the long-term administration of topical anesthetics are discussed later in this chapter.

Anesthetics used for eyelid infiltration or nerve block can be toxic to the extraocular muscles. Myotoxic effects are uncommon but have been reported following injection of 2% lidocaine with 1:100,000 epinephrine.[42] Ptosis, horizontal rectus muscle palsy, and lagophthalmos have been attributed to inadvertent infiltration of anesthetic into the levator, horizontal rectus, and orbicularis muscles, respectively. Spontaneous remission usually occurs in 8 to 12 weeks.[42]

SYSTEMIC

With the exception of one case of grand mal seizure possibly associated with the topical application of benoxinate,[31] no cases of serious systemic reactions caused by topically instilled ocular anesthetics have occurred. However, since 98% or more of systemic reactions to local injectable anesthetics are due to drug overdose,[43,44] such systemic toxic reactions can potentially occur with the excessive administration of topical anesthetics to the eye. Topically applied anesthetics are rapidly absorbed into the systemic circulation, and their blood levels rise almost as rapidly as they do following intravenous injection.[32,45] Systemic absorption of topical anesthetics can result in high blood levels by any of the following mechanisms[43]: (1) too large a dosage of the local anesthetic; (2) unusually rapid absorption of the drug, as in patients with marked conjunctival hyperemia; (3) unusually slow drug detoxification, as in patients with liver disease; and (4) slow elimination of drug, as in patients with kidney disease.

High blood levels following topical application or injection of anesthetics may potentially cause systemic reactions.[20] Toxic effects may appear in the central nervous system (CNS), cardiovascular system, or respiratory system.[23] CNS toxicity appears initially as stimulation and may manifest itself clinically as nervousness, tremors, or convulsions. CNS depression, observed clinically as loss of consciousness and depression of respiration, usually follows.

The earliest signs of cardiovascular involvement are hypertension, tachycardia, and, occasionally, cardiac arrhythmias.[20] Late cardiovascular signs are hypotension, absent pulse, and weak or absent heart beat.[20] The effects on the cardiovascular system can develop simultaneously with CNS depression, or they may develop alone.[20] If allowed to continue, such cardiac depression and resultant peripheral vasodilation is followed by secondary respiratory failure.[23]

Since large doses of local anesthetics can be rapidly metabolized by the liver, usually in 30 to 60 minutes, CNS stimulation or depression is frequently short-lived.[46] Management objectives should therefore center around temporary respiratory and cardiovascular support. Administration of supplemental oxygen usually rapidly restores normal CNS function.[43] In patients in whom cardiovascular collapse is evident, vasopressor therapy may take the form of metaraminol bitartrate 1% (Aramine) given intramuscularly or intravenously. The effect of this potent, short-acting vasopressor lasts about 20 to 60 minutes, depending on route of administration.[46] The diagnosis and management of cardiovascular emergencies are discussed further in Chapter 38.

Hypersensitivity

OCULAR

Although local allergy to topical anesthetics can develop in some patients because of routine diagnostic use over many months or years (e.g., for tonometry), these reactions are extremely uncommon. Allergic episodes occur only with use of the ester groups of anesthetics, that is, the commonly employed anesthetics for topical ocular use, and are virtually nonexistent with the use of the amide group of anesthetics for local injection, such as lidocaine, mepivacaine, and bupivacaine.[19] The usual clinical presentation following topical anesthesia is that of a mild, transient blepharoconjunctivitis characterized by conjunctival hyperemia and chemosis, swelling of the eyelids, lacrimation, and itching (Fig. 6.5).[17,24] These signs and symptoms usually appear 5 to 10 minutes following instillation of the anesthetic.[24] Such reactions may

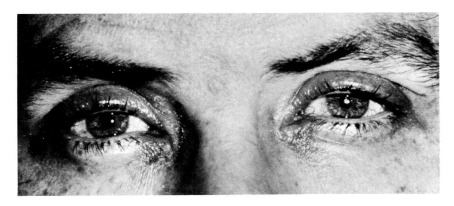

FIGURE 6.5   **Allergic blepharoconjunctivitis following instillation of proparacaine 0.5%. Conjunctival hyperemia, swelling of the eyelids, lacrimation, and itching occur.**

be treated with topical decongestants and cold compresses. Practitioners should record the event in the patient's chart and avoid using the same anesthetic on subsequent patient visits. Since there is apparently little cross-sensitivity between classes of local anesthetics, practitioners can usually change from proparacaine to an ester of PABA, or vice versa, with little risk of local allergy.[20] Unfortunately, no topical anesthetics approved for ocular use have an amide linkage. Such anesthetics, because of their extremely low allergenic potential, would serve as ideal topical ocular anesthetics.

SYSTEMIC

Type I allergic reactions have been estimated to account for less than 1% of all adverse reactions to local anesthetics.[44] Moreover, no life-threatening allergic responses to anesthetics applied topically to the eye have been reported. The small amounts of anesthetic absorbed systemically following topical instillation are usually not sufficient to cause systemic reactions.[19] However, topical anesthetics can cause systemic reactions if enough drug is absorbed into the systemic circulation. Most minor drug-induced systemic allergies are characterized by angioneurotic edema, urticaria (hives), bronchospasm, and hypotension. Joint pain and pruritus occur less commonly.[47,48] Treatment should be directed toward symptomatic relief by the use of systemically administered antihistamines, bronchodilators, or epinephrine.[20,48] Prophylaxis of type I reactions may be difficult, since intradermal skin testing is not an entirely satisfactory method of detecting drug allergy. Prick testing followed by incremental subcutaneous provocative testing has been recommended in lieu of intradermal evaluation.[44] A history of extensive drug allergies should alert practitioners to such a possible consequence of anesthetic administration, but Chandler and associates[44] found no evidence of immediate hypersensitivity reactions when patients with a history of anesthetic allergy were rechallenged, suggesting the relative safety of anesthetic use in such individuals.

Anaphylactoid reactions to local injectable anesthetics are extremely rare. Although these reactions are usually immediate, they may be delayed as long as 15 to 30 minutes.[38,39] Anaphylactoid reactions are characterized by a sudden circulatory collapse following drug administration. Urticaria, respiratory distress, cyanosis, and hypotension usually occur.[38,48] Treatment directed at correcting the circulatory collapse and respiratory failure must be initiated promptly, because even a short delay can be fatal. The diagnosis and management of drug-induced systemic allergy, including anaphylaxis, are discussed in Chapter 38.

Psychomotor Reactions

Psychomotor reactions such as vasovagal syncope (fainting) may be readily mistaken for an adverse drug-related systemic reaction. However, such responses are not drug related and usually occur from anxiety related to the office visit.[23,39] Accordingly, they may occur before, during, or after drug administration. If fainting occurs, patients should be reclined so that the head is low, tight clothing around the neck should be loosened, and patients must be protected from falling or otherwise injuring themselves. Although recovery is usually spontaneous within a few seconds, the inhalation of aromatic spirits of ammonia usually hastens recovery. Respiration and cardiovascular status should be monitored to eliminate drug-induced anaphylaxis as a possible etiology of the collapse.

Prevention of Adverse Systemic Reactions

Although it is unlikely that serious systemic reactions will occur from local ocular anesthetics, practitioners must limit the dosages of the drugs to those compatible with effective anesthesia without substantial risk of systemic toxicity. The determination of exact dosage limits of local anesthetics is impossible, but it has been suggested that the total dose applied topically to mucous membranes such as the conjunctiva should not exceed one-fourth of the maximum allowed for injection.[39] Table 6.4 shows suggested maximum dosages of topical anesthetics based on this formula. It has been reported[24,49] that the toxicity of local anesthetics increases geometrically rather than arithmetically with increases in concentration. Thus, while a given dose of a 1% solution would be four times as toxic as an equal amount of 0.5% solution, a 2% solution would be approximately 16 times as toxic as an equal dose of 0.5% solution.

Contraindications

The commonly employed local anesthetics can generally be used with little risk of significant adverse local or systemic effects. The following specific contraindications should help ensure the safe and effective ocular use of these anesthetics.

TABLE 6.4
Suggested Maximum Dosages of Topical Anesthetics

Anesthetic	*Dosage (mg)*
Cocaine	20 (about 5 drops to each eye of the 4% solution)
Tetracaine	5 (about 7 drops to each eye of the 0.5% solution)
Proparacaine	10 (about 14 drops to each eye of the 0.5% solution)

Modified from Lyle WM, Page C. Possible adverse effects from local anesthetics and the treatment of these reactions. Am J Optom Physiol Opt 1975; 52:736–744.

Hypersensitivity

Allergic reactions to local anesthetics are rare.[15,47,50] These reactions are virtually limited to the ester-linked anesthetics (see Table 6.1).[1,15] Allergy to the amide-linked anesthetics such as lidocaine is extremely rare. Unfortunately, intradermal skin tests as well as conjunctival and patch tests are not reliable for predicting the possibility of allergic reactions.[50] Before administering a topical anesthetic, it is advisable to use a drug from a different chemical family if a patient reports a history of hypersensitivity to a specific anesthetic. For example, an allergic reaction to a para-aminobenzoate drug such as procaine should alert the practitioner to avoid using a similar drug such as tetracaine or benoxinate.[51] In such cases proparacaine can usually be administered safely without causing an allergic reaction.[51] Lidocaine, an amide-linked drug, may be used topically on the eye, but it is not currently approved by the FDA for such use.

Hypersensitivity to benzalkonium chloride has been reported in association with the use of ophthalmic medications.[15] Since several of the commonly used topical ocular anesthetics contain benzalkonium as a preservative, it is reasonable to assume that some of the local allergic reactions to anesthetics may be due to this preservative.

Liver Disease

Local anesthetics containing an amide linkage are metabolized principally by the liver. Thus, patients with hepatic disease may be more likely to exhibit toxic effects from the injectable anesthetics. Local tissue infiltration or nerve blocks should be avoided or performed using minimally effective anesthetic doses in patients with hepatitis, cirrhosis, extrahepatic obstruction (e.g., lithiasis), or other clinically significant hepatic dysfunction.[46]

Concomitant Medications

Local anesthetics containing an ester linkage are metabolized in plasma by pseudocholinesterases. Thus, patients using anticholinesterase medications may be predisposed to exhibit toxic effects from high doses of topical anesthetics. Multiple applications of topical anesthetics are not usually necessary and should be avoided in patients taking systemic anticholinesterase agents such as physostigmine (Antilirium) and pyridostigmine (Mestinon). Glaucoma patients using echothiophate are also at increased risk.[46]

Dry Eye Testing

Topical anesthetics can cause instability of the tear film and diminish reflex aqueous tear production.[41] Because they disrupt the surface microvilli of the corneal epithelium, anesthetics decrease mucous adherence and can contribute to a reduced tear breakup time (BUT).[41,52] Preservatives present in topical anesthetics, such as benzalkonium chloride, can also shorten the tear BUT.[52] These anesthetic-induced changes may affect the examination by masking or otherwise confusing the corneal or conjunctival signs of dry eye. Thus, when the use of sodium fluorescein or rose bengal is anticipated for staining of ocular tissues, the practitioner must avoid instilling an anesthetic until after the vital staining and associated evaluation procedures have been performed.

Perforating Ocular Injury

Topically applied anesthetics may cause corneal endothelial toxicity when used following perforating ocular trauma.[41] When injected intracamerally, benzalkonium chloride, the primary preservative employed in topical ocular anesthetics, can cause irreversible corneal edema in rabbits.[53]

Cultures

Whenever possible, culture specimens from the lid margins or conjunctiva should be obtained without the prior instillation of an anesthetic.[17,54] Preservatives in topical anesthetics exhibit varying degrees of antibacterial and antifungal activity. Moreover, the anesthetic agent itself is often toxic to microorganisms. Tetracaine 0.05% has been shown to inhibit the growth of *Staphylococcus aureus* and *Monilia*.[55] In a 0.5% concentration tetracaine is toxic to *Pseudomonas*.[56] Furthermore, proparacaine 0.5% and tetracaine 0.5% have been shown to have a greater inhibitory effect on bacterial growth than does benoxinate 0.4% or cocaine 5%.[57] However, Kleinfeld and Ellis[54] have shown that when proparacaine is used without preservative, it fails to inhibit the growth of *Staphylococcus albus*, *Pseudomonas aeruginosa*, and *Candida albicans*. Accordingly, these investigators have suggested that proparacaine, in single-dose containers without preservative, should be used when topical anesthesia is desired before obtaining material for culture. Proparacaine would appear to be the best topical anesthetic for use before obtaining culture specimens, and a preservative-free formulation is commercially available.

Self-Administration of Topical Anesthetics

When evaluating an acute injury of the cornea, the practitioner is sometimes tempted to prescribe a topical anesthetic for administration at home by the patient for relief of ocular pain. This practice, however, is extremely dangerous and has led, in numerous instances, to severe infiltrative keratitis and even loss of the eye from anesthetic misuse or abuse by the patient.[58–61] *Topical anesthetics must be used only for the purpose of obtaining initial relief of ocular pain and never as part of a prolonged therapeutic regimen.* The potential corneal toxicity of topical anesthetics precludes their use as self-administered drugs.

A syndrome has been described resulting from the frequent use of topical anesthetics over prolonged periods ranging from 6 days to 6 weeks.[61] Severe corneal lesions and permanent reduction of visual acuity can occur in any eye that has been subjected to prolonged application of topical anesthetics as a means of relieving the pain of minor injuries. Although cocaine-induced corneal injury is well known, it is now recognized that virtually all topical ocular anesthetics can cause corneal damage when used for prolonged periods.[59]

This syndrome has occurred in patients using topical anesthetics on their own initiative and in patients who have received prescriptions for anesthetics as part of their initial treatment. Most of these patients continue to instill the drugs despite advice from practitioners to discontinue their use. Furthermore, many of the patients in whom the syndrome has occurred have a medical or paramedical background and thus have easy access to the offending anesthetic.

The numerous signs and symptoms characterizing the syndrome develop over days or weeks.[59–61] The continuous use of anesthetics, even for only a few days, may cause loss of the corneal epithelium and inhibit the healing of existing epithelial defects. Loss of the epithelial microvilli results in instability and rapid breakup of the tear film, which compounds the drying effect from the decreased blinking secondary to the anesthetic-induced corneal hypoesthesia. Clinically, these changes result in a chronic, nonhealing epithelial defect with a rolled edge. In the earliest stages, the cornea may assume an appearance similar to that observed in neuroparalytic keratitis.[59] As the condition progresses, deeper

manifestations can include stromal edema with folds in Descemet's membrane, disciform cellular infiltrations into the corneal stroma, keratic precipitates, anterior uveitis, hypopyon, and hyphema. Additional findings may include eyelid edema, conjunctival hyperemia and papillary hypertrophy, mucopurulent discharge, and corneal vascularization.

The primary sign allowing objective diagnosis of this disease appears to be a yellowish-white, dense stromal ring surrounding the primary disease process (Fig. 6.6).[61] A history of topical anesthetic abuse, if obtainable, also serves to confirm the diagnosis, but patients often attempt to conceal use of the drug. In some cases patients may exhibit bizarre or combative behavior in efforts to maintain use of the anesthetic. Continued use of the anesthetic serves only to accelerate the development of drug tolerance,[60] creating a cyclical problem of corneal damage, increased corneal pain, and further corneal damage from the more frequent instillation of the drug (with progressively less effect on the relief of pain).[59] The drug-induced corneal changes create an environment that is susceptible to infection by opportunistic microorganisms. Drug allergy may occur in addition to these manifestations of corneal toxicity. Allergies of the immediate type are characterized by the relatively rapid onset of eyelid edema, conjunctival hyperemia and chemosis, and itching. Delayed hypersensitivity, on the other hand, becomes manifest as a slowly developing eczematoid contact dermatitis of the eyelids and surrounding skin.

It has been proposed that the mechanism for these corneal changes may involve depressed respiration and glycolysis, increased epithelial cell permeability, and damage to membranous cytoplasmic structures.[62] In addition, Gipson and Anderson[63] have suggested, on the basis of studies of rat corneal epithelial cells, that topical anesthetics may disrupt the cytoskeletal systems that are responsible for generating the forces necessary to allow corneal epithelial cells to

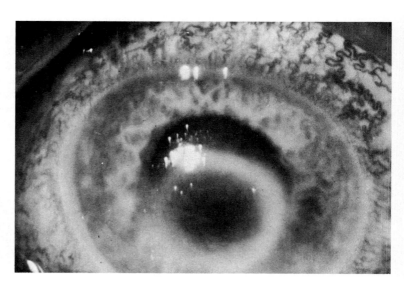

FIGURE 6.6 **Dense corneal stromal ring associated with abuse of topical anesthetics. (From Burns RP, Forster RK, Laibson P, Gipson IK. Chronic toxicity of local anesthetics on the cornea. In: Leopold IH, Burns RP, eds. Symposium on ocular therapy. New York: John Wiley & Sons, 1977;10:31–44.)**

migrate to cover abrasions. Recent investigations[36,64–66] have led to better understanding of the molecular basis for these effects. Because of the ring shape of the corneal stromal infiltration, a possible allergic mechanism has also been suspected.[61] This stromal lesion resembles a Wessely ring, which has been shown in experimental animals to be of immune origin. However, eosinophils, which would suggest an immediate hypersensitivity reaction, have not been isolated from conjunctival or corneal scrapings taken from these patients.

Prevention of this disorder involves better education of the primary physician, who occasionally uses topical anesthetics, as well as of the optometrist and ophthalmologist, who routinely use these drugs.

Maurice and Singh[67] have shown with rabbit cornea that 0.05% proparacaine eyedrops can be used repeatedly to maintain anesthesia without causing corneal toxicity. Bisla and Tanelian,[36] also using a rabbit model, have suggested that low-dose ($\leq$100 μg/ml) lidocaine may be used safely for prolonged periods without inhibiting corneal healing. Thus, the frequent instillation of dilute solutions of proparacaine or lidocaine may be of some value to obtain prolonged local anesthesia in selected patients. It must be emphasized, however, that the safety of this approach has not been evaluated in clinical practice.

Although the syndrome is easily treated once the etiology is known, its recognition may be delayed by deceit on the part of patients. The most important requirement in the management of these patients is discontinuation of the topical anesthetic. Treatment consists of cycloplegic agents, broad-spectrum antibiotics, and firm pressure-patching. Pain must be controlled with systemic analgesics (see Chapter 7). Occasionally therapeutic soft contact lenses may be required to promote corneal healing. In some cases of severe drug tolerance and serious corneal lesions, hospitalization may be required. Once the topical anesthetic has been discontinued, remarkable corneal clearing can occur for as long as 6 months.[60]

References

1. Ritchie JM, Green NM. Local anesthetics. In: Gilman AG, Rall TW, Nies AS, et al, eds. Goodman and Gilman's The pharmacological basis of therapeutics, ed. 8. New York: Pergamon Press 1990;311–331.
2. Covino BG, Vassalo HG. Chemical aspects of local anesthetic agents. In: Local anesthetics–mechanism of action and clinical uses. New York: Grune and Stratton, 1976, Chap 1.
3. Altman AJ, Albert DM, Fournier GA. Cocaine's use in ophthalmology: Our 100-year heritage. Surv Ophthalmol 1985; 29:300–306.
4. Liljestrand G. Carol Koller and the development of local anesthesia. Acta Physiol Scand 1967;30:252–303.
5. Stoelting RK. Local anesthetics. In: Pharmacology and physiology in anesthetic practice. ed. 2. St. Louis: J.B. Lippincott, 1991, Chap 7.
6. Ritchie JM, Greengard P. On the mode of action of local anesthetics. Ann Rev Pharmacol 1966;6:405–430.
7. Bryant JA. Local and topical anesthetics in ophthalmology. Surv Ophthalmol 1969;13:263–283.
8. Wood M. Local anesthetic agents. In: Wood M, Wood AJJ, eds. Drugs and anesthesia. Pharmacology for anesthesiologists, ed. 2. Baltimore: Williams & Wilkins, 1990; Chap. 11.
9. Bloom LH, Scheie HG, Yanoff M. The warming of local anesthetic agents to decrease discomfort. Ophthalmic Surg 1984;15:603.
10. Morsman CD, Holden R. The effects of adrenaline, hyaluronidase and age on peribulbar anesthesia. Eye 1992;6:290–292.
11. Simonson D. Retrobulbar block: A review for the clinician. AANA Journal 1990;58:456–461.
12. Chin GN, Almquist HT. Bupivacaine and lidocaine retrobulbar anesthesia. A double-blind clinical study. Ophthalmology 1983;90:369–372.
13. Vettese T, Breslin CW. Retrobulbar anesthesia for cataract surgery: Comparison of bupivacaine and bupivacaine-lidocaine combinations. Can J Ophthalmol 1985;20:131–134.
14. Nicoll JMV, Treuren B, Acharya PA, et al. Retrobulbar anesthesia: The role of hyaluronidase. Anesth Analg 1986;65:1324–1328.
15. Smith RB, Everett WG. Physiology and pharmacology of local anesthetic agents. Int Ophthalmol Clin 1973;13:35–60.
16. Webster RB. Local anesthetics for ophthalmic use. Aust J Optom 1974;57:399–401.
17. Havener WH. Ocular pharmacology. St. Louis: C.V. Mosby Co, 1983;5:72–119.
18. Meyers EF. Cocaine toxicity during dacryocystorhinostomy. Arch Ophthalmol 1980;98:842–843.
19. Local anesthetics. In: Drug evaluations annual 1993. Chicago: American Medical Association, 1993;153–167.
20. Bryant JA. Local and topical anesthetics in ophthalmology. Surv Ophthalmol 1969;13:263–283.
21. Walsh FB. Clinical neuro-ophthalmology. Baltimore: Williams & Wilkins, 1957;2.
22. Bartlett JD, Wood JW. Optometry and the Drug Enforcement Administration. J Am Optom Assoc 1981;52:495–498.
23. Norden LC. Adverse reactions to topical ocular anesthetics. J Am Optom Assoc 1976;47:730–733.
24. Leopold IH, ed. Ocular therapy; complications and management. St. Louis: C.V. Mosby Co, 1966.
25. Linn JG, Vey EK. Topical anesthesia in ophthalmology. Am J Ophthalmol 1955;40:697–704.
26. Jose JG, Basta M, Cramer KJ, et al. Lack of effects of anesthetic on measurement of intraocular pressure by Goldmann tonometry. Am J Optom Physiol Opt 1983;60:308–310.
27. Vaughn DG. The contamination of fluorescein solutions, with special reference to *Pseudomonas aeruginosa (Bacillus pyocyaneus)*. Am J Ophthalmol 1955;39:55–61.
28. Yolton DP, German CJ. Fluress, fluorescein and benoxinate: Recovery from bacterial contamination. J Am Optom Assoc 1980;51:471–474.
29. Polse KA, Keener RJ, Jauregui MJ. Dose-response effects of corneal anesthetics. Am J Optom Physiol Opt 1978;55:8–14.
30. Jauregui MJ, Sanders TL, Polse KA. Anesthetic effects from low concentrations of proparacaine and benoxinate. J Am Optom Assoc 1980;51:37–41.

31. Cohn HC, Jocson VL. A unique case of grand mal seizures after Fluress. Ann Ophthalmol 1981;13:1379–1380.

32. Wilson RP. Local anesthesia in ophthalmology. In: Tasman W, Jaeger EA, eds. Duane's clinical ophthalmology. Philadelphia: J.B. Lippincott, 1992; vol. 6, Chap 2.

33. Ward B, McCulley JP, Segal RJ. Dermatologic reaction in Stevens-Johnson syndrome after ophthalmic anesthesia with proparacaine hydrochloride. Am J Ophthalmol 1978;86:133–135.

34. Wilson GS, Fullard RJ. Proparacaine sloughs cells. J Am Optom Assoc 1988;59:701–702.

35. Fullard RJ, Wilson GS. Investigation of sloughed corneal epithelial cells collected by noninvasive irrigation of the corneal surface. Curr Eye Res 1986;5:847–856.

36. Bisla K, Tanelian DL. Concentration-dependent effects of lidocaine on corneal epithelial wound healing. Invest Ophthalmol Vis Sci 1992;33:3029–3033.

37. Liu JC, Steinemann TL, McDonald MB, et al. Topical bupivacaine and proparacaine: A comparison of toxicity, onset of action, and duration of action. Cornea 1993;12:228–232.

38. Patterson RW, Yarberry H. Severe drug reactions and their emergency treatment as related to ophthalmology. Am J Ophthalmol 1964;58:1048–1054.

39. Lyle WM, Page C. Possible adverse effects from local anesthetics and the treatment of these reactions. Am J Optom Physiol Opt 1975;52:736–744.

40. Householder JR, Harris JE. Anesthetic drugs in ophthalmology. In: Leopold IH, ed. Ocular therapy, complications and management. St. Louis: C.V. Mosby Co, 1966:100.

41. Rosenwasser GOD. Complications of topical ocular anesthetics. Int Ophthalmol Clin 1989;29:153–158.

42. Rao VA, Kawatra VK. Ocular myotoxic effects of local anesthetics. Can J Ophthalmol 1988;23:171–173.

43. Moore DC, Bridenbaugh LD. Oxygen: The antidote for systemic toxic reactions from local anesthetic drugs. JAMA 1960;174:102–107.

44. Chandler MJ, Grammer LC, Patterson R. Provocative challenge with local anesthetics in patients with a prior history of reaction. J Allergy Clin Immunol 1987;79:883–886.

45. Adriani J, Campbell D. Fatalities following topical application of local anesthetics to mucous membranes. JAMA 1956;162:1527–1530.

46. Sobol WM, McCrary JA. Ocular anesthetic properties and adverse reactions. Int Ophthalmol Clin 1989;29:195–199.

47. Cooley RL, Cottingham AJ. Ocular complications from local anesthetic injections. Gen Dent 1979;27:40–43.

48. Laskin DM. Diagnosis and treatment of complications associated with local anesthesia. Int Dent J 1984;34:232–237.

49. Sadove MS, Wyant GM, Gittelson LA, Kretchmer HE. Classification and management of reactions to local anesthetics. JAMA 1952;148:17–22.

50. Leopold IH. Advances in anesthesia in ophthalmic surgery. Ophthalmic Surg 1974;5:13–23.

51. Molinari JF. Adverse systemic drug reactions acquired from topical ocular drugs. South J Optom 1978;20:11–15.

52. Burstein NL. Corneal cytotoxicity of topically applied drugs, vehicles and preservatives. Surv Ophthalmol 1980;25:15–30.

53. Britton B, Hervey R, Casten K, et al. Intraocular irritation evaluation of benzalkonium chloride in rabbits. Ophthalmic Surg 1976;7:46–55.

54. Kleinfeld J, Ellis PP. Effects of topical anesthetics on growth of microorganisms. Arch Ophthalmol 1966;76:712–71.

55. Erlich H. Bacteriologic studies and effects of anesthetic solutions on bronchial secretions during bronchoscopy. Ann Rev Respir Dis 1961;84:414–421.

56. Murphy JT, Allen HF, Mangiaracine AB. Preparation, sterilization, and preservation of ophthalmic solutions: Experimental studies and a practical method. Arch Ophthalmol 1955;53:63–78.

57. Burns RP. Laboratory methods in diagnosis of eye infection. In: Infectious disease of the conjunctiva and cornea (Symposium of the New Orleans Academy of Ophthalmology). St. Louis: C. V. Mosby Co, 1963:15.

58. Henkes HE, Waubke TN. Keratitis from abuse of corneal anesthetics. Br J Ophthalmol 1978;62:62–65.

59. Epstein DL, Paton D. Keratitis from misuse of corneal anesthetics. N Engl J Med 1968;279:369–396.

60. Michaels RH, Wilson FM, Grayson M. Infiltrative keratitis from abuse of anesthetic eyedrops. J Indiana State Med Assoc 1979;72:51–54.

61. Burns RP, Forster RK, Laibson P, Gipson IK. Chronic toxicity of local anesthetics on the cornea. In: Leopold IH, Burns RP, eds. Symposium on ocular therapy. New York: John Wiley & Sons, 1977;10:31–44.

62. Grant WM. Toxicology of the eye. Springfield, IL: Charles C Thomas, 1974;2:137–139.

63. Gipson IK, Anderson RA. Actin filaments in normal and migrating corneal epithelial cells. Invest Ophthalmol Vis Sci 1977;16:161–166.

64. Higbee RG, Hazlett LD. Topical ocular anesthetics affect epithelial cytoskeletal proteins of wounded cornea. J Ocular Pharmacol 1989;5:241.

65. Dass BA, Soong SK, Lee B. Effects of proparacaine on actin cytoskeleton of corneal epithelium. J Ocular Pharmacol 1988;4:187.

66. Hirikata A, Gupta AG, Proia A. Protein kinase C inhibitors hinder migration of rat corneal epithelial cells. Invest Ophthalmol Vis Sci 1990;31(suppl):316.

67. Maurice DM, Singh T. The absence of corneal toxicity with low-level topical anesthesia. Am J Ophthalmol 1985;99:691–696.

68. Boljka M, Kolar G, Videnšek J. Toxic side effects of local anaesthetics on the human cornea. Br J Ophthalmol 1994;78:386–389.

CHAPTER 7

Analgesics for Treatment of Acute Ocular Pain

Nicky R. Holdeman
Jimmy D. Bartlett

Primary eyecare practitioners often encounter patients who present with substantial pain accompanying the underlying ocular disease process. For example, patients with corneal or conjunctival foreign bodies, superficial abrasions, or traumatic hyphema usually complain of pain as their primary symptom. Unfortunately, clinicians often have inadequate knowledge of analgesics,[1,2] and there is little information on the management of ocular pain. Practitioners may not understand how patients differ in analgesic requirements, and they often fail to prescribe higher than usual doses of analgesics when justified according to patient symptoms.[1,3,4]

Inadequate knowledge of pain management has led to misconceptions among both clinicians and patients, especially regarding the use of narcotic analgesics. The fear of addiction is a major reason for undertreatment of pain.[5,6] The belief that narcotics should be used only sparingly is erroneous.[7]

This chapter considers the basic mechanisms of pain and its pharmacologic relief. In addition, it offers guidelines for the selection and use of analgesics in various clinical situations as well as the management of side effects associated with commonly employed nonnarcotic and narcotic analgesics in outpatient ophthalmic practice.

Mechanisms of Pain and Analgesia

Pain is an unpleasant sensory and emotional experience associated with actual or potential damage to tissues.[8] Although pain is a subjective experience, it has both biological and psychological components that must be addressed if a satisfactory clinical response to pain management is to be achieved. Pain can be described in both acute and chronic terms, and each is a very different clinical entity, requiring different approaches to therapy. This chapter discusses only acute ocular pain, which generally has a specific and obvious predisposing factor such as acute trauma or surgery. Such pain is predictable, of limited duration, and resolves when the source of the pain is detected and treated.

The pain signal is initiated at specialized pain endings in peripheral tissues known as *nociceptors*. These nerve endings are found in the skin, blood vessels, fascia, subcutaneous tissue, and periosteum, including those of the eye.[9] Nociceptors can be activated not only by strong mechanical stimulation, such as trauma, but also by chemical substances released in response to injury. These chemical mediators include substances such as acetylcholine, serotonin, bradykinin, histamine, and prostaglandins.[1] Prostaglandins sensitize the nociceptors to other substances but do not directly stimulate these nerve endings. Several prostaglandins sensitize the nociceptors to mediators such as bradykinin or histamine, which then interact with substance P to stimulate the nerve endings.[10] Figure 7.1 illustrates the sensitization of nociceptors by prostaglandins and other inflammatory mediators to produce pain and inflammation in ocular tissues.

Once the pain signals are initiated at the nociceptive nerve endings in ocular tissue, they are conveyed through the trigeminal nerve system to the brainstem. There they impinge on cells of the sensory and spinal nuclei of the trigeminal nerve. The trigeminal nucleus cells in turn send the pain messages to the opposite side of the brainstem, where they

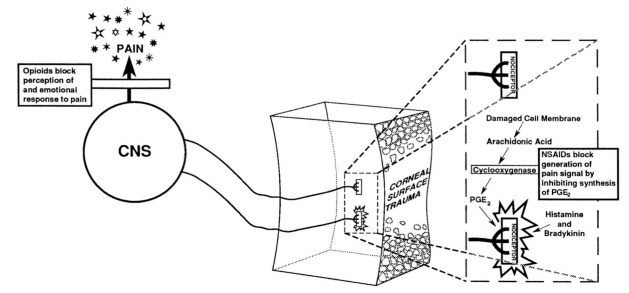

FIGURE 7.1 Sensitization of nociceptors by prostaglandins and other inflammatory mediators to produce pain and inflammation in ocular tissues. Clinically useful analgesics act either in peripheral tissues by inhibiting prostaglandin production or centrally by interrupting the pain signal and its emotional consequences.

ascend to one of the thalamic nuclei and ultimately to the somatosensory cortical areas of the brain where the degree and location of the pain are perceived. Pain produced by stimulation of nerve endings in the uveal tract is quite diffuse in character and cannot easily be localized to one part of the eye or another. This is a direct consequence of the sparse, diffuse pattern of innervation. The cornea, however, is densely innervated by several thousand nerve fibers (with several hundred thousand nerve endings), and pain can often be attributed correctly to a particular region of the cornea. To a lesser extent, the same can be said of the conjunctiva.

Although much attention is given to the emotional effects of the pain process, the physiologic consequences of pain can be quite significant and can lead to harmful cardio-respiratory responses, including tachycardia, systemic hypertension, and tachypnea. Increased peripheral vasoconstriction, blood pressure, and workload of the heart can create a dangerous situation for patients with preexisting cardiovascular disease.[11,12] These physiologic changes mandate that the pain be rapidly terminated, not only to make the patient more comfortable but also to moderate the increased cardiovascular risks. Moreover, pain that is inadequately relieved can lead to protective reflex muscle spasms.[1] Such tonic muscle contractions stimulate muscle nociceptors, which subsequently feed back to the central nervous system. This creates a vicious cycle in which muscle spasms are sustained, causing pain more severe than that of the original injury. If not appropriately relieved, pain can also lead to emotional distress manifested by poor sleep patterns, anxiety, and even uncooperativeness, all of which may result

in slow and unsatisfactory healing of the ocular condition initiating the pain.[13,14]

Acute ocular pain almost always responds to pharmacologic intervention. Analgesic drugs act in three principal ways:[8,15,16]

1. *Peripherally acting agents.* These drugs act on the peripheral pain receptors and prevent sensitization and discharge of the nociceptors. Nonsteroidal anti-inflammatory drugs (NSAIDs), including aspirin, block the formation of inflammatory and pain mediators such as prostaglandins.[17]
2. *Anesthetic agents.* The nociceptive signal can be interrupted between its peripheral source and its central target in the brain or spinal cord. The long-term use of topical anesthetics for treatment of acute ocular pain can lead to serious complications and is thus discouraged.
3. *Centrally acting agents.* These drugs act on opioid receptors in the brain, interrupting both the pain message and its emotional responses. Patients who take centrally acting analgesics are usually indifferent to perceived pain. The opioid (narcotic) analgesics act in this manner.

A fourth class of analgesics, known as the *adjuvants*, do not have direct analgesic effects but can enhance the effects of narcotic agents in certain conditions.[16]

The peripherally acting and centrally acting agents are the mainstay of clinical analgesic practice. The most useful agents in each class are discussed in the following sections.

TABLE 7.1
Commonly Used Aspirin Products

Trade Name	Formulation	Dosage Unit (mg)
Aspirin (generic)	Tablet	325
Genuine Bayer	Tablet	325
Empirin	Tablet	325
Maximum Bayer	Tablet	500
Ecotrin	Enteric-coated tablet	325
Ecotrin Maximum Strength	Enteric-coated tablet	500
8-Hour Bayer Timed-Release	Timed-release tablet	650
Aspirin (generic)	Suppository	120, 200, 300, 600
Buffered Aspirin (generic)	Buffered tablet	325
Ascriptin A/D	Coated, buffered tablet	325
Bufferin	Coated, buffered tablet	325
Ascriptin Extra Strength	Coated, buffered tablet	500

Nonnarcotic Analgesics

The nonnarcotic analgesics are the drugs of choice for treating mild to moderate pain in the outpatient setting.[1,16,18] Among these, the NSAIDs are the most effective[1] and are usually safe for short-term use. Although some clinicians regard the NSAIDs as generally less effective but safer than narcotic analgesics, this presumption is misleading because both types of analgesics have significant side effect potential. The NSAIDs are effective for many types of acute ocular pain, especially when the pain is associated with inflammation.[18] Acetaminophen is also useful as an analgesic for mild to moderate pain but has no effect on inflammation.

Salicylates

PHARMACOLOGY

The salicylate aspirin (acetylsalicylic acid, ASA) is the oldest nonnarcotic analgesic. In addition to analgesic effects, the salicylates have important anti-inflammatory and antipyretic properties. Acting primarily in peripheral tissues, aspirin reduces pain by inhibiting synthesis of the prostaglandin PGE_2 by irreversible acetylation and inactivation of cyclo-oxygenase (see Fig. 7.1).[19] The pharmacologic properties of aspirin are predominantly analgesic at lower doses but assume anti-inflammatory effects at higher doses.[20] Full anti-inflammatory effects, however, generally require doses of at least 3 to 4 grams daily.[16]

Although aspirin relieves pain primarily through its activity in peripheral tissues (e.g., cornea or conjunctiva), it is also believed to have central activity by influencing the perception of pain in the hypothalamus.[21–24] The central mechanisms of action of aspirin have not been elucidated,[25] but it is clear that when used in therapeutic doses, the salicylates generally produce no clinically significant changes in sensorium or mood.[24] This central activity probably accounts for the analgesic efficacy of aspirin in pain states not associated with inflammation.[23]

All nonnarcotic analgesics, including the salicylates, have a "ceiling effect," that is, a dosage beyond which no further analgesia occurs.[15,24] Since the salicylates and other nonnarcotic analgesics do not produce tolerance or physical or psychological dependence,[17,26] they are relatively safe and nonaddicting.

CLINICAL USES

The salicylates are particularly useful for pain associated with inflammation, but their use has now been generally supplanted by other NSAIDs with more favorable safety profiles, largely because of associated gastrointestinal (GI) side effects. Nevertheless, the salicylates are effective for treatment of mild to moderate pain and may produce analgesic effects comparable to those of weak narcotics such as propoxyphene hydrochloride.[20] When used in combination with narcotics the salicylates can be effective for severe pain accompanying acute ocular trauma or inflammation.

Aspirin is commercially available in numerous formulations (Table 7.1). It is compounded as a tablet, enteric-coated tablet, controlled-release tablet, and as a suppository. Enteric-coated aspirin, which decreases GI tract irritation, is recommended for chronic use but is rarely required for the treatment of acute ocular pain, which usually resolves over several days. Likewise, controlled-release aspirin, because of its relatively long onset of action, is not recommended for treatment of acute ocular pain.[27]

Aspirin is often given in a buffered form. The addition of small amounts of antacids decreases GI irritation and increases the dissolution and absorption rate of the aspirin.[27]

TABLE 7.2
Nonacetylated Salicylates

Trade Name	Generic Name	Formulation
Disalcid	Salsalate	500 mg capsule; 500 mg, 750 mg tablet
Sodium salicylate (generic)	Sodium salicylate	325 mg, 650 mg enteric-coated tablet
Arthropan	Choline salicylate	870 mg/5 ml liquid
Original Doan's	Magnesium salicylate	325 mg caplet
Extra-Strength Doan's	Magnesium salicylate	500 mg caplet
Trilisate	Choline-magnesium salicylate	500 mg, 750 mg, 1000 mg tablet; 500 mg/5 ml liquid

Nonacetylated salicylates, including salsalate, sodium salicylate, choline salicylate, magnesium salicylate, and various salicylate combinations, can be effective (Table 7.2). Although these aspirin substitutes are generally somewhat less effective than aspirin, they exhibit minimal antiplatelet properties and have fewer GI side effects.[28,29] They can therefore be useful for patients who cannot tolerate aspirin or other NSAIDs.[24]

The adult dosage of aspirin is 325 to 650 mg every 4 hours as required for treatment of mild to moderate pain.[27] Patients should be advised to take aspirin with food or after meals to decrease GI upset. It should be taken with a full glass of water to reduce the risk of lodging the medication in the esophagus. Aspirin products that have a strong vinegar-like odor should be avoided.[27]

SIDE EFFECTS

GI disturbances are the most common adverse effects observed with therapeutic doses of salicylates. However, their short-term (less than one week) use does not usually cause any significant side effects.[22]

Prostaglandins inhibit gastric acid secretion and have a protective effect on the mucosal lining. Aspirin-induced inhibition of prostaglandin synthesis results in increased gastric acid secretion and a more vulnerable gastric mucosa. As a result, dyspepsia, gastric irritation, and GI bleeding can occur.[15,16] Uncoated aspirin can also injure the stomach through a direct effect on the gastric mucosa. Enteric-coated aspirin or buffered preparations may help to minimize this problem.

All NSAIDs interfere with platelet aggregation, and since aspirin inactivates cyclo-oxygenase irreversibly, its effect is to prolong bleeding time (12 to 15 days).[15,22] The production of a gastric ulcer or erosion with profuse bleeding is potentially a serious problem with aspirin and other NSAIDs. Evidence indicates that choline-magnesium salicylate (Trili-

sate) does not inhibit platelet function and may therefore be indicated in some patients.[30]

Aspirin hypersensitivity can occur in two ways[17]: (1) a respiratory reaction, which is more profound in patients with rhinitis, asthma, or nasal polyps; (2) a typical type I hypersensitivity reaction, including urticaria, wheals, angioedema, itching, rash, bronchospasm, laryngeal edema, hypotension, shock, or syncope.[16] This response occurs within 1 hour of aspirin ingestion. Such aspirin intolerance occurs in 4% to 19% of patients with asthma.[27] Patients who are sensitive to aspirin should not be given any other NSAID because of possible cross-sensitivity reactions. Aspirin cross-sensitivity, however, does not appear to occur with the nonacetylated salicylates such as sodium salicylate or choline salicylate.[27] Aspirin hypersensitivity is more prevalent in patients with asthma, chronic urticaria, or nasal polyposis. This syndrome, consisting of the association of asthma, nasal polyps, and aspirin intolerance, has been termed the "aspirin triad."[27]

Central nervous system (CNS) effects are possible, including confusion in some elderly patients, especially those over age 70.[31] Headache, tinnitus, dizziness, and deafness may occur.[16] In addition, aspirin can cause the retention of salt and water and may reduce renal function, inducing hypertension and increasing congestive heart failure.[32] Aspirin also binds tightly to plasma proteins, which can displace other drugs from protein-binding sites, thereby increasing pharmacologic effects related to the unbound drug. Patients on anticoagulant or oral hypoglycemic therapy, for example, must be monitored closely (see Chapter 36).[16]

Use of aspirin during an antecedent viral infection, such as influenza or chickenpox, has been associated with Reye's syndrome in a small but significant number of children and teenagers.[33] Reye's syndrome is a potentially fatal disease of unknown etiology, characterized by vomiting, lethargy, fatty liver degeneration, encephalopathy, and variable hypoglyce-

TABLE 7.3
Contraindications to Aspirin and Nonsalicylate NSAIDs

- Active upper gastrointestinal disease (peptic ulcers, hiatal hernia, dyspepsia, esophagitis)
- History of bronchial asthma, nasal polyps, or aspirin hypersensitivity
- Bleeding disorders or anticoagulant therapy
- Following cataract or other invasive surgery
- Chronic renal or hepatic disease
- Hypertension or congestive heart failure
- Pregnancy, especially third trimester

mia.[34] Given effective alternatives such as acetaminophen, use of aspirin as an antipyretic and analgesic in children should generally be avoided.

CONTRAINDICATIONS

The most important contraindications to salicylate therapy are listed in Table 7.3.[16] As a general rule, when aspirin is contraindicated or is not tolerated, acetaminophen or a nonacetylated salicylate may be effective as an alternative analgesic while minimizing the risk of side effects.[16]

Salicylates are contraindicated in patients with upper GI disease or a history of adult onset asthma. They should also be avoided in patients with bleeding problems such as hemophilia or those taking anticoagulants such as coumarin or heparin. Since aspirin or aspirin-containing products may lead to prolonged bleeding, it is prudent to limit or avoid their use in patients who have had recent intraocular surgery or invasive surgery of the eyelids.[35] Likewise, aspirin should generally be avoided for treatment of pain associated with hyphema since the incidence of rebleeding can be considerably increased.[36] Aspirin is also contraindicated in patients who are sensitive to aspirin or to nonsalicylate NSAIDs.

Aspirin ingestion during pregnancy can produce adverse effects in the mother, including anemia, prolonged gestation, and prolonged labor. During the later stages of pregnancy aspirin can produce adverse effects in the fetus, including low birth weight, increased incidence of intracranial hemorrhage in premature infants, and even neonatal death. Because salicylates may be teratogenic, they should be avoided during pregnancy, especially in the third trimester.[27] Salicylate use during breastfeeding appears to be safe, because it has not been reported to cause adverse effects on platelet function in nursing infants.

Nonsalicylate NSAIDs

The analgesic efficacy and safety profiles of the nonsalicylate NSAIDs make them appropriate alternatives to aspirin for treatment of mild to moderate pain. Most NSAIDs are used primarily for their anti-inflammatory effects, but they are also effective analgesics to relieve pain associated with a variety of ocular conditions. The nonsalicylate NSAIDs consist of the propionic acid derivatives, indoleacetic acids, anthranilic acids, and several other less commonly used agents (Table 7.4).

PHARMACOLOGY

Like the salicylates, the nonsalicylate NSAIDs produce analgesic effects primarily by inhibiting cyclo-oxygenase in injured or inflamed tissues and thus reduce or eliminate production of the sensitizers for peripheral nociceptors (see Fig. 7.1).[37] In the central nervous system, a less well understood effect occurs whereby the recognition of pain is diminished.[23] The analgesic activity of the nonsalicylate NSAIDs, like the salicylates, is characterized by a ceiling effect, and repeated or chronic use causes neither drug tolerance nor addiction.

The largest class of NSAIDs with both anti-inflammatory and analgesic uses are the propionic acid derivatives (see Table 7.4). These drugs are metabolized in the liver and excreted in the urine. Each has approximately equivalent analgesic effects but has varying systemic absorption to achieve peak plasma levels. Naproxen (Anaprox) was developed specifically to facilitate absorption to reach a rapid peak plasma level.[15]

The indoleacetic acids include indomethacin, sulindac, and tolmetin. These drugs are metabolized in the same way as the propionic acids but with some tendency to biliary excretion as well as enterohepatic circulation. The enterohepatic circulation of sulindac (Clinoril) tends to result in diarrhea.[15]

Although studies are lacking in evaluating analgesic efficacy in painful ocular conditions, the results of other studies may be helpful to indicate the relative usefulness of various NSAIDs for treatment of ocular pain. Table 7.5 summarizes the comparative analgesic efficacy of the commonly used NSAIDs relative to aspirin.[17] Izzo and associates[23] contend that meclofenamate provides significantly faster pain relief compared with other NSAIDs. Cooper[38] has studied ketoprofen, ibuprofen, aspirin, and placebo in postoperative dental surgery patients. Compared with aspirin 650 mg, ketoprofen 25, 50, or 100 mg was found to have superior analgesic effects. Comparing ketoprofen 25 and 100 mg with ibuprofen 400 mg, ketoprofen 100 mg had a faster onset of analgesic effect, the highest peak effect, and the longest duration of action.[38] Cooper[38] concluded that the propionic acid derivatives are superior to aspirin in analgesic efficacy and appear to have a lower incidence and severity of side effects. In the dental surgery patients, both ibuprofen and ketoprofen were more effective than aspirin 650 mg, and ketoprofen 100 mg was significantly more effective than ibuprofen 400 mg.

TABLE 7.4
Nonsalicylate NSAIDs

Classification	Trade Name	Generic Name	Formulation	Adult Analgesic Dosage (mg)[17]
Propionic acids	Motrin, Advil, Nuprin	Ibuprofen	200, 300, 400, 600, 800 mg tablets; 100 mg/5 ml suspension	200–400 q 4–6 h
	Naprosyn	Naproxen	250, 375, 500 mg tablets; 125 mg/5 ml suspension; 375, 500 mg enteric-coated, delayed release tablet	500 initial dose followed by 250 q 6–8 h
	Anaprox, Aleve	Naproxen sodium	220, 275, 550 mg tablets	550 initial dose followed by 275 q 6–8 h
	Nalfon	Fenoprofen	200, 300 mg capsules; 600 mg tablet	200 q 4–6 h
	Orudis	Ketoprofen	25, 50, 75 mg capsules	25–50 q 6–8 h
Indoleacetic acids	Indocin	Indomethacin	25, 50 mg capsules; 75 mg sustained-release capsule; 25 mg/5 ml suspension	25 q 8–12 h
	Toradol	Ketorolac tromethamine	10 mg tablet	10 q 4–6 h
Anthranilic acids	Ponstel	Mefenamic acid	250 mg capsule	500 initial dose followed by 250 q 6 h

During the early 1990s ketorolac tromethamine became the first NSAID to become approved for both oral and intramuscular management of acute pain. This agent has rapidly become accepted as an alternative to opioid analgesics because of its safety and efficacy demonstrated in numerous clinical trials. Oral dosage of 10 mg ketorolac appears to provide an analgesic effect superior to aspirin 650 mg, acetaminophen 600 mg, or acetaminophen 600 mg combined with codeine 60 mg.[96,97] Maslanka and associates[98] have shown that 10 mg ketorolac given orally may have an analgesic effect comparable to 5 or 10 mg intramuscular morphine. The recommended dosage of ketorolac is

TABLE 7.5
Comparative Analgesic Efficacy of Commonly Used NSAIDs[17,96]

NSAID	Analgesic Efficacy Compared to Aspirin (650 mg)
Diflunisal	500 mg superior to aspirin, but has slower onset and longer duration; initial 1000 mg dose shortens time to onset
Choline-magnesium salicylate	Longer duration of action
Ibuprofen	Superior
Naproxen sodium	275 mg comparable to aspirin, but has slower onset and longer duration; 550 mg superior to aspirin
Fenoprofen	Comparable
Ketoprofen	Superior
Indomethacin	Comparable
Ketorolac tromethamine	Superior

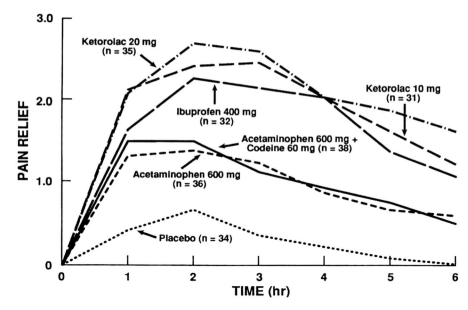

FIGURE 7.2 **Comparative analgesic effects of ketorolac, acetaminophen, acetaminophen-codeine, ibuprofen, and placebo in postoperative oral surgery pain. (Reproduced with permission from Forbes JA, Kehm CJ, Grodin CD, et al. Evaluation of ketorolac, ibuprofen, acetaminophen, and acetaminophen-codeine combination in postoperative oral surgery pain. Pharmacotherapy 1990;10 (6 Pt 2):945–1055.)**

10 mg every 4–6 hours, not to exceed 40 mg daily. A significant analgesic effect occurs by 1 hour, lasting up to 6 hours (Fig. 7.2).

CLINICAL USES

Variability in patient response to the NSAIDs in terms of efficacy and toxicity may relate to differences in binding affinity with cyclo-oxygenase in various tissues.[23] Consequently, no definitive guidelines can be given in selecting the most appropriate NSAID analgesic for a given patient. The choice should be based on clinical experience, patient convenience or preference, past history of favorable analgesic use, side effects, and cost.[27] The primary indications include painful conditions associated with inflammation, including postoperative and posttraumatic pain. The most effective analgesics tend to be those with rapid onset of action so that fast analgesia is achieved for the time corresponding to the acute phase of pain.[23]

Although the NSAIDs are most useful for relief of mild to moderate pain, their analgesic effects are often underestimated. Izzo and associates[23] report that use of nonsalicylate NSAIDs can be effective for intensely painful conditions, including postoperative pain, and can often avoid or delay use of narcotic analgesics. Clinicians should note, however, that patients vary in their responses to individual analgesics. Thus, if patients do not respond to a particular drug at the maximum therapeutic dose, an alternative analgesic should be used.[17]

When instituting NSAID therapy, patients should be advised of the following[27]: (1) the side effects of therapy, which can include GI discomfort and, rarely, more serious events such as GI bleeding; (2) to avoid aspirin and alcoholic beverages; (3) to take the medication with food, milk, or antacids if GI upset occurs. For GI upset with tolmetin, antacids other than sodium bicarbonate should be used, and food and milk should be avoided because drug bioavailability can be affected.

The commercially available formulations and dosage recommendations are summarized in Table 7.4.

SIDE EFFECTS

Side effects associated with the nonsalicylate NSAIDs are essentially those caused by salicylate therapy. NSAIDs occasionally cause CNS dysfunction, including decreased attention span, loss of short-term memory, confusion in elderly patients, and headache.[15,17] Indomethacin appears to have a higher incidence of confusion and headache than do other NSAIDs.[15]

The adverse GI effects seen with aspirin can also occur with nonsalicylate NSAIDs. Although nonsalicylate NSAIDs may be tolerated in some patients who experience GI side effects with aspirin, these patients should be monitored carefully for signs and symptoms of ulceration and bleeding.[27] Patients with ulcers, debilitating diseases, and advanced age appear to be most susceptible.[17] It is not uncommon for patients to experience minor GI complaints such as dyspepsia even after several days of therapy. Serious events such as ulceration, bleeding, or perforation can occur at any time with or without warning symptoms.[17] Susceptible patients who require NSAID therapy should be given the lowest possible therapeutic doses to avoid aggravating or precipitating adverse GI symptoms.[17] Several of the propionic acid derivatives, including ibuprofen, ketoprofen, and naproxen, appear to cause fewer GI effects than do other nonsalicylate NSAIDs.

All nonsalicylate NSAIDs inhibit platelet function by reversibly inhibiting prostaglandin synthesis. However, in contrast to aspirin, which has an irreversible effect on platelets, the nonsalicylate NSAIDs inhibit platelet aggregation only as long as an effective serum drug concentration exists.[17,19,39]

The nonsalicylate NSAIDs can also cause renal insufficiency. Risk factors for NSAID-induced acute renal failure include congestive heart failure, chronic renal insufficiency, systemic lupus erythematosus, diabetes, significant atherosclerotic disease in the elderly, and use of diuretics.[17]

CONTRAINDICATIONS

Contraindications for nonsalicylate NSAID therapy are the same as for aspirin (see Table 7.3). The formation of an ulcer or erosion that may bleed profusely is a serious potential problem with NSAIDs, so any of the nonsalicylate NSAIDs should be used with great caution in patients with active peptic ulcer disease.[15,16] In addition, because of potential cross-sensitivity to other NSAIDs, the nonsalicylate NSAIDs should not be given to patients in whom aspirin or other NSAIDs have caused symptoms of asthma, rhinitis, urticaria, angioedema, bronchospasm, or other symptoms of allergic reactions.[27]

Since the safe use of NSAIDs during pregnancy has not been established, these agents should be avoided during pregnancy, especially in the third trimester. Likewise, these drugs should generally be avoided in nursing mothers because most NSAIDs are excreted in breast milk and may have adverse effects on the cardiovascular system of nursing infants.[27]

Acetaminophen

Acetaminophen is among the most commonly used analgesics in the United States. It is often the first drug used for management of mild to moderate pain, but it can also be of benefit in more severe pain when used as an adjunct to narcotic analgesics. It differs substantially from the NSAIDs in its pharmacologic action and side effect profile.

PHARMACOLOGY

The site and mechanism of the analgesic action of acetaminophen are unclear, but activity in the central nervous system has been postulated.[27,40] The analgesic effects of acetaminophen and aspirin are comparable, but aspirin is superior to acetaminophen for treating pain associated with inflammatory conditions since the latter analgesic has little or no anti-inflammatory properties.[17,20,27] Acetaminophen, however,

does not inhibit platelet aggregation, affect prothrombin time, or produce GI irritation as does aspirin.[20,27]

CLINICAL USES

The superior safety profile of acetaminophen provides the opportunity to use this analgesic when aspirin or therapy with nonsalicylate NSAIDs is contraindicated. The use of acetaminophen is indicated for patients who are allergic to aspirin, because there is no cross-sensitivity between the NSAIDs and acetaminophen.[16,27] In addition, acetaminophen is generally devoid of GI effects, which means it can be used in patients with upper GI disease (e.g., ulcers, gastritis, hiatal hernia). Since acetaminophen does not inhibit platelet function, it is suitable for patients with bleeding disorders (including hemophilia) or for use following cataract extraction or other invasive surgical procedures.[20] Unlike aspirin, acetaminophen has not been associated with Reye's syndrome and can thus be used more safely in children and adolescents.

The safety of acetaminophen during pregnancy or breast-feeding is especially noteworthy. When used on a short-term basis in therapeutic doses, it appears to be safe during all stages of pregnancy. Although acetaminophen is excreted in breast milk in low concentrations, it has no known adverse effects in nursing infants.[27] Thus, acetaminophen is the analgesic of choice for mild to moderate pain during pregnancy or lactation.[27]

Table 7.6 lists commercially available acetaminophen formulations commonly used in clinical practice. A wide range of products, all nonprescription, is available including suppositories, chewable tablets, regular tablets, capsules, elixirs, liquids, and pediatric solutions. The vast array of products facilitates drug selection in individual patients who may prefer or require a specific form of treatment. The typical adult dosage is 325 to 650 mg every 4 to 6 hours, or 1000 mg 3 to 4 times daily.[27] Daily dosage for short-term therapy should not exceed 4 g.

SIDE EFFECTS

When used in recommended doses, acetaminophen rarely causes significant side effects.[27] Overdosage (10–15 g) can lead to serious liver toxicity, but liver damage may also occur at therapeutic doses in chronic alcoholics with pre-existing liver impairment.[41–43] In the usual therapeutic doses, acetaminophen is generally well tolerated, does not affect the gastric mucosa, or induce nephropathy.[17,24]

CONTRAINDICATIONS

Acetaminophen should be used with caution in patients with chronic alcoholism or those with severe liver impairment, because liver toxicity and even severe liver failure can occur following therapeutic doses.[27,41]

TABLE 7.6
Commonly Used Acetaminophen Products

Trade Name	Formulation	Dosage Unit (mg)
Acetaminophen Unisert	Suppository	120, 325, 650
Children's Tylenol	Chewable tablet	80
	Elixir	160/5 ml
Junior Strength Tylenol	Tablet	160
Tylenol Regular Strength	Tablet	325
Tylenol Extended Relief	Dual-layer caplet	650
Anacin-3	Tablet	325
Acetaminophen (generic)	Tablet	325, 500, 650
Tempra Syrup	Liquid	160/5 ml
Acetaminophen Drops (generic)	Solution	100/ml
Bromo Seltzer	Buffered effervescent granules	325

Nonnarcotic Combinations

Many commercial products have been developed that combine various nonnarcotic analgesics with other agents. Although data are lacking to support the efficacy of most of these formulations, many have proven popular among patients who use them for self-treatment of minor painful conditions such as headache.

Nonnarcotic analgesic combinations usually consist of one or more of the following agents: acetaminophen, salicylates, salsalate, and salicylamide. Some of the products contain barbiturates, meprobamate, or antihistamines to produce a sedative effect, and antacids may be included to minimize gastric upset associated with the salicylates. Caffeine, a traditional component of many analgesic combinations, may be beneficial in certain vascular headache syndromes. Some belladonna alkaloids may be incorporated for their antispasmodic properties. Pamabrom, a diuretic, and cinnamedrine, a sympathomimetic amine, are sometimes included in products for premenstrual syndrome.

Some of the more commonly used combination products are listed in Table 7.7. The typical adult dose is 1 or 2 capsules or tablets, or 1 powder packet, every 2 to 6 hours as needed for pain.[27]

Narcotic Analgesics

The narcotic analgesics are also known as *opiates* or *opioids*. These drugs encompass generally all compounds with morphine-like effects, whether synthetic or naturally occurring.[7,24] The terms *opiate* and *opioid* refer specifically to the phenanthrene alkaloids such as morphine and codeine, but the definition has broadened to include drugs with both agonist and antagonist activity at opioid receptors.[24,44] The term "narcotic" is commonly used to refer to the opioid analgesics, but some authors[24] recommend avoiding it because of its negative social, cultural, and legal connotations.

The opioids are generally recognized as the drugs of first choice for the treatment of severe acute pain.[8,24] However, numerous misconceptions surrounding use of these agents have limited their effectiveness. Many clinicians erroneously fear drug-induced complications. As a result, the appropriate use of opioid analgesics may be needlessly denied to patients for whom these analgesics could clearly be beneficial.[45]

Pharmacology

The opioids produce analgesia by binding to various opioid receptors in the brain, brainstem, and spinal cord, thus mimicking the effects of endogenous opioid peptides (endorphins).[24,27] Opioids appear to affect both the sensation of noxious stimulation (pain) and the emotional component of subjective distress (suffering).[24]

The narcotic analgesics are classified as agonists, partial agonists, or mixed agonist-antagonists based on their activity at various opioid receptors. The action of opioids at receptor sites in the central nervous system is highly complex, and the precise role of different receptor subtypes in the modulation of pain remains unclear.[46] Although numerous opioid receptors have been identified,[44] five major receptor groups are recognized and are designated as mu, kappa, sigma, delta, and epsilon. Most of the clinically useful

TABLE 7.7
Commonly Used Nonnarcotic Combinations

Trade Name	Analgesic Components (mg)
Trigesic tablets	Acetaminophen (125)
	Aspirin (230)
	Caffeine (30)
Vanquish caplets	Acetaminophen (194)
	Aspirin (227)
	Caffeine (33)
	Buffers
Excedrin caplets and tablets	Acetaminophen (250)
	Aspirin (250)
	Caffeine (65)
Excedrin P.M. tablets	Acetaminophen (500)
	Diphenhydramine (38)
Anacin caplets and tablets	Aspirin (400)
	Caffeine (32)
Anacin Maximum Strength tablets	Aspirin (500)
	Caffeine (32)
BC Powder	Aspirin (650)
	Salicylamide (195)
	Caffeine (32)

opioid analgesics are agonists acting primarily at the mu and kappa receptors, and they exhibit similar clinical effects.[8] Unlike the nonnarcotic analgesics, the opioids generally do not have a ceiling effect.[16,20] Increased doses produce additional analgesia, but the primary clinical factor that limits dosage is the occurrence of adverse side effects.[16]

Morphine is the standard opioid against which other narcotic analgesics are compared.[7] Its potential side effects, however, along with potential for abuse and addiction, usually make it unsuitable for use in outpatients. Other opioids are preferred for the treatment of moderate to severe pain in most patients. Pharmacologic properties of the commonly employed opioids are summarized in Table 7.8.

Codeine, the most commonly prescribed oral narcotic analgesic in the United States,[15,18] is usually administered in combination with acetaminophen or aspirin (Table 7.9). When given orally, codeine undergoes less first-pass metabolism than other opioids and thus retains about two-thirds of its parenteral potency.[18] Analgesic effects occur as early as 20 minutes following oral ingestion and reach a maximum after 60 to 120 minutes.[7] Codeine undergoes almost complete metabolism in the liver before being excreted in the urine.[47] Since the potential for addiction is extremely low when used in recommended doses for treatment of acute ocular pain,[48] codeine has gained widespread acceptance as an oral narcotic analgesic. However, it produces a relatively

high degree of sedation and results in a high incidence of GI side effects.[18] Codeine also appears to have a ceiling effect, whereby increasing the dosage provides little additional analgesia but markedly increases the incidence of side effects.

Oxycodone is a codeine congener that appears to be 10 to 12 times more potent than codeine.[49] When taken orally, oxycodone is as potent as parenteral morphine,[15] and like codeine, oxycodone retains most of its parenteral potency when given orally.[50] When compared with codeine, morphine, or pentazocine, oxycodone may also have a lower incidence of side effects,[51] but it produces euphoria and thus has potential for abuse.[52] Oxycodone is commercially available only in combination with either acetaminophen or aspirin (see Table 7.9), and it is generally regarded as an excellent oral narcotic analgesic for treatment of moderate to severe pain on an outpatient basis.[18]

Hydrocodone, another codeine congener, is about 6 times more potent than codeine.[53] This agent appears to cause less constipation and less sedation than codeine.[18,54] Clinically hydrocodone may lead to more euphoria than codeine, but this effect has not been substantiated in clinical studies.[18]

Propoxyphene is an analogue of methadone[18] that is widely used as an analgesic. However, single-dose studies[55,56] have shown that the analgesic properties of propoxyphene are no better than those of placebo. When propoxyphene is used alone in usual analgesic doses (32 to 65 mg of the hydrochloride salt, or 50 to 100 mg of the napsylate salt), it is no more effective and possibly less effective than 30 to 60 mg of codeine or 600 mg of aspirin. When combined with other analgesics (codeine or aspirin), however, propoxyphene appears to be more effective than propoxyphene used alone.[27] The marked sedative properties of the drug may account for much of its therapeutic benefit.[18] Propoxyphene is a relatively weak opioid, and it is best reserved for treatment of mild to moderate rather than severe pain.[27] Propoxyphene is commercially available in two salt forms, the hydrochloride or napsylate. Although the napsylate form (Darvon N) is more easily absorbed from the GI tract, its tolerance-producing and addicting effects are similar to those of the hydrochloride salt.[15]

Pentazocine is the only agonist-antagonist opioid analgesic available in an oral preparation in the United States.[18] This drug acts as a partial agonist at the kappa receptor and as a weak mu antagonist.[46] This mixed agonist-antagonist activity was originally developed to maintain powerful analgesia while reducing serious adverse effects, including potential for drug abuse. However, this unique pharmacologic activity of pentazocine is not generally regarded as a major clinical advance.[46] Pentazocine appears to have a ceiling effect for respiratory depression and causes less respiratory depression than do the opioid agonists.[15,18] Due to its antagonist properties, however, pentazocine can reverse opioid analgesia and can precipitate withdrawal when given to patients who are taking opioid agonists.[17,18] The clinical

TABLE 7.8
Pharmacologic Properties of Commonly Used Opioids

Drug	Analgesia	Sedation	Nausea or Vomiting	Constipation	Euphoria
Codeine	+	++	++	++	+
Oxycodone	+++	++	+	+	+++
Hydrocodone	+	+	+	+	++
Propoxyphene	±	++	+	++	+
Pentazocine	++	+	+	+	+

Adapted from Turturro MA, Paris PM. Oral narcotic analgesics. Choosing the most appropriate agent for acute pain. Postgrad Med 1991;90:89–95.

TABLE 7.9
Commonly Used Opioid Analgesics

Opioid	Trade Name	Formulation (mg)	Federal Controlled Substance Schedule	Adult Dosage
Codeine	Tylenol w/Codeine no. 3 tablets	Codeine (30) Acetaminophen (300)	C-III	1–2 q 4 h
	Tylenol w/Codeine no. 4 tablets	Codeine (60) Acetaminophen (300)	C-III	1 q 4 h
	Empirin w/Codeine no. 3 tablets	Codeine (30) Aspirin (325)	C-III	1–2 q 4 h
	Acetaminophen w/Codeine elixir (generic)	Codeine (12)[a] Acetaminophen (120)[a]	C-V	15 ml q 4 h
Oxycodone	Percocet tablets	Oxycodone (5) Acetaminophen (325)	C-II	1 q 6 h
	Tylox capsules	Oxycodone (5) Acetaminophen (500)	C-II	1 q 6 h
	Percodan tablets	Oxycodone HCL (4.5) Oxycodone terephthalate (0.38) Aspirin (325)	C-II	1 q 6 h
Hydrocodone	Lortab liquid	Hydrocodone (2.5)[a] Acetaminophen (120)[a]	C-III	5 ml q 4 h
	Lortab 5/500 tablets	Hydrocodone (5.0) Acetaminophen (500)	C-III	1–2 q 4–6 h
Propoxyphene	Darvon capsules	Propoxyphene HCL (65)	C-IV	1 q 4 h
	Darvon-N tablets	Propoxyphene napsylate (100)	C-IV	1 q 4 h
	Darvocet-N 100 tablets	Propoxyphene napsylate (100) Acetaminophen (650)	C-IV	1 q 4 h
Pentazocine	Talwin NX tablets	Pentazocine (50) Naloxone (0.5)	C-IV	1–2 q 3–4 h
	Talacen caplets	Pentazocine (25) Acetaminophen (650)	C-IV	1 q 4 h

[a] Content given per 5 ml.

advantages of pentazocine include less respiratory depression, lower abuse liability, and less rapid development of tolerance to the analgesic effect compared to the opioid agonists,[57] but it may cause confusion, hallucinations, or other psychotomimetic effects even in patients not taking opioids.[16,17] These reactions can occur in up to 10% of patients taking the drug.[58] Although the theoretical advantages of pentazocine are attractive, Hoskin and Hanks[46] contend that oral pentazocine is closer in analgesic efficacy to that of aspirin and acetaminophen than to the weak opioid analgesics such as codeine. Its tendency to cause dysphoria has also reduced its clinical usefulness as an opioid analgesic.

Occasionally, pentazocine is abused in combination with the antihistamine tripelennamine (known as "Ts and blues"). To offset the abuse potential, pentazocine is now commercially available in combination with low-dose naloxone (Talwin NX). The narcotic antagonist naloxone is ineffective after oral administration but is an effective narcotic antagonist when injected. Any attempt to convert the combination oral product into an injectable form with intent to abuse the drug is thus frustrated.[15]

Table 7.8 summarizes the comparative analgesic efficacy of the commonly used narcotic agonists. Clinicians should note that the indicated analgesic effects for each drug are only an approximation and can vary widely among patients due to individual differences in both the sensitivity of opioid receptors and the efficiency of drug metabolism and elimination. Bioavailability of the analgesic can vary following oral administration, and the analgesic effects of the centrally-acting agents can be clinically unpredictable.[38] Moreover, some of the opioid analgesics have metabolites that, in turn, have additional analgesic activity.[16] It must be expected that individual patients will respond differently or even uniquely to opioids.[17]

Although few studies have directly compared the analgesic efficacy of the various opioids, clinical experience and extrapolation from controlled studies have led to a better understanding of the comparative analgesic efficacy of some of the commonly used agents, both opioid and nonnarcotic. Ketoprofen in doses of 50 and 150 mg has been compared to the analgesia provided by acetaminophen 650 mg combined with codeine 60 mg for the management of moderate to severe postoperative pain.[59] The results suggest that ketoprofen may have a superior analgesic effect and longer duration of analgesia compared with the acetaminophen-codeine combination.

Clinical Uses

Many clinicians are reluctant to prescribe narcotic analgesics because of the perceived risk of iatrogenic addiction. However, short-term use of opioids for management of acute pain in patients without a previous history of addiction rarely results in drug abuse.[60] The opioid analgesics are generally safe for short-term treatment of acute ocular pain as long as the clinical use is appropriate and a rational approach is taken to drug selection. Potential opioid side effects can be more problematic compared with those of nonnarcotic analgesics, but opioids may actually be safer for some patients with contraindications to NSAIDs (e.g., patients with renal failure or peptic ulcer disease).[18]

In the outpatient setting the oral route of administration is preferred for the opioids because of convenience and relatively steady drug plasma levels. For treatment of severe acute pain, the peak drug effect usually occurs after 1½ to 2 hours.[17] Evidence indicates that the addition of a peripherally acting analgesic such as an NSAID to the opioid regimen provides an additive or synergistic analgesic effect.[26,61] Increasing the dose of the narcotic may improve analgesia, but only at the expense of substantially increasing the incidence of side effects. Thus, most oral opioid analgesics are commonly used only in combination with a nonnarcotic analgesic (see Table 7.9).

When opioid analgesic therapy is instituted, patients should be advised of the following[27]:

1. Drowsiness, dizziness, or blurred vision can occur. Patients should be cautious when driving or performing other tasks requiring alertness.
2. Drug-induced nausea, vomiting, or constipation can occur.
3. If GI upset occurs, the medication should be taken with food to decrease GI irritation.
4. Alcohol or other CNS depressants should be avoided because they can exacerbate opioid-induced sedation.
5. Breathing difficulty or shortness of breath can occur.

Commonly employed commercial formulations and dosage recommendations are listed in Table 7.9. A rational approach to opioid analgesic dosing requires recognition that patients vary considerably in their response to analgesic therapy. In general, doses should be titrated to the clinical needs of particular patients and should not necessarily be prescribed at fixed intervals. Opioid analgesics are commonly prescribed in doses that are too small and at intervals that are too long for relief of pain.[7,16] They should instead be administered regularly as needed for pain control, especially if pain is present continually.[17] The opioid analgesics must be given with constant reassessment of efficacy, and dosages should be altered when required.[24] Since patients are the best judge of the efficacy and duration of action of an analgesic, practitioners should maintain flexibility in dosing requirements for individual patients.

Various medications can be administered along with the opioids to enhance the analgesic effects. These drugs are known as *adjuvants* and include tricyclic antidepressants, antihistamines, benzodiazepines, dextroamphetamine, phenothiazines, and anticonvulsants.[17] The adjuvants do not

---

TABLE 7.10
Side Effects of Opioid Analgesics

Central Nervous System
  Sedation
  Light-headedness
  Dizziness
  Drowsiness
  Euphoria
Gastrointestinal System
  Nausea
  Vomiting
  Constipation
Respiratory System
  Respiratory depression

---

possess major analgesic properties but are used to enhance the analgesic effects of other drugs and to counteract side effects. Although most adjuvants are inappropriate for the primary care of ocular pain, caffeine, in doses of at least 65 mg, has been shown to increase analgesia when given with NSAIDs or opioids.[17] The optimal daily dosage of caffeine has not been established, but 100 to 200 mg/day appears to be well tolerated by most patients.[62]

Side Effects

Since the pharmacologic action of the opioids is complex and can result in either CNS depression or stimulation, it is difficult to predict side effects in given patients.[1,8] Clinicians should note that at equipotent analgesic doses, all commonly used opioids produce similar degrees of side effects. However, these side effects are usually mild and do not necessitate discontinuing opioid therapy.[18] The most commonly encountered adverse effects include light-headedness, dizziness, sedation, nausea, vomiting, constipation, and respiratory depression (Table 7.10).[17,27,63] These occur more often in ambulatory patients, in patients without severe pain, and in patients with kidney or liver dysfunction.[27]

Although the opioid analgesics can produce mood elevation (euphoria) in some patients and sedation in others, the more common side effect is CNS depression manifested as sedation or drowsiness. Pentazocine produces subjective effects quite different from those of the other opioids, however.[64] This drug occasionally induces dysphoria, which can contribute to reduced patient acceptance, but it is not uncommon for patients given pentazocine to experience feelings of floating or dissociation.[64] An effective strategy for the treatment of sedation or drowsiness is to reduce the analgesic dose and shorten the interval between doses.[16,17] Clinicians should note that the sedative effect of opioid analgesics is additive with the sedative effects of hypnotics such as alco-

hol and barbiturates. These latter agents must be avoided when opioids are prescribed.

The incidence of opioid-induced nausea and vomiting is markedly increased in ambulatory patients,[16] but appears to be lower with the use of agonist-antagonist drugs such as pentazocine.[64] If narcotic analgesic therapy must be continued, nausea and vomiting can be treated with hydroxyzine or a phenothiazine antiemetic.[65]

The opioids inhibit intestinal tract motility, which causes constipation. This is one of the most common side effects encountered with the narcotic analgesics.[16] Constipation appears to occur less often with the agonist-antagonist pentazocine.[64] If constipation becomes problematic, it can often be relieved by a regimen consisting of docusate sodium (Colace) 50 to 300 mg/day and senna, 2 tablets twice daily.[17]

The most serious side effect of the opioids is respiratory depression. The narcotic agonists suppress the brainstem respiratory centers and thus alter respiratory rate, rhythmicity, minute volume, and responsiveness to CO_2.[44] When used in equianalgesic doses, the opioids, with the exception of pentazocine, produce similar degrees of respiratory depression.[57,66,67] Therapeutic doses of opioid analgesics are unlikely to produce significant respiratory depression in most healthy patients.[24,64,68] The opioids must be used with caution, however, in patients with preexisting pulmonary disease, especially patients with airway compromise such as chronic obstructive pulmonary disease (COPD).[24] Discontinuation of opioid therapy or simple physical stimulation may be sufficient to prevent significant respiratory depression in patients who have received a relative overdose of an opioid analgesic. No deaths due to respiratory depression in patients who remained awake have been reported.[17]

Contraindications

Opioid analgesics are contraindicated in patients with a history of hypersensitivity to narcotics, since there is risk of cross-sensitivity among the various opioids.[27] In addition, they are contraindicated in patients with acute bronchial asthma and in patients with COPD.[27] They should be used cautiously in patients with kidney or liver dysfunction because these conditions increase the risk of drug accumulation and subsequent toxicity.

Use of pentazocine should be avoided in patients with a significant prior exposure to opiates since this drug can precipitate withdrawal syndrome. Pentazocine should also be avoided in patients with myocardial ischemia or infarction; this agent can increase heart rate, systemic and pulmonary arterial pressure, and cardiac work.[64,69]

When used in excessive doses propoxyphene can be a major cause of drug-related death.[27] This can occur when the drug is used either alone or in combination with other CNS depressants such as alcohol. It is prudent to avoid propoxyphene or other opioid analgesics in depressed or suicidal patients and, instead, use nonnarcotic analgesics as tolerated for pain relief.

The safety of narcotic analgesics during pregnancy has not been established, but an association between congenital birth defects and exposure to codeine during the first trimester has been reported.[27] When given near term, opioids can also cause respiratory depression in neonates.[27] Most of the opioid analgesics appear in small quantities in breast milk, but drug effects in nursing infants appear to be insignificant. If possible, breastfeeding should be deferred for at least 4 to 6 hours after opioid analgesics are taken.[27]

Narcotic Antagonists (Naloxone)

Naloxone is a pure opioid antagonist that antagonizes effects of the opioid agonists as well as the mixed agonist-antagonist drugs.[70] Not only does naloxone reverse sedation, respiratory depression, and constipation, but it also interrupts opioid-induced analgesia. The antagonism of agonist effects must be approached with great caution, especially in patients who have received prolonged opioid therapy, those who exhibit opioid dependence, or in patients with extreme pain, because overt withdrawal symptoms can be elicited. Occasionally a life-threatening "overshoot" phenomenon occurs with tachypnea, tachycardia, systemic hypertension, nausea, vomiting, and even sudden death.[71] For these reasons the use of naloxone should be limited to life-threatening opioid side effects such as severe respiratory depression.[24] A safer approach to treatment is the use of mechanical ventilation, patient stimulation, and careful monitoring until respiration returns to normal.[7,24]

Naloxone is supplied only as a parenteral solution. Following intravenous administration, it reverses opioid effects virtually instantaneously.[7] Due to its relatively short plasma half-life, however, its duration of action is much shorter than the agonists it reverses.[72] Thus, when naloxone is administered for treatment of opioid-induced respiratory depression, patients must be monitored carefully for return of the depression following elimination of the naloxone. Treatment may require repeated intravenous doses, intramuscular injection, or a continuous intravenous infusion.[7]

General Strategies for Pain Management

Most patients who present with acute ocular pain have a readily identifiable disease process toward which treatment can be directed. Anterior uveitis, corneal abrasion, superficial ocular foreign bodies, or traumatic hyphema are easily recognized, and treatment of the underlying problem usually restores comfort. In general, analgesia should not be offered to patients in whom the cause of pain is unknown. A comprehensive diagnostic examination should be completed prior to administering analgesics so that objective findings are not masked. Chronic pain or acute pain of unknown etiology must not be treated without regard to its cause. It is extremely important to perform a careful history and physical examination directed toward the disease process responsible for the ocular pain. In some cases laboratory or other diagnostic evaluations may be required. Depending on the site of involvement, these tests may include x-rays, computed tomography or magnetic resonance imaging scans, visual fields, or other tests as appropriate.

The following general guidelines are the basis for a rational approach to analgesic therapy for most patients with acute ocular pain:

- A diagnosis should be made and specific treatment of the underlying disease process should be undertaken.
- Analgesic therapy should be adjusted according to severity of the pain rather than to the extent of objective findings.[73]
- A careful medical and drug history is essential to exclude contraindications to various analgesics, such as peptic ulcer disease, medication allergies, or pregnancy.
- Pain should be treated by the simplest and safest means to achieve patient comfort.
- Analgesic therapy should be provided on a 24-hour schedule to prevent the return of pain.[24]
- The oral route of administration is preferred because of its simplicity and convenience.
- The use of nonprescription analgesics, such as acetaminophen or ibuprofen, reduces the cost of therapy.
- Opioid analgesics should be used with discrimination but should not be withheld if nonopioid agents prove ineffective.
- Various adjuvants can have an additive analgesic effect when used together with peripherally acting or centrally acting agents.

It is helpful to consider analgesic therapy in a stepwise fashion. NSAIDs and acetaminophen should be used for treatment of mild to moderate pain and opioids should be reserved for treatment of moderate to severe pain. This approach is clinically effective, reduces the incidence and severity of side effects, and is well accepted by most patients. For example, a nonopioid analgesic such as ibuprofen 400 mg or acetaminophen 650 mg can be given every 4 to 6 hours. The analgesic ceiling effect for aspirin and acetaminophen is about 1300 mg/dose. Although the duration of analgesia can be increased by exceeding this dosage amount, it does not increase the peak analgesic effect. Thus, if patients do not respond satisfactorily to a particular NSAID at the maximum therapeutic dose, an alternative NSAID in the same therapeutic class should be selected.[16,17] NSAIDs that often provide greater analgesia than aspirin or acetaminophen include ibuprofen, ketoprofen, naproxen, and diflunisal.[17] All NSAIDs except the nonacetylated salicylates should be avoided in the thrombocytopenic or surgical patient because of their antiplatelet effects.[17]

If additional analgesia is required beyond that afforded by the nonnarcotic analgesics, an opioid such as oxycodone or codeine should be used. The narcotic analgesic of first choice for many practitioners is a combination of acetaminophen with 15 to 60 mg of codeine or 5 to 30 mg of oxycodone.[20] If opioid side effects are unacceptable or become problematic, the narcotic dose is reduced or an alternative opioid is selected.

Various adjuvants can be used to enhance the analgesic effect of the nonopioid and opioid agents. In ophthalmic practice the treatment of acute trauma may involve pressure patching, bandage (disposable) contact lenses, cold compresses, or cycloplegics as required for treatment of corneal abrasions, external ocular foreign bodies, or anterior uveitis. These ancillary procedures have inherent analgesic properties and are extremely useful to enhance the pain-relieving effects of the analgesics.[74] Furthermore, orally administered caffeine can be effective not only to enhance analgesia but also to overcome drowsiness and sedation associated with the opioid analgesics.[17] Continuous or long-term topical anesthetics should never be used to augment orally administered analgesics. The risks of local complications far outweigh the benefits to be achieved from the self-administration of topical anesthetics by patients[75] (see Chapter 6).

Analgesic Use in Children

The perception of pain depends on many factors, including age, developmental level, previous pain experience, and emotional state. The assessment of pain in children can be even more difficult than in adults because children often lack the verbal or cognitive ability to express their feelings.[63] Many behavioral cues can be helpful in assessing pain in preverbal or nonverbal children. These include facial expression, body positioning, jerking of limbs, crying, or whimpering.[63]

Unfortunately, children often suffer needlessly because their pain is not treated appropriately. Several studies[76–78] have documented that children in pain receive fewer analgesic doses than adults, and opioids are less likely to be used for children than for adults. Several misconceptions have perpetuated the mismanagement of pain in children.[63] Respiratory depression is extremely rare and, indeed, children over the age of 6 to 8 months have no greater susceptibility to narcotic-induced respiratory depression than adults.[79] Furthermore, short-term opioid use for acute pain relief in children does not lead to psychological addiction or physical dependence.[63]

Although many analgesics are available for clinical use, few opioid and nonopioid analgesics have widely accepted

TABLE 7.11
Analgesics Commonly Used in Children

Class	Drug	Dosage
Nonopioids	Acetaminophen	10–15 mg/kg PO q 4 h 15–20 mg/kg PR q 4 h
	Ibuprofen	4–10 mg/kg PO q 6–8 h
	Naproxen	5–7 mg/kg PO q 8–12 h
	Tolmetin	5–7 mg/kg PO q 6–8 h
	Choline-magnesium Salicylate	10–15 mg/kg PO q 6–8 h
Opioids	Codeine	0.5–1.0 mg/kg PO q 4 h

PO = oral; PR = rectal.

pediatric dosage guidelines. Drugs listed in Table 7.11 are the most commonly used,[17,24] and it is recommended that the FDA-approved dosage schedules be used. In clinical practice, however, children 12 years of age or older often receive the full recommended adult dose, children 7 to 12 years of age generally require 50% of the adult dose, and children 2 to 6 years of age are given 20 to 25% of the adult dose.[17]

Treatment of Mild to Moderate Pain

As in adults, mild pain in children is initially treated using nonopioids. Because of its association with Reye's syndrome, aspirin has now been abandoned in pediatric practice in favor of safer agents such as acetaminophen and the nonsalicylate NSAIDs.[2,24] Acetaminophen is as effective as aspirin for treatment of pain in children and produces very few serious side effects when given in therapeutic doses.[2] Recommended dosage is 10 to 15 mg/kg orally every 4 hours or 15 to 20 mg/kg rectally every 4 hours, with a maximum of 5 doses (every 4 hours) in a 24-hour period. Rectal absorption may be inconsistent.[80] Because of its favorable safety profile,[81] acetaminophen is often the first agent used for most children with mild to moderate pain, but it can also be of benefit in more severe pain as an adjunct to opioid analgesia.

The nonsalicylate NSAIDs are especially useful for pain of inflammatory origin. However, studies of these agents in younger children are relatively few. Nevertheless, these analgesics are preferred by many pediatricians because the NSAIDs are relatively safe, have few cardiopulmonary side effects, and are nonaddictive.[2] NSAIDs that have been used effectively in children include ibuprofen, naproxen, and tolmetin.[82,83] Because all these drugs can cause gastritis, they should be taken with meals. If GI side effects occur with one NSAID, an alternative agent should be selected.[24]

Children who do not tolerate nonsalicylate NSAID therapy may do well with choline-magnesium salicylate (Trilisate). Therapeutic doses of this agent cause much less gastritis than the commonly used NSAIDs. The recommended individual dose for children is 10 mg/kg three times daily, and this dose can be doubled if tolerated.[24]

Treatment of Moderate to Severe Pain

Treatment of moderate to severe pain requires use of opioid analgesics combined with nonopioids such as acetaminophen. The oral route of administration should always be used, because parenteral analgesics can produce even more pain. Children often suffer in silence to avoid painful injections.[84]

Codeine is the most commonly prescribed opioid analgesic for treatment of moderate to severe pain in ambulatory children over 2 years of age.[7,24] The recommended initial pediatric dose is 0.5 to 1.0 mg/kg orally along with acetaminophen, 10 mg/kg every 4 hours, administered concurrently.[7,24]

Although it has been used occasionally for treatment of moderate to severe pain in children, pentazocine has no currently established indications for the pediatric patient.[24] Likewise, oxycodone and propoxyphene are not recommended for pediatric use.[27]

Management of Side Effects

Stool softeners and cathartics can be used in children, as in adults, to relieve symptoms of constipation. Nausea and vomiting generally diminish as opioid therapy is continued, but antihistamines with antiemetic effects, such as hydroxyzine or promethazine, may be helpful as adjuvants to diminish unpleasant GI symptoms.[63,85] Reducing the opioid dose to minimal analgesic levels may help to limit sedation or drowsiness.

Mild respiratory depression, an uncommon side effect in children, may require only that the opioid dose be reduced. Moderate symptoms of respiratory depression can be treated by administering oxygen, stimulating the patient, or encouraging deep breathing. Serious respiratory depression should be treated with naloxone beginning with a dose of 0.01 mg/kg, with subsequent doses of 0.02 mg and 0.04 mg until the desired clinical response is achieved.[24,63,86]

Analgesic Use in Elderly Patients

Prescribing analgesics for elderly ophthalmic patients can be difficult. Older patients are much more likely than younger ones to experience GI and other side effects of drug use. In addition, they are generally taking more medications that may interact with the prescribed analgesic. Other factors, such as reduced renal and hepatic function, can also affect

the efficacy and accumulation of the analgesic, thus increasing the risk of drug toxicity.[20]

Practitioners must therefore take a careful medical and drug history to determine potential contraindications to analgesic use. Prior analgesic use should be reviewed to determine, if possible, what analgesics were effective and what side effects, if any, occurred. This review is a very practical initial step in selecting the proper analgesic for all patients, especially elderly ones.

Acute renal failure induced by the NSAIDs is more common in elderly patients, especially in those who are taking diuretics or who have congestive heart failure, liver disease, or kidney disease.[87] Safer analgesics for these patients include sulindac (Clinoril) or a nonacetylated salicylate. Acetaminophen is another alternative because it rarely causes acute renal failure when used on a short-term basis.[20]

One of the major problems with use of NSAIDs in elderly patients, especially women, is the increased incidence of gastric mucosal damage (NSAID gastropathy).[88] This can lead to significant GI bleeding and even death.[88] Options for preventing or treating this problem include[20]: (1) use of drugs that produce less gastric irritation, such as nonacetylated salicylates (salsalate, diflunisal, choline-magnesium salicylate), enteric-coated aspirin, and acetaminophen; (2) use of an H_2 blocker, such as ranitidine or famotidine prophylactically; and (3) use of misoprostol (Cytotec), a synthetic prostaglandin E_1 analogue. This drug may be useful when NSAIDs are required for patients who are prone to peptic ulcer disease.[99] Misoprostol inhibits gastric acid secretion while possessing mucosal protective properties.[33]

Most patients undergoing cataract extraction are elderly, and many may have bleeding problems. Acetaminophen and the nonacetylated salicylates affect platelet aggregation only minimally, and these analgesics are preferred for postoperative use.

Treatment of Mild to Moderate Pain

In general, nonopioid analgesics used in elderly patients should produce minimal gastric irritation, have a short to intermediate half-life to prevent drug accumulation and toxicity, and have proven analgesic efficacy. Analgesics that are consistent with these goals include acetaminophen, moderate-dose ibuprofen, diflunisal, and salsalate. Several other nonopioids have significant side effect potential that make them less desirable for use in the elderly ophthalmic patient.[15,20] The most useful nonopioid analgesics for treatment of pain in the elderly are listed in Table 7.12.[20]

For treatment of mild to moderate acute pain, a practical approach is to initiate therapy with acetaminophen 650 to 1000 mg to a maximum of 4000 mg per day. If pain continues, an NSAID should be substituted. If pain still persists, an alternative NSAID, preferably from a different therapeutic class, should be selected. If the alternative

TABLE 7.12
Preferred Analgesics for Use in the Elderly

Nonopioids
  Acetaminophen
  Ibuprofen
  Diflunisal
  Salsalate
  Choline-magnesium salicylate

Opioids
  Codeine with acetaminophen
  Oxycodone with acetaminophen

NSAID is ineffective, full-dose acetaminophen combined with an NSAID should be considered.[26,89] Combinations of several NSAIDs, however, should not be used.[20] This approach is often effective without resorting to the use of opioid analgesics.

Treatment of Moderate to Severe Pain

Elderly patients in moderate to severe pain may require narcotic analgesics, but the use of opioids can be associated with significant toxicity due to the unique metabolic and physiologic alterations in aging patients. Opioids are detoxified in the liver. The metabolic capacity of the liver declines with age, however, reducing drug clearance and thus enhancing the cumulative effects of narcotics.[90] This is of special concern in elderly patients with congestive heart failure or liver disease. In addition, the degree of analgesia and CNS depression produced by opioids is enhanced by normal aging, especially in patients with preexisting CNS dysfunction such as stroke or dementia.[91] Furthermore, opioid-induced respiratory depression is enhanced in the elderly[92] and in persons with depressed CO_2 drives associated with obesity or COPD.[93] Urinary retention can also be a problem in elderly men with preexisting benign prostatic hypertrophy.[20]

Thus, opioid analgesics used in elderly patients should generally have a short half-life to prevent drug accumulation. In addition, they should be limited to the pure agonists, because the mixed agonist-antagonists such as pentazocine can often produce delirium, agitation, and confusion in the elderly.[44] Pentazocine can also increase heart rate, systemic blood pressure, and cardiac work,[69] which makes it a poor choice for use in patients with ischemic heart disease or infarction.[64] The opioid analgesics of choice for use in the elderly are listed in Table 7.12.

For treatment of moderate to severe pain an effective opioid regimen consists of a combination of acetaminophen with 15 to 60 mg of codeine or acetaminophen with 5 to 30 mg of oxycodone.[20] If pain persists, an alternative opioid analgesic should be selected. Adjuvants such as caffeine may enhance the analgesic activity of the opioid.[20]

Management of Side Effects

Opioid-induced constipation is more troublesome in older patients,[91] and it should be anticipated by instituting laxative therapy along with the narcotic. A typical laxative regimen consists of psyllium and a stool softener. A mild stimulant laxative such as bisacodyl (Dulcolax) can be added if constipation becomes problematic.[94]

Nausea and vomiting is another opioid-induced problem that is more significant in elderly patients. Nausea can result from vestibular stimulation, so limiting physical activity may be useful to reduce symptoms. If drug therapy is needed, hydroxyzine is preferable to a phenothiazine.[95] Since the antihistamines have significant anticholinergic effects that can be troublesome in elderly individuals, these drugs should not be routinely given with the opioid unless absolutely needed.

Analgesic Use in Substance Abusers

Substance abusers represent a unique situation that warrants special attention in the treatment of acute ocular pain. These patients often have deranged drug absorption and deficient drug metabolism. These inefficiencies, together with opioid tolerance, can make prescribing for pain especially difficult. Because of the underlying drug addiction, special precautions are necessary to minimize withdrawal symptoms when opioid analgesics are discontinued.[1] The pharmacologic and psychosocial complexities involved in using opioid analgesics to treat pain in substance abusers necessitate that nonopioid analgesics be used whenever feasible. When narcotic analgesics become necessary, optometrists or ophthalmologists should generally consult with the patient's primary physician.

References

1. Tucker C. Acute pain and substance abuse in surgical patients. J Neurosci Nurs 1990;22:339–349.
2. Yaster M, Deshpande JK, Maxwell LG. The pharmacologic management of pain in children. Compr Ther 1989;15:14–26.
3. Angell M. The quality of mercy. N Engl J Med 1982;306:2.
4. Beaver WT. Management of cancer pain with parenteral medication. JAMA 1980;244:2653–2657.
5. Meinhart N, McCaffery M. Pain: A nursing approach to assessment and analysis. Norwalk, Conn: Appleton-Century-Crofts, 1983.
6. Stimmel B. Pain, analgesia and addiction: The pharmacological treatment of pain. New York: Raven Press, 1983.

7. Yaster M, Deshpande JK. Management of pediatric pain with opioid analgesics. J Pediatr 1988;113:421–429.

8. Mather LE, Cousins MJ. The pharmacological relief of pain—contemporary issues. Med J Australia 1992;156:796–802.

9. Tanelian DL, Brunson DB. Anatomy and physiology of pain with special reference to ophthalmology. Invest Ophthalmol Vis Sci 1994;35:759–763.

10. Ferriera SM. Prostaglandins, aspirin-like drugs and analgesia. Nature 1972;240:200–203.

11. Bryan-Brown C. Development of pain management in critical care. In: Cousins M, Phillips G, eds. Acute pain management. New York: Churchill Livingstone, 1986:1–20.

12. Cousins M, Phillips G. Neurological mechanisms of pain and the relationship of pain, anxiety, and sleep. In: Cousins M, Phillips G, eds. Acute pain management. New York: Churchill Livingstone, 1986:21–48.

13. Moyer S, Howe C. Pediatric pain interventions in the PACU. Crit Care Nurs Clin North Am 1991;3:49–57.

14. Eland J. Pharmacologic management of acute and chronic pediatric pain. Issues Compr Pediatr Nurs 1988;11:93–111.

15. Kantor TG. The management of pain by pharmacological agents. Clin J Pain 1989;5:121–127.

16. Coyle N. Analgesics and pain. Current Concepts. Nurs Clin North Am 1987;22:727–741.

17. American Pain Society. Principles of analgesic use in the treatment of acute pain and chronic cancer pain, ed. 2. Clin Pharm 1990;9:601–611.

18. Turturro MA, Paris PM. Oral narcotic analgesics. Choosing the most appropriate agent for acute pain. Postgrad Med 1991;90: 89–95.

19. Koch-Weser J. Nonsteroidal anti-inflammatory drugs. N Engl J Med 1980;302:1179–1185.

20. Egbert AM. Help for the hurting elderly. Safe use of drugs to relieve pain. Postgrad Med 1991;89:217–228.

21. Abu-Saad H, Tesler M. Pain. In: Carrieri VK, Lindsey AM, West CN, eds. Pathophysiological phenomena in nursing. Philadelphia: W.B. Saunders, 1986:235–269.

22. Dahl JB, Kehlet H. Nonsteroidal anti-inflammatory agents: Rationale for use in severe postoperative pain. Br J Anaesth 1991;66:703–712.

23. Izzo V, Pagnoni B, Rigoli M. Recent acquisitions in pain therapy: Meclofenamic acid. Clin J Pain 1991;7 (suppl 1:S49–S53.

24. Shannon M, Berde CB. Pharmacologic management of pain in children and adolescents. Pediatr Clin North Am 1989;36:855–871.

25. Jurna I, Brune K. Central effect of the nonsteroid anti-inflammatory, indomethacin, ibuprofen, and diclofenac, determined in C fibre-evoked activity in single neurons of the rat thalamus. Pain 1990;41:71–80.

26. Beaver WT. Impact of nonnarcotic oral analgesics on pain management. Am J Med 1988;84 (suppl 5A):3–15.

27. Drug facts and comparisons. St. Louis: J.B. Lippincott, 1995: 242–252.

28. Higgs GA, Salmon JA, Henderson B, Vane JR. Pharmacokinetics of aspirin and salicylates in relation to inhibition of arachidonate cyclo-oxygenase and anti-inflammatory activity. Proc Natl Acad Sci USA 1987;84:1417–1420.

29. Ehrlich GE, ed. The resurgence of salicylates in arthritis therapy. Norwalk, CT: Scientific Media Communications, Inc. 1983:75–90.

30. Zucker MD, Rothwell KG. Differential influences of salicylate compounds on platelet aggregation and serotonin release. Curr Res 1978;23:194–199.

31. Goodwin JS, Ragan M. Cognitive dysfunction associated with naprosyn and ibuprofen. Arthritis Rheum 1982;25:1013–1015.

32. Kimberly RP, Bowden RE. Reduction of renal function by newer NSAIDs. Am J Med 1978;64:804–807.

33. Katzung BG. Anti-inflammatory drugs, drugs used in gout and antipyretic analgesics. In: Katzung BG, ed. Drug therapy, ed 2. Norwalk, CT: Appleton & Lange, 1991:247–262.

34. Silverman A, Roy CC. Liver and pancreas. In: Kempe HC, Silver HK, O'Brien D, eds. Current pediatric diagnosis and treatment, ed 8, Los Altos: Lange Medical Publications, 1984:570–571.

35. Newell FW. Aspirin, bleeding and ophthalmic surgery. Am J Ophthalmol 1972;74:559–560.

36. Crawford JS, Lewandowski RL, Chan W. The effect of aspirin on rebleeding in traumatic hyphema. Am J Ophthalmol 1975;80:543–545.

37. Vane JR. Prostaglandins and the aspirin-like drugs. Hosp Pract 1972;7:61–71.

38. Cooper SA. Ketoprofen in oral surgery pain: A review. J Clin Pharmacol 1988;28:S40–S46.

39. Cronberg S, Wallmark E, Soderberg I. Effect on platelet aggregation of oral administration of 10 nonsteroidal analgesics to humans. Scand J Haematol 1984;33:155–159.

40. Amadio P. Peripherally acting analgesics. Am J Med 1984;77 (suppl 3A):17–26.

41. Seeff LB, Cuccherini BA, Zimmerman HJ, et al. Acetaminophen hepatotoxicity in alcoholics. Ann Intern Med 1986;104:399–404.

42. Insel PA. Analgesic-antipyretics and antiinflammatory agents; drugs employed in the treatment of rheumatoid arthritis and gout. In: Gilman AG, Rall TW, Nies AS, Taylor P, eds. Goodman and Gilman's The pharmacological basis of therapeutics, ed 8, New York: Pergamon Press, 1990:638–681.

43. Kantor TG. Peripherally acting analgesics. In: Kuhar M, Pasternak G, eds. Analgesics: Neurochemical, behavioral, and clinical perspectives. New York: Raven Press, 1984:289–309.

44. Martin WR. Pharmacology of opioids. Pharmacol Rev 1984; 35:283–323.

45. Jaffe JH, Martin WR. Opioid analgesics and antagonists. In: Gilman AG, Rall TW, Nies AS, Taylor P, eds. Goodman and Gilman's The pharmacological basis of therapeutics, ed 8, New York: Pergamon Press, 1990:485–521.

46. Hoskin PJ, Hanks GW. Opioid agonist-antagonist drugs in acute and chronic pain states. Drugs 1991;41:326–344.

47. Way EL, Alder TK. The pharmacologic implications of the fate of morphine and its surrogates. Pharmacol Rev 1960;12: 383–446.

48. Beaver WT. Mild analgesics. Am J Med Sci 1966;252:576–599.

49. Beaver WT, Wallenstin SL, Rogers A, et al. Analgesic studies of codeine and oxycodone in patients with cancer. II. Comparisons of intramuscular oxycodone with intramuscular morphine and codeine. J Pharmacol Exp Ther 1978;207:101–108.

50. Kalso E, Vainio A. Morphine and oxycodone hydrochloride in the management of cancer pain. Clin Pharmacol Ther 1990;47: 639–646.

51. Kantor TG, Hopper M, Laska E. Adverse effects of commonly ordered oral narcotics. J Clin Pharmacol 1981;21:1–8.

52. Halpern LM. Analgesic drugs in the management of pain. Arch Surg 1977;112:861–869.

53. Hopkinson JH. Hydrocodone: A unique challenge for an established drug. Comparison of repeated oral doses of hydrocodone (10 mg) and codeine (60 mg) in the treatment of postpartum pain. Curr Ther Res 1978;24:503–516.

54. Turturro MA, Paris PM, Yealy DM, Menegazzi JJ. Hydrocodone versus codeine in acute musculoskeletal pain. Ann Emerg Med 1991;20:1100–1103.

55. Miller RR, Feingold A, Paxinos J. Propoxyphene hydrochloride: A critical review. JAMA 1970;213:996–1006.

56. Moertel CG, Ahmann DL, Taylor WF, et al. A comparative evaluation of marketed analgesic drugs. N Engl J Med 1972;286:813–815.

57. Inturrisi CE, Foley KM. Narcotic analgesics in the management of pain. In: Kuhar M, Pasternak G, eds. Analgesics: Neurochemical, behavioral, and clinical perspectives. New York: Raven Press, 1984:263.

58. Taylor M, Galloway DB, Petrie JC, et al. Psychomimetic effects of pentazocine and dihydrocodeine tartrate. BMJ 1978; 2(6146):1198.

59. Sunshine A, Olson NZ. Analgesic efficacy of ketoprofen in postpartum, general surgery, and chronic cancer pain. J Clin Pharmacol 1988;28:S47–S54.

60. Porter J, Jick H. Addiction rare in patients treated with narcotics. N Engl J Med 1980;302:123.

61. Cooper SA, Precheur H, Rauch D, et al. Evaluation of oxycodone and acetaminophen in treatment of postoperative dental pain. Oral Surg Oral Med Oral Pathol 1980;50:496–501.

62. Laska EM, Sunshine A, Mueler F, et al. Caffeine as an analgesic adjuvant. JAMA 1984;251:1711–1718.

63. Waters L. Pharmacologic strategies for managing pain in children. Orthopaedic Nurs 1992;11:34–40.

64. Rosow CE. The clinical usefulness of agonist-antagonist analgesics in acute pain. Drug Alcohol Depend 1987;20: 329–337.

65. Foley KM. Adjuvant analgesic drugs in cancer pain management. In: Aronoff GM, ed. Evaluation and treatment of chronic pain. Baltimore: Urban and Schwartzenberg; 1985:425–434.

66. Vandam LD. Drug therapy: Butorphanol. N Engl J Med 1977; 296:266–271.

67. Economou G, Ward-McQuaid JN. A cross-over comparison of the effect of morphine, pethidine, pentazocine, and phenazocine on biliary pressure. Gut 1971;12:218–221.

68. Slack J, Faut-Callahan M. Pain management. Nurs Clin North Am 1991;26:463–476.

69. Alderman EL, Barry WH, Graham AF, Harrison DC. Hemodynamic effects of morphine and pentazocine differ in cardiac patients. N Engl J Med 1972;287:623–627.

70. Johnstone RE, Jobes DR, Kennell EM, Behar MG, Smith TC. Reversal of morphine anesthesia with naloxone. Anesthesiology 1974;41:361–367.

71. Nutt JG, Jasinski DR. Methodone-naloxone mixtures for use in methadone maintenance programs. I. An evaluation in man of their pharmacological feasibility. II. Demonstration of acute physical dependence. Clin Pharmacol Ther 1974;15:156–166.

72. Ngai SH, Berkowitz BA, Yang JC, Hempstead J, Spector S. Pharmacokinetics of naloxone in rats and in man: Basis for its potency and short duration of action. Anesthesiology 1976;44:398–401.

73. Melzack R, Wall P. The challenge of pain. New York: Basic Books, 1982.

74. Clompus RJ. Ocular pressure patching. In: Eskridge JB, Amos JF, Bartlett JD, eds. Clinical procedures in optometry. Philadelphia: J.B. Lippincott, 1991:410–413.

75. Henkes HE, Waubke TN. Keratitis from abuse of corneal anesthetics. Br J Ophthalmol 1978;62:63–65.

76. Eland J. Pain in children. Nurs Clin North Am 1990;25:871–883.

77. Beyer J, Aradine C. Content validity of an instrument to measure young children's perception of the intensity of their pain. J Pediatr Nurs 1986;1:386–395.

78. Schechter N, Allan DA, Hanson K. Status of pediatric pain control: A comparison of hospital analgesic usage in children and adults. Pediatrics 1986;77:11–15.

79. Berde C. Regional analgesia in the management of chronic pain in children. J Pain Symp Manag 1989;4:232–237.

80. Gaudreault P, Guay J, Nicol O, Dupuis C. Pharmacokinetics and clinical efficacy of intrarectal solution of acetaminophen. Can J Anaesthesiol 1988;35:149–152.

81. Rumack BH. Aspirin versus acetaminophen: A comparative view. Pediatrics 1978;62:943–946.

82. Bender L, Weaver K, Edwards K. Postoperative patient-controlled analgesia in children. Pediatr Nurs 1990;16:549–554.

83. Levin R. Management of pain in the emergency department. In: Grossman M, Dieckmann R, eds. Pediatric emergency medicine. New York: J.B. Lippincott, 1991:192–195.

84. Eland JM, Anderson JE. The experience of pain in children. In: Jacox A, ed. Pain: A source book for nurses and other health professionals. Boston: Little, Brown, 1977:453–476.

85. Berde C, Albin A, Glazer J. Report of the subcommittee of disease-related pain in childhood cancer. Pediatrics 1990;86:818–825.

86. Yaster M, Deshpande J. Management of pediatric pain with opioid analgesics. J Pediatr 1988;113:421–427.

87. Schlegel SI, Paulus HE. Nonsteroidal and analgesic therapy in the elderly. Clin Rheumatic Dis 1986;12:245–273.

88. Griffin MR, Ray WA, Schaffner W. Nonsteroidal anti-inflammatory drug use and death from the peptic ulcer in elderly persons. Ann Intern Med 1988;109:359–363.

89. Beaver WT. Combination analgesics. Am J Med 1984;77 (suppl 3A):38–53.

90. Kaiko F. Age and morphine analgesia in cancer patients with postoperative pain. Clin Pharmacol Ther 1980;28:823–826.

91. Portenoy RK, Foley, KM. Clinical and pharmacological considerations in the use of narcotic analgesics in the elderly. Geriatr Med Today 1985;4:34–37.

92. Arunasalam K, Davenport HT, Painter S, et al. Ventilatory response to morphine in young and old subjects. Anaesthesia 1983;38: 529–533.

93. Catley DM, Thornton C, Jordan C, et al. Pronounced, episodic oxygen desaturation in the postoperative period: Its association with ventilatory pattern and analgesic regimen. Anesthesiology 1985;63:20–28.

94. Levy MH. Pain management in advanced cancer. Semin Oncol 1985;12:394–410.

95. Hupert C, Yacob M, Turgeon LR. Effect of hydroxyzine on morphine analgesia for the treatment of postoperative pain. Anesth Analg 1980;59:690–696.

96. Forbes JA, Butterworth GA, Burchfield WH, et al. Evaluation of ketorolac, aspirin, and an acetaminophen-codeine combination in

postoperative oral surgery pain. Pharmacotherapy 1990;10 (6 Pt 2):775–935.

97. Forbes JA, Kehm CJ, Grodin CD, et al. Evaluation of ketorolac, aspirin, and an acetaminophen-codeine combination in postoperative oral surgery pain. Pharmacotherapy 1990;10(6 Pt 2): 945–1055.

98. Maslanka MA, de Andrade JR, Maneatis T, et al. Comparison of oral ketorolac, intramuscular morphine, and placebo for treatment of pain after orthopedic surgery. South Med J 1994;87:506–513.

99. Graham DY, White RH, Moreland LW, et al. Duodenal and gastric ulcer prevention with misoprostol in arthritis patients taking NSAIDs. Ann Intern Med 1993;119:257–262.

CHAPTER 8

Mydriatics and Mydriolytics

Siret D. Jaanus
Neal Nyman

Drugs that stimulate the adrenergic division of the autonomic nervous system (ANS), referred to as *sympathomimetics* or *adrenergic agonists*, can affect various ocular functions including pupil size, width of the palpebral fissure, diameter of ocular blood vessels, and aqueous flow.[1–3] In clinical practice these agents are used for pupillary dilation (see Chapter 21), pharmacologic testing for oculosympathetic lesions (Horner's syndrome) (see Chapter 23), vasoconstriction of conjunctival vessels and relief of minor allergic reactions (see Chapters 13 and 26), and on occasion, treatment of ptosis (see Chapter 24). When used for dilating the pupil, they are usually referred to clinically as *mydriatics*.

Drugs that block action of the sympathetic nervous system are known as *adrenergic receptor antagonists*, *antiadrenergics*, or *adrenergic-blocking agents*.[4] Drugs that block β receptors are used clinically to control intraocular pressure (IOP) (see Chapters 10 and 35). Alpha-receptor blocking agents, also referred to clinically as *mydriolytics*, can be useful to reverse the effects of mydriatic drugs.[5]

This chapter presents an overview of the adrenergic innervation to the eye and considers the pharmacologic actions, uses, side effects, and contraindications of mydriatics and mydriolytics in current clinical use.

Adrenergic Innervation to the Eye

The sympathetic innervation to the eye originates from the posterior and lateral nuclei of the hypothalamus. Fibers descend through the lateral aspects of the brainstem to the intermediolateral columns in the cervical cord. Myelinated preganglionic neurons emerge from the thoracic section (C8–T2) of the spinal cord through the anterior roots. They then ascend over the apex of the lung through the stellate ganglion and the cervical sympathetic chain to synapse in the superior cervical ganglion (Fig. 8.1). This part of the pathway comprises the preganglionic portion.[1]

Unmyelinated fibers emerge from the superior cervical ganglion and course toward the cavernous sinus by following the carotid plexus adjacent to the carotid artery. There the fibers cross over the sixth cranial nerve and join the ophthalmic division of the fifth nerve. The fibers then bypass the ciliary ganglion and accompany the long ciliary nerves to the iris dilator muscle and Mueller's muscle of the eyelid, thus completing the postganglionic portion of the oculosympathetic pathway (see Fig. 8.1).[1]

Sympathetic neuronal control of human ciliary muscle activity is less well established. Sympathetic nerves reach the ciliary muscle through the uveal blood vessels in close association with arteries and terminal arterioles. The distribution of the adrenergic fibers in the ciliary muscle appears to vary in different species.[6] In primates, sympathetic nerve terminals can generally be found in the anterior portion of the ciliary muscle. Some evidence indicates that the sympathetic nervous system has an antagonistic effect on accommodation in the human eye.[7] Stephens[8] observed that the accommodative amplitude significantly decreased in human subjects following instillation of phenylephrine or hydroxyamphetamine. Hurwitz and associates[9] reported a marked reduction in accommodative amplitude in monkeys with the β-receptor agonist, isoproterenol. This response was completely eliminated if the eye was pretreated with the β-blocking agent propranolol. Such observations provide evidence that both divisions of the ANS can affect accommodation and further suggest that the adrenergic effects on accommodation may be mediated, at least in part, via β-receptor sites.

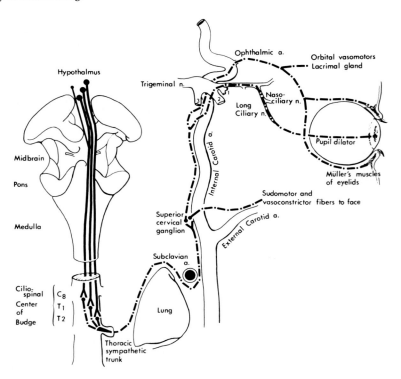

FIGURE 8.1   **The oculosympathetic pathway. Note its origin in the hypothalamus and its course through the brainstem and cervical spinal cord (central or first-order neuron), the upper thorax and lower neck (preganglionic or second-order neuron), and upper neck, middle cranial fossa, cavernous sinus, and orbit as it finally reaches Mueller's muscle of the lid and the iris dilator muscle (postganglionic or third-order neuron). (From Glaser JS. The pupils and accommodation. In: Duane TD, Jaeger EA, eds. Clinical ophthalmology. Hagerstown, MD: Harper & Row, 1987, with permission of the author and publisher.)**

The posterior half of the trabecular meshwork and the inner wall of Schlemm's canal also contain adrenergic nerve terminals.[6] Certain orbital muscles also receive adrenergic innervation. The tonic contraction of the tarsal smooth muscle of the upper lid (Mueller's muscle) is under adrenergic control. The convergence mechanism through the lateral rectus muscle is also at least partially controlled by adrenergic innervation.[10]

In addition to the control exerted on intraocular and orbital muscles, adrenergic receptors are also present in the cornea, lens, and retina.[11–19]

Adrenergic Receptors

The localization of adrenergic receptor types in ocular tissue has been investigated in several species including humans, using primarily isolated ocular muscle strips.[20–24] The distri-bution of receptor types exhibits certain species specificity (Table 8.1).

The human dilator muscle has predominantly α-adrenergic receptors and very few β. Pharmacologically it responds to α-receptor stimulators as well as mixed α- and β-receptor agonists. Mydriasis, however, is inhibited by pharmacologic agents classified as α-receptor antagonists.

The sphincter muscle appears to contain both α and β receptors in equal amounts. *In vitro,* sphincter muscle strips respond poorly to catecholamines, but both contraction and relaxation can be elicited. It has been proposed that adrenergic stimulation produces an α activation of the dilator, resulting in dilator contraction, and β activation of the sphincter, relaxing the latter muscle fibers.

In the epithelium and core of the ciliary processes, β-receptor types appear to dominate, although evidence exists for the presence of a few α receptors.[20] Stimulation with adrenergic agonists results in ciliary muscle relaxation and reduction of IOP.

TABLE 8.1
Distribution of Adrenergic Receptors in Humans and Other Species

	Iris Dilator	Iris Sphincter	Ciliary Muscle
Cat	Mainly α, some β	Mainly β, some α	Mainly β, some α
Rabbit	Mainly α, few β	Mainly β, few α	Mainly α, few β
Monkey	Mainly α, very few β	Mainly α, perhaps β	Exclusively β, no α
Man	Mainly α, very few β	α and β in equal amounts	Mainly β, very few or no α

Adapted from van Alphen GWHM. The adrenergic receptors of the intraocular muscles of the human eye. Invest Ophthalmol 1976; 15:502–505.

Evidence has accumulated indicating that each of the two types of adrenergic receptors may exist in more than one subtype.[3] Although both α_1-, α_2-, and β_1-, β_2-receptor sites have been postulated in the eye, the receptor subtypes are not well defined in ocular tissue. Studies on human ciliary processes from donor eyes indicate a predominance of β_2-adrenergic receptors.[22] Little data are presently available that clarify the distribution of α-receptor subtypes in ocular tissue. However, there is now some evidence that α_2 receptors may possibly exist in the vertebrate retina, since radioactive α_2-receptor agonists show greater affinity for [^{3}H] ligand-binding sites than do compounds known to have α_1-receptor affinity.[25] It is therefore possible that norepinephrine may play a transmitter role in the retina.

Mydriatics

Phenylephrine

PHARMACOLOGY

Phenylephrine is a synthetic sympathomimetic amine structurally similar to epinephrine. It differs chemically from the natural amine only in lacking one hydroxyl group in position 4 on the benzene ring. It acts primarily on α_1 receptors and has little or no effect on β receptors. A minor part of its pharmacologic effects may be attributed to release of norepinephrine from adrenergic nerve terminals.[3]

Following topical application, phenylephrine contracts the iris dilator muscle and smooth muscle of the conjunctival arterioles, causing pupillary dilation and blanching of the conjunctiva, respectively.[26] Mueller's muscle of the upper lid is stimulated, which widens the palpebral fissure.[27,28] IOP may decrease in normal eyes and in eyes with open-angle glaucoma.[29]

More recent fluorophotometric studies[30,31] have confirmed that phenylephrine affects aqueous flow in the human eye. After single instillations, a significant increase in aqueous flow occurs for the first 2 hours, followed by a significant decrease at 4 hours.[31] The change in aqueous flow is accompanied by a concomitant biphasic change in protein entry into the anterior chamber. Thus, it appears that phenylephrine can alter permeability of the blood-aqueous barrier and thereby may cause changes in aqueous flow. Topical phenylephrine, however, does not seem to affect macular blood flow in humans.[32]

Preparations of phenylephrine used for mydriasis are available in 2.5% and 10% solutions (Table 8.2).[33] In solu-

TABLE 8.2
Mydriatic and Mydriolytic Agents

Generic Name	Trade Name	Manufacturer	Concentration (%)
MYDRIATICS			
Phenylephrine HCl	AK-Dilate	Akorn	2.5, 10
	Mydfrin	Alcon	2.5
	NeoSynephrine	Sanofi Winthrop	2.5, 10
	NeoSynephrine Viscous	Sanofi Winthrop	10
	Phenoptic	Optopics	2.5
Hydroxyamphetamine HBr	Paredrine	Pharmics	1
	Paremyd[a]	Allergan	1
MYDRIOLYTICS			
Dapiprazole HCl	Rev-Eyes	Storz	0.5

[a]Also contains 0.25% tropicamide.

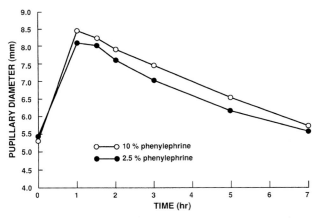

FIGURE 8.2   **Mydriasis induced by 2.5% and 10% phenylephrine (n = 112 eyes). (Reprinted with permission from Paggiarino DA, Brancato LJ, Newton RE. The effect on pupil size and accommodation of sympathetic and parasympatholytic agents. Ann Ophthalmol 1993;25:244–253.)**

tion phenylephrine is clear and is colorless to slightly yellow. Like all adrenergic agonists, it is subject to oxidation on exposure to air, light, or heat. To prolong its shelf life, an antioxidant, sodium bisulfite, is frequently added to the vehicle.

CLINICAL USES

For mydriasis, concentrations of 2.5% or 10% are available. Maximum dilation occurs in 45 to 60 minutes depending on the concentration instilled (Fig. 8.2). Recovery from mydriasis occurs in about 6 to 7 hours.[34–38]

Accommodative amplitude measurements following in-

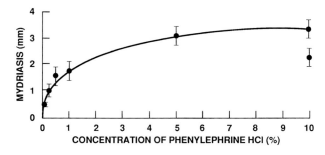

FIGURE 8.3   **Dose-response curve of mydriasis obtained with varying concentrations of freshly prepared phenylephrine hydrochloride. The lower point at 10% concentration represents response to a 10% commercial solution of phenylephrine hydrochloride. (Reprinted with permission from Am J Ophthalmol 1970;70:729–733. Copyright by the Ophthalmic Publishing Company.)**

stillation of 2.5% or 10% phenylephrine generally indicate that the effect is far less than the decrease observed with cycloplegic agents such as tropicamide[38,39] (see Chapter 9). Paggiarino and associates[38] reported a loss of approximately 2.00 D (7.93D from 9.95 D) at 1 hour with 2.5% phenylephrine. Prior to drug instillation the average accommodation was 9.31 D, and with 10% phenylephrine residual accommodation was 7.64 D. Two hours after instillation, an average loss of 1.52 D was reported for both concentrations of drug.

Dose-response curves for phenylephrine indicate an increasing mydriatic effect with concentrations up to 5%.[36] Between 5% and 10% the curve begins to plateau, and little additional effect is observed by increasing the concentration to 10% (Fig. 8.3).

Dilation of the pupil with 2.5% and 10% commercial preparations has been studied in patients selected at random and not controlled for age or color of irides.[38,40,41] The results indicate that the higher concentration does not necessarily produce a significantly greater mydriasis. The data also appear to indicate that the 10% concentration may be a more effective mydriatic in blue irides than is the 2.5% concentration, although no statistically significant difference was observed.[41] Other investigators have reported that dark irides dilate more poorly than do light irides with adrenergic mydriatics.[34,36]

In certain instances phenylephrine may also dilate the pupil at concentrations much lower than 2.5%. The mydriatic effect of 0.125% phenylephrine has been compared in unabraded and posttonography eyes.[42] Three of 10 patients with unabraded corneas showed significant pupillary dilation of 1.0 to 1.5 mm following instillation of 2 drops of 0.125% phenylephrine as compared with the saline control eye. In posttonography patients, however, the test eye was dilated in all instances as compared with the control eye.

Mechanical procedures that alter corneal epithelial integrity, thereby enhancing corneal drug penetration, can affect the response to certain ophthalmic drugs such as phenylephrine.[43] Corneal trauma from procedures such as tonometry or gonioscopy can compromise corneal epithelial integrity and facilitate the pharmacologic effects.

The mydriatic response of phenylephrine can also be enhanced by the prior instillation of a topical anesthetic.[44–46] Using commercially available solutions of phenylephrine, Jauregui and Polse[44] found that prior instillation of 0.5% proparacaine enhanced the mydriatic effect of 2.5% phenylephrine by 2 mm (Fig. 8.4). The time to produce 1 mm of dilation was reduced by 10 to 15 minutes, and the duration of mydriasis was increased by one hour. Kubo and associates[45] studied the effects of 0.125, 0.5, 1.0, and 2.0% phenylephrine with and without prior instillation of 0.5% proparacaine in four subjects (Fig. 8.5). The anesthetic enhanced the mydriatic effects of 0.5, 1.0, and 2.0% concentrations. The 0.125% concentration produced little or no dilation with or without prior instillation of the anesthetic.

Since tonometry was not performed prior to instillation of phenylephrine and the sample size was small, it is difficult to draw conclusions applicable to clinical practice.

Lyle and Bobier[46] compared the effects of anesthetics on mydriasis with 1.0% and 10% phenylephrine. Applying a topical anesthetic to one eye before applying 1.0% phenylephrine to both eyes caused more dilation in the eye that received the anesthetic. The magnitude of the response appeared to vary with iris color. Light irides were generally more responsive in both the presence and absence of the anesthetic. Prior application of 1 drop of 0.5% proparacaine, 0.4% benoxinate, or 0.5% tetracaine followed by 1 drop of 10% phenylephrine resulted in somewhat less mydriasis (1.22 mm average increase with proparacaine) than was produced by the 1% concentration and anesthetic (2.5 mm more dilation in eyes receiving both drugs). No significant differences were observed among the effects of the three different anesthetics.

In addition to its usual mydriatic effect for diagnostic purposes, phenylephrine has several other clinical uses. The drug can be a valuable aid in breaking posterior synechiae. Application of the 10% solution to the cornea preceded by a topical anesthetic is usually recommended to help break the adhesion.[26]

The drug can also be used concomitantly with echothiophate to prevent the formation of miotic cysts during treatment of open-angle glaucoma or accommodative esotropia. Addition of the 2.5% concentration to the echothiophate regimen is recommended.[47] The mechanism whereby phen-

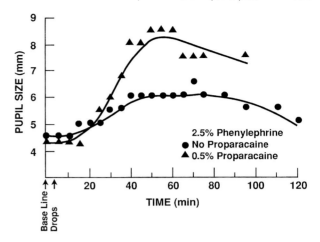

FIGURE 8.4 **Mydriatic effect of 2.5% phenylephrine hydrochloride with and without prior instillation of 0.5% proparacaine. (Reprinted with permission from Jauregui MJ, Polse KA. Mydriatic effect using phenylephrine and proparacaine. Am J Optom Physiol Opt 1974;51:545–549.)**

ylephrine prevents cyst formation is not known. However, inhibition of the intense miosis may account, at least in part, for the beneficial effect.

Ptosis resulting from sympathetic denervation such as in Horner's syndrome may respond to topical phenylephrine.

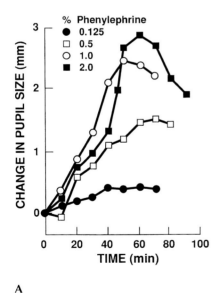

A

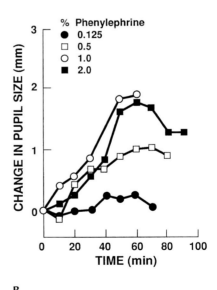

B

FIGURE 8.5 **Dose-response curves showing mydriasis with varying concentrations of phenylephrine with and without prior instillation of 0.5% proparacaine. (A) Phenylephrine and proparacaine. (B) Phenylephrine alone. (Reprinted with permission from Kubo DJ, Wing TW, Polse KA, et al. Mydriatic effects using low concentrations of phenylephrine hydrochloride. J Am Optom Assoc 1975;46:817–822.)**

Dramatic effects on the uneven palpebral apertures are sometimes observed (see Fig. 24.15).

Individuals with poor vision due to cataracts may sometimes benefit from topical phenylephrine. In patients who are unable or unwilling to undergo surgery, phenylephrine-induced pupillary dilation may improve vision (see Chapter 21).

Phenylephrine can also be used as a diagnostic test for Horner's syndrome.[48] Phenylephrine in the 1% concentration can markedly dilate the pupil with postganglionic sympathetic denervation. It causes minimal or no dilation in the normal eye. If the lesion is central or preganglionic, the affected pupil responds in a manner similar to the normal eye, since denervation hypersensitivity is minimal or absent.

SIDE EFFECTS

Topical instillation of phenylephrine can be accompanied by clinically significant adverse local and systemic events.

Ocular Effects (Table 8.3).   Local adverse events can include transient pain, lacrimation, and keratitis.[49] The effect of commercial 2.5% and 10% phenylephrine has been studied in intact and denuded rabbit and cat corneas.[50,51] Topical application to denuded corneas caused a significant increase in corneal thickness and ultrastructural changes in the endothelium. With the epithelium intact, corneal thickness did not change, but the epithelium and anterior stroma demonstrated some structural changes. Although the corneal edema and cytotoxic effect of phenylephrine was more pronounced in corneas with the epithelium removed, these results are obscured by the fact that in both instances a topical anesthetic was used before application of phenylephrine.

Phenylephrine eyedrops have been reported to cause allergic dermatoconjunctivitis.[52,53] The reaction consists of a "scalded" appearance around the eye.

Phenylephrine can cause the release of pigmented granules from the iris.[54,55] The pigment appears in the aqueous

(aqueous floaters) 30 to 40 minutes following instillation of the 2.5% or 10% concentration. These floaters usually disappear within 12 to 24 hours. The release of pigment is related to age and color of the iris, occurring more frequently in older individuals with brown irides. Further investigation has revealed that the pigmented granules have the same characteristics as melanin derived from the pigmented epithelium of the iris. It has been postulated that phenylephrine may cause rupture of the pigmented epithelial cells of the iris. Since this phenomenon has been observed primarily in older patients, it may be due to aging changes in the neuroepithelium.[54]

In patients over age 50 years, phenylephrine also appears to cause a rebound miosis the day after drug administration. Moreover, instillation of phenylephrine at that time causes a diminished mydriatic response.[36] Similarly, with chronic use of the drug reduced dilation frequently occurs, making long-term, frequent use clinically unsatisfactory. Chronic use of phenylephrine at low concentrations for ocular vasoconstriction can result in rebound congestion of the conjunctiva.[49]

Phenylephrine has also been shown to decrease conjunctival PO_2.[56,57] Following instillation of 1 drop of 2.5% phenylephrine into the inferior conjunctival fornix, a 46% reduction in PO_2 was observed for approximately 80 minutes. It has been suggested that the mechanism for the induced hypoxia is a reduction in blood flow caused by the vasoconstrictor effect of phenylephrine and compression of the iris vasculature induced by pupillary dilation.[57] Ciliary vasoconstriction has also been observed following topical application of phenylephrine.[58] These observations suggest that conjunctival hypoxia could occur with long-term use of this agent in clinical situations such as prevention of miotic-induced iris cysts and sustained pupillary dilation.

Systemic Effects (see Table 8.3).   Systemic hypertension following administration of topical ocular phenylephrine was first observed in animals by Heath in 1936.[59] Since then numerous case reports have described acute hypertensive episodes and associated complications with the 10% ophthalmic preparation.[26,60–66]

McReynolds and associates[60] reported an increase in blood pressure in 6 of 100 patients administered topical 10% phenylephrine. In each of the six subjects the increase in pressure was less than 10 mm Hg. Samantary and Thomas[65] studied 60 patients following three applications of the 10% solution in each eye at 10-minute intervals. Thirty minutes following the last drop, systolic elevations of 10 to 40 mm Hg and diastolic elevations of 10 to 30 mm Hg occurred in all subjects. In each case pulse rate decreased 10 to 20 beats per minute.

In contrast to these observations, other investigators have reported a lack of systemic vasopressor response with the 10% concentration.[40,67] In one study,[40] a group of subjects ranging in age from 21 to 53 years received 2 drops of 10% phenylephrine in one eye every 15 minutes for 90 minutes. No rise in blood pressure occurred 90 minutes after the last

TABLE 8.3
Side Effects of Topical Phenylephrine

Ocular Effects	Systemic Effects
Transient pain	Systemic hypertension
Lacrimation	Occipital headache
Keratitis	Subarachnoid hemorrhage
Pigmented aqueous floaters	Ventricular arrhythmia
	Tachycardia
Rebound miosis	Reflex bradycardia
Rebound conjunctival congestion	Blanching of skin
Conjunctival hypoxia	

drop. Brown and associates[67] conducted a double-masked study comparing the systemic hypertensive effects of topical 10% phenylephrine with 1% tropicamide, a drug with no known vasopressor effect, in patients of both sexes with an age range of 13 to 89 years. A total of 6 drops of each drug was administered over a 4-minute period to each eye of all subjects. No statistically significant differences between the two groups with respect to drug effects on blood pressure or pulse rate were observed. The percentage of individual blood pressure elevations greater than 15 mm Hg at 5, 15, and 30 minutes following drug instillation in both the phenylephrine and tropicamide groups is shown in Figure 8.6.

Data collected by the National Registry of Drug-Induced Ocular Side Effects suggest that in the general population, a group of patients may have certain risk factors for side effects from topical ocular 10% phenylephrine.[66] Of 15 patients with myocardial infarcts, 11 died following topical application of 10% phenylephrine. The average age of these patients was 71 years, and nine individuals had a history of cardiovascular disease.

The effects of 2.5% phenylephrine on systemic blood pressure and pulse have also been investigated.[68–70] Jennings and Sullivan[70] observed no significant change in systolic and diastolic blood pressures in a group of 252 patients ranging in age from 3 to 92 years. Kumar and associates[69] reported two cases of acute systemic hypertension following instillation of 2.5% phenylephrine. Both patients, who were 69 and 71 years of age, were scheduled for surgery, and each received multiple drops of the phenylephrine. The medical history of one patient included diabetes and cardiac disease.

It is likely that age as well as physical status determines patients' responses to topical ocular phenylephrine. Neonates respond to 10% phenylephrine with significant increases in blood pressure.[63] Patients who are insulin-dependent diabetics may demonstrate increased systolic and diastolic blood pressure in response to topical 10% phenylephrine.[71] Similarly, individuals with idiopathic orthostatic hypotension respond to low concentrations of phenylephrine with marked blood pressure elevations. In one group of patients, a significant increase in blood pressure occurred following instillation of 1 drop of 2.5% phenylephrine solution in each eye. Heart rate was unaffected.[72]

Other systemic reactions reported with topical ocular phenylephrine include severe occipital headache, subarachnoid hemorrhage,[60] ventricular arrhythmias,[66] tachycardia,[65] reflex bradycardia,[73] ruptured aneurysm, and blanching of the skin.[60]

Patients taking certain systemic medications are also more sensitive to the pressor effects of phenylephrine. In individuals taking atropine, the pressor effect of phenylephrine is augmented and tachycardia can occur.[73] Tricyclic antidepressants (TCAs) and monoamine oxidase (MAO) inhibitors also potentiate the cardiovascular effects of topical phenylephrine.[74] The concomitant use of phenylephrine is contraindicated with these agents, even up to 21 days

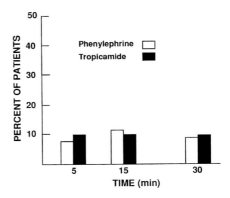

FIGURE 8.6 **Percentage of individual blood pressure elevations greater than 15 mm Hg at 5, 15, and 30 minutes in subjects receiving 10% phenylephrine or 1% tropicamide. (Reprinted with permission from Brown MM, Brown GC, Spaeth GL. Lack of side effects from topically administered 10% phenylephrine eye drops. Arch Ophthalmol 1980;98:487–489. Copyright 1980, American Medical Association.)**

following cessation of MAO inhibitor therapy. Similarly, patients taking reserpine, guanethidine, or methyldopa are at increased risk for adverse pressor effects from topical phenylephrine[71] because of denervation hypersensitivity accompanying the chemical sympathectomy.

Systemic reactions to 2.5% phenylephrine following topical ocular application to an intact eye have rarely been reported in adults.[66] However, an acute rise in systolic blood pressure has occurred in a one-year-old child following the instillation of 0.5 ml of 2.5% phenylephrine during nasolacrimal duct probing.[75] A few seconds following application of the drug to the conjunctiva to clear the surgical field, systolic blood pressure increased to 200 mm Hg. The pressure returned to normal within 20 minutes with no adverse sequelae. In this situation a relatively high dose of drug was applied to an eye already hyperemic and irritated due to probing. This most likely enhanced systemic absorption of the drug. Since the patient weighed only 10 kg, the dose relative to body size was also large.

The threshold dosage of phenylephrine in the average adult has been estimated to be 0.4 mg intravenously, 2 mg subcutaneously, and 50 mg orally.[73] The upper limit for safe dosage in normal adults is about 1.5 mg intravenously and 300 mg subcutaneously. Since a 50 μl drop of 10% phenylephrine contains 5 mg of drug, multiple applications can result in overdosage, especially if absorption from the site of administration is enhanced or if the patient is compromised by age, body size, concomitant medications, or trauma.

It is not known to what extent topical ocular phenylephrine is absorbed into the systemic circulation. However, since the drug causes local vasoconstriction,[3,57,58] this can possibly diminish flow to receptor sites for the drug.

CONTRAINDICATIONS

Based on data submitted to the National Registry of Drug-Induced Ocular Side Effects and those acquired by other investigators, the following guidelines for the clinical use of 10% phenylephrine are suggested.[66,71,72]

- Use phenylephrine 10% with caution in patients with cardiac disease, idiopathic orthostatic hypotension, hypertension, aneurysms, insulin-dependent diabetes, and advanced arteriosclerosis.
- Give only one application of the 10% concentration per hour to each eye.
- The drug is contraindicated in patients taking MAO inhibitors, TCAs, reserpine, guanethidine, or methyldopa.
- Concomitant use of topical phenylephrine is discouraged in atropinized patients, since tachycardia and hypertension can occur.
- Prolonged irrigation, application with a conjunctival pledget, or subconjunctival injection of the 10% solution is not recommended.
- Only the 2.5% solution is recommended for infants and the elderly.

Since the 10% concentration appears to be associated with an increased risk of significant adverse ocular and systemic events, the 2.5% solution, with appropriate precautions, is recommended for routine use.[66] Because phenylephrine in solution can lose its pharmacologic activity over time or with improper use or storage, the manufacturer's instructions should be followed concerning expiration date and

proper handling of the drug. Loss of drug effect can occur even without visible color change.

Hydroxyamphetamine

PHARMACOLOGY

Hydroxyamphetamine (β-4-hydroxyphenylisopropylamine) is similar in chemical structure to norepinephrine. It is classified as an indirect-acting adrenergic agonist since its primary pharmacologic action is thought to be due to release of norepinephrine from adrenergic nerve terminals. Guanethidine, an agent known to deplete norepinephrine, abolishes its adrenergic stimulatory effects.[76] In addition, hydroxyamphetamine has been shown to inhibit MAO as well as the reuptake of norepinephrine into the nerve terminal.[77,78] It may also directly stimulate α- and possibly β-receptor sites, although this effect has been considered minimal and probably clinically insignificant.[79]

Hydroxyamphetamine has little if any effect on accommodation or the refractive state.[39,80] It also does not raise IOP in eyes with open anterior chamber angles.[80]

CLINICAL USES

Topical instillation of a 1% solution in eyes with normal adrenergic innervation causes mydriasis and vasoconstriction.[34,35,80] However, hydroxyamphetamine is used only as a mydriatic agent. Maximum dilation occurs within 60 minutes, and the duration of mydriasis is about 6 hours (Fig. 8.7).

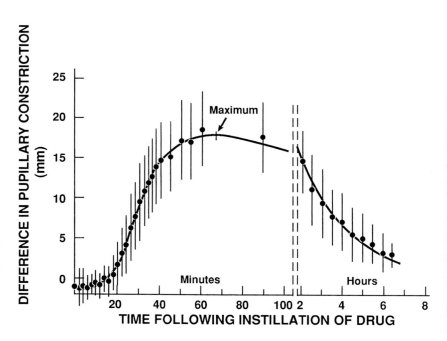

FIGURE 8.7 **Time course of mydriasis following instillation of 1% hydroxyamphetamine. (Reprinted with permission from Gambill HD, Ogle KN, Kearns P. Mydriatic effect of four drugs determined by pupillograph. Arch Ophthalmol 1967;77:740–746. Copyright 1967, American Medical Association.)**

Several investigators have compared the mydriatic effects of phenylephrine and hydroxyamphetamine. Gambill and associates[35] compared 10% phenylephrine with several drugs, including 1% hydroxyamphetamine. The time to maximum dilation was similar (70.2 minutes for phenylephrine and 64.8 minutes for hydroxyamphetamine). The amount of mydriasis produced was somewhat greater with 10% phenylephrine, 2.42 mm as compared to 1.93 mm with hydroxyamphetamine. Barbee and Smith[34] also found similar mydriatic effects for 10% phenylephrine and 1% hydroxyamphetamine in normal subjects ranging in age from 16 to 60 years.

Semes and Bartlett[81] compared the mydriatic effect of 2.5% phenylephrine to 1% hydroxyamphetamine in a group of 28 young adult subjects without ocular disease. The two agents produced a nearly equal pupillary dilation (Fig. 8.8). The maximum effect with both drugs occurred at about 45 minutes.

Hydroxyamphetamine is clinically useful for differentiating between central or preganglionic and postganglionic sympathetic denervation.[48,79,82] Since the drug stimulates release of endogenous norepinephrine from its stores in adrenergic nerve terminals, it fails to dilate a pupil with postganglionic sympathetic denervation depending on the extent of damage. However, if the lesion causing a Horner's syndrome is central or preganglionic, hydroxyamphetamine should cause normal mydriasis, since the nerve endings of the postganglionic fibers should contain normal amounts of norepinephrine and thus respond normally.[48,79,82]

SIDE EFFECTS

When used for routine mydriasis, hydroxyamphetamine appears to be effective while causing little if any ocular irritation. It has been suggested that this drug may be a safe mydriatic to use in eyes with shallow anterior chambers, since because of its indirect action, it may be more readily counteracted with miotics.[83] In patients with open-angle glaucoma hydroxyamphetamine elevates IOP minimally if at all. Reductions of IOP have also been reported.[84]

The actions of hydroxyamphetamine on the cardiovascular system differ in certain respects from those of phenylephrine. The drug can raise blood pressure, but unlike phenylephrine the pressor response is characterized by tachyphylaxis.[85] The drug can also produce sinoauricular tachycardia and ventricular arrhythmia following systemic administration.[86]

Other adverse events observed with subcutaneous or oral doses of hydroxyamphetamine include headache, sweating, nausea, and vomiting. In all instances relatively large doses were administered.[80]

CONTRAINDICATIONS

Contraindications to the topical use of hydroxyamphetamine for routine mydriasis are similar to those of phenylephrine.

However, because of its tachyphylaxis and ineffectiveness in postganglionic denervation, hydroxyamphetamine may be a safer mydriatic for use in patients with insulin-dependent diabetes, idiopathic orthostatic hypotension, or chemical sympathectomy produced by therapy with systemic guanethidine, reserpine, or methyldopa. Thus, hydroxyamphetamine seems to be less strongly contraindicated than phenylephrine in certain high-risk patients.

Cocaine

PHARMACOLOGY

Cocaine is a naturally occurring alkaloid present in the leaves of the shrub *Erythroxylon coca* and other species of trees indigenous to Peru and Bolivia. Chemically it is an ester of benzoic acid with a nitrogen-containing base.[87]

Cocaine exhibits several pharmacologic effects. Following local application it acts as an anesthetic by blocking the initiation and conduction of nerve impulses. It also blocks neuronal reuptake of norepinephrine, thus potentiating adrenergic activity. Moderate doses increase heart rate and cause vasoconstriction. The most striking systemic effect of cocaine is central nervous system (CNS) stimulation.[87]

The ocular effects of cocaine include anesthesia (see Chapter 6), mydriasis, and vasoconstriction. Topical application of a 1 to 4% solution produces anesthesia within 1 minute. Depending on the concentration used, the effect

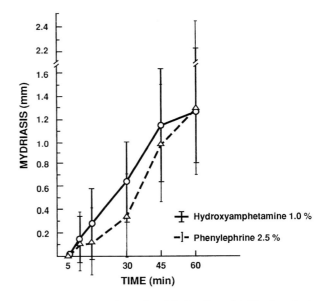

FIGURE 8.8 Comparison of mydriatic effect of 2.5% phenylephrine and 1% hydroxyamphetamine in young adult subjects. (Reprinted with permission from Semes LP, Bartlett JD. Mydriatic effectiveness of hydroxyamphetamine. J Am Optom Assoc 1982;53:899–904.)

can last up to 20 minutes or longer.[88] The mydriatic effect of cocaine depends on the presence of a functioning adrenergic innervation. Following topical application to the eye, the pupil begins to dilate within 15 to 20 minutes.[89] The maximum effect, which is typically less than 2 mm of dilation, occurs within 40 to 60 minutes, and the pupil may remain dilated for 6 or more hours. The mydriasis is accompanied by vasoconstriction that causes blanching of the conjunctiva.[88]

Topical ocular application of cocaine can result in serious corneal epithelial damage.[90] Cocaine is also readily absorbed through the mucous membranes into the systemic circulation.[89]

CLINICAL USES

Because of its deleterious effects on the corneal epithelium, the clinical uses of cocaine are limited. Although it is no longer used for such routine ophthalmic procedures as tonometry, the drug can be helpful in the diagnosis of Horner's syndrome (see Chapter 23). In addition, due to its ability to loosen the corneal epithelium, it can be helpful in the debridement of herpetic corneal ulcers.[88]

SIDE EFFECTS

The most striking effect of systemic absorption of cocaine is CNS stimulation. Signs and symptoms can include excitement, restlessness, rapid and irregular pulse, dilated pupils, headache, gastrointestinal upset, delirium and convulsions. Death usually results from respiratory failure.[87] Moderate doses of cocaine can also raise body temperature.[88] Systemic absorption through mucous membranes is rapid and has been compared to that of intravenous administration.[88]

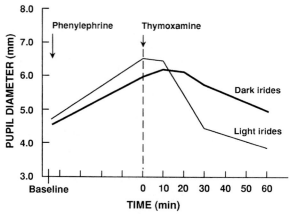

FIGURE 8.9 **Effects of 0.1% thymoxamine on pupil diameter in eyes with light and dark irides following dilation with 2.5% phenylephrine. (Reprinted with permission from Relf SJ, Gharagozloo NZ, Skuta GL, et al. Thymoxamine reverses phenylephrine-induced mydriasis. Am J Ophthalmol 1988;106: 251–255.)**

The most significant effect of topical ocular cocaine is damage to the ocular tissue.[90] Grossly visible grayish pits and corneal epithelial irregularities can occur, especially with repeated application. The corneal epithelium may loosen, leading to large areas of erosion.

CONTRAINDICATIONS

Because of its peripheral adrenergic and CNS stimulatory effects, cocaine should be used with caution in patients with cardiac disease or hyperthyroidism.[33]

Mydriolytics

With few exceptions, the clinical usefulness of these agents is limited in ophthalmic practice. They have been used in the therapy of glaucoma and the reversal of mydriasis produced by diagnostic pharmaceutical agents. Recently, attention has focused on thymoxamine as well as dapiprazole, which has become commercially available in the United States for clinical use to reverse diagnostic mydriasis.

Thymoxamine

PHARMACOLOGY

Thymoxamine hydrochloride is a competitive antagonist of α-adrenergic receptors.[4] When given intravenously, it antagonizes the hypertensive effects of norepinephrine and epinephrine. It dilates human arteries *in vitro* and therefore has been used in various vasopastic conditions such as Raynaud's disease, femoral artery occlusion, and chilblain.[91] When used topically in the eye, it produces postsynaptic blockade of α_1-adrenergic receptors in the iris dilator muscle, leaving the sphincter muscle unopposed and thus producing miosis.[92]

Pau[93] first reported the topical ocular use of thymoxamine in 1955. He applied a 5% solution topically to the eye and observed pupillary constriction and extreme ocular discomfort. Thirteen years later, Turner and Sneddon[5] observed that pretreatment with 0.1% thymoxamine prevented the mydriatic response to 10% phenylephrine and 2% ephedrine. Thymoxamine also rapidly reversed the pupillary dilation caused by 1% hydroxyamphetamine. Relf and associates[94] and Wright and associates[95] conducted randomized, double-masked comparisons of 0.1% thymoxamine and placebo for the reversal of 2.5% phenylephrine-induced mydriasis. The pupils of thymoxamine-treated eyes returned to baseline in 2.2 hours, compared to 5.2 hours for the placebo-treated group.[95] Light and dark irides appear to respond differently to thymoxamine.[94,96] Eyes with dark irides exhibit a significantly slower onset and lesser magnitude of response to thymoxamine than do pupils of light eyes dilated with phenylephrine (Fig. 8.9). While no studies have demonstrated that thymoxamine reverses the reduction in accommodative amplitude produced by tropicamide, it does reverse the effects on accommodation produced by adrenergic agonists such as ephedrine.[97]

The pupillary constriction produced by thymoxamine, unlike the cholinergic miotics, is not accompanied by a shallowing of the anterior chamber[98,99] (Fig. 8.10). Since thymoxamine has no apparent effect on the ciliary body, it should not alter the size or position of the lens.

CLINICAL USES

In recent years, attention has focused on developing noncholinergic miotic agents that safely and effectively reverse the effects of mydriatics without the risks or side effects associated with traditional pilocarpine miosis. Mapstone[100] has presented theoretical evidence that the use of a cholinergic stimulatory agent such as pilocarpine to induce miosis, following the use of an adrenergic mydriatic such as phenylephrine, increases the risk of angle-closure glaucoma. Not only does spasm of accommodation occur with pilocarpine, but in addition, stimulation of the dilator and sphincter muscles simultaneously is most likely to produce shallowing of the anterior chamber and to result in pupillary block.

Unlike pilocarpine, thymoxamine appears to be a safe miotic for reversing phenylephrine-induced mydriasis.[94,101] Moreover, the miosis is maintained long after the phenylephrine effect has dissipated.[101,102] In addition, thymoxamine acts almost as rapidly as pilocarpine in reversing phenylephrine-induced mydriasis. One drop of 0.5% thymoxamine reverses the mydriasis of 10% phenylephrine to the premydriatic pupillary diameter within 30 minutes.[102] Comparing 0.1% thymoxamine to a placebo following dilation with 1 drop of 2.5% phenylephrine, Relf and associates[94] observed a reversal of mydriasis within 1 hour. In comparison, the mean time for reversal of phenylephrine-induced mydriasis with 1.0% pilocarpine is 22 minutes.[103] In a study by McKinna and associates[104] local instillation of 0.5% thymoxamine completely reversed mydriasis produced by 0.5% tropicamide and partially reversed the mydriasis produced by 1.0% tropicamide. Shah and associates[105] also demonstrated that 0.5% thymoxamine partially reverses the mydriasis produced by a combination of 0.5% tropicamide and 2.5% phenylephrine.

Since the miotic effect of thymoxamine appears to occur without an accompanying shallowing of the anterior chamber, it may be useful for the treatment of acute angle-closure glaucoma. Ten patients with angle-closure glaucoma were treated with 0.5% thymoxamine every minute for 5 minutes and then every 15 minutes for up to 3 hours. Of the 10 patients, eight were successfully treated with thymoxamine alone.[106]

Thymoxamine has also been evaluated and appears to be of value as a diagnostic agent for differentiating between angle-closure glaucoma and open-angle glaucoma with narrow angles.[91] Since thymoxamine produces miosis without affecting IOP, facility of outflow, rate of aqueous formation,

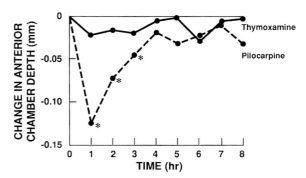

FIGURE 8.10 **Mean change in anterior chamber depth in 11 patients following instillation of 0.5% thymoxamine or 2% pilocarpine. Asterisks indicate values that are significant at P < 0.05. (Reprinted with permission from Saheb NE, Lorenzetti D, Salpeter CS. Effect of thymoxamine and pilocarpine on the depth of the anterior chamber. Can J Ophthalmol 1980;15:170–171.)**

or permeability of the blood-aqueous barrier,[107,108] the angle can be opened for a sufficient time without affecting the ciliary muscle. Thus, if elevated IOP is reduced to normal following instillation of thymoxamine, the diagnosis is angle closure. If the IOP is only partially reduced, the diagnosis is combined mechanism glaucoma (combination of angle-closure and open-angle glaucoma). If the IOP remains elevated, the diagnosis is open-angle glaucoma with narrow angles, where the narrow angles do not contribute to the elevated pressure.

More recently, thymoxamine 0.1% in a buffered solution has been administered intracamerally during extracapsular cataract extraction.[109] Thymoxamine 0.1%, when administered with acetylcholine, produces a more profound and prolonged miosis than does acetylcholine alone.

SIDE EFFECTS

The topical ocular use of thymoxamine is accompanied by a transient stinging and burning sensation.[94,101,106] The burning sensation is less intense with the 0.5% solution compared with the 1.0% solution. Conjunctival hyperemia may last several hours following application, and chemosis and ptosis have also been observed with topical thymoxamine. Two cases of drug-induced Horner's syndrome have been reported.[91,101]

Thymoxamine appears to be relatively free of side effects when administered by the oral, intravenous, or subcutaneous routes. Reported effects have included facial flushing, vertigo, headaches, nausea, and diarrhea.[91]

CONTRAINDICATIONS

Thymoxamine is contraindicated in circumstances where pupillary constriction is undesirable, such as acute anterior uveitis, and in patients having hypersensitivity to any component of the preparation.

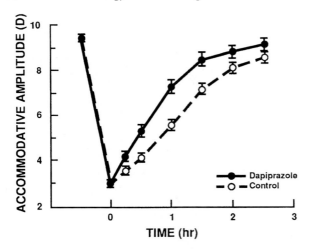

FIGURE 8.11 **Amplitude of accommodation after instillation of 0.5% dapiprazole (0 hour) in eyes dilated with 0.5% tropicamide. (Reprinted with permission from Nyman N, Reich L. The effect of dapiprazole on accommodative amplitude in eyes dilated with 0.5% tropicamide. J Am Optom Assoc 1993;64:625–628.)**

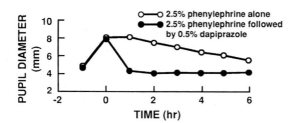

FIGURE 8.12 **Reversal of mydriasis with 0.5% dapiprazole following pupillary dilation induced by 2.5% phenylephrine. (Adapted from Nyman N, Keates EU. Effects of dapiprazole on the reversal of pharmacologically induced mydriasis. Optom Vis Sci 1990;67:705–709.)**

Dapiprazole

PHARMACOLOGY

A more recently developed α-receptor antagonist, dapiprazole, produces miosis and reduces IOP following instillation in the eye.[110–113] Like thymoxamine, dapiprazole reverses mydriasis by blocking α receptors in the iris dilator muscle. Concentrations ranging from 0.12 to 1.5% significantly reduce pupil size in both normal and glaucomatous eyes.[110,111] The miotic effect is concentration-dependent and can last up to 6 hours following instillation. IOP can be reduced for up to 6 hours.[110] In patients with decreased amplitude of accommodation associated with tropicamide-induced cycloplegia, dapiprazole may partially increase the accommodative am-

plitude (Fig. 8.11).[114–117] Studies in rabbits indicate that systemic absorption is minimal following topical application.[116]

CLINICAL USES

Dapiprazole can produce nearly complete reversal of a phenylephrine-dilated pupil (Fig. 8.12).[117,118] Partial reversal of pupils dilated with tropicamide has been reported as well.[117–119,126] A tropicamide-dilated pupil returns to within 0.5 mm or 1.0 mm of its premydriatic diameter in less than 2 hours. Pupils dilated with combinations of phenylephrine and tropicamide or hydroxyamphetamine and tropicamide have been studied, and partial reversal of pupillary dilation occurs within 2 hours, with a significant reduction in pupil size after 1 hour (Fig. 8.13).[118–120,124] Despite the reduction in pupil size, however, dapiprazole may have only limited usefulness in the prepresbyopic population, because the drug may induce little improvement in functional vision as measured by changes in accommodation and near visual acuity.[125] This seems to depend on the agent used for pupillary dilation.

Dapiprazole 0.25% and 0.5% are effective in cases of angle-closure glaucoma.[110–112] In patients with gonioscopically narrow angles, the drug has been effective in preventing angle-closure glaucoma.[112]

The miosis produced by 0.5% dapiprazole begins 10 minutes following instillation and results in a significant reduction in pupil size, compared with the contralateral eye treated with 1% tropicamide alone.[113,119] Since the miosis is due to α-receptor blockade in the iris dilator muscle, no shifting of the iris-lens diaphragm with subsequent shallowing of the anterior chamber occurs.

Intraocular dapiprazole has been shown to be clinically effective for reversing mydriasis during extracapsular cataract extraction (ECCE) with IOL implantation.[113,121] A study by Ponte and associates[121] compared intraocular 0.25% dapiprazole to 1% acetylcholine. They found that after

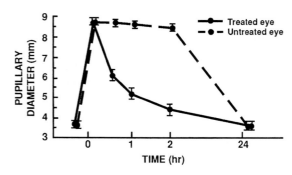

FIGURE 8.13 **Reversal of mydriasis with 0.5% dapiprazole following pupillary dilation induced by a combination of 2.5% phenylephrine and 1% tropicamide. (Reprinted with permission from Allinson RW, Gerber DS, Bieber S, Hodes BL. Reversal of mydriasis by dapiprazole. Ann Ophthalmol 1990;22:131–138.)**

ECCE with posterior chamber IOL implantation, 0.25% dapiprazole was effective in producing a more persistent miosis without side effects. The drug also reduced the transient postoperative IOP increase.

As with thymoxamine, eye color can affect the rate of pupillary constriction.[94,119,122] In patients with brown irides, the rate of pupillary constriction may be slower than in individuals with blue or green irides.[94]

The only FDA-approved use for dapiprazole at present is in the reversal of iatrogenically induced mydriasis produced by adrenergic (phenylephrine or hydroxyamphetamine) or anticholinergic (tropicamide) agents.[122] The drug is currently under investigation in clinical trials that are evaluating other ophthalmic indications. Dapiprazole is commercially available as Rev-Eyes in a kit consisting of one vial of the drug (25 mg), one vial of diluent (5 ml), and a dropper for dispensing. Once the solution has been mixed, the eyedrops are clear, colorless, and slightly viscous and can be stored at room temperature for 21 days.[33] The recommended dosage per eye is 2 drops followed 5 minutes later by an additional 2 drops. When 2.5% phenylephrine is used alone for pupillary dilation, a single drop of dapiprazole has a clinical effect equivalent to the multiple-drop regimen.[127]

SIDE EFFECTS

Transient burning and conjunctival hyperemia following topical ocular application of dapiprazole are common.[110,118] Other mild to moderate ocular side effects include superficial punctate keratitis, corneal edema, chemosis, ptosis, lid erythema and edema, itching, dry eye, and brow ache.[33,110,118] Many of these are the result of the dilation of conjunctival blood vessels, which is a pharmacologic action of α-receptor antagonists. Ptosis (Fig. 8.14) can also be attributed to α-receptor blockade in Mueller's muscle. Blood pressure and pulse rate are not significantly affected by topical use of dapiprazole. A recent study[123] concluded that topical application of dapiprazole produces no corneal endothelial toxicity, but intracameral use postsurgically may result in adverse corneal endothelial effects.

CONTRAINDICATIONS

Dapiprazole is contraindicated in circumstances where pupillary constriction is undesirable, such as acute anterior uveitis, and in patients having hypersensitivity to any component of the preparation.

References

1. Zinn KM. The pupil. Springfield, IL: Charles C Thomas, 1972; Chap. 2.
2. Langham ME, Diggs EM. Adrenergic responses in the human eye. J Pharmacol Exp Ther 1971;179:47–55.
3. Hoffman BB, Lefkowitz RJ. Catecholamines and sympathomi-

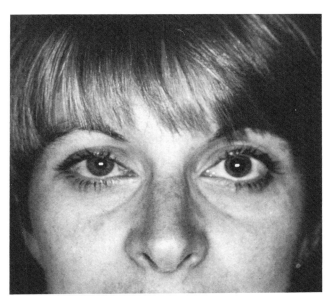

FIGURE 8.14 **Right ptosis, miosis, and conjunctival hyperemia induced by 0.5% dapiprazole instilled into right eye following bilateral pupillary dilation with 2.5% phenylephrine.**

metic drugs. In: Gilman AG, Rall TW, Nies AS, et al, eds. Goodman and Gilman's The pharmacological basis of therapeutics. New York: McGraw-Hill, 1993; Chap. 10.
4. Hoffman BB, Lefkowitz RJ. Adrenergic receptor antagonists. In: Gilman AG, Rall TW, Nies AS, et al, eds. Goodman and Gilman's The Pharmacological basis of therapeutics. New York: McGraw-Hill 1993; Chap. 11.
5. Turner P, Sneddon JM. Alpha-receptor blockage by thymoxamine in the human eye. Clin Pharmacol Ther 1968;9:45–59.
6. Ehinger B. A comparative study of the adrenergic nerves to the anterior eye segment of some primates. Z Zellforsch 1971; 116:157–177.
7. Cogan DC. Accommodation and the autonomic nervous system. Arch Ophthalmol 1937;18:739–766.
8. Stephens KG. Effect of the sympathetic nervous system on accommodation. Am J Optom Physiol Opt 1985;62:402–406.
9. Hurwitz BS, Davidowitz J, Chin NB, et al. The effect of the sympathetic nervous system on accommodation. 1. Beta sympathetic nervous system. Arch Ophthalmol 1972;87:668–674.
10. Lowenfeld IE. Mechanisms of reflex dilation of the pupil; historical review and experimental analysis. Doc Ophthalmol (Den Haag) 1958;12:185–448.
11. Laties A, Jacobowitz D. A histochemical study of the adrenergic and cholinergic innervation of the anterior segment of the rabbit eye. Invest Ophthalmol 1964;3:592–600.
12. Neufeld AH, Zawistowski KA, Page ED, Bromberg BB. Influences on the density of beta adrenergic receptors in the cornea and iris-ciliary body of the rabbit. Invest Ophthalmol 1978;17:1069–1075.
13. Butterfield LC, Neufeld AH. Cyclic nucleotides and mitosis in the rabbit cornea following superior cervical ganglionectomy. Exp Eye Res 1977;25:427–433.

14. Waltman SR, Yarian D, Hart W, Becker B. Corneal endothelial changes with long-term topical epinephrine therapy. Arch Ophthalmol 1977;95:1357–1358.

15. Zadunaisky JA, Lande MA, Chalfie M, Neufeld AH. Ion pumps in the cornea and its stimulation by epinephrine and cAMP. Exp Eye Res 1973;15:577–584.

16. Walkenback RJ, Le Grand RD. Adenylate cyclase activity in bovine and human corneal endothelium. Invest Ophthalmol Vis Sci 1982;22:120–124.

17. Kahan A. Effects of adrenergic activators and inhibitors on the eye. In: Szekeres L, ed. Adrenergic activators and inhibitors. Handbuch Pharm 1981;8:319–344.

18. Voaden MS. A chalone in the rabbit lens. Exp Eye Res 1968; 7:326–331.

19. Kramer SG. Dopamine: A retinal neurotransmitter. I. Retinal uptake, storage, and light-stimulated release of H_3-dopamine in vivo. Invest Ophthalmol 1971;10:438–452.

20. Van Halpern GWHN, Kern R, Robinette SL. Adrenergic receptors of the intraocular muscles. Arch Ophthalmol 1965;74:253–259.

21. Langham ME, Diggs E. β-adrenergic responses in the eyes of rabbits, primates and man. Exp Eye Res 1974;19:281–295.

22. Nathanson JA. Human ciliary process adrenergic receptor: Pharmacological characterization. Invest Ophthalmol Vis Sci 1981;21:798–804.

23. Neufeld AH, Page ED. In vitro determination of the ability of drugs to bind to adrenergic receptors. Invest Ophthalmol Vis Sci 1977;16:1118–1124.

24. Bhargava G, Mahman MH, Katzman R. Distribution of β-adrenergic receptors and isoproterenol-stimulated cyclic AMP formation in monkey iris and ciliary body. Exp Eye Res 1980; 31:471–477.

25. Osborne NN. Binding of (–)³H noradrenaline to bovine membrane retina. Evidence for the existence of α_2-receptors. Vis Res 1982; 22:1401–1407.

26. Heath P, Geiter CW. Use of phenylephrine hydrochloride (Neosynephrine) in ophthalmology. Arch Ophthalmol 1949;41:172–177.

27. Felt DP, Frueh BR. A pharmacologic study of the sympathetic eyelid tarsal muscles. Ophthalmic Plast Reconstr Surg 1988; 4:15–21.

28. Munden PM, Kardon RH, Denison CE, et al. Palpebral fissure responses to topical adrenergic drugs. Am J Ophthalmol 1991;111:706–710.

29. Lee PF. The influence of epinephrine and phenylephrine on intraocular pressure. Arch Ophthalmol 1958;60:863–867.

30. Van Genderen MM, Best JA van, Oosterhuis JA. The immediate effect of phenylephrine on aqueous flow in man. Invest Ophthalmol Vis Sci 1988;29:1469–1473.

31. Araie M, Mori M, Oshika T. Effect of topical phenylephrine on the permeability of the blood-aqueous barrier in man. Graefe's Arch Clin Exp Ophthalmol 1992;230:171–174.

32. Robinson F, Petrig BL, Sinclair SH, et al. Does topical phenylephrine, tropicamide or proparacaine affect macular blood flow? Ophthalmology 1985;92:1130–1132.

33. Ophthalmic drug facts. St. Louis: Facts and Comparisons 1995; Chap. 4.

34. Barbee R, Smith WA. A comparative study of mydriatic and cycloplegic agents. Am J Ophthalmol 1957;44:617–622.

35. Gambill HD, Ogle KN, Kearns TP. Mydriatic effect of four drugs determined by pupillograph. Arch Ophthalmol 1967;77:740–746.

36. Haddad NJ, Moyer NJ, Riley FC. Mydriatic effect of phenylephrine hydrochloride. Am J Ophthalmol 1970;70:729–733.

37. Doughty MJ, Lyle W, Trevino R, et al. A study of mydriasis produced by topical phenylephrine 2.5% in young adults. Can J Optom 1988;50:40–60.

38. Paggiarino DA, Brancato LJ, Newton RE. The effect on pupil size and accommodation of sympathetic and parasympatholytic agents. Ann Ophthalmol 1993;25:244–253.

39. Roth N. Refractive state after instillation of paredrine and neosynephrine. Br J Ophthalmol 1968;52:763–767.

40. Smith RB, Read S, Oczypik PM. Mydriatic effect of phenylephrine. Eye Ear Nose Throat Monthly 1976;55:133–134.

41. Neuhaus RW, Hepler RS. Mydriatic effect of phenylephrine 10% vs phenylephrine 2.5% (aq). Ann Ophthalmol 1980;12:1159–1160.

42. Weiss DI, Shaffer RN. Mydriatic effects of one-eighth percent phenylephrine. Arch Ophthalmol 1962;68:727–729.

43. Marr WG, Wood R, Senterfit, L, Sigelman S. Effect of topical anesthetics on regeneration of corneal epithelium. Am J Ophthalmol 1957:606–610.

44. Jauregui MJ, Polse KA. Mydriatic effect using phenylephrine and proparacaine. Am J Optom Physiol Opt 1974;51:545–549.

45. Kubo DJ, Wing TW, Polse KA, Jauregui M. Mydriatic effects using low concentrations of phenylephrine hydrochloride. J Am Optom Assoc 1975;46:817–822.

46. Lyle WM, Bobier WR. Effects of topical anesthetics on phenylephrine-induced mydriasis. Am J Optom Physiol Opt 1977; 54:276–281.

47. Chiri NB, Gold AA, Breinin G. Iris cysts and miotics. Arch Ophthalmol 1964;71:611–616.

48. Thompson HS, Menscher JH. Adrenergic mydriasis in Horner's syndrome; hydroxyamphetamine test for diagnosis of postganglionic defects. Am J Ophthalmol 1971;72:472–480.

49. Meyer SM, Fraunfelder FT. Phenylephrine hydrochloride. Ophthalmology 1980;87:1177–1180.

50. Edelhauser HF, Hine JE, Pederson H, Van Horn D, Schultz RO. The effect of phenylephrine on the cornea. Arch Ophthalmol 1979;97:937–947.

51. Cohen KL, Van Horn DL, Edelhauser HF, Schultz RO. Effect of phenylephrine on normal and regenerated endothelial cells in cat cornea. Invest Ophthalmol Vis Sci 1979;18:242–249.

52. Hanna C, Brainard J, Augsburger KD, Roy RH, et al. Allergic dermatoconjunctivitis caused by phenylephrine. Am J Ophthalmol 1983;95:703–704.

53. Geyer O, Lazar M. Allergic blepharoconjunctivitis due to phenylephrine. J Ocular Pharmacol 1988;4:123–126.

54. Mitsui Y, Takagi Y. Nature of aqueous floaters due to sympathomimetic mydriatics. Arch Ophthalmol 1961;65:626–631.

55. Fraunfelder FT, Meyer SM, eds. Drug-induced ocular side effects and drug interactions. Philadelphia: Lea & Febiger, 1989: Chap. 6.

56. Isenberg SJ, Green BF. Effect of phenylephrine hydrochloride on conjunctival PO_2. Arch Ophthalmol 1984;102:1185–1186.

57. Pakalnis VA, Wolbarsht ML, Landers MB. Phenylephrine-induced anterior chamber hypoxia. Ann Ophthalmol 1988;20:267–270.

58. Van Buskirk EM, Bacon DR, Fahrenbach WH. Ciliary vasoconstriction after topical adrenergic drugs. Am J Ophthalmol 1990;109:511–517.

59. Heath P. Neosynephrine hydrochloride. Some uses and effects in ophthalmology. Arch Ophthalmol 1936;16:839–846.

60. McReynolds W, Havener W, Henderson J. Hazards of the use of sympathomimetic drugs in ophthalmology. Arch Ophthalmol 1956;56:176–179.

61. Lanche R. Systemic reactions to topical epinephrine and phenylephrine. Am J Ophthalmol 1966;61:95–98.

62. Solosko D, Smith R. Hypertension following 10% phenylephrine ophthalmic. Anesthesiol 1972;36:187–189.

63. Borromeo-McGrail V, Borduik J, Keitel H. Systemic hypertension following ocular administration of 10% phenylephrine in the neonate. J Pediatr 1973;51:1032–1036.

64. Wilensky J, Woodward H. Acute systemic hypertension after conjunctival instillation of phenylephrine hydrochloride. Am J Ophthalmol 1973;76:156–157.

65. Samantary S, Thomas A. Systemic effects of topical phenylephrine. Ind J Ophthalmol 1975;23:16–17.

66. Fraunfelder FT, Scafidi AF. Possible adverse effects from topical ocular 10% phenylephrine. Am J Ophthalmol 1978;85:862–868.

67. Brown MM, Brown GC, Spaeth GL. Lack of side effects from topically administered 10% phenylephrine eyedrops. Arch Ophthalmol 1980;98:487–488.

68. Fraunfelder FT, Meyer SM. Possible cardiovascular effects secondary to topical ophthalmic 2.5% phenylephrine. Am J Ophthalmol 1985;99:362–363.

69. Kumar V, Packer AJ, Choi WW. Hypertension following 2.5% phenylephrine ophthalmic drops. Glaucoma 1985;7:131–132.

70. Jennings BJ, Sullivan DE. The effect of topical 2.5% phenylephrine and 1% tropicamide on systemic blood pressure and pulse. J Am Optom Assoc 1986;57:382–389.

71. Kim JM, Stevenson CE, Mathewson HS. Hypertensive reactions to phenylephrine eyedrops in patients with sympathetic denervation. Am J Ophthalmol 1978;85:862–868.

72. Robertson D. Contraindication to the use of ocular phenylephrine in idiopathic orthostatic hypotension. Am J Ophthalmol 1979;87:819–822.

73. Keys A, Violante A. The cardiocirculatory effects in man of Neo-Synephrine. J Clin Invest 1942;21:1–21.

74. Stack DDC. Effects of giving vasopressors to patients on monoamine oxidase inhibitors. Lancet 1962;1:1405–1406.

75. Wellwood M, Goresky GV. Systemic hypertension associated with topical administration of 2.5% phenylephrine HCL. Am J Ophthalmol 1982;93:369–374.

76. Sneddon JM, Turner P. The interaction of local guanethidine and sympathomimetic amines in the human eye. Arch Ophthalmol 1969;81:622–627.

77. Rutledge CO. The mechanism by which amphetamine inhibits oxidative elimination of norepinephrine in man. J Pharmacol Exp Ther 1970;171:188–196.

78. Caldwell J, Sever PS. The biochemical pharmacology of abused drugs. I. Amphetamines, cocaine and LSD. Clin Pharmacol Ther 1974;16:625–638.

79. Cremer SA, Thompson HS, Digre KB, et al. Hydroxyamphetamine mydriasis in Horner's syndrome. Am J Ophthalmol 1990;110:71–76.

80. Abbott WO, Henry CM. Paredrine (β-4-hydroxyphenylisopropylamine): A clinical investigation of a sympathomimetic drug. Am J Med Sci 1937;193:661–673.

81. Semes LP, Bartlett JD. Mydriatic effectiveness of hydroxyamphetamine. J Am Optom Assoc 1982;53:899–904.

82. Motameni M, Jaanus SD. Pediatric Horner's syndrome. Case report and review. Clin Eye Vis Care 1992;4:103–107.

83. Gartner S, Billet E. Mydriatic glaucoma. Am J Ophthalmol 1957;43:975–976.

84. Kronfeld PC, McGarry HI, Smith HE. The effect of mydriatics upon the intraocular pressure in so called primary wide-angle glaucoma. Am J Ophthalmol 1943;26:245–252.

85. Hanna C. Tachyphylaxis. Some cardiovascular actions of hydroxyamphetamine and related compounds. Arch Int Pharmacodyn 1960;128:469–480.

86. Aviado DM. Cardiovascular effects of some commonly used pressor amines. Anesthesiology 1959;20:7197.

87. Ritchie JM, Greene NM. Local anesthetics. In: Gilman AG, Rall TW, Nies AS, et al, eds. Goodman and Gilman's The pharmacological basis of therapeutics. New York: McGraw-Hill 1993; Chap. 15.

88. Altman AJ, Albert DM, Fournier GA. Cocaine's use in ophthalmology: Our 100-year heritage. Surv Ophthalmol 1985;29:300–306.

89. Friedman JR, Whiting DW, Kosmorsky GS, et al. The cocaine test in normal patients. Am J Ophthalmol 1984;98:808–810.

90. Smith RB, Everett WG. Physiology and pharmacology of local anesthetic agents. Int Ophthalmol Clin 1973;13:35–43.

91. Wand M, Grant WM. Thymoxamine hydrochloride: An alpha-adrenergic blocker. Surv Ophthalmol 1980;25:75–84.

92. Lee DA, Rimele FJ, Brubaker RF, Nagataki S, Van Loutte PM. Effect of thymoxamine on the human pupil. Exp Eye Res 1983;36:655–662.

93. Pau H. Sympathikolyse durch lokale konjuncktivale Opilon. Applikation am auge. Klin Monastbl Augenheil Kd 1955;126:171–176.

94. Relf SJ, Gharagozloo, Skuta GL, et al. Thymoxamine reverses phenylephrine-induced mydriasis. Am J Ophthalmol 1988;106:251–255.

95. Wright MM, Skuta GL, Drake MV, et al. Time course of thymoxamine reversal of phenylephrine-induced mydriasis. Arch Ophthalmol 1990;108:1729–1732.

96. Diehl DLC, Robin AL, Wand M. The influence of iris pigmentation on the miotic effect of thymoxamine. Am J Ophthalmol 1991;111:351–355.

97. Mayer GL, Stewart-Jones JH, Turner P. Influence of alpha adrenoreceptor blockade with thymoxamine on changes in pupil diameter and accommodation produced by tropicamide and ephedrine. Curr Med Res Opinion 1977;4:660–664.

98. Susanna R, Drance S, Schulzer M, Douglas G. The effects of thymoxamine on anterior chamber depth in human eyes. Can J Ophthalmol 1978;13:250–251.

99. Saheb NE, Lorenzetti D, Salpeter-Carlton S. Effect of thymoxamine and pilocarpine on the depth of the anterior chamber. Can J Ophthalmol 1980;15:170–171.

100. Mapstone R. Mechanics of pupil block. Br J Ophthalmol 1968;52:19–25.

101. Mapstone R. Safe mydriasis. Br J Ophthalmol 1970;54:690–692.

102. Saheb NE, Lorenzetti D, East D, Salpeter-Carlton S. Thymoxamine versus pilocarpine in the reversal of phenylephrine-induced mydriasis. Can J Ophthalmol 1982;17:266–267.

103. Anastasi LM, Ogle KN, Kearns TP. Effect of pilocarpine in counteracting mydriasis. Arch Ophthalmol 1968;79:710–715.

104. McKinna H, Stewart-Jones JH, Edgar DF, Turner P. Reversal of tropicamide-induced mydriasis by thymoxamine eyedrops. Curr Med Res Opinion 1988;11:1–3.

105. Shah B, Hubbard B, Stewart-Jones JH, Edgar DF, Turner P. Influence of thymoxamine eyedrops on the mydriatic effect of tropicamide and phenylephrine alone and in combination. Ophthal Physiol Opt 1989;9:153–155.

106. Rutkowski PC, Fernandes JL, Galin MA, Halasa AM. Alpha adrenergic receptor blockade in the treatment of angle-closure glaucoma. Trans Am Acad Ophthalmol Otolaryngol 1973;77:137–142.

107. Wand M, Grant WM. Thymoxamine hydrochloride: Effects on the facility of outflow and intraocular pressure. Invest Ophthalmol 1976;15:400–403.

108. Lee DA, Brubaker RF, Nagataki S. Effect of thymoxamine on aqueous humor formation in the normal human eye as measured by fluorophotometry. Invest Ophthalmol Vis Sci 1981;21:805–811.

109. Grehn F. Intraocular thymoxamine for miosis during surgery. Am J Ophthalmol 1987;103:709–711.

110. Iuglio N. Ocular effects of topical application of dapiprazole in man. Glaucoma 1984;6:110–116.

111. Reibaldi A. A new alpha-blocking agent. Glaucoma 1984;6:255–257.

112. Brogliatti B, Rolle T, Messelod M, Carenini BB. A new alpha blocking agent in treatment of glaucoma: Dapiprazole. Glaucoma 1985;7:232–236.

113. Prosdocimo G, De Marco D. Intraocular dapiprazole to reverse mydriasis during extracapsular cataract extraction. Am J Ophthalmol 1988;105:321–322.

114. Doughty MJ, Lyle WM. A review of the clinical pharmacokinetics of pilocarpine, moxisylyte (thymoxamine), and dapiprazole in the reversal of diagnostic pupillary dilation. Optom Vis Sci 1992;69:358–368.

115. Nyman N, Reich L. The effect of dapiprazole on accommodative amplitude in eyes dilated with 0.5% tropicamide. J Am Optom Assoc 1993;64:625–628.

116. Lati AM, Veleria P, Catanese B, et al. Pharmacokinetics and bioc mistry of dapiprazole. In: Dapiprazole: A new alpha blocking ent in ophthalmology. Amsterdam: Kugler Publications, 198

117. Bor i L, Marchini G, De Feo G, Piccinelli D, Beltini A. On the reve l of diagnostic mydriasis with dapiprazole. Curr Ther Res 198 8:945–952.

118. Ny N, Keates EU. Effects of dapiprazole on the reversal of pha cologically induced mydriasis. Optom Vis Sci 1990;67:705 9.

119. Buc MG, D'andrea D, Bettini A, De Gregorio M. Dapiprazole for reversal of mydriasis due to tropicamide. Glaucoma 198 :94–98.

120. All n RW, Gerber DS, Bieber S, Hodes BL. Reversal of my sis by dapiprazole. Ann Ophthalmol 1990;22:131–138.

121. Po F, Cillino S, Faranda F, Cassanova F, Cucco F. Intraocular dap azole for the reversal of mydriasis after cataract extraction wit ntraocular lens implantation. J Cataract Refract Surg 19 7:785–789.

122. Ba t JD, Classé JG. Dapiprazole: Will it affect the standard of car r pupillary dilation? Optom Clin 1992;2:113–120.

123. Ch s L, Chapman JM, Green K. Corneal endothelial toxicity of iprazole hydrochloride. Lens Eye Toxicity Res 1992;9(2):79

124. Joh n ME, Molinari JF, Carter J. Efficacy of dapiprazole with hy xyamphetamine hydrobromide and tropicamide. J Am Op n Assoc 1993;64:629–633.

125. Co r CG, Campbell JB, Tirey WW. The clinical efficacy of Re yes in reversing the effects of pupillary dilation. J Am Op n Assoc 1993;64:634–636.

126. M ari JF, Johnson ME, Carter J. Dapiprazole. Clinical efficacy fo ounteracting tropicamide 1%. Optom Vis Sci 1994;71:31 22.

127. Ba tt JD, Hogan T, McDaniel D, et al. Study of three different tre ent regimens of dapiprazole HCl in the reversal of mydriasis duced by 2.5% phenylephrine. Invest Ophthalmol Vis Sci 19 35(suppl):1546.

CHAPTER 9

Cycloplegics

Siret D. Jaanus
John H. Carter[a]

Drugs discussed in this chapter inhibit the actions of acetylcholine (ACh) both on effector sites innervated by autonomic nerves and on smooth muscle cells that lack cholinergic autonomic innervation. Since they block muscarinic receptor sites, these agents are referred to as *antimuscarinics, cholinergic antagonists, cholinergic-blocking agents,* or *anticholinergics.* These drugs influence various ocular functions, including pupil size and accommodation. In clinical practice they are commonly referred to as *cycloplegics.* These agents are useful diagnostically for pupillary dilation and cycloplegic refraction, and therapeutically as part of the comprehensive management of anterior uveitis. Since these drugs dilate the pupil, they are also known as *mydriatics* or *mydriatic-cycloplegics.*

A brief overview of the cholinergic innervation to the eye is followed by discussion of the pharmacologic actions, clinical uses, adverse effects, and contraindications to drugs in current use. The adrenergic mydriatics are discussed in Chapter 8.

Cholinergic Innervation to the Eye

The cholinergic innervation to the eye originates in the Edinger-Westphal nucleus (EWN) located within the mesencephalon. Preganglionic parasympathetic fibers emerge from the EWN, exit the central nervous system (CNS) through the third cranial nerve (oculomotor), and proceed to the ciliary ganglion. There they synapse with postganglionic fibers, enter the globe through the short ciliary nerves, and pass to and terminate on the iris sphincter muscle and ciliary body[1] (Fig. 9.1). The neurotransmitter at the ciliary ganglion synapse is ACh. The neurotransmitter at the effector cell junction, that is, the sphincter and ciliary muscle, is also ACh.

Because of its varying size, the pupil controls the amount of light reaching the retina. Pupil size is determined predominantly by varying degrees of parasympathetic innervation to the sphincter muscle, which contracts accordingly, resulting in a corresponding degree of pupillary constriction. Sympathetic innervation, which is secondary, maintains a persistent tone in the dilator muscle, aiding relaxation of the sphincter and resulting in dilation. The degree of parasympathetic innervation to the sphincter muscle is governed by two important pupillary reflexes: the light reflex and the near reflex. The near reflex consists of the accommodation and convergence reflexes. Afferent pathways of both light and near reflexes terminate in the EWN. The efferent pathway from the EWN is the same for both the light reflex and the near reflex (see Fig. 9.1).

The lacrimal gland also receives parasympathetic innervation. Preganglionic fibers originate near the superior salivary nucleus in the pons. They travel with the seventh nerve until they join and synapse with the sphenopalatine ganglion. The postganglionic fibers become part of the fifth nerve and pass to the lacrimal gland through the lacrimal nerve (see Fig. 9.1).[2] Although the mechanism of neural control over normal tear secretion is poorly understood, parasympathetic innervation is clearly responsible for tear production in weeping.[2]

---

[a] Deceased.

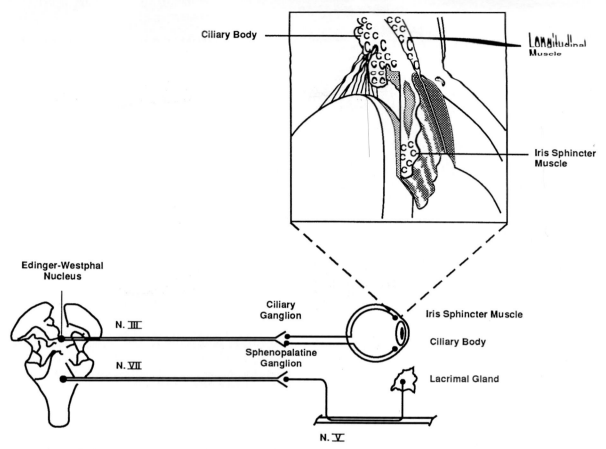

FIGURE 9.1   **Cholinergic innervation to the eye (iris sphincter muscle and ciliary body) and lacrimal gland. "C"'s represent populations of muscarinic receptor sites.**

Other potential targets of cholinergic stimulation or blockade by drugs include the cornea, lens, and retina. The corneal epithelium contains the neurotransmitter ACh and the enzymes choline acetylase and acetylcholinesterase. Experimental evidence indicates that the cholinergic system may play a role in corneal hydration that involves epithelial ionic transport.[3] The lens capsule also exhibits cholinesterase activity, and cholinergic neurons have been demonstrated in the human retina.[4,5]

Cholinergic Receptors

Cholinergic receptors have been identified in ocular tissue by the use of pharmacologic and biochemical procedures.

In both human and nonhuman mammalian iris sphincter tissue[6-9] and ciliary body,[10-13] these receptors have been shown to be of the muscarinic type. Muscarinic agonist action at these receptor sites constricts the pupil, contracts the ciliary muscle, and, in general, lowers intraocular pressure (IOP). Conversely, inhibition of these receptors by cholinergic antagonists induces pupillary dilation (mydriasis), paralysis of accommodation (cycloplegia), and may elevate IOP.

In the human retina, evidence has been offered for a population of both muscarinic and nicotinic receptors in the inner plexiform layer,[14] which suggests that cholinergic neurotransmission occurs in the retina. One related clinical implication is that cholinergic agonists and antagonists may have the potential to affect human vision.

TABLE 9.1
Mydriatic and Cycloplegic Properties of Anticholinergic Agents

Drug	Strength of Solution[a] (%)	Mydriasis		Paralysis of Accommodation	
		Maximal (minutes)	Recovery[b] (days)	Maximal (minutes)	Recovery[c] (days)
Atropine sulfate	1.0	30–40	7–10	60–180	7–12
Homatropine hydrobromide	1.0[d]	40–60	1–3	30–60	1–3
Scopolamine hydrobromide	0.5	20–30	3–7	30–60	5–7
Cyclopentolate hydrochloride	0.5–1.0	20–45	1	20–45	1
Tropicamide	0.5–1.0	20–35	0.25	30–45	0.25

[a]One instillation of 1 drop of solution.
[b]To within 1 mm of original pupillary diameter.
[c]To within 2 diopters of original amplitude of accommodation; ability to read fine print is possible by the third day after atropine and scopolamine and by 6 hours after homatropine instillation.
[d]Full mydriasis and loss of accommodation require instillation of a 5% solution.
Adapted from Brown JH. Atropine, scopolamine, and related antimuscarinic drugs. In: Gilman AG, Rall TW, Nies AS, et al., eds. Goodman and Gilman's The pharmacological basis of therapeutics. New York: McGraw-Hill, 1993; Chap. 8.

Cholinergic Antagonists

Atropine

PHARMACOLOGY

Atropine, a naturally occurring alkaloid, was first isolated from the belladonna plant, *Atropa belladonna,* in its pure form in 1831.[15] The stability of atropine is both pH and temperature dependent. At 20°C, the half-life of atropine is 2.7 years in a pH 7 solution and 27.0 years at pH 6. At 30°C, its stability is reduced to 0.61 years at pH 7 and 6.1 years at pH 6.[16] At the physiologic pH, atropine with a pK_a of 9.8 is partially un-ionized.[17] This enhances intraocular absorption of the drug following its topical application to the eye. Atropine is the most potent mydriatic and cycloplegic agent presently available. Depending on the concentration used, mydriasis may last up to 10 days and cycloplegia, 7 to 12 days (Table 9.1). Atropine is available commercially as a sulfate derivative in concentrations of 0.5% and 1% in ointment form and in 1%, 2%, and 3% solutions (Table 9.2).

The intraocular distribution of atropine has been studied following subconjunctival injection of the radioactive drug in rabbits.[18] At 90 minutes significant radioactivity is exhibited by the cornea, aqueous, and vitreous. Lower concentrations are present in the iris, ciliary body, and retina. By 5 hours, 95% of the radioactivity has left the ocular tissues as the atropine is excreted in the urine.

Lussana,[19] in 1852, was the first to study the effect of atropine on the eyes as part of a general study of its systemic actions. Following oral ingestion of atropine, the pupil dilated, vision became blurred, and the ability to do near work was lost.

Feddersen[20] is credited with the first extended study of the ocular effects of atropine sulfate following topical application of a 1% solution. Following the instillation of 1 drop, the mydriatic effect began at 12 minutes and reached a maximum in 26 minutes. The pupil began to return to normal in 2 days and reached preinstillation size by the tenth day. The cycloplegic effect began in 12 to 18 minutes and reached maximum by 160 minutes. Accommodation began to return in 42 hours, and full accommodative ability was usually attained within 8 days.

Wolf and Hodge[21] observed a similar time course of action for 1% atropine sulfate in a series of 46 eyes (Fig. 9.2). In addition, these authors reported wide variations in individual responses to topical ocular atropine. Drug-pigment binding has been suggested to explain, at least in part, this effect. When applied to heavily pigmented eyes, atropine exhibits a relatively slow onset and prolonged duration of cycloplegic effect. Moreover, the degree of mydriasis obtained is less, particularly in eyes of black patients.[22] Salazar and associates[23] reported that pigmented rabbit and human irides accumulate greater amounts of radioactive ³H-atropine than nonpigmented irides in vitro. On repeated washing, the atropine blockade of nonpigmented iris could be easily removed, whereas that in the pigmented iris was retained. Thus, the smaller magnitude of the mydriatic effect with atropine in humans may be explained, at least in part, by the initial loss of administered drug to pigment cells. The prolonged effect in the more heavily pigmented eye is attributed to the subsequent release of accumulated drug over time onto the muscarinic receptors of the iris and ciliary body.

In addition to pigment binding, the actions of atropine can be affected by the enzyme atropinase (atropinesterase) pres-

TABLE 9.2
Mydriatic-Cycloplegic Preparations

Generic Name	Trade Name	Manufacturer	Formulation and Concentration (%)
Atropine sulfate	Atropine Sulfate Ophthalmic	(Various)	Ointment 1
	Isopto Atropine Ophthalmic	Alcon	Solution 0.5, 1, 3
	Atropisol Ophthalmic	Ciba Vision	Solution 1
	Atropine Sulfate S.O.P.	Allergan	Ointment 0.5, 1
	Atropine-Care Ophthalmic	Akorn	Solution 1
	Atropine-Care	Akorn	Ointment 1
Homatropine HBr	AK-Homatropine	Akorn	Solution 5
	Homatropine Ophthalmic	(Various)	Solution 5
	Isopto Homatropine	Alcon	Solution 2, 5
	Homatropine HBr	Ciba Vision	Solution 5
Scopolamine HBr	Isopto Hyoscine	Alcon	Solution 0.25
Cyclopentolate	Cyclogyl	Alcon	Solution 0.5, 1, 2
	AK-Pentolate	Akorn	Solution 0.5, 1
	Cyclopentolate	(Various)	Solution 1
Tropicamide	Mydriacyl Ophthalmic	Alcon	Solution 0.5, 1
	Tropicacyl	Akorn	Solution 0.5, 1
	Tropicamide	B&L	Solution 0.5, 1
	Paremyd	Allergan	Solution 0.25 with 1% hydroxyamphetamine

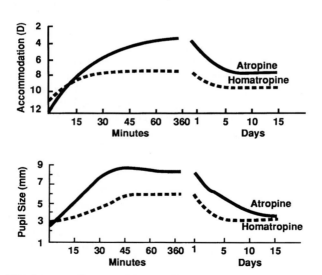

FIGURE 9.2 **Changes of accommodation and pupil size after administration of 1% solution of atropine sulfate and 1% solution of homatropine hydrobromide. (Modified from Wolf AV, Hodge HC. Effects of atropine sulfate, methylatropine nitrate [Metropine], and homatropine hydrobromide on adult human eyes. Arch Ophthalmol 1946;36:293–301.)**

ent in certain species of rabbits, which hydrolyzes the drug and thereby limits its duration of action.[24] Rabbits with and without the enzyme present in the serum exhibit an average half-life for recovery of atropine mydriasis of 12.4 and 96 hours, respectively. Atropinase-negative rabbits show a prolonged effect with atropine, similar to the time course in humans, who lack the enzyme.

CLINICAL USES

Refraction.   Atropine is useful for cycloplegic refraction, particularly for younger, actively accommodating children with suspected accommodative esotropia (see Chapter 22). It should never be used for cycloplegic refraction of adults because other, short-acting agents are as effective and the prolonged paralysis of accommodation renders patients visually handicapped.

For purposes of cycloplegic refraction atropine solution is usually administered 2 to 3 times per day for up to 3 days before refraction, with an additional drop instilled on the morning of the examination. There is no particular justification for this dosage regimen, which may lead to overdosage in some cases. More recent studies, based on retinoscopic findings, indicate that 4 instillations of 1% atropine solution, 3 drops one day before and 1 drop on the morning of the examination, achieve maximal cycloplegia in hyperopic children 4.5 months to 11 years of age.[25] The drug is usually administered at home by an individual who has been instructed in the proper method of drug instillation. To prevent excessive systemic absorption of atropine by the nasal mucosa, nasolacrimal occlusion is advised immediately following drug instillation in the lower cul-de-sac (see Fig. 3.6).

Treatment of Uveitis.   Atropine is extremely useful in the treatment of anterior uveal inflammation. It relieves the pain associated with the inflammatory process by relaxing the ciliary muscle spasm and helps prevent posterior synechiae by dilating the pupil. With the pupil dilated, the area of posterior iris surface in contact with the anterior lens capsule decreases. Moreover, the cycloplegia produced by atropine is of additional value in reducing both the thickness and convexity of the lens. If posterior synechiae should develop even when the pupil is dilated, there is less chance of iris bombé.[26]

Atropine may also help to restore toward normal the excessive permeability of the inflamed vessels and thereby reduce cells and protein in the anterior chamber (aqueous flare).[26]

Treatment of Myopia.   It has been suggested that topical ocular use of atropine may prevent the progression of myopia.[27] By placing the ciliary muscle at rest, accommodation is relaxed, and the tension that produces elongation of the eye may be reduced. However, clinical trials using atropine for myopia control are difficult to interpret due to variations in patient selection and differences in mode and duration of treatment. With administration of 1% atropine for 1 to 8 years, the decrease in myopia in treated eyes of children has usually been less than 0.5 D.[28,29] Sampson[30] reported that instillation of 1% atropine for 20 months to children 7 to 14 years of age seemed to prevent the progression of myopia, but on discontinuation of the drops only 12% of children maintained improvement for more than 6 months. Additional studies with better control are needed to evaluate the efficacy of atropine and other cholinergic antagonists in myopia control.

Treatment of Amblyopia.   Use of atropine can be an alternative to patching of the normal eye in the treatment of suppression amblyopia. The resultant cycloplegic blur in the eye with normal vision may force fixation with the amblyopic eye.

Since therapy with anticholinergics is successful only if the reduction in visual acuity of the normal eye exceeds that of the amblyopic eye, multiple daily instillations may be required.[31,32] Although pharmacologic occlusion can improve visual acuity in amblyopic eyes, care is needed because penalization can result in amblyopia in eyes with normal acuity.[33,34]

Provocative Testing for Glaucoma.   Atropine and other cholinergic antagonists can be useful in inducing acute angle-closure glaucoma in eyes with suspected narrow anterior chamber angles. Since mydriasis can lead to pupillary block, a narrow angle may be occluded. However, not all eyes with suspected narrow angles or a history of angle-closure attacks respond positively to cholinergic blocking agents[35] (see Chapter 35).

SIDE EFFECTS

Ocular Effects.   Ocular reactions include direct irritation from the drug preparation itself, allergic contact dermatitis, risk of angle-closure glaucoma, and elevation of IOP in patients with open angles.[36]

The allergic reaction to atropine generally involves the eyelids and manifests itself as an erythema, with pruritus and edema. Allergic papillary conjunctivitis and keratitis have also been reported.[37]

In general, topical atropine as well as other cholinergic antagonists increase patients' risk for angle-closure glaucoma. However, the risk of inducing angle closure in eyes without previous history of attacks is remote. Keller[38] reviewed the literature on this subject and concluded that with proper precautions, the risk of precipitating an angle-closure attack is at most 1 in 183,000 in the general population and 1 in 45,000 in the population over age 30 years. It has also been argued that a pharmacologically provoked attack of angle closure may be in patients' best interests, since a diagnosis can be made immediately and appropriate treatment provided before a spontaneous attack occurs.

Patients with open-angle glaucoma may experience an elevation of IOP. The effect is unpredictable because not all patients respond to cholinergic antagonists with IOP elevations. The mechanisms involved in the pressure rise are not completely understood. The pressure elevation appears to be related not to the degree of mydriasis attained but rather to a decrease in facility of aqueous outflow.[26,38]

Systemically administered atropine may also cause mydriasis and raise IOP in patients with open-angle glaucoma. Following intramuscular injection of 0.6 to 0.8 mg of atropine, three of eight patients developed 0.5 to 1.5 mm mydriasis.[39] A mean increase of 8 cm in the near point of accommodation following atropine administration was also reported. In another study, 100 patients ranging in age from 16 to 40 years were given atropine intramuscularly (0.016 mg/kg body weight). Thirteen subjects developed pupillary dilation of 2 mm or less, and nine developed ocular pressure elevations of 3 mm Hg or less.[40]

Eyes with open-angle glaucoma respond variably to systemic atropine. In one study 34 eyes with open-angle glaucoma were maintained on glaucoma therapy while atropine 0.01 mg/kg body weight was injected intramuscularly. In 12 eyes the IOP increased from 2 to 5 mm Hg. However, the

TABLE 9.3
Systemic Reactions to Atropine in Children

- Diffuse cutaneous flush
- Thirst
- Fever
- Urinary retention
- Tachycardia
- Somnolence
- Excitement and hallucinations
- Convulsions

overall differences observed in both pupil size and IOP were not statistically significant.[41]

Systemic Effects. Systemic reactions from the topical administration of atropine have also occurred (Table 9.3).[42–45] Following its application to the eye, systemic absorption of drug occurs primarily from the conjunctival vessels and the nasal mucosa.

The adverse systemic reactions appear to be dose dependent, although patients vary in susceptibility.[15] Systemic peripheral effects occur with low doses, which generally do not produce central symptomatology. Depression of salivation and drying of the mouth are usually the first signs of toxicity. Slightly higher dosages produce facial flushing and inhibit sweating. At 20 times the minimum dose where adverse systemic symptoms begin to appear, CNS manifestations can occur.[43] Convulsions have been associated with topical ocular atropine instillation, particularly in children.[45,46] The elderly are also more susceptible to anticholinergic toxicity, including cognitive impairments and delirium.[47,48]

Deaths have been attributed to topical ocular atropine. Six reported cases in the literature have occurred in children 3 years of age and under. The dosages applied ranged from 1.6 mg to 18 mg, but the cases are rather poorly documented. All the children were either ill or had motor and mental retardation.[46,49] However, what these cases imply is that care must be taken not to overdose small children. Caution must be exercised particularly with children who are lightly pigmented individuals or have Down's syndrome, spastic paralysis, or brain damage.[43,44]

The treatment of atropine overdosage is largely symptomatic, with prevention of hyperpyrexia and dehydration. Sedation with diazepam has been advocated. The specific antidote for CNS toxicity is physostigmine (Antilirium) in a subcutaneous dose of 0.25 mg in children and 1 to 2 mg in adults. The initial dose can be supplemented as needed every 15 minutes by doses of similar magnitude.[26]

CONTRAINDICATIONS

Atropine is contraindicated in patients who are hypersensitive to the belladonna alkaloids, have open-angle or angle-closure glaucoma, or have a tendency toward IOP elevations. Manufacturer's recommended dosages should not be exceeded, particularly in infants, small children, and the elderly. Children with Down's syndrome demonstrate a hyperreactive pupillary response to topical atropine.[44,50] Safety guidelines for use during pregnancy or lactation have not been established. Very small amounts of the drug have been detected in breast milk.[50]

Homatropine

PHARMACOLOGY

Homatropine is about one-tenth as potent as atropine and has a shorter duration of mydriatic and cycloplegic action (see Table 9.1). It is partly synthetic and partly, like atropine, from the plants of the Solanaceae family.[51] It is quite stable in solution. At physiologic pH, homatropine with a pK_a of 9.9 is approximately 0.32% un-ionized.[52] Homatropine is commercially available as the hydrobromide salt in concentrations of 2% and 5% (see Table 9.2).

Following topical instillation of a 1% solution, maximum mydriasis occurs by 40 minutes. Recovery requires about 1 to 3 days.[21] The amount and duration of cycloplegia produced by homatropine are significantly less than that produced by a comparable dose of atropine (see Fig. 9.2).

CLINICAL USES

Due to its prolonged mydriatic and cycloplegic effect and relatively weak cycloplegic action, particularly in darkly pigmented irides, homatropine is not a drug of choice for fundus examination or cycloplegic refraction. Its primary clinical usefulness is in the treatment of anterior uveitis where its effects are similar to those of atropine. It also serves as a substitute for atropine in patients with known sensitivities to that drug.[51]

SIDE EFFECTS

The toxic effects of homatropine are indistinguishable from those of atropine, and the treatment is the same.[53]

CONTRAINDICATIONS

Contraindications for homatropine are essentially the same as for atropine. As with topical administration of atropine, homatropine can also induce CNS toxicity in the elderly.[47,48]

Scopolamine (Hyoscine)

PHARMACOLOGY

The antimuscarinic potency of scopolamine on a weight basis is greater than that of atropine. Except for a shorter duration of mydriatic and cycloplegic action at the dosage levels used clinically, its effects are similar to those of atropine (see Table 9.1). Although previously available in both ointment and solution, scopolamine is currently available as the hydrobromide salt in solution at 0.25% concentration (see Table 9.2).

Marron[54] studied the mydriatic and cycloplegic effects of 0.5% solution of scopolamine in subjects ranging from 15 to 37 years of age. Maximum pupillary dilation occurred at 20 minutes. This effect lasted for 90 minutes, and the pupil returned to its preinstallation size by the eighth day. The maximum cyloplegic effect occurred at 40 minutes, with residual amplitude of accommodation at 1.6 D. This effect lasted for at least 90 minutes, and accommodation gradually returned by the third day to a level where the average patient could read.

Lower concentrations of scopolamine have similar effects on pupil size and accommodation.[55] Instillation of 3 drops of 0.025% solution at 5-minute intervals to adult subjects caused a mean increase in pupillary diameter of approximately 4.1 mm at 30 minutes. A marked mydriasis persisted until day 2, after which the pupil size gradually returned to control values. Amplitude of accommodation fell rapidly from a mean of 9.1 D prior to scopolamine to 5.4 D at 16 minutes, and by 75 minutes all subjects had accommodative amplitudes less than 2 D. Residual accommodation remained below 2 D for days 1 and 2. By day 4 accommodative amplitude was 7.1 D and returned to 9.1 D by day six.

CLINICAL USES

Since patients tend to exhibit a higher incidence of toxic reactions to scopolamine[26] than to other anticholinergic agents, it is not a drug of first choice for cycloplegic refraction or treatment of anterior uveal inflammations. Its use is reserved primarily for patients who exhibit sensitivity to atropine.

SIDE EFFECTS

Although adverse reactions from scopolamine are quite similar to those from atropine, CNS toxicity appears to be more common with scopolamine. In a series of several hundred patients whose pupils were dilated with 1% scopolamine, 7 cases of confusional psychosis were observed. The reactions included restlessness, confusion, hallucinations, incoherence, violence, amnesia, unconsciousness, spastic extremities, vomiting, and urinary incontinence.[56] However, no deaths have been reported from topical ocular use of scopolamine. Treatment of toxic reactions is the same as that for atropine toxicity.

Scopolamine is available as a transdermal drug delivery system for prevention of motion sickness. When placed behind the ear, the system delivers 0.5 mg of scopolamine for 3 days. Mydriasis and blurred vision can occur if scopol-

amine from the patch comes in contact with the eyes (see Chapter 23).

CONTRAINDICATIONS

The contraindications for scopolamine are essentially the same as for atropine.

Cyclopentolate

PHARMACOLOGY

Cyclopentolate was introduced into clinical practice in 1951.[57] A stable, water-soluble ester with a pK_a of 8.4, cyclopentolate is primarily in an ionized state at physiologic pH.[17] It is commercially available in 0.5, 1, and 2% solutions (see Table 9.2).

The mydriatic and cycloplegic properties of cyclopentolate have been studied and compared with other anticholinergic agents by several groups of investigators.[58–62] Essentially the same techniques have been used in these studies for determining onset, intensity, and duration of action. Usually the 0.5% or 1% concentration was used, and the subjects were classified according to age, iris color, and race.

In whites, two drops of 0.5% cyclopentolate instilled 5 minutes apart, or 1 drop of 1% solution, produces maximum mydriasis within 20 to 30 minutes. The average pupil size is usually 7.0 to 7.5 mm. In blacks, 2 instillations of 0.5% produce a 6.0 mm pupil in 30 minutes and a 7.0 mm pupil at 60 minutes following instillation of the first drop.[57,59] Cyclopentolate is also a less effective mydriatic in whites with dark irides. (Fig. 9.3).[61]

Maximum cycloplegia in whites occurs 30 to 60 minutes following instillation of 2 drops of 0.5% solution or 1 drop of 1% solution. The residual accommodation ranges between 1.00 D and 1.75 D, with an average of 1.25 D.[57] Manny and associates,[61] however, have recently reported that in patients with light irides, clinically useful cycloplegia may occur as early as 10 minutes following instillation of 1 drop of 1% cyclopentolate. In a group of children with light irides, the residual accommodation measured 0.59 D at 10 minutes. In contrast, individuals with dark irides may require 30 to 40 minutes before accommodation is at an acceptable level for cycloplegic refraction (Fig. 9.4). Lovasik[62] has also shown that eyes with blue irides lose accommodation at a faster rate and also recover in less time as compared to brown eyes. For all eyes the cycloplegic effect usually dissipates within 24 hours.

In groups of black patients ranging in age from 9 to 40 years, 1% cyclopentolate has been reported to produce satisfactory cycloplegia in 98% of patients. The 0.5% concentration was effective in only 66% of the same individuals. The average residual accommodation was 1.75 D following use of 1% cyclopentolate.[58]

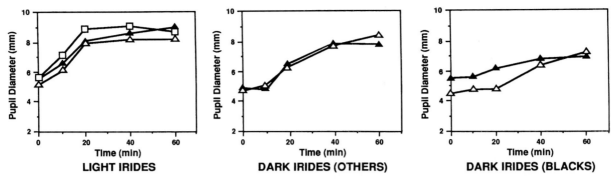

FIGURE 9.3   **Time course of mydriasis induced by 1% cyclopentolate HCl. Solid symbols represent measurements when stimuli to parasympathetic system were minimized; open symbols represent results when accommodation, convergence, and proximal cues were present. Open squares in left panel represent results from one child. (Modified from Manny RE, Fern KD, Zervas HJ, et al. 1% cyclopentolate hydrochloride: Another look at the time course of cycloplegia using an objective measure of the accommodative response. Optom Vis Sci 1993;70:651–665.)**

Cyclopentolate does not generally alter IOP in normal eyes. Tonometry performed in a series of patients ranging in age from 4 to 93 years before and after instillation of 0.5% and 1% cyclopentolate revealed no statistically significant differences in the readings.[57,59]

CLINICAL USES

Cyclopentolate is the cycloplegic agent of choice for routine cycloplegic refractive procedures in nearly all age groups, especially infants and young children. Its cycloplegic effect is superior to that of homatropine[57,58] and closely parallels that of atropine in older children and adults, but with a relatively faster onset and shorter duration (see Table 9.1). Pupils dilated with cyclopentolate do not constrict when exposed to intense light such as that of the binocular indirect ophthalmoscope or during fundus photography. Although full recovery from mydriasis and cycloplegia generally occurs within 24 hours, most patients have sufficient recovery of accommodative amplitude to permit reading in 6 to 12 hours. Moreover, unlike with atropine and homatropine, onset of maximum cycloplegia generally approximates the onset of maximum mydriasis.[57]

Cyclopentolate is also useful in the treatment of anterior uveitis, particularly in patients sensitive to atropine. If the inflammation is severe, more frequent instillations may be necessary, since its duration of action is less than that of atropine.

SIDE EFFECTS

Ocular Effects.   The most common ocular side effect is transient stinging on initial instillation.[37] The degree of irritation appears to be concentration dependent, with the 0.5% solution causing the least amount of burning and tearing.

Allergic reactions to cyclopentolate are quite rare and may go unrecognized by the practitioner. However, several cases of redness and discomfort in eyes of patients following in-office use of cyclopentolate have been reported.[63] Symptoms consist of irritated, diffusely red eyes and a facial rash that develop within minutes to hours of drug instillation. Lacrimation, stringy white mucous discharge, and blurred vision are prominent, but itching is not a significant complaint.

Toxic keratitis has also been reported following abuse of cyclopentolate.[64] Instillation of 100 to 400 drops of the 1% solution for several months caused a diffuse epithelial punctate keratitis with marked conjunctival hyperemia. As expected, the pupils were widely dilated and unresponsive to light.

Topically applied cyclopentolate can increase IOP in patients with primary open-angle glaucoma, and it may precipitate an attack of acute glaucoma in patients with narrow angles.[65,66] Harris[66] reported that 1 of 4 eyes with open-angle glaucoma responds to topical 1% cyclopentolate with a significant elevation of IOP, whereas only 1 out of 50 normal eyes responds in a similar manner. The IOP rise usually begins within 1 hour, reaches a maximum at 2 hours, and returns to preinstillation levels by 4 hours.

Systemic Effects.   Systemic cyclopentolate toxicity is dose related and evolves in a manner similar to that of atropine.[67] However, unlike atropine, cyclopentolate causes more CNS effects.[67–71]

Analysis of blood samples by radioreceptor assay indicates that cyclopentolate is rapidly absorbed following topical ocular application of the 1% solution.[72] Peak plasma concentrations are reached in 5 to 15 minutes. Individuals show a wide variation in the amount of drug absorbed, with peak concentrations ranging from 3.3 to 15.5 ng/ml. These observations are similar to studies with ophthalmic atropine,

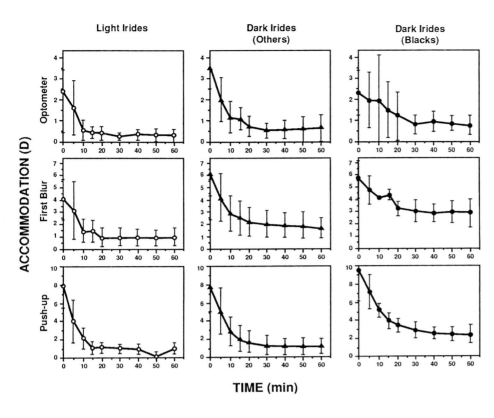

ACCOMMODATION (D)

TIME (min)

FIGURE 9.4 **Time course of cycloplegia induced by 1% cyclopentolate HCl. Values represent means ± SD for subjects with light irides, dark irides, and dark irides in blacks for each measurement technique (objective optometer, subjective first blur, and subjective push-up). (Reprinted with permission from Manny RE, Fern KD, Zervas HJ, et al. 1% cyclopentolate hydrochloride: Another look at the time course of cycloplegia using an objective measure of the accommodative response. Optom Vis Sci 1993;70:651–665.)**

where drug plasma concentrations also peaked at about 10 minutes following topical application of the drug.[73]

The CNS disturbances are characterized by signs and symptoms of cerebellar dysfunction and visual as well as tactile hallucinations. These can include drowsiness, ataxia, disorientation, incoherent speech, restlessness, and emotional disturbances (Table 9.4). The CNS effects are particularly common in children with use of the 2% concentration,[66,67] but multiple instillations of the 1% solution may also cause the same symptoms.[67,68] Binkhorst and associates[68] evaluated 40 children before and after use of the 2% solution. Of these children, five exhibited transient psychotic reactions within 30 to 45 minutes following instillation of the drops. The symptoms included restlessness with aimless wandering, irrelevant talking, visual hallucinations, memory loss, and faulty orientation as to time and place. Psychotic reactions have been reported with the 1% concentration following instillation of 2 drops in each eye in children and adults.[67,70,71] In addition, adults have also complained of drowsiness, nausea, or weakness. All reactions subside usually within 2 hours in adults and 4 to 6 hours in children without permanent sequelae. However, cyclopentolate is not without possible serious toxic effects. Grand mal seizures have been reported with use of both the 1 and 2% solution.[74,75]

Peripheral effects typical of atropine, such as flushing or dryness of the skin or mucous membranes, have not been observed with cyclopentolate in children or adults. Moreover, temperature, pulse, blood pressure, and respiration are generally not affected.[67–71] Treatment of cyclopentolate toxicity is the same as that for atropine toxicity. Since toxic reactions occur more commonly with the 2% solution or with multiple instillations of 1%, the smallest possible dose should be used.

CONTRAINDICATIONS

Since increased susceptibility to the side effects of cyclopentolate has been reported in infants, young children, and children with spastic paralysis or brain damage, use of concentrations higher than 0.5% is not recommended in these patients.[63,75] The potential for systemic absorption of cyclopentolate, like other topically applied ocular drugs, may be reduced with nasolacrimal occlusion.

Tropicamide

PHARMACOLOGY

A synthetic derivative of tropic acid, tropicamide became available for ocular use in 1959. With a pK_a of 5.37, it is only about 2.3% ionized at physiologic pH. The un-ionized molecules can readily penetrate the corneal epithelium, and thus a greater concentration of drug can reach the muscarinic re-

TABLE 9.4
Side Effects of Cyclopentolate

Ocular Effects	Systemic Effects
Irritation and lacrimation	Drowsiness
Conjunctival hyperemia	Ataxia
Allergic blepharoconjunctivitis	Disorientation
Elevated intraocular pressure	Incoherent speech
	Restlessness
	Visual hallucinations

ceptor sites than is the case with atropine, homatropine, and cyclopentolate, with pK_a values of 9.8, 9.9, and 8.4, respectively.[17] The relatively greater diffusibility of tropicamide may also account for its faster onset and shorter duration of action compared with those of other anticholinergic agents. Tropicamide is commercially available as 0.5% and 1% solutions (see Table 9.2).

Merrill and associates[76] were first to report the effects of 0.5% and 1% solution of tropicamide in human eyes. Maximum mydriasis occurred in 25 to 30 minutes following instillation of either the 0.5% or the 1% concentration. The 1% produced an average increase of 4.0 mm in pupil size at 30 minutes. Thereafter, the pupil diameter began to decrease, reaching preinstillation size at 6 hours. The effect of the 0.5% solution on mydriasis was only slightly less than that of the 1% concentration.

Tropicamide has been reported to provide sufficient mydriasis for routine ophthalmoscopy at concentrations as low as 0.25%. Gettes[77] reported that 1 drop of 0.25% tropicamide

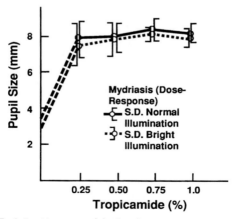

FIGURE 9.5 **Mean mydriatic dose-response curves for tropicamide 0.25, 0.5, 0.75, and 1% under normal and bright illuminance. (Reprinted with permission from Pollack SL, Hunt JS, Polse KA. Dose-response effects of tropicamide HCl. Am J Optom Physiol Opt 1981;58:361–366.)**

provided a 5 mm or greater dilation in most subjects except for blacks, whose eyes dilated to a lesser degree. Pollack and associates[78] observed no significant differences in pupil size under normal or bright illumination in eight white males aged 22 to 32 years following instillation of 1 drop of tropicamide 0.25%, 0.5%, 0.75%, or 1% (Fig. 9.5).

Since, in general, the pupils of diabetic patients are resistant to dilation with anticholinergic agents, adequate mydriasis with tropicamide alone is usually not achieved in these patients. A combination of tropicamide and phenylephrine produces adequate dilation in most cases, particularly since the pupil of diabetic patients shows supersensitivity to adrenergic agonists.[79]

The maximum cycloplegic effect also occurs at 30 minutes following instillation. Unlike the mydriatic effects, there may be a difference on accommodation between the two commercially available concentrations of tropicamide, the 1% producing a somewhat greater loss of accommodation.[76] The average residual accommodation with 1% tropicamide was 1.60 D at 30 minutes and 2.40 D at 40 minutes. Gettes[77] studied the cycloplegic effect of 1% tropicamide and found it to be clinically effective in 90% of the eyes tested, provided that a second drop was instilled 5 to 25 minutes after the first, and provided also that the examination was performed 20 to 35 minutes following instillation. Accommodation returns to preinstillation values within 6 hours.

Pollack and associates[78] studied the cycloplegic effects of 0.25%, 0.5%, 0.75%, and 1% tropicamide. Some inhibition of accommodation occurred with each concentration, and the effects were dose related. The maximum residual accommodation ranged from 3.17 D for the 0.25% concentration to 1.30 D for the 1% concentration. The maximum cycloplegic effects for all subjects occurred 30 to 35 minutes following instillation. Significant differences in cycloplegic effects were found between the 0.25% and 1% solutions but not among 0.5%, 0.75%, or 1% concentrations. Figure 9.6 illustrates the residual accommodation during the period of maximum cycloplegia for all concentrations of tropicamide tested. Two diopters or less of residual accommodation were present for at least 40 minutes with the 0.75% and 1% concentrations and for about 15 minutes with the 0.5% concentration. A mean residual accommodation of 2.2 D was present following the application of 0.25% tropicamide. This effect was sufficient to incapacitate the subjects for most near vision tasks for 40 to 60 minutes.

The mydriatic effect of tropicamide has been compared to that of homatropine and of cyclopentolate.[63,76,80–82] Merrill and associates[76] reported that whereas tropicamide 0.5% or 1% produced maximum mydriasis within 30 minutes, cyclopentolate 1%, homatropine 5%, or phenylephrine 10% did so in 60 to 90 minutes. Moreover, the degree of mydriasis at 30 minutes was greater with tropicamide than with the other drugs tested.[76] Gambill and associates[83] compared the mydriatic effects of tropicamide 0.5%, homatropine 2%, phenylephrine 10%, and hydroxyamphetamine 1%. Tropicamide had the fastest onset and greatest intensity of mydriatic action (Fig. 9.7).

The cycloplegic effectiveness of tropicamide has been compared to that of cyclopentolate and homatropine.[76,80–82] Merrill and associates[76] observed that the maximum cycloplegic effect of 1% tropicamide at 30 minutes was greater than that obtained from 1% cyclopentolate or 5% homatropine but was much shorter, with clinically effective cycloplegia maintained only up to 35 minutes following instillation of a single drop. Gettes and Belmont[80] compared the effects of tropicamide 1%, cyclopentolate 1%, and homatropine 4% combined with hydroxyamphetamine 1%. Two instillations of each drug were given 5 minutes apart, and measurement of accommodation was performed 20 to 40 minutes after the second drop. Figure 9.8 summarizes the results. Although the initial intensity of the cycloplegic effect of tropicamide was nearly equal to that of cyclopentolate, accommodation rapidly returned after 35 minutes. Cyclopentolate remained consistently effective after 25 minutes for the duration of the measurement. The homatropine-hydroxyamphetamine combination exhibited a slower onset, reaching clinically effective levels of cycloplegia for refraction at 45 to 55 minutes. In similar studies using tropicamide 1%, cyclopentolate 1%, or homatropine 5%, two drops to each eye, Milder[81] observed that cyclopentolate and homatropine were superior to tropicamide in 92% and 80% of patients, respectively. Moreover, the magnitude of residual accommodation was inversely related to age, being greater than 2.5 D with tropicamide in patients under 40 years of age (Table 9.5).

Lovasik[62] studied the time course of cycloplegia for tropicamide and cyclopentolate in adult subjects ages 20 to 30 years. His data indicate that 1 drop of 0.5% or 1.0% tropicamide leaves as much as 28 to 40% of baseline accommodation active at 20 minutes following drug instillation. In contrast, cyclopentolate 0.5% or 1.0% induced a deeper and more stable level of cycloplegia within the same period.

Prior application of a topical anesthetic appears to prolong the mydriatic and cycloplegic actions of tropicamide.[84] Mordi and associates[84] reported that prior instillation of proparacaine 0.5% in blue-green eyes prolonged both the time required for 50% recovery to normal pupil size and the time during which mydriasis is maintained within 90% of maximum. In brown-hazel eyes the time for recovery to 50% was lengthened by 30 minutes, but the time during which mydriasis remained 90% of maximum was not lengthened by prior application of the anesthetic. The time during which cycloplegia was maintained within 90% of maximum was extended by 3 to 4 minutes in all eyes, regardless of degree of pigmentation. Lovasik[62] has also observed that the depth of cycloplegia at 20 minutes following instillation of 0.5% or 1.0% tropicamide is greater in eyes pretreated with 0.5% proparacaine than in eyes receiving tropicamide alone.

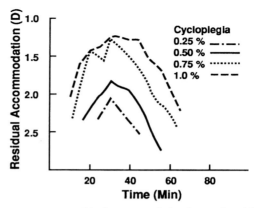

FIGURE 9.6   **Mean residual accommodation for tropicamide over the period of maximum cycloplegia. (Reprinted with permission from Pollack SL, Hunt JS, Polse KA. Dose-response effects of tropicamide HCl. Am J Optom Physiol Opt 1981;58:361–366.)**

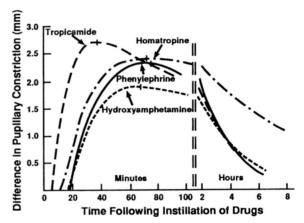

FIGURE 9.7   **Onset, intensity, and duration of mydriasis for tropicamide 0.5%, homatropine 2%, phenylephrine 10%, and hydroxyamphetamine 1% measured by electronic pupillography. (Reprinted with permission from Gambill HD, Ogle KN, Kearns TP. Mydriatic effect of four drugs determined by pupillograph. Arch Ophthalmol 1967;77:740–746. Copyright 1967, American Medical Association.)**

CLINICAL USES

Due to its relatively fast onset, short duration, and sufficient intensity of action, tropicamide is considered the drug of choice for ophthalmoscopy and other procedures where mydriasis is desirable. Moreover, unlike with atropine, homatropine, or cyclopentolate, pupillary dilation with tropicamide appears to be less dependent on iris pigmentation. Dillon and associates[85] achieved a minimum of 6 mm pupil size with 0.5% tropicamide in subjects with either light

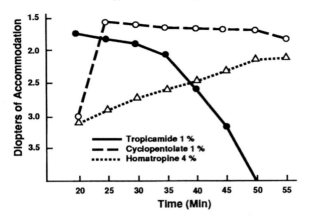

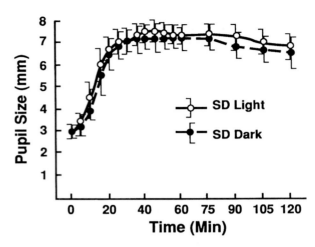

FIGURE 9.8   **Average residual accommodation with tropicamide 1%, cyclopentolate 1%, and homatropine 4% in adult patients.** (Reprinted with permission from Gettes BC, Belmont O. Tropicamide: Comparative cycloplegic effects. Arch Ophthalmol 1961;66:336–340. Copyright 1961, American Medical Association.)

FIGURE 9.9   **Comparison of mean pupillary dilation with 0.5% tropicamide in subjects with light and dark irides.** (Reprinted with permission from Dillon JR, Tyhurst CW, Yolton RL. The mydriatic effect of tropicamide on light and dark irides. J Am Optom Assoc 1977;48:653–658.)

or dark irides. No significant differences in amplitude of dilation occurred with respect to iris pigmentation or race of subjects (Fig. 9.9). Other studies have reported similar results.[62]

For clinical situations where only mydriasis is necessary, it is desirable to obtain pupillary dilation with minimum paralysis of accommodation so as not to interfere with near vision tasks. To achieve clinically useful mydriasis with minimal accommodative paralysis, various combinations of drugs have been investigated.[82,86–92] Priestly and associates[86] evaluated a combination of cyclopentolate 0.2% and phenylephrine 1% (Cyclomydril). This combination produced satisfactory mydriasis 30 minutes following instillation. However, the effect on accommodation with Cyclomydril is equal to or greater than with tropicamide 1%.[87,88]

Other investigators have tested various concentrations of tropicamide with adrenergic agonists.[82,87,89–93] Gettes[82] reported that a combination of 0.1% tropicamide and 1% hydroxyamphetamine was effective for routine ophthalmoscopic examinations. Larkin and associates[91] evaluated various concentrations of tropicamide combined with 1% hydroxyamphetamine to find a clinically useful mydriatic with minimal accommodative effects. When combined with 1% hydroxyamphetamine, 0.05%, 0.1%, 0.25%, or 0.5% tropicamide produced mean pupillary diameters 3.5 to 3.8 mm greater than baseline values (Fig. 9.10). The differ-

TABLE 9.5
Residual Accommodation Following Instillation of Tropicamide 1%, Homatropine 5%, or Cyclopentolate 1%

Age (yr)	Number of Subjects	Tropicamide (30 min)	Homatropine or Cyclopentolate (60 min)
0–9	6	6.25 D	2.50 D
10–14	20	3.65	2.40
15–19	7	3.20	1.40
20–29	7	3.10	1.40
30–39	7	2.60	2.00
40+	3	1.70	1.10

Reprinted with permission from Milder B. Tropicamide as a cycloplegic agent. Arch Ophthalmol 1961; 66:60. Copyright © 1961, American Medical Association.

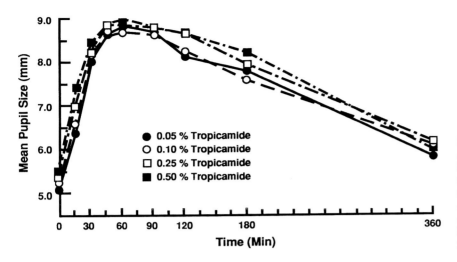

FIGURE 9.10 **Mydriatic dose-response curve for hydroxyamphetamine 1% combined with one of four concentrations of tropicamide. (Modified from Larkin KM, Charap A, Cheetham JK, Frank J. Ideal concentration of tropicamide with hydroxyamphetamine 1% for routine pupillary dilation. Ann Ophthalmol 1989; 21:340–344.)**

ences in pupillary diameter among the concentrations tested were not statistically significant. The effect on accommodation, however, was directly related to the concentration of tropicamide (Fig. 9.11). The mean loss of accommodation was 3.8 D for 0.05% tropicamide and 5.5 D for the 0.5% concentration. Most eyes returned to baseline values at 6 hours. By 24 hours, both pupil size and accommodation were at predrug instillation levels.

Brown and Hanna[87] compared 0.1% tropicamide and 1% phenylephrine suspended in 1% methylcellulose to 1% tropicamide and 10% phenylephrine administered as drops. Both combinations produced nearly equal dilation at 30 minutes. The average residual accommodation measured 1.8 D at 45 minutes with the methylcellulose mixture.

The mydriatic effect of a mixture of 0.75% tropicamide and 2.5% phenylephrine has been compared to that of the separate instillation of 1% tropicamide and 10% phenylephrine in 100 white patients ranging in age from 14 to 85 years.[89] Both direct and indirect ophthalmoscopy were performed on each patient. The low-concentration mixture produced average pupil sizes of 7.4 mm and 7.5 mm in blue and brown irides, respectively, compared with an average dilation of 7.6 mm in all subjects with the separate instillation of 10% phenylephrine and 1% tropicamide. Cycloplegic effects were not evaluated, but based on the data of Pollack and associates,[78] one could presume that accommodation was reduced with both drug regimens.

Several investigators[92,93] have compared the mydriatic and cycloplegic effects of 5% phenylephrine combined with 0.8% tropicamide (Phenyltrope) with 1% tropicamide in young adults. The combination formulation did not differ in its mydriatic effect from 1% tropicamide. Although the rate of accommodative loss was similar for both drug groups, the resultant cycloplegia at 20 minutes was greater for Phenyl-

trope. The tropicamide and the combination formulation did not differ significantly in mydriatic or cycloplegic efficacy between different iris color groups.

The advantage of tropicamide as compared to other mydriatic-cycloplegic agents is its fast onset and relatively short duration of action. Practitioners should note that, clinically, tropicamide has a greater mydriatic than cycloplegic effect, and thus, unlike with cyclopentolate and other anticholinergics, mydriasis does not necessarily indicate adequate cycloplegia for refraction.

SIDE EFFECTS

Tropicamide, especially at the 1% concentration, can produce transient stinging on instillation. As with the other mydriatic-cycloplegics, it can raise IOP in eyes with open-angle glaucoma. The pressure elevation is insignificant in most patients, since it subsides in several hours without damaging the optic nerve.[94,95] However, in open-angle glaucoma patients, dilation can sometimes result in significant increase in IOP. Dilation with 1.0% tropicamide and 2.5% phenylephrine has resulted in pressure elevations of 5 mm Hg or more in 32% and 10 mm Hg or more in 12% of patients with open-angle glaucoma. The incidence of pressure elevations appears to be highest in eyes receiving miotic therapy.[94,95] Thus, to reduce the risk associated with iatrogenic pressure elevations, it seems prudent to recheck IOP following dilation with tropicamide in glaucoma patients.

Adverse systemic reactions to tropicamide are quite rare. Wahl[96] has reported one such reaction in a 10-year-old white male. Immediately following instillation of 1 drop of 0.5% tropicamide into each eye, the patient fell from the chair to the floor unconscious. This was followed by generalized muscular rigidity, pallor, and cyanosis. Within a few minutes

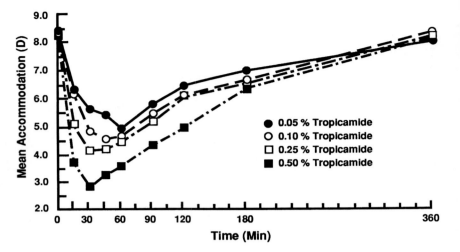

FIGURE 9.11 **Cycloplegic dose-response curve for hydroxyamphetamine 1% combined with one of four concentrations of tropicamide. (Modified from Larkin KM, Charap A, Cheetham JK, Frank J. Ideal concentration of tropicamide with hydroxyamphetamine 1% for routine pupillary dilation. Ann Ophthalmol 1989; 21:340–344.)**

the patient became flaccid and regained consciousness, but he remained in a state of generalized weakness and drowsiness. About 1 hour after the onset of the episode, his vital signs were normal and he was fully recovered. Wahl classified this reaction as acute hypersensitivity manifested by anaphylactic shock. The spontaneous recovery, however, argues against an anaphylactic mechanism. Others have suggested the possibility that psychomotor factors may play a role in such reactions. Yolton and associates[97] and Applebaum and Jaanus[98] have observed no adverse reactions associated with the use of tropicamide in over 12,000 drug applications in patients undergoing ophthalmoscopy. The rarity of systemic reactions to tropicamide may be explained by this drug's low affinity for systemic muscarinic receptors following topical application to the eye.[99]

Since tropicamide is devoid of vasopressor effect,[100] it is one of the safest mydriatic agents for use in patients with systemic hypertension, angina, or other cardiovascular disease.

CONTRAINDICATIONS

Patients with hypersensitivity to belladonna alkaloids may also exhibit cross-sensitivity to topical ocular tropicamide. Tropicamide is also contraindicated in patients with narrow anterior chamber angles, where angle-closure glaucoma may be iatrogenically induced.

References

1. Zinn KM. The pupil. Springfield, IL: Charles C Thomas, 1972; Chap. 2.
2. McEwen WK, Goodner EK. Secretion of tears and blinking. In: Davson H, ed. The eye. New York: Academic Press, 1969;3:341.
3. Zadunaisky JA, Spinowitz B. Drugs affecting the transport and permeability of the corneal epithelium. In: Dikstein S, ed. Drugs and ocular tissue. New York: Krager, 1977;69.
4. Michon J, Kinoshita JH. Cholinesterase in the lens. Arch Ophthalmol 1967;77:807–808.
5. Hutchins JB, Hollyfield JG. Cholinergic neurons in the human retina. Exp Eye Res 1987;44:363–375.
6. Lund KR. Muscarinic receptor binding and the effect of atropine on the guinea pig iris. Exp Eye Res 1979;27:577–583.
7. Smith EL, Edburn DA, Harwerth RS, Macquire GW. Permanent alterations in muscarinic receptors and pupil size produced by chronic atropinization in kittens. Invest Ophthalmol Vis Sci 1985;25:239–243.
8. Kaumann AJ, Hennekes R. The affinity of atropine for muscarinic receptors in human sphincter pupillae. Arch Pharmacol 1979;306:209–239.
9. Hutchins JB, Hollyfield JG. Autoradiographic identification of muscarinic receptors in human iris smooth muscle. Exp Eye Res 1984;38:515–521.
10. Barany E, Berie CP, Birdsall NJ, et al. The binding properties of the muscarinic receptors of the cynomolgus monkey ciliary body and the response to the induction of agonist subsensitivity. Br J Pharmacol 1982;77:731–739.
11. Konno F, Takayangi I. Muscarinic acetylcholine receptors in the rabbit ciliary body smooth muscle: Spare receptors and threshold phenomenon. Jpn J Pharmacol 1984;38:91–99.
12. Polansky JR, Zlock D, Brasier A, Bloom E. Adrenergic and cholinergic receptors in isolated nonpigmented ciliary epithelial cells. Curr Eye Res 1985;4:517–522.
13. Lograno MD, Reibaldi A. Receptor responses in fresh human ciliary muscle. Br J Pharmacol 1986;87:379–385.
14. Hutchins JB, Hollyfield JG. Acetylcholine receptors in the human retina. Invest Ophthalmol Vis Sci 1985;26:1550–1557.
15. Brown JH. Atropine, scopolamine and related antimuscarinic drugs. In: Gilman AG, Rall TW, Nies AS, et al, eds. Goodman and Gilman's The pharmacological basis of therapeutics. New York: McGraw-Hill, 1993; Chap 8.
16. Kondritzer AA, Zvirblis P. Stability of atropine aqueous solution. J Am Pharmacol Assoc 1957;46:53–56.

17. Smith SE. Dose-response relationship in tropicamide-induced mydriasis and cycloplegia. Br J Clin Pharmacol 1974;1:37–40.

18. Janes RC, Stiles JF. The penetration of C[14]-labeled atropine into the eye. Arch Ophthalmol 1959;62:69–74.

19. Lussana F. Dell'azione e delle virtu terapeutiche dell' atropina e della belladonna. Ann Univ di Med 1852;140:514.

20. Feddersen IM. Beitrag zur Atropinvergiftung. Inaug Dissert Berlin; Francke O. 1884, as cited by: Manon J. Cycloplegia and mydriasis by use of atropine, scopolamine and homatropine-paredrine. Arch Ophthalmol 1940;23:340–350.

21. Wolf AV, Hodge HC. Effects of atropine sulfate, methylatropine nitrate (Metropine) and homatropine hydrobromide on adult human eyes. Arch Ophthalmol 1946;36:293–301.

22. Emiru VP. Response to mydriatics in the African. Br J Ophthalmol 1971;55:538–543.

23. Salazar M, Shimada K, Patie PN. Iris pigmentation and atropine mydriasis. J Pharmacol Exp Ther 1976;197:79–88.

24. Cauther SE, Ellis RD, Larrison SB, Kidd MR. Resolution, purification and characterization of rabbit serum atropinesterase and cocainesterase. Biochem Pharmacol 1976;25:181–185.

25. Stolovitch C, Loewenstein A, Nemmet P, Moshe L. Atropine cycloplegia: How many instillations does one need? J Pediatr Ophthalmol Strabismus 1992;29;175–176.

26. Mindel JS. Cholinergic pharmacology. In: Duane TD, Jaeger EA, eds. Biomedical foundations of ophthalmology. Philadelphia: Harper & Row 1982;3 (Chap. 26).

27. Grimbel HV. The control of myopia with atropine. Can J Ophthalmol 1973;8:527–532.

28. Dyer JA. Role of cycloplegics in progressive myopia. Ophthalmology 1979;86:692–694.

29. Bedrossian RH. The effect of atropine on myopia. Ophthalmology 1979;86:713–717.

30. Sampson WG. Role of cycloplegia in the management of functional myopia. Ophthalmology 1979;86:695–697.

31. Gugersen E, Pontoppidan M, Rindziunski E. Optic drugs penalization and favouring in the treatment of squint amblyopia. Acta Ophthalmol 1974;52:60–72.

32. Repka MX, Ray JM. The efficacy of optical and pharmacological penalization. Ophthalmology 1993;100:769–774.

33. Von Noorden GK. Amblyopia caused by unilateral atropinization. Ophthalmology 1981;88:131–133.

34. North RV, Kelley ME. Atropine occlusion in the treatment of strabismic amblyopia and its effect upon the nonamblyopic eye. Ophthalmic Physiol Opt 1991:11:113–117.

35. Sugar HS. The provocative test in the diagnosis of the glaucomas. Am J Ophthalmol 1948;31:1193–1202.

36. Abraham S. Mydriatic glaucoma—a statistical study. Arch Ophthalmol 1933;10:757–762.

37. Cramp J. Reported cases of reactions and side effects of the drugs which optometrists use. Aust J Optom 1976;59:13–25.

38. Keller JT. The risk of angle closure from use of mydriatics. J Am Optom Assoc 1975;46:19–21.

39. Leopold IM, Comroe JH. Effects of intramuscular administration of morphine, atropine, scopolamine, and neostigmine on the human eye. Arch Ophthalmol 1948;40:285–290.

40. Mehra KS, Chandra P. The effects on the eye of premedication with atropine. Br J Anesth 1965;37:133–137.

41. Tammisto T, Castren JA, Marttila I. Intramuscularly administered atropine and the eye. Acta Ophthalmol 1964;42:408–417.

42. Davidson SI. Systemic effects of eye drops. Trans Ophthalmol Soc UK 1974;94:487–495.

43. Eggers HM. Toxicity of drugs used in diagnosis and treatment of strabismus. In: Srinivasan DB, ed. Ocular therapeutics. New York: Masson, 1980; Chap. 15.

44. North RV, Kelly ME. A review of the uses and adverse effects of topical administration of atropine. Ophthal Physiol Opt 1987; 7:109–114.

45. Wright BD. Exacerbation of akinetic seizures by atropine eye drops. Br J Ophthalmol 1992;76:179–180.

46. Morton HG. Atropine intoxication: Its manifestations in infants and children. J Pediatr 1939;14:755–760.

47. Tune LE, Bylsma FW, Hilt DC. Anticholinergic delirium caused by topical homatropine ophthalmologic solution: Confirmation by anticholinergic radioreceptor assay in two cases. J Neuropsych 1992;4:195–197.

48. Jaanus SD. Pharmacologic aspects of aging. In: Rosenbloom AA, Morgan MW, eds. Vision and aging. Boston: Butterworth-Heinemann, 1993; Chap 5.

49. Heath WE. Deaths from atropine poisoning. BMJ 1950;2:608.

50. Ophthalmic drug facts. St. Louis: Facts and Comparisons, 1995; Chap 4.

51. Shutt LE, Bowes JB. Atropine and hyoscine. Anesthesia 1979; 34:476–490.

52. Smith SA. Factors determining the potency of mydriatic drugs in man. Br J Clin Pharmacol 1976;3:503–507.

53. Hoefnagel D. Toxic effects of atropine and homatropine eye drops in children. N Engl J Med 1961;264:168–171.

54. Marron J. Cycloplegia and mydriasis by use of atropine, scopolamine and homatropine-paredrine. Arch Ophthalmol 1940; 23:340–350.

55. Morrison JD, Reilly J. The effects of 0.025% hyoscine hydrobromide eyedrops on visual function in man. Ophthal Physiol Opt 1989;9:41–45.

56. Freund M, Merin S. Toxic effect of scopolamine eye drops. Am J Ophthalmol 1970;70:637–639.

57. Priestly BS, Medine MM. A new mydriatic and cycloplegic drug. Am J Ophthalmol 1951;34:572–575.

58. Gettes BD, Leopold IH. Evaluation of five new cycloplegic drugs. Arch Ophthalmol 1953;49:24–27.

59. Abraham SV. A new mydriatic and cycloplegic drug: Compound 75 GT. Am J Ophthalmol 1953;36:69–73.

60. Milder B, Riffenburgh R. An evaluation of Cyclogyl (compound 75 GT). Am J Ophthalmol 1953;36:1724–1726.

61. Manny RE, Fern KD, Zervas HJ, et al. 1% cyclopentolate hydrochloride: Another look at the time course of cycloplegia using an objective measure of the accommodative response. Optom Vis Sci 1993;70:651–665.

62. Lovasik JV. Pharmacokinetics of topically applied cyclopentolate HCL and tropicamide. Am J Optom Physiol Opt 1986;63:787–803.

63. Jones LW, Hodes DT. Possible allergic reaction to cyclopentolate hydrochloride: Case report and literature review of uses and adverse reactions. Ophthal Physiol Opt 1991;11:16–21.

64. Sato EH, DeFreitas D, Foster CS. Abuse of cyclopentolate hydrochloride (Cyclogyl) drops. N Engl J Med 1992;326:1363–1364.

65. Gartner S, Billet E. Mydriatic glaucoma. Am J Ophthalmol 1957;43:975–976.

66. Harris LS. Cycloplegic-induced intraocular pressure elevations. A

study of normal and open-angle glaucomatous eyes. Arch Ophthalmol 1968;79:242–246.

67. Simcoe CW. Cyclopentolate (Cyclogyl) toxicity. Arch Ophthalmol 1962;67:406–408.

68. Binkhorst RD, Weinstein GW, Baretz RM, Glahane MS. Psychotic reaction induced by cyclopentolate. Am J Ophthalmol 1963;56:1243–1245.

69. Praeger DL, Miller SN. Toxic effects of cyclopentolate (Cyclogyl). Am J Ophthalmol 1964;58:1060–1061.

70. Awan KJ. Adverse systemic reactions of topical cyclopentolate hydrochloride. Ann Ophthalmol 1978;8:695–698.

71. Shihab ZM. Psychotic reaction in an adult after topical cyclopentolate. Ophthalmologica 1980;181:228–230.

72. Kaila T, Huupponen R, Salminen L, Iisalo E. Systemic absorption of ophthalmic cyclopentolate. Am J Ophthalmol 1989;107:562–563.

73. Lahdes K, Kaila T, Huupponen R, et al. Systemic absorption of topically applied ocular atropine. Clin Pharmacol Ther 1988;44:310–317.

74. Kennerdell JS, Wucher FP. Cyclopentolate associated with two cases of grand mal seizure. Arch Ophthalmol 1972;87:634–635.

75. Fitzgerald DA, Hanson RM, West C, et al. Seizures associated with 1% cyclopentolate eyedrops. J Paediatr Child Health 1990;26:106–107.

76. Merrill DL, Goldberg B, Zavell S. bis Tropicamide, a new parasympatholytic. Curr Ther Res 1960;2:43–50.

77. Gettes BD. Tropicamide, a new cycloplegic mydriatic. Arch Ophthalmol 1961;65:48–52.

78. Pollack SL, Hunt JS, Polse KA. Dose-response effects of tropicamide HCL. Am J Optom Physiol Opt 1981;58:361–366.

79. Huber MSE, Smith SA, Smith SE. Mydriatic drug for diabetic patients. Br J Ophthalmol 1985;69:425–427.

80. Gettes BC, Belmont O. Tropicamide: Comparative cycloplegic effects. Arch Ophthalmol 1961;66:336–340.

81. Milder B. Tropicamide as a cycloplegic agent. Arch Ophthalmol 1961;66:70–72.

82. Gettes BC. Tropicamide; comparative mydriatic effects. Am J Ophthalmol 1963;55:84–87.

83. Gambill HD, Ogle KN, Kearns TP. Mydriatic effect of four drugs determined by pupillograph. Arch Ophthalmol 1967;77:740–746.

84. Mordi JA, Lyle WM, Mousa GY. Does prior instillation of a topical anesthetic enhance the effect of tropicamide? Am J Optom Physiol Opt 1986;63:290–293.

85. Dillon JR, Tyhurst CW, Yolton RL. The mydriatic effect of tropicamide on light and dark irides. J Am Optom Assoc 1977;48:653–658.

86. Priestly BS, Medine MM, Phillips CC. Cyclomydril: A new mydriatic agent. Am J Ophthalmol 1960;49:1033–1034.

87. Brown C, Hanna C. Use of dilute drug solutions for routine cycloplegia and mydriasis. Am J Ophthalmol 1978;86:820–824.

88. Jaanus SD, Saulles H, Col PR. A comparative study of diagnostic agents used for mydriasis (abstr.). Am Acad Optom 1979;15.

89. Forman AR. A new low-concentration preparation for mydriasis and cycloplegia. Ophthalmology 1980;87:213–215.

90. Sinclair SH, Pelham V, Gioranoni R, et al. Mydriatic solutions for outpatient indirect ophthalmoscopy. Arch Ophthalmol 1980;98:1572–1574.

91. Larkin KM, Charap A, Cheetham JK, Frank J. Ideal concentration of tropicamide with hydroxyamphetamine 1% for routine pupillary dilation. Ann Ophthalmol 1989;21:340–344.

92. Kergoat H, Lovasik JV, Doughty MJ. A pupillographic evaluation of a phenylephrine HCl 5%-tropicamide combination mydriatic. J Ocular Pharmacol 1989;5:199–216.

93. Lovasik JV, Kergoat H. Time course of cycloplegia induced by a new phenylephrine-tropicamide combination drug. Optom Vis Sci 1990;67:352–358.

94. Portney GL, Purcell TW. The influence of tropicamide on intraocular pressure. Ann Ophthalmol 1975;7:31–34.

95. Shaw DA, Lewis RA. Intraocular pressure elevation after pupillary dilation in open angle glaucoma. Arch Ophthalmol 1986;104:1185–1188.

96. Wahl JW. Systemic reaction to tropicamide. Arch Ophthalmol 1969;82:320–321.

97. Yolton DP, Kandel JS, Yolton RL. Diagnostic pharmaceutical agents: Side effects encountered in a study of 15,000 applications. J Am Optom Assoc 1980;51:113–117.

98. Applebaum MA, Jaanus SD. Use of diagnostic pharmaceutical agents and incidence of adverse effects. Am J Optom Physiol Opt 1983;60:384–388.

99. Vuori M-L, Kaila T, Iisalo E, Saari KM. Systemic absorption and anticholinergic activity of topically applied tropicamide. J Ocular Pharmacol 1994;10:431–437.

100. Brown MM, Brown GC, Spaeth GL. Lack of side effects from topically administered 10% phenylephrine eyedrops. Arch Ophthalmol 1980;98:487–488.

CHAPTER 10

Antiglaucoma Drugs

Jimmy D. Bartlett
Gary D. Novack
Jeffrey A. Hiett
Siret D. Jaanus
Mordechai Sharir

Glaucoma can be a devastating disease, often leading to visual impairment and even blindness. Although great progress has been made in defining the spectrum of diseases known collectively as "glaucoma," their etiopathogenesis is still poorly understood. A common element seems to be intraocular pressure (IOP) in excess of physiologic limits. Management of these disorders is almost always directed at lowering the existing IOP. This can be accomplished either pharmacologically or surgically by decreasing aqueous production or by increasing aqueous outflow.

A myriad of pharmacologic agents is available to decrease IOP through distinctly different mechanisms. Because of their unique mechanisms of action, these drugs are used both alone and in combination in attempts to reduce IOP to acceptable levels that will forestall further damage to the optic nerve or visual field. This chapter considers the most clinically useful ocular hypotensive agents as well as some adjuncts to glaucoma surgery (Table 10.1). Chapter 35 addresses how these drugs are used in the context of specific glaucomatous conditions.

β-Adrenergic Antagonists

The potential ocular hypotensive effects of β-adrenoceptor antagonists (β blockers) were first evaluated over a quarter of a century ago. Phillips and associates[1] found intravenous propranolol, a non-cardioselective agent, to be an effective ocular hypotensive agent in glaucoma patients. Somewhat later Bucci and associates[2] reported its efficacy for lowering IOP upon topical instillation. Unfortunately, concerns over corneal anesthesia following topical propranolol limited its general acceptance.[3] However, the plethora of systemic β blockers has provided ophthalmic researchers with a host of compounds to evaluate for ocular hypotensive efficacy and ocular safety. This section highlights five agents currently marketed in the United States: timolol, levobunolol, betaxolol, metipranolol and carteolol (Table 10.2).

Timolol

PHARMACOLOGY

Timolol is a non-cardioselective β blocker without intrinsic sympathomimetic activity (ISA) and with pharmacologic actions similar to those of propranolol. When used orally for systemic hypertension, timolol is several-fold more potent than propranolol. Ocular metabolism of timolol is not apparent, and its systemic metabolites have no significant β-adrenoceptor antagonistic effect.[4] Within the first hour following topical instillation in humans, the concentration of timolol in the anterior chamber measures 1 to 2 μM (8–100 ng/ml).[5] This level is approximately one-thousand times the

TABLE 10.1
Ocular Hypotensive Agents and Surgical Adjuncts

β-adrenergic antagonists (β blockers)
Timolol
Levobunolol
Betaxolol
Metipranolol
Carteolol

Cholinergic agonists (Miotics)
Pilocarpine
Carbachol
Echothiophate

Adrenergic agonists
Epinephrine
Dipivefrin
Apraclonidine
Brimonidine

Carbonic anhydrase inhibitors
Acetazolamide
Methazolamide
Dichlorphenamide
Sezolamide
Dorzolamide

Hyperosmotic agents
Mannitol
Urea
Glycerin
Isosorbide

Antimetabolites
5-fluorouracil (5-FU)
Mitomycin-C (MMC)

Prostaglandins
Latanoprost

Ethacrynic acid (ECA)

minimum amount required for binding at the ocular β_2-adrenoceptor.[6] Most concur that antagonism of the β_2-adrenoceptor at the ciliary body is primarily responsible for the ocular hypotensive efficacy of timolol,[7,8] although alternate theories exist.[9]

Given topically to humans with elevated IOP, timolol induces a profound and long-lasting ocular hypotension. Table 10.3 shows selected concentrations tested in the first published dose-response, time-response study of timolol in patients.[10] Mean IOP decreases in excess of 30% were observed. The maximal efficacy of 0.1%, 0.25% and 0.5% timolol were similar. Twelve hours after dosing, however, a large apparent diurnal effect occurred, with a 28% reduction in IOP in both the vehicle group and 0.1% timolol group. Both 0.25% and 0.5% timolol were more effective than vehicle at both 12 and 24 hours.

The ocular hypotensive activity of timolol has been compared to pilocarpine in a double-masked, randomized study lasting 10 weeks. Although the timolol group had a higher mean baseline IOP (34.0 vs. 28.0 mm Hg), timolol brought about a greater decrease in IOP than did pilocarpine (Table 10.4). In the timolol group the heart rate decreased approximately 10 beats per minute, and a slight increase in heart rate occurred in the pilocarpine group.[11]

Early in the development of timolol, some reports indicated the relatively rapid development of tolerance to the drug's ocular hypotensive effects, referred to as "escape."[11–13] Krupin and associates[14] investigated several aspects of timolol efficacy in a study of 25 ocular hypertensive patients. The patients received a single drop of 0.25% timolol in one eye, and IOP was measured one hour later. They then used 0.25% timolol twice daily for 3 to 4 weeks, again returning for measurement of IOP. The patients then were titrated up to 0.5% timolol, twice daily, in the same eye for 3 to 4 weeks. Table 10.5 summarizes the results. The IOP was lower acutely with 0.25% timolol than chronically with

TABLE 10.2
Ophthalmic β-Adrenoceptor Antagonists

Generic name	Trade Name(s)	Concentrations	Predominant Receptor Blockade		
			β_1	β_2	ISA[a]
Timolol	Timoptic, Timoptic in Ocudose, Timoptic-XE	0.25%, 0.5%	+	+	−
Levobunolol	Betagan, Levobunolol HCl	0.25%, 0.5%	+	+	−
Betaxolol	Betoptic, Betoptic-S	0.5% (solution) 0.25% (suspension)	+	−	−
Metipranolol	Optipranolol	0.3%	+	+	−
Carteolol	Ocupress	1%	+	+	+

[a]ISA = intrinsic sympathomimetic activity

TABLE 10.3
Acute Ocular Hypotensive Effects of Timolol (mm Hg)

			Dose					
	Vehicle		0.1%		0.25%		0.5%	
Time (hr)	Mean	%	Mean	%	Mean	%	Mean	%
0	22.0		26.2		23.7		28.0	
2	1.0	4.5%	8.5	32.4%	7.8	32.9%	8.7	31.1%
12	6.1	27.7%	6.5	24.8%	9.0	38.0%	11.0	39.3%
24	2.0	9.1%	6.6	25.2%	6.6	27.8%	11.1	39.6%

Treated eye only, selected times and doses.
Modified from Zimmerman TJ, Kaufman HE. Timolol: dose-response and duration of action. Arch Ophthalmol 1977;95:605–607.

TABLE 10.4
Chronic Ocular Hypotensive Effect of Timolol[a]

	Dose			
	Timolol		Pilocarpine	
Time (wk)	Mean IOP	% Change	Mean IOP	% Change
0	34.0		28.0	
2	−13.0	38%	−7.5	27%
6	−13.5	40%	−7.0	25%
10	−13.0	38%	−7.0	25%

[a]Mean IOP, and mean and percent change from baseline (mm Hg).
Adapted from Boger WP, Steinert RF, Puliafito CA, et al. Clinical trial comparing timolol ophthalmic solution to pilocarpine in open-angle glaucoma. Am J Ophthalmol 1978;86:8–18.

TABLE 10.5
Ocular Hypotensive Effect of Timolol (mm Hg)

	Baseline	0.25% Timolol, 1 hr	0.25% Timolol, 3–4 wks	0.5% Timolol, 3–4 wks
Treated eye	28.1 ± 5.3	18.5 ± 4.5	21.1 ± 4.2	20.4 ± 3.5
Control eye	26.7 ± 4.8	23.8 ± 4.9	25.0 ± 5.1	24.0 ± 3.9

Reprinted with permission from Krupin T, Singer PR, Perlmutter J, et al. One-hour intraocular pressure response to timolol: Lack of correlation with long-term response. Arch Ophthalmol 1981;99:840–841. Copyright © 1981, American Medical Association.

either 0.25% or 0.5% timolol, but IOP results were similar with chronic use of either 0.5% timolol or 0.25% timolol. In addition, the fellow, untreated control eye showed a decrease in IOP, which may result from either a consensual (contralateral) effect[15,16] or from changes in the severity of the disease.

Consensual effects, due to systemic drug absorption, can be significant, and some workers have suggested that these effects may allow for unilateral treatment of patients with bilateral disease.[17,18]

Boger and associates[11,12,19] also described a longer term

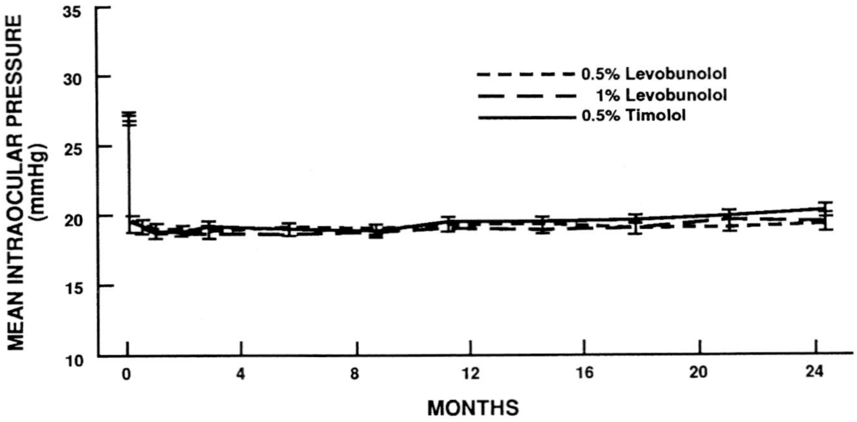

FIGURE 10.1   **Mean IOP throughout first two years of treatment with 0.5% timolol and 0.5% and 1.0% levobunolol, each instilled twice daily. (Reprinted with permission from Levobunolol Study Group. Levobunolol. A beta-adrenoceptor antagonist effective in the long-term treatment of glaucoma. Ophthalmology 1985;92:1271–1276.)**

"drift," or tolerance. After one year of open-label experience with timolol, 7 of 20 patients in one group initially controlled with timolol required additional therapy. These observations may also result from changes in disease state or noncompliance in certain patients, rather than as tolerance to timolol per se. In a controlled four-year study timolol gave a failure rate less than 15% per year.[20]

The use of 0.5% timolol as a comparative agent in the Levobunolol Study Group[20] provides us with long-term controlled data on timolol in a population of 391 patients with open-angle glaucoma or ocular hypertension. In this study, the ocular hypotensive efficacy of timolol was approximately 7 mm Hg, or a 26% reduction (Fig. 10.1). Progressive visual field loss occurred in approximately 18% of patients over a four-year period, or 4% to 5% per year. The incidence of inadequate ocular hypotensive effect, as judged by the need to add additional ocular hypotensive medications, was approximately 5% to 10% per year.

Silverstone and associates[21] have investigated the efficacy of timolol throughout the day with chronic therapy. Both levobunolol and timolol used twice daily provided a consistent ocular hypotensive effect throughout the day. Since the IOP was reduced for at least 12 hours during chronic therapy, the instillation of a second drop provided little additional lowering of IOP.

In controlled studies of timolol, or timolol versus levobunolol, once-daily therapy with timolol appears to be an effective ocular hypotensive regimen. The ocular hypotensive effect of once-daily 0.25% or 0.5% timolol ranged from 17 to 28%, which overlaps with that of twice-daily timolol.[22–25] Aqueous flow shows a diurnal variation, and the ability of timolol to reduce this flow is greatest during the day.[26]

Serendipitously, most of the chronic studies of once-daily instillation of timolol selected a morning instillation. Because timolol decreases aqueous flow after daytime, but not nighttime instillation,[27] and compliance may be greater with a morning rather than evening dose,[28] the morning instillation is probably the better time for once-daily use. However, a more recent study with diurnal, at-home, measurement of IOP suggests that the time of instillation may not be critical in achieving maximal efficacy.[29]

As noted previously in the short-term study of Krupin and associates,[14] little evidence exists for a greater ocular hypotensive effect of 0.5% timolol than for 0.25% timolol with chronic use. A longer term study compared the ocular hypotensive efficacy of twice-daily 0.25% timolol to that of 0.5% timolol in 60 patients for one year.[30] Although the mean baseline IOP was greater in the 0.25% timolol group (26.9 mm Hg vs. 24.8 mm Hg), this group had the greater mean reductions of IOP (22% to 32% vs. 17% to 27%) as well as the greater percentage of successfully treated patients (90% vs. 83%). When 0.25% timolol was compared to 0.25% levobunolol in 55 patients for one year,[31] both agents were similarly effective, decreasing IOP an average of 19% to 20%. Treatment was considered successful in 70% to 71% of patients. Of those failed patients titrated to the 0.5% concentration of their respective agents, no greater mean IOP decrease was observed. Although the response of individual patients may vary, long-term controlled clinical trials provide little data suggesting that 0.5% timolol is more effective than the 0.25% concentration.

The efficacy of even lower concentrations of timolol has been evaluated. A one-year study evaluated the efficacy of 0.1% timolol, twice daily.[32] The mean IOP at baseline was 25.4 mm Hg, which decreased 24% to 19.3 mm Hg. Approximately 70% of the patients were satisfactorily controlled on this treatment. In another study,[33] 18 of 26 timolol patients (69%) were satisfactorily controlled for three months on 0.125% timolol given twice daily. From a mean baseline pressure of 27.8 mm Hg, mean overall reduction was 7.2 mm Hg (25.9%).

The goal of therapy for glaucoma or ocular hypertension is to prevent additional damage to the optic nerve or loss of visual field. This goal is based on observations showing an increased risk of functional and anatomical loss with increasing IOP. This risk is a probability function and does not imply that there is a given physiologic IOP at which loss will occur.[34-36] Some controlled studies support the view that timolol retards the rate of further visual field loss, while others do not.[37-40] For a variety of ethical, scientific and logistical reasons, these studies are difficult to conduct.

The efficacy of timolol has been compared to that of laser trabeculoplasty.[41] For both treatments, additional medications could be added as required. Adequate ocular hypotensive efficacy was observed in 89% of the eyes receiving laser plus medications, in contrast to 66% of the eyes receiving medication only. Based on the first treatment to the eye, laser was effective in 44% of eyes, and timolol was effective in 51% of eyes.[41]

As demonstrated using fluorophotometry,[42,43] timolol acts predominantly by decreasing the production of aqueous humor and does not significantly alter facility of outflow.[44]

The ocular hypotensive effect of timolol is additive to most other therapies, including outflow agents (e.g., pilocarpine) and inflow agents (e.g., acetazolamide, apraclonidine). The additivity of timolol to epinephrine, or to dipivefrin, is more problematic. Conceptually, one would question the rationale for combining a β blocker, timolol, with α- and β-adrenergic agonist, epinephrine. However, for many years, using both drugs has been viewed as effective combination therapy. The twice-daily regimen of each agent, as well as the relative lack of untoward ocular symptoms, makes this a relatively easy two-drug therapy for patients to use. Separating the instillation of timolol and dipivefrin by 3 hours, rather than 10 minutes, while of theoretical benefit, does not seem to alter the efficacy of this combination. However, the additivity is sometimes less than complete and relatively short-lived.[45-57]

Schenker and associates[55] investigated the aqueous humor dynamics supporting the additivity of timolol and epinephrine. They confirmed earlier work that timolol reduced aqueous humor production. They also observed that, by itself, epinephrine both slightly increases aqueous humor production and increases uveoscleral outflow. As the increase in outflow was greater than the increase in production, a net decrease in IOP occurred. When timolol and epinephrine were administered together, the net effect was a decrease in IOP, a decrease in aqueous humor production, and an increase in uveoscleral outflow. However, the variable ocular hypotensive effects of epinephrine when added to various β blockers[45,58] has led to re-evaluation of the mechanism of interaction between these two agents. Clearly, understanding the mechanism of action of epinephrine and its interaction with timolol requires additional research.

CLINICAL USES

Following its introduction into clinical practice in the United States in 1978, timolol quickly became the drug of first choice for the treatment of elevated IOP in most patient populations. This popularity is largely due to its ocular hypotensive efficacy, a duration of action that requires only once- or twice-daily instillation, and a relative lack of untoward ocular symptoms. In addition to its utility in the treatment of primary open-angle glaucoma and ocular hypertension, timolol is effective in the treatment of many secondary glaucomas. Timolol is also effective for the prophylactic treatment of elevations in IOP following laser iridotomy or posterior capsulotomy,[59-62] and cataract surgery.[63,64]

One of the significant advantages of timolol compared with pilocarpine solutions is its less frequent instillation and fewer treatment-related ocular symptoms, which has the potential for better patient compliance. As measured by electronic monitoring in a chronic study, the overall compliance rate with twice-daily timolol was 83%, with great variation among patients.[28] This rate was somewhat higher than the 76% compliance observed with pilocarpine in a separate study.[65]

When topical timolol is administered to patients already receiving oral β-blocking agents for the treatment of systemic hypertension, a significant further reduction of IOP may occur.[66] In patients treated with systemic β blockers, topical adrenoceptor antagonists such as timolol are not absolutely contraindicated.

Timolol is supplied as a 0.25% and 0.5% sterile ophthalmic solution of the levo-isomer of the maleate salt (see Table 10.2). A formulation of timolol in a Gelrite vehicle (Timoptic XE) is also available. A single daily instillation of this formulation in the morning has an ocular hypotensive effect comparable to that of timolol solution used every 12 hours.[67] Multiuse containers of timolol are preserved with benzalkonium chloride 0.01%, and a unit-of-use, nonpreserved product is available (Ocudose). The ocular hypotensive effect of the nonpreserved formulation is the same as the preserved. Timolol is approved for either once- or twice-daily use.

SIDE EFFECTS

Ocular Effects.   The untoward ocular effects of timolol are much less than those of miotics, including pilocarpine. Timolol does not possess the potential for muscarinic-receptor mediated miosis, spasm of accommodation, and browache. Stinging upon instillation, while reported with timolol,[68] is much less frequent or severe than with pilocarpine. Furthermore, since timolol is instilled only once or twice daily, there is less occasion for any untoward symptoms than with the usual 4-times daily dose of pilocarpine. The differential between patient acceptance of pilocarpine and timolol is most apparent in patients under 40 years of age, as they are the most likely to suffer from pilocarpine-induced accommodative spasm. Since timolol has no significant miotic effect, it has advantages over pilocarpine in patients with pre-existing cataracts.

Timolol, however, may cause some untoward ocular ef-

TABLE 10.6

Adverse Effects Possibly Associated with Topical Ophthalmic β Blockers

Cardiovascular system
  Bradycardia
  Conduction arrhythmias
  Hypotension
  Raynaud's phenomenon
  Fluid retention

Pulmonary system
  Bronchoconstriction/Bronchospasm
  Asthma
  Dyspnea

Neurologic system
  Amnesia
  Depression
  Confusion
  Headache
  Migraine prophylaxis
  Impotence
  Insomnia
  Myasthenia gravis

Gastrointestinal system
  Diarrhea
  Nausea

Dermatologic system
  Alopecia
  Nail pigmentation
  Urticaria

Other systemic effects
  Hypoglycemia

Ocular effects
  Allergic blepharoconjunctivitis
  Dry eye / decreased tear break-up time
  Corneal anesthesia
  Macular edema (aphakics)
  Macular hemorrhage / Retinal detachment
  Uveitis
  Cataract progression

Adapted from Novack GD, Leopold IH. The toxicity of topical ophthalmic beta-blockers. J Toxicol—Cut Ocular Toxicol 1987;6:283–297.

fects (Table 10.6).[69–71] A local allergic reaction, somewhat similar to that reported for topical adrenoceptor agonists,[72–74] has been reported.[75] This allergic reaction manifests as a blepharoconjunctivitis, with erythema and edema of the lids. The reaction can occur as early as in the first month of therapy. Management may include changing to another β blocker.[76]

The ability of β blockers to stabilize membrane excitability has been exploited therapeutically in the treatment of selected cardiac arrhythmias. However, when these agents are given topically, such a property can induce corneal anesthesia. Van Buskirk[77,78] reported significant decreases in corneal sensitivity in several patients. In comparative studies using a quantitative esthesiometer, timolol ranks low among β blockers in its corneal anesthetic effects,[3] and corneal sensitivity is not a major clinical problem for timolol.[79] In some patients, timolol can induce superficial punctate keratitis.[78] If this condition becomes chronic and is not treated, it could lead to additional staining and possible corneal epithelial erosions.[80] Topical timolol may reduce tear breakup time,[81] elicit some dry eye symptoms,[82] or decrease tear flow,[83] but it does not appear to induce the severe ocular pemphigoid reaction reported with practolol.[84] Less frequently reported adverse ocular events include macular edema in aphakics, macular hemorrhage, retinal detachment, uveitis, and progressive cataracts.[78,85] None of the commonly used β blockers, including timolol, appears to inhibit corneal epithelial wound healing.

Systemic Effects.   When timolol is given by the topical route, the possibility of systemic β blockade must be considered (see Table 10.6). Within the first few hours after topical instillation of 0.5% timolol, the mean drug plasma level is approximately 1 ng/ml.[5,86–88] This level can be as high as 20 ng/ml in newborns[86] and can be reduced in adults with nasolacrimal occlusion or simple eyelid closure (mean of 0.4 ng/ml).[88] For comparison, therapeutic doses of oral timolol result in levels of 5 to 50 ng/ml, in which the cardiac β blockade is log-linear.[89] Since topical timolol results in mean drug plasma levels less than 5 ng/ml, it is somewhat puzzling that bradycardia is a frequently associated side effect of topical timolol.[90] However, it appears that even with systemic administration, plasma levels of β-blocking agents are not always indicative of systemic β blockade.[91] One should also consider that ocularly instilled medications may reach the heart directly, via nasolacrimal and pharyngeal absorption, without the potential for inactivation by hepatic metabolism or dilution in total body plasma.

The presence of pharmacologically effective plasma levels of timolol after topical instillation dictates that the clinician consider the risk of systemic β blockade when administering any β blocker for glaucoma. Antagonism of β-adrenoceptors can thus result in bradycardia, systemic hypotension, congestive heart failure, heart block, bronchospasm, diarrhea, and amnesia.[92] β-adrenergic antagonists of both subtypes may adversely affect memory consolidation and retrieval.[93–95] All of these adverse effects have occurred with topical timolol therapy (see Table 10.5). In some cases, these adverse events have been serious, life threatening, and even fatal. Systemic adverse events may be more frequent in the elderly because these patients may be more variable in under- and overdosing of medication, have a greater propensity for co-existing systemic conditions, and, as a result of flaccid lids, have the propensity for greater storage of instilled volumes in the lower cul-de-sac.[96]

Mean resting heart rate may decrease 3 to 10 beats per minute during use of timolol.[20] Other cardiovascular effects include palpitations, systemic hypotension, and syncope.[85] Similar to oral β blockers, topical timolol may reduce exercise- or isoproterenol-induced tachycardia. This decrease may be a problem not only in patients with compromised cardiovascular status, but also in patients who normally engage in strenuous exercise.[90,97-100]

Timolol use can bring on wheezing, dyspnea, bronchospasm, and other signs and symptoms of decreased respiratory function.[78] Acute bronchospasm can occur in previously asymptomatic asthmatic patients following the topical use of timolol.[101,102] Timolol elicits an average decrease of 25% in forced expiratory volume (FEV_1) in patients with chronic obstructive pulmonary disease (COPD) (Fig. 10.2).[103] Scharrer and Ober[104] evaluated the safety of timolol in 26 patients with relative cardiovascular and pulmonary contraindications to timolol. While 58% of the patients showed untoward reactions to timolol, 42% did not. This study demonstrates that not all patients expected to have a negative response to timolol actually do so when challenged. Thus, when one reads reports of apparent lack of toxicity of a new β-blocking agent, one should realize the potential for false negatives.[105]

Topical β blockers have been associated with adverse central nervous system (CNS) effects, including depression, emotional lability, and sexual dysfunction. Complaints of lethargy, lightheadedness, weakness, fatigue, mental depression, dissociative behavior, and memory loss are most common. The onset of symptoms varies from a few days to months following initiation of therapy. In most cases these symptoms are mild and transient. In certain patients, however, timolol must be discontinued because of these CNS effects.[85,106]

Timolol may also elicit dermatologic signs and symptoms that include rashes, alopecia, urticaria, and discoloration of nails.[23,78,107] Other systemic effects reported after topical timolol treatment include myasthenia gravis and retroperitoneal fibrosis.[108-111] When treating a nursing mother, clinicians should also be aware that topically applied timolol may find its way to breast milk.[112]

Topical timolol may alter the plasma lipid profile. In hepatic fat cells, stimulation of β-adrenoceptors activates hormone-sensitive lipase, leading to the release of free fatty acids into the circulation as an energy source for exercising muscle. While systemic β-adrenergic antagonists can attenuate the release of free fatty acids from adipose tissue, nonetheless, non-cardioselective β blockers can elicit modest elevations in plasma concentrations of triglycerides and modest decreases in high-density lipoprotein (HDL) cholesterol. This observation is less common with systemic β blockers that are cardioselective or those with intrinsic sympathomimetic activity (ISA).[113] Coleman and associates[114] reported that chronic use of timolol in normal volunteers reduced triglycerides by 12% and HDL by 9%. The clinical relevance of this open-label, uncontrolled trial has been questioned.[115] Freedman and associates[264] have shown that timolol 0.5% used twice daily without nasolacrimal occlusion decreases HDL by 8.0% and raises the ratio of total to HDL cholesterol by 10.0% in normolipidemic adult men. Despite this evidence, however, chronic use of topical timolol does not appear to increase the risk of coronary artery disease.

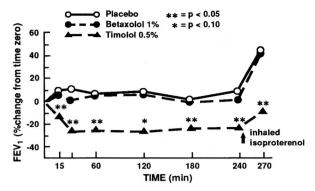

FIGURE 10.2 **Mean change in FEV_1 after instillation of timolol, betaxolol, or placebo (vehicle). Timolol induced a significant decrease in airflow, whereas betaxolol produced values no different from placebo. (Published with permission from the American Journal of Ophthalmology 97:86–92,1984. Copyright by the Ophthalmic Publishing Company.)**

CONTRAINDICATIONS

Timolol is contraindicated in patients with bronchial asthma, a history of bronchial asthma, or severe COPD. It is similarly contraindicated in patients with bradycardia, severe heart block, overt cardiac failure, and hypersensitivity to any of its components (Table 10.7).

More broadly, timolol therapy should be considered with caution in patients with any significant sign, symptom, or history for which systemic β blockade would be medically unwise. This includes disorders of cardiovascular or respiratory origin (e.g., asthma, chronic bronchitis, and emphysema), as well as many other conditions.[116] Spirometric evaluation following institution of timolol therapy may help to identify patients in whom bronchospasm develops following commencement of therapy.[103] In general, however, patients with asthma and other obstructive pulmonary diseases should avoid this drug. Sympathetic stimulation may be essential to support the circulation in individuals with diminished myocardial contractility, and its inhibition by β-adrenoceptor antagonists may precipitate more severe failure.

As may occur with topical timolol, β-adrenoceptor blockade may mask the signs and symptoms of thyrotoxicosis or

TABLE 10.7
Contraindications to Topical Ophthalmic β Blockers

Bronchial asthma
History of bronchial asthma
Severe COPD
Bradycardia
Severe heart block
Overt cardiac failure
Children and infants

acute hypoglycemia. Thus, timolol should be used with caution in patients prone to such disorders, including diabetes.[117,118]

Using two topical β blockers has no potential for added ocular hypotensive efficacy, and such a combination can only increase the possibility of an untoward event. Since the use of timolol in children and infants may result in a relative systemic overdose, its use in these patients should be avoided.

Careful patient histories and examinations are critical prior to using this drug.[119] For many patients, the eye care specialist should contact the patient's internist or primary physician regarding the use of topical timolol or any other topical β blocker. Although this warning is most important for chronic use, some of the reports of serious adverse reactions to timolol involve a single drop of medication.

Levobunolol

PHARMACOLOGY

Similar to timolol, levobunolol is a non-cardioselective β blocker without significant local anesthetic activity or ISA. Like timolol, it is more potent than propranolol when used orally as a treatment for systemic hypertension.[79,120] Its metabolic fate, however, is unlike that of timolol. Levobunolol is metabolized to dihydrobunolol, a compound with equipotent β-blocking effects both systemically and ocularly.[121-123] Topically applied, levobunolol readily penetrates the cornea in rabbits and is metabolized to dihydrobunolol.[124] The potency of levobunolol at the ocular β_2-adrenoceptor is similar to that of timolol.[6]

When given topically to humans with elevated IOP, levobunolol induces a profound and long-lasting ocular hypotension. Levobunolol, 0.5% and 1%, given twice daily for three months reduced mean IOP 9 mm Hg from a baseline pressure of 27 mm Hg.[125] In a large four-year controlled comparison with timolol, the mean reduction in IOP over four years with twice-daily 0.5% and 1% levobunolol was 7 mm Hg, equivalent to that of timolol (see Fig. 10.1). Progressive visual field loss occurred in approximately 18% of patients over a four-year period, or 4% to 5% per year. Inadequate ocular hypotensive effect, as judged by the need to add additional ocular hypotensive medications, was approximately 5% to 10% per year.[20] Levobunolol is similar to timolol in controlling IOP throughout the day.[79,126-129]

As with timolol, the predominant mechanism of levobunolol's ocular hypotensive action is a decrease in the production of aqueous humor, with no significant effect on facility of outflow.[130,131] When pilocarpine and levobunolol are used concomitantly, levobunolol decreases aqueous humor flow while pilocarpine increases trabecular outflow.[132]

Once-daily therapy with levobunolol can be an effective ocular hypotensive regimen. The hypotensive effect of once-daily 0.25% or 0.5% levobunolol is similar to that reported for twice-daily dosing.[23-25,133] Indeed, in one double-masked study where the regimens of once-daily and twice-daily 0.5% levobunolol were directly compared, they were found equivalent.[134] On a single-drop basis, concentrations of levobunolol greater than 0.5% may have enhanced efficacy.[135] Chronic therapy, however, apparently increases the potency of levobunolol. When given chronically once or twice daily, 0.5% and 1% levobunolol are virtually equivalent in ocular hypotensive efficacy.[20,23,125,129,136] The 0.25% and 0.5% concentrations used twice daily are also equally effective.[31] Thus, as with timolol, one may consider using lower concentrations less frequently.

CLINICAL USES

Levobunolol was introduced in the United States in 1985 and is generally available world-wide. Levobunolol is used for the chronic treatment of elevated IOP in ocular hypertension and glaucoma. Levobunolol has a profile similar to timolol in its use with dipivefrin, pilocarpine, or acetazolamide.[130,132,137-139] Also like timolol, levobunolol is effective for prophylactic treatment of elevations in IOP following cataract surgery and Nd:YAG laser capsulotomy.[140] In a study[141] on the use of various agents prophylactically for IOP control following cataract surgery, levobunolol was found the most effective, followed by timolol, with betaxolol not significantly different from placebo. In a separate study[65] in which carbachol was the most effective in controlling postoperative IOP, levobunolol was equieffective to timolol, oral acetazolamide, and pilocarpine gel. Betaxolol was less effective, and apraclonidine was not significantly better than the control.

Levobunolol is supplied as a 0.25% and 0.5% sterile ophthalmic solution of the levo-isomer of the hydrochloride salt, together with the viscosity agent, 1.4% polyvinyl alcohol and preserved with benzalkonium chloride 0.004% (see Table 10.2). All U.S. containers are currently marketed with a passive compliance device, the "C-Cap" (see Chapter 35). In one study,[142] patients who reported that their compliance increased using this device had a greater ocular hypotensive response.

SIDE EFFECTS

Ocular Effects.   Since levobunolol has the same pharmacologic activity as timolol, it has the same advantages over pilocarpine as well as propensity for the same untoward ocular effects as timolol. The ocular comfort of levobunolol is similar to that of timolol,[79] although one report indicates that it is slightly less comfortable than timolol.[68] Corneal anesthesia is not a significant problem with levobunolol, nor does it seem to elicit dry eye symptoms or mydriasis.[3,79,126-129] Although allergic blepharoconjunctivitis can occur with levobunolol, it may also be tolerated in patients in whom timolol elicits an allergic reaction.[76] Dendritic keratopathy, resolving after cessation of treatment, has been reported with levobunolol.[143]

Systemic Effects. Since levobunolol is a potent and effective β_1 and β_2 blocker, it shares with timolol the same potential for systemic β blockade. Mean resting heart rate may decrease 3 to 10 beats per minute during use of levobunolol, and some reduction in blood pressure may occur.[20] Therapeutic dosing with ocular levobunolol results in plasma levels of approximately 1 ng/ml.[144] As with timolol,[97] 0.5% levobunolol, in either a single 20, 35 or 50 μl (commercial) drop, reduces maximal exercise-induced heart rate by approximately 9 beats per minute in normal volunteers.[145] A three-month study using 0.5% levobunolol twice daily showed no difference in either efficacy or safety among these three drop sizes.[145]

CONTRAINDICATIONS

The contraindications for levobunolol are the same as for timolol. Levobunolol is contraindicated in patients with bronchial asthma, a history of bronchial asthma, or severe COPD. It is contraindicated in patients with bradycardia or severe heart block, overt cardiac failure, and in patients with hypersensitivity to any of its components. As with timolol, caution should be used when considering levobunolol therapy in patients with any significant sign, symptom, or history for which systemic β blockade would be medically unwise.

Betaxolol

PHARMACOLOGY

Betaxolol is a β blocker with relative specificity for the β_1-adrenoceptor (cardioselective). At the ocular β_2-adrenoceptor, betaxolol is nearly two orders of magnitude less potent than timolol.[6] Betaxolol (Kerlone) is also available for oral use in the treatment of systemic hypertension.[146]

β_1-adrenoceptors are typically thought of as involved in cardiac rate, rhythm and force; β_2-adrenoceptors are usually thought of as involved in pulmonary function. However, β-receptors are also present in the vascular system. In the skeletal muscular regions in dogs, 85% of the β-adrenoceptors belong to the β_1-subtype. In contrast, in arterioles, nearly all of the β-adrenoceptors belong to the β_2-subtype. Approximately 10% to 30% of the β-adrenoceptors in the mammalian cardiac ventricles are of the β_2-subtype,[147] but most of the β-adrenoceptors in the heart are of the β_1-subtype.[148] In the human lung, the ratio of β_2-adrenoceptors to β_1-adrenoceptors is 3:1.[149] This distribution suggests that the role of the various adrenoceptor subtypes is probably more complex than generally thought. In addition, this means that agents that exhibit a wide separation of selectivity in pre-clinical experiments may be less selective in actual clinical use.

Animal studies suggest that a certain relaxing effect of betaxolol on peripheral vascular beds may contribute to both the systemic and ocular hypotensive effects of the drug.[150–153]

In rabbits receiving single, topical ocular doses of phenylephrine, timolol, or betaxolol, all three agents caused substantial, localized constriction in the arterioles that supply the ciliary processes but did not affect the downstream bore of the same vessels. After receiving a once-daily dose for 7 weeks, tolerance reduced the response to betaxolol to insignificant levels and the response to phenylephrine substantially, whereas timolol continued to produce levels of vasoconstriction identical to those seen with single-dose administration.

Clinical doses of oral betaxolol result in plasma levels of 10–40 ng/ml,[154,155] with a half-life of 12 hours.[156] Given topically, 0.5% betaxolol solution results in plasma levels of approximately 0.5 ng/ml, or half that of timolol 0.25%.[157] Betaxolol, at least when administered systemically, appears to be metabolized to inactive compounds.[158,159]

As with other β blockers, the ocular hypotensive mechanism of betaxolol is a reduction in aqueous production.[160] In this regard, controlled studies have shown that, while effective in reducing aqueous humor production, betaxolol is less effective and in one instance less potent than levobunolol or timolol, and similar in efficacy to carteolol.[161,162] Many research studies have focused on the ocular hypotensive efficacy of betaxolol relative to other topical β blockers. Initial studies found 0.25% betaxolol more effective than its vehicle.[163–167] Subsequent studies evaluated the drug at a concentration of 0.5%. Twice-daily 0.5% betaxolol gave results similar to 0.5% timolol in studies using patient populations up to approximately 20 patients per group.[168–171] Unfortunately, the sample size of these studies combined with the patient selection criteria did not allow for a powerful comparison of equivalency of these two agents. A study of similar size did report that timolol was a more effective ocular hypotensive agent than betaxolol by approximately 2 mm Hg.[172]

In a large three-month study,[173] twice-daily instillations resulted in mean reductions in IOP of 6 mm Hg with 0.25% and 0.5% levobunolol, and 4 mm Hg with 0.5% betaxolol solution. Whereas the difference in efficacy between levobunolol and betaxolol was statistically significant, no such difference was noted in systemic safety measures. Also, the duration of action of betaxolol was less than that of levobunol. In a very large (353 patient) study, patients successfully controlled on timolol therapy were either switched to betaxolol or remained on timolol therapy for three months. Those patients switched to betaxolol solution had a significant increase in both IOP and ocular side effects (burning, stinging and tearing) when compared with patients who continued to receive timolol.[174] Betaxolol appears similar to dipivefrin in its ocular hypotensive efficacy.[175]

Betaxolol may be used in combination with pilocarpine, dipivefrin or acetazolamide.[176] Dipivefrin or epinephrine seems to provide a greater additional pressure reduction when added to betaxolol than to timolol,[58,177] but this observation may relate more to the fact that timolol is a more effective ocular hypotensive agent than is betaxolol.[178] In other studies, however, the additivity of dipivefrin to either timolol or betaxolol occurs only in some patients.[179]

The effect of long-term betaxolol treatment on visual fields has been compared to timolol.[180–183] Although the ocular hypotensive efficacy of timolol was greater than that of betaxolol, there was a small (1–2 dB) difference in mean sensitivity of the visual field in favor of betaxolol, a difference that may not be clinically significant. A study of normal volunteers demonstrated that neither betaxolol, epinephrine, pilocarpine, nor timolol had any influence on visual function as determined by high-pass, resolution perimetry.[184]

CLINICAL USES

Topical betaxolol is indicated in the chronic treatment of ocular hypertension and open-angle glaucoma. Given its relative cardioselectivity, it may be used successfully in patients with coexistent glaucoma and pulmonary disease.[185,186] Note, however, that topical betaxolol may still elicit adverse cardiovascular and pulmonary effects.

Overall, the selection of betaxolol is a relative benefit-risk decision. In head-to-head studies against non-cardioselective agents, betaxolol is generally a less effective ocular hypotensive agent. From a safety perspective, however, betaxolol induces less, although not nil, systemic β blockade than these other agents. While some evidence indicates that betaxolol may differ from timolol in its effects on visual fields and vasculature, the clinical relevance of these observations is not yet clear.

Betaxolol is less effective than timolol or levobunolol in preventing post-cataract surgery elevations in IOP, especially when a viscoelastic agent is used.[65,141,187] Thus, it is probably not the agent of choice for this indication. Betaxolol is supplied in two ophthalmic formulations, a sterile solution of 0.5% betaxolol HCl (Betoptic), and a sterile suspension of 0.25% betaxolol HCl (Betoptic-S). The suspension is a unique formulation containing a polyacrylic acid polymer (carbomer 934P) and a cationic exchange resin, which is believed to increase the drug residence time in the human eye (see Chapter 2).[188] Both products are the racemic compound, preserved with 0.01% benzalkonium chloride, and approved for twice-daily use. The 0.25% suspension is equivalent in efficacy to the 0.5% solution.

SIDE EFFECTS

Ocular Effects.   The prevalence of ocular discomfort upon topical instillation is significantly lower for 0.25% betaxolol suspension than for 0.5% betaxolol solution.[189] The stinging elicited by 0.5% betaxolol solution is significantly greater than any discomfort elicited with timolol or levobunolol.[168,171,190,191] Some studies suggest that betaxolol reduces corneal sensitivity, in some cases more than does timolol,[192–194] but in other cases no significant effect occurs.[195]

Systemic Effects.   Systemic betaxolol has, on average, less effect in attenuating pulmonary function than do the

non-cardioselective agents.[196–198] A significant clinical advantage of topical betaxolol in the treatment of elevated IOP is its much reduced potential for inhibiting pulmonary function. Nine patients with reactive airway disease who had at least a 15% reduction of FEV_1 to topical timolol were enrolled in a study of topical 0.5% timolol, 1.0% betaxolol or vehicle. Timolol reduced mean FEV_1 approximately 25%, while betaxolol and placebo had little effect on FEV_1 (see Fig. 10.2).[103] Timolol, levobunolol, pindolol, befunolol and metipranolol are similar in reducing mean pulmonary function, while betaxolol is similar to its vehicle.[199,200] While most of these studies used 0.5% timolol and 0.5% or 1.0% betaxolol solution, a more recent study[201] reported that 0.25% betaxolol suspension has fewer cardiovascular and pulmonary effects than does 0.5% timolol solution in healthy volunteers. Note, however, that the generalizing of these results to patients with coexistent pulmonary disease and glaucoma may be impractical since one can question the statement of safety based on mean effect (little with betaxolol) versus individual patient effect (some patients may respond adversely to topical betaxolol).[202] Nevertheless, these findings have been replicated in many other studies and substantiate the relative safety of betaxolol in patients with coexistent pulmonary disease and glaucoma.[105,203–206]

Thus, a key clinical advantage of betaxolol is in the treatment of patients with coexistent chronic open-angle glaucoma and pulmonary disease. However, some pulmonary physicians strongly caution against the use of any β blocker, irrespective of cardioselectivity or route of administration, in patients with existing respiratory disease. Should such therapy be contemplated, the pulmonary physician should work closely with the eye care specialist, and the objective measurements of pulmonary function should be determined both before and during ocular therapy.[207]

The potential of betaxolol to elicit systemic $β_1$-adrenoceptor blockade has been investigated. In a study on resting cardiovascular function in older patients, topical instillation of timolol (0.25% and 0.5%), carteolol (1% and 2%), and metipranolol (0.3% and 0.6%) decreased mean heart rate 14% to 17%. However, topical betaxolol 0.5% did not have any significant effect. Some patients in all groups did exhibit a 15% to 20% reduction in systolic blood pressure.[208] In a study of exercise-induced tachycardia in normal volunteers, the maximal heart rate obtained upon exercise decreased 9 beats/minute (bpm) with topical timolol and 4 bpm with betaxolol. The effect of betaxolol did not differ significantly from that of its vehicle.[97] Other studies have shown that compared with placebo, all β blockers result in some degree of systemic β blockade, and the increasing order of potency is betaxolol (0.5%), metipranolol (0.6%), and timolol (0.5%).[98,209] Patients who have various adverse experiences with timolol such as dyspnea and bradycardia may often successfully switch to betaxolol. Betaxolol therapy, however, may result in poorer control of IOP.[210,211]

Although betaxolol generally elicits less systemic β blockade than do non-cardioselective agents, it does cause undesirable systemic effects in some patients. Reported adverse experiences include congestive heart failure,[212] myocardial infarction,[213] respiratory difficulties strongly suggestive of obstructive airway disease,[214] weakness with severe sinus bradycardia,[215] and wheezing with objective reduction in pulmonary function.[216] Within its first year of marketing in the United States, the Food and Drug Administration received 56 reports of adverse events associated with betaxolol solution. Nine of these required hospitalization (six for asthma, and one each for respiratory distress, bradycardia with syncope, and respiratory distress).[217] Similar reports in Germany with both oral and ophthalmic betaxolol led to a re-examination of the labeling for these products.[218]

There has been a report of clinical depression associated with the use of topical betaxolol; the depression improved with cessation of betaxolol therapy.[219] Two pilot studies[106,220] performed at one center investigated the relationship of adverse CNS events to timolol and betaxolol therapy in glaucoma patients. In the first study, 18 patients with adverse CNS events to timolol switched to betaxolol. Of the 18 patients, 16 (89%) noted symptomatic improvement with betaxolol. In the second study, seven patients were treated with timolol and betaxolol in two phases of a double-masked, crossover study. In two patients CNS symptoms resolved with betaxolol; in three patients symptoms improved; and in one patient symptoms worsened with betaxolol.[106] Another center compared betaxolol and timolol using the Minnesota Multiphasic Personality Inventory (MMPI). The incidence of insomnia, depression and diarrhea was less with betaxolol than with timolol.[220]

CONTRAINDICATIONS

Betaxolol is contraindicated in patients with sinus bradycardia, greater than first-degree atrioventricular block, cardiogenic shock, or overt cardiac failure. It is also contraindicated in patients with hypersensitivity to any of its components. As noted above, severe respiratory reactions have occurred, and the drug must therefore be used with caution in patients with asthma or COPD. Also, since minor changes in heart rate and blood pressure can occur, this agent must be used with caution, or avoided, in patients with a history of cardiac failure or heart block. Although factors influencing β blockade in the CNS are not well understood, this selective agent may have some advantages.

Metipranolol

PHARMACOLOGY

Like timolol and levobunolol, metipranolol is a non-cardioselective β blocker without significant local anesthetic activity or ISA. Metipranolol has been used worldwide, both orally in the treatment of systemic hypertension and topically for the treatment of elevated IOP.[221-224]

Like levobunolol, metipranolol has an active metabo-

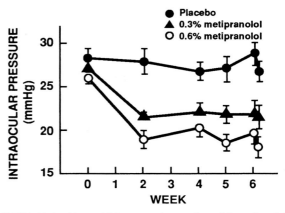

FIGURE 10.3 **Mean IOP over six weeks with twice-daily instillation of 0.3% and 0.6% metipranolol. (Published with permission from the American Journal of Ophthalmology 112:302–307,1991. Copyright by the Ophthalmic Publishing Company.)**

lite, des-acetyl-metipranolol, which is an effective β blocker.[222,225] Metipranolol has been used in concentrations ranging from 0.1% to 0.6% and has ocular hypotensive efficacy within the range of other non-cardioselective agents (Fig. 10.3).[226-234] Metipranolol 0.3% has an ocular hypotensive efficacy comparable to that of 0.1% dipivefrin.[235]

As with other β-adrenoceptor antagonists, metipranolol decreases aqueous humor production.[226] In Germany, a combination product contains both metipranolol and pilocarpine, and combination therapy appears effective.[236-238]

CLINICAL USES

Metipranolol is used for the chronic treatment of elevated IOP in ocular hypertension and glaucoma. Its utility in IOP elevations following laser or cataract surgery, as well as its additivity with other ocular hypotensive agents, have not yet been fully evaluated.

Metipranolol is available in the United States as Optipranolol, a sterile ophthalmic solution of 0.3% racemic metipranolol HCl, preserved with 0.004% benzalkonium chloride and approved for twice-daily use.

SIDE EFFECTS

Ocular Effects. When given twice daily at the 0.6% strength to ocular hypertensive patients, metipranolol elicits greater discomfort than does levobunolol 0.5%.[229,239] Metipranolol therapy has also been associated with allergic blepharoconjunctivitis or periorbital dermatitis[240] similar to that reported for other ophthalmic β blockers.[69,70]

In 1990, approximately 50 cases of anterior uveitis were reported in the United Kingdom (U.K.), where metipranolol has been available since 1986. At one hospital, the incidence of uveitis in patients using 0.6% metipranolol was 14% (15/109). All cases resolved with appropriate management.[241]

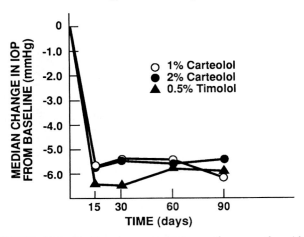

FIGURE 10.4   **Median change in IOP over three months with twice-daily instillation of 1.0% and 2.0% carteolol compared to 0.5% timolol. (Adapted from Stewart WC, Shields MB, Allen RC, et al. A three-month comparison of 1% and 2% carteolol and 0.5% timolol in open-angle glaucoma. Graefe's Arch Clin Exp Ophthalmol 1991;229:258–261.)**

Subsequently, in cooperation with British health authorities, the manufacturer voluntarily withdrew the various concentrations of preserved, multi-dose metipranolol from the United Kingdom market. Non-preserved, unit-dose metipranolol continues to be available in the 0.1% and 0.3% concentrations in the U.K. In Germany, a post-marketing surveillance study indicated newly diagnosed uveitis in only five of 1306 patients (0.4%). None of these cases required cessation of therapy. Thus, there appears to be a low risk of uveitis associated with the use of metipranolol in Germany, in contrast to the reported experience in the United Kingdom, which may result from differences in the formulation.[242] Drug-induced anterior uveitis has also been reported as a rare event in the United States.

Systemic Effects.   Based on its pharmacologic activity, metipranolol theoretically shares with timolol and levobunolol the same potential for systemic β blockade. However, several studies show that the β-adrenoceptor blockade elicited by topical metipranolol may be less than that observed with timolol, although more than that observed with betaxolol.[99,208,209,243,244] As with other reports of greater relative safety, the relevance of this finding bears additional evaluation in the clinical setting.

CONTRAINDICATIONS

The contraindications for metipranolol in the United States are the same as for timolol and levobunolol.

Carteolol

PHARMACOLOGY

Carteolol is a non-cardioselective β blocker similar to timolol, levobunolol and metipranolol. As with levobunolol and metipranolol, a primary metabolite of carteolol, 8-hydroxycarteolol, is also an ocular β blocker.[245,246] In contrast to other topical β-adrenoceptor antagonists, carteolol possesses intrinsic sympathomimetic activity (ISA). In rabbits, topically applied carteolol is well absorbed through the cornea into the aqueous humor.[247] The mechanism of carteolol's ocular hypotensive effect is a reduction in aqueous humor production,[248] without any apparent effect on outflow.[249] In a single-drop study of aqueous humor dynamics in 40 ocular hypertensive patients, timolol induced the greatest decrease of aqueous humor flow (39%), followed by betaxolol (24%) and carteolol (20%).[161]

When given as a single dose, an ocular hypotensive response occurs with concentrations of carteolol ranging from 0.5% to 2%.[250] In an 8-week study, 2% carteolol had ocular hypotensive efficacy similar to that of 0.75% carbachol and to a wide range of pilocarpine concentrations.[251] In a study of 2% carteolol in 12 patients for two weeks, carteolol produced a significant reduction in IOP of approximately 13%.[252]

Several studies have compared the ocular hypotensive efficacy of carteolol and timolol. Overall, some studies have reported equivalency of carteolol to timolol, while others have found timolol either more effective or longer lasting (Fig. 10.4).[253–255] When compared with levobunolol 0.5%, carteolol 2% appears to be less effective as an ocular hypotensive agent.[256] In two separate post-marketing studies involving over 900 patients, carteolol was well tolerated and judged effective and safe in patients switched from other β blockers.[224,257] Chronic treatment with carteolol has been reported to improve retinal sensitivity, similar to timolol,[258] although critical ocular perfusion pressures were reduced more with carteolol than with timolol.[259]

CLINICAL USES

Carteolol is used for the chronic treatment of elevated IOP in ocular hypertension and glaucoma. Its utility in IOP elevations following laser or cataract surgery, as well as its additivity with other ocular hypotensive agents, have not been fully evaluated.

Carteolol is supplied in the United States as Ocupress, a sterile ophthalmic solution of 1.0% racemic carteolol HCl, preserved with 0.005% benzalkonium chloride and approved for twice-daily use.

SIDE EFFECTS

Ocular Effects.   Carteolol 1% and 2% are less irritating than 0.5% timolol.[260] However, unlike other topical β blockers, use of carteolol 1% can cause a moderate corneal anesthesia.[195]

Systemic Effects.   Although the ISA of carteolol might provide some reduced potential for systemic effect, carteolol theoretically shares with other non-cardioselective β blockers the same potential for systemic β blockade. When compared to timolol and levobunolol, carteolol appears similar in its reduction of mean heart rate.[254,256] Various studies evaluating the systemic β-adrenoceptor blockade induced by topical carteolol have found it either similar to, or greater than, that of timolol. In asthmatics, carteolol has slightly less effect on mean FEV_1 than does metipranolol.[243] In normal volunteers, carteolol elicited more $β_1$-adrenoceptor blockade than did timolol or metipranolol in one study,[99] but equivalent effects in another study.[261] In the elderly, carteolol has an effect on resting heart rate similar to timolol and metipranolol, but greater than that of betaxolol.[208] In general, any theoretical advantage of the ISA of topical carteolol has yet to be demonstrated clinically in controlled studies.[262] Administered systemically, carteolol has little effect on plasma lipids.[263] However, Freedman and associates[264] have shown that topical carteolol 1.0% used twice daily without nasolacrimal occlusion decreases high-density lipoprotein (HDL) cholesterol by 3.3% and raises the ratio of total to HDL cholesterol by 4.0% in normolipidemic adult men. The clinical relevance of this observation needs further evaluation.

CONTRAINDICATIONS

The contraindications for carteolol are the same as for timolol and levobunolol.

Cholinergic Agonists (Miotics)

Cholinergic agonists are drugs that produce biologic responses similar to those of acetylcholine. These drugs are also known as *parasympathomimetics* or *cholinomimetics*, and in clinical practice are usually referred to as *miotics*. Cholinergic agonists are classified according to their mechanism of action as direct acting or indirect acting (Table 10.8). The direct-acting drugs activate cholinergic receptors directly at sites on the postsynaptic membranes of nerves or at the neuroeffector junctions of the iris sphincter muscle and ciliary body. The indirect-acting agents exert their cholinergic effects primarily by inhibiting cholinesterase, thereby making increased amounts of acetylcholine available at cholinergic receptors. The cholinesterase inhibitors are subclassified as reversible and irreversible (see Table 10.8). The irreversible cholinesterase inhibitors are exemplified by the organophosphate compound, echothiophate iodide, the cholinesterase inhibitor most commonly used to

TABLE 10.8
Classification of Cholinergic Agonists

Direct-acting
  Acetylcholine
  Methacholine
  Pilocarpine[a]
  Carbachol[a]

Indirect-acting (Cholinesterase inhibitors)
  Reversible
    Physostigmine
    Neostigmine
    Edrophonium
    Demecarium
  Irreversible
    Echothiophate[a]
    Diisopropylfluorophosphate (DFP)

[a]Used to treat glaucoma

treat glaucoma. Pilocarpine and carbachol, both of which are direct acting, and echothiophate, an indirect acting agent, are the miotics most frequently used for treating glaucoma (Table 10.9).

Pilocarpine

PHARMACOLOGY

An alkaloid of natural plant origin, pilocarpine is a direct-acting cholinergic agonist with a dominant action at muscarinic sites both peripherally and centrally. Like other choline esters, it affects the cardiovascular system, exocrine glands, and smooth muscle. The effects of pilocarpine on the cardiovascular system are complex. Small doses injected intravenously briefly reduce blood pressure, as would be anticipated due to stimulation of muscarinic receptors, which relaxes the vasculature. However, some evidence suggests that postsynaptic muscarinic receptors in autonomic ganglia may mediate a vasopressor action.[265] Therefore, under certain circumstances pilocarpine may increase blood pressure.

Exocrine glands are particularly sensitive to pilocarpine. Pilocarpine, 5 to 15 mg administered subcutaneously, has been used both to increase salivation and as a diaphoretic. More recently, an oral preparation of pilocarpine (Salagen) has improved oral dryness in patients with radiation-induced xerostomia who have some residual salivary function. Increased salivation, sweating, and mucous membrane and gastric secretions can also occur as adverse effects of pilocarpine administration.[265]

The cholinomimetic action of pilocarpine on smooth muscle muscarinic receptors generally results in contraction.

TABLE 10.9
Commonly Used Miotics

Generic Name	Trade Name	Manufacturer	Concentration
Pilocarpine HCL solution	Pilocarpine HCL	(Various)	0.5, 1, 2, 3, 4, 6%
	Isopto Carpine	Alcon	0.25, 0.5, 1, 2, 3, 4, 5, 6, 8, 10%
	Pilocar	Ciba Vision	0.5, 1, 2, 3, 4, 6%
	Adsorbocarpine	Alcon	1, 2, 4%
	Akarpine	Akorn	1, 2, 4%
Pilocarpine nitrate solution	Pilagan	Allergan	1, 2, 4%
Pilocarpine insert	Ocusert Pilo-20	Alza	20 µg/hr
	Ocusert Pilo-40		40 µg/hr
Pilocarpine gel	Pilopine H.S. Gel	Alcon	4%
Carbachol, topical	Isopto Carbachol	Alcon	0.75, 1.5, 2.25, 3%
Echothiophate iodide	Phospholine Iodide	Wyeth-Ayerst	0.03, 0.06, 0.125, 0.25%

Pilocarpine enhances the tone and motility in the gastrointestinal tract, ureters, urinary bladder, gallbladder, and ciliary ducts. Since bronchiolar musculature contracts, asthmatic attacks may be precipitated. The response of intraocular smooth muscle to pilocarpine is pupillary constriction, spasm of accommodation, and reduction of IOP.[265]

Although the precise mechanism by which pilocarpine reduces IOP has not been established, the most widely accepted explanation involves direct stimulation of the longitudinal muscle of the ciliary body, which in turn causes the scleral spur to widen the trabecular spaces and increase aqueous outflow.[266] Due to an age-related decline in ciliary muscle mobility, pilocarpine and other miotics may induce a decreasing aqueous outflow response with increasing patient age.[266] However, pilocarpine appears to reduce IOP to the same degree in both healthy and glaucomatous eyes, including those with ocular hypertension. In each case pilocarpine reduces IOP approximately 10% to 40%.[267] On long-term administration pilocarpine has increasing hypotensive effects in concentrations up to 4%, but when used in higher concentrations it appears to have little additional benefit.[268] Ocular pigmentation influences this ocular hypotensive response. Blue eyes demonstrate maximal ocular hypotensive responses, while darkly pigmented eyes demonstrate a relative resistance to IOP reduction (Table 10.10).[269] This dose-response effect should be considered when treating darkly pigmented patients with glaucoma. These patients may require pilocarpine solutions in concentrations exceeding 4%.

As with other ocular hypotensive agents, pilocarpine also exerts a substantial influence in dampening the diurnal IOP variation in patients with glaucoma (Fig. 10.5).[270]

Because of its activity at muscarinic receptor sites on the iris sphincter and ciliary muscles, pilocarpine causes pupillary constriction and varying degrees of accommodative spasm, depending on the patient's age. Long-term therapy with pilocarpine or other miotics alters iris muscle activity and may cause permanent miosis resulting from loss of iris radial muscle tone and from fibrosis of the sphincter muscle.[271]

In addition, most eyes with primary open-angle glaucoma that are treated with pilocarpine demonstrate narrowing of the anterior chamber angle and thickening of the crystalline lens following each instillation of the drug (Figs. 10.6 and 10.7).[272] These effects are measurable within 15 minutes, reach their maximum in one hour, and usually dissipate after two hours.[272] However, in about 15% of eyes with primary open-angle glaucoma undergoing long-term pilocarpine therapy, the drug induces a deepening of the anterior chamber and flattening of the lens, an effect that is not apparently observed in healthy eyes.[272] The reasons for this paradoxical cycloplegia are unknown.

CLINICAL USES

Since its introduction into clinical practice in 1876, pilocarpine has remained the most useful miotic for management of primary open-angle glaucoma, acute angle-closure glaucoma, and many secondary glaucomas. Pilocarpine is commercially available as an ophthalmic solution in concentrations from 0.25% to 10% (see Table 10.9). Although rarely used, it is available in concentrations from 1% to 6% in combination with 1% epinephrine bitartrate (0.5% free epinephrine base). The 2% concentration is available in combination with physostigmine. In some countries, timolol

TABLE 10.10
Mean Applanation Intraocular Pressures after Topical Pilocarpine in Open-Angle Glaucoma Patients with Differing Iris Color (± SEM)

Group	Baseline		1% Solution		4% Solution		8% Solution	
	R	L	R	L	R	L	R	L
Blue[a] (N = 8)	29.28 ± 2.23	29.28 ± 1.84	21.63 ± 1.25	30.63 ±2.48	19.00 ± 0.91	29.37 ± 2.98	18.80 ± 1.41	29.48 ± 2.73
Brown[a] (N = 7)	28.55 ± 1.93	29.05 ± 2.15	24.58 ± 2.24	29.00 ±2.52	20.10 ± 2.10	27.2 ± 2.78	20.14 ± 2.43	28.00 ± 2.46
Black[a] (N = 9)	28.15 ± 2.03	28.29 ± 1.94	24.22 ± 1.41	28.10 ±1.30	22.10 ± 1.60	27.1 ± 1.27	21.11 ± 1.61	27.10 ±1.38

[a]Blue, blue-eyed white patients; Brown, brown-eyed white patients; Black, black patients.
Modified from Harris LS, Galin MA. Effect of ocular pigmentation on hypotensive response to pilocarpine. Am J Ophthalmol 1971;72:923–925.

0.5% is available as a fixed combination with 2% and 4% pilocarpine. These preparations are designed to simplify drug usage when the combination of agents is warranted. In addition, a sustained release, membrane-bound drug delivery system (Ocusert) can deliver pilocarpine at carefully controlled rates of 20 or 40 μg/hr. More recently, pilocarpine has become commercially available as a 4% ophthalmic gel that is supplied in 3.5 g tubes.[273]

The dosage frequency for pilocarpine solutions is usually four times daily. Twice-daily dosage without nasolacrimal occlusion usually results in inadequate control of IOP.[224] Moreover, because patients instructed to use drops four times daily frequently will use them only two or three times per day, it is often unwise to recommend the use of pilocarpine solutions in dosage frequencies less than four times daily. If nasolacrimal occlusion is performed, however, twice-daily dosing may achieve adequate IOP control.[275] Although pilocarpine is available in concentrations exceeding 4%, there is usually no advantage in using these except in black patients and in patients with very darkly pigmented irides.[272,274,276]

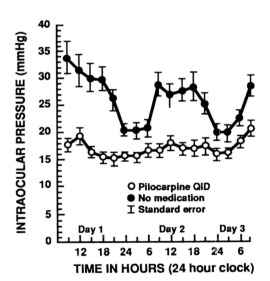

FIGURE 10.5 **Effect of pilocarpine on diurnal variation of IOP in patients with glaucoma. (Reprinted with permission from Worthen DM. Effect of pilocarpine drops on the diurnal intraocular pressure variation in patients with glaucoma. Invest Ophthalmol 1976;15:784–787.)**

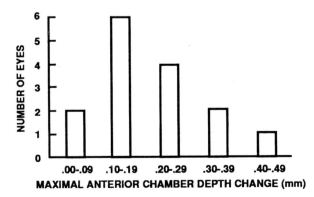

FIGURE 10.6 **Frequency distribution of maximal changes in anterior chamber depth found in 85% of cases following instillation of 1% to 4% pilocarpine. (Reprinted with permission from Abramson DH, Chang S, Coleman J. Pilocarpine therapy in glaucoma. Effects on anterior chamber depth and lens thickness in patients receiving long-term therapy. Arch Ophthalmol 1976; 94:914–918. Copyright © 1976, American Medical Association.)**

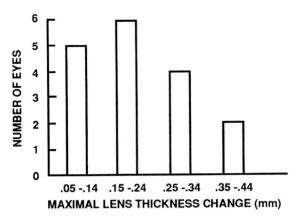

FIGURE 10.7   **Frequency distribution of maximal changes in lens thickness found in 85% of cases following instillation of 1% to 4% pilocarpine. (Reprinted with permission from Abramson DH, Chang S, Coleman J. Pilocarpine therapy in glaucoma. Effects on anterior chamber depth and lens thickness in patients receiving long-term therapy. Arch Ophthalmol 1976;94:914–918. Copyright © 1976, American Medical Association.)**

Pilocarpine remains one of the most useful drugs in the management of glaucoma. Compared with other ocular hypotensive agents, pilocarpine significantly reduces IOP in most patients while causing relatively few adverse effects. It is particularly useful for reducing IOP in patients with primary open-angle glaucoma and for relieving acute angle-closure attacks. When used long term, pilocarpine may be associated with poorer postoperative results in patients having combined cataract and glaucoma filtering surgery than occur in patients who have not received pilocarpine preoperatively.[271] The use of pilocarpine for hastening the resolution of hyphema has been advocated, although such use is of unproved benefit.[272,274]

The maximum ocular hypotensive effect achieved with the Ocusert system occurs about two hours after insertion of the device and lasts about 7 days (see Fig. 3.25). Thus, this device facilitates patient compliance because it requires less frequent application compared with the instillation of pilocarpine drops 4 times daily. The Ocusert Pilo-20 delivers about 20 μg of pilocarpine per hour and has a hypotensive effect approximately equivalent to 1% to 2% pilocarpine solution instilled every 6 hours.[277] The Ocusert Pilo-40 delivers about 40 μg of pilocarpine per hour and has a hypotensive effect approximately equivalent to 2% to 4% pilocarpine solution instilled every 6 hours. The Ocusert is supplied in packages containing 8 individual sterile units. In addition to improved patient compliance, the advantages of the Ocusert compared with pilocarpine solutions include convenience and continuous control of IOP. Disturbances of vision are less pronounced than with the topical solution.[278]

Miosis with the Ocusert is nearly always less intense and less variable than with pilocarpine solutions. In general, the Ocusert provides less frequent, less intense, and fewer fluctuations of vision (refraction, distance vision, near vision, and miosis) compared with pilocarpine solutions.[279]

The visual effects from the Ocusert Pilo-20 do not differ substantially from those of the Ocusert Pilo-40, except for some additional miosis with the latter. Although drug-induced myopic changes may occur with the Ocusert, these are generally low and are more easily corrected with spectacles than are the more highly variable refractive changes associated with pilocarpine drops.[279]

Major disadvantages associated with the Ocusert include difficulty with retention and unnoticed loss of the unit from the eye, rupture of the membrane resulting in excessive medication delivery, and high cost compared with pilocarpine solutions. Several studies[279,280] have shown that only about 50% of patients are successful in wearing the device after three months. The primary reasons for discontinuing the device usually relate to discomfort, difficulty in retaining the device in the eye, and difficulty with insertion and removal. The most critical period of adjustment appears to be the first two weeks. Novak and Stewart[279] found that 71% of the unsuccessful patients discontinued the unit by the end of the first week. Age may also be a significant factor in success, since 74% of the unsuccessful patients were age 60 years or older.[279] Because of the problems of retention, foreign body sensation, difficulty with insertion and removal, and high cost, the Ocusert is rarely used as a drug delivery system for pilocarpine.

The Ocusert may be of particular benefit for the young glaucoma patient (under 40 years of age) who, because of contraindications to β blockers or dipivefrin, requires pilocarpine but who cannot tolerate the drug-induced accommodative spasm and refractive changes associated with pilocarpine solutions or gel. The fact that the Ocusert provides continuous control of IOP may be a significant advantage for elderly patients whose ability to regularly instill pilocarpine solutions may be questionable. On the other hand, since some degree of manual dexterity is required to insert, position, and remove the device correctly, the Ocusert is a poor choice for patients with severe arthritis, tremors, or other fine motor problems unless the patient has some assistance from a spouse, family member, or attendant.

The Ocusert can be used concomitantly with various other antiglaucoma medications. The pilocarpine release rate is not influenced by oral carbonic anhydrase inhibitors or topical solutions of β blockers or dipivefrin. In addition, concomitant therapy with topical antibiotics or steroids may be employed, and topical anesthetics and sodium fluorescein can be used for tonometry without removing the device.[273]

The usual dosage of pilocarpine gel is a one-half-inch ribbon applied in the lower conjunctival sac of the affected eye(s) once a day at bedtime. Adverse effects associated with the once-daily dosage of the 4% gel are not significantly different qualitatively or quantitatively from those associated with the four-times-daily instillation of the 4% drops.[281] Krause and associates,[282] however, have demonstrated that the drops tend to increase myopia and impair nocturnal visual acuity more than does the gel.

Pilocarpine is also indicated, along with other agents, to treat acute angle-closure glaucoma. During an acute angle-closure attack, IOP is often in excess of 60 mm Hg. At those high pressures the ischemic iris sphincter is unresponsive to pilocarpine. Topical β blockers, apraclonidine, or systemic agents are indicated initially to bring the pressure below 50 mm Hg before pilocarpine is administered. The reduction in vitreous volume induced by a systemic hyperosmotic agent helps prevent forward movement of the lens caused by pilocarpine.[283] Pilocarpine is also useful during laser iridotomy to facilitate stretching of the iris.[284]

SIDE EFFECTS

Ocular Effects.   Although pilocarpine is still an important agent for the medical management of many patients with glaucoma, numerous side effects, both ocular and systemic, may be associated with its use in long-term therapy. Adverse ocular events (Table 10.11) are relatively common and necessitate discontinuing the drug in a substantial number of patients. One of the most annoying adverse effects is accommodative spasm, which can last for 2 to 3 hours following instillation of the topical solution. For this reason patients under 40 years of age generally find pilocarpine intolerable.[285] This effect can be minimized by using the lowest concentrations, by changing to the gel[281] or Ocusert, or by treating the symptoms by prescribing a clip-on minus spectacle prescription during the period of blurred vision.[286] Because the accommodative spasm and resulting drug-induced myopia is variable with pilocarpine drops, prescribing permanent spectacles usually does not overcome this problem. Fortunately, these visual disturbances are less frequent and less pronounced in older patients because the ciliary muscle contractile responses to pilocarpine diminish with age.[287]

In addition to accommodative spasm, a significant ocular problem associated with the use of pilocarpine is miosis. The drug-induced pupillary constriction can visually incapacitate patients with nuclear sclerotic and posterior subcapsular cataracts. Moreover, with long-term use, pilocarpine has been implicated in hastening the development of cataracts.[288] The reduction in visual acuity or difficulty in dim illumination associated with the miotic pupil can be overcome by the concomitant use of topical phenylephrine.[289,290] In eyes with open angles, dilation of the pupil with phenylephrine does not adversely affect control of IOP but may provide sufficient improvement in visual acuity to permit the patient to tolerate miotic therapy, which might otherwise prove functionally incapacitating.[289] All topical antiglaucoma medications can be continued while the patient uses 2.5%

TABLE 10.11
Ocular Effects of Miotics

- Accommodative spasm
- Miosis
- Follicular conjunctivitis
- Pupillary block with secondary angle-closure glaucoma
- Band keratopathy[a]
- Allergic blepharoconjunctivitis
- Retinal detachment
- Conjunctival injection[b]
- Lid myokymia[b]
- Anterior subcapsular cataract[c]
- Iris cyst formation[c]

[a]Associated with pilocarpine solutions containing phenylmercuric nitrate as preservative.
[b]Usually subsides within several days or weeks as treatment continues.
[c]Associated with anticholinesterase agents.

phenylephrine in the morning on awakening and then throughout the day and evening as required.[289] The practitioner must be cautious to use only adrenergic mydriatics for this purpose, since anticholinergic mydriatics are well known to elevate IOP (see Chap. 21). In addition, such use of phenylephrine is contraindicated in eyes with narrow angles. The pilocarpine should be regularly discontinued for several days at least twice a year so that the pupils may be pharmacologically dilated for careful stereoscopic examination of the optic disc and retina. Not only does this examination facilitate evaluation of the glaucomatous damage to the optic nerve, but it also prevents permanent miosis, which can result from loss of tone in the iris dilator muscle and fibrosis of the iris sphincter muscle.[288]

Except for accommodative spasm and drug-induced myopia in young patients, the most common adverse effect of pilocarpine therapy is follicular conjunctivitis.[291] Changing the drug to carbachol usually alleviates this condition.

Pilocarpine therapy can also induce pupillary block with subsequent angle closure, which almost always occurs in patients with narrow angles who have advancing cataracts.[292] With forward displacement of the crystalline lens-iris diaphragm associated with the advancing cataract, and the physiologic action of the pilocarpine, angle closure becomes progressively superimposed on the underlying component of open- angle glaucoma, but often in a subacute or chronic manner.[292]

Band keratopathy is rare in patients receiving long-term pilocarpine therapy. It has been associated with pilocarpine solutions containing the preservative phenylmercuric nitrate (PMN).[293] Band keratopathy does not occur in patients using pilocarpine without PMN. Pilocarpine solutions containing PMN are no longer available, but if the disorder is encountered, the calcium deposition can be treated with topical applications of ethylenediaminetetraacetic acid (EDTA).

Occasionally allergic conjunctivitis and dermatitis develop after prolonged therapy.[294] In these instances, the preservative, particularly benzalkonium chloride, is usually implicated. Changing to a formulation with a different preservative often alleviates the problem.[294]

The relationship between miotic therapy and disorders associated with vitreoretinal traction has been a subject of controversy. Although no factual evidence links miotic therapy with retinal detachment, there is circumstantial evidence—the time interval between institution of miotic therapy and retinal detachment and the type of detachment—that pilocarpine and other miotics such as the anticholinesterase drugs may cause retinal detachment.[295,296] The proposed mechanism is anterior displacement of the lens-iris diaphragm, leading to vitreoretinal traction or tractional tears, with or without posterior vitreous detachment.[297,298] This mechanism could also account for the reported cases of macular hole formation[297] and vitreous hemorrhage[298] associated with initiation of topical pilocarpine therapy. It is believed, but not confirmed, that miotics may increase the risk of retinal detachment in patients with myopia, aphakia, or pseudophakia.[299,300] Where horseshoe breaks or dialyses are pre-existing lesions, these should be treated prophylactically prior to miotic therapy. Patients who have no predisposing retinal conditions or who have lattice degeneration or operculated holes should be warned of possible retinal detachment prior to starting miotics.[300] Optimal care entails careful peripheral retinal examination prior to and periodically during miotic therapy. Other ocular side effects include ciliary and conjunctival hyperemia, lid myokymia, frontal headache, and ocular or periorbital pain.[288] Most of these signs and symptoms tend to disappear within several days or weeks as treatment continues.

Systemic Effects. Adverse systemic reactions associated with the cholinergic activity of pilocarpine are rare but do occasionally occur in patients who misuse their medication or who are given frequent instillations of the drug in the treatment of acute angle-closure glaucoma. The systemic toxicity of pilocarpine can be significant and occasionally even life threatening (Table 10.12).[301] Although the symptoms of nausea, diaphoresis, and weakness frequently experienced by patients undergoing attacks of acute angle-closure are often attributed to the glaucoma attack itself, high doses of pilocarpine often cause these symptoms. Other systemic manifestations may include salivation, lacrimation, vomiting, and diarrhea. Bronchiolar spasm and pulmonary edema can occur, possibly initiating an asthmatic attack in patients with pre-existing asthma.[294]

When pilocarpine therapy starts, the patient should be advised of potential minor ocular or systemic side effects, with the suggestion that after 7 to 10 days of continued use, these reactions will either disappear or become tolerable. Providing this information usually improves patient compliance with this medication and improves the patient's confidence in the prescribing practitioner.

CONTRAINDICATIONS

Pilocarpine therapy should be avoided in certain patients (Table 10.13). This drug is contraindicated in patients with cataract, especially nuclear sclerotic and posterior subcapsular, because the drug can affect vision and may accelerate the formation of lens opacities.[294] Pilocarpine is generally contraindicated in patients under 40 years of age because of the intolerable accommodative spasm and refractive changes. Since breakdown of the blood-aqueous barrier occurs with the use of pilocarpine and other miotics,[302] particularly in the presence of neovascular and uveitic glaucoma, pilocarpine should be avoided in these patients.

To prevent retinal detachment, miotic therapy should be instituted gradually in patients with myopia, peripheral retinal disease predisposing to retinal detachment, and in apha-

---

TABLE 10.12
Systemic Effects of Miotics

- Headache
- Browache
- Marked salivation
- Profuse perspiration
- Nausea
- Vomiting
- Bronchospasm
- Pulmonary edema
- Systemic hypotension
- Bradycardia
- Generalized muscular weakness
- Increased tone and motility of gastrointestinal tract (abdominal pain, diarrhea)
- Respiratory paralysis[a]

[a]May occur when anticholinesterase agents are not discontinued before use of succinylcholine during elective surgery.

TABLE 10.13
Contraindications to Miotics

- Presence of cataract
- Patients under 40 years of age
- Neovascular and uveitic glaucoma
- History of retinal detachment
- Asthma or history of asthma
- Phakic eyes[a]
- Surgical procedures employing succinylcholine[a]

[a]Applies only to anticholinesterase agents

kic or pseudophakic patients. This gradual approach to miotic therapy can be accomplished by using low concentrations of pilocarpine and increasing as necessary. Likewise, pilocarpine should be avoided in patients with a history of retinal detachment. Ideally, before initiating pilocarpine therapy, every patient should have a thorough peripheral retinal examination with the binocular indirect ophthalmoscope through widely dilated pupils.[300] During the course of treatment patients should be instructed to report any flashes, spots, or floaters. Such incidents will necessitate prompt reexamination of the peripheral retina with the pupil dilated.

Pilocarpine should generally be avoided in patients with asthma or a history of asthma. In concentrations exceeding 2%, pilocarpine is contraindicated in acute angle-closure glaucoma because these concentrations can lead to further shallowing of the anterior chamber as well as permanent peripheral anterior synechiae and angle-closure.[288] Furthermore, pilocarpine in concentrations of 4% or more should be used with caution in patients with narrow angles, since these concentrations may lead to attacks of acute angle closure.[288]

The necessity of administering pilocarpine solutions four times daily without nasolacrimal occlusion makes this form of therapy a poor choice in patients who are likely to demonstrate poor compliance with this medication schedule. In these instances the practitioner should use a twice-daily dosage with nasolacrimal occlusion,[275] or select an alternative therapy requiring less frequent instillation, such as a β blocker or dipivefrin.

Carbachol

PHARMACOLOGY

Carbachol, another choline ester, is also a direct-acting cholinergic agonist. It is completely resistant to hydrolysis by cholinesterases. Consequently, its bioavailability is prolonged enough so that it becomes adequately distributed to low blood-flow areas and has sustained local effects. Its peripheral actions are both muscarinic and nicotinic (autonomic ganglia in particular), exhibiting a certain degree of selectivity for urinary bladder and gastrointestinal tract. In addition to the drug's direct action, carbachol may act partly through an indirect mechanism involving the displacement of acetylcholine from cholinergic nerve terminals.[265]

In vitro studies have shown carbachol to be considerably more potent in its pupillary effects than pilocarpine.[265] However, when topically applied to the eye, carbachol exerts less miotic action than does pilocarpine.[303] A plausible explanation is that because carbachol is poorly lipid soluble, its intraocular bioavailability is considerably less than the more lipid-soluble pilocarpine.[283] Adding 0.03% benzalkonium chloride (BAK) enhances the corneal penetration of carbachol.

CLINICAL USES

Carbachol is commercially available as the chloride salt for topical ocular application in concentrations of 0.75%, 1.5%, 2.25%, and 3.0% (see Table 10.9). The 3% solution is the most widely prescribed.[275] Although it has been generally stated that carbachol ophthalmic solutions should contain 0.03% BAK to be clinically effective, commercial preparations presently available contain only 0.005% BAK as a preservative. However, these solutions employ 1% hydroxypropyl methylcellulose as a vehicle to promote more prolonged contact of the drug to the ocular surface, thereby enhancing intraocular penetration.[273] It appears that these formulations are clinically effective and less irritating than are those containing 0.03% BAK.[283]

In addition to topical preparations, carbachol is available for intraocular use to produce miosis during surgery. Since carbachol is a potent miotic, this preparation is considerably less concentrated than are the topical solutions. It is available as a 0.01% sterile balanced salt solution with no preservatives and is supplied in 1.5 ml sterile glass disposable vials.[273] The dose is 0.5 ml applied by gentle irrigation. An effective, prolonged miosis ensues 2 to 5 minutes after application.

The topical solutions are indicated for lowering elevated IOP in primary and some secondary open-angle glaucomas. With its prolonged action, carbachol requires less frequent administration than shorter-acting miotics. It is usually instilled every 8 hours. However, when used in conjunction with nasolacrimal occlusion, twice-daily dosing of the 1.5% solution often achieves adequate IOP control.[275] Since carbachol has the disadvantage of having relatively more severe local side effects than does pilocarpine, its use is limited to patients who have become allergic or refractory to pilocarpine. Reichert and associates[304] have suggested, however, that switching from pilocarpine to carbachol may offer a relatively low chance of improving long-term IOP control, while increasing the risk of ocular side effects.

SIDE EFFECTS

Systemic absorption from recommended dosages of carbachol used in the treatment of glaucoma appears insignificant, since systemic toxicity is not common. However, inadvertent increased systemic absorption of carbachol can produce a variety of effects (see Table 10.12). Ocular effects (see Table 10.11) include miosis, transient conjunctival and ciliary injection, and ciliary spasm with a resultant temporary decrease in visual acuity. Allergic reactions to carbachol are rare.

CONTRAINDICATIONS

Conditions precluding the use of carbachol are essentially the same as for pilocarpine (see Table 10.13). The drug should be avoided in anterior uveitis and neovascular glaucoma because its vasodilatory effects cause increased inflammation. Caution should be observed when administering the drug to patients with bronchial asthma, gastrointestinal spasms, peptic ulcers, urinary tract obstructions, acute cardiac failure, and Parkinson's disease. Carbachol should be applied conservatively after procedures that reduce or disrupt the corneal epithelial barrier and conjunctiva, such as gonioscopy or tonometry or after topical anesthesia. These procedures can promote excessive intraocular and systemic absorption of the drug with resultant increased local side effects and increased probability of systemic effects. If extreme miosis occurs, the patient should be advised to be cautious when driving at night or when engaging in hazardous activities in poor illumination.[273]

Echothiophate

PHARMACOLOGY

Echothiophate is an organophosphorous compound that inhibits cholinesterases, thereby enhancing the effects of endogenously released acetylcholine. Its mechanism of enzyme inhibition results in a stable complex that is responsible for the drug's potent and prolonged irreversible activity. Significant spontaneous regeneration of active enzyme requires several hours.

The quaternary nitrogen of the echothiophate molecule imparts the property of low lipid solubility. Consequently, echothiophate's penetration of the blood-brain barrier is theoretically limited. This expectation is corroborated by studies demonstrating that none of the symptoms of toxic doses of echothiophate in animals is attributable to cholinesterase inhibition in the CNS; death was caused by peripheral toxic effects, including paralysis of muscles of respiration and excessive bronchial constriction.[305]

A solution of echothiophate applied topically to the eye results in miosis that begins within 10 to 30 minutes and may last for 1 to 4 weeks. Accompanying reduction of IOP is maximal after 24 hours, lasting for days or weeks.[306] Its ocular hypotensive effect has been attributed to an increase in facility of aqueous outflow similar to that produced by pilocarpine and carbachol.

CLINICAL USES

Echothiophate ophthalmic solutions are commercially available as the iodide salt in concentrations of 0.03, 0.06, 0.125, and 0.25% (see Table 10.9). Because it has a relatively short shelf life, echothiophate must be prepared fresh on dispensing; therefore, it is supplied as a powder in the appropriate amount for reconstitution. A diluent containing a buffer and preservatives is added. After reconstituting, the refrigerated solution is useful for up to six months. Since solutions stored

at room temperature will maintain stability for only one month,[273] it is wise to recommend refrigeration. Due to its low therapeutic index, echothiophate is rarely employed in the treatment of glaucoma. Its main indication is for the treatment of advanced primary and some secondary open-angle glaucomas not controlled by shorter-acting miotics used in combination with dipivefrin, β blockers, or carbonic anhydrase inhibitors.

In the treatment of glaucoma the therapeutic objective is to achieve optimal control of IOP on a diurnal basis, since significant diurnal variations in pressure can cause progressive visual field loss in patients who are inadequately controlled. Echothiophate is advantageous in this respect and is the most widely used anticholinesterase agent for this purpose.[307] The instillation of 0.03% echothiophate at bedtime and in the morning is recommended to obtain as smooth a diurnal pressure curve as possible; however, a single daily dose (at bedtime) or every other day is satisfactory in some patients. The daily dose should always be instilled at bedtime to avoid the inconvenience of drug-induced miosis and accommodative spasm. If results are inadequate, the higher concentrations of echothiophate may be necessary. When used in its highest concentrations, echothiophate has an ocular hypotensive effect that is considerably more pronounced than that of pilocarpine or carbachol. These latter drugs must be discontinued before starting echothiophate therapy because their simultaneous use provides no additional benefit yet increases the risk of both ocular and systemic toxicity.

SIDE EFFECTS

Ocular Effects. The major ocular complication of echothiophate is the development of cataract, usually characterized by anterior subcapsular vacuoles (Fig. 10.8).[291] Moreover, echothiophate may accelerate nuclear sclerosis and posterior subcapsular changes.[308] Thus, echothiophate is more useful in pseudophakic and aphakic than in phakic patients. There is probably a greater risk of retinal detachment with the use of echothiophate than with pilocarpine or carbachol. Reversible iris cysts are a well-known complication of echothiophate (Fig. 10.9). The iris cysts at the pupillary margin occur primarily in young patients and can decrease vision and produce visual field changes that mimic those of glaucoma. The concomitant use of 2.5% phenylephrine can minimize the development of cysts. Patients treated with echothiophate may develop constant tearing associated with stenosis of the puncta, but this tearing usually disappears following discontinuation of the drug.[291]

Systemic Effects. Systemic absorption of echothiophate may lead to intense gastrointestinal symptoms including diarrhea, nausea, and vomiting.[291] These have been attributed to inhibition of cholinesterase. Determination of cholin-

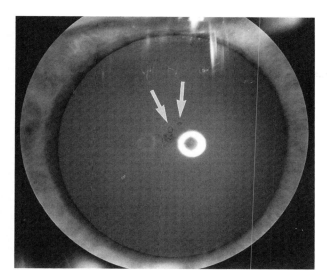

FIGURE 10.8   **Anterior subcapsular cataract (arrows) in a patient treated with anticholinesterase miotics. Pupil has been dilated for photography. The white annular ring is a photographic artifact. (Courtesy David M. Amos, O.D.)**

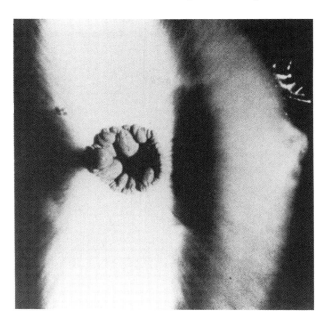

FIGURE 10.9   **Iris cysts associated with topical anticholinesterase therapy. (Reprinted with permission from Sugar HS. Pitfalls in the medical treatment of simple glaucoma. Ann Ophthalmol 1979; 11:1041–1050.)**

esterase levels in red blood cells usually reveals low values in symptomatic patients. Normal values range between 0.6 and 1.1 units. Persons exposed to significant amounts of anticholinesterases have values less than 0.4 units. Although low values are not conclusive regarding a drug-induced effect, normal values rule out a drug-related etiology. Since patients using echothiophate and other anticholinesterase agents have markedly lower plasma and red blood cell cholinesterase, the action of succinylcholine used in general anesthesia may be prolonged, leading to prolonged postoperative respiratory paralysis.[294] The dangers of using echothiophate in patients exposed to organophosphate insecticides or fertilizers and in patients undergoing treatment with anticholinesterase drugs for myasthenia gravis must be emphasized. Under these conditions echothiophate can cause intense intestinal cramps, CNS symptoms, cardiac arrest, hypotension, or respiratory failure. Nasolacrimal occlusion should be mandatory following instillation of the drug to prevent or minimize these systemic effects.

CONTRAINDICATIONS

Conditions precluding the use of echothiophate are the same as for pilocarpine and carbachol (see Table 10.13). In addition, certain precautions should be observed before initiating echothiophate therapy. Gonioscopy should be performed to rule out narrow angles or shallow anterior chambers. The patient should be advised to perform nasolacrimal occlusion (see Fig. 3.6) for at least 3 to 5 minutes following instillation

to minimize systemic absorption. Discontinuation of the medication is indicated if systemic side effects appear. Patients exposed to carbamate or organophosphate insecticides should be warned of their additive effects with anticholinesterases, and preventive measures such as wearing respiratory masks and frequent washing and clothing changes should be recommended.

Anticholinesterases should be used with caution or avoided in patients with illnesses that would be exacerbated by increased cholinergic stimulation; for example, asthma, gastrointestinal disturbances, bradycardia, heart block, recent myocardial infarction, epilepsy, parkinsonism, and history of or predisposition toward retinal detachment.[309]

Echothiophate is contraindicated in phakic glaucoma patients because of the greater risk for the development of cataract compared with the use of the shorter-acting miotics. Echothiophate is also contraindicated in patients with peripheral retinal disease that would predispose to retinal detachment.[290] This drug should be discontinued several weeks before elective surgical procedures employing succinylcholine. It should be discontinued 4 to 6 weeks before intraocular surgery to minimize its inflammatory effects and to diminish conjunctival and episcleral bleeding during conjunctival dissection.[292] As with all miotics, it should be avoided in uveitic glaucoma because of vasodilation and aggravation of the uveitis.

TABLE 10.14
Stepped-Care Approach to Miotic Therapy[a]

Primary Therapy (Group I)	Secondary Therapy (Group II)	Tertiary Therapy (Group III)
Pilocarpine solution 1%–6% q.i.d. Pilocarpine gel 4% h.s. Pilocarpine Ocusert 20–40 μg/h	Carbachol 3.0% t.i.d.	Echothiophate 0.125%–0.25% b.i.d.

[a]Lower concentrations and reduced dosage frequencies may be used if nasolacrimal occlusion is employed.[275]

Stepped-Care Approach to Miotic Therapy

Cholinergic agonists belong to one of three major groups according to their efficacy in reducing IOP (Table 10.14). Each drug in the first group has approximately equal pressure-lowering effects. Changing from one drug to another within a group generally offers no additional ocular hypotensive potential. The practitioner must change from a drug in group I to a drug in group II, or from group II to group III, to achieve a more intense cholinergic (and thus ocular hypotensive) effect. Note, however, that these groupings represent generalizations and that in clinical practice the miotics may respond differently in individual patients. These categorizations lend perspective in the use of miotics in the treatment of glaucoma and allow the practitioner to anticipate therapeutic results more rationally.

Adrenergic Agonists

Since the early 1920s, when Hamburger[310] applied epinephrine topically to the eye to reduce IOP, practitioners have used various adrenergic agonists to control ocular hypertension and glaucoma. Of the agents currently available, epinephrine, dipivefrin, apraclonidine, and brimonidine are in clinical use as ocular hypotensive agents.

Epinephrine

PHARMACOLOGY

Epinephrine, the major hormone secreted by the adrenal medulla, reaches the eye through the systemic circulation. Chemically it resembles norepinephrine, with the addition of a methyl group on the side chain nitrogen. Epinephrine is a direct-acting sympathomimetic amine with combined α- and β-adrenoceptor-stimulating activity. In solution it exhibits both lipid and water solubility, and corneal penetration occurs following topical application to the eye.[311]

Epinephrine is commercially available as the hydrochloride, borate, and in combination with pilocarpine, as the bitartrate salt[312] (Table 10.15). Active concentrations of the bitartrate salt preparations are less than the stated percentage, since a 2% solution contains approximately 1.1% free epinephrine base. However, when administered in equivalent doses of epinephrine base, all three salts are equally effective in lowering IOP.[313] Hydrochloride salt formulations are available in concentrations ranging from 0.1% to 2.0%, with a pH of approximately 3.5. Borate salts are formulated in 0.5%, 1.0%, and 2.0% concentrations, with a pH of 7.4. In addition to the usual additives and preservatives, the hydrochloride formulations also contain sodium bisulfite or sodium metabisulfite as antioxidants to prevent discoloration and to enhance stability of the epinephrine in solution.[312]

Topical administration results in a typical triple response of conjunctival decongestion, slight mydriasis, and reduction of IOP. The effect on ocular pressure outlasts the vasoconstrictor and mydriatic effects. The pupillary dilation is maximum approximately two hours following instillation and gradually diminishes over 12 hours. At low concentrations, epinephrine is a relatively poor mydriatic in the normal eye. The drug's mixed α and β stimulation, its rapid destruction, and the corneal epithelial barrier at least in part explain the clinical effects. The mydriatic effect of epinephrine is enhanced when the cornea is traumatized or when the drug is applied by prolonged contact.[314]

Since the major clinical usefulness of epinephrine lies in its ability to lower IOP in both primary and secondary open-angle glaucoma, this aspect has received the most active investigation. Despite extensive research, however, controversy still remains on the mechanism whereby epinephrine produces its pressure-lowering effects. Species differences among experimental animals, variability in study duration, possible differences in the disease process among patients,

TABLE 10.15
Adrenergic Agonists

Generic Name	Trade Name	Manufacturer	Concentration (%)
Epinephrine hydrochloride	Epifrin	Allergan	0.25, 0.5, 1, 2
	Glaucon	Alcon	1, 2
Epinephrine borate	Epinal	Alcon	0.5, 1, 2
	Eppy/N	Sola/B-H	0.5, 1, 2
Dipivefrin hydrochloride	Propine	Allergan	0.1
Apraclonidine	Iopidine	Alcon	0.5, 1
Brimonidine		Allergan	0.5

Adapted from Bartlett JD, Ghormley NR, Jaanus SD, et al., eds. Ophthalmic drug facts. St. Louis: Facts and Comparisons, 1995.

and inability to use certain techniques in humans restrict experimental comparison.[314]

The effects of epinephrine on IOP have been studied with fluorophotometric techniques combined with tonography and tonometry.[315-319] These studies indicate that epinephrine most likely affects several processes involving aqueous humor formation and outflow. Epinephrine increases both trabecular (conventional) as well as uveoscleral (unconventional) outflow.[315,317-320] Some experimental observations seem to indicate that the effect on uveoscleral outflow may exceed that of conventional outflow mechanisms.[317] Several studies also suggest that epinephrine may, at least initially, increase aqueous humor formation.[315-319] Fluorophotometric studies indicate that epinephrine may stimulate a small increase in aqueous humor production 2 to 5 hours after treatment.[317-319]

Epinephrine's effect on IOP may be mediated via adrenergic receptors, and both α- and β-adrenoceptor subtypes have been implicated.[318,320] A cyclic AMP (cAMP)-dependent mechanism supports the possible effect on β receptors.[321-324] A significant elevation of aqueous cAMP levels occurs in rabbits 30 minutes following epinephrine treatment, with peak levels at 1 to 4 hours.[322] More recently, use of an *in vitro* human eye outflow pathway perfusion model[323] indicates that epinephrine-mediated increases in facility of aqueous outflow correlate in time with epinephrine-induced increases in cAMP levels in the perfusion medium. The elevation in cAMP levels occurs within 30 minutes of perfusion, whereas changes in outflow facility do not occur until 90 minutes. The effect of epinephrine on outflow facility was not altered by the α-receptor antagonist phentolamine. However, two substances completely blocked the effect on outflow: timolol and ICI 118,551, an experimental nonspecific β-blocking agent, at a concentration that preferentially blocks β_2-adrenoceptor sites. Moreover, using isolated

intact human trabecular tissue, the authors reported a similar, time-dependent effect of epinephrine exposure on cAMP levels. These observations seem to indicate that the ocular hypotensive effect of epinephrine is mediated by cAMP, results at least in part from an increase in facility of outflow, and appears to involve β_2 adrenoceptors. The observed delay between the increase in cAMP levels and the increase in outflow facility needs further evaluation. Other cellular events and mediators may have a role in epinephrine-mediated IOP reductions.

In most patients the effect of epinephrine on IOP is proportional to the concentration of the drug, reaching a maximum response at 1% to 2%. However, lower concentrations can also prove effective.[325,326] Since side effects appear to be dose related,[311] the recommended practice is to start with low concentrations, and increasing dosage as necessary to control IOP. Following topical application, the IOP begins to fall within 1 hour, and the maximum effect is reached within 2 to 6 hours.[325]

CLINICAL USES

For some patients epinephrine may be considered an initial drug of choice in the therapy of both primary open-angle glaucoma and, when treated, ocular hypertension.[327] The absence of associated miosis and accommodative spasm makes epinephrine a useful drug in the treatment of glaucoma in prepresbyopic patients who have critical vision requirements: epinephrine allows adequate control of IOP in many patients without impairing visual acuity or inducing refractive changes.[328] Epinephrine has great usefulness for patients who would sustain significant adverse visual effects from pilocarpine solutions or other miotics. However, because of its relatively low therapeutic index, with potential for both ocular and systemic side effects, the prodrug dipivefrin has supplanted epinephrine as the adrenergic agonist of choice for the treatment of most types of glaucoma.

SIDE EFFECTS

Ocular Effects. Following topical application of epinephrine to the eye, various ocular tissues take up and store the drug. The primary sites are the iris, ciliary body, and, to a lesser extent, the choroid. Far less is found in the retina and optic nerve. If the treated eye is aphakic, significantly more epinephrine appears in the choroid, and uptake into the retina and optic nerve is also enhanced.[329] Following topical administration significant amounts are also found in nonocular tissues, particularly those of the heart and spleen.[329]

Numerous adverse events can accompany the topical use of epinephrine in glaucoma therapy (Table 10.16). However, unlike pilocarpine and other miotics, epinephrine does not impair visual acuity, since it has no effect on refractive error and produces little or no mydriasis. Local ocular reactions, such as burning, conjunctival hyperemia, allergy, and irritation, occur in about 25% of patients.[330] Although changing to another salt form of epinephrine often reduces these problems, the associated side effects cause discontinuation of the drug in about 20% to 50% of cases.[331]

Epinephrine may cause true allergic reactions, characterized by lid dermatitis, irritation, lacrimation, and diffuse conjunctival hyperemia.[311] The prevalence of drug-induced allergic blepharoconjunctivitis is as high as 15%. The allergic reactions most likely result from the epinephrine or its oxidation products rather than the vehicle. Patients who demonstrate hypersensitivity reactions have not been sensitive when the vehicle was applied alone.[332]

Injection of epinephrine solution into the anterior chamber can cause increased corneal thickness and loss of corneal endothelial cells.[333] The toxicity appears to result from the formulation's low pH, which results from the presence of the antioxidant, sodium bisulfite. Prolonged use of topical epinephrine can result in localized pigment (adrenochrome) deposits. These occur most frequently in the palpebral conjunctiva (Fig. 10.10), but lid margin pigmentation and, on occasion, corneal pigmentation can occur.[334-336] The black to brown pigment most likely consists of oxidation products of epinephrine. Although adrenochrome deposits within the palpebral conjunctiva are not uncommon, they rarely produce irritation. Deposits in the corneal epithelium can cover the corneal surface by forming a diffuse plaque of adrenochrome, which can resemble a melanoma[335] or uveal prolapse.[336] Diffuse adrenochrome staining of soft contact lenses (Fig. 10.11) may also occur.[337,338] Such staining of soft contact lenses with epinephrine can occur within 2 to 6 weeks of initial topical epinephrine therapy. Soaking the lens for 5 hours in 3% hydrogen peroxide removes the stain.[338]

Epinephrine produces pupillary dilation in some patients. This effect is especially pronounced when epinephrine is used in combination with timolol or other β blockers.[327] Thus, epinephrine may precipitate acute angle-closure glaucoma in patients with narrow angles.

Occasionally, the use of epinephrine may be associated with a significant and prolonged rise of IOP in patients with primary open-angle glaucoma.[339] This rise occurs in the absence of any gonioscopically visible changes in the angle, but tonographic findings show the pressure rise to be associated with impaired outflow facility. The mechanism of this rise is unknown. Because of this IOP rise, practitioners should exercise caution in the use of epinephrine in uniocular patients or in those with advanced glaucoma. This hazard appears to be less significant if miotics are used concomitantly.[339]

Epinephrine maculopathy can occur in aphakic patients.[340] This macular toxicity occurs in 10% to 20% of aphakic eyes undergoing treatment with epinephrine. Experimental evidence indicates that topical epinephrine reaches the retina in significantly higher concentrations in aphakic than in phakic eyes.[329] Epinephrine applied topically to one eye reaches the retina, choroid, and optic nerve of both eyes. If the treated eye is aphakic, the amount reaching the posterior pole of the eye is much greater on that side.[341] The maculopathy is characterized by edema, usually cystic, with or without small flame-shaped hemorrhages.[342] The mechanism by which epinephrine produces cystoid macular edema is unknown. Both the clinical and fluorescein angiographic features of the maculopathy often cannot be distinguished from those observed in other conditions of cystoid macular edema, including the Irvine-Gass syndrome.[342] Clinically, visual acuity may be a poor indicator of epinephrine maculopathy, since some patients have only small acuity changes despite prominent leakage of dye on fluorescein angiography.[343] Thus, if an aphakic glaucoma patient requires treatment with epinephrine, periodic angiography may be advisable.

Systemic Effects. Topical administration of epinephrine can also result in systemic side effects,[344] including severe

TABLE 10.16
Side Effects of Topical Epinephrine

Ocular Effects	Systemic Effects
Irritation and lacrimation	Severe headache
Conjunctival hyperemia	Palpitations
Allergic blepharoconjunctivitis	Tachycardia
Adrenochrome pigmentation	Premature ventricular
Adrenochrome staining of soft contact lenses	contractions
	Hypertensive crisis
Pupillary dilation	Anxiety
Elevation of intraocular pressure	
Cystoid macular edema	

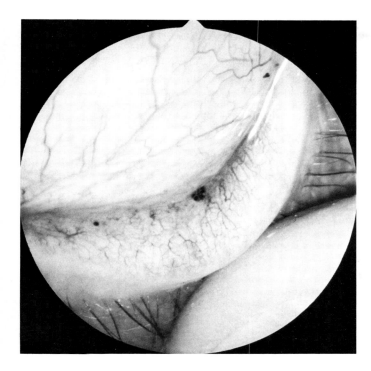

FIGURE 10.10   **Adrenochrome deposits in palpebral conjunctiva of a patient using topical epinephrine for treatment of primary open-angle glaucoma. (Courtesy Lyman C. Norden, O.D.)**

headache, palpitations, tachycardia, premature ventricular contractions, and hypertensive crisis (up to 230 mm Hg systolic).[331,345] The β-adrenoceptor stimulatory effects on the cardiovascular system are responsible for most of these reactions. Instructing the patient to perform nasolacrimal occlusion (see Fig. 3.6) following instillation of the drug may reduce or eliminate these systemic effects.

The amount of epinephrine absorbed systemically from topical glaucoma therapy can be comparable to amounts used parenterally for various conditions. One drop of 2% epinephrine contains approximately 1.0 mg of drug. The usual systemic dose is approximately 0.1 to 0.5 mg.[311,346] Because of possible cardiac effects following systemic absorption of topically applied epinephrine, this agent must be used with caution in patients with cardiovascular disease, as discussed in the following section.

CONTRAINDICATIONS

Table 10.17 summarizes the contraindications to the use of epinephrine.

Because epinephrine may cause pupillary dilation, it should be avoided in patients with narrow angles. Epinephrine should generally be avoided in aphakic or pseudophakic patients because of the risk of cystoid macular edema. In addition, adrenochrome staining of soft contact lenses precludes the simultaneous use of topical epinephrine in patients who wear such lenses.

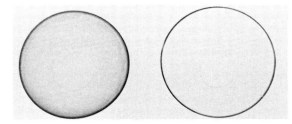

FIGURE 10.11   **Diffuse adrenochrome staining of hydrophilic contact lens (left) compared with normal lens (right).**

It has been suggested that patients with primary open-angle glaucoma, in contrast to those with secondary glaucoma, are more susceptible to the side effects of epinephrine.[345] Therefore, epinephrine should be used with caution in patients with cardiovascular disease, including ischemic heart disease; in patients with marked systemic hypertension; and in patients with hyperthyroidism, who may be sensitized to catecholamines.[347] Epinephrine must be used cautiously in patients treated with monoamine oxidase (MAO) inhibitors or tricyclic antidepressants because these drugs increase the sensitivity of adrenergic receptors, possibly resulting in exaggerated pressor responses such as hypertension or cardiac arrhythmia.[331] The use of epinephrine should be interrupted before general anesthesia with anes-

TABLE 10.17
Contraindications to Epinephrine

- Narrow angles
- Aphakia/pseudophakia
- Hydrophilic contact lens wear
- Cardiovascular disease
- Hyperthyroidism
- Concomitant therapy with MAO inhibitors or tricyclic antidepressants[a]
- General anesthesia with anesthetics that sensitize the myocardium to catecholamines
- Bisulfite allergy

[a]MAO = monoamine oxidase

thetics (e.g., cyclopropane or halothane) that sensitize the myocardium to catecholamines.[348]

Dipivefrin (Dipivalyl Epinephrine)

PHARMACOLOGY

Dipivefrin is an analog of epinephrine formed by the addition of two pivalic acid groups to the hydroxyl groups of epinephrine (Fig. 10.12). This alteration of the epinephrine molecule creates a prodrug that is more lipophilic and better absorbed into the eye than is epinephrine. Subsequent to its corneal penetration, dipivefrin is converted to epinephrine within the eye.[349–352] Comparison of the oil-water partition coefficients of dipivefrin and epinephrine indicates that dipivefrin is 100 to 600 times as lipophilic as epinephrine. In human eyes its corneal penetration is 17 times greater than that of epinephrine.[351]

Dipivefrin is rapidly hydrolyzed to epinephrine by tissue esterases in the cornea and anterior chamber. Human plasma also catalyzes dipivefrin to epinephrine, with a half-life of 18 minutes. Whereas concomitant administration of a cholinesterase inhibitor such as echothiophate blocks the ocular

Pivalic Acid Groups   **Epinephrine**

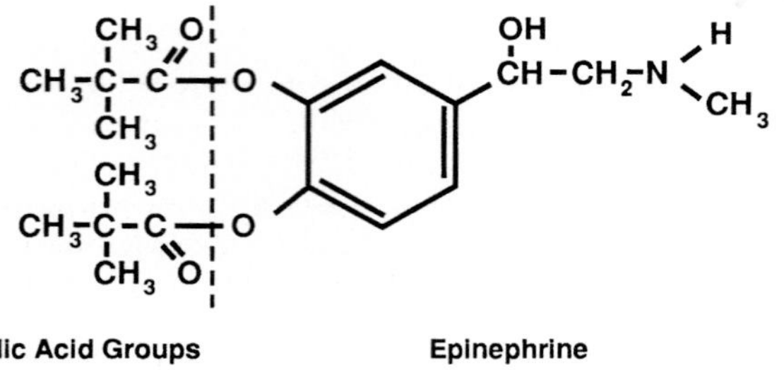

FIGURE 10.12 **Molecular structure of dipivefrin (dipivalyl epinephrine).**

hypotensive effects of dipivefrin in rabbits, this does not occur in human eyes.[353,354]

Following topical application to the eye, dipivefrin lowers IOP when used in concentrations of 0.025%, 0.1%, and 0.5%.[349] The ocular hypotensive response reaches a maximum in 4 to 8 hours and is sustained for about 12 hours. Dipivefrin 0.1% produces an effect approximately equipotent to 2% epinephrine or 2% pilocarpine. With long-term use the ocular hypotensive effect appears to be maintained.[351]

Dipivefrin's mechanism of action in lowering IOP resembles that of epinephrine. Both a reduction of aqueous formation and enhanced aqueous outflow occur.[349] Moreover, as observed with epinephrine, dipivefrin also causes a biphasic response on IOP.[354] An initial hypertensive phase, lasting less than two hours, is followed by a prolonged hypotensive phase. However, the initial hypertensive response is eliminated if an α-adrenergic blocker is also used. In the rabbit eye, an increase in cAMP levels in the aqueous humor accompanies the hypotensive effect of dipivefrin.[349] Michelson and Groh[700] have shown in humans that dipivefrin significantly reduces ciliary body blood flow. This hemodynamic effect may contribute to dipivefrin's ocular hypotensive activity. Dipivefrin also produces a dose-dependent mydriasis.[349] Dilation of the pupil occurs with 0.1% and 0.5% concentrations but not with lower concentrations. In one study[355] the mydriatic effect of the 0.1% solution averaged 0.65 mm as compared to 0.55 mm with 2% epinephrine. These increases in pupil size were statistically significant, and the two drugs did not differ significantly in the degree of pupillary dilation. However, the mydriatic and ocular hypotensive effects of dipivefrin show little correlation.[349] Although dipivefrin is a more potent mydriatic at the 0.25% concentration than at 0.1%, these concentrations appear equipotent in reducing IOP.[350]

CLINICAL USES

Dipivefrin was the first prodrug to become commercially available for use in ophthalmic practice. Its use is limited to the treatment of glaucoma. This drug is presently available as a 0.1% ophthalmic solution (Propine) (see Table 10.15). When employed in its usual dosage schedule of twice daily, it appears to be an effective and safe ocular hypotensive agent. It is especially useful for patients predisposed to adverse systemic side effects from epinephrine.[356] Dipivefrin has become the adrenergic agonist of choice for most glaucoma patients because it can be used concomitantly with topical β-blocker therapy without loss of additivity. Many patients unable to tolerate epinephrine preparations can satisfactorily tolerate dipivefrin, but the converse is not true.[356]

In contrast to epinephrine preparations, patients wearing soft contact lenses can use dipivefrin without significant risk of adrenochrome staining.[357] The addition of two pivalyl groups to form the dipivalyl epinephrine molecule may render the drug less subject to oxidation and therefore may prevent the formation of breakdown products that stain the contact lens. Thus, this epinephrine analog is useful in the treatment of glaucoma patients who must also wear soft contact lenses.

SIDE EFFECTS

Because of the reduced concentration of drug, dose-related side effects, both extraocular and systemic, are also reduced compared with epinephrine preparations. Thus, certain ocular side effects associated with topical epinephrine are minimized with dipivefrin, especially early in therapy.[349,351,354] Patients usually experience minimal ocular discomfort. Tearing, conjunctival hyperemia, corneal edema, and blurred vision are rare. Also, fewer allergic reactions occur. Adrenochrome deposits in the conjunctiva occur less frequently than with epinephrine. The lower incidence of adverse reactions, particularly extraocular side effects, could result from the reduced bioavailability of active drug when applied topically.[354,356,358] Systemic effects are also significantly reduced.[349,351,354,359] Cardiac arrhythmias and elevated systemic blood pressure are less likely to occur with dipivefrin, since these reactions relate to the total amount of epinephrine administered. With dipivefrin, the concentration of epinephrine in the systemic circulation at any given time is much lower.

With long-term use, the incidence of ocular toxicity may increase.[360–363] Follicular conjunctivitis occurs,[360–362] and the associated symptoms can be mild to severe and can include heaviness of the eyes, itching, or irritation.[360] The follicular aggregates contain primarily T-lymphocytes and histiocytes, with a small number of B-lymphocytes.[362] Blepharoconjunctivitis also occurs with dipivefrin therapy.[358,361,363] Patients with a previous history of epinephrine sensitivity may demonstrate cross-reactivity.[358] The condition resolves on withdrawal of the drug.

Although the extraocular effects are generally less with dipivefrin than with epinephrine, intraocular complications would still be expected because the active drug in the eye is epinephrine. However, Borrmann and Duzman[364] reported 20 aphakic and four pseudophakic patients who were treated twice daily with dipivefrin for up to two years. None of the patients developed signs or symptoms of epinephrine-induced maculopathy.

CONTRAINDICATIONS

Contraindications to the use of dipivefrin are the same as for epinephrine (see Table 10.17). However, since the risk of adverse systemic side effects appears considerably less than with epinephrine, the systemic contraindications are considered relative rather than absolute. Dipivefrin, rather than epinephrine, is clearly the adrenergic agonist of choice for glaucoma patients with cardiovascular disease.[311]

Apraclonidine

PHARMACOLOGY

Apraclonidine, a relatively selective α_2-adrenoceptor agonist, is chemically related to clonidine.[365,366] Although topical ocular application of clonidine can lower IOP, a significant reduction in systemic blood pressure can accompany its use.[367] The presence of an amide group at the C-4 position of apraclonidine's benzene ring makes the drug less lipophilic than clonidine and thus decreases its ability to penetrate the CNS.[365,366] Although the increased polarity of apraclonidine also seems to decrease its ability to penetrate the cornea, evidence indicates that it can gain access to the anterior chamber by conjunctival and scleral penetration.[368] Apraclonidine and clonidine appear to have a similar mechanism of action in their effect on IOP. Both drugs decrease aqueous production, with little or no effect on outflow.[369,370] Apraclonidine, however, may also have additional ocular hypotensive effects by influencing vascular tone[371–373] and prostaglandin synthesis.[374–376] Further studies are needed to explain the mechanisms by which apraclonidine lowers IOP.

Apraclonidine lowers IOP in both normal volunteers and patients with elevated pressure.[371,377,378] When compared at 0.5% and 1.0% concentrations, it produces the same percentage decrease in IOP regardless of the initial level of pressure. Although 1% apraclonidine produced a 31% decrease in IOP as compared to a 26% reduction with the 0.5% concentration, no statistically significant difference in the mean percent reduction in IOP occurred with the two concentrations (Fig. 10.13).[371] Most patients treated with apraclonidine show at least a 20% reduction from baseline pressures with the 0.5% or 1.0% solution.[371,378] When given

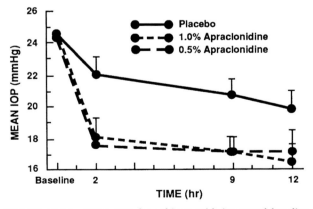

FIGURE 10.13 **Mean IOP for subjects with increased baseline IOP. Both 0.5% and 1.0% apraclonidine lowered IOP significantly more than did the placebo. There was no significant difference between 0.5% and 1.0% apraclonidine. Bars represent one standard error. (Published with permission from the American Journal of Ophthalmology 108:230–237,1989. Copyright by the Ophthalmic Publishing Company.)**

three times daily for three months, apraclonidine 0.5% appears to have an ocular hypotensive effect comparable to that of timolol 0.5% administered twice daily.[395] Neither age, race, nor iris color seem to affect the ocular hypotensive response to apraclonidine.[371,378] In subjects with increased IOP, no differences in response are observed between light and dark irides or white and black individuals.[371]

Apraclonidine also seems to affect the blood-aqueous barrier in normal and postoperative eyes.[379,380] Apraclonidine significantly reduced aqueous flare intensity at six hours in a group of patients undergoing uncomplicated phacoemulsification and posterior chamber intraocular lens implantation.[380] A reduction in the postoperative increase of aqueous protein is clinically desirable since it can help to reduce early postoperative inflammation and associated complications, including elevated IOP.

CLINICAL USES

Apraclonidine is commercially available as apraclonidine hydrochloride 0.5% and 1.0% (Iopidine), preserved with benzalkonium chloride 0.01%.[312] Its currently labeled indications are for control or prevention of postsurgical IOP elevation after anterior segment laser surgery, and for short-term IOP control in open-angle glaucoma prior to filtering procedures. Apraclonidine can also lower IOP in the initial treatment of acute angle-closure glaucoma (see Chap. 35).

Apraclonidine 0.5% can be used three times daily for short-term therapy of patients on maximally tolerated pharmacotherapy who require additional IOP reduction. However, adding apraclonidine to patients already using two inhibitors of aqueous production, such as a β blocker and carbonic anhydrase inhibitor, may not further lower IOP. Moreover, because of the development of tachyphylaxis, the benefit for most patients will not last more than several months.[701] Patients with primary or secondary glaucoma do not appear to differ in either the magnitude or duration of ocular hypotensive response, but patients with developmental or congenital glaucomas tend to respond less well.[701]

Acute rise in IOP is a risk factor in laser iridotomy, trabeculoplasty, and posterior capsulotomy.[381–383] Topical apraclonidine 1.0% can significantly reduce both the incidence and magnitude of IOP increases following anterior segment laser surgery.[371,384–386] Apraclonidine can minimize bleeding associated with ocular surgery. The vasoconstriction induced by the α-adrenoceptor effects of this agent could help to establish hemostasis during various surgical procedures. Apraclonidine's mydriatic effects can also prove advantageous. The induced pupillary dilation could enhance visualization during cataract extraction and vitreoretinal procedures.[365]

Apraclonidine 1.0% has been used for prophylaxis of postcycloplegic IOP spikes. In eyes with open-angle glaucoma dilated with tropicamide 1.0% and phenylephrine 2.5%, apraclonidine both minimized the incidence of spiking and reduced the spike height, as compared to the placebo or miotic treatment.[387]

SIDE EFFECTS

Ocular Effects. Common ocular side effects associated with topical apraclonidine include conjunctival blanching, eyelid retraction, and mydriasis. Although it may be difficult to detect in bilaterally treated patients, conjunctival blanching is the most common side effect, occurring in approximately 85% of patients.[370] The most likely cause is α-adrenoceptor stimulation, similar to that of other adrenergic agonists. However, rebound conjunctival hyperemia does not appear to occur with topical administration. Eyelid retraction most likely results from stimulation of α adrenoceptors on Müller's muscle. It is more readily observed with unilateral treatment, and patients may report that the nontreated eye feels heavy or droopy.[370,376] Pupillary dilation of less than 1 mm occurs in approximately 45% of eyes treated with 0.5% apraclonidine.[370,378] The mydriasis has limited clinical significance since patients usually do not detect it. Patients do sometimes report discomfort, burning, itching, dryness of the eyes, and blurred vision. Allergic reactions to the drug rarely occur following short-term use in laser therapy; however, allergic reactions may require discontinuation of the drug when used long term for treatment of open-angle glaucoma or ocular hypertension.[370,395]

Systemic Effects. The most common nonocular side effect associated with apraclonidine is a sensation of dry mouth or dry nose.[377,378] These symptoms are dose related.[377] Although the increased polarity of apraclonidine as compared to clonidine reduces the drug's potential to be systemically absorbed, cardiovascular and CNS effects can occur with topical application. However, in both normal volunteers and patients with elevated IOP, topical administration appears to cause only minimal effects on resting heart rate and arterial blood pressure.[377,378] Fatigue or lethargy is the most frequently reported CNS effect.[377,378] The reported incidence ranges between 5% and 15% in studies of one-week duration.[377] Other possible side effects include headache, sensation of head cold, chest heaviness, shortness of breath, sweaty palms, and taste abnormalities.[312]

CONTRAINDICATIONS

Apraclonidine is contraindicated in patients sensitive to clonidine and in patients taking monoamine oxidase inhibitors. Caution should be exercised in patients with severe cardiovascular disease, including hypertension. The possibility of vasovagal episodes exists during laser surgery, particularly in patients with a history of such events.

Brimonidine

PHARMACOLOGY

Brimonidine tartrate, a relatively selective α_2-adrenoceptor agonist, is structurally similar to clonidine.[388] Several studies have indicated that following topical instillation brimonidine can penetrate into the aqueous humor and produce a dose-dependent IOP reduction in both normal and glaucomatous eyes.[389-391] The ocular hypotensive effect of 0.2% brimonidine is comparable to that of 0.5% timolol but greater than that of 0.25% betaxolol suspension.[702]

The mechanism of action of brimonidine in lowering IOP in the human eye needs further elucidation, but experimental observations in the primate eye indicate that this agent decreases fluorophotometrically measured aqueous humor production.[391]

CLINICAL USES

Brimonidine 0.5% appears both safe and effective for reducing elevations in IOP following 360° argon laser trabeculoplasty (ALT).[396] Administration of one dose before or after ALT reduced the incidence of pressure elevation of ≥5 mm Hg from 38% to 9% or less.[392] Brimonidine can also lower pressure in patients with chronic elevation of IOP, both when administered alone and as adjunctive therapy in patients taking maximally tolerated medications.[393,394]

SIDE EFFECTS

As with apraclonidine, administration of brimonidine results in conjunctival blanching and eyelid retraction. However, pupil size does not change significantly. Systemic effects associated with topical ocular brimonidine include dry mouth and fatigue.[393] A decrease in systolic blood pressure can also occur,[392,702] but changes in heart rate appear minimal.[392,393]

CONTRAINDICATIONS

The contraindications for brimonidine are the same as for other α_2-adrenergic agonists. Particular care should be exercised in patients with cardiovascular disease.

Carbonic Anhydrase Inhibitors

Mechanism of Action

In 1949, Friedenwald[397] proposed that bicarbonate formation was an essential component of aqueous production. His theory was supported by the discovery of a relatively high concentration of bicarbonate in aqueous humor obtained from the rabbit posterior chamber.[398] Wistrand[399] subsequently demonstrated the presence of carbonic anhydrase in the ciliary processes of the rabbit, and Becker[400] in 1954 reported the ocular hypotensive properties of acetazolamide, a carbonic anhydrase inhibitor (CAI). Tonographic data obtained by Becker[400] suggested that the decrease in IOP induced by acetazolamide results from inhibition of aqueous humor production. Other studies[401] have confirmed this action of CAIs. Since the discovery of their ocular hypotensive properties, CAIs (Table 10.18) have been widely used in the treatment of all types of glaucoma.

All commercially available CAIs are unsubstituted aromatic sulfonamides (ARYL-SO_2NH_2).[402] The resonating heterocyclic side group confers a high inhibitory activity to these agents. Substitutions on the amino nitrogen produce compounds that are inactive as CAIs. These compounds

TABLE 10.18
Carbonic Anhydrase Inhibitors

Drug	Trade Name (manufacturer)	Formulation
Acetazolamide	Diamox (Lederle)	125 and 250 mg tablets 500 mg sustained-release capsules (Sequels) 500 mg vials for injection
Methazolamide	Neptazane (Lederle) MZM (CibaVision)	25 and 50 mg tablets
Dichlorphenamide	Daranide (Merck)	50 mg tablets
Dorzolamide	Trusopt (Merck)	2% ophthalmic solution

produce their primary pharmacologic effects through reversible, noncompetitive binding with the enzyme carbonic anhydrase.[403] Carbonic anhydrase catalyzes the first step (I) in the following reaction:

$$\overset{I}{CO_2 + H_2O} \rightleftharpoons \overset{II}{H_2CO_3} \rightleftharpoons H^+ + HCO_3^-$$

Reaction II is an ionic dissociation reaction that occurs very rapidly and that is not under enzymatic control.[403] Therefore, carbonic anhydrase catalyzes the cellular production of H_2CO_3 and thus the formation of H^+ and HCO_3^-. Although body tissues contain several isoenzymes of carbonic anhydrase, the C-type, sulfonamide-sensitive carbonic anhydrase (also known as type II), is the predominant isoenzyme in the human ciliary processes.[404,405]

Inhibition of carbonic anhydrase activity in the ciliary processes is probably the mechanism responsible for decreased aqueous formation produced by CAIs. The production of bicarbonate in the ciliary epithelium appears to play a key role in the formation of aqueous humor. Although both bicarbonate and chloride are anions present in appreciable concentration in the aqueous humor, Zimmerman and associates[406] found that acetazolamide decreased bicarbonate entry into the posterior chamber of the dog's eye by approximately 50%, while chloride entry was not significantly altered. From this observation, these investigators concluded that bicarbonate is the key anion associated with the decrease in aqueous formation produced by inhibition of carbonic anhydrase. Similar findings in other species further support this conclusion.[407,408]

Inhibition of carbonic anhydrase also decreases sodium entry into the posterior chamber.[409–411] Sodium, transported by Na^+-K^+ adenosine triphosphatase (ATPase), probably acts as the counter-ion for newly formed bicarbonate.[412] These two ions are linked such that inhibition of either carbonic anhydrase or Na^+-K^+ ATPase reduces sodium movement into the posterior chamber.[409,411] In addition, inhibition of both carbonic anhydrase and Na^+-K^+ ATPase produces a net effect on aqueous production no greater than the inhibition of either enzyme individually.[409]

Fluid movement from the stroma of the ciliary processes into the posterior chamber requires the transepithelial movement of several ions. Assuming that Na^+, HCO_3^-, and Cl^- are the major ions involved in secretion, Figure 10.14 illustrates how these ions may function in fluid movement across the nonpigmented ciliary epithelium and into the posterior chamber. Sodium may enter the epithelium from the stromal side either by diffusion or by a Na^+/H^+ exchange system.[413] The intracellular sodium concentration is maintained, since Na^+ is also being transported extracellularly into the lateral intercellular channels of the nonpigmented epithelium by a Na^+-K^+ ATPase-dependent system. HCO_3^- is formed from the hydration of CO_2, a process catalyzed by carbonic anhydrase. Cl^- enters the lateral intercellular channel by a mechanism that is not understood and thereby

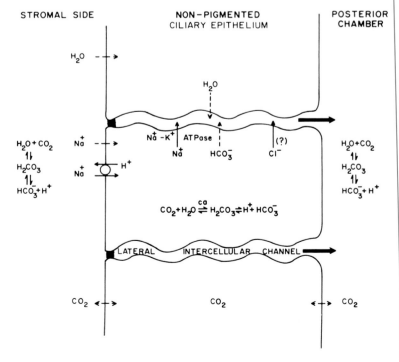

FIGURE 10.14   **Ion and fluid movement in the nonpigmented ciliary epithelium. Na^+ enters the nonpigmented ciliary epithelium from the stromal side either by diffusion or by Na^+/H^+ exchange. Na^+, the main cation involved in aqueous formation, is transported extracellularly into the lateral intercellular channel by a Na^+-K^+ ATPase-dependent transport system. HCO_3^- forms from the hydration of CO_2, a reaction catalyzed by carbonic anhydrase. HCO_3^-, the major anion involved in aqueous formation, balances a portion of the Na^+ being transported into the lateral intercellular channel. Cl^- enters the intercellular space by a mechanism that is not understood. This movement of ions into the lateral intercellular space creates a hypertonic fluid, and water enters by osmosis. Because of the restriction on the stromal side of the channel, the newly formed fluid moves toward the posterior chamber. A rapid diffusional exchange of CO_2 allows for its movement into the posterior chamber. (Adapted from Cole DF. Secretion of aqueous humor. Exp Eye Res (suppl) 1977; 25:161–176.)**

balances a portion of the transported Na⁺. Because of the entry of ions into the lateral intercellular channel, a hypertonic fluid is produced that results in an osmotic water flux.[413] Because of restrictions by the stromal end of the channel, fluid moves by bulk flow toward the posterior chamber. In addition to their ability to decrease bicarbonate formation, carbonic anhydrase inhibitors may also alter the intracellular pH so that ATPase activity is modified and Na⁺ movement is inhibited.[413] Therefore, inhibition of carbonic anhydrase in the ciliary processes probably decreases bicarbonate, sodium, and fluid movement into the posterior chamber, with the net result being decreased aqueous humor formation.

The reduction of intraocular pressure produced by the CAIs has been attributed, at least in part, to the accompanying metabolic acidosis that occurs secondary to the renal effects of these agents.[414,415] This theory receives support from the clinical observation that diabetics in ketoacidosis often have "soft" eyes. In addition, acidosis produced following administration of ammonium chloride has also been shown to decrease IOP.[416,417] Using nephrectomized rabbits, which prevents metabolic acidosis and diuresis, Becker[417] has shown that acetazolamide reduces IOP, thereby illustrating that its renal effects do not contribute significantly to acetazolamide's ocular hypotensive action. Another study[415] using nephrectomized rabbits has confirmed this finding. These investigators demonstrated that acetazolamide (5 mg/kg body weight) can reduce IOP without altering arterial pH, bicarbonate, or pCO₂. However, doses producing metabolic acidosis (> 15 mg/kg) further reduced IOP. Of the carbonic anhydrase inhibitors, acetazolamide has the greatest effect on acid-base balance. Therefore, these experiments have shown that metabolic acidosis produced by CAIs contributes only slightly to their maximal ocular hypotensive effect in animals. In humans, however, metabolic acidosis from acetazolamide does not influence IOP.[418]

Most tissues contain carbonic anhydrase in quantities that exceed physiologic requirements. Because of this excess, at least 99% of carbonic anhydrase activity must be inhibited in order to depress aqueous production significantly.[410,419] Drug levels sufficient to reduce aqueous humor formation are readily achieved following systemic administration of CAIs.[400] However, systemic use has the disadvantage of significantly inhibiting the activity of carbonic anhydrase throughout the body.

Of the currently available CAIs (see Table 10.18), acetazolamide is the prototype drug and has been studied extensively. Other agents within this class include methazolamide and dichlorphenamide. Becker[420] has shown that systemic administration of any of these agents produces a 45% to 55% inhibition of aqueous formation in humans. Recent studies[421] have revealed that acetazolamide decreases aqueous flow by 21% during the day. At night, acetazolamide produces a 24% reduction below the nocturnal flow rate measured during sleep.

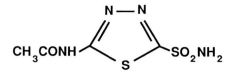

FIGURE 10.15   **Molecular structure of acetazolamide.**

Acetazolamide

PHARMACOLOGY

In the treatment of all types of glaucoma, acetazolamide (Fig. 10.15) is the most widely used orally administered CAI. Acetazolamide (Diamox) is commercially available as 125 and 250 mg tablets, 500 mg sustained-release capsules (Diamox Sequels), and a 500 mg vial formulated for parenteral administration. In long-term antiglaucoma therapy in adults, acetazolamide is usually administered in doses of 250 mg every six hours or a single 500 mg sustained-release capsule twice daily. The recommended acetazolamide dose for children is 5–10 mg/kg body weight, administered every 4 to 6 hours.[422]

Bioavailability studies have shown that generic acetazolamide tablets are equivalent to brand-name acetazolamide (Diamox) tablets.[423] Therefore, patients may use the less expensive generic acetazolamide.

Acetazolamide is readily absorbed from the gastrointestinal tract after oral administration.[424,425] Following ingestion of acetazolamide tablets, the drug attains peak plasma levels within 2 to 4 hours. Peak levels are maintained for 4 to 6 hours.[426] Drug levels are higher after ingesting acetazolamide tablets than after an equivalent dose of the time-release preparation. The time-release capsules produce maximum drug levels in 3 to 4 hours, and levels of 10 μg/ml are maintained for about 10 hours.[427]

The time course of acetazolamide's ocular hypotensive effect parallels its plasma concentration.[428] Oral acetazolamide tablets, in dosages greater than 63 mg, produce a significant ocular hypotensive response within two hours, and the effects last beyond six hours (Table 10.19).[428] The ocular hypotensive effect of the sustained-release capsules begins within two hours, and the maximum reduction in IOP occurs 6 to 18 hours after oral administration.[429] Although a 500 mg capsule administered once daily produces a substantial decrease in IOP lasting at least 24 hours, the magnitude of the pressure drop is greater when the drug is administered twice daily.[430] The sustained-release capsules, administered in dosages of 500 mg twice daily, are as effective in reducing IOP as are 250 mg acetazolamide tablets administered every six hours.[430]

Plasma levels sufficient to decrease IOP occur only minutes after intravenous administration of acetazolamide,[431,432] but this route of administration is generally reserved for

TABLE 10.19
Pharmacokinetic Properties of Carbonic Anhydrase Inhibitors

Drug	Dose	Onset of Ocular Hypotensive Action	Maximum IOP Reduction	Duration of Ocular Hypotensive Action
Acetazolamide tablet	65–250 mg q.i.d.	½–1 hr	2–4 hr	4–6 hr
Acetazolamide capsule	500 mg b.i.d.	1–2 hr	8–12 hr	10–18 hr
Acetazolamide IV	500 mg IV	1 min	20–30 min	4 hr
Methazolamide	25–100 mg b.i.d., t.i.d.	1 hr	7–8 hr	10–14 hr
Dichlorphenamide	25–50 mg b.i.d., t.i.d., q.i.d.	½ hr	2–4 hr	6–12 hr

IOP, intraocular pressure; b.i.d., twice daily; t.i.d., three times daily; q.i.d., four times daily.
Adapted from Flach AJ. Topical acetazolamide and other carbonic anhydrase inhibitors in the current medical therapy of the glaucomas. Glaucoma 1986;8:20–27.

situations, such as in acute angle-closure glaucoma, when vomiting precludes the oral route. Acetazolamide's duration of action after intravenous administration is approximately 4 hours.[433]

In humans, 90% to 95% of acetazolamide in the blood binds to plasma proteins.[419] Therefore, relatively large dosages of acetazolamide are required to produce a significant plasma level of the unbound drug. At plasma pH (7.4), half the unbound acetazolamide ($pK_a = 7.4$) exists in the un-ionized form (Table 10.20), which is the form that penetrates tissues and inhibits carbonic anhydrase.

Acetazolamide is not metabolized; it is excreted, primarily by tubular secretion, into the urine.[425] Due to its action on the kidney, acetazolamide increases urinary excretion of HCO_3^- and produces an alkaline urine. This alteration of urinary pH favors excretion of acetazolamide, since more drug exists in the water-soluble, ionized form.

Acetazolamide therapy is often difficult to optimize due to pharmacokinetic variables and differences in responsiveness.[434] The plasma levels necessary for effective glaucoma therapy reportedly range from 5 to 20 μg/ml.[428,430,434] Fur-

thermore, after a given dose, large interindividual variations in plasma levels often occur. Alm and associates[434] studied plasma concentrations after oral acetazolamide doses of 187.5, 375, 750, and 1000 mg. At all doses, large variations in the plasma drug levels were observed. When the plasma levels achieved following a 1000-mg dose of acetazolamide were analyzed with respect to patients' ages, patients older than 80 years exhibited drug levels that were approximately two to three times higher than patients younger than 60 years (21.6 and 8.3 μg/ml, respectively). Therefore, older patients seem to attain higher serum levels and may require modifications in their doses, especially if renal function is decreased, which may impair excretion.

CLINICAL USES

In the treatment of primary open-angle glaucoma, oral acetazolamide is added to the treatment regimen when topical agents alone do not control IOP satisfactorily (see Fig. 35.9). Acetazolamide produces an additional decrease in IOP when added to drug regimens including miot-

TABLE 10.20
Pharmacologic Properties of Carbonic Anhydrase Inhibitors

Drug	% Bound to Plasma Proteins	pK_a	% Un-ionized in Plasma (pH 7.4)
Acetazolamide	95	7.4	50
Methazolamide	55	7.2	39
Dichlorphenamide	—	8.3	89

Adapted from Wistrand PJ, Rawls JA, Maren TH. Sulfonamide carbonic anhydrase inhibitors and intraocular pressure in rabbits. Acta Pharmacol Toxicol 1960;17:337–355.

ics,[434,435] epinephrine,[436] or β blockers.[437,438] Although both timolol and acetazolamide inhibit aqueous formation, concurrent administration of these agents produces a nearly additive effect on IOP.[437,438] In contrast to timolol, which has no significant effect on aqueous flow in sleeping humans, acetazolamide reduces aqueous flow during sleep.[421] In humans, the aqueous flow rate normally decreases approximately 60% while asleep. Acetazolamide suppresses aqueous flow an additional 24% below the nocturnal flow rate. Thus, administering a dose of acetazolamide just prior to retiring will have a beneficial ocular hypotensive effect. Concurrent timolol administration should be limited to the dose upon awakening.

In acute angle-closure glaucoma, oral or parenteral acetazolamide is often administered soon after making the diagnosis. The combination of acetazolamide, a β blocker, and pilocarpine usually reduces the IOP sufficiently to permit laser iridotomy or surgical peripheral iridectomy. Use of acetazolamide in the management of acute angle-closure glaucoma is frequently limited to the preoperative period, since many patients require no further medication or can be managed with topical agents following surgery.

An additional clinical use of acetazolamide is unrelated to its ocular hypotensive properties. Cox and associates[439] showed that 500 mg of acetazolamide administered daily for 2 weeks produced either a partial or complete resolution of macular edema in many patients with Irvine-Gass syndrome, retinitis pigmentosa, and chronic intermediate uveitis (pars planitis). Macular edema produced by primary retinal vascular diseases (branch and central retinal vein occlusion and macular telangiectasia) did not respond to acetazolamide therapy. Therefore, acetazolamide may improve visual function only if the macular edema stems from retinal pigment epithelial dysfunction.[439–441] Improved macular edema in these conditions may be linked with fluid movement from the retina to the choroid.[439,442] However, acetazolamide does not appear to alter macular blood flow.[443]

SIDE EFFECTS

Systemic Effects. Although acetazolamide is frequently effective as an ocular hypotensive agent, a significant number of side effects limit its clinical usefulness (Table 10.21). Maximal doses of CAIs produce intolerable effects in 30% to 80% of patients.[429,444–447] The incidence of side effects varies with the dose and the formulation; however, when all side effects are considered, the incidence probably approaches 100% in patients taking either acetazolamide tablets or the 500 mg sustained-release capsules. Lichter and associates[447] have shown that only 26% of patients could tolerate acetazolamide tablets beyond six weeks, while 58% of patients could tolerate prolonged use of the time-release preparation. Becker and Middleton[448] have observed a lower incidence of side effects in blacks receiving long-term acetazolamide therapy than in whites.

TABLE 10.21
Side Effects of Acetazolamide

Systemic
  Numbness and tingling of extremities and perioral region[a]
  Metallic taste[a]
  Symptom complex[a]
    Decreased libido
    Depression
    Fatigue
    Malaise
    Weight loss
  Gastrointestinal irritation[a]
  Metabolic acidosis[a]
  Hypokalemia
  Renal calculi
  Blood dyscrasias
  Dermatitis

Ocular
  Transient myopia

[a]Common.

Numbness and tingling of the fingers, toes, and perioral region are among the most common adverse events resulting from use of CAIs.[433] Some patients find this loss of sensitivity quite disconcerting, but rarely is it intolerable. Furthermore, it is usually transient. However, numbness and tingling of the fingers may impair tactile sensation to an unacceptable level for visually impaired patients who use braille.[449] Another common, but tolerable, side effect is an alteration in gustation, resulting in a metallic taste.[433]

Epstein and Grant[446] have described a symptom complex consisting of malaise, fatigue, weight loss, depression, anorexia, and often decreased libido as the side effects most likely to require discontinuation of CAIs. In addition, impotence has been reported in some patients taking acetazolamide. These symptoms may take several months to develop and appear to relate at least partially to serum drug levels.[446,450] The symptom complex also appears to occur more commonly in patients exhibiting marked acidosis.[446] Therefore, sodium bicarbonate (up to 80 mEq/day) has been used in an attempt to decrease the level of acidosis.[446,450] In some patients, supplemental sodium bicarbonate may improve drug tolerance, but this finding has not been associated with significant changes in the level of acidosis.[446]

Symptoms indicating gastrointestinal irritation, including abdominal cramps, nausea, and diarrhea, have been reported following use of acetazolamide.[446] Administering the tablets with food or changing from acetazolamide tablets to the sustained-release capsules may improve these symptoms for some patients.[446] Other patients have obtained relief from gastrointestinal symptoms by using sodium bicarbonate tablets.[446,450] These symptoms, if persistent, can become intolerable and may require an alternative means of IOP control.

CAIs alter renal function primarily by inhibiting carbonic anhydrase in the proximal tubule, which results in decreased bicarbonate reabsorption. Inhibition of intracellular carbonic anhydrase also affects both the distal tubule and the collecting duct. These effects produce decreased secretion of hydrogen ions and increased excretion of sodium, potassium, and bicarbonate ions. The net effect of the renal actions of acetazolamide therapy is alkalinization of the urine and metabolic acidosis. Metabolic acidosis results from the initial bicarbonate loss. Because carbonic anhydrase is inhibited at the level of the distal tubule, normal acidification does not recur. Thus, metabolic acidosis persists with continued acetazolamide use. Moderate metabolic acidosis develops in most patients.[451] This may be useful in determining drug compliance since most patients on acetazolamide will manifest serum CO_2 levels of less than 20 mEq/l.[452] Reabsorption of bicarbonate independent of carbonic anhydrase prevents severe acidosis.[453] Initially, acetazolamide produces diuresis, but urinary output decreases with the development of metabolic acidosis.[454] In addition, decreased urinary citrate excretion follows acetazolamide therapy and has been attributed to the metabolic acidosis it produces.[455] High urinary pH and low urinary citrate concentration are conducive to precipitation of calcium phosphate in both the renal papillae and the urinary tract.[456,457]

Although acetazolamide therapy increases urinary excretion of potassium, problems associated with hypokalemia rarely occur.[446,458] However, this potassium-depleting action may become significant if the patient is also taking a thiazide diuretic[446] or digitalis derivative. Concomitant use of acetazolamide and a thiazide diuretic can lead to drug-induced hypokalemia, and these patients may require potassium supplementation.[446] Since decreased potassium levels also increase the possibility of digitalis toxicity, potassium levels should be monitored closely in patients taking acetazolamide with digitalis derivatives or thiazide diuretics.

The most serious side effects associated with acetazolamide are blood dyscrasias. Thrombocytopenia, agranulocytosis, and aplastic anemia have all occurred in patients taking acetazolamide; however, drug-induced blood dyscrasias are extremely rare.[459,460] Therefore, Fraunfelder and associates[461] have made the following recommendations: (1) complete blood counts should be performed before starting treatment with CAIs and at intervals of every six months thereafter; (2) patients receiving CAI therapy should report a persistent sore throat, fever, fatigue, pallor, easy bruising, epistaxis, purpura, or jaundice; and (3) a decrease in the level of any single, formed blood element should result in immediate termination of CAI therapy. Although strongly recommended by the drug manufacturers and by Fraunfelder and associates,[461] the usefulness of routine hematologic evaluation in patients receiving chronic CAI therapy has been questioned because of its high cost relative to its low detection rate of drug-induced adverse hematologic events.[462,463]

Ocular Effects.   Drug-induced transient myopia has been reported with several sulfonamides.[464–466] Acetazolamide, an unsubstituted heterocyclic sulfonamide, has also been associated with myopic shifts in refractive error.[467–470] Shallowing of the anterior chamber is the only parameter documented to change in eyes exhibiting this increase in myopia following sulfonamide therapy.[471] Myopia probably results from ciliary body edema that produces a forward displacement of the lens-iris diaphragm.[464,471] The myopia subsides upon reducing or discontinuing acetazolamide therapy (see Chap. 37).

CONTRAINDICATIONS

Since long-term use of acetazolamide usually brings on a significant number of side effects, patients who are particularly susceptible to these side effects should avoid acetazolamide (Table 10.22). Because of the significant structural differences between the antibacterial and the carbonic anhydrase-inhibiting sulfonamides, Friedland and Maren[472] believe there is little evidence to suggest overlapping sensitivities between the two classes of drugs. However, Fraunfelder and associates[461] have cited hypersensitivity reactions including exfoliative dermatitis, nonthrombocytopenic purpura, hepatitis, nephropathy, and transient myopia as being linked with sulfonamide compounds and their derivatives. Peralta and associates[473] reported a case of anaphylactic shock and death following a single dose of oral acetazolamide. Thus, patients with known hypersensitivity reactions to sulfonamides should not take CAIs.

Since acetazolamide is excreted unchanged in the urine,[425] patients with impaired renal function may require substantially lower doses and should be monitored closely for side effects. Patients taking potassium-depleting diuretics must use acetazolamide with caution because of the possibility of drug-induced hypokalemia. Since patients taking digitalis preparations are at greater risk of developing digitalis toxicity secondary to hypokalemia, acetazolamide must be used with caution or avoided in these individuals. Patients with cirrhosis of the liver are particularly sensitive

---

TABLE 10.22
Contraindications for Use of Acetazolamide

- Clinically significant liver disease
- Severe chronic obstructive pulmonary disease
- Certain secondary glaucomas[a]
- Renal disease, including kidney stones[a]
- Pregnancy
- Known hypersensitivity to sulfonamides

[a]See text for discussion.

to toxicity associated with acetazolamide use. Alkalinization of the urine decreases urinary trapping of NH_4^+ and may result in increased levels of ammonia in the systemic circulation.[474] An increased level of ammonia in circulation may contribute to the development of hepatic encephalopathy.[474] Therefore, acetazolamide is contraindicated in patients with clinically significant liver disease.

Acetazolamide should be avoided in patients with severe COPD. These patients may be unable to increase their alveolar ventilation enough to compensate for the acid-base alterations induced by acetazolamide. In some patients, especially those with severe pulmonary disease, increased CO_2 gradients or acidosis may lead to acute respiratory failure. However, if acetazolamide is essential to the successful management of glaucoma in such patients, the practitioner should use the lowest effective dose to reduce IOP without completely inhibiting renal or red blood cell carbonic anhydrase activity.[475]

Since medical therapy is often completely ineffective in the management of the closed-angle stage of neovascular glaucoma[476,477] and other secondary glaucomas characterized by severe impairment of aqueous outflow,[478] acetazolamide should not be used routinely because of the systemic side effects it produces.[477] In addition, it is important to remember that CAIs reduce aqueous formation by only 45% to 55%.[420] In glaucomas arising from severe impairment of outflow, as in chronic angle-closure glaucoma, aqueous production will not be inhibited enough to allow long-term control of IOP. Therefore, the clinician may derive a false sense of security from the decrease in IOP produced by CAIs, while the underlying ocular condition progresses.

Black patients with sickle cell hemoglobinopathies and hyphema-induced secondary glaucomas should be administered acetazolamide with caution.[479] Acetazolamide increases the ascorbate concentration in aqueous humor and reduces plasma pH.[479] Both actions can promote sickling of red blood cells in the anterior chamber and within small blood vessels perfusing intraocular structures. Hyphemas containing sickled red blood cells resolve more slowly and elevate IOP more than do hyphemas containing nonsickled red blood cells.[480] Therefore, all black patients with hyphemas should be screened for sickle cell hemoglobinopathies before acetazolamide treatment, as should any black patient requiring long-term acetazolamide therapy.

Since it has been estimated that 5% to 10% of patients receiving long-term acetazolamide therapy either pass urinary calculi or have symptoms indicative of calculi,[481] acetazolamide may precipitate calculi formation in predisposed individuals. Therefore, patients with bacteriuria, previous bladder surgery, or a history suggestive of previous calculus formation should not receive acetazolamide.[481] Furthermore, since high urinary pH and low urinary citrate concentration are conducive to calculus formation, concurrent use of acetazolamide and sodium bicarbonate may increase the risk of calculus formation.[456] In addition, other forms of renal disease should be excluded before long-term acetazolamide therapy. If standard doses of acetazolamide are given to patients with diabetic nephropathy, severe acidosis may result;[482,483] therefore, these patients should have serum electrolytes monitored closely to prevent this complication.

In experimental animals acetazolamide can be teratogenic.[484] Although it has not been linked with birth defects in humans, acetazolamide use should generally be avoided during pregnancy.

DRUG INTERACTIONS

Drug interactions attributable to acetazolamide therapy are uncommon. However, the metabolic acidosis and alkalinization of the urine may alter the activity of several drugs. Amphetamines, quinidine, and tricyclic antidepressants have a prolonged effect and enhanced activity in alkaline urine due to increased renal tubular reabsorption.[485] Another important interaction stems from the increased serum levels of un-ionized salicylic acid that result when aspirin and acetazolamide are used concurrently. The acidosis produced by acetazolamide allows more salicylic acid to become unionized and thereby enhances penetration into the CNS.[486] Therefore, a potential hazard exists in patients with glaucoma who are taking high doses of aspirin for arthritis; arthritic patients requiring CAI therapy should receive low doses of methazolamide, which has a minimal effect on acid-base balance. In addition, these patients should be monitored closely for salicylate intoxication.[487]

Methazolamide

PHARMACOLOGY

During the last several decades, orally administered acetazolamide has been considered the CAI of choice in the treatment of glaucoma. More recently, however, the properties of methazolamide have been re-evaluated, and several studies[455,488,489] indicate possible advantages to its use as an ocular hypotensive agent.

Methazolamide (Fig. 10.16) is structurally similar to acetazolamide. The structure of methazolamide was designed to decrease ionization and thereby improve intraocular penetration.[455] After oral administration, methazolamide is well absorbed from the gastrointestinal tract. Average serum levels peak in 2 to 3 hours after an oral 100-mg dose and are

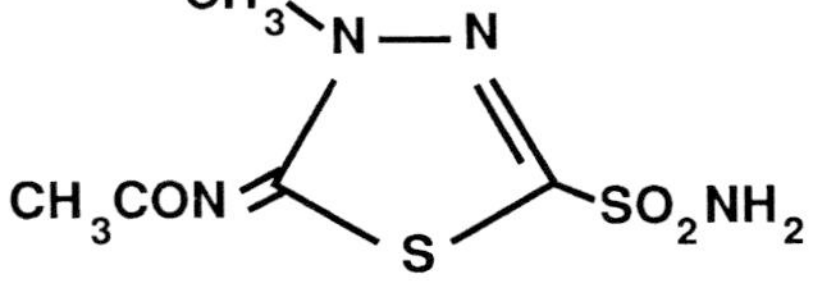

FIGURE 10.16 **Molecular structure of methazolamide.**

maintained nearly constant for at least 8 hours.[489] Methazolamide has higher lipid and water solubilities than does acetazolamide.[490] These properties favor renal tubular reabsorption and increase both its half-life and plasma concentration.[490] Methazolamide has a plasma half-life of approximately 14 hours, compared with five hours for acetazolamide.[455] Since only 25% of methazolamide is excreted unchanged in the urine, the remaining 75% is probably metabolized to an inactive form. However, its precise fate is unknown.[455]

Only 55% of methazolamide binds to plasma proteins, compared with 90% to 95% of acetazolamide.[455] Since only the unbound portion of the drug dose is pharmacologically active, methazolamide can be given at lower doses than acetazolamide to achieve comparable effects. Methazolamide ($pK_a = 7.2$) is 39% un-ionized at plasma pH.

Dose-response studies of methazolamide's ocular hypotensive effect have shown that IOP decreases in a dose-dependent manner for doses of 25, 50, and 100 mg given every 8 hours; the mean decreases in IOP at these doses were 3.3, 4.3, and 5.6 mm Hg, respectively.[489]

CLINICAL USES

Methazolamide, like other CAIs, may be added to the treatment regimen of patients with primary open-angle glaucoma and secondary glaucomas when topical antiglaucoma agents alone provide inadequate pressure control. Because of its ability to decrease IOP with less alteration of acid-base balance, methazolamide is probably a better drug than acetazolamide for use in patients with severe obstructive pulmonary disease.[475]

Methazolamide also alters urinary citrate excretion less than does acetazolamide; therefore, it is recommended for use in patients who require orally administered CAIs but are predisposed to renal calculus formation.[481]

The advantages of methazolamide are numerous enough that many authorities believe it should be the first CAI used for systemic glaucoma therapy.[488,491,492] Methazolamide (Neptazane) is commercially available in 25 and 50 mg tablets. The adult dosage is 25–100 mg three times daily. Zimmerman[491,492] has recommended 25 mg orally adminis-

tered twice daily as the initial dose. This dose usually produces a 4 mm to 5 mm Hg decrease in IOP with minimal side effects. If after one week the IOP remains at an unacceptable level, the dose should be increased to 50 mg orally administered twice daily. The level of IOP reduction should again be evaluated after one week; if the pressure is still not at the desired level, the medication should be changed to acetazolamide 500 mg sequels orally administered twice daily.

SIDE EFFECTS

Methazolamide is one of the best tolerated oral CAIs, especially at low doses.[447,488] However, administration of this drug poses the same general risk as does administration of acetazolamide, and the side effects associated with methazolamide use are essentially those associated with acetazolamide. Compared with acetazolamide, methazolamide generally produces less acidosis and has less effect on urinary citrate levels.[455] Thus, patients who are intolerant of acetazolamide may tolerate methazolamide therapy without difficulty.

Methazolamide is particularly useful in patients predisposed to develop renal calculi.[481] Methazolamide interferes less with excretion of urinary citrate, which may explain why kidney stones have only rarely been associated with its use.[493,494]

Compared with acetazolamide, methazolamide generally causes less paresthesia but often causes more drowsiness.[447] Although extremely rare, aplastic anemia and agranulocytosis have been reported as complications of methazolamide therapy.[461,495] Skin eruptions can also occur.[496]

CONTRAINDICATIONS

Contraindications to the use of methazolamide are essentially those associated with the use of acetazolamide. Methazolamide, however, can be used more safely in patients with a history of kidney stones or renal impairment. Patients with COPD may tolerate methazolamide better than acetazolamide, since the metabolic acidosis is less pronounced.

Dichlorphenamide

PHARMACOLOGY

Dichlorphenamide (Daranide) is a potent CAI. The structure of carbonic acid (H_2CO_3), the substrate for carbonic anhydrase, spatially resembles the sulfonamide portion of those compounds known to inhibit carbonic anhydrase.[420] Since dichlorphenamide (Fig. 10.17) has two sulfamyl ($-SO_2NH_2$) groups, this configuration probably accounts for its unwanted chloruretic effect.[472]

Dichlorphenamide is readily absorbed from the gastrointestinal tract after oral administration. Dichlorphenamide

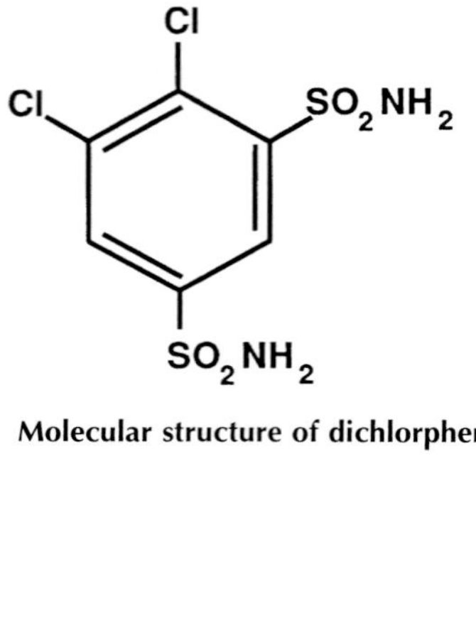

FIGURE 10.17   **Molecular structure of dichlorphenamide.**

($pK_a = 8.3$) is largely un-ionized at plasma pH. The fate of absorbed dichlorphenamide is not known. After oral administration, the decrease in IOP begins within 30 minutes, reaches a maximum within 2 hours, and has a duration of approximately 6 hours.[497] The maximum IOP response during dichlorphenamide therapy is equivalent to that of acetazolamide, although dichlorphenamide produces this effect at lower dosages.[497,498]

CLINICAL USES

The main ocular use for dichlorphenamide is in the treatment of primary open-angle glaucoma and some secondary glaucomas. Dichlorphenamide is generally added to the treatment regimen when the IOP cannot be adequately controlled with topical antiglaucoma agents alone. The drug is available in 50 mg tablets for oral use, and the usual adult dosage range is 25–100 mg administered three times daily. Patients intolerant of acetazolamide and methazolamide may tolerate dichlorphenamide.[497] However, Lichter and associates[447] have reported that only approximately 20% of patients can tolerate dichlorphenamide beyond six weeks. The relatively limited number of patients who can tolerate dichlorphenamide therapy limits the usefulness of this agent.

SIDE EFFECTS

The side effects of dichlorphenamide are similar to those produced by acetazolamide. In addition, dichlorphenamide produces more confusion and anorexia than do other CAIs.[447] The frequency and severity of systemic side effects following dichlorphenamide therapy are greater than with acetazolamide therapy.[447,497]

Unlike acetazolamide, the diuresis produced by dichlorphenamide is not self-limiting. Because dichlorphenamide causes less acidosis, its diuretic action persists with chronic use. Some authors believe that, compared with other CAIs, dichlorphenamide has the greatest potential to deplete potassium.[422,499] The potassium loss associated with dichlorphenamide is linked with its chloruretic effect, a characteristic shared with thiazide diuretics.[472,500] Thus, to detect drug-induced hypokalemia, electrolytes should be monitored in patients taking dichlorphenamide. Potassium supplementation does not alter the drug's ocular hypotensive effectiveness.[478]

Topical Carbonic Anhydrase Inhibitors

Following the introduction of oral acetazolamide, the search began for a topically active CAI that would reduce IOP without the adverse effects associated with the oral CAIs. Initial rabbit studies[501–504] did not show a significant ocular hypotensive effect following topical, subconjunctival, or intracameral administration of acetazolamide. Additional studies[505,506] demonstrated that acetazolamide, dichlorphena-

mide, ethoxzolamide, and methazolamide did not possess the necessary physiochemical properties (pK_a, partition coefficient, solubility, and molecular weight) to allow significant intraocular penetration following topical administration. Several investigators, however, did succeed in reducing IOP under certain circumstances. Friedman and associates[507] found that high-water-content soft contact lenses soaked in acetazolamide and methazolamide delivered a sufficiently high intraocular concentration to lower IOP in rabbits. In addition, Flach[508,509] showed that topical acetazolamide 10% solution administered alone, and in combination with parenteral acetazolamide, significantly reduced the IOP of water-loaded pigmented rabbits. Alpha-chymotryspin-induced ocular hypertensive rabbits also exhibited a reduction in IOP following a single application of dichlorphenamide sodium 10%.[510] These observations resulted in the synthesis of sulfonamides with chemical properties to improve intraocular penetration.

Several compounds have exhibited significant activity as topical CAIs. Trifluormethazolamide, a halogenated derivative of methazolamide, has a pK_a of 6.6, thereby allowing for both lipid and water solubility.[505,511] Preliminary studies indicated that topically applied trifluormethazolamide inhibited intraocular carbonic anhydrase and decreased IOP in cats and rabbits.[506,511,512] Further evaluation of trifluormethazolamide in humans, however, revealed its lack of activity as a topical ocular hypotensive agent.[513] Although several other compounds, including aminozolamide, L-645,151 and L-650,719, demonstrated potential as topical CAIs, these compounds were also found to have limited usefulness as ocular hypotensive agents in humans.[514–517]

The newest group of topical CAIs to be developed are the thienothiopyran-2-sulfonamides.[518] Among the compounds being actively investigated are MK-927, MK-417, and dorzolamide (Table 10.23); these drugs are the first topical CAIs to show significant ocular hypotensive activity in humans, including patients with open-angle glaucoma.[513,519–522] The addition of an alkylamino side group allows these compounds to alternate between an acidic and basic form.[513,520,523,524] This property enhances both lipid and water solubility, thereby allowing increased corneal and scleral penetration.[513,520,523–526] In addition, MK-927, MK-417, and dorzolamide have higher affinity for human carbonic anhydrase II isoenzyme in the nonpigmented ciliary epithelium than did previously tested topical CAIs.[520,524,527]

MK-927

MK-927 is a racemic mixture (50% R-enantiomer and 50% S-enantiomer) formulated as an isotonic aqueous solution in concentrations up to 2.0%.[513,524,528] The amount of the compound needed to double the human carbonic anhydrase II isoenzyme reaction time *in vitro* (IC_{50}) is 1.2 nmol.[528–530]

Initial studies in various animal models showed MK-927 to have significant potential as an ocular hypotensive

TABLE 10.23
Pharmacologic Characteristics of Thienothiopyran-2-sulfonamides

Characteristic	Compound		
	MK-927	MK-417 (Sezolamide)	Dorzolamide
pH	5.2	5.2	4.5–6.0
Vehicle/preservative	0.5% hydroxyethyl cellulose Benzalkonium chloride	0.5% hydroxyethyl cellulose Benzalkonium chloride	0.5% hydroxyethyl cellulose Benzalkonium chloride
Maximum concentration, (%)	2.0	1.8	2.0
IC_{50} (nmol)	1.20	0.54	0.20
IOP reduction* (reported range) (%)	17.7–24.3	19.4–24.7	21.8–26.2
Time to peak IOP reduction, (h)	1–2	1–2	2
Duration,** (h)	8–10	10–12	12
Expected dose frequency	TID	TID	TID

*Values calculated by comparing to equally time-matched prestudy diurnal IOP.
**These values pertain to multiple-dose studies.
Reprinted with permission from Hiett JA, Dockter CA. Topical carbonic anhydrase inhibitors: A new perspective in glaucoma therapy. Optom Clin 1992;2:10.

agent.[531] In human studies, topical MK-927 reduces IOP in both normals and in patients with open-angle glaucoma.[519] The dose-response relationship rises steeply between the 0.5% and 1.0% concentrations; the maximal ocular hypotensive effect occurs at concentrations between 1.0% and 2.0%.[532–536] In single-dose studies, both the 1.0% and 2.0% solutions reduce IOP beyond 8 hours.[532–536] In multiple-dose studies involving open-angle glaucoma patients, maximal IOP reduction occurs within two hours of application. With twice daily administration, the ocular hypotensive effects of the 1% and 2% concentrations are 17.7% to 18.6% and 19.2% to 20.6%, respectively. When administered twice daily, the duration of the ocular hypotensive effect is at least 12 hours. However, the reduction in IOP is considerably less 8 hours after administration. Thus, achieving adequate 24-hour pressure control may require administration three times daily.[529,536,537]

MK-417 (SEZOLAMIDE)

MK-417 (sezolamide) is the S-enantiomer of the racemic mixture, MK-927.[528,529] The S-enantiomer has more *in vitro* activity and greater specificity for carbonic anhydrase isoenzyme II than does the R-enantiomer.[524,528] MK-417's IC_{50} is

0.54 nmol.[520,521,528] As an isotonic solution in 0.5% hydroxyethylcellulose, MK-417 can be prepared in concentrations up to 1.8%.

Clinical trials in humans with open-angle glaucoma have shown encouraging results. A single-dose study comparing 1% MK-417 to 1% MK-927 revealed IOP reductions of 23.9% and 19.8%, respectively.[538] Both compounds produced a peak reduction in IOP 6 hours after topical application. In multiple-dose studies lasting 14 days, 1.8% MK-417 and 2.0% MK-927, administered twice daily, reduced IOP 19.4% to 19.9% and 19.0% to 19.2%, respectively.[529] Both drugs showed a maximal ocular hypotensive response 1 to 2 hours after topical administration. The duration of MK-417's ocular hypotensive effect has been evaluated in several short-term studies.[529] Since the reduction in IOP following 1.8% MK-417 was inadequate 10 hours after the morning dose, twice-daily administration does not seem feasible unless the ocular hypotensive effect becomes more pronounced with prolonged use. More recent studies[520] have demonstrated better IOP control with administration three times daily.

In comparison to other topical inhibitors of aqueous production, 1.8% MK-417 used three times daily appears equivalent to 0.5% timolol used twice daily. With twice-daily administration, 1.8% MK-417 is partially additive to 0.5% timolol; however, this additional ocular hypotensive effect lasts less than 12 hours.[529] Therefore, 1.8% MK-417 would produce more consistent IOP control if administered every 8 hours.

DORZOLAMIDE (TRUSOPT)

Dorzolamide is a very potent inhibitor of human carbonic anhydrase isoenzyme II. Its IC_{50} is 0.2 nmol. If formulated as an isotonic solution and buffered at a pH between 4.5–6.0, dorzolamide can be prepared in concentrations up to 3.0%.[521,522,524,527]

Animal studies revealed dorzolamide to be an effective ocular hypotensive agent.[527,537] The initial dose-response studies demonstrated that the 0.5% and 1.0% concentrations were near the top of the dose-response curve. In animal models dorzolamide produced a greater reduction in IOP than did MK-927.[520]

In human studies, patients with open-angle glaucoma exhibited a marked reduction in IOP following a single dose of 0.7% dorzolamide.[522] The pressure reduction increased with multiple-dose administration. After 12 days of treatment, 0.7% dorzolamide produced an ocular hypotensive effect nearly equal to that of the 2.0% concentration (Fig. 10.18). The 3.0% concentration did not have any greater activity than that of the 2.0%.[539] This finding indicates that 0.7% dorzolamide may be at the top of the dose-response curve, but multiple doses may be required to reach maximal IOP reduction. When administered twice daily and three times daily, 2.0% dorzolamide reduces IOP 21.8% to 24.4% and 22.2% to 26.2%, respectively.[520,522] The maximal ocular hypotensive effect occurs two hours after administration. Although twice-daily administration reduces IOP, dosing three times daily produces better overall ocular hypotensive effect.[50,522,540]

Compared with other ocular hypotensive agents, 2% dorzolamide administered three times daily reduces IOP almost as well as 0.5% betaxolol administered twice daily.[539] Topical 0.7% dorzolamide (twice daily for 5 days, then three times daily for 7 days) is as effective in reducing IOP as is oral methazolamide (100 mg three times daily for 8 days).[541] Furthermore, 2% dorzolamide, twice daily, produces an additional reduction in IOP when added to the drug regimen of patients using 0.5% timolol twice daily.[542]

Dorzolamide is commercially available as Trusopt (Merck) and is supplied as a sterile, isotonic, buffered, slightly viscous aqueous solution with a pH of approximately 5.6. Benzalkonium chloride 0.0075% is added as a preservative. Since a potential exists for an additive systemic effect with other CAIs, the concomitant use of topical dorzolamide with an oral CAI is not recommended. The safety of dorzolamide use has not been established in pregnancy, lactation, or in children. The drug is approved for use three times daily.

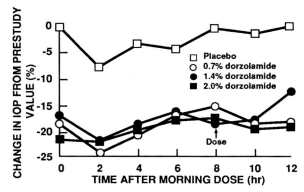

FIGURE 10.18 **Mean percent change in IOP from prestudy day to day 12. Dorzolamide or placebo was administered at 7 AM and 7 PM for the first five days and at 7 AM, 3 PM, and 11 PM for the next 7 days. Hour 0 corresponds to 7 AM. (Reprinted with permission from Lippa EA, Carlson LE, Ehinger B, et al. Dose response and duration of action of dorzolamide, a topical carbonic anhydrase inhibitor. Arch Ophthalmol 1992;110:495–499. Copyright © 1992, American Medical Association.)**

OTHER TOPICAL CARBONIC ANHYDRASE INHIBITORS

L-693,612, a compound structurally similar to dorzolamide, has been tested in glaucomatous monkeys.[543] Its IC_{50} is slightly higher than that of dorzolamide (0.27 nmol and 0.20 nmol, respectively). Although the ocular hypotensive potency of L-693, 612 is similar to that of dorzolamide in monkeys, the duration of action of L-693,612 significantly exceeds dorzolamide at all post-dose times up to 22 hours.[543]

Another topical inhibitor of human carbonic anhydrase II, AL-4333A, has an IC_{50} of 2.6 nmol.[544] This highly water-soluble compound has been tested as a 2% solution. In rabbits, topical 2% AL-4333A lowers IOP for up to five hours following administration. The maximal reduction of IOP (27%) occurs two hours after instillation. Using monkeys, topical 2% AL-4333A lowers IOP for up to six hours. The maximal reduction (25%) is noted three hours after the dose.[544]

PHARMACOLOGY

Conclusive data support the mechanism of action of orally and parenterally administered CAIs. These agents produce widespread inhibition of carbonic anhydrase throughout the body. When at least 99.95% of carbonic anhydrase is inhibited within the ciliary body, aqueous flow rates are suppressed and IOP is decreased.[525] Topical ophthalmic CAIs have been specifically evaluated relative to the IOP effects produced by systemic CAIs. After topical ocular instillation of these agents, drug accumulation has been documented within the ciliary body of the treated eye.[545–547] Topical CAIs alter aqueous humor composition, including lowering pH, decreasing bicarbonate levels, and increasing posterior chamber ascorbate levels limited to the eye receiving the dose.[548] Initially, topical CAIs were thought to gain access to the ciliary body through both local ocular penetration and systemic absorption. Many studies have shown, however, that local penetration is the major route.[505] A recent study[549] found that topical CAIs rapidly enter the uvea, suggesting that intraocular penetration occurs via the translimbal route. Although metabolic acidosis occurs with systemic CAIs, topical CAIs do not appear to produce systemic metabolic changes.[530,549,550] In addition, aqueous flow rates and IOP are decreased only in the eye receiving the topical dose; the contralateral eye is not affected by unilateral administration.[527,531,532-535] Thus, studies seem to indicate that both topical and systemic CAIs act by inhibiting carbonic anhydrase within the ciliary processes.

SIDE EFFECTS

Patients generally tolerate topical CAIs well. MK-927, MK-417, and dorzolamide produce mild to moderate stinging, burning and tearing,[519,520,522,529,532-536] but this local irritation usually lasts only 30 to 60 seconds. Various other ocular side effects occur less frequently, including transient blurred vision, itching, superficial punctate keratitis, conjunctival injection, allergic blepharoconjunctivitis, and foreign body sensation.[519,551] In addition, headaches, bitter taste, and diarrhea have occasionally been linked with the use of topical CAIs.[519,520] Ocular side effects are concentration dependent, increasing with higher concentrations.[520,551] Of the three thienothiopyran-2-sulfonamides, MK-417 produces more ocular side effects than do MK-927 or dorzolamide,[520,529] but some investigators have found no difference between MK-417 and MK-927.[551] In comparison to 0.5% betaxolol, Feicht and associates[552] found 2.0% MK-927 to have a comparable level of intolerance to local side effects. Although other ocular structures contain carbonic anhydrase, including the corneal endothelium, retinal pigment epithelium, and the lens, no ocular toxicity has been reported.[522,553-555] In addition, neither systemic metabolic alterations nor systemic side effects have been linked to topical CAIs.[530,550,556]

CLINICAL USES

Topical CAIs offer distinct advantages over other inhibitors of aqueous humor formation. Compared to β blockers, CAIs reduce the nocturnal flow rate by 25%.[421] β blockers lack the ability to suppress aqueous formation below the already reduced flow rate that occurs during sleep.[421] In contrast to systemic CAIs, topical CAIs lack systemic side effects while producing a comparable ocular hypotensive effect. None of the topical CAIs, however, has the ability to reduce IOP to the level achieved by 500 mg of oral acetazolamide.[557] Thus,

these topical agents should probably be used in place of systemic CAIs only for chronic treatment of primary and secondary open-angle glaucomas.

Systemic Hyperosmotic Agents

Hyperosmotic agents administered by the oral and intravenous routes are particularly useful in the initial management of acute angle-closure glaucoma and before intraocular surgery to reduce IOP.[558] They can also eliminate the need for surgery in cases of transient elevations of pressure, such as occurs with traumatic hyphema.[559]

Following systemic administration, a relatively rapid increase in serum osmolality occurs. The osmotic gradient induced between the ocular fluids (aqueous and vitreous) and the plasma causes fluid to move from the eye into the hyperosmotic plasma, via blood vessels of the retina and uveal tract.[560] The decrease of pressure depends on the degree to which it is elevated and the osmotic gradient induced. When the IOP is elevated, volume changes induced in the eye by loss of water to the hyperosmotic plasma result in a greater effect than when the pressure is at normal levels. Since their mechanism of action is thought to be primarily osmotic, the difference in osmotic pressure between the ocular fluids and the blood will determine the degree of reduction of IOP.[558,561] Agents confined to the extracellular fluid space following administration have a greater effect on plasma osmolality than do those distributed in total body water.[562] Most hyperosmotic agents effectively lower IOP when the serum osmolality is increased by 20 to 30 mOsm/liter.[558] Rates of ocular penetration and route of drug administration play a major role. Agents that enter the eye rapidly produce less of an osmotic gradient than those that penetrate slowly or not at all. In addition, the state of the ocular tissue influences penetration. Inflammation may enhance intraocular penetration of the hyperosmotic agents and decrease the osmotic gradient, thereby reducing the pressure-lowering effect[563] (Fig. 10.19).

Hyperosmotic agents may also lower IOP by a second mechanism, involving osmoreceptors in the hypothalamus. This CNS mechanism is suggested by observations that small doses of hyperosmotic agents administered intravenously can reduce IOP without changing plasma osmolality, and injections of hyperosmotic and hypoosmotic solutions into the third ventricle alter IOP without affecting plasma osmolality.[559,564]

Agents currently in use include the intravenous agents mannitol and urea, and for oral administration, glycerin and isosorbide (Table 10.24). Intravenous administration produces a more rapid onset of action and usually a greater effect on IOP.[565]

Intravenous Agents

MANNITOL

Pharmacology.   Mannitol is one of the most effective agents for reducing IOP, and its distribution is confined to the extracellular fluid compartment.[558,566] Mannitol is stable in solution and can be stored without deterioration. However, the solution should be warmed before use to dissolve crystals that may form during storage. Mannitol is less irritating than urea and does not cause tissue necrosis if the infusion extravasates.[558,567]

Since mannitol exhibits minimal intracellular penetration, it generally reduces IOP significantly. In addition, since it is confined to the extracellular water, it may produce a greater cellular dehydration and diuresis than does urea.[558,566,567] It is not metabolized and is excreted unchanged in the urine.[558] Thus, it may be safely used in diabetic patients.

Clinical Uses.   Mannitol is presently the hyperosmotic agent of choice for intravenous administration. It is available as a 20% solution in water. Intravenous administration in doses of 2.5 to 7.0 ml/kg body weight reduces IOP within 30 minutes. It reaches a maximum effect in 30 to 60 minutes, with a duration of action of approximately six hours.[558,567,568] The full dose is not always necessary, and the infusion can

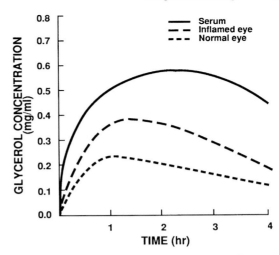

FIGURE 10.19   **Glycerol concentration in serum and aqueous of normal and inflamed rabbit eyes after administration of oral glycerol. (Reprinted with permission from the American Journal of Ophthalmology 62:629–634,1966. Copyright © The Ophthalmic Publishing Company.)**

be terminated when the IOP falls to the desired level.[559] Because mannitol penetrates the eye poorly, it is particularly useful as a hypotensive agent when the eye is inflamed.[565]

TABLE 10.24
Systemic Hyperosmotic Agents

Drug (Conc)	Dosage (gm/kg)	Onset of Effect (min)	Duration (hrs)
Oral Route			
Glycerin (Osmoglyn) 50%	1–1.5 (1.5–3 ml/kg of 50% solution)	15–30	4–5
Isosorbide (Ismotic) 45%	1–3 (1.5–4 ml/kg of 45% solution)	30–60	5–6
Intravenous Route			
Mannitol (Osmitrol) 5%, 10%, 20%, 25%	1–2 (2.5–7 ml/kg of 20% solution, 60 drops/min)	30–60	~6
Urea (Ureaphil) 30%	1–2 (2–7 ml/kg of 30% solution, 60 drops/min)	30–60	4–6

Adapted from Hoskins HD, Kass MA. Hyperosmotic agents. In: Becker-Shaffer's diagnosis and therapy of the glaucomas. St. Louis, CV Mosby, 1989. Chap. 27.

TABLE 10.25
Side Effects of Systemic Osmotherapy

Headache
Pain in upper extremities
Nausea and vomiting
Diuresis
Dehydration
K⁺ deficiency
Hyperglycemia[a]
Fever
Confusion and disorientation
Congestive heart failure
Diarrhea

[a]Can occur with use of glycerin.

Side Effects.   Mannitol is generally less toxic than urea. It is less irritating to tissues should the intravenous infusion extravasate.[558,567] However, diuresis, headache, chills, and chest pain may occur during infusion since mannitol infusion can lead to loss of water and electrolyte imbalances[558,569] (Table 10.25).

Contraindications.   Mannitol should be administered with caution to patients with renal disease.[558,569,570] Urine output should be monitored to maintain a flow of 30 to 50 ml/hr.[570]

UREA

Pharmacology.   In the late 1950s Javid introduced urea for ocular osmotherapy.[571] This compound readily dissolves in water and exerts a relatively strong osmotic effect.[567] Following its administration, urea distributes in all body fluids, including the eye. It diffuses more readily through body water and penetrates the eye more readily than does mannitol, especially if the eye is inflamed.[562] Osmotic alterations occur in both aqueous humor and the vitreous body, causing the anterior chamber to deepen by as much as 0.2 mm.[572] The ability of urea to penetrate cells can result in a rebound effect on IOP if the serum level falls below that of the vitreous.[573] Urea is not metabolized and is excreted unchanged in the urine.[558,567]

Clinical Uses.   Urea is rarely used in clinical practice. Solutions for intravenous infusion must be freshly prepared, since urea decomposes to ammonia on standing. Urea is administered as a 30% solution in 10% invert sugar to prevent hemolysis of red blood cells.[562] Intravenous infusion of 2 to 7 ml/kg body weight reduces IOP within 30 to 60 minutes, with a return to pretreatment levels in 4 to 6 hours.[561,562,572,573] During infusion the site of administration should be frequently observed, since urea can cause tissue

sloughing and phlebitis if the needle becomes dislodged.[567,573]

Side Effects.   The administration of urea causes frequent systemic complications (see Table 10.25).[573] All patients experience a rapid diuresis. Severe headache and arm pain are common. About one-third of patients experience nausea, and some patients become confused and disoriented. Urea may cause depletion of electrolytes, resulting in loss of sodium and potassium.

Contraindications.   Urea should not be administered to patients with impaired renal function, severe liver impairment, or dehydration. The drug should not be infused into the lower extremities of elderly patients.[570]

Oral Agents

GLYCERIN (GLYCEROL)

Pharmacology.   Since 1963 when Virno and associates[574] reported the ocular hypotensive effects of oral glycerin in patients with various types of glaucoma, glycerin has become a commonly used hyperosmotic agent for the initial management of acute angle-closure glaucoma.[575]

Chemically, glycerin is a trivalent alcohol. It is metabolized by the body in a manner analogous to other carbohydrates and produces 4.32 Kcal/g.[574] When glycerin is administered in recommended dosages, the resulting calories do not usually cause any significant problems. However, since hyperglycemia and glycosuria can result following glycerin administration, its caloric value must be considered when repeated administration is necessary.

Following oral administration, glycerin is confined to the extracellular fluid until metabolized and eliminated by the kidneys. It penetrates the eye poorly.[558] However, aqueous levels of glycerin are higher in the inflamed eye due to breakdown of the blood-aqueous barrier, which allows for greater intraocular penetration of the osmotic agent[565] (see Fig. 10.19).

Clinical Uses.   The use of glycerin provides a clinical advantage in that oral administration results in rapid systemic absorption. Although the reduction in IOP is somewhat slower than with intravenous agents, doses of 1.5 to 3.0 ml/kg body weight of a 50% solution reduce pressure within 15 to 30 minutes. The maximum effect is reached within 45 minutes to two hours, with a duration of action of about five hours.[565,574-576] Glycerin is available as a 50% lime-flavored solution (Osmoglyn) preserved with potassium sorbate.[570] The solution should be administered chilled or over ice to reduce potential nausea and vomiting. Figure 10.20 compares the ocular hypotensive effects of oral glycerin with intravenous urea and mannitol.

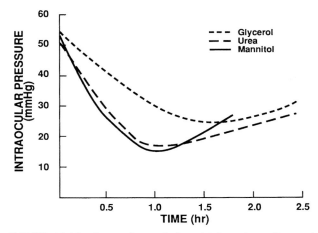

FIGURE 10.20 **Comparison of the IOP-lowering effects of intravenous urea (1 g/kg body weight), intravenous mannitol (3 g/kg), and orally administered glycerol (1.5ml/kg) in humans. (Reprinted with permission from the American Journal of Ophthalmology 62:629–634,1966. Copyright © The Ophthalmic Publishing Company.)**

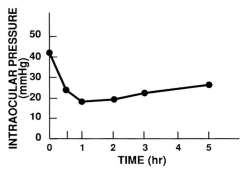

FIGURE 10.21 **A patient with secondary glaucoma shows reduction in IOP following oral administration of isosorbide 2 g/kg. (Reprinted with permission from Becker B, Kolker AE, Krupin T. Isosorbide: an oral hyperosmotic agent. Arch Ophthalmol 1967;78:150. Copyright © 1967, American Medical Association.)**

Side Effects.   Although oral administration simplifies its use, glycerin has several characteristics that may limit its clinical usefulness in acute angle-closure glaucoma and before and after surgery. Since glycerin has a sweet taste, it frequently induces nausea and vomiting. Patients already nauseous or vomiting cannot take glycerin. Extreme caution must be exercised with diabetic patients, since in addition to hyperglycemia, ketoacidosis may be induced. The resultant increase in serum osmolality following administration can cause dehydration, nausea, headache, confusion, and disorientation (see Table 10.25).[570,577,578]

Contraindications.   Glycerin should be administered with caution to patients with congestive heart disease, hypervolemia, and dementia. Caution must also be exercised with elderly, diabetic, or severely dehydrated patients.[570]

ISOSORBIDE

Pharmacology.   Isosorbide is a dihydric alcohol formed by the removal of two molecules of water from sorbitol. It is readily absorbed from the gastrointestinal tract following oral administration. It is distributed in total body water but unlike glycerin, isosorbide can penetrate cells and gain access to the aqueous humor.[558,574] The drug is available as a 45% solution in a vanilla-mint flavored vehicle (Ismotic).

In contrast to glycerin, isosorbide is not metabolized. About 95% of an administered dose is excreted unchanged in the urine.[558] It therefore provides no calories and can be administered to diabetic patients without altering the insulin requirement.[579,580]

Clinical Uses.   Administration of isosorbide reduces IOP within 30 to 60 minutes. The effect lasts for as long as 5 to 6 hours[579] (Fig. 10.21). The recommended dosage ranges from 1–3 g/kg. Indications for use are the same as for glycerin.[570]

Side Effects.   Compared with glycerin, isosorbide generally has a lower incidence of nausea and vomiting.[580] Headache, confusion, and disorientation can occur.[579,580] Rare occurrences of gastric discomfort, dizziness, thirst, and lethargy have been reported.[570]

Contraindications.   As with all hyperosmotic agents, isosorbide must be administered with caution to patients with severe cardiovascular, pulmonary or renal disease, severe dehydration, or hypersensitivity to the drug or to any of the components of the preparation.[570]

Antimetabolites

Approximately 10% of glaucoma patients are unresponsive to medications and adjuvant laser treatments and must undergo filtration surgery. However, 25% of filtering procedures tend to fail due to scarring of the opening created in the sclera.[581,582]

Surgery is usually reserved for patients with little or no response to medical therapy, or where the disease is so advanced that medical treatment alone is inadequate. Improved glaucoma surgical modalities, difficulty in achieving successful long-term medical therapy, and partial and usually transient efficacy of argon laser trabeculoplasty (ALT) have led to a gradual shift toward earlier surgical intervention.[582–585]

Since Cairns[586] introduced his surgical technique over 25 years ago, the risk-benefit ratio of filtering procedures has steadily improved. Although trabeculectomy is generally successful, it is still associated with a high rate of surgical failure. Eyes with a previous failed filter, previous intraocular surgery, glaucoma secondary to uveitis and neovascularization, black patients,[703] children and young adults[704] are at high risk of failure.[587,588] Modulating the processes involved in limbal wound healing is critical to the outcome of glaucoma filtration surgeries.

The major cause of surgical failure is scarring of the ostium and extensive fibrosis, believed to emerge from the neighboring tissues, including Tenon's capsule and conjunctival fibroblasts.[589,590] In a study using rabbits, granulation tissue closed the sclerostomy, and late migration of fibroblasts from episcleral and superior rectus epimysial tissues caused contraction and scarring. As a result, 58% of the blebs had collapsed by 10 days, and 94% by 17 days.[591] In cats, myofibroblasts produced collagen that gradually bridged the incision sites by day 14.[592] In the owl monkey, three phases of wound healing have been distinguished: early healing (days 2 to 6) in which fibroblasts migrated along the wall of the sclerostomy; intermediate healing (days 7 to 9) when 4 of the 10 fistulae were completely occluded. In the late healing phase (days 10 to 14) all but one fistula were completely sealed by granulation tissue.[593] In cynomolgus monkeys the peak cellular proliferation after experimental filtration surgery occurred on the fifth day postoperatively, with contribution from the episclera, cornea, capillary endothelial cells, and conjunctival epithelium.[594] Several authors[595–597] have suggested that aqueous humor may have chemotactic activity that facilitates cicatrization. These observations triggered a detailed evaluation of aqueous humor constituents,[598] the changes occurring in the aqueous humor following glaucoma surgery,[599] and the possible role of ascorbate in modulating wound healing.[600]

To improve duration and success rates of filtering blebs, several antifibrotic agents have been screened *in vitro*. Cytosine arabinoside has been found to reduce the proliferation of human scleral fibroblasts by 50% at 72 hours.[601] Mithramycin, mitomycin, daunorubicin, and bleomycin have prevented human subconjunctival fibroblast attachment and proliferation.[602] Similar effects on Tenon's capsule fibroblasts have been noted with fluorinated pyrimidines.[603] The following compounds may delay wound healing in glaucoma surgery: β-aminopropionitrile,[604] heparin,[605] colchicin, taxol, cytochalasin B,[606] retinoids,[607,608] tissue plasminogen activator,[609,610] Γ-interferon[611] as well as β-irradiation.[612] Two antimetabolites, 5-fluorouracil and mitomycin-C, are currently used clinically as adjuvant therapy to filtration surgery.

5-fluorouracil (5-FU)

PHARMACOLOGY

5-FU is the most extensively investigated and utilized antimetabolite in trabeculectomy.[613–618] This compound, a fluorinated pyrimidine, is a competitive inhibitor of thymidilate synthetase. 5-FU thus interferes with the synthesis of deoxyribonucleic acid (DNA) and to a lesser extent inhibits the formation of ribonucleic acid (RNA). Since both nucleic acids are essential for cell division, unbalanced growth and cell death ensue. Despite its limited lipid solubility, 5-FU diffuses readily across cell membranes. Following systemic absorption, it is metabolized principally by the liver, while approximately 20% of the drug is excreted unchanged in the urine.

CLINICAL USES

5-FU is the first line of adjuvant pharmacologic therapy after surgery, especially in eyes with a substantially higher risk of postoperative failure. 5-FU is injected subconjunctivally usually in divided daily doses over two weeks during the immediate postoperative period. In many instances it is administered together with a steroid. The total dosage ranges from 25 to 200 mg, with a preference toward the lower dosages. The preferred injection site has not been clearly defined. Some surgeons inject 5-FU away from the bleb, usually inferiorly, while others prefer to administer the drug adjacent to the filtration site.

Subconjunctivally administered 5-FU increases the rate of surgical success, decreases the postoperative IOP, and reduces the need for postoperative antiglaucoma medication in eyes with open-angle glaucoma undergoing trabeculectomy.[613] This is especially true for patients with a poor prognosis, such as those who have had a previous cataract extraction or unsuccessful filtering surgery.[617] Adjunctive 5-FU, however, appears to be ineffective when used following filtering surgery combined with extracapsular cataract extraction or phacoemulsification and posterior chamber intraocular lens implantation.[614,615]

Various delivery systems for 5-FU have been evaluated in an effort to increase its therapeutic index and to avoid the necessity for repeated subconjunctival injections. Bleb longevity has been slightly prolonged when bioerodible polymers incorporating 5-FU were placed at the site of filtration surgery in rabbit eyes, but surgical failure occurred after the 17th postoperative day.[619,620] When 5-fluorouridine was incorporated into polyanhydride discs, the duration of surgical success increased significantly in glaucomatous monkeys (26 ± 9 days vs. 8.5 ± 4 days in treated and control groups, respectively).[621] Collagen implants are poor drug delivery systems in glaucoma surgery due to induction of granulomatous reactions.[622]

SIDE EFFECTS

The use of 5-FU has been associated with corneal toxicity, wound leakage, suprachoroidal hemorrhage, retinal detachment, as well as either early or late infection.[587,623–626]

CONTRAINDICATIONS

For postoperative ocular injection, 5-FU treatment is contraindicated in patients with active corneal disease, leaking bleb, infection, flat anterior chamber, or persistent extreme hypotony.

Mitomycin-C (MMC)

PHARMACOLOGY

First introduced by Chen[627] as adjuvant therapy during trabeculectomy, MMC is an antibiotic-antineoplastic agent isolated from *Streptomyces caespitosus*. It inhibits the DNA-dependent RNA synthesis, thereby reducing collagen formation by inhibiting fibroblast proliferation.[705]

CLINICAL USES

For the last three decades MMC has been widely used as a systemic antineoplastic agent as well as adjuvant therapy after pterygium surgery to prevent its recurrence.[628] Recently, MMC has been used as a substitute for 5-FU in glaucoma filtration surgery.[629–631] Yamamoto and associates[632] demonstrated inhibition of fibroblast proliferation in rabbits, with efficacy greater than 100 times that of 5-FU. Even a 48-hour exposure to MMC was sufficient to inhibit 88% of cell growth for as long as 14 days. In another study,[633] a significant increase in bleb duration (from 8.1 to 68 days) was observed with a single intraoperative subconjunctival administration of 0.5 mg/ml MMC solution in Dutch-belted rabbits. Thus, the prospect of avoiding the disadvantages of 5-FU therapy, which include frequent and uncomfortable subconjunctival injections and potential corneal epithelial toxicity, has encouraged clinical studies comparing MMC to 5-FU.

In a preliminary study, Palmer[629] reported an overall success rate of 84% after 6 to 42 months in 33 eyes of high-risk glaucoma patients following intraoperative exposure to a sponge soaked with 0.2 mg/ml MMC solution. Compared to 5-FU in glaucoma patients with poor surgical prognosis, MMC has demonstrated superiority in control of IOP (88% versus 47% in the MMC and 5-FU groups, respectively)[634] and corneal complications (9 of 19 eyes treated with 5-FU and none of the MMC-treated eyes).[635] In these studies,[634,635] MMC was applied only once during trabeculectomy, while 5-FU was injected 10 times in the two weeks after surgery. In contrast to 5-FU, MMC appears to be effective following filtering surgery combined with extracapsular cataract extraction and posterior chamber intraocular lens implantation.[706,707]

SIDE EFFECTS

Retinal toxicity has occurred following intravitreal injection.[636] Intracameral injection of 50 µl MMC (0.5 mg/ml of balanced salt solution) to New Zealand white rabbits has caused a severe inflammatory response within 24 hours. Two days following injection, the corneas opacified and thickened, rapidly progressing to irreversible bullous keratopathy. Histopathologic evaluation revealed complete absence of the nor-

mal corneal endothelium, vascular congestion, and necrosis of the iris and ciliary body.[637] Secondary glaucoma, corneal edema, corneal perforation, cataract, and corectopia have been reported following topical MMC application in patients undergoing pterygium surgery.[638] Severe, persistent hypotony following trabeculectomies using intraoperative MMC can be a serious complication, which can lead to choroidal detachment or hypotony-induced maculopathy.[639,708,709]

Doses of 0.2–0.4 mg/ml MMC with short exposure times of 1 to 3 minutes appear to be relatively safe and effective.[640,710] Unlike 5-FU, however, which appears relatively safe in cases of penetration into the eye through the sclerectomy, it is of critical importance to apply MMC prior to removal of the full-thickness scleral block. Equally important, the exposed tissue must be washed meticulously after the MMC is applied. Accidental access of MMC to the anterior chamber can be extremely toxic to the corneal endothelium.[640]

CONTRAINDICATIONS

As with 5-FU, MMC is contraindicated in patients with active corneal disease, leaking blebs, infection, flat anterior chambers, choroidal hemorrhage, or persistent hypotony.

Recent Developments and Investigational Drugs

Prostaglandins

Prostaglandin (PG) analogs (see also Chap. 12) represent a novel class of topically active ocular hypotensive agents with potential long-term clinical usefulness. Several compounds have demonstrated efficacy at low doses in normal volunteers and patients with open-angle glaucoma. Each drug appears to have a unique and species-specific mechanism of action. Furthermore, dosage is critical since the IOP response may range from pressure rise to pronounced ocular hypotension. The ocular side effects also seem dose dependent. Early experiments used rabbits and focused on the potential efficacy of eicosanoids as ocular hypotensive agents. In retrospect, the rabbit was a poor choice because of its sensitivity to topical preparations. Relatively high doses were applied, causing severe local irritation to the *a priori* hypersensitive rabbit eye.[641,642] In the rabbit model, the main vascular response to high-dose PG was profound vasodilation, an increase in IOP, miosis, iridial hyperemia, and protein leakage into the anterior chamber secondary to disruption of the blood-aqueous barrier.[643] Most of the current PG studies focus on the choice of agent and refinement of the dose to achieve the ideal therapeutic index.

PHARMACOLOGY

PGs were originally discovered in the eye as mediators of the ocular inflammatory response, and most of the preliminary research focused on their potential role in uveitis, iridocyclitis, and other inflammatory processes.[644,645] More recent studies, however, have demonstrated additional roles for PGs in several physiologic processes. When delivered in adequate doses, PGs can either moderate inflammation or lower IOP.[646] Rabbit[647] and human[648] uveal tissues have demonstrated the ability to form various cyclooxygenase and lipoxygenase products.[649,650] Cultured human trabecular meshwork cells can produce PGE_2 and $PGF_{2\alpha}$ as the major cyclooxygenase products, with presumed later metabolic conversion of PGE_2 to $PGF_{2\alpha}$. A small amount of 6-keto $PGF_{1\alpha}$ has also been found, indicating possible *in situ* prostacyclin production as well. High-performance-liquid-chromatography studies have suggested that cultured human trabecular meshwork cells also can form certain lipoxygenase products including LTB_4, 12-HETE, 15-HETE, and small amounts of 5-HETE.[651]

The findings that the normal, uninflamed anterior uvea and conjunctiva have a high capacity to synthesize various cyclooxygenase, and to a lesser extent lipoxygenase products, suggest a physiologic role for the enzymes and their products. Human and animal studies further indicate that certain antiglaucoma medications such as cholinergic and adrenergic agonists, as well as ALT cause a transient elevation of PG levels in the aqueous humor *in vivo*.[652] In addition, cyclooxygenase inhibitors such as indomethacin and flurbiprofen block, or partially inhibit, the reduction in the IOP produced by such pharmacologically diverse compounds as epinephrine, apraclonidine, forskolin, vanadate, verapamil, arachidonic acid as well as ALT. Since the systemic nonsteroidal anti-inflammatory agents are widely prescribed for many common diseases ranging from arthritis to headache, special consideration must be given to potential nonbeneficial interactions with systemic and topical PG preparations.

$PGF_{2\alpha}$

$PGF_{2\alpha}$ has been extensively investigated in both animal and human studies.

Animal Studies.   Topical administration of $PGF_{2\alpha}$ to rabbits in doses ranging from 5–200 μg has been reported to lower IOP,[653] but the hypotensive effect was accompanied by miosis, aqueous flare, and accumulation of cells in the anterior chamber. A profound miotic response also occurred in cats following topical administration of $PGF_{2\alpha}$ in similar dosage ranges.[654] However, when administered to owl monkeys, the IOP remained depressed for three days after $PGF_{2\alpha}$ application, without noticeable side effects.[655] Normotensive cynomolgus and rhesus monkeys responded as the owl monkey in acute studies with topical $PGF_{2\alpha}$.[656]

Both rabbits and cats develop tachyphylaxis to the ocular *hypertensive* effect of some intracamerally injected prostaglandins.[657] Tachyphylaxis also develops to the ocular *hypotensive* effect following topical administration of 5 μg of

$PGF_{2\alpha}$ given three times daily to the rabbit.[658] Thus, the monkey appears a more suitable animal model for evaluating the ocular hypotensive effects of PGs. Both acute[659] and chronic[660] instillation of $PGF_{2\alpha}$ lowered IOP in ocular hypertensive cynomolgus monkeys. When given for two weeks in a dose of 250 μg twice daily, $PGF_{2\alpha}$ lowered IOP consistently in normotensive cynomolgus monkeys, with minimal flare noted in the anterior chamber,[661] and with no histopathologic changes.[662]

Due to the hydrophilic nature of the $PGF_{2\alpha}$ in the free acid form, poor corneal penetration precluded its chronic use.[663] When converted to either a 1-methyl, 1-ethyl or 1-isopropyl ester prodrug form, radioactive assays have demonstrated that the transcorneal movement of $PGF_{2\alpha}$ is greatly enhanced.[664] Once-daily administration of 2.5 μg $PGF_{2\alpha}$ for 4 days in its ester form lowered IOP in cats, but miosis and aqueous flare still occurred.[663]

Human Studies.   Acute application to normotensive volunteers of 200 μg of $PGF_{2\alpha}$ as the tromethamine salt resulted in peak IOP reduction at 7 hours, with the effect lasting up to 24 hours. Pupillary diameter remained unchanged and the anterior chamber remained clear. However, the subjects experienced conjunctival hyperemia and severe foreign body sensation.[665] When administered as a 1-isopropyl ester, 1.1 μg $PGF_{2\alpha}$ induced the same lasting ocular hypotensive effect with no change in aqueous humor outflow.[666] Since a dose of 0.5 μg was effective and tolerated moderately well in glaucoma patients, only doses at the lower end of the dose-response curve have been judged to have potential for future clinical use.

Studies with PhXA34, a $PGF_{2\alpha}$-isopropyl ester analog, have shown promising results in normal volunteers and patients with ocular hypertension.[667,668,677] In normal volunteers, topical application of a single dose of 1, 3 and 10 μg of PhXA34 reduced IOP by about 2, 3 and 4 mm Hg, respectively, 6 to 10 hours after administration. The only side effect was slight conjunctival hyperemia following the 10 μg dose. Once-daily treatment with 10 μg PhXA34 for 7 days induced a sustained ocular hypotensive effect. Unlike other prostaglandins, no initial ocular hypertensive effect occurred. The mean pressure in the treated eye remained below 9 mm Hg 12 hours after dosing throughout the one-week study. Outflow facility showed a small, but statistically significant increase that could explain only approximately one-third of the IOP reduction. Therefore, both the pressure reduction with PhXA34 and its mechanism of action appear similar to those of $PGF_{2\alpha}$-isopropyl ester. However, the side effects are less pronounced.

Continued application of 10 μg PhXA34 resulted in only mild ocular irritation in half the subjects but improved throughout the experimentation period. Fluorescein concentration in the anterior chamber increased by approximately 15% during the first 2 hours after drug instillation. The authors suggest that the 3-μg dose of PhXA34 may be ideal for future use since in normotensive eyes, a 3 mm Hg reduction in IOP occurred with only mild side effects.

PhXA41 (latanoprost), another analog of the prodrug $PGF_{2\alpha}$-isopropyl ester, is the more active R-epimer of PhXA34 and appears to be a more potent ocular hypotensive agent.[680–682] Latanoprost has been evaluated in normal volunteers[678,681] as well as patients with ocular hypertension[678,679,681–683] or open-angle glaucoma.[680,683] When administered either once or twice daily, latanoprost 0.006% decreases IOP 20% to 36%,[678,680,682] and IOP reduction seems to be maintained during the 23 hours following a single daily dose.[680,682] Latanoprost 0.006% appears to be a more effective ocular hypotensive agent than 2% pilocarpine.[679]

Latanoprost 0.005% effectively reduces IOP both during the day and during sleep whether used alone or concomitantly with timolol.[711] The drug has additive ocular hypotensive activity when used with topical β blockers, and the hypotensive effect occurs without regard to iris color. When compared with 0.5% timolol in a large multicenter study involving 268 patients, once-daily latanoprost 0.005% produced a significantly greater IOP reduction (-6.7 ± 3.4 mm Hg vs. -4.9 ± 2.9 mm Hg, respectively). Pulse rate was significantly reduced by timolol, but not by latanoprost. No significant difference between groups occurred in visual acuity, slit-lamp findings, blood pressure, or laboratory values. The results of this study suggest that latanoprost has potential as a new drug of first choice for treatment of glaucoma.[712]

The most significant ocular side effect associated with latanoprost therapy is conjunctival hyperemia,[679,680,682] occurring in about 25% to 35% of patients.[682] A bilateral change in iris color has been reported.[712] This occurred in a patient with concentric iris heterochromia (darker centrally), in which a definite increase in pigmentation made the irides uniformly darker. The increase in iris melanin is considered a benign process.

Most studies[656,661,666] fail to demonstrate any effect of $PGF_{2\alpha}$ on the rate of aqueous humor production. Some studies,[669] but not others,[670,671] have demonstrated a slight increase in the outflow facility of cynomolgus monkeys. However, the slight increases reported in aqueous outflow cannot fully account for the impressive magnitude of the ocular hypotensive effect elicited by $PGF_{2\alpha}$.[669] Either a reduction in the episcleral venous pressure or an increase in uveoscleral outflow ("nonconventional pathway") may account for the ocular hypotensive action of $PGF_{2\alpha}$. The former hypothesis has been dismissed by the argument that an induced decrease in episcleral venous pressure alone cannot account for the large fall in IOP evoked by $PGF_{2\alpha}$.[672] Some indirect evidence indicates that increased uveoscleral outflow is the most likely mechanism of the ocular hypotensive effect in humans and monkeys.[656,671] Pretreatment of cynomolgus monkeys with pilocarpine reduces the ocular hypotensive effect of $PGF_{2\alpha}$. Since pilocarpine contracts the ciliary muscle and obliterates the spaces between the muscle bundles, uveoscleral drainage decreases. Furthermore, pretreatment with atropine antagonizes the effect of pilocarpine. Like other $PGF_{2\alpha}$ analogs, latanoprost's primary mechanism of ocular hypotensive action is increased uveoscleral outflow,[681] although increased trabecular outflow may also contribute to the hypotensive effect.[678]

PGE₂

When administered topically in 10 to 500 μg solution, PGE_2 lowers IOP in rhesus monkeys without major side effects.[654] Repeated instillation to cats of 100 μg PGE_2 for as long as 9 months maintained the ocular hypotensive effect without development of tachyphylaxis or side effects. Clinical studies in normal volunteers have shown that IOP decreased significantly 6 hours following one drop of 0.02% solution of PGE_2, and the effect lasted up to 24 hours.[673] All subjects reported mild ocular pain and photophobia for up to 4 hours. In spite of its efficacy, PGE_2 is not suitable for long-term clinical use due to its very minimal water solubility.[663] Since evidence indicates late metabolic conversion of PGE_2 to $PGF_{2\alpha}$ by trabecular meshwork cells, PGE_2 might also be regarded as a prodrug.

PGD₂, PGD₃, AND BW245C

PGD_2, PGD_3, and BW245C (a potent PGD_2 agonist) have been effective ocular hypotensive agents when given to normotensive rabbits; however, ocular side effects, mainly itching and foreign body sensation, may limit their clinical usefulness as antiglaucoma medications.[674]

ILOPROST

One study indicated that both PGI and its stable analog, iloprost (as an ester), effectively lower IOP in rabbits.[675] The study, however, lasted only six hours, necessitating further evaluation of these agents.

PGA AND PGB

PGA and PGB derive from PGE by dehydration and isomerization. They appear to have greater ocular hypotensive potency than the primary PGs of the E, F and D type. A single application of 1 to 5 μg PGA_2 to the cat eye yielded a greater and more prolonged ocular hypotensive effect than did 100 μg $PGF_{2\alpha}$. Slight conjunctival hyperemia occurred, but the rabbit and the cat showed no miosis following topical administration of PGA_2.[676] PGA_2 retained its ocular hypotensive activity when stored in an aqueous solution at room temperature for 4 months.

Angiotensin-Converting Enzyme (ACE) Inhibitors

Since several antihypertensive agents, including clonidine and β blockers, reduce IOP when given topically,[684–686] ACE inhibitors have been of interest as possible ocular hypotensive agents. Angiotensin-converting enzyme is present in aqueous humor, but its role is unknown.[687] Initial preclinical studies with topical, oral, and intravenous administration of SCH 33861, a potent, reversible ACE inhibitor, did not demonstrate any significant toxicities. A study involving humans used 0.1% and 0.01% ophthalmic solutions of SCH 33861 to measure the effect on IOP.[688] Both single- and multiple-dose effects were measured. The study concluded that SCH 33861 decreased IOP upon acute topical administration, but a significant difference did not occur in the ocular hypotensive effect produced by the 0.1% and 0.01% solutions. Since the ocular hypotensive effect was greater on day 5 than on day 1 of the study, SCH 33861 appeared to have a cumulative effect on IOP. In addition, humans tolerated short-term topical administration of SCH 33861 without significant ocular or systemic side effects. When compared with 0.5% timolol, topical SCH 33861 was much less effective as an ocular hypotensive agent.[688]

Calcium Channel Blockers

Verapamil, a calcium channel blocker, has been used extensively in the treatment of cardiovascular disorders. This agent reduces the entry of extracellular Ca^{++} ions into the myocardium and vascular smooth muscle by inhibiting voltage-sensitive Ca^{++} channels.[689] Topical verapamil has also shown weak activity as an ocular hypotensive agent. In ocular hypertensive human subjects, verapamil (a 40 μl drop of 1.25 mg/ml solution) reduced IOP 3.8 mm Hg beginning two hours after instillation and lasting at least 12 hours. A slight reduction in IOP (1.6 mm Hg) was also noted in the untreated contralateral eye[690] and lasted 6 hours. Possible mechanisms for verapamil's ocular hypotensive effect include:[690] (1) local vasodilation, thereby decreasing the hydrostatic pressure within the ciliary body; (2) altered cellular permeability of the ciliary epithelium; (3) altered cyclic adenosine monophosphate (cAMP) content caused by an effect on the ciliary epithelium. Since subjects tolerated topical ocular administration of verapamil, calcium channel blockers may have potential as ocular hypotensive agents in the future.

Calcium Dobesilate

Calcium dobesilate, an agent administered orally to decrease blood and plasma viscosity, has been studied in patients with both diabetic retinopathy and open-angle glaucoma.[691] After 6 months of therapy using calcium dobesilate 500 mg three times daily, a 24.4% (6.4 mm Hg) reduction in IOP was noted. This ocular hypotensive effect was attributed to a significant increase in aqueous outflow. In addition to enhancing outflow facility, calcium dobesilate reduced retinal hemorrhages in patients with nonproliferative diabetic reti-

nopathy.[691] Further studies are required to elucidate the actions of calcium dobesilate on aqueous humor dynamics, ocular perfusion pressure, and blood viscosity.

Ethacrynic Acid (Xarano)

For many years ethacrynic acid (ECA) has been administered systemically as a loop diuretic, and this compound is currently being investigated as an agent capable of producing pharmacologic trabeculocanalotomy.[692] Since ECA reacts with sulfhydryl groups in cell membranes,[693] it may alter cell shape and cell-to-cell contact within the trabecular meshwork and inner wall of Schlemm's canal.[692] These changes within the cytoskeleton of the trabecular meshwork may increase outflow facility.[692]

In animal studies, ECA increases aqueous outflow following intracameral perfusion in calf and monkey eyes.[694] In addition, intracameral injection of ECA into live monkey eyes reduces IOP and does not produce significant ocular toxicity at anterior chamber concentrations of 0.3 mmol/l or less.[695] However, topical ECA has been associated with epithelial disruption and corneal edema in rabbits.[696] Thus, ECA adducts were created by combining ECA with equimolar cysteine to bind the sulfhydryl-reactive sites.[696] Since ethacrynic acid-cysteine is a thiol adduct of ECA that dissociates rapidly,[697] this compound would ideally penetrate the cornea without producing corneal toxicity. Upon entering the anterior chamber, this adduct may dissociate, thereby liberating free ECA for interaction with sulfhydryl groups in cell membranes within the outflow pathway.[696] Preliminary studies in rabbits and monkeys showed this topically administered ECA adduct to be an effective ocular hypotensive agent that produced less corneal toxicity than did topical ECA.[696] A further reduction of corneal toxicity was noted in rabbits by pretreating the cornea with 2 drops of 100 mmol/l acetylcysteine. Pretreatment with acetylcysteine was used to create a reservoir of sulfhydryl groups within the cornea, thereby providing a site for binding of free ECA other than corneal sulfhydryl sites.[696]

Using human donor eyes, perfusion of the anterior segment with ECA at concentrations from 0.01–0.25 mmol/l increased aqueous outflow from 28% to 105%, respectively.[698] The aged donor eyes did not exhibit any morphologic changes at the 0.01% concentration; at concentrations above 0.01 mmol/l, a loss of cell-to-cell attachments and breaks in the inner-wall endothelial lining of Schlemm's canal were noted by light and transmission electron microscopy.[698] In human eyes with advanced open-angle glaucoma, intracameral injections of ECA creating anterior chamber concentrations of 0.05 mM and 0.15 mM reduced IOP by 9 to 31 mm Hg.[699] This reduction occurred 3 to 24 hours after the intracameral injection, and the hypotensive effect lasted approximately three days with a gradual return to pretreatment IOP within one week. Intracameral ECA did not produce significant intraocular inflammation. Corneal side effects were not noted during this study, and corneal endothelial cell counts remained unchanged two months after intracameral treatment.[699]

References

1. Vale J, Phillips CI. Effect of DL- and D-propranolol on ocular tension in rabbits and patients. Exp Eye Res 1970;9:82–90.

2. Bucci MG, Missiroli A, Pecori-Giraldi J, et al. La somministrazione locale del propranolol nella terapia del glaucoma. Boll d'Ocul 1968;47:51–60.

3. Draeger J. Corneal sensitivity: measurement and clinical importance. Wein/New York: Springer-Verlag, 1984.

4. Novack GD. Ophthalmic beta-blockers since timolol. Surv Ophthalmol 1987;31:307–327.

5. Phillips CI, Bartholomew RS, Levy AM, Grove J, Vogel R. Penetration of timolol eye drops in human aqueous humor: the first hour. Br J Ophthalmol 1985;69:217–218.

6. Wax MB, Molinoff PB. Distribution and properties of beta-adrenergic receptors in human irs/ciliary body. Invest Ophthalmol Vis Sci 1987;28:420–430.

7. Woodward DF, Chen J, Padillo E, Ruiz G. Pharmacological characterization of β-adrenoceptor subtype involvement in the ocular hypotensive response to β-adrenergic stimulation. Exp Eye Res 1986;43:61–75.

8. Elena P, Kosina-Boix M, Moulin G, Lapalus P. Autoradiographic localization of beta-adrenergic receptors in rabbit eye. Invest Ophthalmol Vis Sci 1987;28:1436–41.

9. Polanksy JR. Beta-adrenergic therapy for glaucoma. Int Ophthalmol Clin 1990;30:219–229.

10. Zimmerman TJ, Kaufman HE. Timolol: dose response and duration of action. Arch Ophthalmol 1977;95:605–607.

11. Boger WP, Steinert RF, Puliafito CA, Pavan-Langston D. Clinical trial comparing timolol ophthalmic solution to pilocarpine in open-angle glaucoma. Am J Ophthalmol 1978;86:8–18.

12. Boger WP. Timolol: Short term "escape" and long term "drift". Ann Ophthalmol 1979;11:1239–1242.

13. Boger WP, Puliafito CA, Steinert RF, Langston EP. Long-term experience with timolol ophthalmic solution in patients with open-angle glaucoma. Ophthalmology 1978;85:259–267.

14. Krupin T, Singer PR, Perlmutter J, Kolker AE, Becker B. One-hour intraocular pressure response to timolol: Lack of correlation with long-term response. Arch Ophthalmol 1981;99:840–841.

15. Spinelli D, Montanari P, Vigasio F, Cormanni V. Effects du maléate de timolol sur l'oeil controlatéral sans treatment. J Fr Ophtalmol 1982;5:152–158.

16. Gibbens MV. Sympathetic influences on the consensual ophthalmotonic reaction. Br J Ophthalmol 1988;72:750–753.

17. Kwitko GM, Shin DH, Ahn BH, Hong YJ. Bilateral effects of long-term monocular timolol therapy. Am J Ophthalmol 1987;104:591–594.

18. Shin DH. Bilateral effects of monocular timolol treatment. Am J Ophthalmol 1986;102:275–276.

19. Steinert RF, Thomas JV, Boger WPI. Long-term drift and continued efficacy after multiyear timolol therapy. Arch Ophthalmol 1981;99:100–103.

20. Levobunolol Study Group. Levobunolol: A four-year study of efficacy and safety in glaucoma treatment. Ophthalmology 1989; 96:642–645.

21. Silverstone DE, Arkfeld D, Cowan G, Lue JC, Novack GD. Long-term diurnal control of intraocular pressure with levobunolol and with timolol. Glaucoma 1985;7:138–140.

22. Soll DB. Evaluation of timolol in chronic open-angle glaucoma: once-a-day vs twice-a-day. Arch Ophthalmol 1980;98:2178–2181.

23. Wandel T, Lewis RA, Partamian L, et al. Glaucoma treatment with once-daily levobunolol. Am J Ophthalmol 1986:298–304.

24. Rakofsky S, Lazar M, Almog Y, et al. Once-daily levobunolol for glaucoma therapy. Can J Ophthalmol 1989;24:2–6.

25. David R, Foerster RJ, Ober M, et al. Glaucoma treatment with once-daily levobunolol. Am J Ophthalmol 1987;104:443–444.

26. Topper JE, Brubaker RF. Effects of timolol, epinephrine, and acetazolamide on aqueous flow during sleep. Invest Ophthalmol Vis Sci 1985;26:1315–1319.

27. McCannel CA, Heinrich SR, Brubaker RF. Acetazolamide but not timolol lowers aqueous humor flow in sleeping humans. Graefes Arch Clin Exp Ophthalmol 1992;230:518–520.

28. Kass MA, Gordon M, Morley RE, Meltzer DW, Goldberg JJ. Compliance with topical timolol treatment. Am J Ophthalmol 1987;103:188–193.

29. Letchinger SL, Frochlichstein D, Glieser DK, et al. Can the concentration of timolol or the frequency of its administration be reduced? Ophthalmology 1993;100:1259–1262.

30. Mills KB. Blind randomised non-crossover long-term trial comparing topical timolol 0.25% with timolol 0.5% in the treatment of simple chronic glaucoma. Br J Ophthalmol 1983;67:216–219.

31. Boozman FW, Foerster RJ, Allen RC, et al. The long-term efficacy of twice-daily 0.25% levobunolol and timolol. Arch Ophthalmol 1988;106:614–618.

32. Dausch D, Schad K. Eignet sich 0.1% ige Timolol-maleate augentropflosung zur therapie des chronischen glaukoms?. Klin Mbl Augenheilk 1982;180:141–145.

33. Long D, Zimmerman T, Spaeth G, Novack G, Burke PJ, Duzman E. Minimum concentration of levobunolol required to control intraocular pressure in patients with primary open-angle glaucoma or ocular hypertension. Am J Ophthalmol 1985;99:18–22.

34. Sommer A. Intraocular pressure and glaucoma. Am J Ophthalmol 1989;107:186–188.

35. Armaly MF, Krueger DE, Maunder L, et al. Biostatistical analysis of the collaborative glaucoma study. I. Summary report of the risk factors for glaucomatous visual-field defects. Arch Ophthalmol 1980;98:2163–2171.

36. David R, Livingston DG, Luntz MH. Ocular hypertension—a long-term follow-up of treated and untreated patients. Br J Ophthalmol 1977;61:668–674.

37. Epstein DL, Krug JH, Hertzmark E, Remis LL, Edelstein DJ. A long-term clinical trial of timolol therapy versus no treatment in the management of glaucoma suspects. Ophthalmology 1989;96:1460–1467.

38. Schulzer M, Drance SM, Douglas GR. A comparison of treated and untreated glaucoma suspects. Ophthalmology 1991;98:301–307.

39. Dallas NL, Sponsel WE, Hobley AJ. A comparative evaluation of timolol maleate and pilocarpine in the treatment of chronic angle glaucoma. Eye 1988;2:243–249.

40. Sponsel WE, Hobley A, Dallas NL, Henson DB. Visual Field survival: A comparison of the effects of pilocarpine and timolol in

open angle glaucoma. New Trends in Ophthalmology 1987; II:168–186.

41. The Glaucoma Laser Trial Research Group. The Glaucoma Laser Trial (GLT). 2. Results of argon laser trabeculoplasty versus topical medicine. Ophthalmology 1990;97:1403–1413.

42. Coakes RL, Brubaker RF. The mechanism of timolol in lowering intraocular pressure. Arch Ophthalmol 1978;96:2045–2048.

43. Yablonski ME, Zimmerman TJ, Waltman SR, Becker B. A fluorophotometric study of the effect of topical timolol on aqueous humor dynamics. Exp Eye Res 1978;27:135–142.

44. Sonntag JR, Brindley GO, Shields MB. Effect of timolol therapy on outflow facility. Invest Ophthalmol Vis Sci 1978;17:293–296.

45. Morrison JC, Robin AL. Adjunctive glaucoma therapy. A comparison of apraclonidine to dipivefrin when added to timolol maleate. Ophthalmology 1989;96:3–7.

46. Merkle W. Timolol in combination with other glaucoma drugs. Klin Mbl Augenheilk 1981;178:50–54.

47. Kass MA. Efficacy of combining timolol with other antiglaucoma medications. Surv Ophthalmol 1983;28(suppl):274–279.

48. Knupp JA, Shields MB, Mandell AI, Hurvitz L, Spaeth GL. Combined timolol and epinephrine therapy for open angle glaucoma. Surv Ophthalmol 1983;28:280–285.

49. Airaksinen PJ, Valkonen R, Stenborg T, et al. A double-masked study of timolol and pilocarpine combined. Am J Ophthalmol 1987;104:587–590.

50. Berson FG, Epstein DL. Separate and combined effects of timolol maleate and acetazolamide in open-angle glaucoma. Am J Ophthalmol 1981;92:788–791.

51. Keates EU. Evaluation of timolol maleate combination therapy in chronic open-angle glaucoma. Am J Ophthalmol 1979;88:565–571.

52. Kass MA, Korey M, Gordon M, Becker B. Timolol and acetazolamide. A study of concurrent administration. Arch Ophthalmol 1982;100:941–942.

53. Korey MS, Hodapp E, Kass MA, et al. Timolol and epinephrine: long-term evaluation of concurrent administration. Arch Ophthalmol 1982;100:742–746.

54. Thomas JV, Epstein DL. Study of the additive effect of timolol and epinephrine in lowering intraocular pressure. Br J Ophthalmol 1981;65:596–602.

55. Schenker HW, Yablonski ME, Podos SM, et al. Fluorophotometric study of epinephrine and timolol in human subjects. Arch Ophthalmol 1981;99:1212–1226.

56. Tsoy EA, Meekins BB, Shields MB. Comparison of two treatment schedules for combined timolol and dipivefrin therapy. Am J Ophthalmol 1986;102:320–324.

57. Puustjärvi TJ, Repo LP, the Scandinavian Timpilo Study Group. Timolol-pilocarpine fixed-ratio combinations in the treatment of chronic open angle glaucoma. A controlled multicenter study of 48 weeks. Arch Ophthalmol 1992;110:1725–1729.

58. Allen RC, Epstein DL. Additive effect of betaxolol and epinephrine in primary open angle glaucoma. Arch Ophthalmol 1986;104:1178–1184.

59. Migliori ME, Beckman H, Channell MM. Intraocular pressure changes after neodymium-YAG laser capsulotomy in eyes pretreated with timolol. Arch Ophthalmol 1987;105:473–475.

60. Liu PF, Hung PT. Effect of timolol on intraocular pressure elevation following argon laser iridotomy. J Ocular Pharmacol 1987;3:249–255.

61. Richter CU, Arzeno G, Pappas HR, Arrigg CA, Wasson P, Steinert RF. Prevention of intraocular pressure elevation following neodymium-YAG laser posterior capsulotomy. Arch Ophthalmol 1985;103:912–915.

62. Stilma JS, Boen-Tan TN. Timolol and intra-ocular pressure elevation following Neodymium: YAG laser surgery. Doc Ophthalmol 1986;61:233–239.

63. Packer AJ, Fraioli AJ, Epstein DL. The effect of timolol and acetazolamide on transient intraocular pressure elevation following cataract extraction with alpha-chymotrypsin. Ophthalmology 1981;88:239–243.

64. Fry LL. Comparison of the postoperative intraocular pressure with Betagan, Betoptic, Timoptic, Iopidine, Diamox, Pilopine Gel, and Miostat. J Cataract Refract Surg 1992;18:14–19.

65. Kass MA, Meltzer DW, Gordon M, Cooper D, Goldberg J. Compliance with topical pilocarpine treatment. Am J Ophthalmol 1986;101:515–523.

66. Mare N, Alvan G, Calissendorff BM, et al. Additive intraocular pressure reducing effect of topical timolol during systemic β-blockade. Acta Ophthalmol 1982;60:16–23.

67. Levy NS, Alsbury C. Evaluation of timolol in gellan gum: a new vehicle to extend its duration of action. Ann Opthalmol–Glaucoma 1994;26:166–169.

68. Sharir M, Zimmerman TJ, Crandall AS, Mamalis N. A comparison of the ocular tolerability of a single dose of timolol and levobunolol in healthy normotensive volunteers. Ann Ophthalmol 1993;25:133–137.

69. Novack GD, Leopold IH. The toxicity of topical ophthalmic beta-blockers. J Toxicol—Cut Ocul Toxicol 1987;6:283–297.

70. Akingbehin T, Sunder Raj P. Ophthalmic topical beta blockers: review of ocular and systemic adverse effects. J Toxicol—Cut Ocul Toxicol 1990;9:131–147.

71. Fraunfelder FT, Meyer SM. Systemic side effects from ophthalmic timolol and their prevention. J Ocular Pharmacol 1987;3:177–184.

72. Schwartz JS, Weinstock SM. Side effects of topical epinephrine therapy. Glaucoma 1983;5:21–23.

73. Theodore J, Leibowitz HM. External ocular toxicity of dipivalyl epinephrine. Am J Ophthalmol 1979;88:1013–1016.

74. Flach AJ, Kramer SG. Supersensitivity to topical epinephrine after long-term epinephrine therapy. Arch Ophthalmol 1980;98:482–483.

75. Spaeth GL. Symposium on glaucoma: Transactions of the New Orleans Academy of Ophthalmology. St. Louis: C.V. Mosby, 1981.

76. Lamping K, Gofman J, Duzman E, Leopold IH, Novack GD. Effect of changing beta-blocker treatment in six patients allergic to timolol. J Toxicol—Cut Ocul Toxicol 1987;6:179–181.

77. van Buskirk EM. Corneal anesthesia after timolol maleate therapy. Am J Ophthalmol 1979;88:739–743.

78. van Buskirk EM. Adverse reactions from timolol administration. Ophthalmology 1980;87:447–450.

79. Berson F, Cohen H, Foerster RJ, Lass J, Novack GD, Duzman E. Levobunolol compared with timolol: ocular hypotensive efficacy and ocular and systemic safety. Arch Ophthalmol 1985;103:379–382.

80. Fraunfelder FT, Meyer SM. Corneal complications of ocular medications. Cornea 1986;5:55–59.

81. Herreras JM, Pastor C, Calonge M, Asensio VM. Ocular surface alteration after long-term treatment with an antiglaucomatous drug. Ophthalmology 1992;99:1082–1088.

82. Nielsen NV, Eriksen JS. Timolol in maintenance treatment of ocular hypertension and glaucoma. Acta Ophthalmol 1979;57: 1070–1077.

83. Kuppens EV, Stolwijk TR, de Keizer RJ, van Best JA. Basal tear turnover and topical timolol in glaucoma patients and healthy controls by fluorophotometry. Invest Ophthalmol Vis Sci 1992;33: 3442–3448.

84. Wright P. Untoward effects associated with practolol administration: oculomucocutaneous syndrome. BMJ 1975;1:595–598.

85. McMahon CD, Shaffer RN, Hoskins HD, Hetherington J. Adverse effects experience by patients taking timolol. Am J Ophthalmol 1979;88:736–738.

86. Passo MS, Palmer EA, van Buskirk EM. Plasma timolol in glaucoma patients. Ophthalmology 1984;91:1361–1363.

87. Alvan G, Calissendorff B, Seideman P, Widmark K, Widmark G. Absorption of ocular timolol. Clinical Pharmacokinetics 1980;5: 95–100.

88. Zimmerman TJ, Kooner KS, Kandarakis AS, Ziegler LP. Improving the therapeutic index of topically applied ocular drugs. Arch Ophthalmol 1984;102:551–553.

89. Bobik A, Jennings GL, Ashley P, Korner PI. Timolol pharmacokinetics and effects on heart rate and blood pressure after acute and chronic administration. Eur J Clin Pharmacol 1979;16:243–249.

90. Leier CV, Baker ND, Weber PA. Cardiovascular effects of ophthalmic timolol. Ann Intern Med 1986;104:197–199.

91. Wellstein A, Palm D, Pitschner HF, Belz GG. Receptor binding of propranolol is the missing link between plasma concentration kinetics and the effect-time course in man. Eur J Clin Pharmacol 1985;29:131–147.

92. Hoffman BB, Lefkowitz RJ. Catecholamines and sympathomimetic drugs. In: Gilman AG, Rall TW, Nies AS, Taylor P, eds. Goodman and Gilman's the pharmacological basis of therapeutics. New York: Pergammon Press, 1990, 187–220.

93. Flexner JB, Flexner LB, Church AC, Rainbow TC, Brunswick DJ. Blockade of beta-1 but not of beta-2 adrenergic receptors replicates propranolol's suppression of the cerebral spread of an engram in mice. Proc Natl Acad Sci USA 1985;82:7458–7461.

94. Sternberg DB, Korol D, Novack GD, McGaugh JL. Epinephrine-induced memory facilitation: Differentiation of adrenergic receptors involved as determined by adrenergic antagonists. Eur J Pharmacol 1986;129:189–193.

95. Introini-Collison I, Saghafi D, Novack GD, McGaugh JL. Memory-enhancing effects of post-training dipivefrin and epinephrine: involvement of peripheral and central adrenergic receptors. Brain Res 1992;572:81–86.

96. van Buskirk EM, Fraunfelder FT. Timolol and Glaucoma. Arch Ophthalmol 1981;99:696

97. Atkins JM, Pugh BR, Timewell RM. Cardiovascular effects of topical beta-blockers during exercise. Am J Ophthalmol 1985;99: 173–175.

98. Hernandez HH, Cervantes R, Frati F, Hurtado R, McDonald TO, DeSouse B. Cardiovascular effects of topical glaucoma therapies in normal subjects. J Toxicol—Cut Ocul Toxicol 1983;2:99–106.

99. Berlin I, Marlel P, Uzzan B, Millon D, Hoang PL, Puech AJ. A single dose of three different opthalmic beta-blockers antagonizes the chronotropic effect of isoproterenol in healthy volunteers. Clin Pharmacol Ther 1987;41:622–626.

100. Doyle WJ, Weber PA, Meeks RH. Effect of topical timolol maleate on exercise performance. Arch Ophthalmol 1984;102:1517–1518.

101. Jones FL, Jr., Ekberg NL. Exacerbation of asthma by timolol [letter]. N Engl J Med 1979;301:270

102. Charan NB, Lakshminarayan S. Pulmonary effects of topical timolol. Arch Intern Med 1980;140:843–844.

103. Schoene R, Abuan T, Ward RL, Beasley H. Effects of topical betaxolol, timolol and placebo on pulmonary function in asthmatic bronchitis. Am J Ophthalmol 1984;97:86–92.

104. Scharrer A, Ober M. Kardiovaskulare und pulmonare Wirkungen bei lokaler beta-blockergabe. Klin Mbl Augenheilk 1981;179: 362–363.

105. Vukich JA, Leef DL, Allen RC. Betaxolol in patients with coexistent chronic open angle glaucoma and pulmonary disease. Invest Ophthalmol Vis Sci 1984;26:227

106. Lynch MG, Whitson JT, Brown RH, Nguyen H, Drake MM. Topical β-blocker therapy and central nervous system side effects: A preliminary study comparing betaxolol and timolol. Arch Ophthalmol 1988;106:908–911.

107. Feiler-Ofry V, Godel V, Lazar M. Nail pigmentation following timolol maleate therapy. Ophthalmologica 1981;182:153–156.

108. Coppeto JR. Timolol-associated myasthenia gravis. Am J Ophthalmol 1984;98:244–245.

109. Benitah E, Chatelain C, Cohen F, Herman D. Fibrose retroperitoneale: éffet systemique d'un collyre beta-bloquant. La Presse Médicale 1987;16:400–401.

110. Coppeto JR. Timolol-associated myasthenia gravis [letter]. Am J Ophthalmol 1984;98:244–245.

111. Shaivitz SA. Timolol and myasthenia gravis [letter]. JAMA 1979; 242:1611–1612.

112. Lustgarten JS, Podos SM. Topical timolol and the nursing mother. Arch Ophthalmol 1983;101:1381–1382.

113. Weiner N, Taylor P. Neurohumoral transmission: the autonomic and somatic motor nervous systems. In: Gilman AG, Goodman LS, Rall TW, Murad F, eds. Goodman and Gilman's the pharmacological basis of therapeutics. New York: Macmillan, 1985, 66–99.

114. Coleman AL, Diehl D, Jampel HD, Bachorik PS, Quigley HA. Topical timolol decreases plasma high-density lipoprotein cholesterol level. Arch Ophthalmol 1990;108:1260–1263.

115. Vogel R. Topical timolol and serum lipoproteins. Arch Ophthalmol 1991;109:1341.

116. Burggraf GW, Munt PW. Topical timolol therapy and cardiopulmonary function. Can J Ophthalmol 1980;15:159–160.

117. Velde TM, Kaiser FE. Ophthalmic timolol treatment causing altered hypoglycemic response in a diabetic patient. Arch Intern Med 1983;143:1627

118. Angelo-Nielsen K. Timolol topically and diabetes mellitus [letter]. JAMA 1980;244:2263

119. Fraunfelder FT, Meyer SM. Systemic adverse reactions to glaucoma medications. Int Ophthalmol Clin 1989;29:143–146.

120. Novack GD. Minireview: Levobunolol for the long-term treatment of elevated intraocular pressure. Gen Pharmacol 1986;17: 373–377.

121. DiCarlo FJ, Leinweber F, Szpiech JM, Davidson IWF. Metabolism of 1–bunolol. Clin Pharmacol Ther 1977;22:858–863.

122. Quast U, Vollmer KO. Binding of beta-adrenoceptor antagonists to rat and rabbit lung: Special reference to levobunolol. Arzneimittelforschung 1984;34:579–584.

123. Woodward DF, Novack GD, Williams LS, Nieves AL, Potter DE. The ocular beta-blocking activity of dihydrolevobunolol. J Ocular Pharmacol 1987;3:11–15.

124. Tang-Liu D, Shackleton M, Richman JB. Ocular metabolism of levobunolol. J Ocular Pharmacol 1988;4:269–278.

125. Bensinger R, Keates E, Gofman J, Novack GD, Duzman E. Levobunolol: a three month efficacy study in the treatment of glaucoma and ocular hypertension. Arch Ophthalmol 1985;103:375–378.

126. Cinotti A, Cinotti D, Grant W, et al. 0.5% and 1.0% levobunolol compared with 0.5% timolol for the long-term treatment of chronic open-angle glaucoma and ocular hypertension. Am J Ophthalmol 1985;99:11–17.

127. Ober M, Scharrer A, David R, et al. Long-term ocular hypotensive effect of levobunolol: results of a one-year study. Br J Ophthalmol 1985;69:593–599.

128. Geyer O, Lazar M, Novack GD, Lue JC, Duzman E. Levobunolol compared with timolol for the control of elevated intraocular pressure. Ann Ophthalmol 1987;18:289–292.

129. Geyer O, Lazar M, Novack GD, Shen D, Eto CY. Levobunolol compared with timolol: a four-year study. Br J Ophthalmol 1988;72:892–896.

130. Yablonski ME, Novack GD, Cook D, Batoosingh AL, Lue JC. Aqueous humor dynamics in humans of a combination of drugs affecting inflow and outflow. Invest Ophthalmol Vis Sci 1987;28(3):12

131. Yablonski ME, Novack GD, Burke PJ, Cook D, Harmon G. The effect of levobunolol on aqueous humor dynamics. Exp Eye Res 1987;44:49–54.

132. Hayashi M, Yablonski ME, Novack GD, Cook DJ. True outflow facility determined by fluorophotometry in human subjects. Exp Eye Res 1989;48:621–625.

133. Wandel TA, Fishman D, Novack GD, Kelley EP, Chen K. Ocular hypotensive efficacy of 0.25% levobunolol once-daily. Ophthalmology 1988;95:252–254.

134. Rakofsky S, Melamed S, Cohen JS, et al. A comparison of the ocular hypotensive efficacy of once-daily and twice-daily levobunolol treatment. Ophthalmology 1989;96:8–11.

135. Partamian LG, Kass MA, Gordon M. A dose-response study of the effect of levobunolol on ocular hypertension. Am J Ophthalmol 1983;95:229–232.

136. Duzman E, Ober M, Scharrer A, Leopold IH. A clinical evaluation of the effects of topically applied levobunolol and timolol on increased intraocular pressure. Am J Ophthalmol 1982;94:318–322.

137. David R, Ober M, Masi R, et al. Levobunolol and pilocarpine: Combination therapy for the treatment of elevated intraocular pressure. Can J Ophthalmol 1987;22:208–211.

138. Allen RC, Robin AL, Long D, Novack GD, Lue JC, Kaplan G. A combination of levobunolol and dipivefrin for the treatment of glaucoma. Arch Ophthalmol 1988;106:904–907.

139. Akira Omi C, De Almeida GV, Belfort-Mattos R. Double masked study of levobunolol and timolol maleate in chronic open angle glaucoma or ocular hypertension patients. Arq Bras Oftalmol 1988;51:190–194.

140. Silverstone DE, Novack GD, Kelley EP, Chen KS. Prophylactic treatment of intraocular pressure elevations after neodymium: YAG laser posterior capsulotomies and extracapsular cataract extractions with levobunolol. Ophthalmology 1988;95:713–718.

141. West DR, Lischwe TD, Thompson VM, Ide CH. Comparative efficacy of the β-blockers for the prevention of increased intraocular pressure after cataract extraction. Am J Ophthalmol 1988;106:168–173.

142. Chang JS, Lee DA, Petursson G, et al. The effect of a glaucoma medication reminder cap on patient compliance and intraocular pressure. J Ocular Pharmacol 1991;7:117–124.

143. Wilhelmus KR, McCulloch RR, Gross RL. Dendritic keratopathy associated with beta-blocker eyedrops. Cornea 1990;9:335–337.

144. Novack GD, Tang-Liu D, Glavinos EP, Liu S, Shen D. Plasma levels following topical administration of levobunolol. Ophthalmologica 1987;194:194–200.

145. Charap AD, Shin DH, Petursson G, et al. The effect of varying drop size on the efficacy and safety of a topical beta-blocker. Ann Ophthalmol 1988;21:351–357.

146. Djian J. Clinical evaluation of betaxolol (Kerlone) as a once-daily treatment for hypertension in 4685 patients. Br J Clin Pract 1985;39:188–191.

147. Murphree SS, Saffitz JE. Delineation of the distribution of β-adrenergic receptor subtypes in canine myocardium. Circulation Research 1988;63:117–125.

148. Brodde O. Cardiac beta-adrenergic receptors. In: Anonymous: ISI atlas of science: Pharmacology. Philadelphia: ISI, 1987, 107–112.

149. Carstairs JR, Nimmo AJ, Barnes PJ. Autoradiographic visualization of beta-adrenoceptor subtypes in human lung. Am Rev Respir Dis 1985;132:541–547.

150. van Buskirk EM, Bacon DR, Fahrenbach WH. Ciliary vasoconstriction after topical adrenergic drugs. Am J Ophthalmol 1990;109:511–517.

151. Satoh N, Suzuki J, Bessho H, Kitada Y, Narimatsu A, Tobe A. Effects of betaxolol on cardiohemodynamics and coronary circulation in anesthetized dogs: comparison with atenolol and propranolol. Jpn J Pharmacol 1990;54:113–119.

152. Bessho H, Suzuki J, Kitada Y, Narimatsu A, Tobe A. [Antihypertensive effect of betaxolol, a cardioselective beta-adrenoceptor antagonist, in renal hypertensive dogs]. Nippon Yakurigaku Zasshi 1990;95:355–360.

153. Bessho H, Suzuki J, Narimatsu A, Tobe A. [Antihypertensive effect of betaxolol, a cardioselective beta-adrenoceptor antagonist, in experimental hypertensive rats]. Nippon Yakurigaku Zasshi 1990;95:347–354.

154. Frisk-Holmberg M, Strom G. Exercise during therapeutic beta-blockade: A two-year study in hypertensive patients. Clin Pharmacol Ther 1986;40:395–399.

155. Warrington SJ, Turner P, Kilborn JR, Bianchetti G, Morselli PL. Blood concentrations and pharmacodynamic effects of betaxolol (SL 75212) a new beta-adrenoceptor antagonist after oral and intravenous administration. Br J Clin Pharmacol 1980;10:449–452.

156. Giudicelli JF, Richer C, Ganansia J, Warrington S, Abriol C, Rulliere R. Betaxolol: Beta-adrenoceptor blocking effects and pharmacokinetics in man. In: Morselli PL, Cavero I, Killborn JR, et al, eds. Betaxolol and other beta-1–adrenoceptor antagonists. LERS Monograph Series. New York: Raven Press, 1983, 89–99.

157. Vuori M, Ali-Melkkila T, Kaila T, Iisalo E, Saari KM. Plasma and aqueous humour concentrations and systemic effects of topical betaxolol and timolol in man. Acta Ophthalmol 1993;71:201–206.

158. Morselli PL, Thiercelin JF, Padovani P, et al. Comparative pharmacokinetics of several beta-blockers in renal and hepatic insufficiency. In: Morselli PL, Cavero I, Kilborn JR, et al, eds. Betaxolol and other β1-adrenoceptor antagonists. LERS Monograph Series. New York: Raven Press, 1983, 233–241.

159. Beresford R, Heel RC. Betaxolol: A review of its pharmacody-

namic and pharmacokinetic properties, and therapeutic efficacy in hypertension. Drugs 1986;31:6–28.

160. Reiss GR, Brubaker RF. The mechanism of betaxolol, a new hypotensive agent. Ophthalmology 1983;90:1369–1372.

161. Coulangeon LM, Sole M, Menerath JM, Sole P. [Aqueous humor flow measured by fluorophotometry. A comparative study of the effect of various beta-blocker eyedrops in patients with ocular hypertension]. Ophtalmologie 1990;4:156–161.

162. Gaul GR, Will NJ, Brubaker RF. Comparison of a non-cardioselective beta adrenoceptor blocker and a cardioselective blocker in reducing aqueous flow in humans. Arch Ophthalmol 1989;107: 1308–1311.

163. Caldwell DR, Salisbury CR, Guzek JP. Effects of topical betaxolol in ocular hypertensive patients. Arch Ophthalmol 1984;102: 539–540.

164. Feghali JG, Kaufman PL. Decreased intraocular pressure in the hypertensive human eye with betaxolol, a beta-1–adrenergic antagonist. Am J Ophthalmol 1985;100:777–782.

165. Radius RL. Use of betaxolol in the reduction of elevated intraocular pressure. Arch Ophthalmol 1983;101:898–900.

166. Levy NS, Boone L. Effect of 0.25% betaxolol v placebo. Glaucoma 1983;5:230–232.

167. Berrospi AR, Leibowitz HM. Betaxolol: A new beta-adrenergic blocking agent for treatment of glaucoma. Arch Ophthalmol 1982; 100:943–946.

168. Berry DB, van Buskirk EM, Shields MB. Betaxolol and timolol: a comparison of efficacy and side effects. Arch Ophthalmol 1984; 102:42–45.

169. Feghali JG, Kaufman PL, Radius RL, Mandell AI. A comparison of betaxolol and timolol in open angle glaucoma and ocular hypertension. Acta Ophthalmol 1988;66:180–186.

170. Levy NS, Boone L, Ellis E. A controlled comparison of betaxolol and timolol with long-term evaluation of safety and efficacy. Glaucoma 1986;7:54–62.

171. Stewart RH, Kimbrough RL, Ward RL. Betaxolol vs. Timolol: A six-month double-blind comparison. Arch Ophthalmol 1986;104: 46–48.

172. Allen RC, Hertzmark E, Walker AM, Epstein DL. A double-masked comparison of betaxolol vs timolol in the treatment of open-angle glaucoma. Am J Ophthalmol 1986;101:535–541.

173. Long DA, Johns GE, Mullen RS, et al. Levobunolol and betaxolol: a double-masked controlled comparison of efficacy and safety in patients with elevated intraocular pressure. Ophthalmology 1988;95:735–741.

174. Vogel R, Tipping R, Kulaga SF, Clineschmidt CM. Changing therapy from timolol to betaxolol. Effect on intraocular pressure in selected patients with glaucoma. Timolol-Betaxolol Study Group. Arch Ophthalmol 1989;107:1303–1307.

175. Albracht DC, LeBlanc RP, Cruz AM, et al. A double-masked comparison of betaxolol and dipivefrin for the treatment of increased intraocular pressure. Am J Ophthalmol 1993;116: 307–313.

176. Allen RC, Cagle GD, Bruce LA. Controlled clinical evaluation of betaxolol (0.5%) ophthalmic solution intraocular pressure and adjunctive therapy. Program and Abstracts, Glaucoma Soc Meeting, Turin (XXV Int Cong Oph) 1986;1:20

177. Allen RC, Bruce LA. Clinical evaluation of betaxolol: intraocular pressure and adjunctive therapy. New Trends in Ophthalmology 1987;II:109–113.

178. Bloom HR, Cech JM, Eston AB, et al. Additive effect of betaxolol

179. Clark JB, Brooks AM, Harper CA, Mantzioros N, Gillies WE. A comparison of the efficacy of betaxolol and timolol in ocular hypertension with or without adrenaline. Aust N Z J Ophthalmol 1989;17:173–177.

180. Kaiser HJ, Flammer J, Messmer C, Stumpfig D, Hendrickson P. Thirty-month visual field follow-up of glaucoma patients treated with β-blockers. J Glaucoma 1992;1:153–155.

181. Messmer C, Flammer J, Stumpfig D. Influence of betaxolol and timolol on the visual fields of patients with glaucoma. Am J Ophthalmol 1991;112:678–681.

182. Messmer C, Stumpfig D, Flammer J. Effect of betaxolol and timolol on visual fields in glaucoma patients. Klin Mbl Augenheilk 1991;198:330–331.

183. Collignon-Brach J. Long-term effect of ophthalmic β-adrenoceptor antagonists on intraocular pressure and retinal sensitivity in primary open-angle glaucoma. Curr Eye Res 1992;11:1–3.

184. Martin-Boglind LM, Graves A, Wanger P. The effect of topical antiglaucoma drugs on the results of high-pass resolution perimetry. Am J Ophthalmol 1991;111:711–714.

185. van Buskirk EM, Weinreb RN, Berry DP, Lustgarten JS, Podos SM, Drake MM. Betaxolol in patients with glaucoma and asthma. Am J Ophthalmol 1986;101:531–534.

186. Weinreb RN, van Buskirk EM, Cherniack R, Drake MM. Long-term betaxolol therapy in glaucoma patients with pulmonary disease. Am J Ophthalmol 1988;106:162–167.

187. Vuori M, Ali-Melkkila T. The effect of betaxolol and timolol on postoperative intraocular pressure. Acta Ophthalmol 1993;71: 458–462.

188. Weinreb RN, Jani R. A novel formulation of an ophthalmic beta-adrenoceptor antagonist. J Parenteral Sci Tech 1992;46:51–53.

189. Weinreb RN, Caldwell DR, Goode SM, et al. A double-masked three-month comparison between 0.25% betaxolol suspension and 0.5% betaxolol ophthalmic solution. Am J Ophthalmol 1990;110: 189–192.

190. Kendall K, Mundorf T, Nardin G, Zimmerman TJ, Hesse R, Lavin P. Tolerability of timolol and betaxolol in patients with chronic open-angle glaucoma. Clin Ther 1987;9:651–655.

191. Vogel R, Clineschmidt CM, Kulaga SF, et al. Comparison of the ocular tolerability of two beta-adrenergic antagonists: Timolol and betaxolol. Glaucoma 1988;10:71–75.

192. Hoh H. Hornhautsensibilitat nach einzeldosen von timolol, betaxolol oder placebo bei augengesunden—randomisierte, prospektive doppblindstudie. Fortschr Ophthalmol 1988;85:132–138.

193. Weissman SS, Asbell PA. Effect of topical timolol (0.5%) and betaxolol (0.5%) on corneal sensitivity. Br J Ophthalmol 1990;74: 409–412.

194. Vogel R, Clineschmidt CM, Hoeh H, Kulaga SF, Tipping RW. The effect of timolol, betaxolol, and placebo on corneal sensitivity in healthy volunteers. J Ocular Pharmacol 1990;6:85–90.

195. Brogliatti B, Raveggi F, Moscone F, Gremmo E, Galli R. Draeger's esthesiometer: its employment to evaluate local anesthetic effect of 3 β-blockers (Timolol, Betaxolol, Carteolol). New Trends in Ophthalmology 1986;2:359–363.

196. Huckauf H. Respiratory tolerance of oral betaxolol in partially reversible obstructive airways disease. In: Morselli PL, Kilborn JR, Cavero I, Harrison DC, Langer SZ, eds. Betaxolol and other β1-adrenoceptor antagonists. New York: Raven Press, 1983, 205–211.

197. Hugues FC, Julien D, Marche J. Influence of betaxolol and atenolol

on airways in chronic obstructive lung diseases: comparison with propranolol. In: Morselli PL, Kilborn JR, Cavero I, Harrison DC, Langer SZ, eds. Betaxolol and other β_1-adrenoceptor antagonists. New York: Raven Press, 1983, 195–211.

198. Palminiteri R, Kaik G. Time course of the bronchial response to salbutamol after placebo, betaxolol and propranolol. Eur J Clin Pharmacol 1983;24:741–745.

199. van Buskirk EM. Comparison of ocular and systemic side effects of betaxolol and timolol. New Trends in Ophthalmology 1987; II:140–144.

200. Dunn TL, Gerber MJ, Shen AS, Fernandez E, Iseman MD, Cherniack RM. The effect of topical ophthalmic instillation of timolol and betaxolol on lung function in asthmatic subjects. Am Rev Respir Dis 1986;133:264–268.

201. Pasquale LR, Nordlund JR, Robin AL, et al. A comparison of the cardiovascular and pulmonary effects of brimonidine 0.2%, timolol 0.5%, and betaxolol suspension 0.25%. Invest Ophthalmol Vis Sci 1993;34(suppl)(4):1139.

202. Spiritus EM, Casciari R. Letter to the editor. Am J Ophthalmol 1985;100:492–493.

203. Brooks AMV, Gillies WE, West RH. Betaxolol eye drops as a safe medication to lower intraocular pressure. Aust NZ J Ophthalmol 1987;15:125–129.

204. Pecori-Giraldi J, Collini S, Planner-Terzaghi A, Arrico L, Grechi G. Timolol, betaxolol und befunolol in der glaukombehandlung: Untersuchung uber die bronchopulmonalen effekte. Fortschr Ophthalmol 1988;85:235–238.

205. Bleckmann H, Dorow P. Behandlung mit betaxolol und placebo-augentropfen bei patienten mit glaukom und reaktiven atemwegserkrankungen. Klin Mbl Augenheilk 1987;191:199–202.

206. Bleckmann H, Dorow P. Lokal applizierte kardioselektive beta-blocker und histaminprovokation bei patienten mit obstruktiven atemwegerkrankungen. Fortschr Ophthalmol 1987;84:346–349.

207. Berger WE. Betaxolol in patients with glaucoma and asthma. Am J Ophthalmol 1987;103:600

208. Le Jeunne C, Bringer L, Mondjee-Tahura Z, Munera Y, Hugues FC. Effets cardio-vasculaires des collyres au timolol, au carteolol, au metipranolol, au betaxolol chez le sujet agé. Therapie 1988;43: 89–92.

209. Bauer K, Brunner-Ferber F, Distlerath LM, et al. Assessment of systemic effects of different ophthalmic beta-blockers in healthy volunteers. Clin Pharmacol Ther 1991;49:658–664.

210. De Vries J, Van de Merwe SA, De Heer LJ. From timolol to betaxolol. Arch Ophthalmol 1989;107:634

211. Brooks AM, Burden JG, Gillies WE. The significance of reactions to betaxolol reported by patients. Aust N Z J Ophthalmol 1989;17: 353–355.

212. Ball S. Congestive heart failure from betaxolol. Arch Ophthalmol 1987;105:320

213. Chamberlain TJ. Myocardial infarction after ophthalmic betaxolol. N Engl J Med 1989;321:1342

214. Harris LS, Greenstein MD, Bloom AF. Respiratory difficulties with betaxolol. Am J Ophthalmol 1986;102:274–275.

215. Zabel RW, MacDonald IM. Sinus arrest associated with betaxolol ophthalmic drops. Am J Ophthalmol 1987;104:431

216. Roholt PC. Betaxolol and restrictive airway disease. Arch Ophthalmol 1987;105:1172

217. Nelson WL, Kuritsky JN. Early postmarketing surveillance of betaxolol hydrochloride, September 1985–September 1986. Am J Ophthalmol 1987;103:592.

218. Anonymous. BGA asks for beta-blocker ADR reports. Script 1988;1275:1.

219. Orlando RG. Clinical depression associated with betaxolol. Am J Ophthalmol 1986;102:275.

220. Cohn JB. A comparative study of the central nervous system effects of betaxolol vs. timolol. Arch Ophthalmol 1989;107:633–634.

221. Battershill PE, Sorkin EM. Ocular metipranolol: A preliminary review of its pharmacodynamic and pharmacokinetic properties, and therapeutic efficacy in glaucoma and ocular hypertension. Drugs 1988;36:601–615.

222. Sugrue MF, Armstrong JM, Gautheron P, Mallorga P, Viader MD. A study on the ocular and extraocular pharmacology of metipranolol. Graefes Arch Clin Exp Ophthalmol 1985;22:123–127.

223. Muller O, Knobel HR. Effectiveness and tolerance of metipranolol—results of a multi-center long-term study in Switzerland. Klin Mbl Augenheilk 1986;188:62–63.

224. Schnarr K-D. Vergleichende multizentrische untersuchung von carteolol-augentropfen mit anderen betablockern bei 768 patienten unter alltagsbedingungen. Klin Mbl Augenheilk 1988;192: 167–176.

225. Noack E. Ocular hypotensive action of beta-adrenergic blockers, with special consideration of metipranolol (Beta-Ophthiole). Klin Mbl Augenheilk 1986;189:1–3.

226. Serle JB, Lustgarten JS, Podos SM. A clinical trial of metipranolol, a noncardioselective beta-adrenergic antagonist, in ocular hypertension. Am J Ophthalmol 1991;112:302–307.

227. Mertz M. Results of a 6 weeks' multicenter double-blind trial: Metipranolol vs Timolol. In: Merte H, ed. Metipranolol: Pharmacology of beta-blocking agents and use of metipranolol in ophthalmology. New York: Springer-Verlag, 1984, 93–105.

228. Merkle W. Bericht Ober die ergebnisse mit neuen betarezeptorenblockern in der glakomtherapie. Fortschr Ophthalmol 1983;79: 413–414.

229. Krieglstein GK, Novack GD, Voepel E, et al. Levobunolol and metipranolol: comparative ocular hypotensive efficacy, safety and comfort. Br J Ophthalmol 1987;71:250–253.

230. Kruse W. Metipranolol—ein neuer betarezeptorenblocker. Klin Mbl Augenheilk 1983;182:582–584.

231. Mills KB, Wright G. A blind randomized cross-over trial comparing metipranolol 0.3% with timolol 0.25% in open-angle glaucoma: a pilot study. Br J Ophthalmol 1986;70:39–42.

232. Dausch D, Brewitt H, Edelhoff R. Metipranolol eye drops: Clinical suitability in the treatment of chronic open angle glaucoma. In: Merte H, ed. Metipranolol: Pharmacology of beta-blocking agents and use of metipranolol in ophthalmology. New York: Springer-Verlag, 1983, 132–147.

233. Schmitz-Valkenberg P, Jonas J, Brambring DF. Reductions in pressure with metipranolol 0.1%. Zeitschrift fur Praktische Augenheilkunde 1984;5:171–175.

234. Demailly P, Lecherpie F. Metipranolol 0.1%: Effect of one single dose on nycthermal pressure graph in chronic open angle primitive glaucoma. J Fr Ophthalmol 1987;10:447–449.

235. Levy NS. Effect of metipranolol 0.3% versus dipivefrin 0.1% in eyes with intraocular pressure elevation. Glaucoma 1992;14: 24–30.

236. Schmitz-Valkenberg P, Kessler C. Low-dose combination or high-dose separate solutions in glaucoma. Invest Ophthalmol Vis Sci 1992;33(suppl):1122.

237. Christ T, Kessler C. Single, combination or separate solutions in

glaucoma treatment?. Invest Ophthalmol Vis Sci 1992;33(suppl): 1122.

238. Scharrer A, Ober M. Fixed combination of metipranolol 0.1% and pilocarpine 2% compared with the individual drugs in glaucoma therapy: a controlled randomized study for intraindividual comparison of efficacy and tolerance. Klin Mbl Augenheilk 1986;189: 450–455.

239. Ober M, Scharrer A, Novack GD, Lue JC. Die lokale subjektive Vertraglich keit von Levobunolol und Metipranolol in einer Doppelblink-Vergliechsstudie bie Patienten mit erhohtem intraokularem druck. Ophthalmologica 1986;192:159–164.

240. de Groot AC, Conemans J. Contact allergy to metipranolol. Contact Dermatitis 1988;18:107–108.

241. Akingbehin T, Villada JR. Metipranolol-associated granulomatous anterior uveitis. Br J Ophthalmol 1991;75:519–523.

242. Kessler C, Christ T. The incidence of uveitis in glaucoma patients using metipranolol. J Glaucoma 1993;2:166–170.

243. Hugues FC, Le Jeunne C, Munera Y, Dufier JL. Comparison des effets des collyres au carteolol et au metipranolol sur les fonctions ventilatoires et cardiovasculaires de l'asthmatique. J Fr Ophthalmol 1987;10:485–490.

244. Bacon PJ, Brazier DJ, Smith R, Smith SE. Cardiovascular responses to metipranolol and timolol eyedrops in healthy volunteers. Br J Clin Pharmacol 1989;27:1–5.

245. Mori H, Kido M, Murakami N, Morita S, Kohri H. [Metabolic fate of carteolol hydrochloride [5–(3-tert-butylamino-2–hydroxypropoxy)-3,4–dihydrocarbostyril hydrochloride, OPC-1085], a new beta-blocker. V. Identification of metabolites in rat, dog and human (author's transl)]. Yakugaku Zasshi 1977;97:305–308.

246. Sugiyama K, Enya T, Kitazawa Y. Ocular hypotensive effect of 8–hydroxycarteolol, a metabolite of carteolol. Int Ophthalmol Clin 1989;13:85–89.

247. Fujio N, Kitazawa T. [Intraocular penetration of 14C-Carteolol hydrochloride (beta-blocker) in the albino rabbits]. Nippon Ganka Gakkai Zasshi 1984;88:236–241.

248. Araie M, Takase M. Effects of S-596 and carteolol, new beta-adrenergic blockers, and flurbiprofen on the human eye: a fluorophotometric study. Graefes Arch Clin Exp Ophthalmol 1985;222: 259–262.

249. Krieglstein GK. Carteolol and tonography. European Glaucoma Society Abstracts 1988;L19.

250. Kitazawa Y, Azuma I, Takase M, Koememushi S. Ocular hypotensive effects of carteolol hydrochloride in primary open-angle glaucoma and ocular hypertensive patients: A double-masked cross-over study for the determination of concentrations optimal for clinical use. Acta Soc Ophthalmol Jpn 1981;85:798–804.

251. Ishikawa T, Okisaka S, Hiwatari S. Pilocarpine, carbachol and carteolol on open-angle glaucoma and ocular hypotension. Nippon Ganka Gakkai Zasshi 1981;85:837–842.

252. Duff GR, Graham PA. A double-crossover trial comparing the effects of topical carteolol and placebo on intraocular pressure. Br J Ophthalmol 1988;72:27–28.

253. Duff GR, Newcombe RG. The 12–hour control of intraocular pressure on carteolol 2% twice daily. Br J Ophthalmol 1988;72: 890–891.

254. Scoville B, Mueller B, White BG, Krieglstein GK. A double-masked comparison of carteolol and timolol in ocular hypertension. Am J Ophthalmol 1988;105:150–154.

255. Stewart WC, Shields MB, Allen RC, et al. A 3-month comparison of 1% and 2% carteolol and 0.5% timolol in open-angle glaucoma. Graefe's Arch Clin Exp Ophthalmol 1991;229:258–261.

256. Behrens-Baumann W, Kimmich F, Walt JG, Lue J. A comparison of the ocular hypotensive efficacy and systemic safety of 0.5% levobunolol and 2% carteolol. Ophthalmologica 1994;208:32–36.

257. Schnaudigel O, Becker H, Fuchs H. Carteolol: Praxisgerechte prufung von wirksamkeit und verträglichkeit eines neuen betablockers in der behandlung des glaukoms. Klin Mbl Augenheilk 1988;192:248–251.

258. Collignon-Brach J. Early visual field changes with beta–blocking agents. Surv Ophthalmol 1989;33(suppl):429–430.

259. Stodtmeister R, Pillunat L, Wilmanns I, Neubrand M, Finger B, Tobias G. [Effect of carteolol and timolol eyedrops on the pressure tolerance of the optic nerve head.]. Ophthalmologica 1989;198: 64–77.

260. Scoville B, Krieglstein GK, Then E, Yokoyama S, Yokoyama T. Measuring drug-induced eye irritation: A simple new clinical assay. J Clin Pharmacol 1985;25:210–218.

261. Brazier DJ, Smith SE. Ocular and cardiovascular response to topical carteolol 2% and timolol 0.5% in healthy volunteers. Br J Ophthalmol 1988;72:101–103.

262. Jay JL. Cardiac side effects of beta blocker eyedrops (letter). Br J Ophthalmol 1988;72:240

263. Frishman WH, Covey S. Penbutolol and carteolol: two new beta-adrenergic blockers with partial agonism. J Clin Pharmacol 1990; 30:412–421.

264. Freedman SF, Freedman NJ, Shields MB, et al. Effects of ocular carteolol and timolol on plasma high-density lipoprotein cholesterol level. Am J Ophthalmol 1993;116:600–611.

265. Taylor P. Cholinergic agonists. In: Gilman AG, Rall TW, Nies AS, et al. eds. Goodman and Gilman's The pharmacological basis of therapeutics. New York: Pergamon Press, 1990;122–130.

266. Gabelt BT, Crawford K, Kaufman PL. Outflow facility and its response to pilocarpine decline in aging rhesus monkeys. Arch Ophthalmol 1991;109:879–882.

267. Krill AE, Newell FN. Effects of pilocarpine on ocular dynamics. Am J Ophthalmol 1964;57:34–41.

268. Harris LS, Galin MA. Dose response analysis of pilocarpine-induced ocular hypotension. Arch Ophthalmol 1970;84:605–608.

269. Harris LS, Galin MA. Effect of ocular pigmentation on hypotensive response to pilocarpine. Am J Ophthalmol 1971;72:923–925.

270. Worthen DM. Effect of pilocarpine drops on diurnal intraocular pressure variation in patients with glaucoma. Invest Ophthalmol 1978;15:784–787.

271. Chen HS, Steinmann WC, Spaeth GL. The effect of chronic miotic therapy on the result of posterior chamber intraocular lens implantation and trabeculectomy in patients with glaucoma. Ophthalmic Surg 1989;20:784–789.

272. Abramson DM, Chang S, Coleman J. Pilocarpine therapy in glaucoma. Arch Ophthalmol 1976;94:914–918.

273. Zimmerman TJ. Agents for glaucoma. In: Bartlett JD, Ghormley NR, Jaanus SD, et al. Ophthalmic Drug Facts. St. Louis: Facts and Comparisons, 1995:157–202.

274. Quigley HA, Pollack IP. Intraocular pressure control with twice-daily pilocarpine in two vehicle solutions. Ann Ophthalmol 1977; 9:427–430.

275. Zimmerman TJ, Sharir M, Nardin GF, Fuqua M. Therapeutic index of pilocarpine, carbachol, and timolol with nasolacrimal occlusion. Am J Ophthalmol 1992;114:1–7.

276. Simmons RJ, Greff LJ. Pilocarpine concentrations. Arch Ophthalmol 1991;109:932.

277. Quigley HA, Pollack IP, Harbin TS. Pilocarpine Ocuserts. Long-term clinical trials and selected pharmacodynamics. Arch Ophthalmol 1975;93:771–775.

278. Brown HS, Meltzer G, Merrill RC, et al. Visual effects of pilocarpine in glaucoma. Arch Ophthalmol 1976;94:1716–1719.

279. Novak S, Stewart RH. The Ocusert system in the management of glaucoma. Tex Med 1975;71:63–65.

280. Stewart RH, Novak S. Introduction of the Ocusert ocular system to an ophthalmic practice. Am J Ophthalmol 1978;3:325–330.

281. Mandell AI, Bruce LA, Khalifa MA. Reduced cyclic myopia with pilocarpine gel. Ann Ophthalmol 1988;20:133–135.

282. Krause K, Kuchle HJ, Baumgart M. Comparative studies of pilocarpine gel and pilocarpine eyedrops. Klin Monatsbl Augenheilkd 1984;187:178–183.

283. Havener WH. Ocular pharmacology. St. Louis: C.V. Mosby, 1983; Chap. 12.

284. Fernandez-Bahamonde JL, Alcaraz-Michelli V. The combined use of apraclonidine and pilocarpine during laser iridotomy in a Hispanic population. Ann Ophthalmol 1990;22:446–449.

285. Podos SM, Ritch R. Epinephrine as the initial therapy in selected cases of ocular hypertension. Surv Ophthalmol 1980;25:188–194.

286. Williams TD. Accommodative blur in pilocarpine-treated glaucoma. J Am Optom Assoc 1976;47:761–764.

287. Lutjen-Drecoll E, Tamm E, Kaufman PL. Age-related loss of morphologic responses to pilocarpine in rhesus monkey ciliary muscle. Arch Ophthalmol 1988;106:1591–1598.

288. Zimmerman TJ. Pilocarpine. Ophthalmology 1981;88:85–88.

289. Harris LS. Phenylephrine in miotic-treated eyes. Ann Ophthalmol 1972;10:861–870.

290. Sugar S. The ten commandments for management of primary open-angle glaucoma. Am J Ophthalmol 1979;5:783–791.

291. Schwartz B. Primary open-angle glaucoma. In: Duane TD, ed. Clinical Ophthalmology. Hagerstown, MD: Harper & Row, 1981; 3:1–45.

292. Van Buskirk EM. Hazards of medical glaucoma therapy in the cataract patient. Ophthalmology 1982;89:238–241.

293. Brazier DJ, Hitchings RA. Atypical band keratopathy following long-term pilocarpine treatment. Br J Ophthalmol 1989;73:294–296.

294. Zimmerman TJ, Wheeler TM. Miotics. Side effects and ways to avoid them. Ophthalmology 1982;89:76–80.

295. Alpar JJ. Miotics and retinal detachment. Am J Ophthalmol 1979; 3:395–401.

296. Weseley P, Liebmann J, Ritch R. Rhegmatogenous retinal detachment after initiation of Ocusert therapy. Am J Ophthalmol 1991; 112:458–459.

297. Benedict WL, Shami M. Impending macular hole associated with topical pilocarpine. Am J Ophthalmol 1992;114:765–766.

298. Schuman JS, Hersh P, Kylstra J. Vitreous hemorrhage associated with pilocarpine. Am J Ophthalmol 1989;108:333–334.

299. Kraushar MF. Miotics and retinal detachment. Arch Ophthalmol 1991;109:1659.

300. Kraushar MF, Steinberg JA. Miotics and retinal detachment: upgrading the community standard. Surv Ophthalmol 1991;35: 311–316.

301. Greco JJ, Kelman CD. Systemic pilocarpine toxicity in the treatment of angle closure glaucoma. Ann Ophthalmol 1973;1:57–59.

302. Mori M, Araie M, Sakurai M, Oshika T. Effects of pilocarpine and

303. tropicamide on blood-aqueous barrier permeability in man. Invest Ophthalmol Vis Sci 1992;33:416–423.

303. Yamauchi DN, Patie PN. Relative potency of cholinomimetic drugs on bovine iris sphincter strips. Invest Ophthalmol 1973;12: 80–83.

304. Reichert RW, Shields MB, Stewart WC. Intraocular pressure response to replacing pilocarpine with carbachol. Am J Ophthalmol 1988;106:747–748.

305. Volle RL. Cholinomimetic drugs. In: DiPalma JR, ed. Drill's pharmacology in medicine. New York: McGraw-Hill, 1971;4:604.

306. Reynolds JEF, ed. Martindale. The extra pharmacopoeia. London: The Pharmaceutical Press, 1993, 1114–1115.

307. Klayman J, Taffets S. Low-concentration phospholine iodide therapy in open angle glaucoma. Am J Ophthalmol 1963;55:1233–1237.

308. De Roeth A Jr. A reappraisal of phospholine iodide. In: Srinivasan BD, ed. Ocular therapeutics. New York: Masson, 1980; 157–158.

309. Taylor P. Anticholinesterase agents. In: Gilman AG, Rall TW, Nies AS, et al., eds. Goodman and Gilman's the pharmacological basis of therapeutics. New York: Pergamon Press, 1990;131–149.

310. Hamburger K. Experimentelle glaucoma therapie. Augenheilkd 1923;7:810–823.

311. Hoskins HD, Kass MA. Adrenergic agonists. In: Becker-Shaffer's Diagnosis and therapy of the glaucomas. St. Louis: CV Mosby 1989; Chap. 27.

312. Ophthalmic Drug Facts. St. Louis: Facts and Comparisons, 1995; Chap. 9.

313. Criswick VG, Drance SM. Comparative study of four different epinephrine salts on intraocular pressure. Arch Ophthalmol 1966; 75:768–770.

314. Holland MG. Autonomic drugs in ophthalmology: some problems and promises. III. Sympathomimetic drugs. Ann Ophthalmol 1974;6:875–888.

315. Weekers R, Delmarcelle Y, Gustin J. Treatment of ocular hypertension by adrenaline and diverse sympathomimetic amines. Am J Ophthalmol 1955;40:666–672.

316. Kacere RD, Dolan JW, Brubaker RF. Intravenous epinephrine stimulates aqueous formation in the human eye. Invest Ophthalmol Vis Sci 1992;33:2861–2866.

317. Townsend DJ, Brubaker RF. Immediate effect of epinephrine on aqueous formation in the normal human eye as measured by fluorophotometry. Invest Ophthalmol 1980;19:256–266.

318. Schenker HI, Yablonski ME, Podos SM, Linder L. Fluorophotometric study of epinephrine and timolol in human subjects. Arch Ophthalmol 1981;99:1212–1216.

319. Nagataki S, Brubaker RF. Early effect of epinephrine on aqueous formation in normal eyes. Ophthalmology 1981;88:278–282.

320. Thomas JV, Epstein DL. Transient additive effect of timolol and epinephrine in primary open angle glaucoma. Arch Ophthalmol 1981;99:91–96.

321. Neufeld AH, Jampol LM, Sears ML. Cyclic AMP in the aqueous humor. The effects of adrenergic action. Exp Eye Res 1972;14: 242–250.

322. Neufeld AH, Sears ML. Adenosine 3'5'-monophosphate analogue increases the outflow facility of the primate eye. Invest Ophthalmol 1975;14:688–689.

323. Erickson K, Liang L, Shum P, Nathanson JA. Adrenergic regulation of aqueous outflow. J Ocular Pharmacol 1994;10:241–252.

324. Boas RS, Messenger MJ, Mittag TW, Podos SM. The effects of

topically applied epinephrine and timolol on intraocular pressure and aqueous humor cyclic-AMP in the rabbit. Exp Eye Res 1981; 32:681–690.

325. Garner LL, Johnstone WW, Ballintine EJ, Carroll ME. Effect of 2% levo-rotary epinephrine on the intraocular pressure of the glaucomatous eye. Arch Ophthalmol 1959;62:230–238.

326. Harris LS, Galin MA, Lerner R. The influence of low dose L-epinephrine on intraocular pressure. Ann Ophthalmol 1970;2: 253–257.

327. Podos SM, Ritch R. Epinephrine as the initial therapy in selected cases of ocular hypertension. Surv Ophthalmol 1980;25:188–194.

328. Tredici TJ. Screening and management of glaucoma in flying personnel. Aerospace Med 1980;50:34–41.

329. Kramer SG. Epinephrine distribution after topical administration to phakic and aphakic eyes. Trans Am Ophthalmol Soc 1980;78: 947–981.

330. Durkee D, Bryant BG. Drug therapy in glaucoma. Am J Hosp Pharm 1979;35:682–690.

331. Sugar SH. Pitfalls in the medical treatment of simple glaucoma. Ann Ophthalmol 1979;11:1041–1050.

332. Aronson SB, Yamamoto EA. Ocular hypersensitivity to epinephrine. Invest Ophthalmol 1966;5:75–80.

333. Edelhauser HF, Hyndiuck RA, Zeeb A, Schultz RO. Corneal edema and the intraocular use of epinephrine. Am J Ophthalmol 1981;93:327–333.

334. Fong DS, Frederick AR, Richter CU, Jakobiec FA. Adrenochrome deposit. Arch Ophthalmol 1993;111:1142–1143.

335. Ferry AP, Zimmerman LE. Black cornea: a complication of topical use of epinephrine. Am J Ophthalmol 1964;58:205–210.

336. Kaiser PK, Pineda R, Albert DM, Shore JW. 'Black cornea' after long-term epinephrine use. Arch Ophthalmol 1992;110:1273–1275.

337. Sugar J. Adenochrome pigmentation of hydrophilic lenses. Arch Ophthalmol 1974;91:11–12.

338. Miller D, Brooks SM, Mobilia E. Adrenochrome staining of soft contact lenses. Ann Ophthalmol 1976;8:65–67.

339. Lee PF. The influence of epinephrine and phenylephrine on intraocular pressure. Arch Ophthalmol 1958;60:863–867.

340. Kolker AE, Becker B. Epinephrine maculopathy. Arch Ophthalmol 1968;79:552–562.

341. Becker B, Morton WF. Topical epinephrine in glaucoma suspects. Am J Ophthalmol 1966;62:272–277.

342. Michels RG, Maumenee AE. Cystoid macular edema associated with topically applied epinephrine in aphakic eyes. Am J Ophthalmol 1975;80:379–388.

343. Mackool RJ, Muldoon T, Fortier A, Nelson D. Epinephrine induced cystoid macular edema in aphakic eyes. Arch Ophthalmol 1977;95:791–793.

344. Ballin N, Becker B, Goldman ML. Systemic effects of epinephrine applied topically to the eye. Invest Ophthalmol 1966;5:125–129.

345. Becker B, Montgomery SW, Kass MA, Shin DH. Increased ocular and systemic responsiveness to epinephrine in primary open-angle glaucoma. Arch Ophthalmol 1977;95:789–790.

346. Davidson SI. Systemic effects of eye drops. Trans Ophthalmol Soc UK 1974;94:487–495.

347. Schwartz B. Primary open-angle glaucoma. In: Duane TD, ed. Clinical ophthalmology. Hagerstown, MD: Harper & Row, 1981; 3:52.

348. Van Buskirk EM. Hazards of medical glaucoma therapy in the cataract patient. Ophthalmology 1982;89:238–241.

349. Kaback MB, Podos SM, Harbin TS, et al. The effects of dipivalyl epinephrine on the eye. Am J Ophthalmol 1976;81:768–772.

350. Mandell AI, Podos SM. Dipivalyl epinephrine (DPE): A new prodrug in the treatment of glaucoma. In: Leopold IH, Burns RP, eds. Symposium on ocular therapy. New York: John Wiley & Sons, 1977;10:109–117.

351. Mandell AI, Stentz F, Kitabicki AE. Dipivalyl epinephrine: a new prodrug in the treatment of glaucoma. Trans Am Acad Ophthalmol Otolaryngol 1978;85:268–274.

352. Wei C, Anderson JA, Leopold IH. Ocular absorption and metabolism of topically applied epinephrine and a dipivalyl ester of epinephrine. Invest Ophthalmol 1978;17:315.

353. Mindel JS, Yablonski ME, Tavitian HO, et al. Dipivefrin and echothiophate. Arch Ophthalmol 1981;99:1583–1586.

354. Mindel JS, Koenigsberg AM, Kharlamb AP, et al. The effect of echothiophate on the biphasic response of rabbit ocular pressure to dipivefrin. Arch Ophthalmol 1982;100:147–151.

355. Kohn AN, Moss AP, Hargett NA, et al. Clinical comparison of dipivalyl epinephrine and epinephrine in the treatment of glaucoma. Am J Ophthalmol 1979;87:196–201.

356. Yablonski ME, Shin DH, Kolker AE. Dipivefrin use in patients with intolerance to topically applied epinephrine. Arch Ophthalmol 1977;95:2157–2158.

357. Newton MJ, Nesburn AB. Lack of hydrophilic lens discoloration in patients using dipivalyl epinephrine for glaucoma. Am J Ophthalmol 1979;87:193–195.

358. Theodore J, Leibowitz HM. External ocular toxicity of dipivalyl epinephrine. Am J Ophthalmol 1979;88:1013–1016.

359. Kerr CR, Hass I, Drance SM, et al. Cardiovascular effects of epinephrine and dipivalyl epinephrine applied topically to the eye in patients with glaucoma. Br J Ophthalmol 1981;66:109–114.

360. Liesgang TJ. Bulbar conjunctival follicles associated with dipivefrin therapy. Ophthalmology 1985;92:228–233.

361. Wilson FM. Adverse external ocular effects of topical ophthalmic medications. Surv Ophthalmol 1979/80;24:57–88.

362. Coleiro JA, Sigurdsson H, Lockyer JA. Follicular conjunctivitis on dipivefrin therapy for glaucoma. Eye 1988;2:440–442.

363. Wandel T, Spinak M. Toxicity of dipivalyl epinephrine. Ophthalmology 1981;88:259–260.

364. Borrmann L, Duzman E. Undetected cystoid macular edema in aphakic glaucoma patients treated with dipivefrin. J Toxicol—Cut Ocular Toxicol 1987;6:173–177.

365. Coleman AL, Robin AL, Pollack IP. Apraclonidine hydrochloride. Ophthalmol Clin North Am 1989;2:97–108.

366. Robin AL, Novack GD. Alpha$_2$-agonists in the therapy of glaucoma. In: Drance SM, Van Buskirk EM, Neufeld AH, eds. Pharmacology of Glaucoma. Baltimore: Williams & Wilkins 1991; Chap. 7.

367. Hodapp E, Kolker A, Kass MA et al. The effect of topical clonidine on intraocular pressure. Arch Ophthalmol 1981;99: 1208–1211.

368. Chien D, Tang-Lieu DD, Gluchowski C. Corneal and conjunctival/scleral absorption of alpha$_2$-adrenergic agents in rabbit eyes. Invest Ophthalmol Vis Sci 1990;31(suppl):403.

369. Gharagozloo NZ, Relf SJ, Brubaker RF. Aqueous flow is reduced by the alpha-adrenergic agonist apraclonidine hydrochloride (ALO 2145). Ophthalmology 1988;95:1217–1220.

370. Robin AL. Short-term effects of unilateral 1% apraclonidine therapy. Arch Ophthalmol 1988;106:912–915.

371. Abrams DA, Robin AL, Crandell AS, et al. Dose response evaluation of apraclonidine in subjects with normal and elevated intraocular pressures. Am J Ophthalmol 1989;108:230–237.

372. Robin AL, Coleman AL. Apraclonidine hydrochloride: an evaluation of plasma concentrations, and a comparison of its intraocular pressure lowering and cardiovascular effects to timolol maleate. Trans Am Ophthalmol Soc 1989;729–761.

373. Van Buskirk, Bacon DR, Fahrenbach WH. Ciliary vasoconstriction after topical adrenergic drugs. Am J Ophthalmol 1990;109:511–517.

374. Wang RF, Camras CB, Podos SM, et al. The role of prostaglandins in the paminoclonidine-induced reduction of intraocular pressure. Trans Am Ophthalmol Soc 1989;87:94–104.

375. McCannel C, Koskela T, Brubaker RF. Flurbiprofen pretreatment does not block apraclonidine's effect on aqueous flow. Arch Ophthalmol 1991;109:810–811.

376. Robin AL. The role of apraclonidine hydrochloride in laser therapy for glaucoma. Trans Am Ophthalmol Soc 1989;87:729–761.

377. Abrams DA, Robin AL, Pollack IP, et al. The safety and efficacy of topical ALO 2145 (para-aminoclonidine hydrochloride) in normal volunteers. Arch Ophthalmol 1987;105:1205–1207.

378. Jampel HD, Robin AL, Quigley HA, Pollack IP. Apraclonidine hydrochloride: a one-week dose response study. Arch Ophthalmol 1988;106:1069–1073.

379. Mori M, Araie M. Effect of apraclonidine on blood-aqueous barrier permeability to plasma protein in man. Exp Eye Res 1992;54:555–559.

380. Araie M, Kiyoshi I. Effects of apraclonidine on intraocular pressure and blood-aqueous barrier permeability after phacoemulsification and intraocular lens implantation. Am J Ophthalmol 1993;116:67–71.

381. Weinreb RN, Ruderman J, Juster R, Zweig K. Immediate intraocular pressure response to argon laser trabeculoplasty. Am J Ophthalmol 1983;95:279–286.

382. Richter CU, Arzeno G, Pappas HR, et al. Intraocular pressure elevations following Nd: YAG laser capsulotomy. Ophthalmology 1985;92:636–640.

383. Robin AL, Pollack IP. A comparison of neodymium: YAG and argon laser iridotomies. Ophthalmology 1984;91:1011–1016.

384. Robin AL, Pollack IP, House B, Enger C. Effects of ALO 2145 on intraocular pressure following argon laser trabeculoplasty. Arch Ophthalmol 1987;105:646–650.

385. Brown RH, Stewart RH, Lynch MG, et al. ALO 2145 reduces the intraocular pressure elevation after anterior segment laser surgery. Ophthalmology 1988;95:378–383.

386. Robin AL. Effect of topical apraclonidine on the frequency of intraocular pressure elevations after combined extracapsular cataract extraction and trabeculectomy. Ophthalmology 1993;100:628–633.

387. Hill RA, Minckler DS, Lee M, et al. Apraclonidine prophylaxis for postcycloplegic intraocular pressure spikes. Ophthalmology 1991;98:1083–1086.

388. Cambridge D. UK 14304–18, a potent and selective alpha-$_2$ agonist for the characterization of alpha-adrenoceptor subtypes. Eur J Pharmacol 1981;72:413–415.

389. Burke JA, Potter DE. The ocular effects of a relatively selective alpha-$_2$ agonist (UK 14304–18) in cats, rabbits and monkeys. Curr Eye Res 1986;5:665–675.

390. Chien DS, Homsy JJ, Gluchowski C, et al. Corneal and conjunctival/scleral penetration of p-aminoclonidine, AGN 190342 and clonidine in rabbit eyes. Curr Eye Res 1990;9:1051–1059.

391. Serle JB, Steidl S, Wang RF, et al. Selective alpha-$_2$ agonists B HT920 and UK 14304–18. Effects on aqueous humor dynamics in monkeys. Arch Ophthalmol 1991;109:1158–1162.

392. Barneby HS, Robin AL, Zimmerman TJ, et al. The efficacy of brimonidine in decreasing elevations in intraocular pressure after laser trabeculoplasty. Ophthalmology 1993;100:1083–1088.

393. Derick RJ, Walters TR, Robin AL, et al. Brimonidine tartrate. A one month dose response study. Invest Ophthalmol Vis Sci 1991;32(suppl):929.

394. Serle JB, Podos SM, Abundo GP, et al. The effect of brimonidine tartrate in glaucoma patients on maximal medical therapy. Invest Ophthalmol Vis Sci 1991;32(suppl):929.

395. Nagasubramanian S, Hitchings RA, Demailly P, et al. Comparison of apraclonidine and timolol in chronic open-angle glaucoma. A three-month study. Ophthalmology 1993;100:1318–1323.

396. David R, Spaeth GL, Clerenger CE, et al. Brimonidine in the prevention of intraocular pressure elevation following argon laser trabeculoplasty. Arch Ophthalmol 1993;111:1387–1390.

397. Friedenwald JS. The formation of the intraocular fluid. Am J Ophthalmol 1949;32:9–27.

398. Kinsey VE. A unified concept of aqueous humor dynamics and the maintenance of intraocular pressure: an elaboration of the secretion-diffusion theory. Arch Ophthalmol 1950;44:215–235.

399. Wistrand PJ. Carbonic anhydrase in the anterior uvea of the rabbit. Acta Physiol Scand 1951;24:144–148.

400. Becker B. Decrease in intraocular pressure in man by a carbonic anhydrase inhibitor, Diamox: A preliminary report. Am J Ophthalmol 1954;37:13–15.

401. Dailey RA, Brubaker RF, Bourne WM. The effects of timolol maleate and acetazolamide on the rate of aqueous formation in normal human subjects. Am J Ophthalmol 1982;93:232–237.

402. Maren TH. Relations between structure and biological activity of sulfonamides. Ann Rev Pharmacol Toxicol 1976;16:309–327.

403. Mudge GH. Diuretics and other agents employed in the mobilization of edema fluid. In: Gilman AG, Goodman LS, Gilman A, et al. eds. The pharmacological basis of therapeutics. New York: Macmillan Co, 1980;6:896–899.

404. Dobbs PC, Epstein DL, Anderson PJ. Identification of isoenzyme C as the principal carbonic anhydrase in human ciliary processes. Invest Ophthalmol Vis Sci 1979;18:867–870.

405. Wistrand PJ, Garg LC. Evidence of a high-activity C type of carbonic anhydrase in human ciliary processes. Invest Ophthalmol Vis Sci 1979;18:802–806.

406. Zimmerman TJ, Garg LC, Vogh BP, Maren TH. The effect of acetazolamide on the movements of anions into the posterior chamber of the dog eye. J Pharmacol Exp Ther 1976;196:510–516.

407. Kinsey VE, Reddy DVN. Turnover of carbon dioxide in the aqueous humor and the effect thereon of acetazolamide. Arch Ophthalmol 1959;62:78–83.

408. Maren TH, Wistrand P, Swensen ER, Talalay ABC. The rates of ion movement from plasma to aqueous humor in the dogfish, *Squalus ascanthias.* Invest Ophthalmol 1975;14:662–673.

409. Garg LC, Oppelt WW. The effect of ouabain and acetazolamide on transport of sodium and chloride from plasma to aqueous humor. J Pharmacol Exp Ther 1970;175:237–247.

410. Maren TH. The rates of movement of Na^+, Cl^-, and HCO_3^- from

plasma to posterior chamber: Effect of acetazolamide and relation to treatment of glaucoma. Invest Ophthalmol 1976,15:356–364.

411. Maren TH. Ion secretion into the posterior aqueous humor of dogs and monkeys. Exp Eye Res 1977;25(suppl):245–247.

412. Maren TH. HCO₃⁻ formation in aqueous humor: Mechanism and relation to treatment of glaucoma. Invest Ophthalmol 1974;13: 479–484.

413. Cole DF. Secretion of aqueous humor. Exp Eye Res (Suppl) 1977; 25:161–176.

414. Bietti G, Virno M, Pecori-Giraldi J, Pellegrino N. Acetazolamide, metabolic acidosis, and intraocular pressure. Am J Ophthalmol 1975;80:360–369.

415. Friedman Z, Krupin T, Becker B. Ocular and systemic effects of acetazolamide in nephrectomized rabbits. Invest Ophthalmol Vis Sci 1982;23:209–213.

416. Langham ME, Lee PM. Action of Diamox and ammonium chloride on formation of aqueous humor. Br J Ophthalmol 1957;41: 65–92.

417. Becker B. The mechanism of the fall in intraocular pressure induced by the carbonic anhydrase inhibitor, Diamox. Am J Ophthalmol 1955;39:177–182.

418. Fanous MM, Maren T. Does metabolic acidosis contribute to the IOP effect of acetazolamide? Invest Ophthalmol Vis Sci 1992;33 (suppl):1246.

419. Maren TH. Carbonic anhydrase: chemistry, physiology, and inhibition. Physiol Rev 1967;47:595–781.

420. Becker B. Carbonic anhydrase and the formation of aqueous humor. Am J Ophthalmol 1959;47:342–361.

421. McCannel CA, Heinrich SR, Brubaker RF. Acetazolamide but not timolol lowers aqueous humor flow in sleeping humans. Graefe's Arch Clin Exp Ophthalmol 1992;230:518–520.

422. Kolker AE, Hetherington J Jr. Becker-Shaffer's diagnosis and therapy of the glaucomas. St Louis: C. V. Mosby Co, 1976;339.

423. Ellis PP, Price PK, Kelmenson R, Rendi M. Effectiveness of generic acetazolamide. Arch Ophthalmol 1982;100:1920–1922.

424. Maren TH, Mayer E, Wadsworth BD. Carbonic anhydrase inhibitors. I. The pharmacology of Diamox,2–acetylamino-1,3,4,-thiadiazole-5-sulfonamiae. Bull Johns Hopkins Hosp 1954;95:199–243.

425. Maren TH, Robinson B. The pharmacology of acetazolamide as related to cerebrospinal fluid and the treatment of hydrocephalus. Bull Johns Hopkins Hosp 1960;106:1–24.

426. Yakatan GJ, Frome EL, Leonard RG, et al. Bioavailability of acetazolamide tablets. J Pharm Sci 1978;67:252–256.

427. Bayne WF, Rogers G, Crisologo N. Assay for acetazolamide in plasma. J Pharm Sci 1975;64:402–404.

428. Friedland BR, Mallonee J, Anderson DR. Short-term dose response characteristics of acetazolamide in man. Arch Ophthalmol 1977;95:1809–1812.

429. Garner LL, Carl EF, Ferwerda JR. Advantages of sustained-release therapy with acetazolamide in glaucoma. Am J Ophthalmol 1963;55:323–327.

430. Berson FG, Epstein DL, Grant WM, et al. Azetazolamide dosage forms in the treatment of glaucoma. Arch Ophthalmol 1980;98: 1051–1054.

431. Linner E, Wistrand P. The initial drop of intraocular pressure following intravenous administration of acetazolamide in man. Acta Ophthalmol 1959;37:209–214.

432. Nissen OI. The immediate response in applanation pressure to

433. Shields BM. A study guide for glaucoma. Baltimore: Williams & Wilkins, 1982;429–430.

434. Alm A, Berggren L, Hartvig P, Roosdorp M. Monitoring acetazolamide treatment. Acta Ophthalmol 1982;60:24–34.

435. Kupfer C, Lawrence C, Linner E. Long-term administration of acetazolamide (Diamox) in the treatment of glaucoma. Am J Ophthalmol 1955;40:673–680.

436. Becker B, Ley AP. Epinephrine and acetazolamide in the therapy of the chronic glaucomas. Am J Ophthalmol 1958;45:639–643.

437. Berson FG, Epstein DL. Separate and combined effects of timolol maleate and acetazolamide in open-angle glaucoma. Am J Ophthalmol 1981;92:788–791.

438. Kass MA, Korey M, Gordon M, Becker B. Timolol and acetazolamide: A study of concurrent administration. Arch Ophthalmol 1982;100:941–942.

439. Cox SN, Hay E, Bird AC. Treatment of chronic macular edema with acetazolamide. Arch Ophthalmol 1988;106:1190–1195.

440. Fishman GA, Gilbert LD, Fiscella RG, et al. Acetazolamide for treatment of chronic macular edema in retinitis pigmentosa. Arch Ophthalmol 1989;107:1445–1452.

441. Chen JC, Kitzke FW, Bird AC. Long-term effect of acetazolamide in a patient with retinitis pigmentosa. Invest Ophthalmol Vis Sci 1990;31:1914–1918.

442. Marmor MF, Negi A. Pharmacologic modification of subretinal fluid absorption in the rabbit eye. Arch Ophthalmol 1986;104: 1674–1677.

443. Grunwald JE, Zinn H. The acute effect of oral acetazolamide on macular blood flow. Invest Ophthalmol Vis Sci 1992;33:504–507.

444. Leopold IH, Carmichael PL. Prolonged administration of Diamox in glaucoma. Trans Am Acad Ophthalmol Otolaryngol 1956;60: 210–214.

445. Becker B. Use of methazolamide (Neptazane) in the therapy of glaucoma: comparison with acetazolamide (Diamox). Am J Ophthalmol 1960;49:1307–1311.

446. Epstein DL, Grant WM. Carbonic anhydrase inhibitor side effects. Serum chemical analysis. Arch Ophthalmol 1977;95:1378–1382.

447. Lichter PR, Newman LP, Wheeler NC, Beall OV. Patient tolerance to carbonic anhydrase inhibitors. Am J Ophthalmol 1978;85:495–502.

448. Becker B, Middleton WH. Long-term acetazolamide (Diamox) administration in the therapy of glaucomas. Arch Ophthalmol 1955;54:187–192.

449. Pesin SR, Brandt JD. Paresthesia and numbness due to drugs: the special case of the blind. JAMA 1991;265:1527–1528.

450. Epstein DL, Grant WM. Management of carbonic anhydrase inhibitor side effects. In: Leopold IH, Burns RP, eds. Symposium on ocular therapy. New York: John Wiley & Sons, 1979;11:51–64.

451. Heller I, Halevy J, Cohen S, et al. Significant metabolic acidosis induced by acetazolamide. Arch Intern Med 1985;145:1815–1817.

452. Alward PD, Wilensky JT. Determination of acetazolamide compliance in patients with glaucoma. Arch Ophthalmol 1981;99: 1973–1976.

453. Maren TH. Chemistry of the renal reabsorption of bicarbonate. Can J Physiol Pharmacol 1974;52:1041–1050.

454. Stitzel RE, Irish JM III. Water, electrolyte metabolism, and diuretic agents. In: Craig CR, Stitzel RE, eds. Modern pharmacology. Boston: Little, Brown, 1982;328–329.

455. Maren TH, Haywood JR, Chapman SK, Zimmerman TJ. The pharmacology of methazolamide in relation to the treatment of glaucoma. Invest Ophthalmol Vis Sci 1977;16:730–742.

456. Parfitt AM. Acetazolamide and sodium bicarbonate-induced nephrocalcinosis and nephrolithiasis. Arch Intern Med 1969;124:736–740.

457. Ahlstrand C, Tiselius HG. Urine composition and stone formation during treatment with acetazolamide. Scand J Urol Nephrol 1987;21:225–228.

458. Spaeth GL. Potassium, acetazolamide, and intraocular pressure. Arch Ophthalmol 1967;78:578–582.

459. Grant WM. Antiglaucoma drugs: problems with carbonic anhydrase inhibitors. In: Leopold IH, ed. Symposium on ocular therapy. St. Louis: C. V. Mosby Co, 1973;6:19–38.

460. Shapiro S, Fraunfelder FT. Acetazolamide and aplastic anemia. Am J Ophthalmol 1992;113:328–330.

461. Fraunfelder FT, Meyer SM, Bagby GC, Dreis MW. Hematologic reactions to carbonic anhydrase inhibitors. Am J Ophthalmol 1985;100:79–81.

462. Zimran A, Beutler E. Can the risk of acetazolamide-induced aplastic anemia be decreased by periodic monitoring of blood cell counts? Am J Ophthalmol 1987;104:654–658.

463. Mogk LG, Cyrlin MN. Blood dyscrasias and carbonic anhydrase inhibitors. Ophthalmology 1988;95:768–771.

464. Granstrom K. Transient myopia following the administration of sulphonamides. Acta Ophthalmol 1949;27:59–68.

465. Mattson R. Transient myopia following the use of sulfonamides. Acta Ophthalmol 1952;30:385–398.

466. Hook SR, Holladay JT, Prager TC, Goosey JD. Transient myopia induced by sulfonamides. Am J Ophthalmol 1986;101:495–496.

467. Back M. Transient myopia after use of acetazolamide (Diamox). Arch Ophthalmol 1956;55:546–547.

468. Halpern AE, Kulvin MM. Transient myopia during treatment with carbonic anhydrase inhibitors. Am J Ophthalmol 1959;48:534–535.

469. Galin MA, Baras I, Zweifach P. Diamox-induced myopia. Am J Ophthalmol 1962;54:237–240.

470. Garland M, Sholk A, Guenter K. Acetazolamide-induced myopia. Am J Obstet Gynecol 1962;84:69–71.

471. Bovino JA, Marcus DF. The mechanism of transient myopia induced by sulfonamide therapy. Am J Ophthalmol 1982;94:99–102.

472. Friedland BR, Maren TH. Carbonic anhydrase: pharmacology of inhibitors and treatment of glaucoma. In: Sears ML, ed. Pharmacology of the Eye. New York: Springer-Verlag, 1984:279–309.

473. Peralta J, Abelairas J, Fernandez-Guardiola J. Anaphylactic shock and death after oral intake of acetazolamide. Am J Ophthalmol 1992;114:367.

474. Warnock DG. Diuretics. In: Katzung BG, ed. Basic and clinical pharmacology. Los Altos: LANGE Medical Publications, 1982:157–158.

475. Block ER, Rostand RA. Carbonic anhydrase inhibition in glaucoma: Hazard or benefit for the chronic lunger? Surv Ophthalmol 1978;23:169–172.

476. Nissen SH. Acetazolamide in the treatment of hemorrhagic glaucoma. Ophthalmologica 1979;179:286–290.

477. Weber PA. Neovascular glaucoma. Current management. Surv Ophthalmol 1981;26:149–153.

478. Havener WH. Ocular pharmacology. St Louis: C. V. Mosby Co, 1978;475–496.

479. Goldberg MF. Sickled erythrocytes, hyphema, and secondary glaucoma: the effect of vitamin C on erythrocyte sickling in aqueous humor. Ophthalmic Surg 1979;10:70–77.

480. Goldberg MF. The diagnosis and treatment of secondary glaucoma after hyphema in sickle cell patients. Am J Ophthalmol 1979;87:43–49.

481. Rubenstein MA, Bucy JG. Acetazolamide-induced renal calculi. J Urol 1975;114:610–612.

482. Siklos P, Henderson RG. Severe acidosis from acetazolamide in a diabetic patient. Curr Med Res Opin 1979;6:284–286.

483. Gabay EL. Metabolic acidosis from acetazolamide therapy. Arch Ophthalmol 1983;101:303–304.

484. Maren TH. Teratology and carbonic anhydrase inhibition. Arch Ophthalmol 1971;85:1–2.

485. Leopold IH, Gordon B. Drug interactions. In: Leopold IH, ed. Symposium on ocular therapy. St Louis: C. V. Mosby, 1973;6:103.

486. Hill JB. Experimental salicylate poisoning: observations on the effects of altering blood pH on tissue and plasma salicylate concentrations. Pediatrics 1971;47:658–665.

487. Anderson CJ, Kaufman PL, Sturm RJ. Toxicity of combined therapy with carbonic anhydrase inhibitors and aspirin. Am J Ophthalmol 1978;86:516–519.

488. Stone RA, Zimmerman TJ, Shin DH, et al. Low-dose methazolamide and intraocular pressure. Am J Ophthalmol 1977;83:674–679.

489. Dahlen K, Epstein DL, Grant WM, et al. A repeated dose-response study of methazolamide in glaucoma. Arch Ophthalmol 1978;96:2214–2218.

490. Vogh BP, Doyle AS. The effect of carbonic anhydrase inhibitors and other drugs on sodium entry to cerebrospinal fluid. J Pharmacol Exp Ther 1981;217:51–56.

491. Zimmerman TJ. Acetazolamide and methazolamide. Ann Ophthalmol 1978;10:509–510.

492. Zimmerman TJ. Basic pharmacology of some glaucoma drugs. Ophthalmic Optician 1981;21:286–289.

493. Ellis PP. Urinary calculi with methazolamide therapy. Doc Ophthalmol 1973;34:137–142.

494. Shields MB, Simmons RJ. Urinary calculus during methazolamide therapy. Am J Ophthalmol 1976;81:622–624.

495. Werblin TP, Pollack IP, Liss RA. Blood dyscrasias in patients using methazolamide (Neptazane) for glaucoma. Ophthalmology 1980;87:350–353.

496. Gandham SB, Spaeth GL, DiLeonardo M, Costa VP. Methazolamide-induced skin eruptions. Arch Ophthalmol 1993;111:370–372.

497. Gonzales-Jimeney E, Leopold IH. Effect of dichlorphenamide on the intraocular pressure of humans. Arch Ophthalmol 1958;60:427–436.

498. Garrison L, Roth A, Rundle H, Christensen RE. A clinical comparison of three carbonic anhydrase inhibitors. Trans Pac Coast Oto-ophthalmol Soc 1967;48:137–143.

499. Heilmann K. Special pharmacology. In: Heilmann K, Richardson KT, eds. Glaucoma. Conceptions of a disease. Pathogenesis, diagnosis, therapy. Philadelphia: W. B. Saunders Co, 1978:284.

500. Beyer KH, Baer JE. Physiological basis of action of newer diuretic agents. Pharmacol Rev 1961;13:517–562.

501. Foss RH. Local application of Diamox: an experimental study of its effect on the intraocular pressure. Am J Ophthalmol 1955;39:336–339.

502. Green H, Leopold IH. Effects of locally administered Diamox. Am J Ophthalmol 1955;40:137–139.

503. Kimura R. Effect of long-term subconjunctival administration of Diamox (acetazolamide) on the ocular tension in rabbit. Arch Klin Exp Ophthalmol 1978;205:221–227.

504. Gloster J, Perkins ES. Effect of carbonic anhydrase inhibitor (Diamox) on intraocular pressure of rabbits and cats. Br J Ophthalmol 1955;39:647–658.

505. Maren TH, Jankowska L, Sanyal G, Edelhauser HF. The transcorneal permeability of sulfonamide carbonic anhydrase inhibitors and their effect on aqueous humor secretion. Exp Eye Res 1983;36:457–480.

506. Maren TH, Bar-Ilan A, Caster KC, et al. Ocular pharmacology of methazolamide analogs: distribution in the eye and effects on pressure after topical application. J Pharm Exp Ther 1987;241:56–63.

507. Friedman Z, Allen RC, Raph SM. Topical acetazolamide and methazolamide delivered by contact lenses. Arch Ophthalmol 1985;103:963–966.

508. Flach AJ, Peterson JS, Seligmann KA. Local ocular hypotensive effect of topically applied acetazolamide. Am J Ophthalmol 1984;98:66–72.

509. Flach AJ. Topical acetazolamide and other carbonic anhydrase inhibitors in the current medical therapy of the glaucomas. Glaucoma 1986;8:20–27.

510. Lotti VJ, Schmitt CJ, Gautheron PD. Topical ocular hypotensive activity and ocular penetration of dichlorphenamide sodium in rabbits. Arch Klin Exp Ophthalmol 1984;222:13–19.

511. Maren TH, Jankowska L, Sanyal G, Edelhauser H. Reduction of aqueous humor secretion by topical carbonic anhydrase inhibitors (abstr.). Invest Ophthalmol Vis Sci 1982;22(suppl):39.

512. Stein A, Pinke R, Krupin T, et al. The effect of topically administered carbonic anhydrase inhibitors on aqueous humor dynamics in rabbits. Am J Ophthalmol 1983;95:222–228.

513. Maren TH, Bar-Ilan A, Conroy CW, et al. Chemical and pharmacological properties of MK-927, a sulfonamide carbonic anhydrase inhibitor that lowers intraocular pressure by the topical route. Exp Eye Res 1990;50:27–36.

514. Bar-Ilan A, Pessah NI, Maren TH. Ocular penetration and hypotensive activity of the topically applied carbonic anhydrase inhibitor L-645, 151. J Ocular Pharmacol 1986;2:109–120.

515. Kalina PH, Shetlar DJ, Lewis RA, et al. 6–Amino-2–benzothiazole-sulfonamide: the effect of a topical carbonic anhydrase inhibitor on aqueous humor formation in the normal human eye. Ophthalmology 1988;95:772–777.

516. Bar-Ilan A, Pessah NI, Maren TH. Ocular hypotensive activity and disposition of the topical carbonic anhydrase inhibitor 6–hydroxy-benzo (b) thiophene-2–sulfonamide, L-650, 719, in the rabbit. J Ocular Pharmacol 1989;5:99–110.

517. Werner EB, Gerber DS, Yoder YJ. Effect of a topical carbonic anhydrase inhibitor, 6–hydroxy-benzo [b] thiophene-2–sulfonamide, on intraocular pressure in normotensive subjects. Can J Ophthalmol 1987;22:316–319.

518. Ponticello GS, Freedman MB, Habecker CN, et al. Thienothiopyran-2–sulfonamides: a novel class of water-soluble carbonic anhydrase inhibitors. J Med Chem 1987;30:591–597.

519. Lippa EA, von Denffer HA, Hofman HM, et al. Local tolerance and activity of MK-927, a novel topical carbonic anhydrase inhibitor. Arch Ophthalmol 1988;106:1694–1696.

520. Lippa EA, Schuman JS, Higginbotham EJ, et al. MK-507 versus sezolamide. Comparative efficacy of two topically active carbonic anhydrase inhibitors. Ophthalmology 1991;98:308–313.

521. Podos SM, Serle JB. Topically active carbonic anhydrase inhibitors for glaucoma. Arch Ophthalmol 1991;109:38–40.

522. Lippa EA, Carlson LE, Ehinger B, et al. Dose response and duration of action of dorzolamide, a topical carbonic anhydrase inhibitor. Arch Ophthalmol 1992;110:495–499.

523. Michelson SR, Schwam H, Baldwin JJ, et al. Topically instilled MK-927: lack of correlation between corneal penetration rate constant and ocular hypotensive activity in rabbits. Invest Ophthalmol Vis Sci 1989;30(suppl):24.

524. Baldwin JJ, Ponticello GS, Murcko M, et al. Three-dimensional structure of the carbonic anhydrase inhibitor complex derived from human carbonic anhydrase II and the optical isomers of MK-927. Invest Ophthalmol Vis Sci 1989;30(supp):374.

525. Maren TH. Carbonic anhydrase: general perspectives and advances in glaucoma research. Drug Development Research 1987;10:255–276.

526. Maren TH, Bar-Ilan A. Ocular pharmacology and hypotensive activity of a topically active carbonic anhydrase (CA) inhibitor, a 4–alkylamino-thienothiopyran-2–sulfonamide, MK-927. Invest Ophthalmol Vis Sci 1988;29(suppl):16.

527. Sugrue MF, Mallorga P, Schwam H, et al. A comparison of L-671,152 and MK-927, two topically effective ocular hypotensive carbonic anhydrase inhibitors, in experimental animals. Curr Eye Res 1990;9:607–615.

528. Baldwin J, Ponticello G, Anderson P, et al. Thienothiopyran-2–sulfonamides: novel topically active carbonic anhydrase inhibitors for the treatment of glaucoma. J Med Chem 1989;32:2510–2513.

529. Bron A, Lippa EA, Gunning F, et al. Multiple-dose efficacy comparison of two topical carbonic anhydrase inhibitors MK-417 and MK-927. Arch Ophthalmol 1991;109:50–53.

530. Buclin T, Biollaz J, Lippa EA, et al. Absence of metabolic effects of the topical carbonic anhydrase inhibitors MK-927 and sezolamide during two-week ocular administration to normal subjects. Clin Pharmacol Ther 1991;49:665–673.

531. Sugrue MF, Gautheron P, Grove J, et al. MK-927: a topically active ocular hypotensive carbonic anhydrase inhibitor. J Ocular Pharmacol 1990;6:9–22.

532. Bron AM, Lippa EA, Hofmann HM, et al. MK-927: a topically effective carbonic anhydrase inhibitor in patients. Arch Ophthalmol 1989;107:1143–1146.

533. Pfeiffer N, Hennekes R, Lippa EA, et al. A single dose of the topical carbonic anhydrase inhibitor MK-927 decreases IOP in patients. Br J Ophthalmol 1990;74:405–408.

534. Serle JB, Lustgarten JS, Lippa EA, et al. MK-927, a topical carbonic anhydrase inhibitor: dose response and reproducibility. Arch Ophthalmol 1990;108:838–841.

535. Higginbotham EJ, Kass MA, Lippa EA, et al. MK-927: a topical carbonic anhydrase inhibitor, dose response and duration of action. Arch Ophthalmol 1990;108:65–68.

536. Lippa EA, Aasved H, Airaksinen PJ, et al. Multiple-dose, dose-response relationship of the topical carbonic anhydrase inhibitor MK-927. Arch Ophthalmol 1991;109:46–49.

537. Wang RF, Serle JB, Podos SM, et al. The ocular hypotensive effect of the topical carbonic anhydrase inhibitor L-671,152 in glaucomatous monkeys. Arch Ophthalmol 1990;108:511–513.

538. Diestelhorst M, Bechetoille A, Lippa EA, et al. Comparative

potencies of the topical carbonic anhydrase inhibitors MK-417 and MK-927. Invest Ophthalmol Vis Sci 1989;30(suppl):23.

539. Kass MA, Laibovitz RA, Lippa EA, et al. Comparative activity of 3% MK-507, a topical CAI with betaxolol. Invest Ophthalmol Vis Sci 1991;32(suppl):989.

540. Wilkerson M, Cyrlin M, Lippa EA, et al. Four-week safety and efficacy study of dorzolamide, a novel, active topical carbonic anhydrase inhibitor. Arch Ophthalmol 1993;111:1343–1350.

541. Maren TH. A comparison between topical and oral sulfonamides in treatment of elevated ocular pressure in man. Invest Ophthalmol Vis Sci 1992;33(suppl):1246.

542. Nardin G, Lewis R, Lippa EA, et al. Activity of the topical CAI MK-507 bid when added to timolol bid. Invest Ophthalmol Vis Sci 1991;32(suppl):989.

543. Sugrue MF, Mallorga P, Schwan H, et al. L-693,612, a topical ocular hypotensive carbonic anhydrase inhibitor with a prolonged duration of action in glaucomatous monkeys. Invest Ophthalmol Vis Sci 1992;33(suppl):1246.

544. Dean T, May J, McLaughlin M, et al. AL-4333A: a new carbonic anhydrase inhibitor which is topically active in the rabbit and monkey. Invest Ophthalmol Vis Sci 1991;33(suppl):1246.

545. Eller MG, Schoenwald RD. Determination of ethoxzolamide in the iris/ciliary body of the rabbit eye by high-performance liquid chromatography. Comparison of tissue levels following intravenous and topical administrations. J Pharm Sci 1984;73:1261–1264.

546. Putnam ML, Schoenwald RD, Duffel MW, et al. Ocular disposition of aminozolamide in the rabbit eye. Invest Ophthalmol Vis Sci 1987;28:1373–1382.

547. Grove J, Gautheron P, Plazonnet B, et al. Ocular distribution studies of the topical carbonic anhydrase inhibitors L-643, 799 and L-650, 719 and related alkyl prodrugs. J Ocular Pharmacol 1988;4:279–290.

548. Bar-Ilan A, Pessah NI, Maren TH. The effects of carbonic anhydrase inhibitors on aqueous humor chemistry and dynamics. Invest Ophthalmol Vis Sci 1984;25:1198–1205.

549. Brechue WF, Maren TH. Correlation of drug accession with IOP reduction following local and intravenous carbonic anhydrase inhibitors. Invest Ophthalmol Vis Sci 1991;32(suppl):1256.

550. Gervasoni JP, Lippa EA, Biollaz J, et al. Absence of metabolic effects of methyl-thienothiopyran-2-sulfonamide, a new carbonic anhydrase inhibitor (CAI) during a 2–week ocular administration. Clin Pharmacol Ther 1991;49:192.

551. Pfeiffer N, Gerling J, Lippa EA, et al. Comparative tolerability of topical carbonic anhydrase inhibitor MK-927 and its S-enantiomer MK-417. Arch Klin Exp Ophthalmol 1991;229:111–114.

552. Feicht B, Hofmann HM, Lippa EA, et al. A new topical carbonic anhydrase inhibitor (MK-927). Tolerance comparison with betaxolol in healthy probands. Klin Monatsbl Augenheilkd 1990;197:254–257.

553. Doughty MJ. Prognosis for long-term topical carbonic anhydrase inhibitors and glaucoma management. Topics in Ocular Pharmacology and Toxicology 1985;11:1.

554. Cyrlin M, Wilkerson M, Lippa EA, et al. Four week safety study of the topical CAI MK-507. Invest Ophthalmol Vis Sci 1991;32(suppl):989.

555. Wistrand PJ, Schenholm M, Lonnerholm G. Carbonic anhydrase isoenzymes CA I and CA II in the human eye. Invest Ophthalmol Vis Sci 1986;27:419–428.

556. Serle JB, Lustgarten J, Lippa EA, et al. Six week safety study of 2% MK-927 administered twice daily to ocular hypertensive volunteers. J Ocular Pharmacol 1992;8:1–9.

557. Lichter PR, Musch DC, Medzihrndsky F, et al. Intraocular pressure effects of carbonic anhydrase inhibitors in primary open-angle glaucoma. Am J Ophthalmol 1989;107:11–17.

558. Becker B, Kolker AE, Krupin T. Hyperosmotic agents. In: Leopold IH, ed. Symposium on ocular therapy. St. Louis: CV Mosby Co, 1968;3:42–53.

559. Hoskins HD, Kass MA. Hyperosmotic agents. In: Becker-Schaffer's Diagnosis and therapy of the glaucomas. St. Louis, CV Mosby 1989;Chap. 27.

560. Galin MA, Brinkhorst RD, Kwitko ML. Ocular dehydration. Am J Ophthalmol 1968;66:233–235.

561. Kolker AE. Hyperosmotic agents in glaucoma. Invest Ophthalmol 1970;9:418–423.

562. Galin MA, Aizawa F, McLean JM. A comparison of intraocular pressure reduction following urea and sucrose administration. Arch Ophthalmol 1960;63:281–286.

563. Galin MA, Davidson R. Hypotensive effect of urea in inflamed and noninflamed eye. Arch Ophthalmol 1962;68:633–635.

564. Krupin T, Podos SM, Becker B. Alteration of intraocular pressure after third ventricle injection of osmotic agents. Am J Ophthalmol 1973;76:948–952.

565. Galin MA, Davidson R, Schachter N. Ophthalmological use of osmotic therapy. Am J Ophthalmol 1966;62:629–634.

566. Spaeth GI, Spaeth EB, Spaeth PG, Lucier AC. Anaphylactic reaction to mannitol. Arch Ophthalmol 1967;78:583–584.

567. Becker B. Use of hyperosmotic agents in the treatment of the glaucomas. Trans New Orleans Acad Ophthalmol 1967;170–174.

568. Smith EW, Drance SM. Reduction of human intraocular pressure with intravenous mannitol. Arch Ophthalmol 1962;68:734–737.

569. Weaver A, Sica A. Mannitol-induced acute renal failure. Nephron 1987;45:233–235.

570. Ophthalmic Drug Facts. St. Louis: Facts and Comparisons, 1995: chap. 10.

571. Javid M. Urea—new use of an old agent; reduction of intracranial and intraocular pressure. Surg Clin North Am 1958;38:907–928.

572. Robbins R, Galin MA. Effect of osmotic agents on the vitreous body. Arch Ophthalmol 1969;82:694–699.

573. Tarter RC, Linn JG. A clinical study of the use of intravenous urea in glaucoma. Am J Ophthalmol 1961;52:323–331.

574. Virno M, Cantore P, Bietti C, Bucci MG. Oral glycerol in ophthalmology: a valuable new method for the reduction of intraocular pressure. Am J Ophthalmol 1963;55:1133–1142.

575. Drance SM. Effect of oral glycerol on intraocular pressure in normal and glaucomatous eyes. Arch Ophthalmol 1964;72:491–493.

576. Thomas RP. Glycerin: An orally effective osmotic agent. Arch Ophthalmol 1963;70:625–628.

577. McCurdy DK, Schneider B, Scheie H. Oral glycerol: The mechanism of intraocular hypotension. Am J Ophthalmol 1966;61:1244–1249.

578. D'Alena P, Ferguson W. Adverse effects after glycerol orally and mannitol parenterally. Arch Ophthalmol 1966;75:201–203.

579. Becker B, Kolker AE, Krupin T. Isosorbide: An oral hyperosmotic agent. Arch Ophthalmol 1967;78:147–150.

580. Wisznia KI, Lazar M, Leopold IH. Oral isosorbide and intraocular pressure. Am J Ophthalmol 1970;70:630–634.

581. Quigley HA. A reevaluation of glaucoma management. Int Ophthalmol Clin 1984;24:1–11.

582. Sharir M, Zimmerman TJ. Initial treatment of glaucoma: surgery or medications. II. Medical therapy. Surv Ophthalmol 1993;37:299–304.

583. Watson PG, Grierson I. The place of trabeculectomy in the treatment of glaucoma. Ophthalmology 1981;88:175–96.

584. Jay JL, Murray SB. Early trabeculectomy versus conventional management in primary open-angle glaucoma. Br J Ophthalmol 1988;72:881–9.

585. Spaeth GL, Baez KA. Argon laser trabeculoplasty controls one third of cases of progressive, uncontrolled, open angle glaucoma for 5 years. Arch Ophthalmol 1992;110:491–4.

586. Cairns JE. Trabeculectomy: preliminary report of a new method. Am J Ophthalmol 1968;66:673–9.

587. Franks WA, Hitchings RA. Complications of 5–fluorouracil after trabeculectomy. Eye 1991;5:385–9.

588. Skuta GL, Parrish, RK II. Wound healing in glaucoma filtering surgery. Surv Ophthalmol 1987;32:149–70.

589. Tahery MM, Lee DA. Review: pharmacologic control of wound healing in glaucoma filtration surgery. J Ocular Pharmacol 1989;5:155–79.

590. Joseph JP, Miller MH, Hitchings RA. Wound healing as a barrier to successful filtration surgery. Eye 1988;2(suppl.):113–23.

591. Miller MH, Grierson I, Unger WI, Hitchings RA. Wound healing in an animal model for glaucoma fistulizing surgery in the rabbit. Ophthalmic Surg 1989;20:350–7.

592. Reddick R, Merritt JC, Ross G, Avery A, Pfeiffer RL. My-ofibroblasts in filtration operations. Ann Ophthalmol 1985;17:200–3.

593. Desjardins DC, Parrish RK II, Folberg R, Nevarez J, Heuer DK, Gressel MG. Wound healing after filtration surgery in owl monkeys. Arch Ophthalmol 1986;104:1835–9.

594. Jampel HD, McGuigan LJ, Dunkelberger GR, Hernault NL, Quigley HA. Cellular proliferation after experimental glaucoma filtration surgery. Arch Ophthalmol 1988;106:89–94.

595. Joseph JP, Grierson I, Hitchings RA. Chemotactic activity of aqueous humor. A cause of failure of trabeculectomies? Arch Ophthalmol 1989;107:69–74.

596. Joseph JP, Grierson I, Hitchings RA. Partial characterization of the fibroblast chemotactic constituents of human aqueous humor. Int Ophthalmol 1989;13:125–30.

597. Joseph JP, Grierson I, Hitchings RA. Normal rabbit aqueous humor, fibronectin, and fibroblast conditioned medium are chemoattractant to Tenon's capsule fibroblasts. Eye 1987;1:585–92.

598. Herschler J, Claflin AJ, Fiorentino G. The effect of aqueous humor on the growth of subconjunctival fibroblasts in tissue culture and its implications for glaucoma surgery. Am J Ophthalmol 1980;89:245–9.

599. Radius RL, Herschler J, Claflin A, Fiorentino G. Aqueous humor changes after experimental filtering surgery. Am J Ophthalmol 1980;89:250–4.

600. Jampel HD. Ascorbic acid is cytotoxic to dividing human Tenon's capsule fibroblasts. A possible contributing factor in glaucoma filtration surgery success. Arch Ophthalmol 1990;108:1323–5.

601. Hajek AS, Parrish RK II, Mallick KS, Gressel M. *In vitro* inhibition of ocular cell proliferation with ara-C: blockage of the antiproliferative effect with 2'-deoxycytidine. Invest Ophthalmol Vis Sci 1986;27:1010–2.

602. Lee DA, Lee TC, Cortes AE, Kitada S. Effects of mithramycin, mitomycin, daunorubicin, and bleomycin on human subconjunc-tival fibroblast attachment and proliferation. Invest Ophthalmol Vis Sci 1990;31:2136–44.

603. Lee DA, Shapourifar-Tehrani S, Stephenson TR, Kitada S. The effects of the fluorinated pyrimidines FUR, FUdR, FUMP, and FdUMP on human Tenon's fibroblasts. Invest Ophthalmol Vis Sci 1991;32:2599–609.

604. Moorhead LC, Smith J, Stewart R, Kimbrough R. Effects of β-aminopropionitrile after glaucoma filtration surgery: pilot human trial. Ann Ophthalmol 1987;19:223–5.

605. Del-Vecchio PJ, Bizios R, Holleran LA, Judge TK, Pinto GL. Inhibition of human scleral fibroblast proliferation with heparin. Invest Ophthalmol Vis Sci 1988;29:1272–6.

606. Joseph JP, Grierson I, Hitchings RA. Taxol, cytochalasin B and colchicine effects on fibroblast migration and contraction: a role in glaucoma filtration surgery? Curr Eye Res 1989;8:203–15.

607. Joseph JP, Grierson I, Hitchings RA. The effect of retinoids on the migration of Tenon's capsule fibroblasts. Eye 1988;2:529–32.

608. Kim RY, Stern WH. Retinoids and butyrate modulate fibroblast growth and contraction of collagen matrices. Invest Ophthalmol Vis Sci 1990;31:1183–6.

609. Fourman S, Vaid K. Effects of tissue plasminogen activator on glaucoma filter blebs in rabbits. Ophthalmic Surg 1989;20:663–7.

610. Strauss GH, Dunn ET, Dunn RC, Bodiford GB, Christie J. Sub-conjunctival high dose plasminogen activator in rabbit filtration surgery. J Ocular Pharmacol 1991;7:9–19.

611. Latina MA, Belmonte SJ, Pak C, Crean E. Gamma-interferon effects on human fibroblasts from Tenon's capsule. Invest Ophthalmol Vis Sci 1991;32:2806–15.

612. Khaw PT, Ward S, Grierson I, Rice NS. Effects of β radiation on proliferating human Tenon's capsule fibroblasts. Br J Ophthalmol 1991;75:580–3.

613. Goldenfeld M, Krupin T, Ruderman JM, et al. 5-Fluorouracil in initial trabeculectomy. A prospective, randomized, multicenter study. Ophthalmology 1994;101:1024–1029.

614. Wong PC, Ruderman JM, Krupin T, et al. 5-Fluorouracil after primary combined filtration surgery. Am J Ophthalmol 1994;117:149–154.

615. O'Grady JM, Juzych MS, Shin DH, et al. Trabeculectomy, phacoemulsification, and posterior chamber lens implantation with and without 5-fluorouracil. Am J Ophthalmol 1993;116:594–599.

616. Smith MF, Sherwood MB, Doyle JW, et al. Results of intraoperative 5-fluorouracil supplementation on trabeculectomy for open-angle glaucoma. Am J Ophthalmol 1992;114:737–741.

617. The Fluorouracil Filtering Surgery Study Group. Three-year follow-up of the fluorouracil filtering surgery study. Am J Ophthalmol 1993;115:82–92.

618. Hefetz L, Keren T, Naveh N. Early and late postoperative application of 5-fluorouracil following trabeculectomy in refractory glaucoma. Ophthalmic Surg 1994;25:715–719.

619. Lee DA, Flores RA, Anderson PJ, Leong KW, Teekhasaenee C, de-Kater AW, Hertzmark E. Glaucoma filtration surgery in rabbits using bioerodible polymers and 5-fluorouracil. Ophthalmology 1987;94:1523–30.

620. Lee DA, Leong KW, Panek WC, Eng CT, Glasgow BJ. The use of bioerodible polymers and 5-fluorouracil in glaucoma filtration surgery. Invest Ophthalmol Vis Sci 1988;29:1692–7.

621. Jampel HD, Leong KW, Dunkelburger GR, Quigley HA. Glaucoma filtration surgery in monkeys using 5-fluorouridine in poly-anhydride disks. Arch Ophthalmol 1990;108:430–5.

622. Hasty B, Heuer DK, Minckler DS. Primate trabeculectomies with 5-fluorouracil collagen implants. Am J Ophthalmol 1990;109: 721–25.

623. Heuer DK, Parrish RK II, Gressel MG, et al. 5-Fluorouracil and glaucoma filtration surgery: III. Intermediate follow-up of a pilot study. Ophthalmology 1986;93:1537–46.

624. Knapp A, Heuer DK, Stern GA, Driebe WT Jr. Serious corneal complications of glaucoma filtering surgery with postoperative 5-fluorouracil. Am J Ophthalmol 1987;103:183–7.

625. Lee DA, Hersh P, Kersten D, Melamed S. Complications of subconjunctival 5-fluorouracil following glaucoma filtering surgery. Ophthalmic Surg 1987;18:187–90.

626. Wolmer B, Liebman JM, Sassani JW, Ritch R, Speaker M, Marmor M. Late bleb-related endophthalmitis after trabeculectomy with adjunctive 5-fluorouracil. Ophthalmology 1991;98: 1053–60.

627. Chen CW. Enhanced intraocular pressure controlling effectiveness of trabeculectomy by local application of mitomycin-C. Trans Asia-Pacific Acad Ophthalmol 1983;9:172–7.

628. Hayasaka S, Noda S, Yamamoto Y, Setogawa T. Postoperative instillation of low-dose mitomycin C in the treatment of primary pterygium. Am J Ophthalmol 1988;106:715–8.

629. Palmer SS. Mitomycin as adjunct chemotherapy with trabeculectomy. Ophthalmology 1991;98:317–21.

630. Lamping KA, Belkin JK. 5-Fluorouracil and mitomycin C in pseudophakic patients. Ophthalmology 1995;102:70–75.

631. Kupin TH, Juzych MS, Shin DH, et al. Adjunctive mitomycin C in primary trabeculectomy in phakic eyes. Am J Ophthalmol 1995; 119:30–39.

632. Yamamoto T, Varani J, Soong KH, Lichter PR. Effects of 5-fluorouracil and mitomycin C on cultured rabbit subconjunctival fibroblasts. Ophthalmology 1990;97:1204–10.

633. Bergstrom TJ, Wilkinson WS, Skuta GL, Watnick RL, Elner VM. The effects of subconjunctival mitomycin-C on glaucoma filtration surgery in rabbits. Arch Ophthalmol 1991;109:1725–30.

634. Kitazawa Y, Kawase K, Matsushita H, Minobe M. Trabeculectomy with mitomycin. A comparative study with fluorouracil. Arch Ophthalmol 1991;109:1693–8.

635. Skuta GL, Beeson CC, Higginbotham EJ, et al. Intraoperative mitomycin versus postoperative 5-fluorouracil in high-risk glaucoma filtering surgery. Ophthalmology 1992;99:438–44.

636. Peyman GA, Greenberg D, Fishman GA, Fiscella R, Thomas A. Evaluation of toxicity of intravitreal antineoplastic drugs. Ophthalmic Surg 1984;15:411–3.

637. Derick RJ, Pasquale L, Quigley HA, Jampel H. Potential toxicity of mitomycin C. Arch Ophthalmol 1991;109:1635.

638. Rubinfeld RS, Pfister RR, Stein RM, et al. Serious complications of topical mitomycin-C after pterygium surgery. Ophthalmology 1992;99:1647–54.

639. Geijssen HC, Greve EL. Mitomycin, suturelysis and hypotony. Int Ophthalmol 1992;16:371–4.

640. Nuyts RM, Pels E, Greve EL. The effects of 5-fluorouracil and mitomycin C on the corneal endothelium. Curr Eye Res 1992;11: 565–70.

641. Bito LZ. Species differences in the responses of the eye to irritation and trauma: a hypothesis of divergence in ocular defense mechanisms, and the choice of experimental animal for eye research. Exp Eye Res 1984;39:807–29.

642. Eakins KE. Prostaglandin and non-prostaglandin mediated break- down of the blood-aqueous barrier. Exp Eye Res 1977;25(suppl): 483–98.

643. Stjernschantz J, Nilsson SF, Astin M. Vasodynamic and angiotensic effects of eicosanoids in the eye. Prog Clin Biol Res 1989;312: 155–70.

644. Samuelson B. An elucidation of the arachidonic acid cascade discovery by prostaglandins, thromboxane, and leukotrienes. Drugs 1987;33(suppl):2–9.

645. Hammarstrom S. Leukotrienes. Ann Rev Biochem 1983;52:355–77.

646. Bito LZ. Prostaglandins and other eicosanoids: their ocular transport, pharmacokinetics, and therapeutic effects. Trans Ophthalmol Soc UK 1986;105:162–70.

647. Bhattacherjee P, Kulkarni PS, Eakins KE. Metabolism of arachidonic acid in rabbit ocular tissues. Invest Ophthalmol Vis Sci 1979;18:172–8.

648. Kulkarni P. Synthesis of cyclooxygenase products by human anterior uvea from cyclic prostaglandin endoperoxide (PGH_2). Exp Eye Res 1981;32:197–204.

649. Kulkarni PS, Fleischer L, Srinivasan BD. The synthesis of cyclooxygenase products in the ocular tissues of various species. Curr Eye Res 1984;3:447–52.

650. Kulkarni PS, Rodriguez AV, Srinivasan BD. Human anterior uvea synthesizes lipoxygenase products from arachidonic acid. Invest Ophthalmol Vis Sci 1984;25:221–3.

651. Polansky JR, Kurtz RM, Alvarado JA, Weinreb RN, Mitchell MD. Eicosanoid production and glucocorticoid regulatory mechanisms in cultured human trabecular meshwork cells. Prog Clin Biol Res 1989;312:113–38.

652. Camras CB, Podos SM. The role of endogenous prostaglandins in clinically-used and investigational glaucoma therapy. Prog Clin Biol Res 1989;312:459–75.

653. Camras CB, Bito LZ, Eakins KE. Reduction of intraocular pressure by prostaglandins applied topically to the eyes of conscious rabbits. Invest Ophthalmol Vis Sci 1977;16:1125–34.

654. Stern FA, Bito LZ. Comparison of the hypotensive and other ocular effects of prostaglandins E_2 and $F_{2\alpha}$ on cat and rhesus monkey eyes. Invest Ophthalmol Vis Sci 1982;22:588–98.

655. Camras CB, Bito LZ. Reduction of intraocular pressure in normal and glaucomatous primate (Aotus trivirgatus) eyes by topically applied prostaglandin $F_{2\alpha}$. Curr Eye Res 1981;1:205–9.

656. Crawford K, Kaufman PL, Gabelt BT. Effect of topical $PGF_{2\alpha}$ on aqueous humor dynamics in cynomologus monkeys. Curr Eye Res 1987;6:1035–44.

657. Beitch BR, Eakins KE. The effects of prostaglandins on the intraocular pressure of the rabbit. Br J Pharmacol 1969;37:158–67.

658. Bito LZ, Draga A, Blanco J, Camras CB. Long-term maintenance of reduced intraocular pressure by daily or twice daily topical application of prostaglandins to cat or rhesus monkey eyes. Invest Ophthalmol Vis Sci 1983;24:312–19.

659. Lee PY, Podos SM, Howard-Williams JR, Severin CH, Rose AD, Siegel MJ. Pharmacological testing in the laser-induced monkey glaucoma model. Curr Eye Res 1985;4:775–81.

660. Lee PY, Podos SM, Serle JB, Camras CB, Severin CH. Intraocular pressure effects of multiple doses of drugs applied to glaucomatous monkey eyes. Arch Ophthalmol 1987;105:249–52.

661. Camras CB, Bhuyan KC, Podos SM, Bhuyan DK, Master RW. Multiple dosing of prostaglandin $F_{2\alpha}$ or epinephrine on cynomolgus monkey eyes. II. Slit-lamp biomicroscopy, aqueous humor

analysis, and fluorescein angiography. Invest Ophthalmol Vis Sci 1987;28:921–6.

662. Camras CB, Friedman AH, Rodriguez MM, Tripathi BJ, Tripathi RC, Podos SM. Multiple dosing of prostaglandin $F_{2\alpha}$ or epinephrine on cynomolgus monkey eyes. III. Histopathology. Invest Ophthalmol Vis Sci 1988;29:1428–36.

663. Bito LZ. Comparison of the ocular hypotensive efficacy of eicosanoids and related compounds. Exp Eye Res 1984;38:181–94.

664. Bito LZ, Baroody RA. The ocular pharmacokinetics of eicosanoids and their derivatives. 1. Comparison of the ocular eicosanoid penetration and distribution following the topical application of $PGF_{2\alpha}$, $PGF_{2\alpha}$-1-methyl ester, and $PGF_{2\alpha}$-1–isopropyl ester. Exp Eye Res 1987;44:217–26.

665. Giuffre G. The effects of prostaglandin $F_{2\alpha}$ in the human eye. Graefe's Arch Clin Exp Ophthalmol 1985;222:139–41.

666. Kerstetter JR, Brubaker RF, Wilson SE, Kullersrand LJ. Prostaglandin $F_{2\alpha}$-1-isopropyl ester lowers intraocular pressure without decreasing aqueous humor flow. Am J Ophthalmol 1988;105:30–4.

667. Villumsen J, Alm A. Ocular effects of two different prostaglandin $F_{2\alpha}$ esters: A double masked cross-over study on normotensive eyes. Acta Ophthalmol 1990;68:341–3.

668. Alm A, Villumsen J. PhXA34, a new potent ocular hypotensive drug. A study on dose-response relationship and on aqueous humor dynamics in healthy volunteers. Arch Ophthalmol 1991; 109:1564–8.

669. Lee PY, Podos SM, Severin C. Effect of prostaglandin $F_{2\alpha}$ on aqueous humor dynamics of rabbit, cat and monkey. Invest Ophthalmol Vis Sci 1984;25:1087–93.

670. Kaufman PL. Effects of intracamerally infused prostaglandins on the outflow facility in cynomolgus monkey eyes with intact or retrodisplaced ciliary muscle. Exp Eye Res 1986;43:819–27.

671. Hayashi M, Yablonski ME, Bito LZ. Eicosanoids as a new class of ocular hypotensive agents. 2. Comparison of the apparent mechanism of the ocular hypotensive effects of A and F type prostaglandins. Invest Ophthalmol Vis Sci 1987;28:1639–43.

672. Bito LZ. Prostaglandins. Old concepts and new perspectives. Arch Ophthalmol 1987;105:1036–9.

673. Flach AJ, Eliason JA. Topical prostaglandin E_2 effects on normal human intraocular pressure. J Ocular Pharmacol 1988;4:13–8.

674. Goh Y, Nakajima M, Azuma I, Hayaishi O. Prostaglandin D_2 reduces intraocular pressure. Br J Ophthalmol 1988;72:461–4.

675. Hyong PF, Groeneboer MC. The effects of prostacyclin and its stable analog on intraocular pressure. Prog Clin Biol Res 1989; 312:369–78.

676. Bito LZ, Baroody RA, Miranda OC. Eicosanoids as a new class of ocular hypotensive agents. 1. The apparent therapeutic advantages of derived prostaglandins of the A and B type as compared with primary prostaglandins of the E, F and D type. Exp Eye Res 1987; 44:825–37.

677. Camras CB, Schumer RA, Marsk A, et al. Intraocular pressure reduction with PhXA34, a new prostaglandin analogue, in patients with ocular hypertension. Arch Ophthalmol 1992;110:1733–1738.

678. Ziai N, Dolan JW, Kacere RD, Brubaker RF. The effects on aqueous dynamics of PhXA41, a new prostaglandin $F_{2\alpha}$ analogue, after topical application in normal and ocular hypertensive human eyes. Arch Ophthalmol 1993;111:1351–1358.

679. Fristrom B, Nilsson SEG. Interaction of PhXA41, a new prostaglandin analogue, with pilocarpine. A study on patients with elevated intraocular pressure. Arch Ophthalmol 1993;111:662–665.

680. Racz P, Ruzsonyi MR, Nagy ZT, et al. Maintained intraocular pressure reduction with once-a-day application of a new prostaglandin $F_{2\alpha}$ analogue (PhXA41). An in-hospital, placebo-controlled study. Arch Ophthalmol 1993;111:657–661.

681. Toris CB, Camras CB, Yablonski ME. Effects of PhXA41, a new prostaglandin $F_{2\alpha}$ analog, on aqueous humor dynamics in human eyes. Ophthalmology 1993;100:1297–1304.

682. Nagasubramanian S, Sheth GP, Hitchings RA, et al. Intraocular pressure-reducing effect of PhXA41 in ocular hypertension. Ophthalmology 1993;100:1305–1311.

683. Alm A, Villumsen J, Tornquist P, et al. Intraocular pressure-reducing effect of PhXA41 in patients with increased eye pressure. A one-month study. Ophthalmology 1993;100:1312–1317.

684. Harrison R, Kaufman CS. Clonidine: effects of a topically administered solution on intraocular pressure and blood pressure in open-angle glaucoma. Arch Ophthalmol 1977;95:1368–1373.

685. Hadapp E, Kolker AE, Kass MA, et al. The effect of topical clonidine on intraocular pressure. Arch Ophthalmol 1981;99: 1208–1211.

686. Williamson J, Young JD, Atta H, et al. Comparative efficacy of orally and topically administered β blockers for chronic simple glaucoma. Br J Ophthalmol 1985;69:41–45.

687. Weinreb RN, Sandman R, Ryder MI, et al. Angiotensin-converting enzyme activity in human aqueous humor. Arch Ophthalmol 1985;103:34–36.

688. Constad WH, Fiore P, Samson C, et al. Use of an angiotensin converting enzyme inhibitor in ocular hypertension and primary open-angle glaucoma. Am J Ophthalmol 1988;105:674–677.

689. Murad F. Drugs used for the treatment of angina: organic nitrates, calcium-channel blockers and β-adrenergic antagonists. In: Gilman AG, Rall TW, Nies AS, Taylor P, eds. Goodman and Gilman's The pharmacological basis of therapeutics. New York: Pergamon Press, 1990:774–780.

690. Abelson MB, Gilbert CM, Smith LM. Sustained reduction of intraocular pressure in humans with the calcium channel blocker verapamil. Am J Ophthalmol 1988;105:155–159.

691. Vojnikoavic B. Doxium (calcium dobesilate) reduces blood hyperviscosity and lowers elevated intraocular pressure in patients with diabetic retinopathy and glaucoma. Ophthalmic Res 1991; 23:12–20.

692. Kaufman PL. Pharmacologic trabeculocanalotomy. Arch Ophthalmol 1992;110:34–36.

693. Koechel D, Cafruny E. Synthesis and structure-activity relationship of some thiol adducts of ethacrynic acid. J Med Chem 1973; 16:1147–1152.

694. Epstein DL, Freddo TF, Bassett-Chu S, et al. Influence of ethacrynic acid on outflow facility in the monkey and calf eye. Invest Ophthalmol Vis Sci 1987;28:2067–2075.

695. Tingey DP, Ozment RR, Schroeder A, et al. The effect of intracameral ethacrynic acid on the intraocular pressure of living monkeys. Am J Ophthalmol 1992;113:706–711.

696. Tingey DP, Schroeder A, Epstein MPM, et al. Effects of topical ethacrynic acid adducts on intraocular pressure in rabbits and monkeys. Arch Ophthalmol 1992;110:699–702.

697. Koechel D, Cafruny E. Thiol adducts of ethacrynic acid: a correlation of the rate of liberation of ethacrynic with the onset and magnitude of the diuretic. J Pharmacol Exp Ther 1975;192:179–194.

698. Liang L, Epstein DL, de Kater AW, et al. Ethacrynic acid increases facility of outflow in the human eye *in vitro*. Arch Ophthalmol 1992;110:106–109.

699. Melamed S, Kotas-Neumann R, Barak A, et al. The effect of intracamerally injected ethacrynic acid on intraocular pressure in patients with glaucoma. Am J Ophthalmol 1992;113:508–512.

700. Michelson G, Groh MJM. Dipivefrin reduces blood flow in the ciliary body in humans. Ophthalmology 1994;101:659–664.

701. Cardakli UF, Smythe BA, Eisele JR, et al. Effect of chronic apraclonidine treatment on intraocular pressure in advanced glaucoma. J Glaucoma 1993;2:271.

702. Nordlund JR, Pasquale LR, Robin AL, et al. The cardiovascular, pulmonary, and ocular hypotensive effects of 0.2% brimonidine. Arch Ophthalmol 1995;113:77–83.

703. Egbert PR, Williams AS, Singh K, et al. A prospective trial of intraoperative fluorouracil during trabeculectomy in a black population. Am J Ophthalmol 1993;116:612–616.

704. Bansal RK, Gupta A. 5–Fluorouracil in trabeculectomy for patients under the age of 40 years. Ophthalmic Surg 1992;23:278–280.

705. Jampel HD. Effect of brief exposure to mitomycin C on viability and proliferation of cultured human Tenon's capsule fibroblasts. Ophthalmology 1992;99:1471–1476.

706. Munden PM, Alward WLM. Combined phacoemulsification, posterior chamber intraocular lens implantation, and trabeculectomy with mitomycin C. Am J Ophthalmol 1995;119:20–29.

707. Joos KM, Bueche MJ, Palmberg PF, et al. One-year follow-up results of combined mitomycin C trabeculectomy and extracapsular cataract extraction. Ophthalmology 1995;102:76–83.

708. Shields MB, Scroggs MW, Sloop CM, et al. Clinical and histopathologic observations concerning hypotony after trabeculectomy with adjunctive mitomycin C. Am J Ophthalmol 1993;116:673–683.

709. Nuyts RMMA, Felten PC, Pels E, et al. Histopathologic effects of mitomycin C after trabeculectomy in human glaucomatous eyes with persistent hypotony. Am J Ophthalmol 1994;118:225–237.

710. Megerand GS, Salmon JF, Scholtz RP, et al. The effect of reducing the exposure time of mitomycin C in glaucoma filtering surgery. Ophthalmology 1995;102:84–90.

711. Bito LZ, Racz P, Ruzsony MR, et al. The prostaglandin analogue, PhXA41, significantly reduces daytime and nighttime intraocular pressure (IOP) by itself, and in timolol-treated eyes. Invest Ophthalmol Vis Sci 1994;35(suppl):2178.

712. Camras CB. USA Latanoprost Study Group. Latanoprost, a new prostaglandin analogue, compared to timolol for the treatment of glaucoma (abstract). Annual Meeting of the Association for Ocular Pharmacology and Therapeutics. New Orleans, LA; January 26–29, 1995.

CHAPTER 11

Anti-Infective Drugs

Diane P. Yolton

Humans are constantly exposed to a variety of microorganisms, including bacteria, viruses, and fungi. In most cases, these microorganisms do not produce infection because the skin and mucous membrane surfaces provide effective barriers against invasion. A few microorganisms, however, can invade directly through these barriers, and others can cause infection if introduced into the body through lesions from surgery or trauma. If microorganisms penetrate the body's outer barriers, the immune system usually deals with them quite effectively. However, some microorganisms possess special properties that allow them to overcome this system. In addition, patients' immune systems do not always function optimally, allowing microorganisms that would normally not pose a problem to cause an infectious disease. When the immune system is depressed, the term *immunocompromised* is used. Two of the many situations that can cause the immune system to become compromised involve the use of drugs that depress the immune response, such as corticosteroids, and infection with human immunodeficiency virus (HIV), which causes acquired immunodeficiency syndrome (AIDS).

Over the years, many different compounds have been used to assist the body's immune system in killing microorganisms. An especially important property that an anti-infective drug must possess is selective toxicity. The drug must be more toxic for the microorganism than for the host. An ideal anti-infective drug kills the microorganisms while causing minimal or no adverse reaction in the host.

Each of the major categories of microorganisms that cause disease (bacteria, viruses, and fungi) has a unique physical structure and metabolism. The differences among them are so broad that drugs that are toxic for organisms in one category will usually not be active against members of the other two categories. Thus, anti-infective drugs are classified into antibacterial, antiviral, or antifungal groups.

Although an anti-infective drug is assigned to one group on the basis of its selective toxicity, it is usually not toxic for all species within that group. The species against which a drug shows intrinsic activity is referred to as the drug's *spectrum of activity*. A narrow-spectrum anti-infective drug is active against only a few species, while a broad-spectrum drug is active against a wide variety of microorganisms. Knowledge of a drug's spectrum of activity is useful in determining clinical applications for the drug.

As the anti-infective drugs are used to treat diseases, microorganisms evolve various strategies to resist them. Resistance occurs when a microorganism that was originally in an anti-infective drug's spectrum of activity is no longer sensitive to that drug. As microorganisms become drug-resistant, new drugs that have the resistant organism in their spectrum of activity must be isolated from other microorganisms or developed in the laboratory.

This chapter describes the mechanisms of action, spectra of activity, resistances, and potential adverse reactions for each of the major antibacterial, antiviral, and antifungal drugs. Antiprotozoal drugs of interest in ocular pharmacotherapy are also discussed. This basic knowledge provides a foundation for the appropriate clinical application of the antimicrobial drugs in the treatment of infectious ocular disease.

Guidelines for Effective Antimicrobial Therapy

The clinical process of selecting an anti-infective drug for the treatment of disease can be complex, and many factors must

TABLE 11.1
Guidelines for Effective Antimicrobial Therapy

Establish accurate clinical and laboratory diagnosis
Select anti-infective drug to which the microorganism is sensitive
Select least toxic anti-infective drug
Establish adequate drug levels at site of infection
    Select optimum route(s) of administration
    Use appropriate dosage regimen
    Prescribe drug for appropriate length of time
Augment drug therapy with physical procedures

be considered (Table 11.1). First, the patient's history, symptoms, and signs must be evaluated to establish a tentative diagnosis, and then a best "guess" regarding the causative microorganism(s) must be made. Based on the "guess," an anti-infective agent (or combination of agents) can be selected and therapy planned. Appropriate patient care often requires that samples of tissue or body fluids be obtained for laboratory culture and identification so that the clinician's "guess" can be confirmed and susceptibility of the isolated microorganisms(s) to the anti-infective drugs can be assessed. Since laboratory identification and susceptibility testing require several days, the clinician often must initiate anti-infective therapy before this process is complete.

After the clinician has selected a drug for use, he or she must determine which route(s) of administration will best ensure a therapeutic concentration at the site of infection. For different types of ocular infections, topical application, subconjunctival injection, oral administration, intravitreal injection, or a combination of routes may be appropriate (Table 11.2). Topical instillation of anti-infective drugs is usually the preferred mode for local therapy of ocular infections. Solution formulations are usually chosen over ointments for adults, particularly during the waking hours, since ointments tend to blur vision following application. Ointments, on the other hand, are often preferred in the therapy of infants and young children because of the prolonged contact time between the drug and eye and the resistance to tear washout.

When planning antibiotic therapy, the clinician should estimate the length of time that the drug should be administered, since an appropriate period will eradicate the microorganisms while minimizing adverse events; excessive use of topically applied anti-infective drugs can cause hypersensitivity or toxicity reactions. In addition, using an antibacterial drug longer than necessary to eradicate the microorganism or using it inappropriately facilitates the development of resistant strains of bacteria. The risk of superinfection, which is an overgrowth of microorganisms that are usually held in check by the normal flora, also exists with the use of any antibacterial drug, especially with excessive use of multiple antibacterial drugs.

A final factor to consider in developing a treatment plan is

to determine which physical procedures might augment the drug therapy. Such procedures can be especially useful when appreciable quantities of purulent exudate or necrotic tissue are present and must be removed from the site of infection. As examples, the application of hot compresses to improve circulation and to remove crusting deposits on the lashes is especially useful in the treatment of lid infections with staphylococci; local massage, such as meibomian gland expression, facilitates the drainage of inflammatory products and allows better penetration of antibacterial drugs; and mechanical debridement of infected corneal epithelial cells in cases of herpetic keratitis removes much of the virus and may allow better penetration of the antiviral drug.

When a patient with an ocular disease fails to respond to anti-infective therapy even though an appropriate treatment plan was developed and followed, a variety of explanations is possible. Table 11.3 outlines these explanations.

Antibacterial Drugs

Bacteria are a diverse group of single-celled microorganisms that, in most cases, can produce their own energy and cellular components. The largest division of bacteria can be subdivided by shape and gram stain reaction. Of the many species of bacteria, only a few are pathogenic in humans. Table 11.4 shows the most common pathogenic bacteria and the infections they cause. In addition, several groups of bacteria that have a unique structural morphology or metabolism also include pathogens that can cause ocular disease. The *Rickettsia* and *Chlamydia* mimic viruses in that they are intracellular parasites that must grow and multiply inside other living cells. The *Rickettsia* occur as harmless parasites in insects such as lice, ticks, and mites but, when transmitted to humans through bites, they cause diseases such as typhus and Q fever.

The *Chlamydia* are transmitted through direct contact with an infected person; *Chlamydia trachomatis* can cause sexually-transmitted disease, inclusion conjunctivitis, and trachoma. The spirochetes, which have a special morphology consisting of flexible spirals, include *Treponema pallidum*, which can cause syphilis with possible ocular complications.

The mycobacteria are characterized by large quantities of lipid in their cell walls, which makes them acid-fast. A member of this group, *Mycobacterium tuberculosis*, can cause tuberculosis with the ocular complications of granulomatous uveitis, phlyctenular keratoconjunctivitis, optic neuritis, and Eales disease. The *Actinomyces* are bacteria characterized by filamentous branching, which closely resembles the hyphae produced by fungi. This group includes *Actinomyces israelii*, which can cause chronic conjunctivitis and canaliculitis, and *Nocardia asteroides*, which can cause chronic corneal ulcers and endophthalmitis.

TABLE 11.2
Antibacterial Drugs of Choice for Initial Treatment of Ocular Infections

Ocular Infection	Antibacterial Drugs	Route of Administration
Blepharitis		
Acute/Chronic staphylococcal	Bacitracin, erythromycin, or gentamicin	Topical
Angular	Bacitracin, erythromycin, gentamicin, or zinc sulfate	Topical
Seborrheic	Bacitracin or erythromycin	Topical (prophylactic)
Acne Rosacea	Tetracycline[a] or doxycycline	Oral
Conjunctivitis		
Acute mucopurulent	Gentamicin, tobramycin, trimethoprim/polymyxin B, ciprofloxacin, norfloxacin, or ofloxacin	Topical
Hyperacute purulent	Bacitracin or gentamicin and	Topical
	Ceftriaxone	Parenteral
Chlamydial	Doxycycline, tetracycline, or erythromycin	Oral
Hordeolum		
External	Bacitracin, gentamicin, or erythromycin	Topical (prophylactic)
Internal	Cloxacillin or dicloxacillin	Oral
Dacryocystitis		
Acute	Cephalexin or oxacillin[b,c] or	Oral
	Cefazolin or oxacillin and	Parenteral
	Erythromycin or gentamicin[c]	Topical (prophylactic)
Neonatal	Gentamicin or erythromycin[b]	Topical (prophylactic)
Preseptal Cellulitis	Cloxacillin, dicloxacillin, erythromycin, or amoxicillin-clavulanate[d] or	Oral
	Cefuroxime, cefonicid, ceftriaxone, cefotaxime, or ceftizoxime	Parenteral
Keratitis	Cefazolin and gentamicin or tobramycin[c] or ciprofloxacin[f]	Topical[e]
		Topical
Endophthalmitis	Vancomycin and gentamicin, tobramycin[g] or ceftazidime and	Topical
	Cefazolin or vancomycin and gentamicin or ceftazidime and	Subconjunctival
	Vancomycin and ceftazidime and	Intravenous
	Vancomycin and amikacin[h]	Intravitreal

[a]Brown SI, Shahinian L. Diagnosis and treatment of ocular rosacea. Ophthalmology 1978;85:779–786.
[b]Tanenbaun M, McCord CD. The lacrimal drainage system. In: Tasman W, Jaeger EA, eds. Duane's clinical ophthalmology. Philadelphia: Lippincott, 1994;4(13):22.
[c]Baum JL. Antibiotic use in ophthalmology. In: Tasman W, Jaeger EA, eds. Duane's clinical ophthalmology. Philadelphia: Lippincott, 1994;4(26):6.
[d]Jones DB, Steinkuller PG. Microbial preseptal and orbital cellulitis. In: Tasman W, Jaeger EA, eds. Duane's clinical ophthalmology. Philadelphia: Lippincott, 1994;4(25):21–22.
[e]Leibowitz HM, Ryan WJ, Kupferman A. Route of antibiotic administration in bacterial keratitis. Arch Ophthalmol 1981;99:1420–1423.
[f]Leibowitz HM. Clinical evaluation of ciprofloxacin 0.3% ophthalmic solution for treatment of bacterial keratitis. Am J Ophthalmol 1991;112:34S–47S.
[g]Forster RK. Endophthalmitis. In: Tasman W, Jaeger EA, eds. Duane's clinical ophthalmology. Philadelphia: Lippincott, 1994;4(24):17.
[h]Doft BH, Barza M. Ceftazidime or amikacin: Choice of intravitreal antimicrobials in the treatment of postoperative endophthalmitis. Arch Ophthalmol 1994;112:17–18.

Bacteria can become resistant to the antibacterial drugs used to treat infections.[1] This resistance can result from chromosomal mutation or can be transmitted by extrachromosomal plasmids. Spontaneous chromosomal mutations occur naturally in the bacterial population, and the presence of an antibacterial agent allows drug-resistant mutants to multiply. Extrachromosomal plasmids carry mutated genes that produce resistance, and these plasmids can easily be transferred from one bacterium to another. Drug resistance produced by chromosomal mutations or extrachromosomal plasmids may take many forms. Perhaps the most common form involves the bacterial production of enzymes that can inactivate the antibacterial drug itself.

Because of bacterial drug resistance, information about a pathogen's pattern of resistance/susceptibility is essential to the choice of a successful antibacterial agent. For purposes of *in vitro* testing, an organism is generally considered susceptible if the concentration of antimicrobial agent necessary to inhibit its growth is lower than that attainable in body fluids, particularly blood. Two types of laboratory tests are available to determine resistance/susceptibility to antibacterial drugs.[2] In diffusion testing, filter-paper discs con-

TABLE 11.3
Reasons for Antimicrobial Failure

Inaccurate diagnosis
Resistant microorganism
Inadequate drug dosage (size, frequency, or duration)
Patient noncompliance
Inadequate supplemental physical procedures
Inadequate patient immune system response

taining fixed amounts of the antibacterial drugs are applied to the surface of an agar plate that has been previously streaked with the test organism. The antibacterial drug diffuses into the medium and either inhibits the growth of or kills the organism. When done as a standardized test, the size of the inhibition zone can then be translated into one of three categories: susceptible, resistant, or intermediate susceptibility. In the second type of susceptibility testing, the dilution test, serial dilutions of the antibacterial drug are inoculated with the test organism to determine the minimal inhibitory concentration (MIC), which is the lowest concentration without apparent growth. The MIC is directly compared with the concentration of the antibacterial drug attainable in the blood to determine resistance or susceptibility. Since the results of these *in vitro* tests correlate closely with *in vivo* results, they are useful in determining the most appropriate antibacterial drug for a systemic infection.

Comparison of the MIC to the attainable blood level to determine the susceptibility breakpoint may be only marginally useful when managing external ocular infections because of the much higher drug levels that can be achieved by local drug delivery. Ormerod and associates[3] found that 10 patients with resistant (as defined using conventional criteria) pseudomonal infections of the cornea responded to fortified gentamicin. Thus, susceptibility breakpoints based on achievable drug concentrations in the ocular tissues should be established to provide a more logical basis for antibiotic choice.

Several differences exist between bacterial and human cells, and these differences form the basis for selective toxicity of the antibacterial drugs (Fig. 11.1). First, bacteria have a unique outermost layer, a cell wall, that is not found in any human cell. The bacterial cell wall is necessary for the bacterium's structural integrity; without it, the bacterium usually undergoes lysis and dies. Several antibacterial drugs act by inhibiting synthesis of the cell wall, thus causing death of the bacteria* (Table 11.5).

A second structure in which bacterial and human cells

---

*Drugs that kill bacteria are termed *bactericidal. Bacteriostatic* implies that growth of the bacteria is inhibited.

may differ is their cell membranes. However, because the membranes of both cell types are so similar, only a few compounds have been found that can selectively disrupt bacterial cell membranes while leaving those of the host cell intact (see Table 11.5).

A third difference between bacterial and human cells involves their ribosomes. Bacterial ribosomes are not the same size, nor do they have the same composition, as human ribosomes. Thus, drugs that bind more to bacterial than to mammalian ribosomes can inhibit bacterial protein synthesis and have a selective toxicity for these cells (see Table 11.5).

A fourth difference between bacterial and human cells involves specific biosynthetic pathways (intermediary metabolism). Bacterial cells usually synthesize their own folic acid, while humans receive folic acid preformed in their food. Thus, drugs that can inhibit folic acid synthesis are selectively toxic for bacteria (see Table 11.5).

A fifth difference between bacterial and human cells involves the enzyme DNA gyrase. DNA gyrase prevents the supercoiling of DNA during replication and transcription. Drugs that inhibit bacterial gyrase and not the corresponding human enzyme have a selective toxicity for bacteria (see Table 11.5).

Drugs Affecting Cell Wall Synthesis

Antibacterial drugs that affect cell wall synthesis include two large families, the penicillins and cephalosporins, and two individual drugs, bacitracin and vancomycin.

Penicillins

PHARMACOLOGY

All penicillins contain a common nucleus composed of a thiazolidine ring and a β-lactam ring connected to a side chain. An intact β-lactam ring is necessary for biologic activity, but the side chain primarily determines the antibacterial spectrum, susceptibility to gastric acid and β-lactamases, and pharmacokinetic properties.

The penicillins act by inhibiting synthesis of the bacterial cell wall (Fig. 11.2). The rigid structure of the cell wall is due to peptidoglycan, which is a mucopeptide made up of linear, cross-linked polysaccharide chains. Bacterial cell wall synthesis is a complex process involving at least 30 enzymes.[4] Penicillins inhibit the terminal step in this process, which is the cross-linking of the polysaccharide chains through peptide bond formation (see Fig. 11.2). The cell walls thus develop abnormally, ultimately resulting in death of the organism. Penicillins exert their bactericidal effect

TABLE 11.4
The Most Common Pathogenic Bacteria and the Infections They Cause

Bacteria	Systemic Infection	Ocular Infection
Gram-positive cocci		
Staphylococcus aureus	Skin abscesses, impetigo, wound infections, pneumonia and other systemic infections; enterotoxin-producing strains cause food poisoning; toxic-shock syndrome	Acute and chronic blepharitis, angular blepharoconjunctivitis, acute and chronic mucopurulent conjunctivitis, dacryocystitis, hordeola, central and marginal corneal ulcers, preseptal and orbital cellulitis, endophthalmitis
Staphylococcus epidermidis	Wound and systemic infections	Acute and chronic blepharitis, acute and chronic conjunctivitis, dacryocystitis, central corneal ulcers, endophthalmitis
Streptococcus pyogenes	Pharyngitis, impetigo, erysipelas, scarlet fever, puerperal fever, glomerulonephritis, rheumatic fever, cellulitis, wound and burn infections	Pseudomembranous and membranous conjunctivitis, dacryocystitis, central corneal ulcers, preseptal and orbital cellulitis, endophthalmitis
Streptococcus pneumoniae	Pneumonia, meningitis, otitis media, sinusitis, upper respiratory infections	Acute mucopurulent conjunctivitis, central corneal ulcers, chronic dacryocystitis, preseptal and orbital cellulitis, endophthalmitis
Streptococcus faecalis (enterococcus)	Endocarditis, urinary tract infections	Acute conjunctivitis, central corneal ulcers
Viridans group of streptococci	Endocarditis, dental caries	Acute mucopurulent, pseudomembranous, and membranous conjunctivitis, central corneal ulcers
Gram-positive rods		
Corynebacterium diphtheria	Diphtheria	Pseudomembranous, membranous conjunctivitis
Corynebacterium species		Acute conjunctivitis, corneal ulcers
Gram-negative cocci		
Neisseria gonorrhoeae	Gonorrhea	Hyperacute, purulent conjunctivitis
Neisseria meningitidis	Meningitis	Hyperacute, purulent conjunctivitis
Gram-negative rods		
Moraxella lacunata		Angular blepharoconjunctivitis, central and peripheral corneal ulcers
Haemophilus influenzae	Upper respiratory tract infections, otitis media, sinusitis, pneumonia, meningitis	Acute mucopurulent conjunctivitis, dacryocystitis, preseptal and orbital cellulitis, endophthalmitis
Pseudomonas aeruginosa	Burn, wound, and systemic infections	Central corneal ulcers, endophthalmitis
Escherichia species Enterobacter species Salmonella species Proteus species Klebsiella species Serratia marcescens Acinetobacter species	Gastrointestinal, urinary tract, wound, and respiratory tract infections	Acute or chronic conjunctivitis, central corneal ulcers, endophthalmitis

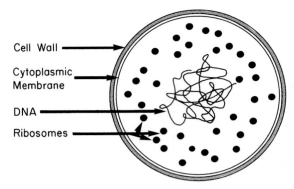

FIGURE 11.1 **Simplified diagram of a sphere-shaped bacterium showing its cell wall, cytoplasmic membrane, ribosomes, and nuclear material. Bacteria do not have a nuclear membrane surrounding the DNA.**

most strongly on actively dividing cells that are synthesizing new cell walls.

The basic penicillin nucleus has been and continues to be chemically modified, and new penicillins with unique advantages frequently become available. Based on their spectra of antibacterial activity and their clinical applications, the penicillins can be divided into four categories (Table 11.6).

CLINICAL USES

Penicillins Effective Against Gram-Positive Bacteria.

The two most important drugs in this category are penicillins G and V. The G form of the drug was originally derived from the fungus *Penicillium notatum*, while the V form is a semisynthetic derivative of penicillin G. Although penicillin G may be administered orally, its instability in gastric acid limits its absorption. Therefore, when therapy indicates an

TABLE 11.5
Classification of Antibacterial Drugs

Drugs affecting cell wall synthesis
  Penicillins
  Cephalosporins
  Bacitracin
  Vancomycin

Drugs affecting the cytoplasmic membrane
  Polymyxin B
  Colistin
  Gramicidin

Drugs affecting protein synthesis
  Aminoglycosides
    Streptomycin
    Neomycin
    Gentamicin
    Tobramycin
    Amikacin
    Kanamycin
  Tetracyclines
  Macrolides
    Erythromycin
    Clarithromycin
    Azithromycin
  Chloramphenicol
  Clindamycin

Drugs affecting intermediary metabolism
  Sulfonamides
  Pyrimethamine
  Trimethoprim

Drugs affecting bacterial DNA synthesis
  Nalidixic acid
  Fluoroquinolones
    Ciprofloxacin
    Norfloxacin
    Ofloxacin

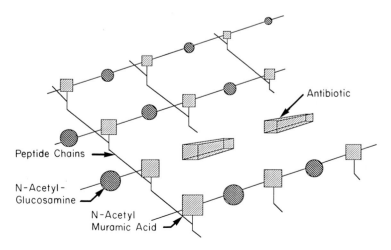

FIGURE 11.2 **Structure of the peptidoglycan of the bacterial cell wall showing the mechanism of action of penicillins and cephalosporins.**

TABLE 11.6
Commonly Used Penicillins

Drug/Additive	Trade Name	Route of Administration	Clinically Useful Spectra of Activity
Penicillins effective against gram-positive bacteria			
Penicillin G	Generic Bicillin Crysticillin Pentids Permapen Pfizerpen Wycillin	IV, IM	Streptococci, gram-positive rods, anaerobes except *Bacteroides fragilis,* spirochetes including *Treponema* and *Borrelia, Neisseria meningitidis*
Penicillin V	Penicillin VK Beepen VK Betapen-VK Ledercillin VK Pen-V Pen Vee K Robicillin VK V-Cillin K Veetids	PO	
Penicillins resistant to penicillinase			
Methicillin	Staphcillin	IV, IM	*Staphylococcus aureus, Staphylococcus epidermidis*
Oxacillin	Generic Bactocill Prostaphlin	PO, IV, IM	
Cloxacillin	Generic Cloxapen Tegopen	PO	
Dicloxacillin	Generic Dycill Dynapen Pathocil	PO	
Nafcillin	Generic Nafcil Nallpen Unipen	PO, IV, IM	
Penicillins with extended spectra of activity			
Ampicillin	Generic D-Amp Omnipen Omnipen-N Polycillin Polycillin-N Principen Totacillin Totacillin-N	PO, IV, IM	Streptococci including the viridans group, certain gram-negative rods such as *Haemophilus influenzae, Escherichia coli, Proteus mirabilis, Salmonella, Shigella*
Ampicillin and Sulbactam	Unasyn	IV, IM	
Bacampicillin (Ampicillin)	Spectrobid	PO	

(continued)

TABLE 11.6
Commonly Used Penicillins (*continued*)

Drug/Additive	Trade Name	Route of Administration	Clinically Useful Spectra of Activity
Amoxicillin	Generic Amoxil Biomox Polymox Trimox Wymox	PO	
Amoxicillin and Clavulanate	Augmentin	PO	
Penicillins with antipseudomonal activity			
Carbenicillin Indanyl	Geocillin	PO	*Pseudomonas aeruginosa, Enterobacter, Proteus*
Ticarcillin	Ticar	IV, IM	
Ticarcillin and Clavulanate	Timentin	IV	
Piperacillin	Pipracil	IV, IM	*Pseudomonas aeruginosa, Enterobacter,* many *Klebsiella,* *Escherichia coli, Serratia, Proteus, Citrobacter*
Mezlocillin	Mezlin	IV, IM	

IV, intravenous; IM, intramuscular; PO, oral.

orally effective penicillin in this category, penicillin V is used, which is not activated by gastric acid. Both penicillins G and V are highly active against gram-positive cocci and are the antibiotics of choice for systemic infections caused by *Streptococcus pneumoniae, Streptococcus pyogenes,* and other streptococci except enterococci. Since *Treponema pallidum* is sensitive to penicillin G, this antibiotic is the drug of choice for treatment of syphilis. Penicillin G is ineffective against gram-negative rod-shaped organisms such as *Pseudomonas* because it cannot penetrate their cell walls.[5]

The most important mechanism of acquired resistance to the penicillins is bacterial production of drug-inactivating enzymes such as β-lactamases or penicillinases. Since most strains of *Staphylococcus aureus* produce penicillinase, penicillins G and V are not effective against this gram-positive bacterium. Gram-negative *Neisseria gonorrhoeae* is within the spectrum of activity of penicillin G, but recent data[6] indicate a nationwide distribution of penicillinase-producing strains of this organism. Since therapy is typically administered before antibacterial susceptibilities are known, the recommended treatment for gonococcal infections is the cephalosporin, ceftriaxone, which gonococcal penicillinase cannot inactivate.[7]

Topical use of the penicillins for the treatment of minor ocular infections such as blepharitis and conjunctivitis is limited by the high incidence of allergic reactions to the drug.[8] Because of this, other ocular antibacterial drugs are used as agents of choice in the local treatment of minor, surface ocular infections. However, for the treatment of more serious ocular infections such as corneal ulcers caused by penicillin-sensitive staphylococci and micrococci, streptococci (including the pneumococcus), *Corynebacterium, Neisseria gonorrhoeae, Neisseria meningitidis,* and anaerobic gram-negative rods, penicillin G is still administered in the form of fortified (concentrated) eyedrops, subconjunctival injection, and if warranted, intravenous injection.[9] Although most strains of *Streptococcus pneumoniae* are sensitive to penicillin G, resistant strains are becoming increasingly prevalent; one such strain has been isolated from a bacterial keratitis.[10]

Penicillins Resistant to Penicillinase. Modification of the penicillin structure has produced a group of drugs including methicillin, oxacillin, cloxacillin, dicloxacillin, and nafcillin, which staphylococcal penicillinase cannot hydrolyze. Their appropriate use is in the treatment of infections caused by strains of *Staphylococcus aureus* and *S. epidermidis* that produce penicillinase. These include the majority of strains isolated from hospital settings and the general community.[11] The initial therapy for infections in which *S. aureus* or *S. epidermidis* is a suspected cause must therefore include a penicillinase-resistant penicillin or a cephalosporin. Since preseptal cellulitis and internal hordeolum are commonly caused by *S. aureus* or *S. epidermidis*, oral cloxacillin or dicloxacillin are often used as initial therapy (see Table 11.2).

The widespread prevalence of methicillin-resistant strains of *S. aureus* and, to a greater extent, *S. epidermidis,* is becoming a problem, especially in nosocomial infections. As commonly used, the term "methicillin-resistant" denotes resistance of these bacteria to all of the penicillinase-resistant penicillins. Such strains are usually cross-resistant to the cephalosporins, aminoglycosides, and erythromycin and, therefore, vancomycin is the drug of choice against these organisms.

Penicillins with Extended Spectra of Activity. Further modification of the basic penicillin structure has produced drugs including ampicillin and amoxicillin with broader spectra of activity than the original penicillins. Ampicillin and amoxicillin are less effective against bacteria that are sensitive to penicillin G, but their range of antimicrobial activity includes gram-negative bacteria such as *Haemophilus influenzae*, *Escherichia coli*, and *Proteus mirabilis*. Both drugs are destroyed by penicillinase.

The addition of a β-lactamase inhibitor to the penicillin preparation can protect a penicillin from inactivation by penicillase or β-lactamase. Potassium clavulanate (clavulanic acid) and sulbactam are potent inhibitors of bacterial β-lactamases. Both these compounds have a structure similar to the penicillins and cephalosporins but have only weak antibacterial properties. Potassium clavulanate and sulbactam are used in fixed-ratio combinations with penicillins that, when administered alone, are susceptible to β-lactamase inactivation. Amoxicillin/clavulanate, ampicillin/sulbactam, and ticarcillin/clavulanate are commercially available (see Table 11.6). Amoxicillin/clavulanate is a reasonable alternative for preseptal cellulitis, orbital cellulitis associated with paranasal sinusitis, and dacryocystitis, all of which can be caused by β-lactamase-producing gram-positive cocci or *H. influenzae*.

Penicillins with Antipseudomonal Activity. The chief advantage of the antipseudomonal penicillins—carbenicillin, mezlocillin, piperacillin, and ticarcillin—is that they act against *Pseudomonas aeruginosa* and certain *Proteus, Enterobacter*, and *Acinetobacter* species not susceptible to most other penicillins. Patients with septicemia, burn infections, pneumonia, severe urinary tract disease, and meningitis caused by these organisms have often dramatically improved with use of carbenicillin, piperacillin, or ticarcillin. Clinicians also use these three drugs to treat patients with serious ocular infections caused by gram-negative bacteria, especially *Pseudomonas aeruginosa*. Carbenicillin or ticarcillin may be used along with an aminoglycoside for the topical and subconjunctival treatment of bacterial corneal

ulcers caused by gram-negative rods including *Pseudomonas aeruginosa*.[12]

SIDE EFFECTS

The major adverse reactions to the penicillins are hypersensitivity responses. The overall chance of developing such a reaction per course of therapy is approximately 2%.[13] Manifestations of hypersensitivity include urticaria, angioedema and anaphylaxis (type I reaction), hemolytic anemia (type II reaction), interstitial nephritis, vasculitis and serum sickness (type III reaction), and contact dermatitis or Stevens-Johnson syndrome (type IV reaction). Once a patient has had a hypersensitivity response to one penicillin, it is probable, but not certain, that a reaction will occur with repeated exposure to the same penicillin or to any other penicillin.[11] Intradermal skin tests can predict whether a patient is at risk for developing a hypersensitivity reaction to the penicillins.[11] If the results are positive, the penicillins should generally be avoided.

The penicillins, per se, are essentially nontoxic to humans. Most nonhypersensitivity reactions are caused by irritant effects produced by excessive concentration in a small area of the body or by responses to another ingredient in the drug mixture. Most common among the irritative responses are pain and sterile inflammatory reactions at the site of intramuscular injection, with the severity of these reactions typically related to drug concentration. The most serious consequences of penicillin's irritant properties involve the nervous system. Accidental injection into a peripheral nerve can cause pain and dysfunction of the body part innervated by the affected nerve. High concentrations of penicillin in the central nervous system (CNS) can cause arachnoiditis, seizures, or fatal encephalopathy.[11]

Administration of large doses of any penicillin in the form of a potassium salt may cause hyperkalemia, and large doses of other penicillins (most often carbenicillin and ticarcillin) can result in hypokalemia. Injection of penicillin G prepared with procaine may result in an immediate reaction characterized by dizziness, tinnitus, headache, hallucinations, and sometimes seizures due to the rapid liberation of toxic concentrations of procaine. Hematologic toxicity produced by penicillins is rare, but granulocytopenia has been reported.[14] Large doses of carbenicillin and ticarcillin can prevent normal platelet aggregation, but significant bleeding disorders are relatively uncommon. Some individuals who receive penicillin intravenously develop phlebitis or thrombophlebitis.[11]

Penicillins alter the normal bacterial flora in areas of the body such as the respiratory and intestinal tracts. Many patients who take penicillin preparations by mouth experience nausea, vomiting, or diarrhea. This is usually of little clinical significance, since the normal microflora reestablish themselves quickly after cessation of therapy. However, serious superinfection with resistant organisms such as

Pseudomonas, *Proteus*, or *Candida* may follow long-term therapy with any penicillin. Superinfection with *Clostridium difficile* can lead to pseudomembranous colitis.[15]

CONTRAINDICATIONS

The penicillins are contraindicated in patients who are allergic to any penicillin. Since the penicillins, cephalosporins, and carbapenems have a common chemical structure, cross-allergies occur with these drugs. Thus, before initiating therapy with a penicillin, careful inquiry should be made concerning previous hypersensitivity reactions to any cephalosporin or carbapenem.

Cephalosporins

PHARMACOLOGY

Like the penicillins, cephalosporins contain the β-lactam ring that is necessary for antimicrobial activity. However, whereas the penicillins are derivatives of 6-aminopenicillanic acid, the parent nucleus of the cephalosporins is 7-aminocephalosporanic acid.

Penicillins and cephalosporins have similar mechanisms of action. They both interfere with the terminal step in bacterial cell wall formation by preventing proper cross-linking of the peptidoglycan (see Fig. 11.2). The cephalosporins also bind to enzymes associated with the cell membrane, triggering a complex series of reactions that may alter bacterial permeability, inhibit protein synthesis, and cause the bacteria to release autolysins. Some cephalosporins cause the bacteria to lyse, and others cause the bacteria to grow into long filamentous forms by preventing cellular division.

The important mechanisms of acquired resistance to cephalosporins include drug inactivation by β-lactamases, to which the cephalosporins have variable susceptibility. For example, the β-lactamases produced by *S. aureus* are considered true penicillinases and do not affect the cephalosporins.[16] Thus, the cephalosporins are usually active against penicillinase-producing *S. aureus*. In contrast, gram-negative bacteria produce β-lactamases that inactivate many of the cephalosporins.

Adding different side chains has extensively modified the parent cephalosporin compound and created a whole family of cephalosporin antibiotics. For the sake of convenience, these drugs are considered as first-, second-, or third-generation compounds based on their spectra of bacterial activity and their clinical uses (Table 11.7). Progression from first to third generation generally produces a declining gram-positive spectrum, a broadening gram-negative spectrum, greater resistance to β-lactamase, and increasing cost.

CLINICAL USES

First-Generation Cephalosporins. First-generation cephalosporins include cephalothin, cefazolin, cephapirin, cephradine, cephalexin, and cefadroxil. All act effectively against gram-positive bacteria but have relatively modest activity against gram-negative bacteria. These drugs are, in addition, sensitive to many of the β-lactamases produced by gram-negative bacteria; this sensitivity partially accounts for their somewhat limited range of clinical application.

Cephalosporins are frequently used clinically for surgical prophylaxis. Several first-generation cephalosporins have been successfully employed as prophylactic agents in certain cardiovascular, orthopedic, head and neck, gastroduodenal, biliary tract, and gynecologic procedures.

Cefazolin has become a drug of first choice for treating bacterial corneal ulcers, either as part of a broad-spectrum approach[12,17] or as a more specific treatment when gram-positive cocci are known to be present.[17] Cefazolin is a drug of choice for several reasons.[18] First, its spectrum of activity encompasses penicillin-resistant staphylococci, *Proteus mirabilis*, streptococci including S. pneumoniae, and *E. coli*.[19] Second, it possesses greater activity against staphylococci and streptococci than do other drugs such as bacitracin. Third, cefazolin is more soluble than other cephalosporins, which is important in making the specially prepared fortified solutions necessary for topical treatment of bacterial corneal ulcers. Finally, cefazolin may be used, with caution, in selected patients who are allergic to penicillin. Cefazolin is administered both topically as specially prepared eyedrops or by subconjunctival injection.

When administered orally, these agents can be useful for the therapy of internal hordeolum and preseptal cellulitis.[20,21] The recommended therapeutic regimen for the initial treatment of endophthalmitis also includes cefazolin along with an aminoglycoside[22] (see Table 11.2).

Second-Generation Cephalosporins. The second-generation cephalosporins include cefamandole, cefaclor, ceforanide, cefuroxime, cefonicid, cefmetazole, cefprozil, cefoxitin, and cefotetan. These drugs are generally more active against gram-negative enteric bacteria than are first-generation analogs but are much less active against these organisms than are third-generation agents. Cefaclor, a commonly prescribed second-generation cephalosporin, is used to treat bacterial infections of the middle ear, lung, and urinary tract. It can also be used to treat internal hordeolum and preseptal cellulitis.[20,21]

Third-Generation Cephalosporins. Third-generation cephalosporins include cefotaxime, cefixime, ceftizoxime, ceftriaxone, cefoperazone, and ceftazidime. These drugs are much more active against gram-negative organisms than are first- or second-generation drugs but are less active against gram-positive bacteria. The primary advantage of ceftazidime when compared to the other currently available third-generation cephalosporins is its excellent activity against gram-negative bacteria including *Pseudomonas aeruginosa*.[19] Because of this, ceftazidime is used topically, subconjunctivally,

TABLE 11.7
Commonly Used Cephalosporins

Drug	Trade Name	Route of Administration	Clinically Useful Spectra of Activity
First Generation			
Cephalothin	Keflin	IV	Gram-positive cocci except enterococci,
Cefazolin	Ancef	IV, IM	*Escherichia coli, Klebsiella, Proteus*
	Kefzol		*mirabilis*
	Zolicef		
Cephapirin	Cefadyl	IV, IM	
Cephradine	Velosef	PO, IV, IM	
Cephalexin	Cefanex	PO	
	Keflet		
	Keflex		
	Keftab		
	Biocef		
Cefadroxil	Duricef	PO	
	Ultracef		
Second Generation			
Cefamandole	Mandol	IV, IM	Gram-positive cocci except enterococci,
Cefaclor	Ceclor	PO	*Haemophilus influenzae, Enterobacter,*
Ceforanide	Precef	IV, IM	*Proteus mirabilis, Escherichia coli,*
Cefuroxime	Ceftin	PO, IV, IM	*Klebsiella,* anaerobes such as *Bacteroides*
	Kefurox		and *Clostridium*
	Zinacef		
Cefonicid	Monocid	IV, IM	
Cefmetazole	Zefazone	IV	
Loracarbef	Lorabid	PO	
Cefprozil	Cefzil	PO	
Cefoxitin	Mefoxin	IV, IM	All of the above plus *Neisseria gonorrhoeae*
Cefotetan	Cefotan	IV, IM	
Third Generation			
Cefotaxime	Claforan	IV, IM	*Escherichia coli, Klebsiella, Proteus,*
Cefixime	Suprax	PO	*Haemophilus influenzae, Serratia,*
Ceftizoxime	Cefizox	IV, IM	*Enterobacter*
Ceftriaxone	Rocephin	IV, IM	All of the above plus *Neisseria gonorrhoeae*
Cefoperazone	Cefobid	IV, IM	*Escherichia coli, Klebsiella, Proteus,*
Ceftazidime	Fortaz	IV, IM	*Haemophilus influenzae, Serratia, Enterobacter,* plus
	Tazicef		*Pseudomonas aeruginosa*
	Tazidime		
	Ceptaz		

IV, intravenous; IM, intramuscular; PO, oral.

and intravenously for the treatment of endophthalmitis[23] (see Table 11.2). Ceftazidime has also been suggested for intravitreal treatment of endophthalmitis.[23,24]

Second-generation cephalosporins, particularly cefoxitin, and most of the third-generation derivatives are considerably more resistant to β-lactamase activity than are the first-generation drugs. Thus, they are especially useful for treating infections caused by gram-negative bacteria that produce β-lactamase or that have become resistant to the aminoglyco-sides. These infections include gram-negative bacillary meningitis, pelvic and abdominal sepsis, lower respiratory tract infections, septicemia, and serious *Klebsiella* infections. With a nationwide distribution of penicillinase-producing *Neisseria gonorrhoeae,* the recommended regimen for treating gonococcal infections is intramuscular ceftriaxone, a third-generation cephalosporin.[7] Intramuscular or intravenous ceftriaxone is also the recommended treatment of gonococcal ophthalmia neonatorum.[7]

SIDE EFFECTS

As with the penicillins, hypersensitivity reactions are the most common systemic adverse events caused by cephalosporins. Maculopapular rash, urticaria, fever, bronchospasm, anaphylaxis, and eosinophilia have been associated with the use of cephalosporins. Because the molecular structures of the penicillins and cephalosporins are similar, patients who are allergic to penicillins may manifest a cross-sensitivity to a cephalosporin. Immunologic studies[25] have found cross-reactivity in as many as 20% of penicillin-allergic patients, but clinical reports[26] suggest a lower range (5% to 10%) of cephalosporin reactions in penicillin-allergic patients. This risk is greatly influenced by the severity of the prior reaction to penicillin. Therefore, a cephalosporin may be an effective substitute for penicillin in patients with an equivocal history of penicillin allergy or a history of mild reactions, but a cephalosporin should not be used for patients who have experienced a severe, immediate hypersensitivity reaction. Like penicillins, cephalosporins alter the normal microflora of the intestinal tract and can cause anorexia, nausea, vomiting, and diarrhea. In some cases the diarrhea can become severe enough to warrant discontinuation of the drug. Antibiotic-associated pseudomembranous colitis due to *Clostridium difficile* can also occur with the cephalosporins[27,28]; therefore, this condition should be considered in the differential diagnosis of diarrhea associated with cephalosporin use. Overgrowth of resistant organisms, such as *Acinetobacter*, *Candida*, and enterococci, can occur after long-term use of the cephalosporins. If therapy is prolonged, a patient should be closely monitored for signs of superinfection, especially if the patient is severely ill or if invasive devices such as catheters have been used. In some patients, cephalosporins destroy certain components of the intestinal microflora, and a vitamin K deficiency leading to bleeding episodes can result. The administration of vitamin K can reverse bleeding.[29] Administration of cephalosporins can lead to reversible renal impairment.[30,31] When a cephalosporin and an aminoglycoside are administered concomitantly, an additive nephrotoxicity may occur. This reaction is most likely to occur in the elderly and in patients with decreased renal function.

CONTRAINDICATIONS

The cephalosporins are contraindicated in patients with known allergies or intolerances to any of the cephalosporins. Since the penicillins, cephalosporins, and carbapenems have a common chemical structure, cross-allergies occur with these drugs. Thus, before initiating therapy with a cephalosporin, careful inquiry should be made concerning previous hypersensitivity reactions to the other drugs. Since a secondary vitamin K deficiency can develop with cephalosporin use, the cephalosporins are contraindicated in patients with hemophilia.[32]

Bacitracin

PHARMACOLOGY

Bacitracin inhibits bacterial cell wall synthesis but acts at a different step in the process than do the β-lactam antibiotics. It prevents the formation of polysaccharide chains that would normally be cross-linked to form the rigid peptidoglycan of the cell wall. Most gram-positive bacteria such as staphylococci, streptococci, and *Clostridium difficile* are susceptible to bacitracin. Although this agent is active against *Neisseria*, most gram-negative bacteria are resistant.

CLINICAL USES

Bacitracin is seldom used parenterally because renal necrosis has occurred after systemic use and because safer, more effective drugs with similar antibacterial spectra, such as the penicillins, are available. Bacitracin is primarily employed topically to treat skin and mucous membrane infections caused by gram-positive organisms because only a few of these bacteria have become resistant to it.[33] A recent report,[34] however, has suggested that bacitracin may have poor activity against many strains of staphylococci and streptococci. If this finding becomes widespread, the general use of bacitracin for gram-positive infections should be reconsidered.

Bacitracin is available in topical preparations either as a single-entity product or as a component of fixed-combination products. Because bacitracin is unstable in solution, it is available only in ointment form in either type of product. The rationale for compounding drugs containing bacitracin along with other antibacterial agents, such as neomycin and polymyxin B, is that by judicious selection, combinations can be produced with complementary antibacterial spectra covering most of the common pathogens. The antibacterial spectrum of bacitracin is mostly gram-positive, while the spectrum of polymyxin B is gram-negative, including *Acinetobacter*. The spectrum of neomycin includes many gram-positive and gram-negative organisms, but not *Acinetobacter*. Thus, bacitracin complements either of the other two agents. Topical fixed-combination ointments containing bacitracin are effective for a variety of dermatologic infections such as ulcers, external otitis, sycosis, and superficial folliculitis or impetigo. These topical combination products are also available as over-the-counter (OTC) preparations for use as skin prophylactics.

Topical ophthalmic preparations containing bacitracin (Tables 11.8 to 11.10) are effective for superficial infections of the eye, especially for staphylococcal blepharitis, since most staphylococci are still sensitive to bacitracin.[35]

SIDE EFFECTS

Hypersensitivity reactions, usually presenting as contact dermatitis, are rare but can occur with topically applied

TABLE 11.8
Antibacterial Drugs for Topical Ocular Therapy

Generic Name	Formulation	Concentration	Trade Name (Manufacturer)
Bacitracin	Ointment	500 U/g	Generic (Various) AK-Tracin (Akorn)
Chloramphenicol	Solution	0.5%	Generic (Various) Chloroptic (Allergan) AK-Chlor (Akorn) Chloromycetin (Parke-Davis)
	Ointment	1%	Generic (Various) Chloroptic (Allergan) AK-Chlor (Akorn) Chloromycetin (Parke-Davis)
Ciprofloxacin	Solution	0.3%	Ciloxan (Alcon)
Chlortetracycline	Ointment	1%	Aureomycin (Storz/Lederle)
Erythromycin	Ointment	0.5%	Generic (Various) Ilotycin (Dista) AK-Mycin (Akorn)
Gentamicin	Solution and ointment	0.3%	Generic (Various) Genoptic (Allergan) Gentacidin (Ciba Vision) Garamycin (Schering) Gentak (Akorn)
Norfloxacin	Solution	0.3%	Chibroxin (Merck)
Ofloxacin	Solution	0.3%	Ocuflox (Allergan)
Polymyxin B	Powder	500,000 U/vial	Polymyxin B sulfate (Burroughs)
Tetracycline	Suspension and ointment	1%	Achromycin (Storz/Lederle)
Tobramycin	Solution and ointment	0.3%	Tobrex (Alcon)

bacitracin.[36] Superinfections have been observed after the use of mixtures containing bacitracin,[37] and this possibility should be considered if a relapse of signs or symptoms follows a period of initial improvement.

CONTRAINDICATIONS

Bacitracin is contraindicated in patients with known hypersensitivity or intolerance to the drug.

Vancomycin

PHARMACOLOGY

Like the other drugs discussed in this section, vancomycin acts by inhibiting biosynthesis of peptidoglycan during bac-

terial cell wall formation. It is highly active against gram-positive cocci, including staphylococci and streptococci, as well as Clostridium, *Corynebacterium diphtheriae*, and *Neisseria gonorrhoeae*.

CLINICAL USES

Because of its toxicity, vancomycin is reserved for serious infections in which less toxic antibiotics are ineffective or not tolerated. Oral vancomycin is the drug of choice for treating patients with pseudomembranous colitis caused by *Clostridium difficile*. Vancomycin, either alone or with an aminoglycoside, is used to treat bacterial endocarditis and for short-term prophylaxis against this condition in penicillin-allergic patients who are undergoing certain dental or surgical procedures. Vancomycin is an acceptable alternative to penicillins or cephalosporins for the treatment of

TABLE 11.9
Combination Antibacterial Drugs for Topical Ocular Therapy

Generic Name	Concentration	Trade Name (Manufacturer)
Solutions		
Polymyxin B	10,000 U/ml	Generic (Various)
Neomycin	0.175%	AK-Spore (Akorn)
Gramicidin	0.0025%	Ocutricin (Bausch & Lomb)
		Neosporin (Burroughs)
		Neocidin (Major)
Trimethoprim	0.1%	Polytrim (Allergan)
Polymyxin B	10,000 U/ml	
Ointments		
Polymyxin B	10,000 U/g	AK-Poly-Bac (Akorn)
Bacitracin	500 U/g	Polysporin (Burroughs)
Polymyxin B	10,000 U/g	Terramycin w/Polymyxin B
Oxytetracycline	0.5%	(Roerig)
Polymyxin B	5,000 U/g	Triple Antibiotic (Various)
Neomycin	0.5%	Neonatal (Hauck)
Bacitracin	400 U/g	
Polymyxin B	10,000 U/g	Generic (Various)
Neomycin	0.35%	Neosporin (Burroughs)
Bacitracin	400 U/g	AK-Spore (Akorn)
		Ocutricin (Bausch & Lomb)

serious infections caused by staphylococci, streptococci, or enterococci and is the drug of choice for treating infections caused by methicillin-resistant staphylococci. A case of blepharitis caused by a methicillin-resistant strain of *S. epidermidis* resolved after treatment with topical vancomycin.[38] Because of its excellent activity against gram-positive bacteria including methicillin- and cephalothin-resistant staphylococci, vancomycin is recommended for topical, subconjunctival, intravenous, and intravitreal therapy in bacterial endophthalmitis[23,39] (see Table 11.2).

SIDE EFFECTS

The use of vancomycin in large oral doses, with prolonged therapy, in concomitant or sequential use with other ototoxic or nephrotoxic drugs, or in patients with impaired renal function has caused permanent deafness and fatal uremia. Hearing and renal function should thus be monitored frequently when administering systemic vancomycin.

CONTRAINDICATIONS

Vancomycin is contraindicated in patients with known hypersensitivity or intolerance to the drug.

Drugs Affecting the Cytoplasmic Membrane

Antibacterial drugs that affect the bacterial cytoplasmic membrane include polymyxin B, colistin, and gramicidin.

Polymyxin B and Colistin

PHARMACOLOGY

Of the large number of compounds that affect the bacterial cytoplasmic membrane, only a few have sufficient selective toxicity to be therapeutically useful. Polymyxin B and colistin (polymyxin E) are cationic detergents or surfactants that interact with the phospholipids of the cell's membranes, disrupting the osmotic integrity of the cell. This, in turn, increases the bacterial cells' permeability and causes leakage of intracellular molecules. The polymyxins are bactericidal and can kill non-dividing cells without necessarily lysing them.

CLINICAL USES

Both drugs are effective against gram-negative bacteria, but with the development of more effective, less toxic antibiot-

TABLE 11.10
Antibiotic-Steroid Combinations for Topical Ocular Therapy

Antibiotic	Steroid	Trade Name (Manufacturer)
Solutions and Suspensions		
Neomycin 0.35%	Dexamethasone 0.1%	Generic (Various) NeoDecadron (Merck) Neodexair (Bausch & Lomb) Neo-Dexameth (Major) AK-Neo-Dex (Akorn)
Neomycin 0.35% Polymyxin B 10,000 U/ml	Dexamethasone 0.1%	Generic (Various) AK-Trol (Akron) Maxitrol (Alcon) Dexacidin (Ciba Vision) Dexasporin (Various)
Neomycin 0.35% Polymyxin B 10,000 U/m	Hydrocortisone 1%	Generic (Various) Cortisporin (Burroughs) Bacticort (Rugby)
Neomycin 0.35% Polymyxin B 10,000 U/ml	Prednisolone 0.5%	Poly-Pred Suspension (Allergan)
Gentamicin 0.3%	Prednisolone 1%	Pred-G (Allergan)
Tobramycin 0.3%	Dexamethasone 0.1%	TobraDex (Alcon)
Oxytetracycline 0.5%	Hydrocortisone 1.5%	Terra-Cortril (Roerig)
Chloramphenicol 0.25%	Hydrocortisone 0.5%	Chloromycetin Hydrocortisone (Park-Davis)
Ointments		
Neomycin 0.35% Neomycin 0.35% Polymyxin B 10,000 U/g	Dexamethasone 0.05% Dexamethasone 0.1%	NeoDecadron (Merck) Generic (Various) AK-Trol (Akorn) Maxitrol (Alcon) Dexacidin (Ciba Vision) Dexasporin (Various)
Neomycin 0.5% Bacitracin 400 U/g Polymyxin B 10,000 U/g	Hydrocortisone 1%	Coracin (Hauck)
Neomycin 0.35% Bacitracin 400 U/g Polymyxin B 10,000 U/g	Hydrocortisone 1%	Generic (Various) Cortisporin (Burroughs) Neotricin HC (Bausch & Lomb) AK-Spore HC (Akorn)
Gentamicin 0.3%	Prednisolone 0.6%	Pred-G (Allergan)
Chloramphenicol 1% Polymyxin B 10,000 U/g	Hydrocortisone 0.5%	Ophthocort (Park-Davis)

ics, indications for the polymyxins have become limited. Currently, polymyxins are systemically administered primarily for serious infections caused by strains of *Pseudomonas aeruginosa* that are resistant to the antipseudomonal penicillins, the third-generation cephalosporins, and the aminoglycosides. They are also used for gram-negative bacillary infections caused by organisms resistant to more preferred antibiotics or for patients who cannot tolerate the preferred drugs.

In combination with other antibacterial drugs or steroids,

polymyxin B is used to prevent and treat skin infections and external otitis. It is also a popular antibiotic for treating common bacterial infections of the conjunctiva and lids. Polymyxin B is commercially available alone as an ophthalmic preparation (see Table 11.8) or in combination with other antibiotics (see Table 11.9) or with steroids (see Table 11.10). Topical application or subconjunctival injection of polymyxin B has been used to treat corneal ulcers caused by *Pseudomonas aeruginosa*,[40] but the newer and less toxic penicillins or aminoglycosides are now the drugs of choice for this condition.

SIDE EFFECTS

The two most important side effects associated with systemic administration of polymyxins are neurotoxicity and nephrotoxicity. Polymyxin B and colistin cause essentially the same incidence and severity of neurotoxicity, but the risk of nephrotoxicity is greater with polymyxin B. Neurotoxic effects include dizziness, vertigo, ataxia, blurred vision, confusion, paresthesias, and numbness of the extremities. Muscular weakness, paresis, and complete paralysis also have been reported.[41] At appropriate systemic dosages, approximately 20% of patients experience nephrotoxicity as evidenced by a rising serum creatinine level, and 1% to 2% develop tubular necrosis. Anuria and tubular necrosis with serious renal failure are particularly common in patients who have received excessive doses or in whom drug use is continued despite impaired renal function.

Adverse reactions to topical application of polymyxins, including irritation and allergic reactions of the eyelids and conjunctiva, are infrequent and typically mild. When administered by subconjunctival injection, however, polymyxin B may cause pain, chemosis, and tissue necrosis.

CONTRAINDICATIONS

Polymyxin B and colistin are contraindicated in patients with known hypersensitivity or intolerance to either drug.

Gramicidin

Like polymyxin B and colistin, gramicidin changes the permeability characteristics of the cell membrane, killing the cell. However, in contrast to polymyxin B and colistin, gramicidin is effective against gram-positive bacteria and replaces bacitracin in some fixed-combination antibacterial solutions used topically for ocular infections (see Table 11.9).

Drugs Affecting Protein Synthesis

Antibacterial drugs that affect bacterial protein synthesis include the aminoglycosides, tetracyclines, macrolides, and the single drugs, chloramphenicol and clindamycin.

Aminoglycosides

Since the isolation of streptomycin from *Streptomyces griseus* in the 1940s, one or another of the aminoglycosides has contributed significantly to the treatment of infections caused by gram-negative bacilli such as *P. aeruginosa*, *Proteus*, *Klebsiella*, *E. coli*, *Enterobacter*, and *Serratia*. Aminoglycosides are also effective against many strains of staphylococci; however, they are not often used for systemic staphylococcal infections because numerous alternative antibiotics, such as penicillinase-resistant penicillins and cephalosporins, are effective and less toxic. In contrast to the other aminoglycosides, neomycin is a broad–spectrum antibacterial drug active against gram-positive as well as gram-negative bacteria. An important exception in its spectrum of activity is its ineffectiveness against *P. aeruginosa*.

PHARMACOLOGY

The aminoglycoside family of antibiotics includes neomycin, gentamicin, tobramycin, and amikacin. These drugs inhibit bacterial protein synthesis by binding to the 30S subunit of the bacterial ribosome (Fig. 11.3). The conse-

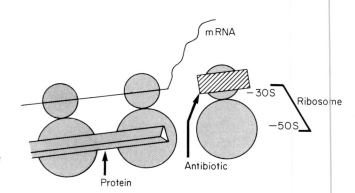

FIGURE 11.3 **Bacterial ribosomes showing the mechanism of action of the aminoglycosides, antibacterial drugs that inhibit protein synthesis.**

quences of this interaction include inhibition of bacterial protein synthesis and an infidelity in correctly reading the genetic code.

Gram-negative bacilli show widespread resistance to the aminoglycosides. This resistance is achieved by one or more of the following three mechanisms: alteration of the bacterial ribosomes, decreased antibiotic uptake, and enzymatic inactivation of the drugs. Enzymatic inactivation is the most common type of resistance and results in production of a modified form of the drug that is not only inactive but that also blocks further uptake of the active drug into the cell. Gram-negative bacilli produce many different aminoglycoside-inactivating enzymes, with some enzymes inactivating certain drugs but not others. Cross-resistance among aminoglycosides that are susceptible to the same inactivating enzymes is often complete. For example, bacteria resistant to gentamicin are usually also resistant to tobramycin.[42] Thus, known resistance patterns are helpful only in the initial selection of an aminoglycoside. The specific sensitivity to each drug must be determined for the individual pathogen.

The aminoglycosides are poorly absorbed from the gastrointestinal tract and must therefore be given parenterally when used systemically. Note that penicillins may inactivate aminoglycosides if mixed together in the same solution for injection or for topical application; each must be administered separately.

CLINICAL USES

Neomycin.   Neomycin is the oldest aminoglycoside. It is available for oral, topical, and parenteral administration, but there are almost no indications for parenteral use. Oral administration is employed chiefly to prepare the bowel for surgery and as an adjunct to hepatic coma therapy.

The most common form of neomycin administration is topical. The drug is available in combination with other antibiotics or steroids in numerous ophthalmic (see Tables 11.9 and 11.10), otic, and dermatologic preparations designed to treat a variety of skin and mucous membrane infections. Topical ocular application of neomycin frequently results in sensitization to the drug, which leads to contact dermatitis in approximately 4% of patients (Fig. 11.4).[37,43] Therefore, routine use of topical preparations containing neomycin is not recommended, and other individual drugs or combinations, such as bacitracin-polymyxin B, should generally be substituted.

Gentamicin.   Gentamicin remains a mainstay in the treatment of serious gram-negative bacillary infections. Systemic uses include complicated urinary tract infections, bone and joint infections, pneumonia, meningitis, and peritonitis in which the causal organism is a gram-negative bacillus sensitive to the drug. In addition, aminoglycosides such as gentamicin are frequently used for empiric therapy in presumed gram-negative bacillary infections before the identification and susceptibility of the causative organism are known.

Topical dermatologic preparations of gentamicin are commonly used for the treatment of infected burns. Topical ophthalmic gentamicin (see Table 11.8) is used to treat a variety of bacterial infections of the external eye and adnexa such as conjunctivitis, blepharitis, keratoconjunctivitis, and dacryocystitis. Since most of the bacteria that cause these infections (staphylococci, *H. influenzae*, and other gram-negative rods) are still sensitive to this antibiotic, gentamicin is efficacious for the treatment of these diseases. This has been substantiated in several clinical studies of external infections in which a favorable therapeutic response to a 0.3% solution or ointment was demonstrated.[44-46] Several investigators[47,48] have found gentamicin as effective as a combination of neomycin, bacitracin, and polymyxin B for treating external ocular infections. In one study,[49] the clinical improvement was 93% and the microbiologic improvement, eradicated or controlled, was 67%. Currently, gentamicin is generally considered an antibiotic of choice for the initial treatment of bacterial infections of the external eye.

Gentamicin is also an antibiotic of choice for the initial treatment of bacterial corneal ulcers,[12,18] but the commercially available strength of ophthalmic gentamicin solution is considered inadequate for the initial treatment of bacterial keratitis.[50] Consequently, solutions containing fortified con-

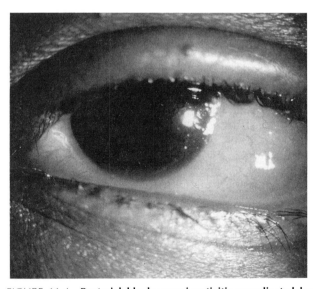

FIGURE 11.4 **Bacterial blepharoconjunctivitis complicated by hypersensitivity to neomycin. Patient was treated with gramicidin-neomycin-polymyxin B (Neosporin). There is erythema and edema of eyelids, chemosis, and intense itching. (Reprinted with permission from Jennings B. Mechanisms, diagnosis, and management of common ocular allergies. J Am Optom Assoc 1990; 61(suppl):S32–S41.)**

centrations are prepared from sterile products intended for parenteral use. Empiric therapy with fortified gentamicin or tobramycin drops along with a penicillinase-resistant penicillin or cephalosporin is useful until the causative organism and susceptibility are known. An initial loading dose (1 drop every minute for 5 minutes) increases the antibiotic concentrations in the cornea rapidly.[51] Drops then can be applied every 15 to 30 minutes for the first 24 to 48 hours. Gentamicin, sometimes in combination with a penicillin having antipseudomonal activity (such as ticarcillin), is a specific treatment of choice for *Pseudomonas aeruginosa* corneal ulcers.[12] Adjunctive subconjunctival injections of antibiotics are controversial for the treatment of bacterial ulcers since it is unknown whether this route offers additional benefit. Nevertheless, subconjunctival injections may be useful when compliance is questionable or in infants or young children, whose crying dilutes topically applied medication.

As in the initial treatment of bacterial corneal ulcers, the initial treatment of bacterial endophthalmitis usually includes two antibiotics: an antibiotic to which penicillinase-producing staphylococci are sensitive, and another drug, such as gentamicin or tobramycin, to which gram-negative bacilli are sensitive.[22] The practitioner may choose to use these antibiotics systemically, topically, subconjunctivally, or intravitreally.

Tobramycin. The antibacterial activity and pharmacokinetic properties of tobramycin resemble those of gentamicin, and tobramycin's therapeutic uses for treating gram-negative bacillary infections are essentially identical to those for gentamicin. Among the gram-positive cocci, staphylococci are susceptible to tobramycin whereas the streptococci, including *S. pneumoniae*, have such high MICs that they are often found to be resistant using conventional susceptibility testing. However, when the tear concentration produced by topical administration of tobramycin is determined, the drug level is usually above the MICs of ocular pathogens, including *S. pneumoniae*.[52a] Thus, tobramycin can be used to treat external surface infections of the eye even when *S. pneumoniae* is a suspected pathogen.

Bacteria resistant to tobramycin are usually also resistant to gentamicin, but some gentamicin-resistant *Pseudomonas* strains still remain sensitive to tobramycin.[42] In contrast to *Pseudomonas*, however, cross-resistance is common between gentamicin and tobramycin for most strains of *Klebsiella*, *Enterobacter*, *E. coli*, and *Serratia*.[42] Amikacin is usually effective for infections caused by organisms resistant to both gentamicin and tobramycin.

Although generally similar in pharmacologic properties, one difference between gentamicin and tobramycin is that, *in vitro*, tobramycin is more potent against *Pseudomonas aeruginosa*.[42] For this reason, tobramycin is often preferred, sometimes in combination with an antipseudomonal penicillin (such as ticarcillin), for infections caused by this organism. However, there is no conclusive proof to indicate whether tobramycin is clinically superior to gentamicin against *P. aeruginosa*.

Another pharmacologic difference between tobramycin and gentamicin is that, when used systemically, tobramycin is less nephrotoxic.[52] However, the use of tobramycin over gentamicin for all patients does not appear warranted since the nephrotoxicity associated with both gentamicin and tobramycin therapy is usually mild and reversible.[52]

Tobramycin is available as a topical ophthalmic solution and ointment (see Table 11.8). The topical uses of ophthalmic tobramycin are similar to those of ophthalmic gentamicin (see Table 11.2).[53] Because tobramycin is more potent *in vitro* against *Pseudomonas aeruginosa*, some clinicians prefer tobramycin over gentamicin for bacterial keratitis.[54] Tobramycin may also be less toxic than gentamicin when injected into the vitreous, and this may make it a more desirable drug for treatment of bacterial endophthalmitis.[55]

Concern about the possibility that widespread use of a clinically important antibacterial drug like tobramycin could facilitate emergence of bacteria resistant to the drug has resulted in the suggestion that tobramycin use should be limited. Although several reports[56,57] have correlated the development of progressive resistance to the aminoglycosides with greater aminoglycoside use, other reports[58,59] have not documented this association. In one study[59] the resistance to tobramycin closely paralleled gentamicin resistance despite limited and controlled use of tobramycin; the restricted use of tobramycin did not prevent or delay the development of resistance to it. Certainly, strategies that limit the emergence of bacterial strains resistant to the aminoglycosides must be considered, but restricting the use of tobramycin has not been proven a worthwhile strategy.

Amikacin. Amikacin was the first semisynthetic aminoglycoside marketed. Because a chemical modification present in amikacin protects the molecule from aminoglycoside-inactivating enzymes, it has become the preferred drug for treatment of gram-negative bacillary infections in which resistance to both gentamicin and tobramycin is encountered.[60] At the clinical level, however, evidence is lacking that amikacin is more efficacious than gentamicin or tobramycin for infections caused by susceptible organisms.

Since amikacin is active *in vitro* against many gram-negative bacilli that are resistant to other aminoglycosides, and since amikacin is less toxic when injected intravitreally, it has become a primary antibiotic, along with vancomycin, for treatment of bacterial endophthalmitis.[24,61]

SIDE EFFECTS

The side effects encountered with topical gentamicin are rare but include corneal and conjunctival toxicity. Punctate epithelial erosions, delayed re-epithelialization, and corneal ulceration characterize the corneal toxicity,[45] while chemosis, hyperemia, and necrosis characterize the conjunctival toxicity.[62] One case has been reported of periocular skin and conjunctival paresthesia.[63] Allergic reactions to topical gentamicin occur infrequently, but approximately 50% of patients who are allergic to neomycin also prove to be allergic to gentamicin.[64]

Topical administration of tobramycin can cause reversible tearing, burning, photophobia, eyelid edema, conjunctival hyperemia and chemosis, and punctate epithelial erosions.[53]

Intravitreally injected aminoglycosides have been widely used for the treatment and prophylaxis of endophthalmitis to cover the gram-negative bacteria. However, Campochiaro and Conway[65] reported 101 cases of retinal damage in the form of macular infarction related to the intravitreal administration of aminoglycosides, mainly gentamicin. In response, lower doses of gentamicin or amikacin have been used to treat endophthalmitis, but even low doses of intravitreal gentamicin have been shown to cause toxic retinal effects.[66] Therefore, the current recommendation for the treatment of postoperative endophthalmitis is to use intravitreal vancomycin as a single agent if laboratory studies rule out gram-negative infection. In the absence of laboratory support, amikacin should also be administered.[39] As an alternative to amikacin, ceftazidime, a cephalosporin with good gram-negative coverage, can be used.[24]

Both vestibular and auditory dysfunction resulting from progressive destruction of vestibular or cochlear sensory cells can follow systemic administration of any of the aminoglycosides. Initial symptoms of cochlear damage include tinnitus or a sensation of pressure or fullness in the ears. Vestibular dysfunction is manifest by nystagmus, vertigo, nausea, vomiting, or acute Meniere's syndrome. Patients receiving systemic aminoglycosides must be carefully monitored for ototoxicity, since only the early symptoms may be reversible on discontinuation of the drug. If the drugs are used long enough or at high dosages, resultant toxicity can produce sensory cell death, and the dysfunction, in most cases, becomes irreversible. A dynamic illegible E test has been proposed as a sensitive screening procedure for detecting aminoglycoside ototoxicity.[67] During the test, the patient's best visual acuity is measured using the illegible E chart. The patient then oscillates his or her head from left to right and back at a frequency of 1 Hz and is asked to read the chart again. A deterioration in visual acuity suggests an infidelity of the vestibulo-ocular reflex that can be associated with aminoglycoside toxicity.

The high concentrations of aminoglycosides that can accumulate in the kidney and urine correlate with the potential for these drugs to cause nephrotoxicity in the form of acute tubular necrosis. Usually discontinuing the drug can reverse early changes.[68] Since the incidence and severity of nephrotoxicity and ototoxicity relate directly to the aminoglycoside concentration in the body and to the length of exposure to the drug, these antibiotics should be used only when less toxic antibiotics are not effective. Plasma drug levels should be monitored, and the dosage for patients with impaired renal function should be reduced. Careful drug selection and control of plasma concentrations can minimize toxicity. Systemic aminoglycoside administration has been associated with neuromuscular blockade. Respiratory depression and possible cardiac arrest characterize this syndrome. The pupils may become dilated, and a myasthenic effect may occur with generalized muscular weakness of the extremities, paralysis of the extraocular muscles, and ptosis.[69] Calcium gluconate can reverse neuromuscular blockade. Systemic gentamicin also causes another rare, visually-related side effect: pseudotumor cerebri with secondary papilledema.[70]

CONTRAINDICATIONS

The aminoglycosides are contraindicated in patients with hypersensitivity or intolerance to any drug within the family.

Tetracyclines

PHARMACOLOGY

Tetracyclines are a family of antibiotics that have been both isolated from species of *Streptomyces* and produced in the laboratory. The tetracyclines are broad-spectrum antibacterial drugs active against gram-positive, gram-negative, aerobic, and anaerobic bacteria as well as spirochetes, *Mycoplasma*, *Rickettsia*, *Chlamydia*, and some protozoa. Based on differences in pharmacokinetics, tetracycline analogs are usually divided into 3 groups: short-acting analogs (half-lives of 6 to 9 hours); intermediate-acting analogs; and long-acting analogs (half-lives of 17 to 20 hours) (Table 11.11). All the analogs are closely related chemically and in general have similar patterns of bacterial susceptibility and resistance.

Tetracyclines gain entry into bacteria by an energy-dependent process. Once inside, they bind to the 30S subunit of the ribosome, blocking the attachment of aminoacyl-tRNA to the receptor site on the messenger RNA-ribosome complex. Tetracyclines also inhibit protein synthesis in human cells but do not accumulate within these cells by an active process. This difference may explain the difference in degree of protein inhibition in host cells versus microorganisms. The difference in active transport, however, does not account for the high sensitivity of various intracellular organisms such as *Chlamydia* and *Rickettsia* to the tetracyclines; other factors appear to be involved.[71]

In addition to its antibiotic action against pathogenic microorganisms, tetracycline also appears to have other properties that can change the course of disease progression. When patients with acne vulgaris,[72] acne rosacea,[73] or primary meibomianitis,[73] all non-infectious inflammatory diseases, receive tetracycline, two changes occur: amelioration of the symptoms and reduction of free fatty acids in the

TABLE 11.11
Tetracyclines: Classes, Oral Doses, and Relative Costs

Generic Name	Trade Name	Oral Preparations	Usual Adult Dosage	Relative Cost Compared with Tetracycline (per capsule)
Short-Acting				
Tetracycline	Generic	100, 250, 500 mg capsules	250–500 mg q.i.d.	250 mg (1)
	Achromycin V	250, 500 mg tablets		
	Ala-Tet	125 mg/5 ml suspension		
	Nor-Tet			
	Panmycin			
	Robitet			
	Sumycin			
	Teline			
	Tetracap			
	Tetralan			
	Tetram			
Oxytetracycline	Generic	250 mg capsules	250–500 mg. q.i.d.	250 mg (2–3)
	E. P. Mycin	250 mg tablets		
	Terramycin			
	Uri-Tet			
Intermediate-Acting				
Methacycline	Rondomycin	150, 300 mg capsules	150 mg q.i.d. or 300 mg b.i.d.	150 mg (90)
Demeclocycline	Declomycin	150 mg capsules	150 mg q.i.d. or	150 mg (70)
		150, 300 mg tablets	300 mg b.i.d.	
Long-Acting				
Doxycycline	Generic	50, 100 mg capsules	200 mg, then	100 mg (3–5)
	Doxy	50, 100 mg tablets	100 mg q.d.	
	Doxychel	50 mg/5 ml solution	or b.i.d.	
	Vibramycin			
	Doryx			
	Vibra-Tabs			
Minocycline	Minocin	50, 100 mg capsules	200 mg, then	100 mg (65)
		50, 100 mg tablets	100 mg b.i.d.	
		50 mg/5 ml suspension		

Modified from Salamon SS. Tetracyclines in ophthalmology. Surv Ophthalmol 1985;29:265–275.

surface sebum. Since normal bacterial flora probably produce the free fatty acids, possibly tetracycline is therapeutically effective in these disorders due to its interactions with normal bacteria, not pathogens. In addition to its antimicrobial properties, tetracycline also has anticollagenase activity, and this action may account for its effectiveness in treating certain noninfectious diseases.[74]

CLINICAL USES

Although the tetracyclines are broad–spectrum, their usefulness against some of the more common microbial patho-gens, such as *S. aureus*, is decreasing due to resistance.[75] The number of clinical indications for the tetracyclines has declined due to increasing resistance and the development of newer anti-infective drugs that are more effective for specific infections. Tetracyclines, however, remain drugs of choice, or very effective alternative therapy, for a wide variety of infections caused by less common pathogens. These include brucellosis; rickettsial infections such as Rocky Mountain spotted fever, typhus, and Q fever; *Mycoplasma* pneumonia; cholera; plague; *Ureaplasma* urethritis; Lyme disease; and chlamydial infections such as sexually-transmitted disease, trachoma, and inclusion conjunctivitis.

One percent tetracycline suspension and ointment, 1% chlortetracycline ointment, and a fixed-combination ointment containing oxytetracycline and polymyxin B are available for topical ocular use (see Tables 11.8 and 11.9). The Centers for Disease Control (CDC) recommends ophthalmic ointments containing a tetracycline or erythromycin as an effective alternative to silver nitrate for prophylaxis of gonococcal ophthalmia neonatorum.[7] A major advantage of using one of the tetracyclines is that they do not cause the chemical conjunctivitis typically produced by silver nitrate, while they decrease the risk of infection with *Neisseria gonorrhoeae* and *Chlamydia trachomatis*.[76]

Although chlamydial ophthalmia neonatorum has been treated with topical tetracycline, topical application does not totally eradicate *Chlamydia* from the body.[77] Systemic tetracycline could be used, but it causes side effects in children under age 8 years. For these reasons, oral erythromycin, an equally effective agent, is the drug of choice for this disease.[77,78]

In adults with ocular infections with *Chlamydia,* such as inclusion conjunctivitis or trachoma, treatment with oral doxycycline or tetracycline is recommended.[79] Doxycycline can be taken without regard to meals, and the twice daily regimen enhances patient compliance. Topical treatment with oxytetracycline ointment, twice daily for 6 weeks, can also reduce trachomatous inflammation, but incomplete cure and subsequent disease transmission can result.[80] Therefore, an oral tetracycline is the most effective treatment for these conditions.

Some surface ocular infections, such as conjunctivitis and keratitis caused by susceptible microorganisms, respond well to topical tetracyclines. However, many of the organisms that cause these infections are either resistant or unresponsive to tetracyclines. One-third or more of staphylococcal strains may be resistant, and *Pseudomonas aeruginosa* is rarely responsive.[75,81] Thus, when the microorganism responsible for a surface ocular infection is unknown, a topical tetracycline is not usually the drug of choice. Tetracycline can be an effective therapy for noninfectious conditions involving the eye. Oral tetracycline has been effective for recalcitrant (i.e., resistant to corticosteroid therapy) cases of nontuberculous phlyctenular keratoconjunctivitis.[82] The treatment resulted in rapid relief of symptoms and apparent arrest of the disease. Phlyctenular keratoconjunctivitis is considered a delayed hypersensitivity reaction to foreign protein, especially the proteins associated with bacteria. The manner in which systemic tetracycline affects the ocular flora or alters the antigenically-stimulated immune response remains unclear.

Oral tetracycline may also be effective for resolving noninfected corneal ulcers or "corneal melting" in which progressive necrosis of stromal tissue occur despite the absence of a positive culture.[83] This form of sterile ulceration may occur by the action of tissue collagenases, and the anticollagenolytic activity of systemic tetracycline may ex-

plain its effectiveness.[74] Similarly, the anticollagenolytic activity of tetracycline may prove clinically useful in treating persistent corneal epithelial defects. Perry and associates[84] gave oral tetracycline to 18 patients with persistent epithelial defects. The defects healed in 14 of the patients, while the other four showed either no improvement or worsened.

Both tetracycline and doxycycline are effective in improving the ocular manifestations of acne rosacea, including irritation, blepharitis, keratitis, meibomianitis, and chalazia.[85,86] While some patients may discontinue medication without recurrence of symptoms, others must continue on low maintenance doses for extended periods. Many patients who had eyelid cultures positive for *S. aureus* at the initiation of tetracycline treatment continued to have positive cultures even though the signs and symptoms of ocular rosacea disappeared.[85] This finding suggests that *S. aureus* does not have a prominent role in the etiology of the condition.

SIDE EFFECTS

Hypersensitivity reactions to tetracyclines, including anaphylaxis, urticaria, periorbital edema, and morbilliform rashes, can occur but are uncommon. Photosensitivity reactions, manifested as an exaggerated sunburn, are common in patients receiving demeclocycline but can occur with all tetracycline analogs.[75,81]

At the usual dosage levels, all tetracyclines have relatively low toxicity, but oral administration can produce varying degrees of gastrointestinal irritation. Anorexia, heartburn, nausea, vomiting, flatulence, and diarrhea commonly occur. Although not usually disabling, these reactions may become severe enough to require discontinuation or interruption of therapy. When diarrhea persists or becomes severe, pseudomembranous colitis caused by *Clostridium difficile* must be considered. The administration of tetracycline with food may ameliorate its irritative effects, but food can adversely affect the drug's absorption. In contrast, the absorption of doxycycline is only slightly affected by the presence of food, including dairy products. Since all tetracyclines can form complexes with divalent cations, the absorption of tetracyclines is markedly decreased when they are administered with iron-containing tonics or antacids containing calcium, magnesium, or aluminum. Sodium bicarbonate also adversely affects tetracycline absorption.[87]

Tetracyclines can produce a negative nitrogen balance and increased blood urea nitrogen (BUN) levels.[88] This condition has little clinical importance when patients with normal renal function receive the usual doses. However, tetracyclines may cause azotemia in patients with impaired renal function. Thus, the only tetracycline recommended for use in such patients is doxycycline because it exits the body mainly via the intestinal tract rather than through the kidneys.

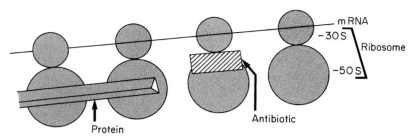

FIGURE 11.5   **Bacterial ribosomes showing the mechanism of action of erythromycin, an antibacterial drug that inhibits protein synthesis.**

Tetracyclines are attracted to embryonic and growing bone tissue, in which they form a tetracycline-calcium orthophosphate complex, temporarily depressing bone growth. They can also cause changes in both deciduous and permanent teeth during the time of tooth development; these changes include dysgenesis, staining, and an increased tendency to caries. Discoloration may be progressive and can vary from yellowish brown to dark gray. Because of bone growth depression and tooth discoloration, women in the last half of pregnancy, lactating women, and children under 8 years of age should avoid tetracyclines.[89]

Intracranial hypertension (pseudotumor cerebri) secondary to the use of many tetracycline analogs can occur in infants and adults.[90,91] When the antibiotic is discontinued, cerebral fluid pressure and any accompanying visual and ophthalmoscopic changes usually return to normal over days or weeks.[90,91]

Rarely, tetracycline causes blood dyscrasias such as hemolytic anemia, thrombocytopenia, neutropenia, and eosinophilia.[75]

Vestibular toxicity appears to be unique to minocycline.[75] Lightheadedness, loss of balance, dizziness, nausea, and tinnitus usually begin 2 to 3 days after starting therapy and occur in up to 70% of patients. Although these side effects are usually reversible after discontinuing the drug, they have severely limited the use of minocycline.

Tetracyclines can interact significantly with other drugs, and these interactions should be considered when the patient is taking concomitant medications (see Chapter 36). Tetracyclines can potentiate the effects of coumarin-type anticoagulants and seriously interfere with blood clotting. They may also interfere with the bactericidal action of the penicillins after concomitant parenteral administration, and such use should be avoided. By increasing hepatic drug metabolism, carbamazepine, diphenylhydantoin,[92] and barbiturates[93] decrease by approximately 50% the half-life of doxycycline. Doxycycline dosages must therefore be increased to compensate for this factor or a different antibiotic selected.

CONTRAINDICATIONS

Tetracyclines are contraindicated in patients with known hypersensitivity or intolerance to any member of the tetracycline family. The use of tetracyclines during tooth development may cause permanent discoloration of teeth and is thus contraindicated in pregnant or breast-feeding women and in children 8 years of age or less.

Macrolides

The macrolide antibiotics include erythromycin, clarithromycin, and azithromycin.

PHARMACOLOGY

The macrolides inhibit bacterial protein synthesis by binding to the 50S ribosomal subunit and preventing elongation of the peptide chain (Fig. 11.5). They have low toxicity because they do not bind to mammalian ribosomes. Erythromycin was previously considered only bacteriostatic, but it is now believed to have bactericidal properties that depend on the organism and the drug concentration.

The spectrum of activity of the macrolides includes gram-positive cocci (streptococci and staphylococci), gram-positive bacilli, *Neisseria*, *Mycoplasma*, *Treponema*, *Rickettsia*, and *Chlamydia*. The macrolides have variable activity against *Haemophilus influenzae*.

Erythromycin.   Erythromycin is a widely used macrolide antibiotic because of its relative lack of toxicity and good activity against susceptible organisms. It is available in topical, oral, and intravenous preparations. Only the free base has biological activity *in vivo*. When given orally, however, gastric acid inactivates the erythromycin base, resulting in decreased absorption. Thus, a large number of formulations and derivatives have been prepared to optimize stability and absorption (Table 11.12). One approach provides a protective coating to shield the erythromycin base

TABLE 11.12
Oral Erythromycin Preparations

Preparation	Trade Name (Manufacturer)	Formulation*
Base	Generic (Various)	250 mg tablets
	Erythromycin Filmtab (Abbott)	333 mg tablets
	E-Mycin (Boots)	500 mg tablets
	ERYC (Parke-Davis)	
	Ery-Tab (Abbott)	
	PCE Dispertab (Abbott)	
	Erythromycin Delayed Release (Abbott)	
	Robinmycin (Robins)	
Stearate	Generic (Various)	250 mg tablets
	Erythrocin Stearate (Abbott)	500 mg tablets
	Erythromycin Stearate (Mylan)	
	Eramycin (Wesley)	
	Wyamycin S (Wyeth-Ayerst)	
Ethylsuccinate	Generic (Various)	200 mg tablets
	E.E.S. (Abbott)	400 mg tablets
	EryPed (Abbott)	200 mg/5 ml suspension
		400 mg/5 ml suspension
Estolate	Generic (Various)	250 mg tablets
	Ilosone (Dista)	500 mg tablets
		125 mg/5 ml suspension
		250 mg/5 ml suspension

*Contains equivalent of erythromycin base

from acid degradation in the stomach. Another approach chemically modifies the erythromycin molecule to decrease acid inactivation. Chemical modification consists of preparing the stearate salt, the ethylsuccinate ester, and the lauryl sulfate salt to the propionyl ester (estolate).

When oral erythromycin preparations are administered in the correct dose and with proper timing in relation to food intake, no one type of preparation appears to offer a significant therapeutic advantage in treating mild to moderate infections. Erythromycin estolate usually is not recommended for adults because of the increased risk of cholestatic hepatitis. In children, however, this derivative rarely causes hepatitis, and some pediatric specialists prefer this formulation because of better availability.

Staphylococcal infections of the eyelid are commonly treated with erythromycin ointment (see Table 11.8) applied on the lid margins. Warm, moist compresses should be applied to the lid, and then the lid margins should be gently cleaned with dilute baby shampoo or a commercial lid cleanser before applying the drug. Erythromycin ointment can be applied at bedtime or more often if the severity of the infection requires.

As discussed earlier, the CDC recommends erythromycin or tetracycline ointment as an alternative to silver nitrate for the prophylaxis of ophthalmia neonatorum.[7] Like silver nitrate, erythromycin is effective for prophylaxis of gonococcal ophthalmia neonatorum.[94] An early study suggested that prophylaxis with erythromycin ointment prevented chlamydial conjunctivitis of the newborn, while silver nitrate did not.[95] Subsequent studies[96,97] demonstrate that silver nitrate is equally effective as erythromycin in preventing chlamydial neonatal infection. For prophylaxis, an approximately 0.5 to 1 cm ribbon of ointment is instilled into each conjunctival sac and is not flushed from the eyes following application.

Chlamydia trachomatis infections in infants and children are primary indications for the use of oral erythromycin. This antibiotic is as effective as the tetracyclines for chlamydial infections and is safer for pregnant women, nursing mothers, and children under 8 years of age.

Erythromycin is also an effective alternative to tetracycline for the treatment of adult chlamydial venereal disease. Adults should receive 2 g of erythromycin daily in 4 divided doses for at least 7 days.[98] Trachoma and inclusion conjunctivitis in the older child or adult can also be effectively treated with oral erythromycin with a 3-week course of 2 g daily in 4 divided doses.[79] Patients receiving full oral therapeutic doses of antibiotic do not need topical antimicrobial treatment with ophthalmic erythromycin ointment. Topical treatment alone is extremely slow, is usually only partially effective in treating adult or neonatal chlamydial disease, and allows frequent relapses.[79]

Clarithromycin.   Clarithromycin, a more recently developed macrolide antibiotic, is the 6-O-methyl derivative of erythromycin. It is stable in gastric acid and is well absorbed. Since the half-life of clarithromycin is approximately twice that of erythromycin, patients take clarithromycin only twice daily compared to 4 times a day for erythromycin. When combined with its active metabolite, 14-hydroxyclarithromycin, clarithromycin is active against *H. influenzae*. Clarithromycin is considerably more active than erythromycin against *Chlamydia*.[99]

Clarithromycin is indicated for the treatment of mild to moderate infections of the upper and lower respiratory tract and skin with susceptible strains of *Streptococcus pyogenes*, *S. pneumoniae*, *H. influenzae*, *Legionella pneumophilia*, and *Mycoplasma pneumoniae*. The usual dosage is 250 to 500 mg twice a day for 7 to 14 days.

Clarithromycin may be an effective topical or systemic antibiotic for the treatment of ocular infections caused by nontuberculous mycobacteria, especially *M. chelonae* and *M. fortuitum* keratitis.[100]

Azithromycin.   Azithromycin is another recent macrolide antibiotic. Following oral administration, azithromycin is rapidly absorbed and widely distributed throughout the body.[99] Because azithromycin has an extended half-life, once-daily dosing is effective and encourages patient compliance.[99] Compared with erythromycin, azithromycin is more active against gram-negative bacteria such as *H. influenzae* and *Moraxella catarrhalis*.

Azithromycin is indicated for mild infections of the respiratory tract and skin caused by susceptible strains of *S. pneumoniae*, *H. influenzae*, and *S. pyogenes*. Treatment is 500 mg as a single dose on the first day followed by 250 mg once daily on days 2 through 5. A single 1-gram dose of azithromycin is effective in the treatment of Chlamydia urethritis and cervicitis.[101] A single 1-gram dose may also prove effective for the treatment of Chlamydia conjunctivitis.[100] Recent studies have suggested that azithromycin may effectively treat toxoplasma infection.[102]

SIDE EFFECTS

Erythromycin is one of the safest antibiotics in clinical use. Gastrointestinal irritation including abdominal cramps, nausea, vomiting, and diarrhea is the most common adverse event produced by erythromycin and is usually associated with oral administration.[103] Irritation is dose related and more common with doses of 2 g or more daily. Some brands of enteric-coated tablets and the ester derivatives (e.g.,

ethylsuccinate) can be taken with food to minimize these adverse effects.

Like erythromycin, the most common side effects of azithromycin and clarithromycin are gastrointestinal, with diarrhea, nausea, and abdominal pain being the most frequently reported.[99] Other side effects of azithromycin include palpitations, vaginitis, headache, dizziness, fatigue, and hypersensitivity reactions. Clarithromycin can cause headache and dyspepsia.

The most serious toxicity of erythromycin involves cholestatic hepatitis, which occurs mainly in adults and only when the estolate preparation of erythromycin is used.[104] Symptoms of nausea, vomiting, and abdominal pain followed by jaundice, fever, and abnormal liver function tests consistent with cholestatic hepatitis can begin after approximately 10 days of therapy. The abnormalities generally resolve within days to a few weeks after discontinuing the drug but may return rapidly on rechallenge. The syndrome appears to be a hypersensitivity reaction to the specific structure of the estolate compound; thus, despite the rarity of this reaction, erythromycin estolate should be used with caution.

Mild allergic reactions such as urticaria and other rashes, fever, and eosinophilia have occurred occasionally with erythromycin use. Sensorineural hearing loss, although extremely rare, has been reported following the use of large doses of erythromycin or the use of erythromycin in the presence of renal failure.[105] The hearing loss usually improves gradually on discontinuation of the drug.

CONTRAINDICATIONS

The macrolide antibiotics are contraindicated in patients with known hypersensitivity or intolerance to any macrolide. Since clarithromycin can have adverse effects on embryo-fetal development in animals, this drug should be avoided in pregnant women unless no other therapy is appropriate.

Chloramphenicol

PHARMACOLOGY

Chloramphenicol acts by binding to the 50S subunit of the bacterial ribosome and blocking peptidyl transferase, thereby inhibiting protein synthesis. This inhibition of protein synthesis produces a bacteriostatic effect on sensitive organisms.

CLINICAL USES

Chloramphenicol is active against most gram-positive and gram-negative bacteria, *Rickettsia*, *Chlamydia*, spirochetes, and *Mycoplasma*; *Pseudomonas aeruginosa* is resistant. However, despite its broad antibacterial spectrum, generally good tolerance by patients, and desirable pharmacokinetic characteristics, chloramphenicol's ability to cause fatal aplastic anemia limits its usefulness, even when administered topically to the eye. Indications for chloramphenicol include severe or life-threatening infections caused by susceptible organisms that are not responsive to less toxic drugs.[106] Systemic use of chloramphenicol for ocular infections has been limited to the treatment of endophthalmitis following penetrating trauma or surgery. Because of chloramphenicol's high lipid solubility, the drug can cross the blood-aqueous barrier. Since it also has a reasonably broad spectrum, it would seem an ideal drug for treatment of endophthalmitis. However, concern about its ability to cause aplastic anemia has shifted the drugs of choice for intraocular infections to a penicillinase-resistant penicillin or a cephalosporin combined with an aminoglycoside.[22]

Topical application of chloramphenicol ointment or solution (see Table 11.8) is effective against the majority of bacterial infections of the external eye.[107,108] However, because aplastic anemia has occurred following topical ocular use of chloramphenicol,[109–111] its use should be limited to infections for which less toxic antibiotics prove ineffective.

SIDE EFFECTS

Chloramphenicol causes two types of hematopoietic abnormalities. The first is a dose-related toxic effect causing a reversible bone marrow depression associated with inhibition of mitochondrial protein synthesis. Reticulocytopenia, anemia, elevated serum iron and iron-binding capacity, and decreased erythrocytic uptake of iron characterize this toxicity. It is more likely to occur in patients receiving 6 g or more daily or in patients with serum levels of approximately 25 mg/ml. Usually discontinuing use of the antibiotic reverses this toxicity.[112]

A second, more serious type of bone marrow depression consists of aplastic anemia. Considered an idiosyncratic reaction rather than a drug toxicity, aplastic anemia occurs most commonly weeks to months following completion of therapy and is not dose-related. It can occur after either systemic or topical drug use[109,111,113] but is more common after systemic administration. In the most severe form of aplastic anemia, pancytopenia with an aplastic marrow is present. Prognosis is thus very poor, since the anemia is usually irreversible. This condition develops in approximately one in 25,000 patients who receive systemic chloramphenicol.[114] Before administering chloramphenicol, even topically, baseline blood counts should be obtained. Thereafter, routine blood studies (every 48 hours) may reveal early changes, and the dosage of the drug can be reduced or discontinued if bone marrow depression occurs.

A high plasma concentration of chloramphenicol in premature infants and neonates can occur because of the immature liver's inability to conjugate the drug or because the immature kidney cannot excrete the active form of the drug. This accumulation can cause a toxic reaction known as the "gray baby syndrome," which is characterized by abdominal distention, vomiting, flaccidity, cyanosis, circulatory collapse, and death. Because the gray baby syndrome can prove fatal, infants should not receive chloramphenicol during the first 2 weeks of life except under unusual circumstances.

Both mild and relatively severe neurologic complications can occur following the use of systemic chloramphenicol. Confusion, depression, or delirium, sometimes associated with headache or mild fever, are not uncommon. Patients receiving prolonged chloramphenicol therapy may develop optic neuropathy resulting in decreased visual acuity,[115,116] and the visual problems associated with the neuropathy do not always resolve on discontinuation of the drug.

Adverse gastrointestinal reactions following use of systemic chloramphenicol include nausea, vomiting, glossitis, stomatitis, diarrhea, and enterocolitis. Rash, angioedema, and urticaria can also follow the administration of chloramphenicol. Sensitization to the drug can occur with topical ocular use, but hypersensitivity reactions to chloramphenicol are rare.

CONTRAINDICATIONS

Because serious and fatal blood dyscrasias can occur after the administration of chloramphenicol, it should be used only in serious infections for which less potentially dangerous drugs are ineffective or contraindicated. Chloramphenicol is contraindicated in patients with known hypersensitivity or intolerance to chloramphenicol, a blood cell or bone marrow disorder, and in patients undergoing dialysis who have other complications, such as cirrhosis.[117]

Clindamycin

PHARMACOLOGY

Like erythromycin and chloramphenicol, clindamycin binds to the 50S ribosomal subunit and inhibits protein synthesis. Clindamycin is active against most gram-positive and anaerobic gram-negative bacteria. It is available for oral, intramuscular, and intravenous administration.

CLINICAL USES

Clindamycin can cause serious or even fatal pseudomembranous colitis. Considering that safer alternative antibiotics are available, this limits the use of clindamycin to only a few conditions. Clindamycin is often the drug of choice for treating anaerobic infections. It is effective for infections outside the CNS that involve *B. fragilis* or other penicillin-resistant anaerobic bacteria; usually these are intraabdominal or gynecologic/pelvic infections. Clindamycin may be useful for the treatment of ocular toxoplasmosis. The recurrent, necrotizing lesions of toxoplasmic retinochoroiditis result from the multiplication of previously encysted *Toxoplasma gondii* in the ocular tissues.[118] Although several antimicrobial drugs, such as the sulfonamides and pyrimethamine, can interfere with growth of the proliferative form of the parasite, their efficacy against the encysted form is limited. Drugs that destroy the parasite within the cysts would have great value, since eradication of the encysted organisms would prevent recurrent episodes. Clindamycin may have this potential. An animal study[119] involving treatment of "healed" toxoplasmic retinochoroiditis demonstrated that clindamycin is effective in reducing the number of cysts and viable organisms in the ocular structures. It did not, however, sterilize all the specimens obtained from chronically infected eyes.

Clindamycin alone or in combination with sulfadiazine also appears effective for the treatment of active recurrent toxoplasmic retinochoroiditis in humans. Ferguson[120] has reported that clindamycin therapy produced rapid resolution of the inflamed toxoplasmic lesions and hastened healing. Final evaluation of clindamycin for the treatment of both active and quiescent ocular toxoplasmosis must, however, await the outcome of controlled, double-masked studies since the active lesions usually heal even without treatment. Clindamycin is expensive and has not yet been approved by the Food and Drug Administration (FDA) for treatment of toxoplasmosis.

SIDE EFFECTS

Clindamycin is usually well tolerated. A common gastrointestinal side effect is mild to moderate diarrhea.[121] More importantly, this antibiotic can allow overgrowth of *Clostridium difficile* in the intestinal tract, causing potentially fatal pseudomembranous colitis.[122] If severe diarrhea occurs while a patient is taking clindamycin, the drug should be discontinued, and, if appropriate, the patient should be treated with vancomycin. Although pseudomembranous colitis is treatable, is not unique to clindamycin, and is relatively uncommon, clindamycin should be prescribed only when specifically required and then with knowledge of the potential for this adverse reaction.

Hypersensitivity reactions can occur during clindamycin treatment; pruritus, rash, and urticaria have been the most commonly observed manifestations. Transient changes in liver function have also occurred during clindamycin administration, but serious hepatotoxicity is rare.

CONTRAINDICATIONS

Clindamycin therapy has been associated with severe pseudomembranous colitis, which can be fatal. Therefore, this drug should be reserved for serious infections where less toxic antimicrobial drugs are ineffective or not tolerated. Patients receiving clindamycin should be carefully monitored for indications of pseudomembranous colitis. Clindamycin is contraindicated in patients with known hypersensitivity or intolerance to the drug or with a history of Crohn's disease or ulcerative colitis.[123]

Drugs Affecting Intermediary Metabolism

Antibacterial drugs that affect the intermediary metabolism of bacteria include the sulfonamides, pyrimethamine, and trimethoprim.

Sulfonamides

PHARMACOLOGY

The sulfonamides were the first group of chemotherapeutic agents used for the prevention or treatment of bacterial infections in humans. They are broad-spectrum compounds effective against gram-positive and gram-negative bacteria as well as *Actinomyces, Chlamydia,* plasmodia, and *Toxoplasma.* Since, in general, the sulfonamides exert only a bacteriostatic effect, cellular, and humoral immune mechanisms must assume responsibility for eradicating the infecting bacteria.

The sulfonamides act by inhibiting the bacterial synthesis of folic acid, a chemical required for synthesis of nucleic acid and protein. Because bacterial cells are impermeable to folic acid, they synthesize it from para-aminobenzoic acid (PABA). The sulfonamides are structural analogs of PABA, and they competitively inhibit the first step in synthesis of folic acid—the conversion of PABA into dihydropteroic acid (Fig. 11.6). Because humans absorb preformed folic acid from food, sulfonamide inhibition has only a minimal effect on host cells.

Sulfonamide-induced inhibition of folic acid synthesis can be reversed by several antagonistic compounds, of which PABA is the most prominent. Local anesthetics such as procaine, tetracaine, and benoxinate, which are esters of PABA, also antagonize these drugs *in vitro* and *in vivo.*[124] The antibacterial action of the sulfonamides can further be inhibited by blood, pus, and tissue breakdown products because the bacterial requirement of folic acid decreases in media that contain purines and thymidine. Thus, sulfonamide therapy is contraindicated for infections with marked purulent exudation (Fig. 11.7).

Because acquired resistance to the sulfonamides is widespread, other antibacterial agents have replaced sulfonamides as drugs of first choice for the treatment of all but a few major infections. Mechanisms of resistance include an overproduction of PABA by the bacteria, decreased enzyme affinity for the sulfonamide, decreased bacterial permeability to the drug, and increased inactivation of the drug by the bacteria. Cross-resistance between sulfonamides is common.

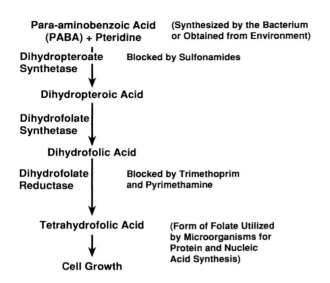

FIGURE 11.6 **Mechanism of action of sulfonamides, trimethoprim, and pyrimethamine.**

The diagram shows:

Para-aminobenzoic Acid (PABA) + Pteridine — (Synthesized by the Bacterium or Obtained from Environment)

↓ Dihydropteroate Synthetase — Blocked by Sulfonamides

Dihydropteroic Acid

↓ Dihydrofolate Synthetase

Dihydrofolic Acid

↓ Dihydrofolate Reductase — Blocked by Trimethoprim and Pyrimethamine

Tetrahydrofolic Acid — (Form of Folate Utilized by Microorganisms for Protein and Nucleic Acid Synthesis)

↓

Cell Growth

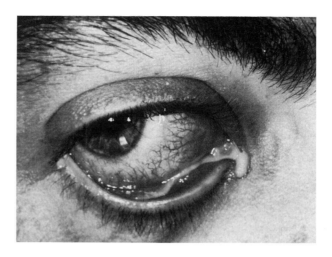

FIGURE 11.7 **Bacterial conjunctivitis with marked purulent exudation. Purulent exudation is a contraindication to topical sulfonamide treatment. (Courtesy Jimmy D. Bartlett, O.D.)**

CLINICAL USES

Clinically the sulfonamides can be divided into three groups: short-acting (administered every 4–6 hours), intermediate-acting (administered every 6–12 hours), and topically applied (Table 11.13).

Short- and Intermediate-Acting Sulfonamides.   These drugs include sulfisoxazole, sulfamethizole, sulfacytine, sulfamethoxazole, and sulfadiazine (see Table 11.13). Sulfamerazine and sulfamethazine together with sulfadiazine can form a short-acting mixture termed *trisulfapyrimidines*. A combination of sulfonamides has the advantage of improved solubility. The older sulfonamides are less soluble than the newer ones and cause urinary tract injury due to precipitation of acetylated drug crystals. Sulfonamide mixtures can circumvent this problem. In the combination, each drug can coexist in solution without interfering with the solubility of the others. Thus, the total concentration of sulfonamides in the mixture is equal to a high dose of a single sulfonamide, but none of the individual drugs has a high enough concentration to precipitate in the kidney. However, because newer, more soluble sulfonamides, such as sulfisoxazole, are available, the use of combinations has declined sharply.

Sulfonamides are sometimes used to treat chlamydial diseases. Topical sulfonamide therapy has occasionally been used to treat chlamydial neonatal conjunctivitis,[77] but this infection is best treated with systemic erythromycin.[78] The treatment of choice for adult inclusion conjunctivitis is an oral tetracycline or erythromycin, with the sulfonamides reserved as a third choice.[79] Patients receiving oral therapeutic doses of any of these drugs do not require topical antimicrobial treatment of the eye.

Trachoma has been treated with oral sulfamethoxazole[125] and with oral or topical sulfacetamide,[125,126] but the preferred treatment is an oral tetracycline, with oral erythromycin a second choice.[79] Oral sulfonamides are also used to treat chlamydial venereal disease, but an oral tetracycline or erythromycin is the drug of choice.[98]

TABLE 11.13
Clinical Uses of Selected Sulfonamides

Drug	Clinical Uses
Short- and Intermediate-Acting	
Sulfisoxazole	Urinary tract infections,
Sulfamethizole	*Nocardia* infections,
Sulfacytine	prophylaxis of rheumatic
Sulfamethoxazole	fever or otitis media,
Sulfadiazine	lymphogranuloma
Trisulfapyrimidines	venereum, *Pneumocystis*
Sulfamerazine	*carinii* infections,
Sulfamethazine	toxoplasmosis, malaria
Sulfadiazine	
Poorly Absorbed	
Sulfasalazine	Ulcerative colitis, regional enteritis
Topically Applied	
Sulfacetamide	Blepharitis, conjunctivitis
Sulfisoxazole	
Silver Sulfadiazine	Prevention of burn infections
Mafenide	

The sulfonamides, particularly sulfadiazine and *trisulfa-pyrimidines*, can be used to treat toxoplasmic retinochoroiditis. The severe damage of the retina and adjacent tissues can be attributed to several factors. Direct infection of retinal cells and multiplication of the parasite are probably the most important of these, but hypersensitivity reactions by the host to toxoplasmic antigens as well as to antigens released from the photoreceptors can also cause retinal damage.[127] Corticosteroids alone have been used successfully to treat this condition, but treatment with steroids may also weaken the host's natural cellular defenses and increase the risk of uncontrolled parasite proliferation. For this reason, steroids should not be used to treat toxoplasmic retinochoroiditis without the cover of at least one antitoxoplasmic agent.[128] Although pyrimethamine and sulfonamides constitute the classic agents for treatment of toxoplasmosis, newer drugs such as clindamycin may eventually substitute for them or be used concomitantly.[120,129] Some authors[130] consider that if only one drug is chosen, trisulfapyrimidines should be the first choice because of minimal expense, good tolerance, lack of spoilage, and simplicity of use.

Topically Applied Sulfonamides.   Topical ophthalmic preparations of sulfonamides include sodium sulfacetamide and sulfisoxazole (Table 11.14). Sodium sulfacetamide is available in 10%, 15%, and 30% solutions; in 10% ointment; and in combination with the steroids prednisolone acetate, prednisolone phosphate, and fluorometholone alcohol (Table 11.15). The 10% solution is the most common preparation for treatment of routine bacterial conjunctivitis because the 30% concentration causes significant stinging on instillation.[131] The ointment may be used instead of the solution, but it is typically reserved for application at bedtime or for use in children. Sulfisoxazole is available as a 4% ophthalmic solution and ointment, and it too can be used to treat conjunctivitis and blepharitis caused by susceptible bacteria.

Combinations of sodium sulfacetamide and prednisolone acetate or phosphate are commercially available and have been an effective treatment for chronic blepharitis. In a comparison study, Aragones[132] investigated patients with clinically diagnosed blepharitis, with an infectious component sensitive to sodium sulfacetamide. Patients were treated using either sulfacetamide alone or the sulfacetamide-prednisolone combination. Results indicated that topical 10% sulfacetamide eliminated culturable evidence of the causative bacteria and cleared the patient's symptoms in approximately 6 to 8 days. Administration of anti-inflammatory therapy along with the anti-infective treatment reduced by half the time required for relief of symptoms without adversely affecting the anti-infective action of the combination. In addition, a few patients who had been treated with

TABLE 11.14
Sulfonamide Preparations for Topical Ocular Therapy

Trade Name	Manufacturer
Sulfacetamide Solutions—10%	
Generic	Various
AK-Sulf	Akorn
Bleph-10	Allergan
Sulf-10	Ciba Vision
Sodium Sulamyd	Schering
Ocusulf-10	Optopics
Sulfacetamide Solutions—15%	
Generic	Various
Isopto Cetamide	Alcon
Sulfacetamide Solutions—30%	
Generic	Various
Sodium Sulamyd	Schering
Sulfacetamide Ointments—10%	
Generic	Various
AK-Sulf	Akorn
Cetamide	Alcon
Bleph-10	Allergan
Sodium Sulamyd	Schering
Sulfisoxazole Solution and Ointment—4%	
Gantrisin	Roche

TABLE 11.15
Sulfacetamide[a]-Steroid Combinations

Steroid	Trade Name (Manufacturer)
Solutions and Suspensions	
Prednisolone acetate 0.5%	Predsulfair (Bausch & Lomb) Metimyd Suspension (Schering) Sulphrin (Bausch & Lomb)
Prednisolone acetate 0.25%	Isopto Cetapred (Alcon)
Prednisolone phosphate 0.25%	Vasocidin (Ciba Vision)
Prednisolone acetate 0.2%	Blephamide (Allergan) Sulfacort (Rugby)
Fluorometholone 0.1%	FML-S (Allergan)
Ointments	
Prednisolone acetate 0.5%	Sulphrin (Bausch & Lomb) Vasocidin (Ciba Vision) Metimyd (Schering) AK-Cide (Akorn)
Prednisolone acetate 0.25%	Cetapred (Alcon)
Prednisolone acetate 0.2%	Blephamide (Allergan)

[a]10% concentration

sulfacetamide alone had persistent symptoms of inflammation even after "bacteriologic cure." When a steroid was added to their antibiotic regimen, the patients experienced a dramatic improvement.[132]

Although the treatment of chronic blepharitis with sulfacetamide or with the combination of sulfacetamide and prednisolone can be clinically useful, an additional factor must be considered. In one study,[133] 50% of patients with clinical "staphylococcal blepharitis" were culture-positive for *S. aureus*. The remainder were positive for *S. epidermidis*. Possibly due to overuse of sulfonamides in the treatment of chronic blepharitis, only 29% of the *S. aureus* isolates and 33% of the *S. epidermidis* isolates were sensitive to sulfonamides. With the large number of strains of *S. aureus* and *S. epidermidis* resistant to sulfonamides, a sulfonamide alone or in combination with a steroid is no longer considered the appropriate therapy for this condition.

In contrast to the resistance found among isolates of *S. aureus* and *S. epidermidis*, *Streptococcus pneumoniae* and *H. influenzae* remain sensitive to the sulfonamides. Thus, topical sodium sulfacetamide or sulfisoxazole is still useful for some forms of bacterial conjunctivitis presenting with minimal purulent discharge.

SIDE EFFECTS

The sulfonamides can produce a wide variety of side effects, and an adverse reaction to one sulfonamide frequently precludes the use of other sulfonamide derivatives. Anorexia, nausea, vomiting, and diarrhea are common side effects of systemic sulfonamide therapy. Blood dyscrasias such as acute hemolytic anemia, aplastic anemia, agranulocytosis, thrombocytopenia, and leukopenia occur only rarely, but the consequences of these conditions are potentially serious.[134] Because sulfonamides cross the placenta and compete with bilirubin for albumin binding, they can cause high levels of free bilirubin in infants born to mothers who have taken sulfonamides close to term. Since sulfonamides are also excreted in breast milk, nursing mothers or pregnant women close to term should not be prescribed these drugs.

Sulfonamides administered by any route, including topical, may cause hypersensitivity reactions, including urticaria and rashes often accompanied by pruritus and fever. Other hypersensitivity reactions include malaise and a serum sickness-like syndrome.[134] A case has been reported of an immune corneal ring formation after administration of sulfamethoxazole.[135] Contact dermatitis is common with topical application of these drugs, and they have caused more serious dermatologic problems such as erythema nodosum, erythema multiforme (Stevens-Johnson syndrome), and exfoliative dermatitis. Rubin[136] reported a patient who experienced a skin reaction after taking an oral sulfonamide and subsequently developed Stevens-Johnson syndrome after topical ophthalmic use of sodium sulfacetamide. Perhaps the most common ocular side effect in patients taking systemic sulfonamides is transient myopia, with or without induced astigmatism.[137,138] The myopia is usually bilateral and may exceed several diopters, but the refractive state usually returns to normal when the serum drug level decreases (see Chapter 37).

In addition to hypersensitivity reactions, topical administration of sulfonamides can lead to other problems. When sulfonamide ointments are applied for treatment of staphylococcal blepharitis, local photosensitization may result in sunburning of the lid margins, which can mimic an allergic reaction.[139] Topical use of sulfadiazine ointment for 1 year has caused formation of multiple small white concretions of sulfadiazine within cysts in the palpebral conjunctiva,[140] and topical use of sulfacetamide has caused white plaques to form on the cornea.[141] Topical sulfacetamide in the 30% concentration has been reported to produce a significant decrease in corneal sensitivity, while the 10% concentration produced no change compared with the control.[142]

CONTRAINDICATIONS

Sulfonamides are contraindicated in patients with known hypersensitivity or intolerance to any member of this family of drugs. Sulfonamides are also contraindicated in pregnancy at term, nursing mothers, and infants less than 2 months old because sulfonamides can promote kernicterus in the newborn by displacing bilirubin from plasma proteins.[143] The sulfonamides are contraindicated in patients with documented blood dyscrasias.[144]

Caution should be used in prescribing sulfonamides for patients taking oral hypoglycemic drugs, such as tolbutamide or chlorpropamide, since the sulfonamides can potentiate the hypoglycemic effect of these drugs. Sulfonamides can enhance the action of coumarin anticoagulants and should be used with caution in patients taking these drugs. PABA-containing compounds and PABA analogs, such as the ester-type local anesthetics, can reduce the effectiveness of sulfonamides by competing with the antibiotic for the enzyme dihydropteroate synthetase, thereby allowing bacteria to synthesize more folic acid from the available PABA substrates.

Pyrimethamine and Trimethoprim

PHARMACOLOGY

Pyrimethamine and trimethoprim are 2 of many 2,4-diaminopyrimidines that were synthesized and tested for antimicrobial activity. Both pyrimethamine and trimethoprim bind to and reversibly inhibit the enzyme dihydrofolate reductase, which catalyzes the reduction of dihydrofolic acid to tetrahydrofolic acid (see Fig. 11.6). The trimethoprim-binding affinity is much stronger for the bacterial enzyme than the corresponding mammalian enzyme and thereby manifests true selective toxicity.[145] A powerful synergism exists between either of these drugs and the sulfonamides. The sulfonamides inhibit dihydropteroate synthetase, the enzyme that converts PABA to dihydropteroic acid, the immediate precursor of dihydrofolic acid, while pyrimethamine and trimethoprim block a sequential step in the pathway, the conversion of dihydrofolic acid to tetrahydrofolic acid (see Fig. 11.6). This sequential blockage of the same biosynthetic pathway results in a high degree of synergistic activity against a wide spectrum of microorganisms.

CLINICAL USES

Pyrimethamine was initially selected for its antimalarial properties. In combination with a sulfonamide such as sulfadiazine, it is useful for the treatment of acute attacks of chloroquine-resistant *P. falciparum* malaria, and it is also used as a prophylactic and suppressive drug for *P. vivax* malaria.

Administered concurrently with sulfadiazine or with triple sulfonamides (sulfadiazine, sulfamerazine, and sulfamethazine), pyrimethamine is effective for the treatment of toxoplasmosis.[130] The synergism of the combined drugs greatly enhances the therapeutic effect; combined therapy requires only one-eighth as much sulfonamide and one-twenty-fourth as much pyrimethamine as would be necessary if either drug were used alone.[146]

Trimethoprim is used in combination with sulfamethoxazole for treatment of *Pneumocystis carinii* pneumonitis in the immunologically impaired patient and for treatment of adults with shigellosis, urinary tract infections, acute otitis media, and acute exacerbations of chronic bronchitis associated with *H. influenzae* or *S. pneumoniae*. It is also used as the sole drug for initial episodes of uncomplicated urinary tract infections. A combination of trimethoprim (0.1%) and polymyxin B (10,000 units/ml) is available as a topical ophthalmic solution (see Table 11.9), which has a broad spectrum of activity for treatment of surface ocular infections. Trimethoprim has significant *in vitro* activity against gram-positive and gram-negative organisms including staphylococci, streptococci, *Haemophilus* and gram-negative enterics. However, since it is not active against *Pseudomonas*, polymyxin B is included in the combination to cover gram-negative bacteria, including *Pseudomonas*.

The effectiveness of trimethoprim-polymyxin B has been evaluated against a combination of trimethoprim, sulfacetamide, and polymyxin B for the treatment of blepharitis, conjunctivitis, and blepharoconjunctivitis.[147] Trimethoprim-polymyxin B alone proved effective, and sulfacetamide did not enhance the clinical or bacteriologic efficacy of the combination. Topical trimethoprim-polymyxin B is as effective as a combination of gramicidin-neomycin-polymyxin B or chloramphenicol alone for the treatment of blepharoconjunctivitis or conjunctivitis.[148,149] In addition, topical trimethoprim-polymyxin B has been shown to be as effec-

tive as topical gentamicin or sulfacetamide in treating 158 patients with culture proven *H. influenzae* or *S. pneumoniae* conjunctivitis.[150]

SIDE EFFECTS

When the recommended dosage of 25 mg pyrimethamine once weekly is used for prophylaxis of malaria, no significant toxic effects occur. Higher dosages, however, as needed for the treatment of toxoplasmosis, can result in white blood cell and platelet depression or megaloblastic anemia caused by drug-induced folic acid deficiency.

When given in the recommended dosages, trimethoprim-sulfamethoxazole usually does not produce folate deficiency in normal individuals. For a patient deficient in folic acid, however, this drug combination may precipitate hematologic reactions associated with a deficiency of this nutrient. Administering folinic (*not* folic) acid may counteract the toxicity induced by pyrimethamine or trimethoprim. Use of folinic acid bypasses the need for dihydrofolate reductase by supplying the fully reduced folate.

Skin reactions typical of those produced by the sulfonamides have an increased incidence when the trimethoprim-sulfamethoxazole combination is used compared with a sulfonamide alone.[151]

Trimethoprim-polymyxin B is well tolerated with few reported serious adverse reactions with topical ophthalmic use. The most frequent adverse event (about 4%) is local irritation, including transient burning or stinging, itching, or redness following instillation.[152] Less than 2% of patients experience a hypersensitivity reaction consisting of lid edema, itching, increased redness, tearing, or periocular rash.[152] Since no cross-allergic reactions occur between the sulfonamides and trimethoprim, trimethoprim-polymyxin B is especially useful for patients allergic to the sulfonamides.[153]

CONTRAINDICATIONS

Pyrimethamine and trimethoprim are contraindicated in patients with known hypersensitivity to these drugs. Both drugs are contraindicated in patients with documented megaloblastic anemia due to folate deficiency. Although the presence of thymine and thymidine in pus could allow some bacteria to escape the blockage of dihydrofolate reductase produced by trimethoprim, clinical studies suggest that a purulent discharge is not a contraindication to the use of trimethoprim-polymyxin B.[147,150] This clinical effectiveness seems to depend on the high concentration of trimethoprim overcoming the effect of thymine on the surface of an infected eye.[154] Moreover, with some bacteria, a synergistic action may occur between trimethoprim and polymyxin B. This appears to enhance the antibacterial effect of this combination.[155]

TABLE 11.16
Commonly Used Fluoroquinolones for Topical Ocular Therapy

Generic Name	Trade Name	Indication	Formulation
Ciprofloxacin	Ciloxan	Conjunctivitis and keratitis	0.3% solution
Norfloxacin	Chibroxin	Conjunctivitis	0.3% solution
Ofloxacin	Ocuflox	Conjunctivitis	0.3% solution

Drugs Affecting Bacterial DNA Synthesis

Drugs that inhibit bacterial DNA synthesis include a new generation of fluorinated quinolones (fluoroquinolones) structurally related to nalidixic acid: norfloxacin, ofloxacin, ciprofloxacin, lomefloxacin, temafloxacin, and enoxacin. Temafloxacin was marketed in 1991 but withdrawn when serious adverse reactions were reported, such as hemolytic anemia and renal failure. The other fluoroquinolones have proven both efficacious and safe in clinical use.

Pharmacology

The fluoroquinolones interfere with DNA synthesis during bacterial replication by inhibiting DNA gyrase activity.[156] During bacterial DNA replication or transcription, DNA gyrase cuts and reseals the DNA strands to prevent excessive supercoiling. Bacterial gyrase, unlike the comparable human enzyme, is susceptible to inhibition by the fluoroquinolones, and this inhibition kills the bacteria.

Oral nalidixic acid has been used for many years to treat urinary tract infections because it is bactericidal for most of the gram-negative bacteria that cause these infections. The drug is less active against gram-positive bacteria, and *Pseudomonas* is resistant. In contrast, the new fluoroquinolones are broad-spectrum antibacterial drugs. These drugs demonstrate low MICs against both gram-positive and gram-negative bacteria, but fluoroquinolone activity against anaerobes and mycobacteria is variable.

Despite initial claims of a low frequency of resistance to the quinolones, including ciprofloxacin,[156] staphylococcal strains are developing a relatively high rate of clinical resistance against ciprofloxacin.[157] Strains of methicillin-resistant staphylococci have also become rapidly resistant to ciprofloxacin despite initial *in vitro* indications of susceptibility.[158] Other organisms developing resistance include *Pseudomonas aeruginosa*, *Klebsiella pneumoniae*, *Citrobacter* species, and *Enterobacter* species.[159] *Staphylococcus epidermidis* and *Xanthomonas maltophia* resistant to ciprofloxacin have been isolated from corneal ulcers.[160]

Clinical Uses

Oral ciprofloxacin, norfloxacin, enoxacin, lomefloxacin, and ofloxacin are indicated for the treatment of urinary tract infections, including those that are complicated and recurrent.[161,162] Norfloxacin, ciprofloxacin, enoxacin, and ofloxacin have been effective in the treatment of patients with uncomplicated gonorrhea.[163–165] Oral ciprofloxacin and norfloxacin are also effective in the treatment of acute diarrhea caused by enterotoxic *E. coli*, *Salmonella*, *Shigella*, and *Campylobacter*.[163] Following oral administration, ciprofloxacin, and ofloxacin achieve therapeutic levels in most tissues and thus can be used to treat gram-negative infections of the respiratory tract, bones, joints, and skin.

Ciprofloxacin, norfloxacin and ofloxacin are available as topical ophthalmic solutions (Table 11.16). Studies comparing the *in vitro* effectiveness of ciprofloxacin, norfloxacin, and ofloxacin against ocular pathogens with the effectiveness of antibacterial drugs such as bacitracin, erythromycin, tobramycin, and gentamicin have demonstrated that the fluoroquinolones have the greatest potency and broadest spectrum of activity.[32,166,167] In these studies, the flouroquinolones proved active against *S. aureus, S. epidermidis, Streptococcus pneumoniae, P. aeruginosa, H. influenzae,* and most other gram-negative bacteria.

Topical ciprofloxacin is effective for bacterial conjunctivitis. Clinical trials have demonstrated that ciprofloxacin 0.3% is as effective as tobramycin 0.3%[167] and chloramphenicol 0.5%[168] in eradicating or reducing the concentration of various bacterial pathogens. Limberg and Bugge,[169] using normal volunteers, have shown that ciprofloxacin tear concentrations are significantly greater than the MICs for 90% of bacterial strains of most potential pathogens 4 hours after a single application of the 0.3% solution.

Ciprofloxacin 0.3% solution and 0.3% ointment have been used successfully to treat bacterial keratitis caused by a variety of pathogens.[170–172] In one study,[170] 148 patients with culture-proven bacterial keratitis were treated with either ciprofloxacin 0.3% or standard therapy consisting of fortified cefazolin and fortified gentamicin or tobramycin. Treatment with ciprofloxacin yielded a 92% success rate, whereas standard therapy yielded an 88% success rate. In addition, 50 patients with bacterial keratitis unresponsive to initial therapy with other antibacterial drugs were treated with ciprofloxacin; the corneal ulcers resolved in 46 (92%) of the cases. Bacterial keratitis caused by methicillin-resistant strains of *Staphylococcus aureus* that were unresponsive to other antibiotics has also been successfully treated with 0.3% topical ciprofloxacin.[173] Atypical mycobacteria such as *Mycobacterium chelonae* and *M. fortuitum* are rare causes of keratitis. Topical ciprofloxacin has been effective against both organisms in a rabbit model[174] and in human keratitis.[175]

Like ciprofloxacin, norfloxacin can be used for treatment of bacterial conjunctivitis. Miller and associates[176] compared norfloxacin and gentamicin for the treatment of culture-positive conjunctivitis. After seven days, complete eradication of the pathogen occurred in 87 of 120 patients (72%) treated with norfloxacin and 101 of 133 patients (76%) treated with gentamicin. There was no significant difference in the effectiveness of the two drugs. In a similar study, Jacobson and associates[177] compared norfloxacin with tobramycin for treatment of external ocular infections. Bacteriologic outcomes were comparable in the two treatment groups. In two studies,[178,179] norfloxacin was compared with chloramphenicol for treatment of bacterial conjunctivitis and blepharoconjunctivitis. Norfloxacin was as effective as chloramphenicol in eradicating the pathogens, and its use avoided the potentially dangerous side effects of chloramphenicol. Topical norfloxacin can also be a useful alternative to gentamicin in the prophylaxis of conjunctivitis during conservative treatment of dacryocystitis in adults.[180]

Norfloxacin is not indicated for the treatment of bacterial keratitis. Despite the good *in vitro* activity of norfloxacin against ocular pathogens,[34] the commercially available concentration of norfloxacin has less ability to penetrate the cornea, and thus it might not achieve levels adequate for the eradication of bacteria.[181] However, Vajpayee and associates[182] have used topical norfloxacin 0.3% in the successful treatment of 12 patients with *Pseudomonas* corneal infections.

Ofloxacin has similar *in vitro* activity against ocular pathogens as do ciprofloxacin and norfloxacin.[166] In addition, it is clinically effective in the treatment of ocular bacterial infections such as conjunctivitis, blepharitis, and keratitis. The efficacy and safety of 0.3% ofloxacin have been compared to those of 0.5% chloramphenicol,[108] 0.3% tobramycin,[183] and 0.3% gentamicin[49] for the treatment of external bacterial ocular infections. The percentage of patients for whom ofloxacin decreased the clinical signs and symptoms of infection and eradicated the pathogens was similar to the percentage of patients successfully treated with chloramphenicol, tobramycin, or gentamicin. The low incidence of adverse reactions was also similar among the four drugs.

Even though ofloxacin and tobramycin are equally efficacious in the treatment of bacterial conjunctivitis, the signs and symptoms of infection are reduced more rapidly with ofloxacin than with tobramycin.[183] This reduction could be due to the superior tear profile of ofloxacin. Compared to tobramycin, ofloxacin remains in the tears at a concentration above the MICs for most ocular pathogens for a longer time,[52] and this could result in a more rapid eradication of the pathogens.

Studies of intraocular penetration after topical application in human eyes indicate that of the currently available topical fluoroquinolones, ofloxacin achieves the highest aqueous humor concentration.[184,185] Currently, little is known about the oral or IV use of the fluoroquinolones for intraocular infections. However, initial studies on the intraocular penetration and safety of ciprofloxacin suggest that this antibiotic may become useful for the treatment of these infections.[186-188] When ciprofloxacin is injected intravitreally, however, it is eliminated so quickly that it can provide only short-term therapy for endophthalmitis.[189]

Side Effects

As a group, the fluoroquinolones are generally well tolerated with a low incidence of adverse reactions. Following systemic administration, the most common side effects include nausea, headache, dizziness, rash, bitter taste, elevation of liver enzymes, and eosinophilia.[190]

The frequency of adverse reactions to topical ophthalmic ciprofloxacin, norfloxacin, and ofloxacin is low. In a study of over 1500 healthy volunteers and patients, no serious events related to ciprofloxacin occurred.[170] The most frequently reported adverse reactions were local burning or discomfort following instillation (9.7%); bitter taste following instillation (5.0%); white precipitates (3.6%); foreign body sensation (2.0%); itching (1.0%); and conjunctival hyperemia, chemosis and photophobia (less than 1% each). Frequent instillation of ciprofloxacin for treatment of corneal ulceration resulted in white precipitates occurring in 17% of the patients, but the precipitates did not require discontinuation of therapy. One report, however, suggests that the precipitates can form an adherent plaque on the cornea that interferes with healing.[191] Opaque deposits can also form on "bandage" soft contact lenses when ciprofloxacin and prednisolone are used concomitantly.[192] The corneal epithelial cytotoxicity of the fluoroquinolones has been evaluated in animal models, and each drug was found to have minimal toxicity at therapeutic concentrations.[193]

Contraindications

The quinolones are contraindicated in patients with a history of hypersensitivity to any quinolone. Absorption of oral norfloxacin, ciprofloxacin, and ofloxacin is reduced by ferrous sulfate, and thus they should not be taken concomitantly.[194] Oral ciprofloxacin inhibits the metabolism of theophylline, and toxicity can occur when the two drugs are administered concurrently (see Chapter 36). Oral administration of the fluoroquinolones can cause convulsions and should therefore be used with caution in patients with CNS disorders. Erosion of cartilage in the weight-bearing joints and other signs of arthropathy have been reported in several species of immature animals.[156] Although such lesions have not been described in humans, these drugs are not recommended for systemic administration in children, adolescents below the age of 18 years, or pregnant women. Topical administration to immature animals does not cause arthropathy, and the ophthalmic dosage form does not appear to affect the weight-bearing joints in humans.[176] All of the topical ophthalmic fluoroquinolones, including ciprofloxacin, norfloxacin, and ofloxacin, are approved for use in patients one year of age and older.

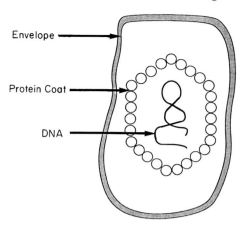

FIGURE 11.8 **Herpes virus particle showing the outer envelope and the nucleocapsid composed of the protein coat and DNA.**

Antiviral Drugs

Viruses are the smallest of the infectious organisms. They are obligate, intracellular organisms that can infect humans, animals, plants, and bacteria. Their simple structure consists of either DNA or RNA as genetic material and a protein coat called a *capsid*. For some viruses, an envelope composed of the nuclear or cell membrane of a previously infected cell surrounds the capsid (Fig. 11.8).

Viruses depend on host cells for multiplication. For a virus to replicate, it must invade (infect) a host cell and take over its metabolic machinery. After new viral nucleic acid and protein are produced, the host cell releases new viruses that can infect other host cells (Fig. 11.9). This type of infection produces an acute disease that is usually limited by the response of the patient's immune system. Alternatively, some viruses can invade cells and then become latent. In these cases, the viral DNA becomes incorporated into the host cell's DNA, where it escapes detection by the host's immune system. At some future time this viral DNA can be stimulated to produce new viruses that cause recurrent disease episodes.

Although the development of antibacterial drugs has progressed quickly over the last several decades, the development of effective antiviral drugs has not been as rapid. This results in large part from the nature of viruses them-

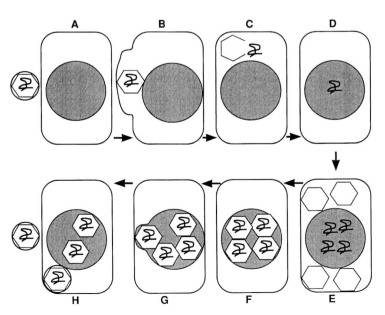

FIGURE 11.9 **Steps in herpes virus replication cycle.** *(A)* **Adsorption of the virus to the human cell.** *(B)* **Fusion of the viral envelope with the human cell membrane.** *(C)* **Release of the viral DNA.** *(D)* **Viral mRNA synthesis.** *(E)* **Viral protein and DNA synthesis.** *(F)* **Viral nucleocapsid assembly in nucleus.** *(G)* **"Budding" of nuclear membrane around viral nucleocapsid to produce infectious particle.** *(H)* **Replication process complete—new virus ready to infect another cell.**

selves. Viruses grow and multiply inside host cells and are integrated into the metabolism of these cells. Consequently, it is difficult to find an antiviral drug that is selectively toxic for the virus while leaving the host cells unaffected. Many of the currently available antiviral drugs are antimetabolites that inhibit nucleic acid synthesis; their usefulness is directly related to their ability to block viral nucleic acid synthesis selectively and leave host nucleic acid synthesis unaffected.

Because of ongoing development and testing of new antiviral drugs, consensus about the uses and therapeutic regimens for these drugs is not as complete as for the antibacterial drugs, and much of the work in this area is still in the investigational stage. The commercially available antiviral drugs are used primarily for the treatment of herpes infections. This virus group includes 4 distinct members: herpes simplex virus (HSV), varicella-zoster virus (VZV), Epstein-Barr virus (EBV), and cytomegalovirus (CMV). Two types of HSV exist: type 1, which is associated with infections involving the eye, mouth, and skin above the waist; and type 2, which usually affects the skin including and surrounding the genitalia. A primary systemic infection with HSV-1 occurs in most children and is often subclinical with mild, flu-like respiratory symptoms. If the primary infection has ocular manifestations, they usually begin as a follicular conjunctivitis. Clusters of vesicles can occur on the periorbital and eyelid skin; corneal involvement in the form of diffuse epithelial keratitis or microdendrites may also be present. Generally, the immune system controls the primary infection, but the virus usually becomes latent in the trigeminal ganglion, allowing for later recurrences of disease. During recurrent episodes, the viruses produced in the trigeminal ganglion move through the sensory nerves to the cornea and can infect the epithelial cells, producing a characteristic dendritic pattern. The virus can also cause stromal keratitis characterized by infiltration and necrosis or can cause disciform keratitis characterized by corneal edema. Besides affecting the eye, HSV-1 can cause recurrent herpes labialis, producing "cold sores" or "fever blisters" on the skin around the mouth. HSV-2 is a sexually transmitted disease that usually causes genital infection. As with HSV-1 infection, the primary HSV-2 infection allows the virus to become latent, and the disease usually becomes recurrent.

In the nonimmunized host, the primary infection with VZV produces chickenpox. Once this infection has occurred, the virus remains latent in sensory ganglia, such as the trigeminal ganglion, for the patient's life. When triggered by stress or other factors, the virus can reactivate, producing the syndrome of zoster (shingles). During a zoster episode, the virus replicates in the sensory ganglion and migrates along the sensory nerves to the skin or eye. Signs and symptoms include vesicular eruption and neuralgic pain in the areas supplied by the sensory nerves from the affected ganglion.

Herpes zoster ophthalmicus usually first manifests as a severe, unilateral, disabling neuralgia in the region innervated by the ophthalmic division of the trigeminal nerve. The virus then produces vesicles on the skin corresponding to the distribution of the nerve. Ocular complications include conjunctivitis, scleritis, keratitis, anterior uveitis, or glaucoma. Treatment should be aggressive, since the disease can have devastating ocular consequences.

The EBV probably causes some or all of the cases of infectious mononucleosis. Ocular involvement can include regional lymphadenopathy, uveitis, dacryocystitis, retinal periphlebitis, and rarely, vitritis. Since the immune system usually limits the disease, treatment is primarily symptomatic.

CMV is the leading cause of congenital viral infections, but the majority of these infections do not manifest themselves clinically. Adults frequently show serologic evidence of previous CMV infections, but clinical illness is rarely recognized in healthy individuals. CMV can cause clinical disease, however, in immunocompromised adults and newborns. CMV retinitis is a necrotizing infection leading to full-thickness destruction of the retina that may result in total loss of vision. This infection is common in patients with AIDS; in one early study,[195] 32% of AIDS patients had CMV retinopathy.

Idoxuridine

PHARMACOLOGY

Idoxuridine (IDU) is a halogenated pyrimidine that resembles thymidine (Fig. 11.10). IDU is phosphorylated by both viral and host cell (human) thymidine kinases to the active triphosphorylated derivative, which, in turn, is incorporated into both the viral and the host cell's DNA chains, thereby creating fraudulent DNA. The result is antiviral activity but with sufficient host cytotoxicity to limit systemic use severely. Such toxicity is less significant, however, when applying the drug topically to the eye.

CLINICAL USES

HSV infection of the cornea is the primary clinical indication for treatment with IDU, which is commercially available as a 0.1% solution and a 0.5% ointment for topical ocular use (Table 11.17). Therapy should continue 3 to 5 days after corneal healing is complete (as demonstrated by absence of fluorescein staining) to ensure that any virus released late in the recurrent episode does not initiate another active corneal infection. Therapy should not last more than 21 days because prolonged treatment increases the risk of corneal toxicity.

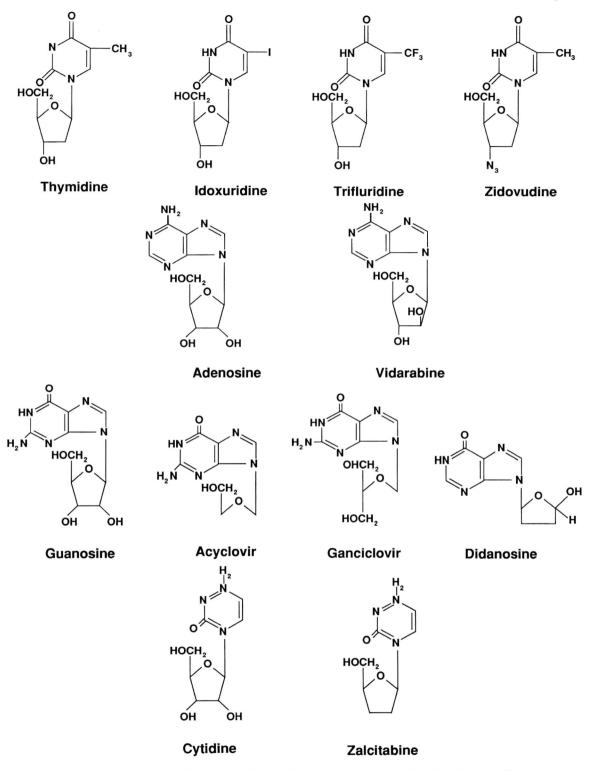

FIGURE 11.10 Chemical structures of antiviral drugs and the DNA nucleosides they resemble.

TABLE 11.17
Antiviral Drugs for Ocular Therapy

Generic Name	Trade Name (manufacturer)	Formulation	Indication
Topical			
Idoxuridine	Herplex (Allergan)	0.1% solution	HSV keratitis
Vidarabine	Vira-A (Parke-Davis)	3% ointment	HSV keratitis
Trifluridine	Viroptic (Burroughs Wellcome)	1% solution	HSV keratitis
Oral			
Acyclovir	Zovirax (Burroughs Wellcome)	200 mg capsules 800 mg tablets 200 mg/5 ml suspension	Herpes zoster ophthalmicus
Ganciclovir	Cytovene (Syntex)	250 mg capsules	CMV retinitis
Intravenous			
Ganciclovir	Cytovene (Syntex)	500 mg/vial	CMV retinitis
Foscarnet	Foscavir (Astra)	24 mg/ml bottles	CMV retinitis

Two weeks of treatment with IDU cures approximately 75% of patients with dendritic or geographic epithelial herpes.[196,197] However, because idoxuridine does not eradicate the latent virus in the trigeminal ganglion, topical therapy with this drug does not decrease the recurrence rate of herpetic keratitis.[198] During recurrent episodes, the acute infection is often controllable, but the infectious process or hypersensitivity reactions to the virus can cause corneal scarring. When HSV keratitis fails to respond to antiviral therapy, as evidenced by a lack of healing after 5 to 7 days or by an enlargement of the epithelial ulceration, several factors can be involved. In addition to the causes outlined in Table 11.3, the disease process or drug toxicity can also disrupt corneal epithelial healing.[199] The result is a persisting epithelial defect or "ghost" dendrite that may mimic an active lesion. Thus, in many cases the corneal herpetic infection is cured, but the persisting lesion gives the appearance of treatment failure.

In addition to using idoxuridine for the treatment of recurrent dendritic keratitis, this drug is also effective for primary herpetic keratitis. The treatment regimen for the primary corneal infection resembles that for the recurrent disease.[200] In the absence of corneal ulceration, a prophylactic antiviral drug such as IDU may be administered until the follicular conjunctivitis or periocular skin lesions resolve. When skin lesions appear as part of the primary HSV infection, they are best treated by sound hygienic measures since IDU is ineffective against HSV infection of the skin.[201]

IDU is relatively insoluble in water and does not penetrate into or through the cornea; it has no demonstrable effect on herpetic stromal disease or anterior uveitis.[202] However, treatment of herpetic stromal keratitis with high-dose steroids usually requires prophylactic use of an antiviral drug such as IDU to reduce the risk of recurrence of the epithelial disease. Patients with herpetic stromal disease often require relatively long-term steroid treatment, and simultaneous use of a topical antiviral agent may lead to substantial epithelial toxicity. Thus, when an antiviral drug is used prophylactically along with steroids, the dosage, tapering, and termination schedules of the antiviral drug remain controversial.[203,204]

SIDE EFFECTS

Although IDU is most active in virus-infected cells, the drug also affects the metabolism of normal cells. Toxic effects associated with the disruption of normal cellular DNA synthesis include changes in the cornea, conjunctiva, and lids. The cornea may show fine, superficial punctate keratopathy, corneal filaments, indolent ulceration, and the combination of slowed epithelial healing and superficial stromal opacification that can give the appearance of a "ghost" dendrite. Inhibition of corneal stromal wound healing with IDU use is well established.[199] These adverse effects have severely limited use of topical IDU in favor of other, less toxic, antiviral agents.

CONTRAINDICATIONS

Idoxuridine is contraindicated in patients who are allergic to the drug. Some strains of HSV are resistant to idoxuridine. If no healing occurs with 14 days of idoxuridine administration, another antiviral drug should be used.

Vidarabine (Adenine Arabinoside)

PHARMACOLOGY

Vidarabine is an analog of the purine nucleoside, adenosine (see Fig. 11.10). Both viral and host cell kinases phosphorylate this agent to the corresponding active vidarabine phosphate. However, because the phosphorylated vidarabine is a more potent inhibitor of the herpes virus DNA polymerase than of host DNA polymerase, viral DNA synthesis is blocked at lower doses and a selective antiviral effect can be achieved. This drug is active against vaccinia virus, HSV, CMV, and VZV.

CLINICAL USES

The primary clinical indication for vidarabine is dendritic or geographic epithelial keratitis caused by HSV. For this infection, the 3% ointment (see Table 11.17) is usually applied 5 times daily for a maximum of 21 days, with treatment continuing 3 to 5 days after the cornea has healed. This regimen is effective for the keratitis associated with both primary and recurrent infection.

Vidarabine is as effective as IDU for the treatment of HSV keratitis.[204,205] Treatment with vidarabine or IDU results in similar improvements in symptoms including lacrimation and photosensitivity, and results in similar rates and times for corneal reepithelialization. The reepithelialization time for dendritic and geographic ulcers is often between 6 and 7 days with each of the drugs. Pavan-Langston and Buchanan[202] have shown that many patients whose ulcers do not respond to IDU have re-epithelialization within 4 weeks of treatment with vidarabine. Thus, vidarabine can be considered an effective alternative in cases of recurrent disease when the patient is intolerant of IDU or when the virus is resistant to that drug.

Vidarabine is approved for the treatment of HSV encephalitis.[206] It decreases over-all mortality and debilitating neurologic sequelae, but comparison studies suggest that acyclovir is the drug of choice for treatment of this infection.[207] Like IDU, vidarabine has not proven useful for herpes simplex labialis or genitalis.

SIDE EFFECTS

Side effects associated with topical use of vidarabine are similar to those seen with IDU.[202] Symptoms include stinging, burning, irritation, lacrimation, and conjunctival hyperemia. Other reactions are follicular conjunctivitis, marked superficial punctate keratitis, corneal edema, corneal erosion, trophic epithelial defects, delay of corneal wound healing, and lacrimal punctal occlusion. Compared with IDU, however, vidarabine is less toxic and less likely to provoke adverse reactions.[199] If a patient demonstrates a reaction to vidarabine, another antiviral drug should be used.

CONTRAINDICATIONS

Vidarabine is contraindicated in patients who have developed hypersensitivity or intolerance to the drug.

Trifluridine (Trifluorothymidine)

PHARMACOLOGY

As with idoxuridine, trifluridine is an analog of thymidine (see Fig. 11.10). It is an effective inhibitor of thymidine synthetase and therefore inhibits DNA synthesis in both virus-infected and normal host cells. Trifluridine is also incorporated into both viral and host DNA, producing a faulty DNA that does not allow replication of the virus.

CLINICAL USES

Like IDU and vidarabine, trifluridine is used to treat HSV keratitis. The 1% solution (see Table 11.17) is used 9 times daily for 14 days or until re-epithelialization has occurred. The medication is then reduced to 1 drop every 4 hours, while the patient is awake, for an additional 7 days. Administration of trifluridine for more than 21 continuous days should be avoided because of the drug's potential for ocular toxicity. As with IDU and vidarabine, trifluridine is effective for both primary and recurrent epithelial keratitis.

When treatment of dendritic and geographic corneal ulcers with trifluridine was compared to treatment with idoxuridine, Wellings and associates[208] found trifluridine to be significantly superior. The mean time for healing of epithelial lesions with trifluridine was 6.3 days, significantly shorter than the 8.2 days with IDU. The number of treatment failures with trifluridine was also significantly less than with IDU, 7.5% with trifluridine compared to 39.5% with idoxuridine. Treatment of dendritic and geographic corneal ulcers with trifluridine has also been compared to treatment with vidarabine, and trifluridine has been shown to be significantly superior.[209,210] Pavan-Langston and Foster[197] demonstrated that when patients failed to respond to either IDU or vidarabine therapy (or were intolerant to either of these agents), substituting trifluridine resulted in healing in the majority of cases. Because of this superior clinical efficacy, trifluridine is now the drug of choice for initial treatment of epithelial HSV keratitis.

Another possible use of trifluridine has been suggested by a report of four patients with Thygeson's superficial punctate keratitis who were successfully treated with this drug.[211]

SIDE EFFECTS

Adverse ocular reactions to trifluridine are often overlooked or assumed to be a worsening of the disease process. Corneal epithelial defects at a location other than the site of the active infection (dendritic or geographic ulceration) can be a sign of drug toxicity.[199] Additional side effects associated with trifluridine are mild transient burning or stinging on instillation, conjunctival hyperemia and chemosis, corneal erosion and edema, keratitis sicca, delayed corneal wound healing, and elevated intraocular pressure. The epithelial defects and other adverse reactions are generally reversible on discontinuation of the drug. However, some cases of ptosis and lacrimal punctual occlusion produced by trifluridine have been permanent.[212] Long-term use of this antiviral agent can also cause conjunctival scarring,[213] but compared with IDU and vidarabine, trifluridine causes the least amount of local irritation and toxicity.[199]

CONTRAINDICATIONS

Trifluridine is contraindicated in patients who are allergic or intolerant to the drug.

Acyclovir (Acycloguanosine)

PHARMACOLOGY

Acyclovir, an analog of guanosine (see Fig. 11.10), is active against HSV and VZV. The selective actions of acyclovir against these herpes viruses are a result of two major factors: the phosphorylation of acyclovir to the active phosphate moiety by the herpes-specified thymidine kinase, and the inhibitory action of acyclovir triphosphate against herpes-specified DNA polymerase, which results in viral DNA chain termination.[214] Acyclovir must be phosphorylated to inhibit DNA replication, and this phosphorylation takes place through the action of thymidine kinase, the enzyme that normally phosphorylates thymidine. Viral thymidine kinase, an enzyme specifically induced by the virus only in infected cells, readily phosphorylates acyclovir, but the uninfected host cell thymidine kinase appears to be more fastidious and does not phosphorylate acyclovir. Thus, acyclovir does not disrupt DNA synthesis nor interfere with the replication of normal cells, but it does disrupt viral DNA replication in virus-infected cells. This highly selective activity makes acyclovir a very potent and effective antiherpetic agent without the toxicity associated with other antiviral drugs.

CLINICAL USES

Acyclovir has proven efficacy in the treatment of both primary and recurrent episodes of genital herpes. During initial episodes, oral acyclovir can decrease the duration of viral shedding from the genital lesions, reduce the development of new lesions, decrease the healing time of lesions, and decrease the severity of symptoms such as pain, adenopathy, dysuria, malaise, and headache.[215] However, after completion of treatment, acyclovir does not alter the time to subsequent recurrence and the rate of recurrence.[215]

In individuals who suffer severe and frequent recurrences of genital herpes, oral acyclovir is effective as a long-term suppressive agent. In several studies,[216,217] fewer recurrences occurred in the acyclovir-treated groups as compared to placebo groups. However, after acyclovir treatment was discontinued, the mean time to recurrence was similar for both groups, indicating that the drug has no permanent effect on the latent virus.[216,217]

Although not practical for most patients with herpes labialis, oral acyclovir may have some value for treating severe lesions by decreasing duration of pain and healing time.[218]

Although vidarabine is effective for the treatment of biopsy-proved HSV encephalitis, acyclovir is now the treatment of choice for this infection because the latter antiviral agent causes less mortality and morbidity.[207] Acyclovir ointment is effective for the treatment of HSV epithelial keratitis. Coster and associates[219] found that 1% IDU ointment and 3% acyclovir ointment produced comparable healing rates and times when used to treat herpetic epithelial keratitis. Collum and associates,[220] however, showed that acyclovir ointment is superior to IDU for treating herpetic dendritic ulceration by producing more rapid corneal healing (4.4 days versus 9.2 days) and an increased healing rate (100% versus 76%). These investigators[220] also demonstrated a higher incidence of toxicity in the form of superficial punctate keratitis in the IDU-treated patients as compared with the acyclovir-treated patients. In two studies,[221,222] topical acyclovir applied as a 3% ointment 5 times daily for 14 days was as effective for the treatment of HSV dendritic and geographic ulcers as was vidarabine ointment applied in the same dosage. No significant differences occurred in healing rates or times between the two patient groups in either study. Lau and associates[223] compared 3% acyclovir ointment to a 2% trifluridine ointment, each used 5 times daily. Both drugs were highly effective and gave 87% (acyclovir) and 82% (trifluridine) success rates. These studies show that although acyclovir ointment is effective for treating HSV epithelial keratitis, it has no clearly demonstrable superiority over the currently available topical antiviral drugs.

Oral acyclovir can be alternative therapy to topical antiviral therapy for the treatment of HSV dendritic keratitis. In two studies,[224,225] patients with dendritic corneal ulceration were treated with either oral acyclovir, 400 mg 5 times daily, or 3% acyclovir ophthalmic ointment 5 times daily. No difference occurred in the proportion of patients healed in either treatment group, and no systemic or significant local side effects were seen in either treatment group. In most cases of HSV epithelial keratitis, a topical antiviral drug, such as trifluridine, is preferable to a systemic drug. However, oral acyclovir might be useful in certain situations such as in patients who find using an eyedrop or ointment difficult or impossible or as an alternative for patients with topical antiviral ocular toxicity.

The role of acyclovir in the treatment of HSV stromal or uveal disease is not clear but is currently under investigation.

Colin and associates[226] used both acyclovir ointment and oral acyclovir to treat 32 patients with herpetic anterior uveitis without active corneal inflammation. The results of this study suggest that oral acyclovir may be effective in the initial treatment of patients with herpetic keratouveitis who have not previously received steroids.

Several investigators in small uncontrolled studies have reported a beneficial effect of acyclovir used concurrently with a topical steroid to treat HSV stromal or uveal disease. Topical acyclovir combined with betamethasone is at least as effective as vidarabine combined with betamethasone for the treatment of herpetic disciform keratitis.[227] In patients with active herpetic disciform keratitis being treated with topical prednisolone, 400 mg oral acyclovir taken 5 times daily was as effective as 3% acyclovir ointment in inhibiting viral replication.[228] Schwab[229] used oral acyclovir in 20 patients with recalcitrant stromal keratitis or keratouveitis; all 20 patients improved with the addition of acyclovir. Patients with previous multiple recurrences remained disease-free as long as oral acyclovir was administered. Because discontinuation led to recurrences, chronic acyclovir treatment might have a role in long-term suppression in HSV ocular disease. Recently a multicenter clinical trial evaluated the efficacy of oral acyclovir in the treatment of herpetic stromal keratitis in patients receiving concomitant topical steroids and trifluridine. The results indicated no statistically or clinically significant benefit of oral acyclovir with regard to time to treatment failure, proportion of patients who failed treatment, proportion of patients whose keratitis resolved, or 6-month best corrected visual acuity.[230]

In addition to activity against HSV, acyclovir is also active against VZV. Oral acyclovir can moderate the course of primary varicella (chickenpox) in immunocompetent children[231,232] and adults,[233] but the clinical usefulness of this treatment is not clear.

Oral acyclovir is effective in the treatment of herpes zoster infections (shingles). In two studies[234,235] using immunocompetent patients with localized cutaneous zoster infections, acyclovir prescribed at 800 mg 5 times daily for 7 to 10 days shortened the times to lesion healing and cessation of pain, and it reduced the duration of viral shedding and of new lesion formation. Treatment also reduced the prevalence of localized zoster-associated neurologic symptoms such as paresthesia, dysesthesia, and hyperesthesia.

Oral acyclovir is beneficial in the treatment of herpes zoster ophthalmicus (HZO). Cobo and associates[236] found that treatment with oral acyclovir, 600 mg 5 times daily for 10 days, resulted in prompt resolution of signs and symptoms and shortened the duration of viral shedding, particularly for patients treated within 72 hours after onset of the skin lesions. The most dramatic effect of oral acyclovir was to decrease the incidence and severity of secondary ocular inflammatory disease. Oral acyclovir significantly reduced the incidence of pseudodendritiform keratopathy, stromal keratitis, and anterior uveitis. However, oral acyclovir did not affect postherpetic neuralgia. It was postulated that although the 600 mg dose was beneficial, it might have just reached the threshold for effect.[236] Other investigators[237,238] using 800 mg 5 times daily for 7 to 14 days have substantiated the previous findings that oral acyclovir reduces the ocular complications of HZO. They have also proposed that clinicians use acyclovir and avoid steroids to treat HZO in immunocompetent patients.

To determine the most cost-effective duration of acyclovir treatment of HZO, Hoang-Xuan and associates[239] compared a 7-day with a 14-day course of treatment using 800 mg 5 times daily. The two groups showed no significant differences in terms of subjective symptoms, skin lesions, and ocular complications. Postherpetic neuralgia was also reduced. Thus, 7 days of therapy appears sufficient.

Aylward and associates[240] detected no beneficial effects of oral acyclovir on the rate of ocular complications in patients with HZO as compared to patients with HZO not treated with acyclovir. However, the number of patients treated early in the disease process with an adequate regimen of acyclovir was small, and this may have influenced the study results.

In summary, oral acyclovir is indicated for all immunocompetent patients with herpes zoster ophthalmicus; it should be used in a dosage of 800 mg 5 times a day for 7 days. The treatment is most effective when started within 72 hours of the onset of skin lesions.[236] The role of topical acyclovir in the management of the ocular complications of HZO is uncertain, especially in light of the recommendation that patients receive oral acyclovir and that steroid therapy should be avoided. Topical acyclovir alone is insufficient for severe ocular inflammation associated with HZO.[241]

Famciclovir (Famvir) is available as an alternative to acyclovir for the treatment of acute herpes zoster.[242] Famciclovir is a prodrug for penciclovir. Like acyclovir, penciclovir selectively inhibits herpesvirus DNA synthesis by interfering with the action of viral DNA polymerase. Unlike acyclovir, which has a low bioavailability, famciclovir is rapidly absorbed from the gastrointestinal tract and converted enzymatically to penciclovir. Famciclovir has some pharmacokinetic advantages and requires fewer doses per day than acyclovir, but whether it has any clinical advantage remains to be established.

Acyclovir has a role in the treatment of acute retinal necrosis syndrome, a disease characterized by the triad of acute confluent peripheral necrotizing retinitis, retinal arteritis and vitritis in otherwise healthy adults.[243] Current evidence implicates HSV and VZV as etiologic agents.[243,244] Intravenous acyclovir has become the mainstay therapy.[243] With this therapy, regression of the retinitis begins in approximately 4 days and is usually complete in approximately 1 month.[245] Despite acyclovir therapy, however, progressive vitritis is common, and the incidence of retinal detachment is high.[243,245]

SIDE EFFECTS

Acyclovir is a remarkably safe drug. During oral therapy the most frequent adverse reactions are nausea, vomiting, diarrhea, headache, and skin rash.[246] Less frequent reactions include anorexia, edema, leg pain, fatigue, sore throat, paresthesia, and lymphadenopathy.[246] The incidence of reported adverse reactions to acyclovir ophthalmic ointment is extremely low; superficial punctate keratopathy and burning or stinging are the most common side effects.[247]

CONTRAINDICATIONS

Acyclovir is contraindicated in patients with a history of hypersensitivity or intolerance to the drug. Patients with renal insufficiency should be monitored carefully, especially if high doses of acyclovir are used.

Ganciclovir (Dihydroxy Propoxymethyl Guanine, DHPG)

Ganciclovir was the first drug approved for treatment of CMV retinitis in AIDS patients. It is also indicated for prevention of CMV disease in transplant recipients. Ganciclovir is a nucleoside analog of deoxyguanine and differs from acyclovir only by the addition of a terminal hydroxy methyl group (see Fig. 11.10). This chemical change makes it 10 to 25 times as active as acyclovir against CMV.[248] As with acyclovir, only the triphosphate form of the drug inhibits viral DNA polymerase. The inhibition is reversible and virus production resumes when ganciclovir is removed.[249] Ganciclovir is administered as an intravenous infusion. In patients who cannot tolerate intravenous therapy because of toxic side effects, the drug is administered intravitreally[250] or as an intravitreal implant.[251] Oral ganciclovir can be used as an alternative maintenance therapy for CMV retinitis after the condition has been stabilized by prior IV induction therapy.

AIDS patients treated with ganciclovir demonstrate regression or disappearance of the exudative, hemorrhagic, and periphlebitic lesions of CMV retinitis.[252–254] However, reactivation occurs in 27% to 50% of patients despite the use of maintenance doses of ganciclovir.[254] This reactivation might be due to drug levels that are inadequate for complete suppression of viral replication[255] or to the development of viral resistance.[256] Retinal detachments also occur in 15% to 20% of patients despite successful long-term maintenance ganciclovir treatment of CMV retinitis.[257] The major toxicity of ganciclovir is bone marrow depression, resulting in neutropenia and thrombocytopenia. Because both ganciclovir and zidovudine cause bone marrow toxicity, zidovudine must be discontinued when ganciclovir therapy begins.[254] Retinal toxicity from intravitreal injections of ganciclovir

has not been reported except in one patient who was inadvertently administered an excessively high dose.[258]

Foscarnet (Phosphonoformic Acid, PFA)

Foscarnet is approved for treatment of CMV retinitis in AIDS patients who are unresponsive to or intolerant of ganciclovir. It differs from ganciclovir in that it is not a nucleoside analog, but rather a pyrophosphate analog. It selectively inhibits viral DNA polymerases and reverse transcriptases (RNA polymerases) at concentrations that do not affect host DNA polymerase.[259] Since foscarnet directly affects the pyrophosphate binding site of DNA polymerase, it does not require phosphorylation to become activated.[260] Foscarnet is administered as an intravenous infusion.

Foscarnet appears as effective as ganciclovir for the initial therapy of CMV retinitis in AIDS patients.[261,262] As with ganciclovir, preventing recurrent retinitis requires chronic maintenance therapy with foscarnet.[263] In patients intolerant of high doses of either foscarnet or ganciclovir, combination therapy using both drugs at lower doses has been reasonably well tolerated, and has prolonged vision in patients with CMV retinitis.[264] Foscarnet therapy prolongs life in AIDS patients more than ganciclovir does, possibly because of its anti-HIV effect and because it can be used in conjunction with zidovudine.[265] Foscarnet is also useful for the treatment of acyclovir-resistant herpetic infections (both HSV and VZV) that occur in patients with AIDS.[266,267]

Because of adverse reactions such as fever and gastrointestinal problems, patients do not tolerate foscarnet as well as they do ganciclovir. The most common serious adverse effect is renal impairment; it is necessary to monitor serum creatinine frequently and to adjust the dose based on changes in renal function.[268] In addition, foscarnet has been associated with changes in serum calcium, phosphorus, and magnesium, leading to seizures; patients should therefore be monitored for changes in plasma electrolyte levels.[269]

Zidovudine (Azidothymidine, AZT)

Zidovudine, a thymidine analog that inhibits HIV replication *in vitro*,[269] was the first drug approved for treatment of patients with AIDS. In the body, cellular enzymes phosphorylate the drug, and as the triphosphate, it inhibits reverse transcriptase. This inhibition terminates viral DNA elongation.[270] Zidovudine delays the progression of asymptomatic HIV infection[271] and early, symptomatic HIV disease.[272] In patients with advanced, symptomatic HIV disease, zidovudine decreases the mortality rate and reduces the risk of acquiring an opportunistic infection.[273] The drug has been used successfully to treat CMV retinitis[274] as well as HIV-induced iridocyclitis and anterior uveitis[275] in patients with

AIDS. Nevertheless, zidovudine is a very toxic drug that can cause bone marrow hypoplasia and leave some patients vulnerable to bacterial infections.[276]

Didanosine (ddl, Dideoxyinosine)

Didanosine is approved for treatment of advanced AIDS patients who are intolerant of or unresponsive to zidovudine treatment. Didanosine is chemically related to zidovudine and must be similarly converted to the triphosphate form to become active (see Fig. 11.10).[277] The major toxic effects are painful peripheral neuropathy and acute pancreatitis.[278] Hyperuricemia, rash, and increased levels of hepatic transaminases can also occur. Unlike zidovudine, however, didanosine is minimally toxic to bone marrow and can be used concurrently with ganciclovir. Pigmentary retinal lesions have been associated with didanosine therapy. These lesions first appear as patches of retinal pigment epithelial mottling and atrophy in the midperiphery and later become circumscribed by a border of pigment. Lesions progress during didanosine treatment, but progression appears to stop when the drug is discontinued.[279]

Zalcitabine (ddC, Dideoxycytidine)

Zalcitabine in combination with zidovudine is indicated for the treatment of adult patients who have advanced HIV infection and who have demonstrated significant clinical or immunologic deterioration.[280] Zalcitabine is an analog of the nucleoside cytidine which, when intracellularly converted to an active triphosphate metabolite, inhibits replication of HIV (see Fig 11.10).[281] Zalcitabine may act by inhibiting reverse transcriptase and terminating the viral DNA chain. The major clinical toxicities of zalcitabine are a painful peripheral neuropathy and, much less frequently, pancreatitis.[282]

Antifungal Drugs

The fungi (molds and yeasts) are an extremely large and diverse group of microorganisms ranging in size and complexity from simple unicellular yeasts (Fig. 11.11) to multicellular molds and mushrooms. The fungi differ from viruses and bacteria in size, structure, and chemical composition. The main structural component of a multicellular fungus is a filamentous tube containing cytoplasm and having nuclei spaced at irregular intervals (see Fig. 11.11). In some fungi, septations or cross-walls interrupt these tubes at numerous points. An individual filament is called a *hypha*, and an entire mat of *hyphae* is referred to as a *mycelium*.

Some of the hyphae in a mycelium can differentiate into reproductive structures that produce reproductive cells called *spores*. Classification of the filamentous fungi into genera and species is based on the morphologic arrangement of the reproductive structures and spores.

Of the nearly 100,000 species of fungi, only a few cause infections in humans. Fungal infections are classified as dermatophytic, mucocutaneous, or systemic. The most common fungal infections, dermatophytic infections, involve the keratinized portions of the body: skin, hair, and nails. Species of *Epidermophyton, Trichophyton,* and *Microsporum* cause these infections, which are known collectively as *tinea* or *ringworm*.

The yeast *Candida* causes most of the mucocutaneous infections, which usually affect moist skin or mucous membranes such as in the oral cavity (thrush), gastrointestinal tract, or perianal or vulvovaginal areas. Patients with diabetes and those receiving steroids or broad-spectrum antibiotics are predisposed to candidiasis of the intertriginous skin folds and mucous membranes. These conditions, as well as pregnancy or use of oral contraceptives, predispose patients to candidal vulvovaginitis.

Systemic mycoses may be either deep or subcutaneous. Fungi causing deep mycoses usually enter the body by inhalation, and the infection may spread hematogenously to other tissues. Fungi causing subcutaneous infections typically enter the body through the skin, usually by trauma, and the infection spreads directly to contiguous tissues. Examples of deep systemic mycoses include aspergillosis, blastomycosis, coccidioidomycosis, cryptococcosis, histoplasmosis, mucormycosis, candidiasis, and paracoccidioidomycosis. Major subcutaneous mycoses include chromoblastomycosis, mycetoma, and sporotrichosis.

Two fungal infections of the eye, fungal keratitis and endophthalmitis, occur most often after injury or surgery or when host resistance is depressed. The increased incidence of fungal corneal ulcers observed in recent years has been attributed to the widespread use of steroids, which depress the immune system, and possibly to broad-spectrum antibiotic use. Although many fungi have been cultured from mycotic corneal ulcers, the most frequent are *Aspergillus, Fusarium solani, Candida albicans,* and *Acremonium* (formerly *Cephalosporium*).[283,284]

Because fungal infections of the cornea occur relatively rarely, pharmaceutical companies have little incentive to develop new therapeutic agents specifically intended for topical use in the eye. Natamycin (pimaricin) is the only antifungal drug commercially available in the United States as a topical ophthalmic product, but dilute solutions or suspensions of some parenteral antifungal drugs such as amphotericin B, nystatin, and miconazole can be used for topical therapy. When administered either topically or systemically, most antifungal drugs penetrate the eye poorly.[285]

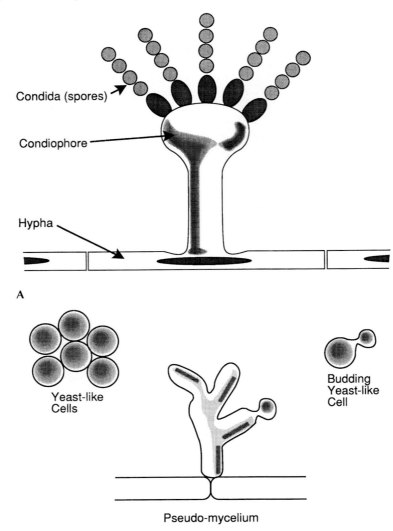

Condida (spores)

Condiophore

Hypha

A

Yeast-like
Cells

Budding
Yeast-like
Cell

Pseudo-mycelium

B

FIGURE 11.11   (*A*) *Aspergillus fumigatus,* a filamentous fungus. (*B*) *Candida albicans,* a yeast.

Therefore, mycotic corneal ulcers are often very difficult to treat successfully.

Amphotericin B

PHARMACOLOGY

Amphotericin B is classified as a polyene (Table 11.18). The polyenes bind to ergosterol present in the fungal cell membrane, and the polyene-sterol complex alters the selective permeability of the membrane, permitting leakage of essen-tial intracellular constituents.[286] An organism's ability to bind amphotericin B depends on the presence of sterol in the cellular membrane, and, because bacterial membranes do not contain the sterol, they do not bind the drug. Bacteria are thus insensitive to amphotericin B.

CLINICAL USES

Amphotericin B is the drug of choice for the treatment of systemic infections resulting from *Coccidioides immitis, Histoplasma capsulatum, Cryptococcus neoformans, Blas-tomyces dermatitidis, Candida,* and many other less com-

Histoplasma capsulatum, Cryptococcus neoformans, Blastomyces dermatitidis, Candida, and many other less common fungi. The period of therapy is usually 6 to 10 weeks, but it can continue as long as 3 to 4 months. Since amphotericin B is not adequately absorbed when given orally for systemic fungal infections, it must be administered intravenously or intrathecally.

For many years, topically administered amphotericin B was the major antifungal therapy for keratomycoses. A 1% solution was made from the commercial preparation intended for systemic use. Although this therapy was effective, it was toxic to the eye due to both the drug concentration and to the desoxycholate present for solubilization purposes in the commercial preparation.[287] A 0.15% solution of amphotericin B has been found to be reasonably well tolerated and effective for the treatment of corneal ulcers caused by *Fusarium, Candida, Aspergillus*, and *Alternaria*.[288] The most common concentration of amphotericin B currently administered for the treatment of keratomycoses is 0.10% to 0.25%.[289] The regimen for treatment of corneal ulcers often involves topical administration of amphotericin B every hour throughout the day and every 2 to 4 hours after bedtime. Since the corneal epithelium is a significant barrier to the penetration of amphotericin B, drug efficacy is reduced if the epithelium is intact.[290]

Amphotericin B has also been given subconjunctivally to treat fungal corneal ulcers. Subconjunctival injection can result in permanent yellowing of the cornea, and, at high doses, can cause salmon-colored conjunctival nodules.[291]

Amphotericin B has been administered systemically, subconjunctivally, and, more recently, intravitreally to treat fungal endophthalmitis.[292] However, amphotericin B is toxic and can cause retinal damage and ocular inflammation.[293] Another form of the drug, amphotericin B methyl ester, which is a water-soluble derivative of amphotericin B, appears less toxic and has been effective for treating experimental fungal endophthalmitis in animals.[294]

SIDE EFFECTS

Unpleasant and potentially dangerous toxic effects are associated with the systemic use of amphotericin B. Headaches, chills, fever, and vomiting are common during infusion of the drug. Toxic reactions can result from the binding of

TABLE 11.18
Antifungal Drugs for Ocular Therapy

Generic Name	Trade Name (Manufacturer)	Route of Administration	Clinically Useful Spectra of Activity
Polyenes			
Amphotericin B	Fungizone (Squibb)	IV, IT	*Candida* (disseminated), *Coccidiodes immitis, Histoplasma capsulatum* (disseminated), *Sporothrix schenckii* (extra-cutaneous), *Aspergillus, Cryptococcus neoformans, Blastomyces dermatitidis*
Nystatin	Nystatin (Various) Mycostatin (Squibb) Nilstat (Lederle) Nystex (Savage)	PO, Topical	*Candida* (cutaneous, vaginal, oral)
Natamycin (Pimaricin)	Natacyn (Alcon)	Topical	Filamentous and yeast fungi (ocular)
Pyrimidines			
Flucytosine	Ancobon (Roche)	PO	*Cryptococcus neoformans, Candida*
Imidazoles			
Miconazole	Monistat (Janssen) Monistat (Ortho)	IV, IT, Topical	*Candida* (cutaneous, vaginal, oral)
Ketoconazole	Nizoral (Janssen)	PO	*Candida* (mucocutaneous), *Histoplasma capsulatum* (pulmonary)
Triazoles			
Fluconazole	Diflucan (Roering)	PO, IV	*Candida* (oropharyngeal/esophageal) *Cryptococcus neoformans* (meningitis)

IV, intravenous; IT, intrathecal; PO, oral

amphotericin B to the sterol moiety of human renal tubular cells and erythrocytes; most patients receiving prolonged high doses of amphotericin B show renal damage, the extent of which depends on the total drug dose. Moderate anemia is also frequently encountered but usually disappears after therapy is discontinued. Other adverse events include gastrointestinal cramps, hypomagnesemia, and hypokalemia. Because of these side effects, amphotericin B should be used only when the patient has a reasonably well-substantiated mycotic infection.

Nystatin

Nystatin is also a polyene (see Table 11.18) and works in a manner similar to that of amphotericin B. It is used for the treatment of *Candida* infections of the skin, mucous membranes, and intestinal tract. Oral, esophageal, gastric, and intestinal candidiasis usually respond to oral administration of nystatin. Vaginitis and stomatitis (thrush) caused by this organism are usually treated using topical therapy.

Topical application of nystatin ointment has also been used successfully to treat corneal infections caused by *Candida* and *Aspergillus*,[295–297] but there is no experimental or clinical evidence indicating that nystatin is more effective than amphotericin B against *Candida* or the filamentous corneal pathogens such as *Aspergillus* or *Fusarium*.

Since oral preparations of nystatin are poorly absorbed, adverse effects are uncommon, but mild and transient nausea, vomiting, and diarrhea may occur. Neither irritation of the skin or mucous membranes nor hypersensitivity reactions have been reported following topical application. Neither the blood nor blood-forming organs show toxic effects.

Natamycin (Pimaricin)

Natamycin (pimaricin) is a small polyene (see Table 11.18) that acts in a manner similar to that of amphotericin B. Clinical trials of the 5% suspension have substantiated the effectiveness of natamycin for treatment of keratitis caused by *Acremonium* and other fungi.[298,299] Natamycin appears more effective than amphotericin B against *Fusarium*.[300]

The 5% natamycin suspension is the only FDA-approved drug for topical treatment of ocular fungal infections; because of its broad spectrum of activity and its commercial availability, it is the drug of choice for initial therapy in fungal keratitis.[289]

Because natamycin does not penetrate the cornea, conjunctiva, or other mucosal surfaces, topical application does not produce effective levels in the deep stroma or the anterior chamber. Natamycin should not be administered by subconjunctival injection because of the potential for producing severe conjunctival inflammation and necrosis.

Only a few adverse reactions have been reported. The suspension often adheres to areas of epithelial ulceration, and one case of conjunctival hyperemia and chemosis, possibly allergic, has been reported.[152]

Flucytosine

Flucytosine is a fluorinated pyrimidine (see Table 11.18) related to fluorouracil. In fungal cells, it is converted to fluorouracil, which is metabolized to 5-fluorodeoxyuridylic acid, an inhibitor of thymidylate synthetase. Since no evidence indicates flucytosine is converted to fluorouracil in normal host cells, toxicity is low with oral administration.

Flucytosine is used orally to treat systemic infections caused by *Candida* or *Cryptococcus neoformans*, including *Candida* endophthalmitis.[301,302] Because the development of drug resistance during therapy is high, the drug is usually used concomitantly with amphotericin B.

Flucytosine is readily absorbed after oral administration and can penetrate the blood-brain barrier. Side effects include bone marrow depression, hepatic damage, nausea, vomiting, diarrhea, and CNS symptoms such as confusion and hallucinations.

Miconazole

Miconazole is an imidazole (see Table 11.18) having two distinct antifungal actions. A fungistatic effect results from the inhibition of ergosterol synthesis in fungal cell membranes, which affects the membrane's permeability.[303] An additional fungicidal effect involves rapid membrane damage. This effect appears unrelated to the imidazole-induced inhibition of ergosterol synthesis.[303] Because in low doses miconazole is only fungistatic, eradication of the fungus may require prolonged treatment.

Miconazole has a broad spectrum of activity against *Candida* and other yeasts, numerous genera of filamentous fungi, and the dermatophytes. Topical application of 2% miconazole ointment is effective for treatment of dermatophytosis, *Candida* vulvovaginitis, and skin infections. Intravenous administration is effective for treatment of deep infections caused by *Candida, Coccidioides, Cryptococcus, Paracoccidioides,* and *Pseudallescheria* organisms.

Miconazole has been used topically, subconjunctivally, and intravenously to treat fungal infections of the cornea.[304–306] For example, topical and subconjunctival miconazole have been used to treat keratomycoses caused by *Candida* and *Aspergillus*.[304] Progressive corneal ulceration stopped in each case, and clinical evidence of corneal infection disappeared. Topical and subconjunctival miconazole have also been combined with oral ketoconazole for successful therapy of keratomycosis.[305] Intravitreal miconazole[307] has been used to treat fungal endophthalmitis with beneficial results. Miconazole appears to cause no major adverse reactions. Minor side effects include pruritus, rash, chills, phlebitis, and gastrointestinal symptoms.

Ketoconazole

Ketoconazole (see Table 11.18) acts similarly to miconazole by interfering with the biosynthesis of ergosterol and causing disorganization of the plasma membrane. Ketoconazole is an effective treatment for chronic superficial candidiasis and chronic dermatophytosis.[308] Limited data suggest that this antimycotic is also useful for the treatment of systemic (deep) mycoses caused by *Paracoccidioides*, *Histoplasma*, *Candida*, and *Coccidioides*.[309,310]

Topical application of ketoconazole has been effective for the treatment of keratitis due to *Aspergillus* and *Fusarium*.[311] A 1% solution does not irritate the conjunctiva or cornea even after prolonged use.[311] Oral ketoconazole used both alone[312] and in combination with topical and subconjunctival miconazole[305] has been successful for treatment of keratomycosis caused by *Fusarium*, *Aspergillus*, *Drechslera*, *Curvularia*, and *Candida*. Nausea and pruritus are the most common adverse effects, with headache, dizziness, abdominal pain, constipation, diarrhea, and nervousness occurring less frequently. Side effects also include hepatic toxicity, which is usually reversible on discontinuation of the drug. In at least one case, however, the liver toxicity led to a fatality.[313] Ketoconazole does not appear to produce ocular toxicity following systemic administration.

Fluconazole

Fluconazole is the first of the new, orally active triazole antifungal agents. Like the imidazoles, fluconazole acts by inhibiting ergosterol biosynthesis in fungal cell membranes. Fluconazole is regarded as the drug of choice for prophylaxis and therapy of oropharyngeal/esophageal candidiasis in both immunocompromised and immunocompetent patients.[314] It is also effective for the treatment of serious systemic candidal infections including urinary tract infection, peritonitis, and pneumonia.

Fluconazole is effective for treating active cryptococcal meningitis in AIDS patients[315]; however, additional studies are required to determine whether fluconazole is superior to amphotericin B. To prevent the recurrence of cryptococcal meningitis in AIDS patients following eradication of active disease, oral fluconazole is clearly superior to placebo[316] and may be superior to amphotericin B.

Fluconazole has also demonstrated efficacy in blastomycosis, coccidioidomycosis, and histoplasmosis. However,

because of limited clinical data, it can be considered only an alternative therapy in these infections.[317] Systemic administration of fluconazole, with or without vitrectomy and intravitreal administration of antifungal agents, has been used to treat patients with endophthalmitis.[318] Topical fluconazole 0.2%, applied with or without systemic therapy, has also been used to treat patients with keratomycosis.[318]

Fluconazole is generally well tolerated. The most common side effects associated with its use are nausea, headaches, and skin rash. Elevated liver enzymes occur in fewer than 5% of patients treated with the drug and are reversible upon discontinuation of therapy.[319]

Antiprotozoal Drugs

Acanthamoeba is a genus of free-living amoebae found in soil, water, and the human throat. The life cycle of the amoebae involves two basic forms: a motile, dividing trophozoite and a resistant cyst.

Acanthamoeba can infect the cornea and cause a chronic stromal keratitis. Five species are known to cause corneal infections: *A. castellani*, *A. cubertsoni*, *A. hatchetti*, *A. polyphagia*, and *A. rhysodes*.[320] Contact lens wearers, especially those who still use distilled water and salt tablets instead of commercially prepared saline solutions, are at particular risk.[321]

Acanthamoeba keratitis is difficult to treat. The biggest single variable affecting the outcome of the disease is the length of time between the appearance of the first symptoms and the institution of an anti-amoebal drug regimen.[322] Upon initial infection, trophozoites are the predominant form, and most of the drugs used can kill them. As the infection continues, however, the organism forms cysts in response to hostile conditions, and these cysts are resistant to standard drug therapy. Ultimately, penetrating keratoplasty might be required to remove the area infested with cysts.

Initial treatment of *Acanthamoeba* keratitis requires a combination of anti-amoebal drugs. Propamidine (Brolene) and neomycin have become the first-line treatment, with various imidazoles (clotrimazole, miconazole, itraconazole) used if the infection does not respond.[322,323] Both neomycin and propamidine have good trophozoidal activity but poor cysticidal activity.[324] Corneal epithelial toxicity can result from the prolonged propamidine therapy usually necessary to treat *Acanthamoeba* keratitis.[325]

A new antiparasitic agent has recently been described. Polyhexamethylene biguanide is a sterilizing agent found in the pool-cleaning product Baquacil. When used on the eye, it is diluted to a 0.02% solution with artificial tears.[326] This concentration kills both trophozoites and cysts *in vitro*.[327] When added to neomycin and propamidine, polyhexamethylene biguanide has been shown to enhance and hasten the treatment of *Acanthamoeba* keratitis.[327,328] Polyhexamethylene biguanide is well tolerated by the corneal and conjunctival epithelium and produces fewer toxic effects than neomycin or propamidine.[327]

References

1. Murray BE, Moellering RC. Patterns and mechanisms of antibiotic resistance. Med Clin North Am 1978;62:899–919.

2. Rosenblatt JE. Laboratory tests used to guide antimicrobial therapy. Mayo Clin Proc 1987;62:799–805.

3. Ormerod LD, Heseltine PNR, Alfonso E, et al. Gentamicin-resistant pseudomonal infection. Cornea 1989;8:195–199.

4. Mandell GL, Sande MA. Penicillins, cephalosporins, and other betalactam antibiotics. In: Gilman AG, Rall TW, Nies AS, et al, eds. Goodman and Gilman's The pharmacological basis of therapeutics, ed. 8. New York: Pergamon Press, 1990;46:1065–1097.

5. Glasser DB, Hyndiuk RA. Antibacterial agents. In: Tabara KF, Hyndiuk RA, eds. Infections of the eye. Boston: Little, Brown, 1986;13:211–238.

6. Schwarcz, SK, Zenilman JM, Schnell D, et al. National surveillance of antimicrobial resistance in *Neisseria gonorrhoeae*. JAMA 1990;264:1413–1417.

7. 1989 Sexually transmitted diseases treatment guidelines. MMWR 1989;38(suppl 8):1–43.

8. Noe CA. Penicillin treatment of eyelid infections. Am J Ophthalmol 1947;30:477–479.

9. Jones DB. Decision-making in the management of microbial keratitis. Ophthalmology 1981;88:814–820.

10. Sutphin JE, Pflugfelder SP, Wilhelmus KR, et al. Penicillin-resistant *Streptococcus pneumoniae* keratitis. Am J Ophthalmol 1984;97:388–389.

11. Wright AJ, Wilkowske CJ. The penicillins. Mayo Clin Proc 1987;62:806–820.

12. Baum JL. Antibiotic use in ophthalmology. In: Tasman W, Jaeger EA, eds. Duane's clinical ophthalmology. Philadelphia: J.B. Lippincott, 1992;4(26):6.

13. Drug evaluations annual 1993. Chicago: American Medical Association, 1992:1320.

14. Vanarsdel PP, Gilliland BC. Anemia secondary to penicillin treatment: Studies on two patients with "non-allergic" serum hemagglutinins. J Lab Clin Med 1965;65:277–285.

15. Bartlett JG, Chang TW, Gurwith M, et al. Antibiotic-associated pseudomembranous colitis due to toxin-producing clostridia. N Engl J Med 1978;298:531–534.

16. Farrar WE, O'Dell NM. Comparative β-lactamase resistance and antistaphylococcal activities of parenterally and orally administered cephalosporins. J Infect Dis 1978;137:490–493.

17. Abbot RL, Abrams MA. Bacterial corneal ulcers. In: Tasman W, Jaeger EA, eds. Duane's clinical ophthalmology. Philadelphia: J.B. Lippincott, 1992;4(28):28.

18. Baum JL. Initial therapy of suspected microbial corneal ulcers. I. Broad antibiotic therapy based on prevalence of organisms. Surv Ophthalmol 1979;24:97–116.

19. Thompson RL. Cephalosporin, carbapenem and monobactam antibiotics. Mayo Clin Proc 1987;62:821–834.

20. Israele V, Nelson JP. Periorbital and orbital cellulitis. Pediatr Infect Dis J 1987;6:404–410.

21. Matoba AY. Acute bacterial infections of eyelids and tarsal plate. Ophthalmol Clin North Am 1992;5:169–176.

22. Forster RK. Endophthalmitis. In: Tasman W, Jaeger EA, eds. Duane's clinical ophthalmology. Philadelphia: J.B. Lippincott, 1992;4(24):10–12.

23. Forster RK. Endophthalmitis. In: Tasman W, Jaeger EA, eds. Duane's clinical ophthalmology. Philadelphia: J.B. Lippincott, 1994;4(25):17.

24. Doft BH, Barza M. Ceftazidime or amikacin: Choice of intravitreal antimicrobials in the treatment of postoperative endophthalmitis. Arch Ophthalmol 1994;112:17–18.

25. Levine BB. Antigenicity and cross reactivity of penicillins and cephalosporins. J Infect Dis 1973;128(suppl):364–366.

26. Sher TH. Penicillin hypersensitivity—a review. Pediatr Clin North Am 1983;30:161–176.

27. Bartlett, JG, Willey SH, Chang TW, et al. Cephalosporin-associated pseudomembranous colitis due to *Clostridium difficile*. JAMA 1979;242:2683–2685.

28. Tan J, Bayne LH, McLeod PJ. Pseudomembranous colitis. A fatal case following prophylactic cephaloridine therapy. JAMA 1979;242:749–750.

29. Bang NU, Kammer RB. Hematologic complications associated with beta-lactam antibiotics. Rev Infect Dis 1983;5(suppl 2):S380.

30. Barza, M. The nephrotoxicity of cephalosporins: An overview. J Infect Dis 1978;137(suppl):S60.

31. Pasternak DP, Stephens BG. Reversible nephrotoxicity associated with cephalothin therapy. Arch Intern Med 1975;135:599.

32. Long JW. The essential guide to prescription drugs: 1992. New York: Harper Collins Publishers, 1992.

33. Kanof NB. Bacitracin and tyrothricin. Med Clin North Am 1970;54:1291–1293.

34. Goldstein EJ, Citron DM, Bendon L, et al. Potential of topical norfloxacin therapy. Comparative *in vitro* activity against clinical ocular bacterial isolates. Arch Ophthalmol 1987;105:991–994.

35. Bellows J, Farmer C. The use of bacitracin in ocular infections. Am J Ophthalmol 1948;31:1211–1216.

36. Binnick AN, Clendenning WE. Bacitracin contact dermatitis. Contact Dermatitis 1978;4:180–181.

37. Fraunfelder FT, Meyer SM. Drug-induced ocular side effects and drug interactions, ed. 2. Philadelphia: Lea & Febiger, 1982.

38. Khan JA, Hoover D, Ide CH. Methicillin-resistant *Staphylococcus epidermidis* blepharitis. Am J Ophthalmol 1984;98:562–565.

39. Donahue SP, Kowalski RP, Eller AW, et al. Empiric treatment of endophthalmitis. Are aminoglycosides necessary? Arch Ophthalmol 1994;112:45–47.

40. Havener WH. Ocular pharmacology, ed. 5. St. Louis: C.V. Mosby Co, 1983.

41. Fekety FR, Norman PS, Cluff LE. The treatment of gram-negative bacillary infections. The toxicity and efficacy in 49 patients. Am Intern Med 1962;57:214.

42. Melby K, Midtvedt T, Dahl O. A comparison of the *in vitro* activity of tobramycin and gentamicin against 6042 clinical isolates. Chemotherapy 1979;25:286–295.

43. Wilson FM. Adverse external ocular effects of topical ophthalmic medications. Surv Ophthalmol 1979;24:57–88.

44. Magnuson RH, Suie T. Gentamicin sulfate in external eye infections. JAMA 1967;199:177–178.

45. Halasa AH. Gentamicin in the treatment of bacterial conjunctivitis. Am J Ophthalmol 1967;63:1699–1702.

46. Magnuson R, Suie T. Clinical and bacteriologic evaluation of gentamicin ophthalmic preparations. Am J Ophthalmol 1970;70: 734–738.

47. Fox SL. Some aspects in the diagnosis and management of external infections of the eye: Experiences of a new antibiotic, gentamicin. South Med J 1970;63:1047–1052.

48. Gordon DM. Gentamicin sulfate in external eye infections. Am J Ophthalmol 1970;69:300–305.

49. Gwon A. Topical ofloxacin compared with gentamicin in the treatment of external ocular infection. Br J Ophthalmol 1992;76: 714–718.

50. Stern GA. Update on the medical management of corneal and external eye diseases, corneal transplantation, and kerato-refractive surgery. Ophthalmology 1988;95:842–854.

51. Glasser DB, Gardner S, Ellis JG, et al. Loading doses and extended dosing intervals in topical gentamicin therapy. Am J Ophthalmol 1985;99:329–332.

52. Drug evaluations annual 1993. Chicago: American Medical Association 1992;1453–1478.

52a. Tang-Liu DD, Schwob DL, Usansky JI, et al. Comparative tear concentrations over time of ofloxacin and tobramycin in human eyes. Clin Pharm Ther 1994;55:284–292.

53. Wilhelmus KR, Gilbert ML, Osato MS. Tobramycin in ophthalmology. Surv Ophthalmol 1987;32:111–122.49.

54. Smolin G, Okumoto M, Wilson FM. The effect of tobramycin on *Pseudomonas* keratitis. Am J Ophthalmol 1973;76:555–560.

55. D'Amico DJ, Caspers-Velu L, Libert J, et al. Comparative toxicity of intravitreal aminoglycoside antibiotics. Am J Ophthalmol 1985;100:264–275.

56. Moellering RC, Wennersten C, Kunz LF, et al. Resistance to gentamicin, tobramycin, and amikacin among clinical isolates of bacteria. Am J Med 1977;62:873–881.

57. Siebert WT, Moreland NJ, Williams TW. Resistance to gentamicin: A growing concern. South Med J 1977;70:289–292.

58. Duncan IBR, Rennie RP, Duncan NH. A long-term study of gentamicin-resistant *Pseudomonas aeuruginosa* in a general hospital. J Antimicrob Chemother 1981;7:147–150.

59. Cross AS, Opal S, Kopecko DJ. Progressive increase in antibiotic resistance of gram-negative bacterial isolates. Arch Intern Med 1983;143:2075–2080.

60. Yu VL, Rhame FS, Pesanti EL, et al. Amikacin therapy. Use against infections caused by gentamicin- and tobramycin-resistant organisms. JAMA 1977;238:943–947.

61. Talamo JH, D'Amico DJ, Kenyon KR. Intravitreal amikacin in the treatment of bacterial endophthalmitis. Arch Ophthalmol 1986; 104:1483–1485.

62. Davison CR, Tuft SJ, Dart JKG. Conjunctival necrosis after administration of topical fortified aminoglycosides. Am J Ophthalmol 1991;111:690–693.

63. Awan KJ. Mydriasis and conjunctival paresthesia from local gentamicin. Am J Ophthalmol 1985;99:723–724.

64. Records RE. Gentamicin in ophthalmology. Surv Ophthalmol 1976;21:49–58.

65. Campochiaro PA, Conway BP. Aminoglycoside toxicity—a survey of retinal specialists. Arch Ophthalmol 1991;109:946–950.

66. Campochiaro PA, Lim JL. Aminoglycoside toxicity in the treatment of endophthalmitis. Arch Ophthalmol 1994;112:48–53.

67. Longridge NS, Mallinson AI. A discussion of the dynamic illegible "E" test: A new method of screening for aminoglycoside vestibulotoxicity. Otolaryngol Head Neck Surg 1984;92:671–677.

68. Learner AM, Reyes MP, Cone LA, et al. Randomized controlled trial of comparative efficacy, auditory toxicity, and nephrotoxicity of tobramycin and netilmicin. Lancet 1983;1:1123–1125.

69. Argov Z, Mastaglia FL. Disorders of neurotransmission caused by drugs. N Engl J Med 1979;301:409–413.

70. Boe R, Conner CS. Pseudotumor cerebri. JAMA 1973;226:567.

71. Tabbara KF. Chlamydial conjunctivitis. In: Tabbara KF, Hyndiuk RA, eds. Infections of the eye. Boston: Little, Brown, 1986;24: 421–436.

72. Freinkel RK, Strauss JS, Yip SY, et al. Effect of tetracycline on the composition of sebum in acne vulgaris. N Engl J Med 1965;273: 850–854.

73. Salamon SM. Tetracyclines in ophthalmology. Surv Ophthalmol 1985;29:265–275.

74. Golub LM, Ramamurthy NS, McNamara TF, et al. Tetracyclines inhibit tissue collagenase activity: A new mechanism in the treatment of periodontal disease. J Periodontal Res 1984;19:651–655.

75. Neu HC. Symposium on the tetracyclines: A major appraisal. Bull NY Acad Med 1978;54:141–155.

76. Laga M, Plummer FA, Piot P, et al. Prophylaxis of gonococcal and chlamydial ophthalmia neonatorum: Silver nitrate versus tetracycline. N Engl J Med 1988;318:653–657.

77. Rotkis WM, Chandler JW. Neonatal conjunctivitis. In: Tasman W, Jaeger EA, eds. Duane's clinical ophthalmology. Philadelphia: J.B. Lippincott, 1992;4(6):3.

78. Sandstrom I. Neonatal conjunctivitis caused by *Chlamydia trachomatis*. Acta Otolaryngol (Stockh) 1984;407(suppl):67–69.

79. Dawson CR, Sheppard JD. Follicular conjunctivitis. In: Tasman W, Jaeger EA, eds. Duane's clinical ophthalmology. Philadelphia: J.B. Lippincott, 1992;4(7):17–18.

80. Darougar S, Jones BR, Viswalingam N, et al. Topical therapy of hyperendemic trachoma with rifampin, oxytetracycline, or spiramycin eye ointments. Br J Ophthalmol 1980;64:37–42.

81. Finland M. The place of the tetracyclines in antimicrobial therapy. Clin Pharmacol Ther 1973;15:3–8.

82. Zaidman GW, Brown SI. Orally administered tetracycline for phlyctenular keratoconjunctivitis. Am J Ophthalmol 1981;92: 173–182.

83. Perry HD, Golub LM. Systemic tetracyclines in the treatment of noninfected corneal ulcers: A case report and proposed new mechanism of action. Ann Ophthalmol 1985;17:742–744.

84. Perry HD, Kenyon KR, Lamberts DW, et al. Systemic tetracycline hydrochloride as adjunctive therapy in the treatment of persistent epithelial defects. Ophthalmology 1986;93:1320–1322.

85. Brown SI, Shahinian L. Diagnosis and treatment of ocular rosacea. Ophthalmology 1978;85:779–786.

86. Frucht-Perry J, Sagi E, Hemo I, et al. Efficacy of doxycycline and tetracycline in ocular rosacea. Am J Ophthalmol 1993;116:88–92.

87. Barr WH, Adir J, Garrettson L. Decrease of tetracycline absorption in man by sodium bicarbonate. Clin Pharmacol Ther 1971;12: 779–784.

88. Boston Collaborative Drug Surveillance Program. Tetracycline and drug attributed changes in blood urea nitrogen. JAMA 1972; 220:377–379.

89. Committee on Drugs, American Academy of Pediatrics. Requiem for tetracyclines. Pediatrics 1975;55:142–143.

90. Giles CL, Soble AR. Intracranial hypertension and tetracycline therapy. Am J Ophthalmol 1971;72:981–982.

91. Pierog SH, Al-Salihi FL, Cinotti D. Pseudotumor cerebri—a complication of tetracycline treatment of acne. J Adolesc Health Care 1986;7:139–140.

92. Penttila O, Neuvonen PH, Aho K. Interaction between doxycycline and some antiepileptic drugs. Br Med J 1974;2:470–472.

93. Neuvonen PJ, Penttila O. Interaction between doxycycline and barbiturates. Br Med J 1974;1:535–536.

94. Christian JR. Comparison of ocular reactions with the use of silver nitrate and erythromycin ointment in ophthalmia neonatorum prophylaxis. J Pediatr 1960;57:55–60.

95. Hammerschlag MR, Chandler JW, Alexander ER, et al. Erythromycin ointment for ocular prophylaxis of neonatal chlamydial infection. JAMA 1980;244:2291–2293.

96. Hammerschlag MR, Cummings C, Roblin PM, et al. Efficacy of neonatal ocular prophylaxis for the prevention of chlamydial and gonococcal conjunctivitis. N Engl J Med 1989;320:769–772.

97. Bell TA, Sandstrom KI, Gravett MG, et al. Comparison of ophthalmic silver nitrate solution and erythromycin ointment for prevention of natally acquired *Chlamydia trachomatis*. Sex Transm Dis 1987;14:195–200.

98. Drug Evaluations Annual 1993. Chicago: American Medical Association. 1992:1276.

99. Stein GE, Havlichek DH. The new macrolide antibiotics. Postgrad Med 1992;92:269–282.

100. Jones DB. New horizons in antibacterial antibiotics. Int Ophthalmol Clin 1993;33:179–186.

101. Martin DH, Mroczkowski TF, Dalieza, et al. A controlled trial of a single dose of azithromycin for the treatment of chlamydial urethritis and cervicitis. N Engl J Med 1992;327:921–925.

102. Kirst HA, Sides GD. New directions for macrolide antibiotics: Structural modifications and *in vitro* studies. Antimicrob Agents Chemother 1989;33:1419–1422.

103. Cater BL, Woodhead JC, Cole KJ, et al. Gastrointestinal side effects with erythromycin preparations. Drug Intell Clin Pharm 1987;21:734–738.

104. Sande MA, Mandell G. Antimicrobial agents: Tetracyclines, chloramphenicol, erythromycin, and miscellaneous antibacterial agents. In: Gilman AG, Rall TW, Nies AS, et al, eds. Goodman and Gilman's The pharmacological basis of therapeutics. New York: Pergamon Press, 1990;48:1117–1145.

105. Karmody CS, Weinstein L. Reversible sensori-neural hearing loss with intravenous erythromycin lactobionate. Ann Otol Rhinol Laryngol 1977;86:9–11.

106. Kucers A. Current position of chloramphenicol chemotherapy. J Antimicrob Chemother 1980;6:1–9.

107. Roberts W. Topical use of chloramphenicol in external ocular infections. Am J Ophthalmol 1951;34:1081–1088.

108. Bron AJ, Leber G, Rizk SNM, et al. Ofloxacin compared with chloramphenicol in the management of external ocular infection. Br J Ophthalmol 1991;75:675–679.

109. Abrams SM, Degnan TJ, Vinciguerra V. Marrow aplasia following topical application of chloramphenicol eye ointment. Arch Intern Med 1980;140:576–577.

110. Rosenthal RL, Blackman A. Bone marrow hypoplasia following use of chloramphenicol eyedrops. JAMA 1965;191:136–137.

111. Fraunfelder FT, Bagby GC, Kelly DJ. Fatal aplastic anemia following topical administration of ophthalmic chloramphenicol. Am J Ophthalmol 1982;93:356–360.

112. Scott JL, Finegold SM, Belkin GA, et al. A controlled double-blind study of the hematologic toxicity of chloramphenicol. N Engl J Med 1965;272:1137–1142.

113. Best WR. Chloramphenicol-associated blood dyscrasias. A review of cases submitted to the American Medical Association Registry. JAMA 1967;201:99–106.

114. Wellerstein RO, Condit PK, Kasper CK, et al. Statewide study of chloramphenicol therapy and fatal aplastic anemia. JAMA 1969; 208:2045–2050.

115. Cocke JG, Brown RE, Geppert LJ. Optic neuritis with prolonged use of chloramphenicol. J Pediatr 1966;68:27–31.

116. Joy RJT, Scaletter R, Sodee DB. Optic and peripheral neuritis. Probable effect of prolonged chloramphenicol therapy. JAMA 1960;173:1731–1734.

117. Suhrland LF, Weisberger AS. Chloramphenicol toxicity in liver and renal disease. Arch Int Med 1963;112:747–754.

118. Frenkel JK, Jacobs L. Ocular toxoplasmosis. Arch Ophthalmol 1958;59:260–279.

119. Tabbara KF, Dy-Liacco J, Nozik RA. Clindamycin in chronic toxoplasmosis. Effect of periocular injections on recoverability of organisms from healed lesions in the rabbit eye. Arch Ophthalmol 1979;97:542–544.

120. Ferguson JG. Clindamycin therapy for toxoplasmosis. Ann Ophthalmol 1981;13:95–100.

121. Lakhanpal V, Schocket SS, Nirankari VS. Clindamycin in the treatment of toxoplasmic retinochoroiditis. Am J Ophthalmol 1983;95:605–613.

122. Tedesco FJ. Clindamycin and colitis: A review. J Infect Dis 1977; 135(suppl):95–99.

123. American hospital formulary service drug information 91. Bethesda: American Society of Hospital Pharmacists 1991:335.

124. Lyle WM, Page C. Possible adverse effects from local anesthetics and the treatment of these reactions. Am J Optom Physiol Opt 1975;52:736–744.

125. Darougar S, Viswalingam N. Trachoma. In: Fraunfelder FT, Roy, FH, eds. Current ocular therapy 2. Philadelphia: Saunders, 1985; 35–36.

126. Agarwal LP, Saxena RP, Gupta BLM. Antibiotic and chemotherapeutic agents in treatment of trachoma. Am J Ophthalmol 1955; 40:553–556.

127. O'Connor GR. The roles of parasite invasion and of hypersensitivity in the pathogenesis of toxoplasmic retinochoroiditis. Ocular Inflam Ther 1983;1:37–46.

128. O'Connor RG. Manifestations and management of ocular toxoplasmosis. Bull NY Acad Med 1974;50:192–210.

129. Tabbara KF, O'Connor GR. Treatment of ocular toxoplasmosis with clindamycin and sulfadiazine. Ophthalmology 1980;87:129–134.

130. Schlaegel TF. Toxoplasmosis. In: Fraunfelder FT, Roy FH, eds. Current ocular therapy 2. Philadelphia: W.B. Saunders Co, 1985; 80–82.

131. Siniscal AA. The sulfonamides and antibiotics in trachoma. JAMA 1952;148:637–639.

132. Aragones JV. The treatment of blepharitis: A controlled double blind study of combination therapy. Ann Ophthalmol 1973;5: 49–52.

133. McCulley JP, Dougherty JM, Deneau DG. Classification of chronic blepharitis. Ophthalmology 1982;89:1173–1982.

134. Parker CW. Drug therapy—drug allergy. N Engl J Med 1975;292: 511–514.

135. Gutt L, Feder JM, Feder RS, et al. Corneal ring formation after

exposure to sulfamethoxazole. Arch Ophthalmol 1988;106:726–727.

136. Rubin Z. Ophthalmic sulfonamide-induced Stevens-Johnson syndrome. Arch Dermatol 1977;113:235–236.
137. Abramowicz M. Adverse ocular effects of systemic drugs. Med Lett Drugs Ther 1976;18:63–64.
138. Rittenhouse EA. Myopia after use of sulfanilamide. Arch Ophthalmol 1940;24:1139–1143.
139. Flach A. Photosensitivity to sulfisoxazole ointment. Arch Ophthalmol 1981;99:609–610.
140. Boettner EA, Fralick FB, Wolter JR. Conjunctival concretions of sulfadiazine. Arch Ophthalmol 1974;92:446–448.
141. Tabbara KF, Veirs ER. Corneal white plaques caused by sulfacetamide eyedrops. Am J Ophthalmol 1984;98:378–380.
142. Chang FW, Reinhart S, Fraser NM. Effect of 30% sodium sulfacetamide on corneal sensitivity. Am J Optom Physiol Opt 1984;61:318–320.
143. Drug evaluations annual 1993. Chicago: American Medical Association; 1992;1479–1497.
144. American hospital formulary service drug information 91. Bethesda: American Society of Hospital Pharmacists 1991:448.
145. Trimethoprim. In: Gennaro AR, ed. Remington's pharmaceutical sciences, ed. 18. Easton PA: Mack Publishing, 1990:1223.
146. Eyles DE, Coleman N. Synergistic effect of sulfadiazine and Daraprim against experimental toxoplasmosis in the mouse. Antibiot Chemother 1953;3:483–490.
147. Lamberts DW, Buka T, Knowlton GM. Clinical evaluation of trimethoprim containing ophthalmic solutions in humans. Am J Ophthalmol 1984;98:11–16.
148. Gibson JR. Trimethoprim-polymyxin B ophthalmic solution in the treatment of presumptive bacterial conjunctivitis—a multicentre trial of its efficacy versus neomycin-polymyxin B gramicidin and chloramphenicol ophthalmic solutions. J Antimicrob Chemother 1983;11:217–221.
149. The Trimethoprim-Polymyxin B Sulphate Ophthalmic Ointment Study Group. Trimethoprim-polymyxin B sulphate ophthalmic ointment versus chloramphenicol ophthalmic ointment in the treatment of bacterial conjunctivitis—a review of four clinical studies. J Antimicrob Chemotherapy 1989;23:261–266.
150. Lohr JA, Austin RD, Grossman M, et al. Comparison of three topical antimicrobials for acute bacterial conjunctivitis. Pediatr Infect Dis J 1988;7:626–629.
151. Arndt KA, Jick H. Rates of cutaneous reactions to drugs. JAMA 1976;235:918–922.
152. Physicians' desk reference for ophthalmology, ed. 21. Montvale, NJ: Medical Economics Data, 1993.
153. Duncan C. Sulfonamide cross-allergenicity—answers to common questions. Hosp Pharm 1989;24:666–667.
154. Then R, Angehrn P. Nature of the bactericidal action of sulfonamides and trimethoprim, alone and in combination. J Infect Dis 1974;128:S498–S501.
155. Penland R, Pyron M, O'Brien T, et al. *In vitro* activity of trimethoprim-polymyxin B (Polytrim) against ocular isolates. Invest Ophthalmol Vis Sci 1992;33(suppl):936.
156. Neu HC. Microbiologic aspects of fluoroquinolones. Am J Ophthalmol 1991;112:15S-24S.
157. Trucksis M, Hooper DC, Wolfson JS. Emerging resistance to fluoroquinolones in staphylococci: An alert. Ann Int Med 1991;114:424–426.
158. Budnick LD, Schaefler S, New York MRSA Study Group.

Ciprofloxacin-resistant methicillin-resistant *Staphylococcus aureus* in New York health facilities, 1988. Am J Pub Health 1990;80:810–813.
159. Acar JF, Francoual S. The clinical problems of bacterial resistance to the new quinolones. J Antimicrob Chemother 1990;26(suppl B):207–213.
160. Synder ME, Katz HR. Ciprofloxacin-resistant bacterial keratitis. Am J Ophthalmol 1992;114:336–338.
161. Wang C, Sabbaj M, Corrado M, et al. World-wide clinical experience with norfloxacin: Efficacy and safety. Scand J Infect Dis (suppl) 1986;48:81–89.
162. Monk JP, Campoli-Richards DM. Ofloxacin. A review of its antibacterial activity, pharmacokinetic properties and therapeutic use. Drugs (New Zealand) 1987;33:346–391.
163. Holmes B, Brogden RN, Richards DM. Norfloxacin: A review of its antibacterial activity, pharmacokinetic properties and therapeutic use. Drugs (New Zealand) 1985;30:482–513.
164. Crider SR, Colby SD, Miller LK, et al. Treatment of penicillin-resistant *Neisseria gonorrhoeae* with oral norfloxacin. N Engl J Med 1984;311:137–140.
165. Oriel JD. Ciprofloxacin in the treatment of gonorrhoea and non-gonococcal urethritis. J Antimicrob Chemother 1986;(suppl):129–132.
166. Osato MS, Jensen HG, Trousdale MD, et al. The comparative *in vitro* activity of ofloxacin and selected ophthalmic antimicrobial agents against ocular bacterial isolates. Am J Ophthalmol 1989;108:380–386.
167. Leibowitz HM. Antibacterial effectiveness of ciprofloxacin 0.3% ophthalmic solution in the treatment of bacterial conjunctivitis. Am J Ophthalmol 1991;112(suppl):29S–33S.
168. Power WJ, Collum LM, Easty DL, et al. Evaluation of efficacy and safety of ciprofloxacin ophthalmic solution versus chloramphenicol. Eur J Ophthalmol 1993;3:77–82.
169. Limberg M, Buggé C. Tear concentrations of topically applied ciprofloxacin. Cornea 1994;13:496–499.
170. Leibowitz HM. Clinical evaluation of ciprofloxacin 0.3% ophthalmic solution for treatment of bacterial keratitis. Am J Ophthalmol 1991;112(suppl):34S-47S.
171. Parks DJ, Abrams DA, Sarfarazi FA, et al. Comparison of topical ciprofloxacin to conventional antibiotic therapy in the treatment of ulcerative keratitis. Am J Ophthalmol 1993;115:471–477.
172. Wilhelmus KR, Hyndiuk RA, Caldwell DR, et al. 0.3% ciprofloxacin ophthalmic ointment in the treatment of bacterial keratitis. Arch Ophthalmol 1993;111:1210–1218.
173. Insler MS, Fish LA, Silbernagel J, et al. Successful treatment of methicillin-resistant *Staphyloccus aureus* keratitis with topical ciprofloxacin. Ophthalmology 1991;98:1690–1692.
174. Lin R, Holland GN, Helm CJ, et al. Comparative efficacy of topical ciprofloxacin for treating *Mycobacterium fortuitum* and *Mycobacterium chelonae* keratitis in an animal model. Am J Ophthalmol 1994;117:657–662.
175. Probst LE, Brewer LV, Hussain Z, et al. Treatment of *Mycobacterium chelonae* keratitis with amikacin, doxycycline and topical ciprofloxacin. Can J Ophthalmol 1992;29:81–84.
176. Miller IM, Vogel R, Cook TJ, et al. Topically administered norfloxacin compared with topically administered gentamicin for treatment of external ocular infections. Am J Ophthalmol 1992;113:638–644.
177. Jacobson JA, Call NB, Kasworm EM, et al. Safety and efficacy of topical norfloxacin versus tobramycin in the treatment of external

ocular infections. Antimicrob Agents Chemother 1988;32:1820–1824.

178. Avisar R, Vender T, Savir H, et al. Norfloxacin ophthalmic versus chloramphenicol in bacterial conjunctivitis and blepharitis (letter). DICP 1990;24:640–641.

179. Miller IM, Wittreich JM, Cook T, et al. The safety and efficacy of topical norfloxacin compared with chloramphenicol for the treatment of external ocular bacterial infections. Eye 1992;6:111–114.

180. Huber E, Steinkigler FJ, Huber-Spitzy V. A new antibiotic in the treatment of dacryocystitis. Orbit 1991;10:33–35.

181. Reidy JJ, Hobden JA, Hill JM, et al. The efficacy of topical ciprofloxacin and norfloxacin in the treatment of experimental *Pseudomonas* keratitis. Cornea 1991;10:25–28.

182. Vajpayee RB, Gupta SK, Angra SK, et al. Topical norfloxacin therapy in *Pseudomonas* corneal ulceration. Cornea 1991;10:268–271.

183. Gwon A. Ofloxacin vs. tobramycin for the treatment of external ocular disease. Arch Ophthalmol 1992;110:1234–1237.

184. Donnenfeld ED, Schrier M, Perry HD, et al. Penetration of topically applied ciprofloxacin, norfloxacin, and ofloxacin into the aqueous humor. Ophthalmology 1994;101:902–905.

185. Von Gunten S, Lew D, Paccolat E, et al. Aqueous humor penetration of ofloxacin given by various routes. Am J Ophthalmol 1994;117:87–89.

186. Stevens SX, Fouraker BD, Jensen HG. Intraocular safety of ciprofloxacin. Arch Ophthalmol 1991;109:1737–1743.

187. Keren G, Alhalel A, Bartov E, et al. The intravitreal penetration of orally administered ciprofloxacin in humans. Invest Ophthalmol Vis Sci 1991;32:2388–2392.

188. Lesk MR, Ammann H, Marcil G, et al. The penetration of oral ciprofloxacin into the aqueous humor, vitreous, and subretinal fluid of humans. Am J Ophthalmol 1993;115:623–628.

189. Pearson PA, Hainsworth DP, Ashton P. Clearance and distribution of ciprofloxacin after intravitreal injection. Retina 1993;13:326–330.

190. Drug evaluations annual 1993. Chicago: American Medical Association 1992:1518–1526.

191. Kanellopoulos AJ, Miller F, Wittpenn JR. Deposition of topical ciprofloxacin to prevent re-epithelialization of a corneal defect. Am J Ophthalmol 1994;117:258–259.

192. Macsai MS, Goel AK, Michael MM, et al. Deposition of ciprofloxacin, prednisolone phosphate, and prednisolone acetate in Seequence disposable contact lenses. CLAO J 1993;19:166–168.

193. Matsumoto SS, Stern ME, Oda RM, et al. Effect of ofloxacin on corneal epithelial wound healing evaluated by *in vitro* and *in vivo* methods. Drug Invest 1993;6:96–103.

194. Lehto P, Kivisto KT, Neuvonen PJ. The effect of ferrous sulphate on the absorption of norfloxacin, ciprofloxacin and ofloxacin. Br J Clin Pharmacol 1994;37:82–85.

195. Holland GN, Pepose JS, Pettit TH, et al. Acquired immune deficiency syndrome. Ophthalmology 1983;90:859–872.

196. Collum LMT, Benedict-Smith A, Hillary IB. Randomized double-blind trial of acyclovir and idoxuridine in dendritic corneal ulceration. Br J Ophthalmol 1980;64:766–769.

197. Pavan-Langston D, Foster CS. Trifluorothymidine and idoxuridine therapy of ocular herpes. Am J Ophthalmol 1977;84:818–825.

198. Carroll, JM, Martola EL, Laibson PR, et al. The recurrence of

199. Rich LF. Toxic drug effects on the cornea. J Toxicol—Cut Ocular Toxicol 1982;1:267–297.

200. Hyndiuk RA, Glasser DB. Herpes simplex keratitis. In: Tabbara KF, Hyndiuk RA, eds. Infections of the eye. Boston: Little, Brown. 1986;20:343–368.

201. Juel-Jensen BE, MacCallum FO. Treatment of herpes simplex lesions of the face with idoxuridine: Results of a double-blind controlled trial. Br Med J 1964;2:987–988.

202. Pavan-Langston D, Buchanan RA. Vidarabine therapy of simple and IDU-complicated herpetic keratitis. Trans Am Acad Ophthalmol Otolaryngol 1976;81:813–825.

203. Pavan-Langston D, Dohlman CH. A double blind clinical study of adenine arabinoside therapy of viral keratoconjunctivitis. Am J Ophthalmol 1972;74:81–88.

204. Hirst LW. Ocular and periocular infections. Sights and sounds in ophthalmology, vol. 6. St. Louis: C.V. Mosby Co, 1985.

205. Pavan-Langston D. Clinical evaluation of adenine arabinoside and idoxuridine in the treatment of ocular herpes simplex. Am J Ophthalmol 1975;80:495–502.

206. Whitley RJ, Soong SJ, Dolin R, et al. Adenine arabinoside therapy of biopsy-proved herpes simplex encephalitis: NIAID collaborative antiviral study. N Engl J Med 1977;297:289–294.

207. Whitley RJ, Alford CA, Hirsch MS, et al. Vidarabine versus acyclovir therapy in herpes simplex encephalitis. N Engl J Med 1986;314:144–149.

208. Wellings PC, Awdry PH, Bors FH, et al. Clinical evaluation of trifluorothymidine in the treatment of herpes simplex corneal ulcers. Am J Ophthalmol 1972;73:932–942.

209. McKinnon JR, McGill JI, Jones BR. A coded clinical evaluation of adenine arabinoside and trifluorothymidine in the treatment of ulcerative herpetic keratitis. In: Langston D, Buchanan RA, Alford CS, eds. Adenine arabinoside: An antiviral agent. New York: Raven Press, 1975.

210. Coster DJ, Jones BR, McGill JI. Treatment of amoeboid herpetic ulcers with adenine arabinoside or trifluorothymidine. Br J Ophthalmol 1979;63:418–421.

211. Nesburn AB, Lowe GH, Lepoff NJ, et al. Effect of topical trifluridine on Thygeson's superficial punctate keratitis. Ophthalmology 1984;91:1189–1192.

212. Lass JH. Antivirals. In: Lamberts DW, Potter DE, eds. Clinical ophthalmic pharmacology. Boston: Little, Brown, 1987;4:107–156.

213. Udell IJ. Trifluridine-associated conjunctival cicatrization. Am J Ophthalmol 1985;99:363–364.

214. Elion GB. The biochemistry and mechanism of action of acyclovir. J Antimicrob Chemother 1983;12(suppl B):9–17.

215. Nilsen AE, Aasen T, Halsos AM, et al. Efficacy of oral acyclovir in the treatment of initial and recurrent genital herpes. Lancet 1982;2:571–573.

216. Thin RN, Jeffries DJ, Taylor PK, et al. Recurrent genital herpes suppressed by oral acyclovir: A multicentre double blind trial. Br J Antimicrob Chemother 1985;16:219–226.

217. Mindel A, Weller IVD, Faherty A, et al. Acyclovir in first attacks of genital herpes and prevention of recurrences. Genitourin Med 1986;62:28–32.

218. Raborn GW, McGaw WT, Grace M, et al. Oral acyclovir and herpes labialis: A randomized, double-blind, placebo-controlled study. J Am Dent Assoc 1987;115:38–42.

219. Coster DJ, Wilhelmus KR, Michaud R, et al. A comparison of acyclovir and idoxuridine as treatment for ulcerative herpetic keratitis. Br J Ophthalmol 1980;64:763–765.

220. Collum LMT, Benedict-Smith A, Hillary IB. Randomized double-blind trial of acyclovir and idoxuridine in dendritic corneal ulceration. Br J Ophthalmol 1980;64:766–769.

221. Collum LMT, Logan P, McAuliffe-Curtin D, et al. Randomised double-blind trial of acyclovir (Zovirax) and adenine arabinoside in herpes simplex amoeboid corneal ulceration. Br J Ophthalmol 1985;69:847–850.

222. Jackson WB, Breslin CW, Lorenzetti DWC, et al. Treatment of herpes simplex keratitis: Comparison of acyclovir and vidarabine. Can J Ophthalmol 1984;19:107–111.

223. Lau C, Oosterhuis JA, Versteeg J, et al. Multicenter trial of acyclovir and triflurothymidine in herpetic keratitis. Am J Med 1982;(suppl):305–306.

224. Collum LMT, Akhtar J, McGettrick P. Oral acyclovir in herpetic keratitis. Trans Ophthalmol Soc UK 1985;104:629–632.

225. Collum LMT, McGettrick P, Akhtar J, et al. Oral acyclovir (Zovirax) in herpes simplex dendritic corneal ulceration. Br J Ophthalmol 1986;70:435–438.

226. Colin J, Malet F, Chastel C, et al. Acyclovir in herpetic anterior uveitis. Ann Ophthalmol 1991;23:28–30.

227. Collum LMT, O'Connor M, Logan P. Comparison of the efficacy and toxicity of acyclovir and of adenine arabinoside when combined with dilute betamethasone in herpetic disciform keratitis: Preliminary results of a double-blind trial. Trans Ophthalmol Soc UK 1983;103:597–599.

228. Porter SM, Patterson A, Kho P. A comparison of local and systemic acyclovir in the management of herpetic disciform keratitis. Br J Ophthalmol 1990;74:283–285.

229. Schwab IR. Oral acyclovir in the management of herpes simplex ocular infections. Ophthalmology 1988;95:423–430.

230. Barron BA, Gee L, Hauck WW, et al. Herpetic eye disease study. A controlled trial study of oral acyclovir for herpes simplex stromal keratitis. Ophthalmology 1994;101:1871–1882.

231. Balfour JJ, Kelly JM, Suarez CS, et al. Acyclovir treatment of varicella in otherwise healthy children. Pediatr 1990;116:633–639.

232. Dunkle LM, Arvin AM, Whitley RJ, et al. A controlled trial of acyclovir for chickenpox in normal children. N Engl J Med 1991;325:1539–1544.

233. Feder HM. Treatment of adult chickenpox with oral acyclovir. Arch Intern Med 1990;150:2061–2065.

234. Huff JC, Bean B, Balfour HH, et al. Therapy of herpes zoster with oral acyclovir. Am J Med 1988;85:85–89.

235. Morton P, Thompson AN. Oral acyclovir in the treatment of herpes zoster in general practice. NZ Med J 1989;102:93–95.

236. Cobo LM, Foulks GN, Liesegang T, et al. Oral acyclovir in the treatment of acute herpes zoster ophthalmicus. Ophthalmology 1986;93:763–770.

237. Harding SP, Porter SM. Oral acyclovir in herpes zoster ophthalmicus. Curr Eye Res 1991;10:177–182.

238. Herbort CP, Buechi ER, Piguet B, et al. High-dose oral acyclovir in acute herpes zoster ophthalmicus: The end of the corticosteroid era. Curr Eye Res 1991;10:171–175.

239. Hoang-Xuan T, Buchi ER, Herbort CP, et al. Oral acyclovir for herpes zoster ophthalmicus. Ophthalmology 1992;99:1062–1071.

240. Aylward GW, Claoue CMP, Marsh RJ, et al. Influence of oral acyclovir on ocular complications of herpes zoster ophthalmicus. Eye 1994;8:70–74.

241. Marsh RJ, Cooper M. Double-masked trial of topical acyclovir and steroids in the treatment of herpes zoster ophthalmicus. Br J Ophthalmol 1991;75:542–546.

242. Famciclovir for herpes zoster. Med Letter 1994;36:97–98.

243. Duker JS, Blumenkranz MS. Diagnosis and management of the acute retinal necrosis (ARN) syndrome. Surv Ophthalmol 1991;35:327–343.

244. Duker JS, Nielsen JC, Eagle RC, et al. Rapidly progressive acute retinal necrosis secondary to herpes simplex virus, type I. Ophthalmology 1990;97:1638–1643.

245. Blumenkranz MS, Culbertson WW, Clarkson JG, et al. Treatment of the acute retinal necrosis syndrome with intravenous acyclovir. Ophthalmology 1986;93:296–300.

246. Physicians desk reference, ed. 47. Montvale, NJ: Medical Economics, 1993.

247. Grant DM. Acyclovir (Zovirax) ophthalmic ointment: A review of clinical tolerance. Curr Eye Res 1987;6:231–235.

248. Cole NL, Balfour HH: *In vitro* susceptibility of cytomegalovirus isolated from immunosuppressed patients to acyclovir and ganciclovir. Diag Microbiol Infect Dis 1987;6:255–261.

249. Rosecan LR, Stahl-Bayliss CM, Kalman CM, et al. Antiviral therapy for cytomegalovirus retinitis in AIDS with dihydroxy propoxymethyl guanine. Am J Ophthalmol 1986;101:405–418.

250. Cantrill HL, Henry K, Melroe NH, et al. Treatment of cytomegalovirus retinitis with intravitreal ganciclovir: Long-term results. Ophthalmology 1989;96:367–374.

251. Martin DF, Parks DJ, Mellow SD, et al. Treatment of cytomegalovirus retinitis with an intraocular sustained-release ganciclovir implant. Arch Ophthalmol 1994;112:1531–1539.

252. Robinson MR, Streeten BW, Hampton GR, et al. Treatment of cytomegalovirus optic neuritis with dihydroxy propoxymethyl guanine. Am J Ophthalmol 1986;102:533–534.

253. Henry K, Cantrill H, Fletcher C, et al. Use of intravitreal ganciclovir (dihydroxy propoxymethyl guanine) for cytomegalovirus retinitis in a patient with AIDS. Am J Ophthalmol 1987;103:17–23.

254. Gross JG, Bozzette SA, Mathews WC, et al. Longitudinal study of cytomegalovirus retinitis in acquired immune deficiency syndrome. Ophthalmology 1990;97:681–686.

255. Kupperman BD, Quiceno JI, Flores-Aguilar M, et al. Intravitreal ganciclovir concentration after intravenous administration in AIDS patients with cytomegalovirus retinitis: Implications for therapy. J Infect Dis 1993;168:1506–1509.

256. Drew WL, Miner RC, Busch DF, et al. Prevalence of resistance in patients receiving ganciclovir for serious cytomegalovirus infection. J Infect Dis 1991;99:716–719.

257. Freeman WR, Henderly DE, Wan WL, et al. Prevalence, pathophysiology, and treatment of rhegmatogenous retinal detachment in treated cytomegalovirus retinitis. Am J Ophthalmol 1986;103:527–536.

258. Saran BR, Maguire AM. Retinal toxicity of high dose intravitreal ganciclovir. Retina 1994;14:248–251.

259. Klintmalm G, Lonnqvist B, Oberg B, et al. Intravenous foscarnet for the treatment of severe cytomegalovirus infection in allograft recipients. Scand J Infect Dis 1985;17:157–163.

260. Oberg B. Antiviral effects of phosphonoformate (PFA foscarnet sodium). Pharmacol Ther 1983;19:387–415.

261. Palestine AG, Polis MA, DeSmet MD, et al. A randomized

controlled trial of foscarnet in the treatment of cytomegalovirus retinitis in patients with AIDS. Ann Intern Med 1991;115:665–673.

262. Studies of Ocular Complications of AIDS Research Group in Collaboration with the AIDS Clinical Trials Group. Foscarnet-ganciclovir cytomegalovirus retinitis trial: 4. Visual outcomes. Ophthalmology 1994;101:1250–1261.

263. Jacobson MA, O'Donnell JJ, Mills J. Foscarnet treatment of cytomegalovirus retinitis in patients with the acquired immunodeficiency syndrome. Antimicrob Agents Chemother 1989;33:736–741.

264. Weinberg DV, Murphy R, Naughton K. Combined daily therapy with intravenous ganciclovir and foscarnet for patients with recurrent cytomegalovirus retinitis. Am J Ophthalmol 1994;117:776–782.

265. Studies of Ocular Complications of AIDS Research Group, in Collaboration with the AIDS Clinical Trials Group. Mortality in patients with the acquired immunodeficiency syndrome treated with either foscarnet or ganciclovir for cytomegalovirus retinitis. N Engl J Med 1992;326:213–220.

266. Safrin S, Grumpacker C, Chatis P, et al. A controlled trial comparing foscarnet with vidarabine for acyclovir-resistant mucocutaneous herpes simplex in the acquired immunodeficiency syndrome. New Engl J Med 1991;325:551–555.

267. Youle MM, Hawkins DA, Collins P, et al. Acyclovir-resistant herpes in AIDS treated with foscarnet. Lancet 1988;II:341–342.

268. LeHoang P, Girard B, Robinet M, et al. Foscarnet in the treatment of cytomegalovirus retinitis in acquired immune deficiency syndrome. Ophthalmology 1989;96:865–874.

269. Mitsuya H, Weinhold KJ, Furman PA, et al. 3'-azido-3'-deoxythymidine (3W A509U): An antiviral agent that inhibits the infectivity and cytopathic effect of human T-lymphotropic virus type III/lymphadenopathy-associated virus in vitro. Proc Natl Acad Sci USA 1985;82:7096–7100.

270. St. Clair MH, Weinhold K, Richards CA, et al. Characterization of HTLV-III reverse transcriptase and inhibition by the triphosphate of BW A509U. In: Program and abstracts of the twenty-fifth interscience conference on antimicrobial agents and chemotherapy, Minneapolis, October 1985. American Society of Microbiology 1985;172.

271. Volberding PA, Lagakos SW, Koch MA, et al. Zidovudine in asymptomatic human immunodeficiency virus infection. A controlled trial in persons with fewer than 500 CD4–positive cells per cubic millimeter. N Engl J Med 1990;322:941–949.

272. Fischl MA, Richman DD, Hansen N, et al. The safety and efficacy of zidovudine (AZT) in the treatment of subjects with mildly symptomatic human immunodeficiency virus type 1 (HIV) infection. A double-blind, placebo-controlled trial. Ann Intern Med 1990;112:727–737.

273. Fischl MA, Richman DD, Grieco MH, et al. The efficacy of azidothymidine (AZT) in the treatment of patients with AIDS and AIDS related complex: A double-blind placedo-controlled trial. N Engl J Med 1987;317:185–191.

274. D'Mico DJ, Skolnik PR, Kosloff BR, et al. Resolution of cytomegalovirus retinitis with zidovudine therapy. Arch Ophthalmol 1988;106:1168–1169.

275. Farrell PL, Heinemann MH, Roberts CW, et al. Response of human-immunodeficiency virus-associated uveitis to zidovudine. Am J Ophthalmol 1988;106:7–10.

276. Richman DR, Fischl MA, Grieco MH, et al. The toxicity of azidothymidine (AZT) in the treatment of patients with AIDS and AIDS related complex: A double-blind placebo-controlled trial. N Engl J Med 1986;317:192–197.

277. Yarchoan R, Mitsuya A, Meyers CE, et al. Clinical pharmacology of 3'-azido-2,3'-dideoxythymidine (zidovudine) and related dideoxynucleosides. N Engl J Med 1989;321:726–738.

278. Yarchoan R, Pluda JM, Tomas RV, et al. Long-term toxicity/activity profile of 2'3'-dideoxyinosine in AIDS or AIDS-related complex. Lancet 1990;336:526–529.

279. Whitcup SM, Dastgheib K, Nussenblatt RB, et al. A clinicopathologic report of the retinal lesions associated with didanosine. Arch Ophthalmol 1994;112:1594–1598.

280. Meng TC, Fischl MA, Boots AM, et al. Combination therapy with zidovudine and dideoxycytidine in patients with advanced human immunodeficiency virus infection. A phase I/II study. Ann Intern Med 1992;116:13–20.

281. Whittington R, Brogden RN. Zalcitabine. A review of its pharmacology and clinical potential in acquired immunodeficiency syndrome (AIDS). Drugs 1992;44:656–683.

282. Berger AR, Arezzo JC, Schaumburg HH, et al. 2', 3'-dideoxycytidine (ddC) toxic neuropathy: A study of 52 patients. Neurology 1993;43:358–362.

283. Polack FM, Kaufman HE, Newmark E. Keratomycosis. Medical and surgical treatment. Arch Ophthalmol 1971;85:410–416.

284. Kolodner H. Fungal corneal ulcers. Int Ophthalmol Clin 1984;24:17–24.

285. Green WR, Bennett JE, Goos RD. Ocular penetration of amphotericin B. Arch Ophthalmol 1965;73:769–775.

286. Butler WT. Pharmacology, toxicity, and therapeutic usefulness of amphotericin B. JAMA 1966;195:127–131.

287. Anderson B, Roberts S, Gonalez C, et al. Mycotic ulcerative keratitis. Arch Ophthalmol 1959;62:169–179.

288. Wood TO, Williford W. Treatment of keratomycosis with amphotericin B 0.15%. Am J Ophthalmol 1976;81:847–849.

289. Jones DB. Diagnosis and management of fungal keratitis. In: Tasman W, Jaeger EA, eds. Duane's clinical ophthalmology. Philadelphia: J.B. Lippincott Company, 1992;4(21):1–19.

290. O'Day DM, Ray WA, Head S, et al. Influence of the corneal epithelium on the efficacy of topical antifungal drugs. Invest Ophthalmol Vis Sci 1984;25:855–859.

291. Bell RW, Ritchey JP. Subconjunctival nodules after amphotericin B injection: Medical therapy for Aspergillus corneal ulcer. Arch Ophthalmol 1973;90:402–404.

292. Perraut LE, Perraut LE, Bleiman B, et al. Successful treatment of Candida albicans endophthalmitis with intravitreal amphotericin B. Arch Ophthalmol 1981;99:1565–1567.

293. Jones DB. Therapy of postsurgical fungal endophthalmitis. Ophthalmology 1978;85:357–373.

294. McGetrick JJ, Peyman GA, Nyberg MA. Amphotericin B methyl ester: Evaluation for intravitreous use in experimental fungal endophthalmitis. Ophthalmic Surg 1979;10:25–29.

295. Mangiaracine AB, Liebman SD. Fungus keratitis (Aspergillus fumigatus): treatment with nystatin (mycostatin). Arch Ophthalmol 1957;58:695–698.

296. McGrand JC. Symposium on direct fungal infection of the eye: Keratomycosis due to Aspergillus fumigatus cured by nystatin. Trans Ophthalmol Soc UK 1969;89:799–803.

297. Roberts SS. Nystatin in monilia keratoconjunctivitis. Am J Ophthalmol 1957;44:108–109.

298. Forster RK, Rebell G. The diagnosis and management of keratomycoses. Arch Ophthalmol 1975;93:1134–1136.

299. Newmark E, Ellison AC, Kaufman HE. Pimaricin therapy of *Cephalosporium* and *Fusarium* keratitis. Am J Ophthalmol 1970; 69:458–466.

300. Jones DB, Forster RK, Rebell G. *Fusarium solani* keratitis treated with natamycin (pimaricin): Eighteen consecutive cases. Arch Ophthalmol 1972;88:147–154.

301. Richards AB, Jones BR, Whitwell J, et al. Corneal and intraocular infection by *Candida albicans* treated with 5-fluorocytosine. Trans Ophthalmol Soc UK 1969;89:867–885.

302. Robertson DN, Riley FC, Hermans PE. Endogenous *Candida* oculomycosis: Report of two patients treated with flucytosine. Arch Ophthalmol 1974;91:33–38.

303. Sud IJ, Feingold DS. Mechanisms of action of the antimycotic imidazoles. Invest Dermatol 1981;76:438–441.

304. Foster CS. Miconazole therapy for keratomycosis. Am J Ophthalmol 1981;91:622–629.

305. Fitzsimons R, Peters AL. Miconazole and ketoconazole as a satisfactory first-line treatment for keratomycosis. Am J Ophthalmol 1986;101:605–608.

306. Ishibashi Y, Matsumoto Y. Intravenous miconazole in the treatment of keratomycosis. Am J Ophthalmol 1984;97:646–647.

307. Fowler BJ. Treatment of fungal endophthalmitis with vitrectomy and intraocular injection of miconazole. J Ocular Ther Surg 1984; 3:43–47.

308. Hay RJ. Ketoconazole in the treatment of fungal infection: Clinical and laboratory studies. Am J Med 1983;74:16–19.

309. Graybill JR, Lundberg D, Donovan W, et al. Treatment of coccidioidomycosis with ketoconazole: Clinical and laboratory studies of 18 patients. Rev Infect Dis 1980;2:661–673.

310. Cuce LC, Wroclawski EL, Sampaio SAP. Treatment of paracoccidioidomycosis, candidiasis, chromomycosis, lobomycosis and mycetoma with ketoconazole. Int J Dermatol 1980;19:405–408.

311. Torres MA, Mohamed J, Cavazos-Adame H, et al. Topical ketoconazole for fungal keratitis. Am J Ophthalmol 1985;100:293–298.

312. Ishibashi Y. Oral ketoconazole therapy for keratomycosis. Am J Ophthalmol 1983;95:342–345.

313. Lake-Bakaar G, Scheuer PJ, Sherlock S. Hepatic reactions associated with ketoconazole in the United Kingdom. Br Med J Clin Res Ed 1987;294:419–422.

314. Cleary JD, Taylor JW, Chapman SW. Imidazoles and triazoles in antifungal therapy. DICP 1990;24:148–152.

315. Statton CW. Antifungal agents: The old and the new. Infect Dis Newslett 1990;9:41–45.

316. Bozzette SA, Larsen RA, Chiu J, et al. A placebo-controlled trial of maintenance therapy with fluconazole after treatment of cryptococcal meningitis in the acquired immunodeficiency syndrome. N Engl J Med 1991;324:580–584.

317. Grant SM, Clissold SP. Fluconazole: A review of its pharmacodynamics and pharmocokinetic properties, and therapeutic use in superficial and systemic mycoses. Drugs 1990;39:877–916.

318. Urbank SF, Degn T. Fluconazole in the management of fungal ocular infections. Ophthalmologica 1994;208:147–156.

319. Grant SM, Clissold SP. Fluconazole: A review of its pharmacodynamic and pharmacokinetic properties, and therapeutic potential in superficial and systemic mycoses. Drugs 1990;39:877–916.

320. Centers for Disease Control. *Acanthamoeba* keratitis associated with contact lenses—United States. MMWR 1986;35:405–408.

321. Stehr-Gree JK, Bailey TM, Visvesvara GS. The epidemiology of *Acanthamoeba* keratitis in the United States. Am J Ophthalmol 1989;107:331–336.

322. Bacon AS, Frazer DG, Dart JKG, et al. A review of 72 consecutive cases of *Acanthamoeba* keratitis, 1984–1992. Eye 1993;7: 719–725.

323. Berger ST, Mondino BJ, Hoft RH, et al. Successful medical management of *Acanthamoeba* keratitis. Am J Ophthalmol 1990; 110:395–403.

324. Elder MJ, Kilvington S, Dart JKG. A clinicopathologic study of in vitro sensitivity testing and *Acanthamoeba* keratitis. Invest Ophthalmol Vis Sci 1994;35:1059–1064.

325. Johns KJ, Head S, O'Day DM. Corneal toxicity of propamidine. Arch Ophthalmol 1988;106:68–69.

326. Yee E, Fiscella R, Winarko TK. Topical polyhexamethylene biguanide (pool cleaner) for treatment of *Acanthamoeba* keratitis. Am J Hosp Pharm 1993;50:2522–2523.

327. Larkin DFP, Kilvington S, Dart JKG. Treatment of *Acanthamoeba* keratitis with polyhexamethylene biguanide. Ophthalmology 1992;99:185–191.

328. Varga JH, Wolf TC, Jensen HG, et al. Combined treatment of *Acanthamoeba* keratitis with propamidine, neomycin, and polyhexamethylene biguanide. Am J Ophthalmol 1993;115:466–470.

CHAPTER 12

Anti-Inflammatory Drugs

Siret D. Jaanus

Gary A. Lesher

Since recognition of the anti-inflammatory activity of adrenal cortical extracts in the early 1940s, hydrocortisone (cortisol), which is the main glucocorticoid secreted by the adrenal cortex, and various synthetic derivatives have proven useful in ocular inflammatory and autoimmune disease states. Although corticosteroids can bring about dramatic clinical results, chronic high-dose therapy can result in undesirable effects in various ocular tissues. Attempts have therefore been made to develop both steroidal and nonsteroidal compounds with effective anti-inflammatory activity but reduced tendency for toxicity. In addition to corticosteroids, two other classes of pharmacologic agents, the nonsteroidal anti-inflammatory drugs, and certain immunosuppressive agents, can modulate ocular inflammatory processes. This chapter considers the ocular applications of the corticosteroids, nonsteroidal anti-inflammatory drugs, and immunosuppressive agents, along with their mechanisms of action, potential adverse reactions and contraindications.

Corticosteroids

More than 40 years following their introduction into ocular therapy by Gordon and McLean,[1] steroids remain frequently used agents for control of both posterior and severe anterior segment inflammatory disease. They can be effective in protecting the ocular structures from many of the deleterious effects accompanying the inflammatory response, particularly scarring and neovascularization.[2-7] They are generally more effective in acute than chronic inflammatory states, and degenerative diseases are usually completely refractory to steroid therapy.[3] The anti-inflammatory effects of steroids appear nonspecific, occurring whether the etiology is allergic, traumatic, or infectious. In most clinical applications they do not act directly to correct a specific disorder, but appear to modify a pre-existing or ongoing response to a foreign or endogenous substance.[7]

Pharmacology

MECHANISMS OF ACTION

Present evidence indicates that specific receptor proteins mediate the effects of steroids.[5-8] Following interaction with its cytoplasmic receptor, the steroid receptor-complex migrates into the cell nucleus and affects protein synthesis (Fig. 12.1). Virtually every tissue has receptors for steroids, which most likely contributes to the many physiologic and pharmacologic effects that occur following steroid administration. This has made it difficult to determine which of the many cellular events that occur following steroid administration relate directly to the observed clinical effects. Experimental observations indicate that at least some of the effects at the cellular level result from altered protein production in immunologically competent cells.[8]

Steroids appear to have an effect on nearly every aspect of the immune system.[7] They inhibit both migration of neutrophils into the extracellular space and their adherence to the vascular endothelium at the site of tissue injury. In therapeutic dosages, steroids also inhibit macrophage access to the site of inflammation and interfere with lymphocyte activity in the immune response.[7]

Evidence indicates that steroids may affect other sub-

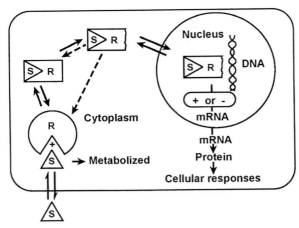

FIGURE 12.1 **Proposed sequence of corticosteroid hormone action. Following entry into the cell, the hormone (S) combines with the receptor (R) followed by a sequence of events resulting in the synthesis of specific proteins that mediate steroid hormone responses. (Adapted from Polansky JR, Weinreb RN. Antiinflammatory agents. In: Sears ML, ed. Pharmacology of the eye. New York: Springer-Verlag, 1984:515.)**

stances that modulate inflammation. Both histamine synthesis and arachidonic acid release, a precursor of prostaglandins, are inhibited.[6,7] Steroids also decrease capillary and fibroblast proliferation and the quantity of collagen deposition, thereby influencing tissue regeneration and repair.[9]

BIOAVAILABILITY

Ophthalmic steroids vary in their ability to penetrate the cornea and subsequently to become distributed in ocular structures. This variability has been attributed to properties of the cornea and physicochemical differences among the individual steroidal compounds.[7] To penetrate the trilayered structure of the cornea, which has both hydrophobic and hydrophilic layers, the ideal steroid should be biphasic in its polarity.[10] This property allows for solubility in both the lipid (hydrophobic) layers of the epithelium and endothelium and the aqueous (hydrophilic) media of the stroma. De-epithelization of the cornea by removal or inflammation alters the hydrophobic properties of the corneal surface and allows water-soluble preparations to penetrate to a greater extent.

Although each steroid has an inherent water or lipid solubility, this characterization can be altered by chemical modification of the steroid base into various derivatives.[5] Acetate and alcohol derivatives of the base compound render the steroid molecule more lipophilic or fat-soluble. Salts, such as sodium phosphate and hydrochloride, are relatively more hydrophilic or water-soluble. The alcohol derivative has intermediate lipophilicity between acetates and salts such as the phosphates.[11]

Modification of a steroid base influences not only ocular penetration through an intact or inflamed cornea, but also formulation of the particular steroid product. The water-soluble salts are generally formulated as solutions, and the more lipid-soluble derivatives are available as suspensions and ointments. Since the acetate, and to a lesser extent the alcohol preparations, are more lipophilic, in theory they should be able to penetrate the intact cornea better than the water-soluble phosphates. Experimental data both in animal models and human subjects seem to support this hypothesis.[12-15] Topical administration of an acetate or alcohol derivative to an uninflamed eye with an intact epithelium produces significantly higher corneal and aqueous steroid levels than does the phosphate derivative of the same steroid base. In the absence of the corneal epithelium in an uninflamed eye, comparison of bioavailability of topically applied acetate and phosphate derivatives shows that the drug level of the phosphate derivative is several times higher than that of the acetate (Table 12.1). In the presence of intraocular inflammation in an eye with an intact epithelium, the acetate derivative again produces the highest corneal concentration. However, some decrease in the hydrophobic epithelial barrier occurs since the phosphate derivative attains somewhat higher levels in the anterior chamber of the inflamed eye with an intact epithelium compared to the uninflamed eye with an intact epithelium.[16]

Although animal models have provided most of the data on bioavailability, Leibowitz and associates[17] have used similar techniques to measure bioavailability of prednisolone acetate in human aqueous humor. Both human and rabbit corneas appear to have similar kinetics of penetration of this steroid into the anterior chamber.

ANTI-INFLAMMATORY EFFICACY

Few well-controlled clinical trials have assessed the efficacy of the available steroids in various ocular inflammatory diseases. Variability in patient signs and symptoms, ethical difficulties, and the number of patients studied make meaningful conclusions difficult.[11]

In addition to variables in clinical signs and symptoms and the ability to penetrate the ocular structures, the derivative of a steroid base also seems to influence its anti-inflammatory efficacy. Using a rabbit corneal model, Leibowitz and associates[13,18] have demonstrated that acetate and alcohol derivatives are more effective than the phosphate derivative in suppressing corneal inflammation both in the presence and absence of corneal epithelium (see Table 12.1). The mechanism by which a derivative affects the anti-inflammatory activity of a steroid base applied topically to the eye is not known, but some data seem to indicate that receptor binding or metabolism may play a role in the observed anti-inflammatory effects.[5,19]

TABLE 12.1

Relationship of the Derivative of an Ophthalmic Corticosteroid Base to Its Corneal Bioavailability and Anti-Inflammatory Efficacy

Corticosteroid	Bioavailability (µg-min/gm)	Anti-Inflammatory Efficacy (%)
Epithelium intact		
Prednisolone acetate 1.0%	2,395	51
Prednisolone phosphate 1.0%	1,075	28
Epithelium absent		
Prednisolone acetate 1.0%	4,574	53
Prednisolone phosphate 1.0%	16,338	47
Epithelium intact		
Fluorometholone alcohol 0.1%		31
Fluorometholone alcohol 0.25%		35
Fluorometholone acetate 0.1%		48
Epithelium absent		
Fluorometholone alcohol 0.1%		37
Epithelium intact		
Dexamethasone acetate 0.1%	111	55
Dexamethasone alcohol 0.1%	543	40
Dexamethasone phosphate 0.1%	1,068	19
Epithelium absent		
Dexamethasone acetate 0.1%	118	60
Dexamethasone alcohol 0.1%	1,316	42
Dexamethasone phosphate 0.1%	4,642	22

Adapted from Leibowitz HM, Kupferman A. Use of corticosteroids in the treatment of corneal inflammation. In: Leibowitz HM, ed. Corneal disorders: Clinical diagnosis and management. Philadelphia: Saunders, 1984.

Ophthalmic Corticosteroids

PREDNISOLONE

A synthetic analog of the major glucocorticoid, hydrocortisone (cortisol), prednisolone has proven an effective anti-inflammatory agent in patients with external as well as intraocular inflammations.[5,7,13,18,19] It is commercially formulated as an acetate and a phosphate (Table 12.2). Experimental models using inflamed rabbit corneas indicate that the mean decrease in corneal inflammation is greater for the prednisolone acetate derivative than for the phosphate, regardless of whether the corneal epithelium is intact or absent[12,13,18] (see Table 12.1). The acetate substitution in the 21 position of the steroid molecule may increase the affinity of the steroid for its receptor, possibly explaining part of the enhanced effect. This increased affinity could enhance its pharmacologic response and also in some way alter its metabolism in ocular tissue.[5,19]

Prednisolone acetate is available at the 0.125% and 1% concentration.[20] Kinetic studies have shown that raising the concentration of prednisolone acetate from 1% to 1.5% or 3% does not enhance its anti-inflammatory effects.[21] The rabbit experimental keratitis model has shown that optimal suppression of corneal inflammation occurs when prednisolone acetate 1% is administered every 15 minutes.[14] However, due to the logistical constraints associated with such frequent instillation, topical dosing of 1% prednisolone acetate at 1-minute intervals for 5 minutes each hour may provide equal clinical suppression of inflammation[8,22] (Table 12.3). When compared with other topical ocular steroids, 1% prednisolone acetate is generally considered the most effective anti-inflammatory agent for anterior segment ocular inflammation.[12]

DEXAMETHASONE

This agent is available as the alcohol or phosphate derivative in the form of a 0.1% ophthalmic suspension or solution. It is also formulated as dexamethasone sodium phosphate ointment, 0.05% (see Table 12.2).[20] Experimental studies indicate that dexamethasone alcohol is superior in anti-

TABLE 12.2
Topical Ocular Corticosteroids

Corticosteroid Base	Derivative	Formulation	Concentration (%)	Trade Name
Prednisolone	Acetate	Suspension	0.125	Econopred (Alcon) Pred Mild (Allergan)
			1.0	Econopred Plus (Alcon) Pred Forte (Allergan)
Prednisolone	Sodium phosphate	Solution	0.125	Inflamase Mild (Ciba Vision) AK-Pred (Akorn)
			1.0	Inflamase Forte (Ciba Vision) AK-Pred (Akorn)
Dexamethasone	Alcohol	Suspension	0.1	Maxidex (Alcon)
Dexamethasone	Sodium phosphate	Solution	0.1	Decadron Phosphate (Merck)
		Ointment	0.05	Decadron Phosphate (Merck) Maxidex (Alcon) AK-Dex (Akorn)
Loteprednol	Etabonate	Suspension	0.5	Lotemax (Pharmos)
Rimexolone		Suspension	1.0	Vexol (Alcon)
Fluorometholone	Alcohol	Ointment	0.1	FML (Allergan)
		Suspension	0.1	FML (Allergan) Fluor-Op (Ciba Vision)
			0.25	FML Forte (Allergan)
Fluorometholone	Acetate	Suspension	0.1	Flarex (Alcon) Eflone (Ciba Vision)
Medrysone	Alcohol	Suspension	1.0	HMS (Allergan)

TABLE 12.3
Anti-Inflammatory Effect of Different Dosage Schedules for Topical Administration of Prednisolone Acetate 1%

Treatment Regimen	Total No. of Doses Delivered	Decrease in Corneal Inflammation (%)
1 drop every 4 hours	6	11
1 drop every 2 hours	10	30
1 drop every hour	18	51
1 drop every 30 minutes	34	61
1 drop every 15 minutes	66	68
1 drop each minute for 5 minutes every hour	90	72

From Leibowitz HM, Kupferman A. Int Ophthalmol Clin 1980; 20:117–134.

inflammatory activity to dexamethasone sodium phosphate, both in the presence or absence of the corneal epithelium[8,16] (see Table 12.1). The poorer performance of the dexamethasone sodium phosphate may result from its binding to the receptor approximately 50-fold less than the alcohol deriva-

tive.[8,19] In contrast, the corneal bioavailability of dexamethasone phosphate is higher than the alcohol derivative with corneal epithelium either intact or absent (see Table 12.1).

The human aqueous humor contains detectable levels of both dexamethasone alcohol and phosphate within 30 minutes of topical application.[23,24] Peak levels occur between 90 and 120 minutes. Thereafter drug levels diminish, but detectable amounts remain 12 hours following administration.[23] Observations such as this seem to indicate that dexamethasone is resistant to metabolism following penetration into the aqueous humor.[19,24]

Although dexamethasone derivatives show similar biologic activity as other steroid bases when applied topically to the eye, dexamethasone acetate is not commercially available as an ophthalmic formulation.[20]

FLUOROMETHOLONE

Unlike prednisolone and dexamethasone, which are structurally related to cortisol, fluorometholone is a fluorinated structural analog of progesterone. Initially formulated as an alcohol, fluorometholone 0.1% (FML) has proven an effective agent in external ocular inflammations, with relatively low potential for elevating intraocular pressure (IOP).[25] Comparative anti-inflammatory studies indicate that the efficacy of fluorometholone alcohol is somewhat less than dexamethasone alcohol and prednisolone acetate (see Table 12.1). Increasing the concentration of fluorometholone alcohol from 0.1% to 0.25% does not significantly increase its anti-inflammatory activity but does enhance its tendency to raise IOP.[26,27] The more recently synthesized 17-acetate derivative of fluorometholone has demonstrated greater anti-inflammatory activity in the experimental rabbit keratitis model than has fluorometholone alcohol.[28,29] Clinical evaluation in patients with conjunctivitis, episcleritis, and scleritis also indicates that fluorometholone acetate improves clinical signs and symptoms of inflammation significantly more than fluorometholone alcohol.[29] Furthermore, when fluorometholone acetate 0.1% was compared to prednisolone acetate 1.0% in patients with moderate inflammation, Leibowitz and associates[29] found no difference in the anti-inflammatory effects of the two steroids.

Following topical application to the eye, fluorometholone alcohol penetrates into the aqueous humor.[30,31] Its ability to do so appears independent of the state of the corneal epithelium or the degree of ocular inflammation.[30] Radiolabeled studies indicate that fluorometholone alcohol is rapidly metabolized within the aqueous humor.[24,32] However, similar studies with fluorometholone acetate show that this derivative metabolizes much more slowly (Fig. 12.2).[19] Thus, it is possible that the 17-acetate substitution to the fluorometholone base not only enhances its anti-inflammatory effects, but also impedes its metabolism. Therefore, in clinical use the benefit/risk ratio of fluorometholone may possibly correlate with the type of derivative used, location of the inflammation, and ocular health status of the patient.

Fluorometholone is commercially available as the alcohol derivative 0.1% suspension and ointment (FML) and 0.25% suspension (FML Forte), and as the 0.1% acetate suspension (Flarex)[20] (see Table 12.2).

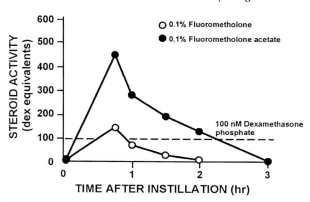

FIGURE 12.2 **Aqueous humor steroid activity using the glucocorticoid receptor assay following administration of topical unlabeled 0.1% fluorometholone and 0.1% fluorometholone acetate in rabbits. (Adapted from Polansky JR. Basic pharmacology of corticosteroids. Current topics in ocular inflammation 1993;1:19.)**

MEDRYSONE

Like fluorometholone, medrysone is a synthetic derivative of progesterone.[19] It is commercially available as a 1% ophthalmic suspension (HMS).[20] Compared to prednisolone, dexamethasone and fluorometholone,[5,7] medrysone exhibits limited corneal penetration and a lower affinity for glucocorticoid receptors. In clinical use, it appears to be the weakest of the available ophthalmic steroids.[33] Medrysone can be useful for superficial ocular inflammations, including allergic and atopic conjunctivitis, but intraocular inflammatory conditions generally do not respond.[34] Clinical experience with medrysone has also indicated that it is less likely to cause a significant rise in IOP.[35,36] However, caution needs to be exercised in patients known to respond to steroids with a rise in IOP (steroid responders), since pressure increases can lead to ocular damage.[37]

LOTEPREDNOL AND RIMEXOLONE

The tendency of ophthalmic steroids to raise IOP has resulted in the synthesis of compounds with anti-inflammatory activity but less propensity for pressure increases. Both in human and animal models, loteprednol etabonate and rimexolone have shown anti-inflammatory effects with reduced potential to raise IOP.[38-41]

Loteprednol was designed as an analog of prednisolone according to the "soft drug" concept proposed by Bodor.[42] Synthesis of a "soft drug" is achieved by starting with a known, inactive metabolite of an active drug. The inactive metabolite is then structurally modified to an active form that *in vivo* undergoes a predictable, one-step transformation back to the inactive metabolite. Loteprednol contains a metabolically-labile ester in the 17-beta position, a stable carbonate group in the 17-alpha position, and lacks a ketone group in position 20.[43,44] Following topical instillation, loteprednol penetrates the cornea but is rapidly transformed to its inactive metabolite in the anterior chamber. Despite its rapid transformation, loteprednol does appear to exert significant anti-inflammatory activity in the rabbit cornea.[44] Bartlett and associates[41] studied the effects of 0.5% loteprednol in patients with giant papillary conjunctivitis and observed that loteprednol improved symptoms and significantly reduced papillae size. The IOP did not rise during the study, and the drug was well tolerated.

Bartlett and associates[38] have also compared the effects of loteprednol 0.5% on IOP in individuals known to be steroid responders to prednisolone acetate 1%. Loteprednol produced less effect on IOP than did prednisolone acetate.

Rimexolone, a synthetic topical steroid, also exhibits minimal effects on IOP.[40] The ocular hypertensive effect of rimexolone 1% appears to be comparable to that of 0.1% fluorometholone alcohol but less than that of prednisolone acetate 1% and dexamethasone phosphate 0.1%. Rimexolone also alleviates signs and symptoms associated with allergic conjunctivitis, including itching and tearing.[45] Rimexolone is commercially available as a 1.0% ophthalmic suspension (Vexol) preserved with 0.01% benzalkonium chloride. It is indicated for the treatment of postoperative inflammation following cataract surgery and for treatment of anterior uveitis.

Principles of Corticosteroid Therapy

Following more than four decades of clinical experience with ocular corticosteroid therapy, the use of these drugs remains largely empirical. Experience, however, has led to some general therapeutic principles:[46]

- The specific type and location of the inflammation determine whether topical, systemic, periocular or multiple routes of administration are appropriate.
- Treatment should be instituted as soon as possible when indicated, and the dose should be high enough to suppress the inflammatory response.
- The appropriate dose for a specific condition is largely determined by clinical experience and must be reevaluated at frequent intervals during the course of treatment.
- Long-term, high-dosage therapy should not be discontinued abruptly. The dose should be gradually reduced over time.
- Short-term, low-dosage topical ocular therapy generally does not produce significant side effects.

Ideally, the minimal effective dose should be used for the shortest time necessary to secure the desired clinical response. The dosage should be individualized as much as possible to the patient and the severity of the condition. The patient's general health must be considered and close supervision maintained to assess the effects of steroid therapy on the course of the disease and possible adverse effects.[47]

With ocular disease the route of steroid administration is an important determinant of the pharmacologic and therapeutic effects observed. Topical ocular therapy is usually satisfactory for inflammatory disorders of the lids, conjunctiva, cornea, iris, and ciliary body. In severe forms of anterior uveitis, topical therapy may require supplementation with systemic or periocular (local injection) steroids. Chorioretinitis and optic neuritis are generally treated with systemic or periocular steroids or both.[49]

The severity and location of the disorder as well as the steroid's inherent anti-inflammatory and toxic effects are important considerations in situations that seriously threaten vision. In such cases, the most efficacious steroid may be indicated despite its potential risks.

TOPICAL OCULAR ADMINISTRATION

Shortly after the introduction of corticosteroids to ocular therapeutics, clinical use indicated that local treatment was equal to or superior to systemic administration, providing that the diseased tissue could be brought in contact with sufficient steroid.[3] Generally speaking, when possible, topical administration is indicated for anterior segment disease. Ease of application, comparatively low cost, and relative absence of systemic complications make it the preferred route of steroid therapy. Selection of a particular topical steroid and the dosage administered varies with the location and severity of the inflammation.

Topical therapy should usually continue at a reduced dosage for several days to several weeks after inflammatory signs and symptoms have disappeared, since prematurely discontinuing treatment can lead to relapse, particularly with high-dosage therapy.[3,4] Corticosteroids reduce the leukocytic elements of the blood. Consequently, white cells proliferate when therapy stops. The immature cells can produce large quantities of antibodies to residual antigen in the ocular tissue. A massive polymorphonuclear leukocytic reaction follows the resultant antigen-antibody reaction. This sequence of events, unless interrupted immediately, can lead to a recurring, serious, necrotizing inflammatory reaction.[3,4] Thus, depending on the response obtained and the dosage used, topical therapy should generally be tapered over several days to weeks.[3,4,47,48]

SYSTEMIC TREATMENT

Inflammations of the posterior segment, optic nerve, or orbit usually require systemic administration of steroids. Selection of the particular steroid preparation and the dosage remains largely an individual choice, but the tendency is to use compounds with minimal mineralocorticoid activity (Table 12.4). Prednisone is a popular agent of choice for oral administration. For intravenous administration (IV), methyl-

TABLE 12.4
Relative Anti-Inflammatory Activity, Sodium-Retaining Activity, and Equivalent Doses of Representative Systemic Corticosteroids

Generic Name	Trade Name	Relative Anti-Inflammatory Activity	Relative Sodium-Retaining Activity	Equivalent Dose (mg)
Hydrocortisone (cortisol)	Cortef, Hydrocortone	1.0	1.0	20.00
Cortisone acetate	Cortisone, Cortone	0.8	0.8	25.00
Prednisone	Prednicen-M, Orasone, Deltasone, Meticorten	4.0	0.8	5.00
Prednisolone	Prednicen, Delta-Cortef, Sterane	4.0	0.8	5.00
Triamcinolone	Aristocort, Kenacort	5.0	0.0	4.00
Methylprednisolone	Medrol	5.0	0.0	4.00
Paramethasone acetate	Haldrone	10.00	0.0	2.0
Fludrocortisone acetate	Florinef	20.0	125.0	0.10
Dexamethasone	Decadron, Hexadrol	25.0	0.0	0.75
Betamethasone	Celestone	25.0	0.0	0.75

prednisolone sodium succinate has proven useful. The Optic Neuritis Treatment Trial (ONTT)[49] indicated that patients receiving a 3-day course of IV methylprednisolone, followed by oral prednisone for 11 days, showed faster improvement in visual acuity compared to the group receiving only oral prednisone.

Since adverse effects are more likely to occur with systemic therapy (Table 12.5), dosage should be individualized for each patient. The minimal effective dose for the shortest possible time is advocated. When long-term therapy is necessary, the lowest possible dose to control the disease must be given.

Some general therapeutic guidelines for systemic steroid therapy have been suggested. For most mild to moderate ocular inflammatory disorders, initial daily dosage of 20 to 40 mg of prednisone or its equivalent is recommended.[46,49] For patients with severe inflammation, initial daily doses of 40 to 60 mg of prednisone or its equivalent should be used. If no improvement occurs within 48 to 72 hours, an increase to 80 mg or more may be necessary.[46,49]

As soon as the clinical response occurs, the dosage should be decreased over days or weeks depending on the length of treatment. Reduction should be in graduated decrements, guided strictly by the clinical course of the disease, usually reducing the daily dosage 10 mg for larger doses and 2 to 5 mg for smaller doses at intervals of 3 to 4 days. Once a dosage level of 15 to 20 mg is reached, the patient should remain at that level for 1 to 2 weeks to prevent recurrent flare-up of inflammation. If exacerbation of the inflammation follows a given dose reduction, the dose of steroid must

TABLE 12.5
Systemic Effects of Corticosteroid Therapy

- Adrenal insufficiency
- Cushing's syndrome
- Peptic ulceration
- Osteoporosis
- Hypertension
- Muscle weakness or atrophy
- Inhibition of growth
- Diabetes
- Activation of infection
- Mood changes
- Delay in wound healing

be immediately raised to the pre-reduction level. As long as evidence of active disease persists, therapy must continue at a level that permits control of signs or symptoms.[49] The available steroids vary in their ability to suppress the inflammatory response. Table 12.4 shows the approximate equivalent doses of systemic steroids in current use. Methylprednisolone is commercially available in a package for programmed delivery of oral steroid tapered during 6 days of therapy. This formulation (Medrol DosePak) is highly convenient for short-term treatment and helps to ensure patient compliance in the tapering schedule.

LOCAL INJECTION

Periocular steroids can be administered by subconjunctival, sub-Tenon's, or retrobulbar injection. A topical anesthetic is often instilled before injection of the steroid. This route of administration can be effective during surgical procedures, as a supplement to topical and systemic steroids in cases of severe inflammation, and in patients not compliant with the prescribed regimen.[50] Experiments using radiolabeled methylprednisolone acetate (Depo-Medrol) indicate that retrobulbar injection can deliver high concentrations of medication to sclera, choroid, retina, and vitreous for a week or longer.[51] Long-term repository vehicles containing triamcinolone acetonide injected beneath Tenon's capsule have proven valuable in several chronic inflammatory conditions, including anterior uveitis.[52] Locally injected methylprednisolone acetate and triamcinolone acetate have been shown effective in the treatment of chalazia.[53,54] The success rate appears greater with chalazia less than 8 mm in size.[55] Combined excision and drainage with intralesional steroid injection is also an option with a high success rate.[56]

The use of periocular steroids has several limitations and complications. The injections are usually somewhat uncomfortable, and thus patients prefer to avoid them. Adverse ocular effects have included retinal detachment, optic nerve atrophy, and preretinal membrane formation.[57] Intraocular pressure can rise, particularly since the drug may remain in the eye for several days to weeks.[58] Some of the observed effects may result from the vehicle rather than from the steroid itself.

Periocular injection of steroids should be reserved for those situations requiring an anti-inflammatory effect greater than that obtainable with topical or systemic administration.[4] Concurrent administration of steroid by both topical and subconjunctival routes does appear to produce an additive therapeutic effect in severe inflammations, but periocular injection alone does not necessarily result in greater anti-inflammatory effects. Experiments comparing equal doses of steroid applied topically or by injection indicate that a greater reduction in polymorphonuclear leukocyte invasion of the cornea occurs following topical use compared with periocular injection.[59] These data suggest that topical administration should be the primary route of steroid therapy for anterior segment inflammations. Table 12.6 com-

pares the advantages and disadvantages of the three routes of steroid administration.[50]

ALTERNATE-DAY THERAPY

In 1963 Harter and associates[60] reported that single-dose alternate-day systemic administration of corticosteroid can be as effective as divided-dosage daily treatment. With this regimen a patient receives the entire total dose that would be given over a 2-day period as a single dose every other morning. This regimen permits metabolic recovery and prevents toxic effects from becoming cumulative. The concept of alternate-day systemic therapy applies only to shorter-acting systemic steroids such as prednisone. Compounds with longer half-lives such as triamcinolone and dexamethasone continue their activity on the off-treatment day.[49]

Since the normal physiologic release of ACTH and cortisol is characterized by episodic secretion with highest levels at 8:00 AM, single-dose as well as the first dose of the day in divided-dosage therapy should occur in the early morning hours.

Alternate-day therapy can prove useful for conditions, such as chronic uveitis, that require long-term systemic administration.[61] This approach has also been advocated for treatment of chronic conditions in children because it minimizes growth suppression. The alternate-day regimen has not been widely accepted, and modifications have been suggested. Clinical experience also indicates that this treatment method is not as effective as divided, daily doses, particularly in severe ocular inflammatory conditions. Adrenal gland suppression and other side effects associated with systemic therapy can still occur with the alternate-day regimen.[49]

Clinical Uses

Table 12.7 lists the primary ocular inflammatory disorders in which steroids may provide a therapeutic benefit.[49]

Steroids are generally contraindicated in most ocular infections because they are not bactericidal and because they reduce resistance to many types of invading microorganisms, including bacteria, viruses, and fungi. In particular, owing to the difficulty in controlling replication of fungi in ocular infection, steroid use can enhance microbial replication in this as well as other types of infection and also can mask evidence of progression of the infection.[7,8] In severe infections having considerable ocular involvement and threatening vision, steroids may be used within 48 hours of starting the appropriate anti-infective therapy.[3,7]

ALLERGY AND HYPERSENSITIVITY REACTIONS

Type I allergic reactions often respond rapidly to topical steroids. For milder reactions such as allergic conjunctivitis due to airborne allergens, cold compresses and vasoconstrictors or antihistamines may suffice. Mast cell

TABLE 12.6
Advantages and Disadvantages of the Three Routes of Corticosteroid Administration

Topical	Periocular	Systemic
	Advantages	
Placed near where it is needed	Placed near where it is needed	Tablets are easy to take
Simple to apply	Can treat one eye and use the other as a control	May be better at reaching all parts of the eye
Can treat uniocular disease	Can treat the worse of two eyes	
Avoids most systemic effects	Can treat uniocular diseases	
	Avoids most systemic effects	
	Of value if patient cannot be trusted to take medication	
	Valuable at time of surgery to help prevent flare-up	
	Disadvantages	
Occasionally patient will develop adrenal suppression	Patient will probably develop some adrenal suppression	Adrenal suppression
Will aggravate a dendritic ulcer	Discomfort with injection	Systemic side effects more likely to occur
May leave white residue	Occasionally, white material is cosmetically objectionable	
Epithelial keratopathy from frequent applications	Subconjunctival adhesions	
Occasional conjunctival infections	Allergy to diluent	
	Occasional orbital infection	
	Occasional intraocular injection of steroid	
	Ulceration of conjunctiva after repeated injections if not given behind the eye	
	Exophthalmos and rugae in fundus	
	Papilledema	

Adapted from Schlaegel TF. Depot corticosteroid by the cul-de-sac route. In: Kaufman HE, ed. Ocular anti-inflammatory therapy. Springfield, IL: Charles C Thomas, 1970; 3:117.

stabilizers and certain nonsteroidal anti-inflammatory agents can also be used with success (see Chapter 13). Severe forms of vernal or atopic keratoconjunctivitis may respond to topical steroids, such as fluorometholone or prednisolone, with dramatic improvement of symptoms.[7] Prescribing the lowest dosage and frequency necessary helps to avoid complications. Use of mast cell stabilizers may decrease the need for prolonged steroid therapy. Contact dermatitis of the eyelids and preservative-induced blepharoconjunctivitis, if not responsive to avoidance of the allergen, may benefit from topical administration of steroids.[62] For certain allergic diseases, such as phlyctenular keratoconjunctivitis, specific antimicrobial therapy may also reduce the need for steroids, possibly by eliminating the antigenic stimuli.[5]

UVEITIS

In both anterior and posterior uveitis, corticosteroids can reduce inflammation, relieve pain, and prevent synechiae.[7] Adjunctive medication such as cycloplegics and antiglaucoma drugs may be necessary. Posterior uveitis often requires periocular or oral steroids along with specific antimicrobial or cytotoxic therapy.[5,7]

HERPES SIMPLEX KERATITIS

The use of corticosteroids in herpes simplex keratitis is controversial, since steroids can disseminate the infectious agent and thus may contribute to a more destructive lesion.[7] Generally steroids should be reserved for stromal involvement and used only in the presence of an intact corneal epithelium. Antiviral coverage should also be provided, and the possibility of superinfection must always be considered.[5] A multicenter, placebo-controlled clinical trial recently demonstrated that topical steroids can reduce persistence and progression of stromal inflammation and shorten the duration of herpes simplex keratitis.[63] Both treatment groups in this study also received topical trifluridine.

OPHTHALMIC SURGERY

Surgical manipulation of the eye can stimulate a wide array of pathways, leading to both anterior and posterior segment

TABLE 12.7
Indications for Use of Corticosteroids in Ocular Disease

Eyelids	Uvea
Allergic blepharitis	Anterior uveitis
Contact dermatitis	Posterior uveitis
Herpes zoster dermatoblepharitis	Sympathetic ophthalmia
Chemical burns	
Neonatal hemangioma	Sclera
	Scleritis
Conjunctiva	Episcleritis
Allergic conjunctivitis	
Vernal conjunctivitis	Retina
Herpes zoster conjunctivitis	Retinal vasculitis
Chemical burns	
Mucocutaneous conjunctival	Optic nerve
lesions	Optic neuritis
	Temporal arteritis
Cornea	
Immune reaction after keratoplasty	Globe
Herpes zoster keratitis	Endophthalmitis
Disciform keratitis	Hemorrhagic glaucoma
Marginal corneal infiltrates	
Superficial punctate keratitis	Orbit
Chemical burns	Pseudotumor
Acne rosacea keratitis	Graves' ophthalmopathy
Interstitial keratitis	
	Extraocular muscles
	Ocular myasthenia gravis

inflammation. The value of corticosteroids in preventing surgically-induced inflammation has been debated.[7,64] Evidence indicates that steroids may be effective in aphakic and pseudophakic cystoid macular edema (CME).[65] Topical steroids, including prednisolone and dexamethasone, may reduce postoperative corneal edema and provide a protective effect for the blood-aqueous barrier following cataract extraction and intraocular lens implantation.[66,67] Recent evidence suggests, however, that the nonsteroidal anti-inflammatory agents may be more effective in preventing breakdown of the blood-aqueous barrier and reduce the incidence of both angiographic and clinical CME in the postoperative period.[68] The effect of topical steroids, particularly long term, in decreasing corneal inflammation and affecting refractive outcome following laser photorefractive keratectomy (PRK) remains to be demonstrated.[69]

MISCELLANEOUS CONDITIONS

Corticosteroids can also be useful in episcleritis, in the initial treatment of some alkali burns, in the early stages of thyroid ophthalmopathy, and along with appropriate antimicrobial therapy in interstitial keratitis associated with syphilis and microbial endophthalmitis.[70] Part III of this book considers many examples of steroid use in specific disease states.

Side Effects

Although the effectiveness of corticosteroids in the treatment of ocular inflammation has stood the test of time, these agents sometimes cause side effects. Adverse events can occur with all routes of administration and all preparations currently available. Systemic absorption of corticosteroid occurs with topical use on the eyes, skin, and mucosa of the upper respiratory tract.[3,28,29] The incidence of side effects appears to rise significantly with long-term, high-dose therapy. However, short-term, high-dosage therapy appears to cause fewer side effects than do prolonged courses with lower dosages.[71] Ocular complications can develop following either local or systemic steroid administration and range from actual physical damage to the ocular tissue to interference with healing and immune mechanisms (Table 12.8).

CATARACTS

Posterior subcapsular cataracts (PSC) occur with all routes of administration, including systemic, topical, cutaneous, nasal aerosols, and inhalation corticosteroids.[71,72] A decade following the introduction of systemic steroid therapy for rheumatoid arthritis, Black and associates[73,74] reported a high incidence of lens opacities in patients receiving long-term systemic therapy. In 44 rheumatoid arthritis patients treated with various steroids, including prednisone and dexamethasone, 17 (39%) developed bilateral PSC cataracts. Interestingly, dosage and duration of therapy appeared to be correlated with the incidence of cataract development. Patients who received prednisone therapy for 1 to 4 years showed an 11% incidence if the dosage range was less than 10 mg/day, a 30% incidence if the dosage was 10 to 15 mg/day, and an 80% incidence if the dosage was greater than 15 mg/day.[74]

Although the early literature contained conflicting reports,[71] additional supporting evidence became available when several investigators observed increased incidence of PSC cataracts in children receiving systemic steroid therapy for rheumatoid arthritis, systemic lupus erythematosus, and the nephrotic syndrome.[75,76] Although in adults steroid-related PSC cataracts do not usually occur within the first

TABLE 12.8
Ocular Effects of Corticosteroid Therapy

- Posterior subcapsular cataracts
- Ocular hypertension or glaucoma
- Secondary ocular infection
- Retardation of corneal epithelial healing
- Uveitis
- Mydriasis
- Ptosis
- Transient ocular discomfort

year of therapy regardless of dose, children can manifest lens changes at lower doses and within shorter periods.[77]

Topical ocular steroid administration also may cause the development of cataracts in both children and adults.[78–80] Possibly the ocular disease itself may cause the observed lens changes. However, the incidence of cataracts following topical ocular steroid use indicates that long-term therapy may indeed result in lens opacities.[79,80] Two females, aged 17 and 20 years, used topical steroids for several years to eliminate redness associated with contact lens wear. Both developed PSC cataract as well as glaucoma and visual field loss.[80] The opacities associated with steroid administration resemble those produced by ionizing radiation and ocular disease such as uveitis, retinitis pigmentosa, and retinal detachment (Fig. 12.3).[71] They differ from opacities associated with diabetes and trauma, but are indistinguishable from lens changes associated with posterior subcapsular age-related cataract.[73]

In most patients, lens changes accompanying steroid therapy do not significantly impair visual acuity. Less than 10% of patients receiving long-term therapy have vision reduced to less than 20/60 (6/18).[81] Patients seldom complain of visual problems unless the practitioner makes a direct inquiry.[71] Photophobia and glare may be complaints. Once vision is affected, reduction or cessation of steroid therapy seldom resolves the opacity, but it does halt progression; in some cases, the area of opacity decreases.[71,72] Although it is now generally accepted that corticosteroids are cataractogenic, the mechanisms for development of the lens opacities have not been fully elucidated. The relationship of total dose, dosage schedule, patient age, associated disease, and the steroid administered requires further study. Possibly glucocorticoids cause cataract formation by gaining entry to the lens fiber cells. After reacting with specific amino groups of lens crystallins, a conformational change occurs within the cells, exposing sulfhydryl groups. These then form disulfide bonds, which subsequently lead to protein aggregation and finally to complexes that refract light.[71] Significant causative factors could include the relationship of the lens changes to total dose, duration of therapy, and individual susceptibility. Several studies have suggested that the most important factor in steroid-induced PSC cataract formation may be individual susceptibility to the side effects of corticosteroids.[77,82,83] An ethnic susceptibility may also exist. Reportedly, Hispanics are more predisposed to PSC cataract development than are whites or blacks.[77] Diabetic patients also appear to be more susceptible with topical steroid administration. In one study,[84] 9 of 11 patients developed cataract in the eye treated with 0.1% dexamethasone. Differences in patient response to dosage, duration of therapy, age, and inherent genetic factors are all likely possibilities to explain the lenticular changes. The factors that influence individual susceptibility to steroid-induced cataract, including therapeutic regimen, require further investigation.

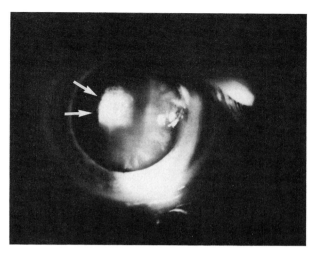

FIGURE 12.3 **Posterior subcapsular (PSC) cataract (arrows) in a 48-year-old white man who had taken oral prednisone 7.5 mg daily for 13 years for the treatment of rheumatoid arthritis. Visual acuity was 20/30 (6/9).**

OCULAR HYPERTENSION OR GLAUCOMA

Following the introduction of corticosteroids for treating ocular inflammatory disease, reports began to appear in the literature implicating topical steroid therapy as a cause for elevation in IOP.[85,86] However, it was not until Goldmann[87] reported his observation with topical steroid therapy in 1962 that it became generally accepted that these agents can produce the clinical picture of open-angle glaucoma.

More conclusive evidence of the ability of steroids to raise IOP comes from controlled studies in which patients showed reversible elevations of pressure with repeated use of topical steroids.[88,89] The hypertensive response can occur in both normal and glaucomatous eyes and usually develops 2 to 8 weeks following initiation of therapy with dexamethasone, betamethasone, prednisolone, hydrocortisone, or fluorometholone. The effects on pressure and the reduction in outflow facility are generally reversible and return to their original levels within 1 to 3 weeks after steroid administration terminates. However, in some cases pressures have not reverted to pretreatment levels, and glaucoma with accompanying vision loss has occurred.[89] The pressure elevations are usually much greater in eyes with open-angle glaucoma and tend to be higher than normal in children of glaucoma patients.[87]

The work of Armaly[90] and Becker[91] has indicated that topically administered steroids tend to produce ocular hypertension in certain susceptible individuals. Statistical analysis of volunteers given topical dexamethasone 0.1% 3 times a day indicated three separate groups of responders in the general population. The largest group in the volunteer population responded with an average pressure elevation of 1.6 mm Hg after 4 weeks of topical dexamethasone. A second group responded with an average elevation of 10 mm Hg. Pressure elevations of 16 mm Hg or greater occurred in the third group. The groups also differed in the timing of their pressure elevation: the second and third groups showed a continued and steady pressure elevation during the 4 weeks of observation compared with the first group. The first group showed a small initial pressure increase that did not continue to rise during subsequent weeks of the study.

The degree of response to topical corticosteroid thus appears genetically determined. Patients may inherit their response to topical steroids in a Mendelian fashion. That is, the offspring of matings of persons with various known degrees of response to topical steroids appear to fit the prediction of Mendelian inheritance.[97] Patients with primary open-angle glaucoma and their relatives show a remarkably high prevalence of pressure elevations with topical steroids. Bartlett and associates[92] have shown that approximately 70% of the first-degree offspring of individuals with glaucoma have IOP elevations of at least 5 mm Hg. Information regarding patient or family history of glaucoma therefore becomes important when considering the use of steroids.

Schwartz[93] has offered an alternative to the Mendelian model of a single genetic locus controlling steroid responsiveness. Based on his studies in twins, Schwartz has proposed a multifactorial or polygenic model for the familial transmission of the ocular hypertensive response. In this model, one locus or gene does not solely determine high responsiveness; rather, the hypertensive response to steroids

results from a complex interaction of multiple genetic and perhaps environmental factors.

In addition to genetic tendencies, other factors can contribute to the pressure elevations resulting from topical steroid administration. These can include patient age, myopia of 5 diopters or more, and Krukenberg's spindles.[94,95] Long-term systemic steroid therapy can also cause IOP elevations. Bernstein and Schwartz[96] found that patients treated with systemic cortisone, 25 mg or its equivalent, for rheumatoid arthritis and other collagen vascular diseases showed significantly higher mean applanation pressures compared with untreated individuals. They also observed lower facility of outflow and changes in ocular rigidity in steroid-treated patients. Other investigators[93] have also observed rises in pressure with systemic steroids. The IOP rose with administration of steroid and fell when intake was reduced or discontinued. If the dosage increased or therapy was reinstituted, the pressure elevations recurred.

Corticosteroid-induced ocular hypertension relates not only to the individual patient, but the specific steroid used may also play a role. In general, dexamethasone 0.1% and betamethasone 0.1% appear more likely to induce significant IOP elevations than do prednisolone acetate, fluorometholone alcohol, or medrysone.[90,91] In one study,[97] 43 patients demonstrated pressure elevation with 0.1% dexamethasone sodium phosphate. Of these individuals, 15 had IOP increases of 5 mm Hg or more while receiving 0.1% fluorometholone, and three patients demonstrated pressure elevations greater than 15 mm Hg. A masked study[36] using male volunteers compared ocular pressure elevations with 0.1% dexamethasone phosphate, 0.1% fluorometholone alcohol, and 1% medrysone applied 4 times a day for 6 weeks. Figure 12.4 shows the relative ability of these steroids to raise IOP. At the end of 6 weeks of treatment the mean pressure increases for dexamethasone, fluorometholone, and medrysone were 63.1%, 33.8%, and 8.3%, respectively. Kass and associates[98] compared the effects of 0.25% fluorometholone alcohol suspension with 0.1% dexamethasone sodium phosphate solution in steroid-responsive patients. Subjects received the medication in 1 eye 4 times daily for up to 6 weeks. Although both drugs elevated IOP, mean pressure increases from baseline in eyes treated with fluorometholone were significantly lower than those in eyes treated with dexamethasone at weeks 2, 4, and 6 (Fig. 12.5). Factors contributing to the reduced propensity of fluorometholone alcohol to raise IOP could include its considerably shorter pharmacokinetic half-life and greater susceptibility to metabolism as compared to dexamethasone phosphate.[24] Further studies are needed to compare the effects of fluorometholone alcohol and fluorometholone acetate on IOP in both nonsteroid and steroid responders. In addition to the individual steroid's effect on IOP, concentration as well as length and frequency of administration may play a role in the observed pressure elevations.[93]

The molecular mechanism whereby corticosteroids in-

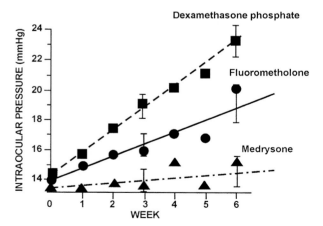

FIGURE 12.4 **Weekly intraocular pressure responses of eyes treated with 1% medrysone, 0.1% fluorometholone, and 0.1% dexamethasone phosphate. Each point represents a mean value (mm Hg) of 12 eyes. (From Mindel JS, Tovitian HO, Smith H, et al. Comparative ocular pressure elevations of topical corticosteroids. Arch Ophthalmol 1980;98:1578. Copyright 1980, American Medical Association.)**

duce pressure elevation is not fully understood. Human trabecular cells possess receptors responsive to steroids.[99] Possibly a direct action on meshwork cells could mediate alterations in outflow facility. Electron microscopic studies of steroid-treated trabecular specimens have indicated the presence of extracellular materials including glycosamino-glycans (GAGs).[100] Their presence may obstruct the mesh-work, thereby causing resistance to aqueous outflow.[101] Alternatively, the presence of excessive GAGs could result in fluid retention.[100]

INFECTION

Since steroids reduce the immunologic defense mechanisms, these drugs lower resistance to many types of infection. In addition, inhibiting the inflammatory response may mask symptoms of disease. Evidence indicates that steroid admin-istration can increase susceptibility to viral, fungal, and bacterial infections.[3]

The use of steroids in ocular infections requires caution to avoid interfering with the reparative processes. If the appro-priate antibiotic is selected and if the course of therapy is relatively short, steroids can help reduce inflammation and prevent possible scarring.[102] In general, however, steroids should be avoided in cases of routine bacterial infections of the lids and conjunctiva because no scarring is anticipated and because steroids provide relatively little benefit in the healing process.

Steroids may prolong the clinical course of dendritic keratitis caused by herpes simplex virus.[103,104] Experiments with rabbits have confirmed these observations. Following inoculation with herpes simplex virus, the group treated with topical prednisolone developed a keratoconjunctivitis earlier than untreated animals, and the condition lasted longer and was more severe than that of the untreated animals.[105] Corti-costeroids also retard the healing of experimental herpes simplex corneal infection. Dexamethasone, methylpredniso-lone, and triamcinolone instilled 3 times a day retarded healing of rabbit corneas inoculated with herpes simplex by as long as 2 weeks depending on the steroid used.[106]

There is general agreement that topical use of steroids enhances ocular susceptibility to fungal infection.[3,107] Minor ocular injuries treated with steroids or steroid-antibiotic combinations have resulted in fungal keratitis. Aggravation of fungal keratitis has also been demonstrated in animals. Inoculation of rabbit corneas with *Candida albicans* resulted in keratitis in 75% of eyes treated with cortisol 1%, while only 37% of eyes not treated with steroid developed the infection.[107] In addition, indirect evidence indicates that steroids decrease human resistance to fungal infections.[3] Therefore, for patients using topical or systemic steroid therapy in whom discontinuation of the steroid is not feasi-ble, elimination of the infection can be difficult and pro-longed.[108]

The enhanced risk of superinfection by bacteria, fungi,

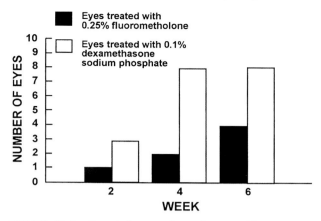

FIGURE 12.5 **Cumulative number of eyes with treatment discontinued because of increased intraocular pressure. (Reprinted with permission from the American Journal of Ophthalmology 1986;102:161. Copyright © the Ophthalmic Publishing Company.)**

and viruses emphasizes the need to maintain a balance between the steroid and the chemotherapeutic agent.[109] Al-though steroids decrease the amount of tissue damage caused by the inflammatory response, preserving the ocular structures requires the use of specific anti-infective therapy to eradicate the replicating organism. It is generally accepted that steroids should never be the sole therapeutic agent in conditions caused by actively replicating microorganisms.[8]

CORNEAL EPITHELIAL HEALING

Both systemic and topical ocular steroid therapy can retard corneal healing.[3,7] Persistent punctate staining of the cornea can indicate epithelial damage by the corticosteroid if the original disease has been eliminated. In experimentally in-duced alkali corneal burns in rabbits, both topical and sys-temic steroid administration can increase by as much as 30% the time required for epithelial regeneration.[110] Effects on collagen synthesis and fibroblast activity have been pro-posed as a possible mechanism.[3,111]

CORTICOSTEROID UVEITIS

It seems paradoxical that the topical use of corticosteroids can lead to acute inflammation of the anterior segment. However, since the first report[112] of the development of anterior uveitis during provocative testing with steroids for glaucoma, additional cases have been reported.[113] The inci-dence is higher in blacks (5.4%) than in whites (0.5%). Symptoms include pain, photophobia, blurred vision, and perilimbal (ciliary) hyperemia; anterior chamber flare and cells can be observed. The corticosteroid itself rather than its vehicle appears to cause the condition. It does not appear to be related to a particular steroid preparation since it can occur with either the sodium phosphate or alcohol derivatives of dexamethasone as well as prednisolone acetate.

MYDRIASIS AND PTOSIS

Dilation of the pupil and ptosis can occur with topical steroid administration.[88] Application of 0.1% dexamethasone in human volunteers has produced mydriasis as early as 1 week following its initial use. The average increase in pupillary diameter was approximately 1 mm. The effect disappears following cessation of drug therapy.[114]

The mydriatic effect of topically applied corticosteroids has been investigated in isolated intraocular muscle preparation[115] as well as in living monkey eyes.[116] The resting tension of the dilator muscle was increased and that of the sphincter decreased in the presence of steroids. Instillation of 0.1% dexamethasone (Decadron) produced pupillary dilation and ptosis as well as elevation of IOP in the monkey eyes. When the steroids were tested without their vehicles, the effects on IOP, pupil size, and upper lid did not occur. Responses to the vehicle alone, however, were identical to steroid-containing drops, whereas corticosteroid in saline did not produce the observed changes. Thus, it has been suggested that an excipient in the vehicle mixture causes the effects, possibly by altering cell membrane permeability.[115,116]

OTHER SIDE EFFECTS

Transient ocular discomfort can ensue following topical application of steroids to the eye. Mechanical effects of the steroid particles in suspension, the vehicle itself, and the severity of the inflammatory condition can all be causative factors.

Steroid-induced calcium deposits in the cornea have been reported.[117] Patients with persistent epithelial defects such as postoperative inflammation, penetrating keratoplasty, and a history of herpetic keratitis and dry eye have developed a calcific band keratopathy following topical use of a steroid phosphate formulation.

Occasional refractive changes, blurring of vision, and increases in corneal thickness occur. Dry eye syndrome in the postinfection period has been reported following topical steroid use for treatment of epidemic keratoconjunctivitis.[118]

SYSTEMIC EFFECTS OF LOCALLY ADMINISTERED CORTICOSTEROIDS

Topical or periocular steroids cause few systemic effects.[7] When Krupin and associates[119] administered topical dexamethasone sodium phosphate 4 times a day for 6 weeks, their subjects showed reduced plasma levels of cortisol. However, elevation of 11-deoxycortisol with the oral metyrapone tartrate test showed that the pituitary-adrenal axis was intact.

Intralesional injection of steroid can lead to adrenal suppression.[120,121] Infants and small children are especially susceptible, since a given amount of steroid is distributed in a smaller volume of fluid and tissue compartments. Infants injected with mixtures of triamcinolone acetonide and betamethasone or dexamethasone for periocular hemangiomas have shown depressed serum cortisol and ACTH levels. The adrenal suppression can last up to 5 months and can result in weight loss and growth retardation. It is not known whether other corticosteroid preparations would produce similar effects or which other factors might influence these results.

In general, topical and periocular use of steroids produce minimal systemic effects. Withdrawal of topical or periocular steroids does not seem to cause adrenal crisis.[7]

Contraindications

Since side effects can complicate the use of corticosteroids, a careful history and certain tests may be advisable, particularly if a patient may require prolonged ocular therapy.[3,8] Steroids should be used with great caution in patients with diabetes mellitus, infectious disease, chronic renal failure, congestive heart failure, and systemic hypertension. Systemic administration is generally contraindicated in patients with peptic ulcer, osteoporosis, and psychoses.[20] Topical steroids must be used with caution and only when necessary in patients with glaucoma.

Patients receiving prolonged systemic therapy usually lack sufficient adrenal reserve to respond appropriately to such stresses as trauma or surgery. These individuals may need supplementary corticosteroid to cover the period of stress.

Concurrent administration of other drugs may interfere with the metabolism and alter the effects of corticosteroids. Some of the effects appear to result from increased metabolism of administered steroid.[122] Barbiturates, phenylbutazone, and phenytoin may enhance metabolism and reduce the anti-inflammatory and immunosuppressive potential of systemic steroids. Additionally, the response to anticoagulant therapy may be reduced by simultaneous administration of steroids.[20]

Patients receiving topical ocular steroids must be examined periodically for corneal, lens, and IOP changes. Slit-lamp examination for punctate, herpetic, or fungal keratitis is necessary. Patients receiving systemic therapy should be monitored for systemic hypertension, glaucoma, and cataracts. If prolonged systemic therapy is necessary, blood glucose levels should be evaluated at appropriate intervals.

Nonsteroidal Anti-Inflammatory Drugs

The nonsteroidal anti-inflammatory drugs (NSAIDs) represent a heterogeneous group of agents, referred to as "nonste-

TABLE 12.9
Topical Ophthalmic Nonsteroidal Anti-Inflammatory Drugs

Class	NSAID	Trade Name (Manufacturer)	Indication
Propionic Acids	Flurbiprofen 0.03%	Ocufen (Allergan)	Inhibition of intraoperative miosis
	Suprofen 1.0%	Profenal (Alcon)	Inhibition of intraoperative miosis Treatment of GPC[a]
Acetic Acids	Diclofenac 0.1%	Voltaren (Ciba Vision)	Treatment of postsurgical inflammation following cataract extraction Treatment of inflammation following ALT[a] Control of pain following RK[a] or excimer laser procedures Treatment of seasonal allergic conjunctivitis
	Ketorolac 0.5%	Acular (Allergan)	Treatment of seasonal allergic conjunctivitis Treatment of postsurgical inflammation following cataract extraction Treatment of CME[a]

[a]GPC = giant papillary conjunctivitis; ALT = argon laser trabeculoplasty; RK = radial keratotomy; CME = cystoid macular edema.

roidal'' because their chemical structures and mechanism of action differ from those of the corticosteroids. The demonstration by Vane[123] that acetylsalicylic acid (aspirin) inhibits the synthesis of prostaglandins, one of the mediators of the inflammatory response, has resulted in the development of other NSAIDs. Several other classes of compounds demonstrate, similar to aspirin, varying degrees of analgesic, antipyretic, and anti-inflammatory effects. With oral as well as topical administration, these agents help alleviate pain and inflammation with relatively few serious toxic effects and generally good patient tolerability. Since side effects can occur with oral use, including frequent gastrointestinal upset, topical ophthalmic preparations that can penetrate the anterior segment have been developed.[124] Of the six major classes of NSAIDs in clinical use, several of the phenylacetic and propionic acids are used for various ocular indications, including prevention of intraoperative miosis, management of postsurgical and nonsurgical inflammation, prevention or treatment of cystoid macular edema (CME) following cataract extraction, and control of ocular pain following corneal abrasions or radial keratotomy (Table 12.9).[125,126,127] These agents may also prove useful when used alone or combined with steroids for control of post-PRK myopic regression.[126] The pharmacologic effects of these drugs appear related to their ability to inhibit cyclooxygenase, the enzyme that catalyzes the rate-limiting step in prostaglandin synthesis in various tissues, including the eye[128] (Fig. 12.6).

Pharmacology

Prostaglandins are present in nearly every organ system, including the eye. Irides of various species contain the biosynthetic pathway for their manufacture. Release of prostaglandins from ocular tissue occurs in response to various stimuli, including stroking the iris, rubbing the fifth cranial nerve, and paracentesis.[123,129]

Historically, the link between prostaglandins and the eye originated from the demonstration that stimulation of the fifth cranial nerve in rabbits causes constriction of the pupil.[130] This observation suggested that a substance other than acetylcholine (ACh) may cause the observed miosis. Subsequently, Ambache1[131] isolated an extract from rabbit irides, which he named *irin*, that caused pupillary constriction. Further studies showed that *irin* was a long-chain unsaturated hydroxy fatty acid that dilated blood vessels and caused miosis in several species. More recent investigations indicate that, in addition to prostaglandins, leukotrienes and substance P may have contributed to the effects initially observed with irin.[132]

Prostaglandins are 20-carbon, unsaturated fatty acid derivatives, each containing a substituted cyclopentane ring structure. They are products of several enzymatic reactions beginning with arachidonic acid, which phospholipase releases from phospholipids. The end products of the prostaglandin biosynthetic pathway include the prostaglandins as well as the prostacyclins and thromboxanes (see Fig. 12.6). In general, these substances are believed to play a role in platelet physiology, smooth muscle contraction, and dilation of ocular blood vessels; in addition, some members of the group may elevate IOP.[133]

Prostaglandins are subdivided into groups depending on the arrangement of ketone and hydroxyl groups. The members of each group are designated by the letters E, F, A, B, C, and D. Table 12.10 summarizes the ocular effects of prostaglandins.

Prostaglandins PGE_2, PGD_2, and PGF_2 have been isolated

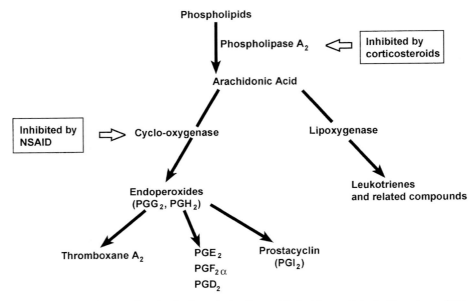

FIGURE 12.6   **Pathways of synthesis of prostaglandins and leukotrienes. (Adapted from Jampol LM. Pharmacologic therapy of aphakic cystoid macular edema. Ophthalmology 1982;89:894.)**

from ocular tissue and aqueous humor.[132] Several prostaglandins have been implicated in IOP elevations resulting from mechanical and chemical trauma to the eye.[129] Arachidonic acid, PGE$_2$, and prostacyclin, a major product of arachidonic acid metabolism, can raise IOP when applied topically or injected intravenously in rabbits.[129]

Contrary to reports that prostaglandins are potent ocular hypertensive agents, studies have demonstrated that several prostaglandins, including PGF$_2$, have ocular hypotensive effects in human eyes (see Chapter 10).[134,135] In addition to the cyclo-oxygenase pathway that leads to the formation of prostaglandins and thromboxane A$_2$, the lipoxygenase pathway is also active in ocular tissues.[132,134] The products of this pathway are referred to as leukotrienes (see Fig. 12.6). Kulkarni and Srinivasan[129] have reported the presence of leukotrienes LTB$_4$ and LTC$_4$ in rabbit aqueous humor following paracentesis. Human tears contain LTB$_4$ during ocular allergy.[136] The exact role of the leukotrienes in ocular inflammation needs further elucidation. If, indeed, the li-

poxygenase pathway participates in ocular inflammatory responses, it may imply that aspirin and other NSAIDs that do not inhibit the lipoxygenase pathway may be ineffective in some forms of ocular inflammation.[136]

Ophthalmic NSAIDs

FLURBIPROFEN

A propionic acid, flurbiprofen is commercially available as a 0.03% ophthalmic solution (Ocufen). Ocular bioavailability studies with labeled flurbiprofen indicate that its ocular penetration suffices to inhibit prostaglandin synthesis.[129] Anderson and Chen[137] have also shown that 3 doses of 0.03% flurbiprofen administered at 30-minute intervals produce higher concentrations in rabbit ocular tissues than does a single dose of 0.03% or 0.1% flurbiprofen. Administration of more than 3 doses, however, did not significantly increase the concentration of flurbiprofen in most ocular tissues. The intraocular penetration of 0.03% flurbiprofen has also been studied in patients prior to cataract surgery.[138] Both flurbiprofen and indomethacin penetrated the cornea, but the amount detected in the aqueous humor was 20 times greater in the subjects receiving flurbiprofen.

Since prostaglandin release from the iris vasculature probably mediates, at least in part, pupillary constriction during cataract extraction, NSAIDs could help in maintaining dilation during surgical procedures by inhibiting prostaglandin activity. Evidence shows that, when used in

TABLE 12.10
Ocular Effects of Prostaglandins

- Pupillary constriction
- Vasodilation
- Increased vascular permeability
- Disruption of ocular blood barriers
- Alteration in intraocular pressure

conjunction with other dilating agents, flurbiprofen can help to maintain pupillary dilation during cataract surgery.[139,140] Keates and McGowan[139] studied 34 patients who received 0.03% flurbiprofen prior to surgery according to the manufacturer's recommended dosage. The flurbiprofen-treated group showed a statistically significant increase in mean pupil size as compared to the control group, which received the vehicle alone. However, most studies indicate that, in general, the effect of flurbiprofen and NSAIDs in maintaining pupillary dilation is small and may vary with dosing regimens, surgical techniques and patient groups (Fig. 12.7).[124,140] In addition, iris color or age may influence the change in pupil area.[139-141] A clinically useful inhibitory effect of flurbiprofen on pupillary constriction has not been observed during vitreoretinal surgery with the 0.03% concentration or in diabetic patients undergoing extracapsular cataract extraction (ECCE) using a higher (0.1%) concentration.[142,143]

Several well-designed studies indicate that flurbiprofen and other NSAIDs may be useful in the management of postoperative inflammation.[124] Flurbiprofen may inhibit postoperative inflammation following intracapsular cataract extraction (ICCE) without implantation of an intraocular lens (IOL).[144] When administered 4 times daily for 2 weeks, starting 24 hours following surgery, flurbiprofen 0.03% reduced the conjunctival hyperemia and anterior chamber cells and flare on postoperative days 3, 7, and 14 as compared to the placebo. However, a statistically significant difference between flurbiprofen and placebo-treated patients was observed only on day 14. Fluorophotometric studies in patients following cataract surgery also indicate that flurbiprofen suppresses the blood-aqueous barrier breakdown.[145] Data from the flurbiprofen-CME study[68] indicate that the incidence and severity of angiographic CME as well as the associated visual dysfunction are reduced early in the postoperative period (days 5 to 240).

The effect of flurbiprofen on postoperative inflammation following argon laser trabeculoplasty (ALT) and cyclocryotherapy has also been evaluated.[146-148] In general, placebo-treated patients showed more conjunctival vasodilation following ALT at 1 hour, 1 day, and 1 week than did flurbiprofen-treated patients.[146] However, the flurbiprofen and the placebo groups did not differ significantly in anterior chamber cells and flare. In contrast to topical corticosteroids, flurbiprofen does not appear to raise IOP following topical application in known high steroid responders.[149] Furthermore, it does not appear to alter the IOP lowering effects of timolol or apraclonidine in normal volunteers or in patients with glaucoma or ocular hypertension.[150,151]

SUPROFEN

Suprofen was the second NSAID approved in the United States for inhibition of intraoperative miosis. A propionic acid derivative, suprofen penetrates the eye in sufficient

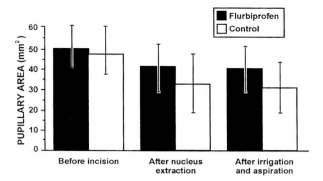

FIGURE 12.7   **Mean pupillary area in 25 patients who received and 25 patients who did not receive flurbiprofen sodium. Vertical bars represent standard deviation. (Reprinted with permission from the Canadian Journal of Ophthalmology 1990;25:240.)**

concentrations to inhibit the release of various prostaglandins.[152] It is available as a 1% ophthalmic solution (Profenal).

Stark and associates[141] investigated the efficacy of suprofen in inhibiting intraoperative miosis in a study involving eight different surgeons. Prior to surgery, 1% suprofen or placebo vehicle was instilled every 4 hours the day before surgery, and 3 additional doses were instilled at hourly intervals just prior to surgery. Each surgeon used his or her normal regimen of mydriatics and cycloplegics before and during surgery. Most surgeons reported a statistically significant increase in pupil size with suprofen as compared to the placebo prior to IOL implantation. Although the final absolute pupil diameters measured only an average of 0.6 mm larger in patients receiving suprofen as compared to placebo, this difference equates to a mean increase in pupil area of 6.3 mm[2] and represents an approximately 20% larger pupil size in patients pretreated with suprofen.

One multicenter study of patients with contact lens-associated giant papillary conjunctivitis (GPC) indicates that suprofen may help reduce the associated signs and symptoms.[153] Patients instilled 2 drops of either suprofen or placebo vehicle into the involved eyes 4 times daily for up to 28 days. All patients discontinued lens wear for the duration of the study. Treatment with suprofen resulted in a greater overall reduction in ocular signs and symptoms compared with placebo. Forty-eight percent of patients had ocular side effects related to suprofen treatment, including burning or stinging, redness, discomfort or irritation, and tearing. Forty percent of patients in the placebo group reported similar signs and symptoms. All ocular side effects occurred immediately following medication instillation and were of short duration.

The anti-inflammatory efficacy of suprofen has not been adequately studied and its postoperative effects remain questionable.[124] Suprofen may be a more potent analgesic than an anti-inflammatory agent, but oral administration can cause serious adverse effects.[152]

DICLOFENAC

A phenylacetic acid derivative, diclofenac sodium 0.1% solution (Voltaren Ophthalmic) is approved for control of inflammation after cataract surgery. Diclofenac significantly reduces prostaglandin levels and may also, at high dosages, partially inhibit leukotriene production.[154–156] It does not inhibit the lipoxygenase enzyme, but appears to decrease arachidonic acid levels by shunting this substance to the triglyceride pool, thereby possibly reducing its bioavailability both for prostaglandin and leukotriene synthesis. Diclofenac significantly reduces prostaglandin E_2 (PGE_2) levels in rabbit corneas undergoing photorefractive keratectomy (PRK) with the 193-nm excimer laser.[155,156] It does not appear to alter levels of LTB_4, a metabolite of the lipoxygenase pathway; moreover, leukocyte infiltration does not decrease in the postablation corneal stroma following diclofenac administration.[155] Diclofenac's ability to decrease PGE_2 levels and prevent a measurable rise in LTB_4 levels may explain, at least in part, both its anti-inflammatory effect and its ability to reduce postsurgical pain in patients following PRK (Fig. 12.8).[157,158] Evidence also suggests that topical ocular application of 0.1% diclofenac to eyes of healthy adults decreases corneal sensation.[159] Diclofenac may possibly exert its analgesic effects by influencing other, presently unidentified, arachidonate metabolites.[158] In addition, diclofenac decreases early epithelialization of corneal scrape wounds but does not appear to affect corneal stromal healing.[160]

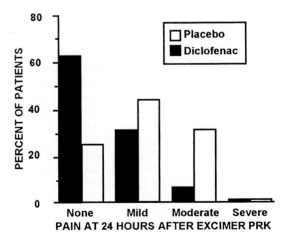

FIGURE 12.8 **Ocular pain assessment at 24 hours after excimer photorefractive keratectomy. Represents summary of categorical scale. (Reprinted with permission from Refractive and Corneal Surgery 1993;9:429.)**

Two clinical trials studied the ability of diclofenac to attenuate ocular inflammation following cataract surgery in 309 patients.[161] Posterior chamber IOLs were implanted in all patients. One drop of diclofenac or placebo vehicle was administered 4 times daily beginning 22 to 24 hours after cataract extraction for up to 16 days. Efficacy evaluations included slit lamp observation of anterior chamber cells and flare and overall assessment of the inflammatory response, including conjunctival hyperemia and ciliary flush. Diclofenac statistically surpassed the vehicle for all parameters tested on days 4, 8, and 15. It appeared to improve distance visual acuity and alleviate eye pain. Diclofenac did not significantly affect IOP.

The anti-inflammatory effect of diclofenac 0.1% has also been compared to dexamethasone phosphate after ECCE and IOL implantation.[162] Anterior chamber inflammation was evaluated by measuring aqueous flare and cells with a laser flare-cell meter at 1, 3, 12, 30, and 60 days following surgery. Flare values did not differ significantly between patients on either drug regimen. Aqueous cell counts also did not differ at 1, 3, 12, and 60 days. At day 30, however, the diclofenac group had a significantly lower cell count. Thus, diclofenac may be as effective as corticosteroids in preventing breakdown of the blood-aqueous barrier following cataract surgery.[163]

Evidence also indicates that diclofenac 0.1% effectively inhibits inflammation following argon laser trabeculoplasty (ALT).[164] Diclofenac 0.1% or a placebo vehicle were administered to patients with pseudoexfoliative or pigmentary glaucoma once before and once immediately after trabeculoplasty. Four daily instillations continued for the next 4 days. Anterior chamber flare measured with a laser flare-cell meter, visual acuity, and IOP were evaluated before trabeculoplasty and up to 14 days after the procedure. Diclofenac blocked immediate post-ALT flare increases and significantly reduced development of flare.

Diclofenac appears as effective as flurbiprofen in preventing intraoperative miosis.[165] As with flurbiprofen, eye color, age, or other factors may influence the pupillary response since mydriasis is often greater for light-colored irides than for dark-colored irides.

Goldberg and associates[166] have recently shown that, despite its ability to inhibit prostaglandin synthesis, diclofenac appears to be ineffective in ameliorating contact lens-induced corneal edema.

KETOROLAC TROMETHAMINE

An acetic acid derivative, ketorolac is available as a 0.5% ophthalmic solution (Acular). When applied topically to the eye, it can reduce conjunctival inflammation and the symptoms, especially itching, associated with seasonal allergic conjunctivitis (see Chapter 13). Despite its anti-inflammatory effect, ketorolac does not appear to impair wound healing significantly as determined by corneal tensile strength, nor does it affect healing of corneal abrasions in rabbits.[167]

The studies of Flach and associates[168–172] indicate that ketorolac can serve as an anti-inflammatory agent following cataract surgery and for the prophylaxis and treatment of CME.

The effect of pre- and postoperative 0.5% ketorolac on signs of anterior ocular inflammation following cataract extraction with and without implantation of an IOL has been compared to placebo.[168,169] In one study, patients without IOL implants were examined with the slit-lamp biomicroscope, and anterior ocular fluorophotometry was performed on days 1, 5, 12, 19, and 21 following surgery.[168] Ketorolac was significantly more effective than the placebo in reducing lid edema, conjunctival vasodilation, and ciliary flush on postoperative days 2, 12, and 19, and was significantly more effective in decreasing anterior chamber cells on day 12. Fluorophotometry showed a favorable effect of ketorolac treatment on all postoperative examination days. A similarly designed study compared postoperative inflammation in patients undergoing ECCE with implantation of a posterior chamber IOL following treatment with ketorolac 0.5% or a placebo.[169] Use of topical corticosteroids was permitted if the observed postoperative inflammation was potentially detrimental. Only 4 of the 60 ketorolac-treated patients, as compared to 25 of 58 placebo-treated patients, required supplemental steroids. Despite inclusion of clinical observations in steroid-treated patients in the final data analysis, ketorolac demonstrated a statistically significant improvement in postoperative inflammation.

The effect of ketorolac 0.5% in reducing postoperative inflammation has also been compared to dexamethasone phosphate 0.1%.[173,174] As assessed by fluorophotometry and slit-lamp examination, ketorolac suppresses postoperative inflammation after cataract surgery as effectively as dexamethasone phosphate.[173]

Topical ketorolac 0.5% may also be effective in the prophylaxis or treatment of angiographic CME and established or chronic symptomatic CME.[170–172] Flach and associates[171] reported a statistically significant reduction in postoperative angiographic CME in patients with cataracts, but no significant difference in visual acuity, when ketorolac was used postsurgically for 3 weeks without concurrent use of steroids.

When used topically for 1 month or longer in chronic aphakic or pseudophakic symptomatic CME, ketorolac has shown a statistically significant improvement in distance visual acuity as compared to placebo-treated patients.[170,172] One study included 120 patients with angiographic evidence of cystoid changes and distance visual acuity of 20/40 (6/12) or less, of at least 6 months' duration. The ketorolac group showed a statistically significant improvement in distance visual acuity of 2 lines or more after 30, 60, and 90 days of treatment. This improvement in visual acuity remained statistically significant for 1 month following cessation of therapy. The clinical benefits of ketorolac and other NSAIDs in CME need further evaluation and comparison to alternative pharmacologic and surgical therapies.[125]

Side Effects

The most common adverse event observed with topical administration of the NSAIDs is transient burning, stinging, and conjunctival hyperemia. To help alleviate some of these effects, suprofen ophthalmic solution is prepared with 1% caffeine since studies in normal volunteers indicated that this formulation is less irritating to the ocular surface.[124] Ketorolac is formulated as the tromethamine salt since addition of the tromethamine moiety both enhances aqueous solubility and reduces ocular irritation.[175]

Although rare, allergies and other hypersensitivity reactions have been associated with use of these agents.[20] Punctate keratitis can also occur.[20] As with steroid therapy, some NSAIDs may delay wound healing, and patients with a history of ocular viral infections should be closely monitored.[20] Unlike therapy with steroids, however, where rapid drug withdrawal can lead to recurrence of signs and symptoms of disease,[111] there is no current evidence to suggest that NSAIDs should be tapered with topical therapy.

Contraindications

Soft contact lens wear is contraindicated since patients have experienced ocular irritation, manifested by redness and burning.[20] All of the presently available topical NSAIDs, with the exception of flurbiprofen, are preserved with benzalkonium chloride. Although the extent of systemic absorption of NSAIDs following topical ocular application to humans has not been fully elucidated, some absorption does occur. NSAIDs increase bleeding time by interfering with platelet aggregation. Therefore, patients with known bleeding tendencies or who are taking medications that may prolong prothrombin time require careful monitoring.[20,124,129]

Since a potential exists for cross-sensitivity with aspirin and other NSAIDs, caution needs to be used with patients who have a history of bronchial asthma accompanied by vasomotor rhinitis, sinusitis and nasal polyps, or who previously exhibited sensitivity to these drugs.[176] Also, since studies are generally lacking in children and pregnant women, caution should be exercised when administering NSAIDs to these patients.[20]

Immunosuppressants

Immunosuppressive agents (Table 12.11) diminish the body's normal physiologic responses to antigenic stimuli.

TABLE 12.11
Immunosuppressive Agents

Drug	Ocular Uses	Side Effects
Azathioprine	Uveitis, Behçet's Syndrome, Sympathetic Ophthalmia, Cicatricial Pemphigoid	Bone Marrow Depression, Nausea, Vomiting
Bromocriptine	Uveitis	Nausea, Vomiting, Dizziness, Headache, Fatigue
Chlorambucil	Behçet's Syndrome, Sympathetic Ophthalmia	Bone Marrow, Depression, Infertility, Teratogenicity, Mutagenicity
Colchicine	Behçet's Syndrome	Nausea, Vomiting, Diarrhea
Cyclophosphamide	Scleritis, Cicatricial Pemphigoid, Behçet's Syndrome, Wegener's Granulomatosis, Mooren's Ulcer, Rheumatoid Arthritis	Alopecia, Thrombocytopenia, Nausea, Vomiting, Hemorrhagic Cystitis, Infertility, Neoplasms
Cyclosporine A (Systemic)	Uveitis, Behçet's Syndrome, Sympathetic Ophthalmia	Nephrotoxicity, Hypertension, Gingival Hyperplasia, Hypertrichosis
Cyclosporine A (Topical)	Chronic Vernal Keratoconjunctivitis, Corneal Graft Rejection	Burning, Itching, Hyperemia
Dapsone	Cicatricial Pemphigoid	Hemolytic Anemia, Methemoglobinemia, Nausea, Vomiting, Anorexia
Methotrexate	Uveitis, Mooren's Ulcer	Bone Marrow Depression, Cirrhosis, Pneumonitis, Teratogenicity, Nausea, Vomiting

These antigens can originate in exogenous sources, such as viruses, bacteria, and foreign macromolecules. Antigens can also be found endogenously, due to recognition of self as antigenic (as in autoimmune disease). These drugs can interact with the immune system at many levels. Corticosteroids can affect synthesis and release of inflammatory mediators, and may also prevent the initiation or activation of some types of immune cells. The steroids continue to be widely used to treat immune disorders. However, in the treatment of some conditions that are resistant to the actions of steroids and NSAIDs, other immunosuppressants may be useful.

Therapeutic actions of the immunosuppressants can occur through several mechanisms. Currently available drugs act as cytotoxic agents to block lymphocyte proliferation (cyclophosphamide, azathioprine, chlorambucil, methotrexate, colchicine) or as immune modulators to block the synthesis of lymphokines (cyclosporine A). Alternatively, immunosuppressants may block the inflammatory effects of the immune response (corticosteroids, colchicine, dapsone, bromocriptine).

Cytotoxic Agents

CYCLOPHOSPHAMIDE

Pharmacology. Cyclophosphamide (Cytoxan, Neosar) is an alkylating agent of the nitrogen mustard type. Once absorbed, cyclophosphamide is metabolically activated to several metabolites with potential therapeutic and toxic effects. The final cytotoxic product is probably phosphoramide; however, 4-OH cyclophosphamide is more effective than phosphoramide. Possibly 4-OH cyclophosphamide may serve as a carrier molecule, transporting phosphoramide across the cell membrane.[177]

Once phosphoramide forms, it reacts with various nucleophilic moieties within the cell. This causes the formation of covalent linkages by alkylation of phosphate, amino, sulfhydryl, carboxyl, and imidazole groups. Its cytotoxic effects relate directly to the alkylation of DNA. The apparent cytotoxic selectivity of cyclophosphamide for rapidly dividing cells may simply reside in the ability of slowly proliferating cells to repair the DNA damage before they are stimulated to divide.[178] Hematopoietic tissue, and lymphocytes in particular, are very susceptible to the actions of cyclophosphamide, and its immunosuppressive action is mediated through antiproliferative effects on lymphocytes and accessory cells.[177] Evidence exists for suppression of both humoral and cell-mediated responses through suppression of both T-suppressor cells and T-helper cells.[179]

Clinical Uses. Cyclophosphamide can be administered orally or by injection. It is well absorbed after oral administration and thus is useful for chronic treatment regimens. It can be given as a single entity or as an essential component of various drug combinations. Cyclophosphamide can be effective for a wide variety of conditions including Hodgkin's disease, other lymphomas, carcinomas, and many inflammatory or immune disorders. Some ocular diseases treated with cyclophosphamide include necrotizing scleritis, cicatricial pemphigoid, Behçet's syndrome, Mooren's ulcer, and the ocular manifestations of rheumatoid arthritis and Wegener's granulomatosis.[179–183]

Tauber and associates[180] reported that cicatricial pemphigoid responds well to cyclophosphamide. In their review of 105 patients initially treated with either dapsone, cyclophosphamide, or azathioprine, these investigators found that cyclophosphamide brought 40% of patients under control (decreased conjunctival inflammation and inhibition of progression of disease). Although this outcome compared favorably to 45% controlled with the use of dapsone, the authors believe cyclophosphamide to be superior to dapsone or azathioprine for the treatment of patients with intense conjunctival inflammation or rapidly progressive disease. Cyclophosphamide treatment was initiated at 2 mg/kg/day but was adjusted individually for each patient based on hematologic tolerance, side effects, and clinical improvement.[180]

For treatment of Behçet's syndrome, Yazici and Barnes[181] recommend the use of cyclophosphamide in a maximum dose of 2 mg/kg/day orally or given intravenously as a bolus injection of 500 mg once a week. However, Kazokoglu and associates[182] reported no significant benefit with cyclophosphamide in 46 patients with ocular symptoms of Behçet's disease. All patients received oral cyclophosphamide (100–150 mg) and prednisolone (5 mg) daily. After a treatment period of 32 months, and a follow-up post-treatment period of 51 months, these patients showed no statistically significant improvement in visual acuity or frequency of attacks. Foster[183] reported that 7 patients with bilateral Mooren's ulcer responded favorably to cyclophosphamide treatment when adequate immunosuppression could be achieved. These patients had not responded to conventional ocular and systemic therapy or surgery. Treatment with 2 to 3 mg/kg/day cyclophosphamide arrested progression of the ulceration, and functional vision was preserved.

Side Effects.   Cyclophosphamide toxicity differs from that of other nitrogen mustards in that the incidence of significant thrombocytopenia is less frequent while alopecia is more frequent.[178] The hair loss is usually reversible, sometimes without discontinuing therapy.[184] Nausea and vomiting commonly occur, especially after IV administration, presumably due to stimulation of the chemoreceptor trigger zone in the central nervous system.[184] Sterile, hemorrhagic cystitis has been reported in 2% to 40% of patients.[182,184] Administration of acetylcysteine or mesna (sodium 2-mercaptoethanesulfonate) greatly reduces the incidence of cystitis.[177] Sterility has occurred in both males and females given cyclophosphamide. The incidence of sterility is dose- and duration-related and may be irreversible in some patients.[185] Cyclophospha-

mide carries a small but definite risk of inducing cancers in nontransplanted patients.[177] The most frequently reported neoplasms are of the lymphoid tissue and skin. Other toxicities occurring infrequently at the doses used in treating ocular disease include mucosal ulcerations, dizziness, increased skin pigmentation, interstitial pulmonary fibrosis, and hepatic damage.

Contraindications.   Contraindications to the use of cyclophosphamide include previous allergic hypersensitivity to the drug and continued use in patients with severely depressed bone marrow function. Since this drug causes teratogenic effects, it is contraindicated during pregnancy.[178]

CHLORAMBUCIL

Pharmacology.   Chlorambucil (Leukeran) is similar to cyclophosphamide in its effects and mechanism of action. However, chlorambucil, the slowest-acting of the nitrogen mustard alkylating agents, does not require activation by liver enzymes. Chlorambucil can cause covalent crosslinking of DNA strands,[178] which prevents DNA strand separation during mitosis and halts cell division. The resulting myelosuppressive action is both moderate and gradual in its development, and rapidly reversible upon discontinuing the drug. A nonspecific suppression of all cellular blood elements and bone marrow occurs, but the rapidly dividing clones of both T and B lymphocytes are affected more than are granulocytes and platelets.[186] Chlorambucil is rapidly and completely absorbed after oral administration, with peak plasma levels reached in 60 minutes. Extensive metabolism occurs in the liver, and only 1% of the drug is excreted unchanged over 24 hours.[185]

Clinical Uses.   Chlorambucil is most frequently employed as an ocular immunosuppressant in the treatment of Behçet's disease and has also been recommended for control of symptoms associated with this condition.[187] Dosages of 0.1 mg/kg/day can control or prevent episodes of uveitis in most patients. Usually after several years of treatment, chlorambucil can be stopped without a major exacerbation in the disease.[187] Other studies have shown success with a short-term but high-dose chlorambucil treatment regimen. Tessler and Jennings[188] reported that 2 mg/day of chlorambucil, increased each week by 2 mg/day until remission of ocular symptoms or blood count parameters below the accepted, safe level of 2,400/mm³, was effective in reducing Behçet's syndrome symptoms. In all six of the patients treated, visual acuities improved to 20/50 (6/15) or better. Daily doses of chlorambucil ranged from 20 to 28 mg/day for 14 to 36 weeks. These authors[188] also reported good results using this dosage regimen in the treatment of five patients with intractable sympathetic ophthalmia. All patients treated with chlorambucil had vision improved to 20/25 (6/8) or better unless macular subretinal neovascularization occurred. BenEzra[189] described a series of patients with endogenous uveitis, including Behçet's disease, treated with a variety of immunosuppressive agents, including chlorambucil. The results showed chlorambucil (maximum 0.2 mg/kg/day) as only moderately effective.

Side Effects.   Only moderate adverse events result from the recommended doses of chlorambucil, and the drug has been given for long periods without serious toxicity to patients with previously compromised bone marrow.[178] However, prolonged therapy does require monitoring for bone marrow toxicity. Chlorambucil has also caused chromatid or chromosomal damage in males, contributing to infertility.[185] Sterility in males is almost inevitable, even after relatively low doses of chlorambucil, necessitating pretreatment sperm banking.[177,188] Both reversible and irreversible azoospermia occur. Amenorrhea and infertility can occur in women and may be as high as 30%.[177] Because of possible mutagenic and teratogenic effects, patients should use contraceptive measures during treatment.[185,188] Mutagenic effects may cause late malignancies in patients treated with chlorambucil for Behçet's disease.[188] This risk apparently increases with chronicity of treatment and large cumulative total doses,[185] but has not yet been observed in patients given the high-dose, short-term therapy (follow-up up to 12 years).[188]

Contraindications.   Contraindications to chlorambucil include known allergic hypersensitivity to the drug and the possibility of cross-allergic reactions to other alkylating agents. In addition, chlorambucil should not be used for conditions having significant resistance to its beneficial effects, which would require administering massive doses of the drug.[185]

METHOTREXATE

Pharmacology.   Methotrexate is classified as a cytotoxic antifolate. The drug is a potent inhibitor of dihydrofolate reductase. This enzyme is critical for maintaining the levels of tetrahydrofolate cofactors necessary for one-carbon transfer reactions in the synthesis of purines and thymidylate. Both are essential components for the replication of DNA and RNA. By interfering with their formation, methotrexate inhibits synthesis of DNA or the S phase of the cell cycle, thus stopping cell division.[190] The cells with the highest mitotic activity are most susceptible to the actions of methotrexate. The immunosuppressant action of methotrexate probably results from the inhibition of T cell and possibly B cell proliferation[178]; however, this explanation is not unanimously accepted. Low-dose methotrexate therapy, used in the treatment of immune disorders, may also reduce the chemotactic response of polymorphonuclear leukocytes, thus preventing some of the inflammatory activity caused by those cells. Methotrexate demonstrates dose-dependent absorption characteristics, with lower oral doses ($<25mg/m^2$) being more completely absorbed than higher doses.[178,190] The kidneys excrete unchanged over 80% of the administered dose of methotrexate. Although liver metabolism may occur, and several toxic metabolites are found after high-dose therapy, the low doses used in immunosuppression would not be expected to produce toxic metabolites.[190]

Clinical Uses.   Several early studies demonstrated that methotrexate was effective in the treatment of various forms of uveitis that were resistant to corticosteroids. These studies, however, showed significant methotrexate-induced toxicity, which has limited use of the drug to patients who have not responded to conventional therapy.[179] Methotrexate may also have arrested the destructive inflammation in a patient with progressive bilateral ulcerative keratitis diagnosed as Mooren's ulcer.[183] This patient had been unresponsive to all previous conventional therapy but showed no recurrent ulceration during a follow-up period of 5 years after only 6 weekly treatments with methotrexate.

Side Effects.   The major sites for toxicity with low-dose methotrexate therapy are the bone marrow, gastrointestinal tract, and liver. The most commonly experienced side effects with low doses of methotrexate are malaise, nausea, vomiting, anorexia, and leukopenia.[190,191] Dividing the single weekly dose into 3 divided doses over 24 hours can reduce the nausea and vomiting.[190] While all the dividing cells of the bone marrow can be affected, severe bone marrow suppression from low doses rarely occurs and is probably the result of decreased elimination of the drug or drug interactions. Patients with decreased renal function are at the greatest risk for severe toxicity. If leukopenia occurs, therapy should be stopped to allow the white blood cell count to recover. Hepatotoxicity is only a major concern in long-term therapy. However, development of cirrhosis appears related to cumulative dose rather than duration of treatment. The weekly dosing schedule, generally employed for immunosuppression, seems to have a low risk of inducing hepatotoxicity.[190] The incidence of cirrhosis and hepatic fibrosis during long-term methotrexate use is highly correlated with the ingestion of ethanol.[192]

Ocular effects during methotrexate therapy may occur in as many as 25% of treated patients. These effects generally consist of ocular irritation, tearing, photophobia, and aggravation of seborrheic blepharitis.[179] Pulmonary toxicity, consisting of acute or chronic nonseptic pneumonitis, can occur with any dose of methotrexate. The mechanism and risk factors for this complication are not known.[192] Since methotrexate is a known teratogen, patients of childbearing age should employ contraceptive measures and continue for 12 weeks after terminating methotrexate therapy. Spermatogenesis is also suppressed, although no mutagenic actions on sperm or ova have been confirmed.[185]

Contraindications.   Methotrexate is contraindicated during pregnancy because of the drug's teratogenic effects. It is contraindicated during breastfeeding because the drug readily passes into the milk of lactating patients, possibly causing myelosuppression in the developing infant.[185] Because of the high correlation of hepatotoxicity with the ingestion of alcohol, alcoholism, alcoholic liver disease, or other chronic liver diseases pose significant risks with use of methotrexate. Since methotrexate can suppress blood cell formation, the drug is contraindicated when there is overt or laboratory evidence of immunodeficiency syndromes, pre-existing blood dyscrasias, or significant anemia.[190]

AZATHIOPRINE

Pharmacology.   Azathioprine (Imuran) is a purine analog that the body converts to 6-mercaptopurine and subsequently metabolizes to mercaptopurine-containing nucleotides. These substances, in turn, exert immunosuppressant effects. Azathioprine causes bone marrow suppression, thus decreasing the lymphocyte proliferation phase of the immune response. While the active metabolites of azathioprine inhibit the synthesis of DNA, RNA and proteins, the exact mechanism of action at the molecular level remains unclear.[193] The immunosuppressive effects of azathioprine likely occur through multiple mechanisms.[178]

Clinical Uses.   Azathioprine is generally used in combination with corticosteroids when steroids alone are ineffective or when the patient cannot tolerate high doses of steroids. Azathioprine frequently allows for a gradual decrease in the amount of steroids needed to control the inflammatory reaction and thus may decrease the toxicity occurring with high steroid doses. Azathioprine can benefit some cases of uveitis,[189] sympathetic ophthalmia,[194] and cicatricial pemphigoid.[180]

BenEzra[189] found that oral azathioprine given alone in doses of 1.0 to 2.0 mg/kg/day proved beneficial in 6 of 12 cases of chronic bilateral uveitis. However, none of the patients was cured, and all needed continued treatment or were switched to other immunosuppressive agents. However, Yazici and associates,[195] using 2.5 mg/kg/day, found that azathioprine prevented the progression of ocular complications of Behçet's disease in 11 of 12 patients, compared to only 5 of 13 patients treated with the placebo. The authors concluded that azathioprine effectively controlled the progression of Behçet's syndrome, especially its most serious manifestation, eye disease. In sympathetic ophthalmia, systemic steroids are the initial drugs of choice. However, in many cases achieving and maintaining good acuity in the sympathizing eye requires toxic doses. Adding azathioprine, usually 50 mg 3 times daily, to the treatment regimen may control the intraocular inflammation at a lower dose of steroid, usually with a concomitant reduction in steroidal side effects.[194] Cases resistant to steroids may respond to the combination treatment and, indeed, some patients may require the addition of other immunosuppressants as well.

Tauber and associates[180] used azathioprine (2 mg/kg/day) to treat cicatricial pemphigoid as either the initial treatment or after treatment with another immunosuppressive agent. When used alone, azathioprine was effective in approximately one-third of patients. The drug was also beneficial when added to treatments initially ineffective with other immunosuppressants. They concluded, however, that azathioprine was least beneficial as compared to cyclophosphamide or dapsone in the treatment of cicatricial pemphigoid.

Side Effects.   Azathioprine, in the doses commonly used for treatment of ocular disease, appears the least toxic of the classic cytotoxic immunosuppressants. Hematologic effects, consisting of bone marrow suppression and leukopenia, are the most frequently reported toxicities that would limit continued treatment. Because of the serious nature of this problem, complete blood cell counts should be performed as often as twice weekly during the initial dosage adjustment and weekly during maintenance therapy.[189] Temporary reduction or cessation of treatment will generally allow recovery from leukopenia.[180,189,195] Anemia and thrombocytopenia have also occurred.[180,192] Gastrointestinal distress, including abdominal pain, nausea, and vomiting, is a common complaint, but seldom limits treatment. Other toxicities with azathioprine include secondary infections, stomatitis, and alopecia.[179] The relatively low doses used for ocular immunosuppression infrequently cause neoplastic disease, generally in the form of lymphoma.[185]

Contraindications.   Contraindications to azathioprine include hypersensitivity to the drug, and pregnancy. Previous treatment with alkylating type immunosuppressant agents, such as chlorambucil or cyclophosphamide, causes a high risk of neoplastic disease with the subsequent use of azathioprine. In addition, concomitant treatment with allopurinol, a xanthine oxidase inhibitor used in gouty arthritis, inhibits the metabolic inactivation of azathioprine. This inhibition dramatically increases the pharmacologic and toxic effects of azathioprine. Reducing the dose of azathioprine to one-third or one-fourth the usual dose is recommended.[192]

COLCHICINE

Pharmacology.   Colchicine is an anti-inflammatory agent used mainly in the treatment of gouty arthritis. This drug has a fairly unique and selective action in that it binds to microtubular protein (tubulin) and interferes with the function of mitotic spindles and thus blocks cell division.[196] Colchicine also inhibits other movements dependent on microtubules. This includes inhibition of granulocyte migration to inflammatory sites, phagocytosis, axonal transport in neurons, and the release of chemical mediators from granules in numerous secretory cells, such as mast cells, pancreatic beta cells, and melanocytes.[196] Due to an enhanced chemotactic response of the polymorphonuclear leukocytes seen with Behçet's disease, some authors believe colchicine may be helpful in that condition as well.[182] Colchicine is rapidly absorbed after oral administration and reaches peak plasma levels within 2 hours. It is metabolized mainly in the liver, and the bile secretes both the active drug and its metabolites.[185]

Clinical Uses.   The use of colchicine in ocular disease has been limited to treatment of Behçet's disease. Although early work with colchicine indicated a beneficial effect and led to its widespread use, controlled studies have been less favorable, showing no benefit over placebo in controlling symptoms of the disease.[181] In a recent report comparing long-term effects of colchicine and cyclophosphamide in the treatment of Behçet's disease, the authors concluded that no statistical improvement in vision or reduction in the frequency of attacks occurred during the period of treatment averaging 27 months.[182] However, patients receiving colchicine at least preserved their initial pretreatment visual acuities. Since the authors' controls were not ideal, they could not equivocally state that colchicine treatment had no effect.[182]

Side Effects.   At the doses of colchicine used for treatment of Behçet's disease (1.0–1.5 mg/day), few toxicities occur.[182] Nausea, vomiting, diarrhea, and abdominal pain are the most common and earliest toxicities occurring with overdosage from colchicine and probably reflect action of the drug on the rapidly proliferating cells of the gastrointestinal tract.[196] Chronic administration of colchicine may cause agranulocytosis, aplastic anemia, myopathy, and alopecia.[196] Since colchicine inhibits cell division, it can cause decreased fertility and azoospermia and can cause fetal harm when given to pregnant women.[185]

Contraindications.   The main contraindication to the use of colchicine is preexisting allergic hypersensitivity. Because of the risk of toxicity to certain tissues, the use of colchicine is contraindicated in preexisting gastrointestinal, renal, hepatic, or cardiac disorders, and blood dyscrasias. Elderly or seriously debilitated patients should be given colchicine only with great caution.[185]

Immune Modulators

CYCLOSPORINE A

Pharmacology.   Cyclosporine A (Sandimmune) may offer a new approach to immunosuppressive therapy. Unlike the cytotoxic agents, cyclosporine A is a reversible and highly selective agent that does not interfere with DNA metabolism and therefore does not produce myelosuppression or mutagenicity. The drug appears mainly to inhibit cytokine production, specifically the production of helper T-cell cytokines, interleukin-2 (IL-2), interleukin-4 (IL-4), interferon gamma, and tumor necrosis factor (TNF).[197] The exact mechanism of action remains unknown, but cyclosporine A appears to bind to cytoplasmic and perhaps nuclear proteins involved in the expression of the genes for IL-2 production and perhaps other cytokines as well.[197]

Cyclosporine A is effective after oral administration, with bioavailability ranging from 20% to 50% of the administered dose. The cytochrome P-450 enzymes of the liver extensively metabolize the drug, and the majority of excretion occurs through the bile. Some of the metabolites may also have immunosuppressive activity.[192] To maintain adequate therapeutic drug levels and reduce dose-related nephrotoxicity, blood levels of cyclosporine A are monitored frequently throughout therapy. Numerous drug interactions can cause changes in cyclosporine A blood levels. Inhibition of cyclosporine A metabolism may occur with erythromycin, ketoconazole, or amphotericin B, leading to increased toxicity. Conversely, stimulation of cyclosporine A metabolism with phenytoin, phenobarbital, or rifampin may decrease its therapeutic effectiveness.[192]

In the continuing effort to utilize the unique immunosuppressant actions of cyclosporine A for ocular disease, studies have focused on the topical ocular administration of cyclosporine A.[198–207] Cyclosporine A is lipid soluble and thus would be expected to penetrate the corneal epithelium after topical administration. Levels of cyclosporine A in rabbit eyes 1 hour after a single topical administration of 10% ointment indicate penetration of the drug into the eye.[199] Levels in the cornea peaked at 3 hours and lasted for at least 24 hours. However, aqueous levels at that time had dropped to less than 10% of the corneal concentration, and the drug was not detected in the blood. In a study comparing the aqueous humor level of cyclosporine A to the blood level after oral administration, patients with uveitis had an intraocular cyclosporine A concentration only 25% to 40% of the blood level.[199] Considering the pharmacokinetics of cyclosporine A—the long-lasting drug levels in the cornea but comparatively short half-life in the aqueous humor and very low levels in posterior ocular tissues after topical administration—topical treatment of intraocular inflammation may not provide the most appropriate route of administration.[199] However, since relatively high corneal concentrations are easily achieved following topical administration with low blood levels of drug, topical cyclosporine A could be a means of reducing rejection in corneal allograft transplants.[199]

Clinical Uses.   Cyclosporine A has been used to treat several ocular immune-mediated diseases, and it has become an important alternative to the traditional treatment of endogenous uveitis.[189,208–214] In a report by BenEzra[189] of 60 patients with severe bilateral uveitis, 22 of 24 patients who had been unsuccessfully treated with steroids or cytotoxic immunosuppressants were successfully treated with cyclosporine A. In another study,[211] low-dose cyclosporine A (average of 4.1 mg/kg/day) alone or combined with oral prednisolone (15 mg/day) was effective in improving vision in 10 of 13 patients with chronic uveitis resistant to previous treatments. When cyclosporine A dosage is reduced or stopped, however, relapse frequently occurs.[208–210] Further studies of 22 patients with various sight-threatening uveitic conditions, previously refractory to other treatments, demonstrated a significant clinical improvement in 19 (86%) of the treated patients. However, the dosage level commonly caused side effects.[209]

Cyclosporine A has been used effectively to treat ocular symptoms of Behçet's disease. One study[215] reported that treatment with doses of 7 to 16 mg/kg/day in 4 patients with ocular symptoms refractory to other treatments produced maintenance or improvement of visual acuity, improvement in color vision, and a reduction in retinal inflammation for up to 18 months. However, adverse reactions frequently occurred, and when doses were decreased or stopped, inflammation recurred. Nephrotoxicity can be minimized by closely monitoring the patients.[197,213] Low-dose cyclosporine A (5 mg/kg/day) gives variable results when used to treat ocular symptoms of Behçet's disease. When compared with cyclophosphamide, low-dose cyclosporine A promoted significant visual improvement during the early phases of treatment. However, a 2-year follow-up indicated that the initial improvement with cyclosporine A was not sustained.[216] As observed in the treatment of idiopathic uveitis, rebound inflammation frequently occurs in Behçet's syndrome when the dose of cyclosporine A is reduced or stopped.[182] Treatment for at least 2 years has been recommended to allow the disease process to run its course and therefore cease to cause tissue damage.[182,210]

Sympathetic ophthalmia responds favorably to adding cyclosporine A (5 mg/kg/day) to the existing systemic steroid therapy. This approach generally allows a reduction in the steroid dose and thus reduces the incidence of systemic toxicity. In addition, some patients not adequately controlled on steroids alone have been controlled with the addition of cyclosporine A or cyclosporine A combined with azathioprine.[194]

Topical cyclosporine A has been advocated for the treatment of corneal graft rejection.[201,203,204] A 2% topical solution was effective in preventing graft rejection in 10 of 11 high-risk patients. After pretreatment and an initial loading dose of 1 drop every 2 hours for the first 4 days, the drug was administered 4 times a day for the first 3 months, 3 times a day for months 3 to 6, and 2 times a day thereafter. Patients also received a topical steroid on the same schedule. Patients were monitored for an average of 16 months. None of the patients was discontinued because of drug toxicity or intolerance.[204] A similar study[201] showed 27 of 44 cases with excellent results using cyclosporine A and dexamethasone

topically after penetrating keratoplasty. The authors stressed the need for HLA matching of donor to high-risk patients to increase the chance of a successful outcome. Both these studies in high-risk patients showed a significant benefit from combined treatment with topical cyclosporine A and a topical steroid, with minimal toxicity over an average of 16 to 19 months of treatment.

To find an alternative to systemic steroids in the treatment of severe chronic vernal keratoconjunctivitis, BenEzra and associates[205] treated 12 children (ages 4–12) with cyclosporine A 2% topical drops. These patients had become refractory to topical treatment and had previously been given systemic steroids to control the disease. One drop of the drug was administered 4 times a day for the first 2 weeks, 3 times a day for the third week, twice a day for the fourth week and once a day for the fifth week. After the first week, 11 of 12 patients showed obvious subjective improvement. Nine of the 11 still demonstrated beneficial effects of the cyclosporine A treatment after 6 weeks. However, the beneficial effects were not sustained and all but three patients demonstrated recurrence of disease within 2 months. Toxicity associated with the topical treatment was minimal; one patient developed maceration of the skin at the lateral canthus during the first week of treatment, which resolved during the second week. In addition, the children responding did not need systemic steroids, and three had remission of symptoms for at least 2 months.

Kervick and associates[202] demonstrated the value of topical cyclosporine A drops for the treatment of paracentral corneal ulcers in six rheumatoid arthritis patients resistant to all other therapies. All patients also had a severe tear deficiency or Sjögren syndrome, and several had significant meibomian gland dysfunction. Topical 2% cyclosporine A, 4 times a day, resulted in arrest of keratolysis and rapid reepithelialization of the ulcer. In a small pilot study of keratoconjunctivitis sicca (KCS), Laibovitz and associates[206] found that 1% cyclosporine ointment relieved a number of subjective symptoms, including foreign body sensation. In addition, one objective finding, rose bengal corneal staining, also decreased. Another masked, placebo-controlled trial with 2% cyclosporine A in olive oil in patients with KCS also indicated beneficial effects on tear break-up time and rose bengal staining after 2 months of treatment.[217] Some evidence in patients with secondary Sjögren syndrome demonstrates that cyclosporine A may have a local immunoregulatory effect on the conjunctiva by affecting T cells.[207] A 6-week course of topical 2% cyclosporine A, 4 times per day, significantly decreased the numbers of CD4+ cells in both the corneal epithelium and substantia propria. However, despite the fact that the specimens taken showed significantly more CD4+ cells following treatment with cyclosporine A, the clinical benefits were not favorable. Local irritation followed use of the drug, and all patients complained of burning. Ocular irritation including burning, redness, and itching occur frequently and may be related to the vehicle used to administer the drug.[206,207]

There is evidence that systemically administered cyclosporine A in renal allograft recipients increases tear flow even when no lacrimal autoimmune disease exists.[218]

Side Effects.

Systemic cyclosporine A has a high risk of nephrotoxicity, occurring in 25% to 75% of patients. Alterations in renal function occur in virtually all patients treated with 10 mg/kg/day.[179,213] Although generally reversible, especially early in treatment, this dose-related nephrotoxicity frequently requires that cyclosporine A therapy be reduced or discontinued.[192] Chronic changes including interstitial fibrosis and renal tubular atrophy have been reported in as many as 22% of patients treated for immunosuppression, including uveitis.[197,213] If the dose does not exceed 5 mg/kg/day, the incidence of histologic changes in the kidney is low.[197] Mild to moderate hypertension (10–15% elevation in blood pressure) occurs in as many as 30% of transplant patients.[192] The incidence seems to be lower (approximately 10% to 15%) in patients treated for autoimmune diseases. The increase in blood pressure develops during the first 6 months of treatment and correlates significantly with kidney dysfunction.[213] Gingival hyperplasia may occur in up to 25% of patients by the third month of treatment[179] but is rarely seen at low doses.[197] Mild to moderate hypertrichosis commonly occurs during the first months of therapy.[179] A high incidence (34–49%) of reversible liver toxicity occurs with the use of high-dose cyclosporine A. This dose-dependent toxicity infrequently occurs with the low doses used for ocular inflammation.[179] Subjective side effects include parasthesias along with hand tremors. These symptoms occur most frequently during the first few weeks of therapy but generally subside without reducing the dose.[197] Gastrointestinal distress, nausea, and vomiting are common (3–10%) but rarely require discontinuing the drug.[185] The overall incidence of withdrawal from cyclosporine A treatment because of side effects was 12% in a series of patients treated for uveitis.[197]

Topical application of 2% cyclosporine A appears relatively nontoxic to corneal epithelium in culture as well as in clinical studies of human allograft recipients. An initial transient punctate epitheliopathy, which cleared in 2 to 9 months, has been reported in corneal transplant patients but may have resulted from the vehicle.[199,201,204] Mild ocular congestion has also been reported with topical cyclosporine A.[201] Since topical administration can lead to measurable plasma cyclosporine A levels,[204] kidney function should be monitored even in patients receiving topical therapy.[202]

Contraindications.

The main contraindication to the use of cyclosporine A is a hypersensitivity to the drug. However, nursing mothers need to be aware that cyclosporine A is excreted in breast milk. A limited number of cases of children born to mothers who used cyclosporine A during pregnancy appear to reflect no major fetal risk in humans. Because of the high risk of renal impairment, patients with preexisting renal disease are poor candidates for treatment and require special caution if cyclosporine A is deemed necessary.[212]

DAPSONE

Pharmacology.

Dapsone is an antibacterial agent related to the sulfonamides. Although its primary clinical use is in the treatment of leprosy, it is also effective for the systemic and ocular inflammatory activity associated with cicatricial pemphigoid.[179,219] Like the sulfonamides, dapsone acts by blocking the synthesis of folate. The mechanism for its proposed benefit in cicatricial pemphigoid is unknown. Some evidence suggests that it may stabilize lysosomal membranes to decrease the release of proteolytic enzymes, or it may interfere with the myeloperoxidase/hydrogen peroxidase-mediated cytotoxic systems found in the polymorphonuclear leukocytes.[220] Others believe it may inhibit inflammation by preventing activation of the complement pathway.[221] Dapsone is slowly but almost completely absorbed after oral administration, with peak plasma levels within 1 to 3 hours. Plasma half-life varies from 10 to 50 hours.[185] The drug is metabolized in the liver.

Clinical Uses.

Dapsone can be of benefit in ocular cicatricial pemphigoid.[179,180,219] Doses can range from 25 mg/day for the first week with an increase to 50 mg/day the second week,[179] to initiating therapy with 2 mg/kg/day and then subsequently adjusting the dose.[180] Tauber and associates[180] reported dapsone to be the most effective agent for the initial treatment of modestly active ocular cicatricial pemphigoid. Conjunctival inflammation resolved, and progressive cicatrization was inhibited in 45% of patients; dapsone successfully treated 93% of the patients with modest conjunctival inflammation. The use of dapsone also decreased both the dose and frequency of systemic steroid in patients who needed steroids to control acute inflammation.

Side Effects.

The toxicity most frequently associated with dapsone is an apparently dose-dependent hemolytic anemia. While patients on doses of 200 to 300 mg/day invariably experience some degree of hemolysis, healthy patients can generally tolerate 50 to 100 mg/day with very little hemolysis.[220] Patients with glucose-6-phosphate (G-6-P) dehydrogenase deficiency are at much higher risk of hemolytic anemia.[179] Red blood cell G-6-P dehydrogenase activity should be measured prior to initiating dapsone therapy to determine any increased risk of hemolysis.[179] In a series of 86 patients treated with dapsone at doses of 2 mg/kg/day or less, 10% had hemolysis and 3% had to discontinue dapsone because of this toxicity.[180] Other side effects include nausea, vomiting, and anorexia in as many as 20% of patients,[180,219,222] and a dose-dependent methemoglobinemia with all patients at 100 mg/day or more showing some signs.[220] Skin rashes, hepatitis, a reversible neuropathy, renal dysfunction, and blurred vision can also occur.[179,181,219,220]

Contraindications.

Previous allergic hypersensitivity to dapsone, sulfones, or sulfonamides are the main contraindications to dapsone. Caution is needed in treating G-6-P dehydrogenase deficient patients due to their greater risk of hemolytic anemia. While extensive experience has not shown an association of dapsone with teratogenic effects, no adequately controlled studies have been performed. Consequently, the drug should be used during pregnancy only if necessary. Dapsone should be avoided during lactation since it is extensively excreted into breast milk, and hemolytic reactions have occurred in neonates.[185]

BROMOCRIPTINE

Pharmacology. Bromocriptine (Parlodel) is an ergot alkaloid derivative that has dopamine (D_2) receptor agonist activity. Its primary clinical use is to control symptoms associated with Parkinson's disease.[223] Recent studies indicate that bromocriptine may also help in the treatment of immune disorders. This appears to result from the proposed action of prolactin as an immune modulator and bromocriptine's ability to inhibit prolactin release.[179] It is also possible, however, that bromocriptine inhibits growth hormone or other factors.[224] Only a small percentage of the administered dose actually reaches the systemic circulation, because the gastrointestinal tract absorbs only 30% of the dose and extensive first-pass metabolism occurs in the liver. Peak plasma concentrations occur within 1.5 to 3 hours after oral administration.[223]

Clinical Uses. Severe endogenous uveitis has been controlled in 4 patients taking bromocriptine either for Parkinson's disease or for hyperprolactinemia.[179] Others have reported decreases in specific autoantibody levels in patients with uveitis treated with bromocriptine alone or in combination with cyclosporine A.[224] The treatment of chronic anterior uveitis with bromocriptine alone was reported to be effective in a small group of 7 patients given 2.5 mg twice daily. Successful outcome was measured by a decrease in the recurrence of inflammation or, if recurrences occurred during treatment, by ease of treatment (with topical vs. systemic steroids). The authors concluded all patients had better results during bromocriptine treatment than in the year prior to treatment.[225] However, in a similar study by Palestine and Nussenblatt,[226] 8 patients with chronic anterior uveitis received no benefit from bromocriptine given in a maximum dosage of 2.5 mg 4 times a day. Thus, in the treatment of chronic anterior uveitis where the course of the disease is highly variable, studies require larger numbers of subjects to demonstrate clearly any beneficial effect from bromocriptine treatment.[226]

Side Effects. Side effects are common (69%) and include nausea, headache, dizziness, fatigue, lightheadedness, vomiting, and abdominal cramping. Most of these effects can be reduced or eliminated by initiating therapy with low dosages, starting with 1.25 mg at bedtime, then slowly increasing by 2.5 mg/day in divided doses until a therapeutic response occurs or the maximum tolerated dose is reached. Taking the drug with food may reduce some gastrointestinal symptoms. A slight systemic hypotensive effect also occurs with this drug, and patients with low blood pressure should be cautioned about sudden changes in position.[185]

Contraindications. Contraindications include any allergic hypersensitivity to the drug or other ergot alkaloids. Patients with severe ischemic heart disease or peripheral vascular disease should not take bromocriptine due to its hypotensive action and the possibility of a "first-dose" phenomenon of cardiovascular collapse. The drug is also contraindicated during pregnancy due to bromocriptine's action to block prolactin release.[185]

References

1. Gordon DM, McLean JM. Effects of pituitary adrenocorticotropic hormone (ACTH) therapy in ophthalmologic conditions. JAMA 1950;142:1271–1276.
2. Duke-Elder S, Ashton N. Action of cortisone on tissue reactions in inflammation and repair with special reference to the eye. Br J Ophthalmol 1951;35:695–707.
3. Leopold IH. The steroid shield in ophthalmology. Trans Am Acad Ophthalmol Otolaryngol 1967;71:273–289.
4. Leibowitz HM, Kupferman A. Anti-inflammatory medications. Int Ophthalmol Clin 1980;20:117–134.
5. Polansky JR, Weinreb RN. Anti-inflammatory agents. Steroids as antiinflammatory agents. In: Sears ML, ed. Pharmacology of the eye. New York: Springer-Verlag, 1984; Chapter 10a.
6. Schleimer RP. The mechanism of antiinflammatory steroid action in allergic disease. Ann Rev Pharmacol Toxicol 1985;85:381–412.
7. Charap AD. Corticosteroids. In: Tasman W, Jaeger EA, ed. Duane's Foundations of clinical ophthalmology. Philadelphia: J.B. Lippincott, 1992; Chap. 31.
8. Frangie JP, Leibowitz HM. Steroids. Int Ophthalmol Clin 1993;33:9–29.
9. Leopold IH, Purnell JE, Camon EJ. Local and systemic cortisone in ocular disease. Am J Ophthalmol 1951;34:361–371.
10. Kupferman A, Pratt MV, Suckewer K, Leibowitz HM. Topically applied steroids in corneal disease: III. The role of drug derivative in stromal absorption of dexamethasone. Arch Ophthalmol 1974;91:373–376.
11. Gardner S. Comparison of topical ophthalmic corticosteroid drops. Ocular Therapeutic Management 1992;3(2):1–14.
12. Leibowitz HM, Kupferman A. Bioavailability and therapeutic effectiveness of topically administered corticosteroids. Trans Am Acad Ophthalmol Otolaryngol 1975;79:78–88.
13. Leibowitz HM, Kupferman A. Antiinflammatory effectiveness in

the cornea of topically administered prednisolone. Invest Ophthalmol 1974;13:757–736.

14. Leibowitz HM, Kupferman A. Use of corticosteroids in the treatment of corneal inflammation. In: Leibowitz HM, ed. Corneal disorders: Clinical diagnosis and management. Philadelphia: Saunders, 1984, Chap. 11.

15. McGhee CNS, Watson DG, Midgeley JM, et al. Penetration of synthetic corticosteroids in human aqueous humor. Eye 1990;4: 526–530.

16. Cox SV, Kupferman A, Leibowitz HM. Topically applied steroids in corneal disease I: The role of inflammation in stromal absorption of dexamethasone. Arch Ophthalmol 1972;8:308–313.

17. Leibowitz HM, Berrospi AR, Kupferman A, et al. Penetration of topically administered prednisolone acetate into human aqueous humor. Am J Ophthalmol 1977;83:402.

18. Leibowitz HM, Lass JH, Kupferman A. Quantitation of inflammation in the cornea. Arch Ophthalmol 1974;92:427–430.

19. Polansky JR. Side effects of topical ophthalmic therapy with antiinflammatory steroids and β-blockers. Curr Opinion Ophthalmol 1992;3:259–272.

20. Ophthalmic drug facts. St. Louis: Facts and Comparisons, 1995; Chap. 6.

21. Leibowitz HM, Kupferman A. Kinetics of topically administered prednisolone acetate. Optimal concentrations for treatment of inflammatory keratitis. Arch Ophthalmol 1977;95:311–314.

22. Leibowitz HM, Kupferman A. Optimal frequency of topical prednisolone administration. Arch Ophthalmol 1979;97:2154–2156.

23. Watson D, Noble MJ, Dutton GN, et al. Penetration of topically applied dexamethasone alcohol into human aqueous humor. Arch Ophthalmol 1988;106:686–687.

24. Polansky JR, Alvarado JA. Isolation and evaluation of target cells in glaucoma research: Hormone receptors and drug responses. Curr Eye Res 1985;4:267–279.

25. Fairbairn WD, Thorson JC. Fluorometholone: Anti-inflammatory and intraocular pressure effects. Arch Ophthalmol 1971;86: 138–141.

26. Leibowitz HM, Ryan WJ, Kupferman A. Comparative anti-inflammatory efficacy of topical corticosteroids with low glaucoma-inducing potential. Arch Ophthalmol 1992;110:118–120.

27. Kass M, Cheetham J, Duzman E, et al. The ocular hypertensive effects of 0.25% fluorometholone in corticosteroid responders. Am J Ophthalmol 1986;102:159–163.

28. Kupferman A, Berrospi AR, Leibowitz HM. Fluorometholone acetate. A new ophthalmic derivative of fluorometholone. Arch Ophthalmol 1982;100:640–641.

29. Leibowitz HM, Hynduick RA, Lindsey C, Rosenthal A. Fluorometholone acetate: Clinical evaluation in the treatment of external ocular inflammation. Ann Ophthalmol 1984;16: 1110–1115.

30. Hull DS, Hine JE, Edelhauser HF, Hynduick RA. Permeability of the isolated rabbit cornea to corticosteroids. Invest Ophthalmol Vis Sci 1974;13:457–459.

31. Leibowitz HM, Kupferman A. Penetration of fluorometholone into the cornea and aqueous humor. Arch Ophthalmol 1975;93: 425–427.

32. Polansky JR, Sandman R, Zlock D, et al. FML vs other ophthalmic steroids. Role of receptor binding and metabolism in determining the IOP response. Invest Ophthalmol Vis Sci 1983; 24(supp):136.

33. Dorsch W, Thygeson P. The clinical efficacy of medrysone. A new ophthalmic steroid. Am J Ophthalmol 1968;65:74–75.

34. Rastogi RK, Mathur A, Raizada IN. Efficacy of medrysone as an antiinflammatory agent. Ind J Ophthalmol 1985;33:295–297.

35. Becker B, Kolker AE. Intraocular pressure response to topical corticosteroids. In: Leopold IH, ed. Ocular therapy: Complications and management. St Louis: C.V. Mosby Co, 1967;79–83.

36. Mindel JS, Tavitian HO, Smith H, Walker EC. Comparative ocular pressure elevations by medrysone, fluorometholone and dexamethasone. Arch Ophthalmol 1980;98:1577–1578.

37. Drance SM, Scott S. A comparison of action of dexamethasone and medrysone on human intraocular pressure. Can J Ophthalmol 1968;3:159–161.

38. Bartlett JD, Horwitz B, Laibovitz R, Howes JF. Intraocular pressure response to loteprednol etabonate in known steroid responders. J Ocular Pharmacol 1993;9:157–165.

39. Howes JF, Baw H, Vered M, Neuman R. Loteprednol etabonate: Comparison with other steroids in two models of intraocular inflammation. J Ocular Pharmacol 1994;10:289–293.

40. Leibowitz HM, Rich R, Crabb JL, et al. Intraocular pressure raising potential of rimexolone 1.0% in steroid responders. Invest Ophthalmol Vis Sci 1994;35(suppl):1508.

41. Bartlett JD, Howes JF, Ghormley NR, et al. Safety and efficacy of loteprednol etabonate for treatment of papillae in contact lens-associated giant papillary conjunctivitis. Curr Eye Res 1993;12: 313–321.

42. Bodor N. The application of soft drug approaches to the design of safer corticosteroids. In: Christophers E, ed. Topical corticosteroid therapy: A novel approach to safer drugs. New York: Raven Press, 1988; pp 13–25.

43. Druzgala PD, Wu WM, Howes JF. Ocular absorption and distribution of loteprednol etabonate: A "soft" steroid. Invest Ophthalmol Vis Sci 1991;32(suppl):735.

44. Leibowitz A, Kupferman A, Ryan WS, et al. Corneal anti-inflammatory efficacy of loteprednol etabonate. A new steroidal "soft drug." Invest Ophthalmol Vis Sci 1991;32(suppl):735.

45. Abelson M, George M, Drake M, et al. Evaluation of rimexolone ophthalmic suspension in the antigen challenge model of allergic conjunctivitis. Invest Ophthalmol Vis Sci 1992;33(suppl):2094.

46. Gordon DM. Diseases of the uveal tract. In: Gordon DM, ed. Medical management of ocular disease. New York: Harper & Row, 1964;245–271.

47. Leopold IH. Pharmacology and toxicology. Arch Ophthalmol 1951;46:159–224.

48. Ellis PP. Corticosteroid therapy in ophthalmology. In: Adriani J, Bernstein HN, eds. Symposium on ocular pharmacology and therapy. St. Louis: C.V. Mosby Co, 1970;49–57.

49. Beck RW, Cleary PA, Anderson MA, et al. A randomized, controlled trial of corticosteroids in the treatment of acute optic neuritis. N Engl J Med 1992;326:581–588.

50. Schlaegel TF. Depot corticosteroid by the cul-de-sac route. In: Kaufman HE, ed. Ocular anti-inflammatory therapy. Springfield, IL: Charles C. Thomas, 1970;117–123.

51. Cloes RS, Krohn DL, Breslin H, Braunstein R. Depo-Medrol in treatment of inflammatory diseases. Am J Ophthalmol 1962;54: 407–411.

52. Sturman RM, Laval J, Sturman MF. Subconjunctival triamcinolone acetonide. Am J Ophthalmol 1966;61:155–166.

53. Leinfelder PS. Depo-Medrol in treatment of acute chalazion. Am J Ophthalmol 1964;58:1078.

54. Pizzarello LD, Jakobiec FA, Hofeldt, AJ, et al. Intralesional corticosteroid therapy for chalazia. Am J Ophthalmol 1978;85: 818–821.

55. Freed D, Walls L. Chalazia treatments using intralesional corticosteroid injections: Clinical studies and literature review. So J Optom 1992;10:28–31.

56. Epstein GA, Putterman AM. Combined excision and drainage with intralesional corticosteroid injection in the treatment of chronic chalazia. Arch Ophthalmol 1988;106:514–516.

57. Schlaegel TF. Nonspecific treatment of uveitis. In: Duane TD, ed. Clinical ophthalmology. Philadelphia: Harper & Row, 1980; 4(43):1–12.

58. Herschler J. Intractable intraocular hypertension induced by repository triamcinolone acetonide. Am J Ophthalmol 1972;81: 788–792.

59. Leibowitz HM, Kupferman A. Periocular injection of corticosteroids. Arch Ophthalmol 1977;95:311–314.

60. Harter JG, Reddy WS, Thorn GW. Studies on intermittent corticosteroids dosage regimen. N Engl J Med 1963;269:591–596.

61. MacGregor RR, Sheagren HN, Lipsett MD, Wolff SM. Alternate day prednisone therapy. N Engl J Med 1969;280:1427–1431.

62. Friedlander MN. Allergy and immunology of the eye. ed. 2. New York: Raven Press, 1993.

63. Wilhelmus RR, Gee L, Hauck WW, et al. Herpetic eye disease study. A controlled trial of topical corticosteroids for herpes simplex stromal keratitis. Ophthalmology 1994;101:1883–1896.

64. Leopold IH. Nonsteroidal and steroidal antiinflammatory agents. In: Surgical pharmacology of the eye. New York: Raven Press, 1984:83–133.

65. Fung WE. Aphakic cystoid macular edema. In: Ryan SJ, ed. Retina, Vol 2. St. Louis: C.V. Mosby Co, 1989; Chap. 111.

66. Diestelhorst M, Aspacher F, Koren W, et al. Effect of dexamethasone 0.1% and prednisolone acetate 1% eye drops on the blood-aqueous barrier after cataract surgery. A controlled randomized fluorophotometric study. Graefe's Arch Clin Exp Ophthalmol 1992;230:451–453.

67. Nissen JN, Ehlers N, Frost-Larsen K, Sorensen T. The effect of topical steroid on postoperative edema and endothelial cell loss after intracapsular cataract extraction. Acta Ophthalmol 1993;71: 89–94.

68. Solomon LD, Flurbiprofen-CME Study Group I. Topical flurbiprofen and indomethacin for the prevention of pseudophakic cystoid macular edema. J. Cataract Refract Surg 1995 (in press).

69. Campos M, Abed HM, McDonnel PJ. Topical fluorometholone reduces stromal inflammation after photorefractive keratectomy. Ophthalmic Surg 1993;24:654–657.

70. Schulman JA, Peyman GA. Intravitreal corticosteroids as an adjunct in the treatment of bacterial and fungal endophthalmitis: A review. Retina 1992;12:336–340.

71. Urban RC, Cotlier E. Corticosteroid-induced cataracts. Surv Ophthalmol 1986;31:102–110.

72. Jaanus SD. Drug-related cataract. Optom Clin 1991;1:143–157.

73. Black RL, Oglesby RB, Von Sallmann L, Bunim JJ. Posterior subcapsular cataracts induced by corticosteroids in patients with rheumatoid arthritis. JAMA 1960;174:166–171.

74. Oglesby RB, Black RL, Von Sallmann L, Bunim JJ. Cataracts in rheumatoid arthritis patients treated with corticosteroids. Arch Ophthalmol 1961;66:519–523.

75. Havre DC. Cataracts in children on long-term corticosteroid therapy. Arch Ophthalmol 1965;73:818–821.

76. Braver DA, Richards RD, Good TA. Posterior subcapsular cataract in steroid treated children. Arch Ophthalmol 1972;286: 160–163.

77. Loredo A, Rodriguez RS, Murillo L. Cataracts after short-term corticosteroid treatment. N Engl J Med 1972;286:160–163.

78. Becker B. Cataracts and topical corticosteroids. Am J Ophthalmol 1964;58:872–873.

79. Bihara JS, Goldberg J, Tavitian HO. Posterior subcapsular cataract related to long-term corticosteroid treatment in children. Am J Dis Child 1968;116:604–608.

80. Burde RM, Becker B. Corticosteroid-induced glaucoma and cataracts in contact lens wearers. JAMA 1970;213:2075–2078.

81. Becker B. The side effects of corticosteroids. Invest Ophthalmol 1964;3:492–497.

82. Forman AR, Loreto JA, Tina LU. Reversibility of corticosteroid-associated cataract in children with nephrotic syndrome. Am J Ophthalmol 1977;84:75–78.

83. Skalka HW, Prchal JT. Effect of corticosteroids on cataract formation. Arch Ophthalmol 1980;98:1773–1777.

84. Yablonski ME, Burde RM, Kolker AE, Becker B. Cataracts induced by topical dexamethasone in diabetics. Arch Ophthalmol 1978;96:474–476.

85. Francisco J. Cortisone et tension oculaire. Ann Oculistique 1954; 187:805–816.

86. Linner E. Adrenocortical steroids and aqueous humor dynamics. Doc Ophthalmol 1959;13:210–222.

87. Goldmann H. Cortisone glaucoma. Arch Ophthalmol 1962;68: 621–626.

88. Armaly MF. Effect of corticosteroids on intraocular pressure and fluid dynamics: I. The effect of dexamethasone in the normal eye. Arch Ophthalmol 1963;70:482–491.

89. Becker B, Mills DW. Corticosteroids and intraocular pressure. Arch Ophthalmol 1963;70:500–507.

90. Armaly MF. Genetic factors related to glaucoma. Ann NY Acad Sci 1968;151:861–875.

91. Becker B. The genetic problem of chronic simple glaucoma. Ann Ophthalmol 1971;3:351–354.

92. Bartlett JD, Woolley TW, Adams CM. Identification of high intraocular pressure responders to topical ophthalmic corticosteroids. J Ocular Pharmacol 1993;9:35–45.

93. Schwartz B. The response of ocular pressure to corticosteroids. Int Ophthalmol Clin 1966;929–989.

94. Akinbekin T. Corticosteroid-induced ocular hypertension. J Cut Ocul Toxicol 1986;5:45–53.

95. Ohji M, Kinoshita S, Ohmi E, Kewayama Y. Marked intraocular pressure response to instillation of corticosteroid in children. Am J Ophthalmol 1991;112:450–454.

96. Bernstein NH, Schwartz B. Effects of long-term systemic steroids on ocular pressure and tonographic values. Arch Ophthalmol 1962;68:742–753.

97. Stewart RH, Kimbrough RL. Intraocular pressure response to topically administered fluorometholone. Arch Ophthalmol 1979; 97:2139–2140.

98. Kass M, Cheetham J, Duzman E, Burke PJ. The ocular hypertensive effect of 0.25% fluorometholone in corticosteroid responders. Am J Ophthalmol 1986;102:159–163.

99. Weinreb RN, Bloom E, Baxter JD, et al. Detection of glucocorticoid receptors in cultured human trabecular cells. Invest Ophthalmol Vis Sci 1981;21:403–407.

100. Francois J. Corticosteroid glaucoma. Ophthalmologica 1984;188: 76–81.

101. Godel V, Rogenbogen L, Stein R. On the mechanism of corticosteroid-induced ocular hypertension. Ann Ophthalmol 1978;10: 191–196.

102. Leibowitz HM, Kupferman A. Topically administered corticosteroids. Effects on antibiotic-related bacterial keratitis. Arch Ophthalmol 1986;98:1287–1290.

103. Leopold IH, Sery TW. Epidemiology of herpes simplex keratitis. Invest Ophthalmol 1963;2:498–503.

104. Pepose J. Herpes simplex keratitis: Role of viral infection versus immune response. Surv Ophthalmol 1991;35:345–352.

105. Kimura SJ, Okumoto M. The effect of corticosteroids on experimental herpes simplex keratoconjunctivitis in the rabbit. Am J Ophthalmol 1957;43:131–134.

106. McCoy G, Leopold IH. Simplex infections of the cornea. Am J Ophthalmol 1960;49:1355–1356.

107. Berson EL, Kobayaski GS, Becker B, Rosenbaum L. Topical corticosteroids and fungal keratitis. Invest Ophthalmol 1967;6: 512–517.

108. O'Day DM, Ray WA, Head WS, et al. Influence of corticosteroid on experimentally induced keratomycoses. Arch Ophthalmol 1991;109:1601–1604.

109. Stern GA, Buttross M. Use of corticosteroids in combination with antimicrobial drugs in treatment of infectious corneal disease. Ophthalmology 1991;98:847–853.

110. Leopold IH, Maylath F. Intraocular penetration of cortisone and its effectiveness against experimental corneal burns. Am J Ophthalmol 1952;35:1125–1134.

111. Durant S, Duval D, Home-De Larch F. Factors involved in the control of fibroblast proliferation by glucocorticosteroids: A review. Endocr Rev 1986;7(3):254–269.

112. Krupin T, LeBlanc RP, Becker B, et al. Uveitis in association with topically administered corticosteroid. Am J Ophthalmol 1970;70: 883–885.

113. Martins JC, Wilensky JT, Asseth CF, et al. Corticosteroid-induced uveitis. Am J Ophthalmol 1974;77:433–437.

114. Spaeth GL. Effects of topical dexamethasone on intraocular pressure and the water drinking test. Arch Ophthalmol 1966;76: 772–783.

115. Kern R, Marci FJ. Steroid eye drops and their components. Arch Ophthalmol 1967;78:794–802.

116. Nesome DA, Wong VG, Cameron TP, Anderson RR. "Steroid-induced" mydriasis and ptosis. Invest Ophthalmol 1971;10: 424–429.

117. Taravella MJ, Stulting RD, Mader TH, et al. Calcific band keratopathy associated with the use of topical steroid-phosphate preparations. Arch Ophthalmol 1994;112:608–613.

118. Trautzellel-Klosinksi S, Sundmacker R, Wigand R. Die wirkung von steroiden bei keratoconjunctivities epidemica. Klin Monatsbl Augenheilk 1980;176:899–906.

119. Krupin T, Mandell AT, Podos SM, Becker B. Topical corticosteroid therapy and pituitary-adrenal function. Arch Ophthalmol 1976;94:919–920.

120. Weiss AH. Adrenal suppression after corticosteroid injection of periocular hemangiomas. Am J Ophthalmol 1989;107:518–522.

121. Glatt HJ, Putterman AM, Van Aalst JJ, Levine MR. Adrenal suppression and growth retardation after injection of periocular capillary hemangioma with corticosteroids. Ophthalmic Surg 1991;22:95–97.

122. Buffington GA, Dominguez JH, Piering WF, et al. Interaction of rifampin and glucocorticoids. JAMA 1976;236:1958–1960.

123. Vane JR. Inhibition of prostaglandin synthesis as a mechanism of action for aspirin-like drugs. Nature [New Biol] 1971;231: 232–235.

124. Flach AJ. Cyclo-oxygenase inhibitors in ophthalmology. Surv Ophthalmol 1992;36:259–284.

125. Flach AJ. Nonsteroidal antiinflammatory drugs in ophthalmology. Int Ophthalmol Clin 1993;33:1–7.

126. Arshinoff S, D'Addario D, Sadler S, et al. Use of topical nonsteroidal anti-inflammatory drugs in excimer laser photorefractive keratectomy. J Cataract Refract Surg 1994;20:216–222.

127. Gwon A, Vaughan ER, Cheetham JK, et al. Ocufen (Flurbiprofen) in the treatment of ocular pain after radial keratotomy. CLAO J 1994;20:131–138.

128. Podos SM. Prostaglandins, nonsteroidal anti-inflammatory agents and eye disease. Trans Am Ophthalmol Soc 1976;74:637–660.

129. Kulkarni PS, Srinivasan BD. Nonsteroidal antiinflammatory drugs in ocular inflammatory conditions. In: Lewis AS, Furst DE, eds. Nonsteroidal antiinflammatory drugs. New York: Marcel Dekker, 1987; Chap. 7.

130. Neufeld AH, Sears ML. Prostaglandins and the eye. Prostaglandins 1973;4:157–168.

131. Ambache N. Irin, a smooth muscle contracting substance present in rabbit iris. J Physiol (Lond) 1955;129:65–66.

132. Bito LZ. Prostaglandins, other eicosanoids and their derivatives as potential anti-glaucoma agents. In: Drance SM, Neufeld AH, eds. Applied pharmacology in medical treatments of glaucoma. New York: Grune & Stratton, 1984; Chap. 20.

133. Leopold IH. Advances in ocular therapy: Noncorticosteroid anti-inflammatory agents. Am J Ophthalmol 1974;78:759–773.

134. Bito LZ. Prostaglandins. Old concepts and new perspectives. Arch Ophthalmol 1987; 105:1112–1116.

135. Kerstetter JR, Brubaker RF, Wilson SE, et al. Prostaglandins F_2a-1–iso-propylester lowers IOP without decreasing aqueous humor flow. Am J Ophthalmol 1988;105:30–34.

136. Bisggard H, Ford-Hutchinson AW, Charleson S. Presence of LTB_4 in human tears. Prostaglandins 1984;28:620–626.

137. Anderson JA, Chen CC. Multiple dosing increases the ocular bioavailability of topically administered flurbiprofen. Arch Ophthalmol 1988;106:1107–1109.

138. Gimbel H, Van Westenbrugge J, Cheetham JK, et al. Intraocular availability and pupillary effect of flurbiprofen compared with indomethacin during cataract surgery. J Cataract Refract Surg 1995 (in press).

139. Keates RM, McGowan KA. Clinical trial of flurbiprofen to maintain pupillary dilation during cataract surgery. Ann Ophthalmol 1984;16:919–921.

140. Heinrichs DA, Leith AB. Effects of flurbiprofen on the maintenance of pupillary dilation during cataract surgery. Can J Ophthalmol 1990;25:239–242.

141. Stark WS, Fagader WR, Stewart RH. Reduction of pupillary constriction during cataract surgery using suprofen. Arch Ophthalmol 1986;104:364–366.

142. Vander JF, Greven CM, Maguire JI, et al. Flurbiprofen sodium to prevent intraoperative miosis during vitreoretinal surgery. Am J Ophthalmol 1989;108:288–291.

143. Tsuchiska H, Takase M. Topical flurbiprofen in intraocular surgery on diabetic and non-diabetic patients. Ann Ophthalmol 1990; 22:15–23.

144. Sabiston D, Tessler H, Sumers K. Reduction of inflammation following cataract surgery by the nonsteroidal antiinflammatory drug, flurbiprofen. Ophthalmic Surg 1987;18:873–877.

145. Araie M, Sawa M, Takase M. Topical flurbiprofen and diclofenac suppress blood-aqueous barrier breakdown in cataract surgery. A fluorophotometric study. Jpn J Ophthalmol 1983;27:535–542.

146. Hotchkiss ML, Robin AL, Pollack IP, et al. Nonsteroidal antiinflammatory agents after argon laser trabeculoplasty: Flurbiprofen and indomethacin. Ophthalmology 1984;91:969–976.

147. Hurvitz LM, Spaeth GL, Zakhour I, et al. Comparison of the effect of flurbiprofen, dexamethasone and placebo on cyclocryotherapy-induced inflammation. Ophthalmic Surg 1984;15:394–399.

148. Weinreb RN, Rohm AL, Baerveldt G, et al. Flurbiprofen pretreatment in argon laser trabeculoplasty for primary open angle glaucoma. Arch Ophthalmol 1984;102:1629–1632.

149. Gieser DK, Hodapp E, Goldberg I, et al. Flurbiprofen and intraocular pressure. Ann Ophthalmol 1981;13:831–833.

150. Sulewski ME, Robin AL, Cummings HL, Arkin LM. Effects of topical flurbiprofen on the intraocular pressure lowering effect of apraclonidine and timolol. Arch Ophthalmol 1991;109:807–809.

151. McCannell C, Koskela T, Brubaker RF. Topical flurbiprofen pretreatment does not block apraclonidine's effect on aqueous flow in humans. Arch Ophthalmol 1991;109:810–811.

152. Todd PA, Heel RC. Suprofen—a review of its pharmacodynamic and pharmacokinetic properties and analgesic efficacy. Drug Eval 1985;30:514–538.

153. Wood TS, Stewart RH, Bowman RW, et al. Suprofen treatment of contact lens-associated giant pupillary conjunctivitis. Ophthalmology 1988;95:822–826.

154. Ku EC, Lee M, Kothari HV, Scholer DW. Effect of diclofenac sodium on the arachidonic acid cascade. Am J Med 1986; 80(suppl):18–23.

155. Phillips AF, Szerenyi K, Campos M, Krueger RR, McDonnell PJ. Arachidonic acid metabolites after excimer laser corneal surgery. Arch Ophthalmol 1993;111:1273–1278.

156. Szerenyi K, Wang XW, Lee M, McDonnell PJ. Topical diclofenac treatment prior to excimer laser photorefractive keratectomy in rabbits. Refract Cornea Surg 1993;9:437–442.

157. Sher NA, Frantz JM, Talley A, et al. Topical diclofenac in the treatment of ocular pain after excimer photorefractive keratectomy. Refract Cornea Surg 1993;9:425–436.

158. Eiferman RA, Hoffman RS, Sher NA. Topical diclofenac reduced pain following photorefractive keratectomy. Arch Ophthalmol 1993;111:1022.

159. Szerenyi K, Sorken K, Garbus JJ, et al. Decrease in normal human corneal sensitivity with topical diclofenac sodium. Am J Ophthalmol 1994;118:312–315.

160. Hersh PS, Rice BA, Baer JC, et al. Topical nonsteroidal agents and corneal wound healing. Arch Ophthalmol 1990;108:577–583.

161. Vickers FF, Mc Guigan LSB, Ford C, et al. The effect of diclofenac sodium ophthalmic on the treatment of post-operative inflammation. Invest Ophthalmol Vis Sci 1991;32(suppl):793.

162. Othenin-Girard P, Tritten SS, Pittet N, Herbort CP. Dexamethasone versus diclofenac sodium eyedrops to treat inflammation after cataract surgery. J Cataract Refract Surg 1994;20:9–12.

163. Kraff MC, Sanders DR, McGuigan L, Raanan MG. Inhibition of blood-aqueous humor barrier breakdown with diclofenac. Arch Ophthalmol 1990;108:380–348.

164. Herbort CP, Mermoud A, Schnyder C, Pittet N. Anti-inflammatory effect of diclofenac drops after argon laser trabeculoplasty. Arch Ophthalmol 1993;111:481–483.

165. Roberts CW. A comparison of diclofenac sodium to flurbiprofen for maintaining intraoperative mydriasis. Invest Ophthalmol Vis Sci 1994;35(suppl):1967.

166. Goldberg MA, McNamara N, Nguyen NT, et al. Effect of diclofenac sodium (Voltaren) on hypoxia-induced corneal edema in humans. CLAO J 1995;21:61–63.

167. Waterbury L, Kunysz EA, Beuerman R. Effect of steroidal and non-steroidal anti-inflammatory agents on corneal wound healing. J Ocular Pharmacol 1987;3:43–54.

168. Flach AJ, Graham J, Druger L, et al. Quantitative assessment of postsurgical breakdown of the blood aqueous barrier following administration of ketorolac tromethamine solution: A double-masked, paired comparison with vehicle-placebo solution study. Arch Ophthalmol 1988;106:344–347.

169. Flach AJ, Lavelle CJ, Orlander KW, et al. The effect of ketorolac tromethamine solution 0.1% in reducing postoperative inflammation after cataract extraction and intraocular lens implantation. Ophthalmology 1988;95:1279–1284.

170. Flach AJ, Dolan BJ, Irvine AR. Effectiveness of ketorolac tromethamine 0.5% ophthalmic solution for chronic and pseudophakic cystoid macular edema. Am J Ophthalmol 1987; 103:479–486.

171. Flach AS, Stegman RC, Graham J, Kruger LP. Prophylaxis of aphakic cystoid macular edema without corticosteroids. A paired comparison, placebo-controlled, double-masked study. Ophthalmology 1990;97:1253–1258.

172. Flach AS, Jampol LM, Weinberg D, et al. Improvement in visual acuity in chronic aphakic and pseudophakic cystoid macular edema after treatment with topical 0.5% ketorolac tromethamine. Am J Ophthalmol 1991;112:514–519.

173. Flach AJ, Jaffe NS, Akers WA. The effect of ketorolac tromethamine in reducing postoperative inflammation: Double-masked parallel comparison with dexamethasone. Ann Ophthalmol 1989;21:407–411.

174. Flach AJ, Kraff MC, Saunders DR, et al. The quantitative effect of 0.5% ketorolac tromethamine solution and dexamethasone sodium phosphate solution on postsurgical blood-aqueous barrier. Arch Ophthalmol 1988;106:480–483.

175. Rooks WH, Malone PJ, Shott LD, et al. The analgesic and antiinflammatory profile of ketorolac and its tromethamine salt. Drugs Exp Clin Res 1985;11:479–492.

176. Probst L, Stoney P, Jeney E, et al. Nasal polyps, bronchial asthma and aspirin sensitivity. J Otolaryngol 1992;21:60–64.

177. Denman AM, Denman DJ, Palmer RG. Alkylating agents. In: Rugstad HE, et al, eds. Immunopharmacology in autoimmune diseases and transplantation. New York: Plenum Press, 1992; Chap. 11.

178. Calabresi P, Chabner BA. Antineoplastic agents. In: Gilman AG, Rall TW, Nies AS, Taylor P, eds. Goodman and Gilman's The pharmacologic basis of therapeutics, ed. 8. New York: Pergamon Press, 1990; Chap. 52.

179. Hemady R, Tauber J, Foster CS. Immunosuppressive drugs in immune and inflammatory ocular disease. Surv Ophthalmol 1991; 35:369–385.

180. Tauber J, de la Maza MS, Foster CS. Systemic chemotherapy for ocular cicatricial pemphigoid. Cornea 1991;10:185–195.

181. Yazici H, Barnes CG. Practical treatment recommendations for pharmacotherapy of Behçet's syndrome. Drugs 1991;42:796–804.

182. Kazokoglu H, Saatci O, Cuhadaroglu H, Eldem B. Long-term effects of cyclophosphamide and colchicine treatment in Behçet's disease. Ann Ophthalmol 1991;23:148–151.

183. Foster CS. Systemic immunosuppressive therapy for progressive bilateral Moorens's ulcer. Ophthalmology 1985;92:1436–1439.

184. Fraiser LH, Kanekal S, Kehrer JP. Cyclophosphamide toxicity. Drugs 1991;42:781–795.

185. Olin BR, Hebel SK, Dombek CE, eds. Drug facts and comparisons. St. Louis: Facts and Comparisons, Inc, 1995.

186. American academy of ophthalmology basic and clinical science course, Section 9: Intraocular inflammation and uveitis. San Francisco: American Academy of Ophthalmology, 1992:129–135.

187. O'Duffy JD. Behçet's syndrome. N Engl J Med 1990;322:326–328.

188. Tessler HH, Jennings T. High-dose short-term chlorambucil for intractable sympathetic ophthalmia and Behçet's disease. Br J Ophthalmol 1990;74:353–357.

189. BenEzra D. Immunosuppressive treatment of uveitis. Int Ophthalmol Clin 1990;30:309–313.

190. Tung JP, Maibach HI. The practical use of methotrexate in psoriasis. Drugs 1990;40:697–712.

191. Endresen L. Pharmacology and general therapeutic principles of methotrexate. In: Rugstad HE, et al, eds. Immunopharmacology in autoimmune diseases and transplantation. New York: Plenum Press, 1992; Chap. 10.

192. Handschumacher RE. Immunosuppressive agents. In: Gilman AG, Rall TW, Nies AS, Taylor P, eds. Goodman and Gilman's The pharmacologic basis of therapeutics, ed. 8. New York: Pergamon Press, 1990; Chap. 53.

193. Bach JF. Mode of action of thiopurines: Azathioprine and 6-mercaptopurine. In: Rugstad HE, et al, eds. Immunopharmacology in autoimmune diseases and transplantation. New York: Plenum Press, 1992; Chap. 9.

194. Hakin KN, Pearson RV, Lightman SL. Sympathetic ophthalmia: Visual results with modern immunosuppressive therapy. Eye 1992;6:453–455.

195. Yazici H, Pazarli H, Barnes CG, Tuzun Y, et al. A controlled trial of azathioprine in Behçet's syndrome. N Engl J Med 1990;322:281–285.

196. Insel PA. Analgesic-antipyretics and antiinflammatory agents; Drugs employed in the treatment of rheumatoid arthritis and gout. In: Gilman AG, Rall TW, Nies AS, Taylor P, eds. Goodman and Gilman's The pharmacologic basis of therapeutics, ed. 8. New York: Pergamon Press, 1990; Chap. 26.

197. Feutren G, von Graffenried B. Cyclosporin A: Pharmacology and therapeutic use in autoimmune diseases. In: Rugstad HE, et al, eds. Immunopharmacology in autoimmune diseases and transplantation. New York: Plenum Press, 1992; Chap. 12.

198. deSmet MD, Nussenblatt RB. Clinical use of cyclosporin in ocular disease. Int Ophthalmol Clin 1993;33:31–45.

199. Belin MW, Bouchard CS, Phillips TM. Update on topical cyclosporin A: Background, immunology, and pharmacology. Cornea 1990;9:184–195.

200. Holland EJ, Olsen TW, Ketchman JM, et al. Topical cyclosporin A in the treatment of anterior segment inflammatory disease. Cornea 1993;12:413–419.

201. Hoffmann F, Wiederholt M. Topical cyclosporin A in the treatment of corneal graft reaction. Cornea 1986;5:129.

202. Kervick GN, Pflugfelder SC, Haimovici R, et al. Paracentral rheumatoid corneal ulceration: Clinical features and cyclosporine therapy. Ophthalmology 1992;99:80–88.

203. Zhao J-C, Jin X-Y, Local therapy of corneal allograft rejection with cyclosporine. Am J. Ophthalmol 1995;119:189–194.

204. Belin MW, Bouchard CS, Frantz S, Chmielinska J. Topical cyclosporine in high-risk corneal transplants. Ophthalmology 1989;96:1144–1150.

205. BenEzra D, Pe'er J, Brodsky M, Cohen E. Cyclosporine eyedrops for the treatment of severe vernal keratoconjunctivitis. Am J Ophthalmol 1986;101:278–282.

206. Laibovitz RA, Solch S, Andriano K, et al. Pilot trial of cyclosporine 1% ophthalmic ointment in the treatment of keratoconjunctivitis sicca. Cornea 1993;12:315–323.

207. Power WJ, Mullaney P, Farrell M, Collum LM. Effect of topical cyclosporine A on conjunctival T cells in patients with secondary Sjögren's syndrome. Cornea 1993;12:507–511.

208. Lightman S. Uveitis: Management. Lancet 1991;338:1501–1504.

209. Wakefield D, McCluskey P. Cyclosporine: A therapy in inflammatory eye disease. J Ocular Pharmacol 1991;7:221–226.

210. Lightman S. Use of steroids and immunosuppressive drugs in the management of posterior uveitis. Eye 1991;5:294–298.

211. Towler HMA, Whiting PH, Forrester JV. Combination low dose cyclosporin A and steroid therapy in chronic intraocular inflammation. Eye 1990;4:514–520.

212. Towler HMA, Cliffe AM, Whiting PH, Forrester JV. Low dose cyclosporin A therapy in chronic posterior uveitis. Eye 1989;3:282–287.

213. Palestine AG, Austin HA, Balow JE, et al. Renal histopathologic alterations in patients treated with cyclosporine for uveitis. N Engl J Med 1986;314:1293–1298.

214. Nussenblatt RB, Palestine AG, Chan CC, et al. Randomized, double-masked study of cyclosporine compared to prednisolone in the treatment of endogenous uveitis. Am J Ophthalmol 1991;112:138–146.

215. Caspers-Velu LE, Decaux G, Libert J. Cyclosporine in Behçet's disease resistant to conventional therapy. Ann Ophthalmol 1989;21:111–118.

216. Ozyazgan Y, Yurdakul S, Yazici H, et al. Low dose cyclosporin A versus pulsed cyclophosphamide in Behçet's syndrome: A single masked trial. Br J Ophthalmol 1992;76:241–243.

217. Gündüz K, Özdemir Ö. Topical cyclosporin treatment of keratoconjunctivitis sicca in secondary Sjörgren's syndrome. Acta Ophthalmol 1994;72:438–442.

218. Palmer SL, Bowen PA, Green K. Tear flow in cyclosporine recipients. Ophthalmology 1995;102:118–121.

219. Foster CS. Cicatricial pemphigoid. Trans Am Ophthalmol Soc 1986;84:527–663.

220. Lang PG. Sulfones and sulfonamides in dermatology today. J Am Acad Dermatol 1979;1:479–492.

221. Hoang-Xuan T, Foster CS, Rice BA. Scleritis in relapsing polychondritis: Response to therapy. Ophthalmology 1990;97:892–898.

222. Mandell GL, Sande MA. Antimicrobial agents: Drugs used in the chemotherapy of tuberculosis and leprosy. In: Gilman AG, Rall

TW, Nies AS, Taylor P, eds. Goodman and Gilman's The pharmacologic basis of therapeutics, ed. 8. New York: Pergamon Press, 1990; Chap. 49.

223. Cedarbaum JM, Schleifer LS. Drugs for Parkinson's disease, spasticity, and acute muscle spasms. In: Gilman AG, Rall TW, Nies AS, Taylor P, eds. Goodman and Gilman's The pharmacologic basis of therapeutics, ed. 8. New York: Pergamon Press, 1990; Chap. 20.

224. Buskila D, Sukenik S, Shoenfeld Y. The possible role of prolactin in autoimmunity. Am J Repro Immunol 1991;26:118–123.

225. Zierhut M, Pleyer U, Waetjen R, et al. Chronic anterior uveitis treated with bromocriptine. In: Usui M, Ohno S, Aoki K, eds. Ocular immunology today. Amsterdam: Elsevier Science Publishers, 1990;463–466.

226. Palestine AG, Nussenblatt RB. The effect of BCP on anterior uveitis. Am J Ophthalmol 1988;106:488–489.

CHAPTER 13

Antiallergy Drugs and Decongestants

Siret D. Jaanus
Sally L. Hegeman
Mark W. Swanson

The eye is a common site of allergic inflammation in both local and systemic hypersensitivity reactions. The vast majority of ocular allergies involve the conjunctiva, and the terms *ocular allergy* and *allergic conjunctivitis* are often used synonymously.[1]

Immunopathology

The immunopathology of ocular allergy involves multiple mechanisms that are influenced, at least in part, by chemical mediators released from mast cells.[2–4] Approximately 50 million mast cells are associated with each human eye and adnexal tissues. Each mast cell contains several hundred vesicles filled with mediators that have been implicated in ocular allergic disease. The surface of the mast cell membrane is estimated to have as many as 500,000 receptors for IgE antibodies, which play a key role in immediate hypersensitivity reactions. Binding of the allergen-IgE antibody with the mast cell results in the activation of a serine esterase enzyme that initiates a change in the Fc portion of the IgE molecule attached to the mast cell membrane.[3] This event leads to an intracellular biochemical cascade resulting in mast cell degranulation and release of mediators, including histamine, prostaglandin D_2, eosinophil chemotactic factors, eosinophil granule major protein, platelet-activating factor, and several other less well-defined preformed or newly synthesized mediators (Fig. 13.1). The release of these mediators causes the signs and symptoms associated with ocular allergy, including itching, tearing, mucous discharge, conjunctival vasodilation, increased vascular permeability, and in more severe cases papillary hypertrophy of the tarsal conjunctiva and ocular surface alterations.[1–3,4]

Traditionally, five forms of ocular allergy are recognized: allergic rhinoconjunctivitis, atopic keratoconjunctivitis, vernal keratoconjunctivitis, giant papillary conjunctivitis and contact allergic conjunctivitis.[1] Although the pathophysiology underlying these conditions is not fully understood, four principal types of hypersensitivity reactions have been identified.[3,5]

Type I, *immediate* or *anaphylactic* reactions occur when allergens attach to two adjacent IgE molecules bound to the surface of a mast cell or circulating basophil, causing physical changes in the cell membrane and subsequent release of mediators and other substances. An individual's immune system may respond to an allergen after one or more exposures by producing IgE antibodies that attach to mast cells and make the cells susceptible to rupture when the antigen is reintroduced. Hayfever allergic conjunctivitis, vernal keratoconjunctivitis (VKC), and giant papillary conjunctivitis (GPC) are examples of ocular allergies with Type I components. Type I reactions also occur in asthma and with reactions to bee stings, penicillin and many other chemicals and toxins.

Type II reactions, also known as *cytotoxic* or *cell-stimulating* or *cytolytic complement-dependent cytotoxicity*, are

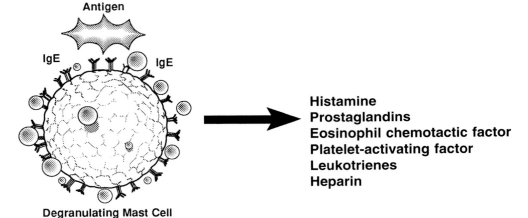

FIGURE 13.1   Release of inflammatory mediators following mast cell degranulation.

triggered by antibody bound to cell membrane. Complement is fixed to the bound antibody, and ultimately lysis of the cells occurs. Examples of Type II reactions include mismatched blood transfusions, early stages of graft rejection, penicillin-induced hemolytic anemia, and possibly ocular cicatricial pemphigoid.

Type III reactions, *toxic complex* or *immune-complex* reactions, occur when circulating antibody-antigen complexes precipitate out of tissues. This results in an acute inflammatory reaction. Particularly vulnerable tissues include joints, kidney, and lung. Serum sickness and some symptoms of rheumatoid arthritis and systemic lupus erythematosus are at least partially caused by Type III reactions. Type III reactions are infrequently encountered in ocular tissue, but intraocular inflammatory disease may be immune-complex mediated.[3]

Type IV reactions, *cell-mediated* or *delayed* reactions, differ from the other three types in that sensitized T-lymphocytes, rather than antibodies, interact with antigen. This interaction injures tissue by causing T-lymphocytes to release a group of biologically active chemicals, the lymphokines.[6] Within 24 to 48 hours of exposure to antigen, the patient develops erythema and perivascular inflammation. Examples of Type IV reactions include most drug allergies, graft rejection, and contact dermatitis. In the eye, atopic keratoconjunctivitis, VKC, GPC, and preservative-induced blepharoconjunctivitis are at least partly induced by cell-mediated hypersensitivity reactions.[3]

In general, treatment of ocular allergic disease is based on symptoms, severity, and characteristics of the allergic reaction. A stepped-care approach to therapy has been advocated, whereby treatment aggressiveness is tailored to the level of disease.[7,8] When possible, avoidance of environmental allergens such as pollen, dust, and grasses is also a key factor in management.

Among the treatment options, topical decongestants, oral and topical antihistamines, mast cell stabilizers, and, more recently, certain nonsteroidal anti-inflammatory agents have proved useful for alleviating the signs and symptoms associated with ocular allergic reactions. Corticosteroids and immunosuppressive agents, representing the most effective agents for severe inflammatory reactions, are discussed in Chapter 12.

Decongestants

Four synthetic adrenergic agonists, phenylephrine, naphazoline, oxymetazoline and tetrahydrozoline are currently available as ocular decongestants (Table 13.1). Following topical application to the eye, constriction of conjunctival blood vessels occurs at drug concentration levels that generally do not cause pupillary dilation. These agents provide only palliative therapy, since they have no effect on the conjunctival response to antigen.[9]

Pharmacology

Phenylephrine, the oldest of the currently available agents, is a synthetic adrenergic agonist. It differs chemically from epinephrine by the absence of the hydroxyl group on position 4 of the benzene ring.[10] At the concentrations used for ocular decongestion, phenylephrine causes vasoconstriction by direct stimulation of alpha receptors on conjunctival vasculature. The resultant clinical effect is usually a decrease in conjunctival hyperemia and edema.[11]

At the 0.12% concentration used for ocular decongestion, phenylephrine can occasionally dilate the pupil.[11] This effect

TABLE 13.1
Ophthalmic Decongestant Preparations

Generic Name	Trade Name	Manufacturer	Concentration (%)
Phenylephrine HCL	AK-Nefrin	Akorn	0.12
	Isopto Frin	Alcon	0.12
	Prefrin Liquifilm	Allergan	0.12
	Relief	Allergan	0.12
Naphazoline HCL	Allerest Eye Drops	Ciba Vision	0.012
	Clear Eyes	Ross	0.012
	Degest 2	Barnes-Hind	0.012
	Estivin 2	Alcon	0.012
	Naphcon	Alcon	0.012
	VasoClear	Ciba Vision	0.02
	Comfort Eye Drops	Barnes-Hind	0.03
	Maximum Strength Allergy Drops	Bausch & Lomb	0.03
	AK-Con	Akorn	0.1
	Albalon	Allergan	0.1
	Opcon	Bausch & Lomb	0.1
	Nafazair	Bausch & Lomb	0.1
	Naphcon Forte	Alcon	0.1
	Vasocon	Ciba Vision	0.1
Oxymetazoline HCL	OcuClear	Schering-Plough	0.025
	Visine LR	Pfizer	0.025
Tetrahydrozoline HCL	Collyrium Fresh	Wyeth-Ayerst	0.05
	Eyesine	Akorn	0.05
	Murine Plus	Ross	0.05
	Optigene 3	Pfeiffer	0.05
	Soothe	Alcon	0.05
	Tetrasine	Optopics	0.05
	Visine	Pfizer	0.05

is most likely to occur if the corneal epithelium is damaged or diseased. Moreover, with chronic use phenylephrine can cause a rebound of conjunctival congestion, resulting in conjunctivitis medicamentosa.[9]

Phenylephrine is chemically compatible with a variety of compounds and can be combined in ophthalmic formulations with various other agents, including antihistamines, corticosteroids, and antibiotics.

Classified chemically as imidazole derivatives, naphazoline, oxymetazoline and tetrahydrozoline differ structurally from other adrenergic agonists by replacement of the benzene ring with an unsaturated ring. In general, these agents exhibit greater alpha than beta adrenergic receptor activities.[10] Following topical application to the eye, they induce a marked vasoconstriction. The imidazole derivatives seem to have a clinical advantage over phenylephrine in that they are less likely to induce rebound congestion and pupillary dilation.[12]

Like phenylephrine, the imidazole derivatives can be combined or used with other agents, including antihistamines.

Clinical Uses

Various investigators have studied the clinical effects of phenylephrine and the imidazole derivatives. Abelson and associates[13] compared the ability of several ocular decongestant formulations to counteract histamine-induced erythema. Phenylephrine 0.12%, tetrahydrozoline 0.05%, and naphazoline ranging in concentrations from 0.012% to 0.1% were tested in a double-masked fashion in human eyes with no ocular disease. All preparations tested produced blanching of the conjunctiva. Naphazoline 0.02%, however, produced blanching of the conjunctiva greater than other nonprescription decongestants containing 0.05% tetrahydrozoline or 0.12% phenylephrine. No significant differences were observed with the 0.02% concentration present in over-the-counter (OTC) formulations and higher concentrations of naphazoline such as 0.1% available by prescription. The blanching effect of 0.02% naphazoline was also comparable to a preparation containing 0.05% naphazoline combined with the antihistamine antazoline phosphate 0.5%.

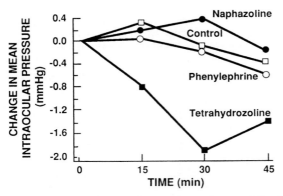

FIGURE 13.2 Mean intraocular pressure changes following instillation of commercially available OTC decongestants containing naphazoline 0.012%, tetrahydrozoline 0.05%, or phenylephrine 0.12%. (From Butler K, Thompson JP, Yolton DP. Rev Optom 1978;11:50.)

Higher concentrations of naphazoline, either alone or in combination with an antihistamine, have been compared to placebo in normal eyes and eyes congested from various causes.[14,15] Hurwitz and Thompson[14] studied the effects of 0.1% naphazoline in over 100 subjects with both normal and congested eyes. Slit-lamp evaluation revealed constriction of the conjunctival vessels, with no effect on the deeper vessels. However, at this concentration, an increase in pupil size occurred in 68 of 120 eyes, and 20 eyes demonstrated an increase in intraocular pressure (IOP) of 3 to 7 mmHg. No accommodative effects were observed with 0.1% naphazoline. In a double-masked fashion with placebo, Miller and Wolf[15] compared the effects of 0.05% naphazoline alone and in combination with 0.5% antazoline phosphate in patients with allergic conjunctivitis. Naphazoline performed better than the placebo in all parameters tested and, except for symptoms of itching, was more effective than antazoline alone. Naphazoline was equally effective as the combination formulation for relief of conjunctival inflammation.

Tetrahydrozoline has also been evaluated in patients with allergic or chronic conjunctivitis.[16,17] Tetrahydrozoline 0.05% produced "good" results in 67% and "fair" results in 30% of the cases.[17] Most eyes blanch within one minute following instillation, and the effect of a single application can last up to four hours. Tetrahydrozoline 0.05% does not appear to alter pupil size or raise IOP.[17]

Butler and associates[18] compared three OTC decongestant formulations containing phenylephrine 0.12%, naphazoline 0.012%, or tetrahydrozoline 0.05% in 40 adult subjects with no apparent ocular disease. No significant changes in pupil size or anterior chamber depth occurred. However, tetrahydrozoline 0.05% significantly lowered IOP at 30 minutes, as compared to phenylephrine 0.12%, which had only a

minimal or no effect. Naphazoline 0.012% produced a somewhat higher average IOP than the control (Fig. 13.2).

Oxymetazoline is available as an OTC ocular decongestant at the 0.025% concentration. Several studies have demonstrated its usefulness in patients with allergic and chlorine-induced conjunctivitis.[19–22] A double-masked, multicenter study compared 0.025% oxymetazoline with placebo in 158 patients with allergic conjunctivitis.[19] Two drops of oxymetazoline or placebo were placed in each eye four times daily for one week. Of the oxymetazoline group, 84% of patients showed improvement as compared with 58% in the placebo group. Oxymetazoline also improves symptoms of burning, itching, tearing and foreign body sensation in patients with moderate to severe conjunctival hyperemia.[22] Onset of action can be as early as 5 minutes following instillation, with peak effects at 60 minutes, and the effect can last up to 6 hours. In patients with chlorine-induced conjunctivitis, oxymetazoline appears to have a faster onset, longer duration of action, and better decongestant effect than OTC concentrations of naphazoline and tetrahydrozoline.[23]

Oxymetazoline 0.025% does not seem to alter IOP or affect pupil size or accommodation.[20,22] However, at higher concentrations of 0.1% to 0.5%, oxymetazoline reduces IOP in a dose-dependent fashion in both monkey and rabbit eyes.[24]

Side Effects

Transient stinging can occur with all decongestant preparations following instillation. Because of the relatively low concentrations required for ocular decongestion, ocular and systemic side effects occur infrequently with the manufacturer's recommended dosage range. Dosage frequency is generally 2 to 4 times daily but should be as infrequent as possible to minimize possible side effects. Pupillary dilation and rebound congestion can occur with extended use.[25] Upper lid retraction has been associated with use of 0.025% oxymetazoline and other decongestants.[19]

Contraindications

Since these agents are adrenergic agonists, they can potentially affect all target tissues innervated by the adrenergic division of the autonomic nervous system. Caution should be exercised in patients with cardiovascular disease, hyperthyroidism, and diabetes.

Use of these agents is contraindicated in patients with angle-closure glaucoma or potentially occludable angles. Application to a diseased or traumatized cornea can result in sufficient absorption to cause a systemic vasopressor response.[25]

Antihistamines

Antihistamines are used to block the actions of endogenously produced histamine. Histamine has numerous effects on cells and tissues, especially when released from mast cells in large quantities as part of a type I allergic reaction. Some of the associated clinical manifestations, such as anaphylactic shock, are life threatening; others, such as rhinitis, itching, tearing, and redness of the eye, are benign although disturbing to the patient.

Two classes of antihistamines, H_1 and H_2, are so designated because of the nature of the histamine receptor to which they bind. H_1 antihistamines prevent histamine-H_1 receptor interaction and thus provide symptomatic relief from histamine activity. H_1 antihistamines have a variety of pharmacologic actions that impart to this class of drugs a wide range of therapeutic uses in addition to the symptomatic relief of allergic reactions. H_2 antihistamines prevent histamine interaction with the H_2 receptor and have therapeutic use in treatment of conditions that involve hypersecretion of gastric acid.

Histamine

Histamine is synthesized and stored in nearly all tissues, with especially high concentrations in the lungs, skin, stomach, duodenum, and nasal mucosa.[26] In normal, nonhuman ocular tissues, histamine occurs in highest concentrations in the lids, conjunctiva, subconjunctiva, episclera, and limbus. Uveal tissue has low but measurable concentrations of histamine, while the lens, aqueous humor, retina, and other internal ocular structures have essentially none.[27] Nowak and Nawrocki[28] analyzed the histamine content of human ocular tissues enucleated because of trauma, uncontrolled glaucoma, or endophthalmitis. Histamine was found in the iris, ciliary body, choroid, retina, sclera, and optic nerve, with the highest levels in the uvea and the lowest levels in the retina and sclera. Tissues from traumatized eyes contained less histamine than eyes with endophthalmitis, although the pattern of high-histamine content in the uvea and low-histamine content in the sclera and retina was consistent in all groups. The tissues from eyes with glaucoma showed intermediate levels of histamine.

Mast Cell Histamine

It has been difficult to ascribe a physiologic function to mast cell histamine, which, when released, produces adverse nonphysiologic symptoms such as severe headache, urticaria (hives), angioneurotic edema, bronchospasm, and anaphylactic shock. However, studies[2,29] suggest that mast cell histamine may be an important modulator of many aspects of the immune response and that the adverse symptoms associated with histamine release occur only when the histamine receptor is somehow deficient or abnormal.

Release of mast cell histamine occurs by direct action of chemical or physical agents on the mast cell membrane, or by allergen-induced sensitization of mast cells.[6] Penicillin most frequently induces histamine release by a Type I hypersensitivity reaction, but procaine, salicylates, folic acid, thiamine, and a variety of protein drugs such as insulin, ACTH, and heparin commonly do so as well.[30]

Besides histamine release (degranulation) by an immune mechanism, some drugs, chemicals, as well as heat and trauma can degranulate mast cells by a direct action on the mast cell membrane. The signs and symptoms resemble a Type I allergic reaction, but because they do not involve the immune system they are called *anaphylactoid*.[30] Drugs are most likely to induce histamine release when administered intravenously, and signs and symptoms usually occur within minutes after drug injection. Some drugs that cause release of histamine by a direct action on the mast cell include morphine, codeine, atropine, curare, hydralazine, and meperidine.[31]

Nonmast Cell (Nascent) Histamine

A number of physiologic roles have been proposed for nonmast cell histamine, the form of histamine synthesized according to cellular demands. Since an increase in the rate of synthesis of histamine occurs during growth and repair of tissue, histamine may participate in tissue growth and repair processes.[32] Because non-mast cell histamine is associated with certain capillary beds, this substance may play a role in regulation of capillary permeability.[33] Some evidence indicates that histamine may serve as a central nervous system (CNS) neurotransmitter,[34] and histamine is known to regulate gastric acid secretion.[35] Nonmast cell histamine is probably not involved in the clinical manifestations associated with mast cell histamine release, such as anaphylaxis and urticaria.

Histamine Receptors

Three types of histamine receptors have been identified: H_1 or "classic," H_2, and H_3. The distinction between the three is based on the chemical structure of the antihistamine that binds to the receptor and on the type of histamine agonist. For example, as shown in Figure 13.3, a methyl group on the C_2 position of the imidazole ring confers H_1 agonist selectivity, while a methyl group on the C_4 position of the imidazole ring confers H_2 agonist selectivity. The H_3 receptor is the most recently described.[36] Currently no therapeutically use-

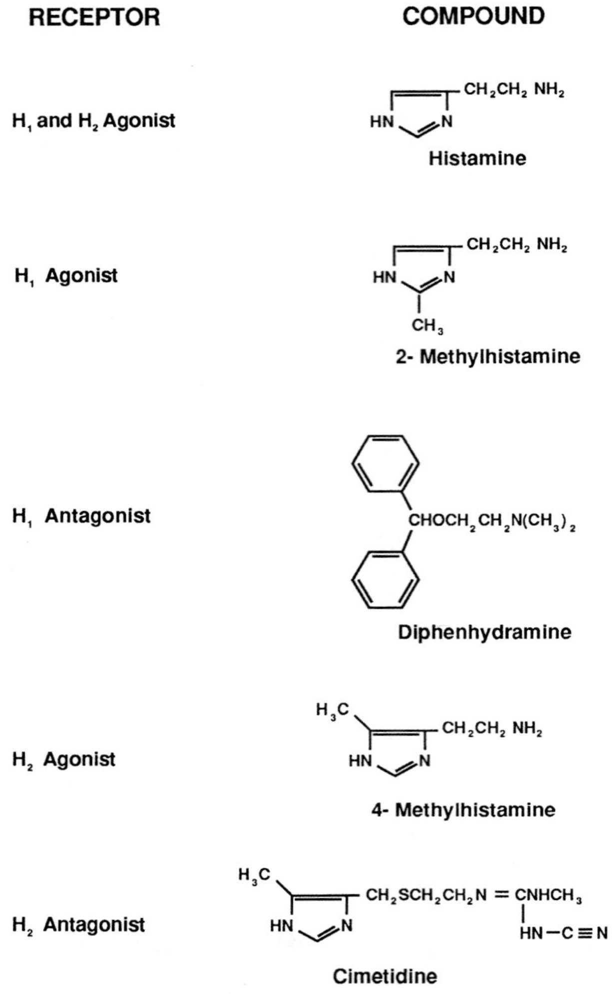

RECEPTOR   **COMPOUND**

H₁ and H₂ Agonist

$$CH_2CH_2\,NH_2$$

Histamine

H₁ Agonist

$$CH_2CH_2\,NH_2$$
$$CH_3$$

2- Methylhistamine

H₁ Antagonist

$$CHOCH_2CH_2N(CH_3)_2$$

Diphenhydramine

H₂ Agonist

$$H_3C$$
$$CH_2CH_2\,NH_2$$

4- Methylhistamine

H₂ Antagonist

$$H_3C$$
$$CH_2SCH_2CH_2N = CNHCH_3$$
$$HN-C\equiv N$$

Cimetidine

FIGURE 13.3   Structures of representative H₁ and H₂ receptor agonists and antagonists.

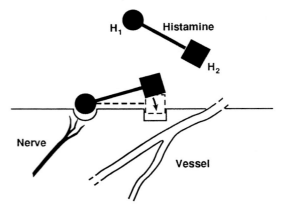

FIGURE 13.4   **Histamine receptor subtype location on neuronal and vascular tissues. Activated H₁ receptors are associated with neuronal tissue and result mainly in itching. H₂ receptors are associated with vascular tissue and result primarily in redness. (Adapted from Abelson MB, Schaefer K. Surv Ophthalmol 1993;38:119.)**

peptic ulcers. Table 13.2 summarizes the distribution of H₁ and H₂ receptors and their common antagonists.

Pharmacologic Actions of Histamine

Histamine is essentially ineffective when given orally. However, when parenterally administered or when massive mast cell disruption occurs, histamine causes significant vascular effects, including transient flushing of the face and neck, reduced blood pressure, and edema. Blood vessels contain H₁ and H₂ histamine receptors that, when stimulated, dilate the small precapillary blood vessels and constrict the larger venules. As a result, passive capillary dilation, pooling of blood, and hypotension occurs.[38] In addition, histamine causes edema by constricting cells of the small venules, thus exposing the basement membrane and allowing plasma to pass into extracellular space. The triple response of Lewis,[39] produced when a small amount of histamine (10 μg) is injected intradermally, illustrates such dilatation and edema. Initially a direct vasodilator action of histamine causes local redness, then a neuronally mediated diffuse redness. A wheal develops at the site of the initial localized erythema caused by increased capillary permeability. A reaction similar to this triple response follows both allergic and physical injury to the skin.

Heart rate and force of contraction increase with histamine administration. H₂ receptor activation causes increased rate and force of contraction, while H₁ receptors produce increased force of contraction and decreased AV conduction. Histamine can also stimulate the heart by releasing norepinephrine from adrenergic nerve terminals.[27]

ful agents, either agonists or antagonists, are known to act selectively on the H₃ receptor.

H₁ receptors occur in many tissues, including the smooth muscle of bronchi, blood vessels, and intestine. Antihistamines commonly used to treat allergies, such as diphenhydramine, are effective blockers of the H₁ receptor. H₂ receptors are present in gastric parietal cells, the heart, pulmonary blood vessels, cells of the immune system, the eye,[37] and other tissues (Fig. 13.4). Many tissues contain both H₁ and H₂ receptors, and the effects of simultaneously stimulating both may be antagonistic or complementary, depending on the specific tissue. H₂ receptors are blocked by the antihistamines cimetidine, ranitidine, nizatidine, and famotidine, drugs used extensively for the treatment of

TABLE 13.2
Distribution of H_1 and H_2 Receptors

Histamine Receptor	Tissue	Representative Antagonists
H_1	Bronchial smooth muscle	Diphenhydramine
	Heart	Chlorpheniramine
	CNS	Pyrilamine
	Mucous membranes	maleate
	Eye (blood vessels)	Promethazine
	Blood vessels	Antazoline
		Cyclizine
		Terfenadine
		Loratadine
H_2	Gastric parietal cells	Cimetidine
	Heart	Ranitidine
	Blood vessels	Nizatidine
	Mast cells	Famotidine
	Eyes (blood vessels)	
	Bronchial smooth muscle	
	CNS	
	White blood cells	

Bronchial smooth muscle constriction is another consequence of histamine injection or mast cell degranulation. Stimulation of the H_1 receptors, in particular, produces constriction, while stimulation of H_2 receptors produces relaxation. In nonasthmatic individuals histamine produces only slight constriction due to the balancing effect of both receptors. In asthmatics, however, histamine injection can provoke severe bronchospasm, probably because these indiviuals have either deficient or abnormal H_2 receptors.[29] Although injected histamine produces some bronchospasm, histamine appears not to be the only bronchoconstrictor involved during an asthmatic attack, since antihistamines will not terminate the attack. Other mast cell substituents, particularly leukotrienes, may be more important mediators of asthma. Certain purified leukotrienes are 100 to 1000 times more potent than histamine in constricting the bronchial tree.[40]

Subcutaneous doses of histamine stimulate gastric acid secretion from parietal cells but produce no other obvious pharmacologic effects. Both gastrin and an intact vagus nerve are required for maximal gastric acid secretion. Cimetidine and other H_2 blockers inhibit gastric acid secretion induced by gastrin, increased vagal activity, histamine, or food. Histamine appears, therefore, to have a key role in gastric acid secretion either by allowing hormones or transmitters to function or by being the final stimulator of the parietal cell.

In the eye, histamine release produces characteristic symptoms of ocular allergy: itching, redness, tearing, and

chemosis. Ocular signs include conjunctival and lid edema, dilation of conjunctival blood vessels, and a papillary reaction.[2] In animal studies topically administered or injected histamine produces hyperemia and edema in the uvea and conjunctiva, increased intraocular pressure, mild pupillary constriction, and in some cases breakdown of the blood-aqueous barrier.[27] Histamine also has a role in the release or synthesis of PGI_2 (prostacyclin), which is implicated as an important mediator of inflammation in allergic conjunctivitis.[41] Blood vessels dilate and leak in structures such as the iris, conjunctiva, and ciliary processes. Histamine, however, has no effect on retinal blood vessels.

Pharmacologic Actions of H_1 Antihistamines

The histamine-blocking properties of the H_1 antihistamines are predictable, based on an appreciation of the biologic actions of histamine. Antihistamines reversibly bind to the histamine receptors, thus preventing the binding of histamine to the receptor sites. The consequence is prevention of the physiologic or pharmacologic actions of histamine and the relief of signs and symptoms associated with histamine release.

H_1 antihistamines can provide considerable symptomatic relief of allergen-induced urticaria, mucosal congestion, and itching. H_1 antihistamines block histamine-induced capillary dilatation, increase in capillary permeability, and the associated itching and pain. If the dilatation and edema have already occurred, administration of these drugs prevents further histamine action but usually does not reverse the clinical manifestations already present.

Although antihistamines may relieve anaphylactic shock and angioedema, which are histamine mediated and often life threatening, the onset of antihistaminic action is slow. These emergencies necessitate subcutaneous administration of the physiologic antagonist, epinephrine. H_1 antihistamines are useful, however, as adjuncts in preventing development of additional symptoms.

Various degrees of cholinergic-blocking actions often accompany the use of H_1 antihistamines. Chlorpheniramine and pyrilamine have minimal blocking effects while diphenhydramine and promethazine have considerable anticholinergic action.[42] Although the anticholinergic actions of H_1 antihistamines are usually considered annoying side effects, the treatment of Parkinson's disease and motion sickness takes advantage of their atropine-like effects. Even though antihistamines with the greatest anticholinergic activity are effective in the treatment of motion sickness, other noncholinergic mechanisms may contribute to the antiemetic properties of this class of drugs.

Although H_1 antihistamines can depress or stimulate the CNS, depression more commonly occurs, especially in adults. Sedation, a common side effect of many H_1 receptor antagonists, may have an anticholinergic basis, but other central mechanisms are presumed to participate as well.

Therapeutic use is made of the sedative properties of diphenhydramine in OTC sleeping medications and of promethazine in prescription sedatives.[42] On the other hand, terfenadine and other minimally sedating agents cannot penetrate the CNS, which makes them useful to relieve mild symptoms of seasonal allergic rhinitis and conjunctivitis in those patients for whom sedation would be dangerous or interfere with activity.[43–45]

Local anesthetic properties probably explain some of the antipruritic effects of topically applied H_1 antihistamines. Topical application to the skin provides therapeutically effective control of allergic symptoms, but since the risk of sensitization is high, this route of administration should be used conservatively.

Topical H_1 Antihistamines

Four antihistamines are currently available for topical ophthalmic use, the three classic antihistamines pheniramine maleate, pyrilamine maleate, and antazoline phosphate; and the second generation agent, levocabastine. Research into ocular allergy has been greatly advanced with the development of the ocular histamine challenge model.[46] The development of this model of ocular allergy has allowed many new agents to be directly tested for antiallergic properties.

PHARMACOLOGY

The classic antihistamines have been used topically since the mid-1940s. Pheniramine is a member of the alkylamine group of antihistaminic drugs, while antazoline and pyrilamine are classified as ethylenediamines. All three agents are similar in action and are specific H_1 receptor antagonists. They differ slightly, however, in their pharmacologic action. Antazoline has some anesthetic properties, but rabbit models have shown that these are insufficient to prevent ocular irritation.[47] Pheniramine and pyrilamine have little effect on IOP, while antazoline has been shown to decrease IOP slightly.[47] Antazoline also has quinidine-like antiarrhythmic properties.[47]

Levocabastine is a cyclohexylpiperidine derivative that has extremely potent antihistaminic properties. It is highly specific for H_1 receptors. Animal studies show it to be 65 times more potent than the most active oral antihistamine, astemizole.[48] Pharmacokinetic studies have demonstrated that the drug is relatively fast acting, with the peak plasma level reached within 1 to 2 hours after oral administration.[49] It has a half-life of 20 to 40 hours, making it ideal for a once- or twice-daily dosing schedule. When given via the topical ocular route, levocabastine is effective within 15 minutes of administration with a high (20% to 40%) bioavailability.

CLINICAL USES

These drugs are indicated for the rapid relief of symptoms associated with seasonal or atopic conjunctivitis. Although

TABLE 13.3
Topical Ocular Antihistamines

Trade Name (manufacturer)	Composition	Concentration (%)
Vasocon-A (CibaVision)	Antazoline phosphate	0.5
	Naphazoline HCl	0.05
Naphcon-A (Alcon)	Pheniramine maleate	0.3
	Naphazoline HCl	0.025
AK-Con-A (Akorn)	Pheniramine maleate	0.3
	Naphazoline HCl	0.025
Opcon-A (Bausch & Lomb)	Pheniramine maleate	0.315
	Naphazoline HCl	0.027
Livostin (CibaVision)	Levocabastine	0.05

they are effective individually, all commercially available classic antihistamine preparations contain the vasoconstrictor agent, naphazoline (Table 13.3). The use of a vasoconstrictor together with the antihistamine is more effective than the use of either agent alone.[15,50] Recommended administration is 1 or 2 drops to each eye 3 or 4 times per day.

The Food and Drug Administration has classified the topical ophthalmic antihistamines into the "less-than-effective" category primarily because of the absence of clinical trial data to document their effectiveness. However, the antazoline-naphazoline combination (Vasocon-A) has proved effective against all major components of the ocular allergic response when compared to placebo, antazoline, or to naphazoline alone.[46]

Levocabastine 0.05% ophthalmic suspension is used 4 times daily to relieve symptoms due to seasonal allergic conjunctivitis. Clinical results indicate that this drug is significantly more effective than placebo in inhibiting itching, hyperemia, eyelid swelling, chemosis, and tearing after an ocular allergen challenge with grass, ragweed, or cat dander.[112] Levocabastine is as effective or more effective than cromolyn sodium in both allergen challenge and natural course clinical trials.[51–59] When used topically, levocabastine appears as effective and well tolerated as oral terfenadine in the treatment of seasonal allergic conjunctivitis.[111]

SIDE EFFECTS

Severe complications can occur with systemic use of the three classic ocular antihistamines, including death, thrombocytopenia, and allergic pneumonitis; no such side effects, however, have been reported with topical use.[60–64] Although these agents are generally well tolerated, burning, stinging and discomfort upon instillation are not uncommon. Studies have shown that pheniramine may produce somewhat less stinging on instillation than does antazoline or pyrilamine.[65] A combination formulation of 0.3% pheniramine with

0.05% tetrahydrozoline has been reported to cause significant mydriasis from 30–120 minutes following topical application to the eye. The effect was more pronounced in patients with light irides.[113] Long-term use of topical antihistamines may induce drug-associated allergy. The antazoline-naphazoline combination has also been implicated as a cause of a verticillate-type keratopathy on long-term administration.[66] Levocabastine produces minimal side effects, with burning and stinging on administration the most common.[54,55] When topically applied, levocabastine produces no CNS side effects.[67–69]

CONTRAINDICATIONS

There are no absolute contraindications to topical antihistamines other than sensitivity to one of the component agents. Since the anticholinergic properties of the antihistamines can produce some degree of mydriasis, these drugs could potentially produce angle-closure glaucoma in patients with narrow angles. The topical antihistamines are thus contraindicated in patients with narrow anterior chamber angles.[25] All antihistaminic compounds have the potential to produce sedation, and caution should be used in combining topical antihistamines with systemic antihistamines.

Topical H₂ Receptor Antagonists

The discovery of H_2 receptors on the ocular surface has sparked interest in the use of H_2 antagonists in combination with H_1 antagonists for the treatment of ocular allergy. The use of both agents in combination would theoretically block all histamine response on the ocular surface. Cimetidine is a selective H_2 antagonist used for a number of years in the treatment of gastric ulcer. Topically applied cimetidine effectively blocks vasodilation produced by histamine agonists.[37] In addition, the combination of cimetidine and pyrilamine is more effective in decreasing vasodilation than either drug applied alone.[70] Currently, no H_2 antagonists are approved for topical ophthalmic use, but research indicates they may play a future role in treatment of allergic conjunctivitis.

Oral H₁ Antihistamines

Many orally administered antihistamines are available either over-the-counter (OTC) or by prescription. They are used to block the actions of histamine and for such other therapeutically useful indications as to produce sedation or anticholinergic effects. Table 13.4 summarizes commonly used oral antihistamines and some of their important pharmacologic properties. Note that these commonly used antihistamines differ little in their H_1-receptor blocking activity.[42] Because the practitioner often prescribes these drugs based on the degree to which they cause sedation, the antihistamines are

classified accordingly. The agents listed in Table 13.4 are formulated as syrups, tablets, or capsules, and several are available in sustained- or timed-release form.[42] In general, antihistamines should be administered orally for patients with moderate to severe eyelid edema (angioedema) and chemosis. The oral route of administration helps to ensure drug delivery deep within the affected ocular tissues where topical antihistamines may not penetrate.

MINIMALLY SEDATING

Terfenadine (Seldane), astemizole (Hismanal), and loratadine (Claritin) are currently available. They are essentially nonsedating at usual therapeutic doses and practically devoid of cholinergic-blocking or antiemetic properties (see Table 13.4). In addition to their histamine-blocking properties, terfenadine and loratadine inhibit the release of histamine, which may account for some of their therapeutic effectiveness.[9] The minimally sedating agents can provide relief of mild to moderate allergic rhinitis and conjunctivitis in patients who need relief while working, operating hazardous equipment, or driving. Studies of terfenadine indicate that therapeutic efficacy is best only for mild to moderate symptoms.[45] All these agents, however, have a relatively long duration of action; astemizole and loratadine are administered once daily on an empty stomach,[9,42] and terfenadine is given every 12 hours.[42] Because of the unique pharmacokinetics of astemizole, its onset of action is slower than that of loratadine or terfenadine and may require 2 to 3 days to achieve maximum effect.[45] The effects of loratadine or terfenadine begin in 1 to 3 hours.[42]

MILDLY SEDATING

Antihistamines in this group (see Table 13.4) are available either alone or in combination with decongestants, analgesics or other agents for the symptomatic relief of colds or type I allergies.[42] The usually mild sedation associated with these antihistamines makes them suitable for daytime use. With the exception of methdilazine, these agents have only moderate cholinergic-blocking properties and consequently fewer problems with drying of secretions, tachycardia, and other anticholinergic effects.

MODERATELY SEDATING

Because these antihistamines are sedating, they should not be used when operating hazardous equipment or when good motor and sensory skills are required. With the exception of tripelennamine, these agents are moderately potent cholinergic blockers, and clemastin, carbinoxamine, and trimeprazine are useful for the treatment of nausea and vomiting due to disturbances of the vestibular apparatus.[42]

STRONGLY SEDATING

Diphenhydramine and promethazine are highly sedating antihistamines, and much of their therapeutic use results from

TABLE 13.4
Oral H₁ Antihistamines

Drug	Trade Name	Anticho-linergic Activity	Antiemetic Activity	Adult Dosage (mg)
Minimally Sedating				
Terfenadine	Seldane	0 to mild	none	60 bid
Astemizole	Hismanal	0 to mild	none	10 daily
Loratadine	Claritin	0 to mild	none	10 daily
Cetirazine	Zyrtec	0 to mild	none	10 daily
Mildly Sedating				
Pyrilamine	Nisaval	mild	none	25–50 tid, qid
Brompheniramine	Dimetane	moderate	none	4 4–6x/day
Chlorpheniramine	Chor-Trimeton	moderate	none	4 qid to q4h
Dexchlorpheniramine	Polaramine	moderate	none	2 qid to q4h
Triprolidine	Actidil	moderate	none	2.5 qid to q4h
Cyproheptadine	Periactin	moderate	none	4 tid
Methdilazine	Tacaryl	strong	very strong	8 bid to qid
Moderately Sedating				
Clemastin	Tavist	strong	strong	1.34–2.68 bid to tid
Carbinoxamine	Clistin	strong	strong	4–8 tid to qid
Tripelennamine	PBZ	mild	none	25–50 qid to q4h
Trimeprazine	Temaril	strong	very strong	2.5 qid
Azatadine	Optimine	moderate	none	1–2 bid
Strongly Sedating				
Diphenhydramine	Benadryl	strong	strong	25–50 tid to qid
Promethazine	Phenergan	strong	very strong	12.5–25 daily to qid

Adapted from Drug Facts and Comparisons, St. Louis: J.B. Lippincott Co. 1995:188a–194a.

their sedating properties. The most widely used, diphenhydramine, is available both OTC and by prescription. Promethazine is available only by prescription. Since these antihistamines are highly sedating, their most appropriate use is to provide relief of allergic symptoms during sleep. They should not be used when the patient is required to be alert or awake. Both are effective antiemetics, but promethazine is stronger and is widely prescribed for this purpose. Both diphenhydramine and promethazine have potent cholinergic-blocking properties, but because these drugs are administered at bedtime, patients are less troubled by them.

OTHER ANTIHISTAMINES

Several agents with histamine-blocking properties have therapeutic uses other than relieving symptoms of Type I allergies. The potent antihistamine hydroxyzine is used as an antianxiety agent, sedative, and antiemetic. It is used to decrease the dose of narcotics and is valuable in relieving itching associated with histamine.[42] H₁ antihistamines such as cyclizine (Marezine) and meclizine (Antivert) are used alone, or in combination with scopolamine, in the treatment of motion sickness.[42]

SIDE EFFECTS

Sedation and depression of reflexes and sensory input are among the most worrisome side effects of the oral antihistamines, especially in patients who drive or operate hazardous machinery. Sedation can be minimized by careful drug selection and dosage, or by changing to another antihistaminic preparation. *Alcohol (or other CNS depressants) and antihistamines must not be taken together.* Serious accidents occur because of the synergistic sedative actions of alcohol and H₁ antihistamines. Because of the many sites of action of the H₁ antihistamines, many other drug interactions can potentially occur (see Chap. 36). In addition to increasing the actions of CNS depressants, H₁ antihistamines are additive with the anticholinergics, adrenergic agonists, phenothiazines, and MAO inhibitors. The actions of adrenergic blockers, corticosteroids, and phenylbutazone, on the other hand, are decreased.[71]

Bothersome systemic side effects include palpitations; drying of secretions in the throat and bronchi; and gastrointestinal and urinary tact disturbances such as anorexia, nausea, vomiting, diarrhea or constipation, urinary frequency, and dysuria. Taking the agents with meals can minimize several of these effects. Adjustment of dose or change of drug may also decrease or eliminate these effects.

Ocular side effects relate primarily to the anticholinergic properties of the H_1 antihistamine. Accordingly, one can anticipate decreased secretion of tears and mucus, and mydriasis with the potential of acute angle-closure glaucoma. Continued use can bring about anisocoria, decreased accommodation, and decreased vision. These atropine-like effects are not common, and usually the antihistaminic therapy can continue, since these effects typically diminish with time.[71]

Allergic reactions to H_1 antihistamines can occur with oral administration but are much more likely following topical use.[72] The ocular allergic signs and symptoms resemble the conditions for which the antihistamine was prescribed. The allergic condition has two etiologic factors—the original allergy and the allergic response to the H_1 antihistamine. Because of the structural diversity of H_1 antihistamines, an allergic reaction to one agent does not imply hypersensitivity to another H_1 drug. Accordingly, the practitioner can change to another, structurally different H_1 antihistamine.

When used in recommended dosages, antihistamines are reasonably safe drugs. Acute toxicity following massive doses is characterized by marked CNS stimulation (convulsions) in children and depression (coma) followed by stimulation (convulsions) in adults. Coma, cardiorespiratory failure, and death follow convulsions in cases of severe toxicity. Treatment is supportive. Phenobarbital or diazepam therapy may be attempted during the convulsive phase.[73]

CONTRAINDICATIONS

H_1 antihistamines are contraindicated in the case of a known hypersensitivity reaction to the agent. Oral preparations are also contraindicated in nursing mothers and in the third trimester of pregnancy because the H_1 antihistamines are secreted in milk and because infants and neonates appear more susceptible to these drugs' adverse effects.[42] As with all medication, extreme caution should be used in prescribing antihistamines to women in the first three months of pregnancy, when the risk of fetal malformation is very high.[30]

Although they are generally well tolerated, terfenadine and astemizole should not be used concurrently with erythromycin, ketoconazole, or itraconazole because of the potential risk of serious cardiac arrhythmias (see Chap. 36).[74,75,114–116] This precaution should probably extend to all macrolides and antifungals. Evidence is accumulating,

however, that these precautions do not apply to loratadine.[117,118]

Methdilazine, a phenothiazine antihistamine, should not be given to patients who are depressed, who are taking antidepressant medications, or who have had an adverse reaction, such as jaundice, to any of the phenothiazines.

Antihistamines that produce sedation should not be used with alcohol or any other sedating drug, such as opioid analgesics.[42,71] Antihistamines with strong anticholinergic effects should be avoided in patients with peptic ulcer disease, prostatic hypertrophy, bladder or pyloroduodenal obstruction, and in patients who have the potential for acute angle-closure glaucoma.[42] Since cyclizine and structurally related compounds are associated with teratogenic effects in animals,[76] these agents should not be administered during pregnancy.

Because of the number of H_1 antihistamines and their diverse pharmacologic properties, and because of potentially dangerous interactions with many medications (see Chap. 36), the clinician prescribing antihistamines should fully understand the actions and side effects of these agents.

Mast Cell Stabilizers

In recent years compounds have been developed that stabilize mast cells following allergen challenge. These have proved useful in the treatment and prophylaxis of a variety of ocular allergic disorders.[77] Included in this group are cromolyn sodium, lodoxamide, and nedocromil.

Cromolyn Sodium

PHARMACOLOGY

Cromolyn sodium was synthesized during a study of the biologic properties of khellin, an extract derived from the seed of the Eastern Mediterranean plant *Ammi visnaga.* Its chemical structure consists of two cromone rings joined by a flexible chain. Each ring contains two polar carboxylic acid groups. It is soluble in water up to 5%, insoluble in alcohol, and sparingly soluble in organic solvents.[78]

Cromolyn sodium has no antihistaminic activity, and it does not interfere with the interaction between IgE antibody and its corresponding antigen on the mast cell surface.[79] The traditional view has been that this agent inhibits mast cell degranulation and release of mediators of allergic disease by preventing calcium influx across mast cell membranes[80] (Fig. 13.5). Evidence however, indicates, that mast cell stabilizers, including cromolyn sodium, may also act via other mechanisms. *In vitro* studies have shown that it inhibits the activation of other cell types, including neutrophils, monocytes, and eosinophils.[78,81]

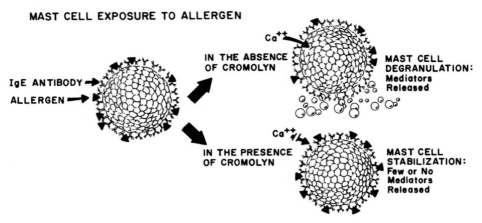

MAST CELL EXPOSURE TO ALLERGEN

FIGURE 13.5   **Inhibition of calcium ion influx and prevention of mast cell degranulation in the presence of cromolyn sodium. (From Cromolyn sodium. Clinical considerations. Excerpta Medica 1987, p. 5.)**

Cromolyn sodium may also prolong the tear break-up time in patients with chronic conjunctivitis. Felius and van Bijsterveld[82] observed a mean increase from a baseline value of 5.95 seconds to 9.0 seconds after treatment, a statistically significant change. Mikuni[83] conducted provocative tests with Japanese cedar pollenosis and observed an increase in the refractive index of tears. When 2% cromolyn sodium was instilled in the eye 5 minutes prior to testing, a significant decline in the index occurred within 5 to 20 minutes. The patients also showed improvement in signs and symptoms such as hyperemia and itching.

Since experience with cromolyn sodium shows a lag period in its clinical effects, patients need to be strongly advised that effective therapy depends on administering the drug at recommended time intervals and continued as long as needed to sustain improvement.

Pharmacokinetic studies indicate minimal ocular or systemic absorption following topical application to the eye.[78] When multiple doses are instilled to rabbit eyes, less than 0.07% of the administered dose is absorbed into the systemic circulation. Less than 0.01% of the dose penetrates into the aqueous humor. Clearance is complete, both from the anterior chamber of the eye and plasma, within 24 hours. In human subjects, analysis of drug excretion after instillation of 4% cromolyn sodium ophthalmic solution indicates that the eye absorbs approximately 0.03% of the administered dose. With topical ocular application, cromolyn sodium does not appear to accumulate in daily wear or extended wear contact lenses.[84]

CLINICAL USES

Cromolyn sodium is effective in ocular allergic reactions in which mast cell degranulation plays a major role.[2,78,85] Studies have indicated that both 2% and 4% concentrations are effective in relieving ocular signs and symptoms associated with seasonal allergic and allergen challenge conjunctivitis.[119,120] Patients often obtain relief within 7 days of initiation of therapy. In cases of chronic allergic conjunctivitis, the results can be less satisfactory. A trial period of 10 to 14 days is recommended before evaluating the effectiveness of therapy.[85]

Easty and associates[86] first demonstrated the usefulness of cromolyn in vernal keratoconjunctivitis (VKC). Both symptoms and clinical signs can be alleviated.[86,87] Cromolyn sodium may be effective when used alone in VKC, but with severe clinical signs and symptoms corticosteroids and other agents may also be required.[85]

Cromolyn administration has generally been less beneficial in giant papillary conjunctivitis (GPC),[88] but improvement in symptoms can occur. Donshik and associates[89] reported that patients whose symptoms were not controlled by changing lenses, were better able to tolerate lens wear with use of cromolyn four times daily. Buckley[90] conducted a double-masked comparison of cromolyn and placebo in patients with GPC. The cromolyn group showed a significant reduction in hyperemia, mucus production, and diffuse infiltration. Some reduction in size of papillae of the upper tarsal conjunctiva was observed after three weeks of treatment.

Cromolyn sodium is formulated as a 4% solution (Crolom) preserved with benzalkonium chloride 0.01% and EDTA 0.1%.

SIDE EFFECTS

Few side effects follow topical ocular administration of cromolyn. Since plasma levels of drug are very low, no adverse systemic reactions have been reported with ocular use.[78]

The most frequently observed ocular reaction is transient

stinging or burning following instillation.[25] Other infrequently reported side effects include conjunctival injection, watery or itchy eyes, dryness around the eye, puffy eyes, and styes.[25,78]

CONTRAINDICATIONS

Cromolym sodium should not be administered to patients sensitive to cromolyn ophthalmic solution or any of its components.

Lodoxamide

PHARMACOLOGY

Lodoxamide, like cromolyn sodium, inhibits mediator release from mast cells during an allergic reaction. Although its mechanism of action is similar to that of cromolyn sodium, this compound is 2,500 times more potent in its ability to inhibit mediator release.[91] Since eosinophil infiltration occurs in VKC and other allergic disease states, part of lodoxamide's action may result from its ability to block mediator release from these cells.[92]

CLINICAL USES

Lodoxamide has shown efficacy in the treatment or prevention of several types of allergic conjunctivitis, notably VKC.[92-96] A three-month study of lodoxamide 0.1% in patients with allergic conjunctivitis demonstrated significant improvement in all major signs and symptoms by two weeks.[94] A randomized, double-masked, placebo-controlled clinical trial of 118 patients age 2 to 71 years evaluated the safety and efficacy of 0.1% lodoxamide in VKC.[92] Lodoxamide or placebo was instilled four times daily for 90 days. Lodoxamide significantly reversed the corneal complications (Fig. 13.6). Discomfort associated with limbal changes and conjunctival discharge where also relieved. Itching decreased to a significantly greater extent in the lodoxamide-treated group. Caldwell and associates[96] compared the efficacy of 0.1% lodoxamide with 4% cromolyn sodium in a 28-day study of 120 patients with VKC. Patients were instructed to instill one drop of the masked medication 4 times daily. Lodoxamide gave a significantly greater and earlier improvement in signs and symptoms compared to cromolyn sodium.

Lodoxamide is available as a 0.1% ophthalmic formulation under the trade name of Alomide (Alcon).

SIDE EFFECTS

Ocular discomfort following instillation can occur. A rare instance of nausea has been reported.[92,96]

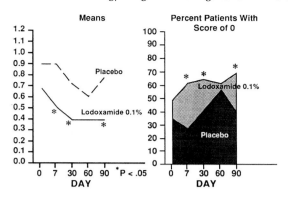

FIGURE 13.6 **Effect of lodoxamide vs placebo on signs of epithelial disease and corneal staining in patients with VKC. (Adapted from Santos C, et al. Invest Ophthalmol Vis Sci 1993; 34(suppl):1492.)**

CONTRAINDICATIONS

Like cromolyn sodium, lodoxamide ophthalmic solution should not be administered to patients sensitive to any components of the product.

Nedocromil Sodium

PHARMACOLOGY

Nedocromil, a disodium salt of the pyranoquinoline dicarboxylate, was developed as a result of research for new compounds to control asthma.[97] Its activity has been studied *in vitro* in a variety of inflammatory cells, including mast cells, eosinophils, and polymorphonuclear leukocytes. Nedocromil appears to be more potent than cromolyn sodium in its ability to inhibit immunologic release of mast cell mediators.[98,99] It can also modify the actions of eosinophils, neutrophils, monocytes, macrophages, and platelets. It appears that nedocromil can inhibit secretion from inflammatory cells and also antagonize the action of mediators involved in the allergic process.[100] Pharmacokinetic studies indicate that ocular penetration of nedocromil sodium is slow, and clearance from the eye is relatively rapid.[100]

CLINICAL USES

Nedocromil has been evaluated against placebo in seasonal allergic conjunctivitis.[101-104] Blumenthal and associates[104] assessed the efficacy and safety of 2% nedocromil sodium administered twice daily in a group of 140 patients with seasonal allergic conjunctivitis. Statistically significant improvement in itching, conjunctival injection, and overall disease severity occurred with nedocromil as compared to placebo.

Nedocromil 2% may be more effective for symptoms of perennial allergic conjunctivitis not fully controlled by cromolyn sodium.[121] In patients with bilateral perennial allergic conjunctivitis recalcitrant to 2% cromolyn, nedocromil demonstrated statistical superiority in relieving symptoms such as itching, burning, grittiness, and tearing that persisted during treatment with cromolyn.

Nedocromil sodium may also be useful in contact lens–induced giant papillary conjunctivitis.[105] Compared to placebo, the medication reduces itching and mucous discharge.

Nedocromil sodium is formulated as a 2% preserved ophthalmic solution under the trade name of Tilavist (Fisons Corporation).

SIDE EFFECTS

Topical ocular administration of nedocromil can cause transient burning and stinging. Another reported side effect is an unpleasant taste sensation following administration of the drops.[104,105]

CONTRAINDICATIONS

Like other mast cell stabilizers, nedocromil sodium ophthalmic solution should not be administered to patients sensitive to any of its components.

Nonsteroidal Anti-Inflammatory Drugs

Various nonsteroidal anti-inflammatory drugs (NSAIDs) have been studied for potential clinical use in allergic conjunctivitis.[4] Ketorolac tromethamine has proved beneficial in seasonal allergic conjunctivitis. Diclofenac (see Chap. 12) may also reduce the signs and symptoms associated with acute seasonal allergic conjunctivitis.[122,123]

Pharmacology

Ketorolac tromethamine is a member of the pyrrolo-pyrolle group of NSAIDs.[106] Its primary action in ocular inflammatory disease may result from its ability to affect prostaglandin synthesis by inhibiting the activity of cyclooxygenase, one of the enzymes responsible for the conversion of arachidonic acid to prostaglandins[107](see Chap. 12). Prostaglandins have been shown to be potent itch-producing substances in the conjunctiva, and the antipruritic efficacy of ketorolac appears to involve inhibition of conjunctival prostaglandins.[124]

Pharmacokinetic data indicate that ketorolac penetrates the cornea following topical ocular administration and reaches concentrations that reduce prostaglandin E levels in the aqueous humor.[108] Plasma levels of ketorolac following topical ocular application are usually below detectable limits as compared to oral administration. Ketorolac does not affect IOP, pupillary response, or visual acuity.

Clinical Uses

The efficacy of ketorolac has been compared to that of placebo in double-masked, controlled trials in patients with ocular allergic disease.[109,110] Ketorolac 0.5% applied four times daily for one week in patients with allergic conjunctivitis was significantly more effective than placebo in relieving itching. Improvement also occurred in clinical signs, including erythema, edema, and mucous discharge.[109] A second trial in patients with acute allergic conjunctivitis compared mean scores for various symptoms before, during, and at the end of one week of treatment.[110] Both ketorolac- and placebo-treated eyes showed a decrease in conjunctival inflammation and a reduction in itching, but the decrease was greater in patients using ketorolac.

Ketorolac (Acular) is formulated as a 0.5% solution with benzalkonium chloride 0.01% and edetate sodium 0.1%. The pH of the solution is 7.4.

Side Effects

The most frequent adverse event reported is transient stinging and burning following instillation of the ophthalmic solution. Rarely, allergic reactions and superficial keratitis have occurred.[108]

Contraindications

The drug is contraindicated in patients while wearing soft contact lenses. Caution should be used with patients who have previously exhibited sensitivity to acetylsalicylic acid, phenylacetic acid derivatives, and other NSAIDs since a potential exists for cross-sensitivity.[108]

References

1. Friedlaender MH. Conjunctivitis of allergic origin: Clinical presentation and differential diagnosis. Surv Ophthalmol 1993;38: 105–114.
2. Allansmith MR, Ross RN. Ocular allergy and mast cell stabilizers. Surv Ophthalmol 1986;30:229–244.
3. Allansmith MR. Immunology of the external ocular tissues. J Am Optom Assoc 1990;61(suppl):16–22.
4. Abelson MB, Schaefer K. Conjunctivitis of allergic origin: immu-

nologic mechanisms and current approaches to therapy. Surv Ophthalmol 1993;38:115–132.

5. Gell PGH, Coombs RRA, eds. Clinical aspects of immunology. Oxford: Blackwell Scientific, 1968.

6. David JR, Davis RR. Cellular hypersensitivity and immunity. Inhibition of macrophage migration and lymphocyte mediators. Prog Allergy 1971;16:300–449.

7. Greiner JV, Ross RN, Allansmith MR. Ocular allergy. In: Samter M, ed. Immunological diseases. Boston: Little Brown, 1989: 1917–1943.

8. Bartlett JD. Pharmacology of allergic eye disease. J Am Optom Assoc 1990;61(suppl):23–31.

9. Ciprandi G, Buscaglia S, Cerqueti PM. Drug treatment of allergic conjunctivitis. Drugs 1992;43:154–176.

10. Hoffman BB, Lefkowitz RJ. Catecholamines and sympathomimetic drugs. In: Gilman AG, Rall TW, Nies AS, et al. eds. Goodman and Gilman's The pharmacological basis of therapeutics. New York: McGraw-Hill, 1993; Chap. 10.

11. Weiss DI, Shaffer RN. Mydriatic effects of one-eighth percent phenylephrine. Arch Ophthalmol 1962;68:727–729.

12. Abelson MB, Butrus SI, Weston JH, Rosner B. Tolerance and absence of rebound vasodilation following topical ocular decongestant usage. Ophthalmology 1984;91:1364–1367.

13. Abelson MB, Yamamoto GK, Allansmith MR. Effects of ocular decongestants. Arch Ophthalmol 1980;98:856–858.

14. Hurwitz P, Thompson JM. Use of naphazoline (Privine) in ophthalmology. Arch Ophthalmol 1950;43:712–717.

15. Miller J, Wolf EM. Antazoline phosphate and naphazoline hydrochloride, singly and in combination for the treatment of allergic conjunctivitis. A controlled double-blind clinical trial. Ann Allergy 1975;35:81–86.

16. Grossman EE, Lehman RH. Ophthalmic use of tyzine. Am J Ophthalmol 1956;42:121–123.

17. Menger HC. New ophthalmic decongestant tetrahydrozoline hydrochloride. JAMA 1958;170:178–179.

18. Butler K, Thompson JP, Yolton DP. Effects of non-prescription ocular decongestants. Rev Optom 1978;115:49–52.

19. Samson CR, Danzig MR, Sasovetz D, Thompson HS. Safety and toleration of oxymetazoline ophthalmic solution. Pharmatherapeutica 1980;2:347–352.

20. Breaky AS, Cinotti AA, Hirshman M, et al. A double-blind, multicenter controlled trial of 0.25% oxymetazoline ophthalmic solution in patients with allergic and non-infectious conjunctivitis. Pharmatherapeutica 1980;2:353–356.

21. Duzman E, Anderson J, Vita JB, et al. Topically applied oxymetazoline. Arch Ophthalmol 1983;101:1122–1126.

22. Duzman E, Warman A, Warman R. Efficacy and safety of topical oxymetazoline in treating allergic and environmental conjunctivitis. Ann Ophthalmol 1986;18:28–31.

23. Personal communication. Schering Laboratories, July 1987.

24. Wang RF, Lee PY, Taniguchi T, et al. Effect of oxymetazoline on aqueous humor dynamics and ocular blood flow in monkeys and rabbits. Arch Ophthalmol 1993;111:535–538.

25. Ophthalmic Drug Facts. St Louis: Facts and Comparisons, 1995.

26. Van Arsdel PP Jr, Beall GN. The metabolism and functions of histamine. Arch Intern Med 1960;106:714–733.

27. Stjernschantz J. Autocoids and neuropeptides. In: Sears ML, ed. Pharmacology of the eye. Handbook of experimental pharmacology, Vol. 69 Berlin: Springer-Verlag, 1984:311–332.

28. Nowak JJ, Nawrocki J. Histamine in the human eye. Ophthal Res 1987;19:72–75.

29. Chand N. Distribution and classification of airway histamine receptors: the physiological significance of histamine H_2 receptors. Adv Pharmacol Chemother 1980;17:103–131.

30. Cluff LE, Caranasos GJ, Stewart RB. Clinical problems with drugs. Philadelphia: W.B. Saunders Co, 1975.

31. Lagunoff D, Martin TW. Agents that release histamine from mast cells. Ann Rev Pharmacol Toxicol 1983;23:331–345.

32. Kahlson G, Rosengren E. Biogenesis and physiology of histamine. London: Arnold, 1971.

33. Schayer RW. Induced synthesis of histamine, microcirculatory regulation and the mechanism of action of the adrenal glucocorticoid hormones. Prog Allergy 1963;7:187–212.

34. Schwartz JC. Histaminergic mechanisms in brain. Ann Rev Pharmacol Toxicol 1977;17:325–339.

35. Soll A, Welch JH. Regulation of gastric acid secretion. Ann Rev Physiol 1979;41:35–53.

36. Arrang JM, Garbarg M, Lancelot JC, et al. Highly potent and selective ligands for histamine H_3 receptors. Nature 1987;327: 117–123.

37. Abelson MB, Udell IJ. H_2 receptors in the human ocular surface. Arch Ophthalmol 1981;99:302–304.

38. Owen DAA, Poy E, Woodward DF. Evaluation of the role of histamine H_1 and H_2 receptors in cutaneous inflammation in the guinea-pig produced by histamine and mast cell degranulation. Br J Pharmacol 1980;69:615–623.

39. Lewis T. The blood vessels of the human skin and their responses. London: Shaw and Sons, 1927.

40. Lewis RA, Austen KF, Drazen JM, et al. Slow-reacting substances of anaphylaxis: identification of leukotrienes C_1 and D from human rat sources. Proc Natl Acad Sci USA 1980;77:3710–3714.

41. Helleboid L, Khatami M, Wei ZG, Rockey JH. Histamine and prostacyclin. Primary and secondary release in allergic conjunctivitis. Invest Ophthalmol Vis Sci 1991;32:2281–2289.

42. Drug Facts and Comparisons. St. Louis: J.B. Lippincott Co, 1993: 188a–194a.

43. Kemp JP, Buckley CE, Gershwin ME, et al. Multicenter, double-blind, placebo-controlled trial of terfenadine in seasonal allergic rhinitis and conjunctivitis. Ann Allergy 1985;54:502–509.

44. Johansen LV, Bjerrum P, Illum P. Treatment of seasonal allergic rhinitis—a double-blind, group comparative study of terfenadine and dexchlorpheniramine. Rhinology 1987;25:35–40.

45. Choice of antihistamines for allergic rhinitis. Med Lett 1987;29: 105–108.

46. Abelson MB, Paradis A, George MA, et al. Effects of Vasocon-A in the allergen challenge model of acute allergic conjunctivitis. Arch Ophthalmol 1990;108:520–4.

47. Krupin T, Silverstein B, Feitl M, Roshe R, Becker B. The effect of H_1-blocking antihistamines on intraocular pressure in rabbits. Ophthalmology 1980;87:1167–72.

48. Zuber P, Pecoud A. Effect of levocabastine, a new H_1 antagonist, in a conjunctival provocation test with allergens. J Allergy Clin Immunol 1988;82:590–4.

49. Dechant KL, Goa KL. Levocabastine: A review of its pharmacological properties and therapeutic potential as a topical antihistamine in allergic rhinitis and conjunctivitis. Drugs 1991;41:202–9.

50. Abelson MB, Allansmith MR, Friedlaender MH. Effects of topically applied ocular decongestant and antihistamine. Am J Ophthalmol 1980;90:254–7.

51. Abelson MB, George MA, Smith LM. Evaluation of 0.05% levo-cabastine versus 4% sodium cromolyn in the allergen challenge model. Ophthalmology 1995;102:310–316.

52. Davis BM, Mullins J. Topical levocabastine is more effective than sodium cromoglycate for prophylaxis and treatment of seasonal allergic conjunctivitis. Allergy 1993;48:519–524.

53. Azevedo M, Castel-Branco MG, Oliveira JF, et al. Double-blind comparison of levocabastine eye drops and sodium cromoglycate and placebo in the treatment of seasonal allergic conjunctivitis. Clin Exp Allergy 1991;21:689–694.

54. Ciprandi G, Cerqueti PM, Sacca S, Cilli P, Canonica GW. Levo-cabastine versus cromolyn sodium in the treatment of pollen-induced conjunctivitis. Ann Allergy 1990;65:156–8.

55. Odelram H, Bjorksten B, Af Klercker T, et al. Topical levocabas-tine versus sodium cromoglycate in allergic conjunctivitis. Allergy 1989;44:432–6.

56. Rimas M, Kjellman NIM, Blychert LO, Bjorksten B. Topical levocabastine protects better than sodium cromoglycate and pla-cebo in conjunctival provocation tests. Allergy 1990;45:18–21.

57. Feinberg G, Stokes TC. Application of histamine-induced con-junctivitis to the assessment of a topical antihistamine, levocabas-tine. Int Arch Allergy Appl Immunol 1987;82:537–8.

58. Bende M, Pipkorn U. Topical levocabastine, a selective H_1-antagonist, in seasonal allergic rhinoconjunctivitis. Allergy 1987; 42:512–515.

59. Pipkorn U, Bende M, Hedner J, Hedner T. A double-blind evalua-tion of topical levocabastine, a new specific H_1-antagonist in patients with allergic conjunctivitis. Allergy 1985;40:491–496.

60. Petrusewicz J, Kaliszan R. Blood platelet adrenoceptor: aggrega-tory and antiaggregatory activity of imidazole drugs. Pharmacol-ogy 1986;33:249–55.

61. Pahissa A, Guardia J, Bofill JM, Bacardi R. Antazoline-induced allergic pneumonitis. Br Med J 1979;2:1328.

62. Bengtsson U, Ahlstedt S, Aurell M, Kaijser B. Antazoline-induced immune hemolytic anemia, hemoglobulinuria, and acute renal failure. Acta Med Scand 1975;198:223–7.

63. Neilsen JL, Dahl R, Kissmeyer-Nielsen F. Immune thrombocyto-penia due to antazoline. Allergy 1981;36:517–9.

64. Ogbuihi S, Audick W, Bohn G. Sudden infant death—fatal intoxi-cation with pheniramine. Z Rechtsmed 1990;103:221–5.

65. Berdy GJ, Abelson MB, George MA, Smith LM, Giovanoni RL. Allergic conjunctivitis—a survey of new antihistamines. J Ocular Pharmacol 1991;7:313–24.

66. Herman DC, Bartley GB. Corneal opacities secondary to topical naphazoline and antazoline (Albalon-A). Am J Ophthalmol 1987; 108:

67. Rombaut N, Bhatti JZ, Curran S, Hindmarch I. Effects of topical administration of levocabastine on psychomotor and cognitive function. Ann Allergy 1991;67:75–79.

68. Tasaka K, Kamei C, Tsujimoto S, et al. Central effect of the potent long-acting H_1 antihistamine levocabastine. Arzneimittel-Forschung 1990;40:1295–1299.

69. Arriaga F, Rombaut N. Absence of central effects with levocabas-tine eye drops. Allergy 1990;45:552–554.

70. Leon J, Charap A, Duzman E, Shen C. Efficacy of cimetidine/pyrilamine eyedrops. A dose response study with histamine chal-lenge. Ophthalmology 1986;93:120–123.

71. Fraunfelder FT. Drug-induced ocular side effects and drug inter-actions. 3rd ed. Philadelphia: Lea & Febiger, 1989:363–365.

72. Mosko MM, Peterson WL. Sensitization to antistine. J Invest Dermatol 1950;14:1–2.

73. Friedman PA. Common poisons. In: Isselbacher KJ, Adams RD, Braunwald E, et al, eds. Harrison's principles of internal medicine, 9th ed. New York: McGraw-Hill, 1981:953–954.

74. Hismanal—new warning. Facts and Comparison's Drug Newslet-ter 1992;11:96.

75. New boxed warnings added for Seldane, Hismanal. FDA Medical Bulletin 1992;22:2–3.

76. Sadusk JF Jr, Palmisano PA. Teratogenic effect of meclizine, cyclizine, and chlorcyclizine. JAMA 1965;194:987–989.

77. Wiens JJ, Jackson WB. New directions in therapy for ocular allergy. Int Ophthalmol Clin 1988;28:332–337.

78. Cromolyn sodium. Clinical considerations. Excerpta Medica Monograph, 1987.

79. Cox JSC. Disodium cromoglycate: A specific inhibitor of reaginic antibody/antigen mechanism. Nature 1967;216:1328–1329.

80. Foreman JG, Garlano LG. Cromoglycate and other antiallergic drugs: a possible mechanism of action. Br Med J 1976;1:820–821.

81. Kay AB, Barns BJ. Pharmacologic modulation of the asthmatic response. In: Kay AB, Goetzl EJ, eds. Current perspectives in the immunology of respiratory diseases. New York: Churchill Living-stone, 1985:30–38.

82. Felius K, van Bijsterveld OP. Effect of sodium cromoglycate on tear film break-up time. Ann Ophthalmol 1987;17:80–82.

83. Mikuni I. Efficacy of 2% DSCG ophthalmic solution for allergic conjunctivitis from Japanese cedar pollinosin. Jpn J Clin Ophthal-mol 1980;34:1655–1659.

84. Iwasaki W, Kosaka Y, Momose T, et al. Absorption of topical disodium cromoglycate and its preservatives by soft contact lens. CLAO J 1988;14:155–158.

85. Sorkin EM, Ward A. Ocular sodium cromoglycate. An overview of its therapeutic efficacy in allergic eye disease. Drugs 1986;31: 131–148.

86. Easty DL, Rice NSA, Jones BR. Clinical trials of topical sodium cromoglycate in allergic conjunctivitis. Clin Allergy 1972;2:99–107.

87. Foster CS. Evaluation of topical cromolyn sodium in the treatment of vernal keratoconjunctivitis. Ophthalmology 1988;95:194–201.

88. Allansmith MR. Pathology and treatment of giant papillary con-junctivitis I: The U.S. perspective. Clin Ther 1987;9:443–450.

89. Donshik PC, Ballow M, Luistro A, Samartino L. Treatment of contact lens-induced giant papillary conjunctivitis. Contact Lens J 1984;10:346–349.

90. Buckley RI. Pathology and treatment of GPC II. The British perspective. Clin Ther 1987;9:451–457.

91. Johnson HG, VanHout CA, Wright JB. Inhibition of allergic reactions by cromoglycate and a new antiallergy drug U-42,585EI. Activity in rats. Int Arch Allergy Appl Immunol 1978; 56:416–421.

92. Santos C, Huang AJ, Hartwich-Young R, et al. Efficacy of lodox-amide 0.1% ophthalmic solution (Alomide) in resolving corneal epitheliopathy associated with vernal keratoconjunctivitis. Invest Ophthalmol Vis Sci 1993;34(suppl):1492.

93. Verin PC, Fritsch DS. Lodoxamide. A maintenance preventive agent for treatment of vernal keratoconjunctivitis. Ophthalmology 1989;96(suppl):120

94. Collum LMT. A three-month clinical evaluation of topical lodox-amide tromethamine for control of allergic conjunctivitis. 26 Internat Congr Ophthalmol 1990;SP-177.

95. Fahy G, Easty DL, Collum L, et al. Double-masked efficacy and safety evaluation of lodoxamide 0.1% ophthalmic solution versus Opticrom 2%. A multicenter study. Ophthalmology Today 1988: 341–342.

96. Caldwell DR, Verin P, Hartwich-Young R, et al. Efficacy and safety of lodoxamide 0.1% vs cromolyn sodium 4% in patients with vernal keratoconjunctivitis. Am J Ophthalmol 1992;113: 632–637.

97. Allergic conjunctivitis and the use of nedocromil sodium. Second International Symposium 1992. Fison Pharmaceuticals.

98. Gonzalez JP, Brogden RN. Nedocromil sodium: a preliminary review of its pharmacodynamic and pharmacokinetic properties and therapeutic efficacy in the treatment of reversible obstructive airway disease. Drugs 1987;34:560–567.

99. Moqbel R. Walsh GM, MacDonald AJ, Kay AB. The effect of nedocromil sodium on the activation of human eosinophils, neutrophils and histamine release from mast cells. Allergy 1988;43: 268–276.

100. Dahlen SE, Bjorck T, Kumlin M, et al. Dual inhibitory action of nedocromil sodium on antigen-induced inflammation. Drugs 1989;37:63–68.

101. Hirsch SR, Melamed J, Schwartz RH. Efficacy of nedocromil sodium 2% ophthalmic solution in the treatment of ragweed seasonal allergic conjunctivitis. J Allergy Clin Immunol 1988;81: 173.

102. Melamed J, Schwartz RH, Hirsh SR, et al. Evaluation of nedocromil sodium 2% ophthalmic solution for treatment of seasonal allergic conjunctivitis. Ann Allergy 1994;73:57–64.

103. Leino M, Jaanio E, Koivunen T, et al. A multicenter double-blind group comparative study of 2% nedocromil sodium eye drops (Tilavist) with placebo eye drops in the treatment of seasonal allergic conjunctivitis. Ann Allergy 1990;64:398–402.

104. Blumenthal M, Casale T, Dockhorn R, et al. Efficacy and safety of nedocromil sodium ophthalmic solution in the treatment of seasonal allergic conjunctivitis. Am J Ophthalmol 1992;113:56–63.

105. Bailey CS, Buckley BJ. Nedocromil sodium in contact lens-associated papillary conjunctivitis. Eye 1993 (suppl):29–33.

106. Rooks WH. Pharmacologic activity of ketorolac tromethamine. Pharmacotherapy 1990;10:308–311.

107. Abelson MB, Butrus SI, Kliman GH, et al. Topical arachidonic acid: a model for screening anti-inflammatory agents. J Ocular Pharmacol 1987;3:63–75.

108. Acular (ketorolac tromethamine) 0.5%. Product monograph, Allergan Pharmaceuticals, 1993.

109. Tinkelman DG, Rupp G, Kaufman H, et al. Double-masked, paired-comparison clinical study of ketorolac tromethamine 0.5% ophthalmic solution compared with placebo eyedrops in the treatment of seasonal allergic conjunctivitis. Surv Ophthalmol 1993; 38:133–140.

110. Ballas Z, Blumenthal M, Tinkelman DG, et al. Clinical evaluation of ketorolac tromethamine 0.5% ophthalmic solution for the treatment of seasonal allergic conjunctivitis. Surv Ophthalmol 1993; 38:141–148.

111. The Livostin Study Group. A comparison of topical levocabastine and oral terfenadine in the treatment of allergic rhinoconjunctivitis. Allergy 1993;48:530–534.

112. Abelson MB, George MA, Schaefer K, Smith LM. Evaluation of the ophthalmic antihistamine 0.05% levocabastine, in the clinical allergen challenge model of allergic conjunctivitis. J Allergy Clin Immunol 1994;94:458–464.

113. Gelmi C, Occuzzi R. Mydriatic effect of ocular decongestants studied by pupillography. Ophthalmologica 1994;208:243–246.

114. Monahan BP, Ferguson CL, Killeavy ES, et al. Torsades de pointes occurring in association with terfenadine use. JAMA 1990;264:2788–2790.

115. Simons FE, Kesselman MS, Giddins NG, et al. Astemizole-induced torsades de pointes. Lancet 1988;2:624.

116. Honig P, Woolsey RL, Zamani K, et al. Changes in the pharmacokinetics and electrocardiographic pharmacodynamics of terfenadine with concomitant administration of erythromycin. Clin Pharmacol Ther 1992;52:231–238.

117. Brannan MD, Reidenberg P, Radwanski E, et al. Evaluation of pharmacokinetic and electrocardiographic parameters following 10 days of concomitant administration of loratadine with ketoconazole (abstract). J Clin Pharmacol 1994;34:1009–1033.

118. Brannan MD, Affrime MB, Reidenberg P, et al. Evaluation of the pharmacokinetics and electrocardiographic pharmacodynamics of loratadine with concomitant administration of erythromycin (abstract). J Clin Pharmacol 1994;34:1009–1033.

119. Leino M, Montan P, Njå F. A double-blind group comparative study of ophthalmic sodium cromoglycate, 2% four times daily and 4% twice daily in the treatment of seasonal allergic conjunctivitis. Allergy 1994;49:147–151.

120. Montan P, Zetterström O, Eliasson E, Strömquist LH. Topical sodium cromoglycate (Opticrom(R)) relieves ongoing symptoms of allergic conjunctivitis within 2 minutes. Allergy 1994;49:637–640.

121. Van Bijsterveld OP, Moons L, Verdonck M, Kempeneers HP. Nedocromil sodium treats symptoms of perennial allergic conjunctivitis not fully controlled by sodium cromoglycate; a double-masked placebo controlled group comparative study. Ocular Immunol Inflamm 1994;2:177–186.

122. Laibovitz RA, Zimmermann KE, Friley CK. A placebo-controlled trial of 0.1% diclofenac ophthalmic solution in acute seasonal allergic conjunctivitis. Invest Ophthalmol Vis Sci 1994; 35(suppl):1291.

123. Tauber J, Abelson M, Ostrov C, Laibovitz R, et al. A multicenter comparison of diclofenac sodium 0.1% to ketorolac tromethamine 0.5% in patients with acute seasonal allergic conjunctivitis. Invest Ophthalmol Vis Sci 1994;35(suppl):1291.

124. Nieves AL, Spada CS, Woodward DF. The pruritogenic and inflammatory effects of prostanoids on the conjunctiva: a rationale for the clinical efficacy of Acular (ketorolac) in allergic conjunctivitis (abstract). Annual Meeting of the Association for Ocular Pharmacology and Therapeutics, New Orleans, LA, January 26–29, 1995.

CHAPTER 14

Lubricants and Other Preparations for Ocular Surface Disease

Siret D. Jaanus

Keratoconjunctivitis sicca (KCS), generally known as dry eye, has been recognized since antiquity as a condition often difficult to alleviate.[1,2] The acronym KCS, or katarrhus siccus, as termed by Peters in 1891, also implies a chronic inflammation of the conjunctiva and was meant to encompass the most severe of eye conditions prevalent at that time.[1] Since an abnormal tear film invariably leads to ocular surface damage, the preferred terminology today is *ocular surface disease*, which includes dry eye conditions ranging from marginal to severe, with alterations in tear film stability or composition as the precipitating cause.

During the eighth century AD, Paul of Aegina suggested bathing the eye with warm water, applying egg white or goose fat, and observing healthy living conditions as a cure for dryness of the eye. Galen and his contemporaries, and later Boerhave in 1750, used elixirs of herbs boiled in wine or vinegar to ameliorate dry eye conditions.[3]

During the nineteenth century, aqueous salt solutions, glycerin, and various oils came into use. Early in this century a more balanced salt solution, Locke's solution, with gelatin added to impart viscosity, became a popular remedy.[4] The introduction of a synthetic cellulose ether, methylcellulose, by Swan[5] proved a major advance in the search for a suitable substitute for ocular secretions lubricating the eye. Over the years, other synthetic colloids have been used to enhance viscosity of artificial tear solutions. Although viscous agents enhance the ocular retention time of tear substitutes, high viscosity itself does not provide relief for all dry eye conditions.[6] Thus, other less viscous hydrophilic substances such as polyvinyl alcohol (PVA) and polyvinylpyrrolidone (PVP)

have been included as the polymeric ingredients of many artificial tear formulations.[7]

Despite advances in understanding the mechanisms involved in tear film formation and rupture, the role of tears in maintaining a normal conjunctival and corneal surface is not completely understood.[8] The availability of synthetic polymers suitable for ocular use has resulted in the development of various artificial tear solutions and other formulations to help alleviate dryness of the ocular surface.

Current strategies consist of ways to formulate products that are physiochemically more compatible with the precorneal tear film and ocular tissues, but similarities between the ancient and modern formulations remain. Water-soluble polymeric systems and bland ointment formulations remain the mainstay of therapy for dry eye conditions, but other products such as solid, water-soluble inserts (Lacrisert) and lacrimal drainage plugs may also be of value in some patients.

Tear Film Physiology

Through the Middle Ages, tears were thought to be excrements of the brain. Approximately 50 years ago Eugene Wolff[9] described in clinical terms the basic concepts governing tear film composition and structure. The tear film is usually described as a three-layered structure consisting of a superficial lipid layer, a middle aqueous layer, and a deep mucoid layer (Fig. 14.1). This relatively thin fluid film

355

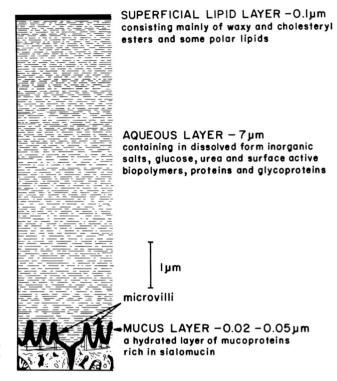

SUPERFICIAL LIPID LAYER −0.1μm consisting mainly of waxy and cholesteryl esters and some polar lipids

AQUEOUS LAYER − 7μm containing in dissolved form inorganic salts, glucose, urea and surface active biopolymers, proteins and glycoproteins

1μm

microvilli

MUCUS LAYER −0.02 −0.05μm a hydrated layer of mucoproteins rich in sialomucin

FIGURE 14.1   Structure and composition of the tear film. (Modified from Holly FJ, Lemp MA. Tear physiology and dry eyes. Surv Ophthalmol 1977;22:70.)

covering the cornea and conjunctiva is approximately 7 μm thick and is commonly referred to as the pre-corneal tear film.[10]

The lipids of the outermost layer are fluid at body temperature and consist primarily of low-polarity lipids such as waxy and cholesteryl esters. This layer, which measures approximately 0.1 to 0.2 μm in thickness, derives from the meibomian glands and covers the entire free surface of the tear fluid. The lipid layer prevents evaporation of the underlying aqueous component of the precorneal tear film, and interacts with the aqueous layer to promote tear film stability.[10,11]

The aqueous layer, supplied by the main and accessory lacrimal glands, measures 7 to 8 μm in thickness, and constitutes the thickest portion of the precorneal tear film. Dissolved in this layer are inorganic salts, glucose, urea, some trace elements, and various surface active biopolymers in the form of proteins and glycoproteins.[10–14] Lactoferrin and lysozyme are the main protein constituents in human tears. Both are considered to play important roles in defense against bacteria.[14] The presence of proteins and bicarbonate ions adds buffering capacity to the tears.[10,11] The aqueous layer also contains immunoglobulins, primarily IgA, lactate dehydrogenase, epidermal growth factor (EGF), and several inhibitors of proteolytic activity.[12–14]

The most posterior layer of the precorneal tear film consists of mucus, which coats the superficial epithelium of the cornea and conjunctiva. Conjunctival goblet cells are most likely one source of the mucoid material. The motion of blinking distributes the material over the preocular surface. A highly hydrated, semisolid layer of glycoproteins of varying molecular weight, the mucous layer may play a vital role in tear film stability through its interactions with both the epithelial surface of the cornea and conjunctiva and the overlying tears.[15,16] Mucin has at least a two-fold function in controlling tear film stability. First, it lowers the surface tension of the tear fluid and the interfacial tension of the tear-epithelium boundary by providing a layer capable of hydrogen bond formation with water. Mucin, therefore, acts as a wetting as well as a stabilizing agent for the thin precorneal tear film between blinks. Second, it plays a role in the removal of excessive lipid contaminants in the form of mucous threads and fibrils.[10,17]

Currently the clinical measurement reflecting relative stability of the tear film is tear breakup time (TBUT or BUT).[4] This test requires instillation of sodium fluorescein and measures the time elapsed between the last complete blink and the appearance of the first randomly formed dry spot on the corneal surface.[16] It is thought to reflect the functional integrity of the tear film. Chapter 25 discusses further the clinical procedure and uses of the test.

Tear Film Abnormalities

Based on our present knowledge of tear film physiology and clinical observations of dry eye states, clarification of tear film abnormalities has become possible. The various dry eye conditions may be divided into groups according to the type of abnormality responsible for the clinical symptoms.[2,10] Ocular surface disease can result from abnormalities in one or more of the tear film components, but ocular and systemic disease, various drugs, and even environmental factors can also play a significant role.[18] Clinical awareness of possible causes can aid the clinician in the diagnosis as well as selection of available dry eye products to help alleviate signs and symptoms associated with ocular surface problems (Table 14.1).

Aqueous Deficiency

Continuous production and drainage of the aqueous tear layer maintains the corneal and conjunctival epithelium in a moist state, supplies nutrients and bacteriostatic agents, and clears the ocular surface by the flushing action of tear movement.[11] Deficiencies in the aqueous tear layer can be partial or absolute. Symptoms can progress from mild foreign body sensation to constant burning or irritative sensation of such degree that the patient can find the condition debilitating.[10] Clinically this condition is most commonly referred to as KCS (see Chap. 25). Instillation of tear substitutes to enhance fluid volume of the eye remains the mainstay in the treatment of aqueous deficiencies, but occlusion of lacrimal puncta, particularly with punctal plugs, can prolong the action of natural as well as artificial tear preparations.[8]

Mucin Deficiency

Diminished secretion of soluble surfactant mucin despite sufficient aqueous volume results in an unstable tear film.[16] Mucin deficiency usually arises from a reduction of goblet cells in the conjunctiva. Conditions that alter goblet cell function affect the integrity of the mucin layer overlying the cornea, resulting in the appearance of nonwetting areas on the corneal and conjunctival surfaces.[10] A clinical sign of mucin deficient dry eye is an abnormally rapid breakup of the tear film (TBUT). In normal patients without ocular disease the TBUT usually ranges between 15 and 45 seconds. Breakup times of less than 10 seconds are considered

TABLE 14.1

Classification of Tear Film Abnormalities and the Possible Role of Lubricants and Other Dry Eye Preparations

Tear Film Abnormality	Treatment Options
Aqueous tear deficiency	Acetylcysteine
	Artificial tears
	Sodium hyaluronate
	Lacrisert
	Lacrimal plug
Mucin deficiency	Artificial tears
	Lacrisert
Lipid abnormality	Artificial tears
	Ointments
Impaired lid function	Artificial tears
	Ointments
Epitheliopathy	Artificial tears
	Ointments
	Vitamin A

Adapted from Farris RL. The dry eye: Its mechanism and therapy, with evidence that contact lens is the cause. CLAO J 1986;12:234–246.

clinically significant. Conditions that diminish goblet cell density such as hypovitaminosis A, ocular pemphigoid, Stevens-Johnson syndrome, and chemical burns all result in an unstable tear film as indicated by decreased TBUT.[10]

Lipid Abnormality

Alterations in lipid composition of tears have been associated with chronic blepharitis.[10,19] Evidence has accumulated indicating that certain microbes can secrete the enzyme lipase that hydrolyzes meibomian lipids to free fatty acids. These free fatty acids are highly surface active, spreading so rapidly as to cause instantaneous dry spot formation in the preocular tear film.[20] A characteristic of avid lipid-mucin interaction is a decrease in the rate of spreading of the tear film, resulting in a rapid TBUT. A rapid TBUT occurs in chronic blepharitis as well as in acne rosacea.[4]

Impaired Lid Function

Shear forces produced by the moving lids play a vital role in the maintenance of a normal tear film.[15,16] Compromise of normal lid-globe contact or an abnormality in the blinking process can adversely affect mucus distribution and turnover.[15] Seventh cranial nerve paresis and symblepharon formation are among the conditions that can restrict lid movement, resulting in exposure keratitis due to localized nonwetting of the corneal epithelium.[10]

Epitheliopathy

Alterations in normal epithelial morphology can affect tear film stability. Electron microscopic studies appear to indicate an intimate relationship between the microvilli of the corneal epithelium and the mucous layer[21] (see Fig. 14.1). The tear film becomes thin and retracts near areas of epithelial irregularity.[10] Dry, nonwetting areas are commonly found associated with both old and active corneal lesions producing an irregular epithelial surface. Nervous innervation may play a role in corneal epithelial integrity, and acetylcholine (ACh) and cholinesterase have been demonstrated in the corneal epithelium.[22] Thus, neurohumoral influences may play an important role in regulating epithelial turnover,[10] and this may explain, in part, the role of certain drugs and chemicals in causing dry eye syndromes.

Gilbard and associates[23,24] have also demonstrated that exposure of the ocular surface to ophthalmic solutions in general, and particularly those that raise tear osmolarity, can alter the normal cell surface and decrease both goblet cell density and corneal epithelial glycogen. Adams and associates[25] found that corneal epithelial cell viability in cultures decreased, compared to controls, when various commercially available artificial tear formulations were added to the medium. Possibly, then, the treatment of dry eye conditions may adversely affect the ocular surface and exacerbate the clinical signs or symptoms.

Composition of Tear Substitutes

Ideally the ingredients of artificial tear formulations should fulfill the physiochemical role of a normal tear film. This implies compatibility with the natural components of tears and no alteration in the clarity of the aqueous layer. An ideal tear subsitute should neither disturb corneal metabolism nor be toxic, even with frequent use.[2] Ideally, it should lower the surface tension of the tear film, aid in the formation of a hydrophilic layer that is compatible with adsorbed mucin, and enhance tear volume when necessary. In the absence of functional mucin, it should form a hydrophilic layer and mimic the functional properties of a normal mucin layer.[1,4] Preferably, the topical application of a well-formulated tear substitute and lubricating agent should provide relief for both aqueous and mucin deficient dry eyes. Moreover, functions associated with the lipid layer of the precorneal tear film should not be altered by artificial tears. In addition, minor epitheliopathies may be aided if the tear substitute also thickens the tear film.[1,4,26] Although preparations cur-

rently available for the dry eye, including solutions, ointments, artificial tear inserts and punctal plugs, help the patient with ocular surface problems, none is presently capable of replacing the normal human tear layer.

Artificial Tear Solutions

Ocular lubricants formulated as solutions are the most frequently used products for symptoms associated with dry eye. They consist of inorganic electrolytes similar to natural tears to achieve tonicity and maintain pH. Those formulated for multidose use contain preservatives to prevent growth of bacteria. To enhance their role in tear film substitution, artificial tear solutions contain various polymers that increase wettability of the hydrophobic corneal surface, extend adhesion, and increase conjunctival sac retention time.[2,27] Polymers in current use include semisynthetic cellulose derivatives, polyvinyl alcohol, dextran and polycarbophil. Viscoelastic agents, such as hyaluronic acid and chondroitin sulfate, have also been evaluated for various dry eye states.[28,29]

Table 14.2 lists representative formulations currently available.[30] They are usually administered in dosage frequencies of 3 to 4 times daily but, depending on the patient's clinical needs and response to therapy, may be administered as often as hourly or only occasionally. Since Chapter 2 discusses the role of electrolytes and preservatives in ophthalmic preparations, this chapter will emphasize the polymeric ingredients found in the various artificial tear solutions.

SUBSTITUTED CELLULOSE ETHERS

Since their introduction for ophthalmic use, methylcellulose (MC) and other substituted cellulose ethers such as hydroxyethylcellulose (HEC), hydroxypropylcellulose (HPC), hydroxypropylmethylcellulose (HPMC), and carboxymethylcellulose (CMC) have been used as artificial tear formulations.[4] These colloids dissolve in water to produce colorless solutions of varying viscosity. They have the proper optical clarity and a refractive index similar to the cornea, and they are nearly inert chemically.[5,6,31] In the past, the most frequently used representative of this group was methylcellulose.

In ocular use since 1945, methylcellulose is a synthetic, granular white substance that forms a viscous solution when added to water. It is stable in the pH range tolerated by the eye and seems unaffected by light or aging of the solution. High temperatures (100° C or above) produce coagulation, but on cooling the methylcellulose redissolves. Heat sterilization is therefore possible. Solutions containing only pure methylcellulose do not support growth of microorganisms. Methylcellulose is available in varying degrees of viscosity. For ocular use a concentration range of 0.25% to 1.0% is

TABLE 14.2
Composition of Selected Preserved Artificial Tear Preparations

Trade Name (manufacturer)	Active Ingredient	Preservative
Adsorbotear (Alcon)	HEC, povidone	Thimerosal 0.004%, EDTA 0.1%
Akwa Tears (Akorn)	PVA, NaCl	Benzalkonium chloride 0.01%, EDTA
Artificial Tears (Rugby)	PVA 1.4%	Benzalkonium chloride, EDTA
Comfort Tears (Barnes-Hind)	HEC, 0.005%	Benzalkonium chloride, 0.02% EDTA
Dakrina (Dakryon)	PVA 0.6%, povidone 5%, vitamin A palmitate 350 IU, vitamin C	Potassium sorbate 0.2%, EDTA 0.05%
Dwelle (Dakryon)	PVA, poly N-glucose	Potassium sorbate 0.05%, 0.2%, EDTA
Eye-Lube-A (Optopics)	Glycerin 0.25%	Benzalkonium chloride, EDTA
Hypotears (Ciba Vision)	PVA 1%, PEG 400, dextrose	Banzalkonium chloride 0.01%, EDTA
Isopto Alkaline (Alcon)	HPMC 1%	Benzalkonium chloride 0.01%
Isopto Tears	HPMC 0.5%	Benzalkonium chloride 0.01%
Lacril (Allergan)	HPMC gelatin A, 0.01, polysorbate 80, dextrose	Chlorobutanol 0.5%
Liquifilm Forte (Allergan)	PVA 3%	Thimerosal 0.002%, EDTA
Liquifilm Tears (Allergan)	PVA 1.4%	Chlorobutanol 0.5%
Lubri Tears (Bausch & Lomb)	HPMC 0.3%, dextran 70 0.1%	Benzalkonium chloride 0.01%, EDTA
Moisture Drops (Bausch & Lomb)	HPMC 0.5%, dextran 0.1%, glycerin 0.2%	Benzalkonium chloride 0.01%
Murine (Ross)	PVA 0.5%, povidone 0.6%	Benzalkonium chloride, EDTA
Murocel (Bausch & Lomb)	MC 1%, propylene glycol	Methylparaben 0.02%, propylparaben 0.01%
Nu-Tears (Optopics)	PVA 1%, PEG-400	Benzalkonium chloride, EDTA
Nutra Tear (Dakryon)	PVA, vitamin B_{12} 0.05%	Benzalkonium chloride 0.001%, EDTA 0.08%
Tear Gard (Medtech)	HEC	Sorbic acid, 0.25%, EDTA 0.1%
Tearisol (CibaVision)	HPMC 0.5%	Benzalkonium chloride, EDTA
Tears Naturale (Alcon)	HPMC 0.34, dextran 70 0.1%	Benzalkonium chloride 0.01%, EDTA 0.05%
Tears Naturale II (Alcon)	HPMC 0.3%, dextran 70 0.1%	Polyquaternium 0.001%, EDTA
Tears Plus (Allergan)	PVA 1.4%, povidone 0.6%	Chlorobutanol 0.5%
Tears Renewed (Akorn)	HPMC, dextran 70	Benzalkonium chloride 0.05%, EDTA
Ultra Tears (Alcon)	HPMC	Benzalkonium chloride 0.01%

HEC, hydroxyethylcellulose; HPMC, hydroxypropylmethylcellulose; MC, methylcellulose; PVA, polyvinyl alcohol; EDTA, ethylenediaminetetraacetic acid.

preferred. At concentrations above 2%, methylcellulose becomes sufficiently viscous to be classified as an ointment.[5,6]

Over the years, the other substituted cellulose ethers, particularly hydroxyethylcellulose and hydroxypropylmethylcellulose, have become frequently used. They are somewhat less viscous than methylcellulose but possess cohesive and emollient properties equal or superior to those of methylcellulose.[26] Like methylcellulose, these ethers also mix well with other polymers and substances present in artificial tear formulations and are compatible with many drugs and chemicals used on the eye.[4]

More recently, carboxymethylcellulose, a polymer with strong anionic characteristics, provided significant improvement in ocular symptoms, fluorescein staining and impression cytology grades in a randomized, double-masked, 8-week comparison study in patients with KCS.[42] The polymer was formulated as a 1% unpreserved artificial tear solution containing calcium chloride, potassium chlo-ride, sodium chloride and sodium lactate (Celluvisc). The significance of this electrolyte combination, and the presence of sodium lactate in particular, is difficult to interpret. Lack of preservative, electrolyte supplementation, and characteristics of carboxymethylcellulose such as its chemical structure and high viscosity may be responsible for the observed therapeutic effects. Studies comparing this polymer with other unpreserved artificial tear supplements are required.

In addition to their use as tear substitutes, cellulose ethers are also used to moisten contact lenses (see Chap. 18); also, as discussed in Chapter 2, they are added to ophthalmic drug formulations to prolong contact time of the active drug with the eye.[6] More viscous solutions are also used for application of gonioscopic lenses to the eye[30] (Table 14.3). The viscous properties of the colloid aid in contact of the lens with the cornea and also prevent damage to the corneal epithelium.[21] When used for this purpose, the solution is

TABLE 14.3
Lubricants Used with Gonioscopic Prisms

Trade Name (manufacturer)	Composition
Goniosol (CibaVision)	Hydroxypropylmethylcellulose
Gonak (Akorn)	2.5%, boric acid, EDTA, benzalkonium chloride 0.01%
Gonioscopic Prism Solution (Alcon)	Hydroxyethylcellulose, thimerosal 0.004%, EDTA 0.1%
Celluvisc (Allergan)	Carboxymethylcellulose 1%, (preservative-free)

EDTA, ethylenediaminetetraacetic acid.

often referred to as *goniogel*. Goniogels should be allowed to flow slowly into the bowl of the gonioscope to minimize annoying bubbles that may subsequently interfere with the diagnostic procedure. Storing goniogels inverted also reduces bubble formation (see Fig. 3.3).

Although the cellulose ethers enhance viscosity and prolong the ocular retention time of solutions, they may also exert other effects, less well understood. For example, cellulose ethers and other water-soluble polymers may adsorb at the cornea-aqueous tear layer interface, thereby stabilizing a thicker layer of fluid adjacent to the adsorbing surface.[8,26,27] The observation that these compounds can prolong TBUT supports such assumptions.[32,33] Norn[32] reported that in the presence of methylcellulose the precorneal film seemed thicker, and wetting time was prolonged by 5 to 42 seconds. Lemp and associates[34] tested the effects of commercial artificial tear solutions on TBUT. A significant increase in TBUT occurred with several of the preparations tested. However, this study used normal subjects with no clinical symptoms of tear deficiencies. Thus, the observed effects may not apply in all cases of dry eye syndromes.

The cellulose ethers are generally nonirritating and nontoxic to the ocular tissues.[35,36] Pfister and Burstein[35] observed no effects on plasma membranes following application of 0.5% methylcellulose in normal saline to rabbit eyes. Concentrations of methylcellulose present in artificial tear solutions do not appear to inhibit the healing of corneal epithelial wounds.[35]

Their relative lack of toxicity, their viscous properties, and their beneficial effects on tear film stability have made cellulose ethers useful components of artificial tear preparations.

POLYVINYL POLYMERS

Polyvinyl alcohol (PVA) is a suspending agent and emulsifier. It has been used since 1964 in topical ocular solutions to enhance ocular contact time of ophthalmic medications. It is also a wetting agent for contact lenses (see Chap. 18). Most frequently used in a 1.4% concentration, it is much less viscous than methylcellulose. A 0.5% solution of methylcellulose has a viscosity of 50 centipoise as compared to 1.4% PVA with a viscosity of 4 centipoise. It lowers the surface tension of water 46 degrees/cm as compared to 47 to 53 degrees/cm for methylcellulose. The refractive index approximates that of distilled water. Like methylcellulose, PVA is transparent and colorless in solution.[7,21,26] Solutions of PVA can be easily sterilized, since they can withstand high temperatures. They can also be autoclaved or filter sterilized through a millipore filtering system.

At the concentration used in ophthalmic preparations, PVA is nonirritating to the eye.[37] Moreover, it does not appear to interfere with normal plasma membrane integrity[35] or corneal epithelial regeneration.[7]

Like methylcellulose and hydroxypropylmethylcellulose, PVA may also enhance stability of the precorneal tear film.[7,11,37] Norn and Opauszki[38] reported that 1.4% PVA increased TBUT by a factor of 1.89. Higher concentrations of PVA further prolonged TBUT. With 3% PVA a 2.96 increase in TBUT occurred. A maximum increase in TBUT occurred with 10.0% PVA. At this concentration the TBUT was prolonged by a factor of 7.16.

Although PVA is compatible with many commonly used drugs and preservatives, certain agents can thicken or gel solutions containing PVA. These include sodium bicarbonate; sodium borate; and the sulfates of sodium, potassium, and zinc.[7] The reasons for these reactions are not well understood. The clinical use of solutions containing PVA with solutions containing any of these agents requires caution to avoid incompatibility. For example, some extraocular irrigating solutions containing sodium borate can cause such a reaction when used to irrigate from the eye contact lens wetting solutions containing PVA.

OTHER POLYMERIC SYSTEMS

Polyvinylpyrrolidone (povidone, PVP) exhibits surface active properties similar to the cellulose ethers. However, it appears to have less ability than the cellulose ethers to lower the interfacial tension at a water-oil interface.[31] Nevertheless, in contrast to the cellulose ethers, PVP appears capable of forming hydrophilic coatings in the form of adsorbed layers.[27,31] Since conjunctival mucin is thought to interact with the ocular surface to form an adsorbing surface for aqueous tears, the formation by artificial means of a hydrophilic layer, that would mimic conjunctival mucin (mucomimetic) seems clinically desirable. Since the wetting ability of the corneal surface would be enhanced, both mucin- and aqueous-deficient dry eyes would benefit.[27,39]

More recently, polycarbophil, an insoluble polymer present in the artificial tear preparation, Aquasite, has demonstrated a longer ocular retention time in the tear film than formulations containing PVA or carboxymethylcellulose.[40] In addition, this formulation has been reported to improve objective abnormalities in impression cytology in patients with dry eye syndrome.[41]

As previously mentioned, of commercial artificial tear formulations can prolong TBUT in humans.[34,39] Lemp and Hamill[39] evaluated the effect of 12 artificial tear preparations on TBUT in normal subjects. Significant prolongation of TBUT occurred with Adapt, Adapette, Adsorbotear, and Tears Naturale. Certain preparations in current use, such as Neo-Tears and Hypotears, were not tested. Geeting and Bakar[33] evaluated four artificial tear solutions (Hypotears, Liquifilm Tears, Neo-Tears, Tears Naturale) in 8 patients having an initial TBUT of not more than 8 seconds. All four preparations prolonged TBUT for approximately 60 to 90 minutes. The greatest mean increase in TBUT occurred with Neo-Tears, which also had the longest duration of action, prolonging TBUT for nearly two hours.

Other parameters of surface chemistry that have been evaluated–surface tension, interfacial tension at the water-oil interface, contact angle of solutions on clean cornea or polymethylmethacrylate (PMMA)—show similarities among cellulose ethers, PVA, and the polymeric systems.[31,38] Surface tension measurements indicate that all are less surface active than mucin.[15,31] Moreover, with artificial tear preparations exhibiting surface activity, their action resulted from the presence of other ingredients, particularly the preservative benzalkonium chloride.[27] These observations indicate that subtle interactions may occur between the various ingredients present in artificial tear formulations. The effects could further extend to interactions among synthetic polymers, preservatives, tear film constituents, and the epithelial surface.[25,42,43] Questions remaining are numerous and can be answered only as better and less ambiguous testing procedures, both *in vitro* and *in vivo*, are developed. Clinical results as well as patient acceptance remain the final criteria of *in vivo* efficacy of specific artificial tear solutions. No single formulation has yet been identified that universally provides improvement in clinical signs and symptoms while allowing patient comfort and acceptance.

Vitamin A Derivatives

Vitamin A deficiency can affect a variety of epithelial-lined organs, including the eye. Epidermal keratinization and squamous metaplasia of the mucus membranes, including the cornea and conjunctiva, respond to both oral and topical vitamin A therapy.[44] Recent evidence suggests that retinol is secreted by the lacrimal gland and is metabolized in the cornea to retinoic acid.[45] Topical use of tretinoin (all-trans retinoic acid), retinol, the alcohol form of vitamin A, and a synthetic retinoic acid analog have been advocated for treatment of various dry eye disorders.[46–51]

Tseng and associates[46,47] evaluated in a noncontrolled fashion the clinical efficacy of tretinoin ointment in various dry eye disorders including KCS, Stevens-Johnson syndrome, pemphigoid, and surgery- or radiation-induced dry eye. Depending on the severity of the condition, doses of 0.01% or 0.1% were applied to affected eyes 1 to 3 times daily for two months. Patients continued to use their previous medications as prescribed. All patients in this study showed clinical improvement in symptoms, including visual acuity, rose bengal staining, and Schirmer testing. Impression cytology performed before and after treatment indicated that vitamin A reversed the squamous metaplastic changes of the surface epithelium observed before treatment. Use of artificial tears and lubricants could be reduced or discontinued. The therapeutic efficacy observed in these patients has been attributed to the restoration of cellular differentiation, with goblet cell regeneration and enhanced mucin production, which normalize the interactions between epithelial cell surface and tear film.[49,51]

Soong and associates[52] evaluated in a controlled study the efficacy and safety of topical tretinoin ointment 0.01% and found it ineffective in improving symptoms and clinical signs in patients with noncicatricial dry eyes. The drug, however, was able to reverse conjunctival keratinization in patients with conjunctival cicatricial diseases, although clinical symptoms and signs showed no significant improvement with tretinoin therapy compared with placebo. The presence of squamous metaplasia thus appears to be a requirement for potentially treatable cases.[49,52]

Others, however, have found vitamin A ointment of no benefit in KCS. In an open-label crossover study, Gilbard and associates[53] reported vitamin A ointment to be no more effective than placebo in patients with KCS.

Other studies using vitamin A (retinol) in solution with polysorbate 80 (ViVA-Drops) have reported improvement in patients with various dry eye disorders.[54] Both subjective and objective improvement was associated with topical application 2 to 3 times daily in patients with complaints of "dry, irritated or burning eyes." Patients with giant papillary conjunctivitis related to contact lens wear reported subjective improvement in symptoms.[55]

Side effects associated with use of topical tretinoin ointment include transient hyperemia, irritation, or burning. Ocular pharmacokinetic studies in rabbits show low levels of drug in the aqueous humor, approximately 1/1000 that of tears, following topical application of [³H]-tretinoin. Major tissue uptake occurs in the surface epithelium and the iris.[50]

Other vitamins, including B$_{12}$ and C, have also been included in various artificial tear formulations (see Table 14.2). Controlled clinical studies are presently lacking regarding the clinical efficacy of these products in patients with ocular surface disease.

Viscoelastic Agents

SODIUM HYALURONATE

A polysaccharide polymer (glycosaminoglycan), hyaluronate is a structural component of vertebrate connective tissue matrices. It is also present in the vitreous and aqueous humor of the eye. At physiologic pH, it is a viscoelastic solution, with a viscosity over 500,000 times that of physiologic saline. Sodium hyaluronate has been used with success in intraocular surgical procedures such as cataract extraction, intraocular lens implantation, corneal transplantation, glaucoma filtration, and procedures to repair retinal detachment.[56]

Polack and McNiece[57] first studied the effects of a 0.5% solution in patients with severe dry eye syndromes. They observed a decrease in pain shortly following instillation, improved vision, and reduced redness within the first week of treatment in patients for whom conventional artificial tear preparations had failed. Since then other investigators have reported similar results in clinical trials with a 0.1% concentration.[58–62] A variety of dry eye syndromes, including KCS, show subjective as well as objective improvement including decreased itching and burning, reduced foreign body sensation, and reduction of mucus strands.

Rose bengal staining of cornea and conjunctiva decreases, and corneal luster appears to increase. Tear film stability may improve[58,60,63] The beneficial effects of sodium hyaluronate follow from to its viscoelastic properties, which lubricate as well as protect the ocular surface.[59] Most patients achieve control of symptoms with topical instillation up to four times daily. Subjective relief of symptoms such as burning and "grittiness" is usually immediate following drug instillation, and these effects can last up to 60 minutes or longer.[58,62]

Sodium hyaluronate is synthesized from rooster coombs and is commercially available as Amvisc or Healon. It is supplied in a disposable glass syringe as a sterile preparation of sodium hyaluronate dissolved in physiologic sodium chloride-phosphate buffered solution with a pH range of 7.0 to 7.5. When prepared as a 0.1% saline solution (Healon tears) it must be vigorously shaken before use. Current limitations to its use as an artificial tear are the absence of a commercial preparation for the dry eye, and its cost, which makes it considerably more expensive than other dry eye preparations for long-term use.

Sodium hyaluronate appears free of adverse ocular or systemic effects when used topically on the eye at the 0.1% concentration. It is nonantigenic and does not cause inflammatory or foreign body reactions.[61]

CHONDROITIN SULFATE

A polysaccharide of D-glucuronic acid and N-acetylgalactosamine, chondroitin sulfate is 350,000 times as viscous as saline. Limberg and associates[64] compared solutions of hyaluronic acid 0.1%, chrondoitin sulfate 1%, and a mixture of chondroitin sulfate 0.38% and hyaluronic acid 0.3% with an artificial tear solution containing PVA and polyethylene glycol. All solutions were instilled at 2-hour intervals for two weeks. All four solutions appeared equally effective in alleviating symptoms of itching, burning, and foreign body sensation in patients with KCS. However, patients with low Schirmer test scores uniformly preferred a solution containing chondroitin sulfate. Since only 20 patients took part in this study, it may be premature to conclude that patients with severe dry eyes derive greater benefit from frequent instillation of chrondroitin sulfate compared with other viscous agents present in artificial tear products.

Chondroitin sulfate is commercially available as Viscoat, a mixture of sodium chondroitin sulfate 40 mg/ml and sodium hyaluronate 30 mg/ml.[30]

Mucolytic Agents

ACETYLCYSTEINE

An N-acetyl derivative of the naturally occurring amino acid L-cysteine, acetylcysteine has been clinically useful as a mucolytic agent in acute and chronic bronchopulmonary conditions. It is believed to exert its action by opening up disulfide linkages in mucus, thereby lowering the viscosity of mucus.[65]

Available as Mucomyst in a 10% or 20% solution as the sodium salt of acetylcysteine, it is usually administered by nebulization for its local effect on the bronchopulmonary tree. Since the product also contains disodium edetate and sodium hydroxide, a slight odor can accompany its administration.[30]

Absolon and Brown[66] compared the effects of an artificial tear solution with a 20% solution of acetylcysteine in a double-masked study in patients with KCS. They observed a greater objective improvement in signs such as conjunctival and corneal staining, mucus threads and filaments by slit-lamp examination in patients using the acetylcysteine solution. However, no subjective differences occurred between the two groups. Acetylcysteine solutions produce a stinging sensation on instillation, which may in part explain the subjective results.[66,67]

When used on the eye, Mucomyst can dissolve mucus threads as well as decrease tear viscosity.[66] A commercial artificial tear preparation containing acetylcysteine is presently not available, but it can be prepared for topical ocular use by diluting the commercial preparation to 2% to 5% in artificial tears or physiologic saline.

Non-Preserved Tear Preparations

A recent advance in artificial tear preparations is the introduction of preservative-free formulations. Of primary con-

TABLE 14.4
Non-Preserved Artificial Tear Preparations

Trade Name (manufacturer)	Active Ingredients
AquaSite (Ciba Vision)	Polycarbophil, PEG-400, dextran 70, EDTA
Bion Tears (Alcon)	HPMC 0.3%, dextran 70 0.1%
Celluvisc (Allergan)	CMC 1%, lactate
Dry Eye Therapy (Bausch & Lomb)	Glycerin 0.3%
HypoTears PF (CibaVision)	PVA 1%, PEG-400, EDTA
Lacrisert (Merck)	HPC 5 mg
OcuCoat PF (Storz)	HPMC 0.8%, dextran 70 0.1%
Refresh (Allergan)	PVA 1.4%, povidone 0.6%
Refresh Plus (Allergan)	CMC 0.5%, lactate
Tears Naturale Free (Alcon)	HPMC 0.3%, dextran 0.1%
Viva Drops (Vision Pharm)	Polysorbate 80, retinyl palmitate, mannitol, sodium citrate, pyruvate

EDTA, ethylenediaminetetraacetic acid; HPMC, hydroxypropylmethylcellulose; CMC, carboxymethylcellulose; PVA, polyvinyl alcohol; HPC, hydroxypropyl cellulose.

TABLE 14.5
Preservative-Free Ointments

Trade Name (manufacturer)	Composition
Akwa Tears (Akorn)	White petrolatum, mineral oil, lanolin
Duolube (Bausch & Lomb)	White petrolatum, mineral oil
DuraTears Naturale (Alcon)	White petrolatum, anhydrous liquid lanolin, mineral oil
HypoTears (CibaVision)	White petrolatum, light mineral oil
Lacri-Lube NP (Allergan)	White petrolatum, mineral oil, petrolatum/lanolin alcohol
Ocu-Lube (Bausch & Lomb)	White petrolatum, mineral oil
Refresh PM (Allergan)	White petrolatum, sodium chloride, mineral oil, petrolatum/lanolin alcohol

Tips of ointment tubes should not come in contact with the eyes during instillation.

Ointment Formulations

Another approach for lubrication and stabilization of the precorneal tear film is the use of nonmedicated, semisolid preparations of petrolatum and mineral oil to which lanolin may be added (see Table 14.5). Although these preparations melt at the temperature of the ocular tissue and disperse with the tear fluid, they appear to be retained longer than other ophthalmic vehicles.[71,72]

Several explanations have been offered as to why the tear fluid retains ointments longer. Because of their molecular size, petrolatum and mineral oil are not as easily removed by the lacrimal drainage system by blinking. Another significant factor appears to be the physiochemical relationship between the components of the ointment and the cornea. The precorneal tear film and the ointment bases both have nonpolar components, allowing the adsorption of the oil bases to the cornea.[73]

Patient acceptance of ointment preparations is highly variable. Blurred vision is a frequent complaint following the daytime instillation of ointment. This problem can usually be resolved by decreasing the amount instilled or using it only at bedtime.[74] Ointment preparations are generally nonirritating to ocular tissue. In addition, ointment vehicles presently used do not appear to interfere with corneal or conjunctival wound healing. Ointment use, however, should be avoided in eyes with impending corneal perforations, deep or flap-like corneal abrasions, or severe corneal lacerations because of the possibility of ointment entrapment.[74]

cern with frequent or prolonged use of tear substitutes is the potential for epithelial toxicity and disruption of tear film stability, particularly by preservatives present in the formulation.[42,43,68,69] Using computerized subjective fluorophotometry, Gobbels and Spitznas[69] compared the effect of artificial tears containing 2% PVP with and without the preservative benzalkonium chloride in dry-eye patients. They demonstrated that the epithelial permeability decreased significantly in patients treated with unpreserved tears, whereas patients treated with preserved tears showed an increase in permeability. Other studies[25,42] have also compared the effects of preserved and unpreserved artificial tears on symptoms and signs in dry eyes. These observations indicate that patients using unpreserved artificial tear products can achieve both subjective and clinical improvement, including a reversal in squamous metaplasia in patients with KCS.

Another clinical use for the more viscous preservative-free artificial tear products is the application of gonioscopic lenses to the eye.[70] Celluvisc, a formulation of 1% carboxymethylcellulose, has sufficient viscosity to allow contact of the lens with the corneal surface without damage to the epithelium. This and other unpreserved formulations are available as unit-dose packages of artificial tear solutions (Table 14.4) or as preservative-free ointments (Table 14.5).

The clinical disadvantages of these formulations is that the unit-dose preparations usually cost more, and they can easily become contaminated by the patient during use. Strict hygienic procedures for instillation must be followed, and any excess solution must be discarded after 12 hours of use.

Since ointments do not mix readily with the tear film, they can reduce tear breakup time and are not generally recommended for daytime use in patients with aqueous-deficient dry eyes.[75]

Artificial Tear Inserts

Another approach to the treatment of moderate to severe dry eye syndromes is the use of water-soluble inserts that provide a constant release of polymer.[75-77] When placed in the inferior cul-de-sac, the insert dissolves over a period of hours while releasing its polymeric contents.

The artificial tear insert (Lacrisert) is a cylindrical rod approximately 1 mm wide and 4 mm long containing 5 mg of hydroxypropylcellulose without preservative. When placed in the inferior cul-de-sac it imbibes fluid and swells to several times its original volume (Fig. 14.2). Following the initial swelling, the insert dissolves over 6 to 8 hours.[78] It is designed to be replaced every 24 hours, although some patients require more frequent replacement.[78]

Measurement of the TBUT in human subjects indicates that the insert prolongs breakup time. The effect lasts longer than with tear substitutes applied as drops.[79] The insert produces a tear film that is clinically thicker than normal and that appears to retain fluid within it.[80,81]

Clinical studies indicate that the insert can be beneficial in the treatment of certain dry eye syndromes such as KCS. Some patients may experience relief of symptoms of burning, photophobia, and foreign body sensation. Corneal abnormalities may also decrease, and rose bengal staining of cornea and conjunctiva may decrease.[81,82]

The device is generally comfortable and well accepted by many patients, but its use does have some disadvantages. Placing the insert properly into the lower cul-de-sac requires a moderate amount of dexterity. The most common patient complaint is blurred vision associated with the intense release of polymer after the first 4 to 6 hours following instillation, resulting in a thickened tear film.[81] Adding fluid such as drops of 0.9% NaCl or artificial tear solution can reduce the tear film viscosity and minimize the visual complaints. As the insert dissolves, it releases debris that can also blur vision and cause irritation. Most patients with only mild signs and symptoms of dry eye do not appreciate improvement with use of the insert compared with use of conventional artificial tear solutions. In fact, complaints of blurred vision and foreign body sensation often limit usefulness of the insert. In addition, absence of measurable tear secretion, as detected by a very low Schirmer test, seems to predict treatment failure with artificial tear inserts.[82]

Lacrimal Occlusive Devices

Occlusion of the lacrimal drainage system has been used to preserve existing tears since Beetham[83] first advocated electrocautery of the canaliculi in 1936. Since cautery may be an irreversible procedure, plugs have been developed to block tear drainage and thus prolong the action of natural tears as well as artificial tear preparations.

Two general types of plugs are in current use. The temporary, water-soluble collagen rods include the Collagen Implant (Lacrimedics) and Temporary Intracannalicular Collagen Implant (Eagle Vision). These plugs are 2 mm long, of varying diameters, and dissolve within 4 to 7 days following insertion into the puncta. Two silicone-based plugs, the Freeman Punctum Plug (Eagle Vision) and the Herrick Lacrimal Plug (Lacrimedics), are more permanent but can be removed when necessary.[84,85]

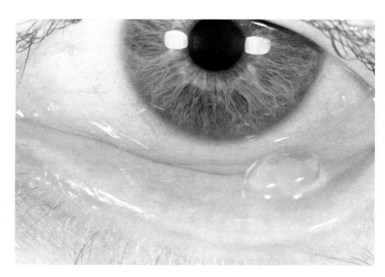

FIGURE 14.2   **Artificial tear insert (Lacrisert). Following placement of insert into the inferior conjunctival sac with specially designed applicator (see Fig. 3.24), the insert swells to several times its original volume and begins to release the nonmedicated polymer to the eye.**

The silicone plugs are usually inserted directly into both inferior puncta. The procedure may require topical anesthesia and dilation of the punctal opening. In some cases insertion can be difficult, and the Freeman plug can be expelled, especially if the patient rubs the eyelid.

The temporary collagen implants range from 0.2 to 0.6 mm in diameter and are packed on the edge of a foam strip (see Fig. 25.12). The implant is grasped from the package with a jeweler's forcep and, with the aid of magnification, is placed halfway into the punctal opening. It is then nudged until flush with the punctum and then further advanced into the horizontal canaliculus. Topical anesthetics may be used to minimize eyelid reaction, but the procedure can be performed without anesthesia. The aqueous environment of the canaliculus causes the collagen implant to swell, impeding tear flow by as much as 60% to 80%. Tear drainage can be blocked for up to 14 days before the implants are totally absorbed.[84–88]

Lacrimal occlusion can benefit patients who have symptoms of dryness or other ocular abnormalities that topical therapy alone does not resolve.[86,88] The procedures are indicated in moderately severe to severe dry eye patients to prevent drainage and thereby conserve natural tears as well as instilled tear substitutes.[89] Although rare, punctal occlusion can lead to epiphora. Tearing secondary to chronic dacryocystitis with mucopurulent discharge is a contraindication to the use of lacrimal plugs. Chapter 25 considers in further detail the use of lacrimal occlusion in dry eye syndromes.

Future Perspectives in Dry Eye Therapy

Based on knowledge gained from the physiology, pathophysiology and diagnosis of dry eye, Lemp[90] has reviewed possible future strategies in treatment of ocular surface disease. Currently in development are artificial tear solutions with unique electrolytes, viscous agents and components that retard surface evaporation and treat the ocular surface directly to manage diseased epithelium. Pharmacologic stimulation of the lacrimal gland to increase tear secretion is also being investigated. Both bromhexine and eledoisin have been used orally in Europe for severe forms of KCS, with varying success.[1] Other possibilities include immunologic modulation with immunosuppressive agents such as cyclosporine (Sandimmune), use of hormonal agents such as the estrogens, and development of substances that will influence meibomian gland or goblet cell secretions.

References

1. Marquardt R. Therapy of the dry eye. In: Lemp MA, Marquardt R, eds. The dry eye. Berlin: Springer-Verlag, 1992; Chap. 6.

2. Holly FJ. Tear film physiology. Int Ophthalmol Clin 1987;27:2–6.

3. Boerhave H. De morbis oculum. Gottingen, 1750.

4. Holly FJ. Artificial tear formulations. Int Ophthalmol Clin 1980; 20:171–184.

5. Swan KC. Use of methylcellulose in ophthalmology. Arch Ophthalmol 1945;33:378–380.

6. Blaug SM, Canada AT. Relationship of viscosity, contact time, and prolongation of action of methyl-cellulose-containing ophthalmic solutions. Am J Hosp Pharm 1965;22:662–666.

7. Krishna N, Brow F. Polyvinyl alcohol as an ophthalmic vehicle: Effect on regeneration of corneal epithelium. Am J Ophthalmol 1964;57:99–106.

8. Lemp MA. Recent developments in dry eye management. Surv Ophthalmol 1987;94:1299–1304.

9. Wolff E. The muco-cutaneous junction of the lid-margin and the distribution of the tear fluid. Trans Ophthalmol Soc UK 1946; 66:291–308.

10. Holly FJ, Lemp MA. Tear physiology and dry eyes. Surv Ophthalmol 1977;22:69–87.

11. Mishima S. Some physiological aspects of the precorneal tear film. Arch Ophthalmol 1965;73:233–241.

12. MacKay C, Abramson DH, Ellsworth RM, et al. Lactate dehydrogenase in tears. Am J Ophthalmol 1980;90:385–387.

13. Anderson JA, Leopold IH. Antiproteolytic activities found in human tears. Ophthalmology 1981;88:82–84.

14. Smolin G. The role of tears in the prevention of infections. Int Ophthalmol Clin 1987;27:25–26.

15. Holly FJ, Patten JT, Dohlman CH. Surface activity of aqueous tear components in dry eye patients and normals. Exp Eye Res 1977; 24:479–491.

16. Holly FJ. Formation and rupture of the tear film. Exp Eye Res 1973; 15:515–525.

17. Adams AD. The morphology of human conjunctival mucus. Arch Ophthalmol 1979;97:730–736.

18. Farris RL. The dry eye: Its mechanism and therapy, with evidence that contact lens is the cause. CLAO J 1986;12:234–246.

19. McCulley JP, Sciallis GF. Meibomian keratoconjunctivitis. CLAO J 1983;9:130–132.

20. McDonald JE. Surface phenomena of tear films. Trans Am Ophthalmol Soc 1968;66:905–939.

21. Pfister RR. The normal surface of the corneal epithelium. A scanning electron microscopic study. Invest Ophthalmol Vis Sci 1973; 12:654–668.

22. Van Alphen GWHM. Acetylcholine synthesis in corneal epithelium. Arch Ophthalmol 1957;58:449–451.

23. Gilbard JP, Carter JB, Sang DN, et al. Morphologic effect of hyperosmolarity on rabbit corneal epithelium. Ophthalmology 1985;92:717–727.

24. Gilbard JP, Rossi SR, Heyda KG. Ophthalmic solutions, the ocular surface and a unique therapeutic artificial tear formulation. Am J Ophthalmol 1989;107:348–355.

25. Adams J, Wilcox MJ, Trousdale, MD, et al. Morphologic and physiologic effect of artificial tear formulations on the corneal epithelial derived cells. Cornea 1992;11:234–241.

26. Benedetto DA, Shah DO, Kaufman HE. The instilled fluid dynamics and surface chemistry of polymers in the preocular tear film. Invest Ophthalmol Vis Sci 1975;14:887–902.

27. Lemp MA, Szymanski ES. Polymer adsorption at the ocular surface. Arch Ophthalmol 1975;93:134–136.

28. Hammer ME, Burch TG. Viscous corneal protection by sodium

hyaluronate, chondroitin sulfate and methylcellulose. Invest Ophthalmol Vis Sci 1984;25:1329–1334.

29. Nelson JD, Farris RL. Sodium hyaluronate and polyvinyl alcohol artificial tear preparations. Arch Ophthalmol 1988;106:484–487.

30. Bartlett JD, Ghormley NR, Jaanus SD, et al., eds. Ophthalmic drug facts. St. Louis: Facts and Comparisons, 1995.

31. Lemp MA, Holly FJ. Ophthalmic polymers as ocular wetting agents. Ann Ophthalmol 1972;4:15–20.

32. Norn MS. Desiccation of the precorneal film. I. Corneal wetting time. Acta Ophthalmol 1969;47:865–880.

33. Geeting DG, Baker SR. In vivo comparison of ocular lubricants in patients having reduced tear film break-up times. J Am Optom Assoc 1980;8:757–780.

34. Lemp MA, Goldberg M, Roddy MR. Effect of tear substitutes on tear film breakup time. Invest Ophthalmol 1975;14:225–258.

35. Pfister RR, Burstein N. The effects of ophthalmic drugs, vehicles, and preservatives on corneal epithelium. A scanning electron microscope study. Invest Ophthalmol 1976;15:246–259.

36. Bigar F, Gloor B, Schimmelpfennig B, et al. Die vertraglichkeit von hydroxypropylmethylcellulose bei der implantation von hinterkammer linsen. Klin Monatsbl Augenheilk 1988;193:21–24.

37. Krishna N, Mitchell B. Polyvinyl alcohol as an ophthalmic vehicle: Effect on ocular structures. Am J Ophthalmol 1965;59:860–864.

38. Norn MS, Opauszki A. Effects of ophthalmic vehicles on the stability of the precorneal film. Acta Ophthalmol 1977;55:23–34.

39. Lemp MA, Hamill JR. Factors affecting tear film breakup in normal eyes. Arch Ophthalmol 1973;89:103–105.

40. Bowman LM, Abelson MB, Doane MG, et al. An evaluation of the retention time of artificial tear treatments in dry eye patients using tear film interferometry. Invest Ophthalmol Vis Sci 1993;34(suppl): 1472.

41. Tauber J, Crosser VA, Mardelli PG. Improvement in squamous metaplasia following Aquasite treatment in patients with dry eye syndrome and in normal volunteers. Invest Ophthalmol Vis Sci 1993;34(suppl):1472.

42. Grene RB, Lankston P, Mordaunt J, et al. Unpreserved carboxymethylcellulose artificial tears evaluated in patients with keratoconjunctivitis sicca. Cornea 1992;11:294–301.

43. Bernal DL, Ubels JL. Artificial tear composition and promotion of recovery of the damaged corneal epithelium. Cornea 1993;12:115–120.

44. Sommer A. Treatment of corneal xerophthalmia with topical retinoic acid. Am J Ophthalmol 1983;95:349–352.

45. Ubels JI, Foley KM, Rismondo V. Retinol secretion by the lacrimal gland. Invest Ophthalmol Vis Sci 1986;27:1261–1262.

46. Tseng SCG, Maumenee AE, Stark WS, Maumenee IH, et al. Topical retinoid treatment of various dry-eye disorders. Ophthalmology 1985;92:717–727.

47. Tseng SCG. Topical retinoid treatment for dry eye disorders. Trans Ophthalmol Soc UK 1985;104:489–495.

48. Wright P. Topical retinoic acid therapy for disorders of the outer eye. Trans Ophthalmol Soc UK 1985;104:869–874.

49. Tseng SCG. Topical tretinoin treatment for dry-eye disorders. Int Ophthalmol Clin 1987;27:47–53.

50. Vidaurri LJ, Huang ASW, Tseng SCG. Pharmacokinetics of topical tretinoin in normal rabbit eyes. Invest Ophthalmol Vis Sci 1986; 27:24.

51. Driot JY, Bonne C. Beneficial effect of a retinoic acid analog, CBS-211A on an experimental model of keratoconjunctivitis sicca. Invest Ophthalmol Vis Sci 1992;33:190–195.

52. Soong HK, Martin NF, Wagoner MD, et al. Topical retinoid therapy for squamous metaplasia of various ocular surface disorders. A multicenter, placebo-controlled, double-masked study. Ophthalmology 1988;95:1442–1446.

53. Gilbard JB, Huang AJ, Belldegreen R, et al. Open-label crossover study of vitamin A ointment as a treatment for keratoconjunctivitis sicca. Ophthalmology 1989;96:844–848.

54. Westerhout DI. Treatment of dry eyes with aqueous antioxidant eye drops. CLJ 1991;19:165–173.

55. Butts BL, Rengstorff RH. Antioxidant and vitamin A eyedrops for giant papillary conjunctivitis. CLJ 1990;18:40–43.

56. Miller D, Stegman R. Healon: A comprehensive guide to its use. In: Ophthalmic surgery, New York: John Wiley & Sons, 1983.

57. Polack RM, McNiece MT. The treatment of dry eyes with Na hyaluronate (Healon). Cornea 1982;1:133–136.

58. DeLuise VP, Peterson WS. The use of topical Healon tears in the management of refractory dry-eye syndrome. Ann Ophthalmol 1984;16:823–824.

59. Stuart JC, Linn JG, Dilute sodium hyaluronate (Healon) in the treatment of ocular surface disorders. Ann Ophthalmol 1985; 17:190–192.

60. Mengher LS, Pandher KS, Bron AJ, et al. Effect of sodium hyaluronate (0.1%) on break-up time (NIBUT) in patients with dry eyes. Br J Ophthalmol 1986;70:442–447.

61. Richter W, Ryde M, Zetterstrom O. Nonimmunogenicity of a purified sodium hyaluronate preparation in man. Int Arch Appl Immunol 1979;59:45–48.

62. Sand BB, Marner K, Norn MS. Sodium hyaluronate in the treatment of keratoconjunctivitis sicca: a double-masked clinical trial. Acta Ophthalmol 1989;67:181–183.

63. Snibson A, Greaves JL, Soper NDW, et al. Ocular surface residence times of artificial tear solutions. Cornea 1992;11:288–293.

64. Limberg MB, McCaa C, Kissling GE, et al. Topical application of hyaluronic acid and chondroitin sulfate in treatment of dry eyes. Am J Ophthalmol 1987;103:194–197.

65. Webb WR. Clinical evaluation of a new mucolytic agent acetylcysteine. J Thorac Cardiovasc Surg 1962;44:330–335.

66. Absolon MJ, Brown CA. Acetylcysteine in keratoconjunctivitis sicca. Br J Ophthalmol 1968;52:310–316.

67. Messner K, Leibowitz HM. Acetylcysteine therapy of keratitis sicca. Arch Ophthalmol 1971;86:357–359.

68. Laflamme MY, Swieca R. A comparative study of two preservative-free tear substitutes in the management of severe dry eye. Can J Ophthalmol 1988;23:174–177.

69. Gobbels M, Spitznas M. Corneal epithelial permeability of dry eyes before and after treatment with artificial tears. Ophthalmology 1992;99:873–878.

70. Moffett DG. A new lubricant (carboxymethylcellulose) for contact lens examination. Arch Ophthalmol 1991;109:173.

71. Norn MS. Role of vehicles in local treatment of the eye. Acta Ophthalmol 1964;42:727–734.

72. Hardberger R, Hanna C, Boyd CM. Effect of drug vehicles on ocular contact time. Arch Ophthalmol 1975;93:42–45.

73. Stenbeck A, Ostholm I. Ointments for ophthalmic use. Acta Ophthalmol 1954;43:405–423.

74. Hanna C, Fraunfelder FT, Cable M, Hardberger RE. Effect of ophthalmic ointments on corneal wound healing. Am J Ophthalmol 1973;76:193–200.

75. Bloomfield SE, Dunn MW, Miyata T, et al. Soluble artificial tear inserts. Arch Ophthalmol 1977;95:247–250.

76. Beslin CW, Katz J, Kaufman HE, Katz I. Slow release artificial tears. In: Leopold IH, Burns RP, eds. Symposium on ocular therapy. New York: John Wiley & Sons, 1977;10:77–83.

77. Katz MK, Blackman WM. A soluble sustained-release ophthalmic delivery unit. Am J Ophthalmol 1977;83:728–734.

78. Lamberts DW, Langston DP, Chu W. A clinical study of slow-releasing artificial tears. Ophthalmology 1978;85:794–800.

79. Gautheron PD, Lotti YJ, Le Douraree JC. Tear film breakup time prolonged with unmedicated cellulose polymer inserts. Arch Ophthalmol 1979;97:1944–1947.

80. Katz JI, Kaufman HE, Breslin C, Katz IM. Slow-release artificial tears and the treatment of keratitis sicca. Ophthalmology 1978; 85:778–793.

81. Werblin TP, Rheinstrom SD, Kaufman HE. The use of slow-release artificial tears in the long-term management of keratitis sicca. Ophthalmology 1981;88:78–81.

82. Lindahl G, Calissendorff B, Carle B. Clinical trial of sustained-release artificial tears in kerataconjunctivitis sicca and Sjogren's syndrome. Acta Ophthalmol 1988;66;9–14.

83. Beetham WP. Filamentary keratitis. Trans Am Ophthalmol Soc 1936;33:413–435.

84. Freeman JM. Punctal plug: Evaluation of a new treatment for dry eyes. Trans Am Acad Ophthalmol Otolaryngol 1975;79:874–879.

85. Herrick RS. Collagen implants said to help Dx of keratoconjunctivitis sicca. Ophthalmol Times 1985;10:3.

86. Dohlman CH. Punctal occlusion in keratoconjunctivitis sicca. Ophthalmology 1978;85:1277–1281.

87. Tuberville AW, Frederick WR, Wood TO. Punctal occlusion in tear deficiency syndromes. Ophthalmology 1982;89:1170–1172.

88. Willis RM, Folberg R, Krachmer JH, Holland EJ. The treatment of aqueous-deficient dry eye with removable punctal plugs. Ophthalmology 1987;94:514–518.

89. American Academy of Ophthalmology: Punctal occlusion for the dry eye (Information Statement). Ophthalmology 1992;99:639–640.

90. Lemp MA. Tear film, pharmacology of eye drops, and toxicity. Curr Opinion Ophthalmol 1993;4:14–19.

CHAPTER 15

Anti-Edema Drugs

Siret D. Jaanus

Osmotherapy was first introduced into ocular therapeutics in 1904 with the use of oral hypertonic saline to reduce elevated intraocular pressure.[1] Since then, several other agents have proven clinically useful when administered systemically or applied topically to the eye. Topical ocular application of hyperosmotic agents can prove valuable in the treatment of corneal edema, particularly when caused by endothelial dysfunction.

This chapter considers agents currently available for topical ocular osmotherapy.

Corneal Hydration

The cornea, a five-layered avascular structure, is bathed on its anterior surface by the tear film and on its posterior surface by the aqueous humor. Under normal physiologic conditions, the cornea is approximately 78% hydrated. The relatively high hydration may result from the water-holding capacity of the proteoglycans that fill the spaces between the collagen fibrils.[2] When excess fluid gains access to the stroma, the ability of the proteoglycans to expand may cause corneal edema. Among the factors controlling corneal hydration are the barrier functions of the epithelium and endothelium, the swelling pressure of the stroma, and the endothelial water-pumping mechanism. Intraocular pressure and fluid evaporation from the corneal surface appear to be of lesser importance[2] (Fig. 15.1).

The endothelium plays a key role in maintaining normal corneal deturgescence, since it bars fluid movement into the cornea from the anterior chamber. It also provides an active transport system for the flow of water from the stroma to the aqueous.[3] When the cornea is exposed to certain drugs, such as ouabain, that affect this transport mechanism, the cornea takes up water and swells.[4]

Intraocular pressures within the normal limits exert minimal influence on corneal thickness. However, with a sudden elevation of intraocular pressure, the stroma becomes compressed and water moves toward the epithelium. The relatively high resistance of the epithelium to water flow, compared with that of stroma and of endothelium, causes retention of water, resulting in epithelial edema.[3]

In addition to intraocular pressure effects, the eyelids and tear film influence epithelial hydration. Changes in corneal thickness occur with the eyelids open and closed.[4] The tear film contributes to the optical surface of the cornea by interaction with the epithelial microvilli. It also influences the state of corneal hydration: when the lids are open, the tear film becomes hypertonic, and the resultant osmotic gradient allows the outward flow of water from the cornea across the epithelium.[5]

Causes of Corneal Edema

A variety of clinical situations can give rise to corneal edema[6,7] (Table 15.1). Since the endothelium is the main structure involved in maintaining normal corneal deturgescence, it must play a role in stromal hydration and compensate for the driving force of intraocular pressure. Also, the active transport system involved in the movement of water and electrolytes from the cornea to aqueous must be maintained to prevent fluid retention. Endothelial failure, a frequent cause of corneal edema, can occur due to defects in the transport system or stromal compression resulting from elevation of intraocular pressure. This can result in water movement toward the epithelium.[3,6]

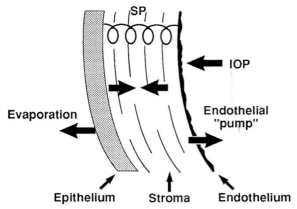

FIGURE 15.1 **Factors affecting corneal hydration. The stromal swelling pressure (SP) is balanced by epithelial and endothelial barriers and the endothelial pumping mechanism. Evaporation and intraocular pressure (IOP) play minor roles. (Adapted from Dohlman CH. Physiology. In: Smolin G, Thoft RA. The cornea, 2nd ed. Boston: Little Brown, and Co, 1987;3–8.)**

TABLE 15.1
Causes of Corneal Edema

Endothelial decompensation
    Birth trauma
    Congenital hereditary corneal dystrophy
    Fuch's dystrophy
    Keratoconus and hydrops
    Mechanical trauma
    Surgical trauma
    Inflammation

Increased intraocular pressure
    Acute angle-closure glaucoma
    Chronic glaucoma

Adapted from Boruchoff SA. Clinical causes of corneal edema. Int Ophthalmol Clin 1968;8:581–600.

Whenever swelling takes place, transparency is lost in the region where the edema occurs.[6] Since the corneal epithelium and tear film constitute the most anterior optical surface of the eye, epithelial edema exerts a major detrimental influence on vision because it induces anterior irregular astigmatism. It is clinically useful to consider corneal edema as epithelial, stromal, or a combination of both.[8] In general, epithelial edema is more responsive to topical hyperosmotic therapy.[9]

The following discussion considers the pharmacologic properties of hyperosmotic agents available for topical use. Chapter 27 discusses in detail the clinical uses of topical osmotherapy in the diagnosis and management of conditions characterized by corneal edema.

Topical Hyperosmotic Agents

The clinical objective of topical osmotherapy is to increase the tonicity of the tear film and thereby enhance the rate of movement of fluid from the cornea. All the currently available hyperosmotic preparations are hyperosmolar to the ocular tissue fluid. When they are applied to the eye, water is drawn from the cornea to the more highly osmotic tear film and is eliminated through the usual tear flow mechanisms. Patients with minimal to moderate epithelial edema often achieve subjective comfort and improved vision with use of these agents.[6,8,9]

Various agents can reduce corneal edema, including corn syrup, glucose, gum cellulose, sodium chloride, and glycerin.[8] Only a few of these have proved clinically useful and acceptable to most patients. Among those presently available, sodium chloride and glycerin (Table 15.2) are the most widely used in clinical practice.

Sodium Chloride

PHARMACOLOGY

Sodium chloride is a component of all body fluids, including tears. A solution of 0.9% is approximately isotonic with tears.[3] Of the various concentrations tested, the 5% formulation has proved the most effective and has an irritation level acceptable to most patients.

Studies comparing various hyperosmotics in human subjects have confirmed the usefulness of hypertonic sodium chloride in the treatment of corneal edema. Luxenberg and Green[10] studied a series of hyperosmotic preparations including sodium chloride in various formulations. These investigators concluded that 5% sodium chloride in ointment form was most effective in reducing corneal thickness and improving vision. A maximum reduction in corneal thickness of approximately 20% occurred 3 to 4 hours following instillation of the ointment (Fig. 15.2).

The usefulness of sodium chloride solutions in edematous corneas with a traumatized epithelium appears limited. The intact corneal epithelium exhibits limited permeability to inorganic ions.[8] In the absence of an intact epithelium, however, the cornea imbibes salt solutions, thereby reducing the osmotic effect. Thus, in the management of corneal edema associated with traumatized epithelium, hypertonic saline solutions may have only limited value due to their increased ability to penetrate the epithelial barrier.

CLINICAL USES

Sodium chloride is commercially available in 2% and 5% solutions and as 5% ointment (see Table 15.2). In clinical

TABLE 15.2
Topical Hyperosmotic Preparations

Trade Name (manufacturer)	Composition
Sodium Chloride	
Adsorbonac Solution, 2% and 5% (Alcon)	NaCl, povidone and other water soluble polymers, thimerosal 0.004%, EDTA 0.1%
Muro-128 Solution, 2% and 5% (Bausch & Lomb)	NaCl, hydroxypropyl methylcellulose, methylparaben, propylparaben, boric acid
Muro-128 Ointment, 5% (Bausch & Lomb)	NaCl, anhydrous lanolin, mineral oil, white petrolatum
AK-NaCl 5% Ointment (Akorn)	NaCl, anhydrous lanolin, mineral oil, white petrolatum
Glycerin (Glycerol)	
Ophthalgan[a] (Wyeth-Ayerst)	Anhydrous glycerin, chlorobutanol 0.55%
Glucose	
Glucose-40[a] (CibaVision)	Glucose 40%, white petrolatum, anhydrous lanolin, methylparaben, propylparaben

[a]Available only by prescription. EDTA, ethylenediaminetetraaceticacid.

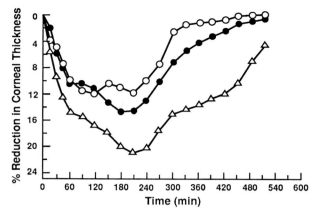

FIGURE 15.2 **Percent reduction in corneal thickness following application of 5% NaCl ointment (△, central; o, nasal; •, temporal). (Modified from the American Journal of Ophthalmology 71:847–853, 1971. Copyright © The Ophthalmic Publishing Company.)**

practice the 5% concentration appears somewhat more effective.[10]

Sodium chloride is useful for reducing corneal edema of various etiologies, including bullous keratopathy. Generally, 1 to 2 drops are instilled in the eye every 3 to 4 hours.[11] Sodium chloride ointment requires less frequent instillation and is generally reserved for nighttime use.[6]

The way in which hyperosmotic preparations are administered may affect the clinical results.[6,8] Since vision is usually worse on arising, several instillations during the first waking hours can prove helpful. On hot, dry days, eyes may require less medication, since tear film evaporation is enhanced.

SIDE EFFECTS

Sodium chloride, especially in the 5% concentration, can cause discomfort upon instillation.[11] Stinging, burning, and irritation are common complaints, but patients generally tolerate the therapy, especially if vision is improved. A case of epistaxis has been associated with use of 2% NaCl solution. The patient complained that the drops irritated the nasolacrimal system, but changing to the ointment form overcame the problem.[12]

Hypertonic saline is nontoxic to the cornea and conjunctiva, and allergic reactions are uncommon.[6]

Glycerin (Glycerol)

PHARMACOLOGY

Glycerin is a clear, colorless, syrupy liquid with a sweet taste. It is miscible with both water and alcohol. When in contact with water, glycerin will absorb water and thereby exert an osmotic effect.[13] When placed on the eye its hydroscopic action will clear the haze of corneal epithelial edema.[13] The osmotic effects of topically applied glycerin are transient. Since the molecules mix readily with water, the osmolality of the applied solution decreases rapidly as water is imbibed from the cornea.[14]

CLINICAL USES

Glycerin is useful to permit ophthalmoscopic and gonioscopic examination of the eye in such clinical conditions as acute angle-closure glaucoma, bullous keratopathy, and Fuch's endothelial dystrophy.[11] Significant reduction of edema occurs within 1 to 2 minutes. Since application to the eye is painful, a topical anesthetic must be instilled before use.[13]

Because its action is transient and its application to the eye painful, glycerin is used primarily for diagnostic purposes. It is valuable for permitting gonioscopy and ophthalmoscopy through edematous corneas when used in concentrations of 50% to 100%. In acute angle-closure glaucoma, additional glycerin may be used as the gonioscopic bonding solution to prolong the hyperosmotic effect during gonioscopy.[11]

SIDE EFFECTS

When applied topically to the eye without prior instillation of an anesthetic, glycerin causes significant stinging and burning. Reflex tearing follows, and dilation of conjunctival vessels may occur. These effects are transient, and no significant toxic effects occur with acute use.[13,14]

Glucose

PHARMACOLOGY

Glucose solutions ranging from 30% to 50% have been used topically on the eye to treat corneal edema. The clinical effectiveness of 40% glucose is comparable to that of 5% sodium chloride.[9]

CLINICAL USES

The dehydrating action of a 30-minute glucose bath eliminates corneal epithelial edema and reduces corneal thickness. The effect lasts 3 to 4 hours.[15] Since it is difficult to maintain sterility of the solution unless a preservative is added, a commercial preparation containing 40% glucose, preserved with methylparaben and propylparaben, is available as an ophthalmic ointment (see Table 15.2).

SIDE EFFECTS

Glucose in the 30% to 50% concentrations is nontoxic to the eye. However, transient stinging and irritation of the conjunctiva may result following instillation.[15]

References

1. Cantonnet A. Essai de traitement du glaucome par les substances osmotiques. Arch D'Ophtalmol 1904;24:1–25.
2. Dohlman CH. Physiology. In: Smolin G, Thoft RA, eds. The cornea. 2nd ed. Boston: Little, Brown and Co, 1987:3–8.
3. Mishima S, Hedbys BO. Physiology of the cornea. Int Ophthalmol Clin 1968;8:527–560.
4. Brown SI, Hedbys BO. The effect of ouabain on the hydration of the cornea. Invest Ophthalmol 1965;4:216–221.
5. Cogan DG, Kinsey VE. The cornea. V. Physiologic aspects. Arch Ophthalmol 1942;28:661–669.
6. Levenson JE. Corneal edema: Cause and treatment. Surv Ophthalmol 1975;20:190–204.
7. Boruchoff SA. Clinical causes of corneal edema. Int Ophthalmol Clin 1968;8:581–600.
8. Lamberts DW. Topical hyperosmotic agents and secretory stimulants. Int Ophthalmol Clin 1980;20:163–169.
9. Payrau P, Dohlman CH. Medical treatment of corneal edema. Int Ophthalmol Clin 1968;8:601–610.
10. Luxenberg MN, Green K. Reduction of corneal edema with topical hypertonic agents. Am J Ophthalmol 1971;71:847–853.
11. Jaanus SD. Hyperosmotic agents. In: Bartlett JD, Ghormley NR, Jaanus SD, et al. Ophthalmic Drug Facts. St. Louis: Facts and Comparisons, 1995:203–214.
12. Kushner FH. Sodium chloride eye drops as a cause of epistaxis. Arch Ophthalmol 1987;105:1634.
13. Cogan DG. Clearing of edematous corneas by glycerine. Am J Ophthalmol 1943;26:551.
14. Hine CH, Anderson HH, Moon HD, et al. Comparative toxicity of synthetic and natural glycerin. Arch Ind Hyg 1953;7:282–291.
15. Bietti GB, Pecori J. Topical osmotherapy of corneal edema. Ann Ophthalmol 1969;1:40–49.

CHAPTER 16

Irrigating Solutions

David R. Whikehart

Originally, the term *irrigating solution* in clinical practice referred to any aqueous solution that could be used to cleanse a tissue while maintaining its moisture. Although extraocular irrigating solutions achieve this purpose, intraocular irrigating solutions must also supply nutrients to the anterior segment, particularly the sensitive corneal endothelium. Accordingly, extraocular solutions may be referred to as true irrigators, while intraocular solutions take on the role of perfusion media. An understanding of these two kinds of irrigating solutions and their respective functions depends on knowledge of the physiologic chemistry of the cornea, lens, uvea and retina.

Desirable Properties of Irrigating Solutions

Nearly any aqueous medium can, in theory, be used to wash debris from the eye. However, the physiologic limitations of ocular tissues must be considered in the design of an appropriate solution. Consequently, the osmolality, pH, and sterility of such solutions are important. Moreover, irrigating solutions must have a sufficiently low concentration of any chemicals toxic to the eye.[1] Nutrient components must be supplied to dependent tissues when irrigation takes place over an extended period, as occurs with intraocular surgery.[2,3]

Metabolic Demands of Anterior Segment Ocular Tissues

CORNEA

The cornea consists of three cellular and two noncellular layers. The most anterior cellular layer, the epithelium, consists of epithelial cells that are normally five to six deep across the entire cornea. These cells act as a barrier to the external environment for the cornea and are nourished by glucose primarily from the aqueous humor and secondarily from the limbal vessels.[4] In contrast, the oxygen supply for cells of the epithelium originates from atmospheric air dissolved in the precorneal tear film. Although epithelial cells are superficially located in the cornea, it appears peculiar that they do not also receive glucose from the precorneal tear film. Evidence against this, however, stems from the paucity of glucose in the tear film compared with that in the aqueous humor. Glucose is generally present in a ratio of approximately 1:12 to 1:15 of tear film to aqueous humor in humans.[4,5] Glucose flux across the cornea from the endothelium toward the epithelium, as studied in rabbits, decreases to less than 10% when silicon blocks the posterior corneal surface.[6] Glucose metabolism in epithelial cells normally does not depend on high amounts of oxygen due to the predominantly anaerobic use of glucose in these cells,[4,7,8] as shown in Table 16.1. These cells also store glucose in the form of glycogen. The corneal epithelium, therefore, can survive quite well with extraocular irrigating solutions that do not contain glucose. During ocular surgery the epithelium can rely on its store of glycogen and on communication with those limbal vessels with which contact remains intact.

The metabolism of stromal keratocytes, the second cellular layer of the cornea, has been difficult to study. This difficulty results, in part, from the stroma's great bulk of collagen and proteoglycans, which interfere with a direct comparison of other corneal tissues on the basis of wet weight and protein. Keratocytes occupy only approximately 10% of the volume of the stroma.[9] Waltman[10] has stated that if correction factors are applied to allow for the small percentage of keratocytes in stroma, then the metabolic rate

373

TABLE 16.1
Glucose Metabolism in Corneal Epithelial Cells[4,7,8]

Pathway	%
Aerobic glycolysis	8
Anaerobic glycolysis	57
Pentose shunt	35

of the stroma would be comparable to that of the epithelium. Present evidence indicates that these cells participate in both aerobic and anaerobic glycolysis; however, the cells lack a key enzyme involved in pentose shunt metabolism.[7] Since glucose destined for the epithelium passes through the stroma, the amount is sufficient for the needs of the stromal cells. Oxygen partial pressure varies from 40–120 mmHg depending on relative anterior-posterior location.[11] This pressure is adequate for the small percentage of cells present in this layer. Keratocytes would not be dependent on a glucose-containing extraocular fluid (irrigating fluid). However, their dependence on a glucose-containing intraocular irrigating fluid during surgery has yet to be established.

The most posterior cellular layer of the cornea, the endothelium, has a comparatively higher percentage of aerobic glycolysis than does the epithelium. Although not specifically measured, the pentose shunt studies of Geroski and associates suggest the higher percentage of aerobic glycolysis in the endothelium.[12] These investigators concluded that 63% of all glucose metabolism occurs by glycolysis in the endothelium compared with 34% in the epithelium. In both cases the remaining CO_2 is formed through the pentose shunt. Riley,[13] by comparison, suggests that 93% of all glucose is processed through the Embden-Meyerhof pathway, of which 23% is aerobic. Endothelial cells can also be inferred to have a high rate of aerobic glycolysis by their numerous mitochondria, more than those of any other cell type except retinal photoreceptors.[14] The endothelium receives both glucose and oxygen directly from the aqueous humor, which bathes their apical cellular membranes. Gaasterland and associates[15] have reported an average value of 53 mg/dL (2.94 mM) of glucose in the aqueous humor of fasting Rhesus monkeys. The partial pressure of oxygen in the aqueous measures approximately 50 mmHg.[11] The endothelial layer causes a drop of approximately 10 mmHg as oxygen diffuses past the endothelium into the stroma.

Endothelial cells are especially vulnerable to interruptions in their source of nourishment. This is unfortunate, since this cellular layer is dominant in controlling the relative hydration and clarity of the cornea.[16,17] Accordingly, the nature of the intraocular irrigating solution used in the course of anterior segment surgery may affect these cells.[18]

CONJUNCTIVA

The conjunctiva generally contains several layers of epithelial cells whose number of mitochondria exceeds that of the corneal epithelial cells.[4] Goblet cells, which secrete tear film mucus, are also present. Conjunctival cells as well as goblet cells receive their supply of glucose and oxygen directly from numerous supporting conjunctival vessels.[19] Consequently, their metabolic needs do not depend on any irrigating solution.

LENS

The lens as a whole has a low metabolic rate.[20] Fiber cells, which make up the bulk of the lens, are largely devoid of both nuclei and mitochondria. In these cells glucose undergoes predominately anaerobic processing. Epithelial cells and the very superficial fiber cells of the lens are, by contrast, quite active metabolically. However, these cells occur only on the anterior surface of the lens. Although the lens can survive quite well anaerobically,[21] the deprivation of glucose may ultimately lead to the formation of cataracts. The time course of this process in humans as well as the detailed mechanism remain unknown. However, Chylack and Schaefer[22] have shown that in rat lens an irreversible shift of lens hexokinase from the soluble to the insoluble form takes place after 8 hours without glucose. This shift drastically reduces the ability of the metabolically active surface cells to phosphorylate glucose and essentially shuts down glucose metabolism. The lens, like corneal endothelium, receives both glucose and oxygen solely from the aqueous. However, an intraocular deprivation of glucose is not a matter of concern in the time course of surgery and apparently, the presence of glucose in an irrigating solution is of no import for the lens. In the diabetic state, however, the osmotic stress due to changes in glucose metabolism is important. This will be considered later.

UVEA

All tissues of the uvea—iris, ciliary body, and choroid—are nourished directly from ocular blood vessels. Consequently, their metabolism does not depend on an intraocular irrigating solution.

RETINA

Ocular blood vessels nourish all tissues of the retina. However, some evidence[23,24] suggests that perfused glucose is important for maintaining the amplitude of the electroretinogram (ERG) when the vitreous is surgically removed.

Physiologic Constraints of the Anterior Segment

Both extraocular and intraocular irrigating solutions must be formulated to fall within the physiologic limitations of the cells with which they come in contact. A hypertonic solution

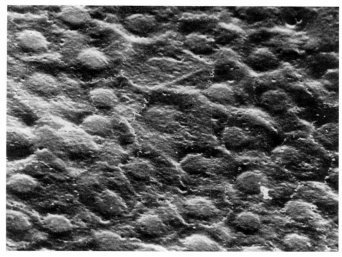

A

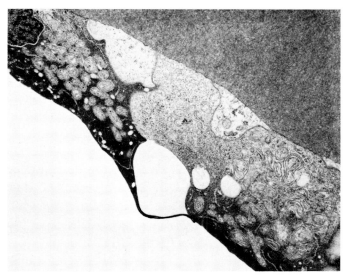

FIGURE 16.1   *(A)* Scanning electron microscopy of the human corneal endothelium following 2-hour perfusion with 200 mOsm salt solution. Nuclear bulges are prominent, and endothelial cells are swollen at junctions ($\times$ 1,000). *(B)* Transmission electron microscopy of the same cornea. There is dilation of intracellular spaces and vacuolization and swelling of cytoplasm ($\times$ 9,500). (Reprinted with permission from Edelhauser HF, Hanneken AM, Pederson HJ, VanHorn DL. Osmotic tolerance of rabbit and human corneal endothelium. Arch Ophthalmol 1981;99:1281-1287. Copyright © 1981, American Medical Association.)

B

will cause cell shrinkage due to water loss, while a hypotonic solution causes swelling and even destruction of cells. Normally at 37°C extracellular and intracellular fluids exert equivalent forces of 5.79×10^3 mmHg at a chemical activity of 300 mOsm.[25] Despite this, Edelhauser and associates[26] have shown that the vulnerable corneal endothelium can withstand a perfusion medium with a range from 200 to 400 mOsm of chemical activity. Figures 16.1 to 16.4 demonstrate effects on the endothelium over a range of 200 to 500 mOsm. A 100 mOsm range above or below 300 mOsm implies a negative or positive pressure on these cells as high as 193 mmHg. However, tolerance to these pressures exists only in the presence of ions known to strengthen cellular adhesion, particularly calcium. Solutions and drugs have been formulated, especially for use within the eye, with an osmolality between 78–440 mOsm. Consequently, the practitioner or surgeon should be cautioned about using agents that introduce cellular stress to ocular regions. Corneal edema has been reported, for example, when acetylcholine (ACh) was used for miosis after removal of the lens in cataract surgery. The osmolality of ACh when reconstituted with sterile saline is in the high range of 388–440 mOsm.[27] Virtually all commercial ophthalmic irrigating solutions, both intraocular and extraocular, are isotonic; that is, they

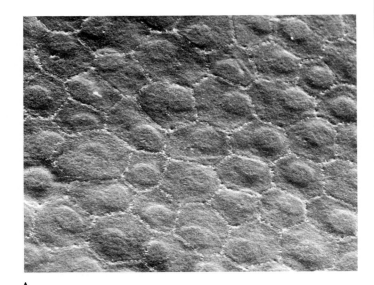

A

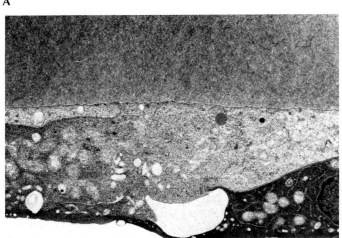

B

FIGURE 16.2   *(A)* Scanning electron microscopy of the human corneal endothelium perfused with balanced salt solution (BSS Plus) (300 mOsm) for 3 hours. Normal mosaic-like pattern of endothelial cells is present (× 1,000). *(B)* Transmission electron microscopy of the same cornea showing intact junctions, normal cell organelles, and some intracellular and extracellular vacuoles (× 10,300). (Reprinted with permission from Edelhauser HF, Hanneken AM, Pederson HJ, VanHorn DL. Osmotic tolerance of rabbit and human corneal endothelium. Arch Ophthalmol 1981;99:1281-1287. Copyright © 1981, American Medical Association.)

are formulated with an osmolality of approximately 300 mOsm. A report by Briggs and McCartney,[28] however, found an exception. Although the composition of salts used is not critical at a chemical activity of 300 mOsm for extraocular irrigating solutions, the composition is important with solutions used for intraocular surgery. Specific salts should be added that not only maintain cells, but also maximize cell adhesion, cell-to-cell junctions, and cellular transport during surgery. The salts included should contain ions of sodium, potassium, calcium, magnesium, chloride and bicarbonate.[3,18,29] Topical hypertonic or hyperosmolar preparations are available to reduce corneal edema, but such

preparations should not be considered as normal physiologic irrigants,[30] and their use should be regarded with the above-mentioned precautions.

Another important physiologic limitation is the hydrogen ion concentration, commonly expressed as pH. Normal serum or plasma extracellular pH is 7.4, with a tolerable range of 7.35–7.45.[31] The precorneal tear film has a pH of 7.4 with a range of 7.3–7.7,[32] while the aqueous humor (in Rhesus monkeys) has been reported at 7.49.[15] Gonnering and associates[33] have shown that both structural and functional alterations occur to the human corneal endothelium outside the pH range 6.5–8.5. These alterations consist of swelling, pits at

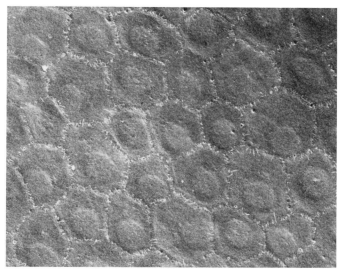

A

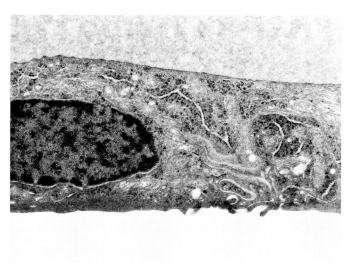

B

FIGURE 16.3   *(A)* Scanning electron microscopy of the human corneal endothelium after 2-hour perfusion of 400 mOsm salt solution. Cells are intact, and tight junctions are present ($\times$ 1,000). *(B)* Transmission electron microscopy of the same cornea. Intercellular junctions are intact, cytoplasm is condensed, and cell organelles are normal ($\times$ 14,350). (Reprinted with permission from Edelhauser HF, Hanneken AM, Pederson HJ, VanHorn DL. Osmotic tolerance of rabbit and human corneal endothelium. Arch Ophthalmol 1981;99:1281-1287. Copyright © 1981, American Medical Association.)

cellular junctions, as well as loss of plasma membrane and recognizable subcellular components (i.e., cell death), as shown in Figures 16.5 to 16.8. A normal corneal endothelium is shown in Figure 16.7 after perfusion at pH 7.2. As mentioned previously regarding osmotic pressure anomalies, drugs and vehicles that are made up without regard to pH buffering capacity, or that are buffered outside the physiologic range, can also destroy ocular tissue. This statement is qualified, however, by the consideration that some drugs must be formulated outside the normal pH range (e.g., pilocarpine HCl) to remain stable before topical administra-

tion. The amount of vehicle contact time at an abnormal pH in topical administration is so small that it involves only momentary discomfort (e.g., stinging) to the patient and is without damage to tissues. When an irrigating solution for intraocular surgery is used, especially for prolonged periods, the potential for cellular destruction exists if the solution is either unbuffered or buffered in preference to a particular medication. Although the pH values of commercially available extraocular irrigating solutions are not stated,[27,34,35] these solutions are generally either neutral or buffered toward neutrality and constitute virtually no pH risk for the

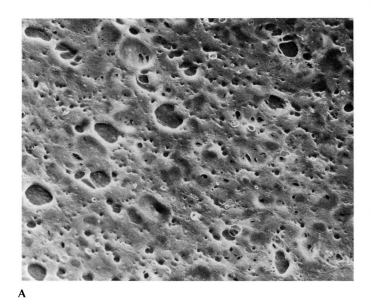

A

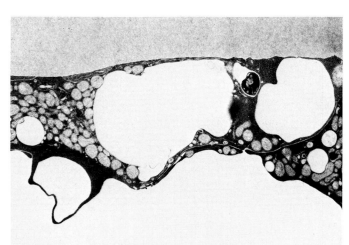

FIGURE 16.4 *(A)* Scanning electron microscopy of the human corneal endothelium after 2-hour perfusion of 500 mOsm salt solution. Mosaic-like pattern has disappeared, and cells are pulling apart (× 1,000). *(B)* Transmission electron microscopy of the same cornea. Posterior surface is wavy, and large intercellular vacuoles are present. Junctions between cells are connected by thin bridges of cytoplasm, and cytoplasm is condensed (× 8,100). (Reprinted with permission from Edelhauser HF, Hanneken AM, Pederson HJ, VanHorn DL. Osmotic tolerance of rabbit and human corneal endothelium. Arch Ophthalmol 1981;99:1281–1287. Copyright © 1981, American Medical Association.)

B

outer ocular surface. Intraocular irrigating solutions are designated as being either pH adjusted or at approximately pH 7.4. Briggs and McCartney,[28] however, have noted one exception.

The Use of Preservatives

Irrigating solutions contain antimicrobial agents to prevent microbial growth and to preserve the composition of the solutions from microbial attack. As such they are often designated as preservatives[36] or disinfectants.[37] Due to their toxic effects on intraocular tissues, their use is limited to extraocular irrigants. Coles[38] has shown that 12 different commonly used therapeutic antimicrobial agents (antibiotics) have some deleterious effects on rabbit corneal endothelia. These effects manifested as increasing corneal thickness and interference with cell membrane or junctional integrity (Fig. 16.9). Lower limits for toxicity have apparently not been adequately demonstrated. Although Leopold[39] has sug-

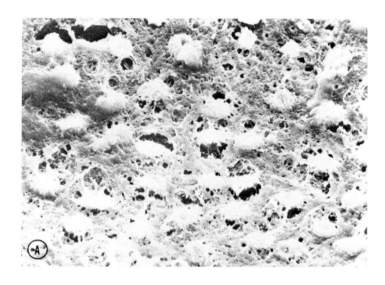

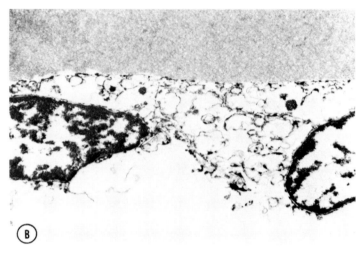

FIGURE 16.5   *(A)* **Scanning electron micrograph of the endothelium of a human cornea perfused at pH 5.50 for 1 hour. The nuclei of most cells are exposed due to the collapse of the outer plasma membrane (× 1000).** *(B)* **Transmission electron micrograph of endothelial cells from the same cornea displaying completely necrotic cells. There are no recognizable organelles, and the outer plasma membrane is completely disrupted (× 11,200). (Reprinted with permission from Gonnering R, Edelhauser HF, VanHorn DL, Durant W. The pH tolerance of rabbit and human corneal endothelium. Invest Ophthalmol Vis Sci 1979;18:373–390.)**

gested dosage schedules for therapeutic agents that may be injected into the anterior chamber, the risks are great. Havener[40] states that irrigation of the anterior chamber with antibiotics can produce endothelial cell death with concomitant corneal opacity, destructive iritis with neovascularization, and cataract induction.

The preservatives used in extraocular irrigating solutions should ideally be effective against both gram-negative and gram-positive bacteria without ocular toxicity. Furthermore,

they should not compromise the components of the solution. Practically, irrigating solutions are formulated to make the best compromise between antimicrobial action and corneal epithelial deterioration. Table 16.2 gives an overview of the preservatives and their use in extraocular irrigating solutions. In general, the preservatives are used at concentrations that are bacteriostatic rather than bactericidal. Assuredly the prevention of bacterial growth is aided by refrigerating these solutions.

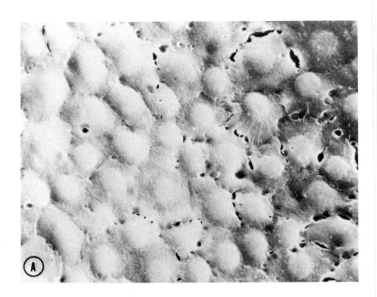

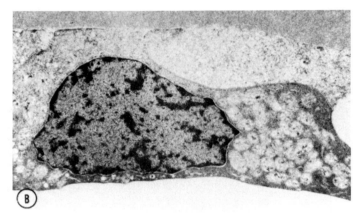

FIGURE 16.6   *(A)* **Scanning electron micrograph of the endothelium of a human cornea perfused at pH 6.50 for 3 hours. The cells appear swollen, and pits are present at many of the junctions (× 1000).** *(B)* **Transmission electron micrograph of endothelial cells from the same cornea displaying both cytoplasmic and mitochondrial swelling and some clumping of the nuclear chromatin. The junctional complexes have partially broken down, leaving large spaces between many cells (× 8600). (Reprinted with permission from Gonnering R, Edelhauser HF, VanHorn DL, Durant W. The pH tolerance of rabbit and human corneal endothelium. Invest Ophthalmol Vis Sci 1979;18:373–390.)**

Extraocular Irrigating Solutions

The previous section has demonstrated that extraocular irrigating solutions must be physiologically balanced with respect to pH and osmolality but do not require nutrients or specific ions. Their short-term use and the fact that cells with which they come in contact obtain nutrients elsewhere render them quite safe as formulated. Their role is primarily that of clearing away unwanted materials from the outer ocular surface. Prolonged extraocular irrigation is uncommon. When and if it exceeds two hours, then specific ions such as calcium and magnesium become important to prevent excessive epithelial cell sloughing and edema.[41,42]

Components

A general and detailed discussion of the components of extraocular irrigating solutions appears in the previous section. Table 16.3 lists the components of three typical extraocular irrigating solutions.

Clinical Uses

These solutions are used primarily for washing away debris and liquids that are foreign to the extraocular surface. The solutions are available over the counter, without prescription, and so may be used by patients and practitioners alike.

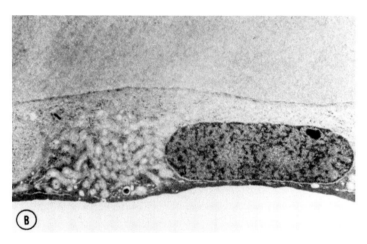

FIGURE 16.7   *(A)* Scanning electron micrograph of the endothelium of a human cornea perfused at pH 7.2 for 3 hours. The normal mosaiclike cellular pattern is preserved (× 1000). *(B)* Transmission electron micrograph of endothelial cells from the same cornea displaying normal ultrastructure except for some clarification of the cytoplasm between the nucleus and Descemet's membrane (× 8600). (Reprinted with permission from Gonnering R, Edelhauser HF, VanHorn DL, Durant W. The pH tolerance of rabbit and human corneal endothelium. Invest Ophthalmol Vis Sci 1979;18:373–390.)

In the practitioner's office they are useful following tonometry (removal of fluorescein) and gonioscopy (removal of methylcellulose) as well as foreign body removal and for the removal of routine, diagnostic fluorescein. They serve an important function in diagnostic nasolacrimal duct irrigation in patients with chronic epiphora. These solutions have further use in washing out mucus or purulent discharge. They are also used at the hospital bedside to clean out eyes between dressing changes.[34]

Irrigating solutions should not be used with contact lenses in place. The solutions tend to cause contact lens irritation by reducing natural, lubricating mucin and, in the case of a rigid lens, by reducing the hydrophilicity of the lens surface.[36] The absorption of benzalkonium chloride by hydrogel lenses can potentially lead to corneal epithelial damage if sufficient amounts of preservative are released to the eye. Although irrigating solutions may be used to wash out the eyes after contact lens wear, these solutions have no value as contact lens solutions per se for wetting, cleansing, or cushioning.

First-Aid Irrigating Solutions

Undoubtedly, one of the worst ocular disasters is a chemical insult to the outer ocular surface. Penetrating chemicals

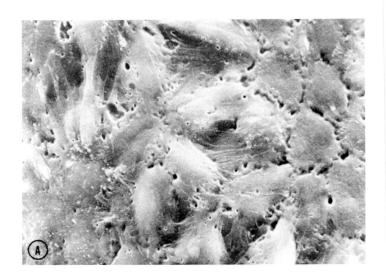

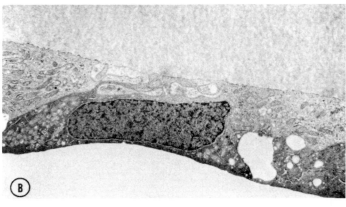

FIGURE 16.8   *(A)* **Scanning electron micrograph of the endothelium of a human cornea perfused at pH 8.50 for 3 hours. Some of the cells appear swollen, whereas others appear quite normal. Pits are present at many of the cellular junctions (× 1000).** *(B)* **Transmission electron micrograph of the endothelial cells from the same cornea showing normal ultrastructure except for varying degrees of cytoplasmic swelling. The junctional complexes have partially broken down, leaving large spaces between many cells (× 6800). (Reprinted with permission from Gonnering R, Edelhauser HF, VanHorn DL, Durant W. The pH tolerance of rabbit and human corneal endothelium. Invest Ophthalmol Vis Sci 1979;18:373–390.)**

require that the eyes receive an immediate copious lavage and that the patient be transported to an emergency room or appropriate treatment facility as soon as possible. Although the ideal irrigating solution for the immediate accident is physiologic saline, water is nearly always the only available substance. Alkali burns are particularly harmful to the cornea, since they cause the saponification and dissociation of cell membrane fatty acids, hydrolysis of proteoglycans, and swelling of collagen fibers[45,46] accompanied by rapid penetration to the aqueous humor with possible similar damage to other ocular tissues. Paterson and associates[47] studied the effects of alkali on the pH of rabbit aqueous humor. They found that with the application of 100 μl of 2N sodium hydroxide, the aqueous pH rose to 12 within 5 minutes and fell to only 11 after 90 minutes. A similar rapid penetration was shown with enucleated human eye-bank eyes. When

rabbit eyes were topically irrigated 2 minutes after the alkali burn with physiologic saline at a rate of 30 drops per minute, the aqueous pH dropped to only 10 after 90 minutes, indicating the inadequacy of this procedure alone for treating alkali burns. The next section will discuss the use of paracentesis of the anterior chamber combined with the intracameral injection of buffer for enhanced treatment.

Intraocular Irrigating Solutions

History

Ophthalmologists once used normal saline routinely as an intraocular irrigating solution in surgery. Merrill and associ-

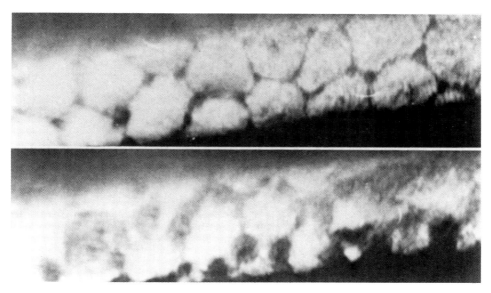

FIGURE 16.9   **Rabbit corneal endothelium showing examples of enlarging intercellular spaces seen with erythromycin and bacitracin. The upper segment represents early changes and the lower segment late changes. Intercellular swelling seems to have pushed the cell substance to the side. Eventually recognizable cell morphology was completely lost. (From Coles WH. Effects of antibiotics on the in vitro rabbit corneal endothelium. Invest Ophthalmol 1975;14:246–250.)**

TABLE 16.2
Preservatives Used in Some Extraocular Irrigating Solutions

Preservative	Epithelial Toxicity Level[a]	Antimicrobial Level[b]		Irrigating Solution Level[c]	
Benzalkonium chloride (BAK)	0.01%[1,38] 0.02%[43]	0.0029%	*Staphylococcus aureus*[38] *Salmonella typhosa*	0.013% 0.005%	AK-Rinse Blinx
		0.0025%	*Eschericha coli*	?	Dacriose[d,e]
		0.0014%	*Cryptococcus neoformans*	0.013%	Eye Stream
		0.0011%	*Streptococcus pyogenes*	0.01%	Eye Wash (Goldline)
		0.02%	*Pseudomonas aeruginosa* (may be partially resistant)	0.005%	Eye Wash (Lavoptik)
Thimerosal	>0.01%[1] >2%[31]	0.01%	*Pseudomonas aeruginosa*[44] *Staphylococcus aureus* *Candida albicans*	0.002%	Collyrium

[a]Concentration at which epithelial cell damage has been reported.
[b]Concentration necessary for bacteriostatic action against the named microorganisms.
[c]Concentration used in the following commercial preparations.
[d]Concentration not given in the pharmacology literature.
[e]Used in combination with ethylenediaminetetraacetic acid (EDTA).
It should be noted that one product (Eye Wash [Bausch & Lomb]) uses 0.1% sorbic acid, which has weak bacteriostatic and antifungal activity.

ates,[48] however, showed in 1960 that such solutions are inadequate for the physiologic well-being of isolated iris and conjunctival tissues after 35-minute perfusion. A balanced salt solution was reported to be significantly less traumatic.

One serious problem that occurs with the use of saline is corneal swelling, which results from rapidly developing abnormalities of the endothelium.[48] Edelhauser and associates[3] demonstrated that lactated Ringer's solution, used in

TABLE 16.3

Components of Some Commercial Extraocular Irrigating Solutions[a]

Solution	Components	
Eye-Stream (Alcon)	0.64%	sodium chloride
	0.075%	potassium chloride
	0.03%	magnesium chloride
	0.048%	calcium chloride
	0.39%	sodium acetate
	0.17%	sodium citrate
	0.013%	benzalkonium chloride
Eye Wash (Lavoptik)	0.49%	sodium chloride
	0.4%	sodium bisphosphate
	0.45%	sodium phosphate
	0.005%	benzalkonium chloride
Eye Irrigating Wash (Hauck)	1.2%	boric acid
	0.38%	potassium chloride
	0.014%	sodium carbonate (dry)
	0.05%	EDTA[b]
	0.01%	benzalkonium chloride

[a]Data from Bartlett JD, Ghormley NR, Jaanus SD, et al., eds. Ophthalmic drug facts. St. Louis: Facts and Comparisons, 1993;237–238.

[b]ethylenediaminetetraacetic acid.

some vitrectomy surgery, and Plasma-Lyte 148, used in some phacoemulsification surgery, are also unacceptable as irrigating solutions for intraocular tissues. Both solutions principally cause early breakdown of corneal endothelial cells. These irrigating solutions lack ions of either calcium, magnesium, or both, which earlier sections in this chapter described as necessary for cell adhesion and cell-to-cell junctions. As early as 1960, a balanced salt solution (BSS, Alcon) containing calcium and magnesium became available for intraocular surgery.[50]

Although a balanced salt solution is apparently acceptable for short-term intraocular surgery,[51,52] it is only marginally acceptable for protracted intraocular surgery since some corneal swelling continues to occur.[3] Glasser and associates[53] have shown the development of polymegathism and pleomorphism in cat corneal endothelial cells after 1 hour in a balanced salt solution. Araie[54] has indicated that endothelial barrier function is compromised with a solution containing only salts.

One report to the contrary[55] indicated that a balanced salt solution (lacking glucose and bicarbonate) caused only corneal swelling. It stated that no cytotoxic damage occurred beyond occasional air bubble destruction. The solution was tested for a period of 2.5 hours. However, the investigator never demonstrated whether the cornea could recover from the swelling (by perfusion in a complete medium). More-

over, the investigator also did not show whether any permanent biochemical effects occurred or whether the cornea suffered subsequent toxic effects. McDermott and associates,[56] however, have demonstrated that a complete medium can deswell human corneas that had been swollen for 2-4 days in eye bank storage solutions in comparison to an incomplete medium (balanced salt solutions), which could not deswell the corneas. Several investigations during the 1970s had already indicated the need for other components in intraocular irrigating solutions. Hodson[57] demonstrated a need for bicarbonate ions, and this has recently been confirmed by Riley and associates.[74] Dikstein and Maurice[58] showed that glucose, adenosine, and glutathione could each thin a swollen cornea, albeit to different degrees. It has never been adequately explained how bicarbonate ions work. Hodson[59] proposed that bicarbonate ions were pumped into the aqueous to aid deturgescence. However, neither Riley and Peters[60] nor Whikehart and Soppet[61] were able to locate a bicarbonate transporting ATPase in the plasma membranes of the corneal endothelial cells. Whikehart and Soppet[62] demonstrated stimulation of membrane-bound Na$^+$K$^+$ ATPase in these cells by glutathione, but not by adenosine. Zagrod and Whikehart[63] demonstrated that adenosine may act as a substitute for glucose by supplying metabolic intermediates via the pentose shunt. In the retina, work by Winkler and associates[29] has shown the importance of bicarbonate in maintaining both the retinal ERG and lactate production. The work of other researchers supports this finding.[23,24] Recently, Li and associates[64] have shown that the complete commercial medium (BSS Plus) containing bicarbonate was best able to preserve the corneal transendothelial electrical potential difference. However, the medium's mechanism is still elusive.

Edelhauser and associates[49] had prepared and perfused rabbit corneas with a modified basic salt solution ("GBR") containing bicarbonate, glucose, adenosine, and glutathione. They found essentially no swelling of rabbit corneas over a 3- to 6-hour period. This compared better than earlier preparations with only partial components of GBR[2,3] in which corneas were always observed to swell in various amounts. However, when Christiansen and associates[65] prepared equivalents of GBR using fresh solutions of D5W and sodium bicarbonate with either lactated Ringer's or Ringer's injection solution and used them in studies of the monkey lens, they found it difficult to control the pH of the solution.

Attempts to prepare GBR and similar intraocular solutions fresh for use in the operating room were met with the same instability. A stable commercial formulation (BSS Plus, Alcon) appeared in 1981 that contained bicarbonate, glucose and glutathione in addition to balanced salts.[50] Maintaining some of the components in a separate dry container prior to use keeps the preparation stable. Adenosine was not included due to problems of maintenance in storage. This commercial formulation has successfully stabilized both the cornea and the lens in nondiabetic patients during long-term ocular surgery (1 to 3 hours).

Components

For comparative purposes Table 16.4 lists the formulations of some commercial intraocular irrigating solutions, past and present. However, even present formulations have limitations, as discussed in the next section. BSS Plus and AMO Endosol Extra have their components divided into two containers that must be premixed before use. Note that BSS Plus, part I, has a pH of 7.4 while Endosol Extra, part I, has a pH of only 2.6. Once mixed, they have the composition given in Table 16.4 and remain stable for the period of surgery.

Use of Intraocular Drugs

It was previously mentioned that preservatives and antibiotic therapeutic agents may have deleterious effects on the cells exposed to the anterior chamber. However, intraocular miotics and mydriatics may be used in intraocular irrigating solutions if sufficiently diluted and free of preservatives as well as antioxidants.[66] Miotics help to minimize postoperative IOP increases while mydriatics assist in the mainte-

nance of a dilated pupil. Viscoelastic agents also help to protect the corneal endothelium from mechanical damage.[67]

Surgical Uses

The metabolic stress to which ocular tissues will be exposed during surgery determines the use of simple (BSS or AMO Endosol) or complete (BSS Plus or AMO Endosol Extra) intraocular irrigating solutions.[68] Factors related to that stress are listed below.

Time: If surgery is to proceed for periods of longer than 60 min (e.g., pars plana vitrectomy; anterior segment reconstruction), then a complete irrigating solution should be used. Sixty minutes is considered the maximum time past which the presence of nutrients becomes critical.

Compromised corneal endothelium: Data suggest that compromised corneas, such as in bullous keratopathy, have a higher likelihood of postoperative edema.[69] A complete irrigating solution would therefore decrease the trauma of surgery.

Surgery without a viscoelastic agent: The corneal endothelium is more prone to damage when a viscoelastic agent is omitted. Under these circumstances a complete irrigant reduces corneal endothelial damage.[70]

Accordingly, the less complete media might be used in ophthalmic surgery when the procedure is less than one hour in patients who have no compromised corneas (endothelia) and during which viscoelastic agents are used.[68] There are

TABLE 16.4
Components of Commercial Intraocular Irrigating Solutions[a] Compared with Physiologic Saline, Lactated Ringer's Solution and Plasmalyte 148

Components (mmoles/L)	Physiologic[b] Saline[3] 308 mOsm/L pH = 7.0	Lactated[b] Ringer's[3] 277 mOsm/L pH = 6.6	Plasmalyte[b] 148[3] 299 mOsm/L pH = 7.4	BSS	AMO Endosol	BSS+	AMO Endosol Extra
				[------------------------ 305 mOsm/L -----------------------]			
				[------------------------pH = 7.4------------------------]			
Sodium chloride	154	102	85.9	109.5	109.5	122.2	109.4
Potassium chloride		4	5	10.1	10.1	5.1	4.6
Calcium chloride		3		4.3	4.3	1.1	1.2
Magnesium chloride			1.5	1.5	1.5	1.0	1.9
Sodium phosphate						2.8	2.7
Sodium bicarbonate						25	22.4
Glucose						5.1	4.6
Glutathione disulfide						0.3	0.3
Sodium acetate			2.7	28.6	28.6		
Sodium citrate				5.8	5.8		
Sodium lactate		28					
Sodium gluconate			16.9				

[a]BSS and BSS+ are products of Alcon. AMO Endosol and AMO Endosol Extra are products of Allergan.
[b]Physiologic saline, lactated Ringer's and Plasmalyte solutions are no longer recommended as intraocular irrigants. The compositions of these solutions are obtained from reference 3 and the manufacturers' literature.

cases, however, in which endothelial damage has occurred with the use of BSS.

Surgical Use Among Diabetics

A different problem that occurs with pars plana vitrectomy is the development during surgery of a posterior subcapsular lens opacification in diabetic patients. The opacification blocks the appearance of both the vitreous cavity and retina. A lensectomy to clear the view may, in turn, double the risk of postoperative neovascular glaucoma. An investigation by Haimann and associates[71] demonstrated that a long-term intraocular irrigating solution was not able to protect against posterior subcapsular cataract formation in diabetic rabbits. It was found, however, that glucose fortification of the solution to 335 mOsm prevented cataract formation during perfusion while performing vitrectomies on rabbits. Perfusions were carried out for 2 hours. The increased osmolarity acts as a guard against osmotic stress, which is worsened with the use of solutions of normal osmolarity. The reason for this is that diabetic lenses have trapped within their cells polyols that cause osmotic stress.[72] This is ameliorated by the high glucose content of a diabetic aqueous. Haimann and associates[71] describe how 50% dextrose (in sterile water, without preservatives) may be added to BSS Plus to obtain a higher osmolar, complete irrigation solution for diabetic vitrectomy.

First-Aid Irrigating Solutions

A continuation of the study by Paterson and associates,[43] mentioned earlier in this chapter, showed that paracentesis of the rabbit anterior chamber following the application of 100 μl of 2N sodium hydroxide to the corneal surface reduced aqueous pH from 12 to 10 in 5 minutes. This compared with the same decrease in pH over 90 minutes with external irrigation using physiologic saline. The same workers, furthermore, demonstrated that the simultaneous introduction of pH 7.2 phosphate buffer, intracamerally injected, can lower aqueous pH to 8.5 in 30 minutes. The pH at 30 minutes with paracentesis alone was still 10. Recall that Gonnering and associates[33] reported structural and functional alterations to the human corneal endothelium outside of the pH range 6.5–8.5. This indicates that immediately following extraocular lavage of an alkali burn the two-fold techniques of paracentesis and intracameral buffer may restore the aqueous to a pH nearly acceptable to the cornea and other ocular tissues. These procedures have been recommended[44,45] in cases of moderately severe and severe alkali burns, using sterile phosphate buffer or other compatible irrigating solutions. In view of the preceding discussions, the solution of choice should be a complete physiologic solution. Herr and associates have recently confirmed this choice.[73]

References

1. Pfister RR, Burstein N. The effects of ophthalmic drugs, vehicles, and preservatives on corneal epithelium: A scanning electron microscope study. Invest Ophthalmol 1976;15:246–259.
2. Whikehart DR, Edelhauser HF. Glutathione in rabbit corneal endothelia: The effects of selected perfusion fluids. Invest Ophthalmol Vis Sci 1978;17:455–464.
3. Edelhauser HF, VanHorn DL, Schultz RO, Hyndick RA. Effects of intraocular irrigating solutions on the cornea. In: Leopold IH, Burns RP, eds. Symposium on ocular therapy. New York: John Wiley & sons, 1977;10:45–60.
4. Friend J. Biochemistry of ocular surface epithelium. Int Ophthalmol Clin 1979;19:73–91.
5. Daum KM, Hill RM. Human tear glucose. Invest Ophthalmol Vis Sci 1982;22:509–514.
6. Thoft RA, Friend J. Corneal epithelial glucose utilization. Arch Ophthalmol 1971;88:58.
7. Edelhauser HF, VanHorn DL, Records RE. Cornea and sclera. In: Records RE, ed. Physiology of the human eye and visual system. Hagerstown, MD: Harper & Row, 1979;68–97.
8. Kinoshita JH. Some aspects of the carbohydrate metabolism of the cornea. Invest Ophthalmol 1962;1:178.
9. Kaye Gl. Stereologic measurement of cell volume fraction of rabbit corneal stroma. Arch Ophthalmol 1969;82:692–794.
10. Waltman SR. The cornea. In: Moses RA, ed. Adler's physiology of the eye. St. Louis: C. V. Mosby Co, 1981;47.
11. Fatt I. Physiology of the eye. Boston: Butterworths, 1987;160–161.
12. Geroski DH, Edelhauser HF, O'Brien WJ. Hexose-monophosphate shunt activity in the component layers of the cornea: Its response to thiol oxidation. Exp Eye Res 1978;26:611–619.
13. Riley MV. Transport of ions and metabolites across the corneal endothelium. In: McDevitt DS, ed. Cell biology of the eye. New York: Academic Press, 1982;53–95.
14. Hogan MJ, Alvarado JA, Weddel JE. Histology of the human eye. Philadelphia: W.B. Saunders Co, 1971;102–109.
15. Gaasterland DE, Pederson JE, MacLellan HM, Reddy VN. Rhesus monkey aqueous humor composition and a primate ocular perfusate. Invest Ophthalmol Vis Sci 1979;18:1139–1150.
16. Maurice D. The location of the fluid pump in the cornea. J Physiol 1972;221:43–54.
17. Green K. Ion transport in isolated cornea of the rabbit. Am J Physiol 1965;209:1311–1316.
18. Edelhauser HF, VanHorn DL, Schultz RO, Hyndick RA. Comparative toxicity of intraocular irrigating solutions on the corneal endothelium. Am J Ophthalmol 1976;81:473–481.
19. Records RE. Conjunctiva and lacrimal system. In: Records RE, ed. Physiology of the human eye and visual system. Hagerstown, MD: Harper & Row, 1979;25–46.
20. Zagrod ME, Whikehart DR. Cyclic nucleotides in anatomical subdivisions of the bovine lens. Curr Eye Res 1981;1:49–52.
21. Kinoshita JH, Kern HL, Merola LO. Factors affecting the cation transport of calf lens. Biochem Biophys Acta 1961;47:458.
22. Chylack LT, Schaefer FL. Mechanism of "hypoglycemic" cataract

formation in the rat lens. II. Further studies on the role of hexokinase instability. Invest Ophthalmol 1976;15:519–528.

23. Negi A, Honda Y, Kawano S-I. Effects of intraocular irrigating solutions on the electroretinographic B-wave. Am J Ophthalmol 1981;92:28–37.

24. Textorious O, Nilsson SEG, Anderson B-E. Effects of intraocular perfusion with two alternating irrigation solutions on the simultaneously recorded electroretinogram of albino rabbits. Doc Ophthalmol 1986;63:349–358.

25. Jenson D. The principles of physiology. New York: Appleton-Century-Crofts, 1980.

26. Edelhauser HF, Hanneken AM, Pederson HJ, VanHorn DL. Osmotic tolerance of rabbit and human corneal endothelium. Arch Ophthalmol 1981;99:1281–1287.

27. Fraunfelder FT. National drug registry of drug-induced ocular side effects. Case reports 1545, 1878, 2016, 2226. Portland: University of Oregon, 1980.

28. Briggs RB, McCartney DL. Balanced salt solution infusion alert. Arch Ophthalmol 1988;106:718.

29. Winkler BS, Simson V, Benner J. Importance of bicarbonate in retinal function. Invest Ophthalmol Vis Sci 1977;16:766–768.

30. Kastrup EK, Olin BR, Connell SI, eds. Drug facts and comparisons. St. Louis: J.B. Lippincott Co., 1988.

31. Siggaard-Anderson O. Blood gases. In: Tietz NW, ed. Fundamentals of clinical chemistry. Philadelphia: W.B. Saunders Co, 1976: 854–944.

32. Milder B. The lacrimal apparatus. In: Moses RA, ed. Adler's physiology of the eye. St. Louis: C. V. Mosby Co, 1981;16–37.

33. Gonnering R, Edelhauser HF, VanHorn DL, Durant W. The pH tolerance of rabbit and human corneal endothelium. Invest Ophthalmol Vis Sci 1979;18:373–390.

34. Henkind P, Walsh JB, Berger AW, eds. Physicians desk reference for ophthalmology. Oradell, NJ: Medical Economics, 1982.

35. Bartlett JD, Ghormley NR, Jaanus SD, Rowsey JJ, Zimmerman TJ, eds. Ophthalmic drug facts. St. Louis: Facts and Comparisons, 1993:237–238.

36. Hales RH. Contact lenses. A clinical approach to fitting. Baltimore: Williams & Wilkins, 1978:32–50.

37. Harvey SC. Antiseptics and disinfectants; fungicides; ectoparasiticides. In: Gilman AG, Goodman LS, Rall TW, Murad F, eds. The pharmacological basis of therapeutics. 7th ed. New York: Macmillan Co, 1985;959–979.

38. Coles WH. Effects of antibiotics on the vitro rabbit corneal endothelium. Invest Ophthalmol 1975;14:246–250.

39. Leopold IH. Antibiotics and antifungal agents. Invest Ophthalmol 1964;3:510–511.

40. Havener WH. Ocular pharmacology. St. Louis: C. V. Mosby Co, 1983.

41. Bachman WG, Wilson G. Essential ions for maintenance of the corneal epithelial surface. Invest Ophthalmol Vis Sci 1985;26: 1484–1488.

42. O'Leary DJ, Wilson G. Tear-side regulation of desquamation in the rabbit corneal epithelium. Clin Exp Optom 1986;69:22–26.

43. Zand LM. Review: The effect of non-therapeutic ophthalmic preparations on the cornea and tear film. Aust J Optom 1981;64:44.

44. Wade A, ed. Martindale, the extra pharmacopoeia. London: Pharmaceutical Press, 1977.

45. Grayson M. Diseases of the cornea. St. Louis: C. V. Mosby Co, 1979.

46. Pfister RR, Koski J. Alkali burns of the eye: Pathophysiology and treatment. South Med J 1982;75:417–422.

47. Paterson CA, Pfister RR, Levinson RA. Aqueous humor pH changes after experimental alkali burns. Am J Ophthalmol 1975; 79:414–419.

48. Merrill DL, Fleming TC, Girard LJ. The effects of physiologic balanced salt solutions and normal saline on intraocular and extraocular tissues. Am J Ophthalmol 1960;49:895–989.

49. Edelhauser HF, VanHorn DL, Hyndiuk RA, Schultz RO. Intraocular irrigating solutions. Arch Ophthalmol 1975;93:648–657.

50. Alcon Laboratories. A brief history of intraocular irrigating solutions. (Form No. 098116A). Fort Worth, TX: Alcon Laboratories, 1981.

51. Rosenfeld SI, Waltman SR, Olk RJ, Gordon M. Comparison of intraocular irrigating solutions in pars plana vitrectomy. Ophthalmology 1986;93:109–115.

52. Kramer KK, Thomassen T, Evoul J. Intraocular irrigating solutions: A clinical study of BSS Plus (and dextrose bicarbonate lactated Ringer's solution. Ann Ophthalmol 1991;23:101–105.

53. Glasser DB, Matsuda M, Ellis JG, Edelhauser HF. Effects of intraocular irrigating solutions on the corneal endothelium after in vivo anterior chamber irrigation. Am J Ophthalmol 1985;99:321–328.

54. Araie M. Barrier function of corneal endothelium and the intraocular irrigating solutions. Arch Ophthalmol 1986;104:435–438.

55. Doughty MJ. Quantitative evaluation of the effects of a bicarbonate and glucose-free balanced salt solution on rabbit corneal endothelium in vitro. Optom Vis Sci 1992;69:846–857.

56. McDermott M, Snyder R, Slack J, Holley G, Edelhauser H. Effects of intraocular irrigants on the preserved human corneal endothelium. Cornea 1991;10:402–407.

57. Hodson S. Evidence for a bicarbonate-dependent sodium pump in corneal endothelium. Exp Eye Res 1971;11:20–29.

58. Dikstein S, Maurice DM. The metabolic basis to the fluid pump in the cornea. J Physiol 1972;221:29–41.

59. Hodson S. The bicarbonate ion pump in the endothelium which regulates the hydration of rabbit cornea. J Physiol 1976;263;563–577.

60. Riley MV, Peters MI. The localization of the anion-sensitive ATPase activity in corneal endothelium. Biochem Biophys Acta 1981;644:251–256.

61. Whikehart DR, Soppet DR. Activities of transport enzymes located in the plasma membranes of corneal endothelial cells. Invest Ophthalmol Vis Sci 1981;21:819–825.

62. Whikehart DR, Soppet DR. The effects of glutathione and adenosine on plasma membrane ATPases of the corneal endothelium. An hypothesis on the stimulatory mechanism of perfused glutathione upon deturgescence. Curr Eye Res 1981;1:451–455.

63. Zagrod ME, Whikehart DR. Adenosine-stimulated production of sugar-phosphates in bovine corneal endothelium. Invest Ophthalmol Vis Sci 1985;26:1475–1483.

64. Li J, Akiyama R, Kuang K, Fischborg J. Effects of BSS and BSS+ irrigation solutions on rabbit corneal transendothelial electrical potential difference. Cornea 1993;12:199–203.

65. Christiansen JM, Kollarits CR, Fukui H, Fishman ML, Michels RG, Mikuni I. Intraocular irrigating solutions and lens clarity. Am J Ophthalmol 1976;82:594–597.

66. MacRae S. Intraocular drugs used in cataract surgery and their effect on the corneal endothelium. Refract Corneal Surg 1991;7: 249–251.

67. Liesegang TJ. Viscoelastic substances in ophthalmology. Surv Ophthalmol 1990;34:268–293.

68. Closson RG, Biggio CA, Childress L, Cox T, Leonard JH, Proffitt DF, Raymond LA, Schleider EM, Teeter ME, Yee EM. Multi-institutional drug-use evaluation of intraocular irrigating solutions. Am J Hosp Pharm 1990;47:2255–2259.

69. Rao GN, Aquavella JV, Goldberg SH, Berk SL. Pseudophakic bullous keratopathy: Relationship to preoperative corneal endothelial status. Ophthalmology 1984;91:1135–40.

70. Kline OR, Symes DJ, Lorenzetti OJ, de Faller JM. Effect of BSS Plus on the corneal endothelium with intraocular lens implantation. J Toxicol Cut Ocul Toxicol 1983;2:243–247.

71. Haimann MH, Abrams GW, Edelhauser HF, Hatchell DL. The effect of intraocular irrigating solutions on lens clarity in normal and diabetic rabbits. Am J Ophthalmol 1982;94:594–605.

72. Kinoshita JH, Kador P, Catiles M. Aldose reductase in diabetic cataracts. JAMA 1981;246:257–261.

73. Herr RD, White GL, Bernhisel K, Mamalis N, Swanson E. Clinical comparison of ocular irrigation fluids following chemical injury. Am J Emerg Med 1991;9:228–231.

74. Riley MV, Winkler BS, Czajkowski CA, et al. The roles of bicarbonate and CO_2 in transendothelial fluid movement and control of corneal thickness. Invest Ophthalmol Vis Sci 1995;36:103–112.

CHAPTER 17

Dyes

Cristina M. Schnider

The use of dyes as ophthalmic diagnostic agents was first reported in the late 1800s following Baeyer's synthesis of fluorescein in 1871.[1] Since that time, numerous agents have been employed externally for assessing the integrity of the ocular surface, lacrimal system patency, and for certain diagnostic procedures such as Goldmann tonometry. Sodium fluorescein has also been used intravenously for assessing anterior segment and retinal vascular function, while a relatively new dye, indocyanine green, has greatly enhanced observation of the choroidal circulation.

Fluorescein Sodium

Fluorescein has been used as a diagnostic agent since Ehrlich's discovery in 1882 that it can enter the anterior chamber of the eye following subcutaneous injection.[2] Ehrlich further observed that following intravenous administration, the dye appears in the anterior chamber as a vertical yellow-green line behind the cornea, and he later used this observation to study aqueous flow. It was, however, Straub[3] who in 1888 popularized the clinical application of fluorescein for the detection of corneal ulcers. In 1910 Burk[4] first reported the use of fluorescein to detect retinal disease.

Pharmacology

Fluorescein is a yellow acid dye of the xanthene series. Its molecular weight is 376, and its solubility in water at 15°C is 50%. It is generally formulated as its sodium salt[5] (Fig. 17.1).

When exposed to light, fluorescein absorbs certain wavelengths and emits fluorescent light of a longer specific wavelength. The absorbed and emitted wavelengths of light can be measured spectrophotofluorimetrically. Figure 17.2 ilustrates the resultant excitation and emission spectra. An overlap occurs between the wavelengths of light absorbed and those emitted. For dilute concentrations of fluorescein, light of wavelength 530 nm produces the maximum intensity of fluorescence.[5]

Since fluorescein is a weak acid, depending on the pH of the solution, it can exist in various ionic states. Below pH 2, the cationic form predominates and a weak blue-green fluorescence occurs. Between pH 2–4, the cations dissociate to neutral molecules. At pH 7, negative ions prevail and are associated with a brilliant yellow-green fluorescence.[5]

Several factors can alter the fluorescence of fluorescein in solution: its concentration, the pH of the solution, the presence of other substances, and the intensity and wavelength of the absorbed light. Increasing the concentration to a maximum of approximately 0.001% results in increased intensity. Likewise, the intensity of fluorescence increases

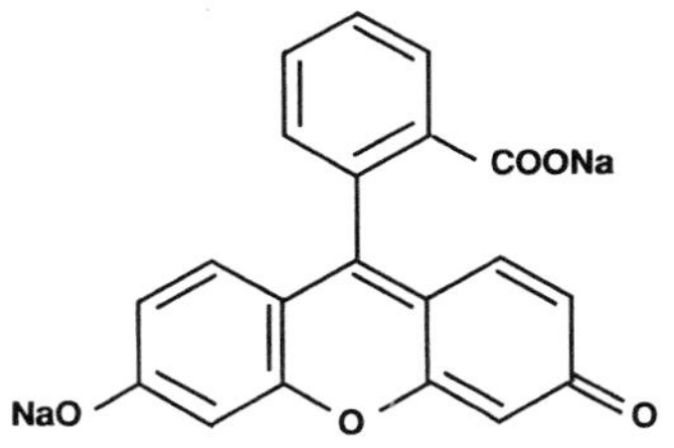

FIGURE 17.1   **Molecular structure of fluorescein sodium.**

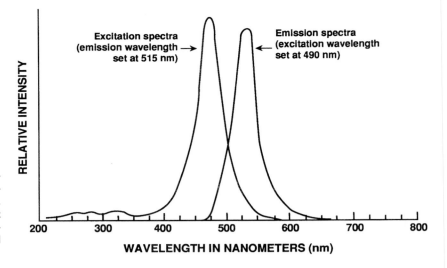

FIGURE 17.2 **Excitation and emission spectra of a 0.00005% solution of sodium fluorescein in KH₂PO₄-K₂HPO₄ buffer at pH 8.** (Reprinted with permission from Romanchuk KG. Fluorescein. Physiochemical factors affecting its fluorescence. Surv Ophthalmol 1982;26:269–283.)

with increasing pH, reaching a plateau at approximately pH 8. Thus, at physiologic pH the fluorescence is nearly maximum. Further increases in pH above 8 reduce the intensity of fluorescence.[5,6]

Clinical Uses

Fluorescein may be applied topically to the eye in the form of a solution or by fluorescein-impregnated filter paper strips (Table 17.1). It is also available in injection form for intravenous use (Table 17.2).

Fluorescein in solution is highly susceptible to bacterial contamination, especially by *Pseudomonas aeruginosa*.[7] This organism grows easily in the presence of fluorescein. Several methods have been devised to reduce the possibility of bacterial growth. Kimura[8] developed fluorescein-impregnated filter paper strips. On wetting the strip, the dye is released and can be applied to the eye. Commercially available fluorescein strips have proved clinically useful for applanation tonometry, contact lens fitting, and other ocular diagnostic procedures requiring topical fluorescein.

The need for sterile fluorescein has also resulted in the development of sterile, combination fluorescein-anesthetic solutions.[9,10] An example of such a preparation is Fluress, which was developed in 1967 (see Table 17.1). Fluress is a combination of sodium fluorescein and a local anesthetic, benoxinate hydrochloride. The preparation contains chlorobutanol 1% as a preservative. The solution is buffered with boric acid to pH 5.[11]

Fluress is remarkably resistant to bacterial contamination.[8–10,12] Bacteriologic studies to determine the bacteriostatic and bactericidal activity, as well as self-sterilization rate of the solution, have been carried out. Using select

organisms to determine maximum dilution for bacteriostatic and bactericidal activity, Fluress has been found to be bactericidal against pathogenic organisms known to infect ocular tissues[10,14] (Table 17.3). The self-sterilization rate of Fluress has been studied by inoculation of the solution with various microorganisms.[12,14] Quickert[10] observed resterilization times of 5 to 120 minutes, depending on the concentration and type of organisms used. The bacterial count declined

TABLE 17.1
Fluorescein Preparations for Topical Ocular Use

Fluorescein Sodium Solutions	
Fluorescein sodium (various manufacturers)	2%; 1, 2, 15 ml
Fluress (Pilkington/ Barnes-Hind)	0.25% with 0.4% benoxinate HCl, boric acid, povidone, 1% chlorobutanol; 5 ml
Fluorocaine (Akorn)	0.25% with 0.5% proparacaine HCl, povidone, glycerin, 0.01% thimerosal
Proparacaine Fluorescein (Bausch and Lomb)	0.25% with 0.5% proparacaine HCl
Fluorescein Strips	
Ful-Glo (Pilkington/ Barnes-Hind)	0.6 mg; sterile
Fluor-I-Strip (Wyeth-Ayerst)	9 mg; with buffers, 0.5% chlorobutanol, polysorbate 80
Fluor-I-Strip-A.T. (Wyeth-Ayerst)	1 mg, with buffers, 0.5% chlorobutanol, polysorbate 80
Fluorets (Akorn)	1 mg
Fluorexon	
Fluoresoft (Akorn, Holles)	0.35% in 0.5 ml pipettes

TABLE 17.2
Fluorescein Preparations for Intravenous Use

Fluorescite (Alcon)	10% in buffered sterile solution; 5 ml ampules
Funduscein-10 (Ciba Vision)	10% in sterile water; 5 ml ampules
AK-Fluor (Akorn)	10% in sterile water; 5 ml ampules
	25% in buffered sterile solution; 2 ml ampules
Fluorescite (Alcon)	25% in buffered sterile solution; 2 ml ampules
Funduscein-25 (Ciba Vision)	25% in sterile water; 3 ml ampules

TABLE 17.3
Resterilizing Time Studies for Fluress

Organisms	Range of Organisms Inoculated Per Tube	Time (min) Required to Kill All Organisms (range)
Klebsiella	6.8×10^4–1.7×10^6	15–120
Pseudomonas aeruginosa μ-21-A	1.9×10^5–1.9×10^6	15–60
P. aeruginosa 7700	4.2×10^4–7.7×10^5	5–120
Escherichia coli K-12	2.6×10^4–7.5×10^5	30–120
E. coli 931	5.7×10^4–1.3×10^6	30–120
Staphylococcus aureus FDA-209	1.8×10^4–2.9×10^5	120–180[a]
S. aureus 6538P	8.4×10^3–6.8×10^4	90>180[a]
Proteus vulgaris	6.1×10^4–7.7×10^5	30–120
Candida albicans	1.5×10^4–1.1×10^5	75–120[a]

[a]In some experiments the exposure time required exceeded 180 minutes. In these instances specific kill times were not determined. However, the organisms were all killed when examined at 24 hours.
From Quickert MH. A fluorescein-anesthetic solution for applanation tonometry. Arch Ophthalmol 1967;77:736. Copyright © 1967. American Medical Association.

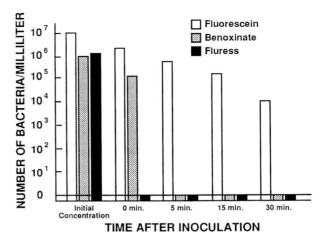

FIGURE 17.3 **Number of *Pseudomonas aeruginosa* present at various times following contamination of fluorescein, benoxinate, and Fluress. (Adapted from Yolton DP, German CJ. Fluress, fluorescein, and benoxinate: recovery from bacterial contamination. J Am Optom Assoc 1980;51:471–474.)**

significantly from the moment the inoculum was added to the Fluress. Yolton and German[12] reported that no organisms could be recovered in even the zero-time sample of Fluress incubated with *P. aeruginosa* or *Staphylococcus aureus*. Figure 17.3 shows the results with *P. aeruginosa*. No detectable bacteria were present in the zero-time sample. Similar data were reported with *S. aureus*. In addition, no microorganisms have been recovered from open bottles of Fluress in routine clinical use for one month or more.[13]

The preservatives used to prevent growth of microorganisms in fluorescein solutions include chlorobutanol and thimerosal. Fluorescein inactivates others, such as benzalkonium chloride, and forms a precipitate. Since fluorescein solutions can support the growth of bacteria,[7] care must be exercised with nonpreserved preparations. Sterile single-dose vials of fluorescein solutions or filter paper strips are recommended for topical use if a preservative is clinically contraindicated. Solutions of fluorescein may be sterilized by autoclaving.

Topical Ocular Applications

ASSESSMENT OF OCULAR SURFACE INTEGRITY

Fluorescein is frequently used in clinical practice to detect lesions of the ocular surface. Because of its high degree of ionization at physiologic pH, fluorescein does not penetrate the intact corneal epithelium, nor does it form a firm bond with any vital tissue.[6,16] Breakdown of the epithelium allows for stromal penetration, and, depending on the extent of the lesion, fluorescein may appear in the anterior chamber as a greenish "flare."[15]

Instillation of the dye in the cul de sac allows detection of corneal and conjunctival lesions such as abrasions, ulcers, and edema and aids in the detection of foreign bodies. When observed with the cobalt blue filter of the slit lamp, the epithelial defect usually appears outlined in vivid green fluorescence, since the yellow-orange dye diffuses freely through the intercellular spaces and accumulates in the defect.[6] However, the addition of a golden yellow barrier filter over the observation system of the slit lamp, Burton lamp or camera will greatly enhance visibility of the stained areas, especially on the conjunctiva.[17] The conjunctiva's

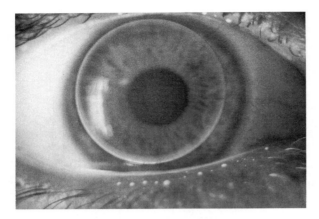

FIGURE 17.4 **Fluorescein photograph of rigid lens fit taken without barrier filter.**

natural fluorescence tends to obscure all but the most severe staining without the barrier filter enhancement. Kodak Wratten #12 or #15 photographic filters or Tiffen #2 photographic filters are relatively inexpensive and serve well in this capacity (Figs. 17.4 and 17.5). The yellow barrier filter must be placed over the optics of the instrument, and not in the path of the blue excitation light. Cox and Fonn[18] have described a system for fluorescein photography that incorporates a band-pass interference filter over the flash attachment, with the barrier filter over the camera lens, to excite and view the fluorescein optimally, while masking annoying flash reflections.

Korb and Herman[19] have suggested that sequential instillations of fluorescein (up to 6 times, 5 minutes apart) may have value as a mildly provocative test of corneal integrity.

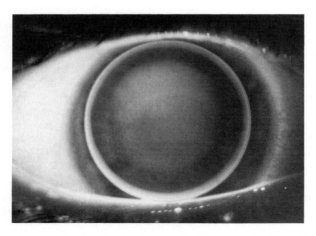

FIGURE 17.5 **Fluorescein photograph of rigid lens fit taken with a Wratten #12 yellow barrier filter in place.**

They found that although only 19% of patients showed fluorescein staining following a single instillation of fluorescein, an additional 23% exhibited staining following repeated instillations. They also noted that the severe degrees of staining appeared to be correlated with contact lens intolerance.

Fluorescein does not actually stain tissues but rather, demonstrates its green coloration because of its fluorescent properties.[5] The reason for the observed color change from orange-yellow to green is not fully understood. Havener[16] suggests that a break in the epithelial barrier permits penetration of fluorescein into Bowman's layer and stroma whereby the dye makes contact with an alkaline interstitial fluid derived from the aqueous humor, and the fluorescein turns bright green due to its pH indicator properties. Romanchuk,[5] however, believes that the change in color of fluorescein when applied following cataract extraction results from its dilution by the leaking of aqueous humor from the anterior chamber. He further suggests that the staining seen with corneal lesions could result from fluorescence of the intracellular contents of groups of cells after fluorescein has gained entry into a damaged cell and is then transferred to the interior of adjacent cells. The exact mechanism of staining of corneal lesions by fluorescein requires further study before a definitive conclusion can be reached.

Fluorescein is useful during corneal surgical procedures such as corneal transplantation.[16] Topical administration of the dye during trephining can detect aqueous leakage from the anterior chamber. When the cornea has been penetrated and the aqueous begins to leak, the dye appears bright green. The dye may also be used to perform Seidel's test,[20] in which a drop of fluorescein is placed on the superior bulbar conjunctiva in an attempt to detect a surgical wound leakage following cataract extraction. If a leak is present, a bright green rivulet of aqueous flows through the fluorescein on the cornea. This line of fluorescence can be traced to its origin and is best seen with cobalt blue light or the cobalt blue filter of the slit lamp (see Fig. 31.1).[5]

CONTACT LENS FITTING AND MANAGEMENT

Vital staining of the tear film is a major aid in the fitting of rigid gas-permeable contact lenses.[21] Following topical application of fluorescein to the eye, the tear layer becomes visible, with a characteristic pattern of green fluorescence. By observing the fluorescein-stained tear film with an ultraviolet light or the cobalt blue filter of the slit lamp, the fit of the lens may be determined. However, it should be noted that more recently developed contact lens materials may contain polymers that block the transmission of light in the ultraviolet region. Therefore, when using an ultraviolet light source such as a Burton lamp, the fluorescein behind the lens may not be visible. Visualizing the fluorescein necessitates changing to a blue light source in the visible region. This may be accomplished by fitting the Burton lamp or other

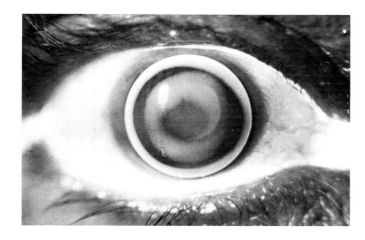

FIGURE 17.6 **Contact lens fluorescein pattern in eye with keratoconus. Central, dark area reflects the absence of fluorescein, indicating central contact lens bearing (touch). There is also bearing in the intermediate area surrounded by peripheral clearance indicated by the pooling of fluorescein. (Courtesy A. Christopher Snyder, O.D.)**

ultraviolet light with a white light source covered with a deep blue excitation filter such as a Kodak Wratten #47, #47A or #47B photographic filter. Areas where the lens makes corneal contact show minimal fluorescence or absence of the fluorescein dye (Fig. 17.6).

In addition to its usefulness during contact lens fitting procedures, fluorescein is essential for assessing the integrity of the cornea in contact lens wearers. Since fluorescein penetrates the corneal epithelium only at sites of interrupted epithelial integrity, the dye will disclose areas where the contact lens may be disrupting the corneal epithelium.[22]

The practitioner should be cautious when interpreting apparent fluorescein staining in a contact lens wearer, since areas of indentation, which do not represent cellular damage, will also demonstrate increased fluorescence. Indentation may result from the accumulation of bubbles (known as *dimple veil*), or from compression by a lens edge or poorly finished junction, which often results in an arcuate pattern of fluorescein pooling. In the case of soft lenses, pooling of fluorescein around the limbus, a condition described by Kame[23] as limbal epithelial hypertrophy (LEH), may be a precursor to neovascularization and/or infiltrative keratitis. Altering lens design or switching solutions, as in the case of trapped bubbles, can solve the problem.

LACRIMAL SYSTEM EVALUATION

Topical ocular fluorescein can be used to evaluate the integrity of the precorneal tear film[24–26] and the patency of the lacrimal drainage system.[27,28]

Assessment of tear breakup time (TBUT), defined as the interval between the last complete blink and the development of the first randomly distributed dry spot in the tear film, is commonly used for determining tear film stability.[25] A wet fluorescein strip is applied to the superior or superotemporal aspect of the bulbar conjunctiva. Using the cobalt blue filter of the slit lamp, the cornea is scanned during the

interval from the last complete blink to the appearance of the first dry spot (see Fig. 25.5). TBUTs of less than 10 seconds suggest an unstable tear film.[29] The determination of TBUT is used clinically as a diagnostic aid in dry eye syndromes and for testing the efficacy of tear replacement products. However, the clinical validity of the test has been questioned, since wide variations in TBUT have been reported.[24] The volume and concentration of fluorescein administered, properties of the precorneal tear film itself, and problems inherent in the technique of measuring TBUT may contribute to the lack of reproducibility in the test.[30,31]

Fluorescein is also useful clinically in evaluating epiphora. Fluorescein testing for lacrimal obstruction usually involves instilling the dye into the conjunctival cul de sac followed by observing for the presence of fluorescein in the nose. Appearance of the dye in the nose or posterior oropharynx indicates that the lacrimal drainage system of that eye is functional.[27,28] Generally a 2% fluorescein solution is used, and this test can be employed in conjunction with other procedures for diagnosis of lacrimal obstruction (see Chapter 25).

APPLANATION TONOMETRY

The use of topical fluorescein is an important component in the measurement of intraocular pressure with the Goldmann applanation tonometer. The dye permits accurate visualization of the 3.06 mm² applanated area.[32]

Measurement of intraocular pressure with the Goldmann applanation tonometer requires that the meniscus of tear fluid surrounding the flattened corneal surface be sufficiently stained with fluorescein so that the apex of the wedge-shaped meniscus is visible. If the fluid apex is not visible, intraocular pressure will be underestimated.[33]

The measurable thickness of a wedge of fluorescein-stained fluid is inversely proportional to the concentration of fluorescein and directly proportional to the concentration of a

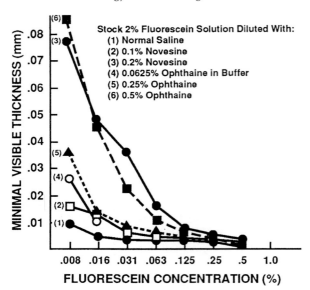

FIGURE 17.7 **The thickness of fluid minimally visible as fluorescent for different fluorescein concentrations and solvents.** (Published with permission from the American Journal of Ophthalmology 49:1149–1155, 1960. Copyright The Ophthalmic Publishing Company.)

substance that can suppress fluorescence.[4] Moses[33] measured the thickness of a minimally visible fluorescent solution at varying concentrations of fluorescein. The vehicle for dilution of the dye was either (1) normal saline alone, (2) equal parts of saline with the anesthetics benoxinate (Novesine) or proparacaine (Ophthaine), or (3) anesthetic solution combined with fluorescein solution. The data indicate that at low fluorescein concentrations, the fluid apex becomes less visible. Although both topical anesthetics impaired fluorescence in a concentration-dependent manner, the quenching effect was least with 0.1% benoxinate (Fig. 17.7).

The effect of anesthetics on the fluorescence of fluorescein can be explained in part by the acidity of the anesthetic solutions (pH 4–4.5), since fluorescein loses its ability to fluoresce in acid solutions.[34] However, since fluorescence is only slightly greater in the presence of a buffer, the anesthetic base must also be able to reduce the fluorescence to some degree.

The concentration of fluorescein that is most satisfactory for applanation tonometry appears to be 0.25% solution.[35] Previous instillation of an anesthetic does not interfere with the fluorescence, provided the anesthetic has been absorbed and is not present in the cul de sac.[9]

It has been suggested that Goldmann applanation tonometry can be performed without fluorescein.[36,37] With the white light of a biomicroscope, intraocular pressure can be measured following the application of an anesthetic alone,

when the two mires are aligned to the point of touch. However, several investigators have compared ocular tension measurements with Goldmann applanation tonometry in the presence and absence of fluorescein.[38–40] The results indicate that readings using white light without fluorescein are significantly lower than those obtained using cobalt blue light with fluorescein. Roper[38] found an underestimation of 5.62 mm Hg when fluorescein was not used. Bright and associates[40] found that readings without fluorescein were lower by an average of 7.01 mm Hg (Table 17.4). The mean reading with Fluress was 18.03 mm Hg as compared to 11.02 mm Hg with the anesthetic, Ophthetic, in the absence of fluorescein. By performing a regression analysis, these investigators further suggest that the difference in intraocular pressure readings with and without fluorescein becomes even greater as the pressure rises.

The lower readings observed in the absence of fluorescein can result from difficulties in viewing the applanated area. The apex of the tear film meniscus, which defines the applanated area, is not clearly visible without fluorescein. The applanated area may be less than 3.06 mm², thus resulting in underestimation of intraocular pressure (Fig. 17.8).[40]

Although there could be certain advantages to performing Goldmann tonometry without fluorescein, including avoidance of possible contamination of the eye or soft contact lens, the differences in the readings at higher pressures can cause significant clinical problems.

Intravenous Applications

The introduction of fluorescein angiography by Novotny and Alvis[41] in 1961 provided a useful method for studying various parameters of ocular function. Intravenous fluorescein is used extensively to delineate vascular abnormalities of the fundus and occasionally to evaluate anterior segment blood and aqueous flow.[42,43]

FLUORESCEIN ANGIOGRAPHY

In the bloodstream fluorescein is excited by a wavelength of 465 nm and emits a wavelength of 525 nm. Circulating fluorescein binds to albumin and red blood cells. It is also metabolized to a weakly fluorescent conjugate, fluorescein monoglucoronide, which exhibits less plasma protein binding than fluorescein. The amount of binding can affect the penetration of fluorescein through blood-ocular barriers.[43,44] Following injection of 10 ml of a 5% solution in the antecubital vein, the dye usually appears in the central retinal artery in 10 to 15 seconds.[45] Both circulation time and integrity of the retina and choroid may be examined.

Fluorescein angiography shows retinal blood vessels in high contrast. Nonvascularized, pigmented retinal and subretinal lesions appear as dark areas against the green fluorescing background.[46] The abnormal fluorescence of various

TABLE 17.4
Results of Intraocular Pressure Readings (mm Hg) from *N* = 100 Eyes for Ophthetic and Fluress

	Mean Tonometric Readings (mm Hg)	Standard Deviation	Standard Error	R	Regression
Fluress	18.03	4.27	0.427	0.552	y = 0.45 + 0.59x
Ophthetic	11.02	4.53	0.453		

From Bright DC, Potter JW, Allen DC, et al. Goldmann applanation tonometry without fluorescein. Am J Optom Physiol Optics 1981;58:1120–1126, with permission of the authors and publisher.

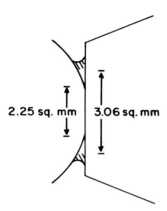

FIGURE 17.8 **Cornea partially flattened by applanation tonometer. The apices of the fluorescein-stained wedges above and below the flattened area are too dilute to be visible. The 3.06 mm² end point of applanation appears to have been reached but in reality consists of a smaller flattened area. (Modified from Moses RA. Fluorescein in applanation tonometry. Am J Ophthalmol 1960;49:1149–1155.)**

retinal and choroidal lesions has been explained by several mechanisms, including (1) some abnormalities in the retina allow for greater visibility of choroidal fluorescence; (2) neovascularization produces enhanced fluorescence due to new vascular channels, and (3) pathologic processes resulting in enhanced capillary permeability allow for leakage of fluorescein into the lesions.[47] These types of abnormalities may often be differentiated by time of onset of fluorescence. Choroidal fluorescence appears early and usually precedes the arterial phase. Depending on the origin of the new vessels, neovascular fluorescence coincides with the arteriolar or venous phase of fluorescence. Enhanced capillary permeability (leakage) delays fluorescence, followed by a slow increase in fluorescence as the dye recirculates and stains the affected tissues.

Fluorescein angiography has proven helpful in the diagnosis of a variety of pathologic conditions of the fundus.

Various macular lesions, central serous choroidopathy,[48] diabetic retinopathy,[49] and disciform macular degeneration show typical fluorescein patterns.

Fluorescein angiography can also differentiate early papilledema from pseudopapilledema. In papilledema, fluorescein angiography shows capillary dilation, microaneurysms, and leakage of the dye into extravascular tissue. The abnormal fluorescence may last for hours. In contrast, no leakage occurs in pseudopapilledema, and the residual fluorescence is insignificant after 10 minutes.[50]

Malignant melanomas, metastatic tumors, and hemangiomas of the choroid also fluoresce. However, since choroidal melanomas and hemangiomas have similar patterns, fluorescein angiography alone cannot differentiate these conditions.[51]

Chapter 32 discusses the clinical procedure and interpretation of fluorescein angiography.

CIRCULATION TIME

Fluorescein can be used to evaluate arm-to-retina circulation time. A fluorescein solution is rapidly injected into the antecubital vein. The appearance of the dye in the central retinal artery of each eye is observed by indirect ophthalmoscopy and is recorded with stopwatches.[52,53]

The normal arm-to-retina circulation time is 11 to 13 seconds, depending on the speed of injection, cardiovascular factors, and intraocular pressure.[53] The time should not differ by more than one second between the two eyes. A prolonged circulation time indicates occlusive carotid disease.

Because the determination of circulation time requires three experienced observers, it is subject to technical error. Although rarely performed today, the determination of circulation time can yield information in support of other clinical findings

IRIS ANGIOGRAPHY

Intravenous injection of fluorescein can be useful for visualization of iris tumors and vessel infarcts.

Following injection into the antecubital vein, the dye first appears in the radial vessels of the iris between 9 and 20 seconds.[54] The amount of iris pigmentation as well as the pattern of its distribution affects the amount of detail observed in a normal iris angiogram. Blue irides generally show the vessels in greater detail than do brown ones.[54] More recently, an adapter mounted in front of a fundus camera lens has made possible more complete visualization of the vascular structure in heavily pigmented irides.[55]

AQUEOUS FLOW

In 1950 Goldmann first measured changes in the concentration of fluorescein in the anterior chamber following intravenous injection.[56] Using a slit-lamp fluorophotometer, the time course of the fluorescence in the circulating blood and the anterior chamber was determined in humans. Goldmann calculated the rate of aqueous flow to be approximately 1.5% to 2% of the volume of the anterior chamber per minute. Since then several other methods have been devised to measure aqueous turnover, and all have given comparable results.[57]

VITREOUS FLUOROPHOTOMETRY

Vitreous fluorophotometry (VFP) is a noninvasive quantitative method for measuring small amounts of fluorescein in various ocular compartments. Cunha-Vaz and associates[58] first introduced this technique to study the blood-retinal barrier. The technique is based on the slit-lamp fluorophotometer method designed by Maurice[59] in 1963.

Since the normal blood-retinal barrier resists various substances, including fluorescein, the presence of fluorescein in the vitreous humor should indicate a functional breakdown of this barrier. Although physiologic factors and instrument artifacts can influence vitreous fluorescence, this technique has been used to detect retinal vascular disease, especially in diabetes.[58,60,61] The procedure has also been used to study the integrity of the blood-retinal barrier in various other diseases, including retinitis pigmentosa,[62] optic neuritis,[63] and essential hypertension.[64]

Oral Fluorescein Angioscopy

Since the integrity of the normal ocular physiologic barriers to fluorescein depends less on dye administration velocity than on certain other parameters, such as retinal circulation time, fluorescein has also been administered by mouth to study certain lesions of the fundus.[65-70] The oral procedure in adults usually involves administering 1 to 2 g of fluorescein powder or 3 vials of 10% injectable fluorescein mixed in a citrus drink over ice.[65,69] In children, fruit juice containing 1 ml of a 10% fluorescein solution/20 ml juice/5 kg body weight has been used to determine macular leakage following removal of congenital cataracts.[67] The dye begins to appear in the fundus in approximately 15 minutes, but maximal fluorescence is not obtained until 45 to 60 minutes following ingestion.[65] Fasting can enhance the serum concentration of the dye.[69]

Oral fluorescein has been used to study disorders characterized by late leakage of dye, such as cystoid macular edema in both children and adults,[65,67-69] and has been used to study retinal vascular abnormalities in young diabetic patients.[70] It is also useful to document other disorders characterized by late leakage, such as retinal pigment epithelial detachment, central serous choroidopathy, and optic disc edema.[69] In the diagnosis of these conditions the arterial and early venous phases of the angiogram are not critical. Note that even in mild cases the oral use of fluorescein can demonstrate late leakage of dye.[65] Oral fluorescein, however, does not clearly outline critical vascular details such as may be needed for photocoagulation.[65]

The use of oral fluorescein thus appears to be a feasible method for evaluating certain clinical conditions in both children and adults. The oral route of administration has the advantage that side effects are rare.[69-71]

Side Effects

Studies in humans indicate that approximately 10% of patients receiving intravenous fluorescein experience adverse effects.[72,73] The most common reaction is nausea, accompanied less frequently by vomiting.[157] The nausea usually occurs 15 to 30 seconds following injection and subsides within several minutes. The incidence of nausea appears to be higher in women. Schatz and Farkos[74] reported that in 400 consecutive patients undergoing intravenous fluorescein angiography, 9.4% of the females experienced nausea compared with 6.1% of male patients. The incidence of post-injection nausea may relate to the concentration of fluorescein used.[75] Intravenous injection of 25% fluorescein resulted in nausea in 23% of patients. Ten percent fluorescein caused nausea in only 11% of patients. With 5% fluorescein the incidence of nausea was only 2%. The speed of injection may also play a role. A slower injection permits more protein binding of the fluorescein in the plasma and thereby reduces the bolus of free fluorescein.[76] Reportedly, the incidence of nausea decreases in susceptible patients by giving 50 mg promethazine orally 1 hour before injecting the dye.[74]

Allergic reactions have also occurred, including urticaria and pruritus. Less frequently, more serious respiratory effects include laryngeal or pulmonary edema.[77,78]

Cardiovascular toxicity in the form of severe hypotension and shock as well as myocardial infarction and basilar artery ischemia have rarely occurred.[78] Other adverse effects reported with intravenous fluorescein include pain at the site of injection, dizziness with rare episodes of fainting, and paresthesia of the tongue and lips.[77]

Patients should be advised that intravenous fluorescein temporarily discolors both skin and urine.

Several investigators have studied the pathophysiologic changes observed during administration of intravenous fluorescein. An allergic reaction of the immediate hypersensitivity type (type I) resulting from an immunologic response of the host to a hapten (drug)-protein combination, or the release of histamine has been proposed as causative factors.[77,79] Studies for cell-mediated immunity reactions have given negative results with fluorescein.[77]

Following infusion of fluorescein, plasma histamine concentrations increase within the first few minutes and remain high up to 10 minutes.[79] Increased histamine has been found in 66% of patients with adverse reactions to fluorescein and in 15% of patients with no reactions. Possibly the occurrence of reactions to fluorescein depends not on the concentration of histamine but, rather, on the individual's susceptibility to respond to histamine in the circulation.[79] Fluorescein also appears in breast milk for up to 76 hours following intravenous administration.[80]

Adverse effects associated with topical fluorescein and anesthetic-fluorescein combinations are usually limited to transient irritation of the cornea or conjunctiva.[10,81] Fluress has been associated with vasovagal responses in three young adults during applanation tonometry. Loss of consciousness was not associated with any other symptoms.[82]

A unique case of grand mal seizure following instillation of Fluress has been reported in one patient.[83] Less than 1 minute following instillation of Fluress into each conjunctival sac, the patient lost consciousness and had a generalized clonic seizure, lasting less than 1 minute. He was placed on the floor and regained consciousness. While lying supine, he had another seizure lasting approximately 1 minute and again regained consciousness. No erythema or edema of the lids or conjunctiva was noted. The patient showed normal findings on follow-up neurologic examination. Note, however, that the fluorescein could not be definitely implicated as the causative factor, since Fluress also contains benoxinate as the anesthetic and a preservative, chlorobutanol. Hypersensitivity testing with each of these ingredients was not performed.

Contraindications

Because of the possibility of adverse reactions, a family and personal history of allergies should be obtained from every patient undergoing fluorescein angiography. Appropriate medications such as epinephrine (1:1000 ampules) should be available in case of allergic responses.[16,79] Other recommended safety precautions include a pressure ventilation device, an airway, corticosteroids, and sedatives[16,76] (see Chap. 38).

Since the topically administered dye will discolor soft contact lenses, the eye should be thoroughly irrigated with

an extraocular irrigation solution or sterile saline until the tears show no discoloration. Two thorough rinses of the upper and lower fornices is recommended. Alternatively, soft lenses should not be reinserted for 1 to 2 hours after fluorescein instillation.

Fluorexon

Since fluorescein sodium can penetrate into soft contact lenses, the lenses become discolored, which is cosmetically objectionable. In addition, the boundary between lens and tears becomes obscured, which precludes the use of fluorescein in soft contact lens fitting. Fluorexon, a molecule similar to that of fluorescein, is less readily absorbed by the soft lens material, which makes it more useful in fitting and evaluating soft and hybrid design lenses.[84]

Pharmacology

Fluorexon, N,N-bis(carboxymethyl)-aminoethylfluorescein tetrasodium salt, has a molecular weight of 710 (Fig. 17.9).[84] Compared with fluorescein sodium, fluorexon has a paler, yellow-brown color. Its staining properties are similar to those of fluorescein sodium. The dye stains epithelial defects but, unlike fluorescein sodium, it does stain devitalized tissue.[85]

Like fluorescein sodium, fluorexon is vulnerable to bacterial contamination,[84] but it appears to support bacterial growth longer than a comparable solution of fluorescein sodium (Table 17.5). For clinical use it is therefore dispensed in single-dose sterile pipettes (see Table 17.1).

Clinical Uses

Fluorexon can aid in the fitting of soft contact lenses and is particularly useful in evaluating hybrid designs such as the SoftPerm lens (Pilkington/Barnes-Hind, Sunnyvale, CA), which consists of a rigid gas permeable center with a hydrogel surround. The use of fluorexon allows visualization of the tear film under the rigid portion of the lens without discoloring the hydrogel portion. Similarly, in a piggy-back

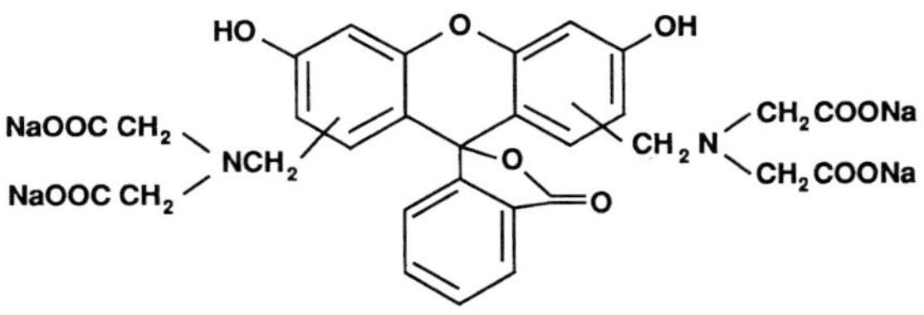

FIGURE 17.9   **Molecular structure of fluorexon.**

TABLE 17.5

Time Course of Contamination of Fluorexon and Fluorescein Following Inoculation with *Pseudomonas aeruginosa*

Contaminant: P. aeruginosa	1 hr	2 hr	24 hr	Meat Broth 24 hr
Control	+[a]	+	+	+
Fluorescein 0.25%	+	+	−[a]	−
Fluorescein 0.25% with benoxinate 0.4%	−	−	−	−
Fluorescein 2.2%	+	+	−	−
Fluorexon 0.25% in normal saline	+	+	+	+

[a]+ means positive culture for organism; −, no growth.

From Refojo MF, Miller D, Fiore AS. A new fluorescent stain for soft hydrophilic lens fitting. Arch Ophthalmol 1972;87:277. Copyright 1972, American Medical Association.

lens system where a rigid lens is placed on a hydrogel lens for fitting special cases such as advanced keratoconus, the use of fluorexon can be a valuable adjunct to the fitting process. It can be applied to the eye with the lens in place, but it is more effective when placed in the posterior bowl of the lens before insertion.

Side Effects

Fluorexon will stain the soft lens if it remains in contact with the lens for more than a few minutes. However, repeated rinsing with saline will usually remove the dye from the lens.

Topical application to the eye may produce a mild stinging sensation. Occasional conjunctival injection has been reported.[84] In clinical use fluorexon has proven nontoxic to ocular tissue. However, it is not widely employed because the observation of dye-stained tears in evaluating soft contact lens fitting is not significantly more effective than evaluating the lens without dye.[85] In addition, observation of the fluorescence requires enhancement by a special yellow filter, which makes the procedure cumbersome.

Contraindications

Fluorexon is not recommended for use with highly hydrated soft lenses with water content of 60% or higher. In such cases the lens can absorb significant amounts of dye resulting in unwanted lens discoloration.

Rose Bengal

Widely identified as a vital dye that stains only degenerated or dead cells and mucous strands,[86] rose bengal has been most frequently used in the diagnosis of ocular surface disease. However, new evidence suggests that it is not truly a vital dye, but one that may actually cause toxicity and cell death under certain circumstances.[87]

Pharmacology

Rose bengal is the 4,5,6,7-tetra-chloro-2′,4′,5′,7′-tetraiodo derivative of fluorescein (Fig. 17.10) and is a commonly used dye for ophthalmic applications. Tissues stained with rose bengal display a vivid pink or magenta color when viewed with white light.[88] It has been formulated as a 1% solution and in the form of sterile impregnated paper strips that require moistening with sterile saline or extraocular irrigation solution.[11]

Rose bengal is a photoreactive compound. When combined with 550 nm wavelength light and oxygen, it generates singlet oxygen,[89,90] which can inactivate enzymes[91,92] and damage single-stranded DNA[93,94] and cell membranes.[95,96] This effect may be responsible for the ability of rose bengal to kill a variety of microorganisms such as viruses,[97] including herpes simplex virus (HSV-1),[98] bacteria[99,100] and protozoa.[101]

More recent studies[87,102] have also demonstrated that cells need not be devitalized or necrotic to display rose bengal staining. In fact, rose bengal will stain numerous types of healthy cultured cells, including rabbit and human corneal epithelial cells in a dose-dependent manner. Furthermore, these studies have also confirmed Norn's[86] earlier observations that the nucleus of the cell retains the dye. Feenstra and Tseng[87] observed a toxic response to rose bengal. Cells exposed to the dye demonstrated instantaneous morphologic changes, loss of cellular motility, cell detachment, and cell death. Exposure to light further augmented this effect, indicating that photosensitivity may be an additional factor in

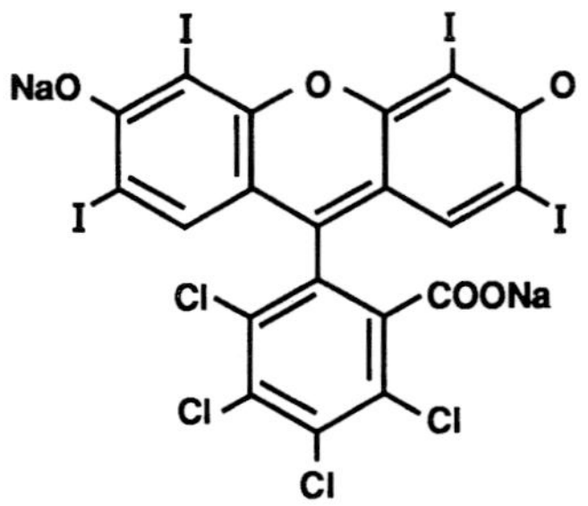

FIGURE 17.10   **Molecular structure of rose bengal.**

the dye's intrinsic toxicity on unprotected epithelial cells. However, this staining could be blocked by the addition of albumin and mucin to the culture medium. This strongly suggests that rose bengal staining results not from a lack of cell vitality but rather from the lack of the protective preocular tear film. This theory appears consistent with the clinical disorders traditionally associated with rose bengal staining, such as keratoconjunctivitis sicca.

Clinical Uses

TOPICAL APPLICATIONS

Marx[103] reported that the first ophthalmic use of rose bengal was a therapeutic one, by Römer, Gebb and Löhlein in 1914. They combined rose bengal with safranine and victoria yellow to treat pneumococcal infection. Marx also credited Kleefeld as the first to use rose bengal as a vital stain in evaluating a corneal ulcer, and himself described punctate staining of the conjunctiva near the lid margin in healthy subjects. Sjögren has been credited with first routinely using the dye in the diagnosis of keratoconjunctivitis sicca (KCS), as described in his M.D. thesis.[104] According to Norn,[86] in normal individuals rose bengal always stains a punctate line on the inferior tarsal conjunctiva along the ciliary margin (Marx's line), a less pronounced line on the superior tarsal conjunctiva, and often the caruncle and the plica semilunaris.

Traditionally, the most frequent use of rose bengal is in the differential diagnosis of dry eye syndromes.[104] However, based on the original concept that the dye does not stain healthy epithelial cells, but only devitalized cells and mucous strands, rose bengal has also found other uses in clinical practice. Rose bengal has been recommended in the evaluation of most types of corneal and conjunctival lesions including abrasions, ulcerations and foreign bodies,[105] as well as dendrites[106] and conjunctival dysplasia or metaplasia.[107] However, when used as the sole agent, its effectiveness in establishing the presence of a clinically significant dry eye has been debated. Golding and Brennan[108] showed that rose bengal staining had a 93% sensitivity and 93% specificity in differentiating between a group of 15 control and 15 dry eye subjects. They suggest combining the use of rose bengal and fluorescein tear break-up time with administration of the McMonnies Dry Eye Questionnaire[109] to improve the ability to diagnose dry eye problems. Others have suggested a combination of laboratory tear function tests such as lactoferrin and lysozyme test, with clinical tests such as rose bengal staining and Schirmer tests, to aid in discriminating between Sjögren's and non-Sjögren's KCS.[110] George and associates[111] have developed a grading scale for quantifying rose bengal staining and suggest that this system may help to assess the severity of dry eye as well as measure treatment effects (Fig. 17.11). Table 17.6 outlines the assessment system. With the knowledge of rose bengal's staining mechanism, the combination of sodium fluorescein and rose bengal may indeed improve the ability to differentiate between cellular damage and disruption of the preocular tear film.[112]

The use of rose bengal in the evaluation of treatment effectiveness has also been variable. Most studies have shown minimal utility when using rose bengal alone,[113] but some have reported success using rose bengal staining with other findings as part of a statistical analysis.[114] Gilbard and associates[115] have demonstrated decreases in rose bengal staining with the use of punctal occlusion[115] and an experimental artificial tear solution[116] but could not show improvement with a vitamin A ointment.[117] It is unclear whether these disparities result from actual treatment effectiveness or inadequacy of the rose bengal staining technique. Therefore, rose bengal should be employed as only one measure in a battery of tests to determine whether a treatment is effective, and controlled clinical trials should be performed to evaluate a potential treatment modality for KCS.

INTRAVENOUS APPLICATIONS

Rose bengal has been used intravenously in animal studies as an initiator for photothrombosis, a novel technique for facilitating the occlusion of blood vessels. Photothrombosis results in vascular occlusion by aggregating platelets responding to photochemically-induced endothelial damage.[118,119] This approach contrasts with the current technique of argon laser photocoagulation, which causes occlusion as a consequence of thermal damage to the vessels. In studies of experimental lipid keratopathy, Mendelsohn and associates[120,121] caused occlusion of corneal neovasculature with photothrombosis using 8 times less intensity and 27 times less energy than with photocoagulation. Huang and associates[122] demonstrated the effectiveness of intravenous rose bengal with argon laser irradiation to occlude long-standing corneal neovascularization in rabbits. They postulated that the long-lasting effect of photothrombosis may result from the fact that thrombi induced by rose bengal consist largely of platelets that contain little or no fibrin and thus resist fibrinolysis by tissue-type plasminogen activator. They also demonstrated that the efficiency of the occlusive effect is dose-dependent. In rabbits, a dose of 8 mg/kg body weight was sufficient for treating corneal neovascularization.

These early animal studies demonstrate the potential for using rose bengal in photothrombosis for treatment of anterior segment neovascularization and possibly the posterior segment as well.[119] Proposed uses include treating ocular surface disorders with conjunctival overgrowth, such as chemical burns, Stevens-Johnson syndrome, and some contact lens-induced vascularization; exudative keratopathy; and as an adjunct treatment for vascularized corneas before penetrating keratoplasty to prevent graft rejection.[122]

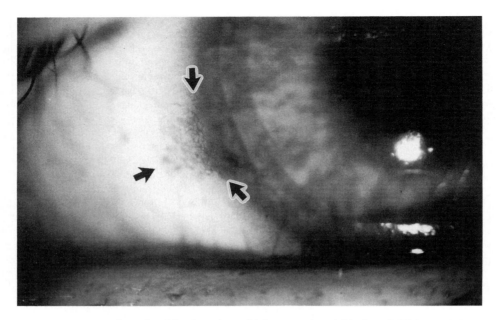

FIGURE 17.11   **Rose bengal staining in patient with keratoconjunctivitis sicca (KCS) (arrows). Note the typical triangular shape and location in the area of lid gap of the cornea and conjunctiva. (Courtesy Mark Williams, O.D.)**

TABLE 17.6
Proposed Grading Scale for Rose Bengal Staining

Grade	Description of Severity	Punctate Dots
0	Absent	0
1	Minimal	3–10
2	Mild	11–30
3	Moderate	31–80
4	Severe	>80

Adapted from George MA, Abelson MB, Mooshian ML, et al. Development of a precise method using rose bengal in the evaluation of dry eye severity and the detection of potential treatment effects. Invest Ophthalmol Vis Sci 1993; 34(suppl):1472.

Side Effects

As noted previously, rose bengal is not truly a vital stain in that it actually contributes to the death of cells unprotected by a coating of mucin and albumin. The ability of rose bengal to stain cells is dose-related.[86,87,102,123] Smarting or stinging commonly occurs with rose bengal and is often proportional to the degree of epithelial damage observed.[123–125] Topical anesthetics, which appear to have a negligible effect on the observed staining, may be employed prior to instilling the rose bengal to reduce the stinging.

Intravenously administered rose bengal (100 mg) is uniformly nontoxic in humans when used for colorimetric liver function studies.[126] However, because the liver metabolizes rose bengal, a potential risk of intravenously delivered rose bengal is altered liver function. Huang and associates[122] reported only transient alteration of liver enzymes with a dose of 40 mg/kg, the highest dose tested. A slight pinkish discoloration of the mucosal surfaces was observed during the first 24 hours following rose bengal injection.

Contraindications

Since rose bengal will also stain skin, clothing, and contact lenses, contact with these should be avoided. In the soft contact lens wearer, thorough irrigation of the ocular surface and fornices should be performed before resuming contact lens wear.

A dilemma exists with the use of rose bengal in the differential diagnosis of dendritic lesions of the cornea. Rose bengal is particularly useful in identifying epithelial herpetic corneal ulcers, by virtue of the characteristic staining of the edges of the dendritic lesion, while fluorescein stains the center. However, due to its potent antiviral activity, the use of rose bengal on a suspected herpetic ulcer may preclude a positive culture result, thus delaying the appropriate course of therapy. Therefore, the severity of the corneal lesion and the importance of positive identification of the causative organism must be carefully considered when making the decision whether to use rose bengal. A false-negative culture result can lead to inappropriate treatment.

The use of intravenous rose bengal is contraindicated in patients with a history of liver disease or dysfunction.[88,126]

Lissamine Green

Lissamine green is a vital stain that stains degenerate cells, dead cells, and mucus in much the same way as does rose bengal.[127] It is also widely used in the food industry as a colorant.

Pharmacology

Lissamine green has a chemical formula of $C_{27}H_{25}N_2NaO_7S_2$ and a molecular weight of 576.6. Figure 17.12 shows the molecular structure of lissamine green B.

Clinical Uses

Lissamine green 1% stains identically to 1% rose bengal.[127] It may be useful when a red dye is not desirable or when another red dye is used simultaneously.[127] Other authors have reported the use of lissamine green along with rose bengal in assessing dry eye conditions.[128,129] Chodosh and associates[130] have demonstrated that lissamine green stains membrane-damaged epithelial cells as well as corneal stroma, in a manner similar to fluorescein, and, like rose bengal, also binds to the nuclei of severely damaged cells. These investigators also reported an antiviral effect *in vitro* with lissamine green B concentrations as low as 0.06%.

Side Effects

Instillation of lissamine green B into the conjunctival sac appears to cause no ocular irritation; no other adverse effects have been reported. Clinical experience suggests the staining effect of lissamine green to be longer lasting than rose bengal.

Contraindications

There appear to be no known contraindications for the topical ocular use of lissamine green B.

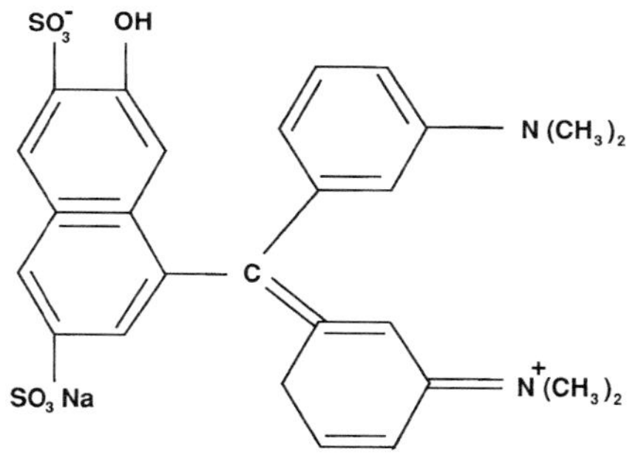

FIGURE 17.12   **Molecular structure of lissamine green B.**

Sulforhodamine B

Sulforhodamine B, also known as *sulphorhodamine B,* can enhance viewing of the conjunctival tear film by separating the green natural fluorescence of the ocular tissues from that of the tear film.[130,131]

Pharmacology

Sulforhodamine B, molecular weight 559, has a chemical structure and properties similar to those of fluorescein but is less lipid soluble. Its fluorescence is orange and is most readily excited by green light, with peak absorption and emission wavelengths of 556 and 572 nm, respectively. It is usually supplied as an acid and must be dissolved in alkali, with solubility achieved up to approximately 20 g/l at pH 7.[130]

Clinical Uses

Due to the strong natural fluorescence of the sclera and crystalline lens, sodium fluorescein does not always permit optimal visualization of corneal and conjunctival staining. Sulforhodamine B fluoresces at longer wavelengths and does not suffer this limitation. Illuminating by green light and viewing through an orange filter can completely eliminate the background fluorescence of the sclera, allowing observation of the tear film over even the conjunctival surface. This approach increases the sensitivity of detecting subtle staining on the conjunctival epithelial surface.[130,131]

Clinically, use of a band pass filter for excitation with wavelengths between 520 and 550 nm, and a Wratten #25 filter (for slit lamp observation) or Wratten #22 (for photography) over the objective allows visualization of the tear film and ocular surface in the presence of sulforhodamine B. Eliason and Maurice[131] compared staining using 0.5% to 2% sulforhodamine B with that of fluorescein and rose bengal in both normal and pathologic eyes, and found that this dye had a greater sensitivity for identifying tear film discontinuities and conjunctival staining than either rose bengal or fluorescein. Chodosh and associates[130] found that sulforhodamine B, like fluorescein, does not stain epithelial cells *in vitro* but does stain corneal explant stroma. They also found that, as with rose bengal, 1% sulforhodamine B inhibits herpes simplex virus plaque formation *in vitro*.

Side Effects

The topical ocular use of sulforhodamine B appears to cause no side effects. Doses of up to 1 g/kg could be injected intraperitoneally in the mouse without causing death, and 50 μg of the saturated solution injected into the stroma of a rabbit cornea had as little effect as an equal volume of saline.[131]

Contraindications

There appear to be no known contraindications for the topical ocular use of sulforhodamine B.

Indocyanine Green

Although the possibility of using indocyanine green (ICG) to observe vasculature of the human choroid was first introduced in the early 1970s,[132–134] not until nearly 20 years later did it gain widespread recognition as a clinical diagnostic tool. Modifications to the original technique[135–137] and availability of commercial ICG angiographic instrumentation were primary factors leading to its emergence into clinical practice.

Pharmacology

ICG is a water-soluble, tricarbocyanine dye with its peak absorption in the near infrared spectrum at 805 nm and maximal emission at 835 nm (Fig. 17.13). This feature constitutes an important difference between ICG and fluorescein angiography. In the 800 nm region of ICG absorp-

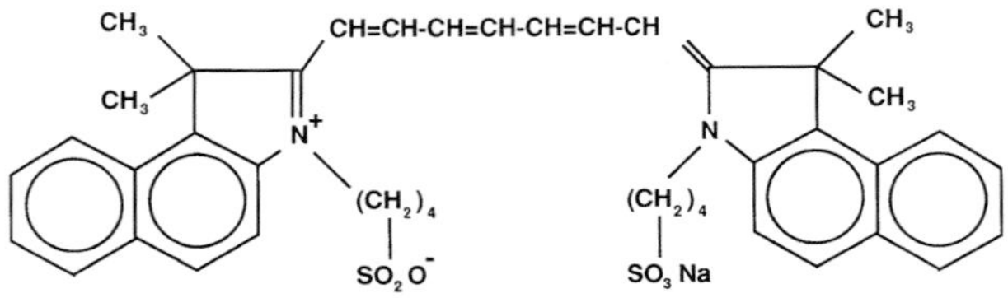

FIGURE 17.13 **Molecular structure of indocyanine green.**

tion, the pigment epithelium and choroid absorb only 21% to 38% of the light, compared to 59% to 75% in the 500 nm region with fluorescein.[138] Photography in the near infrared region also enhances angiogram viewing in the presence of media opacities and subretinal exudation of fluid or blood.[139] Moreover, unlike fluorescein, after intravenous injection ICG is rapidly and completely bound to plasma proteins in blood (especially albumin), so that it does not leak through the fenestrated capillaries of the choriocapillaris to obscure underlying details.[140]

Clinical Uses

Although it has been used in the past to assess viability of rabbit corneal endothelial cells before keratoplasty,[141] ICG's primary use is as a fluorescent dye for retinal and choroidal angiography. Its low fluorescence property initially limited its use in angiography studies.[142] Improvements in video technology,[135] the introduction of appropriate excitation and barrier filters,[134,135] and the development of the scanning laser ophthalmoscope with a modification to permit infrared recording[143] finally allowed choroidal angiograms with high temporal and spatial resolution.

Indocyanine green videoangiography (ICGV) is useful in studying a variety of choroidal abnormalities, including congenital anomalies as well as ischemic, inflammatory, and degenerative disorders. It is used most frequently to identify and characterize choroidal neovascularization (CNV) in age-related macular degeneration (ARMD).[158–160] The collaborative work of the Macular Photocoagulation Study Group has shown that laser photocoagulation is of value in treating CNV.[144–146,158,159] However, fewer than half of newly diagnosed patients with ARMD are eligible for laser therapy based on the results of fluorescein angiography alone.[139] Cases of ill-defined or occult CNV on the fluorescein angiogram are generally associated with poorer results with laser photocoagulation. The efficacy of angiography could be improved with the ability of the ICGV technique to locate and image more accurately the vessels targeted for photocoagulation.

ICG is available commercially as Cardio-Green (Becton-Dickinson).[11] Yannuzzi and associates'[139] technique of administration consisted of dissolving the dye in an aqueous solvent supplied by the manufacturer to a concentration of 12.5 mg/ml, for a total dose of 50 mg. It was administered via injection into the antecubital vein at a rate of 1 cc per second. Images were then obtained at 1 or 2 second intervals until the retinal and choroidal circulations were at maximum brightness, and at increasing intervals over 30 to 40 minutes until fluorescence subsided. Destro and Puliafito[136] used an ICG concentration of 50 mg/ml and injected 3.0 mg/kg followed by a 5.0 ml flush of sterile saline. They found this dose to be well tolerated.

ICGV studies have demonstrated that visualization of the

choroid is greater than with fluorescein angiography, and they allow imaging of rapid choroidal filling not captured by fluorescein angiography.[136,161,162] Moreover, the ICG remains in the area of the CNV long after the dye has cleared from the surrounding retinal and choroidal circulation. Thus, the ICGV technique appears to be particularly beneficial for visualizing poorly defined membranes, especially those with overlying hemorrhage and those near the edge of previously treated areas.[139,162] Use of the infrared scanning laser ophthalmoscope can provide the high resolution required to make the ICGV technique even more successful.[143] Yoneya and Noyori[156] have recently suggested, moreover, that binding ICG with autologous serum prior to injection may further enhance the angiographic results.

Side Effects

Intravenous ICG has proven essentially as safe as sodium fluorescein.[73,147,163] No toxic effects have occurred with ICG doses of 6 mg/kg to 11 mg/kg,[148] but severe allergic reactions have been reported.[149,150,164] In one study,[139] ICG was generally well tolerated and caused fewer reactions than did fluorescein. However, two patients developed hives, and one experienced transient nausea and vomiting. In another series of ICG angiograms of 32 eyes with suspected choroidal neovascularization,[136] patients generally found the near-infrared illumination of the technique more comfortable than that used in fluorescein angiography. Patients did not experience nausea or other adverse effects from ICG. Since ICG remains bound to proteins in the blood and is rapidly metabolized by the liver, discoloration of the urine, skin, or mucous membranes does not occur.

Contraindications

Because ICG contains a small amount of sodium iodide, it should not be used in patients with sensitivities to iodine or shellfish,[88,139] or in patients at high risk for anaphylactic reaction. The safety of this agent in pregnancy has not been established.

Methylene Blue

This vital stain has properties similar to those of rose bengal. It can stain devitalized cells as well as mucus and corneal nerves. It is not a specific stain when applied to the eye because the blue areas may be either cells or mucus. Norn,[151] therefore, does not recommend its use on the cornea. Methylene blue is useful for staining the lacrimal sac before dacryocystorhinostomy (DCR),[16] and it may prove useful in gonioscopic ab interno laser sclerostomy.[152]

Pharmacology

Methylene blue is an aniline dye with an absorption peak of 660 nm. It has bacteriostatic properties against microorganisms.[124] The dye is usually employed as a 5% solution, and benzalkonium chloride may be added to the dye solution to enhance sterility. Methylene blue precipitates in alkaline solutions.

Clinical Uses

Vital staining of corneal nerves requires up to three instillations at 5-minute intervals.[16] The bluish ocular discoloration may remain for 24 hours.

For staining of the lacrimal sac before surgery, the sac is irrigated with methylene blue. The dye should remain in the sac for several minutes. Before beginning surgery the dye should be washed out of the sac, since it can spill out on incision and stain the surrounding tissues.[16]

Side Effects

When topically applied, methylene blue can be quite irritating to ocular tissue. A topical anesthetic may be used, since it enhances penetration of the drug at the same time as it relieves the discomfort.[124]

Contraindications

Methylene blue is contraindicated in patients allergic to the dye.

Trypan Blue

This stain has proven useful as an indicator of corneal endothelial integrity.

Pharmacology

Trypan blue is an anionic acid dye. It appears to stain only damaged or dead endothelial cells.[153]

Clinical Uses

Vital staining with trypan blue has been advocated for determining the suitability of human donor corneal material for grafting.[153,154] The dye has also been injected as a 1%

solution into the human anterior chamber during cataract extraction to identify corneal endothelial damage.[155]

Side Effects

Trypan blue appears to be free of any adverse effects on human corneal cells.

References

1. Baeyer A. Uber eine neue klasse von farbstoffen. Ber Deutsch Chem Ges 1871;4:555–558.
2. Ehrlich P. Uber provozierte fluorescenz sersheinungen am auge. Deutsch Med Wochnschr 1882;8:35–36.
3. Straub A. 1888. As quoted by Campbell FW, Boyd TAS. Use of sodium fluorescein in assessing the rate of healing in corneal ulcers. Br J Ophthalmol 1950;34:545–549.
4. Burk A. Die klinische physiologische und pathologische Bedeutung der Fluoreszenz in Auge nach Darreichung von Uranin. Klin Montagsbl Augen–heilkund 1910;48:445–454.
5. Romanchuk KG. Fluorescein: Physiochemical factors affecting its fluorescence. Surv Ophthalmol 1982;26:269–283.
6. Maurice DM. The use of fluorescein in ophthalmological research. Invest Ophthalmol 1967;6:464–477.
7. Vaughan DG. The contamination of fluorescein solutions-with special reference to Pseudomonas aeruginosa. Am J Ophthalmol 1955;39:55–61.
8. Kimura SJ. Fluorescein paper; a simple means of insuring the use of sterile fluorescein. Am J Ophthalmol 1951;34:446–447.
9. Hales RH. Combined solution of fluorescein and anesthetic. Am J Ophthalmol 1967;64:158–160.
10. Quickert MH. A fluorescein-anesthetic solution for applanation tonometry. Arch Ophthalmol 1967;77:734–739.
11. Jaanus SD. Ophthalmic dyes. In: Bartlett JD, Ghormley NR, Jaanus SD, et al. Ophthalmic drug facts. St. Louis: Facts and Comparisons, 1995; Chap. 2.
12. Yolton DP, German CJ. Fluress, fluorescein and benoxinate: Recovery from bacterial contamination. J Am Optom Assoc 1980; 51:471–474.
13. Lee H. Prolonged antibacterial activity of a fluorescein-anesthetic solution. Arch Ophthalmol 1972;88:385–387.
14. Palmberg R, Gutierrez YS, Miller D, et al. Potential bacterial contamination of eyedrops used for tonometry. Am J Opthalmol 1994;117:578–582.
15. Bourne WM. The permeability of the corneal endothelium to fluorescein in normal human eye. Curr Eye Res 1984;3:509–513.
16. Havener WH. Ocular pharmacology. St. Louis: C.V. Mosby Co, 1983; Chap. 17.
17. Justice J, Soper JW. An improved method of viewing topical fluorescein. Trans Am Acad Ophthalmol Otolaryngol 1976;81:927–928.
18. Cox I, Fonn D. Interference filters to eliminate the surface reflex and improve contrast during fluorescein photography. Int Contact Lens Clin 1991;18:178–181.
19. Korb DR, Herman JP. Corneal staining subsequent to sequential fluorescein instillations. J Am Optom Assoc 1979;50:361–367.
20. Seidel E. Weitere experimentelle utersuchungen uber die quelle und den verlauf der intrakularen saftromung XII. Uber den manometrischen nachweis des physiologischen druckfalles zwischen voderkammer and schlemmschen kanal. Arch Ophthalmol 1921; 107:101–104.
21. Young G. Fluorescein in rigid lens fit evaluation. Int Contact Lens Clin 1988;15:95–100.
22. Norn MS. Micropunctate fluorescein staining of the cornea. Acta Ophthalmol 1970;48:108–118.
23. Kame RT. When does LEH become evident? Contact Lens Spectrum 1993;8:14.
24. Norn MS. Dessication of the precorneal tear film. I. Corneal wetting time. Acta Ophthalmol 1969;47:865–880.
25. Lemp MA, Hamill JR. Factors affecting tear breakup in normal eyes. Ophthalmology 1973;89:103–105.
26. Benedetto DA, Clinch TE, Laibson PR. In vivo observation of tear dynamics using fluorophotometry. Arch Ophthalmol 1984;102:410–412.
27. Jones LT. The lacrimal secretory system and its treatment. Am J Ophthalmol 1966;62:47–60.
28. Flach A. The fluorescein appearance test for lacrimal obstruction. Ann Ophthalmol 1979;11:237–242.
29. Lemp MA, Dohlman CH, Kuwabarat T, et al. Dry eye secondary to mucus deficiency. Trans Am Acad Ophthalmol Otol 1971;75:1223–1227.
30. Vanley GT, Leopold IH, Gregg TH. Interpretation of tear film breakup. Arch Ophthalmol 1977;95:445–448.
31. Mengher LS, Bron AJ, Tonge SR, Gilbert DJ. Effect of fluorescein instillation on the pre-corneal tear film stability. Curr Eye Res 1985;4:9–12.
32. Goldmann H. Applanation tonometry. In: Newell FW, ed. Glaucoma. New York: Josiah Mach, Jr. Foundation 1956;167–220.
33. Moses RA. Fluorescein in applanation tonometry. Am J Ophthalmol 1960;49:1149–1155.
34. The Merck Index, ed. 9. Rahway, NJ: Merck & Co. Inc., 1967; 4042–4043.
35. Grant WM. Fluorescein for applanation tonometry: more convenient and uniform application. Am J Ophthalmol 1963;55:1252–1253.
36. Smith R. Applanation tonometry without fluorescein. Am J Ophthalmol 1979;87:583.
37. Weinstock FJ. Applanation tonometry without fluorescein. Ophthalmology 1979;84:797.
38. Roper DL. Applanation tonometry with and without fluorescein. Am J Ophthalmol 1980;90:668–671.
39. Rosenstock T, Breslin CW. The importance of fluorescein in applanation tonometry. Am J Ophthalmol 1981;92:741.
40. Bright DC, Potter JW, Allen DC, Spruance RD. Goldmann applanation tonometry without fluorescein. Am J Optom Physiol Optics 1981;58:1120–1126.
41. Novotny HR, Alvis DL. A method of photographing fluorescence in circulating blood in human retina. Circulation 1961;24:82–86.
42. Bron AJ, Easty DL. Fluorescein angiography of the globe and anterior segment. Trans Ophthalmol Soc UK 1980;100:388–399.
43. Meyer PAR, Watson PG. Low dose fluorescein angiography of the conjunctiva and episclera. Br J Ophthalmol 1987;72:2–10.
44. Nagataki S, Matsunaga I. Binding of fluorescein monoglucuronide to human serum albumin. Invest Ophthalmol Vis Sci 1985; 26:1175–1178.

45. Smith J, Lawton D, Noble J, et al. Hemangioma of the choroid. Arch Ophthalmol 1963;69:51–54.

46. Lebensohn JE. Fluorescein in ophthalmology. Am J Ophthalmol 1969;67:272–274.

47. Kearns TP, Hollenhorst RW. Chloroquine retinopathy. Arch Ophthalmol 1966;76:378–384.

48. Norton EWD, Gutman F. Fluorescein in the study of macular disease. Trans Am Acad Ophthalmol Otol 1965;69:631–642.

49. Norton EWD, Gutman F. Diabetic retinopathy studied by fluorescein angiography. Ophthalmologica 1965;150:5–17.

50. Kearns TP. Neuro-ophthalmology. Arch Ophthalmol 1966;76:729–755.

51. Norton EWD, Gutman F. Fluorescein angiography and hemangiomas of the choroid. Arch Ophthalmol 1967;78:121–125.

52. David NJ, Saito Y, Heyman A. Arm to retina fluorescein appearance time. A new method of diagnosis of carotid artery occlusion. Arch Neurol 1961;5:165–170.

53. Pernberton JW, Britton WA. The arm-retina circulation time. Arch Ophthalmol 1964;71:364–370.

54. Kottow MH. Fundamentals of angiographic interpretation: the normal anterior segment fluorescein angiogram. In: Anterior segment fluorescein angiography. Baltimore: Williams & Wilkins; 1978, Chap. 3.

55. D'Anna SA, Hochheimer BF, Joondeph HC, Graebner KE. Fluorescein angiography in the heavily pigmented iris and new dyes for iris angiography. Arch Ophthalmol 1983;101:289–293.

56. Golmann H. Uber fluorescein in der menschlichen vorderkammer. Das kammer-wasser-minutevolumen des menschen. Ophthalmologica 1950;120:65–79.

57. Brubaker RF. Flow of aqueous humor in humans. Invest Ophthalmol Vis Sci 1991;32:3145–3166.

58. Cunha-Vaz J, De Abreau JRF, Campos AJ. Early breakdown of the blood-retinal barrier in diabetes. Br J Ophthalmol 1975;59:649–656.

59. Maurice DM. A new objective flurophotometer. Exp Eye Res 1963;2:33–48.

60. Cunha-Vaz J. The blood ocular barriers. Surv Ophthalmol 1979;23:279–296.

61. Waltman SR. Sequential vitreous fluorophotometry in diabetes mellitus. A five year prospective study. Trans Am Ophthalmol Soc 1984;82:827–849.

62. Fishman GA, Cunha-Vaz J, Salazano T. Vitreous fluorophotometry in patients with retinitis pigmentosa. Arch Ophthalmol 1981;99:1202–1206.

63. Braude LS, Cunha-Vaz JG, Goldberg MF, et al. Diagnosing acute retrobulbar neuritis by vitreous fluorophotometry. Am J Ophthalmol 1981;91:764–773.

64. Kayazawa F, Miyake K. Ocular fluorophotometry in patients with essential hypertension. Arch Ophthalmol 1984;102:1169–1170.

65. Kelley JS, Kincaid M. Retinal fluorography using oral fluorescein. Arch Ophthalmol 1979;97:2331–2332.

66. Hunter JE. Oral fluorography in retinal pigment epithelial detachment. Am J Optom Physiol Optics 1982;59:908–910.

67. Morgan KS, Franklin RM. Oral fluorescein angioscopy in aphakic children. J Pediatr Ophthalmol Strabismus 1984;21:33–36.

68. Noble MJ, Cheng H, Jacobs PM. Oral fluorescein and cystoid macular edema: detection in aphakic and pseudophakic eyes. Br J Ophthalmol 1984;68:221–224.

69. Potter JW, Bartlett JD, Alexander LJ, et al. Oral fluorography. J Am Optom Assoc 1985;56:784–792.

70. Nuzzi G, Vanelli M, Venturini I, et al. Vitreous fluorophotometry in juvenile diabetes after oral fluorescein. Arch Ophthalmol 1986;104:1630–1631.

71. Nayak BK, Ghose S. A method for fundus evaluation in children with oral fluorescein. Br J Ophthalmol 1987;71:907–909.

72. Marcus DF, Etienne C. Adverse effects of sodium fluorescein as used in fluorescein angiography. Presented at the Ocular Toxicology Symposium, Little Rock, Arkansas, 1977.

73. Yannuzzi LA, Rohrer KT, Tindel LJ, et al. Fluorescein angiography complications survey. Ophthalmology 1986;93:611–617.

74. Schatz H, Farkos WS. Nausea from fluorescein angiography. Am J Ophthalmol 1982;93:370–371.

75. Willerson D, Tate GW, Baldwin HA, Hernsberger PL. Clinical evaluation of fluorescein 25%. Ann Ophthalmol 1976;8:833–842.

76. Charzan BI, Balodimos ML, Konez L. Untoward effects of fluorescein retinal angiography in diabetic patients. Ann Ophthalmol 1971;3:42–49.

77. Lipson BK, Yannuzzi LA. Complications of intravenous fluorescein injections. Int Opthalmol Clin 1989;29:200–205.

78. Hess JB, Pacuraria RI. Acute pulmonary edema following intravenous fluorescein angiography. Am J Ophthalmol 1976;82:567–570.

79. Arroyave CM, Wolbers R, Ellis PP. Plasma complement and histamine changes after intravenous administration of sodium fluorescein. Am J Ophthalmol 1979;84:474–479.

80. Maguire AM, Bennett J. Fluorescein elimination in human breast milk. Arch Ophthalmol 1988;106:718–719.

81. Applebaum M, Jaanus SD. A study of utilization of diagnostic pharmaceutical agents and incidence of adverse effects. Am J Optom Physiol Optics 1983;60:3384–388.

82. National registry of drug-induced ocular side effects. Case reports 404a, 4046, 421. Portland: University of Oregon Health Sciences Center, 1979.

83. Cohn CH, Jocson VL. A unique case of grand mal seizures after Fluress. Ann Ophthalmol 1981;13:1379–1380.

84. Refojo MF, Miller D, Fiore AS. A new fluorescent stain for soft hydrophilic lens fitting. Arch Ophthalmol 1972;87:275–277.

85. Norn MS. Fluorexon vital staining of cornea and conjunctiva. Acta Ophthalmol 1973;51:670–678.

86. Norn MS. Vital staining of cornea and conjunctiva. Acta Ophthalmol 1962;40:389–401.

87. Feenstra RGP, Tseng SCG. What is actually stained by rose bengal? Arch Ophthalmol 1992;110:984–993.

88. Norn MS. Rose bengal vital staining. Acta Ophthalmol 1970;48:546–559.

89. Gandin E, Lion Y, Van de Vorst A. Quantum yield of singlet oxygen production by xanthene derivatives. Photochem Photobiol 1983;37:271–278.

90. Paczkowski J, Lamberts JJM, Paczkowska B, Neckers DC. Photophysical properties of rose bengal and its derivatives. J Free Rad Bio Med 1985;1:341–351.

91. Stern AM, D'Aurora V, Sigman DS. Inhibition of Escherichia coli DNA polymerase 1 by rose bengal. Arch Biochem Biophys 1980;202:525–532.

92. Thompson A, Nigro J, Seliger HH. Efficient singlet oxygen inactivation of firefly luciferase. Biochem Biophys Res Commun 1986;140:888–894.

93. Epe B, Mutzel P, Adam W. DNA damage by oxygen radicals and excited state species: a comparative study using enzymatic probes in vitro. Chem Biol Interact 1988;67:149–165.

94. DiMascio P, Wefers H, Do-Thi H, et al. Singlet molecular oxygen causes loss of biological activity in plasmid and bacteriophage DNA and induces single-strand breaks. Biochem Biophys Acta 1989;1007:151–157.

95. Valenzeno DP, Trudgen J, Hutzenbuhler A, Milne M. Singlet oxygen involvement in photohemolysis sensitized by merocyanine-540 and rose bengal. Photochem Photobiol 1987;46:985–990.

96. Matthews EK, Cui ZJ. Photodynamic action of rose bengal on isolated rat panreatic acini: Stimulation of amylase release. FEBS Lett 1989;256:29–32.

97. Wallis C, Melnick JL. Irreversible photosensitization of viruses. Virology 1964;23:520–527.

98. Roat MI, Romanowski E, Acaullo-Cruz T, Gordon YL. The antiviral effects of rose bengal and fluorescein. Arch Ophthalmol 1987;105:1415–1417.

99. Banks JG, Board RG, Carter J, Dodge AD. The cytotoxic and photodynamic inactivation of microorganisms by rose bengal. J Appl Bacteriol 1985;58:391–400.

100. Dahl TA, Midden WR, Neckers DC. Comparison of photodynamic action by rose bengal in gram-positive and gram-negative bacteria. Photochem Photobiol 1988;48:607–612.

101. Joshi P, Misra RB. Evaluation of chemically-induced phototoxicity to aquatic organisms using Paramecium as a model. Biochem Biophys Res Commun 1986;139:79–84.

102. Chodosh J, Banks MC, Stroop WG. Rose bengal inhibits herpes simplex virus replication in vero and human corneal epithelial cells in vitro. Invest Ophthalmol Vis Sci 1992;33:2520–2527.

103. Marx E. Über vitale Färbungen am Auge und an den Lidern, I: über anatomie, Physiologie und Pathologie des Augenlidrandes und der Tränenpunkte. Albrecht Graefe Arch Ophthalmol 1924;114:465–482.

104. Sjogren H, Bloch KJ. Keratoconjunctivitis sicca and the Sjögren syndrome. Surv Ophthalmol 1971, 16:145–159.

105. Yolton DP. Topical ophthalmic dyes. In: Eskridge JB, Amos JF, Bartlett JD, eds. Clinical procedures in optometry. Philadelphia: JB I ippincott Co., 1991;358–363.

106. Marsh RJ, Fraunfelder FT, McGill JI. Herpetic corneal disease. Arch Ophthalmol 1976;94:1899–1902.

107. Wilson FM II. Rose bengal staining of epibulbar squamous neoplasms. Ophthalmic Surg 1976;7:21–23.

108. Golding TR, Brennan NA. Diagnostic accuracy and inter-correlation of clinical tests for dry eye. Invest Ophthalmol Vis Sci 1993;34(suppl):823.

109. McMonnies CW. Patient history in screening for dry eye conditions. J Am Optom Assoc 1987;58:296–301.

110. Klaassen-Broekema N, Makor AJ, van Bijsterveld OP: The diagnostic power of the tests for tear gland related keratoconjunctivitis sicca. Neth J Med 1992;40(3–4):113–116.

111. George MA, Abelson MB, Mooshian ML, et al. Development of a precise method using rose bengal in the evaluation of dry eye severity and the detection of potential treatment effects. Invest Ophthalmol Vis Sci 1993;34(suppl):1472.

112. Feenstra RP, Tseng SC. Comparison of fluorescein and rose bengal staining. Ophthalmology 1992;99:605–617.

113. Nelson JD, Gordon JF. Chiron Keratoconjunctivitis Sicca Study Group. Topical fibronectin in the treatment of keratoconjunctivitis sicca. Am J Ophthalmol 1992;114:441–447.

114. Klaassen-Broekema N, van Bijsterveld OP. Changes in the diag-

nostic parameters during keratoconjunctivitis sicca therapy. Doc Ophthalmol 1992;80:317–321.

115. Gilbard JP, Rossi ST, Azar DT, et al. Effect of punctal occlusion by Freeman silicone plug insertion on tear osmolarity in dry eye disorders. CLAO J 1989;15:216–218.

116. Gilbard JP, Rossi ST, Heyda KG. Ophthalmic solutions, the ocular surface, and a unique therapeutic artificial tear formulation. Am J Ophthalmol 1989;107:348–355.

117. Gilbard, JP, Hyang AJ, Belldegrun R, et al. Open-label crossover study of vitamin A ointment as a treatment for keratoconjunctivitis sicca. Ophthalmology 1989;96:244–246.

118. Watson BD, Dietrich WD, Busto R, Wachtel MS. Ginsberg MD. Induction of a reproducible infarction by photochemically initiated thrombosis. Ann Neurol 1985;17:497–504.

119. Nanda SK, Hatchell DL, Tiedeman JS, et al. A new method for vascular occlusion: photochemical initiation of thrombosis. Arch Ophthalmol 1987;105:1121–1124.

120. Mendelsohn AD, Stock EL, Lo GG, et al. Laser photocoagulation of feeder vessels in lipid keratopathy. Ophthalmic Surg 1986;93:1304–1309.

121. Mendelsohn AD, Watson BD, Alfonso EC, et al. Amelioration of experimental lipid keratopathy by photochemically induced thrombosis of feeder vessels. Arch Ophthalmol 1987;105:983–988.

122. Huang AJW, Watson BD, Hernandez E, Tseng SCG. Photothrombosis of corneal neovascularization by intravenous rose bengal and argon laser irradiation. Arch Ophthalmol 1988;106:680–685.

123. Norn MS. Rose bengal vital staining: staining of cornea and conjunctiva by 10% rose bengal, compared with 1%. Acta Ophthalmol 1970;48:546–559.

124. Passmore JW, King JH. Vital staining of conjunctiva and cornea. Arch Ophthalmol 1955;53:568–574.

125. Forster HW. Rose bengal test in diagnosis of deficient tear formation. Arch Ophthalmol 1951;45:419–424.

126. Epstein NN, Delprat GD, Kerr WJ. The rose bengal test for liver function: an historical sketch and an improved technique. J Lab Clin Med 1931:16:923–925.

127. Norn MS. Lissamine green. Vital staining of the cornea and conjunctiva. Acta Ophthalmol 1973;51:483–491.

128. Khurana AK, Chaudhary R, Ahluwalia BK, et al. Tear film profile in dry eye. Acta Ophthalmol 1991;69:79–86.

129. Khurana AK, Sunder S, Ahluwalia BK, et al. Tear film profile in Graves' ophthalmopathy. Acta Ophthalmol 1992;70:346–349.

130. Chodosh J, Dix RD, Howell RC, Stroop WG. Staining characteristics and antiviral activity of sulforhodamine B and lissamine green B. Invest Ophthalmol Vis Sci 1994;35:1046–1058.

131. Eliason JA, Maurice DM. Staining of the conjunctiva and conjunctival tear film. Br J Ophthalmol 1990;74:519–522.

132. Kogure K, David NJ, Yamanouchi U, et al. Infrared absorption angiography of the fundus circulation. Arch Ophthalmol 1970;83:209–214.

133. Hochheimer BF. Infrared absorption angiography of the retina with indocyanine green. Arch Ophthalmol 1971;86:564–565.

134. Flower RW, Hochheimer BF. A clinical technique and apparatus for simultaneous angiography of the separate retinal and choroidal circulation. Invest Ophthalmol 1973;12:248–261.

135. Hayashi K, Hasegawa Y, Tokoro T. Indocyanine green angiography of central serous chorioretinopathy. Int Ophthalmol Clin 1986;9:37–41.

136. Destro M, Puliafito CA. Indocyanine green videoangiography of choroidal neovascularization. Ophthalmology 1989;96:846–853.

137. Scheider A, Schroedel C. High resolution indocyanine green angiography with scanning laser ophthalmoscope. Am J Ophthalmol 1989;108:458–459.

138. Geeraets WJ, Berry ER. Ocular spectral characteristics as related to hazards from lasers and other light sources. Am J Ophthalmol 1968;66:15–20.

139. Yannuzzi LA, Slakter JS, Sorenson JA, et al. Digital indocyanine green videoangiography and choroidal neovascularization. Retina 1992;12:191–221.

140. Cherrick GR, Stein SW, Leery CM. Indocyanine green: observation on its physical properties, plasma decay, and hepatic function. J Clin Invest 1960;39:592–601.

141. McEnerney JK, Peyman GA. Indocyanine green. A new vital stain for use before penetrating keratoplasty. Arch Ophthalmol 1978; 96;1445–1447.

142. Hochheimer BF, D'Anna SA. Angiography with new dyes. Exp Eye Res 1978;27:1–16.

143. Scheider A, Kaboth A, Neuhauser L. Detection of subretinal neovascular membranes with indocyanine green and an infrared scanning laser ophthalmoscope. Am J Ophthalmol 1992;113:45–41.

144. Green WR. Clinicopathologic studies of treated choroidal neovascular membrane. Retina 1991;11:328–356.

145. Yannuzzi LA, Friedman R. Age-related macular degeneration. NY Acad Med J 1988;6:995–1013.

146. Macular Photocoagulation Study Group. Subfoveal neovascular lesions in AMD: guidelines for evaluation and treatment. Arch Ophthalmol 1991;109:1242–1258.

147. Cashi TR, Staller BJ, Hepner G. Adverse reactions after administration of indocyanine green dye. JAMA 1978;240:635.

148. Fox IS, Wood EH. Indocyanine green: physical and pathological properties. Proc Mayo Clinic 1960;35:732–744.

149. Iseki K, Onogana K, Fujioni S. Shock caused by indocyanine green dye in chronic hemodialysis patients. Clin Nephrol 1986;14:210.

150. Speich R, Saesseli B, Hoffman U, et al. Anaphylactoid reactions after indocyanine green administration. Ann Intern Med 1988;15:345–346.

151. Norn MS. External eye. Methods of examination. Copenhagen: Scriptor, 1974; Chap. IV.

152. Latina MA, Melamed S, March WF et al. Gonioscopic ab interno laser sclerostomy. Ophthalmology 1992;99:1736–1744.

153. Stocker FW, King EH, Lucas DO, Georiade N. Clinical test for evaluating donor corneas. Arch Ophthalmol 1970;84:2–7.

154. Taylor MS, Hunt CJ. Dual staining of corneal endothelium with trypan blue and alizarin red S: Importance of pH for the dye-lake reaction. Br J Ophthalmol 1981;65:815–819.

155. Norn MS. Preoperative trypan blue vital staining of corneal endothelium. Eight year's follow-up. Acta Ophthalmol 1980;58:550–555.

156. Yoneya S, Noyori K. Improved visualization of the Choroidal circulation with indocyanine green angiography. Arch Ophthalmol 1993;111:1165–1166.

157. Jennings BJ, Mathews DE. Adverse reactions during retinal fluorescein angiography. J Am Optom Assoc 1994;65:465–471.

158. Guyer DR, Yannuzzi LA, Slakter JS, et al. Digital indocyanine-green videoangiography of occult choroidal neovascularization. Ophthalmology 1994;101:1727–1734.

159. Regillo CD, Benson WE, Maguire JI, et al. Indocyanine green angiography and occult choroidal neovascularization. Opthalmology 1994;101:280–288.

160. Slakter JS, Yannuzzi LA, Sorenson AJ, et al. A pilot study of indocyanine green videoangiography—guided laser photocoagulation of occult choroidal neovascularization in age-related macular degeneration. Arch Ophthalmol 1994;112:465–472.

161. Quaranta M, Cohen SY, Krott R, et al. Indocyanine green videoangiography of angioid streaks. Am J Ophthalmol 1995;119:146–142.

162. Guyer DR, Yannuzzi LA, Slakter JS, et al. Digital indocyanine green videoangiography of central serous chorioretinopathy. Arch Ophthalmol 1994;112:1057–1062.

163. Obana A, Mike T, Hayashi K, et al. Survey of complications of indocyanine green videoangiography in Japan. Am J Ophthalmol 1994;118:749–753.

164. Hope-Ross M, Yannuzzi LA, Gragoudas ES, et al. Adverse reactions due to indocyanine green. Ophthalmology 1994;101:529–533.

CHAPTER 18

Contact Lens Solutions and Care Systems

Gerald E. Lowther

Numerous formulations have been developed for use in conjunction with contact lenses. New products are continually being developed to overcome specific problems and to be compatible with new lens polymers. The safety of solutions and lens care systems is of constant concern. In the United States the U.S. Food and Drug Administration (FDA) regulates contact lens solutions for new lens polymers. Most new contact lens solutions, except those used with polymethylmethacrylate (PMMA) lenses, must undergo laboratory tests, including toxicology studies and clinical trials before being placed on the market. This testing does not mean, however, that they are safe and effective for all patients under all conditions. To prescribe the correct solutions and to diagnose problems that they may cause, the practitioner must understand the products in current use, their formulation strategies, interactions, sensitivities, toxicities, and potential for abuse by the patients.

Physiochemical Properties of Contact Lens Solutions

Osmolarity (Tonicity)

The osmolality of a solution affects water flow across a semipermeable membrane. For example, if a hypotonic solution is placed on the cornea, water flows from the solution, which has a low concentration of ions, into the cornea, which has a higher ion concentration. This causes corneal

swelling (edema). Likewise, if the solution has a higher concentration of ions (is more hypertonic) than the corneal tissue, water flows from the cornea into the solution, causing the cornea to deturgesce. In order to maintain normal corneal thickness contact lens solutions should be isotonic with the normal tear film. With the eye open the tear film has a tonicity of 0.95% to 1.0% equivalent NaCl.[1–3] With the eye closed, as during sleep, the tonicity drops to 0.90% equivalent NaCl or less.[1] Variations from 0.5% to 2.0% equivalent sodium chloride solutions usually do not cause discomfort if placed directly onto the eye.

With hydrogel lenses, the tonicity of the solution in which the lens is soaked affects the lens dimensions. If a hydrogel lens is placed in distilled water, a very hypotonic solution, the lens will swell.[4] Conversely, if it is placed in a hypertonic solution, it shrinks. In addition, if a hydrogel lens is soaked in a hypotonic solution and placed on the eye, the lens adheres to the cornea. The greater the difference in tonicity between the lens and cornea, the tighter is the adhesion.[5] If the patient then attempts to remove the lens, corneal epithelium also may be removed. However, if the patient waits a few minutes after placing the lens on the eye, the tears will have time to equilibrate with the solution in the lens, ensuring easy removal.

Because of the tonicity effect on the integrity of ocular tissue, contact lens solutions should be adjusted to a tonicity of 0.9% to 1.0% equivalent NaCl by adding an appropriate amount of a salt, such as sodium or potassium chloride. Contact lens solutions, however, have tonicity values varying from 0.14% to 1.4% equivalent NaCl.[6]

Hydrogen Ion Concentration

This property is specified by the notation pH, where the pH is the logarithm of the inverse of the hydrogen ion concentration. If the pH is 7.0, the solution is neutral; if less than 7.0, it is acidic; and if greater than 7.0, it is alkaline. A change in pH of 1.0 unit is a 10 times change in H^+ concentration. The average pH of the normal tear film is approximately 7.35, with most ranging between 7.0 and 7.4. With the eye closed, the pH often decreases by 0.1 to 0.3 pH units.

A solution that is too acidic (pH 6.6) or too alkaline (pH 7.8) may cause ocular discomfort.[7] Some of the problems include tearing, burning for the first few minutes after lens placement, conjunctival injection, stringy mucus formation, and lens filming.[8]

The pH of a solution is important for the optimum effectiveness of preservatives. Certain preservatives, such as chlorobutanol, are most effective and stable at an acidic pH. Others, like benzalkonium chloride, exert their maximum anti-bacterial effect in an alkaline environment. Thus, fluctuations in pH can inactivate a preservative and increase the chance of microbial contamination. Such changes can occur if CO_2 from the air diffuses into the solution, forming carbonic acid. CO_2 can diffuse through polyethylene storage bottles or rubber stoppers used on some hydrogel lens vials. Such decreases in pH may cause ocular discomfort indicating the importance of using buffers to maintain solution pH.

The pH of contact lens solutions varies, possibly explaining why some patients complain of discomfort on initial lens placement and why patients often prefer one brand of solution to another.

Buffering

Buffers are used to maintain a solution at a desired pH. The more strongly a solution is buffered, the more acid or base can be added before the pH changes. Buffers are either acid or alkaline salts and include phosphates, borates, citrates, acetates, and bicarbonates. Bicarbonates are relatively volatile and unstable, and may be incompatible with other compounds.[9] The type of buffer used often depends on the preservative. For example, borate buffer is incompatible with the preservative benzalkonium chloride.[10] Likewise, if used with alkaline contact lens solutions or solutions containing polyvinyl alcohol (PVA), borates can form a gel or gummy deposit.[9] This points out the importance of not mixing solutions that may be incompatible. For example, using a wetting solution from one manufacturer with a soaking solution from a different manufacturer may result in such a reaction.

If a contact lens solution requires an acidic pH to maintain an active preservative or to prevent the breakdown of other compounds while stored in the bottle, it may be buffered at the optimum pH for the preservative. However, since the tear film is basic, the application of a highly buffered acidic solution to the eye might cause discomfort or corneal damage. Thus, any solution that is destined for the eye and requires an acidic environment should be only minimally buffered, so that the tear film's buffering capacity can bring the solution to the tear film pH. If the solution has an alkaline pH near 7.3 to 7.4, it can be strongly buffered since the pH will not have to change when the solution is introduced on the eye.

If saline solutions are unbuffered, the pH may drop to 5 and 6 due to the formation of carbonic acid from the diffusion of carbon dioxide from the atmosphere. Buffered solutions, however, remain at their initial pH values.[11]

Preservatives and Disinfectants

The major concern with contact lens fitting is maintenance of ocular health. A potential problem is ocular infection from contaminated lenses. Likewise, accessory solutions for use with lenses can become contaminated in the bottle if these solutions are not properly packaged or preserved. Due to contamination from the environment and favorable growth factors offered by the nutrients from the tear film, if a lens is removed from the eye and placed in water or unpreserved saline, organisms usually thrive (Fig. 18.1).

In an attempt to overcome the problem of microorganism contamination, numerous procedures and chemicals have been used. This section discusses some of these chemicals, often called preservatives. Later sections of this chapter

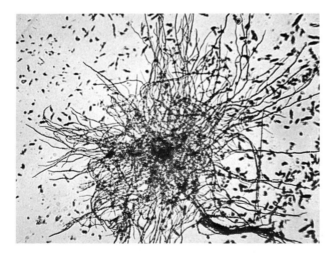

FIGURE 18.1   **Fungal and bacterial organisms on a hydrogel lens.**

consider other methods of preventing growth or killing organisms.

Benzalkonium Chloride

Benzalkonium chloride (BAK), known by a number of proprietary names including Zephiran Chloride and Roccal, is a quaternary ammonium compound. It was employed extensively in solutions for use with PMMA contact lenses. This surface active agent is a cationic detergent compound having a hydrophilic end group and a hydrophobic (lipophilic) end group (Fig. 18.2). Thus, it acts as a soap and attaches to surfaces, such as lens and cell surfaces, and acts at lipid-water interfaces. A detrimental effect of this compound is that the hydrophilic end groups align on the lens surface, exposing the lipophilic end groups. This causes the lens to become hydrophobic. Thus, this preservative requires the use of an effective wetting agent to maintain lens wettability.[12]

Benzalkonium chloride acts against microorganisms by adsorbing on the cell membrane, increasing its permeability, and eventually causing it to rupture. In addition, the compound may penetrate the cell wall and precipitate respiratory and glycolytic enzymes.[13] It is used in concentrations of 0.001% (1:100,000) to 0.01% (1:10,000). As with any preservative, the concentration must be high enough to prevent microbial growth but not cause significant toxicity to the eye. Numerous studies[12,14] have shown that BAK can cause corneal damage in concentrations as low as 0.005%, although it may require a longer exposure time than would normally occur with a solution used on a hydrophobic contact lens.[15,16] At concentrations of 0.0075% to 0.01% major corneal epithelial damage can occur within several minutes of continuous exposure.

Since hydrogel lenses absorb and concentrate significant amounts of BAK,[9,17,18] it cannot be used in soaking solutions for these lenses.

Benzalkonium chloride is most effective at an alkaline pH of approximately 8.0.[19] Phospholipids inactivate this preservative, and it is strongly absorbed by organic matter, rubber, fibers, and sponge material.[20] Therefore, all tear film debris must be cleaned from the lens before placing the lens in a storage solution containing BAK. In addition, cases that contain absorbent material should be avoided. Likewise, since soap inactivates BAK,[21] soap must be well rinsed off the hands before handling lenses.

Ions such as magnesium, calcium, and potassium have an inhibitory effect on the action of BAK by competing for active sites on the bacterial cell membrane. To overcome this problem the chelating agent, ethylenediaminetetraacetic acid (EDTA) which can bind divalent ions, is usually used with BAK to increase its effectiveness.[12,19]

BAK's use in contact lens solutions has decreased dra-

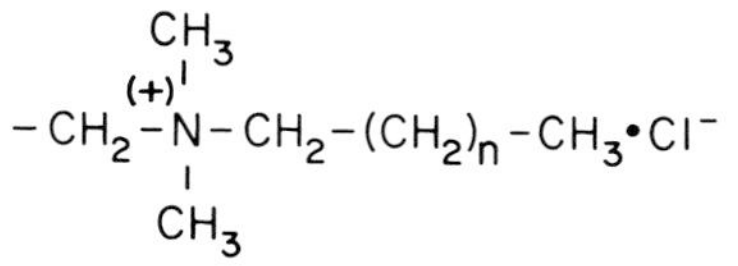

FIGURE 18.2   **The chemical structure of benzalkonium chloride.**

matically because of the incompatibility with new lens materials, especially with hydrogels and because of its potential adverse effect on the cornea.

Chlorobutanol

Some solutions for use with PMMA lenses contain chlorobutanol. A volatile compound having a characteristic odor, it is easily inactivated.[22] Chlorobutanol is effective at acidic pH but not alkaline pH. It is also easily deactivated by heat. Because of its instability and low bacteriostatic effect, it is used infrequently. It is combined with other preservatives such as BAK in concentrations of 0.3% to 0.5%. Chlorobutanol cannot be used with hydrogel lenses.

Phenylmercuric Nitrate

This compound has slow antimicrobial activity but has been used to a limited extent in some rigid contact lens solutions in combination with other preservatives.

Thimerosal

Thimerosal is an organic mercury compound (Fig. 18.3) used in both rigid and hydrogel lens solutions. It does not bind significantly to hydrogel lenses,[23] but the negatively charged ion may bind with proteins.

Thimerosal must be maintained in a neutral or alkaline pH since it may precipitate in an acid environment. In addition, it should be stored in an opaque container, since light breaks it down.[20] It acts by forming covalent bonds with SH-groups of microbial cell enzymes, thereby inhibiting enzyme function and killing microorganisms. Thi-

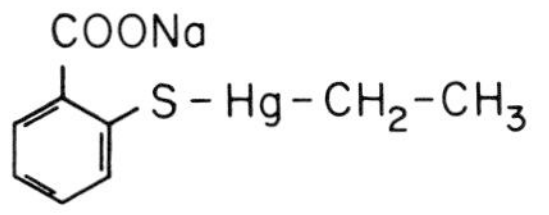

FIGURE 18.3   **The chemical structure of thimerosal.**

merosal also inhibits cell membrane processes by this mechanism.[13]

Thimerosal does not seem to have as great an effect on corneal integrity as does BAK,[24] but at least under some conditions corneal tissue can absorb it, causing corneal damage.[25]

Thimerosal is usually used in concentrations of 0.001% to 0.2% in combination with other preservatives such as EDTA or chlorhexidine. It is not chemically compatible with BAK.

As many as 25% to 50% of patients wearing hydrogel lenses develop sensitivities and toxicities to the compound. For this reason, the use of thimerosal in contact lens solutions has decreased dramatically.

Chlorhexidine

Chlorhexidine (Fig. 18.4) has been used as a preservative in both rigid and hydrogel lens solutions. Chlorhexidine gluconate and chlorhexidine diacetate have both been employed, with the former causing less ocular irritation. Chlorhexidine does bind to hydrogel lenses and is only slowly released.[18,26,27] It also binds to proteins and other tear film substances. This adherence to surface deposits on lenses may cause some of the observed toxicities. This preservative can cause ocular surface damage but usually not to the extent demonstrated by BAK.[16]

Chlorhexidine interferes with cell membrane function. It inhibits both cation transport and membrane-bound adenosine triphosphate (ATP) in the microbial cell membrane.[13] Chlorhexidine is not very effective against certain bacteria and fungi. For example, strains of *Serratia marcescens* have become resistant to this compound and have grown to high levels in bottles of solution preserved with chlorhexidine.[28,29] It is usually used in combination with another preservative such as thimerosal. It is less stable in alkaline than acidic solutions and should be maintained in a neutrally buffered solution.

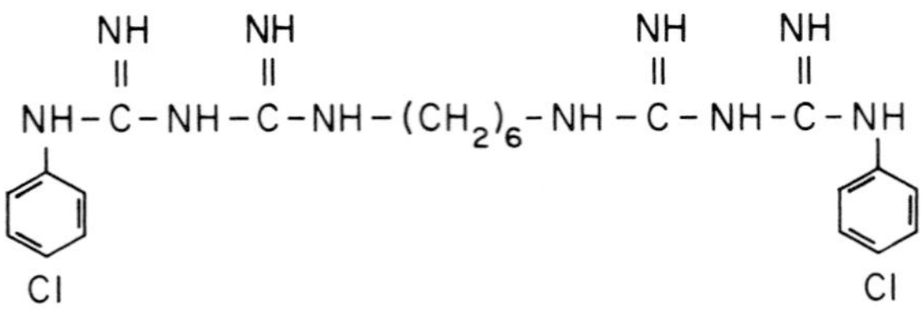

FIGURE 18.4 **The chemical structure of chlorhexidine.**

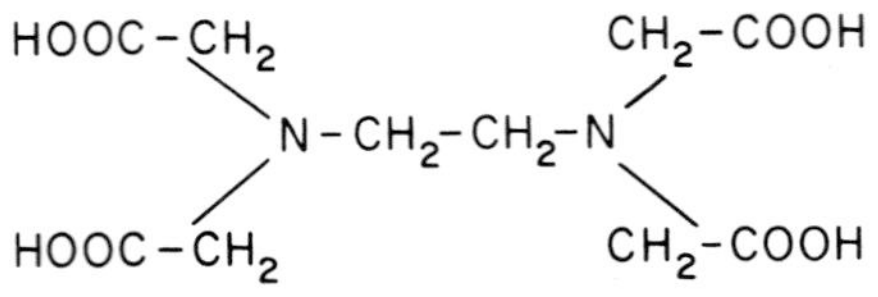

FIGURE 18.5 **The chemical structure of EDTA.**

Ethylenediaminetetraacetic Acid (EDTA) and Disodium Edetate

EDTA (Fig. 18.5) is a chelating agent that binds bivalent or trivalent metal ions. Disodium edetate is the same compound in solution as EDTA. Since bacteria need trace amounts of metal ions, this compound slows or prevents cell growth. An ineffective antimicrobial agent when used alone, EDTA is used only in combination with other preservatives. When used with other preservatives, a synergistic effect increases the combination's effectiveness. Most contact lens preparations contain EDTA or disodium edetate.

Sorbic Acid

Sorbic acid (Fig. 18.6) or its salt, sorbate, is a preservative used in hydrogel contact lens solutions. Its greatest advantage is that it can be used with hydrogel lenses since it is associated with a very low incidence of allergic or toxic reactions. Sorbic acid is most effective at a pH of 4.5 and is not effective above a pH of 6.5.[30] It is usually used in concentrations of 0.1% to 0.2% and is employed in combination with EDTA. Sorbic acid is a weak preservative. As a bacteriostatic agent it can be used as a preservative in saline for heat disinfection or as a lens rinse, but not as a chemical disinfection solution. It can cause a discoloration of hydrogel lenses.

Tris (2-hydroxyethyl) Tallow Ammonium Chloride

This preservative has been used in conjunction with thimerosal as a hydrogel lens disinfecting solution since it is not sufficiently strong to be used alone as a disinfectant. The solution (Allergan Hydrocare Cleaning and Disinfection Solution) contains other polymeric compounds to aid in the formation of micelles, large groups of molecules that minimize absorption of the preservatives into the lens and thus decrease allergic or toxic reactions.

$$CH_3-CH=CH-CH=CH-COOH$$

FIGURE 18.6 **The chemical structure of sorbic acid.**

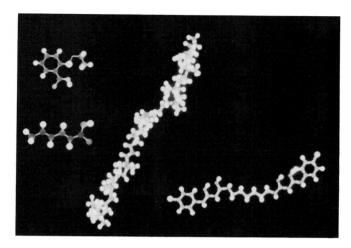

FIGURE 18.7 **Relative sizes of different preservative molecules, thimerosal (upper left), sorbic acid (left), alkyl triethanol ammonium chloride (lower right) and Polyquad (center). The Polyquad molecule is shown at one-quarter the size of the other molecules. (Courtesy Alcon Laboratories.)**

Polyquad

This compound, as well as Dymed, was developed for use with hydrogel lenses to overcome the toxic and allergic reactions common with thimerosal and chlorhexidine solutions. Polyquad is a high molecular weight quaternary compound. Because of its large molecular size (Fig. 18.7) it is not absorbed into most hydrogel lenses and thus toxic or allergic reactions are rare.

Polyaminopropyl Biguanide (Dymed)

The molecule consists of chains of six carbon groups with biguanide groups between them (Fig. 18.8), resulting in a long chain molecule. The molecule is positively charged and reacts with the negatively charged phospholipid groups in the cell walls of the microorganisms causing damage to the membrane and cell death. It is used in very low concentrations (0.00005%). Polyaminopropyl biguanide belongs to the same family of compounds as chlorhexidine but does not have the parachloroaniline end group that may degrade, causing the toxic problem occasionally found with chlorhexidine.

Polyhexamethylene Biguanide Hydrochloride and Tromethamine (COMPLETE Multi-Purpose Solution by Allergan)

This disinfection system appears similar in action and use to the DYMED system.

Hydrogen Peroxide

Use of hydrogen peroxide was one of the earliest methods for disinfecting hydrogel lenses.[31] The early systems utilized

sodium bicarbonate and required multiple steps to neutralize the low pH (3–5) of the hydrogen peroxide. Today, more effective methods of neutralization are used.

High concentrations of hydrogen peroxide, for example the 3% hydrogen peroxide used in disinfecting solutions, can cause severe discomfort in the eye. It will also cause a chemical keratitis seen as fine stipple staining across the cornea. The concentration at which most patients do not report discomfort varies with different studies. Concentrations as high as 250 to 300 ppm hydrogen peroxide have been reported not to cause discomfort.[32–33] Other studies indicate 100 ppm as the threshold.[34] Since it is a strong oxidizing agent, hydrogen peroxide might cause ocular damage even at the low concentrations found following neutralization of the systems used to disinfect contact lenses. The naturally occurring catalase in tissues neutralizes the small concentration of hydrogen peroxide that occurs in the ocular tissues as a result of normal metabolism. When concentrations as high as 2000 ppm were applied to the anterior surface of the eye, no increase in the aqueous levels occurred.[35] When applied to the cornea alone, where the conjunctival tissues cannot neutralize it, some penetration occurred with concentrations above 600 ppm.[35] Riley and Kast[36] found no penetration through the cornea when up to 680 ppm were applied to the corneal surface. No corneal swelling occurred with 10 minute exposures of the rabbit cornea for concentrations up to 240 ppm, although swelling appeared when concentrations between 70 to 150 ppm were

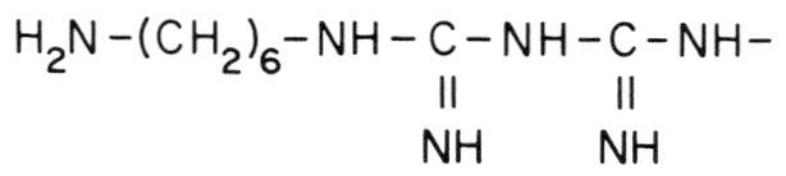

$$H_2N-(CH_2)_6-NH-\underset{\underset{NH}{\|}}{C}-NH-\underset{\underset{NH}{\|}}{C}-NH-$$

FIGURE 18.8 **The chemical structure of polyhexamethylene biguanide (Dymed).**

$$2\,H_2O_2 \longrightarrow 2\,H_2O + O_2$$

FIGURE 18.9 **The chemical reaction for the breakdown of hydrogen peroxide.**

$$Na_2SO_3 + H_2O_2 \longrightarrow Na_2SO_4 + H_2O$$

FIGURE 18.11 **Sodium sulfite neutralization of hydrogen peroxide.**

sustained for 2.5 hours.[37] Since the amount of hydrogen peroxide remaining in solution after neutralization is less than 60 ppm, no clinical problems should ensue.

Hydrogen peroxide is a highly reactive oxidizing agent with the advantage that it can be broken down into water and oxygen (Fig. 18.9). It apparently kills organisms by the oxidizing action of the free radicals that form. Its effectiveness relates to the concentration and time of exposure to the organism. Since it is a very reactive substance, it can break down in the bottle if not properly stabilized. Small quantities of inorganic sodium stannate and sodium nitrate stabilize most hydrogen peroxides used with contact lenses. Some hydrogel peroxides not specifically formulated for contact lenses may be stabilized with other compounds that can cause brownish, pink, yellow or other lens discoloration.

Numerous methods of neutralizing hydrogen peroxide are available. One of the first commercially viable methods was the use of a platinum catalyst to accelerate the breakdown of hydrogen peroxide to water and oxygen. A small amount of platinum is coated on a plastic disk. When the hydrogen peroxide contacts the disk, the peroxide is neutralized but the platinum is not consumed in the reaction. However, with time the disk may become coated, requiring replacement. Some time is required for all the hydrogen peroxide to come in contact with the catalytic disk, as it must diffuse from the lens and through the solution to the disk.

Patients' sensitivity to hydrogen peroxide varies, but if the level is less than 30 to 60 ppm, the majority of patients have no discomfort.[37–39] If the disk becomes coated and is not as effective in neutralizing the hydrogen peroxide discomfort can occur.

With the catalytic system (AOSept) the lens and 3% hydrogen peroxide (30,000 ppm) are placed in the case with the catalytic disk. Since it takes some time for the hydrogen peroxide to break down (Fig. 18.10), it is present for a sufficient time to kill most organisms.

Another system of neutralization uses an enzyme, catalase, which breaks down the hydrogen peroxide.[40] Derived from bovine liver, catalase is used in the OxySept and Lensept systems. Catalase in solution neutralizes the added hydrogen peroxide in approximately 1 minute. Unfortunately, using catalase involves two steps: dumping out the hydrogen peroxide solution and replacing it with the catalase solution. This is not convenient for the patient and decreases patient compliance.

An improved catalase system (UltraCare) uses a hydroxypropyl methylcellulose coated catalase tablet to breakdown the H_2O_2. The coating allows the tablet to be placed in the case at the same time as the 3% H_2O_2, resulting in a one-step procedure. The coating takes some time to dissolve, during which the hydrogen peroxide remains at full strength to disinfect the lenses. Once the coating is dissolved, the catalase is released and neutralizes the hydrogen peroxide.

Sodium pyruvate is also used to neutralize the hydrogen peroxide in 5 to 6 minutes.

Sodium sulfite is another compound used to break down hydrogen peroxide rapidly. The chemical reaction is shown in Figure 18.11. Sodium thiosulfate, used in the Consept system, also neutralizes hydrogen peroxide (Fig. 18.12) but apparently takes a longer time than catalase and sodium pyruvate. It is a two-step system.

The concentration of hydrogen peroxide can also be decreased by dilution. Multiple rinses with saline decrease the levels of hydrogen peroxide sufficiently for some patients not to notice stinging on lens placement, but this technique is not sufficient for many patients.

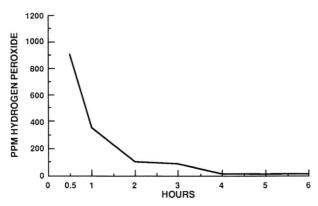

FIGURE 18.10 **Rate of decomposition of hydrogen peroxide when 3% hydrogen peroxide is placed in with the catalytic disk (AOSept system) (adapted from Gyulai et al[38]).**

$$2\left[S_2O_3\right]^{-2} + H_2O_2 \longrightarrow \left[S_4O_6\right]^{-2} + 2\left[OH\right]^{-1}$$

FIGURE 18.12 **Thiosulfate neutralization of hydrogen peroxide.**

Sodium Dichloroisocyanurate and p-(dichlorosulfamoyl) Benzoic Acid (halazone)

Sodium dichloroisocyanurate (DCIC) and halazone in effervescent tablet form are used for hydrogel lens disinfection outside the U.S. A tablet is placed in saline with the lens and breaks down giving off chlorine, which is an oxidative disinfectant. The resulting chlorine concentration is 4 ppm for DCIC and 8 ppm for halazone.[41] Disfection requires 2 to 4 hours. Following disinfection the lenses must be thoroughly rinsed with saline.

Alcohol

Alcohol can disinfect as well as clean. One solution uses 20% isopropyl alcohol as a cleaner (MiraFlow) and effectively reduces microbial growth. If the solution is not sufficiently rinsed from the lens, it causes considerable discomfort. One system uses this cleaner as a disinfectant and then soaks the lens in a preserved saline.

Benzyl alcohol in low concentrations (0.1%) is also being used in both rigid lens solutions. It is reported to be very effective in killing organisms.[42–44] A system (Sherman Laboratories) that has been well accepted by patients.[45]

Effectiveness of Preservatives

Many factors that influence the effectiveness of a preservative against microorganisms must be taken into account in clinical practice. For example, with time many compounds break down so should not be used beyond their expiration date. Increased heat can alter compounds. For example, if a patient keeps solutions on a heater or leaves them in a hot car, their decomposition will be accelerated. Leaving the container open allows evaporation, affecting the concentration of the solution. Some preservatives are absorbed into the bottle surfaces and to any organic contaminates that get into the bottle or lens case, decreasing the amount of preservative available to work against microorganisms.

The amount of preservative in a solution does not necessarily determine the solution's antimicrobial activity. Other components in the system such as viscosity-increasing agents, wetting agents, buffers, salts, and other ingredients can affect the activity. Figure 18.13 shows the effect of two formulations of 0.001% chlorhexidine against *Staphylococcus aureus*.[46]

Hydrogel lenses both absorb and adsorb preservatives. Figure 18.14 shows the effect of having lenses present in a solution of 0.001% chlorhexidine on the time required to kill *Staphylococcus aureus*.[46] As can be seen, the presence of the lenses increases the time considerably. The presence of

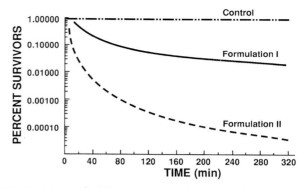

FIGURE 18.13 **The kill rate of two different formulations of the same concentration of chlorhexidine against *S. aureus* (adapted from Meakin[46]).**

foreign material, such as proteins, increases the time required to kill microorganisms.

The temperature of disinfection can also be a factor. Some patients may soak lenses in solutions in very warm climates or bathrooms while others may have them in much cooler locations and climates. Figure 18.15 shows the difference in kill times between two very feasible environmental temperatures.[42]

In the U.S., the FDA requires numerous tests for new solutions and preservatives. These include the effectiveness against a challenge of a series of bacteria at a level of 10[6] colony forming units (CFU)/ml of challenge solution and a rechallenge after 2 weeks to see if the preservative remains effective.

The ability of a disinfecting system to kill organisms is often reported as a D-value. The D-value is the time required to decrease the number of organisms 1 log unit, i.e., to kill

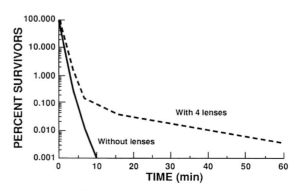

FIGURE 18.14 **Effect of the presence of lenses on the kill rate of chlorhexidine (adapted from Meakin[46]).**

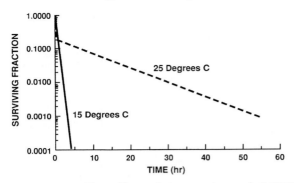

FIGURE 18.15 **The effect of temperature of 0.001% chlorhexidine against *P. aeruginosa* (adapted from Meakin[46]).**

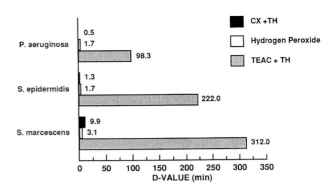

FIGURE 18.17 **The relative kill times of three organisms for a chlorhexidine-thimerosal (CX+TH) solution, and a 3% hydrogen peroxide and alkyl triethanol ammonium chloride-thimerosal (TEAC+Th) solution (adapted from Houlsby et al[47]).**

90% of the organisms present. Therefore, the shorter the D-value, the faster the solution kills the organism.

Not only must the disinfectant itself be tested, but the effect of the entire system must be taken into account. This approach can result in different effectivenesses being reported for the same preservative. For example, cleaning and rinsing a lens prior to placing it in the disinfecting solution is important. If a lens is taken from a solution of organisms and cleaned with a contact lens cleaner and rinsed with saline, many organisms are removed prior to going into the disinfectant. Figure 18.16 shows the effect of the cleaning and rinsing.[47] Thus, it is important to educate the patient about proper cleaning and rinsing not only to prevent deposits, but also to help prevent infections. Since many patients may not clean lenses prior to disinfecting, a system reported as safe may not be in actual use.

Different compounds and systems have different kill rates. Figure 18.17 shows the effect of three different preservative systems on three different organisms.[47] Another

study[48] under different conditions showed somewhat different times but the same general relationship.

Most of the disinfecting systems are effective against *P. aeruginosa* and *Staphylococcus*. However, *Serratia marcescens* is more difficult to kill. Dymed and Polyquad are not totally effective against *S. marcescens*.[49]

Bacteria are killed more quickly than are fungi. In one study[47] the D-value for *Candida albicans* was 3.7 minutes for the chlorhexidine-thimerosal solution, 27.9 for the hydrogen peroxide, and 98.3 for the tallow ammonium chloride and thimerosal solution. For *A. fumigatus* it was 25.1 minutes for hydrogen peroxide, 215 minutes for alkyl triethanol ammonium chloride and thimerosal solution and undetermined for the chlorhexidine-thimerosal solution due to a nonlinear disinfection rate. Penley and associates[48] found that the chlorhexidine-thimerosal and the alkyl triethanol ammonium chloride-thimerosal solutions gave adequate disinfection against three different fungi, but the dichloroisocyanurate dihydrate tablet system and a povidone-iodine system did not give adequate disinfection. Richardson and associates[50] found that 3% hydrogen peroxide (UltraCare, AOSEPT, and OxyTab) was very effective in killing the fungi *Beauveria bassiana*, but ReNu and Opti-Free were not. Shih and associates[49] found that Dymed and Polyquad were not effective against *Candida albicans* or *A. fumigatus*.

Another area of concern and controversy has been the effective disinfection time for hydrogen peroxide. With the AOSept system the hydrogen peroxide starts to undergo neutralization immediately on placement in the case and then decreases, reaching less than 400 ppm after one hour as compared to the 30,000 ppm initially. With the chemical neutralization methods the disinfection ends within seconds or minutes after introducing the neutralizer. Is the 10- or 20-minute recommended time sufficient to kill organisms that

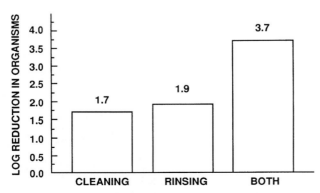

FIGURE 18.16 **The effect of cleaning and rinsing a lens prior to disinfection on the removal of microoganisms (adapted from Houlsby et al[47]).**

may be present? Studies[37,51] have indicated that bacteria such as *P. aeruginosa*, *S. aureus*, and *S. epidermidis* have D-values less than 5 minutes, so a 10- or 20-minute soak will usually suffice. Conversely, most fungi require much longer D-values in 3% hydrogen peroxide. Figure 18.18 shows the D-values for several fungi. Note that the tests used high levels of fungi; but on the other hand, the D-value is the time to kill 90% of all organisms, not 100%. Seldom would properly cared for lenses have such high levels of organisms. However, for safety, longer disinfecting times could be recommended. In general, no adverse lens effects occur with 1 hour or overnight disinfection time, with the exception of some high water ionic lenses that have a temporary change in parameters.[52,53]

There has been particular concern about the possibility of transmitting the human immunodeficiency virus (HIV), which causes acquired immunodeficiency syndrome (AIDS), through contaminated contact lenses, especially diagnostic lenses used in the office on more than one patient. A 5- to 10-minute soak in 3% hydrogen peroxide kills the virus on both hydrogel and rigid lenses.[54] Likewise, standard heat disinfection as used by patients with hydrogel lenses kills the virus. A study[55] has also indicated that using chlorhexidine-preserved solutions following normal cleaning kills the virus. Cleaning the lens with MiraFlow immediately kills the virus. This virus is very fragile outside the body, and most contact lens care systems apparently kill it. Just rinsing with saline alone, however, does not affect the virus.

Acanthamoeba keratitis is a rare infection but can prove devastating to the cornea. The lack of effective drug therapy results in most cases progressing to corneal grafts. *Acanthamoeba*, a free-living protozoan, can exist in two forms, the motile trophozoite form and a dormant cyst. The majority of cases have occurred in hydrogel contact lens wearers.[56,57] Many of the early cases of the disease involved patients improperly using salt tablet-prepared saline or using distilled water for enzymatic cleaning. Exposure to contaminated water, such as soaking in hot tubs or swimming in stagnate water, can be a source of the infection. Lenses should not be rinsed in anything except sterile or preserved contact lens solutions.

Standard heat disinfection kills both forms of *Acanthamoeba*.[58] Miraflow, the cleaner containing isopropyl alcohol, is very effective in killing the organism.[59,60] Reports on the effectiveness of other compounds against the organisms disagree. One report states that alkyl triethanol ammonium chloride-thimerosal and 3% hydrogen peroxide chemical disinfection are ineffective against the organism.[58] The chlorhexidine-thimerosal system was effective against some strains of *Acanthamoeba* but not against others.[58] Conner and associates[60] reported that solutions containing thimerosal were 89% effective compared with all other preservatives tested (chlorhexidine, BAK, hydrogen peroxide, and polyaminopropyl biguanide appeared relatively in-

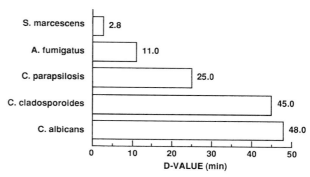

FIGURE 18.18   **Kill rates (minutes) for different organisms in 3% hydrogen peroxide (adapted from Penley et al[48]).**

effective). In contrast, Silvany and associates[61] concluded that chlorhexidine (0.001% and 0.005%), polyaminopropyl biguanide (0.0015%), BAK (0.001% and 0.004%), thimerosal (0.004%) in combination with EDTA, and hydrogen peroxide (3%) were very effective. They indicated that thimerosal (0.0001% and 0.004%), sorbic acid (0.1%), potassium sorbate (0.13%), EDTA (0.1%), polyaminopropyl biguanide (0.00005%) and polyquaternium-1 (0.001%) were not effective. Penley and associates[59] found chlorhexidine and BAK ineffective against the cysts.

The buildup of biofilms (both tear film components and material secreted by bacteria) on the lens and storage case surface can enhance bacterial growth and decrease the effectiveness of disinfection systems. Therefore, frequent replacement of the lens case is important, as well as cleaning.

In addition, a system's effectiveness depends on patient compliance with the required techniques. Simplifying the techniques helps compliance. Patient education with respect to hand washing, lens cleaning, daily replacement of solution in the case, and cleaning and drying the case is important.

Wetting Agents

Solutions used with contact lenses can be placed into general categories based upon their function. With rigid contact lenses some type of wetting solution is normally used. Such a solution forms a uniform film over the lens surface so that when the lens is placed on the cornea, the lens is compatible with the ocular tissue. If the lens surface is dry when the eyelid moves over the lens, it will be quite irritating and cause tearing. Likewise, tear film breakup on the front of the lens will cause blurred vision. If the relative wettability of the surface is adequate, a thin mucoid layer forms on the lens surface after the lens has been on the eye a few minutes, and the tear film wets the lens. This natural wetting by the tears is necessary since any solution placed on the lens dissipates within a few minutes. If the polymer surface is quite hydrophobic ("water-hating"), the tear film does not form and the lens becomes unwearable. Conversely, a hydrophilic ("water-loving") surface becomes wetted with a uniform film.

With nonhydrogel lenses a wetting or viscosity-increasing agent helps to obtain an initial liquid film over the hydrophobic lens surface to improve comfort and vision following lens placement. Pharmaceutical companies have taken two approaches to overcoming the hydrophobic surface: (1) to use a wetting agent that interacts with the surface, and (2) to use a viscosity agent that coats the surface simply by thickening the tear film.

The most commonly used wetting agent is polyvinyl alcohol (PVA). It adheres to the surface of the lens and reportedly remains on the lens considerably longer than do viscosity-increasing agents.[62] PVA is a synthetic, long-chain polymer with a very low viscosity. Partially acetylated PVA is often used since it has the better surface-wetting properties. However, partially acetylated PVA will hydrolyze to yield PVA and acetic acid in an alkaline solution. Excessive acetic acid acts as a buffer and prevents the pH of the solution from adjusting to the pH of the tears, thus causing stinging. Therefore, solutions with PVA must be kept at an acidic pH (5–6).

PVA is compatible with most preservatives. It also does not retard corneal epithelial healing.[14,62] The use of solutions of PVA may lessen the symptoms of some patients who produce an excessive amount of mucus.[10]

Polysorbate 80 is another wetting agent used in some contact lens-wetting solutions. It is an oleic acid ester of sorbitol. Because of the ester linkage, insoluble oleic acid and several alcohol species may result from hydrolytic breakdown of wetting solutions containing polysorbate 80.

Lubricants

Other solutions may also be used in conjunction with contact lens wear. One category is the lubricating, comfort, or rewetting solutions placed onto the eye while the lenses are being worn. Sometimes lens surfaces dry, particularly in low humidity or windy conditions. These solutions rewet the surface and in some cases help prevent and remove surface deposits. They may make the lenses temporarily more comfortable and extend the wearing time. Solutions with high viscosity tend to coat a lens surface heavily and stay on the lens until mechanically wiped or washed off the lens by lid action and tearing. Since these substances are inert, no chemical interaction occurs between these solutions and the lens.

The most common viscosity agents used in contact lens solutions are methylcellulose and its derivatives, hydroxyethylcellulose, and hydroxypropylcellulose. Solutions of these compounds form a thicker film on the lens than does PVA, but the contact angle (measure of the wettability of the lens material) does not correlate with the film thickness.[63] Increased film thickness may be a detrimental factor, since a thick film can cause blurred vision and a sticky sensation and may coat the lid margins and dry, forming a white coating on the lids.

Polyvinylpyrrolidone (povidone, PVP) is another viscosity agent that is finding increasing usage in contact lens solutions. A polymer, it can be produced in varying molecular weights.

Soaking (Storage) Agents

In the early years of rigid contact lens fitting, eye care specialists could not agree over whether contact lenses should be stored dry or in solution when not being worn. At that time only water or poorly preserved solutions were available for lens storage. Thus, the lenses maintained in these media had an increased chance of microbial contamination and ocular infection. Organisms do not normally thrive on a clean, dry surface. However, if lenses are stored dry, the dimensions, particularly the base curve radius, change as the lens rehydrates, even though only approximately 1.5% to 2.5% water is absorbed.[64,65] Moreover, the dry surface does not wet well, even if a wetting solution is used, until the surface layers of the polymer become hydrated. Since solutions are currently formulated to prevent growth of organisms, soaking solutions are now universally used. Not only do they keep the lens hydrated, but they also prevent tear film debris from drying on the lens surface.

Soaking solutions are used with hydrogel lenses to maintaining lens hydration and softness. Since growth of microorganisms is also a concern with these lenses, the solution used must contain a chemical agent to prevent microbial growth. Alternatively, the system must employ another method of killing contaminating organisms, such as heat. A separate wetting agent is not necessary with hydrogel lenses due to the hydrophilic nature of the lens material. The same solution used for soaking is usually used on the lens prior to placement on the eye. In some cases, a rinsing solution, with less or no preservative, is used prior to lens placement to decrease the amount of preservative introduced onto the eye.

Cleaning Agents

Since proteins, mucus, and lipids from the tear film, and foreign material such as oils, hand creams, and make-up can contaminate the lens surface, cleaning solutions must be used. These help to maintain a clean, wettable surface and good optics. Coatings develop on both rigid and soft lenses, and are usually more difficult to remove from soft lenses. To prevent coating, daily cleaning is necessary. More effective cleaning methods or surface polishing may be required periodically.

The daily use of surfactant cleaners is routinely recommended for all daily lens wearers of either rigid or soft lenses. Surfactant cleaners remove microbes, reduce surface tension, emulsify lipids, and solubilize other contaminants. Mechanical rubbing of the lens is required and is a very important step in cleaning. Nonionic surfactants are often used so no interaction occurs between the solution and the lens. Octoxynol, a macrogel ether, is an example of a surfactant. Such cleaners often have a high pH because proteins are more soluble in alkaline solutions. Chelating agents may also be used to remove ionic materials. Some surfactant cleaners contain mild abrasive compounds to enhance cleaning. Some cleaners include isopropyl and other alcohols to remove lipids. Other surfactant cleaners are hypertonic to help remove deposits from hydrogel lenses. The osmotic pressure is thought to force water out of hydrogel lenses, lifting debris from the lens surface.

Anionic surfactants (detergents) have been used with rigid lenses. The rationale focuses on ionic change. Since lens surfaces are negatively charged, positively charged debris attaches to the surface. Negatively charged (anionic) cleaners, therefore, should remove the debris. However, the cleaner may adhere to the lens surface, forming an insoluble film.

Patients and some practitioners have used household cleaners such as dish washing compounds, laundry soaps, shampoos, toothpaste, scouring compounds, and skin cleaners. These should not be used because many contain anionic detergents and contain perfuming agents, solvents, reoiling agents, or abrasives. Such compounds may form insoluble films and craze or scratch the lens surface, thereby adversely affecting the cornea. Anionic detergents are not compatible with cationic preservatives such as BAK.

A variety of enzymatic cleaners in the form of tablets remove deposits from hydrogel lens surfaces. Papain, derived from the papaya fruit, was the first enzyme used with hydrogel lenses and acts by breaking the peptide bonds in the proteins.[66–70] The tablets contain an activator that gives the resulting solution a characteristic odor. Cysteine hydrochloride is added to the tablet (Allergan Enzymatic and Extenzyme) to act as a substrate modifier. Cysteine breaks disulfide bonds in the denatured lysozyme, which should then expose more of the peptide bonds to the proteolytic action. Heat and hydrogen peroxide deactivate the enzyme. Another enzyme in common use is the pancreatic enzyme (from the hog pancreas). It contains lipase and amylase as well as protease.

Subtilisin A and B enzymes (produced by microorganisms) are being used extensively. They are in effervescent formulations, as are the papain or pancreatic enzymes. Since subtilisin is not deactivated quickly in hydrogen peroxide

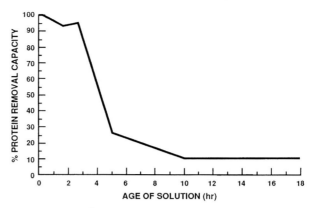

FIGURE 18.19 **Cleaning capacity of subtilisin in 3% hydrogen peroxide (courtesy of Allergan Pharmaceuticals).**

(Fig. 18.19), it can be used during hydrogen peroxide disinfection, decreasing the number of steps required in lens care, thus increasing compliance (Ultrazyme-Allergan). The enzyme's cleaning ability is apparently enhanced in hydrogen peroxide as compared to saline. The enzyme appears to enhance the microbiological effectiveness of hydrogen peroxide (Fig. 18.20). Dissolving enzyme tablets in chemical disinfecting solutions achieves enzyme cleaning simultaneous with disinfection. The subtilisin enzyme has also been formulated to use with heat disinfection by placing the tablet in the case and enzyme treating the lenses at the same time as the lenses undergo heat disinfection (ReNu Thermal Enzymatic Cleaner-Bausch and Lomb). However, this procedure has not proven as effective as the effervescent formulations.

Most of the enzyme formulations contain an effervescent

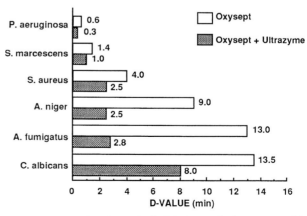

FIGURE 18.20 **The effect of subtilisin in 3% hydrogen peroxide (Oxysept) on shortening the kill times for various organisms (courtesy of Allergan Pharmaceuticals).**

compound for more rapid dissolving of the tablets. Since these enzymes degrade in the presence of moisture, they are supplied in foil wrappers. The significant advantage of enzymatic cleaners is that they remove denatured proteins from the lens surface, whereas most surfactant cleaners do not.

Polishing Compounds

A number of different polishing compounds polish lens surfaces during manufacture and clean and polish patients' rigid contact lenses. Contact lens laboratories commonly use polishes such as tin oxide and precipitated calcium carbonate. One commercial product is XPAL (WR Grace Co, Davison Chemical Division, Pompton Pines, NJ), which is available from most contact lens laboratories that finish rigid lenses. The commercially available powder is mixed with water for use as a lens polish. Sil-O_2-Care (Optacryl Inc, 2890 S. Tejon, Englewood, CO 80110) and the Boston Polish (Polymer Technology, 33 Industrial Way, Wilmington, MA 01887) are polishes formulated for use with rigid gas permeable lenses. In the past, one of the most common polishes used in office practice was Silvo (RT French Co, Rochester, NY), which is formulated as a polish for silver. It performs well as a polish for PMMA lenses. However, it should not be used with the RGP polymers since the ammonia it contains may damage these materials.

Decongestant Agents

Ocular decongestants, such as phenylephrine or naphazoline, are occasionally used with contact lens wear. In some cases they may be justified; however, they should not be used routinely as they may mask irritation and signs of a poorly performing lens. The underlying cause of persistent redness and irritation should be diagnosed and corrected. Decongestants and artificial tears are discussed in Chapters 13 and 14.

Clinical Use of Solutions with Nonhydrogel Lenses

Wetting Solutions

A wetting solution should be used on nonhydrogel lenses before lens placement. This provides a film on the surface that increases the lens comfort and provides good visual acuity following lens placement. Such solutions must be formulated for comfort and compatibility with ocular tissues. This requires that they be nearly isotonic and pH compatible. Sodium chloride or potassium chloride salts can usually achieve isotonicity. The pH of the solution should be near physiologic pH, or only lightly buffered so that the pH will rapidly adjust to that of the tear film. A borate or phosphate buffer is commonly used. With polyvinyl alcohol (PVA) as the wetting agent, the pH is in the acidic range, but the solution must not be highly buffered. As previously discussed, a wetting agent is used either with or without a viscosity agent; alternatively, a viscosity agent is used alone to obtain the surface coating on the lens. If a wetting agent only (e.g., PVA) is used, the solution will not be viscous but will be very thin, like water. Incorporating a viscosity agent increases the thickness of the solution even though the viscosity agent is not needed to wet the surface. In cases in which only a viscosity agent is used, the wetting solution will be thick. In addition to the these ingredients, preservative(s) must be used to prevent contamination.

In using the wetting solution, the patient should remove the lenses from the soaking solution, place a few drops of the wetting solution on the lens, and gently rub the lens surfaces between the thumb and forefinger. Some patients will put a drop or two of the solution on the lens before placement. As a result, excessive solution often spills onto the lids and lashes and then dries, leaving a white residue, especially with solutions containing a viscosity agent. When indicated, lightly rinsing the lens with a saline solution prior to placement prevents this problem.

Patients have different sensitivities to the pH, tonicity, and preservatives used in solutions. Some patients report that a certain wetting solution stings or burns immediately following lens placement. Patients having mild discomfort following lens placement should change to another wetting solution. If a solution with a low pH is being used, substituting another with a higher pH or lower buffering capacity may eliminate the problem. A solution with a different preservative may be required if the patient has a sensitivity to the preservative. In some cases corneal infiltrates occur with rigid lens wetting solutions if the patient has an allergy to the solution.[71] Aging of solutions can result in the breakdown of compounds, pH changes,[72] and changes in tonicity.[73]

Prosthetic eyes are manufactured from PMMA, and solutions formulated for rigid lenses can be used on them. Enuclene (Alcon) is formulated for use with prosthetic eyes. It contains benzalkonium chloride (0.02%), hydroxpropylethyl cellulose, tyloxapol (0.25%), boric acid, and sodium phosphate.

Soaking Solutions

A soaking solution maintains lens hydration, prevents contamination of the lens with microorganisms, and helps to maintain a clean lens by solubilizing debris from the surface. This solution is not intended for instillation onto the eye, but it nevertheless must not cause ocular damage, since it might accidentally be used as a wetting solution. A soaking solution should not be viscous, since this hampers solubilization of surface debris. Likewise, it should have a high enough concentration of preservatives to prevent the growth of microorganisms if a relatively large number are introduced into the solution with the lens, or if considerable organic matter, such as tear film debris, is introduced.

Patients should clean the lenses well following removal, using a cleaning solution, and then place the lenses in the storage case with fresh soaking solution. The importance of using fresh soaking solution each day must be emphasized, since the preservative's effectiveness is rapidly lost when it becomes bound to proteins and other debris.

Controversy exists over the use of BAK-preserved solutions with gas permeable lenses. Some reports[74,75] have indicated that BAK adsorbs onto the lenses and can create clinical problems. Others,[76–78] however, indicate that the adsorption of BAK to these materials is no greater than to PMMA lenses. Many patients wearing silicone/acrylate lenses have used solutions containing BAK without problems. However, some patients may develop a sensitivity, and the clinician should not hesitate to change to solutions not containing BAK. Likewise, if hyperemia, superficial punctate keratitis, or infiltrates occur, a solution with a different preservative may alleviate the problem.

Cleaning Solutions

These solutions contain cleaners that are usually nonionic surfactants (Table 18.1). EDTA may be used not only to enhance the antimicrobial activity of other preservatives, but also to soften the water by removing ions, thereby enhancing the solution's cleaning action. Mild abrasive compounds may also be added. Because of their nature and the fact that they are not intended for instillation onto the eye, these compounds usually cause considerable discomfort if inadvertently used as a wetting solution. Punctate epithelial keratitis may occur.

Patients should clean the lenses well upon removal by placing each lens in the palm of the clean hand along with a few drops of the cleaner. The lens should then be rubbed, both front and back surfaces, for several seconds. The

TABLE 18.1
Representative Cleaning Solutions for Nonhydrogel Lenses

Solution	Manufacturer	Preservative	Other Ingredients
Opti-Clean	Alcon	thimerosal (0.004%) edetate disodium (0.1%)	Tween 21 polymeric cleaning agents hydroxyethylcellulose
Opti-Clean II	Alcon	Polyquad (0.01%) disodium edetate (0.01%)	Tween 21 polymeric cleaning agents hydroxyethylcellulose
LC-65	Allergan	thimerosal (0.001%) disodium edetate	cleaning agent
Concentrated Cleaner	Bausch & Lomb	none	ionic and other surfactants friction enhancing agents sodium chloride
Lobob	Lobob	none	nonionic surfactant
Sereine	Optikem	benzalkonium chloride (0.1%) EDTA (0.1%)	surfactants viscosity agents
Titan	Paragon	Potassium Sorbate (0.13%) disodium edetate (2.0%)	nonionic surfactants
Gas Permeable Daily Cleaner	Paragon	Potassium Sorbate (0.13%) disodium edetate (2.0%)	nonionic cleaning agents buffers
SLC Hard Lens Cleaner	Permeable Tech	sorbic acid (0.1%) EDTA (0.1%)	surfactants abrasives
Boston Lens Cleaner	Polymer Tech	none	sodium chloride anionic sulfate surfactant friction enhancing agents (silica gel)
Boston Advance Cleaner	Polymer Tech	none	surfactants silica gel

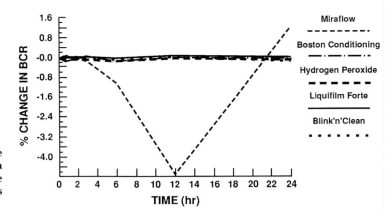

FIGURE 18.21 **Effect of solutions on the base curve radius of Boston IV (silicone/acrylate) lenses following a 24-hour soak. Miraflow was the only solution to change the BCR. A similar change occurred with Equalens (fluorosiloxane/acrylate) lenses (From Lowther[82]).**

cleaner should be thoroughly rinsed from the lens, using soaking solution or saline, before the lens is placed in fresh soaking solution for storage. Often deposits will build up on the back surface of the lens and not be sufficiently cleaned with normal rubbing. Such coating can cause superficial punctate keratitis and discomfort. Patients developing this problem should be taught to clean the back surface by rubbing it with a cotton tipped applicator coated with the surfactant cleaner.

The lens should not be cleaned with the surfactant cleaner in the morning before placement or during a break in wearing during the day but, rather, after removal at the end of the wearing period. Overnight soaking dilutes any residual cleaner and prevents discomfort.

Some cleaners contain abrasive particles (OptiFree Cleaner, Boston Cleaner, and SLC Cleaner) to enhance cleaning. These products are suspensions and should therefore be shaken before use to ensure even distribtion of particles. Patients must be particularly careful to rub and rinse the cleaner from the lens because any residue left on the lens can cause discomfort. Over-zealous cleaning with abrasive cleaners can change the lens power and decrease the thickness. Changes of 1 to 3 diopters in power with a corresponding decrease in lens thickness of up to 0.08 mm have been reported.[79–81]

Alcohol is a good solvent for lipid and other nonaqueous deposits and is present in Miraflow. One must exercise caution in using alcohol with gas permeable lenses and instruct patients not to soak lenses in it. Soaking for several hours causes swelling and changes the base curve.[82] Minus lenses will steepen initially and then flatten (Fig. 18.21). They may also become toric and/or distorted and not regain their original dimensions when returned to the proper solution.

Enzymatic cleaners can also effectively remove protein deposits from rigid lenses and, thus, increase wearing time and comfort. The same enzymes used with hydrogel lenses can be used with rigid lenses. One enzyme cleaner,

PROFREE/GP (Allergan), is a papain enzyme specifically packaged for rigid lens patients. Enzyme cleaning once a week usually suffices. More frequent use does not adversely affect the lens.

One cleaning system (ComfortCare-Barnes-Hind) for RGP lenses utilizes a tablet containing subtilisin enzyme and a surfactant cleaner. A cleaning tablet is dissolved in the soaking solution each night and the lenses allowed to soak in the solution overnight.

Combination Solutions

For patient convenience manufacturers have developed combination solutions. These can be wetting-soaking (Table 18.2), cleaning-soaking (Table 18.3), or wetting-soaking-cleaning combinations. The problem with combination solutions is that compromises in function must be made.

A wetting-soaking solution may be more viscous than desired for a soaking solution, and thus it will not solubilize and clean the lens surface or be as effective against microorganisms as will a separate soaking solution. The concentration of preservative and buffering capacity may not be as adequate as the separate soaking solution because the combination solution must be capable of being placed on the eye without discomfort. Furthermore, the combination solution may be less viscous than a separate wetting solution.

The soaking-cleaning solution may represent less of a compromise since neither of the separate solutions is intended for placement on the eye. However, the strength of the cleaner must be compromised, since some of the soaking solution may get into the eye if not fully rinsed from the lens with wetting solution. With this combination no soaking solution dilutes the stronger cleaner.

The all-in-one solutions require the greatest compromise. These solutions cannot be as effective as a separate cleaner because the combination must be compatible with ocular

TABLE 18.2
Representative Wetting and Soaking Combinations for Nonhydrogel Lenses

Solution	Manufacturer	Preservative	Other Ingredients
Soaclens	Alcon	thimerosal (0.004%) disodium edetate (0.1%)	buffers
Wet-N-Soak PLUS	Allergan	BAK (0.003%) disodium edetate	polyvinyl alcohol buffers
Wetting & Soaking	Bausch & Lomb	chlorhexidine (0.006%) EDTA (0.05%)	hydrophilic polyelectrolyte polyvinyl alcohol hydroxyethylcellulose other hydrophilic polymers
Sereine Wetting & Soaking	Optikem	benzalkonium chloride (0.1%) EDTA (0.1%)	viscosity agents
ComfortCare	Paragon	chlorhexidine (0.005%) edetate disodium (0.1%)	octylphenoxy ethanol hydroxyethylcellulose
BH Wetting & Soaking	Paragon	chlorhexidine (0.005%) edetate disodium (0.02%)	polyvinyl alcohol
Boston Lens Conditioning Solution	Polymer Tech	chlorhexidine (0.006%) EDTA (0.05%)	hydrophilic polyelectrolyte polyvinyl alcohol hydroxyethylcellulose other hydrophilic polymers
Boston Advance Conditioning	Polymer Tech	polyaminopropyl biguanide (0.0015%) edetate Disodium	cellulose polymer
Stay-Wet 3	Sherman	benzyl alcohol (0.1%) trisodium edetate (0.1%) sodium bisulfite (0.02%)	polyvinyl pyrrolidone polyvinyl alcohol hydroxyethylcellulose

TABLE 18.3
Representative Cleaning and Soaking Combinations for Nonhydrogel Lenses

Solution	Manufacturer	Preservative	Other Ingredients
Clean-N-Soak	Allergan	phenylmercuric nitrate (0.004%)	cleaning agent buffers
Cleaning-Soaking	Paragon	BAK (0.01%) disodium edetate (0.1%)	
Sereine Soaking & Cleaning	Optikem	BAK (0.01%) edetate disodium	surfactants
de-Stat 3	Sherman	benzyl alcohol (0.01%) edetate tresodium (0.5%)	lauryl sulfate salt of imidazoline octylphenoxypoly-ethoxyethanol

tissue. It must contain a wetting or viscosity agent if it is to act as a wetting solution, and these agents interfere with the soaking and cleaning functions.

Combination solutions represent a compromise. However, the majority of systems available today are combinations due to ease of use and improved patient compliance.

Lubricating (Rewetting or Comfort) Solutions

Occasionally while wearing contact lenses the patient will experience dehydration of the lens surface, causing blurred vision, or drying of the peripheral cornea and conjunctiva. This condition may lead to burning, stinging, conjunctival hyperemia, and ocular discomfort. When this occurs, the practitioner must first attempt to find and alleviate the underlying cause. Potential causes include a poorly fitted lens, inadequate lens oxygen permeability, or a poorly shaped or thick edge that results in infrequent blinking. If none of these problems exists, and the signs and symptoms appear due to low humidity or a dry eye, then lubricating drops may be used.

Lubricating solutions (Table 18.4) are usually isotonic or slightly hypertonic to enable water to be removed from the cornea in cases of edema. Lubricating solutions usually contain a viscosity agent and/or wetting agent to keep the eye

TABLE 18.4
Representative Lubricating/Rewetting Solutions

Solution	Manufacturer	Preservative	Other Ingredients
Adapettes for Sensitive Eyes	Alcon	sorbic acid edetate disodium	absorbase
Opti-Free Rewetting Drops	Alcon	Polyquad (0.001%) edetate disodium	citrate buffer dextran, NaCl, KCl
Opti-Tears	Alcon	Polyquad (0.1%) edetate disodium	hydroxypropylmethylcellulose dextran, NaCL, KCl
Clerz 2	Alcon	sorbic acid edetate disodium	hydroxyethylcellulose Polxomer 407, NaCl potassium chloride sodium borate, boric acid
Lens Fresh	Allergan	sorbic acid (0.1%) edetate disodium (0.2%)	hydroxyethyl cellulose sodium chloride sodium borate, boric acid
Lens Plus Rewetting Drops	Allergan	none	boric acid, NaCl
Lens-Wet	Allergan	thimerosal (0.002%) disodium edetate	polyvinyl alcohol sodium phosphates sodium chloride
Lens Lubricant	Bausch & Lomb	thimerosal (0.004%) disodium edetate (0.1%)	povidone polyoxyethylene
Sensitive Eyes Drops	Bausch & Lomb	sorbic acid (0.1%) edetate disodium	sodium chloride borate buffer
RENU Rewetting Drops	Bausch & Lomb	sorbic acid (0.15%) edetate disodium	boric acid poloxamine sodium borate
Lens Lubricant	Blairex Lab	sorbic acid (0.25%) edetate disodium (0.1%)	hydroxypropylmethylcellulose glycerin, borate buffer, NaCl
Charter Lens Lubricant for Sensitive Eyes	Charter Labs	boric acid (0.25%) edetate disodium	glycerin hydroxypropylmethylcellulose sodium borate, NaCl, KCl
Ciba Vision Drops	Ciba Vision	sorbic acid (0.1%) edetate disodium (0.2%)	hydroxyethylcellulose sodium borate, boric acid sodium chloride
Soft Mate Comfort Drops	Paragon	potassium sorbate (0.13%) disodium edetate (0.1%)	sodium chloride borate buffer
Boston Advance Rewetting Drops	Polymer Tech	chlorhexidine (0.006%) EDTA	hydrophilic polyelectrolyte polyvinyl alcohol hydroxyethylcellulose other hydrophilic polymers
Stay-Wet "In-Eye" Lubricant	Sherman Labs	benzalkonium chloride (0.01%) EDTA (0.25%)	polyvinyl alcohol hydroxyethylcellulose PVP

moist as long as possible between instillations. The solutions also contain preservatives to prevent contamination.

These preparations should not be used excessively because they contain preservatives and other agents detrimental to the cornea.[83] In addition, the patient may have or develop a sensitivity to an ingredient in the solution. The practitioner should determine if the patient is using such drops when other solutions are changed in response to a suspected solution reaction. If the patient continues to use the lubrication drops after discontinuing other solutions, the signs and symptoms may continue.

Clinical Use of Solutions and Systems with Hydrogel Lenses

Hydrogel lenses present unique problems in care, cleaning, and disinfection. Since hydrogel lenses are hydrophilic and absorb water and water soluble substances, they also absorb compounds in solutions used with these lenses. If the absorbed substances are toxic, such as preservatives in suffi-

cient concentration, then corneal and ocular damage might occur during lens wear as the preservative is released onto the cornea. The situation worsens if the preservative concentrates in the lens. In some cases the concentration of preservative in the lens may be much higher than is its concentration in the solution in which the lens is soaked. For this reason many preservatives, especially benzalkonium chloride and chlorobutanol, cannot be used with hydrogel lenses.

The water content of the hydrogel lens may also be a factor in the method of care or solution used. Most high-water content lenses are more susceptible to deterioration from heating. Likewise, they may absorb or adsorb more foreign material such as preservatives. Some cleaning systems, such as enzymes, might cause a toxic reaction when used with high-water content lenses due to absorption of the enzyme, which may remain active if the lens is not heat or hydrogen peroxide disinfected. The FDA has classified hydrogel lenses into four categories (Table 18.5) for purposes of testing new solutions and care systems. This classification can be useful clinically. If a patient is having deposit, discoloration, or solution problems with a lens, the practitioner can

TABLE 18.5
Classification of Some Representative Hydrogel Lenses

Group 1	Group 2	Group 3	Group 4
Low Water (<50% H_2O)	High Water (>50% H_2O)	Low Water (<50% H_2O)	High Water (>50% H_2O)
Nonionic	Nonionic	Ionic	Ionic
Polymers	Polymers	Polymers	Polymers
Telfilcon (38%)	Lidofilcon B (79%)	Bufilcon A (45%)	Bufilcon A (55%)
Cibasoft	CW 79	Hydrocurve II$_{45}$	Hydrocurve II$_{55}$
Cibathin	Surfilcon A (74%)	Soft Mate	Soft Mate
Ciba STD	Permaflex	Sport Mate	Perfilcon A (71%)
Torisoft	Lidofilcon A (70%)	Deltafilcon A (43%)	Permalens
Tetrafilcon A (43%)	B&L 70	Amsoft	Etafilcon A (58%)
Aquaflex	Q&E 70	Q&E	AcuVue
Illusions Vantage	Medalist Toric	Softact	SureVue
Preference		Droxifilcon A (47%)	Ocufilcon B (53%)
Crofilcon (39%)		Accugel	Ocu-Flex
CSI		Phemfilcon A (38%)	Phemfilcon A (55%)
Hefilcon A&B (43%)		Durasoft 2	Durasoft 3
Alges			Methafilcon (55%)
Unilens			Hydracon
Isofilcon (36%)			HydraSoft
AL-47			Hydracon Toric
Polymacon (38%)			Sunsoft
Echelon			Vifilcon A (55%)
Edge III			Focus
Medalist			NewVues
Occasions			Softcon
Optima			Spectrum
Seequence			
Softlens			
Zero-4			
Zero-6			

minimize chances of recurrence by changing to a lens in a different group instead of another one in the same group.

The use of improper solutions can also result in discolored, coated, or otherwise damaged lenses. If a hydrogel lens is heat disinfected in some solutions formulated for rigid lenses[84,85] or solutions formulated for cold disinfection, the lens may become white due to crystallization of material in the lens. The use of water contaminated with certain salts or minerals will cause crystal formation on and in the lenses.[86–88]

Since hydrogel lenses absorb the soaking solution, the solution must be compatible with the eye. The tonicity must be near that of the tear film to maintain proper lens parameters and to prevent an osmotic pressure difference between the lens and the cornea. A significant difference may cause the lens to adhere to the eye and be uncomfortable. To maintain proper tonicity, a sterile saline solution, either unpreserved or preserved, is used.

Saline solution is an effective medium for growth of microorganisms and can be the source of ocular infection.[89,90] If lenses are stored in saline without disinfection or preservatives, growth of bacteria or fungi commonly occurs. To prevent this, the lenses must be disinfected by heat or by the use of chemicals. Disinfection kills most vegetative organisms, but may spare spores. Thus, if lenses remain in the solution for several days, spores may become vegetative. In the case of sterilization (usually by heating to 120° C under a pressure of 15 lb/sq in. for 15 minutes) all organisms are killed. As long as the container remains sealed, the lenses should remain sterile indefinitely.

Heat Disinfection

Disinfecting lenses with heat avoids use of preservatives that cause toxic or allergic reactions. Saline is used with no preservatives or only sufficient preservative to prevent contamination of the solution in the bottle. The heat system is effective even in the presence of considerable contaminating organic matter such as tear film components or exceptionally large numbers of organisms. In such cases chemical systems may prove ineffective because the chemicals bind to organic material and become unavailable to act against organisms. Heat kills the organisms very rapidly, usually within 15 to 20 minutes, whereas many chemical systems may require several hours.

The primary disadvantage of heat disinfection is that it may shorten the useful lens life. Heat denatures proteins and other contaminants and crystallizes materials on the lens surface that may not be removed with cleaners. Heat disinfection cannot be used with high water content lenses. Heat systems are not continuous disinfection systems; that is, if the patient disinfects the lens, opens the case and handles the lens thereby contaminating it, then places the lens back in the case, the introduced organisms may thrive. With chemi-cal systems, except hydrogen peroxide systems, the chemicals would still be present to counteract the contamination after the lens handling. Transportation of the disinfection unit, and the availability of electricity when camping and of appropriate current when traveling overseas, can also present problems for heat disinfection systems.

Present heat-disinfecting units are easy to use, reliable, and readily transportable. Since the units automatically turn off following the disinfection cycle, the patient can place the lens in the unit, activate it, and leave it until the next morning, when the lenses are ready to be worn again. The patient should occasionally check the unit to be sure that it is heating. Most of the units are low-temperature systems with the temperature reaching only 80 to 90° C. This temperature kills the organisms but minimizes lens damage.

Other Disinfection Techniques

Microwave irradiation of lenses was suggested a number of years ago and research continues on this technique.[91] Microwave irradiation of contact lenses in saline is effective; however, presently no such systems are on the market.[92–94]

Ultraviolet radiation is another system effective in killing bacteria, fungi, and *Acanthamoeba* within less than 5 minutes without lens damage; however, effective patient systems have not been marketed in the U.S.[95–100]

A commercial ultrasound unit (Sonasept Ultrasonic Contact Lens Cleaner and Disinfector) and a standing wave unit (Soft Mate Professional Cleaning Unit) have been tested for their efficacy in killing bacteria and fungi. Neither unit killed enough organisms to be used with saline alone as a means of lens disinfection.[101,102]

Salt Tablet Saline

One of the early systems required the patient to put salt tablets in distilled water to formulate saline. This approach created many problems, particularly with respect to bacterial contamination. Salt tablets are seldom used today and should be avoided.

Unpreserved Saline

Various methods of packaging prepared saline have been used. One method is unit-dose packages that contain only enough solution in each package for one use. The top of the container is broken off or the package torn open, the solution used, and the package discarded. The main problem with the unit dose is its high cost. Because of the price, some patients attempt to retain the opened container for later use, with the potential problem of contamination. This practice must be discouraged.

Another method uses saline in a can under positive pressure. The advantages of such systems are that the solution is sterile and does not contain minerals to damage the lens. Buffers are added to most of these solutions to maintain the proper pH.

Some practitioners and patients use prepared saline in 1-liter bottles obtained from a hospital supply outlet. This practice is discouraged because such solutions can become contaminated after opening. Also, saline packaged in such containers is sometimes preserved, which can cause hypersensitivity reactions.

Preserved Saline

To overcome many of the potential problems with unpreserved saline, a preservative is commonly used in a concentration that is bacteriostatic and not bactericidal (Table 18.6).

The first preservatives used were thimerosal (0.001%) and EDTA (0.1%). Although many patients find these satisfactory, some develop an allergic or toxic reaction to the thimerosal.[103–110] The signs and symptoms as well as the time course of such reactions vary with each patient. If patients have previously been sensitized to thimerosal, they can develop a very injected and irritated eye within minutes after the lens, soaked in the solution, is placed on the eye. A relatively severe reaction also occurs in such patients by irrigating the eye with a thimerosal-preserved irrigating solution. A more common history is that the patient seems to do well with the lenses for weeks to months, and then the eyes become injected and irritated immediately upon lens placement. These patients had not been previously sensitized to the thimerosal but develop the allergy during use. Skin patch tests are often positive to thimerosal (see Fig. 28.3).[111,112] With the other type of reaction, the signs and symptoms become progressively worse. In addition to the conjunctival inflammation, the patient may develop corneal subepithelial infiltrates, limbal infiltrates, punctate epithelial keratitis, or swollen lids. With long-term use, neovascularization can occur. The patient may complain of itching, burning, dryness, photophobia, pain, and decreased visual acuity. Due to these problems, thimerosal-preserved contact lens solutions are seldom used.

Sorbate- and sorbic acid-preserved salines alleviate or avoid many of these adverse reactions. Patients sensitive to thimerosal-preserved saline do not appear sensitive to the solution containing sorbic acid. A small number of patients will report mild discomfort or stinging with sorbic acid or sorbate-preserved solutions. Sorbate and sorbic acid may cause a slight lens yellowing or discoloration of high-water-content lenses. Higher concentrations (0.3% or greater) of sorbate or sorbic acid than normally used in preserved solutions commonly cause discoloration. The discoloration apparently comes from the breakdown of sorbic acid to aldehydes, which in turn react with amino acids from proteins coating the lens to give the coloration.[113] It must be emphasized that sorbate and sorbic acid are weak preservatives. If contamination level is high, they may not prevent microbial growth.

A preserved saline system that does not seem to cause reactions uses three borate buffers that produce a trace

TABLE 18.6
Representative Preserved Salines for Hydrogel Lenses

Solution	Manufacturer	Preservative	Other Ingredients
Opti-Soft	Alcon	Polyquad (0.001%) edetate disodium (0.1%)	borate buffer NaCl
Saline Solution for Sensitive Eyes	Alcon	sorbic acid (0.125%) edetate disodium (0.1%)	borate buffer NaCl
Soft Mate	Paragon	potassium sorbate (0.13%) disodium edetate (0.025%)	borate buffer NaCl
ReNu Saline	Bausch & Lomb	Dymed (0.00003%) edetate disodium	boric acid NaCl
Sensitive Eyes	Bausch & Lomb	sorbic acid (0.1%) disodium edetate	borate buffer NaCl
Sensitive Eyes Saline/Cleaning	Bausch & Lomb	sorbic acid (0.1%) edetate disodium (0.1%)	borate buffer NaCl surfactant
SoftWear Saline	Ciba Vision	sodium perborate	boric acid sodium borate phosphoric acid

amount of hydrogen peroxide (SoftWear Saline). The level of hydrogen peroxide is so low that it does not cause discomfort but with the buffers is bacteriostatic and has been shown to have a good kill rate.[114,115]

When changing from a preserved saline or chemical disinfection system, due to sensitivity to preservatives, it may be necessary to purge the lenses of the chemicals.[116] Purging is accomplished by thoroughly cleaning the lens with a surfactant cleaner not containing the offending chemical, and rinsing the lens well with unpreserved saline. The lenses should be soaked in several changes of saline or other disinfecting solution.

Chemical (Cold) Disinfection

Some of the problems and inconveniences of heat disinfection can be overcome with the use of chemical (nonthermal) disinfection systems (Table 18.7). Since no heat or electric-ity is required, this method is more convenient for travel. It minimizes the problem of deposits and lens deterioration. Disinfection occurs constantly as long as the lens is in the disinfecting solution.

As with preserved saline solutions, a major concern is hypersensitivity to the solutions. Patient compliance with multiple step disinfection systems can also prove a problem. Patients must follow the proper procedures including cleaning the lenses prior to disinfection, changing the solution each day, and soaking the lenses in the solutions for at least 4 to 6 hours.

THIMEROSAL-CHLORHEXIDINE SYSTEMS

The first chemical disinfecting systems employed thimerosal (0.001%), chlorhexidine gluconate (0.005%), and EDTA (0.1%) as preservatives in saline with appropriate buffers. The sensitivity reactions that occur are the same as with the thimerosal-preserved salines.

TABLE 18.7
Representative Chemical Disinfecting Solutions for Hydrogel Lenses

Solution	Manufacturer	Preservative	Other Ingredients
Opti-Free	Alcon	Polyquad (0.001%) edetate disodium (0.1%)	citrate buffer sodium chloride
Flex-Care for Sensitive Eyes	Alcon	chlorhexidine (0.005%) disodium edetate (0.1%)	sodium borate boric acid sodium chloride
Opti-Soft	Alcon	Polyquad (0.001%) edetate disodium (0.1%)	borate buffer sodium chloride
Hydrocare Cleaning & Disinfection	Allergan	thimerosal (0.002%) Tris and bis (2-hydroxyethyl) tallow ammonium chloride	sodium bicarbonate sodium phosphate propylene glycol polysorbate 80 soluble poly-hema hydrochloric acid buffers
ReNu Multi-Purpose	Bausch & Lomb	Dymed (0.00005%) edetate disodium	sodium borate sodium chloride poloxamine
Disinfecting Solution	Bausch & Lomb	thimerosal (0.001%) disodium edetate (0.1%) chlorhexidine (0.005%)	sodium borate boric acid sodium chloride
Quick Care Starting Solution	Ciba Vision	isopropanol	polyoxypropylene block copolymer sodium lauroampho-diacetate
Soft Mate Disinfection (Thimerosal free)	Paragon	chlorhexidine (0.005%) edetate disodium (0.1%)	povidone octylphenoxyl (oxyethylene) ethanol borate buffer sodium chloride

CHLORHEXIDINE

Chlorhexidine (0.005%) with disodium edetate has also been used as a disinfecting solution. It has decreased antimicrobial activity over the combination with thimerosal but has greatly reduced sensitivity reactions. However, sensitivities to it can occur. The chlorhexidine may bind to tear film components on the lens surface and become a source of irritation. Chlorhexidine may make the lens surface hydrophobic increasing the adherence of lipids.[117] Decomposition of chlorhexidine may turn the lens yellow to yellow-green.

A novel form of chlorhexidine disinfection uses chlorhexidine in a tablet form (OptimEyes). The tablet dissolves in tap water to form the disinfecting solution.[118] The solution formulated is reported effective against the normally tested bacteria, fungi, and *Acanthamoeba* when used with numerous sources of tap water from Great Britain.[119]

ALKYLTRIETHANOL AMMONIUM CHLORIDE-THIMEROSAL SOLUTION

This disinfecting system, introduced by Allergan, contains Tris (2-hydroxyethyl) tallow ammonium chloride (0.013%), bis (2-hydroxyethyl) tallow ammonium chloride, thimerosal (0.002%), polymers, and surfactants including a soluble HEMA, propylene glycol, and polysorbate 80 as well as buffers and salts to adjust tonicity. Due to sensitivity reactions, this solution is not widely used.

POLYQUAD-PRESERVED SOLUTION

This large quaternary ammonium molecule (molecular weight approximately 5000) does not significantly invade the lens polymer and therefore seldom causes toxic reactions. Patients who have sensitivities to thimerosal solutions normally do not have problems with this solution. The Alcon OptiSoft and OptiFree solutions use this compound, which can be employed as a preserved saline for heat as well as chemical disinfection. As previously discussed, this preservative alone is not totally effective, especially at killing fungi. Therefore, the cleaning and rinsing steps are very important.

POLYAMINOPROPYL BIGUANIDE (DYMED)

Developed to overcome the problems of preservative sensitivity and toxic reactions, this is a relatively large molecule (molecular weight about 2000) with few reported reactions. The Bausch and Lomb ReNu Disinfecting and Multi-Purpose solutions employ it. As with the previous system, the disinfectant is not totally effective, and the cleaning and rinsing steps are critical.

HYDROGEN PEROXIDE

Hydrogen peroxide (H_2O_2) does not result in clinically significant sensitivity problems when used properly because it breaks down into water and oxygen. As an oxidizing agent, hydrogen peroxide may have some small effect in keeping the lenses clean but does not eliminate the need for cleaners. Early disadvantages of H_2O_2 were patient compliance and instability of the hydrogen peroxide. Present formulations of hydrogen peroxide are stable, and numerous systems have been devised to make patient compliance easier (Table 18.8).

Only hydrogen peroxide formulated for contact lenses should be used. Over-the-counter hydrogen peroxide may have stabilizers that are not compatible, have colorants that might discolor lenses, have a pH well below that of the manufacturer's hydrogen peroxide (especially with AOSept),[120] and lack the salts required with some systems for a proper saline solution following neutralization.

The lenses must soak in the 3% hydrogen peroxide solution for at least 10 minutes (see previous discussion of microbial effectiveness). Since hydrogen peroxide causes considerable discomfort if placed on the eye, it must be neutralized.

The first neutralization procedure consisted of rinsing and soaking in a 0.5% sodium bicarbonate neutralizing solution followed by placing the lenses in preserved saline. This proved too time consuming for daily use by the patient. Next a platinum catalytic disk was introduced to break down any residual hydrogen peroxide. With this system (Septicon) the lens soaks in the hydrogen peroxide for 10 minutes, is then transferred to the case with the catalyst and filled with preserved saline. The lens soaks in this case for at least 3 to 4 hours, at which time the residual hydrogen peroxide breaks down. This approach is still a two-step procedure and requires that a preserved saline be used as the last solution, which introduces potential preservative reactions.

A further refinement of this system eliminates the step of removing the lens from the hydrogen peroxide and placing it in the second case with saline. In the AOSept system the hydrogen peroxide is placed in the case with the catalytic disk and the lens. The disk immediately begins to break down the hydrogen peroxide to water and oxygen. After 6 hours the lens can be removed and worn. The AOSept hydrogen peroxide solution contains NaCl and phosphate buffer so the lens ends up in normal saline. Since oxygen is given off as the hydrogen peroxide is decomposed, the case has vent holes to allow the gas to escape. If the patient uses a surfactant cleaner before disinfecting with AOSept and does not properly rinse the cleaner off, excessive foaming of the solution may result in foam exuding from the case. The surfactant is a soap and will form bubbles. The catalytic disk must be replaced periodically to prevent complaints of burning or stinging on lens placement in the morning. Replacement should occur after a hundred or so uses of the system (3 months).

Another method of neutralizing the hydrogen peroxide uses a chemical neutralizer (sodium pyruvate or sodium thiosulfate) or an enzyme (catalase). These systems result in

TABLE 18.8
Hydrogen Peroxide Disinfection Systems

System	Company	Disinfection	Neutralization
MiraSept	Alcon	MiraSept Disinfection 3% hydrogen peroxide sodium stannate sodium nitrate phosphoric acid (10 minutes minimum)	MiraSept Rinsing & Neutralization 0.5% sodium pyruvate boric acid sodium borate edetate disodium sorbic acid (0.1%) (10 minutes minimum)
Lens Plus Oxysept	Allergan	Oxysept I 3% hydrogen peroxide sodium stannate sodium nitrate phosphate buffer (10 minutes minimum)	Oxysept II catalase edetate disodium mono & dibasic sodium phosphate NaCl (10 minutes minimum)
UltraCare System	Allergan	3% hydrogen peroxide sodium stannate sodium nitrate (at least 15 minutes)	catalase tablets hydroxypropylmethylcellulose (10 minutes)
AOSept	Ciba Vision	3% hydrogen peroxide sodium stannate sodium nitrate phosphate buffer 0.85% NaCl (6 hours)	catalytic disc (6 hours total)
Lensept	Ciba Vision	3% hydrogen peroxide sodium stannate sodium nitrate phosphate buffer (55 minutes)	catalase (5 minutes)
Consept	Paragon	3% hydrogen peroxide sodium nitrate (10 minutes)	0.5% sodium thiosulfate polyoxyl 40 stereate borate buffer (10 minutes)

rapid neutralization, less than 5 minutes. One advantage of such systems is that the patient can clean and disinfect lenses in less than 30 minutes. This may be important for extended wear patients who want to disinfect the lenses without leaving them out overnight. Most companies recommend that the lenses be placed in the 3% hydrogen peroxide for 10 to 20 minutes prior to the neutralization. Another way to use such a system is to allow the lenses to soak overnight in the hydrogen peroxide and neutralize them prior to wearing in the morning. This system has two advantages: (1) the patient does not have to wait 10 to 20 minutes following lens removal to change the solution before going to bed, and (2) the longer disinfection time is more effective against some organisms. The disadvantage is that some polymers (the high water lenses) may change shape and take an hour or longer to return to the pre-hydrogen peroxide soak dimensions.[52,53]

An addition to the hydrogen peroxide armamentarium is a catalase tablet system (UltraCare-U.S. and Oxysept "One Step" outside the U.S.). At the time the lenses are placed in the 3% hydrogen peroxide, the tablet is also placed in the solution. Hydroxypropyl methylcellulose (HPMC) coats the tablet and initially prevents the release of the catalase. Over time the coating dissolves, releasing the catalase and neutralizing the hydrogen peroxide. Therefore, the lens is in the full strength hydrogen peroxide for a period of time allowing full antimicrobial effect, but the approach has only one step for the patient. This system is well accepted.[121]

Another way to eliminate the hydrogen peroxide after disinfection is simply to rinse and dilute it. Rinsing once or twice with preserved saline and then allowing the lenses to soak in saline so the residual hydrogen peroxide will diffuse out results in a low enough level of hydrogen peroxide that it will not be a problem for many patients. However, the rinsed lense has enough residual hydrogen peroxide that many patients complain of burning and stinging on lens placement.

Hydrogen peroxide systems can fade some tinted hydrogel lenses over time.[122] Where possible, it is best to use another chemical system. However, if necessary, hydrogen peroxide can be used, since it fades most tints only slightly.

ISOPROPYL ALCOHOL

A cleaning solution with 20% isopropyl alcohol (Miraflow) very effectively kills organisms. Using this concept a disinfection system using the alcohol cleaner (called Starting Solution) followed by soaking in a preserved saline (the same as SoftWear but called Finishing Solution) has been introduced in the United States as Quick Care by Ciba Vision (outside the U.S. it is called InstaCare). This system quickly and simply disinfects as the patients clean their lenses.

IODINE SYSTEMS

Iodine is a disinfecting compound that has been used to disinfect hydrogel lenses.[123,124] Polyvinylpyrrolidone iodine (also termed povidone-iodine) (0.1%) systems are marketed outside the United States. This method is an effective disinfectant and apparently does not cause many sensitivity reactions. If the patient inadvertently places the lens on the eye before the solution decolorizes, discomfort and corneal damage can occur. Iodine systems may cause lens yellowing.

Cleaning of Hydrogel Lenses

A variety of surface coatings and deposits develop on hydrogel lenses as a result of surface drying during wear, heat disinfection, lens handling, and exposure to the environment.[87,88,125–127] The most common deposit is a relatively uniform surface coating (Fig. 18.22) of tear film components, mainly proteins. These coatings are limited to the surface or surface layers of the polymer.[126] Soft silicone lenses can also develop surface coatings that appear similar to hydrogel coatings but have cracks in the deposits due to the elasticity of the material. Lipids can coat the surfaces of both types of lenses. If ions or minerals are present in the solution used with heat disinfection, crystalline formation will occur on and in the hydrogel lens.[87,126,127] These usually consist of calcium carbonate or calcium phosphate along with other tear film components. In some cases lenses will turn brown, possibly due to the formation of a melanin-like pigment from aromatic compounds in the tears.[128]

Discrete spots, probably lipids and calcium salts, can develop on extended-wear lenses (Fig. 18.23). These invade the polymer and will leave a surface defect if removed.

MECHANICAL CLEANING

Hydrogel lenses can be cleaned of many substances by simply rubbing the lens surface between the fingers or in the palm of the hand using only saline or surfactant cleaners. However, denatured or crystallized material is not removed. The use of lens rubbing is important in conjunction with most of the cleaning solutions and systems.

Polishing the lens surface using XPAL in water and a soft pad will also remove some deposits.[129,130]

ULTRASONIC CLEANING

Ultrasonic cleaning of contact lenses has been suggested.[131] Phillips and associates[102] found that using an ultrasonic unit with a surfactant cleaner was more effective than the surfactant alone. However, the use of an enzyme appeared as effective as the ultrasound and surfactant. Ultrasonic cleaning was less effective than manual lens rubbing.[101] Fatt [132]

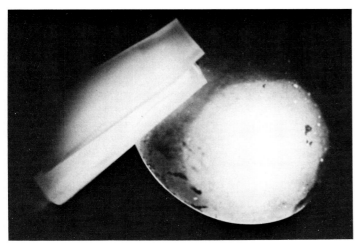

FIGURE 18.22 **Surface coating of tear film components on a hydrogel lens.**

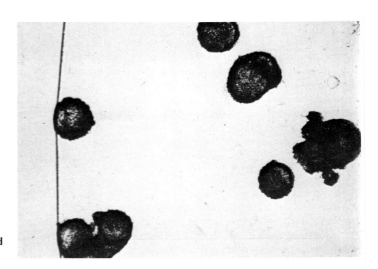

FIGURE 18.23   **Deposits on a high water content extended wear lens.**

has indicated that ultrasonic cleaners have little chance of being effective with hydrogel lenses due to the small difference between the properties of the lens material and the water in which it is submersed. When the two are so similar, little energy is generated at the interface and thus little cleaning occurs.

SURFACTANT CLEANERS

Many surfactant cleaners are available for use with hydrogel lenses (Table 18.9). Surfactants lower surface tension and emulsify lipids, oils, and other materials. In addition to nonionic surfactants these cleaners contain salts, buffers, and preservatives. Most of the surfactants are prophylactic cleaners that must be used daily to prevent deposits. Once material is denatured on the surface, these cleaners will not sufficiently remove it. There are some exceptions. For example, Opti-Free Cleaner contains abrasive particles (Fig. 18.24). All the surfactants depend on mechanical rubbing of the surface for cleaning. Since various cleaners employ different surfactants and formulations, they may have varying effectiveness against different contaminants. Some contain other cleaners, such as isopropyl alcohol (MiraFlow), to dissolve lipids.

OXIDIZING CLEANERS

These cleaners act by breaking down proteins and other contaminants into small molecules that can be removed. Some cleaners are quite strong oxidizing agents (such as sodium perborate, high concentrations of hydrogen peroxide, or chlorine) and with repeated use can damage lens polymers. Due to the possibility of ocular damage if the cleaner is not neutralized or properly rinsed, these cleaners are not generally available in the United States. Frequent

replacement and disposable lenses have lessened the need for such cleaners.

ENZYMATIC CLEANERS

Enzymatic cleaners (Table 18.10) are effective in removing proteinaceous coatings from hydrogel lenses. Papain, the first proteolytic enzyme used, derives from the papaya and also functions as a meat tenderizer.[133,134] The enzyme cleaners are provided in tablet form. Disinfecting solution, preserved saline, or sterile unpreserved saline should be used to dissolve the tablets and not tap or distilled water. This approach minimizes the possibility of microorganism contamination. The dirty lens soaks in the solution for a period of time, depending on its type. With low water content lenses, a period of at least 2 hours and commonly overnight has been recommended. Leaving the lens in the solution longer than 8 to 12 hours does not result in additional cleaning since the enzyme denatures in the aqueous solution. Since the solution does not disinfect, either in conjunction with or following the enzyme soak, the lenses must be disinfected. Heat and hydrogen peroxide disinfection will denature any residual enzyme but other chemical disinfection systems will not. Papain tablets have an added activator that gives a characteristic odor.

Since moisture will slowly deactivate the enzyme, patients should discard any tablets in open foil packages. The enzyme is normally quite safe and can be used repeatedly without lens or ocular damage. Although once-weekly enzyming usually maintains the lenses clean of protein deposits, enzyme cleaners do not remove inorganic deposits.[135,136]

If the papain enzyme is not removed or denatured, it may cause an allergic hypersensitivity or bind preservatives, causing discomfort. For this reason there has been debate over whether this enzyme should be used with chemical

TABLE 18.9
Representative Surfactant Cleaning Solutions for Hydrogel Lenses

Solution	Manufacturer	Preservative	Other Ingredients
Opti-Clean	Alcon	thimerosal (0.004%) disodium edetate (0.1%)	Tween 21 polymeric cleaning agents hydroxyethylcellulose
Opti-Free Daily Cleaner (also Opti-Clean II)	Alcon	Polyquad (0.01%) edetate disodium (0.1%)	hydroxyethylcellulose Tween 21 polymeric cleaning agents
Preflex for Sensitive Eyes	Alcon	sorbic acid (0.2%) disodium edetate (0.2%)	hydroxyethyl cellulose polyvinyl alcohol tyloxapol phosphate buffer
LC-65	Allergan	thimerosal (0.001%) disodium edetate	undisclosed cleaner
Lens Clear	Allergan	sorbic acid (0.1%) edetate disodium	surfactants
Lens Plus Daily Cleaner	Allergan	edetate disodium	cocoamphocarboxyglycinate sodium lauryl sulfate hexylene glycol sodium phosphate
Soft Mate Daily II (or ps Daily) (or Hands Off Daily Cleaner)	Paragon	potassium sorbate (0.13%) edetate disodium (0.2%)	octylphenoxyl ethanol hydroxyethylcellulose
Sensitive Eyes Daily Cleaner	Bausch & Lomb	sorbic acid (0.25%) disodium edetate (0.5%)	sodium chloride borate buffer hydropropylmethylcellulose surfactant
Sterile Daily Cleaner	Bausch & Lomb	thimerosal (0.004%) disodium edetate (0.2%)	hydroxyethyl cellulose polyvinyl alcohol tyloxapol sodium phosphates
DURAcare	Blairex	thimerosal (0.004%) EDTA (0.1%)	detergents salt buffers
Ciba Vision Cleaner	Ciba Vision	sorbic acid (0.1%) edetate disodium (0.2%)	sodium lauryl sulfate hexylene glycol cocoamphocarboxyglycinate
Mira Flow	Ciba Vision	none	isopropyl alcohol (20%) poloxamer 407 (15%) amphoteric 10 (10%)
Pliagel	Alcon	sorbic acid (0.25%) trisodium edetate (0.5%)	poloxamer 407 (15%) potassium chloride
Sof/Pro Clean S.A.	Sherman	sorbic acid (0.1%) EDTA (0.1%)	lauryl sulfate salt of imidazoline octylphenoxypolyethoxyethanol sodium bisulfite

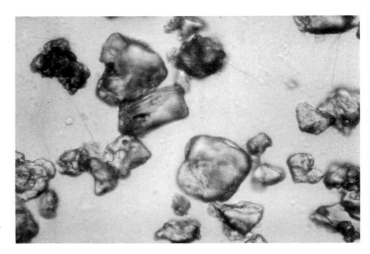

FIGURE 18.24 **Particles found in Opti-Free as seen under the microscope.**

disinfection systems.[137,138] Many patients can use the enzyme with chemical disinfection, but some patients may develop conjunctival injection and discomfort. With high water content lenses and extended-wear lenses, the soaking time decreases to 15 to 60 minutes to minimize the diffusion of the enzyme into the lens matrix. In cases where a reaction still occurs, an alternate enzyme must be used or enzyme cleaning should be discontinued.

Pancreatin is another enzyme used to remove deposits from lenses. It derives from the hog pancreas and has lipase and amylase action as well as protease activity. This enzyme is used in the same fashion as the papain enzyme. The tablet (Opti-Free Enzymatic Cleaner) can be dissolved in Opti-Free Disinfecting Solution so that disinfecting and enzyming can be done at one time.[139]

Subtilisin is an enzyme effective against a wide variety of proteins and over a wide range of temperatures and pHs. Therefore, it can be used during a thermal disinfection cycle (ReNu Thermal) or with hydrogen peroxide (Allergan Ultrazyme or ReNu Effervescent). This approach decreases cleaning time and hopefully increases compliance with cleaning. It does not require an activator and thus does not have an odor. It is 90% neutralized by an overnight soak in 3% hydrogen peroxide. As an added advantage, the combination of enzyme and hydrogen peroxide disinfects more effectively than hydrogen peroxide alone. The ReNu thermal enzymatic cleaner should not be used with CSI lenses as it will tend to make the lenses stiff and change their shape. Returning to normal condition and shape may require more than 1 hour once placed back into saline.

Most of the tablets are effervescent to shorten the time for the tablet to dissolve and thus decrease the cleaning time.

Disinfecting and Storing Diagnostic Lenses

Maintaining a stock of diagnostic lenses can create special challenges and concerns. Should rigid diagnostic lenses be stored dry or in solution? The advantages of storing the lenses in solution is that the hydration and wettability of the

TABLE 18.10
Enzymatic Cleaners

Solution	Manufacturer	Ingredients
Opti-Free Enzymatic Cleaner	Alcon	purified pork pancreatin
Opti-zyme	Alcon	purified pork pancreatin
Enzymatic Soft Lens Cleaner	Allergan	stabilized papain, NaCl, sodium carbonate, sodium borate edetate disodium
Extenzyme Protein Cleaner	Allergan	same as above
ProFree/GP Weekly Enzymatic Cleaner	Allergan	same as above
Ultrazyme	Allergan	subtilisin A
ReNu Effervescent Enzymatic Cleaner	Bausch & Lomb	stabilized subtilisin polyethylene glycol sodium carbonate tartaric acid, sodium chloride
ReNu Thermal Enzymatic Cleaner	Bausch & Lomb	stabilized subtilisin boric acid, sodium carbonate, NaCl

surfaces of the lenses are maintained. The disadvantages include the solution drying up in the case and leaving a residue on the lenses between usages and the potential for contamination. One study found some contamination in rigid lens cases for both wet and dry storage with a lower percentage of contaminated lenses with dry storage.[140] For wet storage, the lenses should be cleaned well prior to placing them in solution. In addition, the solution in the case should be changed periodically. For dry storage, the lens should be cleaned well and the lens and case dried with a soft tissue or cloth. Leaving tears, solution, or water on the lens defeats the advantage of dry storage. Few organisms survive on a perfectly dry lens. RGP lenses can be disinfected with hydrogen peroxide prior to storage.[141] Most practitioners store their rigid diagnostic lenses dry.

Storing hydrogel lenses also presents problems. Because of the days or weeks between uses, one either must be sure that all the organisms on the lenses are killed prior to storage or that disinfection is continuous. A safe method, which the manufacturer employs prior to sending lenses out, is to sterilize the lenses with autoclaving. Autoclaving kills all organisms. As long as the lens vial is not opened, it will not become contaminated. A few offices and clinics use this technique, but it is costly, and time-consuming. In addition, repeated use can damage lenses, especially high water lenses. Heat disinfecting the lenses is effective but has some of the same drawbacks as autoclaving. The common alternative to heat disinfection is a chemical disinfection system. Because microbial growth can occur with the present chemical systems in use with hydrogel lenses,[142] precautions must be taken. Prior to storage, the lenses should be cleaned well, preferably with a cleaner containing alcohol (MiraFlow), which kills organisms. Likewise, re-cleaning and storing with new disinfecting solution periodically is helpful. Cleaning with the MiraFlow and rinsing prior to using the lens is an added precaution. Infection from diagnostic lenses has not been reported but is of concern and proper precautions should be taken. Using disposable lenses as diagnostic lenses overcomes this problem.

Medications and Contact Lens Wear

Ocular Medications

The use of topical ocular medications with nonhydrogel (such as rigid and silicone) lenses is permissible in some cases since the lenses do not absorb the drugs. However, the lens may impede the drug from reaching the cornea. Alternatively, once under the lens, medication may be held against the cornea for longer than normal. Since contact lenses may compromise the corneal epithelium, reduce the blink rate, and impair tear circulation, topically applied drugs are likely to penetrate the cornea in greater quantity. Ointments will cause blurred vision if instilled with contact lens wear. When possible, topical medications should be instilled without the lenses in place.

Hydrogel lenses, however, present a different situation because they will absorb water soluble compounds. If a hydrogel lens is placed in a drug solution, the drug usually concentrates in the lens. This absorption ability of hydrogel lenses has been used to treat various ocular conditions.[143–149] The amount of drug absorbed depends upon the lens material, the drug, the concentration of the drug in the solution, and the length of time the lens is soaked.[143] Chapter 3 discusses the use of hydrogel lenses as drug delivery devices.

Because of the exaggerated effect of many drugs when used in conjunction with hydrogel lenses, it is best not to soak lenses in the medication or to use drops while wearing hydrogel lenses, unless such an effect is desired. However, there has been some controversy whether placing a drop of medication on the eye while wearing a lens results in significant drug absorption or adverse effect.[149–151] Due to the small volume of instilled medication and the rate at which tears wash it away, there appears to be little risk. The preservatives in artificial tears and other topically applied solutions also present little risk.

Soaking lenses in or repeated instillations of epinephrine, phenylephrine, dopa, or related oxidizable adrenergic drugs can stain lenses gray, black, or brown.[149,152,153] Therefore, glaucoma patients using topical epinephrine should not wear hydrogel lenses. Once such lens staining has occurred, however, hydrogen peroxide or other oxidizing agent may clear the lens.

Systemic Medications

Numerous systemic medications can affect contact lens wear or discolor hydrogel lenses. Most of the effects on lens wear result from changes in the tear film. Some antihistamines, anticholinergic drugs, tricyclic antidepressants, and antianxiety agents may decrease tear production and result in discomfort with lens wear and drying of the lens surface, ultimately causing blurred vision.[154] Propranolol (Inderal), a β-adrenergic blocking agent commonly prescribed to treat hypertension and some cardiovascular diseases, can also cause decreased tearing as well as conjunctival allergic reactions.[155] Diuretics such as Dyazide (hydrochlorothiazide and triamterene) and Lasix (furosemide) also cause decreased lacrimation as well as conjunctival allergic reactions and photophobia. Gold injections for rheumatoid arthritis and Accutane used for acne can cause inflammation and affect contact lens wear.[156] Acetylsalicylic acid (aspirin) taken orally is excreted into the tears.[157] This drug might be absorbed into a hydrogel lens and cause corneal epithelial irritation, since aspirin is a known irritant.[158]

Oral contraceptives have been implicated in contact lens-wearing problems.[159] Possible etiologic mechanisms include changes in tear production and in corneal thickness. However, other evidence indicates that the prevalence of contact lens problems associated with this class of drugs is probably less than previously reported.[158,160]

Numerous drugs can be excreted into the tear film and discolor hydrogel lenses. These include phenazopyridine, tetracycline, phenolphthalein, and nitrofurantoin.[155] Rifampin, a drug used in the treatment of meningococcal disease and tuberculosis, is excreted into the tears and has been reported to stain hydrogel lenses orange.[161]

Disulfiram (Antabuse), a drug used in the management of chronic alcoholism, has caused a reaction with rigid lens wear similar to that which would occur if alcohol were imbibed. The reaction, reportedly related to the polyvinyl alcohol in the wetting solution,[162] consists of flushing, dry mouth, a prickly sensation, dizziness, nausea, vomiting, and weakness.

For the above reasons, one must carefully question the contact lens patient about the concurrent use of ocular and systemic drugs.

References

1. Terry J, Hill RM. Human tear osmotic pressure. Arch Ophthalmol 1978;96:120–122.
2. Mishima S. Corneal thickness. Surv Ophthalmol 1978;13:57–96.
3. Hill RM. Osmotic vulnerability. Int Contact Lens Clin 1977;4:31–33.
4. Gumpelmayer T. Absorption and diffusion of small molecules in hydrophilic materials. Optician 1976; Spec Supp:44–48.
5. Mandell RB. Sticking of gel contact lenses. Int Contact Lens Clin 1975;2:28–29.
6. Hill RM, Young WH. Ophthalmic solutions. J Am Optom Assoc 1973;44:263–270.
7. Moses RA, ed. Adler's physiology of the eye: clinical application. ed. 6. St. Louis: Mosby, 1975.
8. Alder I, Wlodyga RJ, Rope SJ. The effects of pH on contact lens wearing. J Am Optom Assoc 1968;39:1000–1001.
9. MacKeen DG, Bulle K. Buffers and preservatives in contact lens solutions. Contacto 1977;21:33–36.
10. Phillips AJ. Contact lens plastics, solutions and storage: Some implications. Ophthalmic Optician 1968;8:1058, 1075–1076.
11. Demas GN. pH consistency and stability of contact lens solutions. J Am Optom Assoc 1989;60(10):732–734.
12. Dabezies DH. Contact lenses and their solutions: A review of basic principles. Eye, Ear, Nose, Throat Monthly 1966;45:39–44, 68–72, 82–84.
13. Kreiner CF. Biochemical aspects of ophthalmic preservatives. Contacto 1979;23:10–14.
14. Zand ML. The effect of non-therapeutic ophthalmic preparation on the cornea and tear film. Aust J Optom 1981;64:44–67.
15. Burstein NL, Klyce SD. Electrophysiologic and morphologic effects of ophthalmic preparations on rabbit corneal epithelium. Invest Ophthalmol Vis Sci 1977;16:899.
16. Burstein NL. Preservative cytotoxic threshold for benzalkonium chloride and chlorhexidine digluconate in cat and rabbit corneas. Invest Ophthalmol Vis Sci 1980;19:308–313.
17. Ganju S, Cordrey P. Proceedings: reversible uptake of preservatives by soft contact lenses. J Pharm Pharmacol 1975;27 (suppl 2):25.
18. Kaspar H. Binding characteristics and microbiological effectiveness of preservatives. Aust J Optom 1976;59:4–9.
19. Weir NW. Do the varying pHs of contact lens solutions affect their bacterial action against *Pseudomonas aeruginosa*? Ophthalmic Optician 1977;17:311–313.
20. Riegelman S. Bacterial testing of contact lens solutions. Am J Ophthalmol 1967;64:485–486.
21. Stone J. Notes on the after-care of contact lens patients. Ophthalmic Optician 1967;10:966–976.
22. Hopkins CJ. Contact lens solutions and preservatives. Ophthalmic Optician 1980;20:626.
23. Sibley MJ, Yung G. A technique for the determination of chemical bindings to soft contact lenses. Am J Optom Physiol Opt 1973;50:710–714.
24. Burton GD, Hill RM. Aerobic responses of the cornea to ophthalmic preservatives measured in vivo. Invest Ophthalmol Vis Sci 1981;21:842–845.
25. Winder AF, Astbury NJ, Sheraidah GAK, Ruben M. Penetration of mercury from ophthalmic preservatives into the human eye. Optician 1981;181:22–24.
26. Refojo M. Reversible binding of chlorhexidine gluconate to hydrogel contact lenses. Contact Intraocular Lens Med J 1976;2:47–31.
27. Riedhammer TM. A simple chemical test for chlorhexidine in hydrophilic contact lenses. Int Contact Lens Clin 1979;6:26–30.
28. Snyder C. A microbiological assessment of rigid contact lens wet and dry storage. Int Contact Lens Clin 1990;117(2):83–87.
29. Gandhi PA, Sawant AD, Wilson LA, Ahearn DG. Adaptation and growth of *Serratia marcescens* in contact lens disinfectant solutions containing chlorhexidine gluconate. Applied Environ Microbio 1993;59(1):183–188.
30. Lum VJ, Lyle WM. Chemical components of contact lens solutions. Can J Optom 1981;43:136–151.
31. Isen A. The Griffin lens. J Am Optom Assoc 1972;43(3):275–286
32. McNally JJ. Clinical aspects of topical application of dilute hydrogen peroxide solutions. CLAO J 1990;16(1 suppl):S46–S51.
33. Riley MV, Wilson G. Topical hydrogen peroxide and the safety of ocular tissues. CLAO J 1993;19(3):186–190.
34. Holden B. A report card on hydrogen peroxide for contact lens disinfection. CLAO J 1990;16(1 suppl):S61–S64.
35. Wilson G, Riley MV. Does topical hydrogen peroxide penetrate the cornea? Invest Ophthalmol Vis Sci 1993;34(9):2752–2760.
36. Riley MV, Kast M. Penetration of hydrogen peroxide from contact lenses or tear-side solutions into the aqueous humor. Optom Vis Sci 1991;68(7):546–551.
37. Wilson GS, Chalmers RL. Effect of H_2O_2 concentration and exposure time on stroma swelling: An epithelial perfusion model. Optom Vis Sci 1990;67:252–255.
38. Janoff LE. The Septicon system: A review of pertinent scientific data. Int Contact Lens Clin 1984;11(5):274–279.
39. Gyulai P, et al. Relative neutralization ability of six hydrogen peroxide disinfection systems. Contact Lens Spectrum 1987;2:61–66.
40. Gyulai P, et al. Efficacy of catalase as a neutralizer of a hydrogen peroxide disinfecting solution for soft contact lenses. Int Eyecare 1986;2(8):418–422.

41. Beekhuis WH, Eggink FA, Vreugdenhil W, Platenkamp GJ, Buitenwerf J. Disinfection of trial mid water content soft contact lenses in the practice: The efficacy of sodium dichloroisocyanurate. J Br Cont Lens Assoc 1992;15(3):103–107.

42. Feldman GL. Benzyl alcohol—New life as an ophthalmic preservative. Cont Lens Spectrum 1989;4(5):41–44.

43. Feldman GL, Krezanoski JZ, Costerton JW. Is benzyl alcohol effective against biofilms on RGP's? Cont Lens Spectrum 1992; 7(3):29–33.

44. Feldman GL, Krezanoski JZ, Ellis B. Control of bacterial biofilms on rigid gas permeable lenses. Cont Lens Spectrum 1992; 7(10):36–39.

45. Lowther GE, Pole J, Biolo M. Comparison of two care systems when used with low Dk and high Dk silicone/acrylate materials. Int Cont Lens Clin 1990;17(11&12):276–279.

46. Meakin, BJ. Contact lens solutions in the United Kingdom. J Br Cont Lens Assoc 1984;7(4);192–203.

47. Houlsby RD, Ghajar M, Chavez G. Microbiological evaluation of soft contact lens disinfecting solutions. J Am Optom Assoc 1984; 55(3):205–211.

48. Penley CA, et al. Laboratory evaluation of chemical disinfection of soft contact lenses. Contact Intraocular Lens Med J 1981; 7(2):101–110.

49. Shih KL, et al. Disinfecting activities of non-peroxide soft contact lens cold disinfection solutions. CLAO J 1991;17(3):165–168.

50. Richardson LE, Begley CG, Keck GK. Comparative efficacies of soft contact lens disinfection systems against a fungal contaminant. J Am Optom Assoc 1993;64(3):210–214.

51. Penley CA, et al. Efficacy of hydrogen peroxide disinfection systems for soft contact lenses contaminated with fungi. CLAO J 1985;11(1):65–68.

52. Janoff LE. The exposure of various polymers to a 24-hour soak in Lensept™: The effect on base curve, J Am Optom Assoc 1985; 56(3):222–225.

53. Jones L, Davies I, Jones D. Effect of hydrogen peroxide neutralization on the fitting characteristics of group IV disposable contact lenses. J Br Cont Lens Assoc 1993;16(4):135–140.

54. Recommendations for preventing possible HTLV-III/LAV virus from tears, MMWR 1985;34(34):1429.

55. Vogt MW, et al. Safe disinfection of contact lenses after contamination with HTLV-III. Ophthalmology 1986;93(6):771–774.

56. Moore MB, et al. *Acanthamoeba* keratitis associated with soft contact lenses. Am J Ophthalmol 1985;100(3):396–403.

57. Dornic DI, et al. *Acanthamoeba* keratitis in soft contact lens wearers, J Am Optom Assoc 1987;58(6):482–486.

58. Ludwig IH, et al. Susceptibility of *Acanthamoeba* to soft contact lens disinfection systems. Invest Ophthalmol Vis Sci 1986; 27(4):626–628.

59. Penley CA, Willis SW, Sickler SG. Comparative Antimicrobial Efficacy of Soft and Rigid Gas Permeable Contact Lens Solutions against *Acanthamoeba*. CLAO J 1989;15(4):257–60.

60. Conner CG, Hopkins SL, Salisbury RD. Effectivity of contact lens disinfection systems against *Acanthamoeba culbertsoni*. Optom Vis Sci 1991;68(2):138–141.

61. Silvany RE, Dougherty JM, McCulley JP. Effect of contact lens preservatives on *Acanthamoeba*. Ophthalmology 1991;98(6): 854–857.

62. Krishna N, Brown F. Polyvinyl alcohol as an ophthalmic vehicle: Effect on regeneration of corneal epithelium. Am J Ophthalmol 1964;57:99–106.

63. Benedetto D, Shah D, Kaufman H. The dynamic film thickness of cushioning agents on contact lens materials. An Ophthalmol 1978; 10:437–442.

64. Gordon S. Dimensional stability of contact lenses. J Am Optom Assoc 1971;42:239.

65. Pearson RM. Dimensional stability of several hard contact lens materials. Am J Optom Physiol Opt 1977;54:826–833.

66. Lloyd DJ. Enzyme cleaners: The structure, properties and mode of action of enzymes. Ophthalmic Optician 1979;19:833–839.

67. Phillips AJ. The cleaning of hydrogel contact lenses. Ophthalmic Optician 1980;20:375–388.

68. Josephson JE, Caffery BE. Selecting an appropriate hydrogel lens care system. J Am Optom Assoc 1981;52:227–234.

69. Kleist FD. Soft lens cleaners compared. Contact Lens Forum 1980;5:47–51.

70. Dea D, Huth SW. The effect of reducing agents on enzymatic cleaning efficacy. Int Contact Lens Clin 1988;15:256–259.

71. Bellows R, Lowther GE. Subepithelial infiltrates. Int Contact Lens Clin 1979;6:73.

72. Hill RM. Escaping the sting. Int Contact Lens Clin 1979;6:27.

73. Hill RM. Aging ophthalmic solutions. Int Contact Lens Clin 1978; 5:124.

74. Rosenthal P, et al. Quantitative analysis of chlorhexidine gluconate and benzalkonium chloride adsorption on silicone/acrylate polymers. CLAO J 1986;12(1):43–50.

75. Sterling J, Hecht A. BAK adsorption in silicone/acrylates. Contact Lens Forum 1987;12(6):80.

76. Walters K, Gee H, Meakin B. The interaction of benzalkonium chloride with Boston contact lens material. Part I. Basic interaction studies, J Br Contact Lens Assoc, 1983;6(2):42–50.

77. Wong, et al. Adsorption of benzalkonium chloride by RGP lenses. Contact Lens Forum 1986;11(5):25–32.

78. Hoffman W. Ending the BAK-RGP controversy. Int Contact Lens Clinic 1987;14(1):31–35.

79. Friedman DM. Too much lens cleaning can also be destructive. Contact Lens Forum 1989;14(9):80.

80. Boltz KD. The overzealous contact lens cleaner. Contact Lens Spectrum 1989;4(12):53–54.

81. Bennett ES, Henry VA. RGP lens power change with abrasive cleaner use. Int Cont Lens Clin 1990;17(3):152–153.

82. Lowther G. Effect of some solutions on HGP contact lens parameters. J Am Optom Assoc 1987;58(3):188–192.

83. Zand ML. The effect of non-therapeutic ophthalmic preparation on the cornea and tear film. Aust J Optom 1981;64:44–67.

84. Bailey N. Wrong solutions to the cleaning problem. Contact Lens Forum 1976;1:10–15.

85. Jurkus JM, Cedarstaff TH, Nuccio RS. Solution confusion: Photodocumentation of what can happen. Int Contact Lens Clin 1981;8:47–56.

86. Krezanoski JZ. Water and the care of soft contact lenses. Int Contact Lens Clin 1975;2:48–55.

87. Lowther GE, Hilbert J. Deposits on hydrophilic lenses: Differential appearance and clinical causes. Am J Optom Physiol Opt 1975;52:687–692.

88. Hilbert J, Lowther GE, King J. Deposition of substances within hydrophilic lenses. Am J Optom Physiol Opt 1976;53:51–54.

89. Wilson LA, Schlitzer RL, Aearn DG. *Pseudomonas* corneal ulcers associated with soft contact lens wear. Am J Ophthalmol 1981;92: 546–554.

90. Dada VK, Agarwal LP, Seger KR. Preventable hazard of soft lens wear. Am J Optom Physiol Opt 1976;53:431–432.

91. Rohrer, MD, et al. Microwave sterilization of hydrophilic contact lenses. Am J Ophthalmol 1986;101(1):49–57.

92. Harris MG, Kirby JE, Tornatore CW, Wrightnour JA. Microwave disinfection of soft contact lenses. Optom Vis Sci 1989;66(2):82–86.

93. Harris MG, Rechberger J, Grant T, Holden BA. In-office microwave disinfection of soft contact lenses. Optom Vis Sci 1990; 67(2):129–132.

94. Harris MG, Gan CM, Grant T, Lycho T, Holden BA. Microwave irradiation and soft contact lens parameters. Optom Vis Sci 1993; 70(10):843–848.

95. Dolman PJ, Dobrogowski MJ. Contact lens disinfection by ultraviolet light. Am J Ophthalmol 1989;108(6):665–669.

96. Harris MG, Fluss L, Lem A, Leong H. Ultraviolet disinfection of contact lenses. Optom Vis Sci 1993;70(10):839–842.

97. Harris MG, Buttino LM, Chan JC, Wang M. Effects of ultraviolet radiation on contact lens parameters. Optom Vis Sci 1993; 70(9):739–742.

98. Palmer W, Scanlon P, McNulty C. Efficacy of an ultraviolet light contact lens disinfection unit against microbial pathogenic organisms. J Br Cont Lens Assoc 1991;14(1):13–16.

99. Kilvington S, Scanlon P. Efficacy of an ultraviolet light contact lens disinfection unit against *Acanthamoeba* keratitis isolates. J Br Cont Lens Assoc 1991;14(1):9–11.

100. Bartolomei A, Alcaraz L, Bottone E, Asbell P et al. Clinical evaluation of Purilens, an ultraviolet light contact lens care system. CLAO J 1994;20(1):23–26.

101. Efron M, Lowe R, Vallas V, Gruisner E. Clinical efficacy of standing wave and ultrasound for cleaning and disinfecting contact lenses. Int Cont Lens Clin 1991;18(1):24–29.

102. Phillips AJ, Bakenoch P, Copley C. Ultrasound cleaning and disinfection of contact lenses: A preliminary report. Trans J Br Cont Lens Assoc 1989;12:20–23.

103. Pedersen N. Allergy to chemical solutions for soft contact lenses. Lancet 1976;2:1363.

104. Wilson L. Thimerosal hypersensitivity in soft contact lens wearers. Contact Lens J 1981;9:21–24.

105. Neill JC, Hanna JJ. A study of the effect of various media on the radii of microcorneal contact lenses. Contacto 1963;7:10–13.

106. McMonnies CU. Allergic complications in contact lens wear. Int Contact Lens Clin 1978;5:182–189.

107. Josephson JE, Caffery BE. Infiltrative keratitis in hydrogel lens wearers. Int Contact Lens Clin 1979;6:47–71.

108. Rudner EJ. Epidemiology of contact dermatitis in North America. 1972. Arch Dermatol 1973;108:537–540.

109. Rudner EJ, et al. The frequency of contact sensitivity in North America 1972–74. Contact Dermatitis 1975;1:277–280.

110. Lepine EM. Results of routine office patch testing. Contact Dermatitis 1976;2:89–91.

111. Molinari JF, Nash R, Badham D. Severe thimerosal hypersensitivity in soft contact lens wearers. Int Contact Lens Clin 1982;9:323–329.

112. Mondino B, Salamon S, Zaidman G. Allergic and toxic reactions in soft contact lens wearers. Surv Ophthalmol 1982;26:337–344.

113. Sibley M, Chu V. Understanding sorbic acid preserved contact lens solutions. Int Contact Lens Clin 1984;9(11):531–542.

114. Christensen B, James JA. Clinical investigation of the new SoftWear saline. Contact Lens Spectrum 1990;5(11):37–40.

115. Zigler LG. SoftWear saline and the sensitive patient. Contact Lens Spectrum 1990;5(12):50–51.

116. Josephson J. The "Multi-purge Procedure" and its application for hydrophilic lens wearers utilizing preserved solutions. J Am Optom Assoc 1978;49:280–281.

117. Kleist FD. Appearance and nature of hydrophilic contact lens deposits–Part 2: Inorganic deposits. Int Contact Lens Clin 1979;6: 177–186.

118. Davies D, Meakin B, Anthony Y. A new concept in contact lens disinfection. Optician 1990;199:21–24.

119. Anthony Y, Davies DJG, Meakin BJ, Halliday J, et al. A chlorhexidine contact lens disinfection tablet: Design criteria and antimicrobial efficacy in potable tap water. J Br Cont Lens Assoc 1991; 14(3):99–108.

120. Harris MG, Gan CM, Long DA, Cushing LA. The pH of over-the-counter hydrogen peroxide in soft lens disinfection system. Optom Vis Sci 1989;66(12):839–842.

121. Kershaw J, Legerton J, Neweman AR, Schultz JE, Schwab G. Clinical acceptability of hydrogen peroxide disinfection: Ultra-Care vs. AOSept. Contact Lens Spectrum 1992;7(8):55–58.

122. Lowther GE. A review of transparent hydrogel tinted lenses. Contax 1987, March pp 6–9.

123. Siberman HI. An investigation of a method of cold sterilization of hydrogel contact lenses by polyvinylpyrrolidone-iodine complex. J Am Optom Assoc 1973;44:1040–1046.

124. Conn H, Langer R. Iodine disinfection of hydrophilic contact lenses. Ann Ophthalmol 1981;13:361.

125. Hathaway R, Lowther GE. Factors influencing the rate of deposit formation on hydrophilic lens. Aust J Optom 1978;61:92–96.

126. Lowther GE, Hilbert J, King J. Appearance and location of hydrophilic lens deposits. Int Contact Lens Clin 1975;2:30–34.

127. Lowther GE. The relationship between the chemistry of the tear film and hydrophilic lens deposits. In: Soft contact lenses: Second National Research Symposium Proceedings. Amsterdam, Excerpta Medica, 1977. (International Congress Series, 398).

128. Kleist FD. Appearance and nature of hydrophilic contact lens deposits. Part 1: Protein and organic deposits. Int Contact Lens Clin 1979;6:120–130.

129. Bailey N. Cleaning of coated soft lenses. J Am Optom Assoc 1974;45:1049–1052.

130. Bier N, Lowther GE. Contact lens correction. Boston: Butterworth, 1976:410–424.

131. Roetzheim WH. Ultrasonic C.L. cleaning. Contact Lens Forum 1983;8(11):29–35.

132. Fatt I. Physical limitation to cleaning soft contact lenses by ultrasonic methods. J Br Cont Lens Assoc 1991;14(3):135–136.

133. Phillips AJ. The cleaning of hydrogel contact lenses. Ophthalmic Optician 1980;20:375–388.

134. Lloyd DJ. Enzyme cleaners: The structure, properties and mode of action of enzymes. Ophthalmic Optician 1979;19:833–839.

135. Lowther G. Effectiveness of an enzyme in removing deposits from hydrophilic lens. Am J Optom Physiol Opt 1977;54:76–84.

136. Hathaway R, Lowther GE. Soft lens cleaners: Their effectiveness in removing deposits. J Am Optom Assoc 1978;49:259–266.

137. Fichman S, Baker VV, Horten H. Iatrogenic red eyes in soft contact lens wearers. Int Contact Lens Clin 1978;5:202–206.

138. Bellemare F. Compatibility of enzymatic cleaning with cold contact lens disinfection. Int Contact Lens Clin 1979;6:219–222.

139. Cedrone RM, Meisel R, Saxton SR, Toscano FR, Woloschak MJ.

One-step enzymatic cleaning for better compliance. Contact Lens Spectrum 1992;7(7):39–41.

140. Snyder C. A microbiological assessment of rigid contact lens wet and dry storage. Int Cont Lens Clin 1990;17(2):83–87.

141. Boltz RL, Leach NE, Piccolo MG, Peltzer B. The effect of repeated disinfection of rigid gas permeable lens materials using 3% hydrogen peroxide. Int Cont Lens Clin 1993;20(6):215–221.

142. Barr JT. Trial lens disinfection roundtable. Contact Lens Spectrum 1993;8(1):47–53.

143. Podos SM, et al. Pilocarpine therapy with soft contact lenses. Arch Ophthalmol 1972;73:336–341.

144. Maddox YT, Bernstein HN. An evaluation of the bionite hydrophilic contact lens for use in a drug delivery system. Ann Ophthalmol 1972;4:789–802.

145. Waltman SR, Kaufman HE. Use of hydrophilic contact lenses to increase ocular penetration of topical drugs. Invest Ophthalmol 1970;9:250–255.

146. Mizutane Y, Miwa Y. On the uptake and release of drugs by soft contact lenses. Contact Intraocular Lens Med J 1975;1:177–183.

147. Marmion VJ. Role of soft contact lenses and delivery of drugs. Trans Ophthalmol Soc UK 1976;96:319–321.

148. Gasset AR. Therapeutic applications. In: Mandell RB. Contact lens practice, ed. 3. Springfield, IL: Thomas, 1981;607–618.

149. Krezanoski JZ. Topical medications. Int Ophthalmol Clin 1981; 21:173–176.

150. Bronson L, Koetting RA, Janoff L, Williams T, Katz I, Egan DJ. Use of Timoptic with soft lenses. Collected Letters, Int Corr Soc Optom 1980;4:2–6.

151. Hales RH. Contact lenses: A clinical approach to fitting. Baltimore: Williams & Wilkins, 1978;32–56.

152. Sugar J. Adrenochrome pigmentation of hydrophilic lenses. Arch Ophthalmol 1974;91:11–12.

153. Miller D, Brooks S, Mobilia E. Adrenochrome staining of soft contact lenses. Ann Ophthalmol 1976;6:65–66.

154. Aucamp A. Drug excretion in human tears and its meaning for contact lens wearers. S Afr Optom 1980;39(3):128–136.

155. Wartman, RH. Contact lens-related side effects of systemic drugs. Contact Lens Forum 1987;12(8):42–44.

156. Shovlin JP. Systemic medications and their interaction with soft contact lenses. Int Cont Lens Clin 1990;17(5):250–251.

157. Valentic JP, Leopold IH, Dea FJ. Excretion of salicylic acid into tears following oral administration of aspirin. Ophthalmology 1980;87:815–820.

158. Miller D. Systemic medications. Int Ophthalmol Clin 1981; 21(2):177–183.

159. Koetting RA. The influence of oral contraceptives on contact lens wear. Am J Optom Physiol Opt 1966;43(4):268–274.

160. Soni PS. Effects of oral contraceptive steroids on the thickness of human cornea. Am J Optom Physiol Opt 1980;57:825–834.

161. Lyons RW. Orange contact lenses from rifampin. N Eng J Med 1979;300:372–373.

162. Newson SR, Hayer BS. Disulfiram alcohol reactions caused by contact lens wetting solutions. Contact Intraocular Lens Med J 1980;6(4):407–408.

CHAPTER 19

Adjunctive Agents

Kari E. Blaho

This chapter considers many unrelated substances for which the common thread is that they serve a "helper" role or are used in conjunction with other agents or procedures. Some of these compounds have clear clinical indications, but many are unproven. They are unproven because they are in their infancy, are newly applied for ophthalmic diseases, or simply lack demonstrated efficacy. Some of these agents will fade from use while others will take on a more significant role in future ocular pharmacotherapeutics.

Growth Factors

Growth factors are endogenous polypeptides that are responsible for normal turnover of a variety of cell types including corneal epithelium. Growth factors are produced in response to tissue injury.[1-3] In the eye, these factors are important for proper wound healing after either chemical or mechanical damage.[2-4] Several growth factors currently are being evaluated for clinical use as agents to promote wound healing. Studies suggest that although these growth factors participate in wound healing, they may also act as key factors in stimulating neovascularization in diseases such as diabetic retinopathy.[5] Much of the current knowledge of growth factors is based on results of animal studies, as well as *in vitro* experiments with human, rabbit and bovine cell cultures.

Although many growth factors have been identified, only those that have been evaluated for their effects in ocular healing are discussed here (Table 19.1). Growth factors aid in the repair process by[6-8]:

- Stimulating migration of corneal cells to areas of damage
- Stimulating mitosis of all corneal cell types

- Stimulating the synthesis of extracellular matrices
- Stimulating chemotaxis

Human milk, tears, aqueous humor, plasma, and urine all contain epidermal growth factor (EGF).[9-11] EGF stimulates ocular healing by cAMP (cyclic adenosine monophosphate)-dependent proliferation and differentiation of tissue.[10-20] This effect occurs in both corneal epithelium and endothelium.[21-33] EGF produces dose-dependent corneal wound healing in both rabbit and human models and has a trophic effect in cultured retinal pigment epithelial cells.[34,35] In both clinical and animal trials, EGF reduces the time for corneal healing, except in injuries resulting from penetrating keratoplasty, multiple herpetic lesions, and pseudophakic bullous keratopathy.[11,36,37] In addition to mitogenic properties, EGF has angiogenic properties that may contribute to neovascular disorders.[5,38] Because EGF has not been used

TABLE 19.1
Clinical Uses of Growth Factors

Growth Factor	Proposed Clinical Use
Epidermal growth factor	Corneal wound healing
Fibroblast growth factor	Corneal wound healing Neurotrophic agent
Transforming growth factors	Corneal wound healing Neurotrophic agent Treatment of neovascularization Treatment of macular holes
Insulin-like growth factor	Treatment of neovascularization

extensively, side effects and contraindications have not yet been established. However, potential adverse effects will most likely stem from the lack of specificity of these agents for only corneal epithelial cells. Enhancing growth of other tissue types may not be a desired effect.

Fibroblast growth factor (FGF) is synthesized and released from various types of retinal cells; animal studies show that it enhances corneal wound healing after mechanical and chemical injury.[39-43] The exact mechanism of FGF's pharmacologic activity has not been elucidated, but similar to other growth factors, it stimulates mitosis, chemotaxis, and cell migration via interaction with specific receptors.[2,44-46] Two forms of FGF, acidic and basic, have been isolated. Little is known about their physiologic role, but these factors may be involved in the neovascularization process and may have neurotrophic properties.[47-50] Basic FGF may also be an important neurotrophic factor in photoreceptor degeneration associated with inherited retinal dystrophy.[51] Potential benefits from compounds like FGF could result from either mimicking or antagonizing their actions, depending on the disease or condition being treated.

Transforming growth factors (TGF-α and TGF-β) exist in multiple forms and have been isolated from various ocular tissues.[52,53] These growth factors accelerate tissue healing by stimulating migration, proliferation, and differentiation of many cell types including corneal epithelial cells, stromal fibroblasts, and endothelial cells.[45,52-54] In addition, the transforming growth factors may provoke the immune response in ocular tissue,[45,52] and they have been hypothesized to inhibit neovascularization induced by other growth factors.[55] The exact mechanism of these physiologic actions is unknown. TGF-β appears to enhance the ability to flatten the rim of subretinal fluid and create a chorioretinal adhesion around macular holes. The TGF-β is applied to the macula during vitrectomy. Eyes with successful closure of the macular hole seem to have a small bridge of glial tissue plugging the foveal defect.[56,57]

Insulin-like growth factor (IGF) stimulates mitosis and cell differentiation, and also stimulates several key steps in the neovascularization process.[3,5] IGF may be one of the primary factors responsible for proliferative diabetic retinopathy.[5,39,58-62] IGF-induced neovascularization is mediated by specific IGF receptors located on the retinal microvasculature.[5] When stimulated, these receptors induce several steps in neovascularization including endothelial cell proliferation, endothelial cell migration and the secretion of proteases. IGF may also act as a mitogenic agent in retinal pigment epithelium and may prove important for the processing of vitamin A in the retina.[6,63]

Fibronectin is an endogenous protein that promotes mitosis and adhesion of cells in an area of injury.[64-66] Its precise mechanism of action is unknown. Results from clinical trials designed to characterize its clinical efficacy and indications for use are inconclusive.[67,68] Fibronectin may contribute to the development of secondary cataracts by stimulating the migration of lens epithelial cells.[69]

Botulinum Toxin

Botulinum toxin is produced by the bacterium *Clostridium botulinum.* Several chemically similar forms of Botulinum toxin exist.[70] Botulinum A toxin corrects strabismus and other ocular motor disorders by interfering with the release of acetylcholine from the nerve terminals in extraocular or other muscles (Fig. 19.1).[71] Injecting the toxin into the muscle results in a dose-dependent paralysis that may last up to 9 months. Full recovery of the treated muscle after that time is variable.[71-73]

Once injected into the muscle, botulinum does not diffuse into the systemic circulation.[74] Dosing and administration of botulinum toxin are individualized on a case-by-case basis, and multiple injections may be necessary to achieve the desired effect (see Chaps. 23 and 34).

Botulinum A toxin is indicated for the correction of strabismus, nystagmus, blepharospasm, hemifacial spasms, myokymia, lower lid entropion, and corneal ulcers that result from exposure.[70] Some studies have shown that the success of botulinum toxin treatment depends greatly on the subtype and severity of the disorder.[70,75,76] For example, patients with esotropia may respond better to botulinum injections than do patients with exotropia. Treatment with botulinum is most effective when used for small angle deviations, sensory deviations, transient sixth nerve palsies, subacute dysthyroid ophthalmopathies, overcorrections, residual deviations after strabismus surgery, and strabismus in which the use of anesthesia is prohibited.[70,77-79]

Table 19.2 summarizes adverse effects associated with the use of botulinum toxin. The incidence of these reported adverse events varies somewhat from study to study because of variability in administration technique, degree of ocular deviation, and specific condition treated.

Viscoelastic Agents

Viscoelastic agents (Table 19.3) consist of large macromolecules that exert a protective effect on ocular tissues during surgical procedures. These agents limit the mechanical damage from invasive procedures by separating and lubricating tissues. They decrease corneal endothelial cell loss during surgery.[80,81] Viscoelastic agents are routinely used as adjuncts in cataract surgery, intraocular lens (IOL) implantation, corneal transplantation, and surgery for glaucoma, trauma, and vitreoretinal disorders.

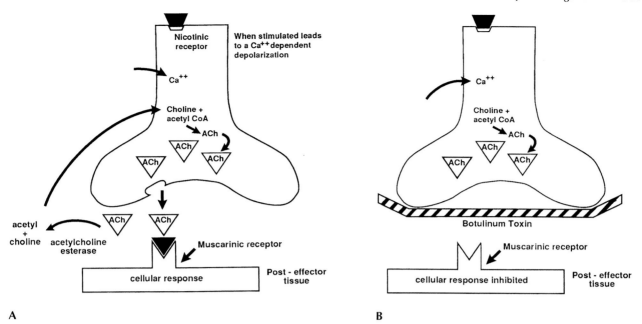

FIGURE 19.1   *(A)* Acetylcholine (ACh) is released from vesicles in the cholinergic neuron upon depolarization. ACh binds to and activates a muscarinic receptor on the innervated tissue. Binding of ACh with the muscarinic receptor elicits a series of intracellular events that result in a tissue-dependent effect such as muscle contraction. *(B)* Schematic of the mechanism of action of botulinum toxin. Botulinum interferes with vesicular release of ACh from the neuron and inhibits cellular responses in the innervated tissue. In muscles innervated by cholinergic neurons, paralysis results.

Sodium Hyaluronate (Hyaluronic Acid)

A main component of vitreous humor, hyaluronic acid is a large macromolecule primarily composed of two monosaccharides. Hyaluronic acid stimulates neutrophil function,[82] cell proliferation, aggregation and migration, and may also facilitate wound healing.[83] Hyaluronic acid has been detected in ocular tissues in various animal models of ocular injury[84–86] and may be a mediator of ocular inflammation. It is indicated for use in anterior and posterior surgical procedures such as IOL implantation, retinal reattachment, corneal transplantation and glaucoma filtering surgery.[87] When formulated for topical use, hyaluronic acid has been successfully employed for the treatment of dry eye.[88]

Adverse effects associated with hyaluronic acid (Healon, Amvisc) include an elevation in postoperative intraocular pressure (IOP), postoperative inflammatory and allergic reactions, and the presence of particulates in the ocular area.[89] Corneal haze formation can occur and may result from distortion of the normal stromal lamellar structure, altering corneal water balance and changing the index of refraction.[85] The increase in IOP postoperatively may result from trabecular meshwork "clogging" as the viscoelastic clears from the eye. Removing the hyaluronic acid after surgery minimizes transient rises in IOP.[90,91] Hyaluronic acid should be removed from the anterior chamber following completion of the surgical procedures, especially when the patient has glaucoma or has had a traumatic injury in which debris could occlude the trabecular meshwork.[90] Residual hyaluronic acid can augment postoperative inflammation.[92] Use of Healon GV, a high-molecular-weight hyaluronate, has been associated with crystalline deposits on intraocular lenses. These deposits can sometimes be visually significant.[264]

Chondroitin Sulfate

Chondroitin sulfate is similar to hyaluronic acid in chemical structure and in mechanism of action. It is a large macromolecule that is a normal constituent of the eye. Chondroitin sulfate in combination with hyaluronate (Viscoat) is indicated for use in anterior segment procedures such as cataract extraction and IOL implantation. Like hyaluronic acid, it is associated with allergic reactions and has potential for transient elevations in postoperative IOP.[93] In concentrations of 20% or greater, a decrease in corneal thickness occurs, most likely resulting from the high osmolarity of the solution.[93] Chondroitin sulfate can remain in the anterior chamber after

TABLE 19.2
Adverse Effects of Botulinum Toxin[70-77]

Adverse Effect	Comment
Diplopia	Patching may be necessary for several weeks after injection
Ptosis	Phenylephrine may correct mild cases by temporarily stimulating Müller's muscle
Undercorrection	
Scleral perforation	May be due to injury during injection
Hemorrhage	
Pupillary dilation	May be caused by injury to ciliary ganglion during injection
Reduced accommodation	
Induced deviations	Vertical deviations most common with administration to medial rectus muscle
Skin rash	Following eyelid injection
Local swelling	Following eyelid injection
Lagophthalmos	Occurs after treatment for facial spasm
Lower facial weakness	Occurs after treatment for facial spasm
Ecchymosis	Occurs after treatment for facial spasm
Ectropion	Occurs after treatment for facial spasm
Entropion	Occurs after treatment for facial spasm
Dry eye	Occurs after treatment of blepharospasm
Motor nerve sprouting	Significance is unknown

TABLE 19.3
Viscoelastic Agents

Drug	Trade Name (manufacturer)	Concentration
Sodium hyaluronate	Amvisc (Ciba Vision)	12 mg/ml
	Amvisc Plus (Ciba Vision)	16 mg/ml
	AMO Vitrax (Allergan)	30 mg/ml
	Healon (Pharmacia)	10 mg/ml
	Healon GV (Pharmacia)	14 mg/ml
	Provisc (Alcon)	10 mg/ml
Chondroitin sulfate plus sodium hyaluronate	Viscoat (Alcon)	40 mg/ml 30 mg/ml
Viscoat plus Provisc	DuoVisc Viscoelastic System (Alcon)	
Hydroxypropyl-methylcellulose	OcuCoat (Storz)	2%

surgery and is eliminated in less than 2 days.[94] Like most viscoelastic solutions, chondroitin sulfate is well tolerated, and there are no contraindications for its use.

Combinations of viscoelastic agents are available (see Table 19.3). Some studies indicate that the combination of hyaluronic acid and chondroitin sulfate provides better protection of anterior segment structures than does hyaluronic acid alone.[95,96]

Hydroxypropylmethylcellulose

Hydroxypropylmethylcellulose resembles other viscoelastic agents in its mechanism of action, protective effects, and therapeutic indications. It is a derivative of cellulose, a natural fiber found in trees. Side effects of hydroxypropylmethylcellulose are the same as those associated with other viscoelastics: postoperative inflammation and increases in postoperative IOP.[96-98]

Collagen

Collagen is a protein found in supporting connective tissues throughout the body. Primarily derived from human placental tissue, type IV collagen is the form used as a viscoelastic agent for anterior segment procedures.[99] Collagen is similar to hyaluronic acid in its therapeutic efficacy and spectrum of adverse effects.

Another agent, silicone oil, has been used as a vitreous replacement and for retinal tamponade in the treatment of retinal detachments and tears.[100-103] It is an effective vitreous substitute because of its refractive index and high viscosity.[103] Long-term use of silicone oil, however, can cause glaucoma, cataracts, keratopathy, proliferation of retinal pigment epithelium, and emulsification of the silicone oil.[103-105] The incidence of adverse effects produced by silicone oil may relate to the purity and viscosity of the preparation used.[101] The adverse effects associated with the oil necessitate that it generally be removed from the eye within one year of surgery. This product is commercially available in the United States under the trade name Adato Sil 5000 (Escalon).

Nutritional Agents

In the United States, the annual sales of vitamins and nutritional supplements represents a $3.3 billion business.[106] Vitamins and minerals are not innocuous medications, and manufacturers of these preparations must now have and make available to the consumer scientific data that offers proof of efficacy.

Vitamins are organic compounds necessary for normal physiologic functioning. The amount required for normal function varies with each vitamin. Most vitamins must be obtained from dietary sources because the body either cannot synthesize them or makes them in insufficient quantities to meet physiologic requirements.[107]

Minerals are trace elements that are required in much smaller quantities than vitamins. In general, minerals perform various physiologic functions such as carrying electrical impulses or functioning as part of enzyme systems. Like vitamins, minerals must be supplied from exogenous dietary sources.

The amount of vitamins and minerals necessary for normal physiologic functioning is known as the recommended dietary allowance (RDA). Based on age and sex, these estimated amounts are designed to provide for the physiologic needs of healthy individuals. Periodically they are reviewed and altered by the Dietary Allowances Committee of the Food and Nutrition Board.[107] The vitamins are generally broken down into two main categories, the *fat-soluble* and the *water-soluble* vitamins.

Not enough scientific data currently exist to determine whether supplementation in the absence of frank deficiency has any therapeutic benefit. Most cases of deficiency have underlying causes such as alcoholism, malabsorption syndromes, drug interactions, or dialysis. Because additional supplementation is not without risk, the clinician should carefully weigh the benefit-to-risk ratio of additional supplementation before prescribing or recommending nutritional agents.

Fat-Soluble Vitamins

VITAMIN A

Vitamin A (retinol) belongs to a class of chemically similar compounds known as the *retinoids*. Dietary sources such as eggs, liver, butter, cheese, whole milk, fish, green leafy or yellow vegetables supply vitamin A and β-carotene (provitamin A).[107,108] Once absorbed, β-carotene is metabolically converted to two molecules of retinol.

Deficiencies of vitamin A occur when the RDA of 375 to 1200 μg/day is not met. These deficiencies rarely occur in the United States unless there are underlying diseases such as chronic pancreatic disease, gastrointestinal disease, lipid

TABLE 19.4
Physiologic Functions of Vitamin A (Retinol)

Retinoid	Tissue	Effect
retinoic acid	epithelia, bone	growth and differentiation
retinal	reproductive organs, mucous membranes	proper functioning
retinol	retina	rhodopsin production

disorders, or severe dietary insufficiency. In Asia, the Middle East, Africa, and South and Central America, vitamin A deficiencies are common and are responsible for an estimated 500,000 cases of irreversible blindness in children each year.[107,109] Vitamin A deficiency during childhood may cause latent epithelial cell changes in the lens and may contribute to the high number of cataracts in third world countries.[110]

Vitamin A, a lipid-soluble vitamin, is stored as an ester in the liver.[107] When administered orally, vitamin A is absorbed with fat. Retinol is carried to the tissues by binding to serum retinol-binding protein. The liver constitutes the greatest store of vitamin A, and it takes many months to deplete these stores and to develop vitamin A deficiency. Ocular tissues are supplied with vitamin A via the tears and through the limbal and corneal blood vessels.[111–114]

Physiologically, the retinoids have several important functions (Table 19.4). The functional and structural integrity of epithelial cells throughout the body depends on an adequate supply of vitamin A. The retinoids appear to control cell growth and differentiation, mucus production, and keratinization of these tissues. Vitamin A also functions in dark adaptation (Fig. 19.2). The retinoids control cell differentiation by glycosylation of proteins and lipids.[115–120] In the eye, the retinoids increase the integrity of the lens membrane and maintain the lens epithelium, a function that helps to prevent cataract formation.[121] The exact mechanism of the retinoids resembles that of steroid and thyroid hormones. The retinoid binds to and activates an intracellular receptor. This vitamin A-receptor complex migrates to the nucleus, where it alters gene transcription and synthesis of various proteins (Fig. 19.3).

Vitamin A and the other retinoids may interfere with the development of certain types of malignancies because of their effect on cell differentiation.[122,123] Certain retinoids, such as β-carotene, also have antioxidant activity beneficial in reducing tissue damage by free radicals.[121,124,125] Free radicals are highly unstable molecules with an unpaired electron. They are generated from UV light, tobacco smoke, organic solvents, pollutants, pesticides, and radiation.[126]

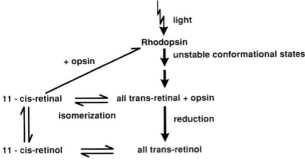

FIGURE 19.2   **The role of retinoids in the visual cycle. When a photon of light interacts with rhodopsin, it breaks down into several unstable mediators, the final one being all trans-retinal. All trans-retinal has two pathways: 1) it may be isomerized to 11-cis retinal, which can then combine with opsin to form rhodopsin; or 2) it can be further reduced to all trans-retinol. All trans-retinol can isomerize to 11-cis-retinol, which can then be converted to 11-cis-retinal and completes the visual cycle. Without vitamin A, the visual cycle would be impaired.**

Free radicals can destroy plasma membranes and other structures with a high fatty acid content. The eye is particularly prone to free radical damage since it has a high concentration of oxygen, is exposed to large amounts of UV light, and has a large amount of fatty acids in rods and cones.[127] Damage from free radicals has been implicated in the etiology of many ocular diseases including malignancies, cataracts, and age-related macular degeneration.[128–134]

Table 19.5 lists clinical manifestations of vitamin A deficiency. In the eye, vitamin A deficiency produces xerophthalmia. The corneal epithelium sloughs due to a decrease in size and number of hemidesmosomes. Loss of hemidesmosomes decreases the basement membrane surface area.[135] A decrease in the goblet cell population, an increase in epithelial cell mitosis, and a decrease in conjunctival wound healing also occur.[136,137] This decrease in wound healing may relate to a reduction in fibronectin, a protein that facilitates healing.[138,139] The corneal and conjunctival epithelial tissue become keratinized and mucus secretion decreases, resulting in an increased risk of infection.[107,140]

Other epithelial surfaces are also affected by vitamin A deficiency. Even mild deficiencies have been associated with an increased risk of and increased mortality from infectious diarrheal and respiratory illnesses in preschool-aged children.[141–145]

Vitamin A administration is indicated for patients with a deficiency or for prophylaxis in patients at risk for developing a deficiency, such as those with chronic liver, pancreatic, or gastrointestinal diseases, or those in periods of high physiologic demand such as pregnancy or lactation.[107,146] The current World Health Organization recommendations for vitamin A treatment of children 1 year of age and older

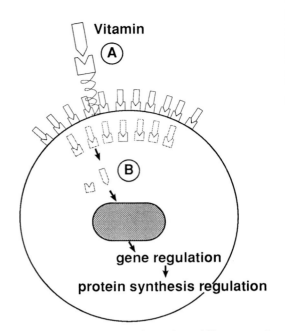

FIGURE 19.3   **Fat-soluble vitamins and steroid hormones share a similar mechanism of action. The vitamin binds to a receptor located on the extracellular membrane (A). The receptor-vitamin complex is internalized (B). The vitamin dissociates from the receptor and migrates to the nucleus, where it alters gene transcription and protein synthesis.**

are one 200,000-IU oral dose every 3 to 6 months of prophylaxis and three of these doses for treatment of xerophthalmia.[265] The results from human studies in which vitamin A has been evaluated for the prevention of cataracts are inconclusive.[147,148]

The use of topical vitamin A treatment in dry eye syndromes such as keratoconjunctivitis sicca or in dry eye produced by irradiation, Stevens-Johnson syndrome, or inactive pemphigoid is controversial and has been shown to be of limited therapeutic benefit;[149–152] however, in one study the use of topical vitamin A drops 500 and 15,000 IU/ml 4 times daily was associated with a reduction in the lesions associated with superior limbic keratoconjunctivitis in 83% of the patients.[153] In patients with common forms of retinitis pigmentosa (RP), 15,000 IU/day of oral vitamin A slowed the progression of retinal decline (as defined by the cone ERG) without producing dose-limiting side effects.[154] The mechanism of this beneficial effect in RP patients has not been elucidated, but it is hypothesized that vitamin A may be of benefit by preserving photoreceptor function or that RP patients may have a reduction in retinal vitamin A concentrations because of the loss of rods and cones. Caution is warranted in the use of vitamin A in RP patients, however, since more studies are needed to establish the efficacy and safety of vitamin A therapy.

TABLE 19.5
Ocular and Systemic Manifestations of Vitamin A Deficiency[108,109,127,136,140]

Ocular	Systemic
Xerophthalmia	Increased mucus secretion and keratinization of the lining of the airway, leading to increased incidence of respiratory infections
Keratomalacia	
Bitot's spot on conjunctiva	
Conjunctival xerosis	
Dry eye	Keratinization and drying of skin, papular eruptions
Corneal perforation	Urinary calculi formation
Perivasculitis	Infertility
Degeneration of rod outer segments	Birth defects
Nyctalopia	Diarrhea
	Sweat gland atrophy and development of keratinizing squamous-cell metaplasia
	Lack of proper bone structure
	Impaired taste and smell
	Impaired hearing
	Development of neuropathies

Vitamin A (retinol) is available in many different oral formulations. Those prepared in aqueous solutions, such as Aquasol A, afford the greatest absorption after oral administration and result in higher plasma concentrations, especially in cases of malabsorption syndromes. The preparations of vitamin A formulated in an oil base result in higher concentrations of the vitamin in the liver.[107] Available ocular preparations of vitamin A include Viva Drops and Dakrina, which also contains vitamin C.

Adverse effects associated with vitamin A result from excess ingestion, known as *hypervitaminosis* A. Approximately 8% of children treated prophylactically with 200,000 IU of oral vitamin A have side effects such as nausea, vomiting, and fever.[265] Chronic retinoid use of greater than 7.5 mg per day can result in skin disorders such as dry skin, pruritic skin, erythematous dermatitis, alterations in hair growth, cracked lips, pain and tenderness of the bones, headache, papilledema, anorexia, edema, fatigue, irritability, and hemorrhage.[107] Liver damage may include fibrosis, sclerosis, and cirrhosis that can result in portal hypertension and ascites. Vitamin A is contraindicated in hypervitaminosis A or in patients allergic to vitamin A. Use should be carefully monitored in pregnant females.

VITAMIN E

Vitamin E is a fat-soluble vitamin that exists in many different chemical forms. Together, the vitamin E-related compounds are known as the *tocopherols*. Alpha-tocopherol is the most important of this group because it has the greatest biologic activity at tissue sites.[107] The RDA for vitamin E ranges from 3 mg/day in infants to 11 mg/day in lactating mothers. Vitamin E is obtained by the consumption of vegetable oils, wheat germ, leafy vegetables, egg yolks, margarine, and legumes. The tocopherols, including vitamin E, exert their pharmacologic effects by acting as antioxidants, and they may also have anti-inflammatory activity.[155,156] Like vitamin A and the steroid and thyroid hormones, the tocopherols bind to and activate a tissue receptor that then alters gene expression and protein synthesis.

The tocopherols occur in retinal tissues that are prone to damage from UV light. Vitamin E intercalates into the cell membrane and protects cellular constituents from the harmful outcomes of free radical oxidation. Vitamin E has been shown in animal studies to offer protection against some drugs, metals, and chemicals that can initiate the formation of free radicals.[156,157] Table 19.6 outlines clinical manifestations of vitamin E deficiency.

The tocopherols are well absorbed from the intestinal tract after oral administration. They are distributed to all tissues and are stored in liver and fat. They undergo liver metabolism and renal excretion of the hepatic metabolites. Available preparations of vitamin E include capsules, tablets, and drops as well as a parenteral formulation that can be used in the emergent treatment of severe vitamin E deficiency.

Vitamin E administration (alpha-tocopherol) is indicated for use when there is a risk of developing a deficiency, such as in pregnancy, cystic fibrosis, cholestatic liver disease, alcoholism, improper diet, and in pre- and post-surgery situations[107,158] The use of vitamin E for prevention and management of retinopathy of prematurity (ROP) has been a subject of much debate. The beneficial effects produced by vitamin E for ROP were first suggested in 1949.[159] Since that time, however, studies have produced contradictory data. Some studies show that vitamin E supplementation helps in the prevention and management of ROP, while others demonstrate no benefit.[130,160–170] Because an increased risk exists

TABLE 19.6
Clinical Manifestations of Vitamin E Deficiency[108,109]

Neurologic abnormalities
  hyporeflexia, gait disturbances, axonal degeneration

Ophthalmoplegia

Pigmented retinopathy leading to visual disturbances

Infertility, spontaneous abortions

Muscular weakness

Cardiac myopathy

Anemias

for the development of necrotizing enterocolitis, sepsis, and intraventricular hemorrhage in premature infants who have received vitamin E, it is not currently indicated for the prevention or management of ROP.[171,172] Some reports indicate that vitamin E may be efficacious in the prevention of cataracts, but no clinical studies have confirmed this hypothesis.[173–194] Vitamin E may also aid in preventing retinopathy associated with abetalipoproteinemia and may decrease the risk of neovascular age-related macular degeneration when used in combination with vitamin C and selenium.[195,196] Although excess vitamin E can be toxic to the lungs, blood, and liver,[197] there are no contraindications for use of vitamin E in therapeutic doses.

VITAMIN D

Vitamin D is necessary in amounts of 7.5 to 10 μg/day to avoid the complications of deficiency. The two forms of vitamin D, cholecalciferol (D_3) and calciferol (D_2), work with parathyroid hormone and calcitonin to regulate calcium and phosphate levels in the body. Vitamin D can be obtained from dietary sources or can be synthesized in the skin when 7-dehydrocholesterol is exposed to UV light and is converted into cholecalciferol. Cholecalciferol is activated to calcitrol by the liver and kidney. Of all the vitamin D-related compounds, calcitrol has the greatest biologic activity. Vitamin D acts through specific receptors to increase plasma calcium and phosphate levels by increasing absorption from the small intestine, mobilizing calcium and phosphate from bone, and decreasing the renal excretion of both. Vitamin D may also regulate the growth and differentiation of certain malignancies, possibly by inhibiting angiogenesis.[198–206] In one animal study,[207] the growth of retinoblastoma was inhibited, but toxicity limited the effectiveness of this treatment. Vitamin D or its analogs may be of future benefit in the treatment protocols for childhood cancers and retinoblastoma.[207]

Deficiencies in vitamin D lead to rickets. Children with rickets fail to mineralize new growth in bone, causing deformation of the bones and joints. In adults, osteomalacia occurs, a generalized decrease in bone density. Available preparations of vitamin D include ergocalciferol, dihydrotachysterol, calcifediol, cholecalciferol, and calcitriol.

Excess vitamin D, as little as 1800 USP units per day, leads to hypercalcemia and is characterized by weakness, fatigue, lassitude, headache, nausea, vomiting and diarrhea, impaired renal function, and calcification of blood vessels, heart, lungs, and skin.[107]

VITAMIN K

Vitamin K (phytonadione) is necessary for the synthesis of clotting factors II, VII, IX, and X. Found in many green vegetables and synthesized by intestinal bacteria, vitamin K has an RDA of 5 to 65 μg/day. The major manifestation of vitamin K deficiency is an increased tendency to bleed.

Ecchymosis, epistaxis, hematuria, gastrointestinal bleeding, and hemorrhage may occur. Deficiencies in vitamin K may result from use of prolonged antibiotic therapy, some antihyperlipidemic agents, and oral anticoagulants. Phytonadione and related compounds are associated with flushing, dyspnea, the formation of blood clots, and cardiovascular collapse. In the newborn these compounds can cause hemolytic anemia, kernicterus, and hyperbilirubinemia. In patients with glucose-6-phosphate dehydrogenase deficiency, menadione, a derivative of vitamin K, can induce hemolysis.[107,208] Vitamin K is indicated for the treatment of oral anticoagulant toxicity or in documented vitamin K deficiency. Administration of phytonadione is contraindicated in patients with a known hypersensitivity to components of vitamin K supplements.

Water-Soluble Vitamins

VITAMIN C

Vitamin C, or ascorbic acid, is a water-soluble vitamin obtained from dietary sources such as citrus fruits, potatoes, tomatoes, strawberries and cabbage. The RDA for ascorbic acid ranges from 30 to 90 mg/day.

Ascorbic acid is well absorbed from the gastrointestinal tract after oral administration. It is distributed to all tissues in the body and is stored in white blood cells. Plasma actively transports vitamin C into the eye which has a 20-fold greater concentration of the vitamin than does plasma.[209,210] Vitamin C facilitates the absorption of iron from the gastrointestinal tract and is therefore often found in combination with iron supplements. The liver metabolizes vitamin C; alternatively, it can be excreted unchanged by the kidney.

Vitamin C supplementation is indicated for cases in which poor diet or gastrointestinal disease has resulted in deficiency. It is also used to protect the natural flavor and color of foods because of its antioxidant properties. No studies conclusively show that vitamin C helps to prevent or treat viral and bacterial illnesses or malignant diseases,[211–213] but anecdotal evidence suggests some benefit.

Ascorbic acid acts as a cofactor in many enzymatic reactions throughout the body. As an antioxidant, vitamin C protects ocular tissue from the damage produced by free radicals. Animal studies show that vitamin C decreases light-induced damage and protects the eye from oxidative damage during inflammation by interrupting the formation or actions of light-induced substances toxic to ocular tissues.[174,214–221] Vitamin C may have some efficacy in decreasing cataract formation in humans and in animals due, in part, to its antioxidant properties.[173,222–225]

A deficiency of vitamin C, known as scurvy, may occur in patients with alcoholism, those with inadequate diets, those with chemical dependencies, and infants with inadequate amounts of vitamin C in their formulas. Table 19.7 lists signs

TABLE 19.7
Clinical Manifestations of Vitamin C Deficiency

Loosening of teeth

Gingivitis

Anemia

Hyperkeratosis

Petechiae

Ecchymosis

Decreased wound healing

and symptoms of scurvy. Like all other water-soluble vitamins, the potential for toxicity is much less than with fat-soluble vitamins because the body can easily eliminate water-soluble vitamins in the urine. Adverse effects associated with vitamin C occur with large doses of the vitamin and are mostly limited to gastrointestinal upset.

VITAMIN B$_1$

Vitamin B$_1$ (thiamine) is an essential component of enzyme systems responsible for the metabolism of carbohydrates. Thiamine also plays a role in the maintenance of neurons. Food sources rich in thiamine include unpolished grains, meats, yeast, and nuts. The RDA for thiamine ranges from 0.3 to 1.6 mg/day. The chronic intake of less than this amount may lead to thiamine deficiency, or beriberi. Manifestations of deficiency include cardiovascular and neurologic aberrations. Cardiovascular signs and symptoms include edema; cardiac failure; and altered blood flow to the kidneys, brain, and skeletal muscle. Neurologic findings in beriberi include Wernicke's encephalopathy and Korsakoff syndrome that present as impaired sensory, motor, and reflex responses; degeneration of myelin sheaths, including those surrounding the optic nerve and optic tract; nystagmus; ophthalmoplegia; ataxia; and mental deterioration.[226,227] Since most cases of thiamine deficiency occur in alcoholics, distinguishing thiamine deficiency from alcohol-induced neuropathies may be difficult. Thiamine is indicated for prophylaxis of deficiency or for the correction of deficiencies that may occur from malabsorption states, chronic malnutrition, and dialysis.

VITAMIN B$_2$

Vitamin B$_2$ (riboflavin) is incorporated into the cofactors flavin mononucleotide (FMN) and flavin adenine dinucleotide (FAD), which are essential for the enzymes that metabolize carbohydrates, fats, and proteins. The RDA for riboflavin is 0.4 to 1.7 mg/ day and can be obtained from dairy products, grains, meats, and green leafy vegetables. As with other vitamins, riboflavin is indicated for the prophy-

laxis or treatment of deficiency states. A deficiency in riboflavin leads to ariboflavinosis, which is characterized by sore throat, angular stomatitis, cheilosis, dermatitis, anemias and neuropathies. Ocular signs of deficiency include photophobia, corneal vascularization, decreased visual acuity, keratoconjunctivitis sicca, and cataract formation.[228]

VITAMIN B$_3$

Vitamin B$_3$ (niacin or nicotinic acid) is found in dietary sources such as cereals, nuts, and legumes. Niacin is converted to nicotinamide adenine dinucleotide (NAD) and nicotinamide adenine dinucleotide phosphate (NADPH), coenzymes for fat and carbohydrate metabolism. An intake of less than 5 to 20 mg/day (RDA) leads to deficiency, or pellagra. Clinical manifestations of pellagra include the "3 Ds": diarrhea, dementia, and dermatitis. Niacin is also used to treat hyperlipoproteinemias and may decrease the absorption of bile acids from the gut, thereby decreasing blood cholesterol and LDL-cholesterol levels. When used for the treatment of lipid disorders, niacin can cause flushing and pruritis, adverse effects that can be attenuated by the concurrent administration of aspirin.[107]

VITAMIN B$_5$

Vitamin B$_5$ (pantothenic acid) is a necessary cofactor in energy metabolism, hemoglobin formation, and steroid hormone synthesis. Food sources that contain pantothenic acid include green vegetables, beef, organ meats, and dry cereals. Deficiency causes neuromuscular degeneration and adrenocortical insufficiency.

VITAMIN B$_6$

Vitamin B$_6$ (pyridoxine) is found in grains, meats, and various vegetables. The active form, pyridoxal phosphate, functions as a coenzyme for hemaglobin formation and for the metabolism of amino acids and proteins. A chronic intake of less than the RDA of 0.3 to 2.1 mg/day of pyridoxine leads to manifestations of deficiency that include anemias, seborrheic dermatitis, cheilosis, glossitis, nausea, vomiting, and dizziness. Deficiency due to poor diet is rare, but the use of isoniazid, an antituberculosis agent, may inhibit formation of the coenzyme form of pyridoxine and produce symptoms of deficiency. Hydralazine, an antihypertensive medication, and penicillamine, an agent used to treat gout, can also lead to drug-induced pyridoxine deficiency.

VITAMIN B$_{12}$

Vitamin B$_{12}$ (cyanocobalamin) is converted to cofactors involved in carbohydrate metabolism and the production of red blood cells, lipids, amino acids, and nucleic acids. Cyanocobalamin is also involved in producing the myelin sheath on neurons. The RDA for vitamin B$_{12}$ is 0.3 to 2.6 µg/day.

Dietary sources rich in vitamin B$_{12}$ include organ meats such as liver, red meat, milk and milk products. Vitamin B_{12} is absorbed from the gastrointestinal tract after binding to intrinsic factor, a protein produced by the parietal cells of the gastric mucosa. In the absence of intrinsic factor, cyanocobalamin cannot be systemically absorbed. Deficiencies of B_{12} most commonly result from lack of intrinsic factor. In these cases, B_{12} must be administered parenterally. Clinical manifestations of vitamin B_{12} deficiency include pernicious anemia (megaloblastic anemia) and, ultimately, permanent neurologic damage. Since megaloblastic anemia is similar to the anemia that results from folate deficiency, it is important that B_{12} deficiency be differentiated from folate deficiency. In B_{12} deficiency, folate administration improves megaloblastic anemia while allowing neurologic damage to continue unchecked.

The neurologic damage seen in B_{12} deficiency is progressive and is characterized by paresthesias of the hands and feet, loss of vibratory senses and deep tendon reflexes, loss of memory, mental confusion, nystagmus, and loss of central vision.[107,229–231] Since these neurologic findings can occur without the classic megaloblastic anemia, vitamin B_{12} deficiency should be considered as a possible diagnosis in elderly patients with dementia and psychiatric disorders.[232]

Administration of vitamin B_{12} is indicated only in the treatment of deficiency. It has little efficacy in the treatment of other neurologic diseases such as trigeminal neuralgia, multiple sclerosis, and psychiatric disorders or for patients who are chronically fatigued. No studies have demonstrated the therapeutic efficacy of cyanocobalamin in any disease except for frank B_{12} deficiency. Allergic reactions have rarely been associated with the administration of vitamin B_{12}.

BIOTIN

Biotin is a vitamin necessary for proper metabolism of oxalocetic acid, amino acids, and fatty acids. It can be obtained by the dietary consumption of organ meats such as liver and kidney, egg yolks, yeast, cauliflower, nuts, and legumes. The RDA for biotin ranges from 10 to 100 μg/day. Deficiency causes loss of hair, dermatitis, atrophic glossitis, and neuromuscular disorders.

FOLIC ACID

Folic acid is found in green leafy vegetables, fruits, organ meats, and dried yeast. Avoiding deficiency requires 25 to 260 μg/day. Folic acid is metabolized into cofactors necessary for the proper synthesis of DNA and hemoglobin. Deficiency causes impaired protein and nucleic acid synthesis and megaloblastic anemia similar to that seen with vitamin B_{12} deficiency. Low levels of folate in women have been associated with an increase in neural tube defects in their children.[233] The most common cause of folate deficiency among adults is chronic alcohol ingestion. Folate supplementation is indicated to prevent deficiency and to treat the signs and symptoms of deficiency. Adverse effects associated with folate administration are minor and include allergic reactions. Folate should not be given for pernicious anemia where there is a deficiency of cyanocobalamin.

Minerals

ZINC SULFATE

Zinc sulfate is used as an antiseptic or preservative agent because it precipitates various bacterial proteins and enzymes.[234] It is sometimes used as a 0.25% solution to treat various types of bacterial conjunctivitis.

Zinc is an essential trace element, present in a variety of dietary sources including seafood, liver, and eggs. It is an integral part of superoxide dismutase and catalase, two antioxidant enzymes, and is necessary for proper wound healing.[235–239] Zinc has been postulated to be an effective treatment for cataracts and may cause cataracts when ocular levels are elevated.[235–246] In populations at risk for developing age-related macular degeneration (ARMD), dietary zinc levels have been shown to be decreased.[247] In a pilot study, zinc supplementation reduced the visual deterioration in ARMD.[248] Zinc deficiency leads to a syndrome similar to vitamin A deficiency because the conversion of retinol to retinal requires zinc. Deficiency may result in night blindness, decreased color perception, hyperkeratinization of lid margins with lacrimal punctal stenosis, blepharitis, conjunctivitis, photophobia,[249–252] anorexia, growth retardation, hypogonadism, dwarfism, and immunologic abnormalities. Since studies have not confirmed any beneficial effects of zinc in preventing cataract formation or reducing the incidence or progression of macular degeneration, zinc supplementation is presently indicated only for documented deficiency.

SELENIUM

Selenium is essential for the proper functioning of the antioxidant enzyme, glutathione peroxidase.[253] Glutathione peroxidase is especially important in catalyzing the breakdown of peroxide, which can produce ocular tissue damage. Low selenium levels have been associated with Keshan disease, which is characterized by myocardial necrosis, arrhythmias, peripheral myopathies, and shock. Selenium has been hypothesized to decrease the incidence of some types of cancer, but its role as an antineoplastic agent has not been confirmed. Selenium may also play a role in the pathogenesis of ARMD.[254]

COPPER

Liver, seeds, and nuts contain copper, an important part of several metalloenzymes including superoxide dismutase. Copper deficiency is rare but can cause anemias, psychomotor dysfunction, and skin and bone lesions. Copper toxicity results when greater than 15 mg is administered and is characterized by abdominal pain, nausea, vomiting, diarrhea, myalgia, metabolic acidosis, coma, and death.[108] Wilson's disease is a genetic abnormality that leads to the progressive accumulation of copper. In addition to the above-mentioned effects of copper, Kayser-Fleischer rings, sunflower cataracts, and renal dysfunction can occur.[108]

Ophthalmic Multivitamin/Mineral Formulations

Several multivitamin preparations are currently targeted for ophthalmic use (Table 19.8). These formulations contain varying doses of both fat- and water-soluble vitamins and minerals. Preparations that contain β-carotene may offer an advantage over products that contain only vitamin A. β-carotene (provitamin A) is an antioxidant, is safer than vitamin A, and is converted to vitamin A in limited quantities.[255,256] Some formulations also contain additional antioxidant compounds such as glutathione.

Although no clear scientific evidence indicates that vitamin and mineral supplementation has any beneficial effect on ocular diseases such as ARMD,[266] supplementation may be beneficial for patient populations such as the elderly who are at risk for deficiency.[257] The choice of supplement should be made on a case by case basis after the clinician has carefully weighed the potential benefits and risks. Since these products contain zinc, they should generally be taken with meals to minimize zinc-related gastrointestinal distress.[255]

The present scientific data are insufficient to support a clinical dosage recommendation or dosage duration to obtain an effect.[267] West and associates[268] have shown that well-nourished individuals seem to demonstrate no protective effect for ARMD from the use of vitamin supplements. The data related to cataract development are also inconclusive. Some preliminary information has suggested a protective effect,[269] but other studies[270,271] suggest that any protective effect for nuclear and cortical opacities may exist only in certain populations. High serum levels of some carotenoids and α-tocopherol may actually increase the risk of nuclear sclerosis, especially in women.[270] In persons without diabetes, the regular use of multivitamin formulations may also increase the risk for cortical cataracts.[271] Clearly, additional research is required before widespread vitamin and mineral supplementation can be recommended.

Chelating Agents

Exposure to heavy metals such as lead, mercury, arsenic, and iron occurs as a by-product of industrialization and pollution. Heavy metals interact with active groups on enzymes, resulting in interference with normal physiologic functions.

Chelating agents are compounds with active sites available to bind a metal ion and form a stable complex. The chelator-metal complex renders the heavy metal inactive and prevents it from interfering with other ligands. The most common use for chelating agents is in systemic poisoning with a heavy metal such as lead or for toxic poisonings with arsenic, calcium, mercury, or iron.

British Anti-Lewisite (BAL, 2,3, dimercapto-1-propanol) is a chelating agent that binds lead, arsenic, and mercury. BAL, or dimercaprol, forms a stable complex between the metal and its sulfhydryl groups.[107] Once the metal-chelator complex has formed, it undergoes renal elimination.

When used as an ophthalmic ointment or in ethylene glycol solution in 5% to 10% concentration, BAL effectively prevents corneal scarring from the arsenic-containing war gas known as Lewisite.[258,259] Arsenic is a component of many herbicides and pesticides[260] and is a by-product of many industrial processes such as smelting. BAL is an ocular irritant and can produce reversible but severe lacrimation, blepharospasm, and conjunctival injection[258] after its topical administration.

Deferoxamine is a chelator that preferentially binds iron. It is indicated for the treatment of systemic overdoses of iron. Because it is poorly absorbed from the gastrointestinal tract, it must be given parenterally. Deferoxamine is eliminated by liver metabolism and renal excretion of both the metabolized and unchanged drug. Adverse effects from deferoxamine administration include severe allergic reactions, fever, tachycardia, diarrhea, fever, leg cramps, and dysuria. Systemic use of deferoxamine[107] has been reported to cause cataract formation. The use of deferoxamine is contraindicated in pregnant patients and those with renal disease. In a 10% solution, deferoxamine has been used for nonsurgical removal of corneal rust rings.[107] Ocular formulations of deferoxamine in concentrations greater than 20% produce ocular irritation.

Ethylenediaminetetraacetate (EDTA) is a chelating agent that binds to calcium, iron, zinc, manganese, lead, and other metals. It is used systemically for the treatment of hypercalcemia and in the treatment of lead poisoning. EDTA can be used topically for the removal of corneal deposits of calcium.[262] Although no preparations of EDTA are commercially available for ophthalmic use, ophthalmic irrigation solutions of EDTA 0.7% can be prepared for removing calcium deposits from the anesthetized cornea.[261] Adverse effects associated with topical administration include conjunctival hyperemia, chemosis, and corneal stromal edema.[262]

Tissue Adhesives

No ocular tissue adhesives are currently approved for use in the United States. The ocular use of tissue adhesives is still experimental, but their potential indications are listed in

TABLE 19.8
Ocular Vitamin Supplements

Brand Name	A	Beta-carotene	B_1	B_2	B_3	B_5	B_6	B_{12}	C	D	E	Cu	Se	Zn	Miscellaneous
Ocuvite	—	5000 IU	—	—	—	—	—	—	60 mg	—	30 IU	2 mg	40 mcg	40 mg	
Ocuvite Extra		6000 IU		3 mg					200 mg		50 IU	2 mg	40 mcg	40 mg	niacinamide, manganese, L-glutathione
Vital Eyes		10,000 IU							200 mg		100 IU	2 mg	40 mcg	40 mg	manganese
Ocucaps		5000 IU							400 mg		200 IU	2 mg	40 mcg	40 mg	glutathione, sodium pyruvate
Antioxidants		5000 IU							400 mg		200 IU	2 mg	40 mcg	40 mg	gluthathione pyruvate
ICAPS-Plus		6000 IU		20 mg	—	—		—	200 mg		60 IU	2 mg	30 mcg	40 mg	manganese
Lipotriad		5000 IU	20 mg	1.2 mg	20 mg	10 mg	2 mg	6 mcg	60 mg		30 IU	2 mg	40 mcg	30 mg	
Ocugard		1000 IU	12.5 mg						375 mg		100 IU	—	25 mcg	6.25 mg	
Nutri-Vision		5000 IU							300 mg		100 IU	1.5 mg	50 mcg	30 mg	chromium
OcuSoft VMS		5000 IU							60 mg		30 IU	2 mg	40 mcg	40 mg	

TABLE 19.9
Potential Indications for Ocular Tissue Adhesives[261,263]

Sealing perforated corneal ulcers

Sealing surgical incisions in corneal surgery

Cataract incision closure

Tarsorrhaphy

Descemetocoeles

Leaking filtering blebs

Progressive corneal thinning

Impending perforations of the cornea

Impending perforations of the conjunctiva

Impending perforations of the sclera

Blepharoplasty

Foreign body localization

Table 19.9. The advantages of an ocular adhesive include use with local anesthesia rather than general anesthesia, and use in a more timely manner to repair ocular damage or trauma.[263]

The adhesives are derivatives of cyanoacrylate, and their adverse effects vary with the chemical structure. Derivatives that contain hexyl, octyl, and decyl moieties are generally well tolerated by ocular tissues when used in small amounts, but they can produce ocular irritation, inflammation, ulceration, neovascularization, and edema.[261] N-butyl cyanoacrylate (Nexacryl) is the only tissue adhesive being considered by the FDA for approval. In one clinical study, N-butyl cyanoacrylate decreased the rate of enucleation in patients with severe injuries or diseased states.[263] Adverse effects associated with N-butyl cyanoacrylate were an increased rate of infection, inflammatory reactions, and local irritation.

Surgical Miotics

Acetylcholine (ACh) is commercially available as an ophthalmic preparation (acetylcholine chloride solution 1:100) (Table 19.10) and is indicated for rapid and complete miosis during surgical procedures such as cataract extraction, penetrating keratoplasty, and iridectomy. Since it is ineffective when applied topically to the cornea, it must be placed directly onto the exposed iris during the surgical procedure. However, ACh ophthalmic solution appears to be safe and effective for intraocular use. ACh exerts its cholinergic-stimulating effects by interacting directly with cholinergic receptors. Its effects are brief due to its susceptibility to cholinesterases. Prolonged miosis may be achieved by applying a longer-acting miotic (e.g., pilocarpine) topically on the cornea before applying a surgical dressing; however, the disadvantages associated with longer-acting agents include increased postoperative pain and inflammation. ACh is not practical in the management of glaucoma and for other therapeutic and diagnostic uses because of its short duration of action and relative ineffectiveness when applied topically to the eye.

In addition to topical preparations (see Chap. 10), carbachol is available for intraocular use to produce miosis during surgery. Since carbachol is a potent miotic, this preparation is considerably less concentrated than are the topical solutions. It is available as a 0.01% sterile balanced salt solution with no preservatives and is supplied in 1.5 ml sterile glass disposable vials. The dose is 0.5 ml applied by gentle irrigation. An effective, prolonged miosis ensues 2 to 5 minutes after application.

References

1. Grant MB, Khaw PG, Schults GS, et al. Effects of epidermal growth factor, fibroblast growth factor and transforming growth factor on corneal cell chemotaxis. Invest Ophthalmol Vis Sci 1992;33:3292–3301.
2. Ie D, Glaser BM, Thompson JT, et al. Retreatment of full-thickness macular holes persisting after prior vitrectomy. A pilot study. Ophthalmology 1993;100:1787–1793.
3. Gills JP, McIntyre LG. Growth factors and their promising future. J Am Optom Assoc 1989;60:442–445.
4. Wilson SE, Lloyd SA, He Y. EGF, basic FGF and FGF beta-1 messenger RNA production in rabbit corneal epithelial cells. Invest Ophthalmol Vis Sci 1992;33:1987–1995.

TABLE 19.10
Surgical Miotics

Drug	Trade Name	Manufacturer	Concentration
Acetylcholine chloride	Miochol	Ciba Vision	Powder, 20 mg, for reconstitution to 1:100 solution
	Miochol-E	Ciba Vision	Powder, 20 mg, for reconstitution to 1:100 solution with electrolyte diluent
Carbachol	Miostat	Alcon	0.01%
	Carbostat	Ciba Vision	0.01%

5. Schultz GS, Grant MB. Neovascular growth factors. Eye 1991;5: 170–180.

6. Leschey KH, Hackett SF, Singer JH, Campochiaro PA. Growth factor responsiveness of human retinal pigment epithelial cells. Invest Ophthalmol Vis Sci 1990;31:839–846.

7. Lynch SE, Noxon JC, Colvin RB, Antoniades HN. Role of platelet-derived growth factor in wound healing: Synergistic effects with other growth factors. Proc Natl Acad Sci USA 1987;84:7696.

8. Sporn MB, Roberts AB. Peptide growth factors and inflammation, tissue repair, and cancer. J Clin Invest 1986;78:329.

9. Happenreijs VPT, Pels E, Vrensen GFJM, et al. Effects of human epidermal growth factor on endothelial wound healing of human corneas. Invest Ophthalmol Vis Sci 1992;33:1946–1957.

10. Parelmann JJ, Nicolson M, Pepose JS. Epidermal growth factor in human aqueous humor. Am J Ophthalmol 1990;109:603.

11. Scardovi C, De Felice GP, Gazzaniga A. Epidermal growth factor in the topical treatment of traumatic corneal ulcers. Ophthalmologica 1993;206:119–124.

12. Cohen S. Isolation of mouse submaxillary gland protein accelerating incisor eruption and eyelid opening in the newborn animal. J Biol Chem 1962;237:155–162.

13. Savage CR, Cohen S. Epidermal growth factor and a new derivative: Rapid isolation procedures and biological and chemical characterization. J Biol Chem 1972;247:7609–7611.

14. Cohen S, Savage CR. Recent studies on the chemistry and biology of epidermal growth factor. Recent Prog Horm Res 1974;30:551–574.

15. Gospodarowicz D, Mescher AL, Birdwell CR. Stimulation of corneal endothelial cell proliferation in vitro by fibroblast and epidermal growth factor. Exp Eye Res 1977;25:75–89.

16. Gospodarowicz D, Greenberg G. The effects of epidermal and fibroblast growth factors on the repair of corneal endothelial wounds in bovine corneas maintained in organ culture. Exp Eye Res 1979;28:147–157.

17. Gospodarowicz D. Fibroblast and epidermal growth factors: Their uses in vivo and in vitro in studies on cell functions and cell transplantation. Mol Cell Biochem 1979;25:79–109.

18. Gospodarowicz D, Moran JS. Growth factors in mammalian cell culture. Rev Biochem 1976;45:531–558.

19. Raymond GM, Jumblatt MM, Bartels SP, Neufeld AH. Rabbit corneal endothelial cells in vitro: Effects of EGF. Invest Ophthalmol Vis Sci 1986;27:474–479.

20. Hongo M, Itoi M, Yamaura Y, et al. Distribution of epidermal growth factor receptors in rabbit lens epithelial cells. Invest Ophthalmol Vis Sci 1993;34:401–411.

21. Chan KY, Lindquist TD, Edenfield MJ, et al. Pharmacokinetic study of recombinant human epidermal growth factor in the anterior eye. Invest Ophthalmol Vis Sci 1991;32:3209–3215.

22. Soong HK, Hassan T, Varani J. Fibronectin does not enhance epidermal growth factor-mediated acceleration of corneal epithelial wound closure. Arch Ophthalmol 1989;107:1052.

23. Ho PC, Davis WH, Elliot JH, Cohen S. Kinetics of corneal epithelial regeneration and epidermal growth factor. Invest Ophthalmol 1974;13:804.

24. Petroutsos G, Courty J, Guimaraes R, et al. Comparison of the effects of EGF, FGF and EDGF on corneal epithelium wound healing. Curr Eye Res 1984;3:593.

25. Arturson G. Epidermal growth factor in the healing of corneal wounds, epidermal wounds and partial-thickness scalds. Scand J Plast Reconstr Surg Hand Surg 1984;18:33.

26. Singh G, Foster CS. Epidermal growth factor in alkali-burned corneal epithelial wound healing. Am J Ophthalmol 1987;103: 802.

27. Reim M, Busse S, Leber M, Schultz C. Effect of epidermal growth factor in severe experimental alkali burns. Ophthalmic Res 1988; 20:327.

28. Chung JH, Fagerholm P. Treatment of rabbit corneal alkali wounds with human epidermal growth factor. Cornea 1989;8:122.

29. Brightwell JR, Riddle SL, Eiferman RA, et al. Biosynthetic human EGF accelerates healing of Neodecadron-treated primate corneas. Invest Ophthalmol Vis Sci 1985;26:105.

30. Schultz GS, Davis JB, Eiferman RA. Growth factors and corneal epithelium. Cornea 1988;7:96.

31. Gospodarowicz D, Rudland P, Linstrom J, Benirsrike K. Fibroblast growth factor: Its localization, purification, mode of action, and physiological significance. Adv Metab Dis 1975;8:301–335.

32. Nayak SK, Samples JR, Deg JK, Binder PS. Growth characteristics of primate (baboon) corneal endothelium in vitro. Invest Ophthalmol Vis Sci 1986;27:607.

33. Raphael B, Kerr NC, Shimizu RW, et al. Enhanced healing of cat corneal endothelial wounds by epidermal growth factor. Invest Ophthalmol Vis Sci 1993;34:2305–2311.

34. Beaubien J, Boisjoly HM, Gagnon P, et al. Mechanical properties of the rabbit cornea during wound healing after treatment with epidermal growth factor. Can J Ophthalmol 1994;29:61–65.

35. Leschey KH, Hackett SF, Singer J, Campochiaro PA. Growth factor responsiveness of human retinal pigment epithelial cells. Invest Ophthalmol Vis Sci 1990;31:839–842.

36. Kandarakis A, Page C, Kaufman H. The effect of epidermal growth factor on epithelial healing after penetrating keratoplasty in human eyes. Am J Ophthalmol 1984;98:411–415.

37. Daniele I, Frati L, Fiore C, Santoni G. The effect of the epidermal growth factor (EGF) on the corneal epithelium in humans. Graefe's Arch Clin Exp Ophthalmol 1979;210:159–165.

38. Gospodarowicz D, Brown KD, Birdwell CR, Zetter BR. Control of proliferation of human vascular endothelial cells. Characterization of the response of human umbilical vein endothelial cells to fibroblast growth factor, epidermal growth factor and thrombin. J Cell Biol 1978;77:774–787.

39. Frank RN. On the pathogenesis of diabetic retinopathy. Ophthalmology 1991;98:586–593.

40. Hanneken A, Lutty GA, McLeod DS, et al. Localization of basic fibroblast growth factor to the developing capillaries of the bovine retina. J Cell Physiol 1989;138:115–120.

41. Baudouin C, Fredj-Reygrobellett D, Caruelle JP, et al. Acidic fibroblast growth factor distribution in normal human eye and possible implications in ocular pathogenesis. Ophthalmic Res 1990;22:73–81.

42. Noji S, Matsuo T, Koyama E, et al. Expression pattern of acidic and basic fibroblast growth factor genes in adult rat eyes. Biochem Biophys Res Commun 1990;168:343–349.

43. Fredj-Reygrobellet D, Plouet J, Delayre TH, et al. Effects of αFGF and βFGF on wound healing in rabbit corneas. Curr Eye Res 1987;6:1205–1208.

44. Gospodarowicz D, Mescher AL, Brown KD, Birdwell CR. The role of fibroblast growth factor and epidermal growth factor in the proliferative response of the corneal and lens epithelium. Exp Eye Res 1977;25:631.

45. Roberts AB, McCune BK, Sporn MB. Kidney Int 1992;41:557–559.

46. Baird A, Bohlen P. Peptide growth factors and their receptors. Springer-Verlag, 1990.

47. Logan A, Berry M. Transforming growth factor-β1 and basic fibroblast growth factor in the injured CNS. Trends Pharmacol Sci 1993;14:337–343.

48. Buntrock P, Buntrock M, Marx I, et al. Stimulation of wound healing using brain extract with fibroblast growth factor (FGF) activity III. Exp Pathol 1984;26:247–254.

49. Dreyer D, Lagrange A, Grothe C, Unsicker K. Basic fibroblast growth faction prevents ontogenetic neuron death in vivo. Neurosci Lett 1989;99:35–38.

50. Ferrari G, Minozzi MC, Toffano G, et al. Electron microscopy, angiography, ultrastructural autoradiography of granulomatous tissue. Basic fibroblast growth factor promotes the survival and development of mesencephalic neurons in culture. Dev Biol 1989; 133:140–147.

51. Faktorovich EG, Steinberg RH, Yasumiera D, et al. Photoreceptor degeneration in inherited retinal dystrophy delayed by basic fibroblast growth factor. Nature 1990;347:83–86.

52. Pasquale LR, Dorman-Pease ME, Lutty GA, Quigley HA, Jampel HD. Immunolocalization of TGF-β1, TGF-β2 and TGF-β3 in the anterior segment of the human eye. Invest Ophthalmol Vis Sci 1993;34:23–29.

53. Postlewaite AE, Koski-Oja J, Moses HL, Kang AH. Stimulation of the chemotactic migration of human fibroblasts by transforming growth factor β. J Exp Med 1987;165:251–256.

54. Del Vecchio PJ, Bizois R, Holleran LA, et al. Inhibition of human scleral fibroblast proliferation with heparin. Invest Ophthalmol Vis Sci 1988;29:1272.

55. Muller G, Behrens J, Nussbaumer U, Bohlen P, Birchmeier W. Inhibitory action of transforming growth factor β on endothelial cells. Proc Natl Acad Sci 1987;84:5600–5604.

56. Smiddy, WE, Glaser BM, Thompson JT, et al. Transforming growth factor-β2 significantly enhances the ability to flatten the rim of subretinal fluid surrounding macular holes. Retina 1993;13:296.

57. Thompson JT, Hiner CJ, Glaser BM, et al. Fluorescein angiographic characteristics of macular holes before and after vitrectomy with transforming growth factor beta-2. Am J Ophthalmol 1994;117:291–301.

58. King GL, Goodman AD, Bosnex S, et al. Receptors and growth promoting effects of insulin and IGF 1 on cells from bovine retinal capillaries and aorta. J Clin Invest 1985;75:1028.

59. Grant M, Jerdan J, Merimee TJ. Insulin like growth factor-1 modulates endothelial cell chemotaxis. J Clin Endocrin Metab 1987;65:370–371.

60. Merimee TJ, Zapf J, Froesch ER. Insulin-like growth factors: Studies in diabetics with and without retinopathy. N Engl J Med 1983;309:527–530.

61. King GL, Buzney SM, Kahn CR, et al. Differential responsiveness to insulin of endothelial and support cells from micro and macro vessels. J Clin Invest 1983;71:974–979.

62. Merimee TJ. Diabetic retinopathy. A synthesis of perspectives. N Engl J Med 1990;322:978–983.

63. Edwards RB, Adler AJ, Claycomb RC. Requirement of insulin or IGF-1 for the maintenance of retinyl ester synthetase activity by cultured retinal pigment epithelial cells. Exp Eye Res 1991;52:51–57.

64. Phan TM, Foster CS, Shaw CD, et al. Topical fibronectin in an alkali burn model of corneal ulceration in rabbits. Arch Ophthalmol 1991;109:414–419.

65. Elger T, Zalik SE. Fibronectin distribution during cell type conversion in newt lens regeneration. Anat Embryol 1989;180:131–142.

66. McCarthy JB, Hagen ST, Furcht LT. Human fibronectin contains distinct adhesion- and motility-promoting domains for metastatic melanoma cells. J Cell Biol 1986;102:179–188.

67. Nishida T, Ohashi Y, Awata T, et al. Fibronectin: A new therapy for corneal trophic ulcer. Arch Ophthalmol 1983;101:1046–1048.

68. Gordon J, Johnson P. Results of a randomized double-masked, multicenter clinical trial of fibronectin in the treatment of persistent epithelial defects (PED). Invest Ophthalmol Vis Sci 1992;33:890.

69. Olivero DK, Furcht LT. Type IV collagen, laminin and fibronectin promotes the adhesion and migration of rabbit lens epithelial cells in vitro. Invest Ophthalmol Vis Sci 1993;34:2825–2833.

70. Osako M, Keltner JL. Botulinum A toxin (Oculinum??) in ophthalmology. Surv Ophthalmol 1991;36:28–46.

71. Scott AB. Clostridial toxin as therapeutic agents. In: Simpson LL, ed. Botulinum neurotoxin and tetanus toxin. New York: Academic Press, 1989;399–412.

72. Gammon JA. Chemodenervation treatment of strabismus and blepharospasm with botulinum toxin. Ocular Therap 1984;1:3–7.

73. Scott AB, Rosenbaum A, Collins CC. Pharmacologic weakening of extraocular muscles. Invest Ophthalmol 1973;12:924–927.

74. Scott AB. Botulinum toxin injection of eye muscles to correct strabismus. Trans Am Ophthalmol Soc 1981;79:734–770.

75. Dunlop D, Pittar G, Dunlop C. Botulinum toxin in ophthalmology. Aust NZ J Ophthalmol 1988;16:15–20.

76. Gammon JA, Gemmill M, Tigges J, Lerman S. Botulinum chemodenervation treatment of strabismus. J Pediatr Ophthalmol Strabismus 1985;22:221–226.

77. Magoon EH. The use of botulinum toxin injection as an alternative to strabismus surgery. Contemp Ophthalmic Forum 1987;5:222–229.

78. Scott AB, Reese PD, Magoon EH. Clinical decisions in ophthalmology. Projects in medicine. New York: Park Row Pub., 1987.

79. Scott AB. Botulinum treatment of strabismus following retinal detachment surgery. Arch Ophthalmol 1990;108:509–510.

80. Balazs EA. Sodium hyaluronate and viscosurgery. In: Miller D, Stegmen R, eds. Healon: A guide to its use in ophthalmic surgery. New York: John Wiley & Sons, 1983;114.

81. Fechner PU, Fechner MU. Methylcellulose and lens implantation. Br J Ophthalmol 1983;67:259.

82. Hakansson L, Venge P. The molecular basis of the hyaluronic acid mediated stimulation of granulocyte function. J Immunol 1987; 138:4347.

83. Inoue M and Katakami C. The effect of hyaluronic acid on corneal epithelial cell proliferation. Invest Ophthalmol Vis Sci 1993;34:2313–2316.

84. Fagerholm P, Fitzsimmons T, Harfstrand A, Schenholm, M. Reactive formation of hyaluronic acid in the rabbit corneal alkali burn. Acta Ophthalmol 1992;70:67.

85. Hassell J, Cintorn C. Kublin C, Newsome D. Proteoglycan changes during restoration of transparency in corneal scars. Arch Biochem Biophys 1983;222A:362.

86. Fitzsimmons TD, Fagerholm P, Harfstrand A, Schenholm M. Hyaluronic acid in the rabbit cornea after excimer laser superficial keratectomy. Invest Ophthalmol Vis Sci 1992;33:3011–3015.

87. Miller D, Stegmann R. Use of Na-hyaluronate in anterior segment eye surgery. Am Intra-Ocular Implant Soc J 1980;6:13.

88. Limberg MB, Kaufman HE. Topical application of hyaluronic acid and chondroitin sulfate in the treatment of dry eyes. Am J Ophthalmol 1987;103:194–197.

89. Pruett RC, Schepens CL, Swann DA. Hyaluronic acid vitreous substitute. A six year clinical evaluation. Arch Ophthalmol 1979; 97:2325.

90. Silver FH, LiBrizzi J. Use of viscoelastic solutions in ophthalmology: A review of physical properties and long-term effects. J Long-term Effects of Med Implants 1992;2:49–66.

91. Agapitos PJ. Cataract surgical techniques and adjuncts. Curr Opin Ophthalmol 1992;3:13–28.

92. Tsurimaki Y, Shimizu H. Effects of residual sodium hyaluronate on postsurgical blood-aqueous barrier. Jpn J Ophthalmol 1991;35: 445–452.

93. MacRae SM, Edelhauser HF, Hyndick RA, et al. The effects of sodium hyaluronate, chondroitin sulfate, and methylcellulose on the corneal endothelium and intraocular pressure. Am J Ophthalmol 1983;95:332.

94. Harrison, SE, Soll DB, Shayegan M, Clinch T. Chondroitin sulfate: a new and effective protective agent for intraocular lens insertion. Ophthalmology 1982;89:1254.

95. Koch DD, Liu JF, Glasser DB, Merin LM, Haft E. A comparison of corneal endothelial changes after use of Healon or Viscoat during phacoemulsification. Am J Ophthalmol 1993;115:188–201.

96. Rafuse PE, Nichols BD. Effects of Healon vs. Viscoat on endothelial cell count and morphology after phacoemulsification and posterior chamber lens implantation. Can J Ophthalmol 1992;27: 125–129.

97. Chumbley LC, Morgan AM, Musallam I. Hydroxypropyl methylcellulose in extracapsular cataract surgery with intraocular lens implantation: Intraocular pressure and inflammatory response. Eye 1990;4:121–126.

98. Sand BB, Work E, Skovbo A, Elboll P. Sodium hyaluronate and methylcellulose in extracapsular cataract extraction. Acta Ophthalmol 1991;69:65–67.

99. Bleckmann H, Vogt R, Garus HJ. Collagel—a new viscoelastic substance for ophthalmic surgery. J Cataract Refract Surg 1992; 18:20–26.

100. Gonvers M. Temporary silicone oil tamponade in the management of retinal detachment with massive proliferative vitreoretinopathy. Am J Ophthalmol 1985;100:239.

101. McCuen BW, deJuan E, Machemer R. Silicone oil in vitroretinal surgery: Part 1. Surgical techniques. Retina 1985;5:189.

102. Eller AW, Gardner TW, D'Antonio JA. A survey of intraocular silicone oil use in the United States. Ophthalmology 1992;99: 1174–1176.

103. Friberg TR, Verstraeten TC, Wilcox DK. Effects of emulsification, purity, and fluorination of silicone oil on human retinal pigment epithelial cells. Invest Ophthalmol Vis Sci 1991;32: 2030–2034.

104. Parel JM. Silicone oils: Physiochemical properties. In: Ryan SJ, Glaser BM, Michels RG, eds. Retina, Vol. 3, St. Louis: C.V. Mosby Co 1989;261–277.

105. Federman JL, Schubert HD. Complications associated with the use of silicone oil in 150 eyes after retina or vitreous surgery. Ophthalmology 1988;95:870.

106. Lear's Magazine, April 1993;103.

107. Marcus R, Coulston AM. The vitamins. In: Gilman AG, Rall TW, Nies AS, Taylor P, eds. Goodman and Gilman's the pharmacological basis of therapeutics. New York: Pergamon Press, 1990;1523–1582.

108. Nutrition—General Considerations. In: Berkow R, Fletcher AJ, eds. Rahway, NJ: Merck Sharp & Dohme Research Laboratories, 1987;Chapter 79.

109. Anonymous. Invest Ophthalmol Vis Sci 1993;34:1.

110. World Health Organization. Global situation—Vitamin A deficiency (Based on reports received by the World Health Organization as of October 1988) In: Expanded Program on Immunization Update. Geneva, Switzerland: World Health Organization: December 1988.

111. Ubels JL, Edelhauser HF. Retinoid permeability and uptake in corneas of normal and vitamin A deficient rabbits. Arch Ophthalmol 1982;100:1828–1831.

112. Ubels JL, Foley KM, Rismondo V. Retinol secretion by the lacrimal gland. Invest Ophthalmol Vis Sci 1986;27:1261–1268.

113. Ubels JL, MacRae SM. Vitamin A is present as retinol in the tears of rabbits and humans. Curr Eye Res 1984;3:315.

114. Rismondo V, Ubels JL. Isotretinoin in lacrimal gland fluid and tears. Arch Ophthalmol 1987;105:416–420.

115. Sporn MB, Roberts AB, Goodman DeW S, eds. The retinoids, Vol I and II. New York: Academic Press, 1984.

116. Kiorpes TC, Kim YR, Wolf G. Stimulation of the synthesis of specific glycoproteins in corneal epithelium by vitamin A. Exp Eye Res 1979;28:23–35.

117. Aydelotte MB. The effects of vitamin A and citral on epithelial differentiation in vitro. J Embryol Exp Morphol 1963;11:621–635.

118. Fuchs, E, Green HJ. Regulation of terminal differentiation of cultured human keratocytes by vitamin A. Cell 1981;25:617–624.

119. Hassell JR, Newsome DA, De Luca LM. Increased biosynthesis of specific glycoconjugates in rat corneal epithelium following treatment with vitamin A. Invest Ophthalmol Vis Sci 1980;19: 642–647.

120. Jayaraj AP, Lella R, Rao PBR. Studies on cornea and conjunctival mucus metaplasia in vitamin A deficient rats. Exp Eye Res 1971; 12:1–5.

121. Kim YC, Wolf G. Vitamin A deficiency and the glycoproteins of rat corneal epithelium. J Nutr 1979;104:710–718.

122. Kartha VMR, Krishnamorthy S. Antioxidant function of vitamin A. Inter J Vit Nutr Res 1977;47:394–401.

123. Moon RC, Itri LM. Retinoids and cancer. In: Sporn MB, Roberts AB, Goodman WS, eds. The retinoids, Vol. II, New York: Academic Press, 1984;327–371.

124. Pirie A, Overall M. Effect of vitamin A deficiency on the lens epithelium of the rat. Exp Eye Res 1972;13:105–109.

125. Pokrovsky AA, Lashneva NV, Kon IY. Study of vitamin A effects on lipid peroxidation in rat liver. Inter J Vitam Nutr Res 1974;44: 477–486.

126. Toufexis A. The new scoop on vitamins. Time, April 6, 1992; 54–59.

127. Handelman GJ, Dratz EA. The role of antioxidants in the retina and retinal pigment epithelium and the nature of prooxidant-induced damage. Adv Free Radical Bio Med 1986;2:1–89.

128. Menkes MS, Comstock GW, Vuilleumier JP, et al. Serum beta-carotene, vitamins A and E, selenium and the risk of lung cancer. N Engl J Med 1986;315:1250–1254.

129. Schneider EL, Reed JD. Modulations of aging processes. Hand-

book of the biology of aging, ed. 2. New York: Van Nostrand Reinhold Co., 1985.

130. Muller DPR. Vitamin E therapy in retinopathy of prematurity. Eye 1992;6:221–225.

131. Sanders DR. Nutritional compliance and macular degeneration. Ocular Surg News Suppl 1991;1:1–15.

132. Young RW. Solar radiation and age-related macular degeneration. Surv Ophthalmol 1988;32:252–269.

133. Varma SD. Scientific basis for medical therapy of cataracts by antioxidants. Am J Clin Nutr 1991;53:335S–345S.

134. Leske MC, Chylack LT, Wu S. The lens opacities case-control study. Arch Ophthalmol 1991;190:244–251.

135. Shams NBK, Hanniner LA, Chaves HV, et al. Effect of vitamin A deficiency on the adhesion of rat corneal epithelium and the basement membrane complex. Invest Ophthalmol Vis Sci 1993;34:2646–2654.

136. Rao V, Friend J, Thoft RA, et al. Conjunctival goblet cells and mitotic rate in children with retinol deficiency and measles. Arch Ophthalmol 1987;195:378–380.

137. El-Ghorab M, Capone-Jr A, Underwood BA, et al. Response of ocular surface epithelium to corneal wounding in retinol-deficient rabbits. Invest Ophthalmol Vis Sci 1988;29:1671–1676.

138. Watanabe K, Frangieh G, Reddy CV, Kenyon K. Effect of fibronectin on corneal epithelial wound healing in the vitamin A deficient rat. Invest Ophthalmol Vis Sci 1991;32:2159–2162.

139. Frargieh GT, Hayashik-Teekhascinee C, Wolf G, et al. Fibronectin and corneal epithelial wound healing in the vitamin A deficient rat. Arch Ophthalmol 1989;107:567–571.

140. Moore T, Holmes PD. The production of experimental vitamin A deficiency in rats and mice. Lab Anim 1971;5:239–250.

141. Sommer A, Katz J, Tarwotjo I. Increased risk of respiratory disease and diarrhea in children with preexisting mild vitamin A deficiency. Am J Clin Nutr 1984;40:1090–1095.

142. Milton R, Reddy V, Maidu A. Mild vitamin A deficiency and childhood morbidity: An Indian experience. Am J Clin Nutr 1987;46:825–829.

143. Sommer A, Tarwotjo I, Hussanini G, Susanto D. Increased mortality in children with mild vitamin A deficiency. Lancet 1983;2:585–588.

144. Sommer A, Tarwotjo I, West KP, et al. Impact of vitamin A supplementation on childhood mortality: A randomized controlled community trial. Lancet 1986;1:1169–1173.

145. Tarwotjo I, Sommer A, West KP, et al. Influence of participation on mortality in a randomized trial of vitamin A prophylaxis. Am J Clin Nutr 1987;45:1466–1471.

146. Gans M, Taylor C. Reversal of progressive nyctalopia in a patient with Crohn's disease. Can J Ophthalmol 1990;25:156–158.

147. Atkinson DT. Malnutrition as an etiological factor in senile cataract. Eye, Ear, Nose, Throat Monthly 1952;31:79–83.

148. Libondi T, Costaglioa C, Della Corte M, et al. Cataract risk factors: Blood level of antioxidative vitamins, reduced glutathione and malondialdehyde in cataractous patients. Metab Pediatr Syst Ophthalmol 1991;14:31–36.

149. Gilbard JP, Huang AJW, Bellegrum R, et al. Open label crossover study of vitamin A ointment as a treatment for keratoconjunctivitis sicca. Ophthalmology 1989;96:244–246.

150. Soong HK, Martin NF, Wagoner MD, et al. Topical retinoid therapy for squamous metaplasia of various ocular surface disorders. Ophthalmology 1988;95:1422–1446.

151. Tseng SCG, Maumenee AE, Stark WJ, et al. Topical retinoid treatment for various dry eye disorders. Ophthalmology 1985;92:717–727.

152. Wright P. Topical retinoic acid therapy for disorders of outer eye. Trans Ophthalmol Soc UK 1985;104:869–874.

153. Ohashi Y, Watanabe H, Kinoshita S, et al. Vitamin A eyedrops for superior limbic keratoconjunctivitis Am J Ophthalmol 1988;105:523–527.

154. Berson EL, Rosner B, Sandbergm MA, et al. A randomized trial of vitamin A and vitamin E supplementation for retinitis pigmentosa. Arch Ophthalmol 1993;111:761–772.

155. Pararajaseguram G, Sevanin A, Rao NA. Suppression of S antigen-induced uveitis by vitamin E supplementation. Ophthamic Res 1991;23:121–127.

156. Hollis A, Butcher WI, Davis H, et al. Structural alterations in retinal tissues from rats deficient in vitamin E and selenium therapy with hyperbaric oxygen. Exp Eye Res 1992:54:671–684.

157. Hafeman DG, Loekstra WE. Lipid peroxidation in vivo during vitamin E and selenium deficiency in the rat as monitored by ethane evolution. J Nutr 107;777–672.

158. Physicians Desk Reference, ed. 47. Montvale, NJ: Medical Economics Data, 1993.

159. Owens WC, Owens EU. Retrolental fibroplasia in premature infants. II. Studies on the prophylaxis of the disease: The use of alpha-tocopherol acetate. Am J Ophthalmol 1949;32:1631–1637.

160. Hittner HM, Rudolph AJ, Kretzner FL. Suppression of severe retinopathy of prematurity with vitamin E supplementation. Ophthalmology 1984;91:1512–1523.

161. Schaffer DR, Johnson L, Quinn GE, et al. Vitamin E and retinopathy of prematurity. Ophthalmology 1985;92:1005–1011.

162. Johnson L, Schaffer D, Boggs TR. The premature infant. Vitamin E deficiency and retrolental fibroplasia. Am J Clin Nutr 1974;27:1158–1173.

163. Johnson L, Quinn GE, Abbasi S, et al. Effect of sustained pharmacological vitamin E levels on incidence and severity of retinopathy of prematurity: A controlled clinical trial. J Pediatr 1989;114:827–838.

164. Phelps DL. Vitamin E and retrolental fibroplasia in 1982. Pediatrics 1982;70:420–425.

165. Phelps DL, Rosenbaum AL, Isenberg SJ, et al. Tocopherol efficacy and safety for preventing retinopathy of prematurity: A randomized, controlled, double-masked trial. Pediatrics 1987;79:489–500.

166. Finner NN, Peters KL, Hayek Z, Merel CL. Vitamin E and necrotizing enterocolitis. Pediatrics 1984;73:387–393.

167. Anon J. Retinopathy of prematurity. Lancet 1991;337:83–84.

168. Watts JL, Milner RA, McCormick AQ. Failure of vitamin E to prevent RLF. Clin Invest Med 1985;8:A176.

169. Pukin JE, Simon RM, Ehrenkranz RA. Influence on retrolental fibroplasia of intramuscular vitamin E administration during respiratory distress syndrome. Ophthalmology 1983;89:96–102.

170. Bremer DL, Rogers GL. The efficacy of vitamin E in retinopathy of prematurity. J Pediatr Ophthalmol Strabismus 1986;23:132–136.

171. Committee on Fetus and Newborn. Vitamin E and the prevention of retinopathy of prematurity. Pediatrics 1985;76:315–316.

172. Lorch V, Murphy D, Hoersten LR, et al. Unusual syndrome among premature infants association with a new intravenous vitamin E product. Pediatrics 1985;75:598–602.

173. Ross WM, Creighton MO, Inch WR, Trevithick JR. Radiation

cataract formation diminished by vitamin E in rat lenses in vitro. Exp Eye Res 1982;36:645–653.

174. Augustin AJ, Breyohol W, Boker T, Wegner A. Evidence for the prevention of oxidative tissue damage in the inner eye by vitamins A and C. German J Ophthalmol 1992;1:394–398.

175. Bhat KS. Nutritional status of thiamin, riboflavin and pyridoxine in cataract patient. Nutr Rep Int 1987;36:685–692.

176. Skalka HW, Prchal JT. Riboflavin deficiency and cataract formation. Metab Pediatr Ophthalmol 1981;51:17–20.

177. Jacques PF, Chylack LT Jr, McGandy RB, Hartz SC. Nutritional status in persons with and without senile cataract: Blood vitamin and mineral levels. Am J Clin Nutr 1988;48:152–158.

178. Jacques PF, Chylack LT Jr, McGandy RB, Hartz SG. Antioxidant status in persons with and without senile cataract. Arch Ophthalmol 1988;106:337–340.

179. Swanson A, Truesdale A. Elemental analysis in normal and cataractous human lens tissue. Biochem Biophys Commun 1971;45:1488–1496.

180. Bhat KS. Plasma calcium and trace minerals in human subjects with mature cataract. Nutr Rep Int 1988;37:157–163.

181. Jacques PF, Chylack LT Jr. Epidemiologic evidence of a role for the antioxidant vitamins and carotenoids in cataract prevention. Am J Clin Nutr 1991;53:352S–355S.

182. Leske MC, Chylack LT Jr, Wu SY. The lens opacities case-control study: Risk factors for cataract. Arch Ophthalmol 1991;109:244–251.

183. Robertson JM. A possible role for vitamins C and E in cataract prevention. Am J Clin Nutr 1991;53:346S–351S.

184. Mansour SA, Richards RD, Kuck JF, Varma SD. Effect of antioxidant (vitamin E) on the progress of emory mice. Invest Ophthalmol Vis Sci 1984;25:138.

185. Creighton MO, Trevithick JR. Cortical cataract formation prevented by vitamin E and glutathione. Exp Eye Res 1979;29:689–693.

186. Devamanoharan P, Henein M, Morris S, et al. Prevention of senile cataract by vitamin C. Exp Eye Res 1991;52:563–568.

187. Varma SD, Richards RD. Light-induced damage to ocular lens cation pump: Prevention by vitamin C. Proc Natl Acad Sci USA 1970;67:3504–3506.

188. Robertson JM, Donner AP, Trevithick JR, et al. Vitamin E intake and risk of cataracts in humans. Ann NY Acad Sci 1989;570:372–382.

189. Ross WM, Creighton MO, Trevithick JR. Radiation cataractogenesis induced by neutron or gamma irradiation in the rat lens is reduced by vitamin E. Scan Micros 1990;4:641–650.

190. Ross WM, Creighton MO, Stewart-Deltan PH, et al. Modeling cortical cataractogenesis. In vivo effects of vitamin E on cataractogenesis in diabetic rats. Can J Ophthalmol 1982;17:61–66.

191. Varma SD, Beacju MA, Rocjards RD. Photoperoxidation of lens lipids: Prevention by vitamin E. Photochem Photobiol 1982;36:623–636.

192. Chuistova IP, Shermet NA, Larmak TD. Experimental morphologic foundation for the usage of zinc in the treatment of cataract. Ophthalmology 1985;7:396.

193. Bravetti G. Preventative medical treatment of senile cataract with vitamin E and anthocyanosides: Clinical evaluation. Ann Ophthalmol 1989;115:109.

194. Bunce GE. Nutrition and cataracts. Nutr Rev 1979;37:337–343.

195. Runge P, Muller DPR, McAllister J, et al. Oral vitamin E supplements can prevent the retinopathy of abetalipoproteinemia. Br J Ophthalmol 1986;70:166–173.

196. Eye Disease Case-Control Study Group. Antioxidant status and neovascular age-related macular degeneration. Arch Ophthalmol 1993;11:194–209.

197. Abdo KM, Roa G, Montgomery CA, et al. Thirteen-week toxicity study of d-α-tocopherol acetate (vitamin E) in Fischer 344 rats. Food Chem Toxicol 1986;24:1043–1050.

198. Albert DM, Saulenas AM, Cohen SM. Verhoeff's query: Is Vitamin D effective against retinoblastoma? Arch Ophthalmol 1988;106:536–540.

199. Frampton R, Omond S, Eisman J. Inhibition of human cancer cell growth by 1,25-dihydroxyvitamin D metabolites. Cancer Res 1983;43:4443–4447.

200. Munker R, Norman A, Koeffler H. Vitamin D compounds: Effect on clonal proliferation and differentiation of human myeloid cells. J Clin Invest 1986;78:424–430.

201. Olsson I, Gullberg U, Ivhed I, et al. Induction of differentiation of the human histiocytic lymphoma cell line U-937 by 1-alpha,25-dihydroxycholecalciferol. Cancer Res 1983;43:5862–5867.

202. Shokravi MT, Marcus DM, Alroy J, et al. Vitamin D inhibits angiogenesis in transgenic murine retinoblastoma. Invest Ophthalmol Vis Sci 1995;36:83–87.

203. Honma Y, Hozumi M, Abe E, et al. 1-alpha,25-dihydroxyvitamin D and 1–alpha-hydroxyvitamin D prolong survival time of mice inoculated with myeloid leukemia cells. Proc Natl Acad Sci USA 1983;80:201–204.

204. Moore M. Biologicals for cancer treatment: Growth and differentiating agents. Hosp Pract 1986;69–80.

205. Eisman J, Barkla D, Tutton D. Suppression of in vivo growth of human cancer solid tumor xenografts by 1,25-dihydroxyvitamin D. Cancer Res 1987;47:21–25.

206. Garland C, Shekelle RB, Barret-Connor E, et al. Dietary vitamin D and calcium and risk of colorectal cancer. A 19-year prospective study in men. Lancet 1985;307–309.

207. Saulinas AM, Cohen SM, Key LL, et al. Vitamin D and retinoblastoma. Arch Ophthalmol 1988;106:533–535.

208. Barash P, Kitahata LM, Mandel S. Acute cardiovascular collapse after intravenous phytonadione. Anesth Ann Curr Res 1976;55:304–306.

209. Becker B. Ascorbate transport in guinea pig eyes. Invest Ophthalmol 1967;6:410–415.

210. Cole DF. The eye: Comparative physiology. In: Davson H, Graham LT, eds. London: Academic Press, 1974;71–162.

211. Pitt HA, Costrini AM. Vitamin C prophylaxis in marine recruits. JAMA 1979;241:908–911.

212. Pauling L. Evolution and the need for ascorbic acid. Proc Natl Acad Sci USA 1970;67:1643–1648.

213. Cameron E, Pauling L. Supplemental ascorbate in the supportive treatment of cancer: Prolongation of survival times in terminal human cancer. Proc Natl Acad Sci USA 1978;73:3685–3689.

214. Varma SD, Kumar S, Richards RD. Light induced damage to ocular lens cation pump: Prevention by vitamin C. Proc Nat Acad Sci 1979;76:3504–3506.

215. Williams RN, Paterson CA. A protective role for ascorbic acid during inflammatory episodes in the eye. Exp Eye Res 1986;42:211–218.

216. Orgnisciak DT, Wang HM, Kous AL. Ascorbate and glutathione levels in the developing normal dystrophic rat retina; Effect of intense light exposure. Curr Eye Res 1984;3:257–267.

217. Organisciak DT, Wang HM, Li AY, Tso MOM. The protective effect of ascorbate in retinal light damage of rats. Invest Ophthalmol Vis Sci 1985;26:1580–1588.

218. Organisciak DT, Wang HM, Noell WK. Aspects of the ascorbate protective mechanism in rats with normal and reduced ROS docosahexaneoic acid. In: Hollyfield J, Anderson R, LaVail M, eds. Progress in clinical and biological research. New York: Alan R. Liss 1987;455–468.

219. Organisciak DT, Jiang Y, Wang H, Bicknell I. The protective effect of ascorbic acid in retinal light damage of rats exposed to intermittent light. Invest Ophthalmol Vis Sci 1990;31:1195–1202.

220. Organisciak DT, Bickness IR, Darrow RM. The effects of L and D ascorbic acid administration on retinal tissue levels and light damage in rats. Curr Eye Res 1992;11:231–241.

221. Li Y, Tso MOM, Wang HM, Organisciak DT. Amelioration of phototoxic injury in rat retina by ascorbic acid: A histopathologic study. Invest Ophthalmol Vis Sci 1985;26:1589–1598.

222. Mutmann V, Re BV, Lachman R. El tratamiento de la cataracta senil incipiente por el acido ascorbico. Arch Oftalmologica 1939; Buenos Aires 14:552–576.

223. Charalampous FC, Hegsted DM. Effect of age and diet on development of cataracts in the diabetic rat. Am J Physiol 1950;161: 540–544.

224. Linklater HA, Dzialoszynski T, McLeod HL, et al. Modeling cortical cataractogenesis XI. Vitamin C reduces γ-crystalline leakage from lenses in diabetic rats. Exp Eye Res 1990;51:241–247.

225. Robertson JM, Donner AP, Trevithick JR. Vitamin E intake and risk of cataracts in humans. Proc NY Acad Sci 1989;570:372–382.

226. Rodger FC. Experimental thiamine deficiency as a cause of degeneration in the visual system pathway of the rat. Br J Ophthalmol 1953;31:11–29.

227. Wilson JD. Vitamin deficiency and excess. In: Wilson JD, Braunwald E, Isselbacher KJ, et al, eds. Harrison's Principles of internal medicine. New York: McGraw-Hill, 1991;434–442.

228. Sydenstriker V, Stebrell W, Cleckley H. The ocular manifestations of ariboflavinosis. JAMA 1940;114:2437.

229. Roach ES, McLean WT. Neurologic disorders of vitamin B_{12} deficiency. AFP 1982;25:111–115.

230. Mayfrank L, Thoden U. Downbeat nystagmus indicates cerebellar or brain-stem lesions in vitamin B_{12} deficiency. J Neurol 1986; 233:145–148.

231. Sandyk R. Paralysis of upward gaze as a presenting symptom of vitamin B_{12} deficiency. Eur Neurol 1984;23:198–200.

232. Lindenbaum J, Healton EB, Savage DG, et al. Neuropsychiatric disorders caused by cobalamin deficiency in the absence of anemia or macrocytosis. N Engl J Med 1988;318:1720–1728.

233. Czeizel AE, Dudas I. Prevention of the first occurrence of neuraltube defects by periconceptional vitamin supplementation. N Engl J Med 1992;327(26):1832–1835.

234. Ellis PP. Ocular therapeutics and pharmacology, ed. 7. St. Louis: C.V. Mosby Co, 1985.

235. Solomons NW. On the assessment of zinc and copper nutriture in man. Am J Clin Nutr 1979;32:856–871.

236. Leure-du Pree AE, McClain CJ. The effect of severe zinc deficiency on the morphology of the rat retinal pigment epithelium. Invest Ophthalmol Vis Sci 1983;23:425–434.

237. Underwood EJ. Trace elements in human and animal nutrition, ed. 4. London: Academic Press, 1977.

238. Hubbard GB, Herron BE, Andrews JS, et al. Influence of topical

239. Tennican P, Carl G, Frey J, et al. Topical zinc in the treatment of mice infected intravaginally with herpes genitalis virus. Proc Soc Ex Biol Med 1980;164:593–597.

240. Heinitz M. Clinical and biochemical aspects of the prophylaxis and therapy of senile cataract with zinc asparate. Klin Monatsbl Augenheikd 1978;172:778–783.

241. Ketola GH. Influence of dietary zinc on cataracts in rainbow trout. J Nutr 1979;109:965–969.

242. Ogino C, Yang GY. Requirements of rainbow trout for dietary zinc. Tenth Session of the European Fisheries Advisory Committee, 1978.

243. Racz, P, Kovaes B, Varga L, et al. Bilateral cataracts in acrodermatitis enteropathica. J Pediatr Ophthalmol Strabismus 1979;16: 180–182.

244. Murata T, Okazawa Y, Hinokuma R. Studies on the trace elements in the crystalline lens. Folia Ophthalmol (Jpn) 1972;23:648.

245. Murata T, Taura Y. Study of trace metallic elements in the lens. Ophthalmol Res 1975;7:8.

246. Racz P, Ordogh M. Investigations on trace elements in normal and senile cataractous lenses. Activation analysis of Cu, Zn, Mn, Co, Ru, Se, and Ni. Arch Klin Exp Ophthalmol 1977;204:67–72.

247. Pennigton JAT, Young BE, Wilson DB, et al. Mineral content of foods and total diets: The selected minerals in foods survey 1982 to 1984. J Am Diet Assoc 1986;86:876–878.

248. Newsome DA, Swartz M, Leone NC, et al. Oral zinc in macular degeneration. Arch Ophthalmol 1988;106:192–198.

249. Matta CS, Flicker GV, Ide CH. Eye manifestations in acrodermatitis enteropathica. Arch Ophthalmol 1975;93:140–142.

250. Wirshing L Jr. Eye symptoms in acrodermatitis enteropathica. Acta Ophthalmol 1962;40:567–574.

251. Karicoglu AZ. Pathology of zinc and copper related disorders in humans and animals. In: Karicoglu AZ, Sarper MR, eds. Zinc and copper in medicine. Springfield, IL: Charles C. Thomas, 1980; 181–223.

252. Warshawsky RS, Hill CW, Doughman DJ, et al. Acrodermatitis enteropathica. Corneal involvement with histochemical and electron microscopic studies. Arch Ophthalmol 1975;93:194–197.

253. Murray RK. Harper's Biochemistry, ed. 22. Norwalk, CT: Appleton & Lange, 1990.

254. Keshan Disease Research Group. Epidemiologic studies on the etiologic relationship of selenium and Keshan disease. Chin Med J 1979;92:477–82.

255. Kaminski MS, Yolton DP, Jordan WT, Yolton RL. Evaluation of dietary antioxidant levels and supplementation with ICAPS-Plus and Ocuvite. J Am Optom Assoc 1993;64:862–870.

256. Bendich A. The safety of β-carotene. Nutr Cancer 1988;11:207–214.

257. Van der Hagen AM, Yolton DP, Kaminski MS, Yolton RL. Free radicals and antioxidant supplementation: A review of their roles in age-related macular degeneration. J Am Optom Assoc 1993;64: 871–878.

258. Leopold IH, Adler FH. Specific treatment of ocular burns due to Lewisite (β-chlorovinyldichloroarsine). Arch Ophthalmol 1947; 38:174.

259. Adler FH, Fry WE, Leopold IH. Pathologic study of ocular lesions due to Lewisite (β-chlorovinyldichloroarsine). Arch Ophthalmol 1947;38:89.

260. Windship KA. Toxicity of inorganic arsenic salts. Adverse Drug React Acute Poisoning Rev 1984;3:129–160.

261. Havener WH. Adhesives. In: Havener WH, ed. Ocular pharmacology, ed. 5. St. Louis: C.V. Mosby Co, 1983;3:47–50.

262. Grant WM. A new treatment for calcific corneal opacities. Arch Ophthalmol 1952;48:681.

263. Leahey AB, Gottsch JD, Stark WJ. Clinical experiences with N-butyl cyanoacrylate (Nexacryl) tissue adhesive. Ophthalmology 1993;100:173–180.

264. Jensen MK, Crandall AS, Mamalis N, et al. Crystallization on intraocular lens surfaces associated with the use of Healon GV. Arch Ophthalmol 1994;112:1037–1042.

265. Sovani I, Humphrey JH, Kuntinalibronto DR, et al. Response of Bitot's spots to a single oral 100,000– or 200,000–IU dose of vitamin A. Am J Ophthalmol 1994;118:792–796.

266. Christen WG. Antioxidants and eye disease. Am J Med 1994; 97(suppl 3A):145–175.

267. Seddon JM, Hennekens CH. Vitamins, minerals, and macular degeneration. Promising but unproven hypotheses. Arch Ophthalmol 1994;112:176–179.

268. West S, Vitale S, Hallfrisch J, et al. Are antioxidants or supplements protective for age-related macular degeneration? Arch Ophthalmol 1994;112:222–227.

269. Seddon JM, Christen WG, Manson JE, et al. The use of vitamin supplements and the risk of cataract among US male physicians. Am J Public Health 1994;84:788–792.

270. Mares-Perlman JA, Brady WE, Klein BEK, et al. Serum carotenoids and tocopherols and severity of nuclear and cortical opacities. Invest Ophthalmol Vis Sci 1995;36:276–288.

271. Mares-Perlman JA, Klein BED, Klein R, et al. Relation between lens opacities and vitamin and mineral supplement use. Ophthalmology 1994;101:315–325.

PART III

Ocular Drugs in Clinical Practice

Experience is the best teacher.

—Anonymous

CHAPTER 20

Topical and Regional Anesthesia

David K. Talley
Jimmy D. Bartlett

Synthetic local anesthetics enable the practitioner to perform numerous diagnostic or surgical procedures in the office while keeping the patient comfortable and avoiding the relative risk from general anesthesia. The advantages of local anesthesia over general anesthesia include minimal physiologic changes, a relatively pleasant postprocedure period with little or no nausea and hangover, and the potential for prolonged relief of pain when long-acting anesthetics are used for regional nerve block. Since most procedures involving the eye and its adnexa are short and can be accomplished with local anesthesia, they present almost no risk to the patient's general health. In addition, local anesthesia has the advantage of simplicity; no cumbersome equipment is required, and minor in-office diagnostic or surgical procedures can usually be performed with little inconvenience or cost to the patient.

Topical Anesthesia

Topical application represents the most common route of administration of local anesthetics for procedures involving the eye. Topically applied anesthetics are surface-acting drugs that produce a reversible inhibition of the sensory nerve endings within the corneal and conjunctival epithelium, producing transient local anesthesia of the corneal and conjunctival surfaces.

Although most of the commonly used topical anesthetics are similar in onset, duration, and depth of anesthesia (see Chapter 6), several important differences exist. Thus, selecting the appropriate topical anesthetic for individual clinical procedures helps in maximizing its effectiveness while minimizing undesirable side effects.

Selecting the Anesthetic

Most of the commonly employed topical ocular anesthetics provide adequate clinical anesthesia within 10 to 20 seconds following instillation, and their anesthetic action lasts about 10 to 20 minutes. Anesthesia can be prolonged, if necessary, by repeated application.

Following the instillation of most topical anesthetics, many patients report a subjective sensation of "heaviness" of the lids that frequently lasts for several minutes following the return of corneal sensation.

Conjunctival hyperemia and mild lacrimation sometimes occur following the application of most topical anesthetics. Even topical cocaine occasionally produces mild hyperemia and lacrimation despite its local vasoconstrictor action.[1] In addition, the reflex action associated with discomfort may cause the fellow eye to become hyperemic when the anesthetic is placed in only one eye.

In addition to these direct effects, many topically applied anesthetics produce various indirect effects including increasing corneal permeability to subsequently applied drugs, occasionally desquamating corneal epithelium, and retarding the mitosis and migration processes associated with corneal epithelial regeneration.[2]

Because the onset, duration of action, and depth of anesthesia of the commonly employed topical anesthetics are quite similar, and since the desirable clinical characteristics of local anesthetics vary only slightly with the ocular procedure to be performed, the clinician should select a single anesthetic that provides effective topical anesthesia for most clinical uses rather than employ different drugs for different purposes.[3] A single topical anesthetic usually serves this purpose, and the other available drugs can be reserved for specialized uses as discussed in the following sections.

When the clinical usefulness of proparacaine is compared with that of the other commonly employed topical anesthetics, this drug has several advantages:

- Rapid onset of surface anesthesia
- Relatively short duration of anesthesia
- Minimal discomfort or pain on instillation
- Absence of associated mydriasis
- Stability at room temperature
- Low incidence of hypersensitivity
- Absence of cross-sensitivity with benoxinate and tetracaine

These advantages make proparacaine the single most useful general-purpose anesthetic for topical use in ophthalmic practice. The other topical anesthetics are usually reserved for specialized uses, as shown in Table 20.1.

Clinical Utilization

The following general guidelines[4-7] should be observed to facilitate the safe and effective clinical use of topical anesthetics.

- For routine diagnostic procedures such as applanation tonometry and gonioscopy, topical anesthetics render the eye vulnerable to accidental damage during the period of anesthesia. The protective blink reflex is inhibited, and abnormal drying of the cornea can occur. Since minute foreign bodies can create severe corneal damage if brushed across the hypoesthetic cornea, the patient should be advised against rubbing the eye during the period of anesthesia, usually lasting 20 to 30 minutes following the diagnostic procedure.
- It is beneficial to instill the topical anesthetic into *both*

eyes before routine diagnostic procedures such as gonioscopy, applanation tonometry, and fundus contact lens biomicroscopy. This approach inhibits the blink reflex of the fellow eye, facilitating the diagnostic procedure on the eye under examination. This practice also reduces examination time, since drug instillation into both eyes occurs before beginning the procedure.
- The mild local stinging or burning sensation following instillation of the anesthetic is transient, and treatment requires only patient reassurance.
- Since topically applied anesthetics frequently cause transient irregularity of the surface of the corneal epithelium, corneal disruption can interfere with subsequent procedures requiring critical visualization inside the eye, such as fundus photography. Ideally, photographic procedures should be performed without application of a topical anesthetic.
- Topical anesthetics are ineffective on skin surfaces and are therefore ineffective for dermatologic procedures such as removal of verrucae.
- Ideally, resumption of contact lens wear should be delayed for at least 60 minutes following application of the anesthetic.[8]
- Epinephrine or other vasoconstrictors have no significant effect on the duration of topical anesthesia and should never be combined with commercially available topical anesthetics. They serve no useful purpose, yet increase the risk of systemic side effects.

Topical ocular anesthetics have many uses in clinical practice. Most commonly they are used to improve patient tolerance of various diagnostic procedures. In addition, these drugs often provide sufficient anesthesia for minor surgical procedures of the cornea and conjunctiva. The following sections discuss the most commonly employed procedures that topical anesthesia facilitates.

Gonioscopy

One or 2 drops of 0.5% proparacaine allows sufficient topical anesthesia to permit gonioscopy for as long as 15 to

TABLE 20.1
Specialized Uses of Topical Anesthetics

Procedure	*Indicated Anesthetic*
Forced duction test	4% cocaine or 4% lidocaine applied with cotton-tipped applicator
Electroretinography	0.5% tetracaine ointment
Goldmann applanation tonometry	0.4% benoxinate-sodium fluorescein or 0.5% proparacaine-sodium fluorescein
Corneal epithelial debridement	4% cocaine

20 minutes. If the anesthetic is instilled into both eyes before beginning the procedure, it need not be reapplied before beginning gonioscopy on the second eye.

Applanation Tonometry

Two techniques are commonly used for ensuring topical anesthesia before Goldmann applanation tonometry: (1) the use of a solution of benoxinate-sodium fluorescein or proparacaine-sodium fluorescein, or (2) a 2-step procedure involving the instillation of a topical anesthetic followed by separate application of sodium fluorescein.

Use of a solution of benoxinate-sodium fluorescein (Fluress) or proparacaine-sodium fluorescein allows simultaneous application of the required anesthetic and sodium fluorescein dye. This method increases the efficiency of the procedure by eliminating the need for separate applications of the anesthetic and dye, but it has the disadvantages of irritation from the benoxinate as well as excessive instillation of dye. Sometimes 30 to 60 seconds must elapse to allow the excess dye to dissipate before accurate tonometry can be performed. In addition, solutions of sodium fluorescein have the inherent risk of overflowing and subsequently staining the patient's lids, cheeks, or clothing. Note, however, that differences in the results of tonometry using either benoxinate or proparacaine are not clinically significant.[9]

Also used is a 2-step procedure involving the instillation of a topical anesthetic such as proparacaine followed by the separate application of sodium fluorescein from either a sterile solution or a dye-impregnated paper strip. The application of sodium fluorescein by moistening the impregnated strip with lacrimal fluid and residual anesthetic contained within the inferior conjunctival sac (Fig. 20.1) allows, with practice, a consistent amount of fluorescein to be applied. This technique permits immediate and accurate tonometry by eliminating the excessive dye often associated with sodium fluorescein solutions.

Regardless of which technique is used, the drugs should be applied to both eyes before beginning tonometry. This approach reduces the blink reflex of the fellow eye and increases the speed and efficiency with which the practitioner can perform the procedure.

Fundus Contact Lens Biomicroscopy

Following topical anesthesia, fundus contact lenses such as the Quadraspheric (Volk Optical)[10,11] are applied to the cornea with appropriate gonioscopic bonding solution. For anesthesia, 1 or 2 drops of 0.5% proparacaine is sufficient. As in gonioscopy and applanation tonometry, applying the anesthetic to both eyes before beginning the procedure increases the speed and efficiency of the procedure.

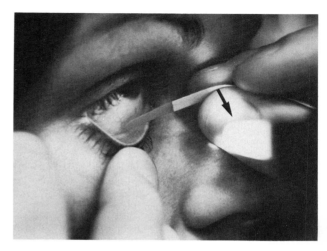

FIGURE 20.1   **Application of sodium fluorescein for applanation tonometry by moistening the dye-impregnated strip with lacrimal fluid and residual anesthetic contained within the inferior conjunctival sac. The sodium fluorescein strip is moistened by placing it within the conjunctival sac, between the bulbar and tarsal conjunctivae. Illumination may be provided by white light on the tonometer prism (arrow).**

Evaluation of Superficial Abrasions

Since repeated applications of a topical anesthetic to an injured cornea may seriously delay or prevent regeneration of the epithelium, the practitioner should refrain from the liberal instillation of topical anesthetics in cases of corneal abrasions, foreign bodies, or other superficial injuries.[12] Often, however, the blepharospasm, lacrimation, and pain accompanying the corneal injury prevent adequate examination of the eye. In such cases, 1 or 2 drops of 0.5% proparacaine frequently relieves the pain enough to allow slit-lamp evaluation of the injury. The patient, however, should *never* be given a topical anesthetic for self-administration at home. Very serious corneal damage may result[13] (see Chapter 6). Instead, the pain associated with the injury should be treated by cycloplegics, pressure-patching, cold compresses, and systemic analgesics (see Chapter 7).

Forced Duction Test

The forced duction test is used to investigate deficient ocular rotations to differentiate between deficiencies due to neurogenic or myogenic weakness and those caused by muscle restrictions such as in Graves' ophthalmopathy.[14] The practitioner can detect a mechanical limitation (restrictive myopathy) if, when attempting to move the globe actively, considerable resistance prevents eye movement. On the

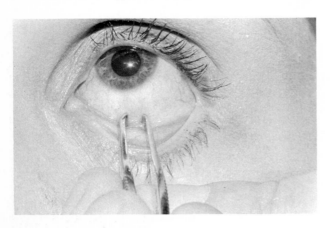
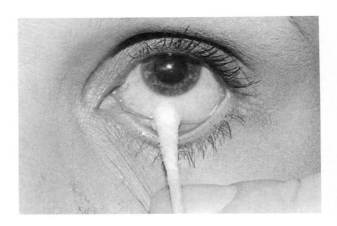

A   **B**

FIGURE 20.2   **Forced duction test.** *(A)* **Traditional technique involving attempted movement of the globe with toothed forceps.** *(B)* **Technique involving attempted movement of the globe with cotton-tipped applicator positioned at limbus.**

other hand, a neurogenic cause is isolated if the globe moves freely on forced duction testing. Two methods of performing this test are commonly used: (1) the traditional technique involving attempted movement of the globe with toothed forceps, or (2) a less traumatic technique involving attempted movement of the globe with a cotton-tipped applicator positioned at the limbus.

In the forceps technique, the practitioner uses the forceps to grasp the insertion of the rectus muscle to be investigated and attempts to move the globe in a direction opposite the field of action of that muscle (Fig. 20.2A). Most of the topical anesthetics commercially available fail to eliminate completely the patient's awareness of the forceps. Although this awareness is not particularly painful, the sensation of the eye being touched often increases patient apprehension, provokes blepharospasm, and prevents adequate investigation of the muscle being tested. Using a 4% solution of lidocaine as the topical anesthetic can greatly reduce or eliminate this problem. A cotton-tipped applicator moistened with this solution should be applied to the surface of the conjunctiva at the site overlying the rectus muscle insertion to be investigated. The applicator should be applied for 1 to 2 minutes. The depth of topical anesthesia achieved using this method has been found to be far more satisfactory than that provided by the more routinely used anesthetics such as tetracaine or proparacaine.[14] Cocaine in a 4% solution applied with a cotton-tipped applicator also provides sufficient local anesthesia to permit traditional forced duction testing.

Smith has described a simpler technique for the forced duction test.[15] Following topical anesthesia with 0.5% proparacaine, movement of the globe is attempted by placing a cotton-tipped applicator at the limbus (Fig. 20.2B). This technique allows the practitioner to detect a mechanical limitation of the globe without subjecting the patient to the discomfort associated with toothed forceps.

Schirmer No. 1 Test

The Schirmer No. 1 test has been used for decades as a quantitative test of aqueous tear production. When performed without topical anesthesia, this test assesses both the basic aqueous secretion from the lacrimal gland and accessory glands of Kraus and Wolfring, as well as neurogenic lacrimal secretion stimulated by irritation of the conjunctiva and lid tissues with the Schirmer strip. To eliminate the neurogenic component of tear secretion, the Schirmer test can be performed following the application of a topical anesthetic, thus allowing a more accurate assessment of basic aqueous secretion. The conjunctival sac should be dried with a cotton-tipped applicator following administration of the anesthetic. This will prevent reflex tearing that may result from irritation by the anesthetic and will also prevent false-negative findings from strip wetting by the anesthetic itself. The average Schirmer test result following topical anesthesia in the patient with a normal lacrimal system is approximately 15 mm of strip-wetting at 5 minutes.[16]

Electroretinography

Depending on the specific protocol used for electroretinography (ERG), the procedure usually lasts from 20 minutes to approximately 1 hour. Placement of the contact lens electrode (Fig. 20.3) is facilitated by the application of 0.5% proparacaine, but the duration of anesthesia does not permit procedures exceeding 20 to 30 minutes. For prolonged procedures, the topical anesthetic of choice is 0.5% tetracaine ointment. This preparation allows prolonged patient comfort and thus facilitates determination of the final scotopic values so critical in electroretinographic evaluations.

Lacrimal Drainage Procedures

Increasing patient comfort during lacrimal dilation and irrigation (see Figs. 25.18 and 25.20), requires the application of a topical anesthetic such as 0.5% proparacaine. One or 2 drops topically instilled is usually sufficient. Normal blinking following instillation of the anesthetic promotes drainage of the drug through the nasolacrimal drainage system. The dilation and irrigation procedures can begin 1 or 2 minutes following instillation of the anesthetic.

Although not always required, 1 or 2 drops of topically applied 0.5% proparacaine will improve patient comfort for the insertion of collagen implants and other forms of punctal and canalicular occlusion (see Fig. 25.11).

Contact Lens Fitting

To evaluate the eye's normal physiologic responses to contact lens wear, contact lenses should be fitted *without* topical anesthesia. However, certain limited circumstances may justify the use of topical anesthetics in contact lens evaluations. These include determining the effect of a rigid contact lens on monocular diplopia when the cornea is suspected to be the etiologic source. Topical anesthesia allows the rigid lens to be easily placed on the eye and readily tolerated by the patient during the initial diagnostic evaluation. Topical anesthesia may also be used when fitting infants and very young children with rigid contact lenses. Topical anesthesia facilitates the molding of scleral shells or contact lenses and also the fitting of rigid contact lenses to mentally retarded patients or other patients unable to cooperate with evaluation procedures. The practitioner, however, should avoid using topical anesthetics in conjunction with hydrogel lenses. These lenses absorb the anesthetic and act as a drug reservoir by gradually releasing the drug to the eye, with the potential complications associated with long-term anesthesia.

Superficial Foreign Body Removal

As with the evaluation of corneal abrasions, the application of 1 or 2 drops of 0.5% proparacaine is often necessary to allow adequate examination of the eye with a corneal or

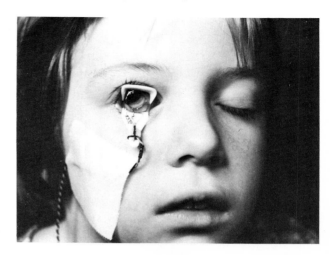

FIGURE 20.3 **Topical anesthesia is necessary to facilitate placement of contact lens electrode for electroretinography.**

conjunctival foreign body. Before removing superficial foreign bodies, an additional 1 to 2 drops of topical anesthetic loosens the epithelium. In some cases, this loosening may be sufficient to permit removal of the foreign object with a cotton-tipped applicator. The additional topical anesthetic also allows somewhat deeper anesthesia for removal of corneal foreign bodies in the deep epithelium or superficial stroma. The limbal area, however, is often difficult to anesthetize, and a solution of 4% to 5% cocaine applied with a cotton-tipped applicator may achieve adequate anesthesia.[17] Topical anesthetics *must never be prescribed for self-administration by the patient at home.* Following foreign body removal, associated pain should be treated by cycloplegics, pressure-patching, cold compresses, and systemic analgesics (see Chapter 7).

If topical anesthesia is needed to examine an eye suspected of having a penetrating or perforating injury, a nonpreserved anesthetic should be used to decrease the risk of corneal endothelial damage.[18] Currently available nonpreserved agents include proparacaine 0.5% in a 1 ml unit-dose formulation.[19]

Minor Surgery of the Conjunctiva

The excision of small, superficial conjunctival lesions such as concretions can usually be achieved with topical anesthesia alone (Fig. 20.4). Two or 3 drops instilled at 1-minute intervals allows sufficient anesthesia for this purpose. Alternatively, a cotton pledget or cotton-tipped applicator soaked in the anesthetic solution may be applied for 1 to 2 minutes

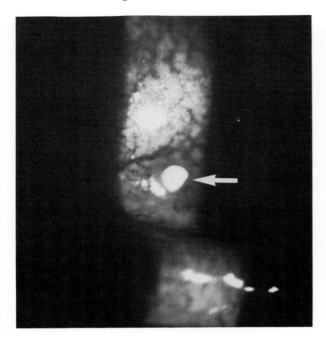
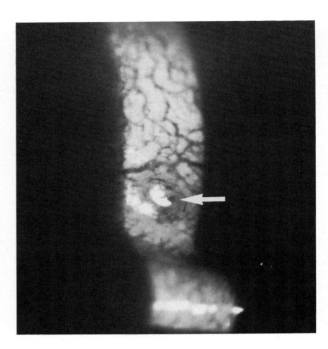

A   B

FIGURE 20.4   **Topical anesthesia permits the removal of symptomatic conjunctival concretion.** *(A)* **Concretion (arrow) before removal.** *(B)* **Conjunctival depression (arrow) at site of removed concretion. (Courtesy Larry J. Alexander, O.D.)**

before surgery. This allows anesthesia of deeper portions of the conjunctiva.

Before routine infiltration anesthesia for chalazion resection, 4% lidocaine solution or 5% lidocaine ointment can be applied to the tarsal conjunctiva using a cotton-tipped applicator. This procedure effectively reduces the pain of chalazion surgery without side effects.[20]

Corneal Epithelial Debridement

At one time mechanical debridement of the corneal epithelium was the only effective treatment for herpetic epithelial keratitis.[21] Although the use of newer antiviral drugs has increased the therapeutic armamentarium against herpetic keratitis, debridement remains a safe, effective, and occasionally preferred treatment of herpetic corneal infection. The mechanical removal of virus-replicating epithelium abolishes a source of infection for other epithelial cells and eliminates an antigenic stimulus to stromal inflammation.[21]

Debridement is performed at the slit lamp following topical anesthesia with 2 to 3 drops of 4% cocaine applied over several minutes. Not only does the cocaine provide excellent surface anesthesia, it also substantially softens and loosens the corneal epithelium, thereby facilitating its re-

moval with a sterile cotton-tipped applicator (Fig. 20.5). A sharp knife blade should not be used because of the risk of damaging Bowman's layer and thus creating a portal of virus entry into the corneal stroma.[21]

Suture Barb Removal

Occasionally suture material may protrude through the surface of the conjunctiva or cornea days, weeks, or even years following cataract surgery or penetrating keratoplasty, giving rise to symptoms such as foreign body sensation, redness, itching, and mucus discharge. Giant papillary conjunctivitis can also occur as a result of suture-induced irritation.[22] Removal of the offending suture is easily achieved following topical anesthesia using 1 or 2 drops of 0.5% proparacaine.

To ensure adequate healing of the surgical wound, it is prudent to delay suture removal for 3 months following cataract extraction and for as long as 6 to 9 months following penetrating keratoplasty. Furthermore, to reduce the risk of serious complications such as endophthalmitis, a broad-spectrum antibacterial agent such as gentamicin or tobramycin may be used topically several times daily for 2 to 3 days before removal of the offending suture.[23]

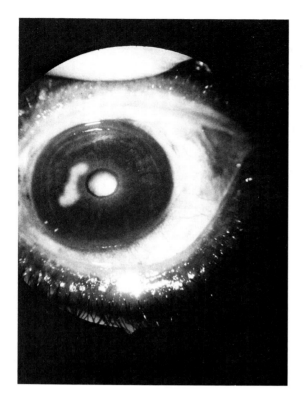
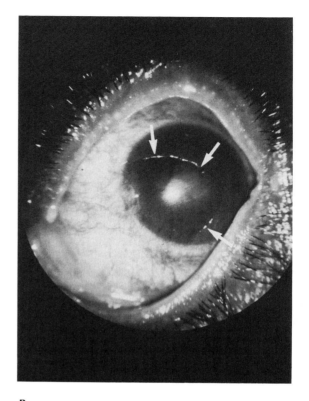

A   B

FIGURE 20.5   **Corneal epithelial debridement. *(A)* Herpetic corneal lesion stained with sodium fluorescein. *(B)* Following the topical application of 4% cocaine, debridement is performed with a sterile cotton-tipped applicator. Edge of debrided area is denoted by arrows. (Courtesy Mark Flora, O.D.)**

The eye should be anesthetized with topically applied 0.5% proparacaine. For deeper anesthesia, 4% lidocaine can be applied with a cotton-tipped applicator held against the suture for 30 to 60 seconds.[24] Broken sutures are removed by firmly grasping the knotted end with jewelers forceps and slowly pulling the suture free. If the suture is intact, the practitioner should grasp the knot with forceps and gently snip the suture using a #11 scalpel or straight blade iris scissors. Following suture removal, the integrity of the surgical wound should be confirmed and the patient given a prophylactic topical antibacterial agent, such as gentamicin or tobramycin, for 3 to 5 days.

Predrug Instillation

Since topical anesthetics increase permeability of the corneal epithelium to subsequently applied drugs,[12] the practitioner may capitalize on this fact to increase the clinical effectiveness of mydriatics and cycloplegics. Moreover, use of a topical anesthetic must precede the application of some drugs to reduce or eliminate severe stinging or burning associated with those drugs.

MYDRIATICS

Several investigators have studied the effect of topical anesthetics on phenylephrine-induced mydriasis.[25–27] These studies have shown that applying proparacaine before phenylephrine reduces the time required to produce maximum dilation, increases the amplitude of maximum dilation, and increases the duration of dilation. The enhancement of mydriasis is similar for benoxinate, proparacaine, and tetracaine.[25] Mordi and associates[28] have shown that the prior instillation of 0.5% proparacaine prolongs both the mydriatic and the cycloplegic effects of 1% tropicamide. The topically applied anesthetic may increase the mydriatic's bioavailability by inhibiting tear flow and thus increasing corneal absorption of the drug.[25,29] Furthermore, the anesthetic-induced inhibition of tear flow, by increasing the amount of mydriatic absorbed through the cornea, decreases the quantity of mydriatic available for systemic absorption. This reduces the risk of systemic side effects.[25] This anesthetic-induced enhancement of mydriasis is helpful in eyes difficult to dilate such as in patients with diabetes or those with darkly pigmented irides. In addition, the reduced risk of systemic side effects is reassuring in patients with diabetes, cardiovascular disease such as hypertension, and hyperthyroidism.

GLYCERIN

The practitioner should precede the topical instillation of glycerin, a hyperosmotic agent, with a topical anesthetic. Since without topical anesthesia the instillation of glycerin causes severe stinging, burning, or ocular pain, the use of topically applied glycerin is limited to the practitioner's office. Patients should never be permitted to self-administer a topical anesthetic at home in conjunction with the use of topical glycerin.

TRICHLOROACETIC ACID

A topical anesthetic should always precede the use of trichloroacetic acid as a chemical cauterizing agent on the cornea. One or 2 drops of 0.5% proparacaine allows sufficient surface anesthesia for such chemical cauterization.

Regional Anesthesia

Some minor surgical procedures involving the eye and surrounding adnexa require a deeper and more prolonged

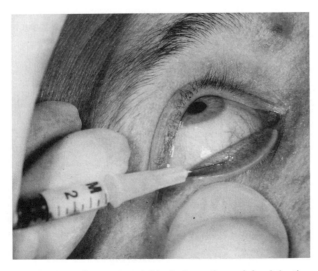

FIGURE 20.6 **A retrotarsal block is performed by injecting anesthetic subconjunctivally along the proximal tarsal border.**

TABLE 20.2
Minor Surgical Procedures Requiring Regional Anesthesia

- Papilloma and lid lesion removal
- Chalazion incision and drainage
- Electrohyfrecation for trichiasis
- Repair of superficial non-marginal eyelid defects

anesthesia than can be achieved with topically applied anesthetics (Table 20.2). Such cases require injectable amide anesthetics such as bupivacaine, etidocaine, lidocaine, or mepivacaine. In addition to their anesthetic effects, these agents also produce a peripheral vasodilation by a direct relaxant effect on vascular smooth muscle.[30] Epinephrine, in a concentration of 1:100,000 or less, can be added to the anesthetic solution to produce a longer-acting block, to decrease systemic side effects of the anesthetic, and to provide for local hemostasis.

The choice of anesthetic for each surgical procedure is a matter of personal preference. Table 6.2 gives the onset, duration of action, and safe dosage for the most commonly used regional anesthetic agents.

Local Infiltration

Infiltration anesthesia is the major type of local anesthesia used in eyelid surgery.[30] It can be subdivided into a pretarsal subcutaneous block and a retrotarsal block. A pretarsal subcutaneous block provides excellent anesthesia to the anterior lamella, including skin, orbicularis muscle, orbital septum, and the anterior tarsal surface. When anesthesia is needed for surgery on the palpebral conjunctiva or posterior tarsal surface, a retrotarsal block is indicated.

In these procedures, approximately 0.5 to 1.0 ml of anesthetic solution is injected subcutaneously or subconjunctivally along the proximal tarsal border using a 27-gauge ½-inch needle (Fig. 20.6). The use of as little anesthetic as possible reduces tissue distortion secondary to the bolus, and massage of the area immediately following injection helps to restore normal anatomy and reduce the chance of hematoma.

Nerve Blocks

In most minor surgical procedures of the eye, local infiltrative anesthesia is adequate. However, patients undergoing multiple lesion removal or exceptionally sensitive to pain, may require a more complete regional anesthesia. This can be accomplished by adding an orbital nerve block. Nerve blocks provide excellent regional anesthesia without distor-

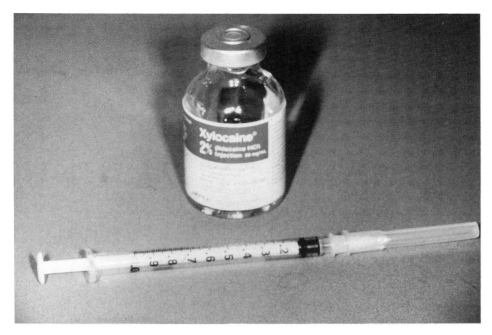

FIGURE 20.7   **Lidocaine 2% and a 27½ G-1 cc syringe used in performing a regional block.**

tion of tissues but do not allow for local epinephrine-induced hemostasis. Injections are usually performed using a 26- to 27-gauge needle of various lengths with approximately 1 ml of anesthetic solution (Fig. 20.7).

V₁ (OPHTHALMIC)

The first two divisions of the trigeminal nerve provide sensation in the eye, orbit, and periorbital tissues (Fig. 20.8). The first (ophthalmic) division divides into the frontal, nasociliary, and lacrimal nerve and enters the orbit through the superior orbital fissure. The frontal nerve divides into the supratrochlear and supraorbital nerves (Fig. 20.9).

The supratrochlear nerve provides sensation to the medial part of the upper eyelid and can be blocked by injecting anesthetic just above the trochlea to a depth of ½ inch (Fig. 20.10).[31]

The supraorbital nerve innervates the central upper lid, the superior conjunctiva, and the supraorbital portion of the forehead. Injecting anesthetic just lateral to the supraorbital notch to a depth of 1¼ inch along the roof of the orbit anesthetizes this region (Fig. 20.11). Placement of the needle in this location effectively blocks both branches of the frontal nerve (supratrochlear and supraorbital) while avoiding orbital hemorrhaging secondary to vessel damage in the supraorbital notch.[31]

The nasociliary nerve divides into the anterior and posterior ethmoidal nerves and the infratrochlear nerve, providing sensation to the inner canthus, the lacrimal sac, and adjacent nasal skin. An injection of anesthetic just above the medial canthal ligament to a depth of 1 inch will blocks branches of the nasociliary nerve (Fig. 20.12).[31]

The lacrimal nerve supplies the lateral upper lid and the lacrimal gland. An injection along the upper outer wall of the orbit to a depth of 1 inch generally provides an adequate block (Fig. 20.13).[31]

V₂ (MAXILLARY)

The second division of the trigeminal nerve enters the orbit through the infraorbital fissure where it becomes the infraorbital nerve. It passes through the infraorbital foramen and supplies sensory fibers to the lower lid, much of the cheek, and part of the inner canthus and lacrimal sac. An infraorbital nerve block is accomplished by injecting 2 ml of anesthetic at the mouth of the infraorbital foramen (Fig. 20.14), which can be located as a palpable, small depression in the maxilla, two-thirds of an inch inferior to the midpoint of the lower lid.[31]

Presurgical Evaluation

Preparing the patient for minor eye surgery is an important aspect of care. Areas of concern that may affect anesthesia are the patient's age, medical history, current medications,

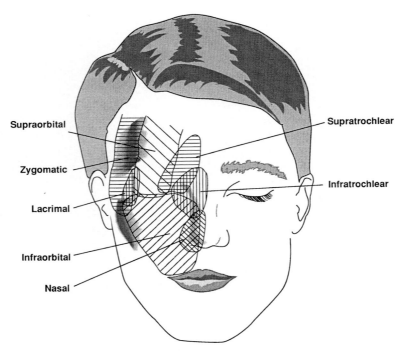

FIGURE 20.8   **Distribution of area for regional anesthesia blocks. (Adapted from Wilson RP. Anesthesia. In: Spaeth GL, ed. Ophthalmic surgery: Principles and practice. Philadelphia: WB Saunders, 1990;81.)**

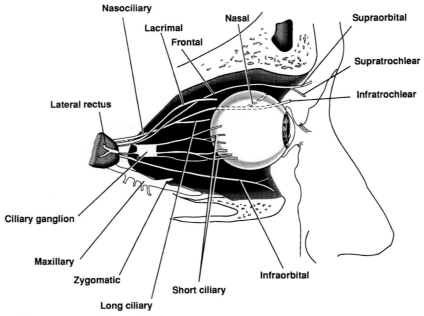

FIGURE 20.9   **Location of nerves supplying the orbital area. (Adapted from Wilson RP. Plastic surgery. In: Spaeth GL, ed. Ophthalmic surgery: Principles and practice. Philadelphia: WB Saunders. 1990;553.)**

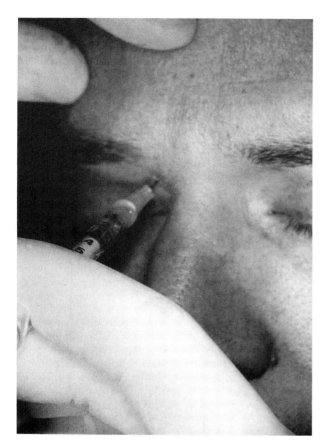

FIGURE 20.10 **A block of the supratrochlear branch of the frontal nerve is obtained by injecting anesthetic just above the trochlea to a depth of ½ inch.**

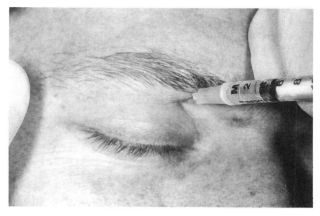

FIGURE 20.11 **Injection of anesthetic just lateral to the supraorbital notch to a depth of 1¼ inch effectively blocks both the supratrochlear and supraorbital nerves.**

result in excessive bleeding. Patients with significant hypertension or cardiac arrhythmia should receive little or no epinephrine. The presence of significant liver dysfunction may increase the risk of anesthesia by limiting drug metabolism. Questions regarding prior anesthesia and any family history of problems with anesthesia will aid in assessing the patient's suitability for local anesthesia.[30,31]

allergies, and the surgical procedure to be performed. In addition, patient apprehension should not be overlooked.

AGE

Local anesthesia required in minor surgical procedures of the eye may be used in cooperative children as young as 6 years of age. Younger or uncooperative patients will require general anesthesia.[30]

MEDICAL HISTORY

The patient's systemic condition should be reviewed to determine the patient's physical status and ability to tolerate local anesthetic procedures. A careful history regarding possible bleeding diatheses (e.g., easy bruising, hemorrhaging during previous surgical procedures or dental extractions) are important considerations. Unstable systemic disease such as hypertension, diabetes, and cardiac arrhythmia may complicate anesthesia. Elevation of blood pressure may

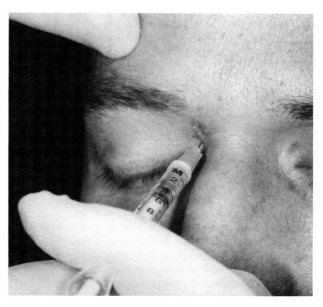

FIGURE 20.12 **Anesthesia to the inner canthus, the lacrimal sac, and adjacent nasal skin can be accomplished using a regional block of the nasociliary nerve.**

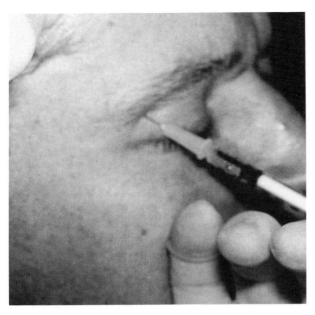

FIGURE 20.13   **Injection of anesthetic along the upper outer wall of the orbit to a depth of 1 inch blocks the lacrimal nerve.**

CURRENT MEDICATIONS

The use of aspirin and other drugs that impair clotting may be discontinued 2 to 3 weeks prior to surgery unless the anticoagulants are otherwise indispensable to the patient's medical care.[30,31]

ALLERGIES

Allergic reactions to commonly used amide anesthetics are rare.[32] To identify patients with true allergic reactions, a careful history should be taken regarding prior anesthesia. In addition to questioning the patient and possibly the previous treating physician, reviewing the medical chart may provide valuable information. Attention should be placed on the offending drug, route of administration, concurrent medications, vasoconstrictors, and preservatives. Patients with a proven history of allergic reaction can probably be safely given a preservative-free anesthetic of unrelated structure.[33] More commonly, adverse reactions relate to systemic toxicity usually secondary to overdosage, rapid systemic absorption, or inadvertent intravascular injection.[34] To reduce the chance of systemic toxicity, the smallest effective dose of the lowest anesthetic concentration should be used. In addition, aspirating before injection and moving the needle during injection will help avoid intravascular injection.

SURGICAL PROCEDURE

The nature and potential length of the operative procedure will influence the anesthesia selected. Excision of a small papilloma will usually require only a pretarsal subcutaneous block, while a chalazion curettage of the upper eyelid may require infiltrative anesthesia with an orbital nerve block.

PATIENT APPREHENSION

Most patients experience some apprehension regarding surgery. Preoperative counseling regarding the anticipated se-

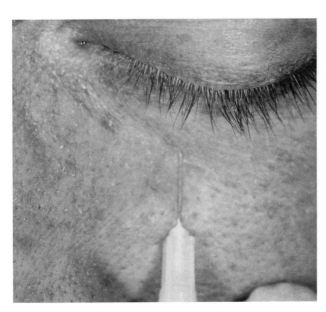

FIGURE 20.14   **The infraorbital nerve is blocked by injecting approximately 2 ml of anesthetic at the mouth of the infraorbital foramen.**

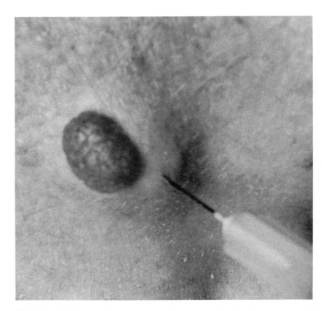

FIGURE 20.15   **Subcutaneous injection of 1% lidocaine with epinephrine at base of papilloma provides adequate anesthesia for excision.**

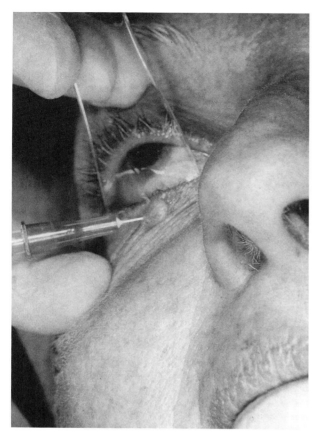

FIGURE 20.16   **Use of a Jaeger lid plate protects the globe from accidental perforation when performing anesthetic injections into the eyelid.**

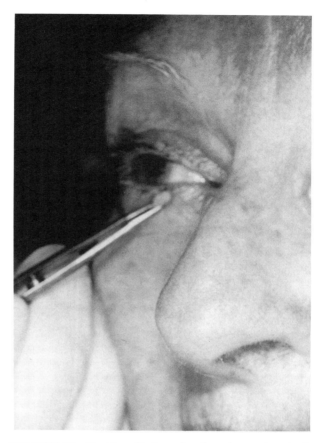

FIGURE 20.17   **Pinching of lesion using tissue forceps is a simple way to determine whether adequate anesthesia is present.**

quence of events can minimize this apprehension. An educational videotape can also help in reassuring the patient. During the procedure the clinician should demonstrate an ongoing calm attitude to reduce the patient's anxiety. Some patients may require a mild sedative, such as 5 to 10 mg diazepam by mouth, 60 minutes prior to surgery.

Minor Surgical Procedures

PAPILLOMA AND LID LESION REMOVAL

Lid lesions are common and usually clinically benign. In most cases, the patient desires their removal for cosmetic reasons, but occasionally they may interfere with the patient's spectacle placement or present with a suspicious history that warrants removal of the lesion for pathological analysis. Anesthesia for the surgical removal of most lid lesions is accomplished using a pretarsal subcutaneous block. A typical anesthetic agent is 1% lidocaine with 1:100,000 epinephrine.

First, a topical anesthetic such as 0.5% proparacaine is instilled in both eyes to reduce reflex tearing. Then approximately 0.3 to 0.6 ml of anesthetic solution is injected subcutaneously at the base of the lesion using a 27-gauge ½-inch needle (Fig. 20.15). Injecting too much anesthetic may distort the lesion, making it more difficult to excise. Gently massaging the area after injection disperses the bolus of anesthetic and helps to restore normal anatomy. Using a Jaeger lid plate (Fig. 20.16) decreases the likelihood of penetrating the globe while performing the injection.

Patient safety and comfort during the procedure must be maximized. This can be accomplished by controlling the patient's movement and continually reassuring the patient. A common injection technique is to recline the patient and to keep one hand against the patient's forehead to prevent any sudden movement. A technician or support staff member should be present to assist with the patient's anesthesia and surgery. Approximately 5 minutes post-injection, the patient's anesthesia should be evaluated by pinching the lesion or area with tissue forceps (Fig. 20.17). The patient should be able to detect the forceps' presence but not experience any discomfort.

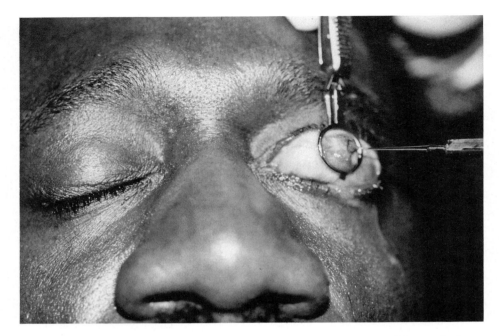

FIGURE 20.18   **Curettage of large chalazion involving the central upper eyelid. Anesthesia was delivered using both retrotarsal infiltration and a supraorbital nerve block.**

CHALAZION INCISION AND DRAINAGE

Anesthesia for chalazion incision and drainage depends on the extent of lipid material and its location (Fig. 20.18). Small to medium size chalazia anterior to the tarsus require a transcutaneous approach warranting a pretarsal subcutaneous block. If the chalazion is located posterior to the tarsus, however, surgery occurs through the palpebral conjunctiva. Anesthesia to this area consists of using topical 4% lidocaine and injectable 1% lidocaine with epinephrine (Fig. 20.19). After instilling 1 drop of 0.5% proparacaine to each eye, the palpebral conjunctiva and lid margin should be anesthetized using a sterile cotton-tipped applicator soaked in 4% lidocaine. This approach decreases pain associated with the retrotarsal injection.

For chalazia in the tarsus, infiltrative anesthesia should be given both subcutaneously and subconjunctivally along the proximal border of the tarsal plate. Large chalazia (greater than 8 mm) and hypersensitive patients may require a regional nerve block at the appropriate branches of the trigeminal nerve as previously discussed.

ELECTROHYFRECATION FOR TRICHIASIS

Electrohyfrecation for trichiasis can eradicate one or several cilia that are threatening or damaging the cornea or conjunctiva. The required anesthesia is administered via a subcutaneous infiltrative block along the lid margin adjacent to the

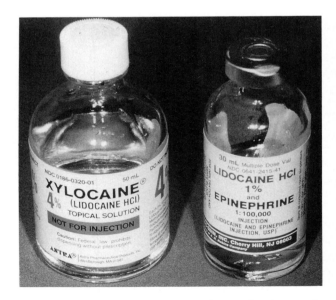

FIGURE 20.19   **Anesthesia to the posterior tarsal surface can be provided using both topical 4% lidocaine and injectable 1% lidocaine with epinephrine. The topical lidocaine decreases pain associated with the retrotarsal injection.**

area to be treated. The use of a Jaeger plate or scleral shell is recommended to prevent injury to the globe.

REPAIR OF EYELID DEFECTS

Trauma to the eye is a common occurrence, and superficial non-marginal lacerations of the eyelid and surrounding tissue often require suturing. The goal is to aid wound healing by restoring the tissue as completely as possible to its presurgical condition. This is done as atraumatically as possible through the use of local anesthetics, and local infiltrative blocks usually provide adequate anesthesia.

References

1. Jervey JW. Topical anesthetics for the eye. A comparative study. South Med J 1955;48:770–774.
2. Webster RB. Local anesthetics for ophthalmic use. Aust J Optom 1974;57:399–401.
3. Linn JG, Vey EK. Topical anesthesia in ophthalmology. Am J Ophthalmol 1955;40:697–704.
4. Local anesthetics. In: Drug evaluations annual 1993. Chicago: American Medical Association, 1993;153–167.
5. Allen ED, Elkington AR. Local anaesthesia and the eye. Br J Anaesth 1980;52:689–694.
6. Lyle WM, Page C. Possible adverse effects from local anesthetics and the treatment of these reactions. Am J Optom Physiol Opt 1975;52:736–744.
7. Adriani J, Zepernick R. Clinical effectiveness of drugs used for topical anesthesia. JAMA 1964;188:711–716.
8. Hill RM. Anesthetic impact. Int Cont Lens Clin 1980;7:199–200.
9. Jose JG, Basta M, Cramer KJ, et al. Lack of effects of anesthetic on measurement of intraocular pressure by Goldmann tonometry. Am J Optom Physiol Opt 1983;60:308–310.
10. Wing JT, Barker FM. Auxiliary lenses in fundus biomicroscopy. A comparison of fields of view. J Am Optom Assoc 1990;61:544–547.
11. Barker FM, Wing JT. Ultra wide field fundus biomicroscopy with the Volk Quadraspheric Lens. J Am Optom Assoc 1990;61:573–575.
12. Bryant JA. Local and topical anesthetics in ophthalmology. Surv Ophthalmol 1969;13:262–283.
13. Duffin RM, Olson RJ. Tetracaine toxicity. Ann Ophthalmol 1984;16:836–837.
14. Raab EL. Traction test (letter). Arch Ophthalmol 1977;95:1649.
15. Smith JL. The optic nerve. Miami: JL Smith, 1975;49.
16. Ingis TM, Hornblass A. Lacrimal function tests: A comparative study. Surg Forum 1977;28:516–517.
17. Newell SW. Management of corneal foreign bodies. Am Fam Physician 1985;31:149–156.
18. Rosenwasser GOD. Complications of topical ocular anesthetics. Int Ophthalmol Clin 1989;29:153–158.
19. Bartlett JD. Local anesthetics. In: Bartlett JD, Ghormley NR, Jaanus SD, et al, eds. Ophthalmic drug facts. St. Louis: Facts and Comparisons, 1995;19–36.
20. Gerde LS, Hanson B. Anesthesia in chalazion surgery. South Med J 1983;76:11.
21. O'Day DM, Jones BR. Herpes simplex keratitis. In: Tasman W, Jaeger EA, eds. Duane's Clinical ophthalmology. Philadelphia: J. B. Lippincott, 1992;vol 4, Chap. 19:1–27.
22. Melore GG. Suture barb syndrome. South J Optom 1987;5:70–73.
23. Gelender H. Bacterial endophthalmitis following cutting of sutures after cataract surgery. Am J Ophthalmol 1982;94:528–533.
24. Dornic DI. How to treat suture barbs. Rev Optom 1987;124:67–68.
25. Lyle WM, Bobier WR. Effects of topical anesthetics on phenylephrine-induced mydriasis. Am J Optom Physiol Opt 1977;54:276–281.
26. Jauregui MJ, Polse KA. Mydriatic effect using phenylephrine and proparacaine. Am J Optom Physiol Opt 1974;51:545–549.
27. Kubo DJ, Wing TW, Polse KA, et al. Mydriatic effects using low concentrations of phenylephrine hydrochloride. J Am Optom Assoc 1975;46:817–822.
28. Mordi JA, Lyle WM, Mousa GY. Does prior instillation of a topical anesthetic enhance the effect of tropicamide? Am J Optom Physiol Opt 1986;63:290–293.
29. Patton TF, Robinson JR. Influence of topical anesthetics on tear dynamics and ocular drug biovailability in albino rabbits. J Pharm Sci 1976;64:267–271.
30. Dutton JJ. Atlas of ophthalmic surgery: vol 2. Oculoplastic, lacrimal and orbital surgery. St. Louis: Mosby-Year Book, Inc, 1992; Chap.1:2–3.
31. Wilson RP. Anesthesia. In: Spaeth GL, ed. Ophthalmic surgery: Principles and practice. Philadelphia: W.B. Saunders Company, 1990;77–88.
32. Stoelting RK. Allergic reactions during anesthesia. Anesth Analg 1983;62:341.
33. Incaudo G, Schatz M, Patterson R, et al. Administration of local anesthetics to patients with a history of prior adverse reaction. J Allergy Clin Immunol 1978;61:339.
34. Wilson RP. Local anesthesia in ophthalmology. In: Tasman W, Jaeger EA, eds. Duane's Clinical ophthalmology. Philadelphia: J B Lippincott, 1992;Vol 6, Chap. 2:1–20.

CHAPTER 21

Dilation of the Pupil

Jimmy D. Bartlett

Since the invention of the direct ophthalmoscope in the 19th century, practitioners have used mydriatic drugs to facilitate examination of the crystalline lens, vitreous, retina, and optic nerve. With the advent of the binocular indirect ophthalmoscope, three-mirror fundus contact lenses, and other diagnostic instrumentation, a panoramic and stereoscopic view of the fundus from ciliary body to optic nerve has been made available to the ophthalmic practitioner. Much of this view, however, is accessible only with the use of mydriatics. The proper use of mydriatics enables the practitioner to identify and diagnose more accurately various abnormalities of the eye that might otherwise go undetected. This chapter considers the incorporation of routine pupillary dilation into office practice, anterior angle evaluation before dilation, dilation drug regimens, clinical procedures facilitated by the use of mydriatics, and pupillary dilation as a therapeutic procedure.

Incorporation of Pupillary Dilation into Examination Routine

The successful incorporation of pupillary dilation procedures into the examination routine improves the clinical effectiveness of mydriatics by allowing the drugs to be used without disrupting normal patient flow in the office. Such use requires attention to certain patient management aspects, the examination routine itself, and the selection of patients for dilation.

Patient Management Aspects

Some practitioners acquiesce to the wishes of their patients who decline to be dilated. Although this is acceptable in some cases, the ability to communicate to patients the desirability of pupillary dilation is largely a matter of practitioner-patient rapport. Many older adult patients may remember being dilated as a child when the standard drug regimen was atropine or scopolamine, the effects of which lasted 1 or 2 weeks. These patients can be reassured that contemporary mydriatics are rapid acting with little debilitating effect on vision. Other patients sometimes have unrealistic conceptions of "dilation" procedures. Thus, to prevent or minimize dilation-related patient apprehension, the effects of the drugs should be explained before dilation, and the benefits of their use should be emphasized. With this approach, most patients are not only willing to be dilated, but they actually desire the procedure once they understand the reasons for it.

Examination Routine

Most clinicians dilate patients only after most other examination procedures have been performed. Complete histories, visual acuities, external examination, pupillary examination, ocular motility, refraction, biomicroscopy, Goldmann tonometry, and other routine evaluations precede instilling the mydriatic(s) (Fig. 21.1). This approach ensures that dilation does not interfere with the refraction, assessment of accommodation or binocularity, or any other refractive find-

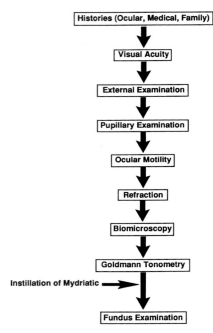

FIGURE 21.1 **Example of examination routine in which the mydriatic is instilled near the conclusion of the examination.**

ing. In most routine cases, ophthalmoscopy or fundus biomicroscopy is the only procedure remaining after dilation. After the drops have been instilled for dilation, the patient may proceed to the reception area, "dilation room," or to the dispensary for spectacle frame selection while the pupils dilate.[1] Frame selection can usually be completed without interference from the mydriatic. While this patient's pupils dilate, the practitioner examines the next scheduled patient. In 20 to 30 minutes, after all procedures except dilation have been performed on the second patient and the pupils of the first patient have dilated, the second patient then proceeds to frame selection or the dilation room while the first patient returns for ophthalmoscopy and any other indicated procedures. Most practitioners who incorporate pupillary dilation as a routine part of their service use this "round robin" or "leap frog" approach (Table 21.1).[2] Note, however, that patient appointment schedules will vary depending on the number and responsibilities of staff personnel and of practitioners in the office.[3]

The placement of dilation procedures toward the conclusion of the routine examination enables the practitioner to perform all the mydriatic preinstillation examination as a standard routine. All the procedures that should be accomplished before instilling the mydriatic—visual acuity, tonometry, anterior angle evaluation, drug sensitivity history—occur in a natural and logical sequence. Thus, the

patient may immediately undergo pupillary dilation if warranted. If the practitioner does not wish to dilate the pupils, direct ophthalmoscopy or monocular indirect ophthalmoscopy can then be performed in the usual manner.

Indications and Contraindications

When the various clinical and legal factors governing patient care are considered, a standard of care (see Chapter 5) appears to be emerging that requires that virtually all "new" patients presenting for comprehensive eye examination undergo dilated fundus examination using binocular indirect ophthalmoscopy. Since pupillary dilation allows a substantially more thorough evaluation of the ocular media, fundus including peripheral retina, and optic disc than is possible without dilation, careful indirect ophthalmoscopy with or without fundus biomicroscopy should be performed through a dilated pupil in a variety of clinical circumstances (Table 21.2).[4–6]

In rare clinical situations, dilation of the pupil may be contraindicated (Table 21.3), but if patient history, signs, or symptoms seem to indicate that dilation is necessary, the practitioner should proceed by following the guidelines given later in this chapter. Legal issues of negligence (failure to dilate) and patient informed consent are extremely important and can play a pivotal role in the selection of patients whose pupils should be dilated (see Chapter 5).[7]

Anterior Angle Evaluation

Acute angle-closure glaucoma is a well-recognized complication of mydriatic use. Since the risk of such a complication is greatest in eyes with shallow chambers and narrow anterior angles, the practitioner should evaluate the anterior angle before instilling the mydriatic. The anterior angle can be assessed by using the shadow test, slit-lamp method, or gonioscopy.

Shadow Test

The easiest and most rapid method of evaluating the anterior angle entails using a penlight to illuminate the iris (Fig. 21.2). This method is less accurate than the slit-lamp or gonioscopic procedures; nevertheless, it is reliable for identifying critically narrow angles that might be predisposed to angle closure. Furthermore, it is useful in the pediatric age group, when slit-lamp examination or gonioscopy may not be permitted.

This method involves directing the penlight beam from the temporal side at the level of the pupil. The entire iris is

TABLE 21.1

Illustration of "Round Robin" Procedure for Incorporating Dilation into Examination Routine[a]

Time (AM)	Patient A	Patient B	Patient C
8:00	(8:00) Arrives for appointment (8:05–8:10) Preliminary work-up by technician (8:10–8:30)		
8:15	Examination by optometrist (8:30)	(8:15) Arrives for appointment (8:20–8:30)	
8:30	Drops instilled for pupillary dilation (8:30–8:50)	Preliminary work-up by technician (8:30–8:50)	
8:45	Frame selection or "dilation room" (8:50–9:00)	Examination by optometrist (8:50)	(8:45) Arrives for appointment (8:50–8:55)
9:00	Ophthalmoscopy and other indicated procedures, patient consultation	Drops instilled for pupillary dilation	Preliminary work-up by technician
		(8:50–9:10) Frame selection or "dilation room" (9:10–9:20)	(8:55–9:10) Examination by optometrist (9:10)
9:15		Ophthalmoscopy and other indicated procedures, patient consultation	Drops instilled for pupillary dilation
			(9:10–9:30) Frame selection or "dilation room" (9:30–9:40)
9:30			Ophthalmoscopy and other indicated procedures, patient consultation

[a]Time allotments represent approximations and may vary according to practitioner requirements, patient punctuality for appointment, and other factors. These suggestions are for illustration purposes only.

TABLE 21.2
Indications for Pupillary Dilation

- Symptoms of floaters or flashes of light
- Visual acuity not correctable to 20/20
- Visual field loss
- Presence of cataract or other media opacities
- Myopia exceeding 6 D
- Episodes of intermittent blurred vision or blackouts
- Ocular contusion injury
- History of diabetes
- Unexplained ocular pain or redness
- History of lattice degeneration, retinal holes, or retinal detachment
- Afferent pupillary defect (Marcus Gunn pupil)
- History of metastatic tumors
- Miotic pupils
- Nystagmus or unsteady fixation
- Unexplained headaches
- History of use of drugs with known toxicity to lens, retina, or optic nerve
- Any symptom suggesting posterior segment involvement
- Elevated intraocular pressure

TABLE 21.3
Contraindications to Pupillary Dilation

- Iris-supported intraocular lens (IOL)
- Subluxated crystalline lens
- Subluxated IOL
- Extremely narrow or closed anterior chamber angles[a]
- History suggesting angle-closure glaucoma, with or without surgical or laser intervention.[a]

[a]Dilate with caution.

Adapted from Alexander LJ, Scholles J. Clinical and legal aspects of pupillary dilation. J Am Optom Assoc 1987;58:432–437.

illuminated if the iris lies in a flat plane (Fig. 21.2A). This is characteristically observed in eyes with deep anterior chambers, such as those in myopia and aphakia, in which the open angle (grade 4) makes a 45° angle between the iris and cornea.[8] When the angle between the iris and cornea measures 20° or less (grade 2 to 0), the lens-iris diaphragm is displaced anteriorly. As a result, the penlight beam illuminates the temporal iris, but a shadow falls on the

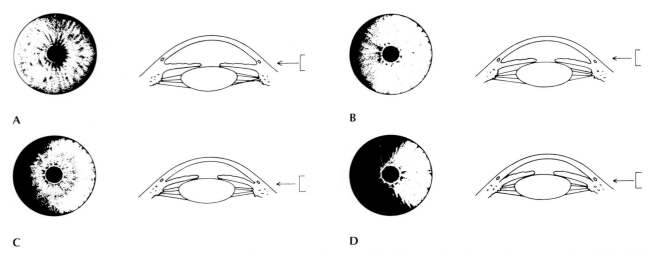

FIGURE 21.2 **Shadow test. The light source illuminates the nasal aspect of the iris to varying degrees depending on the depth of the anterior chamber.** *(A)* Wide open angle (grade 4). *(B)* Open angle (grade 3). *(C)* Moderately narrow angle (grade 2). *(D)* Extremely narrow angle (grade 1).

nasal aspect of the iris in proportion to the convexity of the lens-iris diaphragm.

Although this method of evaluating the anterior angle is reliable in most patients, the practitioner must avoid misinterpretation. It is possible to estimate the angle as being narrower than it actually is because of central shallowing of the anterior chamber. This is especially common in older patients with enlarged lenses. In such eyes, the peripheral iris often recedes from the trabecular meshwork, leaving the angle incapable of closure.[8] Properly positioning the penlight exactly perpendicular to the visual axis enhances the accuracy of this method.[9] If the penlight is positioned too far anteriorly or if the eye is deviated temporally, the penlight may illuminate the nasal aspect of the iris directly, thus giving a false-negative result.

Slit-Lamp Method

A more accurate method for anterior angle evaluation is the slit-lamp technique described by van Herick, Shaffer, and Schwartz.[8] With the patient at the slit lamp, the vertical slit-lamp beam is placed at the temporal limbus just inside the corneoscleral junction. The slit-lamp beam should be as narrow as possible and should be directed toward the eye at an angle of approximately 60° from the direction of the observation microscope (Fig. 21.3). The depth of the anterior chamber at the temporal limbus is compared with the thickness of the cornea through which the beam travels. In the case of a wide open, or grade 4, angle, the depth of the anterior chamber is equal to or greater than the thickness of the cornea. If the depth of the anterior chamber is equal to approximately half the thickness of the cornea, the angle is

classified as grade 3. An anterior chamber depth equal to one-fourth the corneal thickness is classified as a grade 2 angle, and an anterior chamber depth less than one-fourth the corneal thickness is classified as grade 1. Table 21.4 shows the implications of such a classification in terms of the risk for angle closure.

This method is an extremely rapid (requiring only seconds) and accurate technique for estimating the depth of the anterior chamber angle. Also, it tends to correlate well with gonioscopic findings.[8,10] Such slit-lamp grading is based on the findings at the temporal and sometimes nasal limbus and serves as a reliable average of the entire angle.[8]

Using this technique, van Herick and associates[8] found grade 1 narrow angles to have a prevalence of only 0.64% and grade 2 a prevalence of 1%. The prevalence of grades 1 and 2 angles increases with age, but this finding is expected considering the normal increase of lens thickness with age.[8] The practical implication of the slit-lamp method is that assessments of 0.25 or less indicate a risk of angle closure and merit gonioscopic confirmation before dilating the pupil.[10]

Gonioscopy

Gonioscopy provides the most definitive assessment of the anterior angle. This procedure allows direct or indirect visualization of the anterior angle structures and thus indicates with greater accuracy the risk of angle closure associated with pupillary dilation. The most commonly employed techniques involve use of the Goldmann, Zeiss (Posner), or Sussman gonioprisms (Fig. 21.4). Each of these gonioprisms allows an indirect view of the anterior chamber angle by reflection through a mirror.

TABLE 21.1
Illustration of "Round Robin" Procedure for Incorporating Dilation into Examination Routine[a]

Time (AM)	Patient A	Patient B	Patient C
8:00	(8:00) Arrives for appointment (8:05–8:10) Preliminary work-up by technician (8:10–8:30)		
8:15	Examination by optometrist (8:30)	(8:15) Arrives for appointment (8:20–8:30)	
8:30	Drops instilled for pupillary dilation (8:30–8:50)	Preliminary work-up by technician (8:30–8:50)	
8:45	Frame selection or "dilation room" (8:50–9:00)	Examination by optometrist (8:50)	(8:45) Arrives for appointment (8:50–8:55)
9:00	Ophthalmoscopy and other indicated procedures, patient consultation	Drops instilled for pupillary dilation (8:50–9:10)	Preliminary work-up by technician (8:55–9:10)
9:15		Frame selection or "dilation room" (9:10–9:20) Ophthalmoscopy and other indicated procedures, patient consultation	Examination by optometrist (9:10) Drops instilled for pupillary dilation (9:10–9:30)
9:30			Frame selection or "dilation room" (9:30–9:40) Ophthalmoscopy and other indicated procedures, patient consultation

[a]Time allotments represent approximations and may vary according to practitioner requirements, patient punctuality for appointment, and other factors. These suggestions are for illustration purposes only.

TABLE 21.2
Indications for Pupillary Dilation

- Symptoms of floaters or flashes of light
- Visual acuity not correctable to 20/20
- Visual field loss
- Presence of cataract or other media opacities
- Myopia exceeding 6 D
- Episodes of intermittent blurred vision or blackouts
- Ocular contusion injury
- History of diabetes
- Unexplained ocular pain or redness
- History of lattice degeneration, retinal holes, or retinal detachment
- Afferent pupillary defect (Marcus Gunn pupil)
- History of metastatic tumors
- Miotic pupils
- Nystagmus or unsteady fixation
- Unexplained headaches
- History of use of drugs with known toxicity to lens, retina, or optic nerve
- Any symptom suggesting posterior segment involvement
- Elevated intraocular pressure

TABLE 21.3
Contraindications to Pupillary Dilation

- Iris-supported intraocular lens (IOL)
- Subluxated crystalline lens
- Subluxated IOL
- Extremely narrow or closed anterior chamber angles[a]
- History suggesting angle-closure glaucoma, with or without surgical or laser intervention.[a]

[a]Dilate with caution.
Adapted from Alexander LJ, Scholles J. Clinical and legal aspects of pupillary dilation. J Am Optom Assoc 1987;58:432–437.

illuminated if the iris lies in a flat plane (Fig. 21.2A). This is characteristically observed in eyes with deep anterior chambers, such as those in myopia and aphakia, in which the open angle (grade 4) makes a 45° angle between the iris and cornea.[8] When the angle between the iris and cornea measures 20° or less (grade 2 to 0), the lens-iris diaphragm is displaced anteriorly. As a result, the penlight beam illuminates the temporal iris, but a shadow falls on the

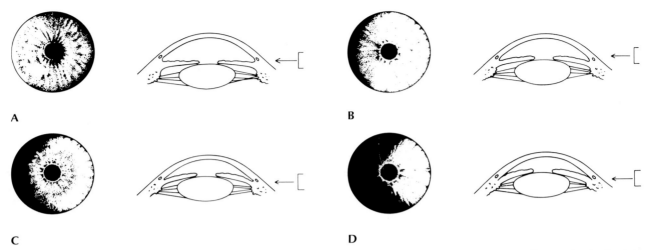

A

B

C

D

FIGURE 21.2   **Shadow test. The light source illuminates the nasal aspect of the iris to varying degrees depending on the depth of the anterior chamber.** *(A)* **Wide open angle (grade 4).** *(B)* **Open angle (grade 3).** *(C)* **Moderately narrow angle (grade 2).** *(D)* **Extremely narrow angle (grade 1).**

nasal aspect of the iris in proportion to the convexity of the lens-iris diaphragm.

Although this method of evaluating the anterior angle is reliable in most patients, the practitioner must avoid misinterpretation. It is possible to estimate the angle as being narrower than it actually is because of central shallowing of the anterior chamber. This is especially common in older patients with enlarged lenses. In such eyes, the peripheral iris often recedes from the trabecular meshwork, leaving the angle incapable of closure.[8] Properly positioning the penlight exactly perpendicular to the visual axis enhances the accuracy of this method.[9] If the penlight is positioned too far anteriorly or if the eye is deviated temporally, the penlight may illuminate the nasal aspect of the iris directly, thus giving a false-negative result.

Slit-Lamp Method

A more accurate method for anterior angle evaluation is the slit-lamp technique described by van Herick, Shaffer, and Schwartz.[8] With the patient at the slit lamp, the vertical slit-lamp beam is placed at the temporal limbus just inside the corneoscleral junction. The slit-lamp beam should be as narrow as possible and should be directed toward the eye at an angle of approximately 60° from the direction of the observation microscope (Fig. 21.3). The depth of the anterior chamber at the temporal limbus is compared with the thickness of the cornea through which the beam travels. In the case of a wide open, or grade 4, angle, the depth of the anterior chamber is equal to or greater than the thickness of the cornea. If the depth of the anterior chamber is equal to approximately half the thickness of the cornea, the angle is

classified as grade 3. An anterior chamber depth equal to one-fourth the corneal thickness is classified as a grade 2 angle, and an anterior chamber depth less than one-fourth the corneal thickness is classified as grade 1. Table 21.4 shows the implications of such a classification in terms of the risk for angle closure.

This method is an extremely rapid (requiring only seconds) and accurate technique for estimating the depth of the anterior chamber angle. Also, it tends to correlate well with gonioscopic findings.[8,10] Such slit-lamp grading is based on the findings at the temporal and sometimes nasal limbus and serves as a reliable average of the entire angle.[8]

Using this technique, van Herick and associates[8] found grade 1 narrow angles to have a prevalence of only 0.64% and grade 2 a prevalence of 1%. The prevalence of grades 1 and 2 angles increases with age, but this finding is expected considering the normal increase of lens thickness with age.[8] The practical implication of the slit-lamp method is that assessments of 0.25 or less indicate a risk of angle closure and merit gonioscopic confirmation before dilating the pupil.[10]

Gonioscopy

Gonioscopy provides the most definitive assessment of the anterior angle. This procedure allows direct or indirect visualization of the anterior angle structures and thus indicates with greater accuracy the risk of angle closure associated with pupillary dilation. The most commonly employed techniques involve use of the Goldmann, Zeiss (Posner), or Sussman gonioprisms (Fig. 21.4). Each of these gonioprisms allows an indirect view of the anterior chamber angle by reflection through a mirror.

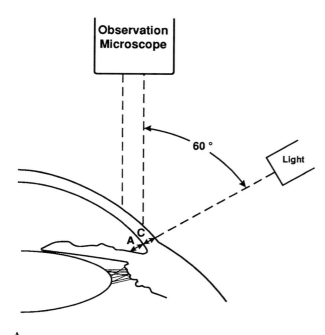

A

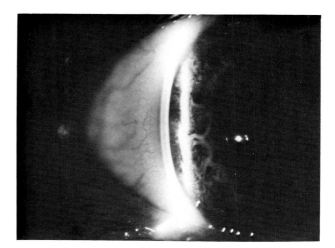

B

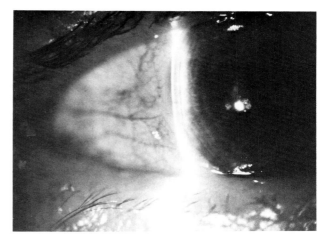

C

FIGURE 21.3   **Slit-lamp method for anterior angle evaluation.** *(A)* **The slit lamp beam should be as narrow as possible and should be directed toward the eye at an angle of approximately 60° from the direction of the observation microscope. The depth of the anterior chamber (A) is compared with the thickness of the cornea (C) through which the beam travels.** *(B)* **Slit-lamp view of a wide open (grade 4) angle in which the depth of the anterior chamber is greater than the thickness of the cornea.** *(C)* **Slit-lamp view of a grade 2 angle in which the depth of the anterior chamber is one-fourth the thickness of the cornea.**

TABLE 21.4
Classification and Implications of Slit-Lamp Assessment of Anterior Angle

Ratio of Anterior Chamber Depth to Corneal Thickness	Grade (van Herick)	Implication
1	4	Angle incapable of closure
0.5	3	Angle incapable of closure
0.25	2	Narrow angle—perform gonioscopy
Less than 0.25	1	Dangerously narrow angle—perform gonioscopy

When viewed gonioscopically, the normal anterior angle most often appears narrower superiorly, widest inferiorly, and has a depth intermediate between these two extremes at the temporal and nasal aspects.[10] Therefore, the major anatomic landmarks of the angle (Fig. 21.5) should be evaluated for the entire 360° and the findings documented by using a recording system such as the one illustrated in Figure 21.6. Table 21.5 summarizes the classification and implications of the gonioscopic observations.

Since the risk of angle closure is inversely proportional to the extent to which the angle structures are visualized during gonioscopy, a conservative estimate is that anterior angles in which the posterior trabeculum is obscured have increased risk of closure.[10] Cockburn[11] found 6.0% of eyes with some or all of the superior trabeculum obscured and 2.0% with

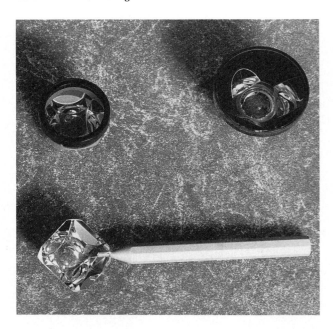

only the anterior half of the trabeculum visible. Thus, about 6% of eyes have significantly narrowed angles and 2% have critically narrowed angles. Using criteria that are generally accepted as defining significantly narrowed anterior angles, other investigators have obtained results that closely agree.

In most instances the slit-lamp method of evaluating the anterior chamber depth correlates well with gonioscopy, except when the angle is extremely narrow.[10] For example, patients having a slit-lamp assessment of 0.3 or less are likely to demonstrate only partial visualization of the trabecular meshwork on gonioscopy.[10] However, it is generally

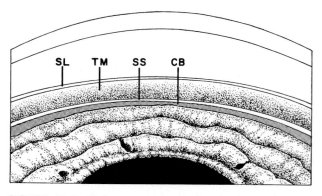

FIGURE 21.5   **Major anatomic landmarks in gonioscopy. Schwalbe's line (SL), trabecular meshwork (TM), scleral spur (SS), and ciliary body (CB).**

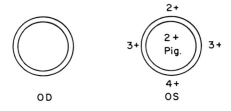

GONIOSCOPY

FIGURE 21.6   **Recording form for gonioscopy. The observations for each of the 4 quadrants of the anterior angle can be quickly and easily recorded by grading each quadrant according to the classification shown in Table 21.5.**

unnecessary to perform gonioscopy on all patients to identify those with significantly narrow angles.[11] The slit-lamp method may be used to select patients in need of gonioscopy—patients having an anterior chamber depth of 0.25 or less should generally undergo gonioscopy. If, during gonioscopy, half or less of the trabeculum is visible in all quadrants, the eye should be considered at risk of angle closure during pupillary dilation.[11] Note, however, that partial angle closure can occur without significant elevation of intraocular pressure or ocular damage.[12] Thus, the widest quadrant of the anterior chamber angle is generally the most critical for evaluation. Furthermore, despite careful gonioscopy, predicting precisely which eyes will sustain angle closure on pupillary dilation is still not possible.[13] Later parts of this chapter discuss methods of dilating pupils of eyes with narrow angles.

General Guidelines

The following general guidelines for the clinical use of mydriatics should enhance the clinical effectiveness of pupillary dilation.

1. Topical anesthesia before instilling the mydriatic enhances pupillary dilation by reducing irritation of the medication and enhancing corneal permeability of the mydriatic.[14,15] By eliminating the stinging sensation produced by the mydriatic, the topical anesthetic diminishes lacrimation and blinking and thus decreases dilution and nasolacrimal drainage of the medication.[14] Benoxinate, proparacaine, and tetracaine produce approximately equal degrees of enhancement of pupillary dilation.[16] If Goldmann applanation tonometry has been performed immediately before dilation, the corneal epithelial disruption provided by the tonometer, together with the effects of the anesthetic, will enhance the dilation, especially in patients with dark irides.[17]

TABLE 21.5
Classification and Implication of Gonioscopic Assessment of Anterior Angle

Visible Angle Anatomy	Grade (Shaffer)	Angular Subtense (°)	Implications
All of ciliary body and trabeculum	4	30–45	Angle incapable of closure
Some ciliary body and all trabeculum	3	20–30	Angle incapable of closure
Most of trabeculum	2	10–20	Narrow angle
Only narrow section of trabeculum	1	10 or less	Dangerously narrow angle
No angle anatomy visible	0	—	Closed angle

2. The goal of dilation should be wide and rapid mydriasis.[2] Installation of a topical anesthetic and use of a combination of adrenergic and anticholinergic agents achieves this goal. The single instillation of tropicamide or phenylephrine alone may result in some pupillary constriction on intense light stimulation provided by binocular indirect ophthalmoscopy. Furthermore, tropicamide alone may prove less effective in the elderly because of decreased sympathetic pupillary tone.[18] Thus, topically administered adrenergic and anticholinergic drugs used in combination produce faster and more complete mydriasis. In most cases pupils obtain maximum mydriasis within 15 to 30 minutes, and virtually all pupils will be maximally dilated within 45 minutes.[19] The combination of phenylephrine and tropicamide is suitable for routine dilation purposes because the drugs have a similar duration of action, and tropicamide is less likely to elevate intraocular pressure than are most other anticholinergic drugs.[20]

3. Various combinations of mydriatics have been investigated for their efficacy in pupillary dilation while minimizing side effects.[20–22] The individual agents (usually tropicamide and phenylephrine, or tropicamide and hydroxyamphetamine) can be instilled in any order, and instilling the second drug immediately after the first does not adversely influence the drugs' additive effects.[23] One commercially available mydriatic combination, 0.2% cyclopentolate with 1% phenylephrine (Cyclomydril), has much too prolonged mydriatic and cycloplegic durations for routine pupillary dilation. Use of this combination requires nearly 8 hours for sufficient accommodation to return to allow reading ability.[24] In contrast, a commercially available combination of 0.25% tropicamide with 1% hydroxyamphetamine (Paremyd) provides satisfactory mydriasis and inhibition of the pupillary light response in young adults, with only minimal paralysis of accommodation.[25]

4. Although mydriatic combinations give more rapid and wider dilation, phenylephrine or hydroxyamphetamine may be used alone for dilation when the patient or practitioner has concerns about the possibility of drug-induced blurred vision. These drugs spare accommodation but usually require more than 1 instillation and more time for adequate dilation to occur.[26]

5. Multiple instillations of mydriatics are rarely required to achieve a wide pupillary dilation. The single instillation of a suitable combination of mydriatics usually achieves rapid and complete mydriasis while minimizing the risk of side effects associated with drug overdosages.[15,27] However, in patients whose pupils may be anticipated to dilate poorly, such as in insulin-dependent diabetes or darkly pigmented irides, 2 drops of the mydriatic applied in rapid succession may potentiate the mydriatic response.[28]

6. A pupillary diameter of 7 mm is usually adequate to permit thorough examination of the fundus, including the peripheral retina.[29] Even smaller pupillary apertures may prove adequate in many instances to allow binocular indirect ophthalmoscopy or other stereoscopic examination procedures.

7. The goal of dilation should be a maximally dilated pupil.[2] Minimally dilated pupils pose a risk of pupillary-block glaucoma that is not present with maximally dilated pupils.[30]

8. Unless specifically contraindicated, the pupils of both eyes should be dilated rather than dilating only the pupil of the eye with the suspected lesion.[2] Failure to dilate the pupil of the contralateral eye causes diagnostic errors because lesions considered normal variants frequently occur bilaterally. Failure to dilate the contralateral eye does not allow comparison with the fellow eye and, thus, may contribute to errors in diagnostic judgment. In addition, the Pulfrich phenomenon that is induced by monocular dilation can annoy patients.[2] Patients may experience dizziness, vertigo, or other uncomfortable symptoms, all of which bilateral pupillary dilation can prevent or minimize.

9. In most patients the degree of mydriasis is consistent and reproducible on consecutive dilations,[31] but some variability can occur with regard to the rapidity or degree of dilation obtainable on different occasions.[29]

10. In patients at risk for systemic side effects from topi-

cally administered adrenergic mydriatics, manual naso-lacrimal occlusion (see Fig. 3.6) is a reasonable procedure to minimize nasolacrimal drainage of drug and subsequent absorption into the systemic circulation.

11. Although rare, mydriatic-induced angle-closure glaucoma can occur in young patients, and the previous use of mydriatics without adverse effects does not necessarily indicate that angle closure will not develop on subsequent pupillary dilation in patients of any age.[29,32]

Dilation Drug Regimens

Routine Dilation

ADULTS

Rapid and effective mydriasis may be obtained in adults by using 1 drop of 0.5% to 1% tropicamide.[22] Another effective regimen is 1 drop each of 2.5% phenylephrine and 0.5% to 1% tropicamide or 1 drop each of 1% hydroxyamphetamine and 0.5% to 1% tropicamide.[2,19,33] These combinations are effective in dilating pupils with age-related miosis in which there is decreased sympathetic pupillary tone, where the use of tropicamide alone is less effective.[18] A commercially available combination of 0.25% tropicamide with 1% hydroxyamphetamine (Paremyd) is effective in young adults and has minimal cycloplegic effects.[25]

CHILDREN

Effective dilation in the pediatric age group is obtained by using no more than 2 drops into each eye of tropicamide 0.5% to 1%, cyclopentolate 0.5% to 1%, and phenylephrine 2.5%, instilled separately. This combination produces wide mydriasis for fundus examination and allows effective cycloplegia for retinoscopy or subjective refraction.[34] These agents can also be administered together as a spray by combining 3.75 ml cyclopentolate 2% with 7.5 ml tropicamide 1% and 3.75 ml phenylephrine 10%. When mixed, the final spray solution contains cyclopentolate 0.5%, tropicamide 0.5%, and phenylephrine 2.5%.[35] The spray is applied to the closed eyelids and produces mydriasis and cycloplegia comparable to those provided by the same combination of mydriatics administered as eyedrops to the open eye.[36,37] Moreover, compared with traditional eyedrop instillation, children usually have less avoidance reaction with the spray.[36]

NEONATES AND INFANTS

Ophthalmoscopic examination of premature infants requires wide pupillary dilation and binocular indirect ophthalmoscopy. Since premature infants treated with oxygen concentrations exceeding room air are at increased risk of developing retinopathy of prematurity, binocular indirect ophthalmoscopy is required to detect early signs of this disease.[38] Other neonates or infants may require dilation to evaluate congenital cataracts or to search for ocular signs of toxoplasmosis, cytomegalovirus, or herpes. Thus, the mydriatics chosen must be effective and safe in allowing examination of the ocular media, posterior pole, and peripheral retina.

Because of the premature infant's small body mass and less mature cardiovascular and cerebrovascular status, prudence dictates using the lowest concentration yet the most effective combination of mydriatics for pupillary dilation. This approach minimizes the risk of systemic side effects, which are especially common with topical phenylephrine. Ten percent aqueous or viscous phenylephrine causes innocuous blanching of the skin around the eyes of newborns but, more important, frequently elevates both systolic and diastolic blood pressure.[39] Rosales and associates[40] showed that 80% of low-birth-weight infants administered 2.5% phenylephrine in combination with 0.5% tropicamide had greater than 20% elevation in systolic blood pressure; 30% of the patients had an elevation of 50% or more. In contrast, several investigators[38,41] have shown that a combination of 2.5% phenylephrine and 0.5% to 1% tropicamide provides sufficient mydriasis without adverse cardiovascular effects in preterm infants. The use of tropicamide alone, however, does not generally produce a sufficient mydriasis in premature babies.[41] Adding cyclopentolate to the tropicamide regimen improves mydriasis but may contribute to elevated blood pressure and heart rate.[41] Moreover, because of possible gastric secretory inhibition and the risk of necrotizing enterocolitis in preterm infants, the concentration of cyclopentolate should be limited to 0.25%.[42,43] A commercially available combination of phenylephrine 1% and cyclopentolate 0.2% (Cyclomydril) has proven effective and has minimal risk of cardiovascular or gastrointestinal effects.[42,44]

To facilitate the application of mydriatics in neonates and infants, a single-instillation solution may be prepared by combining 3.75 ml of cyclopentolate 2% with 7.5 ml of tropicamide 1% and 3.75 ml of phenylephrine 10%. The final solution contains cyclopentolate 0.5%, tropicamide 0.5%, and phenylephrine 2.5%.[35] This combination produces no major side effects and gives an effective pupillary dilation.[35,39] In infants with blue irides, 1 drop in each eye is usually adequate, while in other patients a second instillation within 5 to 10 seconds of the first usually provides consistently adequate mydriasis.[35] The solution can also be applied as a spray (see Chapter 3).[36]

Following dilation of the premature infant's eyes, the absolute pupillary diameter may remain small.[45] The mydriasis, however, compares to that of the adult when expressed as a percentage of corneal diameter; that is, the absolute pupillary size of the premature neonate following dilation may remain small simply because of the small size of the infant eye.[45]

During insertion of the lid speculum, binocular indirect ophthalmoscopy, and scleral depression procedures, care should be taken to recognize any stimulation of the oculocardiac reflex and, if necessary, to institute measures for infant resuscitation immediately.[46]

Systemic Disease

Because of the risk of adverse pressor effects from topical phenylephrine, especially the 10% concentration, this drug should generally be avoided for pupillary dilation in patients with cardiac disease, systemic hypertension, aneurysms, and advanced arteriosclerosis.[47] However, mild hypertension not controlled with guanethidine or reserpine is not necessarily a contraindication to the use of phenylephrine.[48] The use of tropicamide alone for dilation of patients with such cardiovascular disease is probably the safest drug regimen, since tropicamide is virtually free of pressor effect and thus produces little risk of acute hypertensive crisis.[48,49]

Idiopathic orthostatic hypotension is a condition that leads to denervation hypersensitivity.[50] The topical instillation of even 2.5% phenylephrine in patients with this condition often elevates blood pressure dramatically.[50] Thus, because of the increased pressor response to phenylephrine in patients with idiopathic orthostatic hypotension, the practitioner should avoid phenylephrine for dilation in patients with this condition. Instead, hydroxyamphetamine, an indirect-acting adrenergic agent, may provide the desired mydriasis while minimizing the risk of adverse cardiovascular effects.[51] The addition of tropicamide will improve the mydriasis.

Patients with Down's syndrome are hypersensitive to topically applied anticholinergic agents. The pupils often dilate widely in response to tropicamide, reflecting an imbalance between cholinergic and adrenergic autonomic activity in the iris.[52]

Because of increased sensitivity to circulating catecholamines in patients with hyperthyroidism, patients with this disease may have an increased risk of adverse pressor effects from phenylephrine or hydroxyamphetamine. Thus, these drugs should be avoided or used conservatively in patients with hyperthyroidism.

Sympathetic denervation is common in patients with either insulin-dependent or noninsulin-dependent diabetes.[53–55] This sympathetic denervation results from autonomic neuropathy, affects the iris and cardiovascular system, and increases the risk of systemic side effects from adrenergic agonists.[56] Smith and Smith[57] have reported that the pupils of patients with diabetes demonstrate hypersensitivity to phenylephrine but show normal reactions to hydroxyamphetamine. This response is consistent with a partial postganglionic denervation of the iris dilator muscle.[58] Clinical impression,[59] however, is that pupillary dilation of patients with diabetes is difficult, presumably

because of impaired sympathetic innervation to the dilator muscle. This sympathetic autonomic neuropathy may be especially common in female diabetics.[59] An effective mydriatic regimen is tropicamide 0.5% to 1% in combination with phenylephrine 2.5%.[57,60] This regimen usually produces satisfactory dilation with a minimum of systemic side effects.

Concomitant Drug Therapy

Drug interactions can play an important role in causing systemic side effects following pupillary dilation. Since the tricyclic antidepressants (Table 21.6) and monoamine oxidase (MAO) inhibitors increase the pressor effects of phenylephrine, phenylephrine should be avoided in patients taking these medications.[47] Phenylephrine should be avoided even up to 21 days following termination of MAO inhibitor therapy.[47] Furthermore, the use of topical phenylephrine in atropinized patients can enhance the pressor effects and produce tachycardia.[47] Hydroxyamphetamine should also be avoided in these patients. The use of tropicamide alone allows effective mydriasis while minimizing the risk of systemic side effects.

Partial sympathetic denervation with resultant hypersensitivity may occur in patients who are taking reserpine, guanethidine, methyldopa, or other α-adrenergic blocking agents.[51,56] Such pharmacologic sympathectomy following the depletion of norepinephrine gives rise to reduced sensitivity to indirect-acting adrenergic agents but also results in increased sensitivity to catecholamines.[51] The resulting denervation hypersensitivity may cause prolonged mydriasis in patients dilated with phenylephrine.[56] More important, however, the risk of adverse pressor effects from phenylephrine increases. On the other hand, hydroxyamphetamine, an indirect-acting adrenergic, appears to be a safer drug for pupillary dilation in these patients because of a reduced risk of adverse cardiovascular effects in patients with pharmacologic sympathectomy.[51] Depending on the magnitude of the local sympathectomy of the iris dilator muscle, hydroxyamphetamine may have somewhat reduced effectiveness when used alone for dilation in patients taking such drugs. However, adding tropicamide will usually ensure satisfactory mydriasis.

TABLE 21.6
Commonly Prescribed Tricyclic Antidepressants

Generic Name	Trade Name
Imipramine HCl	Tofranil (Geigy)
Amitriptyline HCl	Elavil (Stuart), Triavil (Merck)
Doxepin HCl	Sinequan (Roerig)

Open-Angle Glaucoma

The management of open-angle glaucoma requires periodic dilation of the pupil for fundus, optic nerve, and visual field examination. Pupillary dilation is essential for the following reasons:[2]

- Patients receiving long-term miotic therapy can develop sphincter rigidity and atrophy. Periodic dilation will "rejuvenate" the iris sphincter by allowing it to relax.
- Miotics may cause peripheral retinal tears with subsequent rhegmatogenous retinal detachment. Periodic dilation for peripheral retinal examination can identify these patients.[61]
- Stereoscopic examination of the optic nerve head is essential for the proper long-term management of open-angle glaucoma. Critical judgments are often necessary in establishing the initial diagnosis of glaucomatous disc damage, and monocular viewing can easily overlook subtle changes of the nerve head.
- Accurate evaluation of glaucomatous visual fields requires at least a 3 to 4 mm pupillary aperture so that cataractous changes or miosis do not cause artifactual field loss. Since many glaucoma patients also have progressive lenticular changes, performing serial visual field testing with the same pupillary size may better control this and other variables.[62]

When the pupils of eyes with open-angle glaucoma are dilated with cycloplegics, intraocular pressure (IOP) can rise significantly.[63–67] This effect is transient and occurs in treated as well as untreated open-angle glaucoma. However, it is only rarely observed in healthy patients.[63] The incidence of this cycloplegic response is about 25% to 38% in open-angle glaucoma, 35% in miotic-treated open-angle glaucoma, but only 2% in the general population.[63,64,67] All strong cycloplegics elevate IOP, but those with only a minimal effect on accommodation do not produce this response.[64] Tropicamide may elevate IOP in patients with open-angle glaucoma who are being treated either with or without miotics. Hill and associates[67] found a clinically significant IOP elevation (≥ 6 mmHg) in approximately 38% of patients with open-angle glaucoma dilated with tropicamide 1%. Cyclopentolate causes a 3 to 22 mm Hg elevation of IOP in most eyes with open-angle glaucoma.[65] Miotic treatment of the glaucoma significantly enhances the incidence of pressure elevation with cyclopentolate but does not, however, significantly influence the magnitude of the response.[63]

Cycloplegic-induced pressure elevations appear to to result from a decrease of facility of aqueous outflow. However, no association exists between the magnitude of pupillary dilation and the IOP elevation, nor is there any association between pressure elevation and the initial IOP.[63] Cycloplegic-induced pressure elevations are not necessarily reproducible in a particular eye or a particular patient.[63] Generally responsive eyes may occasionally fail to develop significant elevations of pressure on subsequent dilation. Less commonly, consistently unresponsive eyes may develop significant elevations of pressure. Thus, the use of cycloplegics for dilation of eyes with open-angle glaucoma generally requires some caution.[65,66] Apraclonidine, an α_2-adrenergic agonist, may be used prophylactically to prevent or minimize precipitous elevations of IOP in susceptible patients. One drop of apraclonidine instilled 10 minutes before tropicamide is effective for this purpose.[67]

Unlike cycloplegic agents, adrenergic mydriatics have essentially no effect on IOP in patients with open-angle glaucoma.[64,65,68] Since dilation of the pupil with phenylephrine usually does not elevate the pressure and does not consistently reduce the facility of aqueous outflow, it may be used safely for dilation in patients with open-angle glaucoma.[65] Practitioners can also use phenylephrine to dilate the pupils of patients who have primary open-angle glaucoma and who are being treated with miotics, even strong miotics such as the anticholinesterase agents.[68] In such cases phenylephrine will partially overcome the miosis but may require up to 60 minutes or longer to obtain a pupillary size adequate for optic disc or fundus examination. Thus, the pupils of miotic-treated eyes can be dilated without altering IOP when phenylephrine is used as the mydriatic.

Dilation of eyes with exfoliation or pigmentary glaucoma may liberate pigment into the anterior chamber, which can greatly elevate IOP.[69,70] Profuse pigment liberation during dilation of such eyes may cause transient blocking of the trabecular meshwork, with obstruction of aqueous outflow and subsequent elevation of IOP.[70] This elevation of pressure is transient,[69] but pigment can be liberated during pupillary dilation without a concurrent elevation of pressure.[70] Dilation with cycloplegic rather than adrenergic mydriatics is less likely to liberate pigment, but on the other hand it has a greater tendency to raise IOP because of mechanisms independent of pigment liberation. Thus, no particular mydriatic exhibits clear advantages over another for dilation of eyes with exfoliation or pigmentary glaucoma. Note, however, that the pupils of eyes with exfoliation syndrome generally dilate more poorly than do healthy eyes.[71,72] This situation may result from bonding of the posterior surface of the iris to the preequatorial lens capsule and anterior zonules by exfoliation material,[73] or from iris infiltration and fibrosis.[74]

In summary, phenylephrine or hydroxyamphetamine alone[75] or in combination with tropicamide can be used to dilate most eyes with open-angle glaucoma. The combination of phenylephrine and tropicamide generally permits wide mydriasis while minimizing potential elevation of IOP.[76]

Narrow Angle with Intact Iris

Mydriatic-induced angle-closure glaucoma most commonly occurs in the elderly. It can, however, occur in young patients, and the previous use of mydriatics without adverse

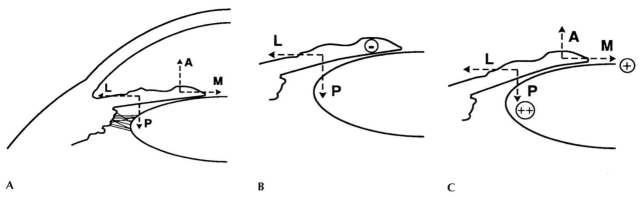

FIGURE 21.7   Mechanics of pupillary dilation. *(A)* Components of iris muscle activity. Anterior component of iris sphincter activity (A), medial component of iris sphincter activity (M), lateral component of iris dilator activity (L), and posterior component of iris dilator activity (P). *(B)* Pupillary dilation with anticholinergic mydriatic. The iris sphincter is inactivated, and the posterior component of the iris dilator acts peripherally. *(C)* Pupillary dilation with adrenergic mydriatic. The iris dilator is stimulated and its posterior component is augmented while the medial component of the iris sphincter persists.

sequelae does not necessarily indicate that angle closure will not develop on subsequent dilation.[29,32] Thus, the practitioner should approach the dilation of eyes with narrow anterior angles with the knowledge that some risk exists for angle closure. Note that gonioscopy has no value in predicting which narrow angles will close on dilation because it allows only a subjective assessment of the magnitude of the narrow angle.[13,30] An understanding of the mechanics of pupillary dilation lends support to the various philosophies governing the dilation of eyes with narrow angles.

MECHANICS OF PUPILLARY DILATION AND ANGLE CLOSURE

Eyes with deep anterior chambers are essentially free of the risk of pupillary block and iris bombé. However, in eyes predisposed to angle-closure glaucoma, the lens is generally displaced anteriorly, which increases the pressure of the iris against the lens. This situation favors pupillary block and iris bombé with subsequent secondary angle closure.[77,78] When the iris rests on an anteriorly positioned lens, the forces of pupillary dilation (iris dilator muscle activity) can be resolved into two components—a posterior and a lateral. Likewise, the force of pupillary constriction (iris sphincter muscle activity) can be resolved into two components—a medial and an anterior[79] (Fig. 21.7A). The total sphincter pupillary blocking force varies according to size and position of the pupil.[30] A miotic pupil is generally associated with a taut iris and small pupillary blocking force; a mid-dilated pupil is associated with a lax iris and large pupillary blocking force; and wide dilation is associated with a compressed iris and small pupillary blocking force. Thus, the position of greatest risk with respect to potential angle closure is mid-dilation.[30] With a mid-dilated pupil, regardless of how it is obtained pharmacologically, the pupillary blocking force is maximum; and, if predisposed to angle

closure, some eyes will undergo acute angle closure because the pupillary block has increased the pressure in the posterior chamber. The increased pressure produces iris bombé, which subsequently leads to secondary angle closure[80] (Fig. 21.8).

DILATION PHILOSOPHIES

Routine Dilation.   A valid approach to the dilation of eyes with extremely narrow angles is to use routine drug regimens such as a combination of tropicamide and phenylephrine. If drug-induced angle closure occurs and is promptly recognized and treated, the patient ultimately benefits from the experience, since the angle-closure attack occurs under controlled conditions in which proper treatment facilities are usually readily available.[81] Thus, the use of routine drug regimens constitutes essentially a "provocative test." However, before proceeding with such an approach, the practitioner should obtain the patient's informed consent (see Chapter 5), dilate only one eye at the initial visit, and postpone dilation of the fellow eye until the response of the initial dilation has been ascertained. Since most angle-closure

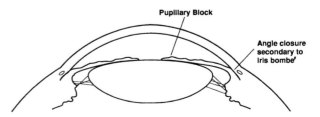

FIGURE 21.8   Pupillary block causes increased pressure in the posterior chamber relative to anterior chamber. This produces iris bombé, which obstructs aqueous outflow and causes secondary angle closure.

attacks occur 4 to 8 hours following instillation of the mydriatics, the dilation should be performed earlier in the day, when appropriate emergency care is more readily available. Ideally, the patient should remain in the office until the pupil has spontaneously returned to normal. Before dismissing the patient, IOP should be determined, and the patient should be informed of the symptoms of acute angle-closure glaucoma and have specific instructions for 21.19 emergency treatment should this become necessary.[49,76]

Anticholinergic Agents Only. Although dilation of the pupil with anticholinergic drugs such as tropicamide can cause angle closure,[80] the risk is generally considered to be much less than from dilation using adrenergic mydriatics. As previously noted, however, reduced aqueous outflow facility may elevate IOP, but this elevation is unrelated to the angle-closure mechanism.[82]

In eyes with intact irides and shallow anterior chambers, dilation with an anticholinergic agent infrequently leads to angle closure because this drug inhibits the force of iris sphincter contraction, while the force of dilator contraction and the force associated with iris tissue stretching retain their normal values.[77] Consequently, the posterior component of the pupillary dilation force is located toward the periphery of the iris, where contact between the lens and iris is less than it is near the pupil. The weakened sphincter will have a reduced medial component, resulting in less contact between the iris and lens at the pupillary margin. This condition allows the aqueous to pass from the posterior to the anterior chamber without obstruction[79] (Fig. 21.7B).

Of the available anticholinergic agents, tropicamide is preferred for routine dilation of eyes with shallow anterior chambers, narrow angles, and intact irides.[79] Homatropine and cyclopentolate do not act as rapidly as tropicamide and therefore appear less safe with regard to precipitating angle closure.[79] However, the disadvantage of using anticholinergic agents is the difficulty in overcoming the dilation with miotics if angle closure occurs.[83] In general, pilocarpine produces little or no miosis following dilation with anticholinergic drugs, and the pupil may remain dilated or partially dilated for a prolonged time.[84] However, dapiprazole or thymoxamine, both α-adrenergic antagonists, may reverse the mydriasis produced by tropicamide, as discussed later in this chapter.

Angle-closure glaucoma following dilation with tropicamide generally occurs within the first hour following instillation of the medication.[30] If the IOP has not risen significantly within 1 hour, the probability of angle closure is extremely low, and the practitioner can dismiss the patient without observation. The use of cholinergic miotics following dilation is discouraged, since it is both unnecessary and may cause angle closure.[30] If angle closure occurs, the IOP is usually readily brought to normal levels because angle closure following dilation with tropicamide is only rarely complete.[30]

Adrenergic Agents Only. Although Shaffer[76] has recommended the use of phenylephrine for routine dilation of eyes with extremely narrow angles, Mapstone[77] and Lowe[79,85] have advised against the use of adrenergic mydriatics based on the model of pupillary dilation shown in Figure 21.7. Adrenergic drugs augment the force of dilator contraction while leaving the force of sphincter contraction unaffected. The posterior component of the pupillary dilation force thus increases at the iris periphery while the medial component of the iris sphincter contraction persists[77,79] (Fig. 21.7C). Consequently, the total force available for causing pupillary block is greater than occurs when using an anticholinergic mydriatic for dilation. The contact between iris and lens at the pupillary margin increases, resulting in pupillary block with subsequent obstruction of aqueous flow from posterior to anterior chamber. This situation produces iris bombé with secondary angle closure.[79]

Although the risk of pupillary block is greater with the use of phenylephrine compared with tropicamide, dilation with the former is much more easily overcome with the use of miotics such as pilocarpine or dapiprazole.[83] The mydriatic effect of most adrenergic mydriatics is rapidly counteracted by pilocarpine in less than 30 minutes.[83] However, pilocarpine-induced miosis following dilation with phenylephrine should generally be avoided because the increased stimulation of the iris sphincter leads to angle closure in a significant proportion of eyes. The stimulation of the iris sphincter enhances the medial vector force and increases the contact between iris and lens.[30,79]

In contrast to the effects of pilocarpine, the use of adrenergic blocking agents following dilation with phenylephrine leaves the force of sphincter contraction unaffected but decreases the vector force of dilator contraction toward the lens. By inhibiting the dilator muscle and decreasing the component of the dilator contraction toward the lens, the total pupillary blocking forces decrease, and iris bombé and secondary angle closure become less probable.[77] Dapiprazole or thymoxamine can be used to counteract mydriasis following phenylephrine administration. The primary advantage of using dapiprazole or thymoxamine following dilation with phenylephrine is that it rapidly constricts the pupil, usually within 30 minutes, and thus prevents the pupil from remaining in the mid-dilated position.[30,86]

Sector Dilation. As an alternative to full dilation of the pupil, a procedure may be used that primarily dilates the inferior aspect of the pupil. Shaffer[76] first described sector dilation in 1967. A small, pear-shaped pupillary dilation can be obtained by placing in the inferior conjunctival sac a cotton pledget moistened with 1:1000 epinephrine or 2.5% phenylephrine. The pledget should remain for only 2 to 3 minutes lest too much drug delivery causes complete dilation of the pupil.[76,87] As the drug penetrates into the inferior aspect of the anterior chamber, it dilates the inferior pupillary zone and leaves the remainder of the pupil essentially

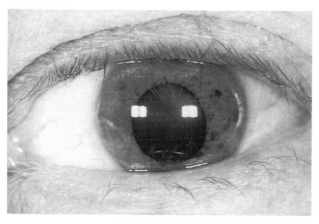

FIGURE 21.9   **Vertically oval pupil produced by sector dilation.**

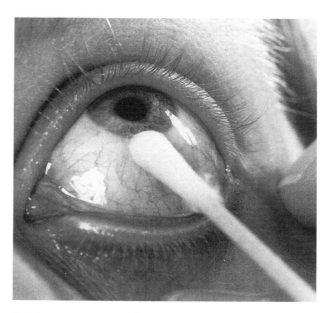

FIGURE 21.10   **Sector dilation technique using cotton-tipped applicator held at inferior limbus. Phenylephrine-moistened swab is applied for about 20 seconds.**

intact. A vertically oval pupil results (Fig. 21.9). Alternatively, the tip of a thin strip of filter paper (Schirmer strip) can be moistened with 2.5% phenylephrine and placed in the inferior conjunctival sac.[87,88] The paper should remain for only 1 minute, since longer contact may dilate the entire pupil. Locke and Meetz [89] have described another technique. After moistening a sterile cotton-tipped applicator with 2.5% phenylephrine, the swab is applied for approximately 20 seconds to the inferior limbus of the anesthetized eye (Fig. 21.10).

Tropicamide cannot be used for sector dilation because it tends to produce complete pupillary dilation even when used in low concentrations.[90]

Before sector dilation, the eye should be anesthetized topically to reduce subsequent lacrimation, which might dilute and spread the mydriatic.[88] The sectorially enlarged pupillary aperture obtained from sector dilation usually allows easy access to the posterior segment of the eye by enabling satisfactory binocular indirect ophthalmoscopy or other procedures requiring stereopsis.

Although this technique may not necessarily prevent angle closure, it does seem to reduce the risk of angle closure because of the minimal and brief focal dilation.[2,88]

Narrow Angle Following Surgical Iridectomy or Laser Iridotomy

Lowe[85] reported that when the pupils of eyes that have undergone peripheral iridectomy for acute angle-closure glaucoma are dilated with anticholinergic mydriatics such as cyclopentolate or tropicamide, 50% to 66% of eyes will develop angle closure. Despite the presence of a patent peripheral iridectomy, the anticholinergic agent induces angle closure by causing peripheral crowding of the iris against the trabeculum.[91] In such cases, the degree of angle closure generally relates to the magnitude of pupillary dilation. In contrast, dilation with phenylephrine or other adrenergic mydriatic does not cause peripheral folding of the iris and thus fails to produce angle closure.[79,85,92] In addition, phenylephrine has a relatively brief duration of action and permits rapid pupillary constriction without the need for a miotic.[79] The practitioner should ascertain, however, that the peripheral iridectomy or iridotomy is of full iris thickness because phenylephrine may induce angle closure if only the anterior portion of the iris has been removed or destroyed.[79]

Harris and Galin[93] have challenged the foregoing hypothesis regarding angle closure following dilation of eyes having undergone peripheral iridectomy. Using cyclopentolate, these investigators dilated numerous eyes following iridectomy for angle-closure glaucoma and found no drug-induced episode of angle closure. Since peripheral iridectomy or iridotomy removes the risk of pupillary block, precipitation of angle closure must be primary rather than secondary to pupillary block and iris bombé.[79,93] Eyes with plateau iris undergo angle closure by a mechanism involving crowding of the iris against the trabeculum rather than by a mechanism involving pupillary block.[93] Thus, mydriatic-induced angle closure despite a patent iridectomy may be associated with the plateau iris syndrome.[94] Wand and associates[94] have reported such cases to be extremely rare. Since the magnitude of pupillary dilation is the crucial factor, one would expect an equal incidence of angle closure with adrenergic and anticholinergic drugs if mydriasis of comparable magnitude is produced.[93] However, until further definitive studies are performed, use of adrenergic rather than anticholinergic mydriatics is probably wise for routine dilation of eyes having undergone surgical iridectomy or laser iridotomy for acute angle-closure glaucoma.[94]

Ectopia Lentis

Ectopia lentis commonly occurs as part of the syndrome of homocystinuria and Marfan's syndrome. Dilation of the pupil is often essential both for establishing the initial diagnosis and for adequate fundus examination. Because of the risk of precipitating pupillary-block glaucoma, these patients should be dilated in a supine position using a weak mydriatic such as 1% hydroxyamphetamine or 2.5% phenylephrine.[95] Wide pupillary dilation should generally be avoided because of the risk of subluxation of the lens into the anterior chamber. Following examination of the crystalline lens and fundus, the position of the lens should be inspected to confirm its position behind the iris plane. Once the lens is confirmed to be behind the iris, and with the patient still in a supine position, the mydriasis can be reversed by using a miotic such as 0.5% dapiprazole.

Effect of Iris Pigmentation

A common clinical impression is that eyes with greater pigmentation (i.e., darker irides) dilate more poorly than do eyes with less pigmentation (i.e., blue irides). Several investigators[96–98] have demonstrated a greater magnitude of mydriasis in eyes with light irides compared with dark irides. Other investigators,[14,27,99–101] however, have failed to find such differences, reporting equal mydriasis in light and dark irides. Richardson[99] has shown that the pupils in light irides are significantly larger than in dark irides before pupillary dilation, which may explain the somewhat larger pupillary diameters following dilation of light irides.

Effect of Cataract Surgery

Patients who have undergone intracapsular cataract extraction or extracapsular extraction with implantation of an intraocular lens often have pupils that dilate less well than preoperatively. The poorer pupillary response probably relates to the amount of iris trauma occurring at surgery.[102] The difference in mydriatic response may have practical importance in evaluating and treating peripheral retinal abnormalities in aphakic and pseudophakic eyes.

Clinical Procedures Facilitated by the Use of Mydriatics

Examination of Ocular Media

Dilation of the pupil allows more complete evaluation of the ocular media posterior to the iris plane by permitting detailed biomicroscopy of the crystalline lens and vitreous. The pupil must be dilated to examine the lens for cataract formation, since cortical spoking (Fig. 21.11), off-axis posterior subcapsular opacities (Fig. 21.12), and other opacities of the lens can be entirely overlooked without an adequately dilated pupil.[103,104] Exfoliation of the lens capsule (see Fig. 35.25) may also be overlooked with the pupil undilated. Posterior vitreous detachment (PVD) (Fig. 21.13) is the

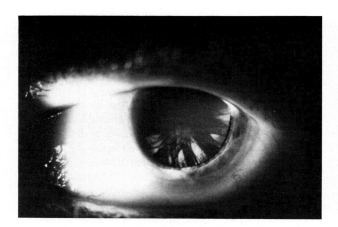

FIGURE 21.11   **Dilated pupil revealing cortical cataract. Visual acuity was 20/20 (6/6).**

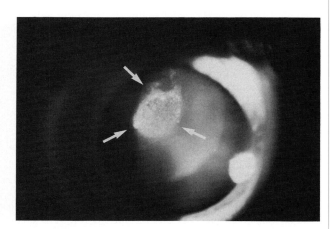

FIGURE 21.12   **Dilated pupil revealing off-axis posterior subcapsular cataract (arrows). Visual acuity was 20/20 (6/6).**

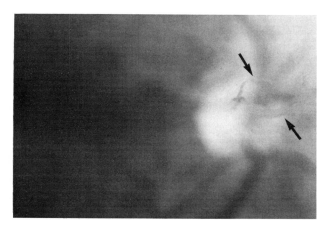

FIGURE 21.13 **Prepapillary glial ring (arrows) characteristic of posterior vitreous detachment.**

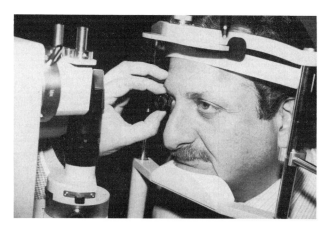

FIGURE 21.14 **Noncontact (90 D) condensing lens positioned near the cornea.**

most common cause of symptoms of flashes or floaters in patients over 50 years of age; pupillary dilation is essential for the diagnosis because it allows adequate stereoscopic examination of the vitreous using binocular indirect ophthalmoscopy or fundus biomicroscopy. Furthermore, the dilation of eyes with extremely dense cataract usually permits a satisfactory fundus evaluation, which might otherwise be impossible because of the small pupillary aperture in association with dense nuclear sclerosis or posterior subcapsular opacities.

Once the pupil has dilated, the practitioner can examine the lens and anterior vitreous directly with the slit lamp; use of a precorneal (60 to 90 D) condensing lens extends the range of the slit lamp into the mid and posterior vitreous.[105-110] The precorneal condensing lens is positioned near the cornea but without ocular contact (Fig. 21.14). Of the available biomicroscopic procedures, the precorneal condensing lens allows more rapid examination of the patient, since it does not require topical anesthesia, the use of gonioscopic bonding solution, or manipulation of the eye for contact lens insertion. The precorneal condensing lens, moreover, provides superior stereopsis and permits a large field of view (Table 21.7).[111] Certain precorneal lenses, such as the Volk Superfield NC, may enhance visualization of the vitreous and vitreoretinal interface.[152]

With the pupil dilated, the practitioner can also evaluate the ocular media by observing the red reflex with the retinoscope, direct ophthalmoscope, or slit lamp. Subtle opacities of the cornea, lens, or vitreous can often be detected more readily than with the pupil undilated. Observing the red reflex with the direct ophthalmoscope allows rapid and effective comparison of each eye with respect to the density of cataractous changes. Use of the binocular indirect ophthalmoscope, because of its large depth of focus, usually permits rapid detection of subtle vitreal changes, including PVD.

TABLE 21.7
Comparison of Fundus Biomicroscopy Techniques

	Hruby Lens	Fundus Contact Lens	90 D Lens
Field of view	Small	Larger	Largest
Image	Virtual erect	Virtual erect	Real inverted and reversed
Surface reflections	Many	Variable	Variable
Patient tolerance	Good	Variable	Good
Stereopsis	Good	Excellent	Excellent
Photography	Poor	Very good	Excellent

Modified from Gutner R, Cavallerano A, Wong D. Fundus biomicroscopy: A comparison of four methods. J Am Optom Assoc 1988; 59:388–390.

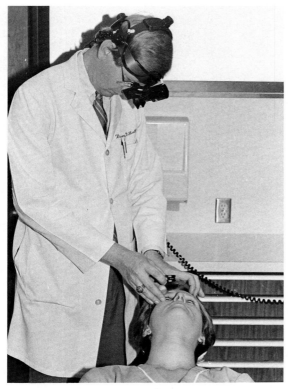

FIGURE 21.15   **Binocular indirect ophthalmoscopy entails use of a hand-held condensing lens and headborne ophthalmoscope. A + 20 D condensing lens is generally adequate, but a + 28 or + 30 D lens may be more satisfactory in patients with only minimal pupillary dilation.**

Fundus Examination

Almost without exception, definitive evaluation and diagnosis of diseases of the retina and choroid require dilation of the pupil. Once the pupil has dilated, stereoscopic observation of fundus lesions can take place, and various procedures may be used to evaluate these lesions fully. Slit-lamp techniques using the precorneal condensing lens help to evaluate lesions of the posterior pole including the macula and optic disc.[105–110] The three-mirror Goldmann lens, precorneal condensing lens, or contact lens system such as the Quadraspheric lens (Volk Optical) may be used to evaluate, using variable magnification and stereopsis, the equatorial and peripheral retina as far anteriorly as the ora serrata and ciliary body processes.[108,111–113] Unlike the direct or monocular indirect ophthalmoscopes, the binocular indirect ophthalmoscope (Fig. 21.15) allows a broad, panoramic view of the fundus while maintaining stereopsis (Table 21.8). These features enable rapid detection and evaluation of subtle changes in tissue texture, color, depth, or elevation. This significantly improves the evaluation and diagnosis of lesions such as retinal detachment, peripheral retinal disease predisposing to retinal detachment, and extensive disease processes such as presumed ocular histoplasmosis and central retinal vein occlusion. Binocular indirect ophthalmoscopy or fundus biomicroscopy also allows differentiation between clinically significant retinal disease and benign processes such as congenital hypertrophy of the retinal pigment epithelium and retinal pigment epithelial window defects. In some instances failure to dilate the pupil for fundus examination has resulted in serious retinal or choroidal disease being overlooked or mismanaged (Fig. 21.16).[114,115]

Fundus photography, including fluorescein angiography, must be performed with the pupil dilated to obtain satisfactory results. Although nonmydriatic cameras are available, these instruments do not consider the necessity for pupillary dilation to formulate a definitive diagnosis. Most fundus cameras are essentially monocular indirect ophthalmoscopes adapted for photographic purposes; dilation of the pupil therefore increases their effectiveness and use.[112,116]

Dilation before electroretinography (ERG) standardizes the results obtained from this electrophysiologic test. Most research and clinical electrophysiologic laboratories, therefore, incorporate pupillary dilation into the examination protocol.

TABLE 21.8
Comparison of Direct, Monocular Indirect, and Binocular Indirect Ophthalmoscopes

	Direct	*Monocular Indirect*	*Binocular Indirect*
Field of view	10° (1½ DD[a])	40° (8 DD[a])	40° (8 DD[a])
Image quality of peripheral fundus	Distorted	Good	Excellent
Stereopsis	Absent	Absent	Present
Image	Erect	Erect	Inverted and reversed
Mydriatic required	No, but helpful	No, but helpful	Yes

[a]DD, Disc diameter.
Modified from Garston MJ. The binocular indirect ophthalmoscope (BIO). J Am Optom Assoc 1977;48:1403–1407.

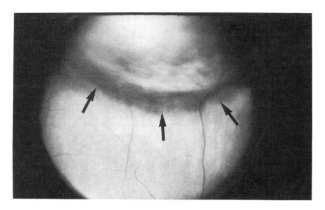

FIGURE 21.16   **Malignant melanoma of choroid (arrows) that was overlooked because the pupil was not dilated.**

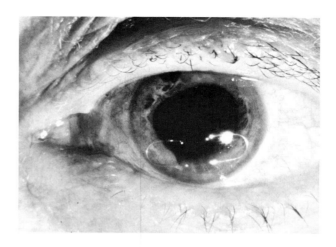

FIGURE 21.17   **Mydriatic-induced dislocation of an intraocular lens. (Copyright 1982, Competency Enhancement Programs. Reprinted with permission from the editors, from the collection of Herbert J. Nevyas, M.D.)**

Examination of Optic Disc

Stereoscopic observation of the optic disc is essential when evaluating abnormalities of the optic nerve head. Following dilation, binocular indirect ophthalmoscopy using the + 20 D condensing lens or, for greater magnification the + 14 D lens, permits satisfactory evaluation in many instances. However, fundus biomicroscopy using the precorneal condensing lens enables higher magnification while maintaining stereopsis.[105–110] These procedures allow detailed evaluation of unusual optic nerve head configurations such as coloboma or tilted disc syndrome. The capability of stereopsis with high magnification is especially important when evaluating subtle abnormalities such as optic disc edema, drusen, optic pits, and various glaucomatous nerve head changes.

Dilation of Pseudophakic Eyes

When the implantation of intraocular lenses (IOLs) became popular during the 1970s, it became clear that eyes with iris-supported lenses (Table 21.9) should not be dilated because of the risk of IOL dislocation (Fig. 21.17).[117,118] Wide dilation is possible, however, with all anterior and posterior chamber lenses (Fig. 21.18),[117,119] and dilation can be safely accomplished even if the IOL appears to be slightly malposi-

tioned. Dilation of the pupil does not change the IOL's position.[104]

Although rare, an important complication of mydriasis in pseudophakia is *pupillary capture*, in which the IOL becomes entrapped within the pupillary aperture and the pupil cannot return to its normal size following dilation (Fig. 21.19).[120] Several conditions can predispose the eye to pupillary capture, including damage to the crystalline lens zo-

TABLE 21.9
Classification of Intraocular Lenses

- Anterior chamber
- Iris supported
- Posterior chamber

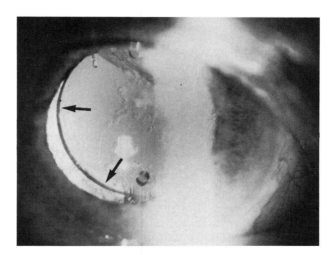

FIGURE 21.18   **Wide pupillary dilation of eye with posterior chamber intraocular lens. Arrows denote edge of lens.**

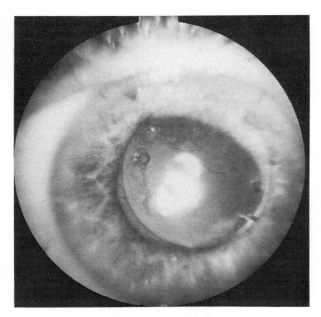

FIGURE 21.19   **Posterior chamber intraocular lens entrapped within the pupillary aperture following dilation. (Courtesy Hernan Benavides, O.D.)**

nules or capsular bag during surgery,[104] IOL fixation into the ciliary sulcus,[121] and the presence of nonangulated IOL haptics. The development of 10-degree haptic angulation has reduced the incidence of pupillary capture by positioning the IOL more deeply into the posterior chamber.[122] The increased flexibility of silicone posterior chamber IOLs may also predispose to forward movement during mydriasis.[123]

If pupillary capture persists, secondary complications can occur, including pupillary block glaucoma;[123] iris chafing; iris sphincter erosion; and disruption of the blood-aqueous barrier with secondary inflammation leading to corneal decompensation, cystoid macular edema, or hemorrhage.[122] Since pupillary capture rarely leads to vision loss, noninvasive corrective procedures should be used initially to reposition the IOL.

Pupillary dilation alone may correct the problem.[121] If the pupillary capture occurs with an anterior chamber lens, the patient should be placed in a supine position, and the pupil should be dilated with phenylephrine and then constricted with dapiprazole or thymoxamine. The force of gravity should maintain the iris behind the lens. Alternatively, a Zeiss four-mirror or Sussman gonioscope or tonometer prism can be forcibly applied to the cornea after the pupil has been dilated. This maneuver may displace the iris posteriorly, behind the plane of the anterior chamber IOL.[124]

To correct an entrapped posterior chamber IOL, the pupil should be dilated, dapiprazole or thymoxamine adminis-

tered, and the patient placed in a prone position, with the face downward. The force of gravity may position the iris in front of the IOL. As an alternative, gentle percussion of the globe can be performed by softly "tapping" the temporal side of the closed eyelids, or by exerting microhydraulic forces to the cornea with a Zeiss four-mirror or Sussman gonioscope. These forces are transmitted to the iris and IOL and may be sufficient to free small adhesions.[122] Other noninvasive procedures include external haptic manipulation with cotton-tipped applicators,[125] and mechanical shock-wave IOL retropulsion using the Nd:YAG laser.[126] Some cases may require direct surgical repositioning of the IOL.[127,128] Even after successful repositioning of the IOL, however, pupillary capture may recur. Consequently, the patient may benefit from long-term, low-dose pilocarpine therapy.[122]

The Plateau Iris

In 1960 Shaffer[129] first proposed and described the concept of plateau iris. Wand and associates[94] subsequently distinguished between *plateau iris configuration* and *plateau iris syndrome.* The former is defined as the preoperative finding of an anterior chamber of normal depth with a flat iris plane as observed directly with the slit lamp, but with an extremely narrow or closed angle by gonioscopy. The latter is defined as the postoperative finding of an anterior chamber of normal depth with a flat iris plane and patent iridectomy or iridotomy by direct slit-lamp examination, but with gonioscopically confirmed angle closure following dilation of the pupil.

Although the prevalence of plateau iris configuration is unknown, most authors believe that it is rare, and the plateau iris syndrome is considered even more uncommon.[94]

Plateau iris configuration results in angle closure by a mechanism independent of pupillary block.[94] Since the anterior chamber has normal depth and the iris plane is flat, little or no pupillary block occurs. Instead, dilation of the pupil causes a peripheral iris roll to approximate and close the angle, thus precipitating an attack of acute angle-closure glaucoma (Fig. 21.20).[91,94] In eyes with plateau iris syndrome, ultrasound biomicroscopy has demonstrated anteriorly positioned ciliary processes.[153] These processes provide structural support beneath the peripheral iris, thus preventing the iris root from falling away from the trabecular meshwork after iridectomy or iridotomy. Since the depth of the anterior chamber in these eyes does not provide a clue to the possible development of angle closure following dilation, gonioscopy is essential for the clinical diagnosis.[94] However, many practitioners and investigators believe that plateau iris configuration is difficult to detect even with carefully performed gonioscopy. In many cases, the diagnosis is made only after an apparently open angle has sustained

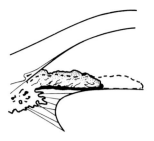

FIGURE 21.20   **Plateau iris. Dilation of the pupil causes the iris to obstruct aqueous outflow, thus causing acute angle-closure glaucoma.**

angle closure following pupillary dilation. Once the diagnosis is made, the practitioner should exercise caution with dilation, since the existence of plateau iris configuration preoperatively suggests a high risk for mydriatic-induced angle closure postoperatively. These eyes should generally be managed using continuous miotic therapy[94] or by laser peripheral iridoplasty.[130]

Postdilation Procedures

Monitoring Intraocular Pressure

The routine measurement of IOP following dilation of the pupil is unnecessary.[2] In nonglaucomatous patients with open angles, dilation with adrenergic mydriatics, such as phenylephrine, would not be expected to elevate IOP,[96] while dilation with relatively weak anticholinergic agents such as tropicamide would be expected to elevate IOP in only approximately 2% of patients.[64] In glaucomatous patients with open angles, approximately 25% to 33% of patients will demonstrate pressure elevations following dilation with anticholinergic drugs.[63,64] As previously discussed, these pressure elevations are associated with reduced aqueous outflow facility and are unrelated to any angle-closure mechanism.[63] Such pressure elevations are clinically insignificant, decline to normal levels within 4 to 6 hours, and do not require monitoring.[64] Thus, patients with open angles can be dismissed following dilation without regard to the IOP.

In contrast, monitoring IOP following dilation of eyes with narrow angles is reasonable and prudent.[2] The patient should remain in the office until the pupils have reached their predilation size, and IOP should be determined before dismissing the patient. If the patient leaves immediately following dilation, he or she should be advised of the symptoms of angle closure and cautioned to return to or telephone the practitioner's office in the event of such an attack.

Use of Miotics

The instillation of pilocarpine to counteract the effects of the mydriatic is inadvisable. When pilocarpine is used following dilation with phenylephrine, the relative pupillary block is likely to increase by the additional stimulation of the iris sphincter, which enhances the medial component of the sphincter force against the lens.[79] In addition, pilocarpine increases aqueous outflow through the trabecular meshwork, which, in the presence of pupillary block, might create a greater differential pressure between the anterior and posterior chambers and lead to iris bombé with secondary angle closure.[86,131] Pilocarpine can also reduce the depth of the anterior chamber, which exacerbates the factors causing angle closure.[132,133] These changes may predispose the eye to angle closure, even in eyes in which closure seems unlikely.[133]

Following dilation with anticholinergic mydriatics such as tropicamide, pilocarpine induces little or no miosis, and the pupil returns to its predilation size no more rapidly than without the miotic.[83,134] In addition, pilocarpine has no beneficial effect on amplitude of accommodation, and the miotic can even have a deleterious effect on distance visual acuity.[134] Thus, pilocarpine is usually ineffective in counteracting the dilation produced by anticholinergic mydriatics.

The use of α-adrenergic antagonists is an effective and safe alternative to cholinergic miotics. Dapiprazole 0.5% (Rev-Eyes) can reverse mydriasis induced by phenylephrine 2.5% or tropicamide 0.5% to 1% used alone or in combination.[135,136] The miosis produced by dapiprazole 0.5% begins 10 minutes after instillation, and almost one-half the pupils of treated eyes achieve their premydriatic diameter within 2 hours following dilation with phenylephrine 2.5% and tropicamide 1%.[135] Unlike miosis induced by pilocarpine, the α-receptor blockade produced by dapiprazole does not shift the lens-iris diaphragm forward; the anterior chamber depth remains constant; and accommodation is not stimulated. The most clinically significant side effects of dapiprazole are transient stinging or burning upon instillation, and conjunctival hyperemia lasting several hours in many patients.[135,137]

Thymoxamine, another α-adrenergic antagonist, can also reverse pharmacologically-induced mydriasis. When used in 0.1% solution, thymoxamine can reverse in about 2 hours the mydriasis produced by phenylephrine 2.5%.[138] Patients with lightly pigmented irides respond more rapidly than do those with dark irides.[138–140] When formulated in 0.5% solution, thymoxamine can completely reverse in 20 minutes the mydriasis induced by phenylephrine 2.5%.[141] It can also reverse the mydriatic effect of tropicamide 0.5%,[141,142] but only incompletely the effect of tropicamide 1%[142] or tropicamide 0.5% combined with phenylephrine 2.5%.[141] As with dapiprazole, the thymoxamine-related side effects of local irritation and conjunctival hyperemia are self-limiting.[140,142]

The use of mydriolytic agents such as dapiprazole or thymoxamine should be considered for patients with narrow

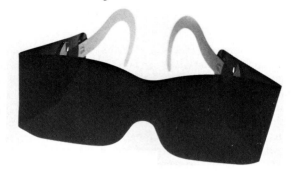

FIGURE 21.21   **Mydriatic spectacles protect the patient from light sensitivity after dilation.**

anterior chambers at risk of angle-closure glaucoma following dilation with phenylephrine.[138,140] These mydriolytics should also be offered for patients who are fearful of dilation or for those who have need of relatively uninterrupted vision immediately following the ocular examination. Mydriolytics are especially useful for patients with cataract or other media opacities, in whom light-induced glare can be problematic, and for patients with significant uncorrected hyperopia, in whom the mydriolytic may restore vision to acceptable levels before these patients attempt potentially hazardous activities such as driving.[137]

Mydriatic Spectacles

Because of increased sensitivity to light and in some instances frank photophobia, patients should have some form of protection while their pupils remain dilated. Commercially available paper sunglasses (Fig. 21.21) are inexpensive and can be discarded after the pupils have returned to normal. Without such protection, patients can be left significantly incapacitated. Patient objections to dilation frequently relate to a previous experience in which they received no protection from light.[2]

Pupillary Dilation as a Therapeutic Procedure

Nuclear Sclerotic or Posterior Subcapsular Cataract

By increasing the pupillary diameter, patients with central lens opacities such as nuclear sclerotic or posterior subcapsular cataract may experience significant improvement in visual acuity. This improvement can be evaluated in the office by determining visual acuity following pupillary dilation. If significant improvement occurs, the use of mydriatic therapy on a long-term basis may forestall the need for

cataract extraction. This approach may prove especially useful in debilitated patients or in patients otherwise at surgical risk because of systemic illness or contraindications to general or local anesthesia.

For this purpose, any mydriatic can be used, but preferably those agents that are less likely to elevate IOP. These include phenylephrine or low concentrations of tropicamide or homatropine. The effect on accommodation is relatively unimportant in elderly patients, but the cycloplegia may be an important consideration in younger patients. It is wise to evaluate IOP periodically during therapy with cycloplegic mydriatics.

Since cycloplegic mydriatics have a greater risk of elevating IOP than do adrenergic agents, it is wise to avoid cycloplegics for long-term dilation of eyes with open-angle glaucoma.[65] Phenylephrine, on the other hand, overcomes the effects of even strong miotics without compromising IOP.[65,68]

During long-term use of phenylephrine in elderly patients, the pupil may become progressively less responsive to the mydriatic effect.[75] This reduction in mydriasis, which is apparently an age-related phenomenon, may result from drug-induced damage to the iris dilator muscle[75] or to drug tolerance.

Uveitis

The primary purpose for pupillary dilation of eyes with anterior uveitis is to prevent the formation of posterior synechiae. Any mydriatic can accomplish this purpose, but the combination of atropine and phenylephrine acts synergistically to produce strong and wide mydriasis. This combination is also helpful in breaking posterior synechiae that have already developed.[75] Although posterior synechiae are less likely to develop with the iris in this fully dilated position because of less contact between iris and lens, nevertheless posterior synechiae can form.[75] Thus, most cases of uveitis should be treated with shorter-acting mydriatics such as homatropine or cyclopentolate rather than the longer-acting atropine. The shorter-acting agents allow the pupil mobility and consequently reduce the risk of developing posterior synechiae.

Complications

Blurred Vision

Patients generally encounter some degree of blurred vision following dilation because glare induced by light, spherical aberration associated with the large pupillary aperture, and accommodative paresis following use of a cycloplegic.[143] In the latter instance, patients likely to encounter blurred distance vision (driving difficulty) are limited to those with uncorrected nonpresbyopic hyperopia. Most other patients should not encounter significant difficulty with distance vision associated with pupillary dilation.[2]

For reading and other near visual activities following dilation, myopic patients remove their spectacles, and presbyopic patients can wear their reading lenses.[143] Thus, with proper instructions to the patient, significantly blurred vision following dilation is relatively uncommon.[2] When tropicamide has been used for dilation, most patients will recover reading ability within 1 to 3 hours, and virtually all patients will completely recover accommodation within 4 to 6 hours.[20,144,145] In many instances, patients never lose the ability to read.[20,100] Patients can therefore be reassured that any postdilation blurred vision will be transient.

Light Sensitivity

Mydriatic-induced light sensitivity can be problematic for many patients, especially those with cataracts or other opacities of the ocular media.[146–148] Troublesome glare and reduced contrast sensitivity function can severely limit visual activities following pupillary dilation. To help reduce sensitivity to light, a mydriolytic agent may be used, and the patient should have some form of protection from bright sunlight and other illuminated environments. Commercially available mydriatic spectacles (see Fig. 21.21) are designed specifically for this purpose.

Acute Angle-Closure Glaucoma

Although the prevalence of significantly narrow angles in the general population range from 2% to 6%,[11] Keller[149] estimates the risks of angle-closure glaucoma from the use of mydriatics at only 1 in 183,000 for the general population and only 1 in 45,000 for the population over 30 years of age. When a practical benefit-risk ratio approach is taken to the problem of potential angle closure following pupillary dilation, the low risk of angle closure should not prevent the practitioner from using mydriatics when necessary. Newell and Ernest[150] suggested that the greater danger is overlooking significant retinal disease by failure to dilate rather than of inducing angle closure by dilating. Halpern's[151] discovery of peripheral retinal breaks in 6% of 250 patients without symptoms supports this statement. By evaluating the anterior angle with slit lamp or gonioscopy, eyes predisposed to angle closure are readily identified, and appropriate mydriatics can usually be satisfactorily administered according to the guidelines previously discussed in this chapter.

Chapter 35 discusses the signs and symptoms as well as the definitive management of acute angle-closure glaucoma.

Systemic Complications

Although adverse systemic reactions to topically administered mydriatics do occur, dilation of the pupil is safe and without adverse sequelae in the vast majority of patients. The risk of adverse systemic reactions is greater in patients with certain systemic illnesses or in those taking certain systemic medications such as tricyclic antidepressants (see Table 21.6). There have been few reports of adverse systemic reactions associated with the use of 2.5% phenylephrine in recommended dosages. The potential for adverse reactions associated with the use of 10% phenylephrine increases in patients with cardiac disease, systemic hypertension, insulin-dependent diabetes, and idiopathic orthostatic hypotension.[50] In such patients who are predisposed to adverse cardiovascular events, the use of tropicamide either alone or in combination with hydroxyamphetamine provides satisfactory mydriasis while minimizing the risks of systemic complications.[19] In addition, the use of low concentrations of drug, single applications, and nasolacrimal occlusion also minimize adverse reactions in susceptible patients.

Chapter 38 considers the diagnosis and management of systemic complications associated with adrenergic mydriatics.

References

1. Barker A. The logia: Waiting room deluxe. Optom Manage 1979;15:147.
2. Bartlett JD. Pitfalls encountered in the clinical utilization of mydriatic drugs. South J Optom 1980;22:8–14.
3. Townsend WW. Incorporating ophthalmic pharmaceuticals into your practice. J Am Optom Assoc 1987;58:426–430.
4. Alexander LJ, Scholles J. Clinical and legal aspects of pupillary dilation. J Am Optom Assoc 1987;58:432–437.
5. Lewandowski PJ, Augsburger A. Frequency of pupil dilation by optometrists. N Engl J Optom 1992;44:7–9.
6. Olsen CL, Gerber TM, Kassoff A. Care of diabetic patients by optometrists in New York state. Diabetes Care 1991;14:34–41.
7. Classé JG. Pupillary dilation: An eye opening problem. J Am Optom Assoc 1992;63:733–741.
8. van Herick W, Shaffer RN, Schwartz A. Estimation of width of angle of anterior chamber. Incidence and significance of the narrow angle. Am J Ophthalmol 1969;68:626–629.
9. Bresler MJ, Hoffman RS. Prevention of iatrogenic acute narrow-angle glaucoma. Ann Emerg Med 1981;10:535–537.
10. Cockburn DM. Slit lamp estimate of anterior chamber depth as a predictor of the gonioscopic visibility of the angle structures. Am J Optom Physiol Opt 1982;59:904–908.
11. Cockburn DM. Prevalence and significance of narrow anterior chamber angles in optometric practice. Am J Optom Physiol Opt 1981;58:171–175.
12. Mapstone R. Outflow change in positive provocative tests. Br J Ophthalmol 1977;61:634–646.

13. Wilensky JT, Kaufman PL, Frohlichstein D, et al. Follow-up of angle-closure glaucoma suspects. Am J Ophthalmol 1993;115:338–346.

14. Apt L, Henrick A. Pupillary dilation with single eyedrop mydriatic combinations. Am J Ophthalmol 1980;89:553–559.

15. Caldwell JBH. Use of dilute drug solutions for routine cycloplegia and mydriasis (letter). Am J Ophthalmol 1979;87:727–728.

16. Lyle WM, Bobier WR. Effects of topical anesthetics on phenylephrine-induced mydriasis. Am J Optom Physiol Opt 1977;54:276–281.

17. Carlson DW, Tychsen L. Touching the cornea enhances pharmacologic dilation of the pupil, mainly in the dark iris. Aviat Space Environ Med 1989;60:994–995.

18. Borthne A, Davanger M. Mydriatics and age. Acta Ophthalmol 1971;49:380–387.

19. Semes LP, Bartlett JD. Mydriatic effectiveness of hydroxyamphetamine. J Am Optom Assoc 1982;53:899–904.

20. Levine L. Mydriatic effectiveness of dilute combinations of phenylephrine and tropicamide. Am J Optom Physiol Opt 1982;59:580–594.

21. Cable MK, Hendrickson RO, Hanna C. Evaluation of drugs in ointment for mydriasis and cycloplegia. Arch Ophthalmol 1978;96:84–86.

22. Molinari JF. A clinical comparison of mydriatics. J Am Optom Assoc 1983;54:781–784.

23. Geyer O, Godel V, Lazar M. The concurrent application of ophthalmic drops. Aust NZ J Ophthalmol 1985;13:63–66.

24. Levine L. Cyclomydril, a combination mydriatic. Oregon Optom 1981;48:5–7.

25. Larkin KM, Charap A, Cheetham JK, Frank J. Ideal concentration of tropicamide with hydroxyamphetamine 1% for routine pupillary dilation. Ann Ophthalmol 1989;21:340–344.

26. Doughty MJ, Lyle W, Trevino R, Flanagan J. A study of mydriasis produced by topical phenylephrine 2.5% in young adults. Can J Optom 1988;50:40.

27. Forman AR. A new low-concentration preparation for mydriasis and cycloplegia. Ophthalmology 1980;87:213–215.

28. Loewenstein A, Geyer O, Blanc A, Lazar M. Dosing problems in the use of topical ophthalmic drops. Graefe's Arch Clin Exp Ophthalmol 1992;230:378–379.

29. Feldman JB. Mydriatics. A clinical observation. Arch Ophthalmol 1949;41:42–59.

30. Mapstone R. Dilating dangerous pupils. Br J Ophthalmol 1977;61:517–524.

31. Maclean H. Reproducibility of mydriasis. Ophthalmic Res 1992;24(suppl 1):36–39.

32. Brooks AMV, West RH, Gillies WE. The risks of precipitating acute angle-closure glaucoma with the clinical use of mydriatic agents. Med J Aust 1986;145:34–36.

33. Levine L. Minimizing risk of adverse reactions to mydriatic agents in binocular indirect ophthalmoscopy. J Am Optom Assoc 1985;56:542–548.

34. Lee PF. Congenital glaucoma. In: Feman SS, Reinecke RD, eds. Handbook of pediatric ophthalmology. New York: Grune & Stratton, 1978:88.

35. Caputo AR, Schnitzer RE, Lindquist TD, et al. Dilation in neonates: A protocol. Pediatrics 1982;69:77–79.

36. Wesson MD, Bartlett JD, Swiatocha J, Woolley T. Mydriatic efficacy of a cycloplegic spray in the pediatric population. J Am Optom Assoc 1993;64:637–640.

37. Ismail EE, Rouse MW, DeLand PN. A comparison of drop instillation and spray application of 1% cyclopentolate hydrochloride. Optom Vis Sci 1994;71:235–241.

38. Reibaldi A, Santocono M, Scuderi A, Pizzo G. Retinopathy of prematurity (ROP): Optimal timing of clinical evaluation and standard procedures. Doc Ophthalmol 1990;74:229–234.

39. Caputo AR, Schnitzer RE. Systemic response to mydriatic eyedrops in neonates: Mydriatics in neonates. J Pediatr Ophthalmol Strabismus 1978;15:109–122.

40. Rosales T, Isenberg S, Leake R, et al. Systemic effects of mydriatics in low weight infants. J Pediatr Ophthalmol Strabismus 1981;18:42–44.

41. Bolt B, Benz B, Korner F, Bossi E. A mydriatic eyedrop combination without systemic effects for premature infants: A prospective double-blind study. J Pediatr Ophthalmol Strabismus 1992;29:157–162.

42. Isenberg SJ, Abrams C, Hyman PE. Effects of cyclopentolate eyedrops on gastric secretory function in pre-term infants. Ophthalmology 1985;92:698–700.

43. Bauer CR, Trottier MCT, Stern L. Systemic cyclopentolate (Cyclogyl) toxicity in the newborn infant. J Pediatr 1973;82:501–505.

44. Isenberg S, Everett S, Parelhoff E. A comparison of mydriatic eyedrops in low-weight infants. Ophthalmology 1984;91:278–279.

45. Carpel EF, Kalina RE. Pupillary responses to mydriatic agents in premature infants. Am J Ophthalmol 1973;75:988–991.

46. Bates JH, Burnstine RA. Consequences of retinopathy of prematurity examinations. Arch Ophthalmol 1987;105:618–619.

47. Fraunfelder FT, Scafidi AF. Possible adverse effects from topical ocular 10% phenylephrine. Am J Ophthalmol 1978;85:447–453.

48. Brown MM, Brown GC, Spaeth GL. Lack of side effects from topically administered 10% phenylephrine eyedrops. A controlled study. Arch Ophthalmol 1980;98:487–489.

49. Chang FW. Pharmacology of mydriasis for modern optometric procedures. J Am Optom Assoc 1977;48:365–368.

50. Robertson D. Contraindication to the use of ocular phenylephrine in idiopathic orthostatic hypotension. Am J Ophthalmol 1979;87:819–822.

51. Sneddon JM, Turner P. The interactions of local guanethidine and sympathomimetic amines in the human eye. Arch Ophthalmol 1969;81:622–627.

52. Sacks B, Smith S. People with Down's syndrome can be distinguished on the basis of cholinergic dysfunction. J Neurol Neurosurg Psych 1989;52:1294–1295.

53. Straub RH, Jeron A, Kerp L. The pupillary light reflex: 2. Prevalence of pupillary autonomic neuropathy in diabetics using age-dependent and age-independent pupillary parameters. Ophthalmology 1992;204:143–148.

54. Clark CV. Ocular autonomic nerve function in proliferative diabetic retinopathy. Eye 1988;2:96–101.

55. Fulk GW, Bower A, McBride K, Boatright R. Sympathetic denervation of the iris dilator in noninsulin-dependent diabetes. Optom Vis Sci 1991;68:954–956.

56. Kim JM, Stevenson CE, Mathewson HS. Hypertensive reactions to phenylephrine eyedrops in patients with sympathetic denervation. Am J Ophthalmol 1978;85:862–868.

57. Smith SA, Smith SE. Evidence for a neuropathic aetiology in the small pupil of diabetes mellitus. Br J Ophthalmol 1983;67:89–93.

58. Thompson HS. 12th pupil colloquium (report). Am J Ophthalmol 1981;92:435–436.

59. Bryant RC. Pupil motility in long-term diabetes (letter). Diabetologia 1980;18:170–171.

60. Huber MJE, Smith SA, Smith SE. Mydriatic drugs for diabetic patients. Br J Ophthalmol 1985;69:425–427.

61. Beasley H. Retinal detachments secondary to miotics. Symposium on drug-induced ocular side effects and ocular toxicology. Little Rock, AR: Sept. 10, 1977.

62. Rebolleda G, Munoz FJ, Fernandez Victorio JM, et al. Effects of pupillary dilation on automated perimetry in glaucoma patients receiving pilocarpine. Ophthalmology 1992;99:418–423.

63. Harris LS, Galin MA. Cycloplegic provocative testing. Effect of miotic therapy. Arch Ophthalmol 1969;81:544–547.

64. Harris LS. Cycloplegic-induced intraocular pressure elevations. A study of normal and open-angle glaucomatous eyes. Arch Ophthalmol 1968;79:242–246.

65. Schimek RA, Lieberman WJ. The influence of Cyclogyl and Neosynephrine on tonographic studies of miotic control in open-angle glaucoma. Am J Ophthalmol 1961;51:781–784.

66. Shaw BR, Lewis RA. Intraocular pressure elevation after pupillary dilation in open angle glaucoma. Arch Ophthalmol 1986;104:1185–1188.

67. Hill RA, Minckler DS, Lee M, et al. Apraclonidine prophylaxis for postcycloplegic intraocular pressure spikes. Ophthalmology 1991;98:1083–1086.

68. Becker B, Gage T, Kolker AE, et al. The effect of phenylephrine hydrochloride on the miotic-treated eye. Am J Ophthalmol 1959;48:313–321.

69. Kristensen P. Mydriasis-induced pigment liberation in the anterior chamber associated with acute rise in intraocular pressure in open-angle glaucoma. Acta Ophthalmol 1965;43:714–724.

70. Valle O. The cyclopentolate provocative test in suspected or untreated open-angle glaucoma. III. The significance of pigment for the result of the cyclopentolate provocative test in suspected or untreated open-angle glaucoma. Acta Ophthalmol 1976;54:654–664.

71. Lundvall A. Zetterstrom C. Exfoliation syndrome and the effect of phenylephrine and pilocarpine on pupil size. Acta Ophthalmol 1993;71:177–180.

72. Carpel EF. Pupillary dilation in eyes with pseudoexfoliation syndrome. Am J Ophthalmol 1988;105:692–694.

73. Dark AJ. Cataract extraction complicated by capsular glaucoma. Br J Ophthalmol 1979;63:465–468.

74. Ghosh M, Speakman JS. The iris in senile exfoliation of the lens. Can J Ophthalmol 1974;9:289.

75. Davidson SI. Mydriatic and cycloplegic drugs. Trans Ophthalmol Soc UK 1976;96:327–329.

76. Shaffer RN. Problems in the use of autonomic drugs in ophthalmology. In: Leopold IH, ed. Ocular therapy: Complications and management. St. Louis: C.V. Mosby Co, 1967;2:18–23.

77. Mapstone R. Mechanics of pupil block. Br J Ophthalmol 1968;52:19–25.

78. Anderson DR, Jin JC, Wright MM. The physiologic characteristics of relative pupillary block. Am J Ophthalmol 1991;111:344–350.

79. Lowe RF. Angle-closure, pupil dilation, and pupil block. Br J Ophthalmol 1966;50:385–389.

80. Mapstone R. The syndrome of closed-angle glaucoma. Br J Ophthalmol 1976;60:120–123.

81. Havener WH. Synopsis of ophthalmology. St. Louis: C.V. Mosby Co, 1975;4:490–494.

82. Mapstone R. Safe mydriasis. Br J Ophthalmol 1970;54:690–692.

83. Anastasi LM, Ogle KN, Kearns TP. Effect of pilocarpine in counteracting mydriasis. Arch Ophthalmol 1968;79:710–715.

84. Ophthalmic drug facts. St. Louis: Facts and Comparisons, 1995.

85. Lowe RF. Primary angle-closure glaucoma. Investigations using 10% phenylephrine eyedrops. Am J Ophthalmol 1965;60:415–419.

86. Bartlett JD, Hogan T, McDaniel D, Voce M. Study of three different treatment regimens of dapiprazole HCl in the reversal of mydriasis induced by 2.5% phenylephrine. Invest Ophthalmol Vis Sci 1994;35(suppl):1546.

87. Chang FW, McCan TA, Hitchcock JR. Sector pupil dilation with phenylephrine and tropicamide. Am J Optom Physiol Opt 1985;62:482–486.

88. Bienfang DC. Sector pupillary dilation with an epinephrine strip. Am J Ophthalmol 1973;75:883–884.

89. Locke LC, Meetz R. Sector pupillary dilation: An alternative technique. Optom Vis Sci 1990;67:291–296.

90. Chang FW, Temme BA, Hitchcock JR. Effects of decreasing concentrations of tropicamide on sector pupil dilation. Am J Optom Physiol Opt 1986;63:804–806.

91. Lowe RF. Persistent symptoms after peripheral iridectomy for angle-closure glaucoma. Aust NZ J Ophthalmol 1987;15:83–87.

92. Mapstone R. Partial angle closure. Br J Ophthalmol 1977;61:525–530.

93. Harris LS, Galin MA. Cycloplegic provocative testing. Arch Ophthalmol 1969;81:356–358.

94. Wand M, Grant WM, Simmons RJ, et al. Plateau iris syndrome. Trans Am Acad Ophthalmol Otol 1977;83:122–130.

95. Hagee MJ. Homocystinuria and ectopia lentis. J Am Optom Assoc 1984;55:269–276.

96. Haddad NJ, Moyer NJ, Riley FC. Mydriatic effect of phenylephrine hydrochloride. Am J Ophthalmol 1970;70:729–733.

97. Gambill HD, Ogle KN, Kearns TP. Mydriatic effect of four drugs determined with pupillograph. Arch Ophthalmol 1967;77:740–746.

98. Emiru VP. Response to mydriatics in the African. Br J Ophthalmol 1971;55:538–543.

99. Richardson RW. Comparing the mydriatic effect of tropicamide with respect to iris pigmentation. J Am Optom Assoc 1982;53:885–887.

100. Dillon JR, Tyhurst CW, Yolton RL. The mydriatic effect of tropicamide on light and dark irides. J Am Optom Assoc 1977;48:653–658.

101. Levine L. Tropicamide-induced mydriasis in densely pigmented eyes. Am J Optom Physiol Opt 1983;60:673–677.

102. Gibbens MV, Goel R, Smith SE. Effect of cataract extraction on the pupil response to mydriatics. Br J Ophthalmol 1989;73:563–565.

103. Dziadul J, Teague B, Oshinskie L, et al. A comparison of lens disorders using undilated and dilated biomicroscopy. N Engl J Optom 1988;40:15–17.

104. Amos JF, Semes LP, Swanson MW, Thurschwell LM. Pupillary dilation for aphakic patients, pseudophakic patients, and patients with cataract. Optom Clin 1991;1:188–194.

105. Gutner R, Cavallerano A, Wong D. Fundus biomicroscopy: A comparison of four methods. J Am Optom Assoc 1988;59:388–390.

106. Cavallerano A, Gutner R, Garston M. Indirect biomicroscopy techniques. J Am Optom Assoc 1986;57:755–758.

107. Barker FM. The Volk steady mount holder for the +90 D lens. J Am Optom Assoc 1988;59:558–560.

108. Barker FM. Vitreoretinal biomicroscopy: A comparison of techniques. J Am Optom Assoc 1987;58:985–992.

109. Jackson JE, Fisher M. Evaluation of the posterior pole with a 90 D lens and the slit-lamp biomicroscope. South J Optom 1987;5:80–83.

110. Lundberg C. Biomicroscopic examination of the ocular fundus with a +60-diopter lens. Am J Ophthalmol 1985;99:490–491.

111. Wing JT, Barker FM. Auxillary lenses in fundus biomicroscopy–a comparison of fields of view. J Am Optom Assoc 1990;61:544–547.

112. Houston G. Peripheral fundus photography using the Volk 90 diopter lens. South J Optom 1988;6:13–15.

113. Barker FM, Wing JT. Ultra wide field fundus biomicroscopy with the Volk Quadraspheric lens. J Am Optom Assoc 1990;61:573–575.

114. Semes L, Gold A. Clinical and legal considerations in the diagnosis and management of ocular tumors. J Am Optom Assoc 1987;58:134–139.

115. Siegel BS, Thompson AK, Yolton DP, et al. A comparison of diagnostic outcomes with and without pupillary dilation. J Am Optom Assoc 1990;61:25–34.

116. Houston G. Fundus photography using the Volk 90 D lens. South J Optom 1988;6:23–26.

117. Phillips LJ. Implants (letter). Rev Optom 1981;118:12.

118. Hamburger HA, Lerner L. Surgical treatment of dislocated iris-plane intraocular lenses. Ann Ophthalmol 1985;17:434–436.

119. Devita VJ, Gentile RS. Examination of the pseudophakic patient. J Am Optom Assoc 1985;56:103–107.

120. Nevyas HJ. How to manage the cataract patient. Rev Optom 1986;123:46–52.

121. Bucci FA, Lindstrom RL. Total pupillary capture with a foldable silicone intraocular lens. Ophthalmic Surg 1991;22:414–415.

122. Bowman CB, Hansen SO, Olson RJ. Noninvasive repositioning of a posterior chamber intraocular lens following pupillary capture. J Cataract Refract Surg 1991;17:843–847.

123. Marcus DM, Azar D, Boerner C, Hunter DG. Pupillary capture of a flexible silicone posterior chamber intraocular lens. Arch Ophthalmol 1992;110:609.

124. Wilcox TK. Release of an iris captured IOL following gonioscopy. South J Optom 1987;5:27.

125. Lindstrom RL, Herman WK. Pupil capture: Prevention and management. Am Intra-Ocular Implant Soc J 1983;9:201–204.

126. Stinert RF, Puliafito CA. New applications of the Nd:YAG laser. Am Intra-ocular Implant Soc J 1984;10:372–376.

127. Panton RW, Sulewski ME, Parker JS, et al. Surgical management of subluxed posterior-chamber intraocular lenses. Arch Ophthalmol 1993;111:919–926.

128. Rollins L. Repositioning of subluxated intraocular lenses. South J Optom 1993;11:19–20.

129. Shaffer RN. Gonioscopy, ophthalmoscopy, and perimetry. Trans Am Acad Ophthalmol Otol 1960;64:112–127.

130. Ritch R, Lowe RF, Reyes A. Therapeutic overview of angle-closure glaucoma. In: Ritch R, Shields MB, Krupin T, eds. The glaucomas. St. Louis: C.V. Mosby Co, 1989;855–864.

131. Gorin G. Angle-closure glaucoma induced by miotics. Am J Ophthalmol 1966;62:1063–1067.

132. Francois J, Goes F. Ultrasonographic study of the effect of different miotics on the eye components. Ophthalmologica 1977;175:328–338.

133. Wilkie J, Drance SM, Schulzer M. The effects of miotics on anterior-chamber depth. Am J Ophthalmol 1969;68:78–83.

134. Nelson ME, Orton HP. Counteracting the effects of mydriatics. Does it benefit the patient? Arch Ophthalmol 1987;105:486–489.

135. Allinson RW, Gerber DS, Biber S, Hodes BL. Reversal of mydriasis by dapiprazole. Ann Ophthalmol 1990;22:131–138.

136. Nyman N, Keats EU. Effects of dapiprazole on the reversal of pharmacologically induced mydriasis. Optom Vis Sci 1990;67:705–709.

137. Bartlett JD, Classe JG. Dapiprazole: Will it affect the standard of care for pupillary dilation? Optom Clin 1992;2:113–120.

138. Wright MM, Skuta GL, Drake MV, et al. Time course of thymoxamine reversal of phenylephrine-induced mydriasis. Arch Ophthalmol 1990;108:1729–1732.

139. Diehl DLC, Robin AL, Wand M. The influence of iris pigmentation on the miotic effect of thymoxamine. Am J Ophthalmol 1991;111:351–355.

140. Relf SJ, Gharagozloo NZ, Skuta GL, et al. Thymoxamine reverses phenylephrine-induced mydriasis. Am J Ophthalmol 1988;106:251–255.

141. Shah B, Hubbard B, Stewart-Jones JH, Edgar DF. Influence of thymoxamine eyedrops on the mydriatic effect of tropicamide and phenylephrine alone and in combination. Ophthal Physiol Opt 1989;9:153–155.

142. McKinna H, Stewart-Jones JH, Edgar DF, Turner P. Reversal of tropicamide-induced mydriasis by thymoxamine eyedrops. Curr Med Res Opin 1988;11:1–3.

143. Montgomery DMI, Macewan CJ. Pupil dilatation with tropicamide. The effects on acuity, accommodation, and refraction. Eye 1989;3:845–848.

144. Pollack SL, Hunt JS, Polse KA. Dose-response effects of tropicamide HCl. Am J Optom Physiol Opt 1981;58:361–366.

145. Gettes BC. Tropicamide, a new cycloplegic mydriatic. Arch Ophthalmol 1961;65:48–51.

146. Adamsons I, Rubin GS, Vitale S, et al. The effects of early cataracts on glare and contrast sensitivity. A pilot study. Arch Ophthalmol 1992;110:1081–1086.

147. Drews-Bankiewicz MA, Caruso RC, Datiles MB, Kaiser-Kupfer MI. Contrast sensitivity in patients with nuclear cataracts. Arch Ophthalmol 1992;110:953–959.

148. Lasa MSM, Datiles MB, Podgor MJ, Magno BV. Contrast and glare sensitivity. Association with the type and severity of the cataract. Ophthalmology 1992;99:1045–1049.

149. Keller JT. The risk of angle closure from the use of mydriatics. J Am Optom Assoc 1975;46:19–21.

150. Newell FW, Ernest JT. Ophthalmology: Principles and concepts. St. Louis: C.V. Mosby Co, 1974;3:150.

151. Halpern JI. Routine screening of the retinal periphery. Am J Ophthalmol 1966;62:99–102.

152. Cavallerano AA, Gutner RK, Semes LP. Enhanced non-contact examination of the vitreous and retina. J Am Optom Assoc 1994;65:231–234.

153. Pavlin CJ, Ritch R, Foster FS. Ultrasound biomicroscopy in plateau iris syndrome. Am J Ophthalmol 1992;113:390–395.

CHAPTER 22

Cycloplegic Refraction

John F. Amos
David M. Amos

Although new methods of refraction have been developed over the years, cycloplegic refraction has remained a time-tested, reliable and valid procedure for obtaining significant data on specific refractive patients. Without cycloplegic drugs, determining the true refractive status of patients with accommodative esotropia, pseudomyopia, or latent hyperopia would be fraught with error. In noncommunicative or uncooperative patients, those with functional vision problems, visual acuity not corrected to an expected level, or inconsistent responses or symptoms, and in patients with aberrations or opacification of the ocular media, cycloplegia often proves essential for the proper diagnosis of refractive errors.

This chapter considers the indications, precautions, and contraindications associated with the use of cycloplegics in refraction. The chapter also discusses selecting the appropriate cycloplegic agent, procedures for refraction, and principles of spectacle prescribing.

Indications and Advantages

Cycloplegia plays a very important role in the refractive examination of young patients. Although certainly not indicated for every child, in numerous clinical situations cycloplegia can supply the practitioner with information that could not otherwise be obtained. For patients who have definite visual symptoms, performing a cycloplegic refraction is almost always advisable.[1]

Cycloplegic refraction is indicated in individuals whose total refractive error does not manifest itself in the course of a subjective noncycloplegic examination. The reasons for determining this latent refractive error are practical ones. In young patients with suspected accommodative esotropia, determining the full amount of hyperopia is vital in order to prescribe plus power lenses to relieve the effort placed on the accommodative-convergence system and, in turn, bring the eyes into alignment. As discussed later in this chapter, the full amount of plus lens correction may not be prescribed, especially for children over 4 to 6 years of age, but the value derived from the cycloplegic examination serves as an initial starting point that is then modified by clinical judgment and experience.

In a more general sense, cycloplegic refraction is also indicated in young patients who demonstrate any problem with ocular motility. Not only does cycloplegia allow the clinician to diagnose correctly any accompanying refractive error, but it prepares the patient for a dilated fundus examination. All young strabismic patients should have such a thorough evaluation, at least when initially examined. This evaluation can rule out an occult etiology of the ocular deviation and can conveniently be incorporated into the examination following the cycloplegic refraction, while the pupils are still dilated.

Nonstrabismic children with latent hyperopia are perhaps less obvious in their presentation, but this is another instance in which information gained by cycloplegic examination is essential to the ultimate management plan. When considering the amount of total hyperopia in conjunction with the patient's signs and symptoms, a successful spectacle prescription can be determined more accurately.

Because patients age 3 years and younger often have unreliable responses during subjective refraction, it is wise to use a cycloplegic-assisted examination in these children. Clearly, as an objective method for determining refractive error in children between the ages of 18 and 48 months, cycloplegic techniques are superior to noncycloplegic ones.[2–4] Not only is cycloplegic retinoscopy of young children and infants more accurate, it is also more easily performed, since the examination does not depend on the patient's position and fixation distance.

The clinician may consider using cycloplegics in all children who exhibit myopia for the first time. This approach allows the practitioner to rule out accommodative spasm (pseudomyopia) as the etiologic source. With the diagnosis of myopia established, future cycloplegic examinations can be excluded for a cooperative child. A still broader recommendation comes from Duke-Elder and Abrams,[5] who advised that nonmyopic patients up to the age of 16 years have a cycloplegic refraction. Many other clinicians disagree. However, since all children should have a thorough funduscopic evaluation, the use of drugs for pupillary dilation that also allow substantial cycloplegia facilitates both the fundus evaluation and the refraction.

Cycloplegic refraction is also indicated for patients with active accommodative systems whose best-corrected visual acuity in each eye is less than 20/20 (6/6) and for whom there is no apparent reason for the decreased vision. It allows the clinician to determine whether an uncorrected refractive error is responsible for the decreased visual acuity.

Patients may benefit from a cycloplegic examination if they demonstrate no known ocular disease but are impaired or handicapped so that they are unresponsive or inconsistent in their responses to subjective refraction. Indeed, this may be the only way the clinician can determine the degree of refractive error, if any. In a similar category are suspected malingering or hysterical patients. The clinician can avoid the unreliable patient's subjective responses and arrive at objective refractive data through the use of cycloplegics.

Finally, patients whose visual signs or symptoms do not correlate with the nature and degree of their manifest refractive error may benefit from cycloplegic refraction. A cycloplegic refraction aids in the differential diagnosis by helping to ensure that the patient's problem is not refractive. The clinician can then concentrate on other aspects of the visual system. Table 22.1 summarizes the indications for cycloplegic refraction.

Disadvantages

Despite the previously mentioned advantages of cycloplegic refraction, it does have some disadvantages. Wide dilation of the pupil can create excessive spherical aberration in the ocular media, resulting in difficult retinoscopy and refraction. This situation is especially true when synergistic agents such as hydroxyamphetamine or phenylephrine are used to

TABLE 22.1
Indications for Cycloplegic Refraction

- Accommodative esotropia (any age)
- All children under 3 years of age
- Suspected latent hyperopia
- Suspected pseudomyopia
- Uncooperative patients
- Noncommunicative patients
- Patients whose subjective responses during the manifest refraction are variable and inconsistent
- Suspected malingering
- Suspected hysterical amblyopia
- Visual acuity not corrected to predicted level
- Strabismic children (other than accommodative esotropia)
- Patients whose symptoms seem unrelated to the nature or degree of the manifest refractive error

permit fundus examination following the retinoscopy. In addition, an allowance for ciliary tonus is usually necessary, and the clinician must consider this allowance to determine the appropriate refractive correction for each patient. The accommodative-convergence relationship must be considered before cycloplegia. Furthermore, since all cycloplegic drugs have potential side effects, caution must be exercised in their use. Cycloplegics may blur vision for 1 to 3 days or longer, and sunlight or any bright light can be extremely annoying even with the use of sunglasses.

Precautions and Contraindications

Before administering a cycloplegic agent, the clinician should perform a preinstillation ocular evaluation. This evaluation not only protects the clinician legally, but also provides valuable information regarding contraindications to the indicated drug(s). Moreover, it furnishes certain baseline clinical information that may be unobtainable after cycloplegia. The following information and procedures are usually obtained as part of the comprehensive eye examination. They constitute the minimum examination recommended before instilling a cycloplegic agent.

- Medical and ocular history, with particular emphasis on present medications, allergies, drug reactions, and previous eye examinations
- Visual acuity at distance and near
- Pupillary examination
- Motility evaluation
- Manifest ("dry") refraction
- Accommodative function, if desired
- Accommodative-convergence relationships, if desired

- Slit-lamp evaluation with particular attention to the anterior chamber depth, and an estimation of the anterior angle by penlight or van Herick's classification[6] (see Chapter 21)
- Tonometry, if possible
- Gonioscopy, if a shallow anterior chamber is observed or suspected[7]

Some of these tests are often not practical or possible with infants or uncooperative children unless performed under general anesthesia. A penlight estimation of the anterior chamber depth (see Chapter 21) can give the practitioner a reasonable idea regarding the safety of pupillary dilation without the necessity of resorting to examination under anesthesia.

Cycloplegia is contraindicated in patients with a history of angle-closure glaucoma. Atropine, in particular, should be used with caution in patients with Down's syndrome and in patients receiving systemic anticholinergic drugs. Any known sensitivity to a specific cycloplegic agent can often be bypassed by substituting another cycloplegic, as discussed below. In addition, some authors recommend obtaining patient or parental consent before administering cycloplegics[8] (see Chapter 5).

Selection and Use of Specific Cycloplegic Agents

All cycloplegics exhibit anticholinergic properties by blocking the response to acetylcholine at the receptor sites on the smooth ocular muscles innervated by post-ganglionic cho-linergic nerves.[9] Clinically this anticholinergic response appears as some degree of pupillary dilation and cycloplegia.

Cycloplegics, to be clinically useful, should ideally possess the following properties:[10,11]

- Rapid onset of cycloplegia
- Complete paralysis of accommodation
- Adequate duration of maximum cycloplegia
- Rapid recovery of accommodation
- Absence of side effects

Although no cycloplegic agent meets all these criteria, the more recently developed agents satisfactorily achieve the desired clinical purpose with a minimum of disadvantages. Table 22.2 lists the common cycloplegic agents in current use. Chapter 9 discusses in greater detail the pharmacologic properties of cycloplegic agents.

Atropine

Atropine, a drug from the order Solanaceae, has been known since biblical times. Its source is the plant *Atropa belladonna*, whose berry ripens to a black color, giving rise to its common name "deadly nightshade." It was used as a cosmetic in Renaissance Italy and as a mydriatic in Spain.[12] The name *belladonna*, "beautiful lady," apparently arose from these uses where cosmetics and dilated pupils were regarded as signs of beauty, perhaps associated with the youthful look of innocence. Atropine's cycloplegic effect was not described until 1811 by Wells. This was the only topical ophthalmic drug available for mydriasis or cyclople-

TABLE 22.2
Clinical Characteristics of Common Cycloplegic Agents

Cycloplegic Agent	Commonly Used Concentration (%)	Dosage	Onset of Maximum Cycloplegic Effect	Duration of Cycloplegic Effect	Relative Residual Accommodation
Atropine sulfate (ointment or solution)	½[a]	1 gt t.i.d.[b] for 3 days before refraction *or*	3–6 hours	10–18 days	Negligible
	1	1 gt t.i.d.[b] for 1 day before refraction (see text)			
Scopolamine hydrobromide	0.25	1 gt, repeated in 20 minutes	60 minutes	5–7 days	Negligible
Cyclopentolate hydrochloride	1[c] 2	1 gt, repeated in 10 minutes	20–30 minutes	8–24 hours	Minimal
Tropicamide hydrochloride	1	1 gt, repeated every 5 minutes for 3 instillations	20–30 minutes	4–8 hours	Moderate

[a]Recommended ointment concentration.
[b]Atropine solution; ointment formulation should be instilled b.i.d.
[c]Recommended concentration for most clinical purposes.

gia until the 1950s. Thus, much of the older population's resistance to dilation may relate to its experience with atropine and the duration of its effect on vision.

Atropine cycloplegia occurs within 1 hour of administration. Maximum cycloplegia is usually achieved within 6 hours, and accommodation is inhibited for 10 to 18 days. As occurs with most cycloplegics, darkly pigmented irides are often more resistant to atropine than are lightly pigmented irides. In addition, atropine produces mydriasis that may last for 14 to 21 days. The degree of mydriasis frequently proves unreliable in judging the degree of cycloplegia. Atropinized patients often exhibit relatively poor mydriasis while sustaining complete paralysis of accommodation. This condition seems especially true for patients with darkly pigmented irides.

Atropine is currently available in 0.5% to 3% solution and 0.5% and 1% ointment. The ointment has the advantage of allowing effective cycloplegia while decreasing systemic drug absorption, which minimizes systemic side effects. The traditional dosage for the refraction of patients with accommodative esotropia is 1% atropine solution 3 times daily or 0.5% atropine ointment twice daily for 3 days before examination. Dosing occurs at home. The drops or ointment are not instilled on the day of refraction, since no additional cycloplegia is obtained and because the ointment tends to interfere with the refractive procedure by introducing distortions of the optical media. Note that this dosage regimen is excessive, since maximum cycloplegia is usually achieved by the second day. However, it does allow for missed instillations at home. If the parents are reliable, 3 instillations of the atropine solution one day before, and 1 instillation on the morning of the examination should be adequate.[13] Table 22.3 shows the typical instructions that the parents may receive for home administration of atropine.

TABLE 22.3
Typical Instructions for Home Administration of Atropine

1. Do not use this medication until _____ (day), _____ (date). This is _____ day(s) before your child's appointment.
2. Place once in each eye as instructed, _____ times a day beginning on the morning of the day noted for the _____ day(s) before the day of appointment. Do not use on the day of appointment.
3. Discontinue medication if child develops a fever or persistent redness of the face.
4. It is normal to notice:
   a. Sensitivity to bright light
   b. Blurred vision
   c. Dilated (enlarged) pupils
5. *Discard medication after the appointment.* This is not "general purpose eye medication."
6. If any problems occur, call our office immediately.

Since atropine provides the most effective cycloplegia of any of the currently available anticholinergic agents, it is an excellent drug for cycloplegic retinoscopy of infants and children up to age 4 years with suspected accommodative esotropia. The use of atropine allows determination of the maximum amount of hyperopia so that plus lenses can more effectively relieve the effort placed on the accommodative-convergence mechanism. The cycloplegic (atropine) examination should be repeated several months after the patient has worn plus lenses. Frequently, the second examination uncovers more hyperopia. Refraction of nonstrabismic children and of adults does not require atropine, since complete cycloplegia is not essential in these patients. Furthermore, atropine cycloplegia is usually unnecessary and impractical in adults because of their already reduced amplitude of accommodation and because they are usually intolerant of the prolonged cycloplegia and dilated pupils.[9]

Scopolamine

Scopolamine, or hyoscine, is derived from *Hyoscyamus niger* or henbane as it is commonly known.[12] It is indicated for cycloplegic retinoscopy only as a substitute for atropine in atropine-sensitive patients. It has an onset of cycloplegia within 1 hour, and maximum cycloplegia occurs within 1 hour. This allows only negligible residual accommodation and has a duration of cycloplegia from 5 to 7 days.

Scopolamine is available in 0.25% solution. Concentrations greater than 0.5% can cause central nervous system manifestations.[9] A 0.25% solution of scopolamine has approximately the same cycloplegic effect as 1% atropine. The usual dosage for cycloplegic refraction is 1 drop of the 0.25% solution, repeated in 15 to 20 minutes.

Cyclopentolate

Because of its quick action and completeness of cycloplegia, cyclopentolate is the cycloplegic agent of choice for most patients. The onset of cyclopentolate cycloplegia begins in 5 to 20 minutes and reaches maximum in 20 to 30 minutes.[24,54] The cycloplegia lasts 8 to 24 hours. Residual accommodation is approximately 1.00 D for white patients but, with the instillation of only 1 drop, can be as high as 5.00 D for black patients.[9]

Cyclopentolate is available in 0.5%, 1%, and 2% solution. One drop of the 0.5% or 1% solution, repeated in 5 or 10 minutes, allows sufficient cycloplegia for most children. However, Miranda[14] found that 1 drop of 1% cyclopentolate alone achieved unsatisfactory cycloplegia in patients with dark brown irides and recommended that a combination of 1% cyclopentolate and 1% tropicamide be used to obtain adequate cycloplegia in such patients. Black children, infants, or children with dark brown irides may require 2 or 3 instillations of the 1% solution to achieve less than 2.00 D residual accommodation. The clinician should avoid use of 2% cyclopentolate because of the increased risk of systemic side effects.

Cyclopentolate has become the drug of choice for the cycloplegic refraction of strabismic patients, particularly those over age 4 years and nonsquinters of any age. Although atropine may be unnecessary in patients under age 4 years with accommodative esotropia, it is required where ocular alignment is not achieved using cyclopentolate to uncover the full amount of hyperopia. However, even in these patients the current trend is to use cyclopentolate before considering atropine.

Tropicamide

Introduced in the early 1960s, tropicamide is used primarily for routine pupillary dilation. However, it may be an effective anticholinergic agent for screening patients who may need a comprehensive cycloplegic examination.

Tropicamide has a rapid onset of cycloplegia of 5 to 20 minutes, with maximum cycloplegia occurring in 20 to 30 minutes and then quickly diminishing. Residual accommodation averages 3.50 D, which makes tropicamide an unreliable cycloplegic.[15] Another problem with tropicamide is the short duration of maximum cycloplegia. If refraction or retinoscopy is not performed within the few minutes of maximum cycloplegia, residual accommodation becomes an unwanted factor and may contribute to errors in refraction. Such timing is often difficult in a busy practice.

Tropicamide is available in 0.5% and 1% solution. One drop of the 1% solution, repeated at least 2 or 3 times at 5-minute intervals, is usually advised for refraction, but even this dosage cannot guarantee adequate cycloplegia. Several authors,[16,52,55] however, have shown that tropicamide may provide effective cycloplegia comparable to that of cyclopentolate, even in young adults and nonamblyopic, nonstrabismic, low to moderately hyperopic children.

Comparison of Cycloplegics

Gettes and Belmont[17] compared the residual accommodation allowed by various cycloplegics relative to 1% atropine. These investigators found cycloplegic efficacies of 92% for 1% cyclopentolate, 80% for 1% tropicamide, and only 54% for 4% homatropine with 1% hydroxyamphetamine. Thus, 1% cyclopentolate produces less residual accommodation than does 1% tropicamide or 4% homatropine and is therefore considered the drug of choice for routine cycloplegic refraction not requiring absolute paralysis of accommodation. Another advantage of cyclopentolate is its shorter duration of action compared with atropine.

Although Havener[9] has reported that 3 drops of 1% cyclopentolate applied at 10-minute intervals will provide the same cycloplegic effect as the traditional 3-day atropine regimen, Ingram and Barr[18] found that 1% cyclopentolate was significantly less effective than 1% atropine in producing cycloplegia in 1-year-old children.

Rosenbaum and associates[19] have shown that refraction with 1% atropine is essential to uncover the maximum amount of hyperopia in esotropic children. In this study, which compared the effects of 1% atropine and 1% cyclopentolate, a difference of an additional +1.00 D or more was uncovered with atropine in 22% of the children. Note that almost all subjects in this subgroup had 2.00 D or more of hyperopia. Therefore, the use of atropine may prove even more important in children with moderate hyperopia whose eyes are not aligned after cycloplegic retinoscopy using cyclopentolate.

Clinical Procedure

Administration of Cycloplegic Agents

Many clinicians prefer to use a topical anesthetic before instilling the cycloplegic. The anesthetic diminishes the local stinging, irritation, and lacrimation that often accompany cycloplegic drops. The anesthetic can also be combined with the cycloplegic. A single-dose combination consisting of equal volumes of 2% cyclopentolate and 0.5% proparacaine can provide effective cycloplegia with minimal discomfort.[53] Several authors[20–22] have reported increased corneal drug penetration and therefore increased effectiveness of phenylephrine following topical anesthesia. Increased effectiveness of cycloplegics may also occur following topical anesthesia.[23]

The cycloplegic can be administered alone or as a combination cycloplegic-mydriatic solution to permit adequate binocular indirect ophthalmoscopy in neonates, infants, and young children following cycloplegic retinoscopy. The combination drugs can be administered individually or as a combination solution prepared by mixing certain volumes of each constituent drug as discussed in Chapter 21 and as shown in Figure 22.1.

The cycloplegic or combination cycloplegic-mydriatic solution can be administered to the eye as a drop, a spray (see Chapter 3), or an ointment (atropine). Clinicians find the spray particularly effective in children, who are often resistant to drop instillation in the usual manner. Several studies have compared the efficacy of administering cycloplegic agents in a spray as compared to conventional eyedrop. Bartlett and associates[24] instilled cycloplegic agents in four matched groups. Eyedrops were instilled in eyes that were opened or closed, and a cycloplegic spray was administered to opened or closed eyes. Residual accommodation was measured using dynamic retinoscopy or the

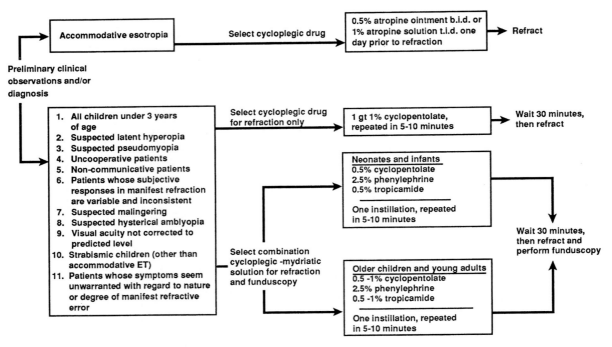

FIGURE 22.1   **Flowchart for cycloplegic refraction.**

push-up method at various times following administration of the medications. These investigators reported no differences in cycloplegic effect among the four groups. Ismail and colleagues[25] found no statistically significant difference between a cycloplegic eyedrop instilled in opened eyes and spray administered to closed eyes based on objective refractive measurements in 37 hyperopic children. These investigators also compared ease of administration of the two formulations and found the spray method significantly better.

The practitioner must observe the recommended dosages for cycloplegic refraction. The dosage for all cycloplegic drugs should be the lowest concentration that satisfactorily achieves the desired cycloplegia. To overmedicate when maximum cycloplegia has been reached increases the probability of systemic drug absorption and the risk of side effects.

Following cycloplegic examination, some clinicians advise the use of a miotic such as pilocarpine to hasten departure of the cycloplegic effect. However, miotic application can cause ciliary spasm, browache, and an increased risk of angle-closure glaucoma by the pupillary-block mechanism. Furthermore, when Nelson and Orton[26] assessed the effects of 2% pilocarpine in countering cycloplegia, they found no significant difference in the decrease of pupil size or the rate of return of accommodation. Distance vision actually worsened in some subjects. Thus, dispensing disposable mydriatic sunglasses to the patient and letting the cycloplegic effect run its natural course appears best.[8,27,28] The patient or parent should be advised regarding the expected dilated pupils, increased sensitivity to light, and blurred vision.

Near Versus Cycloplegic Refraction

In 1975 Mohindra[29] described a procedure of near retinoscopy in which retinoscopy is performed monocularly 50 cm from the patient with the patient fixating the retinoscope light in a dim room. The author devised the technique to avoid the use of cycloplegics, primarily in infants. An adjustment factor of −1.25 D, determined by comparing the "gross" retinoscopic value to the subjective refractive error in adults, is algebraically added to the "gross" retinoscopic value to determine the "net" refraction.[30] Mohindra subsequently compared determination of refractive status using this procedure versus cycloplegic refraction (1% tropicamide) in infants[31] and early elementary school children.[32] Since these reports by Mohindra, several investigators have attempted to replicate her results.

Maino and associates[2] compared refractive errors in 311 hyperopic preschool children utilizing cycloplegic retinoscopy (1% tropicamide) versus near retinoscopy. Although they found good agreement between investigators using the two procedures, they did not find the adjustment factor to yield reliable, objective measurements.

Borghi and Rouse[33] compared refractive error in 22 children using near and cycloplegic retinoscopy (1% cyclopentolate). They found statistically significant differences when comparing values on an absolute basis but good agreement when comparing all meridians, particularly as the amount of hyperopia increased. When ciliary tonicity was taken into account in the cycloplegic retinoscopy values, the two procedures produced essentially the same results.

Wesson and associates[3] compared cycloplegic retinoscopy (1% cyclopentolate) versus near retinoscopy, both monocularly and binocularly, in 10 infants and 10 young children. They found a significant difference between the two procedures in regard to best sphere and cylinder, larger for infants than children. In addition, they reported no difference when the procedure was performed with one or both eyes opened. Because of the significant differences, these investigators cautioned against substituting one procedure for the other.

Saunders and Westall[34] investigated the validity of the two procedures in 31 infants and 43 children. They reported near retinoscopy gave on average a less hyperopic result than did cycloplegic refraction, especially in infants. They suggested changing the adjustment factor to 1.00 D for children and 0.75 D for infants to improve agreement with cycloplegic retinoscopy. Analysis found poorest agreement between the procedures when examining infants and when the examiners had poor confidence in near retinoscopy.

Cruz and associates[35] have also reported the results of cycloplegic versus near retinoscopy in 17 patients with accommodative esotropia. These investigators found good statistical correlation between the two procedures but large variability in the differences. As a result, they did not recommend near retinoscopy in patients with accommodative esotropia.

In summary, it appears that near retinoscopy may have some value as a nonpharmacologic procedure for screening refractive errors in children but not as a reliable substitute for cycloplegic refraction. It appears to produce the least valid results in infants, the very group in which it was designed to assess refractive error. As with any procedure, statistical agreement does not necessarily result in good, clinical agreement on an individual patient. A number of factors may contribute to the variability noted in these studies. Some investigators used tropicamide[2,30–32] to obtain cycloplegia while others used cyclopentolate.[3,33–35] Some studies use an allowance factor for ciliary tonicity to adjust for tonicity not in effect during cycloplegic refraction. Finally, use of different statistical methodology makes comparison of data difficult.

Refractive Techniques

After the cycloplegic has been instilled and the time limit for maximum cycloplegia has been reached, the clinician must decide whether the degree of cycloplegia is adequate to permit reliable refraction. Reinecke and Herm[36] have described two methods of measuring monocular residual accommodation.

1. Lens powers are changed while the patient observes a near accommodative target such as a reading card positioned at a fixed fixation distance. For example, if the eye under cycloplegia cannot read print at 40 cm until a +2.50 D lens is placed over the distance correction, and the print remains clear until the addition of a +4.00 D lens, the residual accommodation is 1.50 D.
2. Another method is to place a +2.50 D lens over the distance correction and then move the print from 40 cm, first away from the eye and then toward the eye, until it blurs in each direction. If the print is clear between 50 cm and 20 cm from the eye, the patient has 3.00 D of residual accommodation.

Of course, these tests are often impossible to perform on the very patients who require cycloplegia, and the experienced clinician quickly learns to use the retinoscope to judge accommodative activity. Completeness of cycloplegia can be ascertained clinically by asking the patient to fixate the light of the retinoscope. If cycloplegia in the emmetropic patient is complete, then a nonfluctuating "with" motion of approximately 2.00 D is observed. If accommodation in the emmetropic patient is active, however, fluctuation of the retinoscopic reflex will be observed. If residual accommodation exceeds 2.00 D, cycloplegic refraction may be unreliable and inaccurate.[17,37–39]

After the cycloplegia has been determined to be clinically satisfactory, retinoscopy should be performed before the child becomes restless. The best guideline for retinoscopy is to neutralize the central 4 mm of the pupil, ignoring the movement in the periphery, which may be confusing and distracting because of spherical aberration associated with the dilated pupil. A retinoscope light of low to medium intensity helps to reduce such aberrations. The patient should fixate a distant target if the cycloplegia is not completely adequate. However, if the cycloplegia is complete, the patient may fixate directly at the retinoscope light without jeopardizing the retinoscopic result. In addition, the retinoscope should be as close to the visual axis as possible to avoid errors associated with spherical aberration. It is often difficult to perform retinoscopy on young children through a phoroptor. Instead, loose, hand-held trial lenses or lens bars can be used to facilitate retinoscopy of the young child or infant (Fig. 22.2).

Following retinoscopy, subjective refraction should be attempted. Although the practitioner often cannot perform a subjective refraction on young patients because of their lack of maturity and cooperation, he or she should attempt it when possible. The practitioner should note that spherical aberration can cause errors in the subjective refraction just as it does in retinoscopy.

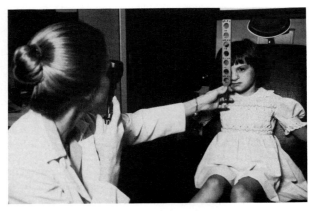

FIGURE 22.2 **Cycloplegic retinoscopy of young child. (Courtesy Jimmy D. Bartlett, O.D.)**

Spectacle Prescribing

Prescribing spectacle lenses from cycloplegic findings is truly an art rather than an exact science and thus places great demands on the clinician's judgment, skill, and experience. In many cases determination of the final spectacle prescription is straightforward, but in other cases it requires considerable thought and judgment. Since the ultimate criterion for a satisfactory and successful prescription is relief of patient symptoms, guidelines for spectacle prescribing are necessarily somewhat broad and imprecise. Nevertheless, the following recommendations represent the most widely accepted approaches to spectacle prescribing.

In accommodative esotropia, the full amount of plus lens correction determined by retinoscopy should be prescribed in children younger than 4 years of age. With older children, the plus power can be reduced as long as fusion is maintained. Chapter 34 considers additional guidelines for prescribing spectacles to patients with accommodative esotropia.

Before prescribing lenses for the nonstrabismic patient, the clinician must consider the patient's symptoms. Conservative prescribing, if any, should be the rule in asymptomatic patients. However, for patients with significant symptoms, such as asthenopia or reading difficulty, the prescribing of lens powers closer to the cycloplegic amount is indicated. In the vast majority of patients over age 20 years, usually very close agreement exists between the cycloplegic and manifest refractive findings, especially in myopic patients. However, in children the cycloplegic refraction nearly always reveals more plus power in hyperopia than does the manifest refraction, while for myopia the two procedures produce more equivalent results.[40] Therefore, for nonstrabismic patients most practitioners usually prescribe the full amount of astigmatic (cylinder power and axis) or myopic correction found by cycloplegic retinoscopy.

In patients with latent hyperopia but no esotropia, the practitioner should prescribe a reduced amount of plus lens power to compensate for intrinsic ciliary muscle tonus.[41] A reduction of plus lens power is essential in hyperopic patients accustomed to accommodating 2 to 3 D or more to compensate for their refractive error, because full correcting lenses result in blurred distance vision and are not readily accepted. The results from the cycloplegic examination can be used as a guide to a postcycloplegic manifest refraction performed on a different day. It is often helpful to determine by binocular refraction or cyclodamic techniques the amount of plus power actually accepted by the patient.

Since considerable judgment is involved in evaluating and prescribing from cycloplegic findings in patients with latent hyperopia but without accommodative esotropia, it is difficult to give specific guidelines for use in individual clinical circumstances. Mitchell[42] recommends reducing the hyperopic prescription 1.00 D on nonstrabismic atropinized patients, while Reinecke and Herm[36] suggest a 2.00 D subtraction for such patients. As a broad general guideline for use with 1% cyclopentolate, a satisfactory prescription may often be derived by simply reducing the dioptric power according to patient age as shown in Table 22.4.[43] Perhaps a more accurate approach, however, is to prescribe not only according to patient age but also by considering the difference between the manifest and cycloplegic findings, as suggested in Table 22.5. The greater the difference between the manifest and cycloplegic refractions, the greater should be the reduction in plus lens correction.

Regardless of the method used to determine the amount of plus lens correction, a further reduction in power can often be made in accordance with the guidelines ordinarily governing the prescribing of corrections for hyperopia. Prepresbyopic hyperopic patients are usually more comfortable with a partial correction than a full correction for their first prescription. In these patients the practitioner can usually prescribe approximately one-half the total hyperopic amount for near work only. As the patient adapts to this prescription over time, the amount of power prescribed and

TABLE 22.4
Amount Deducted in Hyperopia Using 1% Cyclopentolate

Age (yr)	Amount Deducted (D)
0–6	1.00
10	0.75
15	0.50
20	0.25
30	0–0.25
40	0

Adapted from Tait EC. Refraction and heterophoria. In: Harley RD, ed. Pediatric Ophthalmology. Philadelphia: W. B. Saunders Co, 1975;113–131.

TABLE 22.5
Plus Lens Correction Prescribed for Latent Hyperopia

Manifest Refraction (D)	Cycloplegic Refraction (D)		
	1.00	2.50	5.00
Age 5 years			
Plano	1.00	2.00	4.00
1.00	1.00	2.00	4.00
2.00	NA	2.00	4.50
Age 12 years			
Plano	1.00	2.00	3.50
1.00	1.00	2.00	4.00
2.00	NA	2.00	4.00
Age 25 years			
Plano	1.00	1.50	3.00
1.00	1.00	2.00	3.50
2.00	NA	2.00	4.00

NA = Not applicable.

the distances for which worn may increase. This partial correction is advisable for the following reasons[42]:

- When some of the plus lens power is subtracted from the cycloplegic refraction, accommodation can more easily relax and allow the spectacle lens to compensate for the refractive error. Distance visual acuity is less blurred, and patient cooperation is easier to obtain, especially from the young patient.
- A partial correction does not so violently upset the habitual relationship existing between accommodation and convergence. The abrupt changes made in this relationship by full plus lens correction may give rise to as much discomfort as was associated with the original problem.
- A partial correction forces the patient to accommodate to overcome the uncorrected portion of the refractive error. This approach may keep the amplitude of accommodation higher and does not allow the patient to become totally dependent on the hyperopic prescription. This can be a significant advantage when the prescription may not be worn, as in sporting events or social functions.

When the final spectacle prescription is dispensed, a mild cycloplegic, such as 0.5% cyclopentolate or 0.5% to 1.0% tropicamide, may be prescribed if necessary to permit the patient with latent hyperopia to accept the plus lens correction more easily.[44–46] The dosage should gradually be tapered (e.g., 1.0% tropicamide 4 times daily for 1 day, 3 times daily for 1 day, twice daily for 1 day, once daily for 1 day, then discontinued).

Figure 22.1 summarizes the clinical procedure for cycloplegic refraction.

Adverse Reactions

Most reactions to cycloplegic agents can be classified as either drug allergy (hypersensitivity) or toxicity. Hypersensitivity reactions to topically applied cycloplegics are usually unexpected responses[47] and are most commonly seen as dermatologic eruptions of the skin of the eyelids. The sequence of toxic drug reactions, however, often follows a predictable pattern. Although the incidence of adverse events to cycloplegic agents administered in recommended doses is low, local ocular as well as systemic reactions can occur. Chapters 9 and 38 discuss these reactions in detail.

Cycloplegic Refraction for Research Purposes

Many reasons exist for having a benchmark against which one can assess refractive instruments' reliability as well as validity. This benchmark is particularly important when conducting clinical research and comparing one procedure or instrument against the standard. For example, studies assessing various autorefractors require a benchmark. Nayak and associates[48] compared manifest and cycloplegic refraction using the Nikon Auto Refractometer (NR-1000F) compared with clinical refraction using homatropine in young patients with low to moderate refractive errors. These investigators found this instrument to induce instrument myopia during the manifest refraction. Salvesen and Kohler[49] examined 46 eyes with the Nidek 1000-AR autorefractometer to determine variation in measurements between manifest, cyclopentolate, and atropine refractions. The greatest variation occurred in the spherical component, the youngest age group, and between atropine and dry measurements. A more recent development in autorefractors is photorefraction for visual screening. Morgan and Johnson[50] found the Visiscreen 100 to be within 2.50 D in 77% of the 63 children screened compared to the cycloplegic spherical equivalent. Zadnik and associates[51] compared the reliability of retinoscopy, subjective refraction, and Canon R-1 autorefraction (noncycloplegic and cycloplegic using 1% tropicamide). They found that the most reliable measure of refractive error was autorefraction with cycloplegia, followed by cycloplegic subjective refraction and cycloplegic retinoscopy. These studies demonstrate the important role that cycloplegics play in performing clinical research in refractive conditions.

References

1. Augsburger AR. Hyperopia. In: Amos JF, ed. Diagnosis and management in vision care. Boston: Butterworths, 1987;5:110.

2. Maino JH, Cibis GW, Cress P, et al. Noncycloplegic vs cycloplegic retinoscopy in pre-school children. Ann Ophthalmol 1984;16:880–882.

3. Wesson MD, Mann KR, Bray NW. A comparison of cycloplegic refraction to the near retinoscopy technique for refractive error determination. J Am Optom Assoc 1990;61:680–684.

4. Saunders KJ, Westall CA. Comparison between near retinoscopy and cycloplegic retinoscopy in the refraction of infants and children. Optom Vis Sci 1992;69:615–622.

5. Duke-Elder S, Abrams D. System of ophthalmology. Duke-Elder S, ed. St. Louis: C.V. Mosby Co, 1970;5:387.

6. Van Herick W, Shaffer RN, Schwartz A. Estimation of width of angle of anterior chamber. Am J Ophthalmol 1969;68:626–629.

7. Fisch B. Gonioscopy and the glaucomas. Boston: Butterworth-Heinemann, 1993;35–57.

8. Milder B, Rubin M. The fine art of prescribing glasses. Gainesville, FL: Triad Scientific, 1980;3:44–51.

9. Havener WH. Ocular pharmacology. St. Louis: C.V. Mosby Co, 1983;5:261–417.

10. Priestly BS, Medine M. A new mydriatic and cycloplegic drug. Compound 75 GT. Am J Ophthalmol 1951;34:572–575.

11. Beitel RJ. Cycloplegic refraction. In: Tasman W, Jaeger EA, eds. Duane's clinical ophthalmology. Philadelphia: J.B. Lippincott, 1990;1:Chap 41:1–4.

12. Packer M, Brandt JD. Ophthalmology's botanical heritage. Surv Ophthalmol 1992;36:357–365.

13. Stolovitch C, Loewenstein A, Nemmet P, Moshe L. Atropine cycloplegia: How many instillations does one need? J Pediatr Ophthalmol Strabismus 1992;29:175–176.

14. Miranda MN. Residual accommodation. A comparison between cyclopentolate 1% and a combination of cyclopentolate 1% and tropicamide 1%. Arch Ophthalmol 1972;87:515–517.

15. Gettes BC. Tropicamide, a new cycloplegic mydriatic. Arch Ophthalmol 1961;65:632–635.

16. Pollack SL, Hunt JS, Polse KA. Dose-response effects of tropicamide HCl. Am J Optom Physiol Opt 1981;58:361–366.

17. Gettes BC, Belmont O. Tropicamide: Comparative cycloplegic effects. Arch Ophthalmol 1961;66:336–340.

18. Ingram RM, Barr A. Refraction of 1–year-old children after cycloplegia with 1% cyclopentolate: Comparison with findings after atropinisation. Br J Ophthalmol 1979;63:348–352.

19. Rosenbaum AL, Bateman JB, Bremer DL, et al. Cycloplegic refraction in esotropic children. Ophthalmology 1981;88:1031–1034.

20. Keller JT, Chang FW. An evaluation of the use of topical anesthetics and low concentrations of phenylephrine HCl for mydriasis. J Am Optom Assoc 1976;47:753.

21. Kubo DJ, Wing TW, Polse KA, Jauregui MJ. Mydriatic effects using low concentrations of phenylephrine hydrochloride. J Am Optom Assoc 1975;46:817–822.

22. Hopkins GA, Lyle WM. Potential systemic side effects of six common ophthalmic drugs. J Am Optom Assoc 1977;48:1241–1245.

23. Mordi JA, Lyle WM, Mousa GY. Does prior instillation of a topical anesthetic enhance the effect of tropicamide? Am J Optom Physiol Opt 1986;63:290–293.

24. Bartlett JD, Wesson MD, Swiatocha J, Woolley TW. Efficacy of a pediatric cycloplegic administered as a spray. J Am Optom Assoc 1993;64:617–621.

25. Ismail E, Rouse MW, DeLand PN. A comparison of drop instillation and spray application of cyclopentolate. Optom Vis Sci 1992; 69(suppl):101.

26. Nelson ME, Orton DBO. Counteracting the effects of mydriatics. Arch Ophthalmol 1987;105:486–489.

27. Bartlett JD, Classe JG. Dapiprazole: Will it affect the standard of care for pupillary dilation? Optom Clin 1992;2:113–120.

28. Bartlett JD. Administration of and adverse reactions to cycloplegic agents. Am J Optom Physiol Opt 1978;55:229.

29. Mohindra I. A technique for infant refraction. Am J Optom Physiol Opt 1975;52:867–870.

30. Mohindra I. Comparison of "near retinoscopy" and subjective refraction in adults. Am J Optom Physiol Opt 1977;54:319–322.

31. Mohindra I. A non-cycloplegic refraction technique for infants and young children. J Am Optom Assoc 1977;48:518–523.

32. Mohindra I, Molinari JF. Near retinoscopy and cycloplegic retinoscopy in early primary grade school children. Am J Optom Physiol Opt 1979;56:34–38.

33. Borghi RA, Rouse MW. Comparison of refraction obtained by "near retinoscopy" and retinoscopy under cycloplegia. Am J Optom Physiol Opt 1985;62:169–172.

34. Saunders KJ, Westall CA. Comparison between near retinoscopy and cycloplegic retinoscopy in the refraction of infants and children. Optom Vis Sci 1992;69:615–622.

35. Cruz AAV, Sampaio NMV, Vargus JA. Near retinoscopy in accommodative esotropia. J Pediatr Ophthalmol Strabismus 1990;27: 245–249.

36. Reinecke RD, Herm RJ. Refraction. New York: Appleton-Century-Crofts. 1976;2:48–171.

37. Prangen AD. What constitutes satisfactory cycloplegia? Am J Ophthalmol 1931;14:667.

38. Stine GT. Clinical investigation of a new cycloplegic and mydriatic drug. Eye Ear Nose Throat Monthly 1960;22:11–14.

39. Milder B. Tropicamide as a cycloplegic agent. Arch Ophthalmol 1961;66:70–72.

40. Shultz L. Variations in refractive changes induced by Cyclogyl upon children with differing degrees of ametropia. Am J Optom Physiol Opt 1975;52:482–484.

41. Amos DM. Cycloplegics for refraction. Am J Optom Physiol Opt 1978;55:223–226.

42. Mitchell DWA. The use of drugs in refraction. London: The Hereford Times Ltd, 1960;2:57.

43. Tait EC. Refraction and heterophoria. In: Harley RD, ed. Pediatric ophthalmology. Philadelphia: W.B. Saunders Co, 1975;113–131.

44. Milder B, Rubin M. The fine art of prescribing glasses. Gainesville, FL: Triad Scientific, 1980;2:28–30.

45. Duke-Elder S, Abrams D. System of ophthalmology. Duke-Elder S, ed. St. Louis: C.V. Mosby Co, 1970;5:451–486.

46. Silbert J, Alexander A. Cyclotherapy in the treatment of symptomatic latent hyperopia. J Am Optom Assoc 1987;58:40–46.

47. Ellis PP. Ocular therapeutics and pharmacology. St. Louis: C.V. Mosby Co, 1981:6.

48. Nayak BR, Ghose S, Singh JP. A comparison of cycloplegic and manifest refractions on the NR-1000 F (an objective Auto Refractometer). Br J Ophthalmol 1987;71:73–75.

49. Kohler M, Salvesen S. Precision in automated refraction. Acta Ophthalmol 1991;69:338–341.

50. Morgan KS, Johnson WD. Clinical evaluation of a commercial photorefractor. Arch Ophthalmol 1987;105:1528–1531.
51. Zadnik K, Mutti DO, Adams AJ. The repeatability of measurement of the ocular components. Invest Ophthalmol Vis Sci 1992;33: 2325–2333.
52. Mutti DO, Zadnik K, Egashira S, et al. The effect of cycloplegia on measurement of the ocular components. Invest Ophthalmol Vis Sci 1994;35:515–527.
53. Nelson PS, Veith J. Use of a single-dose cycloplegic-anesthetic combination in clinical practice. Clin Eye Vision Care 1992;4:162–165.
54. Manny RE, Fern KD, Zervas HJ, et al. 1% cyclopentolate hydrochloride: Another look at the time course of cycloplegia using an objective measure of the accommodative response. Optom Vis Sci 1993;70:651–665.
55. Egashira SM, Kish LL, Twelker JD, et al. Comparison of cyclopentolate versus tropicamide cycloplegia in children. Optom Vis Sci 1993;70:1019–1026.

Neuro-Ophthalmic Disorders

Larry J. Alexander
Leonid Skorin, Jr.
Jimmy D. Bartlett

The optometrist and ophthalmologist often encounter patients with ophthalmic manifestations of neurologic impairment. Patients with anisocoria, neuromuscular abnormalities, and optic neuropathies can be challenging and may require pharmacologic intervention for either diagnosis or treatment. This chapter considers the most prevalent neuro-ophthalmic disorders of interest to the clinician. The proper diagnostic and therapeutic uses of various pharmacologic agents are described for the management of these conditions.

Anisocoria

Many clinical conditions can exhibit anisocoria as a primary or secondary feature. Table 23.1 lists the most common disorders with unequal pupils as a primary diagnostic sign. Some of these conditions, such as physiologic (essential) anisocoria, are benign and have an excellent prognosis. Others, such as third-nerve palsy, can indicate significant intracranial disease and may have a grave prognosis. Although a discussion of all conditions associated with anisocoria is beyond the scope of this chapter, those disorders that most easily lend themselves to evaluation by clinical and pharmacologic methods will be emphasized. These conditions have in common that *only one* pupil is involved and that the basic underlying abnormality manifests itself as an inability of the affected pupil either to *dilate* or to *constrict*. Consequently, either the sympathetic or the parasympathetic

nervous system can be implicated, and various drugs affecting the autonomic nervous system may pharmacologically differentiate the site of impairment. Table 23.1 identifies the disorders that are most easily evaluated pharmacologically, in which only one pupil is abnormal.

The initial clinical evaluation of the patient with unequal pupils frequently allows diagnosis of the underlying condition without resorting to pharmacologic or other more elaborate methods of examination. Thus, the practitioner must perform the appropriate clinical examination of the patient as the initial phase of the evaluation.

Pupil Size

In addition to the customary evaluation of pupillary function (direct reflexes and evaluation for Marcus Gunn sign), pupil size must be measured accurately. Flash photography can provide this measurement, or it can be accurately estimated using the area of the pupil rather than its diameter.[1] The black semicircles found on rulers and near reading cards are suitable for this purpose and are preferred over simple millimeter rules.

Light Reaction

In testing the response to direct light, one pupil responding poorly clearly indicates the abnormal pupil. Differential diagnosis includes third-nerve palsy, anticholinergic mydri-

TABLE 23.1
Disorders Characterized by Anisocoria

- Physiologic (essential) anisocoria
- Alternating contraction anisocoria
- Claude Bernard syndrome
- Horner's syndrome[a]
- Episodic unilateral mydriasis
- Adie's syndrome[a]
- Third-nerve palsy[a]
- Adrenergic mydriasis
- Anticholinergic mydriasis[a]
- Argyll Robertson pupils
- Local iris disease (sphincter atrophy, posterior synechiae, etc.)
- Hutchinson's pupil
- Angle-closure glaucoma

[a]Disorders that are most easily evaluated pharmacologically, in which usually only one pupil is abnormal.

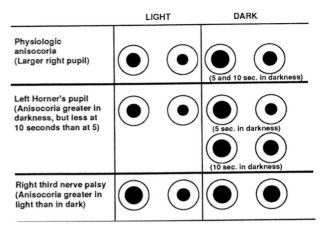

FIGURE 23.1 **Use of light and dark illumination in differentiating the various causes of anisocoria.**

asis, Adie's pupil, or local iris disease. If each eye has a good pupillary light reaction, differential diagnosis includes Horner's syndrome or physiologic anisocoria.

Nature of Anisocoria in Light versus Dark

A comparison of the anisocoria in bright and dim ambient illuminations may help in reaching a diagnosis by clinical means alone. Although use of a semidarkened room facilitates the clinical evaluation of unequal pupils, this method is often self-defeating when the patient has dark irides, since there is poor contrast between the iris and the pupil. Using an ultraviolet light in a completely darkened room can overcome this problem.[2,3] The technique employs the principle of lenticular fluorescence from ultraviolet stimulation and involves instrumentation that is readily available in most ophthalmic and general medical offices. The ultraviolet light source (such as a Burton lamp) should be held 8–12 inches from the patient so that the visible emission will not stimulate pupillary activity.[2] If the anisocoria increases in darkness, the differential diagnosis includes Horner's syndrome or physiologic anisocoria (Fig. 23.1). In Horner's syndrome the oculosympathetic paresis does not allow the iris dilator to function properly in darkness; consequently, the anisocoria increases as the normal pupil dilates in response to darkness. Although no autonomic nervous system abnormalities exist in physiologic anisocoria, this benign condition also exhibits increased anisocoria in darkness.

An anisocoria that is greater in the light than in darkness generally indicates an abnormal parasympathetic innervation to the iris sphincter (see Fig. 23.1). Differential diagnosis includes Adie's pupil, iris sphincter atrophy (possibly associated with previous anterior segment trauma), or any of

the disorders implicated as a "unilateral fixed and dilated" pupil (third-nerve palsy, anticholinergic mydriasis, or Adie's pupil). Since the underlying abnormality is generally associated with the parasympathetic innervation to the iris sphincter, the abnormal (larger) pupil does not appropriately constrict to stimulation by light. The anisocoria is therefore greater in bright light than in dim illumination.

Slit-Lamp Examination

The clinician should carefully examine the physical characteristics of the iris with the biomicroscope for evidence of mechanical restrictions of the pupils. Some patients have iris damage due to previous ocular inflammation or trauma. Careful evaluation may uncover subtle areas of posterior synechiae that immobilize the pupil. Careful biomicroscopic examination can also detect iris sphincter atrophy. Careful examination of the iris, moreover, may reveal sector palsies with associated vermiform movements, indicating Adie's pupil.

Inspection of Photographs

Frequently the question arises whether the anisocoria is recent or long-standing. Patients often insist that their newly found condition is of recent onset. In such cases, examination of personal photographs (both recent and old) may indicate with some certainty the onset and duration of the condition. However, different conditions of lighting and accommodation in old photographs could result in differences between present and past observations of anisocoria.

The use of old photographs appears to be most valid when they agree with current observations of anisocoria.[4]

Associated Ocular or Systemic Findings

Diagnostic physical findings are often associated with the observed anisocoria. For example, ipsilateral ptosis and facial anhydrosis are highly suggestive of Horner's syndrome and allow such a diagnosis without the need for pharmacologic confirmation. In addition, a history of sympathectomy with subsequent unilateral ptosis, anhydrosis, and miosis are all consistent with a diagnosis of Horner's syndrome. On the other hand, the patient with a unilateral sluggish pupil with associated accommodative insufficiency and diminished deep tendon reflexes may be strongly suspected of having Adie's syndrome, especially if these signs and symptoms are of recent onset in a healthy young adult female.

Thus, careful pupillary examination, with special attention paid to the patient's history as well as to other ocular or systemic physical findings, may allow the practitioner to establish the diagnosis without resorting to pharmacologic or other more sophisticated methods of examination. When the findings are ambiguous, however, or if insufficient clinical information is available to establish the diagnosis with certainty, pharmacologic evaluations should be performed as discussed in the following sections.

Guidelines for the Pharmacologic Evaluation of Anisocoria

When the patient's history is incomplete or noncontributory, or when the clinical signs and symptoms are too ambiguous to enable a definitive diagnosis, the practitioner should proceed with pharmacologic testing. Pharmacologic evaluation of unequal pupils is easily and quickly accomplished in the office and frequently obviates further neuroradiologic or laboratory investigations.

Adherence to the following general guidelines will facilitate pharmacologic evaluation and improve the accuracy with which the drugs allow a definitive diagnosis[5-7]:

- One drop of the indicated drug should be instilled into each eye and repeated after several minutes. This ensures adequate drug application if the first drop is removed by tearing.
- The drops should always be instilled into *both* eyes so that the reaction of the affected pupil can be compared with that of the normal pupil. If the condition is bilateral, as in anticholinergic mydriasis caused by systemic agents, the drop should be placed in only *one* eye so that the response of each pupil can be compared.

- The patient's general status can influence the size of the pupils. A change in alertness, either toward arousal or somnolence, can affect the "before" and "after" comparisons. If the patient becomes uncomfortable or anxious while waiting for the drug to act, both pupils may dilate. If the patient becomes drowsy, both pupils may constrict. In the case of Adie's pupil, drowsiness may constrict the normal pupil more than the Adie's pupil. This fact emphasizes the importance of instilling the drug into both eyes so that one pupil always serves as a control when only one pupil is affected.
- The amount of ambient illumination before and after drug instillation must be constant.
- Accommodation should be carefully controlled during the "before" and "after" evaluations so that it can be eliminated as a factor producing the change in pupil size.
- Photography is highly recommended to enable a more accurate evaluation of pupil size both before and after instillation of the indicated drug. Frequently an accuracy of 0.1 mm can be obtained using flash photography.[8] Since appropriate patient management depends on accurate diagnosis, the practitioner should not simply estimate the differences in pupil size because this estimate may lead to an incorrect diagnosis.

Physiologic Anisocoria

The most common condition characterized by unequal pupils is physiologic (essential) anisocoria. Depending on how it is defined, this condition is found in from 1% to more than 50% of the general population.[9,10] It is seldom greater than 1 mm and can be variable, changing from day to day or even from hour to hour.[4,10,11] The clinical and pharmacologic features of physiologic anisocoria are summarized in Table 23.2.

Horner's Syndrome

In 1869 Johann Friedrich Horner, a Swiss physician, described the findings now associated with the syndrome bearing his name.[12] Although the case reported by Horner was

TABLE 23.2
Clinical and Pharmacologic Features of Physiologic Anisocoria

- Constricts briskly to light
- No dilation lag in darkness
- No disturbed psychosensory dilation
- Dilates normally with cocaine
- Exhibits greater anisocoria in darkness than in light

caused by a preganglionic lesion, the term *Horner's syndrome* is now used to refer to any oculosympathetic palsy or paresis.

Etiology

The fibers comprising the oculosympathetic pathway have a long and tortuous course from the hypothalamus to the eye. Since a variety of vascular, traumatic, or neoplastic lesions can interrupt this pathway and produce the signs characteristic of Horner's syndrome, the clinician must understand the clinical anatomy to evaluate and manage appropriately patients with lesions of the oculosympathetic pathway. This sympathetic pathway can be divided into three portions:

1. The central (first-order) neuron originates in the hypothalamus, courses through the brainstem and cervical cord, and terminates at the ciliospinal center of Budge at C8-T2.
2. The preganglionic (second-order) neuron is located in the chest and neck extending from the cervical cord (C8-T2) through the stellate ganglion at the pulmonary apex to the superior cervical ganglion at the bifurcation of the internal and external carotid arteries.
3. The postganglionic (third-order) neuron originates at the superior cervical ganglion (located at the level of the angle of the jaw) and travels through the internal carotid plexus until it penetrates the base of the skull, passes

through the cavernous sinus, and accompanies the long ciliary nerves to the dilator muscle of the iris. Postganglionic sympathetic fibers also innervate Müller's muscle of the upper and lower lids.

The sympathetic fibers for sweating that innervate the face leave the superior cervical ganglion, follow the *external* carotid artery, and are therefore not involved in lesions of the carotid plexus. In some patients, however, a portion of the sympathetic fibers to the sweat glands in the ipsilateral forehead may follow branches of the *internal* carotid artery, allowing a lesion of the postganglionic oculosympathetic pathway to produce a small area of anhydrosis above the brow.[13]

The most common causes of Horner's syndrome are listed in Table 23.3.[13–20] Maloney and associates[21] studied 450 patients retrospectively with Horner's syndrome and were able to determine the cause for the sympathetic paresis in only 60% of the patients. Of the patients for whom no causes were determined, 35% were reexamined from 6 months to 28 years after the initial finding of Horner's syndrome, and the cause was still not discovered in any patient, indicating that whatever the cause, the lesion probably was a benign and stable process. In rare cases congenital Horner's syndrome can be inherited with an autosomal dominant transmission.[22]

Table 23.4 shows the distribution of various tumors causing Horner's syndrome. Although Giles and Henderson[23] identified neoplasia, more often malignant than benign, as the most common cause of Horner's syndrome, Maloney

TABLE 23.3
Etiologies of Horner's Syndrome[13–20, 83–88]

Central	Preganglionic	Postganglionic
Basal meningitis	Spinal birth injury	Abnormalities of the internal carotid artery
Pituitary tumor	Tuberculosis	Unilateral vascular headache syndromes
Tumor of third ventricle	Pancoast's tumor	Direct or indirect trauma
Syphilis of midbrain	Aortic aneurysm	Spontaneous or traumatic occlusion
Tumor of pons	Enlarged mediastinal glands	Aneurysms
Syringobulbia	Enlargement of thyroid	Atherosclerosis
Syringomyelia	Lymphadenopathy	Spontaneous dissection
Cervical cord trauma	Thoracic neuroblastoma	Lesions involving the middle cranial fossa and
and tumors	Pulmonary mucormycosis	cavernous sinus
Spinal tabes	Trauma	Basal skull fractures
Poliomyelitis	Cervical arthritis	Locally invasive neoplasms (meningiomas, etc.)
Stroke	Thoracostomy tube	Metastatic neoplasms
Multiple sclerosis		Inflammation of adjacent structures
		Tolosa-Hunt syndrome
		Otitis media
		Trigeminal herpes zoster
		Sinusitis

TABLE 23.4
Tumors Causing Horner's Syndrome[21,23,40,85]

Benign	Malignant
Neuroma-neurofibroma	Bronchogenic carcinoma
Thyroid adenoma	Metastatic carcinoma
Meningioma	Sarcoma
Dermal cyst	Hodgkin's lymphoma
Osteoma	Thyroid carcinoma
Pituitary adenoma	Neuroblastoma
	Lacrimal gland carcinoma
	Pharyngeal carcinoma

TABLE 23.5
Diagnostic Signs in Horner's Syndrome

- Unilateral ptosis
- Elevation ("upside-down ptosis") of the lower lid
- Narrowed palpebral fissure (apparent enophthalmos)
- Ipsilateral miosis
- Dilation lag
- Absence of dilation to psychosensory stimuli
- Conjunctival hyperemia
- Facial or body anhydrosis
- Heterochromia iridis, if congenital

and associates[21] found fewer than 3% of patients with Horner's syndrome had malignancies.

Most lesions causing Horner's syndrome involve the preganglionic neuron.[23] Patients with such lesions may have a lung or breast malignancy that has spread to the thoracic outlet. The patient may also have a history of surgery or trauma to the neck, chest, or cervical spine. In one study,[23] nonoperative trauma was the etiologic factor in 13% of the cases of preganglionic Horner's syndrome. These cases included injuries to the brachial plexus due primarily to birth trauma or to automobile accidents.

Although most lesions producing postganglionic Horner's syndrome are benign, a variety of potentially serious conditions may interrupt the postganglionic sympathetic pathway (see Table 23.3). Neoplasia as a cause of postganglionic Horner's syndrome is relatively rare. These lesions include nasopharyngeal tumors, meningiomas of the middle cranial fossa, or carcinomas invading from the sphenoid sinus. In one series[13] nearly half the patients with unilateral headache had typical cluster headache. In these patients the Horner's syndrome probably results from compromise of the postganglionic oculosympathetic fibers as they course with the sheaths surrounding a swollen internal carotid artery in the bony petrous canal.

The patient's age at the time of onset is an important aid to the clinician investigating a Horner's syndrome of unknown etiology. From birth to age 20 years, trauma is the leading cause. From 21 to 50 years, almost half the cases result from tumors. In the older age group (51 years of age and older), neoplasia is the most important cause.[23]

Diagnosis

CLINICAL EVALUATION

Table 23.5 lists the primary clinical signs diagnostic of Horner's syndrome. Although the complete syndrome is quite dramatic, it is only rarely encountered. Consequently, diagnosis based on the patient's clinical signs alone can be difficult.

Since Müller's muscle, which is innervated by oculosympathetic fibers, assists in elevating the upper lid, interruption of the sympathetic innervation to this muscle results in some degree of ptosis. The degree of ptosis varies. In some patients ptosis may be completely absent, in others it may be substantial, and in some it can worsen with fatigue. If the lesion is located centrally (i.e., in the first-order neuron), the only sign clinically observable may be pupillary constriction, without ptosis.[3,24] In contrast, if the lesion is in the cervical sympathetic region, all the signs comprising the syndrome, including ptosis, may be present.[3] However, the clinician should not misinterpret the partial ptosis of Horner's syndrome for retraction of the contralateral lid, since the patient can employ the levator or frontalis muscles to elevate the ptotic lid. The practitioner should simply cover the eye that does not appear to display lid retraction, and if the patient has Horner's syndrome, the covered eye will manifest a ptosis.[25]

Since sympathetically innervated smooth muscle fibers also exist in the lower lid, oculosympathetic paresis can produce elevation of the lower lid ("upside-down ptosis"). This condition is often subtle. However, this sign, along with ptosis of the upper lid, contributes to a narrowing of the palpebral fissure, giving the appearance of enophthalmos.[26]

Disruption of the sympathetic innervation to the iris dilator enables the parasympathetically innervated iris sphincter to have the predominant action on the iris, thus producing miosis. The degree of anisocoria, however, may not remain constant in any given patient, since the pupil size can vary with completeness of the syndrome, location of the lesion, patient alertness, ambient illumination, degree of denervation hypersensitivity, patient fixation, and the concentration of neurotransmitter substances.[3]

An extremely helpful sign in the clinical diagnosis of Horner's syndrome is *dilation lag,* in which the pupil fails to redilate quickly to its original size when light is extinguished. This can be easily evaluated by comparing the dilation time in each eye.[24] Following a bright stimulus the normal pupil returns to its original darkness diameter in approximately 12 to 15 seconds, with approximately 90% of the dilation occurring during the first 5 to 6 seconds. This includes pupils manifesting physiologic anisocoria. The Horner's pupil, however, requires approximately 25 seconds to return to its original darkness diameter, reaching about 90% of its final diameter within the first 10 to 15 seconds. The maximum difference between the normal pupil and Horner's pupil on dark dilation occurs after 4 to 5 seconds of

darkness. This difference is an expression of the dilation lag that is pathognomonic of Horner's syndrome. Flash Polaroid photographs should first be taken after the patient has been in bright light for a few minutes, then in darkness 4 to 5 seconds after the light has been extinguished, and then finally in darkness 10 to 12 seconds after the light has been extinguished (Fig. 23.2). The criteria for recognizing dilation lag are (1) poor dilation of the more miotic pupil at 4 to 5 seconds compared with the dilation achieved after 10 to 12

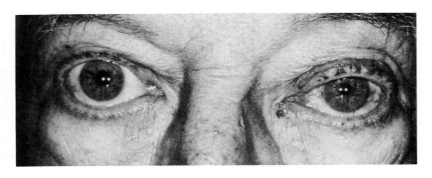

A

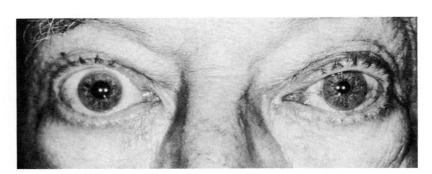

B

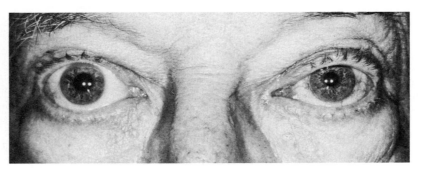

C

FIGURE 23.2   **Dilation lag in 72-year-old male with left Horner's syndrome.** *(A)* **Obvious anisocoria in bright illumination. Note greater anisocoria at 4 to 5 seconds in darkness** *(B)* **compared with the anisocoria at 10 to 12 seconds in darkness** *(C).*

seconds of darkness, and (2) increased anisocoria in darkness, more marked at 4 to 5 seconds than at 10 to 12 seconds.

Conjunctival hyperemia is usually a transient clinical sign and occurs only in the acute phase of Horner's syndrome, usually disappearing after the first several weeks.[27]

Since sweating is mediated by sympathetic innervation, interruption of these fibers results in facial or body anhydrosis or hypohydrosis. However, lesions involving the postganglionic sympathetic pathway generally cause Horner's syndrome without anhydrosis.[24] The presence of asymmetric sweating between each side of the forehead can be easily assessed by performing the friction sweat test.[28] This test assesses sweating by evaluating resistance to the movement of a standard office prism bar across the forehead. After cleaning both the forehead and prism bar with an alcohol pad, the face and bar are allowed to dry. Holding the bar against the forehead, and perpendicular to the floor, the bar is drawn downward while exerting mild pressure against the forehead. The amount of resistance to movement of the bar is compared for each side of the forehead. The anhydrotic side will be almost frictionless, while the normal side will display marked resistance to bar movement.

The finding of heterochromia iridis indicates congenital or neonatal Horner's syndrome. Normal pigmentation of the iris is associated in some way with integrity of the cervical sympathetic nervous system. Pigmentation of the iris is not complete until age 2 years. Hypopigmentation of the iris on the side of the lesion is characteristic of spinal birth injury involving the preganglionic (second-order) neuron.[24] Oculosympathetic paresis occurring after 2 years of age generally does not result in heterochromia, but several cases have been reported in adults.[383]

The term *Raeder's syndrome* designates any painful postganglionic Horner's syndrome.[15] The pain may consist of a unilateral headache or facial pain in the distribution of the trigeminal nerve. Patients with Raeder's syndrome fall into three major groups[15]: (1) those with either multiple parasellar cranial nerve involvement (III, IV, V, VI) or involvement of the second, third, or all three divisions of the trigeminal nerve; (2) those with a typical history of cluster headache; and (3) those with a pain history atypical of cluster headache, who may also have involvement of the first (ophthalmic) division of the trigeminal nerve only. Common to all three groups is the association of unilateral headache with interruption of the postganglionic oculosympathetic fibers along the course of the internal carotid artery.[29] The significance of Raeder's syndrome and its three major subclasses becomes apparent with regard to the strategies used in patient management.

PHARMACOLOGIC EVALUATION

The decision to proceed with pharmacologic testing is based solely on the clinical findings.[3,30] If there is unequivocally no ptosis and no dilation lag, the anisocoria can be considered to be physiologic, and the patient need not undergo pharmacologic evaluation. The patient who has minimal anisocoria with minimal ptosis, but without dilation lag, likewise can be considered to have physiologic anisocoria. If enough clinical findings, however, strongly suggest the possibility of Horner's syndrome, such as definite ptosis but equivocal dilation lag, then the cocaine test is indicated to confirm the diagnosis.[30] If definite miosis exists in association with definite ptosis, and if an unequivocal dilation lag also exists, the diagnosis of Horner's syndrome can be made on clinical grounds, and the practitioner may proceed directly to the hydroxyamphetamine test. In some cases various clinical signs can have significant localizing value, enabling the clinician to identify tentatively the site of the lesion before proceeding with pharmacologic testing (Table 23.6). Table 23.7 summarizes the indications for pharmacologic testing in patients with suspected Horner's syndrome.

Cocaine Test. When topically applied, cocaine produces dilation of the pupil by preventing the reuptake of norepinephrine that has been released into the synaptic junctions of

---

TABLE 23.6
Clinical Localizing Signs in Horner's Syndrome

Central Neuron Lesions	*Preganglionic Neuron Lesions*	*Postganglionic Neuron Lesions*
• Contralateral hypothesia of the body • Loss of sweating on entire half of body • Vertigo • Syringomyelia • Absense of ptosis	• Pain in ipsilateral arm or shoulder • Brachial plexus palsy • Pancoast's syndrome • Anhydrosis of face and neck • Flushing or blanching of face and neck • Thyroidectomy scar and hoarseness • Cervical osteoarthritis • Thoracic surgery	• Facial pain • No loss of sweating, except perhaps in supraorbital area

Modified from Pilley SFJ, Thompson HS. Pupillary "dilation lag" in Horner's syndrome. Br J Ophthalmol 1975;59:731–735.

TABLE 23.7
Indications for Pharmacologic Testing in Suspected Horner's Syndrome

Signs	Presumptive Clinical Diagnosis	Indicated Pharmacologic Testing
No ptosis No dilation lag[a]	Physiologic anisocoria	None
Minimal ptosis No dilation lag[a]	Physiologic anisocoria	None
Definite ptosis Equivocal dilation lag[a]	Horner's syndrome	Cocaine test followed by hydroxyamphetamine test
Definite ptosis Unequivocal dilation lag[a]	Horner's syndrome	Hydroxyamphetamine test

[a]Documented by photography.

the iris dilator muscle in response to a nerve impulse. If the sympathetic innervation to the eye is interrupted at any level (central, preganglionic, or postganglionic), cocaine should theoretically have no mydriatic effect because in each case the flow of nerve impulses has been impeded and no endogenous norepinephrine is released.[6] However, when the lesion is in the brainstem or spinal cord (first-order neuron), mydriasis with cocaine may be impaired but not entirely abolished. This impairment results from incomplete interruption of the descending sympathetic pathway.[6] Thus, as a rule, *dilation with cocaine is reduced or absent in any Horner's pupil regardless of the site of impairment.* Consequently, the cocaine test is useful as a screening procedure to confirm the presence or absence of oculosympathetic paresis, but *this test does not indicate the location of the lesion.*[31]

To perform the test, one drop of cocaine solution should be instilled into each eye and repeated after several minutes, and the pupils should be evaluated after 50–60 minutes[32] (Fig. 23.3). Ten percent cocaine is preferred over 5%, since weaker concentrations may require several hours before significant dilation is recognized in the normal pupil.[6,33] This situation is especially true for patients with dark irides, which may dilate very slowly and poorly.[33] Kardon and associates[32] have found that simply measuring the amount of postcocaine anisocoria provides a better prediction of Horner's syndrome than does calculating the net change in anisocoria. Table 23.8 shows the probability that a given amount of postcocaine anisocoria is associated with an actual diagnosis of Horner's syndrome. In general, a postcocaine anisocoria of at least 1.0 mm is required to confirm the diagnosis.[32]

Hydroxyamphetamine Test. In 1971 Thompson and Mensher[6] first suggested that the failure of hydroxyamphetamine (Paredrine) to dilate the postganglionic Horner's pupil could distinguish patients with postganglionic lesions from patients with central or preganglionic lesions. The pharmacologic rationale for this use of hydroxyamphetamine as a localizing drug is sound, and the value of hydroxyamphetamine in localizing the lesion in Horner's syndrome has been established with some certainty.[6,21,34]

The localizing value of hydroxyamphetamine lies in its

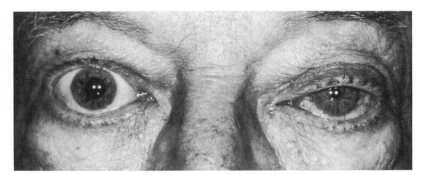

FIGURE 23.3   **Cocaine test for Horner's syndrome (same patient as in Fig. 23.2A). Following instillation of 10% cocaine into each eye, dilation occurs in the normal right pupil but not in the left Horner's pupil.**

TABLE 23.8
Interpretation of the Cocaine Test[a]

Postcocaine Anisocoria (mm)	Probability that Patient Has Horner's Syndrome
0.5	77:1
0.6	185:1
0.7	441:1
0.8	1050:1
0.9	2510:1
1.0	5990:1

[a]Applies only to white patients.
Adapted from Kardon RH, Denison CE, Brown CK, Thompson HS. Critical evaluation of the cocaine test in the diagnosis of Horner's syndrome. Arch Ophthalmol 1990;108:384–387.

indirect pharmacologic action.[35] This drug is an indirect acting α-adrenergic agonist that dilates the pupil only in the presence of endogenous norepinephrine.[36,37] In the case of postganglionic Horner's syndrome, the postganglionic sympathetic pathway is compromised enough to diminish the normal concentration of norepinephrine contained within the presynaptic vesicle. Consequently, hydroxyamphetamine cannot produce mydriasis or produces only incomplete mydriasis[6,36,37] (Fig. 23.4). In the case of central or preganglionic lesions, the postganglionic sympathetic pathway is left undisturbed so that the norepinephrine contained within the presynaptic vesicles may be released by the topically instilled hydroxyamphetamine, thus producing normal mydriasis.[6] Thus, hydroxyamphetamine has a mydriatic effect only when the postganglionic sympathetic pathway to the eye is intact. However, one source of error in hydroxyamphetamine testing is its use in infants with acquired preganglionic lesions. Due to transsynaptic degeneration, the pupil may behave pharmacologically as if a postganglionic lesion were present.[38]

The current clinical usefulness of hydroxyamphetamine lies in its ability to distinguish between central or preganglionic and postganglionic lesions. Hydroxyamphetamine provides a clearer distinction between preganglionic and postganglionic defects than does any other mydriatic test.[6,34,37] Although the hydroxyamphetamine test is not subject to error due to factors that tend to enhance corneal penetration, the results of this test may be somewhat ambiguous when the Horner's syndrome is incomplete.[25,37] Furthermore, since pretreatment with cocaine interferes with the action of hydroxyamphetamine,[6] at least two days should elapse after cocaine administration before proceeding with the hydroxyamphetamine test. Brumberg[3] has proposed a useful mnemonic for the hydroxyamphetamine test—"FAIL-SAFE." This phrase suggests that failure of the pupil to dilate with hydroxyamphetamine indicates a good prognosis (postganglionic lesion). Table 23.9 shows the probability that the lesion causing Horner's syndrome is postganglionic based on results of the hydroxyamphetamine test. The pupils should be observed 45–60 minutes after instilling the medication.

Table 23.10 summarizes the expected responses of the Horner's pupil to cocaine and hydroxyamphetamine. This current schema for drug testing in Horner's syndrome applies only to *complete* lesions of the oculosympathetic pathway and should not be relied on in patients with incomplete lesions. Cocaine is used initially to confirm the presence of Horner's syndrome, while hydroxyamphetamine is employed several days later to localize the lesion to the central preganglionic or postganglionic sympathetic pathway. Note that *presently no pupillary drug test clearly distinguishes central from preganglionic lesions.*[5,39]

Management

It is crucial to differentiate central or preganglionic lesions from postganglionic lesions, since appropriate patient man-

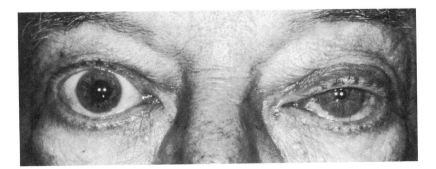

FIGURE 23.4 **Hydroxyamphetamine test in Horner's syndrome (same patient as in Fig. 23.2A). Following instillation of 1% hydroxyamphetamine into each eye, dilation of the normal right pupil occurs but not of the left Horner's pupil, indicating a postganglionic lesion.**

TABLE 23.9
Interpretation of the Hydroxyamphetamine Test

Difference in Dilation to Hydroxyamphetamine[a] (mm)	Probability that Lesion Is Postganglionic (%)
−1.4	0.7
−1.2	1.3
−1.0	2.2
−0.8	3.7
−0.6	6.3
−0.4	10.6
−0.2	17.1
0.0	26.5
0.2	38.7
0.4	52.5
0.6	65.9
0.8	77.1
1.0	85.5
1.2	91.2
1.4	94.8
1.6	96.9
1.8	98.2
2.0	99.0
2.2	99.4
2.4	99.7

[a]Difference in dilation is calculated as the change in diameter of the unaffected pupil minus the change in diameter of the affected pupil.

Adapted from Cremer SA, Thompson HS, Digre KB, Kardon RH. Hydroxyamphetamine mydriasis in Horner's syndrome. Am J Ophthalmol 1990; 110:71–76.

agement depends on accurate localization of the lesion. When the detailed history, clinical examination, and pharmacologic testing indicate a central or preganglionic lesion of unknown etiology, the patient should be referred to a thoracic surgeon or internist because of the risk of malignancy.[27] Because of the risk of neuroblastoma, pediatric patients with early onset Horner's syndrome should also be investigated.[40] Neurologic consultation should be considered when central lesions are strongly suspected.[41]

Postganglionic lesions, however, are most likely associated with a benign vascular headache syndrome. Such patients with unilateral headache and isolated postganglionic Horner's syndrome usually have a benign course and need no further evaluation. However, if the headaches do not spontaneously resolve within several months, or if objective involvement of the trigeminal nerve or other parasellar cranial nerves is documented, then further neurologic investigation should be considered.[29,41] Figure 23.5 summarizes the management of the patient with Horner's syndrome of unknown etiology.

Adie's Syndrome

In 1932, Adie described a syndrome in which usually unilateral defective accommodation and constriction of the pupil were associated with absent or markedly diminished tendon reflexes but without evidence of syphilis.[42] An association between tonic pupils and hyporeflexia is known as *Adie's syndrome,* and the tonic pupil alone without associated hyporeflexia is termed *Adie's pupil.*

Etiology

The etiology of Adie's pupil is usually unknown.[43] It is generally accepted, however, that the lesion is in the ciliary ganglion, with damage to the postganglionic neurons serving the ciliary muscle and iris sphincter.[43,44] Adie's pupil frequently follows a mild upper respiratory infection, and thus in some cases it may be associated with a nonspecific viral illness. In other instances orbital trauma can produce the syndrome, and surgical repair of orbital floor fractures can also cause Adie's pupil due to damage to the ciliary ganglion or postganglionic neurons.[45] Adie's-like pupils with accommodative paresis have occurred as complications following peripheral retinal laser treatment. They result from laser damage to cholinergic nerve fibers, beneath the treated area, that innervate the ciliary body and iris sphinc-

TABLE 23.10
Mydriatic Drug Tests in Horner's Syndrome

Drug	Normal	Central Lesion	Preganglionic Lesion	Postganglionic Lesion
Cocaine 10% (2 drops)	Mydriasis	Impaired dilation	No dilation	No dilation
Hydroxyamphetamine 1% (2 drops)	Mydriasis	Normal dilation	Normal dilation	No dilation

Modified from Thompson HS. Diagnostic pupillary drug tests. In: Blodi FC, ed. Current concepts in ophthalmology. St. Louis: C. V. Mosby Co, 1972;3:76–90, with permission of the author and publisher.

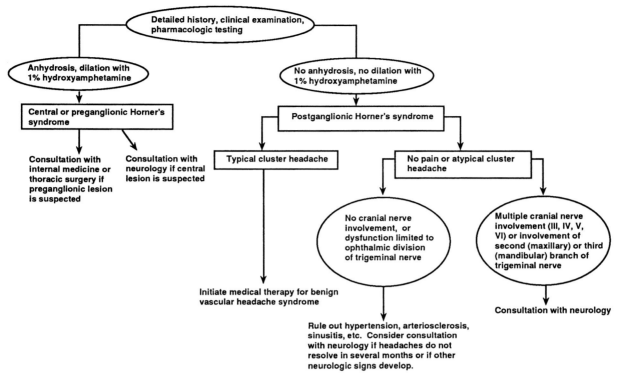

FIGURE 23.5   **Flowchart for the management of the patient with Horner's syndrome of unknown etiology. (Modified from Grimson BS, Thompson HS. Raeder's syndrome. A clinical review. Surv Ophthalmol 1980;24:199–210.)**

ter.[46] An Adie's-like sector palsy, but without accommodative insufficiency, can follow argon laser trabeculoplasty for treatment of primary open-angle glaucoma.[47] Coppeto and associates[48] have reported Adie's pupils following ipsilateral third-nerve palsy, probably caused by misdirection of injured preganglionic parasympathetic fibers. When Adie's pupil occurs bilaterally, it may be associated with orthostatic hypotension, Riley-Day syndrome, or neurosyphilis.[49]

Perhaps the most widely accepted interpretation of Adie's pupil involves the concept of aberrant regeneration of nerve fibers.[25,44] The parasympathetic accommodative fibers in the ciliary ganglion are believed to be far more numerous than those that supply the iris sphincter. Following destructive ciliary ganglion disease, nerve fiber regeneration may occur with some accommodative fibers becoming misdirected and supplying the iris sphincter. This results in attenuation or loss of the pupillary light response but with preservation of the potential for constriction of the pupil in accommodation, so-called light-near dissociation. Although this hypothesis does not explain the hyporeflexia that often accompanies the ocular findings in Adie's syndrome, the syndrome may represent a form of mild polyneuropathy,[50] accounting for the diminished deep tendon reflexes. In rare cases Adie's

syndrome and a *severe* polyneuropathy can be associated with underlying malignant disease.[51] Perhaps the most noteworthy difference between the clinical signs of Adie's pupil and those of isolated third-nerve pupillary palsy is the presence of light-near dissociation in the former and its absence in the latter.[25]

Diagnosis

CLINICAL EVALUATION

Adie's pupil is a benign disorder.[52] However, because the patient is often alarmed by the presence of a sudden unilateral fixed and dilated pupil, prompt and accurate diagnosis is extremely important. A diagnosis of Adie's pupil eliminates the need for elaborate and expensive neuroradiologic investigations. Table 23.11 lists the primary clinical characteristics diagnostic of Adie's syndrome.

Adie's pupil is unilateral in 80% to 90% of all cases.[7,53] Of the unilateral cases being monitored, approximately 4% become bilateral each year.[7]

In the acute stage, the pupil is usually dilated and reacts

TABLE 23.11
Diagnostic Signs in Adie's Syndrome

- Relative mydriasis in bright illumination
- Absent or poor light reaction
- Slow (tonic) contraction to prolonged near effort
- Slow redilation after near effort
- Vermiform movements of pupillary margin (i.e., sector palsies of iris sphincter)
- Accommodative paresis
- Diminished deep tendon reflexes
- Onset in third to fifth decade[a]
- Females affected in 70% of cases

[a]Can rarely occur in children[89]

very poorly to light. The tonic pupil often changes size in a random manner, possibly being larger in the morning or smaller in the afternoon.[53] Adie's pupils tend to become smaller with time.[7] Some patients who have been monitored for several years have shown a strikingly progressive miosis of the affected pupil. The gradual constriction is more marked than the normal miosis of aging. In an extensive review, Thompson[7] collected data suggesting that Adie's pupils are generally larger than normal initially and quickly become smaller. In fact, the dilated pupil usually returns to its previous size within a few months, and after approximately two years a very slowly progressive additional miosis occurs. In some cases, however, the affected pupil may be miotic, without ever passing through the dilated phase.[54] Thus, the diagnosis should be considered in any patient with a poorly reactive pupil, regardless of its size. In darkness most Adie's pupils are smaller than normal. In a patient with an Adie's pupil larger than the normal pupil in darkness, the condition is most likely of very recent onset.[7] The tendency of Adie's pupils to become progressively miotic and to become bilateral with age suggests that many Adie's pupils eventually become disguised as Argyll Robertson-like pupils or simply become inconspicuous among the smaller pupils of the elderly.[7] Furthermore, the patient learns that the condition is benign and seeks no further medical attention.

The reaction of the Adie's pupil to an accommodative stimulus is very sluggish and poor.[53] The typical slow and tonic near response serves as the mechanism for the most distinguishing clinical feature of this syndrome, namely, tonic and sluggish redilation as the patient changes fixation from near to distance.

Of patients with Adie's pupil, 50% to 90% demonstrate significantly impaired or absent deep tendon reflexes, and this sign serves as a helpful clinical confirmation of the diagnosis. In the series of patients reported by Thompson,[7] the majority had tendon reflexes that were abnormal throughout the body, but the ankles and triceps had greater impairment than the knees and biceps. Approximately one-third of patients with Adie's syndrome have entirely normal knee jerks, but about half of patients have completely absent ankle jerks. In Thompson's[7] series, only 10% had entirely normal reflexes.

When observed with the slit lamp, the iris may demonstrate subtle and irregular (vermiform) movements of its sphincter.[7] Segmental palsies of portions of the iris sphincter occur in almost every patient with Adie's pupil. Vermiform movements of the sphincter are nothing more than physiologic pupillary unrest (hippus) of those segments of the sphincter that are intact and still functioning in response to light. Although the affected pupil shows some residual light reaction in most patients, approximately 10% of patients have a total palsy of the iris sphincter.[7,55] Segmental palsies of the iris sphincter characterize Adie's pupil, but they are not pathognomonic.[55,56]

Most patients with Adie's pupil have an accommodative paresis in the involved eye at the onset of the condition, and this paresis is often the primary source of their symptoms.[7] A relative accommodative paresis in the affected eye of 0.50 D or more at initial examination occurred in two-thirds of the patients evaluated by Thompson.[7] However, accommodation tends to recover, and most of this recovery occurs during the first two years.[7]

In summary, the typical patient with acute Adie's syndrome is young (20–40 years of age), otherwise healthy female presenting with a unilateral fixed and dilated pupil, with blurred near vision in the affected eye, and with impaired deep tendon reflexes. Clinical evaluation reveals tonic redilation of the pupil from near to distance. Such a patient can usually be given the diagnosis of Adie's syndrome on clinical grounds alone without the need for pharmacologic, laboratory, or neuroradiologic investigations. In those instances, however, in which the clinical signs are ambiguous or incomplete, pharmacologic testing is indicated.

PHARMACOLOGIC EVALUATION

Pilocarpine Test. Clinicians have known for many years that the denervated iris sphincter in Adie's pupil shows cholinergic hypersensitivity. This response is expected according to the principle of denervation hypersensitivity. Although helpful in confirming the diagnosis, the diagnosis can often be made even when hypersensitivity cannot be demonstrated. Furthermore, the hypersensitivity does not seem to correlate with the amount of sphincter denervation, the duration of the Adie's pupil, or the amount of light-near dissociation.[7] Occasionally an acute Adie's pupil shows very little hypersensitivity during the first few weeks after onset but gradually becomes more hypersensitive several months following the initial episode.[7,53]

Although methacholine became popular to elicit the cholinergic denervation hypersensitivity in Adie's pupil, its usefulness was quite limited because fewer than half of Adie's pupils demonstrated a convincing miosis to the 2.5% solution.[7] Methacholine has not been commercially available for many years, but pilocarpine, when used in very low concentrations, serves as a more useful and more reliable substitute. Clinicians have demonstrated cholinergic hypersensitivity by using pilocarpine in 0.0625%, 0.1%, 0.125%, or 0.25% solution (Table 23.12). The usefulness of the pilocarpine test in eliciting cholinergic hypersensitivity depends on the presence of a standardized concentration of drug at the iris. Thus, any clinical procedure that compromises the corneal epithelium, the use of wetting agents, or other factors that enhance corneal penetration may result in false-positive findings. Although not clinically practical, the pilocarpine should ideally be administered in a vehicle that is not preserved with benzalkonium chloride or another substance that may enhance corneal penetration of the drug.[25]

Younge and Buski[11] have recommended using a 0.1% pilocarpine solution. These investigators report that too many false-positive reactions occur with 0.2% and that too many insufficient responses (false negative) of the Adie's pupil occur with 0.05% pilocarpine solution. These authors found that a 0.1% concentration of pilocarpine performed the best clinically to confirm the Adie's pupil. This concentration of pilocarpine does not usually constrict the normal pupil but does constrict the tonic pupil.

Thompson[7] and Pilley and Thompson,[57] however, have

TABLE 23.12
Dilution of Commercially Available Pilocarpine[a]

Concentration (%) of Commercially Available Pilocarpine	Desired Final Concentration (%)	
	0.1	0.125
1	1/9	1/7
2	1/19	1/15

[a]Dilutions are prepared by mixing the indicated number of drops of commercially available drug (numerator of fraction) with the indicated number of drops of extraocular irrigating solution or normal saline (denominator of fraction). Equal drop sizes should be used.

recommended using pilocarpine as a 0.125% solution. This concentration slightly constricts most normal pupils, with the degree of miosis differing among individuals from just noticeable to several millimeters.[7] Using a concentration that slightly constricts the normal pupil allows the clinician to ascertain whether each eye has received an adequate amount of drug. In the typical patient with Adie's pupil, 0.125% pilocarpine causes a slight constriction of the normal pupil, while the affected pupil becomes even more miotic[5] (Fig. 23.6).

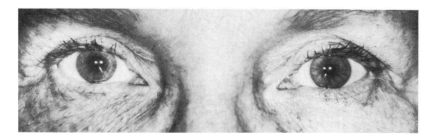

A

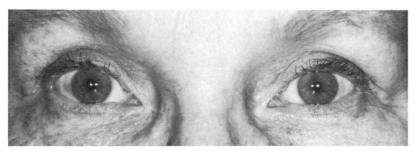

B

FIGURE 23.6 **Pilocarpine test in 57-year-old woman with right Adie's pupil.** *(A)* **Before drug instillation.** *(B)* **Following instillation of 0.125% pilocarpine into each eye, the normal left pupil constricts slightly while the right Adie's pupil constricts significantly.**

When evaluating cholinergic hypersensitivity, it is important to use the lowest ambient illumination possible to reduce the additional miotic influence of light. This approach enhances judgment of pupil size and response to the dilute pilocarpine. Jacobson and Olson[58] have suggested a practical endpoint interpretation of the pilocarpine test. If the patient's larger pupil becomes the smaller pupil in dim illumination after dilute pilocarpine is instilled into both eyes, the reaction of the larger pupil most likely represents a hypersensitive response and thus indicates a diagnosis of Adie's pupil. This endpoint does not apply, however, to suspected bilateral tonic pupils, tonic pupils that are smaller than their normal fellow pupils in dim illumination, or longstanding Adie's pupils that are small in both darkness and normal ambient light.[58]

Management

Since Adie's syndrome is a benign disorder, the most important aspect in patient management is reassurance. The associated accommodative paresis tends to recover during the first several years, and any visual impairment thus improves. The patient should be advised that the second eye may become involved but that the other changes associated with the syndrome (decreased light reaction and diminished deep tendon reflexes) do not represent significant functional impairments. For many patients the chief concern is for the cosmetic appearance of the unequal pupils. Most patients can be reassured that, with time, this should become less noticeable.

In most cases the clinician should *not* prescribe pilocarpine for the affected pupil because the intermittent drug-induced accommodative spasm, which the hypersensitivity of the ciliary muscle aggravates, is not usually tolerated. Symptomatic patients, however, may benefit from the instillation of 0.1% to 0.125% pilocarpine into the affected eye three or four times daily.[59,60] Because of individual variability, various low concentrations of pilocarpine should be attempted to determine the optimum concentration of miotic that alleviates symptoms such as periocular discomfort, headache, photophobia, or blurred vision.[60] If a miotic is used in this fashion, the patient should be carefully monitored in anticipation of modifying the drug regimen if the degree of cholinergic hypersensitivity changes with time.

The practitioner can also prescribe tinted lenses, which not only shield the cosmetic appearance of the unequal pupils but also alleviate perception of the Pulfrich phenomenon produced by the anisocoria. Moreover, when affected patients are presbyopic, unequal bifocal powers are clearly justified and frequently serve to alleviate the asthenopia associated with near vision. Reading lenses may be indicated for patients who are prepresbyopic.

Unilateral Fixed and Dilated Pupil

A unilateral fixed and dilated pupil in an ambulatory and otherwise healthy patient is seldom associated with significant neurologic disease. Yet, historically, the practitioner has been cautioned to consider this a sign of potentially grave intracranial disease. Although the possible causes of a fixed and dilated pupil are numerous and include potentially destructive vascular and neoplastic processes, the clinician is usually able, by a careful history and physical examination, to narrow the possible diagnoses to three[61]: (1) involvement of the intracranial third nerve, (2) Adie's pupil, or (3) anticholinergic mydriasis.

Since the fixed and dilated pupil is clearly the abnormal pupil, the pharmacologic evaluation involves instillation of a miotic, usually pilocarpine, to assess the degree of impairment of the iris sphincter or its parasympathetic innervation. In the majority of cases only one pupil is dilated and fixed, and instilling the drug into both eyes can avoid false-positive or false-negative drug tests. Constriction of the normal pupil thus indicates that enough pilocarpine was instilled. When both pupils are dilated and fixed, the drops should be placed in only one eye so that any constriction can be attributed solely to the drug.[61]

The following sections consider the most common disorders associated with a unilateral fixed and dilated pupil, including third-nerve palsy, anticholinergic mydriasis, iris sphincter atrophy, and adrenergic mydriasis. Since a dilated pupil does not always characterize Adie's syndrome, this disorder has been discussed separately.

Third-Nerve Palsy

The patient presenting with the classic signs of a complete third-nerve palsy (Fig. 23.7) need not undergo pharmacologic testing; the diagnosis can be made on clinical grounds alone. The patient should be referred to a neurologist, since a complete third-nerve palsy of recent onset is of neurologic significance.[62] The most common cause of a sudden unilateral third-nerve palsy in an adult with a dilated and fixed pupil and with headache is an aneurysm at the junction of the ipsilateral internal carotid artery and the posterior communicating arteries.[63] The practitioner should recall, however, that the most common cause of a sudden unilateral third-nerve palsy in an adult with headache but with *spared* pupil is diabetes mellitus.[53,64] The pupillary findings, therefore, are extremely important in the evaluation and management of an acute third-nerve palsy.

If, however, the patient exhibits only a unilateral fixed and dilated pupil without evidence of ptosis or extraocular muscle involvement, the clinician should perform the pilocarpine test, first using a 0.125% solution to reveal any cholinergic hypersensitivity as evidence for Adie's pupil. If

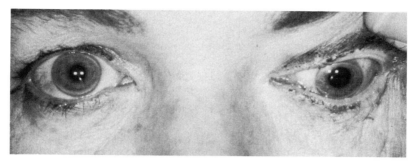

FIGURE 23.7   **Complete third-nerve palsy. Note the left ptosis, exotropia, hypotropia, and dilated pupil.**

there is no local iris damage by slit-lamp examination, no sector palsy of the iris sphincter, and no cholinergic hypersensitivity demonstrated by the 0.125% pilocarpine, then the condition might be associated with interruption of the preganglionic innervation to the iris sphincter (i.e., third-nerve palsy). If the patient has a third-nerve palsy, topically instilled pilocarpine in moderate concentrations will activate the muscarinic receptor sites on the iris sphincter. Therefore, if 0.125% pilocarpine reveals no cholinergic hypersensitivity, the practitioner should subsequently instill pilocarpine in a concentration of 0.5% or 1.0%. This should promptly constrict the affected pupil[8,65] (Fig. 23.8). Several authors[66,67] have shown, however, that many patients with intracranial third-nerve palsy may appear to manifest hypersensitivity to low concentrations of pilocarpine. This occurs due to the greater mechanical reactivity of the larger pupil, and in long-

standing cases may also be caused by actual denervation hypersensitivity of the iris sphincter due to transsynaptic degeneration of postganglionic neurons.[67] Thus, the clinician should carefully evaluate all clinical signs and symptoms before reaching a final diagnosis.

Anticholinergic Mydriasis

ETIOLOGY

Anticholinergic mydriasis, also known as pharmacologic blockade or "atropinic" mydriasis, refers to the fixed and dilated pupil resulting from the accidental inoculation into the eye of drugs or substances with anticholinergic properties. Medical personnel such as doctors, nurses, and pharma-

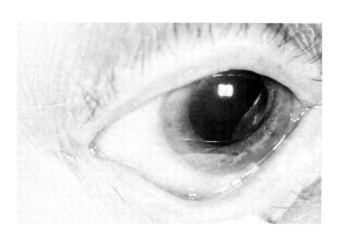

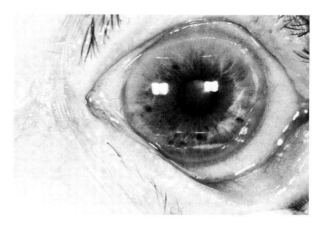

A   B

FIGURE 23.8   **Pilocarpine test in third-nerve palsy.** *(A)* **Before drug instillation.** *(B)* **Following instillation of 1.0% pilocarpine, the pupil promptly constricts.**

cists are particularly susceptible to this condition, since they frequently handle such medications. Often some medication spills over the side of the bottle, and the practitioner or nurse who next handles the bottle comes into contact with the dried medication. The drug is then easily transferred to the eye by simple rubbing. Although such medications commonly include cyclopentolate, homatropine, and atropine, many other drugs or substances with anticholinergic properties have been implicated. On occasion, the patient admits to having placed some drops into the affected eye but often cannot recall the name of the medication. In these cases the practitioner should inquire about the color of the medication cap, since cycloplegics are commercially packaged with red caps. Often patients have instilled into their mildly irritated eye atropine drops previously prescribed for an episode of anterior uveitis.

Other substances have also been implicated in anticholinergic mydriasis. Jimson weed (*Datura stramonium*) grass is found in many parts of the United States, and the entire plant from root to flower contains significant concentrations of belladonna alkaloids including atropine, scopolamine, hyoscine, and hyoscyamine.[68] A farmer working in a dusty field often sustains relatively insignificant ocular foreign bodies, and a particle of jimson weed irritates the eye no more than any other particle of plant origin. The farmer may not notice the drug-induced dilated pupil and blurred vision until the following day, and he or she often does not associate the onset of the condition with an ocular foreign body. Numerous cases of jimson weed mydriasis have been reported.[69–71] Thus, the practitioner should suspect jimson weed mydriasis in farmers, or in children who have been "picking flowers," if these patients present with an acute onset of unilateral mydriasis. Moreover, the dried pods of the plant are often used in floral arrangements for indoor decoration during the winter. This use may contribute to an increased risk of systemic toxicity in the pediatric age group, since children have been known to consume such "berries." In fact, fatal cases have been reported in children whose stomachs contained the seeds at autopsy.[68] In addition to *bilaterally* dilated pupils when the weed is consumed orally, the early symptoms of systemic toxicity are those typical of anticholinergic drugs: blurred vision, dryness of the mouth, extreme thirst, constipation, urinary retention, convulsions, dry and flushed skin, diffuse erythematous rash, tachycardia, and fever.

The practitioner should be alert to the possible inoculation into the eye of *any* drug or substance with anticholinergic properties, including plants, cosmetics, perfumes, or medicines. Several patients have sustained unilateral fixed and dilated pupils following the use of antiperspirants.[72,73] The use of transdermal scopolamine (Transderm Scop) for the prophylaxis of motion sickness can result in the development of unilateral fixed and dilated pupils.[74–77] Scopolamine from the disk placed behind the ear can be inadvertently inoculated into the eye, producing the typical signs of anticholinergic mydriasis. Fixed and dilated pupils have also resulted from direct droplet contamination associated with the use of anticholinergic aerosols for treatment of acute asthma and other airflow obstructions.[78,79]

DIAGNOSIS

Since the pupillary paralysis of neurogenic origin (i.e., third-nerve palsy) is clinically indistinguishable from anticholinergic mydriasis, many practitioners have unnecessarily subjected patients to extensive neurologic, radiologic, and laboratory investigations for possible intracranial disease. Instead, the diagnostic procedure of choice in such instances is one or two drops of 0.5% or 1.0% pilocarpine instilled into each eye (Fig. 23.9). If the muscarinic receptor sites on the affected iris sphincter have been occupied by an anticholinergic drug, the pilocarpine fails to activate the receptors and constrict the pupil. Thus, this simple test quickly and easily differentiates between anticholinergic mydriasis and pupillary paralysis associated with third-nerve palsy; the former does not react to the pilocarpine, while the latter constricts.[8,65,70]

Thompson and associates[61] have recommended using pilocarpine initially in a 0.5% rather than 1.0% concentration because a pupil that is only weakly dilated with an anticholinergic drug might become constricted by the stronger pilocarpine solution, resulting in a false-positive finding. If neither the normal nor the affected pupil constricts when the 0.5% pilocarpine is instilled, the stronger solution should then be used.

MANAGEMENT

Once the diagnosis of anticholinergic mydriasis has been confirmed, the patient should be reassured that with time, usually a few days to a few weeks, the pupil will spontaneously return to its original size, and vision (accommodation) will improve as the effects of the inoculated substance subside.

Damage to the Iris

Damage to the iris sphincter muscle by high intraocular pressure, trauma, or inflammation may impair pilocarpine's ability to constrict the pupil. Clinically, these conditions can usually be ruled out by careful history and physical (biomicroscopic) examination. Mechanical factors associated with malpositioned intraocular lenses[80] or posterior synechiae may also limit movement of the iris. Depending on the extent of iris damage, the pupil may demonstrate constriction ranging from complete to nonexistent.[8,61,65]

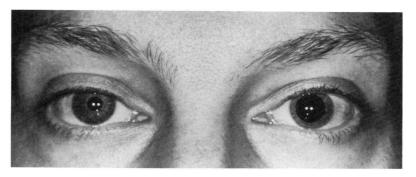

A

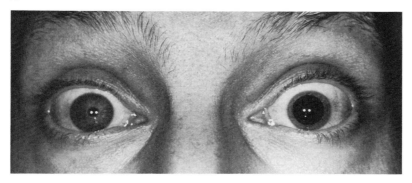

B

FIGURE 23.9 **Pilocarpine test in anticholinergic mydriasis. (A) 27-year-old man with fixed and dilated left pupil. (B) Following instillation of 1.0% pilocarpine into each eye, the right pupil constricts while the left pupil does not.**

Adrenergic Mydriasis

Although the pupil that has become dilated in response to topically instilled adrenergic drugs is often not completely immobile, this condition is included here for the sake of completeness. A patient who is unusually sensitive to adrenergic agonists may sustain a dilated pupil as a consequence of the accidental inoculation into the eye of nose drops, nasal sprays, or other substances with adrenergic properties.[81] In addition, some patients with minor corneal epithelial compromise may sustain a dilated pupil following the instillation of decongestant eyedrops. In these instances, however, the adrenergic mydriasis can usually be distinguished from the dilated pupil of third-nerve palsy or anticholinergic mydriasis by the blanched conjunctiva, the residual pupillary light reaction, and the occasional retracted upper eyelid[25,61] (Fig. 23.10). Although dilation associated with adrenergic agonists is usually incomplete and short-lived, the concomitant use of topical epinephrine and timolol for the treatment of glaucoma may occasionally result in the development of

long-standing fixed and dilated pupils.[82] A careful history and clinical evaluation of the patient will usually eliminate the need for pharmacologic testing.

Figure 23.11 summarizes the clinical and pharmacologic evaluations of the patient with anisocoria in which only one pupil is affected.

Myasthenia Gravis

Myasthenia gravis is an autoimmune disease that affects the neuromuscular junction. A decrease in the number of available acetylcholine receptors due to circulating antibodies results in impaired neuromuscular transmission. This impairment manifests itself clinically as weakness and fatigability of voluntary musculature. Ocular and other muscles innervated by cranial nerves are most often involved. Although different treatment modalities are available, anticholinesterase drugs are still the mainstay of therapy.

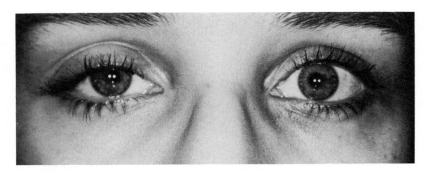

FIGURE 23.10   Retracted left upper lid following instillation of 0.012% naphazoline (Degest 2) as a decongestant.

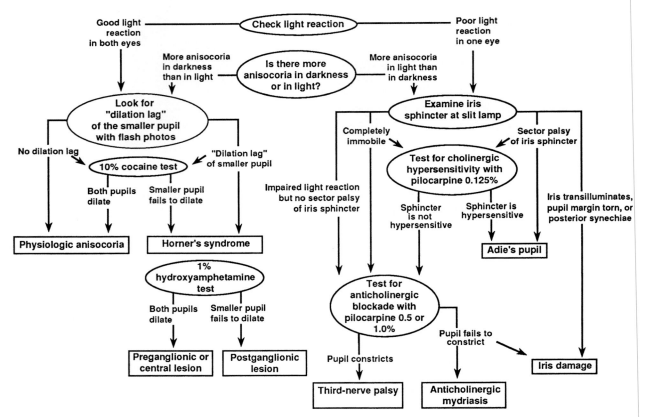

FIGURE 23.11   Flowchart for the clinical and pharmacologic evaluations of the patient with anisocoria in which only one pupil is affected. (Modified from Thompson HS, Pilley SFJ. Unequal pupils. A flow chart for sorting out the anisocorias. Surv Ophthalmol 1976; 21(1):45–48, with permission of the authors and publisher.)

Etiology

Although the originating event is unknown, the presence of antibodies to the acetylcholine receptor reduces the availability of functioning acetylcholine receptors at the neuro-muscular junction, resulting in defective neuromuscular transmission.[90,91] These circulating antibodies can be found in up to 90% of patients with generalized myasthenia gravis and in almost 70% of individuals with only ocular symptoms.[92,93]

Pathologic changes in myasthenia gravis are limited to voluntary (skeletal) muscle and the thymus gland. The most common abnormality in muscle is single fiber atrophy, although lymphocytic infiltration is also prevalent.[94]

Approximately 75% of myasthenic patients have thymus gland abnormalities. Of these, 85% show germinal-center formation or hyperplasia, and encapsulated tumors or thymomas occur in the remaining 15%.[95] The complex relationship between the thymus gland and myasthenia gravis suggests that this organ may play a critical role in both the origin and maintenance of the autoimmune process.[91]

Epidemiology

The prevalence of myasthenia gravis in the United States is 3/100,000, and before age 40 years the disease is three times more common in females. In older individuals, the disease affects males and females equally.[96] Of the 15% of myasthenics who have thymomas, approximately 60% are older males.[97]

Infants born to myasthenic mothers exhibit generalized weakness for several days or weeks, but resolution is usually complete. Congenital myasthenia occurs in children of nonmyasthenic mothers, and these children exhibit ophthalmoplegia from birth. This type of myasthenia is not autoimmune in nature since these patients have no measurable serum acetylcholine receptor antibodies.[90,94,96]

Diagnosis

The diagnostic evaluation of myasthenia gravis includes a complete history and physical examination, objective evidence of circulating acetylcholine receptor antibodies, electrophysiologic evidence of abnormal neuromuscular transmission, and pharmacologic evaluation with anticholinesterase drugs.

CLINICAL FEATURES

The voluntary or skeletal musculature exhibits variable weakness, which can fluctuate during the day or from day to day. Usually the weakness is greater after muscle use and diminishes with rest.

Ocular muscles are affected first in approximately 40% of cases, and these muscles are eventually affected in over 90% of patients.[96,98] Unilateral or bilateral ptosis is often the first presenting sign. Levator weakness can be tested by instructing the patient to blink several times in rapid succession to determine whether the ptosis worsens. The patient should also stare upward at a fixed point so the practitioner can observe the upper eyelids for gradual lowering. Cogan[99] described the lid-twitch sign, in which the patient is directed to look down for 10–15 seconds and then to refixate quickly

in the primary position. Observation of an upward overshoot of the lid with several twitches, followed by repositioning of the lids to the original ptotic state identifies the easy fatigability and rapid recovery of the myasthenic levator muscle.

Diplopia secondary to extraocular muscle involvement may occur separately or accompany eyelid ptosis and can be variable. Variability in measuring phorias and tropias during the same examination or on different examination days is highly suggestive of myasthenia. Extraocular muscle weakness can also mimic internuclear ophthalmoplegia, horizontal or vertical gaze palsies, or oculomotor nerve palsies.

Strength of the orbicularis oculi muscle can be easily tested by instructing the patient to forcefully close the eyes while the examiner attempts to open the eyelids manually. Because of orbicularis muscle fatigue in myasthenics, the eyelids offer little resistance and open easily.

Nonocular muscle involvement is also prevalent, ranging from fluctuating dysarthria to dysphagia. No specific pattern of limb weakness occurs, although the proximal muscles are most often affected.[94]

PHARMACOLOGIC EVALUATION

The most commonly used pharmacologic test for the diagnosis of myasthenia gravis is the edrophonium chloride (Tensilon) test. This anticholinesterase agent acts by inactivating the enzyme acetylcholinesterase. This leads to accumulation of excessive amounts of acetylcholine, resulting in prolonged neurotransmitter activity on the muscle fiber's specialized motor endplate. Tensilon is a reversible agent of rapid onset (30–60 seconds following intravenous injection) and short duration of action, lasting approximately 10 minutes.[100]

The Tensilon test can be performed in the clinician's office if appropriate resuscitation equipment is available (see Chap. 38). The ideal testing protocol involves two examiners, one giving the injection and the other recording the results. Photographing or videotaping the objective findings is also helpful. Although any muscle or muscle groups can be observed for clinical improvement, ptosis appears to respond better than diplopia to Tensilon testing[101] (Fig. 23.12).

Tensilon is available in multiple-dose or single-dose, 10 mg/ml ampules. An accessible vein is found on one of the patient's arms, and a butterfly infusion set with a 27-gauge needle is attached to a 1-ml tuberculin syringe containing 10 mg edrophonium (Tensilon) solution (Fig. 23.13). Initially, 2 mg (0.2 ml) of edrophonium is injected intravenously. A saline flush may follow this injection to confirm appropriate dose administration. If after 1 or 2 minutes definite improvement in ptosis or ocular misalignment occurs, the test is considered positive and no further edrophonium injection is necessary. If no definite improvement occurs, however, another 3 mg (0.3 ml) of edrophonium is injected and the patient is again observed. If no improvement occurs, the remaining 5 mg (0.5 ml) of edrophonium can be given and

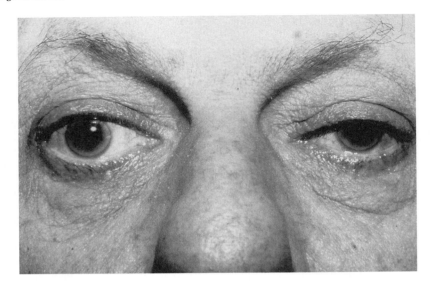

A

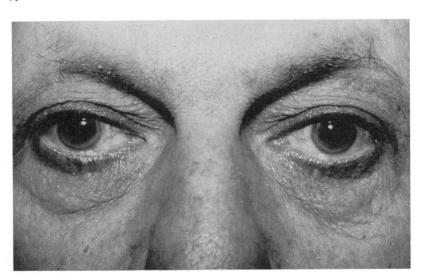

B

FIGURE 23.12 *(A)* **Left eyelid ptosis before Tensilon testing.** *(B)* **Resolution of ptosis after Tensilon injection.**

the patient evaluated for several more minutes. Doses higher than 10 mg do not produce any improvement of symptoms if lower doses failed to elicit improvement.[102]

The practitioner can perform placebo testing with saline solution if he or she suspects that the observed weakness has a functional origin. This may help in evaluating limb weakness but is not necessary in investigating levator or orbicularis muscle weakness because the latter cannot be

simulated.[96] In ocular myasthenia without systemic manifestations, up to 95% of patients will have a positive Tensilon test.[101]

Cholinergic side effects associated with edrophonium include increased salivation, nausea, vomiting, sweating, perioral fasciculations, and diarrhea. These side effects resolve quickly after Tensilon testing has stopped. More serious side effects include systemic hypotension, bradycardia,

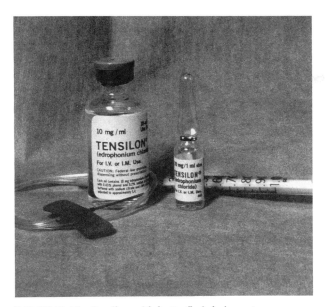

FIGURE 23.13   **Tensilon with butterfly infusion set.**

or increased muscle weakness resulting in respiratory distress. These adverse effects may require treatment with atropine sulfate.[100] Atropine can be administered prophylactically by giving 0.3–0.4 mg intramuscularly 15 minutes before Tensilon testing. Alternatively, 0.3–0.5 mg atropine should be available in a tuberculin syringe for intravenous injection in case Tensilon testing brings on a severe life-threatening reaction.[100]

The neostigmine (Prostigmin) test is used more often to help evaluate limb strength in suspected myasthenics. Neostigmine, a reversible cholinesterase inhibitor with a duration of action longer than that of edrophonium, can be administered either intravenously or intramuscularly.[100] The usual adult dose is 1.5 mg intramuscularly in combination with 0.5 mg atropine to prevent cholinergic-induced side effects.[90]

OTHER DIAGNOSTIC TESTS

Electromyographic response to nerve stimulation is also used to diagnose myasthenia gravis. The characteristic electrodiagnostic abnormality is progressive decrement in the amplitude of muscle action potentials evoked by repetitive nerve stimulation at 3 or 5 Hz.[96] In generalized myasthenia this decremental response occurs in approximately 90% of patients if multiple muscles are tested, and up to 50% of patients with ocular myasthenia.[96,101]

Serum testing reveals circulating antibodies to acetylcholine receptors in approximately 90% of individuals with generalized myasthenia and in almost 70% of those with only ocular symptoms.[92,93] False-positive results are rare,

and the antibody titer does not correlate with the severity of symptoms.[96]

Management

Before initiating treatment, the clinician should rule out the presence of myasthenia-like syndromes such as Eaton-Lambert syndrome, which has clinical features similar to those of myasthenia but typically spares the eyes. Definitive diagnosis is important, since approximately 70% of Eaton-Lambert patients harbor malignant neoplasms, usually bronchogenic carcinoma.[103]

The pharmacologic treatment of myasthenia gravis is based on increasing the amount of available acetylcholine by use of oral cholinesterase inhibitors such as neostigmine, pyridostigmine, or ambenonium. Pyridostigmine bromide (Mestinon) is used most often and effectively relieves myasthenic symptoms in small muscles innervated by cranial nerves, particularly those involved in ptosis, diplopia, and dysarthria.[104]

An analog of neostigmine, pyridostigmine has a longer duration of action and fewer gastrointestinal side effects than neostigmine.[100] In adults, the usual starting dose of pyridostigmine is 60 mg given orally every 4 hours. This dosage may be increased, but additional clinical benefit is not expected in dosages exceeding 120 mg every 2 hours.[100] The drug is also available in a slow-release tablet (Timespan) of 180 mg and as a syrup for children.[100]

Thymectomy, corticosteroids, and other immunosuppressive drugs such as azathioprine and cyclosporine have been used to suppress the disease itself. Thymectomy is beneficial for patients with thymoma and is usually recommended in patients with generalized myasthenia gravis.[96] Of patients with generalized myasthenia, up to 85% may show complete remission or significant improvement following thymectomy.[90] Steroid therapy is usually reserved for patients who have life-threatening or severely disabling myasthenia and who have failed to respond to thymectomy, or in whom thymectomy is contraindicated because of advanced age or debilitating illness.[94]

Plasmapheresis is an intermediate form of therapy for myasthenia gravis, having effects that last longer than those of cholinesterase inhibitors but shorter than those of thymectomy. Although improvement in myasthenic symptoms often occurs, its duration is unpredictable. Moreover, because of its expense, plasmapheresis is usually reserved for patients having severe symptoms resistant to other therapeutic approaches or for patients preparing for thymectomy.[90]

In addition to these medical and surgical therapies, optical management of ptosis using dark lenses or a ptosis crutch may also be indicated. For smaller, constant ocular muscle misalignments, Fresnel press-on prisms may be used. An opaque (occluder) lens may be needed for larger, fluctuating deviations.

Benign Essential Blepharospasm and Hemifacial Spasm

Benign essential blepharospasm (BEB) is a dystonia characterized by involuntary sustained (tonic) and spasmodic (rapid or clonic), repetitive contractions involving the orbicularis oculi, procerus and corrugator musculature.[105–107] When the muscles of facial expression that are innervated by the facial nerve are similarly involved on only one side of the face, a hemifacial spastic dystonia occurs.[108,109]

Etiology

The exact neuroanatomic and neurophysiologic origins of blepharospasm and its related cranial-cervical dystonias are still unknown. Radiologic evidence indicates possible lesions located in the brain. Specific sites identified include the thalamus, basal ganglia, cerebellum and mesencephalon.[110,111]

Adrenergic variability may be a neurochemical cause of blepharospasm. Decreased norepinephrine levels have been identified in the hypothalamus, mamillary bodies and locus ceruleus, while increased norepinephrine levels have been identified in the dorsal raphe nucleus, red nucleus, substantia nigra and thalamus.[112] A neurochemical abnormality, if it exists, appears to result from a loss of inhibitory adrenergic input to the locus ceruleus which supplies information to the cortex, brainstem and spinal cord, resulting in adrenergic excess at the distal sites.[112,113] This neurochemical abnormality may be genetically determined.[107]

The brainstem's role as the origin of blepharospasm has been further tested in two patients with secondary blepharospasm. Both showed abnormal brainstem-evoked and somatosensory-evoked potentials.[114] Abnormal auditory-evoked potentials have also been identified in patients with essential blepharospasm.[115]

Unlike blepharospasm, the origins of hemifacial spasm are much better understood. Hemifacial spasm may occasionally be familial.[116] In most instances, however, the spasm results from microvascular compression or irritation of the facial nerve by an aberrant artery of abnormal vasculature in the posterior fossa or a cerebellopontine tumor.[107]

Diagnosis

A careful history and clinical examination are critical for the definitive diagnosis of blepharospasm. Up to 78% of patients who eventually develop BEB first show variable episodes of increased blinking lasting from seconds to minutes.[117–119] These episodes eventually progress to involuntary spasms of eyelid closure. Other accompanying symptoms include ocular irritation and photophobia, often simulating dry eye syndrome or neurosis.[114]

Remissions and exacerbations are common during the early stages of the disease.[117] Even when symptoms initially affect only one side, bilateral involvement becomes the rule.[120] BEB usually begins in individuals aged 50–70 with a mean age of onset of 56 years.[117,121] Almost two-thirds of these patients are female.[106,120]

Functional incapacitation can be significant,[119] with visual disability as the most incapacitating functional defect. Several assessments and scales have been suggested for more uniform grading of the functional disorder.[122,123] In most patients symptoms become stable within 5 years.[124]

External events can initiate or aggravate the episodes of spasm. These events include stress, driving, especially night driving when there are oncoming headlights, and bright sunlight.[125] Sleep and other stress-relieving forms of relaxation can occasionally alleviate the blepharospasm.

All patients with blepharospasm should receive dry eye testing, since dry eye can exacerbate the spasming. Appropriate dry eye therapy with ocular lubricants or lacrimal occlusion should accompany any other treatment for blepharospasm. The clinician should search for and correct other treatable problems that may exacerbate the disease, such as corneal erosion, foreign bodies, acute glaucoma, uveitis, entropion, eyelash abnormalities, and blepharitis.[126] Emotional problems or neurosis are usually not a significant precipitating cause of blepharospasm in adults but may play a prominent role in younger individuals.[127]

The term *essential blepharospasm* applies specifically to spasms localized to the orbicularis oculi, procerus and corrugator musculature.[128] Similar dyskinesias can occur in muscles other than those innervated by the facial nerve. These dyskinesias can occur in the lower face, mouth, jaw, neck and soft palate.[106] Localized, self-limiting spasm of the orbicularis oculi muscle is termed *eyelid myokymia*. Although this condition can mimic early blepharospasm, the former has a significantly more favorable prognosis (see Chap. 24).

When blepharospasm is accompanied by periodic lower facial movement, the disorder is referred to as Meige's syndrome or idiopathic orofacial dystonia. If the mandible also becomes involved, the disorder is referred to as *Breughel's syndrome* or *oromandibular dystonia*. When several cranial nerves are involved, the disorder is called *segmental cranial dystonia*.[117] Although often discussed as separate entities, these dystonic syndromes may be the same disease process with variable clinical manifestations.

Hemifacial spasm differs from blepharospasm in that the former is unilateral. As mentioned earlier, however, blepharospasm may begin on only one side of the face or one side may have greater involvement than the other, but bilateral involvement eventually occurs.[120] Hemifacial spasm may begin in the orbicularis oculi muscle and then slowly spread to other ipsilateral facial muscles.[106] Unlike blepharospasm, which sleep may relieve, hemifacial spasm continues during sleep.[129,130] As in blepharospasm, hemifacial spasm occurs in middle-aged individuals and is more common in women.[109,131]

Management

Before appropriate treatment for blepharospasm can be administered, a correct diagnosis must be made. In the early stages of the disease, patients are often misdiagnosed, assigned psychogenic disorders such as neurosis, and referred to psychiatrists or psychologists.[117] Other patients attempt hypnosis, acupuncture, faith healing, herbal remedies, biofeedback and relaxation therapy.[132–134] None of these techniques has proved particularly effective. Ophthalmic therapy includes treating any underlying ocular condition and using spectacle-mounted ptosis crutches. Adjunctive pharmacotherapy may include medications such as clonazepam (Klonopin), carbidopa with levodopa (Sinemet), reserpine, baclofen (Lioresal), or haloperidol (Haldol).[114,135] In addition to these measures, emotional or psychological counseling may prove effective for patients having difficulty adjusting to or accepting their condition or its treatment.[a]

BOTULINUM TOXIN TYPE A

The most effective nonsurgical treatment for both BEB and hemifacial spasm is botulinum toxin type A (Botox).[106,136,137] Sixty-nine percent to 100% of patients receiving botulinum toxin injection have had clinically significant improvement.[122,138]

Each vial of Botox contains 100 U of botulinum toxin (Fig. 23.14). In its nonreconstituted form, the toxin can remain stable for up to 4 years.[139] The recommended diluent for reconstitution is sterile nonpreserved 0.9% sodium chloride.[140] The reconstituted toxin deteriorates within a few hours and, if not used immediately, should be refrigerated (2–8°C).[140]

The diluent of sterile normal saline is drawn up in a syringe and gently injected into the vial containing the Botox. Rapid, forceful injection that causes frothing or other mechanical stress is discouraged since this can inactivate the toxin.[140] Table 23.13 gives the recommended dilutions calculated for an injection volume of 0.1 ml.

Without previous anesthesia and avoiding penetration of the orbital septum, the diluted Botox is typically injected subcutaneously or intramuscularly, using a 27–30 gauge needle. The most commonly used dilution is 2.5 U/0.1 ml of volume at each injection site. In patients with blepharospasm the initial injection sites should include the medial and lateral pretarsal orbicularis oculi of the upper lid, and the lateral pretarsal orbicularis oculi of the lower lid[140] (Fig.

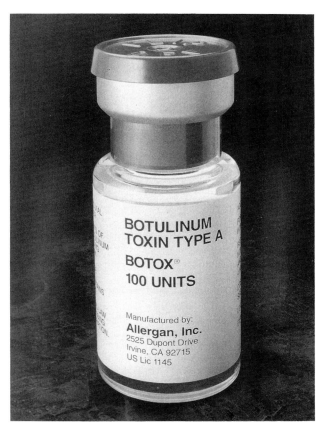

FIGURE 23.14 **Botulinum toxin type A (Botox). (Courtesy of Allergan Pharmaceuticals, Inc.)**

TABLE 23.13
Dilution of Botulinum Toxin

Diluent Added[a] (ml)	Resulting Dose (Units/0.1 ml)
1.0	10.0
2.0	5.0
4.0	2.5
8.0	1.25

[a]diluent = 0.9% NaCl injection
Modified from Oculinum (Botulinum Toxin Type A), Product Information, Allergan, Inc., 1989

23.15). Patients with hemifacial spasm should receive similar injections to any affected muscles of the lower face (Fig. 23.16). The cumulative dose of Botox in a 30-day period should not exceed 200 U.[140]

Muscle mass affects the toxin's response. More toxin is

---

[a]Information on emotional and psychological support can be obtained from Benign Essential Blepharospasm Research Foundation, Inc., P.O. Box 1268, Beaumont, TX 77726–2468.

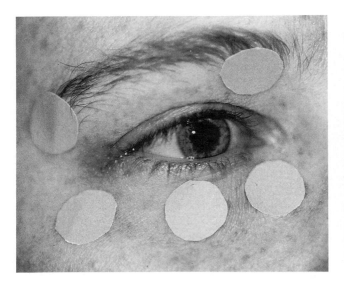

FIGURE 23.15 **Sites of botulinum toxin injections in patient with blepharospasm.**

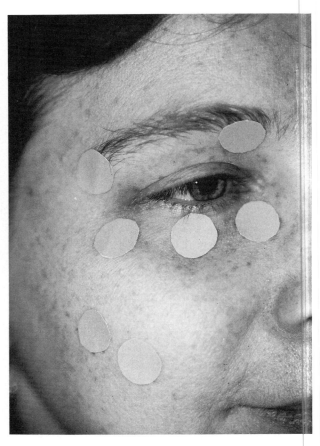

FIGURE 23.16 **Sites of botulinum toxin injections in patient with hemifacial spasm.**

needed locally to produce a desired effect in areas of increased muscle mass.[141,142] Histologic examination of orbicularis oculi musculature after treatment with botulinum toxin shows no evidence of alteration of muscle fiber diameter, disruption of internal muscle architecture, or pathologic changes in the motor endplates.[143,144]

In addition to titrating the injection dose for desired effect, the practitioner can also modify the injection sites. If the corrugator and procerus muscles are affected, the toxin may be injected in the glabellar region. Avoiding injection of the middle of the lower lid or completely eliminating injection of the lower lid has also been suggested.[145–147]

The initial effect of the injections usually occurs within three days and is maximal 1–2 weeks following treatment (Fig. 23.17). The therapeutic effectiveness of botulinum toxin in patients with blepharospasm lasts 6 to 28 weeks, with most patients becoming symptomatic again in approximately 3 months.[138,148] The average interval between injections is longer in patients with hemifacial spasm, sometimes up to 6 months.[138,148] With repeated injections the therapeutic interval decreases in some patients but appears to stabilize in most after the fourth and fifth injection.[149] This reduction in efficacy may result from the toxin's binding to the nonactive large protein chain,[137] a resprouting of motor endplates,[150–153] or the development of an antitoxin.[154]

Botulinum toxin is contraindicated in patients with a known allergy to the drug or with infection or inflammation at the proposed injection sites. Safety for use during pregnancy or lactation has not been established. Other contraindications include poor patient cooperation, coagulopathy

(including pharmacologic anticoagulation), and other neuromuscular diseases such as myasthenia gravis.[155]

The most frequently encountered side effect, occurring in up to 40% of patients, is exposure keratitis resulting from decreased blinking and lagophthalmos.[156] Ptosis is the second most common side effect and results from the toxin's direct effect on the levator palpebrae superioris muscle.[156] Avoiding injection of the middle of the upper eyelid and adjacent eyebrow region can reduce or eliminate this side effect.[129,137]

Other side effects include pain at the injection site, ecchymosis, increased tearing, ectropion, entropion, dry eye symptoms, and diplopia.[122,146,157] Avoiding injection of the middle or all of the lower eyelid may alleviate some of these side effects.[145–147]

Adverse events in patients who receive botulinum toxin injections for hemifacial spasm are virtually identical to those that occur in treatment of BEB. However, diplopia and

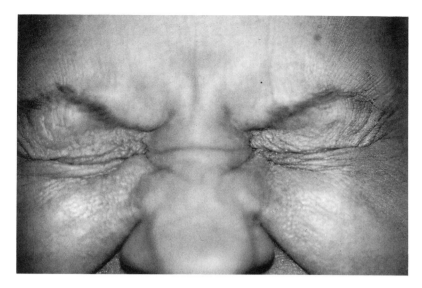

A

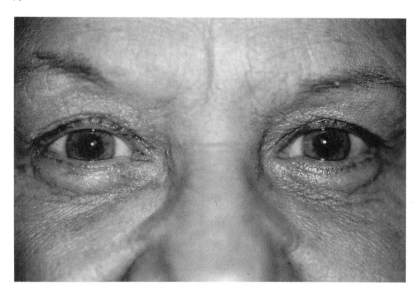

B

FIGURE 23.17   *(A)* **Patient with BEB prior to injection of Botox around both eyes.** *(B)* **After injection, patient had relief for 3 months.**

lower facial weakness are more common in patients with hemifacial spasm.[106]

SURGERY

Surgical treatment is a viable option for patients who cannot tolerate repeated botulinum toxin injections or for those who have an inadequate response. Effective procedures for blepharospasm include selective facial myectomy involving removal of the muscles that close the eyelids, and strengthening the muscles that open the eyelids.[154,158]

Surgery for hemifacial spasm involves microvascular decompression of the facial nerve by placement of a sponge under posterior fossa vessels (Jannetta procedure).[159,160] Surgical intervention, however, can have serious complications such as permanent facial paralysis, deafness, stroke, and even death.[107]

The Optic Neuropathies

Acquired optic nerve disease can result from numerous afflictions. In the past, terms such as optic neuritis and papilledema have erroneously been applied to optic neuropathy. This discussion considers acquired diseases of the optic nerve under the heading of optic neuropathy. Terminology is then applied that specifically defines the pathologic process. The suffix -*itis* refers only to proven inflammatory processes, and the term *optic disc edema* refers to any swelling of the nerve fibers of the optic nerve.

Demyelinizing Optic Neuropathy

ETIOLOGY

Classically referred to as *retrobulbar neuritis,* demyelinizing optic neuropathy is an inflammatory process of the optic nerve posterior to the globe. Although the etiology of this condition remains obscure, the association of retrobulbar neuritis with demyelinizing disease is irrefutable.[161,162] Several studies address the associated progression of isolated idiopathic optic neuritis to an eventual diagnosis of multiple sclerosis (MS). Reports vary from 10.8% in 1 to 5 years,[163] 25% in 12 years,[164] to 45% within 15 years.[165] The risk also seems to increase with the frequency of recurrence of the attacks.

Other conditions have also been implicated in demyelinizing optic neuropathy, especially those of viral origin such as herpes zoster,[166] Epstein Barr virus, and the Guillain-Barré syndrome.[167] In addition, environmental factors such as carbon monoxide poisoning have been reported in a delayed-reaction case of retrobulbar neuritis.[168] Metabolic relationships with diabetes, thyroid disease, inflammatory bowel disease, and vitamin deficiencies also exist.[169] A relationship to Leber's hereditary optic neuropathy has also been suggested as both conditions may be immunologically related.[170]

From an epidemiologic standpoint, retrobulbar neuritis is usually a disease of the young. Viral conditions in the active or postinfectious stage can incite the inflammation in children or young adults. Optic neuritis in an individual under 40 years of age should create some concern about the possibility of a demyelinizing disease. A recent study[171] reported demyelinizing optic neuropathy as the most frequent neurologic problem presenting to an eye hospital.

DIAGNOSIS

Diagnosis in the classic sense—"patient sees nothing, doctor sees nothing"—reflects the absence of ophthalmoscopic changes of the optic nerve head. Retrobulbar neuritis is most often unilateral, presenting as an impairment of vision and progressing to maximum loss after one week. Optic disc edema occurs in approximately one-third of cases of demyelinizing optic neuropathy.[172] Tenderness of the globe, especially above the superior rectus muscle, and pain on gross extraocular muscle excursions may also precede or run concurrently with the vision loss. A Marcus Gunn pupil is usually present as well, as are variable central or centrocecal scotomas.

Abnormalities present in the fellow eye may include reduced visual acuity (13.8%), altered contrast sensitivity (15.4%), altered color vision (21.7%), and visual field defects (48.0%).[173] In the later progressive phase of the disease, pendular nystagmus may also occur.[174]

Efficiency of diagnostic tests in demyelinizing optic neuropathy vary considerably and are related to an associated diagnosis of multiple sclerosis. In one report of neuropathy associated with MS, the visually-evoked potential (VEP) was abnormal in 81.8%, contrast sensitivity abnormal in 72.7%, color vision by Ishihara in 31.8%, and pupillary light reflex in 52.3%.[175]

Other nerve conduction tests such as Pulfrich stereo phenomenon, color comparison test, reduction of chromatic sensitivity, and light comparison test are often abnormal as well.[176]

L'Hermitte's and Uhthoff's symptoms are often present with demyelinizing optic neuropathy. It also appears that Uhthoff's is a prognostic indicator for the early development of MS.[177] Further neurologic assessment such as Romberg's sign may aid in the differential diagnosis. In addition, double-flash resolution tests may be of benefit in detecting subclinical demyelinization of the visual pathway.[178]

Recent advances have improved diagnosis of demyelinizing optic neuropathy, especially as it relates to MS. Magnetic resonance imaging (MRI) has proved a very sensitive tool for detecting demyelinizing plaques both within the optic nerve as well as in secondary sites.[178-183] As mentioned previously, VEP is especially useful in assessing both the affected and the fellow eye.[179] Cerebrospinal fluid analysis is sensitive especially when analyzing the oligoclonal bands (OBs). Pleocytosis and an increase in the IgG-index are of value in the differential diagnosis.[180,184] Elevated titers of anti-myelin basic protein are also correlated with acute idiopathic optic neuropathy and relapses of MS.[185]

MANAGEMENT

Prognosis for return of vision function is good. Vision characteristically begins to improve within 2 to 3 weeks, with stabilization at near normal by the fourth to fifth week.[384] Some patients improve rapidly to a moderate acuity level, stabilize, then experience a return of vision to near normal over a prolonged period. Recurrences characterize the disease, and with each recurrence acuity or visual field become further compromised. If visual acuity drops to no-light-perception (NLP) in the first attack, approximately two-thirds of patients recover vision to 20/400 or better, while one-third maintain dense central scotomas with vision below 20/400.[186] Each attack of retrobulbar neuritis can produce optic atrophy, although the incidence of such optic atrophy is as low as 36%.[187]

One additional consideration in prognosis is neuromyelitis optica (Devic's disease), which is considered a variant of multiple sclerosis in children and young adults. Characterized by a rapid, bilateral loss of vision, this disease has a poorer prognosis for visual recovery.

Differential diagnosis is vital. Although most optic neuropathy in the 20- to 40-year age group results from a demyelinating disease, the clinician must rule out other potential causes.

Multiple sclerosis does not always present systemically after demyelinating optic neuropathy. Reports in the literature vary for the development of multiple sclerosis after a case of retrobulbar neuritis. Some of the discrepancy involves inappropriate diagnoses of either demyelinating optic atrophy or multiple sclerosis.

The criteria for the diagnosis of multiple sclerosis are very controversial. The Medical Research Council Committee has developed a set of criteria for classification of the disease (Table 23.14). Appropriate patient management includes deciding what to tell the patient with an isolated idiopathic attack of optic neuropathy. The proper approach depends upon the individual patient, but at a minimum, the patient deserves a consultation with a neurologist for diagnostic testing with MRI and cerebrospinal fluid assessment. The rate of progression to MS is high enough that either the neurologist or the eyecare specialist should at least discuss the possibility with the patient.[188]

The proponents of therapeutic intervention in the optic neuritides maintain that allowing the edema associated with the inflammation to progress can result in significantly more damage. Photographs after treatment of disc edema in acute papillitis have demonstrated the efficacy of steroid therapy. Reducing edema may lessen the extent of scarring.[189] The "treaters" consider the euphoria-inducing effect of steroids to be beneficial and believe that patients perceive that drugs are necessary in managing a disease that is causing them to "go blind."[190] The medicolegal standards often force the issue toward treatment, since it is often difficult to prove that withholding treatment may be more beneficial than providing it.

The opponents of therapeutic intervention in optic neuritis claim that no clinical model supports the theory that edema or inflammation is implicated in the evolution of optic neuritis. The opponents of treatment hold that if edema were involved, steroid therapy would bring about more dramatic effects. Even proponents admit no statistical significance in ultimate visual acuities achieved with treatment compared with no treatment, although they report that treat-

TABLE 23.14
Diagnostic Classification Criteria for Multiple Sclerosis

Classification	Clinical Signs or Symptoms
Proven	Pathologic proof
Clinically definite	Some physical disability, remissions and relapses greater than two episodes
Early or probable	Signs of lesions at two or more sites
	Age of onset 10–50 years
	No better explanation
	Lesions predominantly in white matter
	Remissions and relapses
	Early single episode suggesting multiple sclerosis with signs of multiple lesions
	Slight or no disability

ment enhances short-term recovery.[191,192] All arguments advocating therapy must be tempered by the inherent risks of adrenocorticotropic hormone (ACTH) or steroid therapy.[193]

Recently the Optic Neuritis Treatment Trial[194] provided important information regarding steroidal intervention in demyelinating optic neuropathy. This randomized clinical trial assessed the effects of oral prednisone (1 mg per kg body weight per day for 14 days); intravenous methylprednisolone (250 mg every 6 hours for 3 days) followed by oral prednisone (1 mg per kg body weight per day for 11 days); or an oral placebo. The oral prednisone group and the oral placebo group had essentially the same outcome at six months except that the oral prednisone group actually had more recurrences than either the IV or placebo group. The IV methylprednisolone group had slightly better visual fields, contrast sensitivity, and color vision than did the oral prednisone or placebo groups but not significantly better visual acuity at six months. The IV group also recovered vision function faster and had fewer recurrences than did the placebo or oral prednisone groups. Thus, the treatment of choice for optic neuropathy appears to be IV methylprednisolone followed by oral prednisone. Oral prednisone alone is not effective. Side effects associated with IV methylprednisolone include psychotic depression, acute pancreatitis, sleep disturbances, mood changes, gastrointestinal distress, facial flushing, and weight gain.[195]

A 1-year follow-up on the trial demonstrated that visual acuity was 20/40 or better in 95% of the placebo group, 94% of the IV methylprednisolone group, and 91% of the oral prednisone group. The recurrence rate at the one-year visit was significantly higher for the oral prednisone group. The use of IV methylprednisolone therefore has only a short-term benefit, but oral prednisone should not be used.[196]

Attempts have also been directed toward treatment of the demyelinating disease at a systemic level. These modalities have often demonstrated transient therapeutic benefit to the patients. Forms of interferon therapy have given equivocal results.[197–200] Plasmapheresis still remains controversial.[201] Use of 4-aminopyridine (4-AP) intravenously appears to have transient benefits.[202] Hyperbaric oxygen therapy has not proved beneficial.[203]

Inflammatory Optic Neuropathy

ETIOLOGY

Inflammatory optic neuropathy, classically referred to as papillitis, occurs when a localized inflammatory process affects the optic nerve and may also secondarily affect the retina (neuroretinitis).

Inflammatory optic neuropathy is the most common form of optic neuropathy in children, with bilateral presentation more common in children than in adults.[204] From an etiologic standpoint, papillitis has been associated with a variety of conditions. Intraocular inflammatory conditions such as juxtapapillary choroiditis, sympathetic ophthalmia, bee sting to the eye,[205] syphilis,[206] toxoplasmosis,[207] and toxocariasis have been implicated. Toxoplasmic papillitis may also be the initial manifestation of acquired immunodeficiency syndrome (AIDS).[208] The development of papillitis can also relate to the acute retinal necrosis syndrome (ARNS), which is associated with both herpes simplex and herpes zoster virus.[209] Causes of papillitis include both acute and chronic meningitis, acute encephalomyelitis, and cat scratch fever.[210–213] Viral syndromes such as measles, mumps, Epstein Barr virus, and Guillain-Barré syndrome have also been linked to inflammatory optic neuropathy.[214–216] Drug-related idiosyncratic reactions also can precipitate inflammatory optic neuropathy.[217,218]

DIAGNOSIS

The clinical characteristics of papillitis make the entity easily distinguishable from other conditions of optic disc edema. Symptoms include a rapid loss of vision (central scotoma) and, at times, ocular or orbital pain. The vision loss in papillitis resembles the pattern experienced in retrobulbar neuritis. A rapid decrease in acuity occurs during the first 2 or 3 days, followed by stabilization over 7 to 10 days, leading to a gradual improvement of vision.[221] Some degree of secondary optic atrophy is always possible 4 to 8 weeks after the inflammation. Signs include:

- Optic disc edema varying from subtle to severe
- Marcus Gunn pupil
- Cells in the vitreous
- Obscuration of the central cup
- Vascular alterations depending on elapsed time

Two distinctive types of papillitis with surrounding retinal changes exist. The type of papillitis associated with viral infections in children (e.g., mononucleosis) exhibits dirty-yellow, globular exudates scattered throughout the papillomacular bundle. These exudates are approximately the size of a retinal vessel and may coalesce to form a macular wing or star. Superficial retinal edema also occurs. This condition carries a good visual prognosis, resolving spontaneously without treatment over weeks to months. The other type of papillitis is nonspecific in origin and is characterized by a yellowish swollen disc. The retinal edema spreads considerably; vessels may be obscured; and small linear hemorrhages can occur adjacent to the disc (Fig. 23.18). This form often resolves with residual perivascular sheathing, gliosis, and disc pallor, but visual acuity is often severely reduced.[169]

MANAGEMENT

Prognosis for return of vision function in inflammatory optic neuropathy varies considerably depending on the underlying causative factors. An aggressive attempt must be made to ascertain the basic precipitating condition. Adjunctive diagnostic tests must be ordered with supplementary tests added when a specific underlying cause is suspected. Basic laboratory diagnostic tests should include a Westergren erythrocyte sedimentation rate (ESR) to rule out arteritic ischemic optic neuropathy, a complete blood count (CBC) to rule out infections, fluorescent treponemal antibody absorption test (FTA-ABS) to rule out syphilis, a collagen vascular screen, and computed tomography (CT) or magnetic resonance imaging (MRI) to rule out a space-occupying lesion. Rapid diagnosis of the underlying cause and proper management often determine the long-term visual prognosis.

The same argument regarding proper therapeutic intervention exists for inflammatory optic neuropathy as for demyelinating optic neuropathy. The decision to initiate local or oral steroid therapy must be tempered by the inherent risks of therapy, keeping in mind the results of the Optic Neuritis Treatment Trial.[194] Conditions such as papillitis secondary to ARNS clearly benefit from steroid or ACTH intervention. Papillitis related to syphilis appears to respond well to local subTenon's triamcinolone injections.[219] Cyclosporine for the treatment of optic neuropathy in Behçet's patients also effectively reduces the inflammatory response.[220] Aggressive management is more sound in inflammatory optic neuropathy than in demyelinating optic neuropathy as the return to normal function without intervention is the exception rather than the rule in the former.

Ischemic Optic Neuropathy

Ischemic optic neuropathy (ION) is a clinical diagnosis that describes an acute compromise of the optic nerve with ensuing vision or visual field loss in the absence of identifiable inflammation, demyelinization, or cranial-orbital com-

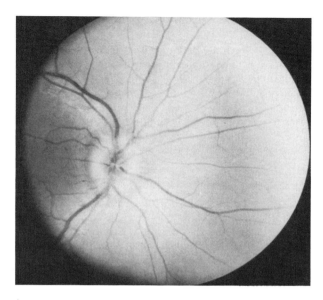

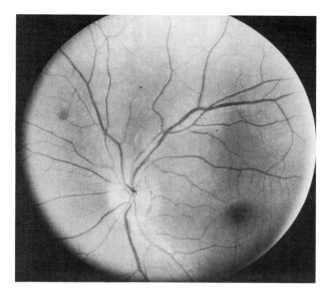

A

B

FIGURE 23.18   Unilateral inflammatory optic neuropathy demonstrating significant optic disc edema in the right eye *(A)* compared with the left *(B)*.

pression by a mass lesion. The condition is usually acute and involves the prelaminar region of the optic nerve, although it may also occur chronically in the retrolaminar position. Although many classifications have been assigned to this condition, three categories are distinct with regard to etiology: (1) non-arteritic ION, (2) temporal or cranial arteritic ION, and (3) diabetic ION or diabetic papillopathy. Two of these conditions will be discussed separately, since management of each differs distinctly.

NON-ARTERITIC ISCHEMIC OPTIC NEUROPATHY

Etiology.   Non-arteritic ION is a small vessel disease causing impaired perfusion in the optic nerve head.[221–223] Hayreh[224] contends that the lesion occurs in the short posterior ciliary arteries that supply the choroid and distal optic nerve. Regardless of the pathogenesis, however, sudden systemic hypotension[225] and a high prevalence of associated systemic hypertension and diabetes[226,227] lend credence to the claim that this condition is simply an acute alteration of the pressure-perfusion ratio at the nerve head.[228] The underlying causes of the altered pressure perfusion include Lyme disease, complications of general surgery, radiation therapy, relapsing polychondritis, and tamoxifen therapy.[229–246] Maintaining nerve head tissue entails precisely balancing intraocular pressure, blood pressure, and cerebrospinal fluid pressure. Altering this balance compromises optic nerve tissue. The corollary for chronically altered pressure-perfusion ratio is low-tension glaucoma.

Diagnosis.   Patients with a broad range of ages present with non-arteritic ION. In general, age may range from 40 to 80 years, but only about 5% of patients are older than age 70 years. The majority of patients are between 55 and 77 years of age.[226]

The clinical presentation includes:

- Acute visual acuity or visual field loss
- Marcus Gunn pupil
- Inferonasal visual field defect, a variety of altitudinal defects, or a central scotoma
- Family history of diabetes or hypertension, but no associated transient ischemic attacks, ischemic cerebral infarction, or complications of large-vessel arteriosclerosis or cardiac disease with embolism[227]
- Optic disc edema that is usually sectorial but rarely extending beyond the edge of the disc when in the early phase
- Hyperemic disc with small, linear, flame-shaped hemorrhages on the disc margin that disappear in 3 to 5 weeks or that may present as pale optic disc edema
- As the condition progresses, optic atrophy with subsequent cupping in some instances

The condition progresses to a decrease of vision over 24 hours to four weeks, but in most cases this loss occurs in less than 9 days without remission. There are usually no systemic complaints associated with the episode.[247] Stabilization of vision then occurs, but optic atrophy ensues within about three months. Visual acuity stabilizes at 20/60 (6/18) or better in 45% to 50% of cases and is worse than 20/200 (6/60) in approximately 40% of cases.[226] Spontaneous recovery of vision can occur in untreated non-arteritic ION.[248,249] The primary concern is subsequent involvement in the fellow eye, which can occur months to years later.[227] The incidence of involvement of the fellow eye varies between 16% and 40%, averaging 35%.[222] The coincident occurrence of central retinal artery occlusion is a possible complication.[250]

Of special interest is the appearance of ION during the cataract postoperative period. The presentation of ION associated with cataract surgery may be secondary to increased intraocular pressure in the immediate postoperative period. The patient presenting with the postoperative ION is at greater risk in the fellow eye should surgery be performed. If cataract extraction is attempted in the fellow eye, presurgical reduction of intraocular pressure is crucial, with special attention given to maintaining reduced pressure in the immediate postoperative period. Intraocular pressure should be maintained at a low level for at least one week postoperatively and should be monitored carefully thereafter.[172]

Management. The management of ION is multifactorial. Recognition and management of the underlying systemic condition is imperative. One other rare but important concern is differentiation of the Foster-Kennedy syndrome from ischemic optic neuropathy. Table 23.15 summarizes the primary differences between the two entities.[251] The success of therapy for the optic nerve lesion depends on the rapidity of diagnosis. Proponents of steroid therapy encourage starting that treatment at the earliest possible moment to reduce optic disc edema. The reduction of edema may help by reducing capillary permeability and thus improving circulation. Note, however, that no therapeutic intervention beyond management of any potential underlying systemic condition is currently thought to have any benefit in the management of non-arteritic ION. This is in contrast to the therapeutic benefits in the management of arteritic ION.

If the ION is not secondary to a frank vasculitis, steroid therapy is often instituted. However, this approach has no proven benefit,[252,253] although some authors argue that therapeutic intervention should occur if optic disc edema is present.[253] In addition, aspirin and urokinase may prove useful in the treatment of ION.[252,253]

Surgery has now been proved of no benefit in cases of non-arteritic ION. Optic nerve decompression in progressive cases has been reported to improve vision function.[254-256] Recent evidence, however, demonstrates that decompression surgery is not effective and may actually be harmful.[257]

ARTERITIC ISCHEMIC OPTIC NEUROPATHY

Etiology. Arteritic ION is a true ocular emergency. Immediate recognition of this condition is crucial to prevent involvement of the fellow eye, with the possible consequence of bilateral blindness. Arteritic ION is associated with giant cell arteritis, a systemic disease with special predilection for arteries of the head and neck, although a similar condition has been reported associated with atrial myxoma.[258] The condition most often occurs in patients over 70 years of age.

Diagnosis. A very sudden loss of vision function characterizes arteritic ION.[259] One to two weeks before actual onset of the condition, the patient may experience prodromal symptoms. These can consist of hazy vision, visual field defects, flashing lights, color vision disturbances, temporal headaches, an unexplained weight loss, suboccipital neck pains, scalp tenderness, and jaw aches associated with chewing and talking. Polymyalgia rheumatica also may be a prodromal symptom complex.[260] An acute vision loss to the 20/60 (6/18) to NLP level heralds the attack.[226] Ophthalmoscopically, the disc shows pallid edema. Approximately 50% of cases show a chalky-white swelling of the disc with an occasional hemorrhage.[261] Patients with arteritic ION may also have larger cup-disc ratios and a delay in fluorescein dye appearance in the choroid and retinal vessels when compared to patients with non-arteritic ION and normals.[262,263] Color Doppler ultrasonography also confirms decreased blood flow in the orbit associated with arteritic

TABLE 23.15
Differential Diagnosis between Foster-Kennedy Syndrome and Ischemic Optic Neuropathy

	Ischemic Optic Neuropathy	Foster-Kennedy Syndrome
Onset	Sudden vision loss or field defect in one eye followed by stabilization	Insidious progression of reduced vision with papilledema in fellow eye
Visual fields	Altitudinal hemianopsia, arcuate scotoma, central scotoma	Central scotoma in eye with optic atrophy and enlarged blind spot in fellow eye
Fundus	Sector optic disc edema followed by sector atrophy	Uniform optic atrophy with optic disc edema in fellow eye
Associated systemic signs and symptoms	May be a family or personal history of hypertension, diabetes, or stroke	Hemiplegia, loss of sense of smell, personality change

ION.[264] Cilioretinal artery occlusion and a high C-reactive protein creating hyperviscosity can occur.[265] Clinically leukocytosis, elevated ESR, serum globulins on serum electrophoresis, decreased hematocrit (HCT), decreased red blood cell filterability, increased plasma viscosity, increased fibrinogen,[266] and a hard nonpulsating temporal artery are reliable indicators of a positive diagnosis. An ESR over 40 (Westergren) should indicate the need for temporal artery biopsy. However, some patients can present with arteritic ION with normal ESRs.[267] A positive temporal artery biopsy provides the definitive diagnosis. However, *the delay for a biopsy should not delay initiation of therapy.* Prompt steroid therapy can have dramatic results, sometimes improving vision from NLP to 20/20.[268]

Prognosis is grim with regard to ocular involvement. Without therapeutic intervention, the process usually involves the fellow eye within one year. Even with therapy some patients proceed to total blindness. The ultimate outcome of an active case is optic atrophy.

Management. Management of arteritic ION involves massive doses of systemic steroids to prevent vision loss in the fellow eye. Vision function in the affected eye may deteriorate,[226] improve, or remain stable after initiation of systemic steroid therapy.[269–272] The true inflammatory nature of this condition makes steroids necessary. Steroids decrease capillary permeability so that the anoxic and toxic destruction by edema of the nerve fiber layer is reduced to a minimum. The typical recommended treatment regimen varies considerably among clinicians. However, most clinicians prescribe high initial dosages of prednisone (80 to 120 mg daily).[273] Relief of symptomatology and reduction of the ESR determine the precise amount. Once the appropriate dosage level has been established, therapy must be maintained and regulated according to the ESR. Therapy may continue for years in the absence of strong contraindications to steroid therapy.

Anticoagulants (heparin, streptokinase) should be given only in cases of confirmed hyperviscosity syndromes and then only in consultation with an internist. The use of anticoagulants in the elderly carries the risk of cerebral hemorrhage. Vasodilators, such as theophylline and nicotinic acid derivatives, apparently offer no benefit in ischemic conditions.[260]

Leber's Hereditary Optic Neuropathy

ETIOLOGY

An enigma, Leber's hereditary optic neuropathy is considered a distinct clinical entity. It is classically defined as a visually debilitating optic atrophy that occurs as a sequel to acute or subacute optic neuritis. The etiology is somewhat obscure, but some authors have proposed that it may be an inherited inability to detoxify cyanide.[274] Further studies have implicated a deficiency of thiosulfate sulfurtransferase (Rhodanese) as a cause for this defect in the detoxification of cyanide.[275] Others have suggested that Leber's optic neuropathy is a mitochondrial disease.[276] The condition has recently been associated with mutations in the mitochondrial genome.[277] Some reports associate this condition with mutations at 11778 (in 50% of families),[278–281] 4216, 4917, 13708,[282] 3460 and 14484. The latter site demonstrates a higher incidence of visual recovery than other mutation sites.[283–285]

The hereditary aspect of this disease is equally obscure. In the United States men are more often affected than women (6.7:1), with age of onset for men at 18 to 30 years and women at 10 to 40 years.[286] Late onset is possible, however, and creates confusion with the diagnosis of arteritic and non-arteritic ION.[287] The following characteristics summarize the inheritance patterns that do not conform to Mendelian principles[288–291]:

- Males are predominantly affected.
- Affected males cannot transmit the disease.
- The sister of an affected male is a carrier.
- Affected females all have normal fathers.
- All women born into families with only females affected are carriers.
- The heterozygous female can transmit the trait to her sons and the carrier state to her daughters.

DIAGNOSIS

Acute or subacute vision loss characterizes the disease. Usually both eyes are affected simultaneously, but an interval of 1 to 6 months can occur between involvement of the two eyes.[292] Preacute signs and symptoms do occur. In some patients atrophy of retinal nerve fibers occurs before the actual attack, as well as an altered Farnsworth-Munsell 100-hue test and visual-evoked potential (VEP).[293–295] When the actual attack occurs, there is mild optic disc edema with early circumpapillary telangiectatic microangiopathy.[296] The disease has a predilection for the nerve fibers of the macula, thereby causing an early vision loss and a central scotoma that can break out to the periphery. This vision loss is to the 20/200 (6/60) to 20/400 (6/120) level, and the condition eventually settles into a permanent optic atrophy that most often affects the temporal sector of the disc. During the active condition, the patient may have headaches associated with meningitis, cerebral edema, swelling of the optic nerves, and opticochiasmatic arachnoiditis. A demonstrable distension of the optic nerve sheaths also occurs in some cases.[297,298]

MANAGEMENT

The prognosis for Leber's optic neuropathy is grim. The condition usually becomes stationary, although the literature contains some reports of spontaneous improvement of vi-

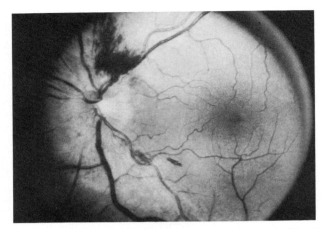

FIGURE 23.19 **Mild optic disc edema associated with dilated tortuous veins and hemorrhage in papillophlebitis.**

sion in 16% to 75% of affected patients, even in 11778 mutations after the declaration of legal blindness.[299] However, the vision loss may progress further even after years of stability.[276] No treatment is effective in symptomatic cases. However, in view of the suspected defect in cyanide metabolism, an effective therapeutic approach may consist of hydroxocobalamin (vitamin B_{12A}) and cyanocobalamin (vitamin B_{12}), 1 mg parenterally daily for 7 days.[300] This vitamin therapy has no side effects, but no proof of its efficacy exists. Advocates of such vitamin therapy cite the similarity of Leber's disease to toxic optic neuropathies that respond favorably to vitamin therapy. Such therapy follows from the belief that a thiamine-dependent transferase catalyzes a step in the pentose shunt. When this step is compromised, nerve fiber loss ensues.[301] In addition, one female patient with concurrent Type 1 diabetes mellitus and confirmed mitochondrial mutations recovered vision after effective control of the diabetes.[302]

The clinician must also consider other mitochondrial mutations of DNA, such as Kearns-Sayre syndrome, which may potentially impact on morbidity and mortality.[303] All cases of optic atrophy of unexplained origin must be considered as potential Leber's hereditary optic atrophy until proven otherwise. Analysis of mitochondrial DNA assists in the diagnosis, but laboratory analysis is currently limited to certain centers and is expensive.

Papillophlebitis

ETIOLOGY

Papillophlebitis is optic disc edema accompanied by venous dilation and tortuosity as well as hemorrhages in young patients. The condition is often associated with a variation of central retinal vein occlusion that was thought to be initiated by a localized phlebitis.[304] Papillophlebitis was previously considered a relatively benign condition occurring in otherwise systemically and ocularly healthy adults. Males are affected approximately 2:1 over females.[305] The condition has also been referred to as a variation of the acute idiopathic blind spot enlargement syndrome.[306,307]

DIAGNOSIS

Hayreh[304] has classified two distinct ophthalmoscopic presentations: (1) type 1, optic disc vasculitis characterized by gross unilateral disc edema without retinal vascular abnormalities; and (2) type 2, optic disc vasculitis characterized by disc edema with hemorrhages on and surrounding the disc in the early stages and with grossly dilated and tortuous retinal veins (Fig. 23.19), more pronounced than one would anticipate in the equivalent stage in the development of papilledema. Other clinical findings include enlarged blind spots with some variability in the central scotoma.[306] In addition, small white dots may appear in the edematous zone and a prolongation of the venous transit time may occur as well as leakage at the optic nerve head with fluorescein angiography.[172]

MANAGEMENT

Papillophlebitis is still considered a benign self-limited condition with none of the complications typically associated with central retinal vein occlusion or other causes of optic disc edema. The condition usually resolves without treatment over a 6- to 18-month period, but recent findings indicate that long-term visual complications may accompany cystoid macular edema; macular pigmentary changes; macular hole formation; retinal, disc, and iris neovascularization; and vitreous hemorrhage. A younger age of onset and no associated systemic conditions appear to afford some protection against severe vision loss.[305] Perivenous sheathing of the large veins may occur many months after the onset of optic disc edema. Dilated venules on the disc surface as well as optociliary shunts can develop to drain the congested disc, and these may remain after the process has subsided.[308]

Active management is controversial: there are both avid proponents of the conservative, "no-treatment" approach as well as those who advocate aggressive steroid therapy. Because papillophlebitis is viewed as a vasculitis, steroid therapy should theoretically be of benefit, especially when one considers the associated optic disc edema. An occasional report indicates dramatic response with steroid therapy similar to that obtained in cases of optic disc edema secondary to optic neuritis. However, no controlled studies exist to substantiate the effectiveness of this therapy.[306] Indeed, case reports often acknowledge that neither steroid nor anticoagulant therapy affects optic disc edema.

Systemic conditions reportedly associated with papillophlebitis must be ruled out. These include pregnancy,[309] hypertension, heart disease, gastrointestinal disease, hyperlipidemia, pulmonary disease, renal disease, arthritis, and HIV. However, over 50% of cases have no associated systemic condition.[306,310] Nonetheless, the practitioner may order CT or MRI scans, blood work including a CBC, lupus erythematosus prep (LE prep), antinuclear antibodies (ANA), sedimentation rate (Westergren ESR), fluorescent treponemal antibody absorption test (FTA-ABS), a possible LP, and a chest X-ray.[306,308] Appropriate interventive therapy, such as retinal photocoagulation, may benefit cases with ocular complications such as neovascularization of the optic disc, retina, or iris.

In summary, steroid therapy appears ineffective in papillophlebitis. Moreover, such therapy can mask a much more serious condition causing the optic disc edema. Patients suspected of having papillophlebitis should be monitored carefully, since unilateral optic disc edema can be secondary to many other conditions. Routine follow-up examination can confirm the stability and subsequent remission of papillophlebitis.

Papilledema

Papilledema is best defined as optic disc edema occurring secondary to increased intracranial pressure (ICP). Although the exact etiopathogenesis is somewhat obscure and may involve both mechanical as well as vascular factors, the mechanical theory proposed by Hayreh seems most plausible.[311,312] Visual symptoms are rare in the early phases of papilledema, since the axoplasmic stasis has little to do with transfer of the nerve impulse along the outer membrane of the nerve fibers.[313] The reduction in vision does not occur until frank ischemia of nerve fibers occurs associated with the vascular phase of the optic disc edema.[312,314]

Etiology

ICP and thus papilledema have many related causes. Any intracranial space-occupying lesion may create increased ICP.[315] Superior sagittal sinus thrombosis is a cause that can prove fatal.[316] Spinal cord tumors and injury may be associated with increased ICP.[317,318] As with traumatic brain injury, which has a 50% to 75% occurrence of increased ICP at some point, spinal cord injuries should be followed with repeat ocular examinations including stereoscopic optic disc observation and visual fields.[319–322] Other associations include intracerebral or subarachnoid hemorrhage,[323] inflammatory polyneuritis,[324] toxic metabolic diseases,[325] lithium treatment,[326] amiodarone,[327] transient erythroblastopenia of childhood,[328] radical neck surgery,[329] empty sella syndrome,[330] AIDS,[331] sleep apnea,[332] Behçet's disease,[333] Lyme

disease,[334] mucopolysaccharidoses,[335] primary open-angle glaucoma,[336] and brucellosis.[337]

Benign intracranial hypertension (BIH) or pseudotumor cerebri (PTC) also has an important relationship to papilledema. This condition is characterized by bilateral papilledema associated with headache, some compromise of visual acuity or fields, occasional sixth-nerve palsy with absence of frank focal neurologic signs, and depressed plasma steroid levels.[338] Although not life threatening, a definite potential for blindness exists.[339,340] Benign intracranial hypertension may occur secondary to middle ear disease, minor head injury, childhood systemic lupus erythematosus,[341] or toxic conditions such as hypervitaminosis A or tetracycline and nalidixic acid toxicity. However, the condition appears to result from poor resorption of the cerebrospinal fluid.[342] The syndrome can also relate to anti-phospholipid antibodies associated with cerebral venous thrombosis.[343] In over 50% of cases, the underlying etiology is unknown. Females aged 10 to 50 years dominate the cases with no apparent etiology.[344]

Diagnosis

The diagnosis of papilledema in the early stages often presents a significant clinical challenge. It involves a combination of stereoscopic observation of the optic disc, visual field analysis, evaluation of focal neurologic signs, and the patient's history of transient obscurations (5–30 *seconds* of blurring or loss of vision usually associated with postural changes). Experimental evidence shows that the optic disc edema itself occurs approximately 1 to 7 days after increased intracranial pressure.[345] However, papilledema can occur much sooner (within 2 to 48 hours) because of intracranial hemorrhage.[346,347] The absence of a venous pulsation may be a sign of increased intracranial pressure,[348] although some investigators have questioned this concept.[349]

Proper patient management requires a successful differential diagnosis between papilledema and pseudopapilledema (Table 23.16, Fig. 23.20). Pseudopapilledema is a congenital anomalous elevation of the optic nerve head that may occur in conjunction with high hyperopia, hyaloid remnants, myelinated nerve fibers, hyaline bodies (drusen), or other, unexplainable, congenital elevations. This condition is often misdiagnosed, resulting in unnecessary invasive and expensive neurologic evaluations.[350] Fluorescein angiography has some value in differentiating true papilledema from pseudopapilledema, but a normal fluorescein angiogram does not rule out papilledema. Stereoscopic fundus photography and observation of the peripapillary reflex with a red-free filter also have value in the differential diagnosis.

Optic disc edema is the first observable sign of papilledema. The swelling of the nerve fibers and subsequent transudation of the debris first appear in the inferior aspect of the disc, followed by the superior then the nasal aspects, with the temporal aspect least susceptible to swelling. This

TABLE 23.16
Differential Diagnosis between Papilledema and Pseudopapilledema

Characteristic	Papilledema	Pseudopapilledema
Abnormal vasculature	No	Yes
Familial patterns	No	Yes
Hemorrhages	Yes	Only when drusen shear vessels
Nerve fiber layer swelling	Yes, into retina	No
Exudates and cotton wool spots	Yes	No
Enlarged blind spot	Yes	No
Transient obscurations of vision	Yes	No
Spontaneous venous pulsation	Usually no	Usually yes
Maintenance of central cup	Yes, until late	No
Buried drusen	No	Yes at times
Headache	Postural and severe	Possibly migraine
Other neurologic signs or symptoms	Yes	No
Fluorescein leakage	Yes	No

swelling eventually spreads into the surrounding retina. The disc margins then blur with later involvement of the small vessels of the disc.[351,352] As the process progresses, hemorrhage on or near the disc may occur at any retinal level, but rarely beyond the radius of the macula. Some reports indicate diffuse hemorrhagic retinopathy similar to venous stasis disease. As the papilledema progresses, vision is maintained. Later, visual field defects occur that progress to involve fixation. The enlarged blind spot may eventually expand to involve fixation.

Other complications that may lead to reduced visual acuity are subretinal pigment epithelial neovascularization,[353] choroidal folds,[354] preretinal macular hemorrhage, choroidal and subretinal hemorrhages, macular star formation, and retinal pigment epithelial disease.[355] Another fundus sign of long-standing papilledema is the development of optociliary shunt vessels most often associated with sphenoid ridge meningiomas.[356]

In the differential diagnosis of papilledema, MRI or CT imaging is an invaluable and necessary adjunct. The MRI is especially sensitive in imaging the distention and any other alterations of the optic nerve.[357]

Management

If left untreated, papilledema can progress to intractable optic atrophy. Clearly the most important aspect of treatment is management of the underlying cause of increased intracranial pressure. A diagnosis of true papilledema should always imply emergency hospital admission. If the practitioner cannot readily determine the underlying cause, medical or surgical intervention must be undertaken.

Medical treatment must be used with caution, since the

papilledema may resolve while the underlying condition continues untreated. Should cerebral edema exist, causing severe neurologic signs and optic disc edema, treatment may be instituted until the underlying cause can be managed. Using 2 to 4 g of acetazolamide daily in addition to 40 to 100 mg (usually 60 mg) of oral prednisone daily can control the edema. Lumbar punctures may also be employed in skilled hands. Should this regimen not alleviate the problem, neurosurgical shunting procedures or optic nerve decompression must be undertaken. Neurosurgical shunting procedures (lumboperitoneal shunt) alleviate the problem of elevated intracranial pressure but may be compromised by infection, plugs, or resultant low intracranial pressure with headache and dizziness. Optic nerve decompression involves invasion of the subarachnoid space of the optic nerve with direct relief of intracranial pressure. Recent efforts at optic nerve sheath decompression associated with PTC have shown a 68% to 97% improvement or stabilization of function in cases with progressive vision loss.[358-361] The treatment may, however, result in complications such as third- and sixth-nerve palsies.[362]

Treatment of benign intracranial hypertension depends on cause, initial severity, and success of long-term controllability. If the cause is amenable to treatment, such as otitis or hypervitaminosis A, that condition must take precedence. Because benign intracranial hypertension is self-limited, usually resolving in 3 to 9 months, there are generally only two reasons to employ treatment—severe headaches or evidence of optic neuropathy.[338] If the plasma steroid level is depressed, daily dosages of oral prednisone—80 to 100 mg, in conjunction with acetazolamide, 250 mg four times daily—may be necessary. Jefferson and Clark[363] advocate abstention from steroid therapy and surgical intervention. These authors favor dehydration therapy and monitor reso-

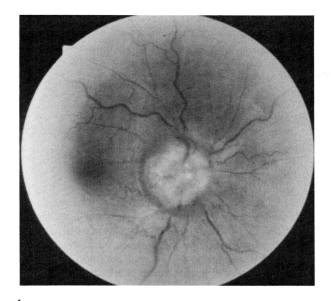

A

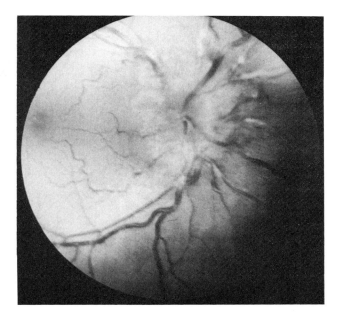

B

FIGURE 23.20 *(A)* **Compensated papilledema in a case of benign intracranial hypertension.** *(B)* **Noncompensated papilledema in a case of acute aqueductal stenosis.** *(C)* **Pseudopapilledema secondary to buried drusen of the optic nerve head.**

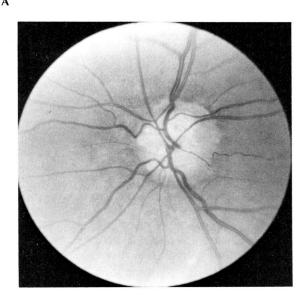

C

lution by measuring the blind spot. The patient must limit fluid intake to 900 ml daily. The dehydrating agents employed may be one or a combination of the following: oral urea (1 g/kg body weight daily until resolution), oral glycerol (1–1.5 g/kg daily until resolution), hydroflumethiazide (100 mg on alternate days until resolution), and chlorthalidone (200 mg on alternate days until resolution). These investigators prefer chlorthalidone because of rapid resolution with a mean time-to-cure of 12 weeks. If medical therapy is unsuccessful in controlling the condition, a theroperitoneal shunt may be needed.[364] Techniques of medical therapy are constantly improving. In-dwelling intracranial pressure monitoring devices allow modifying therapy to maximize results.[365]

Nutritional and Toxic Optic Neuropathy

Etiology

Nutritional and toxic optic neuropathy refers to vision loss secondary to degenerative changes of the optic nerve fibers in response to exogenous metabolic stimuli. This vision loss may occur in deficiency states (thiamine or vitamin B_{12}) or as a toxic response to certain drugs or substances (Table 23.17).[366–374] In most cases one can establish that the patient has been exposed to toxins or has had some dietary deficiency. The precise pathogenesis of the atrophic process is somewhat obscure, although adenosine triphosphate (ATP) formation appears to have undergone a change. This change leads to a stasis of axoplasmic flow with subsequent optic disc edema, eventually resulting in axonal death.[375–377]

TABLE 23.17

Drugs or Substances Associated with the Development of Retinal Changes or Optic Neuropathy

Alcohol	Ethchlorvynol
Barbiturates	Iodide Compounds
Carbon Monoxide	Isoniazid
Chlorambucil	Hexamethonium
Chloramphenicol	Lead
Chloroquine	Lithium
Ciprofloxacin	Methotrexate
Cocaine	Placidyl
Corticosteroids	Phenothiazines
Cyanide	Steroid Compounds
Cyclosporine	Streptomycin
Cyproterone	Tamoxifen
Digitalis	Tobacco
Diiodohydroxyquin	Typarsamide
Disulfiram	Vitamin D
Ethambutol	Vitamin A and Retinoids

Diagnosis

A gradual, bilateral painless reduction of visual acuity with eventual centrocecal scotomas characterizes the atrophies. The scotomas have variable margins that are better defined and much larger with red targets. There are no specific nerve fiber bundle defects, but often a dense scotoma occurs in the area corresponding to the papillomacular bundle. The defects characteristically do not cross the vertical meridian, although ethambutol toxicity may demonstrate a bitemporal hemianopsia, since the chiasm may be implicated in the process. Although somewhat reversible, the visual field changes are usually progressive. Dyschromatopsia occurs, but the patient may remain unaware of the color vision loss. Even though this condition can cause reduced vision, vision generally is not reduced below hand motion. Ophthalmoscopically the optic disc may be edematous with isolated splinter hemorrhages in the early stages, but the nerve head eventually becomes atrophic.

Management

The condition is reversible and has a favorable prognosis if the toxic agent or nutritional deficiency is detected and removed. Occasionally vision function may improve even without treatment.[369] Recognize that patients treated with ethambutol can develop atrophy because of the chelation of zinc and other metals necessary for optic nerve function. Serum zinc levels should be evaluated in these patients. Even children with hereditary optic atrophy may have reduced serum zinc levels.[378] Zinc sulfate, 100 to 250 mg three times daily, may promote reversal of the neuropathy. The

dosage of oral zinc sulfate depends on the individual's ability to absorb the drug as well as the possible side effects such as nausea, vomiting, diarrhea, and bleeding secondary to gastric erosion. Zinc therapy is not yet approved by the Food and Drug Administration.[379,380]

If isoniazid is implicated in optic neuropathy or other neurologic signs, then pyridoxine (vitamin B$_6$), 25 to 100 mg daily, may be used. Prophylactic administration of this agent can occur in combination with isoniazid and monoamine oxidase inhibitor therapy.

The patient with tobacco or alcohol amblyopia usually has either low serum levels of vitamin B$_{12}$ or cannot absorb this vitamin in sufficient amounts. Thus, the treatment for this condition involves supplemental vitamin therapy. After documenting a serum vitamin B$_{12}$ deficiency, the patient should receive 300 mg of oral thiamine each week and 1000 g of intramuscular hydroxocobalamin each week for 10 weeks. The sooner this therapy begins, the better the prognosis. The hydroxocobalamin form of vitamin B$_{12}$ appears more effective than cyanocobalamin.[381] In terms of recovery from the amblyopia, cessation of smoking or drinking does not appear to produce remission unless the patient concurrently improves his or her diet. Thus it is unnecessary and in practice difficult to persuade patients who are habitual abusers of these agents to stop. Improvement of dietary status seems to be the most important factor.[382]

Vitamin B$_{12}$ deficiency can also cause megaloblastic anemia. White-centered hemorrhages can occur in the posterior pole, and disc pallor also may occur. If the ischemia is severe enough, cotton wool spots may occur. A CBC can confirm the diagnosis, but the clinician should realize that visual-neurologic symptoms can occur before the clinical laboratory changes. Serum folate and vitamin B$_{12}$ levels should be determined and appropriate therapy (IM injections of hydroxocobalamin) instituted at the earliest sign of megaloblastic anemia.

The crucial feature of all optic neuropathies that must never be ignored is the possibility of an underlying neoplasm. Visual field analysis at regular intervals aids in excluding the possibility of an optic nerve or chiasmal neoplasm.

References

1. Gray LG. The five-step pupil evaluation. Rev Optom 1981;118:38–44.
2. Alexander LJ. Use of "black light" in assessing pupillary responses. Am J Optom Physiol Opt 1977;54:792–796.
3. Brumberg JB. Horner's syndrome and the ultraviolet light as an aid in its detection. J Am Optom Assoc 1981;52:641–646.
4. Ettinger ER, Wyatt HJ, London R. Anisocoria. Variation and clinical observation with different conditions of illumination and accommodation. Invest Ophthalmol Vis Sci 1991;32:501–509.

5. Thompson HS. Diagnostic pupillary drug tests. In: Blodi FC, ed. Current concepts in ophthalmology. St. Louis: C.V. Mosby Co, 1972;3:76–90.

6. Thompson HS, Mensher JH. Adrenergic mydriasis in Horner's syndrome. Hydroxyamphetamine test for diagnosis of postganglionic defects. Am J Ophthalmol 1971;72:472–480.

7. Thompson HS. Adie's syndrome: some new observations. Trans Am Ophthalmol Soc 1977;75:587–626.

8. Czarnecki JSC, Pilley SFJ, Thompson HS. The analysis of anisocoria. The use of photography in the clinical evaluation of unequal pupils. Can J Ophthalmol 1979;14:297–302.

9. Loewenfeld IE. "Simple, central" anisocoria: a common condition, seldom recognized. Trans Am Acad Ophthalmol Otolaryngol 1977;83:832–839.

10. Lam BL, Thompson HS, Corbett JJ. The prevalence of simple anisocoria. Am J Ophthalmol 1987;104:69–73.

11. Younge BR, Buski ZJ. Tonic pupil: A simple screening test. Can J Ophthalmol 1976;11:295–299.

12. Horner F. Uber eine form von ptosis. Klin Monatsbl Augenheilkd 1869;7:193–201.

13. Grimson BS, Thompson HS. Postganglionic Horner syndrome. In: Glaser JS, ed. Neuro-ophthalmology. St. Louis: C.V. Mosby Co, 1977;9:190–197.

14. Jaffe NS. Localization of lesions causing Horner's syndrome. Arch Ophthalmol 1950;44:710–728.

15. Grimson BS, Thompson HS. Raeder's syndrome. A clinical review. Surv Ophthalmol 1980;24:199–210.

16. Swann PG, Johnson LB. Horner's syndrome: an unusual precursor of occlusive disease of the carotid arterial system. J Am Optom Assoc 1985;56:131–132.

17. Musarella MA, Chan HSL, DeBoer G, et al. Ocular involvement in neuroblastoma: prognostic implications. Ophthalmology 1984;91:936–940.

18. Kline LB, Vitek JJ, Raymon BC. Painful Horner's syndrome due to spontaenous carotid artery dissection. Ophthalmology 1987;94:226–230.

19. Levy H, Sacho H, Feldman C, et al. Pulmonary mucormycosis presenting with Horner's syndrome. S Afr Med J 1986;70:363–365.

20. Smith PG, Dyches TJ, Burde RM. Topographic analysis of Horner's syndrome. Otolaryngol Head Neck Surg 1986;94:451–457.

21. Maloney WF, Younge BR, Moyer NJ. Evaluation of the causes and accuracy of pharmacologic localization in Horner's syndrome. Am J Ophthalmol 1980;90:394–402.

22. Hageman G, Ippel PF, te Nijenhuis FCAM. Autosomal dominant congenital Horner's syndrome in a Dutch family. J Neurol Neurosurg Psych 1992;55:28–30.

23. Giles CL, Henderson JW. Horner's syndrome: an analysis of 216 cases. Am J Ophthalmol 1958;46:289–296.

24. Pilley SFJ, Thompson HS. Pupillary "dilatation lag" in Horner's syndrome. Br J Ophthalmol 1975;59:731–735.

25. Carter JH. Diagnosis of pupillary anomalies. J Am Optom Assoc 1979;50:671–680.

26. Van der Wiel HL, Van Gijn J. No enophthalmos in Horner's syndrome. J Neurol Neurosurg Psych 1987;50:498–499.

27. Thompson HS. Diagnosing Horner's syndrome. Trans Am Acad Ophthalmol Otolaryngol 1977;83:840–842.

28. Rosenberg ML. The friction sweat test as a new method for detecting facial anhidrosis in patient's with Horner's syndrome. Am J Ophthalmol 1989;108:443–447.

29. Castillo M, Kramer L. Rader syndrome; MR appearance. AJNR 1992;13:1121–1123.

30. Thompson BM, Corbett JJ, Kline LB et al. Pseudo-Horner's syndrome. Arch Neurol 1982;39:108–111.

31. Van der Wiel HL, Van Gijn J. The diagnosis of Horner's syndrome. Use and limitations of the cocaine test. J Neurol Sci 1986;73:311–316.

32. Kardon RH, Denison CE, Brown CK, Thompson HS. Critical evaluation of the cocaine test in the diagnosis of Horner's syndrome. Arch Ophthalmol 1990;108:384–387.

33. Friedman JR, Whiting DW, Kosmorsky GS, et al. The cocaine test in normal patients. Am J Ophthalmol 1984;98:808–810.

34. Van der Wiel HL, Van Gijn J. Localization of Horner's syndrome. Use and limitations of the hydroxyamphetamine test. J Neurol Sci 1983;59:229–235.

35. Heitman K, Bode' DD. The Paredrine test in normal eyes. A controlled study. J Clin Neuro-ophthalmol 1986;6:228–231.

36. Cremer SA, Thompson HS, Digre KB, Kardon RH. Hydroxamphetamine mydriasis in normal subjects. Am J Ophthalmol 1990;110:66–70.

37. Cremer SA, Thompson HS, Digre KB, Kardon RH. Hydroxamphetamine mydriasis in Horner's syndrome. Am J Ophthalmol 1990;110:71–76.

38. Weinstein JM, Cutler JI. Observations on transsynaptic changes in acquired Horner's syndrome. Am J Ophthalmol 1983;95:837–838.

39. Lepore FE. Diagnostic pharmacology of the pupil. Clin Neuropharmacol 1985;8:27–37.

40. Woodruff G, Buncic JR, Morin JD. Horner's syndrome in children. J Pediatr Ophthalmol Strabismus 1988;25:40–44.

41. Digre KB, Smoker WRK, Johnston P, et al. Selective MR imaging approach for evaluation of patients with Horner's syndrome. AJNR 1992;13:223–227.

42. Adie WJ. Tonic pupils and absent tendon reflexes: a benign disorder sui generis; its complete and incomplete forms. Brain 1932;55:98–113.

43. Purcell JJ, Krachmer JH, Thompson HS. Corneal sensation in Adie's syndrome. Am J Ophthalmol 1977;84:496–500.

44. Czarnecki JSC, Thompson HS. Spontaneous cyclic segmental sphincter spasms in an Adie's tonic pupil. Am J Ophthalmol 1976;82:636–637.

45. Bodker FS, Cytryn AS, Putterman AM, Marschall MA. Postoperative mydriasis after repair of orbital floor fracture. Am J Ophthalmol 1993;115:372–375.

46. Lifshitz T, Yassur Y. Accommodative weakness and mydriasis following laser treatment at the peripheral retina. Ophthalmologica 1988;197:65–68.

47. Pfeiffer N, Kommerell G. Sector palsy of the sphincter pupillae muscle after argon laser trabeculoplasty. Am J Ophthalmol 1991;111:511–512.

48. Coppeto JR, Monteiro MLR, Young D. Tonic pupils following oculomotor nerve palsies. Ann Ophthalmol 1985;17:585–588.

49. Fletcher WA, Sharpe JA. Tonic pupils in neurosyphilis. Neurology 1986;36:188.

50. Fite JD, Walker HK. The pupil. In: Walker HK, Hall WD, Hurst JW, eds. Clinical methods: The history, physical and laboratory examinations. Boston: Butterworths, 1980;2:577–585.

51. Bell TAG. Adie's tonic pupil in a patient with carcinomatous neuromyopathy. Arch Ophthalmol 1986;104:331–332.

52. Scheinberg IH, Adler RI. Adie's syndrome: case report. Ann Ophthalmol 1979;11:247–248.

53. Smith JL. The pupil. Miami: Smith, 1975.

54. Rosenberg ML. Miotic Adie's pupils. J Clin Neuro-ophthalmol 1989;9:43–45.

55. Thompson HS. Segmental palsy of the iris sphincter in Adie's syndrome. Arch Ophthalmol 1978;96:1615–1620.

56. Cox TA. Spontaneous contractions of the pupillary sphincter in traumatic ophthalmoplegia. Am J Ophthalmol 1986;102:543–544.

57. Pilley SFJ, Thompson HS. Cholinergic supersensitivity in Adie's syndrome: Pilocarpine vs. Mecholyl (abstr.). Am J Ophthalmol 1975;80:955.

58. Jacobson M, Olson KA. Influence of pupil size, anisocoria and ambient light on pilocarpine miosis. Implications for supersensitivity testing. Ophthalmology 1993;100:275–280

59. Flach AJ, Dolan BJ. The therapy of Adie's syndrome with dilute pilocarpine hydrochloride solutions. J Ocular Pharmacol 1985;1:353.

60. Flach AJ, Dolan BJ. Adie's syndrome: a medical treatment for symptomatic patients. Ann Ophthalmol 1984;16:1151–1154.

61. Thompson HS, Newsome DA, Loewenfeld IE. The fixed dilated pupil. Sudden iridoplegia or mydriatic drops? A simple diagnostic test. Arch Ophthalmol 1971;86:27.

62. Teasdale E, Statham P, Straiton J, Macpherson P. Non-invasive radiological investigation for oculomotor palsy. J Neurol Neurosurg Psych 1990;53:549–553.

63. Brodsky MC, Frenkel REP, Spoor TC. Familial intracranial aneurysm presenting as a subtle stable third nerve palsy. Arch Ophthalmol 1988;106:173.

64. Nadeau SE, Trobe JD. Pupil sparing in oculomotor palsy: a brief review. Ann Neurol 1983;13:143–148.

65. Thompson HS, Pilley SFJ. Unequal pupils. A flow chart for sorting out the anisocorias. Surv Ophthalmol 1976;21:45–48.

66. Slamovis TL, Miller NR, Burde RM. Intracranial oculomotor nerve paresis with anisocoria and pupillary parasympathetic hypersensitivity. Am J Ophthalmol 1987;104:401–406.

67. Jacobson DM. A prospective evaluation of cholinergic supersensitivity of the iris shpincter in patients with oculomotor nerve palsies. Am J Ophthalmol 1994;118:377–383.

68. Blattner RJ. Jimson weed poisoning: Stramonium intoxication. J Pediatr 1962;61:941–943.

69. Reader AL. Mydriasis from *Datura wrightii*. Am J Ophthalmol 1977;84:263–264.

70. Thompson HS. Cornpicker's pupil: Jimson weed mydriasis. J Iowa Med Soc 1971;61:475–478.

71. Simmons FH. Jimson weed mydriasis in farmers. Am J Ophthalmol 1957;44:109–110.

72. Nissen SH, Nielsen PG. Unilateral mydriasis after use of propantheline bromide in an antiperspirant (letter). Lancet 1977;2:1134.

73. Silbert PL, Edis RH. Accidental mydriasis due to prantal powder. Aust NZ J Med 1991;21:929.

74. McCrary JA, Webb NR. Anisocoria from scopolamine patches. JAMA 1982;248:353–354.

75. Verdier DD, Kennerdell JS. Fixed dilated pupil resulting from transdermal scopolamine (letter). Am J Ophthalmol 1982;93:803–804.

76. Rosen NB. Accidental mydriasis from scopolamine patches. J Am Optom Assoc 1986;57:541–542.

77. Bienia RA, Smith M, Pellegrino T. Scopolamine skin-disks and anisocoria. Ann Intern Med 1983;99:572–573.

78. Jannum DR, Mickel SF. Aniscoria and aerosolized anticholinergics. Chest 1986;90:148–149.

79. Helprin GA, Clarke GM. Unilateral fixed dilated pupil associated with nebulised ipratropium bromide. Lancet 1986;2:1469.

80. Lippman JI. Pupillary abnormalities associated with posterior chamber lens implantation. Ophthalmic Surg 1982;13:197–200.

81. Stirt JA, Shuptrine JR, Sternick CS, et al. Anisocoria after anaesthesia. Can Anaesth Soc J 1985;32:422–424.

82. Laibovitz RA. The fixed, dilated pupil: a new cause. Tex Med 1980;76:59.

83. Wimalaratna HS, Capildeo R, Lee HY. Herpes zoster of second and third segments causing ipsilateral Horner's syndrome. Br Med J 1987;294:1463.

84. Monteiro MLR, Coppeto JR. Horner's syndrome associated with carotid artery atherosclerosis. Am J Ophthalmol 1988;105:93–94.

85. Gibbs J, Appleton RE, Martin J, Findlay G. Congenital Horner syndrome associated with non-cervical neuroblastoma. Developmental Med Child Neurol 1992;34:642–644.

86. Campbell P, Neil T, Wake PN. Horner's syndrome caused by an intercostal chest drain. Thorax 1989;44:305–306.

87. Fields CR, Barker FM. Review of Horner's syndrome and a case report. Optom Vis Sci 1992;69:481–485.

88. Foster RE, Kosmorsky GS, Sweeney PJ, Masaryk TJ. Horner's syndrome secondary to spontaneous carotid dissection with normal angiographic findings. Arch Ophthalmol 1991;109:1499–1500.

89. Dutton GN, Paul R. Adie syndrome in a child: a case report. J Pediatr Ophthalmol Strabismus 1992;29:126.

90. Wyngaarden JB, Smith LH, eds. Cecil's Textbook of medicine. Philadelphia: WB Saunders, 1985,2211–2215.

91. Drachman DB. Present and future treatment of myasthenia gravis (editorial). N Engl J Med 1987;316:743–745.

92. Vincent A, Newsom-Davis J. Acetylcholine receptor antibody characteristics in myasthenia gravis. I. Patients with generalized myasthenia or disease restricted to ocular muscles. Clin Exp Immunol 1982;49:257–265.

93. Vincent A, Newsom-Davis J. Acetylcholine receptor antibody as a diagnostic test for myasthenia gravis: Results of 153 validated cases and 2,967 diagnostic assays. J Neurosurg Psychiatry 1985;48:1246–1252.

94. Rowland LP, Layzer RB. Muscular dystrophies, atrophies, and related diseases. In: Joynt RJ, ed. Clinical neurology. Philadelphia: JB Lippincott Co, 1988:67–77.

95. Drachman DB. Myasthenia gravis: Part I. N Engl J Med 1978;298:136–142.

96. Penn AS, Rowland LP. Neuromuscular junction. In: Rowland LP, ed. Merritt's Textbook of neurology. Philadelphia: Lea & Febiger, 1989;697–704.

97. Schwab RS, Leland CC. Sex and age in myasthenia gravis as critical factors in incidence and remissions. JAMA 1953;153:1270–1273.

98. Oosterhuis HJGH. The ocular signs and symptoms of myasthenia gravis. Doc Ophthalmol 1982;52:363–378.

99. Cogan DG. Myasthenia gravis: A review of the disease and a description of lid twitch as a characteristic sign. Arch Ophthalmol 1965;74:217–221.

100. Physicians Desk Reference, 49th ed, Montvale, NJ: Medical Economics Co., 1995.

101. Evoli A, Tonali P, Bartoccioni E, et al. Ocular myasthenia: Diag-

nostic and therapeutic problems. Acta Neurol Scand 1988;77:31–35.

102. Seybold ME. The office tensilon test for ocular myasthenia gravis. Arch Neurol 1986;43:842–843.

103. Glaser JS. Infranuclear disorders of eye movement. In: Tasman W, Jaeger EA, eds. Duane's Clinical ophthalmology. Philadelphia: J.B. Lippincott Co., 1990; vol 2, chap. 12:1–56.

104. Osserman KE. Ocular myasthenia gravis. Invest Ophthalmol 1967;6:277–287.

105. Jankovic J, Falin S. Dystonic syndromes. In: Jankovic J, Tolosa E, eds. Parkinson's disease and movement disorders. Baltimore: Urban and Schwartzenberg, 1988, 283–314.

106. Osaka M, Keltner JL. Botulinum A toxin (Oculinum) in ophthalmology. Surv Ophthalmol 1991;36:28–46.

107. Jankovic J, Brin MF. Therapeutic uses of botulinum toxin. N Engl J Med 1991;324:1186–1194.

108. Ferguson JH. Hemifacial spasm and the facial nucleus. Ann Neurol 1978;4:97.

109. Digre K, Corbett JJ. Hemifacial spasm: differential diagnosis, mechanism and treatment. Adv Neurol 1988;49:151–176.

110. Jankovic J. Blepharospasm with basal ganglia lesions. Arch Neurol 1986;43:866–868.

111. Jankovic J, Patel SC. Blepharospasm associated with brainstem lesions. Neurology 1983;33:1237–1240.

112. Jankovic J, Svendesen CN. Brain neuro-transmitters in dystonia. N Engl J Med 1986;316:278–279.

113. Hornykiewicz O, Kish SJ, Becker LE, et al. Brain neurotransmitters in dystonia muscularum deformans. N Engl J Med 1986;315:347–353.

114. Jankovic J, Ford J. Dystonia: clinical and pharmacological findings in 100 patients. Ann Neurol 1983;13:402–411.

115. Holds JB, Creel DJ, Anderson RL. Brainstem auditory potentials in essential blepharospasm. Invest Ophthalmol Vis Sci 1989;30 (suppl):411.

116. Carter JB, Patrinely JR, Jankovic J, et al. Familial hemifacial spasm. Arch Ophthalmol 1990;108:249–250.

117. Jordan DR, Anderson RL. Essential blepharospasm. In: Focal Points 1988: Clinical Modules for Ophthalmologists. San Francisco: American Academy of Ophthalmology, 1988;6:1–10.

118. Jankovic J, Orman J. Blepharospasm: Demographic and clinical survey of 250 patients. Ann Ophthalmol 1984;16:371–376.

119. Jankovic J, Havins WE, Wilkins RB. Blinking and blepharospasm: mechanism, diagnosis and management. JAMA 1982;248:3160–3164.

120. Malinovsky V. Benign essential blepharospasm. J Am Optom Assoc 1987;58:646–651.

121. Savino PJ, Maus M. Botulinum toxin therapy. Neurol Clin 1991;9:205–224.

122. Therapeutics and Technology Assessment Subcommittee of the American Academy of Neurology. Assessment: The clinical usefulness of botulinum toxin A in treating neurologic disorders. Neurology 1990;40:1332–1336.

123. Elston JS. The clinical use of botulinum toxin. Sem Ophthalmol 1988;3:249–260.

124. Scott AB. Botulinum toxin for blepharospasm. In: Spaeth G, Katz LJ, Parker KW, eds. Clinical therapy in ophthalmic surgery. Toronto: BC Decker 1989;322–324.

125. Koster ML. Blepharospasm-patient's perspective. In: Jankovic J, Tolosa E, eds. Facial dyskinesias. New York: Raven Press, 1988, 65–72.

126. Pita-Salorio D, Quintana-Conte R. Ophthalmologic causes of blepharospasm. In: Jankovic J, Tolosa E, eds. Facial dyskinesias. New York: Raven Press 1988;91–102.

127. Borodic G, Cozzolino D. Blepharospasm and its treatment with emphasis on the use of botulinum toxin. Plast Reconstr Surg 1988;83:546–554.

128. Frueh BR, Callahan A, Cortzbach RK, et al. A profile of patients with intractable blepharospasm. Trans Am Acad Ophthalmol Otolaryngol 1976;81:591–594.

129. Frueh BR, Musch DC. Treatment of facial spasm with botulinum toxin. An interim report. Ophthalmology 1986;93:917–923.

130. Montagna P, Imbriaco A, Zucconi M, et al. Hemifacial spasm in sleep. Neurology 1986;36:270–273.

131. Gonnering RS. Treatment of hemifacial spasm with botulinum A toxin: results and rationale. Ophthalmic Plast Reconstr Surg 1986;2:143–146.

132. Cavenar JD, Brantley IJ, Braasch E. Blepharospasm: organic or functional? Psychosomatics 1978;19:623–628.

133. Roxannos MR, Thomas MR, Rapp MS. Biofeedback treatment of blepharospasm with spastic torticollis. Can Med Assoc J 1978;119:48–49.

134. Peck DF. The use of EMG feedback in the treatment of a severe case of blepharospasm. Biofeedback Self Regul 1977;2:273–275.

135. Metzer WS, Nazarian SM. Blepharospasm: Overview and update. In: Smith JL, Katz RS, eds. Neuro-ophthalmology enters the nineties. Miami: Neuro-Ophthalmology Tapes, 1988;343–353.

136. Arthurs B. Treatment of blepharospasm with medication, surgery and type A botulinum toxin. Can J Ophthalmol 1987;22:24–28.

137. Scott AB, Kennedy RA, Stubbs HA. Botulinum A toxin injection as a treatment for blepharospasm. Arch Ophthalmol 1985;103:347–350.

138. American Academy of Ophthalmology. Botulinum toxin therapy of eye muscle disorders: safety and effectiveness. Ophthalmology 1989;96:37–41.

139. Scott AB. Botulinum toxin injection of eye muscles to correct strabismus. Trans Am Ophthalmol Soc 1981;79:734–770.

140. Rowsey JJ. Surgical adjuncts. In: Bartlett JD, Ghormley NR, Jaanus SD, et al. Ophthalmic drug facts. St. Louis: Facts and Comparisons, 1993:213–232.

141. Scott AB. Botulinum treatment for blepharospasm. In: Smith BC, ed. Ophthalmic plastic and reconstructive surgery. St. Louis: CV Mosby, 1987:609–613.

142. Scott AB. Clostridial toxin as therapeutic agents. In: Simpson LL, ed. Botulinum neurotoxin and tetanus toxin. New York: Academic Press, 1989:399–412.

143. Harris CP, Alderson K, Nebeker J, et al. Histologic features of human orbicularis oculi treated with botulinum A toxin. Arch Ophthalmol 1991;109:393–395.

144. Tyler HR. Pathology of the neuromuscular apparatus in botulism. Arch Pathol 1963;76:55–59.

145. Biglan AW, Burnstine RA, Rogers GL, et al. Management of strabismus with botulinum A toxin. Ophthalmology 1989;96:935–943.

146. Dutton JJ, Buckley EG. Long term results and complications of botulinum A toxin in the treatment of blepharospasm. Ophthalmology 1988;95:1529–1534.

147. Frueh BR, Nelson CC, Kapustiak JF, et al. The effect of omitting botulinum toxin from the lower eyelid in blepharospasm treatment. Am J Ophthalmol 1988;106:45–47.

148. Mauriello JA. Treatment of benign essential blepharospasm and

hemifacial spasm with botulinum toxin. A preliminary study of 68 patients. In: Bosniak SG, Smith BG, eds. Advances in ophthalmic plastic and reconstructive surgery-blepharospasm. New York: Pergamon Press, 1985;283–289.

149. Engstrom PF, Arnoult JB, Mazow ML, et al. Effectiveness of botulinum toxin therapy for essential blepharospasm. Ophthalmology 1987;94:971–975.

150. Drachman DB. The role of acetylcholine as a neurotropic transmitter. Ann NY Acad Sci 1974;228:160–176.

151. Duchen LW. The changes in the electron microscopic structure of slow and fast skeletal muscle fibers of the mouse after the local ingestion of botulinum toxin. J Neurol Sci 1971;14:61–74.

152. Elston JS, Russell RW. Effective treatment with botulinum toxin on neurogenic blepharospasm. Br Med J 1985;290:1857–1859.

153. Sellin LC: Botulinum-An update. Milit Med 1984;148:12–16.

154. Jordan DR, Patrinely JR, Anderson RL, et al. Essential blepharospasm and related dystonias. Surv Ophthalmol 1989;34:123–132.

155. The National Institutes of Health. Clinical use of botulinum toxin. NIH Consens Dev Conf Consens Statement. Vol.8, Nov. 12–14, 1990.

156. McLeish WM, Anderson RL. Advances in blepharospasm therapy. Ophthalmol Clin N Am 1991;4:193–199.

157. Kennedy RH, Bartley GB, Flanagan JC, et al. Treatment of blepharospasm with botulinum toxin. Mayo Clin Proc 1989;64: 1085–1090.

158. Jones TW, Waller RR, Samples JR. Myectomy for essential blepharospasm. Mayo Clin Proc 1985;60:663–666.

159. Jannetta PJ, Abbasy M, Maroon JC, et al. Etiology and definitive microsurgical treatment of hemifacial spasm: operative techniques and results in 47 patients. J Neurosurg 1977;47:321–328.

160. Jannetta PJ: Hemifacial spasm. In: Samii M, Jannetta PJ, eds. The cranial nerves. Berlin: Springer-Verlag, 1981;484–493.

161. Burde RM, Keltner JL, Gittinger JW, Miller NR. Optic neuritis-etiology? Surv Ophthalmol 1980;24:307–314.

162. Lessell S. Current concepts in ophthalmology. Optic neuropathies. N Engl J Med 1978;299:533–537.

163. Lana-Peixoto MA, Lana-Peixoto MI. The risk of multiple sclerosis developing in patients with isolated idiopathic optic neuritis in Brazil. Arquivos De Neuro-Psiquiatria 1991;49:377–383.

164. Sandberg-Wollheim M, Bynke H, Cronqvist S, Holtas S, Platz P, Ryder LP. A long-term prospective study of optic neuritis: evaluation of risk factors. Ann Neurol 1990;267:386–393.

165. Mapelli G, Pavoni M, DePalma P, et al. Progression of optic neuritis to multiple sclerosis: a prospective study in an Italian population. Neuroepidemiology 1991;10:117–121.

166. Godel V, Blumenthal M, Regenbogen L. Retrobulbar neuritis and central serous chorioretinopathy. J Pediatr Ophthalmol 1977;14: 296–298.

167. Nikoskelainen E. Symptoms, signs and early course of optic neuritis. Acta Ophthalmol 1975;53:254–271.

168. Reynolds NC Jr, Shapiro I. Retrobulbar neuritis with neuroretinal edema as a delayed manifestation of carbon monoxide poisoning: case report. Milit Med 1979;144:472–473.

169. Walsh FB, Hoyt WF. Clinical neuro-ophthalmology, ed. 3. Baltimore: Williams & Wilkins 1969;1:991.

170. Harding AE, Sweeney MG, Miller DH, et al. Occurrence of a multiple sclerosis-like illness in women who have a Leber's hereditary optic neuropathy mitochondrial DNA mutation. Brain 1992;115:979–989.

171. Simcock PR, Jones NP, Watson AP. Neurological problems presenting to an ophthalmic casualty department. Acta Ophthalmol 1992;70:721–724.

172. Alexander LJ. Primary care of the posterior segment, ed 2. Appleton & Lange: E Norwalk, CT, 1993.

173. Beck RW, Kupersmith MJ, Cleary PA, Katz B. Fellow eye abnormalities in acute unilateral optic neuritis. Experience of the optic neuritis treatment trial. Ophthalmology 1993;100:691–697.

174. Barton JJ, Cox TA. Acquired pendular nystagmus in multiple sclerosis: clinical observations and the role of optic neuropathy. J Neurol Neurosurg Psych 1993;56:262–267.

175. van Diemen HA, Lanting P, Koetsier JC, et al. Evaluation of the visual system in multiple sclerosis: a comparative study of diagnostic tests. Clin Neurol Neurosurg 1992;94:191–195.

176. Russell MH, Murray IJ, Metcalfe RA, Kulikowski JJ. The visual defect in multiple sclerosis and optic neuritis. A combined psychophysical and electrophysiological investigation. Brain 1991; 114:2419–2435.

177. Scholl GB, Song HS, Wray SH. Uhtoff's symptom in optic neuritis: relationship to magnetic resonance imaging and development of multiple sclerosis. Ann Neurol 1991;30:180–184.

178. Pary DW. Magnetic resonance in multiple sclerosis. Curr Opin Neurol Neurosurg 1993;6:202–208.

179. Frederiksen JL, Larsson HB, Olesen J. Correlation of magnetic resonance imaging and CSF findings in patients with acute monosymptomatic optic neuritis. Acta Neurologica Scand 1992;86: 317–322.

180. Optic Neuritis Study Group. The clinical profile of optic neuritis. Experience of the Optic Neuritis Treatment Trial. Arch Ophthalmol 1991;109:1673–1678.

181. Barkhof F, Scheltens P, Valk J, et al. Serial quantitative MR assessment of optic neuritis in a case of neuromyelitis optica, using Gadolinium-"enhanced" STIR imaging. Neuroradiology 1991;33:70–71.

182. Jacobs L, Munschauer FE, Kaba SE. Clinical and magnetic resonance imaging in optic neuritis. Neurology 1991;41:15–19.

183. Christiansen P, Fredriksen JL, Henriksen O, Larsson HB. Gd-DTPA-enhanced lesions in the brain of patients with acute optic neuritis. Acta Neurologica Scand 1992;85:141–146.

184. Martinelli V, Comi KG, Filippi M, et al. Paraclinical tests in acute-onset optic neuritis: basal data and results of a short follow-up. Acta Neurologica Scand 1991;84:231–236.

185. Warren KG, Catz I, Shutt K. Optic neuritis anti-myelin basic protein synthetic peptide specificity. J Neurol Sci 1992;109:88–95.

186. Slamovits TL, Rosen CE, Cheng KP, Striph GG. Visual recovery in patients with optic neuritis and visual loss to no light perception. Am J Ophthalmol 1991;111:209–214.

187. Marshall D. Ocular manifestations of multiple sclerosis and relationship to retrobulbar neuritis. Trans Am Ophthalmol Soc 1950; 48:487–575.

188. Slamovits TL, Macklin R, Beck RW, et al. What to tell the patient with optic neuritis about multiple sclerosis. Surv Ophthalmol 1991;35:47–50.

189. Lubow M, Adams L. The changing management of acute optic neuritis. In: Smith JL, ed. Neuro-ophthalmology. Symposium of the University of Miami and the Bascom Palmer Eye Institute. St Louis: C.V. Mosby Co, 1972;6:44–50.

190. Wray SH. The treatment of optic neuritis. Sight Sav Rev 1972;42: 5–13.

191. Rawson MD, Liversedge LA, Goldfarb G. Treatment of acute

retrobulbar neuritis with corticotrophin. Lancet 1966;2:1044–1046.

192. Rose AS, Kuzma JW, Kurtzke JF, et al. Cooperative study in the evaluation of therapy in multiple sclerosis: ACTH versus placebo. Final report. Neurology 1970;20(5, pt. 2):1–59.

193. Rawson MD, Liversedge LA. Treatment of retrobulbar neuritis with corticotrophin (letter). Lancet 1969;2:222.

194. Beck RW, Cleary PA, Anderson MM, et al. A randomized, controlled trial of corticosteroids in the treatment of acute optic neuritis. The Optic Neuritis Study Group. N Eng J Med 1992;326:581–588.

195. Chrousos GA, Kattah JC, Beck RW, et al. Side effects of glucocorticoid treatment. Experience in the optic neuritis treatment trial. JAMA 1993;269:2110–2112.

196. Beck RW, Cleary PA. The Optic Neuritis Study Group. Optic Neuritis Treatment Trial. Arch Ophthalmol 1993;111:773–775.

197. Panitch HS. Systemic alpha-interferon in multiple sclerosis. Long-term patient follow-up. Arch Neurol 1987;44:61–63.

198. Camenga DL, Johnson KP, Alter M, et al. Systemic recombinant alpha-2 interferon therapy in relapsing multiple sclerosis. Arch Neurol 1986;43:1239–1246.

199. Panitch HS, Hirsch RL, Haley AS, et al. Exacerbations of multiple sclerosis in patients treated with gamma interferon. Lancet 1987;1:893–895.

200. Jacobs L, Salazar AM, Herndon R, et al. Multicentre double-blind study of effect of intrathecally administered natural human fibroblast interferon on exacerbations of multiple sclerosis. Lancet 1986;2:1411–1413.

201. Tindal RS, Rollins JA. Assessment of therapeutic plasmapheresis in demyelinating neurologic disorders. South Med J 1986;79:991–997.

202. Stefoski D, Davis FA, Faut M, et al. 4-Aminopyridine improves clinical signs in multiple sclerosis. Ann Neurol 1987;21:71–77.

203. Harpur GD, Suke R, Bass BH, et al. Hyperbaric oxygen therapy in chronic stable multiple sclerosis: double blind study. Neurology 1986;36:988–991.

204. Kennedy C, Carroll FD. Optic neuritis in children. Trans Am Acad Ophthalmol Otolaryngol 1960;64:700–712.

205. Song HS, Wray SH, Bee sting optic neuritis. A case report with visual evoked potentials. J Clin Neuro-Ophthalmol 1991;11:45–49.

206. Deschenes J, Seamone CD, Baines MG. Acquired ocular syphilis: diagnosis and treatment. Ann Ophthalmol 1992;24:134–138.

207. Friedman AH. Uveitis affecting the retina and posterior pole. In: Freeman WR, ed. Practical atlas of retinal disease and therapy. New York: Raven Press, 1993:37–43.

208. Falcone PM, Notis C, Merhige K. Toxoplasmic papillitis as the initial manifestation of acquired immunodeficiency syndrome. Ann Ophthalmol 1993;25:56–57.

209. Gerling J, Neumann-Haefelin D, Seuffert HM, Schrader W. Diagnosis and management of the acute retinal necrosis syndrome. Ger J Ophthalmol 1992;1:388–393.

210. Miettinen P, Wasz-Hockert O. Ophthalmological aspects of tuberculous meningitis. Acta Ophthalmol Suppl 1960;61:1–54.

211. Okun E, Butler WT. Ophthalmological complications of cryptococcal meningitis. Arch Ophthalmol 1964;71:52–57.

212. Munn R, Farrell K, Cimolai N. Acute encephalomyelitis: extending the neurological manifestations of acute rheumatic fever? Neuroped 1992;23:196–198.

213. Ulrich GG, Waecker NJ, Meister SJ, et al. Cat scratch disease associated with neuroretinitis in a 6-year-old girl. Ophthalmology 1992;99:246–249.

214. Glaser JS. Neuro-ophthalmologic examination: General considerations and special techniques. In: Duane TD, Jaeger EA, eds. Clinical ophthalmology. Philadelphia: Harper & Row, 1987;2: Chap. 2, pp. 1–38.

215. Nadkarni N, Lisak RP. Guillain-Barre syndrome (GBS) with bilateral optic neuritis and central white matter disease. Neurology 1993;43:842–843.

216. Matoba AY. Ocular disease associated with Epstein-Barr virus infection. Surv Ophthalmol 1990;35:145–150.

217. Gupta DR, Strobas RJ. Bilateral papillitis associated with Cafergot® therapy. Neurology 1972;22:793–797.

218. Wollensak J, Grajewski O. Bilateral vascular papillitis following ergotamine medication. Klin Monatsbl Augenheikd 1978;173:731–737.

219. Tomsak RL, Lystad LD, Katirgi MB, Brassel TC. Rapid response of syphilitic optic neuritis to posterior sub-Tenon's steroid injection. J Clin Neuro-Ophthalmol 1992;12:6–7.

220. Chavis PS, Antonios SR, Tabbara KF. Cyclosporine effects on optic nerve and retinal vasculitis in Behçet's disease. Doc Ophthalmologica 1992;80:133–142.

221. Bajandas FJ. Neuro-ophthalmology board review manual. Thorofore, NJ: Charles B. Slack, 1980.

222. Lieberman MF, Shahi A, Green WR. Embolic ischemic optic neuropathy. Am J Ophthalmol 1978;86:206–210.

223. Anderson DR, Davis EB. Retina and optic nerve ater posterior ciliary artery occlusion. Arch Ophthalmol 1974;92:422–426.

224. Hayreh SS. Anterior ischemic optic neuropathy. New York: Springer-Verlag, 1975;126.

225. Drance SM, Morgan RW, Sweeney VP. Shock-induced optic neuropathy: A cause of non-progressive glaucoma. N Engl J Med 1973;288:392–395.

226. Boghen DR, Glaser JS. Ischaemic optic neuropathy. Brain 1975;98:689–708.

227. Ellenberger C Jr. Ischemic optic neuropathy as a possible early complication to vascular hypertension. Am J Ophthalmol 1979;88:1045–1051.

228. Kay MC. Ischemic optic neuropathy. Neurol Clin 1991;9:115–129.

229. Burde RM. Ischemic optic neuropathy. In: Smith JL, Glaser JS, eds. Neuro-opthalmology. Symposium of the University of Miami and the Bascom Palmer Eye Institute. St. Louis: C.V. Mosby Co, 1973;7:38–62.

230. Schechter SL. Lyme disease associated with optic neuropathy. Am J Med 1986;81:143–145.

231. Rizzzo JF, Lessell S. Posterior ischemic optic neuropathy during general surgery. Am J Ophthalmol 1987;103:808–811.

232. Guy J, Schatz NJ. Hyperbaric oxygen in the treatment of radiation-induced optic neuropathy. Ophthalmology 1986;93:1083–1088.

233. Isaak BL, Liesegang TJ, Michet CJ Jr. Ocular and systemic findings in relapsing polychondritis. Ophthalmology 1986;93:681–689.

234. Pugesgaard T, Von Eyben FE. Bilateral optic neuritis evolved during tamoxifen treatment. Cancer 1986;58:383–386.

235. Heafield MT, Carey M, Williams AC, Cullen M. Neoplastic angioendotheliomatosis: a treatable "vascular dementia" occurring in an immunosuppressed transplant patient. Clin Neuropath 1993;12:102–106.

236. Quinlan MF, Salmon JF. Ophthalmic complications after heart transplantation. J Heart Lung Transplant 1993;12:252–255.

237. Fry CL, Carter JE, Kanter MC, et al. Anterior ischemic optic neuropathy is not associated with carotid artery atherosclerosis. Stroke 1993;24:539–542.

238. Coppeto JR, Greco TP. Autoimmune ischemic optic neuropathy associated with positive rheumatoid factor and transient nephrosis. Ann Ophthalmol 1992;24:434–438.

239. Abe H, Sakai T, Sawaguchi S, et al. Ischemic optic neuropathy in a female carrier with Fabry's disease. Ophthalmologica 1992;205:83–88.

240. Borruat FX, Herbort CP. Herpes zoster ophthalmicus. Anterior ischemic optic neuropathy and acyclovir. J Clin Neuro-Ophthalmol 1992;12:37–40.

241. Defer G, Fauchon F, Schaison M, et al. Visual toxicity following intra-arterial chemotherapy with hydroxyethyl-CNU in patients with malignant gliomas. A prospective study with statistical analysis. Neuroradiology 1991;33:432–437.

242. Coutteel C, Leys A, Fossion E, Missotten L. Bilateral blindness in cavernous sinus thrombosis. Int Ophthalmol 1991;15:163–171.

243. Golnik KC, Newman SA. Anterior ischemic optic neuropathy associated with macrocytic anemia. J Clin Neuro-Ophthalmol 1990;10:244–247.

244. Gupta A, Jalili S, Bansal RK, Grewal SP. Anterior ischemic optic neuropathy and branch retinal artery occlusion in cavernous sinus thrombosis. J Clin Neuro-Ophthalmol 1990;10:193–196.

245. Savino PJ, Burde RM, Mills RP. Visual loss following intranasal anesthetic injection. J Clin Neuro-Ophthalmol 1990;10:140–144.

246. Guyer DR, Green WR, Schachat AP, et al. Bilateral ischemic optic neuropathy and retinal vascular occlusions associated with lymphoma and sepsis. Clinicopathologic correlation. Ophthalmology 1990;97:882–888.

247. Von Noorden GK, Burian HM. Visual acuity in normal and amblyopic patients under reduced illumination. I. Behavior of visual acuity with and without neutral density filter. Arch Ophthalmol 1959;61:533–535.

248. Barrett DA, Glaser JS, Schatz NJ, Winterkorn JM. Spontaneous recovery of vision in progressive anterior ischemic optic neuropathy. J Clin Neuro-Ophthalmol 1992;12:219–225.

249. Aiello AL, Sadun AA, Feldon SE. Spontaneous improvement of progressive anterior ischemic optic neuropathy: report of two cases. Arch Ophthalmol 1992;110:1197–1199.

250. Quigley H, Anderson DR. Cupping of the optic disc in ischemic optic neuropathy. Trans Am Acad Ophthalmol Otolaryngol 1977;83:755–762.

251. Limaye SR, Adler J. Pseudo-Foster Kennedy syndrome in a patient with anterior ischemic optic neuropathy and a nonbasal glioma. J Clin Neuro-Ophthalmol 1990;10:188–192.

252. Miller NR. Anterior ischemic optic neuropathy: diagnosis and management. Bull NY Acad Med 1980;56:643–654.

253. Hayreh SS. Anterior ischemic optic neuropathy. III. Treatment, prophylaxis, and differential diagnosis. Br J Ophthalmol 1974;58:981–989.

254. Spoor TC, McHenry JG, Lau-Sickon L. Progressive and static nonarteritic ischemic optic neuropathy treated by optic nerve sheath decompression. Ophthalmology 1993;100:306–311.

255. Flaharty PM, Sergott RC, Lieb W, et al. Optic nerve sheath decompression may improve blood flow in anterior ischemic optic neuropathy. Ophthalmology 1993;100:297–302.

256. Spoor TC, Wilkinson MJ, Ramocki JM. Optic nerve sheath decompression for the treatment of progressive nonarteritic ischemic optic neuropathy. Am J Ophthalmol 1991;111:724–728.

257. The Ischemic Optic Neuropathy Decompression Trial Research Group. Optic nerve decompression surgery for nonarteritic anterior ischemic optic neuropathy (NAION) is not effective and may be harmful. JAMA 1995;273:625–632.

258. Taylor RH, Deutsch J. Myxoma mix-up. A case report. J Clin Neuro-Ophthalmol 1992;12:207–209.

259. Hayreh SS. Ophthalmic features of giant cell arteritis. Baillieres Clin Rheum 1991;5:431–459.

260. Boke W, Voigt GJ. Circulatory disturbances of the optic nerve. Ophthalmologica 1980;180:88–100.

261. Fraunfelder FT, Roy FH. Current ocular therapy. Philadelphia: W.B. Saunders Co, 1980;528–529.

262. Siatkowski RM, Gass JD, Glaser JS, et al. Fluorescein angiography in the diagnosis of giant cell arteritis. Am J Ophthalmol 1993;115:57–63.

263. Mack HG, O'Day J, Currie JN. Delayed choroidal perfusion in giant cell arteritis. J Clin Neuro-Ophthalmol 1991;11:221–227.

264. Williamson TH, Baxter G, Paul R, Dutton GN. Colour Doppler ultrasound in the management of a case of cranial arteritis. Br J Ophthalmol 1992;76:690–691.

265. Hayreh SS. Anterior ischaemic optic neuropathy. Differentiation of arteritic from non-arteritic type and its management. Eye 1990;4:25–41.

266. Wiek J, Krause M, Schade M, et al. Haemorheological parameters in patients with retinal artery occlusion and anterior ischaemic optic neuropathy. Br J Ophthalmol 1992;76:142–145.

267. Neish PR, Sergent JS. Giant cell arteritis. A case with unusual neurologic manifestations and a normal sedimentation rate. Arch Int Med 1991;151:378–380.

268. Diamond JP. Treatable blindness in temporal arteritis. Br J Ophthalmol 1991;75:432.

269. Cohen DN. Temporal arteritis: improvement in visual prognosis and management with repeat biopsies. Trans Am Acad Ophthalmol Otolaryngol 1973;77:Op. 74–85.

270. Mosher HA. The prognosis in temporal arteritis. Arch Ophthalmol 1959;62:641–644.

271. Schneider HA, Weber AA, Ballen PH. The visual prognosis in temporal arteritis. Ann Ophthalmol 1971;3:1215–1230.

272. Whitfield AGW, Bateman M, Cooke WT. Temporal arteritis. Br J Ophthalmol 1963;47:555–566.

273. Eshaghian J. Controversies regarding giant cell (temporal, cranial) arteritis. Doc Ophthalmol 1979;47:43–67.

274. Wilson J, Linnell JC, Matthews DM. Plasma-cobalamins in neuro-ophthalmological diseases. Lancet 1971;1:259–261.

275. Poole CJ, Kind PR. Deficiency of thiosulphate sulphur-transferase (Rhodanese) in Leber's heredity optic neuropathy. Br Med J 1986;292:1229–1230.

276. Novotny EJ Jr, Singh G, Wallace DC, et al. Leber's disease and dystonia: A mitochondrial disease. Neurology 1986;94:213–218.

277. Newman NJ. Leber's hereditary optic neuropathy. New genetic considerations. Arch Neurol 1993;50:540–548.

278. Weiner NC, Newman NJ, Lessell S, et al. Atypical Leber's hereditary optic neuropathy with molecular confirmation. Arch Neurol 1993;50:470–473.

279. Van Caelenberghe E, Meir F, Broux C, et al. Leber's hereditary optic neuropathy: clinical and molecular genetic aspects. Preliminary results in our families. Bulletin De La Societe Belge Ophtalmologie 1992;243:139–146.

280. Cavelier L, Gyllensten U, Dahl N. Intrafamilial variation in Leber hereditary optic neuropathy revealed by direct mutation analysis. Clin Gen 1993;43:69–72.

281. Barboni P, Mantovani V, Montagna P, et al. Mitochondrial DNA analysis in Leber's hereditary optic neuropathy. Ophthalmic Paediatr Genet 1992;13:219–226.

282. Johns DR, Berman J. Alternative, simultaneous complex I mitochondrial DNA mutations in Leber's hereditary optic neuropathy. Biochem Biophys Res Comm 1991;174:1324–1330.

283. Johns DR, Heher KL, Miller NR, Smith KH. Leber's hereditary optic neuropathy. Clinical manifestations of the 14484 mutation. Arch Ophthalmol 1993;111:495–498.

284. Mackey D, Howell N. A variant of Leber hereditary optic neuropathy characterized by recovery of vision and by an unusual mitochondrial genetic etiology. Am J Human Gen 1992;51:1218–1228.

285. Johns DR, Smith KH, Miller NR. Leber's hereditary optic neuropathy. Clinical manifestations of the 3460 mutation. Arch Ophthalmol 1992;110:1577–1581.

286. Francois J. Hereditary optic atrophy. Int Ophthalmol Clin 1968;8:1016–1054.

287. Borruat FX, Green WT, Graham EM, et al. Late onset Leber's optic neuropathy: a case confused with ischaemic optic neuropathy. Br J Ophthalmol 1992;76:571–573.

288. Waardenburg PJ. Some remarks on the clinical and genetic puzzle of Leber's optic neuritis. J Hum Genet 1969;17:47996.

289. Went LN. Leber disease and variants. In: Vinken PJ, Brugn GW, eds. Handbook of clinical neurology. New York: American Elsevier, 1972

290. Seedorff T. Leber's disease IV. Acta Ophthalmol 1969;47:813–821.

291. Seedorff T. Leber's disease V. Acta Ophthalmol 1970;48:186–213.

292. Newman NJ, Lott MT, Wallace DC. The clinical characteristics of pedigrees of Leber's hereditary optic neuropathy with the 11778 mutation. Am J Ophthalmol 1991;111:750–762.

293. Nikoskelainen E, Sogg RL, Rosenthal AR, et al. The early phase in Leber hereditary optic atrophy. Arch Ophthalmol 1977;95:969–978.

294. Crutz-Coke R. Diagnosis in color blindness: an evolutionary approach. Springfield, IL: Charles C Thomas, 1970.

295. Livingstone IR, Mastaglia FL, Howe JW, Aherne GES. Leber's optic neuropathy: clinical and visual evoked response studies in asymptomatic and symptomatic members of a 4-generation family. Br J Ophthalmol 1980;64:751–757.

296. Smith JL, Hoyt WF, Susac JO. Ocular fundus in acute Leber optic neuropathy. Arch Ophthalmol 1973;90:349–354.

297. de Gottrau P, Buchi ER, Daicker B. Distended optic nerve sheaths in Leber's hereditary optic neuropathy. J Clin Neuro-Ophthalmol 1992;12:89–93.

298. Smith JL, Tse DT, Byrne SF, et al. Optic nerve sheath distention in Leber's optic neuropathy and the significance of the "Wallace mutation." J Clin Neuro-Ophthalmol 1990;10:231–238.

299. Stone EM, Newman NJ, Miller NR, et al. Visual recovery in patients with Leber's hereditary optic neuropathy and the 11778 mutation. J Clin Neuro-Ophthalmol 1992;12:10–14.

300. Chew SJ. Leber's hereditary optic atrophy: an atypical case with response to hydroxycobalamine therapy. Singapore Med J 1990;31:293–294.

301. Lessell S. Toxic and deficiency optic neuropathies. In: Smith JL, Glaser JS, eds. Neuro-ophthalmology. Symposium of the University of Miami and the Bascom Palmer Eye Institute. St. Louis: C.V. Mosby Co, 1973;7:21–37.

302. DuBois LG, Feldon SE. Evidence for a metabolic trigger for Leber's hereditary optic neuropathy. J Clin Neuro-Ophthalmol 1992;12:15–16.

303. Phillips CI, Gosden CM. Leber's hereditary optic neuropathy and Kearns-Sayre syndrome: mitochondrial DNA mutations. Surv Ophthalmol 1991;35:463–472.

304. Hayreh SS. Optic disc vasculitis. Br J Ophthalmol 1972;56:652–670.

306. Laibovitz RA. Presumed phlebitis of the optic disc. Ophthalmology 1979;86:313–319.

305. Fong ACO, Schatz H, McDonald HR, et al. Central retinal vein occlusion in young adults (papillophlebitis). Retina 1991;11:3–11.

307. Singh K, de Frank MP, Shults WT, Watzke RC. Acute idiopathic blind spot enlargement; a spectrum of disease. Ophthalmology 1991;98:497–502.

308. Lonn LI, Hoyt WF. Papillophlebitis: A cause of protracted yet benign optic disc edema. Eye Ear Nose Throat Monthly 1966;45:62–68.

309. Humayun M, Kattah J, Cupps TR, et al. Papillophlebitis and arteriolar occlusion in a pregnant woman. J Clin Neuro-Ophthalmol 1992;12:226–229.

310. Walters RF, Spalton DJ. Central retinal vein occlusion in people aged 40 years or less: a review of 17 patients. Br J Ophthalmol 1990;74:30–35.

311. Hayreh SS. Optic disc edema in raised intracranial pressure. VI. Associated visual disturbances and their pathogenesis. Arch Ophthalmol 1977;95:1566–1579.

312. Wirtschafter JD, Rizzo FJ, Smiley BC. Optic nerve axoplasm and papilledema. Surv Ophthalmol 1975;20:157–189.

313. Hayreh SS. Optic disc edema in raised intracranial pressure. Arch Ophthalmol 1977;95:1553–1565.

314. Green GJ, Lessell S, Loewenstein JI. Ischemic optic neuropathy in chronic papilledema. Arch Ophthalmol 1980;98:502–505.

315. Winterkorn JM. Peripapillary hemorrhage. Surv Ophthalmol 1993;37:362–372.

316. Macken P, Arora A, Hipwell G, Hunyor A. Superior sagittal sinus thrombosis—an unexpected cause of papilloedema. Aust NZ J Ophthalmol 1992;20:337–342.

317. Matzkin DC, Slamovits TL, Genis I, Bello J. Disc swelling: a tall tail? Surv Ophthalmol 1992;37:130–136.

318. Hardten DR, Wen DY, Wirtschafter JD, et al. Papilledema and intraspinal lumbar paraganglioma. J Clin Neuro-Ophthalmol 1992;12:158–162.

319. Catz A, Appel I, Reider-Grosswasser I, Grosswasser Z. Late-onset papilledema following spinal injury. Case report. Paraplegia 1993;31:131–135.

320. Bouma GJ, Muizelaar JP. Cerebral blood flow, cerebral blood volume, and cerebrovascular reactivity after severe head injury. J Neurotrauma 1992;9(Suppl 1):S333–S348.

321. Marmarou A. Increased intracranial pressure in head injury and influence of blood volume. J Neurotrauma 1992;9(Suppl 1):S327–S332.

322. Miller JD, Dearden NM, Piper IR, Chan KH. Control of intracranial pressure in patients with severe head injury. J Neurotrauma 1992;9(Suppl 1):S317–S326.

323. Pagani LF. The rapid appearance of papilledema. J Neurosurg 1969;30:247–249.

324. Morley JB, Reynolds EH. Papilloedema and the Landry-Guillain-Barre syndrome. Brain 1966;89:205–222.

325. Lobo A, Pilek E, Stokes PE. Papilledema following therapeutic dosages of lithium carbonate. J Nerv Ment Dis 1978;166:526–529.

326. Levine SH, Puchalski C. Pseudotumor cerebri associated with lithium therapy in two patients. J Clin Psych 1990;51:251–253.

327. Gittinger JW Jr, Asdourian GK. Papillopathy caused by amiodarone. Arch Ophthalmol 1987;105:349–351.

328. Green NS, Garvin JH Jr, Chutorian A. Transient erythoblastopenia of childhood presenting with papilledema. Clin Pediatr 1986;25:278–279.

329. de Vries WA, Balm AJ, Tiwari RM. Intracranial hypertension following neck dissection. J Laryngol Otol 1986;100:1427–1431.

330. Niutta A, Scorcia G, Princi P, et al. Visual disturbances associated with primary empty sella syndrome in patients with chronic renal failure. Ann Ophthalmol 1992;24:56–63.

331. Johnston SR, Corbett EL, Foster O, et al. Raised intracranial pressure and visual complications in AIDS patients with cryptococcal meningitis. J Infect 1992;24:185–189.

332. Doyle KJ, Tami TA. Increased intracranial pressure and blindness associated with obstructive sleep apnea. Otolaryngol-Head Neck Surg 1991;105:613–616.

333. el-Ramahi KM, al-Kawi MZ. Papilloedema in Behçet's disease: value of MRI in diagnosis of dural sinus thrombosis. J Neurol Neurosurg Psych 1991;54:826–829.

334. Lesser RL, Kornmehl EW, Pachner AR, et al. Neuro-ophthalmologic manifestations of Lyme disease. Ophthalmology 1990;97:699–706.

335. Collins ML, Traboulsi EI, Maumenee IH. Optic nerve head swelling and optic atrophy in the systemic mucopolysaccharidoses. Ophthalmology 1990;97:1445–1449.

336. Hayasaka S, Noda S, Sekimoto M, et al. Hyperemic swollen optic disk in patients with primary open-angle glaucoma. Ophthalmologica 1992;205:187–190.

337. Cavallaro N, Randone A, LaRosa L, Mughinin L. Bilateral papilledema in a patient with brucellosis. Metab Ped Syst Ophthalmol 1990;13:115–118.

338. Boddie HG, Banna M, Bradley WG. "Benign" intracranial hypertension: a survey of the clinical and radiological features, and long-term prognosis. Brain 1974;97:313–326.

339. Bowman MA. Pseudotumor cerebri. Am Fam Physician 1987;35:177–182.

340. Bence G, Grala PE. Pseudotumor cerebri. J Am Optom Assoc 1986;57:751–754.

341. DelGiudice GC, Scher CA, Athreya BH, Diamond GR. Pseudotumor cerebri and childhood systemic lupus erythematosus. J Rheumatol 1986;13:748–752.

342. Johnson I, Paterson A. Benign intracranial hypertension. II. CSF pressure and circulation. Brain 1974;97:301–312.

343. Mokri B, Jack CR, Petty GW. Pseudotumor syndrome associated with cerebral venous sinus occlusion and antiphospholipid antibodies. Stroke 1993;24:469–472.

344. Johnson I, Paterson A. Benign intracranial hypertension. I. Diagnosis and prognosis. Brain 1974;97:289–300.

345. Hayreh MS, Hayreh SS. Optic disc edema in raised intracranial pressure. I. Evolution and resolution. Arch Ophthalmol 1977;95:1237–1244.

346. Cogan DC. Neurology of the visual system. Springfield, IL: Charles C Thomas, 1966;142–143.

347. Walsh TJ, Garden JW, Gallagher B. Obliteration of retinal venous pulsations during elevation of cerebrospinal-fluid pressure. Am J Opthalmol 1969;67:954–956.

348. Hayreh SS, Hayreh MS. Optic disc edema in raised intracranial pressure. II. Early detection with flourescein fundus angiography and stereoscopic color photography. Arch Ophthalmol 1977;95:1245–1254.

349. Savino PJ, Glaser JS. Pseudopapilledema versus papilledema. Int Ophthalmol Clin 1977;17:115–137.

350. Mamalis N, Mortenson S, Digre KB, White GL. Congenital anomalies of the optic nerve in one family. Ann Ophthalmol 1992;24:126–131.

351. Tso MOM, Hayreh SS. Optic disc edema in raised intracranial pressure. IV. Axoplasmic transport in experimental papilledema. Arch Ophthalmol 1977;95:1458–1462.

352. Galvin R, Sanders MD. Peripheral retinal haemorrhages with papilloedema. Br J Ophthalmol 1980;64:262–266.

353. Jamison RR. Subretinal neovascularization and papilledema associated with pseudotumor cerebri. Am J Ophthalmol 1978;85:78–81.

354. Bird AC, Sanders MD. Choroidal folds in association with papilloedema. Br J Ophthalmol 1973;57:89–97.

355. Morris AT, Sanders MD. Macular changes resulting from papilloedema. Br J Ophthalmol 1980;64:211–216.

356. Eggers HM, Sanders MD. Acquired optociliary shunt vessels in papilloedema. Br J Ophthalmol 1980;64:267–271.

357. Wiegand W. The optic nerve pathology in magnetic resonance imaging. Metab Ped Syst Ophthalmol 1990;13:60–66.

358. Spoor TC, McHenry JG. Long-term effectiveness of optic nerve sheath decompression for pseudotumor cerebri. Arch Ophthalmol 1993;111:632–635.

359. Hamed LM, Tse DT, Glaser, et al. Neuroimaging of the optic nerve after fenestration for management of pseudotumor cerebri. Arch Ophthalmol 1992;110:636–639.

360. Horton JC, Seiff SR, Pitts LH, et al. Decompression of the optic nerve sheath for vision-threatening papilledema caused by dural sinus occlusion. Neurosurg 1992;31:203–211.

361. Kelman SE, Heaps R, Wolf A, Elman MJ. Optic nerve decompression surgery improves visual function in patients with pseudotumor cerebri. Neurosurg 1992;30:391–395.

362. Smith KH, Wilkinson JT, Brindley GO. Combined third and sixth nerve paresis following optic nerve sheath fenestration. J Clin Neuro-Ophthalmol 1992;12:85–87.

363. Jefferson A, Clark J. Treatment of benign intracranial hypertension by dehydrating agents with particular reference to the measurement of the blind spot area as a means of recording improvement. J Neurol Neurosurg Psychiatry 1976;39:627–639.

364. Keltner JL, Miller NR, Gittinger JW, Burde RM. Pseudotumor cerebri. Surv Ophthalmol 1979;23:315–322.

365. Gucer G, Viernstein L. Long-term intracranial pressure recording in the management of pseudotumor cerebri. J Neurosurg 1978;49:256–263.

366. Yiannakis PH, Larner AJ. Visual failure and optic atrophy associate with chlorambucil therapy. BMJ 1993;306:109.

367. Markus H, Polkey M, Harrison M. Visual loss and optic atrophy associated with cyproterone acetate. BMJ 1992;305:159.

368. Gross EG, Helfgott MA. Retinoids and the eye. Derm Clin 1991;10:521–531.

369. Stelmach MZ, O'Day J. Partly reversible visual failure with methanol toxicity. Aust NZ J Ophthalmol 1992;20:57–64.

370. Johansson BA. Visual field defects during low-dose methotrexate therapy. Doc Ophthalmologica 1992;79:91–94.

371. Good WV, Ferriero DM, Golabi M, Kobori JA. Abnormalities of the visual system in infants exposed to cocaine. Ophthalmology 1992;99:341–346.

372. Avery R, Jabs DA, Wingard JR, et al. Optic disc edema after bone marrow transplantation. Possible role of cyclosporine toxicity. Ophthalmology 1991;98:1294–1301.

373. Vrabec TR, Sergott RC, Jaeger EA, et al. Reversible visual loss in a patient receiving high-dose ciprofloxacin hydrochloride (Cipro). Ophthalmology 1990;97:707–710.

374. Jaanus SD. Ocular side effects of selected systemic drugs. Optom Clin 1992;2:73–96.

375. Martin-Amat G, Tephly TR, McMartin KE, et al. Methyl alcohol poisoning. II. Development of a model for ocular toxicity in methyl alcohol poisoning using the rhesus monkey. Arch Ophthalmol 1977;95:1847–1850.

376. Hayreh MS, Hayreh SS, Baumbach GL, et al. Methyl alcohol poisoning. III. Ocular toxicity. Arch Ophthalmol 1977;95:1851–1858.

377. Baumbach GL, Cancilla PA, Martin-Amat G, et al. Methyl alcohol poisoning. IV. Alterations of the morphological findings of the retina and optic nerve. Arch Ophthalmol 1977;95:1859–1865.

378. Leopold IH. Zinc deficiency and visual impairment? (editorial.) Am J Ophthalmol 1978;85:871–875.

379. Moynahan EJ. Zinc deficiency and disturbances of mood and visual behaviour (letter). Lancet 1976;1:91.

380. Moore R. Bleeding gastric erosion after oral zinc sulphate. Br Med J 1978;1:754.

381. Faigenbaum SJ, Leopold IH. Ophthalmology in nutritional support of medical practice. Hagerstown, NJ: Harper & Row, 1977: 422–431.

382. Lessell S, Coppeto JM. The management of optic neuritis and nutritional amblyopia. In: Srinivasan BD, ed. Ocular therapeutics. New York: Masson, 1980;201–208.

383. Diesenhouse MC, Palay DA, Newman NJ, et al. Acquired heterochromia with Horner syndrome in two adults. Ophthalmology 1992;99:1815–1817.

384. Beck RW, Cleary PA, Backlund JC. The Optic Neuritis Study Group. The course of visual recovery after optic neuritis. Experience of the Optic Neuritis Treatment Trial. Ophthalmology 1994; 101:1771–1778.

CHAPTER 24

Diseases of the Eyelids

Jimmy D. Bartlett
Gerald G. Melore

Disorders of the eyelids are among the most common ocular abnormalities encountered by the optometrist and other primary eyecare practitioners. Because of their widespread prevalence and the fact that eyelid diseases often include conjunctival, corneal, or systemic involvement, the practitioner must be able to recognize and manage specific diseases affecting the eyelids. This chapter considers the pharmacologic management of the most common and clinically significant disorders.

Clinical Anatomy and Physiology

A meaningful discussion of eyelid disease requires knowledge of major anatomic structures and functions of the lids. Figure 24.1 shows the important anatomic features. The eyelid is limited anteriorly by the dermis, which often plays an important role in allergic eyelid manifestations. The seventh cranial nerve innervates the orbicularis muscle, which is primarily responsible for normal involuntary blinking as well as tight eyelid closure. The eyelashes (cilia) emerge from individual follicles, surrounded by the glands of Zeis and Moll. Posterior to the lash line lies the row of meibomian glands. The meibomian glands and glands of Zeis are sebaceous glands, which secrete oil, while the glands of Moll are modified sweat glands. The meibomian glands serve an important function in tear physiology: They supply the lipid layer of the tear film, which prevents evaporation of the underlying aqueous component. Meibomian gland abnormalities may thus play an important role in dry eye syndrome.

The third cranial nerve innervates the levator muscle, which is responsible for elevation of the upper eyelid. Müller's muscle, innervated by the sympathetic division of the autonomic nervous system, augments action of the levator muscle in elevating the upper lid.

Congenital Abnormalities

Coloboma

Congenital eyelid coloboma is a rare clinical entity characterized by absence of a portion of the eyelid. In 90% of cases the upper lid is involved,[1] and the most common position of the coloboma is at the junction of the medial and middle third of the lid.[2] A variety of other orbital, facial, or ocular abnormalities may accompany this abnormality, including limbal dermoids, strabismus, and corneal opacities.[3]

The primary problem caused by congenital eyelid coloboma is exposure keratopathy, which occurs when 30% or more of the upper lid is absent.[4] Management then, depends on the severity of the individual situation. Surgical correction is generally indicated for cosmesis,[5] but can be delayed until the child is 3 to 6 months old, at which time general anesthesia poses a less serious risk. In the meantime, the cornea should be protected by use of topically applied lubricating ointments as well as antibiotic ointments if infection is a significant risk. If four-fifths of the upper lid is absent, corneal exposure and scarring are quite likely, and surgery may be necessary within the first 48 hours of life.[1]

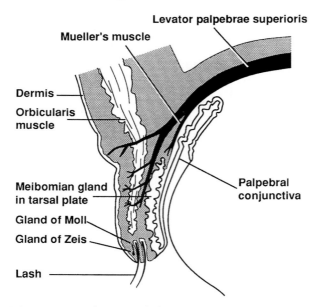

FIGURE 24.1   **Major anatomic features of the eyelids.**

Even topical antibiotics or lubricating ointments often prove unsatisfactory in such cases.

Distichiasis

Congenital distichiasis is a rare condition in which an accessory row of eyelashes lies posterior to the normal lashes (Fig. 24.2). The accessory lashes arise from the meibomian gland orifices.[6] The meibomian glands themselves may be rudimentary, atrophic, or normal.[7] This disorder occurs sporadically or as an autosomal dominant trait.[7,8] The condition displays a wide variation in the number of eyelids involved; the number of abnormal lashes; the diameter, length, or pigmentation of the lashes; and the direction of their shafts. The lashes are often softer, shorter, and more delicate than normal cilia, and the patient may be entirely asymptomatic, especially during early childhood.[9,10]

Associated findings can include corneal hypoesthesia and corneal epithelial staining with sodium fluorescein.[8] In rare instances distichiasis occurs in conjunction with skeletal abnormalities and may occur along with congenital heart disease and peripheral vascular anomalies.[11] Distichiasis has also been reported in association with cleft palate,[10] Milroy's disease (hypoplastic lymphatics), and late-onset hereditary lymphedema (hyperplastic lymphatics).[12] Acquired distichiasis can occur after long-standing inflammation and cicatricial conditions of the mucosa, such as Stevens-Johnson syndrome, ocular pemphigoid, and severe chemical burns. Mechanical or surgical trauma to the tarsus and meibomian

glands can also trigger metaplastic processes within the glands to support a hair-bearing function.[13]

Distichiasis requires no treatment if the patient is asymptomatic, but when the lashes cause corneal irritation, they should be removed. If only a few lashes are involved, they can be removed by epilation or electrolysis. When the condition is extensive, however, surgical correction[14,15] or cryotherapy[16] is indicated. The application of artificial tear solutions or lubricating ointments or, in severe cases, antibiotics may be indicated before surgical intervention.

Abnormalities Associated with Trauma

Thermal Burns

Flame, flash, and scald burns are the most common causes of eyelid burns.[17-19] It is vital to exclude the possibility of ocular damage by exposing and examining the globe for penetrating injury or thermal burns of the cornea and conjunctiva. Once ocular injury has been excluded, first- or second-degree burns of the lids usually result only in temporary loss of lashes and require no more than general supportive care.[17] The eyelids and conjunctival sacs should be irrigated to remove any remaining particulate material. Singed lashes may be removed using a moist sponge or cotton-tipped applicator. Tonometry should be performed since pronounced periorbital edema can raise intraocular pressure to dangerous levels.[20] Initial therapy should include careful lid and lash hygiene with gauze and saline to keep crusting of the lids to a minimum.[21] Topically applied burn creams should be avoided because they can irritate the conjunctiva and impair lid motion.[18] Antibiotic ointments should be applied to the lids 2 to 4 times daily to prevent secondary infection, but these may have little value in managing minor burns involving unbroken skin.[22] If applied soon after the injury, the use of cold compresses or iced-saline gauze over the eyelids is effective in reducing edema.[19] Oral analgesics should be used as required for relief of pain (see Chap. 7). Minor burns may also benefit from the application of topical 1% hydrocortisone cream or ointment to reduce inflammatory signs and symptoms.[22] Healing is generally uncomplicated (Fig. 24.3). Immediately following the injury trichiasis may occur due to charring, distortion of the lashes, or lid edema. Since corneal abrasion can result from the trichiasis, the offending lashes should be epilated, or the cornea and globe should be protected with soft contact lenses or scleral shells.[21]

In cases of severe, third-degree burns of the lids, the cornea should be protected with any combination of artificial tears, bland lubricating ointment, or soft contact lenses. Since structural deformities resulting from extensive lid scarring are likely, immediate consultation with an oculoplastic surgeon is indicated.[17,18]

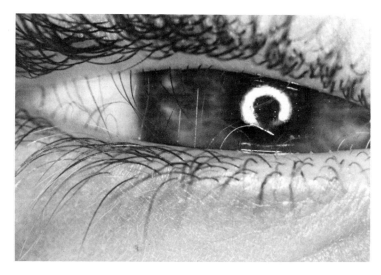

FIGURE 24.2   **Congenital distichiasis. (Courtesy Jerry R. Pederson, O.D.)**

Chemical Burns

The accidental inoculation of foreign chemicals into the eye may result in only minor irritation or serious, destructive burns depending on the chemical involved. Acid burns are generally self-limited, and the resultant injury is usually superficial unless the acid remains in contact with the tissues for a prolonged time. On the other hand, alkaline fluids typically cause more extensive tissue damage because they can penetrate the eyelid or ocular tissue.[19]

Regardless of the type of chemical injury, speed is essential in the initial first-aid of the chemical burn. The eye(s) should be irrigated with copious amounts of clean water or irrigating solution. The irrigation will be more comfortable if a topical anesthetic is first instilled. Most cases require only 1 to 2 minutes of irrigation, except for acid or alkali burns, which should receive prolonged irrigation.[23] In addition, if the contaminant is chemically reactive or has an oily or viscous base, the irrigation should also be extended. Every 5 to 10 minutes during the course of irrigation the conjunctival sac should be tested with a pH test paper. Once the pH has returned to normal, it is unnecessary to continue irrigation. The sticky paste and powder of lime (calcium hydroxide) can be removed from the lids and conjunctival sac by using cotton-tipped applicators that have been soaked in ethylenediaminetetraacetic acid (EDTA), 0.01 M.[24] Following irrigation, the cornea and conjunctiva should be carefully examined for damage. If the eye may be contaminated with solid particles, the entire conjunctival sac must be inspected for any residual particles.

In the case of an alkali burn,[23] the eye or eyelids should be treated with a topical antibiotic, which may include gentamicin or tobramycin solution four times daily or erythromycin or bacitracin ointment four times daily. Cycloplegia with cyclopentolate 1%, homatropine 5%, or atropine 1%, one to several times daily, should be instituted according to the severity of the chemical burn. Elevated intraocular pressure can be treated with acetazolamide, 250 mg four times daily, or a topical β blocker twice daily. For several days following the alkali burn, topical steroids such as dexamethasone 0.1% or prednisolone 1% can be used several times daily along with the topical antibiotic to reduce the severity of any anterior uveitis. However, steroids should not be used for more than 5 to 7 days, since they tend to suppress tissue repair processes.[23,24] If the chemical injury is serious enough to cause potential eyelid, conjunctival, or corneal deformities, immediate consultation with an oculoplastic surgeon is warranted.[24]

Hydrofluoric acid burns represent a special case requiring immediate consultation with a burn team to avoid potentially fatal complications. Even minimal skin exposure to hydrofluoric acid can cause severe, life-threatening metabolic imbalances. Skin exposure involving as little as 8% of body surface area can cause intractable cardiac arrhythmia and death associated with hypocalcemia.[25]

Cyanoacrylate Tarsorraphy

Cyanoacrylate adhesives (e.g., Krazy Glue, Super Glue) are widely used in both industrial and household settings. Occasionally the adhesive can be inadvertently spilled onto the ocular tissues, and in some instances the similarity of containers can lead to accidental instillation into the eye.[26,27] Although chemically induced tarsorraphy or even total ankyloblepharon can result, the condition is temporary and

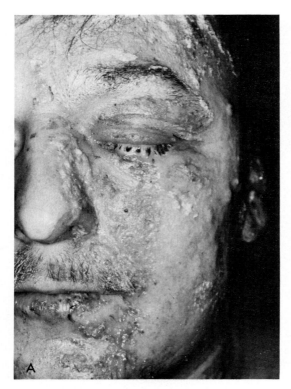
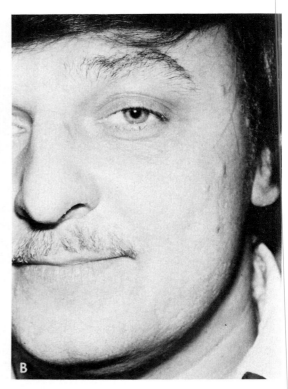

FIGURE 24.3   *(A)* **Burn injuries of the face and eyelid.** *(B)* **The wound healed in two weeks, and the deformity was minimal. (From Huang TT, Blackwell SJ, Lewis SR. Burn injuries of the eyelids. Clin Plast Surg 1978;5:571–581, with permission of the authors and publisher).**

does not cause permanent injury.[28,29] However, the patient will often experience extreme anxiety and functional vision impairment as long as the eyelids are apposed.

In the absence of complicating factors, surgical lysis of the adhesion should not be undertaken. Surgical lysis is unnecessary, since most of the adhesion is between the lashes of the upper and lower lids.[30] Because the glue can be irritative, the involved lashes can be cut, allowing the lids to separate quickly and easily with only mild pressure.[30] A more conservative approach consisting of the application of tap water- or mineral oil-soaked eyepads is effective and results in less eyelid morbidity.[28,31] The moistened eyepads may need to be applied for at least 24 hours. Another approach consists of instilling antibiotic ointment into the conjunctival sac and onto the adhesion, covering the eye with a light pressure dressing. This conservative management often allows easy removal of the glue with forceps 24 hours later.[29] Oral analgesics may be needed for patient discomfort or pain.

Although cyanoacrylate adhesives generally cause no permanent ocular damage, some patients have residual epithelial keratopathy or corneal abrasion,[26,27,29] especially if the glue is not immediately irrigated from the eye.[32,33] This residual condition should be treated in the usual fashion, using topical antibacterial ointment and pressure-patching, if necessary.

Inflammatory Diseases

External Hordeolum

External hordeolum (common stye) is one of the most common eyelid disorders encountered in clinical practice. It is often self-treated by the patient using various home remedies, but the optometrist or other primary care clinician is often consulted because of its painful and cosmetically displeasing course.

ETIOLOGY

An external hordeolum is an acute staphylococcal infection of the glands of Zeis and Moll. The hordeolum is usually a localized area of inflammation, but it may be associated with staphylococcal blepharitis. The lesions are often associated with fatigue, poor diet, and stress and can be recurrent.[34]

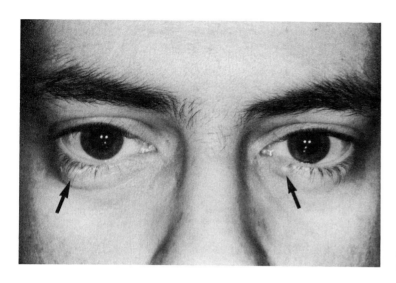

FIGURE 24.4   **Bilateral external hordeola (arrows), presenting as localized areas of redness, tenderness, and swelling near the lid margin.**

DIAGNOSIS

The lesion usually presents as a localized area of redness, tenderness, and swelling near the lid margin (Fig. 24.4). The primary symptom is localized pain of recent onset. Within a few days of onset of redness and tenderness, the localized area develops a yellow point. In most cases the abscess will spontaneously drain within 3 or 4 days following pointing.

MANAGEMENT

The application of hot compresses several times daily will serve to hasten pointing and drainage. Generally this is all that is necessary for resolution. Topically applied antibiotic solutions or ointments several times daily may prevent infection of surrounding lash follicles but will not affect the course of the external hordeolum itself.[35] One of the best methods to hasten drainage of the lesion is simply to epilate 1 or 2 involved lashes, which creates an effective drainage channel.[36]

For lesions resistant to the usual therapy, an incision can be made with a sterile needle or blade into the area of pointing, without using a topical anesthetic.[34,36,37] This will allow the abscess cavity to drain. Following the stab incision, topical antibiotic ointment such as gentamicin or bacitracin-polymyxin B should be applied to the lid margin and conjunctival sac.[36]

Bacitracin or erythromycin ointment applied four times daily during the acute phase and continued twice daily for one week thereafter may prove helpful. Topical steroids are indicated only if inflammation is severe.[37] If staphylococcal infection exists elsewhere in the body, or if the practitioner notes preauricular lymphadenopathy, systemic antibiotics may be necessary. Erythromycin 250 mg or dicloxacillin 125 to 250 mg can be administered orally four times daily for up to two weeks.[37] If recurrence is likely, long-term prophylactic therapy may consist of tetracycline 250 mg administered twice daily one hour before meals for several months.[37] If the hordeolum is recurrent despite such antibiotic therapy, a lid culture should be obtained to identify the organism so that specific antibiotic therapy can be instituted.[34]

Internal Hordeolum

ETIOLOGY

An internal hordeolum is a localized staphylococcal infection of the meibomian gland.[34] The infection usually results from blockage of the gland and is found more frequently in the upper lid.

DIAGNOSIS

Palpation of the affected lid area reveals a localized area of swelling, inflammation, and tenderness within the tarsus (Fig. 24.5). The onset and course of the internal hordeolum are usually more prolonged than that of the external hordeolum.[34]

MANAGEMENT

Because the infection is deep within the lid tissue, the topical application of antibiotics is usually ineffective. In mild cases the application of hot compresses several times daily is sufficient for resolution. However, in moderate to severe cases oral antibiotic therapy is indicated. Since *Staphylococcus* sp. invariably cause infection, primary therapy should consist of a penicillinase-resistant penicillin such as dicloxa-

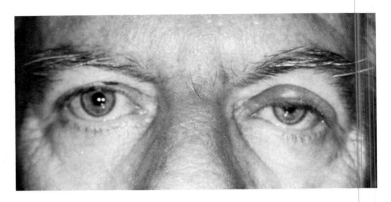

FIGURE 24.5 Internal hordeolum of left upper lid, characterized by swelling, inflammation, and tenderness within a localized area of tarsus. The swelling has caused pseudoptosis.

cillin. Dosages of 125 to 250 mg every 6 hours usually result in prompt resolution of the infection. Patients who have a history of mild penicillin allergy can be given a first- or second-generation cephalosporin. Other second-line therapy may consist of erythromycin or tetracycline. Erythromycin 250 mg four times daily or tetracycline 250 mg four times daily usually allows resolution within 1 to 2 weeks. In cases resistant to such therapy, puncture and drainage using a sterile needle or blade may be necessary. Topically applied antibiotic solution or ointment following drainage will serve to prevent secondary infection.

Chalazion

ETIOLOGY

A chalazion is a chronic, sterile, lipogranulomatous inflammation of the meibomian gland due to retention of normal secretions.[34,38] Such duct obstruction and granuloma formation may occur during *Demodex brevis* invasion of the meibomian glands, but the precise role of this organism in the formation of chalazia has not been established.[39,40] Chalazia occur spontaneously or may follow an episode of acute internal hordeolum.

DIAGNOSIS

The lesion usually develops over several weeks and is more common in the upper lid, appearing as a hard, immobile lump[41] (Fig. 24.6). The lesion can measure as little as 2 mm to as large as 7 or 8 mm in diameter.[41] It is often associated with seborrhea, including seborrheic blepharitis, and rosacea.[41-43] Palpation of the lesion produces no pain or tenderness, an important feature differentiating it from internal hordeolum. If the chalazion enlarges, it may produce mild discomfort, be cosmetically displeasing, or induce corneal astigmatism.[44,45] Cottrell and associates[46] have reported that at least 25% of chalazia resolve spontaneously within six months of onset, but most require treatment.

MANAGEMENT

In most cases chalazia can be treated successfully by the simple application of physical therapy. Topically or systemically administered antibiotics are ineffective and are not justified, because the lesion is sterile.[42] The application of hot compresses followed by vigorous digital massage to the chalazion several times daily for 2 to 4 weeks often leads to resolution, especially when the mass is small.[47] Bohigian[42] found no significant difference in improvement of chalazia using hot moist compresses four times daily as compared with topical sulfonamide four times daily following the hot compress therapy. In each group approximately half the patients improved after 1 month, and the cure rate after one month was approximately 40% with this conservative therapy. Perry and Serniuk[48] employed a different form of conservative therapy that resolved the chalazia in almost 80% of patients. Patients were instructed to apply warm saline soaks to the eyelids a few times daily and to use a moistened cotton-tipped applicator to the base of the eyelashes (Table 24.1). This therapy resolves the condition in approximately three weeks, ranging from two days to four weeks.

Chalazia that fail to respond to such conservative management may be treated with intralesional steroids.[49-53] Ten milligrams per milliliter of triamcinolone acetonide (Kenalog-10) is diluted with normal saline to a concentration of 5 mg/ml.[54] Some clinicians, however, use triamcinolone in a concentration of 10 mg/ml.[50,51] A volume of 0.05 to 0.3 ml of this steroid suspension is injected into the center of the lesion after topical anesthesia, using a 1-ml tuberculin syringe fitted with a 27- or 30-gauge ⅝-inch needle.[54,55] If the chalazion is pointing anteriorly, the injection can be given through the skin of the lid, but if the chalazion points posteriorly, the injection is given through the conjunctiva. After the application of topical anesthetic onto the eye, an appropriate sized chalazion clamp is put in place. The clamp is useful in stabilizing the lid while the needle is inserted into the chalazion. Resistance may be encountered with insertion, especially if the chalazion is long-standing.

The patient is discharged and followed in a week. If the chalazion persists, a second injection is given and a follow-up of one week is again scheduled. Usually, chalazia responsive to steroid injection will have resolved either before or after the second injection. If the chalazion persists after the second injection, surgical excision is indicated.

Although Jacobs and associates[49] have shown poor results with intralesional steroids compared with conventional incision and curettage, most other investigators[56] have demonstrated good to excellent results. Chalazia typically resolve within 1 or 2 weeks following a single injection of steroid, but larger lesions ($\geq$ 6 mm in diameter) often require a second injection 2 to 4 weeks after the first.[51,52] The overall success rate is 77% to 93% after 1 or 2 injections,[56] thus making intralesional steroids a viable treatment alternative in the management of chalazia. It is effective in all age groups and for lesions of both short and long duration.[51] This treatment modality is particularly suitable for use in children and for lesions located near the lid margin or lacrimal drainage apparatus. It is also useful for patients allergic to local anesthetics.[53]

The rationale for the use of locally injected steroid is that chalazia are composed chiefly of steroid-sensitive histiocytes, multinucleated giant cells, lymphocytes, plasma cells, polymorphonuclear leukocytes, and eosinophils.[54] The injected steroid suppresses additional inflammatory cells and impedes chronic fibrosis. The advantages of intralesional steroid therapy over conventional surgery are as follows:[55] (1) the in-office time required is usually less than 5 minutes; (2) since patching the eye is unnecessary, the practitioner can treat multiple chalazia in eyelids of both sides at one sitting; (3) bleeding and pain are minimal; (4) surgical damage to the lacrimal drainage apparatus is avoided in the treatment of chalazia near the medial canthus; and (5) this treatment has a high patient acceptance and reduces the cost of therapy.

Complications from intralesional steroid therapy are usually minimal (Table 24.2) and include depigmentation of the eyelid at the injection site.[57] This depigmentation can be avoided by using a transconjunctival rather than a transepidermal injection in darkly pigmented patients.[58] When depigmentation occurs, it is usually reversible. Thomas and Laborde[59] reported a single case of retinal and choroidal vascular occlusion in an 8-year-old boy that immediately followed steroid injection into a chalazion.

If, after 1 or 2 months of conservative therapy or 2 to 4 weeks of intralesional steroid therapy, the chalazion has not resolved, surgical resection can be recommended.[60] For cases that are atypical or that recur following surgical removal, the chalazion should be submitted for pathologic examination to exclude the possibility of sebaceous gland carcinoma or Merkel cell tumor.[61–63]

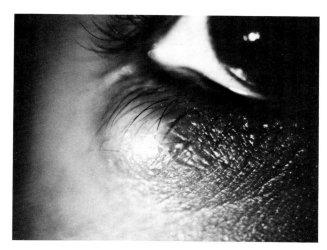

FIGURE 24.6 **A large chalazion located at the lateral aspect of the lower eyelid.**

TABLE 24.1
Instructions for Lid Hygiene

A. Warm Saline Soaks
   1. Prepare a saline solution using ½ teaspoon of table salt in 1 quart of warm water.
   2. Place 1 saline-soaked, sterile cotton ball on each eye with the lids closed until the cotton ball cools.
   3. Replace the cotton balls with fresh ones as they cool, and continue the soak for 10 minutes.
B. Cleaning the Lashes
   1. Gently brush the lashes using a cotton-tipped applicator moistened with the warm salt water.
   2. Clean the lashes twice daily.

Adapted from Perry HD, Serniuk RA. Conservative treatment of chalazia. Ophthalmology 1980;87:218–221.

TABLE 24.2
Complications of Intralesional Steroids for Treatment of Chalazia

- Pain on injection
- Subcutaneous white (steroid) deposits
- Depigmentation of eyelid
- Retinal and choroidal vascular occlusion
- Temporary skin atrophy

TABLE 24.3
Classification of Chronic Blepharitis

Staphylococcal
Seborrheic
  Alone
  Mixed seborrheic/staphylococcal
  Seborrheic with meibomian seborrhea
  Seborrheic with secondary meibomianitis
Primary meibomianitis

Adapted from McCulley JP, Dougherty JM, Deneau DG. Classification of chronic blepharitis. Ophthalmology 1982;89:1173–1180.

Blepharitis

The term *blepharitis* refers to a variety of inflammatory conditions of the eyelid margin. Recent evidence suggests that alterations in meibomian gland lipids may play a prominent role in the etiology of this disease, especially in some patients with chronic blepharitis.[64] Although some authors have maintained that *Demodex folliculorum,* the hair follicle mite, and *Demodex brevis,* found in sebaceous glands including the meibomian glands, are important factors in the development of chronic blepharitis,[65] most investigators[38,66–70] still believe there is no evidence, either histopathologic or pathogenetic, that confirms a role for these organisms in blepharitis. McCulley and associates[66] have developed a classification of chronic blepharitis (Table 24.3) that takes into consideration recent data on the significance of infectious, seborrheic, as well as meibomian gland factors in the production of this disease.[71,72]

STAPHYLOCOCCAL BLEPHARITIS

Etiology.   Groden and associates[73] performed microbiologic evaluations of 332 patients with chronic blepharitis and found the most common organisms to be *Staphylococcus epidermidis* (96%), *Propionibacterium acnes* (93%), *Corynebacterium* sp. (77%), *Acinetobacter* sp. (11%), and *Staphylococcus aureus* (10.5%). *S. epidermidis, P. acnes,* and *Corynebacterium* sp. were present significantly more often than in patients without blepharitis. However, *S. aureus* was not more common in blepharitis patients. Although *S. aureus* is a common etiologic factor in infectious blepharitis, the pathogenic properties and causative role of coagulase-negative staphylococci have only recently been acknowledged.[74] Moreover, patients with acne rosacea appear to have an increased predisposition to staphylococcal infection.[75] In these and other patients with infectious blepharitis, the presence and hydrolysis of cholesterol esters of meibomian secretions may contribute to proliferation of staphylococcal organisms, especially *S. aureus.*[76] In addition, although most retail eye mascaras are initially free of microbial contamination, the cosmetics are subject to contamination during use and may therefore become a significant source of bacterial infection.[77] Hypersensitivity to *S. aureus* may also play a role in the pathogenesis of this condition.[78]

Diagnosis.   Hard, brittle, fibrinous scales surrounding the lashes and on the lid margin characterize the more common, squamous type of staphylococcal blepharitis.[79] These scales are less greasy than those observed in seborrheic blepharitis.[66] A characteristic hyperemia of the lid margin is also present. Symptoms include foreign body sensation, mattering of the lids on awakening, itching, tearing, and burning. Matted, hard crusts surrounding the individual lashes characterize the less common ulcerative type.[79] Removing these crusts often exposes small ulcers, and bleeding may occur. In chronic staphylococcal blepharitis, associated findings may include loss of lashes (madarosis) (Fig. 24.7), trichiasis, or thickened lid margins (tylosis ciliaris).[79]

A chronic, papillary conjunctivitis is almost invariably associated, and the minimal mucopurulent discharge contains a preponderance of polymorphonuclear leukocytes.[79] An epithelial keratitis, due to the liberation of exotoxins from the lid margin, often appears as a superficial punctate keratitis affecting predominantly the inferior quadrant of the cornea.

Management.   Since staphylococcal blepharitis can become chronic and more difficult to treat, it must be treated aggressively to be successful. The patient needs to understand that treatment usually *controls* the condition rather than *cures* it. The first phase of therapy, lasting 2 to 8 weeks, consists of vigorous treatment to bring the condition under control, while the chronic phase of therapy aims at keeping the signs and symptoms in check. However, in contrast to treatment of other forms of blepharitis, staphylococcal blepharitis can sometimes be completely irradicated without the need for long-term maintenance therapy.[80]

The mainstay of therapy should be careful lid hygiene. The patient accomplishes this at home with hot compresses (15 or 20 minutes 2 to 4 times daily), each application followed by lid scrubs using a mild detergent cleanser compatible with ocular tissues. Although use of baby shampoo has been popular, recent experience shows that other commercially available cleansers (see Table 3.3) are as effective with potentially less ocular stinging and toxicity.[81,82] Several authors have shown that Eye-Scrub is effective and well tolerated.[81,82]

Following each session of hot compresses and hygienic scrubs, antibiotics should be applied in the form of a lid scrub directly to the lid margin. Although use of sulfonamides has been popular for many years, McCulley and associates[66] have shown that only approximately 30% of *S. aureus* strains cultured from the lids are sensitive to sulfonamides. These investigators have further shown that 56% of

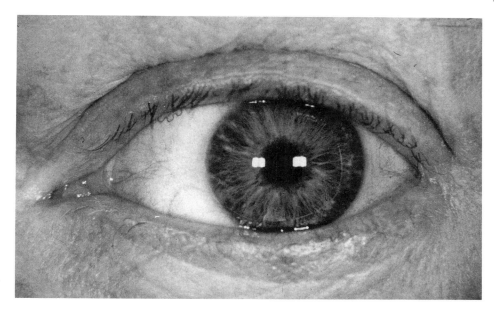

FIGURE 24.7   **Madarosis and hyperemia of eyelid margins characteristic of staphylococcal blepharitis.**

S. epidermidis strains are sensitive to tetracycline, 90% to erythromycin, but only 33% to sulfonamides. Since bacitracin and erythromycin ointment are each effective against both *S. aureus* and *S. epidermidis,* these antibiotics have become the treatment of choice.[83] Aminoglycosides such as gentamicin and tobramycin are also effective and can be administered in solution or ointment form as a lid scrub.[70,80] Note, however, that many staphylococcal isolates are now resistant to gentamicin[75] and that long-term treatment with an aminoglycoside can lead to chemical blepharitis, necessitating withdrawal of the drug.[84] Several investigators[85,86] have reported that the combination of trimethoprim-polymyxin B is effective in the treatment of staphylococcal blepharitis. Whichever antibacterial agent is chosen as initial therapy, it is important to alternate treatment using a different antibiotic on consecutive weeks or months to avoid or minimize the development of resistant organisms.[75]

Yellow mercuric oxide ointment (Stye) is effective for both signs and symptoms of staphylococcal blepharitis. When used twice daily as a lid scrub, 1% yellow mercuric oxide improves the clinical signs and bacterial counts and is well tolerated.[74,87] This medication improves access to care because it is available without prescription.

Since locally applied steroids may be useful for controlling the hypersensitivity component that is often present and for reducing the congestion and irritation that often provoke the patient to rub the eyelids and aggravate the blepharitis, a combination steroid-antibacterial agent may provide the most effective treatment in some cases.[35] Donshik and associates[88] have shown that the combination of gentamicin-betamethasone is more effective than either of its components alone in relieving the signs and symptoms

of staphylococcal blepharitis. Topical steroids are generally not required, however, and, indeed, can lead to serious ocular complications if used indiscriminately by the patient.

In cases that are resistant to the initial antibiotic therapy, discontinuation of contaminated cosmetics sometimes results in marked improvement.[77] Silver nitrate 1% may be effective when applied to the lid margins.[89] The topical application of rifampin, a drug known to kill intraleukocytic staphylococci, may also be considered, although the Food and Drug Administration (FDA) has not approved this route of administration.[79,90] Systemic antibiotic therapy may also prove helpful. Oral erythromycin or tetracycline, 1 g initially then 250 mg daily, can be administered.[91] Tetracycline, however, should not be used in the treatment of children or pregnant women, and the estolate form of erythromycin should be avoided.[79] If the blepharitis is unilateral, the lacrimal drainage system should be carefully examined as the etiologic factor.

If culture and sensitivity studies show that methicillin-resistant *S. epidermidis* is causing the blepharitis, a trial of topical vancomycin should be considered.[92,93] A 50 mg/ml solution can be prepared by mixing a single ampule (500 mg) of vancomycin hydrochloride with 10 ml of phosphate-buffered artificial tears. The patient should shake the bottle vigorously before instilling the medication four times daily. This solution will retain its antibacterial activity for at least 2 weeks without refrigeration.[93]

Dermatologic consultations should be sought for patients who have recalcitrant disease. The signs and symptoms of blepharitis will frequently improve once treatment is begun for seborrheic dermatitis, acne rosacea, or atopy.[75] Patients

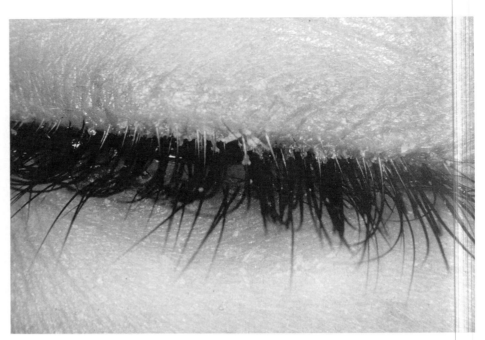

FIGURE 24.8 **Seborrheic blepharitis, characterized by greasy crusts and minimal hyperemia of the eyelid margin.**

with rosacea are treated with oral tetracyline 250 mg four times daily, decreasing to 250 mg per day once the inflammation has been brought under control. Doxycycline, 100 mg twice daily, can be substituted for tetracycline in patients unable to tolerate tetracycline. Pregnant women and children under 12 years of age should be given erythromycin rather than tetracycline.[83]

Patients need to understand the importance of complying with the recommended therapy. Because of complications associated with chronic staphylococcal blepharitis, the importance of early and effective treatment cannot be overemphasized. The practitioner should observe the patient perform lid scrubs to ensure that the patient can properly administer the therapy at home.

Since the incidence of associated keratoconjunctivitis sicca is significantly higher in patients with chronic blepharitis than in healthy patients,[66,80] symptoms of dry eye should be adequately treated with artificial tears and lubricants. Otherwise, symptoms may persist despite adequate treatment of the obvious infection.

Since any associated toxic epithelial keratitis should respond to treatment of the lid infection, the use of topical steroids for the keratitis is unnecessary.[79] However, if symptoms are severe, steroid drops such as prednisolone 0.12% may be used 2 or 3 times daily for a few days. If a hypersensitivity corneal infiltrate occurs, prednisolone drops should be added to the treatment regimen in doses ranging from 0.12% 2 or 3 times daily to 1.0% four or more times daily.[79]

SEBORRHEIC BLEPHARITIS

Etiology. Seborrheic blepharitis is nearly always associated with a more generalized seborrheic dermatitis and probably represents a localized form of a more generalized disorder.[66]

Diagnosis. As in staphylococcal blepharitis, lid and lash crusting characterize seborrheic blepharitis, but in the latter the crusts are more greasy and the lid margins are less inflamed (Fig. 24.8).[66]

Management. The treatment of seborrheic blepharitis involves careful lid hygiene. This can be performed by softening the crusts with warm compresses and then gently cleaning the lid margin with a cotton-tipped applicator moistened with an eyelid cleanser.[34,81,82] The patient should perform this cleaning at home 2 to 4 times daily. In addition, the patient should vigorously clean the hair and scalp, using a shampoo containing selenium sulfide (Selsun). In cases resistant to such therapy, antibiotic lid scrubs may be employed using bacitracin or erythromycin ointment twice daily for three weeks to discourage staphylococcal infection.[80] Any associated keratoconjunctivitis sicca should be treated using an appropriate regimen of artificial tears and lubricants.

MIXED SEBORRHEIC-STAPHYLOCOCCAL BLEPHARITIS

Most cases of blepharitis involve a combination of staphylococcal and seborrheic changes.[34] Thus, the patient should be instructed carefully in adequate lid hygiene techniques, and the application of antibiotics as previously described should be instituted. In addition, the patient should shampoo the scalp and eyebrows with an antiseborrheic product such as selenium sulfide (Selsun). If not treated properly, this form of blepharitis can lead to chronic conjunctivitis, permanent thickening of the lid margin, and madarosis.[80]

SEBORRHEIC BLEPHARITIS WITH MEIBOMIAN SEBORRHEA

Etiology.   Meibomian seborrhea is characterized by an increase of normal meibomian secretions without associated solidification of the secretions or surrounding inflammation.[66,70,80]

Diagnosis.   Patients are often relatively asymptomatic but more often they complain of burning, itching, or tearing. The marked symptoms are typically out of proportion to the observed signs, since frequently no signs of inflammation occur.[66,94] The diagnostic signs, when present, are moderate foam in the tear meniscus and occasionally minimal bulbar conjunctival injection.[66] The slit lamp may show a thickened oily layer of the precorneal tear film as an increased interface phenomenon manifested by multiple colors of the spectrum.[94] Contact lens wearers may develop buildup of this material on the lenses, possibly leading to reduced visual acuity, allergic manifestations, or vague, nonspecific symptomatology associated with lens wear.

Management.   The management of meibomian seborrhea in symptomatic patients is extremely difficult because of the relative inability to reduce normal meibomian secretions. Treating the seborrheic component of the blepharitis as previously described sometimes reduces, but does not eliminate, symptoms. The practitioner can perform digital meibomian gland massage and expression in the office and can instruct the patient in these techniques, to be performed twice daily at home. These procedures "milk" the meibomian glands of their excessive secretions and thus should be performed immediately after the use of hot compresses but before lid scrubs.[80]

SEBORRHEIC BLEPHARITIS WITH SECONDARY MEIBOMIANITIS

Etiology.   A meibomianitis (meibomitis) secondary to the seborrheic blepharitis may manifest as stagnation or solidification of meibomian secretions. This occurs in a spotty pattern involving scattered clusters of meibomian glands.[66]

Diagnosis.   The typical findings of seborrheic blepharitis are observed along with scattered clusters of inflamed meibomian glands, which have orifices plugged with white, stagnant secretions. Digital massage over these isolated areas results in expression of a thick, creamy-white material from the glands.

Management.   Treatment involves attention to lid hygiene and the use of antibiotics as previously described. In addition, the meibomianitis is treated with hot compresses 2 to 4 times daily followed by digital expression of the meibomian glands.

These procedures usually bring the condition under control within 2 to 8 weeks. If, however, the condition seems resistant, a trial of oral tetracycline, 250 mg four times daily, should be considered.[80] Once sufficient improvement has occurred, the dosage of tetracycline can be tapered and discontinued. Rarely is oral drug therapy required beyond 8 weeks.[80]

PRIMARY MEIBOMIANITIS

Etiology.   Primary meibomianitis (meibomitis) is a form of generalized sebaceous gland dysfunction and is therefore frequently found in association with seborrheic dermatitis or rosacea.[43,66] Both clinical as well as cytologic studies indicate that the condition results from obstruction of the meibomian gland orifices by desquamated epithelial cells that tend to aggregate in keratotic clusters.[95] Increases in cellular debris cause thickening of lipids in the gland thus leading to stagnation of the sebaceous secretion. This stagnation alters the contribution of the meibomian gland to the tear film.[96] *Demodex brevis* organisms have been implicated,[39] but cultures fail to yield bacterial pathogens, which implies that this disease is not a primary bacterial disorder.[66,97]

Normal bacterial flora of the lid margin and meibomian glands release free fatty acids from meibomian gland lipids through production of lipase and other hydrolytic enzymes. The free fatty acids can be extremely toxic to the ocular surface, having the capacity to alter the tear film and produce ocular inflammation.[98]

Diagnosis.   In contrast to secondary meibomianitis, primary meibomianitis tends to involve all meibomian glands to a similar degree.[66] The meibomian gland changes are not always accompanied by significant inflammatory signs, and the condition may be easily overlooked.[99] Although the clinical findings can vary considerably, symptoms usually consist of complaints of irritation, chronic burning, stinging, foreign body sensation, or mild conjunctival hyperemia. Signs include inspissated plugs at the orifices of the meibomian glands, cloudy or thickened yellow-white meibomian secretions on gland expression, foamy discharge into the tear film, hyperemia and mild papillary hypertrophy of the palpebral conjunctiva, and thickened, rounded eyelid margins (Fig. 24.9). Special examination techniques, such as transilluminated biomicroscopy and infrared photography, may document morphologic abnormalities of the meibomian glands themselves.[100] Superficial punctate keratopathy, with rose bengal staining of the cornea and conjunctiva in the interpalpebral space, contributes to an unstable tear film.[66,101] Stagnation of the meibomian glands, which produce the

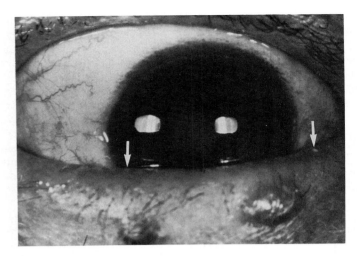

A

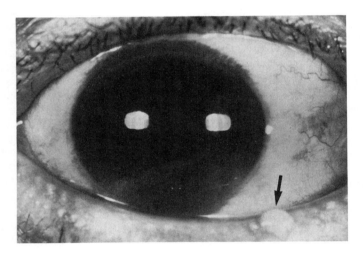

B

FIGURE 24.9   *(A)* **Primary meibomianitis, characterized by inspissated plugs at orifices of the meibomian glands (arrows), and thickened, rounded lid margin.** *(B)* **Digital massage expresses thick, white, creamy material from the meibomian glands (arrow).**

lipid layer of the tear film, may also account for the tear film instability, which is clinically evident by a markedly reduced tear breakup time (TBUT).[102]

Management.   The most effective treatment for primary meibomianitis involves relieving the obstruction of the meibomian ducts and orifices by applying digital massage and gland expression 2 to 4 times daily.[99] The practitioner can perform this treatment in the office and instruct the patient in

the proper technique for meibomian expression at home. The application of hot compresses before gland expression is usually more effective in promoting return of normal meibomian gland flow.

In addition to the use of hot compresses and meibomian gland expression several times daily, antibiotic ointment can be applied to the lid margin twice daily. Although no pathogen is implicated in primary meibomianitis, the use of lid scrubs to deliver bacitracin or erythromycin ointment to the lid margin is recommended and often promotes significant improvement in the condition within 2 to 4 weeks.[80,94] The use of warm compresses and simple hygienic lid scrubs, without antibacterial agents, can increase tear film stability and improve subjective comfort in patients with contact lens intolerance associated with meibomian gland dysfunction.[103]

Oral tetracycline has become the primary therapy for moderate to severe cases of meibomianitis.[98] The drug is given initially in dosages of 1 to 2 g daily. Once the condition is controlled, low maintenance doses of 250 mg daily may be required to ensure long-term control.[98] Tetracycline appears to reduce the quantity of lipolytic enzymes elaborated by bacteria residing on the lid margin, reducing free fatty acids in the sebum and thus stabilizing the tear film. This can be accomplished even without killing the organisms.[98]

Since there is only a minimal increase of inflammatory cells in affected meibomian glands, the use of local steroids is unlikely to have any benefit.[67]

During the course of therapy attention should be given to the keratoconjunctivitis sicca that occurs in nearly every case of primary meibomianitis.[102] The use of artificial tears or lubricating ointments is indicated to ensure improvement in symptoms.

ANGULAR BLEPHARITIS

Etiology. Angular blepharitis is caused by infection with *Moraxella* species, but this condition can also represent a form of eczematoid blepharitis caused by staphylococci.[38] Glasser[104] has described a case apparently caused by gramnegative bacillus DF-2.

Diagnosis. The characteristic signs of angular blepharitis include chronic hyperemia, desquamation, and ulceration of the lateral, and sometimes medial, canthal regions (Fig. 24.10).[38] Simultaneous involvement of the conjunctiva often occurs. Symptoms include irritation and tenderness of the involved area.

Management. Angular blepharitis secondary to *Moraxella* responds well to zinc sulfate 0.25% solution applied with a cotton-tipped applicator several times daily. If this treatment fails, staphylococcal organisms are probably causing the condition. The practitioner should change the therapy to erythromycin or bacitracin ointment.

Preseptal (Periorbital) Cellulitis

ETIOLOGY

Preseptal, or periorbital, cellulitis is an infectious process involving the lid structures anterior to the orbital septum. The condition generally occurs in one of three clinical settings:[105,108] (1) secondary to localized infection or inflammation of the eyelids or adjacent structures, including exter-

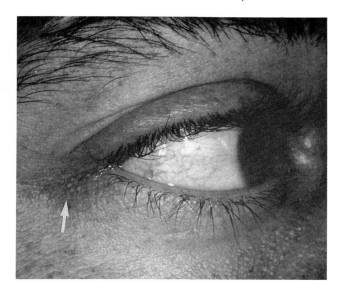

FIGURE 24.10 **Inflammation of temporal bulbar conjunctiva and excoriation of outer canthus (arrow), characteristic of angular blepharoconjunctivitis.**

nal or internal hordeola, acute dacryocystitis, impetigo, herpetic blepharitis, or severe conjunctivitis; (2) secondary to eyelid or facial trauma; and (3) following an upper respiratory tract infection.

Profound inflammation and edema of the preseptal eyelid may accompany infection of the skin of the face and eyelids. In most of these patients, *Staphylococcus aureus* or betahemolytic streptococci causes the local infection.[106] These organisms can accompany infected lacerations and abrasions, infected insect stings or bites, impetigo, infected foreign bodies, or bacterial superinfection of viral lesions caused by herpes simplex or varicella zoster. Impetigo is caused by *S. aureus* or group A *Streptococcus pyogenes*.[107] Erysipelas, a rare form of preseptal cellulitis, is caused by *S. pyogenes* group A. Infection occurs by invasion of the organism to the subcutaneous tissue through an abrasion or inflammatory ulceration.[107] Anaerobic organisms such as *Peptostreptococcus* and *Bacteroides* sp., which are part of the normal oral flora, can be significant causative organisms in patients with preseptal cellulitis associated with human or animal bites.[106] Foul-smelling discharge, necrotic tissue, gas in the tissue, or severe toxemia suggest such anaerobic infections.[107]

In patients without evidence of local infection or trauma, preseptal cellulitis is usually found in conjunction with a recent history of an upper respiratory tract infection with or without evidence of sinusitis.[106] In children under 6 years of age the condition is caused almost exclusively by *Haemophilus influenzae* type B or *Streptococcus pneumoniae*.[107] Although the most likely primary focus of infection is the

TABLE 24.4
Differential Diagnosis between Preseptal Cellulitis and Orbital Cellulitis

Clinical Finding	Bacterial Preseptal Cellulitis	Orbital Cellulitis
Proptosis	Absent	Marked
Chemosis	Rare	Common
Vision	Normal	Often reduced
Pupils	Normal	May be afferent defect
Motility	Usually normal	Usually restricted
Pain on motion	Absent	Present
Intraocular pressure	Normal	May be elevated
Temperature	Normal or slightly elevated	Elevated (102° to 104°F)

Modified from Jones DB, Steinkuller PG. Microbial preseptal and orbital cellulitis. In: Tasman W, Jaeger EA, eds. Duane's Clinical Ophthalmology. Philadelphia: JB Lippincott, 1993; vol. 4, Chap. 25, 1–24.

nasopharynx and sinuses, cellulitis may develop by spread of organisms from the middle ear to the preseptal space via the vascular or lymphatic systems.[107] Serious *H. influenzae* type B infections occur most commonly in children between ages 6 months and 2 years.[107] Preseptal cellulitis due to *H. influenzae* occurs only in children younger than 6 years of age and apparently has not been documented in older children or adults.[106,107] Preseptal cellulitis occurring in older children and adults without trauma or skin infections usually results from spread of organisms from the sinuses, upper respiratory tract,

or middle ear. In these situations the most common causative organisms include streptococci and *S. aureus*.[107]

DIAGNOSIS

The practitioner needs to differentiate preseptal cellulitis from the more serious orbital cellulitis (Table 24.4). Chemosis, conjunctival injection, pain, redness, and swelling of the eyelid occur in both preseptal and orbital cellulitis. When these occur without evidence of proptosis, the diagnosis is invariably preseptal cellulitis (Fig. 24.11). In addition to

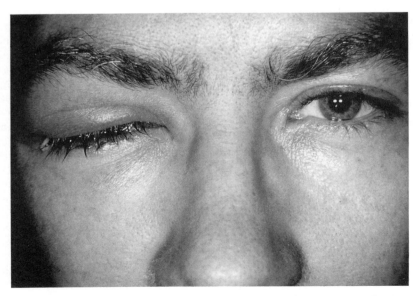

FIGURE 24.11 **Preseptal cellulitis of right upper eyelid. Note generalized swelling and erythema of eyelid. The patient had no pupillary abnormalities and no proptosis, and visual acuity was 20/25.**

evidence of proptosis, other signs of orbital cellulitis include limited extraocular motility, reduced visual acuity, and an afferent pupillary defect.[106,107] Although fever and headache occur in patients with either preseptal or orbital infection, acute fever and prostration are hallmark findings in young children with *H. influenzae* type B preseptal cellulitis.[106]

The eyelid and adnexal tissues should be carefully examined for the presence of puncture wounds, trauma, or infectious lesions of the skin. Facial tenderness, nasal discharge, and malodorous breath are signs of paranasal sinusitis. Focal medial canthal tenderness and tearing may indicate acute dacryocystitis.

In distinguishing preseptal from orbital cellulitis, swelling and inflammation of the eyelid cannot be correlated with the presence or absence of orbital disease. Thus, if the eyelids cannot be separated to examine the globe for the presence of proptosis, limited ocular motility, or vision loss, computed tomography (CT) of the orbit should be considered to rule out the presence of proptosis and orbital congestion. Moreover, CT scanning helps to detect the presence of orbital foreign bodies and sinusitis. A CT scan is recommended if orbital involvement cannot be otherwise excluded on the basis of the routine clinical examination or if there is progression of disease despite antibacterial treatment.[105]

Laboratory evaluation should include a complete white blood cell count with differential as well as a blood culture. Blood cultures are the most common method for establishing the cause. In children younger than 4 years of age, one-third to one-half of blood cultures may be positive, most often yielding *H. influenzae* or *S. pneumoniae*.[106] However, in older children and adults, blood cultures are rarely positive. In these patients or in any patient with skin lesions, specimens should be obtained for culture onto a blood and chocolate agar plate. Although cultures of draining wounds may be useful in cases of preseptal cellulitis related to trauma or local infection, cultures of the conjunctiva, eyelids, and nasal mucosa are generally nonproductive or frequently misleading.[105,106] It is useful to culture puss that has been aspirated or expressed from the lacrimal sac in patients with dacryocystitis, but the associated preseptal cellulitis may not actually represent dissemination of microorganisms into the eyelids. Rather, it may simply represent a nonspecific inflammatory response to the primary focus of infection.[106]

Children with *H. influenzae* type B or *S. pneumoniae* preseptal cellulitis usually have a history of recent or concurrent upper respiratory tract infection.[106,107] The condition is characterized by significant fever (greater than 38°C), leukocytosis, and unilateral hyperemia and edema of the eyelids. *H. influenzae* preseptal cellulitis is characterized by a sharply demarcated, dark purple discoloration of the eyelid skin and adnexal area. Mild conjunctival hyperemia and chemosis may also occur. Unless the patient has received antibiotics, blood cultures are the most effective means of establishing the diagnosis. If meningeal signs are present, a lumbar puncture should be performed; 12% to 25% of patients with *Haemophilus* preseptal or orbital cellulitis have concomitant meningitis.[106]

MANAGEMENT

The initial choice of antimicrobial therapy for treatment of preseptal cellulitis is largely empirical and in many cases remains so because the causative pathogen is not identified. Thus, appropriate therapy must take into consideration the most plausible etiologic associations. Since lesions associated with local trauma or infections are not usually serious, treatment can often consist of oral antibiotics. Mild to moderate infections usually respond to an oral penicillinase-resistant penicillin such as dicloxacillin or to a first-generation cephalosporin such as cephalexin. Therapy should continue for at least 10 days during which topical antibiotic ointment can be applied 2 or 3 times daily.[106,107] In severe cases intravenous nafcillin should be administered; in cases with a history of severe allergic reactions to penicillin, intravenous vancomycin is the preferred antibacterial agent.[106] Additional antimicrobial therapy in patients with bite wounds should include agents with activity against oral anaerobes, such as ampicillin/sulbactam, cefoxitin, clindamycin, or penicillin G.[106] The treatment of choice for preseptal cellulitis associated with erysipelas is intravenous penicillin G for 48 to 72 hours or until there are definite signs of improvement, followed by oral penicillin V for 5 to 7 days.[107]

Infants or young children with no evidence of skin lesions or traumatic wounds should be suspected of having *H. influenzae* or *S. pneumoniae* preseptal cellulitis and should be hospitalized because of the potential rapid progression of the infection and risk of secondary meningitis.[106,107] Cultures should be obtained from both the ipsilateral and contralateral conjunctiva. Blood cultures should also be obtained, and lumbar puncture should be performed in young children with irritability, high fever, and extreme leukocytosis.[107] Because of the increasingly high incidence of β lactamase-producing type B strains of *H. influenzae*, cefuroxime, a second-generation cephalosporin, has become the preferred antibacterial therapy. This antibiotic provides coverage against both *H. influenzae* and aerobic gram-positive cocci.[106,107] Alternatively, a third-generation cephalosporin such as ceftriaxone or cefotaxime provides coverage against these organisms.[105] Systemic chloramphenicol is useful for patients allergic to the cephalosporins.[106] After the child has shown clinical improvement, usually within 24 to 72 hours, oral antibacterial agents can be selected based on the results of culture and sensitivity testing. In the event of a negative culture, empirical therapy can include treatment with oral amoxicillin with potassium clavulanate (Augmentin), trimethoprim with sulfamethoxazole (Bactrim), or cefuroxime (Ceftin). The total duration of antibacterial therapy should be 7 to 10 days. These antibacterial agents can be administered orally as initial therapy for mild infections in older children.[107]

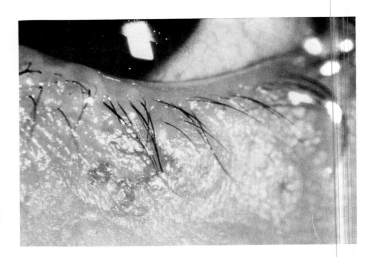

FIGURE 24.12 **Herpes simplex blepharitis with erosions and ulceration along the lid margin. (Courtesy William Wallace, O.D.)**

Herpes Simplex Blepharoconjunctivitis

ETIOLOGY

Blepharoconjunctivitis secondary to herpes simplex virus (HSV) usually occurs as a primary infection in children, but can also occur in adults.[108] HSV type 1 (HSV-1) usually causes this condition, but cases of HSV type 2 (HSV-2) involvement do occur. Primary infection occurs, with or without skin involvement, in the totally nonimmune host,[109] but cases of recurrent HSV blepharitis have been reported as a distinct clinical entity occurring in a previously exposed host.[110] About one-fifth of patients with ocular herpes simplex have lid involvement as the only sign of infection.[108]

DIAGNOSIS

Two forms of clinical involvement have been described. Classically, vesicles along the base of the eyelashes characterize HSV lesions of the eyelids. The vesicles are pinhead in size, have erythematous bases, and may involve the lid margins as well as the periocular skin.[111] These vesicles break and ulcerate, the eyelid margins become edematous, and dermatitis of the eyelids results.[112]

Egerer and Stary[111] have described an erosive-ulcerative form of HSV blepharitis that is much more prevalent than the vesicular herpetic lid lesions. Erosions of the mucocutaneous junction of the lid, skin ulcers located at the lid margins, or a combination of both features characterize this form of HSV blepharitis (Fig. 24.12). This form occurs in the absence of typical vesicular eruptions. The erosions are readily visualized by staining with sodium fluorescein. The involved portion of the lid usually demonstrates mild swelling and tenderness on palpation. Pronounced conjunctival injection may occur adjacent to the lid lesion, and the regional lymph nodes are swollen. Both forms of HSV blepharoconjunctivitis are characterized by the presence of follicular conjunctivitis, occasionally associated with symptoms of a viral illness.

MANAGEMENT

Since topically administered antiviral agents have little or no effect on skin lesions,[113,114] treatment of HSV infection of the eyelid is nonspecific. In the immunologically competent host, the vesicular lesions from primary herpetic infection of the lids remain localized, are generally self-limited, and resolve without scarring, usually within 10 to 14 days.[115,116] In the absence of corneal involvement, antiviral therapy such as trifluridine should be used prophylactically in both eyes several times daily until the skin lesions resolve.[109,114,117] Several authors,[116,118] however, have suggested that prophylactic therapy may be unnecessary, since the risk of corneal involvement appears low. Affected children should be restrained from handling the lid lesions. If corneal involvement occurs, vigorous antiviral therapy should be instituted as described in Chapter 27.

Treatment of the skin lesions themselves requires only warm saline compresses and maintenance of good hygiene.[115] Drying agents can be applied to skin lesions other than those on the lid margins. These agents include Cetaphil lotion, calamine lotion, Unibase, spirits of camphor, or 70% alcohol.[89,113] If the lesions become secondarily infected, topical antibiotic ointment should be applied.[89] Steroids are contraindicated because they may predispose to serious corneal involvement.

Varicella Zoster Blepharoconjunctivitis

ETIOLOGY

The varicella, or chickenpox, virus and the herpes zoster virus are the same organism.[119] The term *varicella zoster*

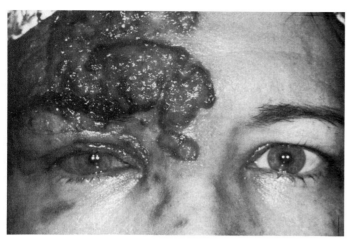

FIGURE 24.13   **Herpes zoster ophthalmicus. Note unilateral nature of vesicular eruptions.**

refers to recurrent infection of the partially immune patient who had previous exposure to chickenpox but who failed to develop an adequate immune system.[120] In recent years the incidence and severity of varicella zoster infection have increased because of the growing number of immunosuppressed patients, including those with Hodgkin's disease, chronic lymphocytic leukemia, and acquired immunodeficiency syndrome (AIDS). Trauma and surgery also increase the risk of zoster infection.[119] Zoster most often occurs in otherwise healthy adults between ages 50 and 70 years.[121] The diagnosis of herpes zoster in patients younger than 45 years warrants testing for HIV since AIDS is now considered a risk factor for zoster infection.[119,120,122,123]

The cranial nerves are frequently affected, but the thoracic dermatomes are most commonly involved, with vesicular skin lesions occurring over the sensory dermatome innervated by the affected dorsal root ganglion.[119] When the first, or ophthalmic, division of the fifth cranial nerve is affected, the resultant disease is referred to as herpes zoster ophthalmicus. One or all nerves of the first division may become involved. The frontal nerve is the most frequently affected, involving the upper lid, forehead, and some superior conjunctiva. The primary sensory nerve to the globe is the nasociliary branch. Its nasal branch innervates the sclera, cornea, iris, ciliary body, and choroid as well as the side and tip of the nose. Characteristic vesicles at the tip of the nose are known as Hutchinson's sign. Involvement of the nasociliary branch thus allows the virus direct access to the intraocular tissues.[119,120]

DIAGNOSIS

The disorder is initially characterized by headache, malaise, fever, and chills, followed in 1 or 2 days by neuralgic pain and 2 or 3 days later by hot, flushed hyperesthesia and edema of the dermatome(s). The skin overlying the affected dermatome then erupts with a single crop of clear vesicles. The vesicles are distributed on only one side of the face and almost never cross more than 1 to 2 mm beyond the midline (Fig. 24.13).[124] These vesicles then become yellow and turbid and by day 7 to 10 form deep eschars, which may leave permanent, pitted scars over the affected dermatome. Although viable virus can be cultured from the vesicles for up to 14 days after appearance of the rash, there is no convincing evidence that zoster can be acquired by contact with patients who have either varicella or zoster.[119]

Some patients experience only relatively minor tingling and numbness, but often excruciating neuralgic pain accompanies the disease.[120] In most cases the severe pain subsides during the first several weeks, but many patients develop postherpetic neuralgia, a chronic condition caused by scarring of the nerves. Such patients experience persistent aching and burning, which can interrupt routine daily activity and in some instances can lead to severe depression or even suicide. Thus, one of the most important aspects of therapy is to prevent scarring and subsequent neuralgia. Although the acute inflammatory stage lasts only 2 to 3 weeks, the skin ulceration may require many weeks to heal and can result in the equivalent of third-degree burns. As a result, serious complications can arise, including total lid retraction, ptosis, madarosis, entropion, or cicatricial ectropion.

MANAGEMENT

In most cases the skin and lid lesions of varicella zoster are self-limited and benign.[113] The primary therapeutic concern should be for any coincident keratitis, and the swollen lids must therefore be carefully separated so that the cornea can be examined. The treatment of corneal lesions is discussed in Chapter 27. Current recommendations for treatment of herpes zoster ophthalmicus are summarized in Table 24.5 and discussed below.[119–121]

TABLE 24.5
Primary Care Management of Herpes Zoster Ophthalmicus

Sign or Symptom	Management
Cutaneous eruption	Oral acyclovir, 800 mg 5 times daily
	Observe for bacterial infection
Acute neuralgia	Oral acyclovir, 800 mg 5 times daily
	Oral analgesics
	Stellate ganglion block
Postherpetic neuralgia	Amitriptyline 10 mg/day, increasing to
	50–75 mg/day as needed, or
	Amitriptyline 25 mg/day plus
	perphenazine 2 mg/day, or
	Amitriptyline 25 mg/day plus
	carbamazepine 200 mg/day
	Capsaicin cream for scalp pain
	Refer for pain management

Modified from Liesegang TJ. Ophthalmic herpes zoster: diagnosis and antiviral therapy. Geriatrics 1991;46:64–71.

- For patients who have little or no pain or mild or no ocular involvement, no therapy is required.
- Topical steroids, such as prednisolone acetate 1.0%, can be administered up to every 3 hours for corneal edema and anterior uveitis.
- During the first 10 days nonopioid or opioid analgesics may be administered for acute neuralgic pain. The acute pain may also be modified by the administration of oral acyclovir if started within 72 hours of onset of the rash.[119] If there is no relief from pain, a chest x-ray film, complete blood count (CBC), and evaluation of immune status should be obtained, followed by prednisone, 20 mg orally four times daily for 7 days, decreasing to 15 mg orally twice daily for 7 days, then decreasing to 15 mg orally every day for 7 days, with continuation of topical steroids and cycloplegics. The patient should be monitored frequently, in consultation with an internist, for dissemination of virus. A stellate ganglion block performed by an anesthesiologist may prove effective for the acute pain if given within 14 days of the rash.[125]
- Postherpetic neuralgic pain can be treated with opioid and nonopioid analgesics, tricyclic antidepressants and antianxiety agents, or anticonvulsants. Finding an effective agent often involves trying several different drugs within a group. Some patients experience pain relief from a phenothiazine, sometimes in combination with antidepressants. A useful combination is amitriptyline 25 to 50 mg orally at bedtime with fluphenazine 1 mg orally twice daily.[126] Although antiviral therapy may help to relieve acute neuralgic pain, neither oral nor intravenous acyclovir is consistently useful in preventing postherpetic pain. Early (within 72 hours of skin rash) and high-dose therapy (800

mg five times daily) seem important in reducing postherpetic neuralgia.[119,127,128]

Capsaicin cream (Zostrix) is reasonably effective when applied 3 to 4 times daily to the area of painful skin.[129–132] Capsaicin's analgesic effect is related to depletion of substance P from local sensory terminals in the skin.[129] Pain relief is usually noted within 2 to 4 weeks of treatment.[130] Approximately 30% of treated patients experience burning, stinging, or redness of the skin on initial application, but with repeated use, these reactions usually diminish or subside.[130]

Considerable attention has been given to the use of acyclovir to prevent complications arising from severe inflammatory changes often associated with varicella zoster infection. This drug has been employed intravenously and orally. The oral route of administration effectively hastens resolution of signs and symptoms, reduces viral shedding and formation of new skin lesions, and decreases both the incidence and severity of ocular complications.[133,134] The beneficial effect of oral acyclovir is most pronounced when the drug is given within 72 hours of initial onset of skin lesions. However, treatment as late as 7 days after onset of the cutaneous lesions may confer a beneficial effect.[135] In the immunocompetent patient, dosage should be 800 mg five times daily for 10 days.[128] Most patients tolerate this dosage regimen well, the most common side effect being gastrointestinal disturbances (nausea and vomiting). Seven days of treatment often suffice and may reduce both the cost and potential side effects associated with acyclovir therapy.[127] Lower doses are indicated for treatment of elderly patients with impaired creatinine clearance.[121] Perhaps the most significant factor in favor of acyclovir use is that it minimizes most of the common complications of the disease, including dendriform keratopathy, stromal keratitis, and anterior uveitis.[133]

In the immunosuppressed patient, the risk of virus dissemination is higher, postherpetic pain can be greater, and systemic complications can be more severe. Thus, hospitalization for intravenous acyclovir ensures higher drug levels compared to oral therapy. Although outpatient therapy with oral acyclovir may be considered for mild localized zoster in some immunosuppressed patients,[121] most authors[121,123,136] favor treatment using intravenous acyclovir in a dosage of 30 mg/kg body weight/day for 7 days. Long-term prophylactic therapy using oral acyclovir may also be appropriate in HIV-infected patients with herpes zoster to reduce the risk of acute retinal necrosis syndrome.[123] These patients should have periodic fundus examinations during the first several months after the initial episode of zoster infection.

Drying lotions should not be used, since they may increase scarring.[121] For the child or adult in whom the skin lesions itch or are irritating, an oral antihistamine such as chlorpheniramine or diphenhydramine may help to prevent scratching, which can predispose to a secondary infection and scarring.[113] In some cases a warm solution of aluminum acetate (Burrow's solution) is effective when applied to the skin and lid lesions for 15 minutes four times a day as supportive therapy.[119] In severe lid involvement, lubricating ointments should be instilled into the eye to prevent complications arising from exposure or trichiasis. An oculoplastic surgeon should manage scarring and contraction of lid tissue that creates cicatricial ectropion, lid retraction, lid margin deformity, or severe corneal complications.

In the management of lid involvement note that the acute lid edema occurring soon after onset of the disorder does not result from bacterial cellulitis. This condition will resolve within a few days without antibiotic therapy.[137]

Steroids have a well-established role in the therapy of herpes zoster ophthalmicus. They act to suppress destructive inflammation while permitting the infection to run its natural course. Recently, however, the usefulness of topical steroid therapy has been questioned. Although topical steroids are indicated for the severe ocular complications of zoster,[138] steroid therapy can prolong the ocular inflammatory complications.[135] Herbort and associates[139] have shown that when oral acyclovir is used in high doses, topical steroids are rarely required. Thus, high-dose acyclovir with avoidance of steroids may virtually eliminate the severe complications of herpes zoster ophthalmicus.

The use of systemic steroids is controversial.[120] Steroid-induced dissemination of virus is possible in patients who are immunologically compromised, such as in lymphoma, AIDS, or leukemia. Elderly patients who have debilitating systemic disease may also respond less satisfactorily. For immunocompetent patients older than 60 years, Liesegang[140] has recommended giving oral prednisone in a dosage of 60 mg daily for five days, tapered over a two-week period. Immunosuppressed individuals, patients with an underlying medical disorder, and younger patients should probably not receive oral steroids.

Phthiriasis Palpebrarum

Phthiriasis palpebrarum is an uncommon eyelid infestation by *Phthirus pubis* (crab louse) and, less commonly, by *Pediculus humanus* species.[141,142] The term pediculosis refers to infestation by *Pediculus corporis* (body louse) or *Pediculus capitis* (head louse) and should not generally be used when referring to eyelid manifestations.

ETIOLOGY

Phthiriasis or pediculosis usually occurs when sanitary conditions are inadequate. Phthiriasis palpebrarum results from lid infestation by the public louse, whose habitat is normally the pubic and inguinal areas.[143] The eyelashes and eyebrows are special sites of predilection for phthiriasis in children.[141] Phthiriasis is usually transmitted by sexual contact, but in children infestation occurs from contact with an infested parent, usually the mother.[141] The lice may also be transferred from bedding and towels contaminated with lice eggs.[143]

The fecal material and saliva excreted by the parasites can be both toxic and antigenic, resulting in an inflammatory response manifested by conjunctivitis, marginal keratitis, and preauricular lymphadenopathy.[144,145]

Pediculosis palpebrarum, on the other hand, occurs only with a florid infestation of the scalp with the head louse.[143] This condition is also transmitted by close contact with an infested individual or by contaminated bedding or clothing.[141]

DIAGNOSIS

Diagnosis is easily accomplished by careful slit-lamp examination, which readily detects the adult lice and eggs (nits). The adult lice vary from 1 to 1.5 mm.[143] The translucent lice are more easily visualized by epilating one or more infested lashes for examination under low power of a light microscope.[38]

Itching and irritation characterize phthiriasis palpebrarum. Blepharoconjunctivitis, blood-stained thickened discharge on the lid margins, and nits and adult parasites on the eyelashes may occur as well (Fig. 24.14). The presence of parasites and their nits, along with tiny, granular, reddish black fecal material matted to the lids and lashes, leads to a dark crusty discoloration of the lid margins.[142] A preauricular lymphadenopathy may also be present.[143]

MANAGEMENT

Treatment is essentially the same for all varieties of lid infestation, whether caused by *Pediculus* or *Phthirus*.[141] The scalp, body, or pubic areas should be treated as well as the lid condition. In addition, for treatment to be effective, thorough investigation and treatment of contacts should be performed, including family members, clothing, and bedding.

In cooperative patients the practitioner can remove the adult parasites with forceps or cotton-tipped applicators using the slit lamp, but this procedure is somewhat uncomfortable, especially in children. Cilia bearing eggs should be epilated. Cryotherapy has been recommended as providing rapid cure.[141] Pharmacologically, a variety of effective treatment modalities are available.[89,141-143] Treatment involving yellow mercuric oxide 1% ophthalmic ointment applied four times daily for 14 days is effective.[146] In addition, bland petrolatum ointment can be thickly applied twice daily for 8 days to smother the parasites. Anticholinesterase agents, such as 0.25% physostigmine ointment, may be applied to the lid margins. These agents, however, have little effect on the nits, and therapy should therefore be continued twice daily for about 10 to 14 days to ensure that all eggs have hatched and that the emerging parasites have been adequately treated. Side effects, such as miosis and browache,

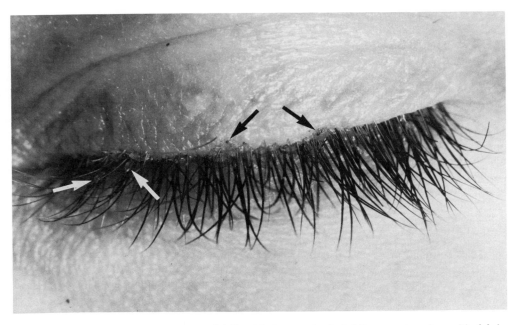

FIGURE 24.14   **Phthiriasis palpebrarum. Adult lice (black arrows), nits (white arrows), and parasitic debris are matted to the base of the lashes. (Courtesy Rodney Nowakowski, O.D.)**

limit the use of such anticholinesterase treatment. The use of gamma benzene hexachloride (Kwell) for the lid condition should be avoided because of potential ocular irritation and chemical conjunctivitis.[142,143] Similarly, pyrethrin gel (A-200 Pyrinate) and other pediculocides should not be used near the eye.[147]

Scalp, body, and pubic hair must be treated with an appropriate pediculocidal agent (Table 24.6) in combination with careful nit removal. Although gamma benzene hexachloride (Kwell) is generally considered the drug of choice for the treatment of head and pubic lice, a pyrethrin-based pediculocide, RID, is equally effective and safe and is available over the counter, without prescription.[148] A single application to the affected areas is usually adequate to eradicate the lice.[143] The application should be repeated in one week if viable nits persist or if new nits appear. Translucent, empty nits are signs of inactive infestation and require no further treatment.[142] Because gamma benzene hexachloride may lead to central nervous system (CNS) toxicity, it must be used cautiously in infants, children, and pregnant women, and excessive application should be avoided.[143] Pubic lice are not resistant to gamma benzene hexachloride.[142] If treat-

TABLE 24.6
Pediculocidal Agents[a]

Active Ingredient	Trade Name	Formulation
Lindane (gamma benzene hexachloride)	Kwell[b]	Cream, lotion, shampoo
Permethrin	Nix	Liquid (creme rinse)
Pyrethrins	Triple X Kit	Liquid
	Barc	Liquid
	A-200	Shampoo
	R&C	Shampoo
	RID	Shampoo

[a]Not for use on or near the eye.
[b]Prescription product. Others are available over-the-counter.

ment appears ineffective, either the patient is noncompliant or reinfestation has occurred.

In addition to treating the lids and body hair, family members or sexual contacts should be examined and treated if infested. This step is important because of the high risk of concurrent sexually transmitted disease in patients with *Phthirus pubis* infestation.[149] Clothing, linens, and grooming instruments should be laundered or sterilized by exposing to dry heat at 140°F (50°C) for 20 to 30 minutes.[142,143] This heat sterilization can usually be accomplished at the highest temperature settings of most household dryers. Contaminated cosmetics should be discarded.

Abnormalities of Motility

Ptosis

ETIOLOGY

Ptosis is present when the margin of the upper eyelid covers more than 2.0 mm of the superior cornea.[150] Although establishing the initial diagnosis of ptosis is not difficult, determining the specific etiology can be challenging. Before the ptosis can be properly managed, the practitioner must identify the underlying etiology.

Both congenital as well as acquired forms of ptosis exist (Table 24.7).[151] In addition, various ocular diseases or abnormalities may simulate ptosis (pseudoptosis). Congenital ptosis can vary from complete closure to only slight asymmetry between sides. It is usually autosomal dominant and is caused by incomplete differentiation of the levator muscle.[35] Acquired ptosis, on the other hand, usually results from abnormality of the levator muscle or its innervation. This may be associated with neurogenic lesions, myogenic problems such as myasthenia gravis, trauma, or mechanical effects. Thiamine deficiency in childhood can also cause ptosis.[152,153] Involutional (age-related) ptosis is common and may be caused by disinsertion of the levator aponeurosis.[154–156]

DIAGNOSIS

The following examination should be performed for the evaluation of ptosis.[151,157]

- The lid level should be measured by instructing the patient to fixate a distant object while the practitioner measures the vertical height of the affected palpebral aperture. The vertical height of the normal palpebral aperture is approximately 10 mm, and in unilateral cases, the fellow eye serves as a control.
- Action of the levator muscle can be assessed by instructing the patient to look up and down while the practitioner's hand stabilizes the frontalis muscle. The prognosis for a successful surgical result is better if the

TABLE 24.7
Classification of Ptosis

Congenital ptosis
  With normal superior rectus function
  With superior rectus weakness
  Blepharophimosis
  Synkinetic ptosis
    Marcus Gunn
    Misdirected third nerve
Acquired ptosis
  Neurogenic
  Myogenic
  Traumatic
  Mechanical
Pseudoptosis
  Microphthalmia, phthisis bulbi, anophthalmia, or enophthalmos
  Hypotropia
  Dermatochalasis
  Lid cellulitis

Adapted from Beard C, Sullivan JH. Ptosis—current concepts. Int Ophthalmol Clin 1978;18:53–73.

levator function is good. Levator function can also be assessed by observing the presence of a lid fold. The presence of a fold at the upper margin of the tarsal plate indicates levator function.
- Congenital ptosis can often be distinguished from acquired ptosis by observing the position of the lids in full downgaze. The inelasticity of the lid in congenital ptosis results in lid lag, whereas in acquired myogenic ptosis, the affected lid usually assumes a lower position on downgaze.
- Orbicularis muscle function should be assessed by observing closure of the lids.
- When the history reveals generalized muscular weakness, the patient should be evaluated for myasthenia gravis, preferably in consultation with a neurologist (see Chap. 23).
- If Horner's syndrome is suspected, one drop of 2.5% phenylephrine can be instilled into each eye and the lid positions compared after 5 minutes. The lid on the affected side elevates when compared with the noninvolved side (Fig. 24.15).[158] This lid retraction results from denervation hypersensitivity of Müller's muscle to the adrenergic agonist. This test must be performed before pupillary dilation with adrenergic mydriatics, because instilling the drops for dilation may cause lid retraction on the noninvolved side.

MANAGEMENT

Surgery represents the most effective treatment modality for most forms of ptosis.[150] In some instances, however, topically applied or systemically administered medications may be of value.

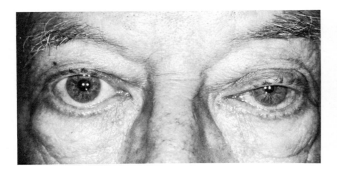
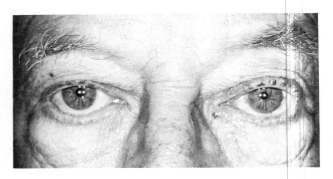

A   **B**

FIGURE 24.15   *(A)* **Ptosis of left upper lid associated with Horner's syndrome.** *(B)* **Marked left upper lid retraction 5 minutes after instillation of 2.5% phenylephrine.**

Surgery for congenital ptosis is usually indicated for cosmetic reasons and can thus be deferred until the child is of school age, at which time the degree of ultimate ptosis is most easily assessed.[35] However, if the ptosis interferes with vision or if compensatory head tilt or furrowed brow become established, surgical correction should be performed earlier.

The treatment of acquired ptosis depends on its cause. Any residual ptosis can be managed by surgical correction.[159] However, if the ptosis is minimal or if surgery is contraindicated or refused, a ptosis crutch attached to the spectacle frame can be employed.[160] Many conventional ptosis crutches do not permit full lid closure, thus necessitating that the patient slide the spectacles down the nose once every 5 minutes to allow lid closure and normal ocular wetting. Failure to do this often results in severe complications from corneal exposure. As an alternative, an ocular prosthesis has been described that permits full lid closure and thus prevents corneal exposure.[161] This prosthetic device is particularly useful for patients with chronic progressive external ophthalmoplegia (CPEO), which is often accompanied by loss of normal corneal protective mechanisms and, consequently, a high risk of postoperative corneal exposure.[162]

The treatment of ptosis associated with myasthenia gravis involves the use of orally administered anticholinesterase agents. Therapy is usually begun with neostigmine bromide (Prostigmin) 15 mg three to five times daily.[35] If neostigmine is unsatisfactory in controlling the systemic manifestations as well as the lid signs, therapy can be changed to pyridostigmine bromide (Mestinon).[163] In addition, thymectomy may be beneficial.[35] Although anticholinesterase therapy frequently controls the systemic manifestations of myasthenia gravis, it is less effective for the lid signs and extraocular muscle palsies.[164] Therefore, for cases that do not adequately respond to such therapy, systemically administered steroids may be required. Following initiation of steroid therapy, the ocular signs may begin to improve within a few days, but substantial improvement may not occur for as long as three

months.[163] The goal of long-term steroid therapy is a maintenance dosage of prednisone 15 or 20 mg every other day.[149] If the ptosis remains refractory to steroid and anticholinesterase therapy, corrective lid surgery may be considered if the ptosis has remained stable for at least 3 to 4 years.[165]

For minimal ptosis, a trial of topical ocular phenylephrine 2.5% or 10% every 4 hours can be used to elevate the lid intermittently for social occasions.[166] The phenylephrine acts on Mueller's muscle to elevate the lid, and the effect may be dramatic within 5 to 10 minutes, especially in patients with Horner's syndrome, where denervation hypersensitivity occurs (see Fig. 24.15).

Ptosis associated with thiamine deficiency often responds rapidly to corrective therapy, sometimes within 2 to 48 hours.[153]

Myokymia

Lid myokymia is a common condition in which mild to moderate fasciculations of the orbicularis muscle cause annoying symptoms, often with no observable eyelid signs.

ETIOLOGY

Etiologic factors include fatigue, stress, tension, anxiety, lack of sleep, irradiated corneal or conjunctival lesions, and occasionally excessive use of alcohol or smoking.[167] The topical ocular use of anticholinesterase agents can also produce lid myokymia,[167] and cases of lid myokymia associated with use of fluphenazine[168] and haloperidol[169] have been reported.

DIAGNOSIS

The patient often complains that the eye "jumps" or "quivers." However, gross external as well as slit-lamp examination fail to uncover any ocular movement abnormality, and the astute clinician soon learns to interpret such complaints to be related to eyelid fasciculations. Rarely, the patient may report associated oscillopsia, correlating with "pseudonys-tagmus" observed on slit-lamp examination.[170] The lower lid is more commonly involved, and the condition is usually unilateral.

MANAGEMENT

In cases that are not drug induced, management involves patient reassurance, since in most cases the myokymia spontaneously resolves. Occasionally, however, the condition is persistent or severe, requiring more specific treatment. Topically administered antihistamines, such as antazoline or pheniramine, are often effective and may give significant relief within 15 to 20 minutes. Antihistaminic therapy relaxes the spasming orbicularis muscle by prolonging its refractory time. The topical medication should be used every 4 hours as needed to abolish symptoms. If this is ineffective, 12.5 to 25 mg of promethazine (Phenergan) can be administered orally one to three times daily, or 75 mg of tripelennamine can be administered orally four times daily.[167] For recalcitrant cases oral quinine, 200 to 300 mg, may be administered one to three times daily either alone or in combination with antihistaminic therapy.[167] Quinine relaxes the orbicularis muscle by a curari-like action, but it must be avoided in pregnant women because of its abortifacient properties.

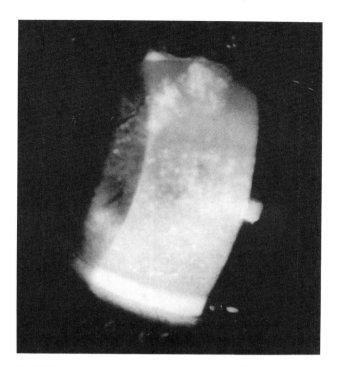

FIGURE 24.16 **Exposure keratitis. Note diffuse superficial punctate staining of central and inferior cornea using sodium fluorescein.**

Lagophthalmos

Lagophthalmos is a condition in which the eyelids cannot fully close.

ETIOLOGY

Lagophthalmos can be classified as:[171–173]

- Physiologic or nocturnal. This form occurs during sleep, and symptoms arising from the condition occur more often in adults than in children, probably because of a reduction of tears in the former group.[174]
- Orbital. This is usually associated with severe proptosis (see Fig. 33.5).
- Mechanical. Scarring of the lid muscles or lids may prevent closure.
- Paralytic. Seventh-nerve palsy is the most common type of paralytic lagophthalmos.

DIAGNOSIS

Symptoms include ocular irritation, especially on awaking. This symptom is accompanied by punctate keratitis of the central or inferior cornea, often in the shape of a horizontal band (Fig. 24.16). If the exposure is severe enough, melting of the inferior cornea can occur.[171] In addition, the conjunc-

tiva is often injected, and the affected portion of the cornea may be hypoesthetic.[171]

The physical examination should confirm the presence of lagophthalmos. This is usually demonstrated easily by instructing the patient to gently close the eyes. In cases of nocturnal lagophthalmos, the presence of lagophthalmos may not be noted until the patient is in a supine position and the closed eyelids are examined carefully with a penlight (Fig. 24.17). Another simple way to determine if nocturnal lagophthalmos is occurring is to query the spouse or parent if the patient sleeps with his or her eyes open. The presence or absence of a Bell's reflex is immaterial, since this phenomenon is unrelated to the position of the globe during gentle lid closure or during sleep.[174]

MANAGEMENT

In cases of acute seventh-nerve palsy, oral steroids may decrease the accompanying pain and the incidence of autonomic synkinesis. Steroid therapy may also hasten recovery and prevent denervation. Treatment should be instituted within 2 to 3 weeks of onset and consist of prednisone 60 mg/day for five days, rapidly tapering over five subsequent days.[175]

When the degree of corneal exposure is mild, bland ocular lubricating ointment applied at bedtime can eliminate symp-

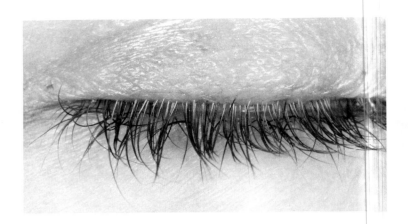

FIGURE 24.17 **Nocturnal lagophthalmos.**

toms. Artificial tears instilled every 2 to 4 hours during the day may also be required according to the severity of the exposure. In addition, the eyelids can be taped closed at bedtime by applying the tape first to the cheek, then pulling the lower lid upward as the tape is attached to the brow and forehead.[171] This form of treatment is usually well tolerated. In cases of severe lagophthalmos, a moisture chamber can be formed of Saran Wrap and placed over the eye at bedtime. Antibiotic ointment may also be indicated if infection seems imminent. Extended wear bandage or disposable contact lenses may also be employed along with antibiotic or lubricant therapy. When these conservative measures fail, or if the condition is long-standing, surgical correction may be necessary.[176,177]

Incomplete Blink

Abelson and Holly[178] have described a condition in which incomplete blinking contributes to inferior punctate keratopathy. Impaired blinking may cause the corneal lesions by producing exposure and inadequate tear film. The condition is treated by blink training,[179] the application of artificial tears or bland lubricating ointment, or bandage soft contact lenses.

Lid Retraction

Lid retraction is most commonly associated with thyroid disease and is considered in Chapter 33.

Abnormalities of Lid Margin Position

Ectropion

Ectropion is a condition in which usually the lower, but sometimes the upper, lid becomes everted, exposing the conjunctiva and cornea and causing irritation and occasionally secondary infection.

ETIOLOGY

Ectropion is classified as involutional (age-related), cicatricial, paralytic, and congenital. By far the most common type is involutional, which results from horizontal laxity of the eyelid tissue components.[180,181] This condition allows gravity to evert the lower lid and expose the conjunctiva and inferior cornea. Complete eversion of the lower lid, termed tarsal ectropion, is caused by disinsertion or dehiscence of the lower eyelid retractors at the inferior tarsal border.[182]

Scarring of the skin of the lids produces cicatricial ectropion. Chemical or thermal burns or chronic dermatoses can cause this condition.[183] Alternatively, it can be secondary to trauma or previous surgery. Cicatricial ectropion has also been reported as a complication of systemic fluorouracil.[184]

Paralytic ectropion results from prolonged paralysis of the orbicularis muscle of the lower lid, most often from Bell's palsy. Failure of the upper lid to protect the cornea aggravates this condition.

Congenital ectropion is usually associated with other eyelid abnormalities. This condition should be distinguished from congenital eversion, which is characterized by protrusion of edematous conjunctiva from everted eyelids.[185,186]

Ectropion can also be caused by hypersensitivity reactions to dipivefrin therapy[186a] or by poorly fitting eyeglass frames.[187]

DIAGNOSIS

In mild or incipient cases of involutional ectropion, no obvious signs of lower eyelid eversion may occur. The lid margin is often in its normal position against the globe, but, if pulled away, it returns slowly rather than briskly. As the ectropion becomes advanced, the patient often complains of tearing or epiphora, since the lower punctum is not in its

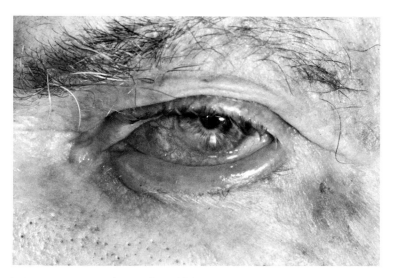

FIGURE 24.18   **Tarsal ectropion with keratinized palpebral conjunctiva.**

normal position to drain the lacrimal lake. Excluding a history of trauma, previous surgery, and burns further confirms the diagnosis. There will be absence of ectropion accentuation on opening the mouth widely, an inability to palpate scar tissue within the eyelid, and the ability to pinch the horizontally redundant, full-thickness eyelid together.[181]

The diagnosis of lower eyelid cicatricial ectropion is made by palpating scar tissue within the eyelid. In addition, opening the mouth widely accentuates the ectropion because the facial skin stretches.[181] In the case of upper eyelid cicatricial ectropion, there is usually evidence of lid lag on downgaze, lid retraction, and lagophthalmos.

MANAGEMENT

In addition to cosmesis, the primary clinical significance of ectropion is resultant exposure of the conjunctiva and cornea, which leads to irritation, secondary infection, and, in some cases, serious complications such as corneal ulceration. Appropriate treatment is therefore indicated.

In mild to moderate ectropion, lubricants can protect the cornea. Bland lubricating ointment should be used at bedtime and artificial tears during the day as needed. In more severe cases extended wear soft contact lenses can be applied for corneal protection, either alone or in combination with a lateral tarsorrhaphy. If epiphora is a major problem, the lower lid can be brought into apposition with the globe by simple lid-taping at the medial canthus.[188] Some cases of cicatricial ectropion may respond to topically applied steroid cream or ointment to the eyelid several times daily.[184] Congenital eyelid eversion is treated by simple mechanical reduction of the eversion, followed by 48 to 72 hours of pressure patching.[185,189]

With failure of such conservative therapy to protect the eye adequately, surgical correction is indicated.[182] Keratinization of the everted palpebral conjunctiva (Fig. 24.18) does not require treatment.[190] Moreover, if the lid is returned to its proper position surgically, this will not damage the cornea, and the conjunctiva will revert to its normal character.

Floppy Eyelid Syndrome

ETIOLOGY

First reported in 1981 by Culbertson and Ostler,[191] the floppy eyelid syndrome refers to the clinical findings of chronic papillary conjunctivitis associated with nonspecific irritative symptoms, along with a soft, rubbery, "floppy," and easily everted upper eyelid. Although the syndrome can occur in women[192] and children,[193] it is usually seen in middle-aged, obese men who may complain of chronic, thick, mucoid discharge and spontaneous eversion of the eyelids during sleep. The condition is usually bilateral but tends to be worse on the side on which the patient sleeps. The mechanism relates to loss of tarsal integrity, causing eyelid eversion during sleep, which creates mechanical irritation to the lids, cornea, and conjunctiva.[194,195,223] In addition, poor contact between the loose upper eyelid and the globe may interfere with distribution of the tear film over the cornea and conjunctiva, creating ocular surface drying and irritation.[196] Since some patients with floppy eyelid syndrome also have keratoconus,[192,197] an underlying connective tissue disorder may be implicated.[198]

DIAGNOSIS

Diagnosis is made by careful history, including sleeping patterns, and the observation of a rubbery upper lid that easily everts on elevation (Fig. 24.19). A mucoid discharge with papillary conjunctivitis may also be seen. In some cases the primary symptoms may result from overriding of a lax upper lid on an often equally lax lower lid, allowing lower

eyelid lashes to rub the upper tarsal conjunctiva.[199] This condition, known as eyelid imbrication, can be difficult to diagnose. Rose bengal staining of the upper lid margin tarsal conjunctiva can greatly aid in its detection.[224]

MANAGEMENT

Treatment consists of discontinuing all previously prescribed medications except those required for concurrent conditions. Symptoms or signs of dry eye, lagophthalmos, and medicamentosa should be managed appropriately. Topical steroids or lubricants alone usually cannot control the symptoms of floppy eyelid. Preventing lid eversion generally requires lid taping or use of a shield at bedtime. The definitive treatment, however, is surgery to correct eyelid laxity and to prevent overriding of the upper eyelid.[199,200]

Entropion

Entropion is a condition in which the lower or upper lid is inverted toward the globe. The primary complication is trichiasis, which can lead to irritation or corneal ulceration.

ETIOLOGY

Entropion is classified as congenital,[201] involutional (age-related), cicatricial, and spastic.[35,154,202] The most common type of entropion is involutional. This condition results from horizontal eyelid laxity, overriding of the preseptal orbicularis muscle, and weakness of the lower eyelid retractors.[203] Atrophy of the orbital tissues creates slight enophthalmos, which enhances the possibility of entropion. Because of the lack of passive resistance provided by the retractors of the

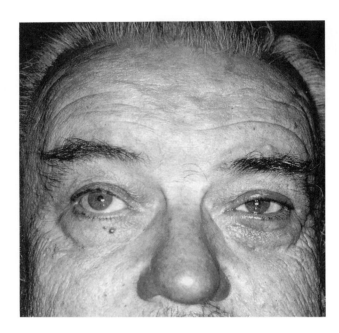

A

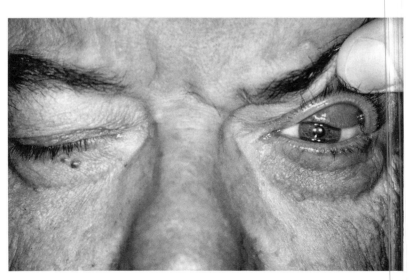

B

FIGURE 24.19 **Floppy eyelid syndrome.** *(A)* **53-year-old obese male with thick, rubbery eyelid tissue.** *(B)* **Eyelid is easily everted with simple upward movement, allowing nocturnal exposure of tarsal conjunctiva and cornea.**

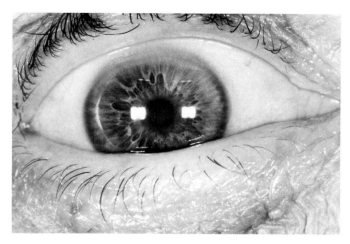 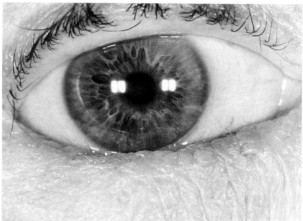

A   B

FIGURE 24.20   **Involutional (age-related) entropion.** *(A)* **Lower lid margin in normal position between blinks.** *(B)* **Entropion evident immediately after tight lid closure.**

lower lid and the combination of horizontal lid laxity, the lower tarsal border moves outward while the upper tarsal border moves inward, resulting in frank entropion.[204] This form of entropion never occurs in the upper lid.[154]

The cicatricial form of entropion occurs as a result of conjunctival scarring. This is sometimes seen in the upper lid as a complication of trachoma.[205]

True spastic entropion occurs only in cases of severe conjunctival and corneal disease, in which irritation of the lid structures provokes lid spasm, resulting in entropion.[154]

DIAGNOSIS

In moderate to severe cases, the diagnosis requires only observing the inverted lid border, with or without trichiasis. Frequently, however, the entropion is not observable early in the course of its development, and pressure from the upper lid on the lower lid margin during tight lid closure is necessary to produce the clinical signs (Fig. 24.20).

MANAGEMENT

Since the primary problem associated with entropion is irritation resulting from trichiasis, the in-turned lashes must be epilated. This treatment often must be repeated every few weeks or months. The eye can be protected with lubricating ointment or artificial tears, and, in cases of severe irritation, prophylactic antibiotic ointment may be indicated. Electrolysis can produce a more permanent cure by destroying the affected lash follicles.

The outer layers of the lower lid can be nonsurgically tightened by applying collodion. As the collodion contracts, it causes mild cicatricial ectropion.[206] Cyanoacrylate adhesive (Krazy Glue) is even more effective in the correction of involutional entropion.[206] The glue can be used to attach a horizontal fold of excess skin of the lower lid to the cheek. Since fumes from the glue may be irritating to the eye, the eyelids must be closed during the application. This form of correction may last from several hours to several weeks, but cleaning the skin well and applying benzoin compound may prolong the adhesion.

If these conservative measures fail, surgical procedures can be undertaken.[203,207]

Trichiasis

Trichiasis is a common clinical problem characterized by the presence of one or more inturning lashes of the upper or lower lid. The misdirected cilia rub against the cornea or bulbar conjunctiva, resulting in a foreign body sensation. These hairs may be so fine and without pigment (lanugo hairs) that they defy detection except by slit lamp examination. In some races, however, particularly orientals, physiologic trichiasis of the lower lids often occurs near the punctum. It requires no treatment unless it causes symptoms.

ETIOLOGY

In most cases trichiasis is the result of aging changes of the lid, and no underlying disease process is present. Other causes include conditions such as trachoma, Stevens-Johnson syndrome, ocular pemphigoid, and trauma, all of which can produce deformity of the lid and conjunctiva. Trichiasis

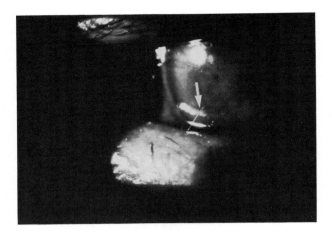

FIGURE 24.21   **Trichiasis (arrow).**

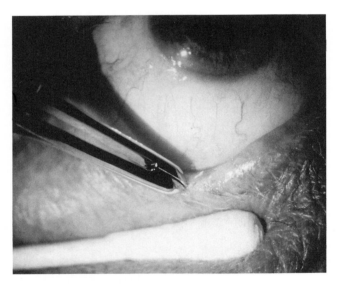

FIGURE 24.22   **Epilation of misdirected eyelash. Forceps are used to firmly grasp the base of the lash before epilating.**

may involve one or several lashes, or the entire row of cilia. The former may be secondary to staphylococcal blepharitis or trauma, while the latter is the result of spastic entropion.

DIAGNOSIS

Diagnosis requires careful physical examination, especially with the slit lamp. One or more inturned lashes is observed (Fig. 24.21), and conjunctival hyperemia or corneal staining in the area of the inturned lash may be evident.

MANAGEMENT

The treatment of one or several misdirected lashes can be achieved by simply removing the offending cilia using epilating forceps. To avoid breakage, the lash should be grasped securely at its base (Fig. 24.22). A firm tug outward will remove the lash by its root. Recurrent trichiasis is common, and the procedure may need to be repeated every few weeks or months since it does not destroy the lash follicle.

The most effective way to eliminate an unwanted lash is to destroy it by use of cryotherapy, argon laser, or electrolysis. Cryotherapy has potential complications including lid notching, corneal ulceration, acceleration of symblepharon formation, xerosis, cellulitis, activation of herpes zoster, skin depigmentation, and severe soft tissue reaction. Laser treatment for trichiasis is more expensive than the other available therapies[208] and is best suited to isolated, aberrant cilia.[209] Perhaps the easiest and least expensive electrolysis method employs the Perma Tweez electrolysis unit.

The Perma Tweez is a small, hand-held, battery-operated instrument that has a thin, blunt spring-loaded stylet at one end (Fig. 24.23). A hand electrode attachment is snapped onto the barrel of the Perma Tweez on one end and held by the patient on the other end. This enables an electric circuit to be completed. Although the instrument is equipped with a tweezer attachment, the stock tweezer attachment should be removed.

With the patient at the slit lamp and holding the hand electrode, the clinician inserts the stylet approximately 1/16 to 1/8 inch into the follicle pore of the targeted lash in the same direction that the hair is growing (Fig. 24.24). With the stylet properly positioned, the battery current starts automatically. White hydrogen bubbles accumulating around the mouth of the follicle are visible evidence of ongoing electrolysis. The current is left on for 30 to 60 seconds after which the stylet is removed from the pore. The lash can then be removed with epilation forceps. Any number of lashes may be treated at one sitting.

Note that the current created to destroy the follicle can cause patient discomfort. Thresholds of sensation vary from patient to patient. To reduce patient discomfort, the patient can loosely hold only the end of the electrode, or most of the electrode can be covered with scotch tape. Since these methods reduce the current generated, more time will be required to destroy the lash follicle. Conversely, to hasten destruction of the follicle, the patient can wet his or her hand and tightly grip the entire electrode. This approach, however, can increase the amount of discomfort experienced. Local infiltrative anesthesia can also eliminate any sensation associated with the procedure. Lidocaine 1% injected subconjunctivally and subcutaneously (see Chap. 20) near the lid margin in the area to be treated renders the procedure painless. Normally, electrolysis causes mild swelling or irritation in the immediate area of treatment. Both will disappear in 1 to 2 days. Even following successful electrolysis, a low incidence of regrowth can occur, especially with coarse or previously tweezed hairs. Stubborn lashes may require several treatments at different intervals before permanent destruction is achieved.

Benign Tumors

Verrucae (Papillomata)

Verrucae, commonly known as warts, are benign skin tumors that can affect any part of the body, including the eyelids. The morphology of these benign lesions is quite characteristic (Fig. 24.25). The verruca vulgaris is a raised, multilobulated, grapelike mass of tissue that is attached to the body by a stalk (pedunculated) of varying thickness. The verruca plana is a round, slightly raised, flat wart (sessile) varying in size from a few millimeters to several centimeters in diameter. It is cauliflower-like and pitted in appearance and may be darkly pigmented. Cutaneous horns are cornified verruca vulgaris. Since they are keratinized and firm, cutaneous horns do not have the fleshy-soft consistency of verruca vulgaris.

ETIOLOGY

Verruca vulgaris, verruca plana and cutaneous horns are forms of viral warts produced by the papillomavirus.[210] Since these lesions are viral in nature, they tend to pour viral toxins and desquamated epithelium onto the conjunctiva, sometimes resulting in a secondary mild chronic conjunctivitis.[211] Verrucae on the eyelids or in close proximity to the globe cause the most symptomatic problems. Of particular importance are warts that occur on the lid margin among the lashes.

DIAGNOSIS

The most common type of wart to occur on the face and lid area is the flat wart (verrucae plana).[212] These are flat-topped, round, slightly raised, 2 to 6 mm in diameter, tan to yellow pink, and with a granular surface. They may be quite numerous and even confluent.

MANAGEMENT

Treatment of verrucae is indicated primarily for cosmetic reasons but also to prevent further dissemination. Since most verrucae resolve spontaneously after several years, therapy should be conservative to avoid scarring. The lesions are limited entirely to the epidermis, and treatment limited to this level should not result in scarring.[212] Specific antiviral therapy is not available, and systemic treatment, including vaccines, is ineffective. Thus, treatment is limited to the topical application of various keratolytic agents or removal by excision.

Chemical cautery entails the use of dichloroacetic acid

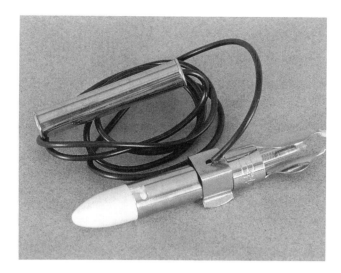

FIGURE 24.23   **Perma Tweez electrocautery instrument.**

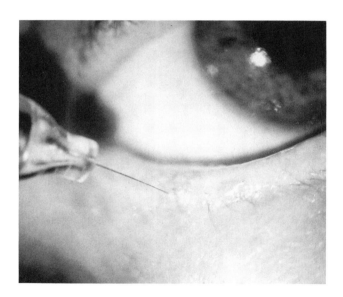

FIGURE 24.24   **Stylus inserted into lash follicle.**

(Bichloracetic Acid). This compound is a potent, clear, colorless liquid cauterant-keratolytic agent and is supplied in a treatment kit (Fig. 24.26). Its cauterizing effect is comparable to that obtained with methods such as electrocautery or freezing. Prior to the use of dichloroacetic acid on verrucae near the eye, a topical anesthetic should be instilled into the cul-de-sac to suppress possible tearing secondary to chemical fumes. Next, petroleum is applied to the skin surrounding the verruca being treated. This ensures

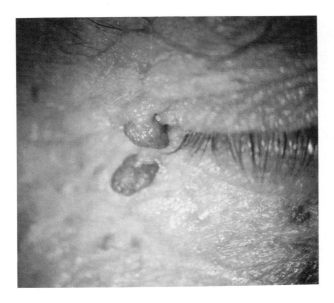

A

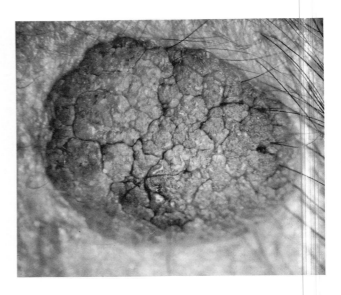

B

FIGURE 24.25 **Types of verruca.** *(A)* **Verruca vulgaris.** *(B)* **Verruca plana.** *(C)* **Cutaneous horn.**

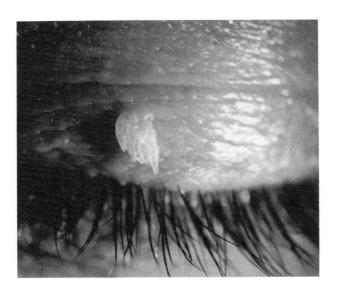

C

protection of the skin surrounding the lesion. Because it is a powerful keratin solvent, the dichloroacetic acid must be used judiciously. The acid is applied to the verruca with care using the pointed end of a wooden stick or a broken cotton-tipped applicator. Application is made exactly to the surface of the verruca and not beyond. The pointed stick should be dipped 2 to 3 mm into the acid and the side of the wetted stick touched to the inside neck of the bottle to drain excess acid before it is applied to the wart. The clinician must not hold the bottle of acid near the patient's face. Rather, the bottle should either remain on a table next to the clinician or be held by an assistant. Also, the acid-dipped stick should never be passed over the face or eyes of the patient. Good lighting and magnification (head loupe) are essential, but use of a slit lamp is discouraged. Placing the patient in a supine position is advantageous because it lessens the possibility of acid dripping once it is applied (Fig. 24.27).

If the lesion is on the lid margin, the lid should be pulled away from the globe while the acid is applied. The patient is also instructed to look in a direction opposite the lesion during acid application. The lid is not released before the acid has dried. If the lid is inadvertently released before the acid has dried, a superficial conjunctival or corneal burn may result. Following copious lavage of the globe, the iatrogenic trauma can be treated as an abrasion, with cyclo-plegic, antibiotic ointment, and pressure patching used as necessary (see Chap. 27). Careful procedural technique, however, can prevent most of these problems. A Jaeger plate can be used not only to pull the lid away from the globe for each application of the acid, but also to protect the globe. The Jaeger plate is a 3-inch long flattened piece of clear lucite or metal with a concave outer surface and convex inner surface (Fig. 24.28). The end of the plate is inserted into the lower cul-de-sac with its concave surface toward the globe.

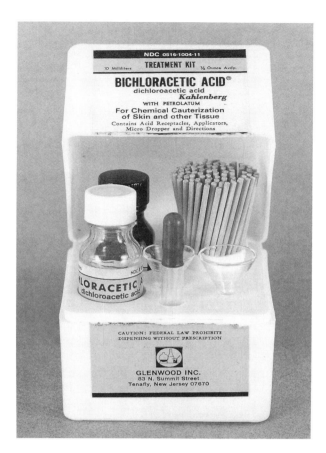

FIGURE 24.26 **Bichloracetic Acid treatment kit.**

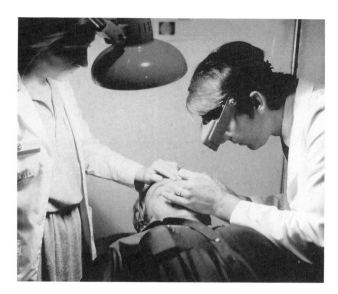

FIGURE 24.27 **Bichloracetic Acid is applied using high magnification, and good illumination, with patient in supine position.**

Immediately after applying the acid, the surface of the verruca turns a milky grayish-white (Fig. 24.29). Within several hours it becomes dark, perhaps even black (Fig. 24.30) In 1 to 2 days an eschar forms which separates in 7 to 10 days. When treating verrucae around or on the thin and delicate skin of the eyelids, slight erythema and mild stinging may accompany application of the acid. These effects usually resolve in a short time. The patient should be cautioned not to touch the resulting scab as infection may result, but normal face washing is permissible.

Pedunculated verrucae can be treated by simple excision. First the area around the verruca is swabbed with alcohol or Betadine. The end of the wart is then grasped with mouse-tooth forceps, and tension is placed on the base of the wart and surrounding skin by pulling. The base of the verruca is snipped with curve-tipped iris scissors. The patient will feel a slight pinching sensation when the verruca is snipped and should be so informed before the procedure is performed. If any bleeding or weeping occurs, pressure can be applied for several minutes using a cotton-tipped applicator soaked in

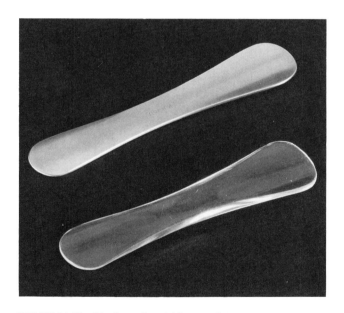

FIGURE 24.28 **Plastic and metal Jaeger plates.**

1:1000 epinephrine. If necessary, when the weeping has stopped the base of the verruca can be treated with dichloroacetic acid as previously described.

Verrucae can affect all races. In dark-skinned people, particularly blacks, verrucae have the same general appear-

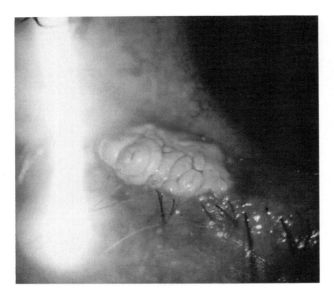

FIGURE 24.29 **White phase immediately after application of Bichloracetic Acid to verruca vulgaris.**

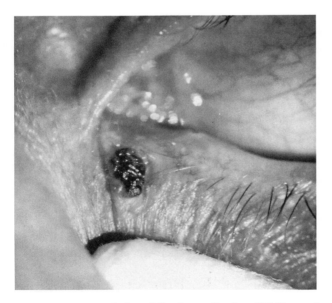

FIGURE 24.30 **Dark phase following application of Bichloracetic Acid.**

ance except that they are darkly pigmented, a result of accumulated melanin. Certain precautionary measures must be taken with darkly pigmented individuals since treatment with dichloroacetic acid can result in hypopigmentation or keloid formation. Keloids are sharply elevated, irregular

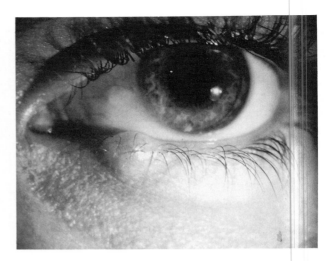

FIGURE 24.31 **Sudoriferous (mucoid) cyst on anterior eyelid margin.**

scars due to the formation of excessive amounts of collagen in the corium during connective tissue repair.[213] Careful questioning of the patient about past injuries will provide information regarding the individual's susceptibility to keloid formation. A verruca on an inconspicuous part of the body, such as the back of the neck, can be treated initially and the healing process carefully observed. If healing is uneventful, other verrucae may be treated without undesirable sequelae.

Sudoriferous (Mucoid) Cysts

Sudoriferous cysts are small, round, translucent, elevated masses caused by blockage of the ducts of the gland of Moll. One or more lesions ranging from 2 to 4 mm in diameter may be observed on the anterior eyelid margin (Fig. 24.31). They are always painless but occasionally can cause irritation or interfere with successful contact lens wear. They are filled with clear, watery fluid.

These lesions tend to reform following puncture, but rarely reappear if the dome of the cyst is excised.[214] After instilling a topical anesthetic into the eye and cleaning the eyelid margin with an antiseptic such as benzalkonium chloride, the area around the cyst should be anesthetized using 1% to 2% lidocaine injected subcutaneously and/or subconjunctivally (see Chap. 20). The cyst is then exteriorized by removing the dome of the cyst (Fig. 24.32). After the area is fully anesthetized, a disposable #9 scalpel is used to make a horizontal incision, parallel to the lid margin, through the midline of the outer surface of the cyst. Once the outer surface is cut, the watery contents of the cyst will flow

A. Incision through dome of mucoid cyst

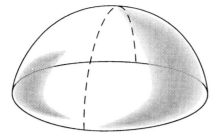

B. Removing anterior half of cyst with forceps and curved-tipped iris scissors

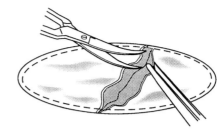

C. Floor of cyst will epithelialize to form new skin

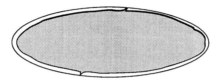

FIGURE 24.32   **Surgical dissection of sudoriferous cyst.**

out. After swabbing the area dry with cotton-tipped applicators or gauze pads, the two halves of the dome can be easily removed using mouse-tooth forceps and curve-tipped iris scissors. After grasping half the dome flap with forceps at the cut edge, slight pulling will create enough space to permit the flap to be cut away with scissors. The second half-moon flap is removed in a similar fashion. Minimal weeping of the excised lesion occurs, and no sutures are required. In approximately a week, the back surface of the cyst reepithelializes without evidence of the former cyst.

Xanthoma Palpebrarum (Xanthelasma)

Xanthoma palpebrarum is an elevated, yellowish discoloration that occurs most commonly in women during the fourth and fifth decades of life. The lesions usually occur bilaterally on the medial aspect of the upper eyelids (Fig. 24.33). The plaque-like character of xanthoma is caused by infiltration of the dermis by xanthoma cells, which are benign histiocytes that imbibe fat.[215] The condition usually occurs independently without associated systemic disease, but some patients may have hypercholesterolemia or other associated disturbance of lipid metabolism.[215–217]

Patients presenting with xanthoma, particularly younger individuals, should first be evaluated for elevated serum lipid levels since 30% to 50% of those with xanthoma have hyperlipoproteinemia.[218] Thus, in addition to cosmetic con-

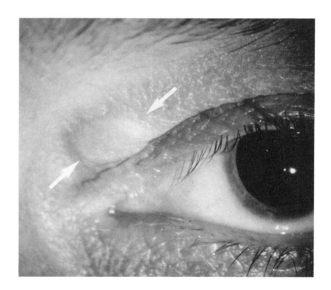

FIGURE 24.33   **Xanthoma (xanthelasma) on medial aspect of upper eyelid (arrows).**

siderations, the major concern in these patients is potential complications of associated atherosclerotic cardiovascular diseases as well as possible systemic disorders such as diabetes and cirrhosis.[219]

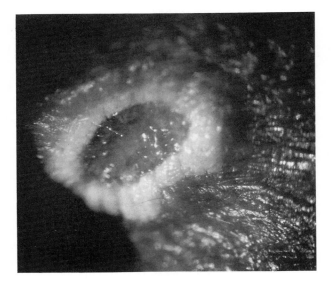

A

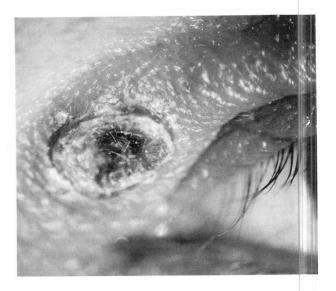

B

FIGURE 24.34 **Treatment of xanthelasma with Bichloracetic Acid.** *(A)* **Note "fried-egg" appearance immediately after treatment.** *(B)* **Eschar formation one week after treatment.** *(C)* **Eschar resolution two weeks after treatment.**

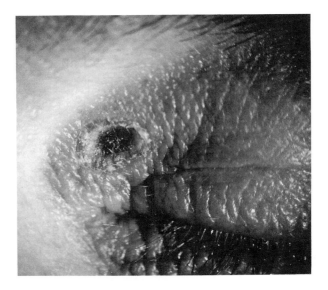

C

will take on a "fried egg" appearance—white borders with a yellow center (Fig. 24.34). In a few days a large eschar forms. This type of eshar resolves more slowly than that formed during verrucae treatment. Once the eschar separates, the skin may appear slightly erythematous or discolored compared to adjacent skin. With time this discoloration disappears and the skin takes on a homogeneous appearance. Since treatment can produce scarring in some patients, much discussion with the patient is advised preceding the commencement of treatment. When carefully done, however, the result is usually a flat, pinkish, pliable scar that blends well with the normal soft, crinkled eyelid skin tissue.[220] Initially, only a small area of the lesion should be treated and the results of healing monitored. Note also that xanthoma, whether treated by chemical cautery or surgically, can recur. This possibility must be carefully explained to the patient.

Sebaceous Cysts

ETIOLOGY

Sebaceous cysts are benign retention cysts of sebum. They often appear in the geriatric population due to aging skin. Milia are small (1–2 mm) round, sebaceous cysts that tend to remain intracutaneous (Fig. 24.35). They are common on the eyelids, are whitish in color, are found away from the lid

Dichloroacetic acid can be used for the cosmetic treatment of xanthoma. The procedure is the same as described for verrucae. The area is first swabbed with alcohol, and petrolatum is applied around the lesion. The acid is applied directly to the lesion using a pointed wooden stick. As the acid is applied, the area becomes "sticky" as the acid reacts with the lipids that are deposited in the histiocytes of the dermis. Following application of the acid, the treated lesion

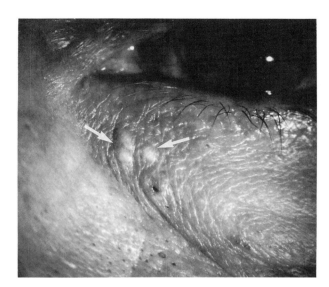

FIGURE 24.35   **Milia (arrows).**

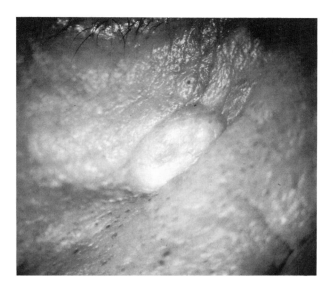

FIGURE 24.36   **Subcutaneous sebaceous cyst.**

margin, and cause little irritation. They are important only from a cosmetic standpoint.

Subcutaneous sebaceous cysts are yellowish in color, may be larger (up to 10–12 mm) than milia, are also asymptomatic, and are firm to the touch. The capsule and its contents are moveable under the overlying skin (Fig. 24.36). Often the plugged orifice of the gland duct is visible. These cysts can occur singly or in groups and are bothersome only from a cosmetic point of view.

MANAGEMENT

Milia are easily removed without the use of anesthesia. A small stab incision is carefully made through the surface of the lesion using the point of a #11 disposable scalpel or of a 25-g or 27-g hypodermic needle. The sebum contained in the cyst is expressed with cotton-tipped applicators or smooth forceps. The interior of the cyst is then cauterized with dichloroacetic acid applied with a sharpened wooden applicator. The removal site is usually invisible in two weeks.[221]

Subcutaneous sebaceous cysts must be removed by total excision since simple incision usually leads to recurrence.[222] After anesthetizing the area surrounding the cyst, a linear incision is made with a #9 disposable scalpel over the cyst with care taken to cut only the overlying skin and not the cyst itself.. The practitioner should study the skin of the patient before making the incision to determine the incision's orientation. The normal creases and wrinkles of the patient's skin should be noted. It is important to make the incision parallel to normal skin folds. This is vital for two reasons. First, after cyst removal, the wound will tend to

close on its own, requiring no sutures and, secondly, no scarring or puckered skin results during wound healing.

Once the incision is made, mouse-tooth forceps should be used to pull the cut edge of one flap while the scalpel is used to cut the fascia and connective tissue connections to the encapsulated gland slowly and carefully. This procedure is followed meticulously on all sides of the gland as well as under it. When the gland is cut free from the connective tissue, it can be removed in its entirety. The skin now comes together naturally if the incision was made properly, and no sutures are necessary. A butterfly bandage can secure the wound.

References

1. Casey TA. Congenital colobomata of the eyelids. Trans Ophthalmol Soc UK 1976;96:65–68.

2. Patipa M, Wilkins RB, Guelzow KWL. Surgical management of congenital eyelid coloboma. Ophthalmic Surg 1982;13:212–216.

3. Miller MT, Deutsch TA, Cronin C, Keys CL. Amniotic bands as a cause of ocular anomalies. Am J Ophthalmol 1987;104:270–279.

4. Bullock JD, Fleishman JA. Eyelid coloboma. In: Fraunfelder FT, Roy GH, eds. Current ocular therapy. Philadelphia: W.B. Saunders Co, 1985;362–363.

5. Hauben DJ, Tessler Z. One-stage reconstruction of a large upper lid defect in a newborn. Plastic Reconstruct Surg 1989;83:337–340.

6. Anderson RL. Surgical repair for distichiasis (letter). Arch Ophthalmol 1977;95:169.

7. Frueh BR. Treatment of distichiasis with cryotherapy. Ophthalmic Surg 1981;12:100–103.

8. Kremer I, Weinberger D, Cohen S, Sira IB. Corneal hypoaesthesia in asymptomatic familial distichiasis. Br J Ophthalmol 1986;70:132–134.

9. Byrnes GA, Wilson ME. Congenital distichiasis. Arch Ophthalmol 1991;109:1752–1753.

10. Bartley GB, Jackson IT. Distichiasis and cleft palate. Plastic Reconstruct Surg 1989;84:129:132.

11. Goldstein S, Qazi QH, Fitzgerald J, et al. Distichiasis, congenital heart defects and mixed peripheral vascular anomalies. Am J Med Genet 1985;20:283–294.

12. Kollin T, Johns KJ, Wadlington WB, et al. Hereditary lymphedema and distichiasis. Arch Ophthalmol 1991;109:980–981.

13. Perusse P. Localized distichiasis after tarsorrhaphy. Am J Ophthalmol 1992;114:104–105.

14. White JH. Correction of distichiasis by tarsal resection and mucous membrane grafting. Am J Ophthalmol 1975;80:507–508.

15. Anderson RL, Harvey JT. Lid splitting and posterior lamella cryosurgery for congenital and acquired distichiasis. Arch Ophthalmol 1981;99:631–634.

16. O'Donnell BA, Collin JRO. Distichiasis: Management with cryotherapy to the posterior lamella. Br J Ophthalmol 1993;77:289–292.

17. Frank DH, Wachtel T, Frank HA. The early treatment and reconstruction of eyelid burns. J Trauma 1983;23:874–877.

18. Edlich RF, Nichter LS, Morgan RF, et al. Burns of the head and neck. Otolaryngol Clin North Am 1984;17:361–388.

19. Huang TT, Blackwell SJ, Lewis SR. Burn injuries of the eyelids. Clin Plast Surg 1978;5:571–581.

20. Evans LS. Increased intraocular pressure in severely burned patients. Am J Ophthalmol 1991;111:56–58.

21. Burns CL, Chylack LT. Thermal burns: the management of thermal burns of the lids and globes. Ann Ophthalmol 1979;11:1358–1368.

22. Covington TR. Management of minor burns. Facts and Comparisons Drug Newsletter 1992;11:1–3.

23. Rost KM, Jaeger RW, deCastro FJ. Eye contamination: A poison center protocol for management. Clin Toxicol 1979;14:295–300.

24. Pfister RR. Chemical injuries of the eye. Ophthalmology 1983;90:1246–1253.

25. Rubinfeld RS, Silbert DI, Arentsen JJ, et al. Ocular hydrofluoric acid burns. Am J Ophthalmol 1992;114:420–423.

26. Morgan SJ, Astbury NJ. Inadvertent self administration of superglue: A consumer hazard. Br Med J 1984;289:226–227.

27. Silverman CM. Corneal abrasion from accidental instillation of cyanoacrylate into the eye. Arch Ophthalmol 1988;106:1029–1030.

28. Bock GW. Skin exposure to cyanoacrylate adhesive. Ann Emerg Med 1984;13:486.

29. Kimbrough RL, Okereke PC, Stewart RH. Conservative management of cyanoacrylate ankyloblepharon: a case report. Ophthalmic Surg 1986;17:176–177.

30. Donnenfeld ED, Perry HD, Nelson DB. More of the conservative management of cyanoacrylate ankyloblepharon. Ophthalmic Surg 1987;18:74–75.

31. Raynor LA. Treatment for inadvertent cyanoacrylate tarsorrhaphy. Arch Ophthalmol 1988;106:1033.

32. Dean BS, Krenzelok EP. Cyanoacrylates and corneal abrasion. Clin Toxicol 1989;27:1169–172.

33. Allar RM. Most cyanoacrylate super-glues should be removed promptly. Ophthalmic Surg 1987;18:156.

34. Alexander KL. Some inflammations of the external eye and adnexa. J Am Optom Assoc 1980;51:142–146.

35. Trevor-Roper PD. Diseases of the eyelids. Int Ophthalmol Clin 1974;14:362–393.

36. Hudson RL. Treatment of styes and meibomian cysts. Practical procedures. Aust Fam Phys 1981;10:714–717.

37. Fraunfelder FT. Hordeolum. In: Fraunfelder FT, Roy FH, eds. Current ocular therapy. Philadelphia: W.B. Saunders Co, 1985;363–364.

38. Jones DB, Liesegang TJ, Robinson NM. Laboratory diagnosis of ocular infections. Washington, DC: American Society for Microbiology, 1981;9–10.

39. English FP, Nutting WB. Demodicosis of ophthalmic concern. Am J Ophthalmol 1981;91:362–372.

40. English FP, Cohn D, Groeneveld ER. Demodectic mites and chalazion. Am J Ophthalmol 1985;100:482–483.

41. Gershen HJ. Chalazion. In: Fraunfelder FT, Roy FH, eds. Current ocular therapy. Philadelphia: W.B. Saunders Co, 1985,354–355.

42. Bohigian GM. Chalazion: A clinical evaluation. Ann Ophthalmol 1979;11:1397–1398.

43. Browning DJ, Proia AD. Ocular rosacea. Surv Ophthalmol 1986;31:145–158.

44. Nisted M, Hofstetter HW. Effect of chalazion on astigmatism. Am J Optom Physiol Optics 1974;51:579–582.

45. Bogan S, Simon JW, Krohel GB, Nelson LB. Astigmatism associated with adnexal masses in infancy. Arch Ophthalmol 1987;105:1368–1370.

46. Cottrell DG, Bosanquet RC, Fawcett IM. Chalazions: The frequency of spontaneous resolution. Br Med J 1983;6405:1595.

47. Catania LJ. Lumps and bumps of the eyelids or "what is that thing?" South J Optom 1979;21:16–19.

48. Perry HD, Serniuk RA. Conservative treatment of chalazia. Ophthalmology 1980;87:218–221.

49. Jacobs PM, Thaller VT, Wong D. Intralesional corticosteroid therapy of chalazia: A comparison with incision and curettage. Br J Ophthalmol 1984;68:836–837.

50. Watson AP, Austin DJ. Treatment of chalazions with injection of a steroid suspension. Br J Ophthalmol 1984;68:833–835.

51. King RA, Ellis PP. Treatment of chalazia with corticosteroid injections. Ophthalmic Surg 1986;17:351–353.

52. Palva J, Pohjanpelto PEJ. Intralesional corticosteroid injection for the treatment of chalazia. Acta Ophthalmol 1983;61:933–937.

53. Castren J, Stenborg T. Corticosteroid injection of chalazia. Acta Ophthalmol 1983;61:938–942.

54. Pizzarello LD, Jakobiec FA, Hofeldt AJ, et al. Intralesional corticosteroid therapy of chalazia. Am J Ophthalmol 1978;85:818–821.

55. Dua HS, Nilawar DV. Nonsurgical therapy of chalazion (letter). Am J Ophthalmol 1982;94:424–425.

56. Freed D, Walls L. Chalazia treatment using intralesional corticosteroid injections: clinical series and literature review. S J Optom 1992;10:28–31.

57. Cohen BZ, Tripathi RC. Eyelid depigmentation after intralesional injection of a fluorinated corticosteroid for chalazion (letter). Am J Ophthalmol 1979;88:269–270.

58. Jakobeic FA, Silvers D. Eyelid depigmentation after intralesional injection of a fluorinated corticosteroid for chalazion-reply (letter). Am J Ophthalmol 1979;88:270.

59. Thomas EL, Laborde RP. Retinal and choroidal vascular occlusion following intralesional corticosteroid injection of a chalazion. Ophthalmology 1986;93:405–407.

60. Gershen HJ. Chalazion excision. Ophthalmic Surg 1974;5:75–76.

61. Bhalla JS, Vashisht S, Gupta VK, et al. Meibomian gland carcinoma in a 20-year-old patient. Am J Ophthalmol 1991;111:114–115.

62. Mamalis N, Medlock RD, Holds JB, et al. Merkle cell tumor of the eyelid: a review and report of an unusual case. Ophthalmic Surg 1989;20:410–414.

63. Kass LG, Hornblass A. Sebaceous carcinoma of the ocular adnexa. Surv Ophthalmol 1989;33:477–490.

64. Shine WE, McCulley JP. Role of wax ester fatty alcohols in chronic blepharitis. Invest Ophthalmol Vis Sci 1993;34:3515–3521.

65. Anderson PH, Jones WL. A recalcitrant case of demodex blepharitis. Clin Eye Vision Care 1988;1:39–43.

66. McCulley JP, Dougherty JM, Deneau DG. Classification of chronic blepharitis. Ophthalmology 1982;89:1173–1180.

67. Gutgesell VJ, Stern GA, Hood CI. Histopathology of meibomian bomian gland dysfunction. Am J Ophthalmol 1982;94:383–387.

68. Roth AM. Demodex folliculorum in hair follicles of eyelid skin. Ann Ophthalmol 1979;11:37–40.

69. Heacock CE. Clinical manifestations of demodicosis. J Am Optom Assoc 1986;57:914–919.

70. McCulley JP, Dougherty JM. Blepharitis associated with acne rosacea and seborrheic dermatitis. Int Ophthalmol Clin 1985;25:159–172.

71. Dougherty JM, Osgood JK, McCulley JP. The role of wax and sterol ester fatty acids in chronic blepharitis. Invest Ophthalmol Vis Sci 1991;32:1932–1937.

72. Shine WE, McCulley JP. The role of cholesterol in chronic blepharitis. Invest Ophthalmol Vis Sci 1991;32:2272–2280.

73. Groden LR, Murphy B, Rodnite J, et al. Lid flora in blepharitis. Cornea 1991;10:50–53.

74. Hydiuk RA, Burd EM, Hartz A. Efficacy and safety of mercuric oxide in the treatment of bacterial blepharitis. Antimicrob Agents Chemother 1990;34:610–613.

75. Huber-Spitzy V, Baumgartner I, Bohler-Sommeregger K, et al. Blepharitis-a diagnostic and therapeutic challenge. A report on 407 consecutive cases. Graefe's Arch Clin Exp Ophthalmol 1991;229:224–227.

76. Shine WE, Silvany R, McCulley JP. Relation of cholesterol-stimulating *Staphylococcus aureus* growth to chronic blepharitis. Invest Ophthalmol Vis Sci 1993;34:2291–2296.

77. Wilson LA, Julian AJ, Ahearn DG. The survival and growth of microorganisms in mascara during use. Am J Ophthalmol 1975;79:596–601.

78. Mondino BJ, Caster AI, Dethlefs B. A rabbit model of staphylococcal blepharitis. Arch Ophthalmol 1987;105:409–412.

79. Smolin G, Okumoto M. Staphylococcal blepharitis. Arch Ophthalmol 1977;95:812–816.

80. McCulley JP. Blepharoconjunctivitis. Int Ophthalmol Clin 1984;24:65–77.

81. Polack FM, Goodman DF. Experience with a new detergent lid scrub in the management of chronic blepharitis. Arch Ophthalmol 1988;106:719–720.

82. Leibowitz HM, Capino D. Treatment of chronic blepharitis. Arch Ophthalmol 1988;106:720.

83. Raskin EM, Speaker MG, Laibson PR. Blepharitis. Infect Dis Clin N Am 1992;6:777–787.

84. Kaufman HE. Chemical blepharitis following drug treatment. Am J Ophthalmol 1983;95:703.

85. Lamberts DW, Buka T, Knowlton GM. Clinical evaluation of trimethoprim-containing ophthalmic solutions in humans. Am J Ophthalmol 1984;98:11–16.

86. Nozik RA, Smolin G, Knowlton G, Austin R. Trimethoprim-polymyxin B ophthalmic solution in treatment of surface ocular bacterial infections. Ann Ophthalmol 1985;17:746–748.

87. Kastl PR, Ali Z, Mather F. Placebo-controlled, double-blind evaluation of the efficacy and safety of yellow mercuric oxide in suppression of eyelid infections. Ann Ophthalmol 1987;19:376–379.

88. Donshik P, Kulvin SM, McKinley P, Skowron R. Treatment of chronic staphylococcal blepharoconjunctivitis with a new topical steroid anti-infective ophthalmic solution. Ann Ophthalmol 1983;15:162–167.

89. Ellis PP. Ocular therapeutics and pharmacology. St. Louis: C.V. Mosby Co, 1985;7:105–120.

90. Smolin G. Staphylococcal blepharitis. In: Fraunfelder FT, Roy FH, eds. Current ocular therapy. Philadelphia: W.B. Saunders Co, 1980;434–435.

91. Salamon SM. Tetracyclines in ophthalmology. Surv Ophthalmol 1985;29:265–275.

92. Khan J, Hoover D, Ide CH. Methicillin-resistant *Staphylococcus epidermidis* blepharitis. Am J Ophthalmol 1984;98:562–565.

93. Fleischer AB, Hoover DL, Khan JA, et al. Topical vancomycin formulation for methicillin-resistant *Staphylococcus epidermidis* blepharoconjunctivitis. Am J Ophthalmol 1986;101:283–287.

94. Flora MR. Meibomianitis and meibomian hypersecretion. South J Optom 1979;21:46–48.

95. Lambert R, Smith RE. Hyperkeratinization in a rabbit model of meibomian gland dysfunction. Am J Ophthalmol 1988;105:703–705.

96. Ong BL, Hodson SA, Wigham T, et al. Evidence for keratin proteins in normal and abnormal human meibomian fluids. Curr Eye Res 1991;10:1113–1119.

97. Seal DV, McGill JI, Jacobs P, et al. Microbial and immunological investigations of chronic non-ulcerative blepharitis and meibomianitis. Br J Ophthalmol 1985;69:604–611.

98. Dougherty JM, McCulley JP, Silvany RE, et al. The role of tetracycline in chronic blepharitis. Inhibition of lipase production in staphylococci. Invest Ophthalmol Vis Sci 1991;32:2970–2975.

99. Korb DR, Henriquez AS. Meibomian gland dysfunction and contact lens intolerance. J Am Optom Assoc 1980;51:243–251.

100. Robin JB, Jester JV, Nobe J, et al. In vivo transillumination biomicroscopy and photography of meibomian gland dysfunction. Ophthalmology 1985;92:1423–1426.

101. McCulley JP, Sciallis GF. Meibomian keratoconjunctivitis. Am J Ophthalmol 1977;84:788–793.

102. Mathers WD. Ocular evaporation in meibomian gland dysfunction and dry eye. Ophthalmology 1993;100:347–351.

103. Paugh JR, Knapp LL, Martinson JR, et al. Meibomian therapy in problematic contact lens wear. Optom Vis Sci 1990;67:803–806.

104. Glasser DB. Angular blepharitis caused by gram-negative bacillus DF-2. Am J Ophthalmol 1986;102:119–120.

105. Malinow I, Powell KR. Periorbital cellulitis. Pediatr Ann 1993;22:241–246.

106. Lessner A, Stern GA. Preseptal and orbital cellulitis. Infect Dis Clin N Am 1992;6:933–952.

107. Jones DB, Steinkuller EG. Strategies for the initial management of acute preseptal and orbital cellulitis. Trans Am Ophthalmol Soc 1988;86:94–112.

108. Liesegang TJ. Epidemiology of ocular herpes simplex. Natural history in Rochester, Minn, 1950–1982. Arch Ophthalmol 1989; 107:1160–1165.

109. Pavan-Langston D. Ocular antiviral therapy. Int Ophthalmol Clin 1980;20:149–161.

110. Liesegang TJ, Melton LJ, Daly PEJ, et al. Epidemiology of ocular herpes simplex. Incidence in Rochester, Minn, 1950–1982. Arch Ophthalmol 1989;107:1155–1159.

111. Egerer I, Stary A. Erosive-ulcerative herpes simplex blepharitis. Arch Ophthalmol 1980;98:1760–1763.

112. Jakobiec FA, Srinivasan BD, Gamboa ET. Recurrent herpetic angular blepharitis in an adult. Am J Ophthalmol 1979;88:744–747.

113. Ostler HB. The management of ocular herpesvirus infections. Surv Ophthalmol 1976;21:136–147.

114. Wander AH. Herpes simplex and recurrent corneal disease. Int Ophthalmol Clin 1984;24:27–38.

115. Chu W, Pavan-Langston D. Ocular surface manifestations of the major viruses. Int Ophthalmol Clin 1979;19:135–167.

116. Simon JW, Longo F, Smith RS. Spontaneous resolution of herpes simplex blepharoconjunctivitis in children. Am J Ophthalmol 1986;102:598–600.

117. Cykiert RC. Spontaneous resolution of herpes simplex blepharo-conjunctivitis in children (letter). Am J Ophthalmol 1987;103: 340.

118. Holland EJ, Mahanti RL, Belongia EA, et al. Ocular involvement in an outbreak of herpes gladiatorum. Am J Ophthalmol 1992; 114:680–684.

119. Liesegang TJ. Diagnosis and therapy of herpes zoster ophthalmicus. Ophthalmology 1991;98:1216–1229.

120. Karbassi M, Raizman MB, Schuman JS. Herpes zoster ophthalmicus. Surv Ophthalmol 1992;36:395–410.

121. Liesegang TJ. Ophthalmic herpes zoster: diagnosis and antiviral therapy. Geriatrics 1991;46:64–71.

122. Netland PA, Zierhut M, Raizman MB. Post-traumatic herpes zoster ophthalmicus as a presenting sign of human immunodeficiency virus infection. Ann Ophthalmol 1993;25:14–15.

123. Sellitti TP, Huang AJW, Schiffman J, et al. Association of herpes zoster ophthalmicus with acquired immunodeficiency syndrome and acute retinal necrosis. Am J Ophthalmol 1993;116:297–301.

124. Pavan-Langston D. Varicella-zoster ophthalmicus. Int Ophthalmol Clin 1975;15:171–185.

125. Currey TA, Dalsania J. Treatment for herpes zoster ophthalmicus: stellate ganglion block as a treatment for acute pain and prevention of post-herpetic neuralgia. Ann Ophthalmol 1991;23:188–189.

126. Mayne GE, Moya F. Herpes zoster/postherpetic neuralgia. Intern Med Special 1987;8:198–212.

127. Hoang-Xuan T, Buchi E, Herbort C, et al. Oral acyclovir for herpes zoster ophthalmicus. Ophthalmology 1992;99:1062–1071.

128. Harding SP, Porter SM. Oral acyclovir in herpes zoster ophthalmicus. Curr Eye Res 1991;10:177–182.

129. Bernstein JE, Bickers DR, Dahl MV, et al. Treatment of chronic post-herpetic neuralgia with topical capsaicin. A preliminary study. J Am Acad Dermatol 1987;17:93–96.

130. Bernstein JE, Korman NJ, Bickers DR, et al. Topical capsaicin treatment of chronic post-herpetic neuralgia. J Am Acad Dermatol 1989;21:265–270.

131. Peikert A, Hentrich M, Ochs G. Topical 0.025% capsaicin in chronic post-herpetic neuralgia: efficacy, predictors of response and long-term course. J Neurol 1991;238:452–456.

132. Bucci FA, Gabriels CF, Krohel GB. Successful treatment of post-herpetic neuralgia with capsaicin. Am J Ophthalmol 1988;106: 758–759.

133. Cobo LM, Foulks GN, Liesegang T, et al. Oral acyclovir in the treatment of acute herpes zoster ophthalmicus. Ophthalmology 1986;93:763–770.

134. Cobo LM, Foulks GN, Liesegang T, et al. Oral acyclovir in the therapy of acute herpes zoster ophthalmicus. An interim report. Ophthalmology 1985;92:1574–1583.

135. Cobo M. Reduction of the ocular complications of herpes zoster ophthalmicus by oral acyclovir. Am J Med 1988;85(suppl 2A):90–93.

136. Seiff SR, Margolis T, Graham SH, et al. Use of intravenous acyclovir for treatment of herpes zoster ophthalmicus in patients at risk for AIDS. Ann Ophthalmol 1988:20:480–482.

137. Marsh RJ. Current management of ophthalmic herpes zoster. Trans Ophthalmol Soc UK 1976;96:334–337.

138. Marsh RJ. Ophthalmic zoster. Br J Ophthalmol 1992;76:244–245.

139. Herbort CP, Buechi ER, Piguet B, et al. High-dose oral acyclovir in acute herpes zoster ophthalmicus: the end of the corticosteroid era. Curr Eye Res 1991;10:171–175.

140. Liesegang TJ. Herpes zoster ophthalmicus. Int Ophthalmol Clin 1985;25:77–96.

141. Awan KJ. Cryotherapy in phthiriasis palpebrarum. Am J Ophthalmol 1977;83:906–907.

142. Chin GN, Denslow GT. Pediculosis ciliaris. J Pediatr Ophthalmol Strabismus 1978;15:173–175.

143. Couch JM, Green WR, Hirst LW, et al. Diagnosing and treating phthirus pubis palpebrarum. Surv Ophthalmol 1982;26:219–225.

144. Kairys DJ, Webster HJ, Terry JE. Pediatric ocular phthiriasis infestation. J Am Optom Assoc 1988;59:128–130.

145. Dornic DI. Ectoparasitic infestation of the lashes. J Am Optom Assoc 1985;56:716–719.

146. Ashkenazi I, Desatnek HR, Abraham FA. Yellow mercuric oxide: a treatment of choice for phthiriasis palpebrarum. Br J Ophthalmol 1991;75:356–358.

147. Pe'er J, BenEzra D. Corneal damage following the use of the pediculocide A-200 pyrinate. Arch Ophthalmol 1988;106:16–17.

148. Smith DE, Walsh J. Treatment of public lice infestation: a comparison of two agents. Cutis 1980;26:618–619.

149. Chapel TA, Katta T, Kuszmar T, et al. Pediculosis pubis in a clinic for treatment of sexually transmitted disease. Sex Transm Dis 1979;6:257–260.

150. Stasior OG, Ballitch HA. Ptosis repair in aesthetic blepharoplasty. Clin Plastic Surg 1993;20:269–273.

151. Beard C, Sullivan JH. Ptosis-current concepts. Int Ophthalmol Clin 1978;18:53–73.

152. Cogan DG, Witt ED, Goldman-Rakic PS. Ocular signs in thiamine-deficient monkeys and in Wernicke's disease in humans. Arch Ophthalmol 1985;103:1212–1220.

153. Varavithya W, Dhanamitta S, Valyasevi A. Bilateral ptosis as a

sign of thiamine deficiency in childhood. Clin Pediatr 1975;14:1063–1065.

154. Beyer CK. Repair of entropion and ectropion. Int Ophthalmol Clin 1978;18:19–52.

155. Martin PA, Rogers PA. Involutional ptosis: recognition and management. Aust NZ J Ophthalmol 1985;13:185–187.

156. Shore JW, McCord CD. Anatomic changes in involutional blepharoptosis. Am J Ophthalmol 1984;98:21–27.

157. Werb A. Ptosis. Trans Ophthalmol Soc NZ 1976;28:29–32.

158. Laibovitz RA, Cain R. Lost lid signs in topical neuro-ophthalmic diagnosis. Tex Med 1977;73:68–69.

159. Linberg JV, Vasquez RJ, Chao GM. Aponeurotic ptosis repair under local anesthesia. Prediction of results from operative lid height. Ophthalmology 1988;95:1046–1052.

160. Cohen MB. Case history: use of a bilateral ptosis crutch. N Engl J Optom 1987;40:26–27.

161. Moss HL. Prosthesis for blepharoptosis and blepharospasm. J Am Optom Assoc 1982;53:661–667.

162. Lane CM, Collins JRO. Treatment of ptosis in chronic progressive external ophthalmoplegia. Br J Ophthalmol 1987;71:290–294.

163. Anderson FG. Treatment of myasthenia gravis ptosis and extraocular muscle palsies. Tex Med 1976;72:84–86.

164. Walsh FB, Hoyt WF. Clinical neuro-ophthalmology. Baltimore: Williams & Wilkins, 1969;3:1292.

165. Castronuovo S, Krohel GB, Kristan RW. Blepharoptosis in myasthenia gravis. Ann Ophthalmol 1983;15:751–754.

166. Beasley H. Ptosis. In: Fraunfelder FT, Roy FH, eds. Current ocular therapy. Philadelphia: W.B. Saunders Co., 1980;432–433.

167. Jaffe NS, Shults WT. Lid myokymia. In: Fraunfelder FT, Roy FH, eds. Current ocular therapy, ed 2. Philadelphia: W.B. Saunders Co., 1985;366.

168. Freed EDD. Rapid tremor of the eyelids after overdose of fluphenazine. Br J Psychiatr 1983;143:525–526.

169. Barbaro AC. Tremor of the eyelids. Br J Psychiatr 1984;144:437–438.

170. Krohel GB, Rosenberg PN. Oscillopsia associated with eyelid myokymia. Am J Ophthalmol 1986;102:662–663.

171. Katz J, Kaufman HE. Corneal exposure during sleep (nocturnal lagophthalmos). Arch Ophthalmol 1977;95:449–453.

172. Harvey JT, Anderson RL. Lid lag and lagophthalmos: a clarification of terminology. Ophthalmic Surg 1981;12:338–340.

173. Jobe RP. Lagophthalmos. In: Fraunfelder FT, Roy FH, eds. Current ocular therapy, ed. 2. Philadelphia: W.B. Saunders Co, 1985; 364–366.

174. Lyons CJ, McNab AA. Symptomatic nocturnal lagophthalmus. Aust NZ J Ophthalmol 1990;18:393–396.

175. Morgenlander JC, Massey EW. Bell's palsy. Ensuring the best possible outcome. Postgrad Med 1990;88:157–161.

176. McNeill JI, Oh Y. An improved palpebral spring for the management of paralytic lagophthalmus. Ophthalmology 1991;98:715–719.

177. Kartush JM, Linstrom CJ, McCann PM, et al. Early gold weight eyelid implantation for facial paralysis. Otolaryngol Head Neck Surg 1990;103:1016–1023.

178. Abelson MB, Holly FJ. A tentative mechanism for inferior punctate keratopathy. Am J Ophthalmol 1977;83:866–869.

179. Collins M, Heron H, Larsen R, Lindner R. Blinking patterns in soft contact lens wearers can be altered with training. Am J Optom Physiol Optics 1987;64:100–103.

180. Stefanyszyn MA, Hidayat AA, Flanagan JC. The histopathology of involutional ectropion. Ophthalmology 1985;92:120–127.

181. Putterman AM. Combined z-plasty and horizontal shortening procedure for ectropion. Am J Ophthalmol 1980;89:525–530.

182. Tse DT, Kronish JW, Buus D. Surgical correction of lower-eyelid tarsal ectropion by reinsertion of the retractors. Arch Ophthalmol 1991;109:427–431.

183. Oestreicher JH, Nelson CC. Lamellar ichthyosis and congenital ectropion. Arch Ophthalmol 1990;108:1772–1773.

184. Hurwitz BS. Cicatricial ectropion: a complication of systemic fluorouracil. Arch Ophthalmol 1993;111:1608–1609.

185. Miller R, Martin F, Allen H. A case of congenital ectropion in Down's syndrome. Aust NZ J Ophthalmol 1988;16:119–125.

186. Sellar PW, Bryars JH, Archer DB. Late presentation of congenital ectropion of the eyelids in a child with Down syndrome: a case report and review of the literature. J Pediatr Ophthalmol Strabismus 1992;29:64–67.

186a. Bartley GB. Reversible lower eyelid ectropion associated with dipivefrin. Am J Ophthalmol 1991;111:650–651.

187. Rubin PAD. Ectropion caused by eyeglasses. Am J Ophthalmol 1992;113:590–591.

188. Miller GR, Tenzel RR, Buffam FV. Lid taping in the preoperative management of tearing or asthenopia. Arch Ophthalmol 1976;94:1289–1290.

189. Kronish JW, Lingua R. Pressure patch treatment for congenital upper eyelid eversion. Arch Ophthalmol 1991;109:767–768.

190. Frueh BR, Schoengarth LD. Evaluation and treatment of the patient with ectropion. Ophthalmology 1982;89:1049–1054.

191. Culbertson WW, Ostler HB. The floppy eyelid syndrome. Am J Ophthalmol 1981;92:568–575.

192. Donnenfeld ED, Perry HD, Gibralter RP, et al. Keratoconus associated with floppy eyelid syndrome. Ophthalmology 1991;98:1674–1678.

193. Eiferman RA, Gossman MD, O'Neill K, et al. Floppy eyelid syndrome in a child. Am J Ophthalmol 1990;109:356–357.

194. Dutton JJ. Surgical management of floppy eyelid syndrome. Am J Ophthalmol 1985;99:557–560.

195. Moore MB, Harrington J, McCulley JP. Floppy eyelid syndrome. Management including surgery. Ophthalmology 1986;93:184–188.

196. Brown MD, Potter JW. Floppy eyelid syndrome: a case report and clinical review. J Am Optom Assoc 1992;63:309–314.

197. Negris R. Floppy eyelid syndrome associated with keratoconus. J Am Optom Assoc 1992;63:316–319.

198. Woog JJ. Obstructive sleep apnea and the floppy eyelid syndrome. Am J Ophthalmol 1990;110:314–315.

199. Karesh JW, Nirankari VS, Hameroff SB. Eyelid imbrication. An unrecognized cause of chronic ocular irritation. Ophthalmology 1993;100:883–889.

200. Bouchard CS. Lateral tarsorrhaphy for a noncompliant patient with floppy eyelid syndrome. Am J Ophthalmol 1992;114:367–369.

201. Bartley GB, Nerad JA, Kersten RC, et al. Congenital entropion with intact lower eyelid retractor insertion. Am J Ophthalmol 1991;112:437–441.

202. Tse DT, Anderson RL, Fratkin JD. Aponeurosis disinsertion in congenital entropion. Arch Ophthalmol 1983;101:436–440.

203. Dresner SC, Karesh JW. Transconjunctival entropion repair. Arch Ophthalmol 1993;111:1144–1148.

204. Rainin EA. Senile entropion. Arch Ophthalmol 1979;97:928–930.

205. Al-Rajhi AA, Hidayat A, Nasr A, et al. The histopathology and the mechanism of entropion in patients with trachoma. Ophthalmology 1993;100:1293–1296.

206. Baylis HI, Hamako C. Office and bedside techniques for treatment of involutional entropion. Trans Am Acad Ophthalmol Otolaryngol 1977;83:663–668.

207. Kersten RC, Kleiner FP, Kulwin DR. Tarsotomy for the treatment of cicatricial entropion with trichiasis. Arch Ophthalmol 1992; 110:714–717.

208. Huneke JW. Argon laser treatment for trichiasis. Ophthalmic Plastic Reconstruct Surg 1992;8:50–55.

209. Bartley GB, Lowry JC. Argon laser treatment of trichiasis. Am J Ophthalmol 1992;113:71–74.

210. Amer M, Tosson Z, Soliman A, et al. Verrucae treated by levamisole. Int J Dermatol 1991;30:738–740.

211. Stenson S, Newman R, Fedukowicz H. Laboratory studies in acute conjunctivitis. Arch Ophthalmol 1982;100:1275–1277.

212. Schmidt LM. Warts: their diagnosis and treatment. Pediatr Ann 1976;5:782–790.

213. Fitzpatrick TB, Eisen AZ, Wolff K, et al. Dermatology in general medicine. 3 ed. New York: McGraw-Hill, 1987:329.

214. Trevor-Roper PD, Curran PV. Diseases of the eyelids. In: The eye and its disorders. 2 ed. Oxford: Blackwell Scientific, 1984:309–340.

215. Depot MJ, Jakobiec FA, Dodick JM, Iwamoto T. Bilateral and extensive xanthelasma palpebrarum in a young man. Ophthalmology 1984;91:522–527.

216. Gladstone GJ, Beckman H, Elson LM. CO_2 laser excision of xanthelasma lesions. Arch Ophthalmol 1985;103:440–442.

217. Parkes ML, Waller TS. Xanthelasma palpebrarum. Laryngoscope 1984;94:1238–1240.

218. Bouste-Blazy P, Marcel YL, Cohen L, et al. Increased frequency of apo E-ND phenotype and hyperpobeta lipoproteinemia in normolipidemic subjects with xanthelasmas of the eyelid. Ann Intern Med 1982;96:164–169.

219. Parkes ML, Waller TS. Xanthelasma palpebrarum. Laryngoscope 1984;94:1238–1240.

220. Stegman SJ, Tromovich TA. Cosmetic dermatology surgery. Arch Dermatol 1992;118:1013–1016.

221. Epstein E. Cysts. In: Common skin disorders. 3 ed. Oradell, NJ: Medical Economics, 1988:78–80.

222. Havener WH. Disorders of the eyelids. In: Synopsis of ophthalmology. 6 ed. St. Louis: C V Mosby 1984:336–350.

223. Netland PA, Sugrue SP, Albert DM, et al. Histopathologic features of the floppy eyelid syndrome. Ophthalmology 1994;101:174–181.

224. Donnenfeld ED, Perry HD, Schrier A, et al. Lid imbrication syndrome. Diagnosis with rose bengal staining. Ophthalmology 1994;101:763–766

CHAPTER 25

Diseases of the Lacrimal System

Leo P. Semes
Richard J. Clompus

Tearing is a common complaint among ophthalmic patients.[1] To pinpoint the offending site within the lacrimal system and to institute appropriate management for these patients requires a logical approach.

Since tears are continually produced and drained, any alteration of this equilibrium can result in tearing. Temporary overproduction of aqueous tears by stimulation of the ophthalmic (first) division of the trigeminal nerve is known as hypersecretion. An example is the reflex tearing resulting from superficial foreign-body irritation. True hypersecretion, resulting from lacrimal nerve stimulation secondary to a mass or lacrimal gland enlargement, is extremely rare.

More frequently encountered is pseudoepiphora. A chronic aqueous deficiency associated with keratoconjunctivitis sicca and Sjögren syndrome results in increased production of reflex (aqueous) tears.

The lacrimal gland produces reflex tears on signals from the lacrimal nucleus. Distinct from continuous (or basic) lacrimal secretions, reflex tears are purely aqueous. Any imbalance in the constituency of the tears can result in an unstable tear film. Some authors[2] believe that such an instability is the major source of tearing complaints.

Obstruction of the lacrimal drainage passageways can result in tearing. A normal tear production rate proves too great for a malfunctioning or blocked drainage system to handle. Tearing usually occurs near the medial canthus.

Management of each patient follows from accurate diagnosis. A careful case history combined with logical testing of the entire lacrimal system, based on its anatomy, usually allows the clinician to provide effective treatment.

Clinical Anatomy and Physiology

A convenient conceptual separation of the lacrimal system can be made based on function. The secretory system produces sufficient quality and quantity of tear film to allow the ocular surface to function normally. A smooth refractive surface, ocular comfort, and resistance to disease and exposure all depend on a healthy tear film.

The lids serve as the distribution system for the tear film. Lid irregularities or disorders can interfere with lid function, resulting in ocular discomfort or compromise.

The excretory system must effectively drain a proper quantity of tears. Deficient access to the lacrimal lake or a blockage within the drainage passageways results in epiphora—classically, tearing secondary to obstruction. The delicate balance among these components of the lacrimal system determines both the comfort and health of the ocular surface (Fig. 25.1).

Secretory System

The secretory portion of the lacrimal system consists of two sets of glands. Reflex (aqueous) secretion comes from the lacrimal gland. Approximately the size and shape of a shelled almond, the lacrimal gland consists of main and accessory portions separated by the aponeurosis of the levator muscle.[1,3] The efferent nerve supply to the lacrimal gland is cholinergic through the anastomosis of the lacrimal and zygomatic nerves. Impulses travel with the seventh cranial

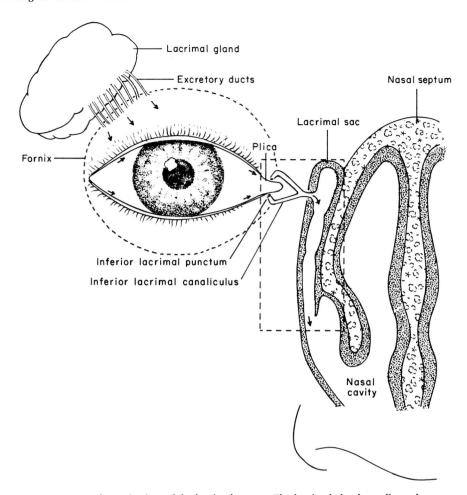

FIGURE 25.1 **Schematic view of the lacrimal system. The lacrimal gland supplies only aqueous (reflex) secretions. Arrows indicate the pathway that tears follow to drainage beginning at the punctum. The area enclosed by dashed lines represents the drainage apparatus. (Adapted from Botelho SY. Tears and the lacrimal gland. Sci Am 1964;211:78–85. Copyright 1964 by Scientific American, Inc. All rights reserved.)**

nerve from the lacrimal nucleus in the pons through the sphenopalatine ganglion and eventually reach the lacrimal gland (see Fig. 9.1).[1,3–5] Drugs that inhibit cholinergic activity, therefore, inhibit aqueous secretion and often cause dry eye signs or symptoms.

Input to the lacrimal nucleus has several sources. The "emotional" center of the frontal cortex, basal ganglion, thalamus, and hypothalamus are all thought to contribute.[4] Irritation of trigeminal nerve endings located in the cornea, conjunctiva, and surface of the face also stimulates reflex tearing.[1,5] In addition, stimulation of the retina by bright light can cause reflex tearing.[5]

Perhaps more important to maintenance of the tear film

and ocular surface integrity are the basic secretors. The three-layer tear film has numerous contributors (Fig. 25.2). The sebaceous meibomian glands of the lids produce the outermost oily or lipid layer. They are located in the tarsus of both the upper and lower eyelids. The glands of Zeis at the palpebral margin of each eyelid and the glands of Moll at the roots of the eyelashes also contribute to this layer. The oily secretions thicken, stabilize, and prevent premature evaporation of the underlying aqueous layer of the tear film.[1,2,5]

The accessory lacrimal glands of Krause and Wolfring are primarily responsible for producing the intermediate, or middle, layer of the tear film. Most of the glands of Krause are located in the superior conjunctival fornix, but a few can

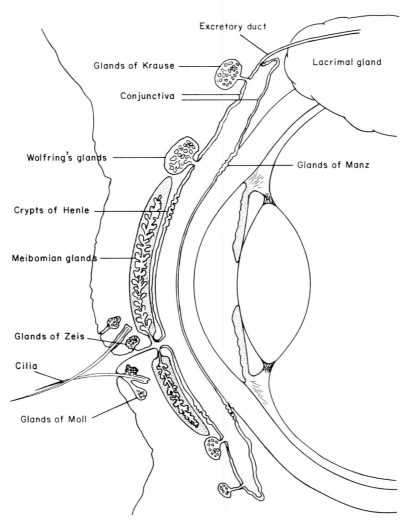

FIGURE 25.2   **Cross-section of the lacrimal secretory system. See text for products of the labelled basal secretors. (Adapted from Botelho SY. Tears and the lacrimal gland. Sci Am 1964;211:78–85. Copyright 1964 by Scientific American, Inc. All rights reserved.)**

be found in the lower fornix. The accessory glands of Wolfring are located posterior to the upper margin of the tarsal plate superiorly and inferiorly.[1,3] These exocrine glands form the bulk of the continuous tear film.

Gillette and associates[6] have pointed out the histologic and immunohistologic similarity of main and accessory lacrimal gland tissue. Combined with their finding of myoepithelial cells among accessory lacrimal gland material, these authors believe that some form of autonomic innervation exists to this tissue.[6] These findings may point to a common source of stimulated (reflex) and unstimulated

(continuous) tears. For practical purposes, continuous tears can be thought of as available on an unstimulated (basal) basis.

The inner layer of the tear film contributes greatly to lubrication of the lids and provides an adsorbing site for the aqueous layer of the tear film to the normally hydrophobic corneal epithelium. The inner layer of tear film is a mucoid layer of polysaccharide (sialomucus)[7] derived primarily from the conjunctival goblet cells located in the fornices. Also contributing to this layer are the tarsal crypts of Henle and limbal glands of Manz[1,3] (see Fig. 25.2).

The basic secretors together produce the continuous flow of tears that bathe the globe. They have no confirmed afferent nerve supply, and their output decreases with age. A basic secretory deficit brings about hyposecretion disorders but has never been implicated in true hypersecretion (reflex tearing).[1,5]

Distribution System

The distribution system for the tear film consists of the lids and the tear meniscus along the lid margins in the open eye.[7] The need to renew the tear film caused by its breakup stimulates the blink reflex.[2] Each blink compresses the super-

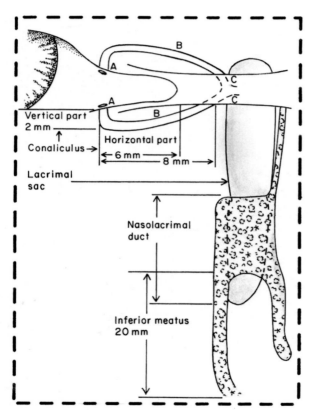

A. PUNCTUM
B. CANALICULUS
C. COMMON CANALICULUS

FIGURE 25.3 **Cut-away view showing the lacrimal excretory system. Tears drain through the punctum and eventually under the inferior turbinate bone of the nose. Dimensions of the canaliculi serve as references for probing and irrigation. (Redrawn with permission from Jones LT. Ophthalmic anatomy: A manual with some clinical applications. I. The orbital adnexa. American Academy of Ophthalmology 1970, 70.)**

ficial lipid layer. The mucous layer acts as a scavenger to pick up any lipid-containing debris and carry it to the fornices. As the eyelid reopens, a new tear-film layer is spread across the ocular surface. Inadequacies of any layer of the tear film increase its instability and may accelerate tear breakup time (TBUT).

The distribution system of the lids also acts as a pumping mechanism to draw tears into the excretory system (see Fig. 25.1). Controversy exists over the exact mechanism for tear fluid dynamics.[2,8–10] It is agreed, however, that the lids direct the lacrimal fluid toward the inner canthi for drainage into the puncta. Whether this mechanism is an active or passive process and whether positive or negative conjunctival pressure propels the tears remain controversial.[1,3,8–10] The most recent endoscopic evidence suggests an active mechanism (negative pressure).[11] The contribution of Daubert and associates[12] supports the contention that the normally functioning lacrimal drainage system is a closed system and re-establishes equilibrium upon occlusion of either punctum.

Excretory System

Blinking is an important factor in tear distribution and also plays a pivotal role in tear drainage.[3,8,10,13] Crucial to proper lacrimal excretory function is the punctum, entry point for lacrimal drainage. Each punctum is located on the posterior eyelid margin at the nasal end of the tarsus about 6 mm from the nasal canthus. Each punctum measures 0.2 to 0.3 mm in diameter and points toward the globe.[3] Proper tear elimination requires that the punctum be apposed to the globe. If it is visible without everting the lid, it is out of position. Should a patient's lower punctum become exposed on upgaze, tear drainage may be adversely affected. Blepharoptosis may cause epiphora. Glatt[14] described a patient whose upper and lower puncta became mutually but reversibly occluded secondary to redundancy of lid tissue.

Anatomically the lacrimal drainage system, except for the punctum, is hidden from direct observation. Understanding its physical characteristics and dimensions is extremely important. Following entry of tears into the punctum, they flow through a 2-mm vertical segment of each canaliculus. Each canaliculus then turns nasalward and runs a horizontal course of approximately 8 mm to reach the lacrimal sac. The lacrimal sac is approximately 12 mm vertically, ballooning above the junction of the superior and inferior canaliculi to form their entrance to the sac, the common canaliculus (Fig. 25.3). The nasolacrimal duct is continuous with the lacrimal sac inferiorly, extends 15 to 20 mm caudalward, narrows, and finally opens into the inferior meatus. Tears are then drained over the nasopharynx and oropharynx to be swallowed.

The drainage pathway may account for up to 90% of the fate of tears. The remainder evaporates. The punctum is essential to proper physiologic drainage of tears.[3,13] Gravita-

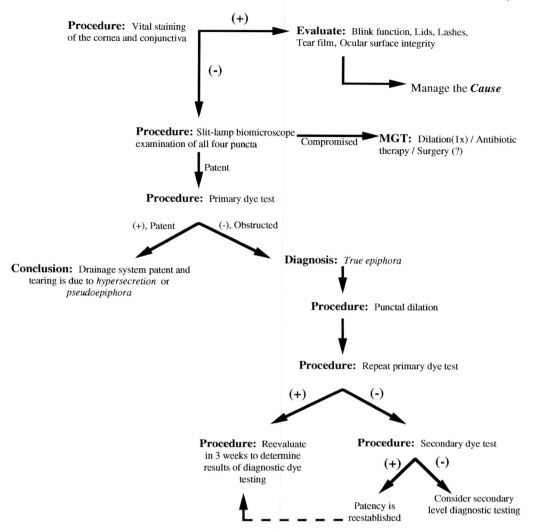

FIGURE 25.4 **A suggested decision-making tree for clinical application to the patient with a complaint of tearing. (Modified from Semes LP. Nasolacrimal testing. In Onofrey BE, ed. Clinical optometric pharmacology and therapeutics. Philadelphia: J.B. Lippincott Company, 1993.)**

tional attraction suggests that the inferior (lower) punctum is the more important in each pair, but a functioning punctum may allow compensatory drainage if the fellow punctum becomes obstructed.[15–17]

General Examination Procedures

Specific examination routines may vary, but the following strategy, with its basis in the anatomic logic of the lacrimal system, can serve as an outline for any patient with a complaint of tearing (Fig. 25.4).

History

A careful patient interview often assists greatly in the diagnosis of lacrimal system disorders before any clinical tests are performed (Table 25.1). McMonnies[18] has proposed a sensitive and specific dry eye questionnaire. The approach discerns information regarding the risk or presence of dry

TABLE 25.1
Subjective Assessment of Lacrimal System Disorders

- Duration and severity (acute, chronic, progressive; seasonal; previous medical or surgical treatment)
- Ocular and visual history
- Systemic health history
- Medication history
- Allergy history
- Occupational or environmental exposures
- Location of tearing (medial/lateral)

eye conditions based on gender and additional information cited in Table 25.1.

Factors such as the patient's sex, age, occupation, and environment may influence differential diagnostic considerations between secretory and excretory abnormalities. For example, infants who present with tearing are more likely to suffer from a drainage problem, while such a "wet" eye in an adult patient whose occupation includes exposure to noxious fumes is likely to be the result of lacrimal gland stimulation. Blink rate decrease, palpebral fissure widening, and increases in ocular surface evaporation have been linked to use of video display terminals.[19]

Pseudoepiphora, resulting from an aqueous deficiency, is most common among postmenopausal women. The dry eye of contact lens wearers may remain sub-clinical and, therefore, asymptomatic for tearing until environmental factors, for example, upset the aqueous equilibrium.

Medications such as anticholinergic agents, antianxiety drugs, and antihistamines can decrease aqueous production and cause a dry eye (see Chap. 37). Patients with obstructed drainage systems may have adapted to carrying a handkerchief or tissue to accommodate the epiphora.

Objective Examination of the Tear Film

Following a comprehensive medical history, the clinician can focus on objective examination of the patient. Physical findings should include fluorescein and rose bengal staining patterns. The presence of fluorescein staining of the cornea or conjunctiva is an indication to examine the blink function, lids, and lashes. Abnormal epithelial cells of the cornea and conjunctiva stain positively with rose bengal dye.[20] Staining in the interpalpebral region (see Fig. 17.11) is generally diagnostic of an aqueous deficiency. Sloughed epithelial cells from the ocular surface do indeed stain with rose bengal, confirming this vital dye's ability to stain dead or devitalized cells. Unfortunately, this explanation fails to account for the presence of intense staining of the ocular surface. Feenstra and Tseng[21] have recently demonstrated the cytotoxic capability of rose bengal as well as its specific-

ity for staining nonmucus-coated epithelial cells. Laroche and Campbell[22] have proposed an elaborate system to quantify rose bengal staining of the exposed ocular surface. They partition the ocular surface into 16 segments and assign a staining score to each. These individual scores are composed of intensity (0–3) as well as area involved (1–100%) within each section.

The diagnosis of lacrimal system disorders begins by observing any staining with sodium fluorescein viewed with cobalt blue light. The presence of fluorescein staining indicates disrupted corneal epithelium.[20] The dye is also used to evaluate tear-film stability when performing the TBUT test.[23] Fluorescein also enhances observation of the tear meniscus, which is reduced in aqueous deficiencies.

The TBUT test quantifies the stability of the pre-corneal tear film using sodium fluorescein as an indicator dye. It must be performed on a cornea that has not been manipulated by earlier tests, including the instillation of a topical anesthetic. A drop of sodium fluorescein is instilled into each inferior cul-de-sac. If a fluorescein strip is used, it should be moistened with saline or irrigating solution rather than more viscous solutions. Increased viscosity may artificially prolong the TBUT and yield misleading results.

The cornea should be scanned under low slit-lamp magnification using cobalt blue light. The patient is instructed to blink once or twice and then stare straight ahead without blinking. The practitioner should note the time it takes for the first randomly formed dry spot to appear (Fig. 25.5). A clinical measurement of 10 seconds or less is consistent with the diagnosis of dry eye.[23] It is important to note that a decreased TBUT finding indicates only tear film instability, not whether the deficiency is mucin or aqueous.[24]

A more sophisticated tear film integrity test is the noninvasive breakup time (NIBUT). This assessment, which is slowly gaining acceptance, involves projecting a fine grid onto the corneal surface and observing the first disruption of the pattern.[25] The normal value for NIBUT may be as long as 40 sec. The practitioner, therefore, needs to specify the method of tear film stability testing.

Recent evidence confirms that preservatives in tear supplements can disrupt the corneal epithelial barrier.[26,27] Use of such products may, therefore, contaminate the results of the tear film stability tests. Factors affecting tear film stability measurements include age,[28] blink rate[29] and tear production,[29,30] and the location on the cornea of the tear film disruption.[31]

Absent from our approach to the evaluation of the lacrimal system is the Schirmer test. Because there is considerable controversy regarding its reliability,[32–36] a review of the components of Schirmer's[37] original strategy will be given with a perspective on its current clinical use.[38,39]

The Schirmer I or "routine" Schirmer test is performed without topical anesthesia. A piece of Whatman No. 41 filter paper is cut into a strip 5 mm X 50 mm, folded, and inserted into the inferior conjunctival fornix about one-third of the

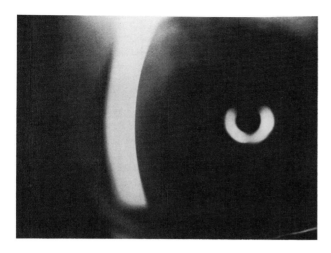

A

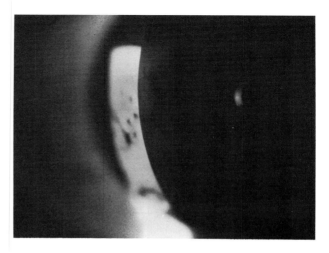

B

FIGURE 25.5   **Tear breakup time (TBUT) test.** *(A)* **Immediately following several complete blinks, there is homogeneous tear film stained with sodium fluorescein.** *(B)* **Randomly formed dry spot signals conclusion of the test and indicates instability of the tear film.**

way from the lateral canthus. The patient is instructed to look slightly above the horizon at a distance. After 5 minutes, the strip is removed, and the extent of wetting from the fold is measured (Fig. 25.6). Some observers obtain useful results under consistently applied conditions. In 1972, a 1-minute variation was shown to be equivalent to the 5-minute test when the amount of wetting was multiplied by 3.[16] Milder[40] suggests that the test be performed simultaneously in both eyes.

The practical clinical information obtained from the Schirmer I test appears to be the confirmation of hyposecretion when less than 5 mm of strip wetting occurs. Greater than 15 mm wetting could indicate decreased, normal, or increased compensatory (reflex) secretion.

When more than 15 mm wetting occurs, the practitioner should differentiate the "basic" from "reflex" contributions to the tear film. Using a topical anesthetic before performing the basic secretion test can eliminate reflex secretion, which can occur secondary to a variety of stimuli. Any residual anesthetic should be wiped from the conjunctival sac using a dry sterile cotton-tipped applicator. When a fresh Schirmer strip is inserted following application of topical anesthetic, the difference between the Schirmer I value and basic secretion test value represents the reflex portion of the tear film.

Less than 5 mm of wetting on the basic secretion test ensures a diagnosis of hyposecretion. Whether this results from an actual deficiency of basic tear-film secretion or "peripheral sensory fatigue block" can be determined using the Schirmer II test. Jones[1,3] proposed that decreased sensory input to the lacrimal nucleus results in the absence of reflex secretion. The Schirmer II test is qualitative and is per-

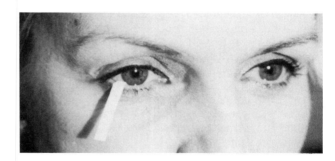

FIGURE 25.6   **Position of filter-paper strip for Schirmer testing. Note that the strip is placed over the lid near the lateral canthus and away from the more sensitive cornea.**

formed immediately following a low value on the basic secretion test. With the same strip in place, mechanical or chemical irritation of the nasal mucosa is carried out. Increased wetting is testimony to integrity of the efferent reflex pathway (peripheral sensory fatigue block[1,3]), while no increase in wetting implies a fault of the reflex secretors.[1,3,40,41] Tsubota[42] has emphasized the importance of nasal stimulation (Schirmer II test) in dry eye patients. He uses this test diagnostically to distinguish Sjögren syndrome dry eye from keratoconjunctivitis sicca (KCS). Lacrimal gland lymphocytic infiltration among Sjögren patients prevents increased reflex tearing, whereas competent lacrimal gland tissue in simple KCS allows tearing provoked by nasal irritation.

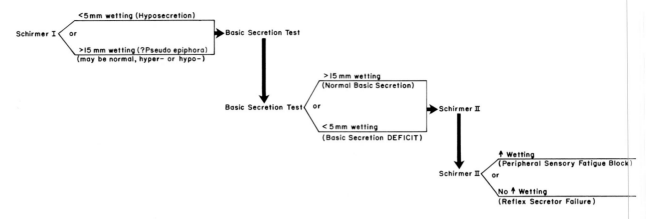

FIGURE 25.7 **Flowchart for Schirmer tests. Complete Schirmer testing includes performing the Schirmer I, basic secretion, and Schirmer II tests sequentially. A small amount of wetting on the Schirmer I test confirms [HYPOSECRETION]; greater than 15 mm wetting is inconclusive. [NORMAL BASIC SECRETION] is indicated by > 15 mm wetting in the basic secretion test (BST). When fewer than 5 mm of the strip is wet on the BST, [BASIC SECRETION DEFICIT] is indicated. The Schirmer II test is now performed to differentiate between [PERIPHERAL SENSORY FATIGUE BLOCK] and [REFLEX SECRETOR FAILURE or LACRIMAL GLAND INFILTRATION].**

Figure 25.7 summarizes the Schirmer test sequence. The objective of Schirmer's tests is the evaluation of tear secretion, but dye tests (sodium fluorescein and rose bengal) can probably evaluate this function more reliably.

Another test available to the clinician is quantitative lysozyme assay.[43] Tear lysozyme level is a useful measure of aqueous tear secretion, since lysozyme constitutes nearly one-fourth of total tear protein. Lysozyme levels are reduced by dilution in hypersecretion and are also reduced in such aqueous-deficient conditions as Sjögren syndrome. The basis for the test is inhibition of bacterial growth using *Micrococcus lysodeikticus*.

Lysozyme concentration in tears has been measured clinically by spectrophotometric[43] and microdiffusion[44] methods. Of these techniques, the immunologic microdiffusion procedure appears to be more applicable to office use.

An alternative to lysozyme assay (which may require sophisticated laboratory facilities) for lacrimal gland function is the measurement of lactoferrin concentration in tears. A clinical comparison between lysozyme and lactoferrin assays among both control and dry eye patients gave consistent results.[28] The strength of lactoferrin measurement lies in its ease of use in the office environment. The commercial version of the test was marketed as Lactoplate (Eagle Vision, Inc., Memphis, TN) (Fig. 25.8) but is no longer available. Contemporary lactoferrin assay may be accomplished using an ELISA-based test requiring only 10 to 15 minutes.[203]

Another sophisticated diagnostic strategy for confirming dry eye is the use of cellulose acetate impressions to investigate ocular surface integrity. Conjunctival impression "cy-tology" is performed to determine goblet-cell density of the bulbar or palpebral conjunctival surface. A strip of commercially available filter paper (MF Millipore Filter VS) is gently pressed against the bulbar or palpebral conjunctiva with a glass rod.[46] Nelson and associates[46] prefer the rougher (versus smooth) side of the paper as the more useful in obtaining specimens. Following staining with Schiff's reagent and counterstaining with hematoxylin, the specimens are graded using a microscope. An alternative stain is Papanicolaou. The results of studies of normal and "dry" eyes (keratoconjunctivitis sicca, ocular pemphigoid, Stevens-Johnson syndrome) indicate normal or decreased goblet-cell counts, respectively.[46,47] Impression cytology has also been applied in monitoring vitamin A deficiency.[48]

Clinical analysis of the tear film has become increasingly sophisticated. Individual test results as well as the findings from a constellation of tests are applied to classify and characterize dry eyes.[21,22,25,49–65] While tear osmolarity measurements may demonstrate the highest positive predictive value among dry eye patients,[51] the dry eye "profile" may be characterized best by results from a battery of tests. Of the noninvasive tests that histologically characterize the ocular surface, cellulose acetate impression cytology may prove the most useful.[155] In fact, Rivas and associates[66] contend that rose bengal and impression cytology are the most sensitive and specific tests for the diagnosis of primary Sjögren syndrome. Lemp,[64] however, uses the results from a group of tests to gauge severity of dry eye and to develop a basis for treatment. The normal values for tear function tests may vary greatly. Table 25.2 lists normal values.

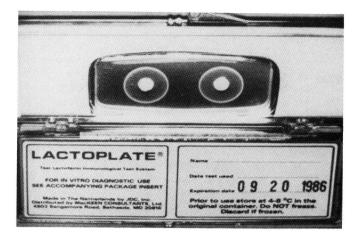

Blink, Lid, and Lash Disorders

Since the lids represent the distribution system for lacrimal fluids, their neural, muscular, and structural components must remain intact for proper maintenance of the tear film. Incomplete or twitch blinking may pose a problem to contact lens wearers or patients with marginal (subclinical) dry eye. Nocturnal lagophthalmos can result in exposure keratitis with characteristic inferior corneal staining observable with sodium fluorescein. Decreased tear osmolarity together with decreased tear volume during sleep may explain the tendency for soft contact lenses to adhere to the corneal surface during overnight wear and may represent the mechanism of recurrent corneal erosion formation.[76]

The seventh cranial nerve is responsible for lid closure during the blink reflex. Bell's palsy can interrupt these impulses, resulting in exposure keratitis. Loss of muscular tone can lead to ectropion, disrupt the "lacrimal pump," and result in impaired tear drainage.

Lid margins are normally smooth and regular. Inflammatory conditions and trauma can distort the lid margins, with potential for disrupted flow of tear film. Blepharoptosis may

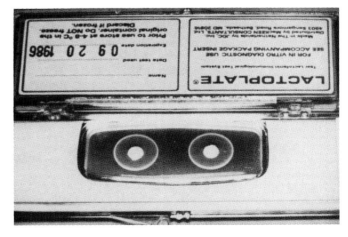

FIGURE 25.8 Lactoferrin immunologic test system (Lactoplate). A tear sample is collected on a filter paper disc and transferred to reagent gel (shown). The results are read after three days of incubation (diffusion) at room temperature. (Courtesy Eagle Vision, Inc., Memphis, TN.)

TABLE 25.2
Tear Function Tests and Normal Values

Test	Significance	Normal Values
Tear meniscus[67]	Aqueous quantity	Range: 0.1–0.6 mm
Schirmer's no. 1[41]	No diagnostic value	>15 mm in 5 min
Basic secretion test	Aqueous deficiency when reduced	>5 mm in 5 min
aLactoferrin[45]	Lacrimal gland function	1.42 mg/mL (<1.00 mg/mL is abnormal)
aTear osmolarity[68]	Lacrimal gland function	>312 mOsm/L
Breakup time (BUT)[23,24]	Tear film stability/mucus deficiency	>10 sec
Noninvasive break-up time (NIBUT)[69]	Microepithelial defects/aqueous adequacy	40 sec
Fluorescein staining[20,70]	Microepithelial defects/mucus deficiency	None visible
aRose bengal staining[41,70,71]	Non-mucus coated epithelium	None visible
aImpression cytology[72]	Epithelial cell appearance/goblet cell density	Normal microscopic appearance
aInterference fringe pattern[23]	Lipid layer integrity	Uniform biomicroscopic appearance
aMeibomian gland expression[74]	Meibomian gland function	Clear
aLysozyme[75]	Lacrimal gland function	TLR <1.0

aAlthough not currently employed in routine clinical practice, these tests have received attention alone as well as in concert with other findings in the diagnosis and management of dry eye states.

Adapted from Semes LP. Keratoconjunctivitis sicca and dry eye. In: Silbert JA, ed. Anterior segment complications of contact lens wear. New York: Churchill Livingstone, 1994.

lead to epiphora.[14] An inturned lash (trichiasis) or blepharitis can disturb the tear film or irritate the cornea to cause physical signs of fluorescein staining and tearing along with symptoms of irritation. Hom and Silverman[77] have recommended a specific evaluation of the meibomian glands of the lids. Expression of the meibomian glands should yield clear fluid; production of cloudy material may indicate dysfunction. Chapter 24 considers lid abnormalities in further detail.

Dacryoadenitis

Etiology

Acute inflammation of the lacrimal gland may accompany local or systemic viral or bacterial infection or be secondary to trauma.[78]

Diagnosis

Pathologic enlargement of the lacrimal gland is characterized by swelling in the temporal one-third to one-half of the upper lid. Milder[78] calls attention to the S curve of the upper lid in lacrimal gland disorders, since it is diagnostic for lacrimal gland disease and is unique among lid abnormalities (Fig. 25.9). Tumors of the lacrimal gland are relatively rare but should be differentiated histopathologically and distinguished clinically from inflammatory disorders of the lacrimal gland.[79-81]

Painless swelling without inflammation in the region should suggest benign mixed tumor (pleomorphic adenoma), while acute onset and pain suggest malignant tumors (carcinoma). Computed tomography following plain x-ray films can be useful in the differential diagnosis of lacrimal gland lesions.[78,82] The role of magnetic resonance imaging (MRI) studies in pre-operative differentiation of benign mixed tumors from carcinoma has yet to be established.[82] Pain or tenderness suggests an acute inflammatory process. Table 25.3 summarizes clinical signs in dacryoadenitis.

Acute dacryoadenitis is an inflammatory process of the lacrimal gland generally seen in infants or children.[82] Aside from age, clinical characteristics include unilateral local tenderness, redness, lid swelling, conjunctival chemosis, discharge or suppuration, and enlarged preauricular nodes.[81,82]

Management

Acute dacryoadenitis usually responds rapidly to systemic corticosteroids.[82] Viral dacryoadenitis associated with acute epidemic parotitis (mumps), infectious mononucleosis, or herpes zoster infection should receive supportive therapy.[79,81] Supportive therapy for mumps should be continued for its typical 2- to 4-week self-limiting course[78] and may take the form of rest, local application of ice, and use of oral analgesics such as acetaminophen.

Bacterial dacryoadenitis should be treated with specific antibiotics following culture and sensitivity testing.[78,79] Broad-spectrum coverage is offered by a combination of gentamicin, 4 mg/kg body weight daily intramuscularly in three divided doses, and a cephalosporin, such as cefazolin, 1 g every 4 hours intravenously with probenecid, 0.5 g orally four times daily.[78] This regimen should be followed for 7 days. Gonorrheal dacryoadenitis is treated with penicillin administered intramuscularly or tetracycline taken orally.[78] Persistent enlargement of the lacrimal gland, when tumor has been ruled out, generally represents chronic dacryoade-

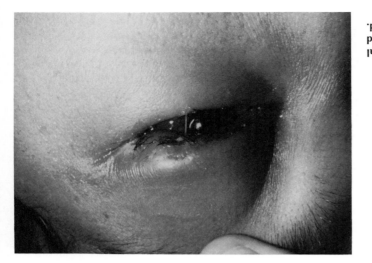

FIGURE 25.9 Dacryoadenitis. Inflammation of the lacrimal gland is characterized by swelling of the superolateral lid and adnexal tissue and the diagnostic S curve of the upper lid. (Courtesy Michael A. Callahan, M.D.)

TABLE 25.3
Clinical Signs in Dacryoadenitis[78–82]

Consistent in All	Associated with Acute Cases or Suggestive of Tumor
Superolateral swelling	Local tenderness
S curve of upper lid	Discharge
	Proptosis
	Diplopia

TABLE 25.5
Differential Diagnosis in Dacryoadenitis[78,79,82]

- Dermoids, dermoid cysts
- Congenital cysts
- Dacryops (lacrimal gland cysts)
- Pseudotumor of lacrimal gland
- Tumor
    Benign mixed (pleomorphic adenoma)
    Malignant (carcinoma)

nitis.[78,79] Biopsy may be necessary when the episode does not follow sarcoidosis, tuberculosis, Graves' ophthalmopathy, Mikulicz syndrome, "sclerosing pseudotumors," or Wegener's granulomatosis.[82] Table 25.4 lists systemic conditions that have been associated with chronic dacryoadenitis. Histopathology studies contribute to the differential diagnosis (Table 25.5).[78,82] Indeed, MacLean and associates[83] have recently emphasized the usefulness of histopathologic investigations in differentiating Mikulicz syndrome from Mikulicz disease. They suggest replacement of the eponymous Mikulicz disease with the more descriptive "benign lymphoepithelial lesion."

Disorders of the Tear Film

Holly and Lemp[2] have arranged tear film abnormalities into five different categories according to physiologic considerations (Table 25.6). This classification is useful for patient management once appropriate examination procedures have led to an accurate diagnosis.

Aqueous Deficiency

ETIOLOGY

The basic secretors decrease their aqueous production with advancing age. Thinning of this, the thickest, segment of the precorneal tear film results in premature contamination of the mucin layer of the tear film and is observed clinically as a rapid TBUT.[23]

Lack of aqueous production at birth is a disorder termed congenital alacrima.[84] This rare condition may result from hypoplasia of lacrimal gland tissue or congenital paresis of cranial nerves.[2] Another congenital and equally rare cause of aqueous deficiency is familial dysautonomia (Riley-Day syndrome),[85] a disorder associated with a short lifespan.

Considerably more common is the aqueous deficiency seen among adults during the fifth and sixth decades of life. Keratoconjunctivitis sicca (KCS) occurs in a disproportionate ratio of women to men (9:1). It has a gradual onset with periods of exacerbation that may be heightened by decreases in ambient humidity. The following discussion will consider only the acquired aqueous deficiencies.

DIAGNOSIS

Symptoms of KCS may include burning, foreign-body sensation, and scratchiness. These symptoms tend to increase in severity during the course of the day. Due to the thinned aqueous, lipid-contaminated mucous strands collect in the fornices.[2] Patients may also complain of increased "mattering" associated with the presence of dried mucus at the nasal canthus on arising. The irritation accompanying the disorder itself combined with excess mucus may prompt the patient

TABLE 25.4
Systemic Conditions Associated with Chronic Dacryoadenitis[78,79,82]

- Sarcoidosis
- Tuberculosis
- Thyroid ophthalmopathy
- Sclerosing pseudotumors
- Wegener's granulomatosis

TABLE 25.6
Tear Film Abnormalities

Disorder	Example
Aqueous deficiency	Keratoconjunctivitis sicca
Mucin deficiency	Cicatricial pemphigoid
Lipid abnormality	Secondary to chronic blepharitis
Impaired lid function	Exposure keratitis secondary to Bell's palsy
Epitheliopathy	Microepithelial irregularity

Adapted from Holly FJ, Lemp MA. Tear physiology and dry eyes. Surv Ophthalmol 1977;22:69–87.

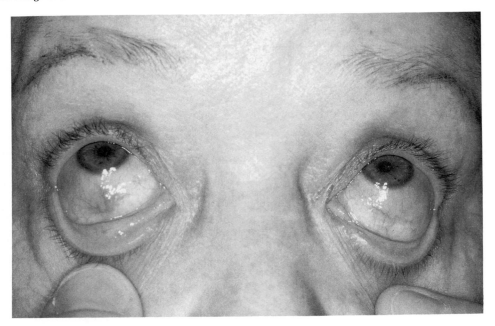

FIGURE 25.10   **Mucus fishing syndrome. Rose bengal staining on the inferior bulbar conjunctiva instead of the expected interpalpebral location. (Courtesy Jimmy D. Bartlett, O.D.)**

to manually attempt to remove the strands. The resulting mechanical irritation can cause further irritation and tearing. This vicious cycle, termed the *mucus fishing syndrome,* is characterized by rose bengal staining of the affected bulbar conjunctiva and cornea[86] (Fig. 25.10).

Clinical signs can include the observation of increased debris in the tear film (due to an increased desquamation rate of the epithelial cells),[2] reduced marginal tear strip, increased mucous strands, rose bengal staining of bulbar conjunctiva or cornea (see Fig. 17.11),[20] filamentary keratitis, reduced TBUT, and corneal staining with sodium fluorescein.[87]

Simple clinical observation and physical findings combined with the history generally confirm the diagnosis. Sophisticated procedures such as tear protein determination are rarely necessary to begin treatment but may be helpful in the early identification of the patient with KCS.[87]

No single disorder causes as much diagnostic confusion and management frustration as Sjögren syndrome. "Primary Sjögren syndrome" (SS) applies to patients manifesting dry eyes (keratoconjunctivitis sicca, KCS) and dry mouth (xerostomia). Additional systemic involvement has been classified as secondary Sjögren syndrome. The most frequently associated systemic disorder is rheumatoid arthritis. The most prevalent ocular manifestation of SS is keratoconjunctivitis sicca (KCS). Due to selective lacrimal and salivary gland involvement, the term *autoimmune exocrineopathy* has been suggested as a synonym for SS.[88]

Because of reduced aqueous volume and concomitant decrease in defensive proteins (lactoferrin, lysozyme, and certain immunoglobulins), a causal relationship may exist between co-existing lid infection among aqueous deficient patients and marked prevalence of blepharitis or conjunctivitis. McGill and associates,[89] however, were unable to document any increase in the aqueous levels of lactoferrin or lysozyme in the presence of supervening infection, suggesting that dry eye patients are unresponsive or underresponsive to such infection. Due to ocular surface compromise, practitioners must exercise continued vigilance for signs and symptoms of infection.

Punctate inferior corneal staining may be potentiated by toxins produced by staphylococcal organisms. Yet McGill and associates [89] could not demonstrate an increase in bacterial population among either blepharitis or dry eye patients with infection. This finding led them to conclude that squamous blepharitis is a sterile condition and that the inferior staining pattern evolves from an alteration of the lid-tear film interface. Tears are not retained, volume drops, and interpalpebral desiccation occurs. The clinical observation of KCS in the presence of a normal tear film supports this concept.

MANAGEMENT

Tear substitutes have been the mainstay of treatment for aqueous-deficient dry eye. The patient generally starts on a regimen of artificial tear solutions 4 to 8 times per day along with the application of a bland ophthalmic ointment at bedtime. Although rare, some artificial tear solutions may contain viscosity-enhancing components (substituted cellulose ethers) that tend to precipitate out of solution and cause crust to form on the eyelids.[90] An alternative approach to the formulation of tear replacements is to substitute polymers (e.g., polyvinyl alcohol) for the cellulose compounds. The treatment strategy, in either case, is to enhance contact time to preserve the scanty aqueous secretion.

Since instability of the tear film represents a keystone in the development of ocular surface disorders and management plans usually include the application of tear supplements to enhance volume or integrity of the tear film, the toxicity of preservatives must not be overlooked. Benzalkonium chloride (BAK) is an effective preservative for ophthalmic solutions, but it can reduce tear breakup time.[91,92] Nonpreserved solutions, however, have been shown in animal studies to be detrimental to the corneal surface.[26,27] Finally, Caffery and Josephson[92a] have demonstrated a subjective preference for non-preserved tear supplements among a group of soft contact lens wearers.

A more significant consequence associated with an unstable tear film may be persistent dry spots. This pattern of persistent dry spots may be associated with abnormalities of the distribution system or reduced tear flow and can in some cases be alleviated by repeated blinking.[92]

One novel formulation in the artificial tear armamentarium is the incorporation of a solubilized lipid component.[93] Since this solution (Tear Gard, Med Tech) has purportedly

been designed to supplement each component of the tear film—lipid, aqueous, and mucin—some believe it to be the ideal physiologic tear replacement. LaMotte and Lesher,[93] however, have reported a slightly negative response by patients due to the increased viscosity the lipid imparts. The transient blurring of vision is often seen as a trade-off for subjective benefits.

The use of a soft contact lens with frequent instillation of saline or artificial tear solution constitutes another level of dry eye treatment. A low-water contact lens is preferred.[94,95] Although agreement is not uniform, such a strategy may prove most useful in treating abnormalities of the tear film, especially those resulting in recurrent corneal erosion.[96]

Another approach to the management of patients with aqueous deficiency and excessive mucous filaments is the topical application of mucolytic agents such as n-acetylcysteine (Mucomyst, Mead Johnson). Initially intended for asthmatics, n-acetylcysteine can be diluted with artificial tears to 2% to 10% concentration for lysing mucous strands in the fornices.[97] However, because this agent has not been FDA-approved for use in the eye, it is not widely employed.

SPECIFIC MANAGEMENT STRATEGIES FOR KERATOCONJUNCTIVITIS SICCA

Traditional approaches to the effects of ocular surface drying consist of volume-enhancing measures or contact-enhancing agents. Few, if any, consistent strategies have emerged to guide the clinician in the management of patients with dry eyes or ocular surface disorders. One staging system,[64] based on severity as measured by four diagnostic tests, advocates tear supplements up to four times daily and lubricating ointments at bedtime (Grade I). Moderate (Grade II) dry eyes would require the addition of sustained release tear inserts or mucolytic agents (Mucomyst, Mead-Johnson). Severe (Grade III) disease may be managed with lacrimal occlusion,[98] bandage contact lenses, estrogen supplementation or moisture chambers.[64] Severe conditions may respond to nonpreserved cellulose compounds or topical bicarbonate-containing supplements.[92] Table 25.7 suggests a stepped-care treatment regimen.

Tear conservation strategies may include moisture-chamber spectacles or lacrimal occlusion (Fig. 25.11). In 1974 Freeman[99] introduced a removable silicone punctal plug. He reported a 50% to 75% subjective success rate in a non-masked clinical trial. Willis and associates[100] evaluated objectively 18 dry eye patients with at least 8 months follow-up after placement of a plug. Decreases in rose bengal and fluorescein staining as well as enhancement of Schirmer values were noted. Interestingly, at 6 week evaluation no changes in conjunctival impression cytology were observed from baseline. Semes and Herrick[101] reported the 6-month follow-up of a patient treated with intracanalicular inserts (Lacrimedics, Inc., Rialto, CA). This Sjögren syndrome patient demonstrated considerable improvement in subjec-

TABLE 25.7
Stepped Primary Care Treatment of Keratoconjunctivitis Sicca

Stage 1 (mild)
- Preserved tear supplements up to qid
- Nonpreserved ointment q hs

Stage 2 (moderate)
- Nonpreserved tear supplements prn
- Nonpreserved ointment q hs
- Sustained-release/prolonged-contact tear supplements qid
- Bicarbonate ion-containing tear supplements prn
- Mucolytic agents

Stage 3 (severe)
- Lacrimal occlusion
- Bandage hydrogel contact lenses
- Moisture chamber spectacles
- Nonpreserved cellulose ether-based tear supplements prn
- Bicarbonate ion-containing tear supplements prn
- Consider secondary level care

Adapted from Lemp MA. General measures in the management of dry eye. Int Ophthalmol Clin 1987;27:36–43; Dohlman CH. Punctal occlusion in keratoconjunctivitis sicca. Trans Am Acad Ophthalmol Otolaryngol 1978;88:1277–1281; Brown SI. Dry spots and corneal erosions. Int Ophthalmol Clin 1973;13:149–156.

tive symptoms as well as fluorescein and rose bengal staining. The use of dissolvable collagen implants (Fig. 25.12) may be helpful diagnostically to predict whether permanent punctal or canalicular occlusion may be effective.

Benson and associates[102] studied the efficacy of argon laser punctal occlusion among 22 patients. They discovered that 19 of 22 (86%) puncta had become patent within 16 months.

Methods other than traditional tear supplementation and conservation measures have been described. LaMotte and associates[103] found no difference in TBUT between topically applied tear supplements and continuously supplied hydroxypropyl cellulose (Lacrisert). Leibowitz and associates[104] reported improvement in objective signs (tear wedge, fluorescein staining) as well as decreased symptoms in response to a long-lasting gel. Gilbard and Kenyon[105] instilled hypotonic saline solutions to determine their effect on lowering tear osmolarity. The hypoosmolar effect lasted a maximum of only 40 minutes following instillation, but rose bengal staining scores improved. Both subjective and objective improvement followed use of extemporaneously prepared viscoelastic materials.[106,109]

The promise of systemic agents to enhance tearing has been reported. Bromhexine decreases symptoms and improves objective dry-eye signs in the treatment of Sjögren syndrome.[110,111]

Since the initial reports of a retinoid ointment in managing severe ocular surface disorders, attention has focused on the use of vitamin A and its structural analogs. Tseng and associates[112] studied 22 selected patients with severe dry eyes. They administered 0.01% or 0.1% all-trans retinoic acid in an ointment formulation and observed clinical improvement in symptoms, visual acuity, rose bengal staining, or Schirmer tests. Moreover, impression cytology documented reversal of squamous metaplasia. These investigators hailed their results as the first nonsurgical attempt to reverse diseased ocular surface epithelium. The postulated mechanism was increased circulation at the conjunctival level.

Using similar compounds, Soong and associates[113] found reversal of conjunctival keratinization but reported little benefit in KCS. Gilbard and associates[114] confirmed these results by determining that 0.01% vitamin A ointment was no more effective than placebo in increasing tear secretion as indicated by the Schirmer test (basic secretion test), tear osmolarity, or in decreasing ocular surface disease as evidenced by the rose bengal score. Interestingly, of the 11 patients studied, seven preferred placebo, two expressed a preference for vitamin A ointment, and the remaining two subjects offered no preference.

Animal studies suggest an immunologic approach to lacrimal gland dysfunction. Topical cyclosporine enhanced tear flow among a group of beagles serving as the animal model for KCS.[115] Subsequently, Laibovitz and associates[116] reported a small series of patients for whom cyclosporine 1%

ophthalmic ointment appeared to benefit the ocular surface in keratoconjunctivitis sicca.

Topical fibronectin,[117] an adhesive glycoprotein, was evaluated with artificial tears for the treatment of KCS. A controlled double-masked clinical trial, comprising 272 patients who were monitored for over two months, failed to demonstrate any statistically significant differences in improvement compared to placebo as measured by self-evaluation of symptoms, rose bengal and fluorescein staining, TBUT, Schirmer testing, and conjunctival impression cytology.

A gastric mucosa protectant, sodium sucrose-sulfate, was evaluated in a group of 22 patients with primary Sjögren syndrome. During 6 months of treatment, statistically significant improvement occurred in rose bengal scores.[118] Although the study used no controls, sucralfate may show promise as a new adsorptive agent for the compromised ocular surface.

Nonpharmacologic methods of treating dry eyes may include the use of home humidifiers or local means of decreasing evaporation of tears. Osmotic infusion pumps and constant flow devices have been proposed and prototypes developed. These, however, remain unpopular.

Mucin Deficiency

ETIOLOGY

The conjunctival mucin produced by goblet cells maintains wettability of the corneal and conjunctival epithelium. Insta-

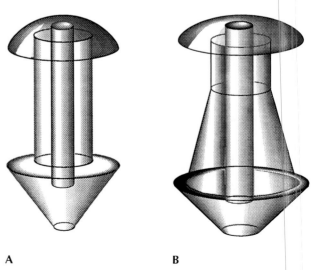

A   **B**

FIGURE 25.11 **Silicone punctal plugs and intracanalicular insert. (A) Original Freeman punctal plug. (B) Tapered-shaft punctal plug (Eagle Vision). (C) Herrick intracanalicular implant (arrow). (D) Schematic insertion of punctal plug. (E) Schematic insertion of intracanalicular implant. (Figure D courtesy Eagle Vision, Inc.; Figures C and E courtesy Lacrimedics, Inc.)**

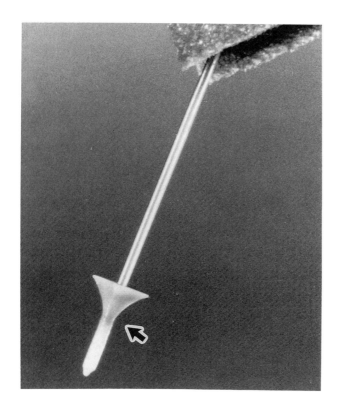

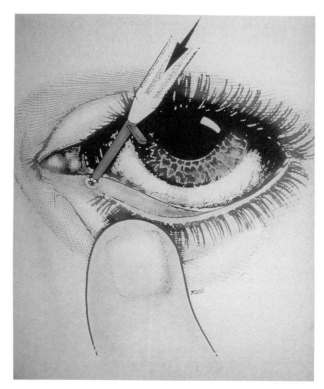

C

D

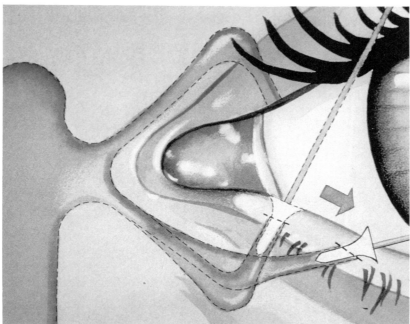

E

FIGURE 25.11   (continued)

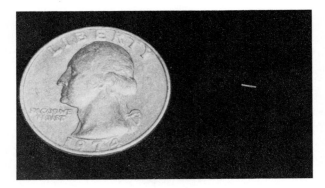

A

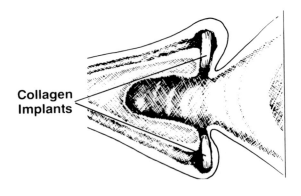

**Collagen
Implants**

B

FIGURE 25.12 **Temporary intracanalicular collagen implants.**
(A) **Photograph illustrating a single implant compared with a U.S.**
quarter dollar. *(B)* **Temporary intracanalicular insert in place.**
(Figure B courtesy Eagle Vision, Inc., Memphis, TN.)

TABLE 25.8
Etiology of Mucin Deficiency[119-123]

Conjunctival destruction (mechanical)
   Ocular cicatricial pemphigoid (OCP)
   Erythema multiforme major (EM); Stevens-Johnson syndrome
   Toxic etiologies
     Chemical burns, irradiation
     Drug-induced (pseudopemphigoid)
       Echothiophate iodide
       Pilocarpine
       Epinephrine
       Systemic practolol
       Topical timolol
Avitaminosis A

has an autoimmune etiology. Support for this concept
comes from a report of 10 patients with pseudopemphigoid[125] (OCP associated with ocular drug administration).
All patients had clinically proven OCP that responded
positively to immunosuppressive therapy.[125] Stevens-Johnson syndrome (erythema multiforme major) manifests similar clinical signs but occurs as acute recurrent episodes
without the chronic relentless progression of OCP.[126]
Thoft[127] argues that ocular surface disorders such as OCP
and Stevens-Johnson syndrome manifest aqueous *and* mucin deficiencies secondary to pathologic changes of the
corneal and conjunctival surface epithelium. For this reason, OCP represents the diagnostic and treatment prototype
for the mechanical forms of mucin deficiency secondary to
conjunctival shrinkage.

DIAGNOSIS

Cicatricial pemphigoid (benign mucosal pemphigoid) is a
subepithelial bullous disease of the aged. It affects the skin
and mucous membranes, leading to shrinkage, scarring, and
adhesions. In the conjunctiva, scar tissue (cicatrization) replaces normal tissue. The prevalence is low (1 in 20,000
ophthalmic patients), with women affected in a 7:3 ratio to
men. The average age at presentation is over 60 years, and
the condition shows no racial predilection.[121]

History of trauma combined with the observation of
persistent dry spots on the cornea should alert the clinician to
consider the possibility of early mucin deficiency. Persistent
dry spots appear as areas of nonwetting or areas of recurrent
tear-film breakup. The loss of corneal surfacing by mucus
causes this clinical picture. Patients with AIDS may have
greater susceptibility to such surface changes.[128]

OCP may begin with typical dry eye complaints in an
elderly patient. The progressive submucosal shrinkage can
also involve the lacrimal and accessory lacrimal gland ducts,
contributing to aqueous deficiency.[129]

Continued progression of conjunctival shrinkage and

bility of the tear film due to mucin deficiency results from
goblet-cell dysfunction. The causes of goblet-cell destruction vary from vitamin A deficiency to direct conjunctival
trauma (chemical burns, radiation) or disease. Table 25.8
lists etiologies of mucin deficiency.[119,120]

Traumatic destruction of conjunctival architecture is generalized; fibrous tissue replaces normal conjunctiva. In contrast, destruction in cases of avitaminosis A appears more
specific. The microcirculation supporting the goblet cells is
lost in this vitamin deficiency, resulting in keratinization.[119,124]

Ocular cicatricial pemphigoid (OCP), a chronic inflammatory disease that can affect the conjunctiva, presumably

scarring can lead to symblepharon formation (Fig. 25.13) with entropion and trichiasis, lagophthalmos and exposure keratitis, and inability to elevate the eyes. Keratinization involving the cornea (see Fig. 26.24) results in decreased visual acuity. Other ocular complications include corneal erosion, corneal neovascularization, and pseudopterygia.[129]

The differential diagnoses of OCP are few. Conjunctival shrinkage and scarring secondary to membranous conjunctivitis of viral etiology (adenovirus types 8 and 9, primary herpetic keratoconjunctivitis) or infection with β-hemolytic *Streptococcus* are acute and self-limiting, in contrast to the chronic and progressive nature of the conjunctival shrinkage in OCP.

MANAGEMENT

As in any tear-film deficiency, treatment of mucin-deficient dry eye with tear supplements plays a major therapeutic role. The strategy involves keeping the patient comfortable rather than attempting to arrest progression of the disorder. Frequent application of tear supplements during the waking hours combined with bland ointment at bedtime may prove useful in early stages or in mild cases. If only clinical signs are present (persistent dry spots) but the patient is asymptomatic, the patient can apply tear supplements 4 times daily in addition to bland ointment at bedtime. This approach is often effective in mild cases. The ointment apparently has a salubrious effect on the corneal epithelium during sleep, and with continuation of the regimen some patients may show reversal of the clinical signs of corneal drying.

Lemp theorizes that mucin deficiency may be the basis for dellen formation.[130] Management may include application of nonpreserved tear supplements, the frequency of application varying with the severity of the clinical signs and symptoms.

In disorders of the mucous membranes with conjunctival shortening secondary to cicatrization, the therapeutic regimen may include topical steroids.[131] Mondino[121] cites the potential for recurrent corneal erosion among patients with OCP. As with other erosive disorders, soft contact lenses may be used judiciously in the management of this complication.[121,132] Because of the increased risk of infection, mucosal scarring disorders may respond better to the limited and indicated use of topical antibiotics rather than to prophylactic antibiotics.[132]

Several investigators have reported the efficacy of oral vitamin A in mucin-deficient dry eyes. Sullivan and associates[133] offered two case reports that illustrate the return of goblet cells following vitamin A therapy. Both alcoholic patients in this series were placed on a 3-week regimen of 25,000 units of oral vitamin A (form not reported). Improvement in goblet cell count and conjunctival appearance occurred, as well as a decrease in keratinization. Singer and associates[134] reported a single case of regeneration of goblet cells following three months of oral vitamin A therapy

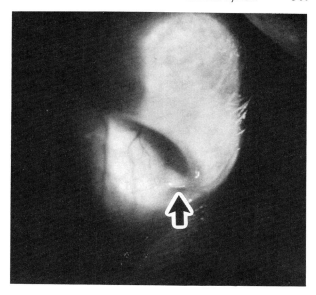

FIGURE 25.13 **Symblepharon formation (arrow) in 72-year-old patient with ocular cicatricial pemphigoid.**

(45,000 IU/day) in a 9-year-old male with Stevens-Johnson syndrome. The response to immunosuppressive therapy may also hold some promise for the future.[135]

In addition to the basic disease process, secondary bacterial infections of the eyelids can complicate the clinical condition. Eyelid scrubs followed by antibiotic ointments are effective for any associated blepharitis (see Chap. 24).

A recent report[131] calls attention to the observation that timolol can potentiate OCP. The authors[131] recommend that elevated intraocular pressure be treated alternatively with carbonic anhydrase inhibitors.

Oculoplastic surgical techniques may correct entropion with trichiasis in the early stages of the disease, but care must be taken not to further shorten the already shrunken conjunctiva.[129] Traditional approaches to the trichiasis may also be used: electrolysis, epilation, and cryoablation.[126,129]

Systemic steroids are useful in the acute stages of OCP.[136] Gardner and associates[129] have suggested that immunosuppressive agents may be promising for selected cases. Mucous membrane transplantation has only limited success.[120]

The treatment of other forms of mucin deficiency resembles that for OCP. Alkali burns are an emergency, and the conjunctival fornices should be copiously flushed with water immediately. Testing the tears in the fornices following lavage can be carried out with pH paper to determine whether all the alkaline material has been flushed. Management of subsequent scarring should follow the same course as treatment of OCP. Table 25.9 summarizes the approach to treatment of mucin-deficient dry eyes.

TABLE 25.9
Treatment Strategies for Mucin Deficiencies

Ocular cicatricial pemphigoid, Stevens-Johnson syndrome
    Tear substitutes
    Consider systemic steroids and immunosuppressive agents
    Treat bacterial infections with appropriate antibiotic
    Manage complications of entropion, trichiasis on an individual
        basis
Chemical burns (acid, alkali, solvents)
    Flush with water or sterile saline *immediately* (first aid)
    Tear substitutes once acute phase has cleared
    Manage complications on an individual basis
Drug-induced (pseudopemphigoid)
    Consider alternative ocular medications
    Consult concerning use of immunosuppressive agents

Another approach to the mucin-deficient eye, the local application of 0.1% or 0.01% all-trans retinoic acid (vitamin A) shows promise. Vitamin A is locally deficient when cicatricial tissue replaces normally vascularized tissue. Since vitamin A is one of the essential factors for epithelial growth and differentiation, its local application may stimulate goblet-cell activity.[124] Tseng and associates[124] studied a series of selected cases. Of 16 patients (27 eyes) with Stevens-Johnson syndrome, OCP, or traumatic goblet-cell loss, all showed improvement in clinical signs and symptoms when treated with local vitamin A. Concentrations used were either 0.01% or 0.1% (weight/weight) of all-trans retinoic acid in ointment form. Spectacular improvements occurred over a relatively short follow-up period (all less than 12 months), but this report[124] may represent the first nonsurgical attempt at treating mucin deficiencies by reversing changes in the diseased ocular surface epithelium. Vitamin A ointment is effective for some surface ocular abnormalities characterized by metaplasia of the surface epithelium.[137]

Lipid Deficiency

ETIOLOGY

Lipid deficiency is extremely rare. Complete absence of meibomian secretion occurs in cases of congenital anhidrotic ectodermal dysplasia.[120] Sebum from the skin of the eyelid then contaminates the aqueous layer. Because of the higher polarity and lower molecular weight of sebum, complete "dewetting" of the ocular surface can result.[120,138]

Meibomian glands contribute secretions to the lipid layer of the precorneal tear film. Ocular diseases and disorders that have the potential to affect the meibomian glands, such as blepharitis, can influence the constituency of the tear film. Such an alteration takes the form of free fatty acid formation associated with the lipase activity of staphylococcal organisms.[133] The causative role of these toxins, however, has been challenged.[139] Other evidence suggests that meibomian secretion rates increase to offset the altered quality.[120] Attendant complications of meibomian dysfunction include increased aqueous tear evaporation from the ocular surface.[140]

A recent investigation of blepharitis focused on the dermatologic aspects of the disorder. Of the 407 cases, only 74 (18.2%) demonstrated reduced TBUT. However, this study[141] found an associated dermatologic disorder (seborrheic dermatitis, acne rosacea, atopic dermatitis) in nearly 75% of cases.

While lipid dysfunction *per se* may be rare, meibomian gland dysfunction may be prevalent. Hom and associates[142] reported that almost 40% of consecutive routine patients demonstrated meibomian gland dysfunction based on the criteria of cloudy or absent expression from meibomian glands.

DIAGNOSIS

Both staphylococcal and seborrheic blepharitis have distinctive clinical signs. Collarettes at the base of the lashes characterize staphylococcal blepharitis. The eyelids show a fibrinous scale and significant inflammation but occasionally can exhibit an ulcerative appearance.[143] Patients with seborrheic blepharitis generally have eyelids with less inflammation combined with more oily or greasy scaling.[143] The two conditions have similar clinical symptoms and may be indistinguishable from keratoconjunctivitis sicca, which may be an associated condition. Among the clinical signs of either tear-film disorder is a reduced TBUT, occurring in about 20% of cases.[141]

The lipase activity of staphylococcal organisms gives rise to the formation of free fatty acids.[133] Clinically this condition may cause "foam" or "soap bubble" accumulation at the outer canthi when viewed with the biomicroscope.

MANAGEMENT

The treatment of lipid deficiency associated with blepharitis consists of a combination of eyelid hygiene, topical antibiotic therapy, and occasionally systemic antibiotic therapy[143] (see Chap. 24). The strategies are designed to reverse the destabilizing effects on the tear film. Typical palliative treatment with tear substitutes during the day and ocular lubricating ointments at bedtime helps to keep the patient comfortable while controlling the supervening blepharitis.

Management should aim at reestablishing normal tear volume as well as ridding the lids of potential sources of infection. Although such lid disease may be considered sterile (the typically cultured organism is *S. epidermidis*, Type IV),[89] treatment measures should be aggressively pursued. Lid margin hygiene consists of warm compresses and lid scrubs. When meibomianitis supervenes, as manifested by frothy discharge, systemic tetracycline (250 mg p.o. qid) should be considered.

Both Jones'[119] and Holly's[120] classifications of tear dysfunction states or lacrimal abnormalities include mechanisms related to disorders of the eyelids. Since the eyelids serve as distributors of the tear film, this inclusion is logical. Management of meibomian gland dysfunction uses warm compresses and massage.[142,143] Chronic blepharitis presents the challenge of gentamicin-resistant bacteria and *Candida* species as causative organisms.[141] Stepped treatment consisting of lid hygiene, meibomian gland expression, topical and systemic antibiotic therapy, and corticosteroid treatment may help in the management of blepharitis (see Chap. 24).

The relationship of ocular surface disease to contact lens wear has been discussed in detail elsewhere.[144]

Disorders of Lacrimal Drainage

Congenital Epiphora

ETIOLOGY

The lacrimal drainage system is generally completely canalized by term. It is generally agreed that the last portion to become patent is the most distal.[145–147] A vestigial remnant of epithelialization of the canal (Hasner's membrane) may occlude this most distal opening, resulting in the most frequent cause of congenital epiphora.

DIAGNOSIS

Any obstruction of lacrimal drainage causes tearing. The clinical characteristics of congenital epiphora include an infant with tearing and possibly a secondary dacryocystitis. The condition may have a prevalence as high as 6%.[148] Congenital epiphora generally appears within the first month of life,[145] and, when accompanied by dacryocystitis, the practitioner must differentiate the purulent discharge from neonatal conjunctivitis. In many cases gently pressing over the nasolacrimal sac and observing mucopurulent reflux from either punctum can confirm the diagnosis of dacryocystitis.[149]

MANAGEMENT

Conservative treatment is a consistent feature of large studies.[145,148–151] However, the exact timing for more aggressive intervention is controversial. Jones[145] has suggested that patients over 1 year of age with epiphora be examined for inflammation and presence of purulent discharge. Topical antibiotics and decongestants are indicated in the presence of inflammatory signs, but in the absence of inflammation, the parents should learn the technique of hydrostatic nasolacrimal massage.[149]

Crigler[152] originally described the hydrostatic technique. It consists of placing the index finger over the common canaliculus to prevent reflux of material through either punctum. A firm downward "stroking" motion increases hydrostatic pressure within the nasolacrimal duct (Fig. 25.14). The objective is to catalyze rupture of membranous obstruction (Hasner's membrane) at the distal end of the nasolacrimal duct. This maneuver should be repeated five times twice a day. Treatment should continue until epiphora stops or until the child is three months old. Use of antibiotic (erythromycin) ointment several times daily is recommended if mucopurulent discharge is present.[149]

Another conservative strategy allows time for a spontane-

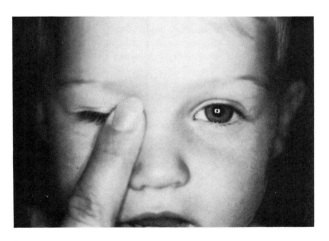

A

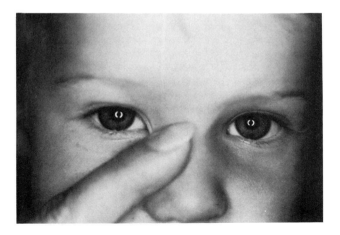

B

FIGURE 25.14   **Sequence illustrating the method for applying digital pressure in congenital dacryocystitis secondary to incomplete distal lacrimal drainage system canalization (see text).**

ous cure. Suckling[150] projected that 94% of infants with obstruction at age 7.5 months resolve if left untreated until 21 months of age. More recently, Nucci and associates[153] reported a spontaneous cure rate of 93% among 59 infants between 1 and 12 months of age. Conservative management may extend to children up to the age of 2 years. The efficacy of delayed intervention beyond 13 months of age has been confirmed in a large series of patients.[151] Almost 95% were cured following a single probing performed under general anesthesia. An alternative approach to probing is high-pressure irrigation.[147]

If irrigation procedures prove unsuccessful, careful probing can be performed. This procedure[154] is best performed in a hospital operating room. An anesthesiologist administers general anesthesia by inhalation. The ophthalmic surgeon uses a Bowman probe of small diameter (usually #1 or #2) (Fig. 25.15) and may coat its tip lightly with a sterile ophthalmic ointment. Once general anesthesia is induced, the ophthalmic surgeon inserts the Bowman probe in the superior punctum of the involved eye. It is then directed downward so that the probe is parallel to the nose. A gentle insertion technique is needed until the tip of the probe exits the ipsilateral nare. In some cases, a cracking sound can be heard as the probe pushes through the structures of the nose. Extreme care should be taken to respect the anatomic structures of the nasolacrimal system. Faulty probing may cause canalicular stenosis.[155]

Accurate diagnosis is mandatory prior to intervention. Infants with nasolacrimal obstruction must have nasolacrimal duct cysts and dacryocystoceles ruled out.[156] More aggressive treatment includes implantation of silicone tubes as surrogate lacrimal drainage pathways. These may be left in place for as few as 6 weeks to prevent complications.[157]

To test the integrity of the lacrimal system after probing, a few drops of 1% sodium fluorescein are instilled into the cul-de-sac of the involved eye. A small clear plastic tube is inserted immediately into the area of the inferior meatus to aspirate the fluorescein. If the nasolacrimal system is patent, the surgeon observes fluorescein in the clear plastic aspiration tube. With the inherent risk of using general anesthesia on an infant, the procedure should be practiced and performed in less than 3 to 4 minutes. The child can recover from the anesthesia in a few more minutes and be back in the parent's arms for recovery. Preoperative preparation and postoperative recovery should require more time than performing the actual procedure.

Failures of probing pose a management dilemma. Bony malformations appear to be the cause of nearly all failures.[147,154,158–162] The inability to pass a probe through the nose or to irrigate saline through the nasolacrimal duct indicates nasal pathology.[158–162]

Regardless of age, the infant should be observed carefully for the presence of true epiphora, and the prospect of parent compliance should play a role in the management decision. Following conservative treatment, lack of spontaneous cure much beyond 1 year of age significantly increases the likelihood of two events: Nasal pathology is more likely to be present, and resolving the tearing problem will probably require more complex procedures.[151,161,162]

Acquired Epiphora

The lacrimal drainage apparatus channels tears from the eye. It plays a vital role in the equilibrium established between tear production and excretion. Except for observation of the

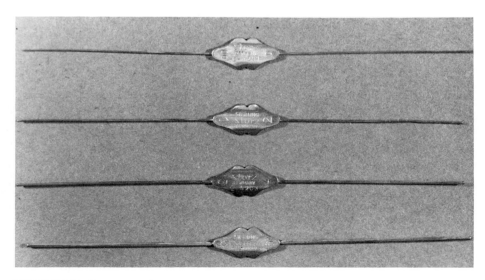

FIGURE 25.15 **Bowman probes.**

punctum, the clinician must rely largely on patient symptoms and evidence from indirect evaluation to arrive at a diagnosis of a lacrimal drainage disorder. Tests for acquired lacrimal drainage dysfunction are based on anatomy of the lacrimal drainage system.

ACQUIRED PUNCTUM OCCLUSION

Etiology.   Occlusion of the lacrimal puncta is called atresia when congenital and stenosis when it is acquired. Each produces true epiphora.

Weil[163] has divided the lacrimal excretory system into upper and lower components conceptually. This separation appears to violate the embryologic, histologic, and anatomic continuity of the system, but it allows consideration of problems of the puncta and canaliculi separate from the more distal portions of the system.

Diseases of the eyelids and lid margins can result in malposition of the punctum. These include blepharitis; seborrheic, atopic, or neurodermatitis; and collagen diseases such as scleroderma.[163] Stenosis (occlusion by flattening) of the punctum can be secondary to lid dermatoses or simply the result of age. The latter is the most frequent cause of acquired epiphora.

Diagnosis.   The diagnosis of true epiphora often occurs before the clinician begins formal examination procedures. A history of persistent tearing and the presence of a handkerchief or tissue in the patient's hand virtually secure the diagnosis.

Apart from direct observation, the clinician may wish to perform the diagnostic dye tests. Controversy exists, however, over interpreting fluorescein as a marker for tear drainage. Jones[164] has suggested instilling fluorescein into the inferior cul-de-sac and awaiting its appearance in the nose after 5 minutes. He favors direct exploration of the inferior meatus of the nose using a cotton-tipped wire applicator. Alternatively, direct observation for fluorescein can be performed with a cobalt-filtered light source (Burton lamp or angioscopy filter in place on a binocular indirect ophthalmoscope headset). Perhaps the most effective method of detecting the fluorescein-stained tears is to incline the patient forward and have the patient clear the nose into a white tissue. This test is performed on one side at a time and reveals particularly dramatic evidence, whether the test is positive or negative.[165] The primary dye test may depend more on the amount of fluorescein placed into the inferior cul-de-sac than on the experience of the clinician. One study involving a resident and two attending physicians suggested that the greater the volume of fluorescein used, the greater the likelihood of a positive primary dye test in a patent nasolacrimal system.[166] Moreover, lacrimal drainage appears to slow with advancing age.[204] Hagele and associates[204] have suggested an upper limit of normal at 6 minutes for patients younger than 45 years and 12 minutes in patients 45 years of age and older.

Other authors[167] have correlated the *dis*appearance of fluorescein from the cul-de-sac with the Jones fluorescein test. The conclusion is that rapid excretion of the fluorescein-stained tears from the marginal tear strip observed with the slit lamp indicates normal physiologic lacrimal drainage. This rapid and easily performed test gives reliable results.[168]

Regardless of the interpretive strategy used, blockage of the lacrimal drainage system does not allow fluorescein to be detected in the nose. This is the Jones No. 1 test, or primary dye test.[164] When fluorescein is present, the test is considered positive (normal lacrimal drainage) and implies physiologic patency of the system. Should the dye remain in the eye or not appear further along the drainage passageways, then a negative test result is recorded, and further diagnostic evaluation is indicated (see Fig. 25.4).

Punctal dilation is the next indicated diagnostic test. Enlargement with a dilator (Fig. 25.16) may open a stenotic punctum, although perhaps only temporarily.[163] If a repeated fluorescein dye test then reveals a positive result, the punctal dilation procedure has solved the patient's problem, even if only temporarily.[163] The patient should be monitored within 2 to 3 weeks.

Punctal dilation can be accomplished easily with little or no patient discomfort. Topical anesthesia can be obtained with the instillation of 1 or 2 drops of 0.5% proparacaine. The following procedure gives deeper anesthesia: A 6-inch sterile cotton-tipped applicator is broken in half and the cotton tip saturated with a few drops of 0.5% proparacaine. The patient should look straight ahead with lids opened as wide as possible. The cotton tip, containing the proparacaine, is then held over the punctum, and the patient closes the lids securely to hold the shortened applicator for about 15 to 30 seconds. The proparacaine can now have longer contact with the lid margin and puncta and provide deeper anesthesia (Fig. 25.17). This method also provides the practitioner with a "patient anxiety index" by observing how much the wooden tip of the applicator wiggles due to lid tension. A rapidly wiggling applicator informs the clinician that the patient may require more support or empathy.

To dilate the inferior punctum, the lower lid is gently pulled away from the globe and the dilator is inserted vertically into the opening of the punctum. The dilator should be rolled slowly between the practitioner's finger and thumb to ease insertion. After traveling about 2 mm inferiorly, the dilator must be lowered to a horizontal position with continued gentle forward motion (Fig. 25.18). The dilator should not exert excessive pressure. As the dilator is inserted further into the canaliculus and the punctal opening dilates, the ring of elastic tissue surrounding the punctum (punctal ring) blanches. If the dilator exerts further pressure against the punctum, the punctum and lower lid begin to turn inward and outward with the turning of the dilator. This turning indicates to the practitioner that he or she is exerting sufficient pressure and that temporary dilation of the punctum is taking place. If a thin layer of epithelial cells occludes

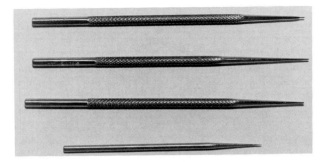

FIGURE 25.16   **Lacrimal dilators (Storz, Inc., St. Louis, MO). Top dilator is the Muldoon instrument; note the medium tip and rapid expansion. The next two are different sizes of the Wilder dilator. The bottom dilator is the Reudemann. It has a very fine tip and narrow taper, making it perhaps the most useful of the group.**

the punctal opening, the needle-tipped dilator (see Fig. 25.16) or a sterilized safety pin can still open it. Most dilation procedures are directed to the lower lid, but the superior punctum can be dilated as well.

If the dye test following punctal dilation still proves negative, then the secondary dye test, or Jones No. 2 test, is indicated. Some preparation is needed before the test is performed. Any remaining fluorescein should be rinsed from the cul-de-sac, and the patient should receive a topical anesthetic. A 2 ml syringe is filled with sterile saline or extraocular irrigating solution and attached to a 23-gauge lacrimal cannula (Fig. 25.19). With the patient inclined forward and holding an emesis basin beneath the nose, the cannula is inserted through the lower punctum into the

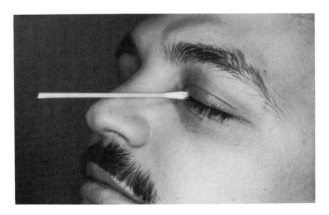

FIGURE 25.17   **Method of obtaining deeper anesthesia for punctum procedures. The cotton-tipped applicator is saturated with topical anesthetic and placed between the superior and inferior puncta. The patient then closes the lids.**

vertical and horizontal portions of the lower canaliculus (Fig. 25.20).

Many clinicians prefer a reinforced 23-gauge straight cannula for this procedure. A metal sleeve reinforces the base of the cannula to prevent the cannula from breaking and lodging in the canaliculus following repeated use. This thickened shaft also occludes the punctum during forced irrigation to prevent saline from regurgitating through the ipsilateral punctum. Other cannulas are available. The 23-gauge West cannula with blunt end and the side opening offers the advantages of easy advancement through the canaliculus and alignment with the nasolacrimal duct, respectively.

Once a hard stop is reached, a distance of approximately 13 mm from the punctum has been traversed. At this point, at least 0.5 ml of solution should be expressed from the syringe. One of four possible outcomes can occur[169]:

1. No fluid appears, indicating complete obstruction of the nasolacrimal duct.
2. Fluorescein-stained fluid appears, indicating partial distal obstruction of the nasolacrimal duct.
3. Clear fluid appears, indicating a negative Jones No. 2 (secondary) dye test. No fluorescein entered the drainage system, and an ectropion or stenosis of the punctum should be ruled out.
4. Regurgitation of saline or discharge appears at the superior punctum. This could indicate an inflammatory or neoplastic process. Table 25.10 summarizes the localizing value of regurgitation by type and site.

An alternative to the classic Jones No. 2 technique places the patient in a reclined position. The patient signals when he or she tastes the salty solution. The clinician can also be alert to observe the swallow reflex. Using only a few milliliters of saline prevents the patient from experiencing an overwhelming gag response.

Management.   Effective management of minor cases of punctal occlusion may require only periodic (or in some cases single) dilation of the stenotic punctum. Some clinicians disdain the transient effects of punctal dilation and favor snip procedures or punch punctumplasty.[163] A one-snip procedure may be augmented by the use of a silicone punctal plug as a temporary conformer. A Freeman punctal plug with the supra punctal lip resting on the eyelid margin remains in place for 2 weeks.[170] Most patients, however, prefer repeated dilation to surgical intervention.

If the punctum is involuted such that it cannot be identified or opened, then a dacryocystorhinostomy is required.[163] This surgical procedure shunts the tears directly from the lacrimal lake to the nasolacrimal duct.

CANALICULAR DISORDERS

Etiology.   Canaliculitis is a relatively rare disorder. In one study[171] only 2% of patients with tearing problems had a

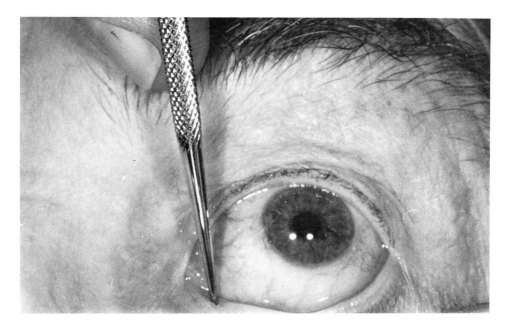

A

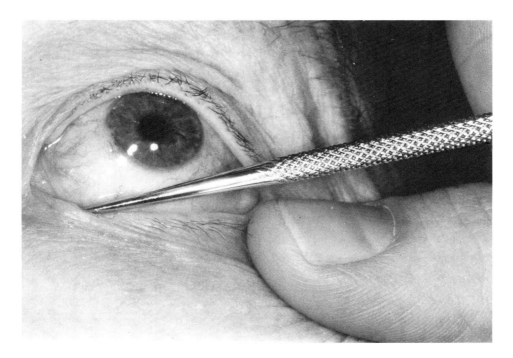

B

FIGURE 25.18   Procedure for lower punctum dilation. *(A)* The dilator is inserted vertically about 2 mm. *(B)* It is then brought near the horizontal plane of the lower lid. The lower lid can be gently pulled laterally to straighten the canaliculus.

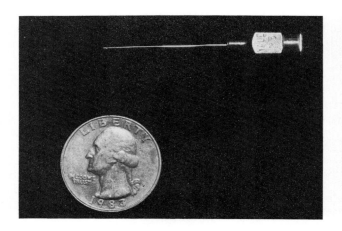

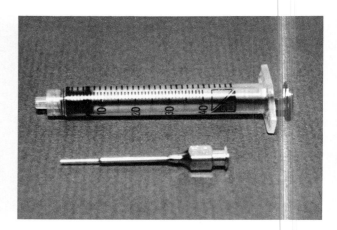

A   B

FIGURE 25.19   **Lacrimal cannulas. (A) The 23-gauge West cannula. The shaft is straight and approximately 25 mm long. The tip is blunt with needle hole in the side. (B) Reinforced 23-gauge cannula and syringe.**

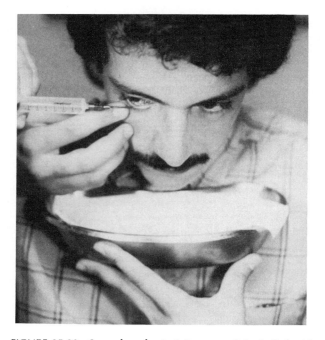

FIGURE 25.20   **Secondary dye test (Jones no. 2 test). Patient is seated and inclined forward for irrigation. Note basin to catch effluent. (From Semes L, Melore GG. Dilation and diagnostic irrigation of the lacrimal drainage system. J Am Optom Assoc 1986;57:518–525. Reprinted with permission of the authors and publisher.)**

final diagnosis of canaliculitis. Actinomycotic and herpetic infections appear the most likely causative agents.[172,173] An allergic etiology has also been reported.[174] Other causes include neoplastic or mechanical factors.[175–177]

Diagnosis.   The patient complains of a smoldering, usually unilateral, red eye that has been resistant to antibiotic therapy.[171,172] Epiphora has a variable association.[174] Diagnostic irrigation may meet with resistance ("soft stop") before reaching the hard stop of the lacrimal bone. An important clinical sign in the diagnosis of obstructed canaliculus has been termed the *wrinkle sign*.[178] When a soft stop is encountered during probing or irrigation, the clinician can observe compression of the medial canthal skin (wrinkling) in the presence of internal obstruction. The visualization of smooth skin and advancement of the instrument to the

TABLE 25.10
Localization of Obstruction by Regurgitation of Irrigating Solution

Site/Type of Regurgitation	Site of Obstruction
Ipsilateral	Ipsilateral canaliculus
Contralateral	Common canaliculus or lacrimal sac
Mucoid	Lacrimal sac
Mucopurulent	Nasolacrimal duct inflammation (dacryocystitis)
Delayed reflux	Nasolacrimal duct

lacrimal bone indicates a patent proximal drainage system. The secondary dye test may be negative.[174]

The initial diagnostic suspicion of canaliculitis may be aided by considering the patient's age. Actinomycotic infections are more likely to appear among patients over age 50 years,[171,172] while primary herpetic infections (herpes simplex, herpes zoster, varicella, and vaccinia) have a distinctly higher prevalence among patients under 20 years of age and will present with cutaneous manifestations of the infectious disease.[173]

Diagnostic testing beyond gram-stained smears or cultures employs sophisticated means. Dacryoscopy (Dyonics, Inc., Woburn, MA) allows direct visualization of lacrimal drainage passages through a needlescope.[179–181] Practitioners can also make use of other endoscopes for diagnostic and surgical procedures.[182,183]

Patients who are patent to irrigation may have incomplete anatomic obstruction demonstrable by intubation dacryocystography with subtraction.[184] Advances in digital subtraction imaging now allow instantaneous high-resolution, magnified, bone-free radiographs of the lacrimal drainage system.[185] A contrast medium is injected before the x-ray film. The advantage of this technique is its dynamic nature, allowing the clinician to interpret the flow of tears as it occurs. Ultrasonographic imaging of the lacrimal drainage system has also been reported. Standardized A-scans as well as the B-scan mode have been employed preoperatively.[186]

Another diagnostic view of the lacrimal drainage pathways makes use of lacrimal scintigraphy.[187,188] In this procedure a radioisotope is instilled into the conjunctival sac and serves as the marker for tear drainage. Some authors[189] believe that this noninvasive imaging medium, when coupled with digital subtraction macrodacryocystography, provides the ultimate in anatomic and physiologic views of the lacrimal drainage system and is useful prognostically.[190]

Canalicular disorders can also be secondary to trauma.[191] Standard primary diagnostic testing should reveal impatencies or lacerations of this nature. Failure to reach a conclusion in the presence of a history of trauma or previous unsuccessful surgery should prompt consideration of higher-level investigations of the lacrimal drainage system.

Management.   Infectious disorders causing canaliculitis should be treated at the direction of the microbiologic tests. Although these tests generally suggest the presence of *Actinomyces,* topical and systemic antibacterial therapy appear to be beneficial. Some authors favor chloramphenicol, while others recommend neomycin, polymyxin B, and bacitracin in combination with systemic penicillin or ampicillin.[171,172] Success in eradicating the infection depends on removal of concretions and purulent material from the involved canaliculi.[171,172]

Herpetic canaliculitis may result from ocular viral infection or may be secondary to its treatment with antiviral agents. Following the recognition of viral blepharoconjunc-

tivitis, especially in the presence of lid vesicles, persistent epiphora should not be ignored. Harley and associates[173] have recommended irrigation of the involved lacrimal drainage apparatus on a bi-weekly schedule. Failure to maintain patency, due to cicatrization, may require a shunt or external dacryocystorhinostomy.[173]

Relief of allergic canalicular obstruction has been reported with use of cromolyn sodium.[174] This report indexed the resolution of intermittent epiphora and eye rubbing to symptomatic relief and lacrimal patency.

Acquired Dacryocystitis

Etiology

When a patient over 1 year of age has swelling over the lacrimal sac, the swelling most often results from acquired dacryocystitis. Culture studies usually identify *Staphylococcus aureus* as the offending organism, with *Haemophilus influenzae* a common pathogen in children.[192]

In the unusual case where chronic dacryocystitis results from infection with *Mycobacterium fortuitum,* surgical management is indicated.[193] Aside from dacryolith formation, *Candida albicans* may be the etiologic agent in nasolacrimal obstruction and subsequent dacryocystitis. Dacryocystorhinostomy appears curative for this fungal infection.[194] In addition, the Epstein-Barr virus may cause acute acquired dacryocystitis.[195] Other signs and symptoms consistent with infectious mononucleosis are present. Finally, implantation of punctal or lacrimal plugs may serve as a vector for infection.[196,197]

Faced with a chronic dacryocystitis, the clinician needs to be aware of masquerade syndromes. Epithelial carcinomas[198] and malignant lymphoma[199] have been reported from histologic and immunohistochemical analysis, respectively, of biopsies of the lacrimal sac taken at dacryocystorhinostomy. Rhabdomyosarcoma has also been identified.[200]

Diagnosis

The swelling characteristic of dacryocystitis is limited in its upward extent by the medial canthal tendon. Mucoceles and solid tumor masses may extend above the tendon and masquerade as dacryocystitis. Although pain and hyperemia are consistent features of acquired dacryocystitis, a mucocele is nontender.[192] Percutaneous aspiration biopsy can provide more sophisticated analysis.[192]

Thermography, which detects subtle temperature differences by infrared scanning devices, can assess lacrimal passageway inflammation.[201] A rudimentary comparison between the affected and normal sides can be made at the primary care level simply by judging the symmetry of temperature on each side.

Management

Hurwitz and Rodgers[192] emphasize the importance of recognizing the stage of acquired dacryocystitis. The presence of a pyocele (pus-filled sac) with orbital cellulitis is a life-threatening condition. Since penicillin-resistant *Staphylococcus* is the most common pathogen, oral cloxacillin or dicloxacillin is the antibiotic of choice. Application of hot compresses minimizes the cellulitis and localizes the infection to the lacrimal sac.[192,201] If the sac enlarges or if cellulitis is absent, hot compresses should be avoided because the risk of spontaneous sac perforation is too great. An initial administration of oral amoxicillin can be attempted while awaiting the results of culture and sensitivity studies.[192] A cephalosporin is an alternative that provides interim coverage.[202] In children, treating for *Haemophilus* is appropriate. However, since reports of amoxicillin-resistant *Haemophilus* are common, third-generation cephalosporins (e.g., cefixime) may be more effective.[202]

After inflammation resolves, diagnostic irrigation should be carried out. The symptomatic patient deserves the very highest level of lacrimal investigation,[192] since any decision concerning surgery should be based on this information.

References

1. Jones LT. The lacrimal secretory system and its treatment. Am J Ophthalmol 1966;62:47–60.
2. Holly FJ, Lemp MA. Tear physiology and dry eyes. Surv Ophthalmol 1977;22:69–87.
3. Jones LT. An anatomical approach to problems of the eyelids and lacrimal apparatus. Arch Ophthalmol 1961;66:111–124.
4. Botehlo SY. Tears and the lacrimal gland. Sci Am 1964;211:78–85.
5. McEwen WK, Goodner EK. Secretion of the tears and blinking. In: Davson H, ed. The eye, ed. 2, vol. 3. New York: Academic Press, 1969:357–359.
6. Gillette TE, Allansmith MR, Greiner JV, et al. Histologic and immunohistologic comparison of main and accessory lacrimal tissue. Am J Ophthalmol 1980;89:724–730.
7. Holly FW, Lamberts DW, Buessler JA. The human lacrimal apparatus: anatomy, physiology, pathology and surgical aspects. Plast Reconstr Surg 1984;74:438–445.
8. Hill JC, Bethell W, Smirmaul HJ. Lacrimal drainage-a dynamic evaluation. I. Mechanics of tear transport. Can J Ophthalmol 1974;9:411–424.
9. Ahl N, Hill JC. Horner's muscle and the lacrimal system. Arch Ophthalmol 1982;100:488–493.
10. Doane MG. Blinking and the mechanics of the lacrimal drainage system. Ophthalmology 1981;88:844–851.
11. Becker BB. Tricompartment model of the lacrimal pump mechanism. Ophthalmology 1992;99:1139–1145.
12. Daubert J, Nik N, Chandeyssoun PA, El-Choufi L. Tear flow analysis through the upper and lower systems. Ophthalmic Plast Reconst Surg 1990;6:193–196.
13. Milder B. Physiology of lacrimal excretion. In: Milder B, Weil BA, eds. The lacrimal system. Norwalk, CT: Appleton-Century-Crofts, 1983;56.
14. Glatt HJ. Epiphora caused by blepharoptosis. Am J Ophthalmol 1991;111:649–650.
15. Canavan YM, Archer DB. Long-term review of injuries to the lacrimal drainage apparatus. Trans Ophthalmol Soc UK 1979;99:201–204.
16. Jones LT, Marquis MM, Vincent NT. Lacrimal function. Am J Ophthalmol 1972;73:658–659.
17. Linberg JV, Moore CA. Symptoms of canalicular obstruction. Ophthalmology 1988;95:1077–1079.
18. McMonnies CW, Ho A. Patient history in screening for dry eye conditions. J Am Optom Assoc 1987;58:296–301.
19. Tsubota K, Nakamori K. Dry eyes and video display terminals. N Engl J Med 1993;328:584–585.
20. Norn MS. Vital staining of the cornea and conjunctiva. Acta Ophthalmol 1972;113(suppl):1–66.
21. Feenstra RPG, Tseng SCG: Comparison of fluorescein and rose bengal staining. Ophthalmology 1992;99:605–617.
22. Laroche RR, Campbell RC: Quantitative rose bengal staining technique for external ocular diseases. Ann Ophthalmol 1988;20:274–276.
23. Lemp MA, Hamill JR. Factors affecting tear film breakup in normal eyes. Arch Ophthalmol 1973;89:103–105.
24. Vanley GT, Leopold IH, Gregg TH. Interpretation of tear film breakup. Arch Ophthalmol 1977;95:445–448.
25. Mengher L Bron AJ, Tonge, Gilbert DJ. A non-invasive instrument for clinical assessment of the pre-corneal tear film stability. Curr Eye Res 1985;4:1–7.
26. Bernal DL, Ubels JL. Quantitative evaluation of the corneal epithelial barrier: Effect of artificial tears and preservatives. Curr Eye Res 1991;10:645–656.
27. Adams J, Wilcox M, Trousdale, et al. Morphologic and physiologic effects of artificial tear formulations on corneal epithelial derived cells. Cornea 1992;11:234–241.
28. Patel S, Farrell JC. Age-related changes in precorneal tear film stability. Optom Vis Sci 1989;66:175–178.
29. Yap M. Tear break-up time is related to blink frequency. Acta Ophthalmol 1991;69:92–94.
30. Patel S, Farrell J, Bevan R. Relation between precorneal tear film stability and tear production rate in normal eyes. Optom Vis Sci 1989;66:300–303.
31. Cho P, Brown B, Chan I, Conway R, Yap M. Reliability of the tear break-up time technique of assessing tear stability and the locations of the tear break-up in Hong Kong Chinese. Optom Vis Sci 1992;69:879–885.
32. Wiggins HE, Karian BK. Evaluation of the lacrimal system: the Schirmer tests and fluorescein dye tests. J Oral Surg 1974;32:622–625.
33. Feldman F, Wood MM. Evaluation of the Schirmer tear test. Can J Ophthalmol 1979;14:257–259.
34. Patton TF. Reliability of the Schirmer tear test (letter). Can J Ophthalmol 1979;15:101.

35. Hornblass A, Ingis TM. Lacrimal function tests. Arch Ophthalmol 1979;97:1654–1655.

36. Shapiro A, Merrin S. Schirmer test and breakup time of the tear film in normal subjects. Am J Ophthalmol 1979;88:752–757.

37. Schirmer O. Studien zur physiologie and pathologie der tranenab-sonderung and tranenabfuhr. Arch Klin Ophthalmol 1903;56:197–291.

38. Cho P, Yap M. Schirmer test. I. A review. Optom Vis Sci 1993;70:152–156.

39. Cho P, Yap M. Schirmer test. II. A clinical study of its repeatability. Optom Vis Sci 1993;70:157–159.

40. Milder B. Diagnostic tests of lacrimal function. In: Milder B, Weil BA, eds. The lacrimal system. Norwalk, CT: Appleton-Century-Crofts, 1983;71–78.

41. van Bijsterveld OP. Diagnostic tests in the sicca syndrome. Arch Ophthalmol 1969;82:10–14.

42. Tsubota K. The importance of the Schirmer test with nasal stimulation. Am J Ophthalmol 1991;111:106–107.

43. de Luise VP, Tabbara KF. Quantitation of tear lysozyme levels in dry-eye disorders. Arch Ophthalmol 1983;101:634–635.

44. Velos P, Cherry PMH, Miller D. An improved method for measuring human tear lysozyme concentration. Arch Ophthalmol 1985;103:31–33.

45. Boersma HGM, van Bijsterveld OP. The lactoferrin test for the diagnosis of keratoconjunctivitis sicca in clinical practice. Ann Ophthalmol 1987;19:152–154.

46. Nelson JD, Havener VR, Cameron JD. Cellulose acetate impressions of the ocular surface. Arch Ophthalmol 1983;101:1869–1872.

47. Nelson JD, Wright JC. Conjunctival goblet cell densities in ocular surface disease. Arch Ophthalmol 1984;102:1049–1051.

48. Natadisastra G, Wittpenn JR, West KP Jr, et al. Impression cytology for detection of vitamin A deficiency. Arch Ophthalmol 1987;105:1224–1228.

49. van Bijsterveld OP: Diagnostic tests in the sicca syndrome. Arch Ophthalmol 1969;82:10–14.

50. Boersma HGM, van Bijsterveld OP: The lactoferrin test for the diagnosis of keratoconjunctivitis sicca in clinical practice. Ann Ophthalmol 1987;19:152–154.

51. Farris RL, Gilbard JP, Stuchell A, Mandell ID. Diagnostic tests in keratoconjunctivitis sicca. CLAO J 1983;9:23–28.

52. Lemp MA, Hammill JR. Factors affecting tear film breakup in normal eyes. Arch Ophthalmol 1973;89:103–105.

53. Vanely LS, Leopold IH, Gregg TH. Interpretation of tear film breakup. Arch Ophthalmol 1977;95:445–448.

54. Norn MS. Vital staining of the cornea and conjunctiva. Acta Ophthalmol 1972;113(suppl):1–66.

55. Nelson JD. Impression cytology. Cornea 1988;7:71–81.

56. Forst G. The precorneal tear film in "dry eyes." Int Contact Lens Clin 1992;19:136–140.

57. Hom MH, Silverman MW. Displacement technique and meibomian gland expression. J Am Optom Assoc 1987;58:223–226.

58. Mackie IA, Seal DV. Quantitative tear lysozyme assay in units of activity per microlitre. Br J Ophthalmol 1976;60:70–74.

59. Taylor HR, Louis WJ. Significance of tear function test abnormalities. Ann Ophthalmol 1980;12:531–536.

60. Mackie IA, Seal DV. Confirmatory tests for the dry eye of Sjögren's syndrome. Scand J Rheumatol 1986;61(suppl):220–223.

61. Goren MB, Goren SB. Diagnostic tests in patient with symptoms of keratoconjunctivitis sicca. Am J Ophthalmol 1988;106:570–574.

62. Lucca JA, Nunez, Farris RL. A comparison of diagnostic tests for keratoconjunctivitis: Lactoplate, Schirmer tests, osmolarity. CLAO J 1990;16:109–112.

63. Yolton DP, Mende D, Harper S, Softing A. Association of dry eye signs and symptoms with tear lactoferrin concentration. J Am Optom Assoc 1991;62:217–223.

64. Lemp MA. General measures in management of the dry eye. Int Ophthalmol Clin 1987;27(1):36–43.

65. Khurana AK, Chaudhary R, Ahluwalia BK, Gupta S. Tear film profile in dry eye. Acta Ophthalmol 1991;69:79–86.

66. Rivas L, Rodriguez JJ, Alvarez MI, et al. Correlation between impression cytology and tear function parameters in Sjögren's syndrome. Acta Ophthalmol 1993;71:353–359.

67. Lamberts DW, Foster CS, Perry HD. Schirmer test after topical anesthetic and tear meniscus height in normal eyes. Arch Ophthalmol 1979;97:1082–1085.

68. Farris RL, Gilbard JP, Stuchell, Mandell ID. Diagnostic tests in keratoconjunctivitis sicca. CLAO J 1983;9:23–28.

69. Mengher L Bron AJ, Tonge, Gilbert DJ. A non-invasive instrument for clinical assessment of the pre-corneal tear film stability. Curr Eye Res 1985;4:1–7.

70. Feenstra RPG, Tseng SCG. Comparison of fluorescein and rose bengal staining. Ophthalmology 1992;99:605–617.

71. Laroche RR, Campbell RC. Quantitative rose bengal staining technique for external ocular diseases. Ann Ophthalmol 1988;20:274–276.

72. Nelson JD. Impression cytology. Cornea 1988;7:71–81.

73. Forst G. The precorneal tear film in "dry eyes." Int Contact Lens Clin 1992;19:136–140.

74. Hom MH, Silverman MW. Displacement technique and meibomian gland expression. J Am Optom Assoc 1987;58:223–226.

75. Mackie IA, Seal DV. Quantitative tear lysozyme assay in units of activity per microlitre. Br J Ophthalmol 1976;60:70–74.

76. Gilbard JP, Cohen GR, Baum J. Decreased tear osmolarity and absence of the inferior marginal tear strip after sleep. Cornea 1992;11.231–233.

77. Hom MH,Silverman MW. Displacement technique and meibomian gland expression. J Am Optom Assoc 1987;58:223–226.

78. Milder B. Diseases of the lacrimal gland. In: Milder B, Weil BA, eds. The lacrimal system. Norwalk, CT: Appleton-Century-Crofts, 1983:105–110.

79. Wright JE, Steward WB, Krohel GB. Clinical presentation of lacrimal gland tumors. Br J Ophthalmol 1979;63:600.

80. Henderson JW, Farrow GM. Primary malignant mixed tumors of the lacrimal gland. Report of 10 cases. Ophthalmology 1979;87:466–475.

81. Wright JE. Lacrimal gland tumors. Trans Ophthalmol Soc NZ 1983;35:101–106.

82. Mafee MF, Haik BG. Lacrimal gland and fossa lesions: role of computed tomography. Radiol Clin North Am 1987;25:767–779.

83. MacLean H, Ironside JW, Cullen JF, Butt Z. Mikulicz syndrome and disease: 2 case reports highlighting the difference. Acta Ophthalmol 1993;71:136–141.

84. Mondino BJ, Brown SI. Hereditary congenital alacrima. Arch Ophthalmol 1976;94:1478–80.

85. Riley CM, Day CL, Greely DM, et al. Central autonomic dysfunction with defective lacrimation. Report of five cases. Pediatrics 1949,3:468–478.

86. McCulley JP, Moore MB, Matoba AY. Mucus fishing syndrome. Ophthalmology 1985;92:1262–1265.

87. Baum J. Clinical manifestations of dry eye states. Trans Ophthalmol Soc UK 1985;104:415–423.

88. Talal N. Overview of Sjögren's syndrome. J Dent Res 1987;66 (special issue): 672–674.

89. McGill J, Laikos G, Seal D, et al. Tear film changes in health and dry eye conditions. Trans Ophthalmol Soc UK 1983;103:313–317.

90. Lemp MA. Artificial tear solutions. Int Ophthalmol Clin 1973;13:221–229.

91. Norn M. The effects of drugs on tear flow. Trans Ophthalmol Soc UK 1985;104:410–414.

92. Brown SI: Dry spots and corneal erosions. Int Ophthalmol Clin 1973;13(1):149–156.

92a. Caffery BE, Josephson JE: Is there a better "comfort drop?". J Am Optom Assoc 1990;61:178.

93. LaMotte J, Lesher G. Relief of dry eye complaints by a lipid-containing tear substitute. Int Eye Care 1986;2:582–585.

94. Baldone JA, Kaufman HE. Soft contact lenses and clinical diseases. Am J Ophthalmol 1983;95:851–852.

95. Mackie IA. Contact lenses in dry eyes. Trans Ophthalmol Soc UK 1985;104:477–483.

96. Farris RL. Contact lens wear in the management of the dry eye. Int Ophthalmol Clin 1987;27:54–60.

97. Messner K, Leibowitz HM. Acetylcystine treatment of keratitis sicca. Arch Ophthalmol 1971;86:357–359.

98. Dohlman CH. Punctal occlusion in keratoconjunctivitis sicca. Trans Am Acad Ophthalmol Otolaryngol 1978;85:1277–1281.

99. Freeman JM. The punctum plug: evaluation of a new treatment for dry eyes. Trans Am Acad Ophthalmol Otolaryngol 1975;79:874–879.

100. Willis RM, Folberg R, Krachmer JH, et al: The treatment of aqueous-deficient dry eye with removable punctal plugs. A clinical and impression-cytology study. Ophthalmology 1987;94:514–518.

101. Semes LP, Herrick RS. The role of nondissolvable intracanalicular implants in the treatment of refractory dry eyes in a patient with Sjögrens syndrome. Proc IV Int Symp Sjögren's Syndrome 1993.

102. Benson DR, Hemady PB, Snyder RW: Efficacy of laser punctal occlusion. Ophthalmology 1992;99:618–621.

103. LaMotte J, Grossman E, Hersch J: The efficacy of cellulosic ophthalmic inserts for treatment of dry eye. J Am Optom Assoc 1985;56:298–302.

104. Leibowitz HM, Chang RK, Mandell AI: Gel tears. A new medication for the treatment of dry eyes. Ophthalmology 1984;91:1199–1204.

105. Gilbard JP, Kenyon KR. Tear diluents in the treatment of keratoconjunctivitis sicca. Ophthalmology 1985;92:646–650.

106. DeLuise VP, Peterson WS: The use of topical Healon tears in the management of refractory dry-eye syndrome. Ann Ophthalmol 1984;16:823–824.

107. Limberg MB, McCaa C, Kissling GE, Kaufman HE: Topical application of hyaluronic acid and chondroitin sulfate in the treatment of dry eyes. Am J Ophthalmol 1987;103:194–197.

108. Nelson JD, Farris RL: Sodium hyaluronate and polyvinyl alcohol artificial tear preparations. A comparison in patients with keratoconjunctivitis sicca. Arch Ophthalmol 1988;106:484–487.

109. Sand BB, Marner K, Norn MS: Sodium hyaluronate in the treat-ment of keratoconjunctivitis sicca. Acta Ophthalmol 1989;67:181–183.

110. Avisar R, Savir H, Machtey I, et al. Clinical trial of bromhexine in Sjögren's syndrome. Ann Ophthalmol 1981;13:971–973.

111. Kriegbaum NJ, von Linstow M, Oxholm P, Prause JU. Keratoconjunctivitis sicca in patients with primary Sjögren's syndrome. A longitudinal study of ocular parameters. Acta Ophthalmol 1988;66:481–484.

112. Tseng SCG, Maumenee AE, Stark WJ, et al. Topical retinoid treatment for various dry-eye disorders. Ophthalmology 1985;92:717–727.

113. Soong HK, Martin NF, Wagoner MD, et al. Topical retinoid therapy for squamous metaplasia of various ocular surface disorders. A multicenter, placebo-controlled double-masked study. Ophthalmology 1988;95:1442–1446.

114. Gilbard JP, Huang AJ, Belldegrun R, et al. Open-label crossover study of vitamin A ointment as a treatment for keratoconjunctivitis sicca. Ophthalmology 1989;96:244–246.

115. Kaswan RL, Salisbury M-A, Ward DA. Spontaneous canine keratoconjunctivitis sicca. A useful model for human keratoconjunctivitis sicca: treatment with cyclosporine eye drops. Arch Ophthalmol 1989;107:1210–1216.

116. Laibovitz RA, Solch S, Andriano K, et al. Pilot trial of cyclosporine 1% ophthalmic ointment in the treatment of keratoconjunctivitis sicca. Cornea 1993;12(4):315–323.

117. Nelson JD, Gordon JF, Chiron Keratoconjunctivitis Sicca Study Group. Topical fibronectin in the treatment of keratoconjunctivitis sicca. Am J Ophthalmol 1992;114:441–447.

118. Prause JU. Beneficial effect of sodium sucrose-sulfate on the ocular surface of patient with severe KCS in primary Sjögren's syndrome. Acta Ophthalmol 1991;69:417–427.

119. Jones DB. Prospects in the management of tear-deficiency states. Trans Am Acad Ophthalmol Otolaryngol 1977;83:693–700.

120. Holly FJ. Tear film physiology. Int Ophthalmol Clin 1987;27:2–6.

121. Mondino B. Cicatricial pemphigoid and erythema multiforme. Ophthalmology 1990;97:939–952.

122. Ohji M, Ohmi G, Kiritoshi A, Kinoshita S. Goblet cell density in thermal and chemical injuries. Arch Ophthalmol 1987;105:1686–1688.

123. Singer L, Brook U, Romen M, Fried D. Vitamin A in Stevens-Johnson syndrome. Ann Ophthalmol 1989;21:209–210.

124. Tseng SCG, Maumence AE, Stark WJ, et al. Topical retinoid treatment for various dry-eye disorders. Ophthamology 1985;92:717–727.

125. Pouliquen Y, Patey A, Foster CS, et al. Drug-induced cicatricial pemphigoid affecting the conjunctiva: light and electron microscopic features. Ophthalmology 1986;93:775–783.

126. Mondino BJ. Cicatricial pemphigoid and erythema multiforme. In: Foulks GN, ed. Noninfectious inflammation of the anterior segment, vol. 23. Boston: Little, Brown, 1983;63–78.

127. Thoft RA. Relationship of the dry eye to primary ocular surface disease. Trans Ophthalmol Soc UK 1985;104:452–457.

128. Belfort R Jr., deSmet M, Whitcup SM, et al. Ocular complication of Stevens-Johnson syndrome and toxic epidermal necrolysis in patients with AIDS. Cornea 1991;10:536–538.

129. Gardner KM, Rajacich GM, Mondino BJ. Ophthalmological manifestations of adult rheumatoid arthritis and cicatricial pemphigoid. In: Callen JP, Eiferman RA, eds. Oculocutaneous diseases, vol. 25. Boston: Little, Brown, 1985;1–34.

130. Lemp MA. The mucin-deficient dry eye. Int Ophthalmol Clin 1973;13(1):185–189.

131. Fiore PM, Jacobs IH, Goldberg DB. Drug-induced pemphigoid: a spectrum of diseases. Arch Ophthalmol 1987;105:1660–1663.

132. Ormerod LD, Fong LP, Foster CS. Corneal infection in mucosal scarring disorders and Sjögren's syndrome. Am J Ophthalmol 1988;105:512–518.

133. Sullivan WR, McCulley JP, Dohlman CH. Return of goblet cells after vitamin A therapy in xerosis of the conjunctiva. Am J Ophthalmol 1973;75:720–725.

134. Singer L, Brook U, Romem M, Fried D. Vitamin A in Stevens-Johnson syndrome. Ann Ophthalmol 1989;21:209–210.

135. Chan LS, Soong HK, Foster CS, et al. Ocular cicatricial pemphigoid occurring as a sequella of Stevens-Johnson syndrome. JAMA 1991;266:1543–1546.

136. Mondino BJ, Brown SI, Lempert S, et al. The acute manifestations of ocular cicatricial pemphigoid: Diagnosis and treatment. Ophthalmology 1979;86:543–552.

137. Soong HK, Martin NF, Wagoner MD, et al. Topical retinoid therapy for squamous metaplasia of various ocular surface disorders. A multicenter, placebo-controlled, double-masked study. Ophthalmology 1988;95:1442–1446.

138. McCulley JP, Sciallis GF. Meibomian keratoconjunctivitis. Am J Ophthalmol 1977;84:788–793.

139. Seal D, Ficker L, Ramakrishnan M, Wright P. Role of staphylococcal toxin in production of blepharitis. Ophthalmology 1990; 97:1684–1688.

140. Mathers WD. Ocular evaporation in meibomian gland dysfunction and dry eye. Ophthalmology 1993;100:347–351.

141. Huber-Spitzy V, Baumgartner I, Bohler-Sommeregger K, Grabner G. Blepharitis—a diagnostic and therapeutic challenge. Graefe's Arch Clin Exp Ophthalmol 1991;229:224–229.

142. Hom MM, Martinson R, Knapp LL, Paugh JR. Prevalence of meibomian gland dysfunction. Optom Vis Sci 1990;67:710–712.

143. Bowman RW, Dougherty JM, McCulley JP. Chronic blepharitis and dry eyes. Int Ophthalmol Clin 1987;27:27–35.

144. Semes LP. Keratoconjunctivitis and ocular surface disease. In: Silbert JA, ed. Complications of contact lens wear. New York: Churchill Livingstone, 1994;221–236.

145. Jones LT. Treatment of lacrimal duct obstructions in the infant. J Pediatr Ophthalmol 1966;3:42–45.

146. Sevel D. Development and congenital abnormalities of the nasolacrimal apparatus. J Pediatr Ophthalmol Strabismus 1981;18:13–19.

147. Busse H, Muller KM, Kroll P. Radiological and histological findings of the lacrimal passages in newborns. Arch Ophthalmol 1980;98:528–532.

148. Baker JD. Treatment of congenital nasolacrimal system obstruction. J Pediatr Ophthalmol Strabismus 1985;22:34–35.

149. Nelson LB, Calhoun JH, Menduke H. Medical management of congenital nasolacrimal duct obstruction. Ophthalmology 1985; 92:1187–1190.

150. Suckling RD. The natural history of congenital epiphora. NZ Med J 1981;93:74–75.

151. El-Mansoury J, Calhoun JH, Nelson LB, et al. Results of late probing for congenital nasolacrimal duct obstruction. Ophthalmology 1986;93:1052–1054.

152. Crigler LW. The treatment of congenital dacryocystitis. JAMA 1923;81:23–24.

153. Nucci P, Capoferi C, Alfarano R, Brancato R. Conservative management of congenital nasolacrimal duct obstruction. J Pediatr Ophthalmol Strabismus 1989;26:39–43.

154. Robb RM. Probing and irrigation for congenital nasolacrimal duct obstruction. Arch Ophthalmol 1986;104:378–379.

155. Lyon DB, Dortzbach RK, Lemke BN, Gonnering RS. Canalicular stenosis following probing for congenital nasolacrimal duct obstruction. Ophthalmic Surg 1991;22:228–232.

156. Grin TR, Mertz JS, Stass-Isren M. Congenital nasolacrimal duct cysts in dacryocystocele. Ophthalmology 1991;98:1238–1242.

157. Migliori ME, Putterman AM. Silicone intubation for the treatment of congenital lacrimal duct obstruction: successful results removing the tubes after six weeks. Ophthalmology 1988;95:792–795.

158. Cibis GW, Jazbi BU. Nasolacrimal duct probing in infants. Trans Am Acad Ophthalmol Otolaryngol 1979;86:1488–1491.

159. Sterk CC. Probing in congenital dacryocystitis or atresia. Doc Ophthalmol 1981;50:321–325.

160. Mittleman D. Probing for congenital nasolacrimal duct obstruction (letter). Arch Ophthalmol 1986;104:1125.

161. Wesley RE. Inferior turbinate fracture in the treatment of congenital nasolacrimal duct obstruction and congenital nasolacrimal duct anomaly. Ophthalmic Surg 1985;16:368–371.

162. Katowitz JA, Welsh MG. Timing of initial probing and irrigation in congenital nasolacrimal duct obstruction. Ophthalmology 1987;94:698–705.

163. Weil BA. Diseases of the upper excretory system. In: Milder B, ed. The lacrimal system. Norwalk, CT: Appleton-Century-Crofts, 1983;125–132.

164. Jones LT, Linn ML. The diagnosis and causes of epiphora. Am J Ophthalmol 1969;67:751–754.

165. Campbell HS, Smith JL, Richman DW, et al. A simple test for lacrimal obstruction. Am J Ophthalmol 1962;53:611–613.

166. Wright MM, Bersani TA, Freuh BR, Musch DC. Efficacy of the primary dye test. Ophthalmology 1989;96:481–483.

167. Zappia RJ, Milder B. Lacrimal drainage function. I: The Jones fluorescein test. Am J Ophthalmol 1972;74:154–159.

168. Meyer DR, Antonello A, Linberg JV. Assessment of tear drainage after canalicular obstruction using fluorescein dye disappearance. Ophthalmology 1990;97:1370–1374.

169. Jones BR. Syndromes of lacrimal obstruction and their management. Trans Ophthalmol Soc UK 1973;93:581–588.

170. Kristan RW. Treatment of lacrimal punctal stenosis with a one-snip canaliculotomy and temporary punctal plugs. Arch Ophthalmol 1988;106:878–879.

171. Demant E, Hurwitz JJ. Canaliculitis: review of 12 cases. Can J Ophthalmol 1980;15:73–75.

172. Smith RL, Henderson PN. Actinomycotic canaliculitis. Aust J Ophthalmol 1980;8:75–79.

173. Harley RD, Stefanyszyn MA, Apt L, et al. Herpetic canalicular obstruction. Ophthalmic Surg 1987;18:367–370.

174. Wojno TH. Allergic lacrimal obstruction. Am J Ophthalmol 1988; 106:48–52.

175. Bartley GB. Acquired lacrimal drainage obstruction: an etiologic classification system, case reports, and a review of the literature. Part 1. Ophthalmic Plast Reconst Surg 1992;8:237–242.

176. Bartley GB. Acquired lacrimal drainage obstruction: an etiologic classification system, case reports and a review of the literature. Part 2. Ophthalmic Plast Reconst Surg 1992;8:243–249.

177. Zapala, J Bartkowski AM, Bartkowski SB. Lacrimal drainage system obstruction: management and results obtained in 70 patients. J Cranio-Maxillo-Fac Surg 1992;20:178–183.

178. Burns JB, Penland WR, Cahill KV. The wrinkle sign in tear duct obstruction. Ophthalmic Surg 1984;15:930–931.

179. Cohen SW, Prescott R, Sherman M, et al. Dacryoscopy. Ophthalmic Surg 1979;10:57–63.

180. Nixon J, Birchall IWJ, Virjee J. The role of dacryocystography in the management of patients with epiphora. Br J Radiol 1990;63:337–339.

181. King SJ, Haigh SF. Technical report: Digital subtraction dacryocystography. Clin Radiol 1990;42:351–353.

182. Fein W, Daykhovsky L, Papaioannou T, et al. Endoscopy of the lacrimal outflow system. Arch Ophthalmol 1992;110:1748–1750.

183. Gonnering RS, Lyon DB, Fisher JC. Endoscopic laser-assisted lacrimal surgery. Am J Ophthalmol 1991:111:152–157.

184. Rosenstock T, Hurwitz JJ. Functional obstruction of the lacrimal drainage passages. Can J Ophthalmol 1982;17:249–255.

185. Galloway JE, Kavic TA, Raflo GT. Digital subtraction macrodacryocystography. Ophthalmology 1984;91:956–962.

186. Dutton JJ. Standardized echography in the diagnosis of lacrimal drainage dysfunction. Arch Ophthalmol 1989;107:1010–1012.

187. Amanat LA, Hilditch TE, Kwok CS. Lacrimal scintigraphy. II. Its role in the diagnosis of epiphora. Br J Ophthalmol 1983;67:720–728.

188. Hanna IT, MacEwen CJ, Kennedy N. Lacrimal scintigraphy in the diagnosis of epiphora. Nuclear Medicine Communications 1992;13:416–420.

189. Millman A, Liebeskind A, Putterman AM. Dacryocystography: the technique and its role in the practice of ophthalmology. Radiol Clin North Am 1987;25:781–786.

190. Mannor GE, Millman AL. The prognostic value of preoperative dacryocystography in endoscopic intranasal dacryocystorhinostomy. Am J Ophthalmol 1992;113:143–137.

191. Jones LT. The cure of epiphora due to canalicular disorders: trauma and surgical failures on the lacrimal passages. Trans Am Acad Ophthalmol Otolaryngol 1962;66:506–524.

192. Hurwitz JJ, Rodgers KJA. Management of acquired dacryocystitis. Can J Ophthalmol 1983;18:213–216.

193. Artenstein AW, Eiseman AS, Campbell GC. Chronic dacryocystitis caused by *Mycobacterium fortuitum.* Ophthalmology 1993:100:666–668.

194. Purgason PA, Hornblass A, Loeffler M. Atypical presentation of fungal dacryocystitis. A report of two cases. Ophthalmology 1992;99:1430–1432.

195. Steele RJ, Meyer DR. Nasolacrimal duct obstruction and acute dacryocystitis associated with infectious mononucleosis (Epstein-Barr virus). Am J Ophthalmol 1993;115:265–266.

196. Glatt HJ. Acute dacryocystitis after punctal occlusion for keratoconjunctivitis sicca. Am J Ophthalmol 1991;111:796–797.

197. Mathews D. Pyogenic granuloma associated with silicone punctal plugs. South J Optom 1990;8(3):17–19.

198. Watts MT, Berman M, Collin JRO. Epithelial carcinoma of the lacrimal sac. Orbit 1992;11:19–21.

199. Karesh JW, Perman KI, Rodrigues MM. Dacryocystitis associated with malignant lymphoma of the lacrimal sac. Ophthalmology 1993;100:669–673.

200. Baron EM, Kersten RC, Kulwin DR. Rhabdomyosarcoma manifesting as acquired nasolacrimal duct obstruction. Am J Ophthalmol 1993;115:239–242.

201. Rosenstock T, Chart P, Hurwitz JJ. Inflammation of the lacrimal drainage system-assessment by thermography. Ophthalmic Surg 1983;14:229–237.

202. Linberg JV. Disorders of the lower excretory system. In: Milder B, Weil BA, eds. The lacrimal system. Norwalk, CT: Appleton-Century-Crofts, 1983;133–143.

203. McCollum CJ, Foulks GN, Bodner B, et al. Rapid assay of lactoferrin in keratoconjunctivitis sicca. Cornea 1994;13:505–508.

204. Hagele JE, Guzek JP, Shavlik GW. Lacrimal testing. Age as a factor in Jones testing. Ophthalmology 1994;101:612–617.

CHAPTER 26

Diseases of the Conjunctiva

Gary E. Oliver
Christopher J. Quinn
J. James Thimons

Conjunctivitis affects patients of any age, race, gender, or socioeconomic level. It is among the most common external ocular diseases diagnosed by eye care practitioners. The National Health Survey conducted in 1970–1971 found that the prevalence rate of conjunctivitis in the United States for patients ages 1 to 74 was 13 cases per 1,000 persons.[1] Conjunctivitis may originate from both infectious organisms and inflammatory etiologies. Potential causes include allergy, bacteria, viruses, dermatologic conditions of the eyelids, mechanical irritation, toxins, trauma, and systemic diseases. Conjunctivitis worldwide often occurs in association with epidemic outbreaks of infectious disease. In many cases, primary conjunctivitis is self-limiting and resolves without intervention. However, successful pharmacologic treatment depends on the eye care practitioner's ability to recognize and diagnose properly the numerous clinical presentations of conjunctivitis. Timely therapy can reduce conjunctival morbidity. This chapter discusses the most frequently encountered forms of conjunctivitis with emphasis on pharmacologic management of each disease.

Anatomy of the Conjunctiva

The conjunctiva is a mucous membrane that lines the inner portions of the eyelids and is reflected onto the globe over the anterior sclera. The membrane consists of nonkeratinized epithelium overlying a substantia propria or stroma containing connective tissue and a vascular network. Anatomically and clinically, the conjunctiva consists of three sections: palpebral or tarsal conjunctiva, fornix conjunctiva, and bulbar conjunctiva (Fig. 26.1). The conjunctiva develops embryologically from surface ectoderm along with the epidermis of the eyelid, corneal epithelium, and lens epithelium. This situation provides an anatomic basis for the clinical relationship of conjunctivitis to dermatologic conditions of the eyelids in addition to certain systemic diseases.[2]

Palpebral Conjunctiva

The palpebral conjunctiva begins at the posterior lid margin and extends posteriorly towards the fornix. The keratinized epithelium of the eyelids gradually transforms into the moist mucous membrane of the conjunctiva.[2] The palpebral conjunctiva adheres tightly to the tarsus over the entire superior lid as compared to the loosely adherent inferior palpebral conjunctiva.[3] Clinically, this anatomic variation accounts for the difference in appearance of papillary hypertrophy between the superior and inferior palpebral conjunctiva.

The palpebral conjunctiva is composed of nonkeratinized stratified epithelium which decreases in thickness as it proceeds from the lid margin. Many mucin-secreting goblet cells are located near the fornix. The epithelium overlies the substantia propria, which consists of delicate connective tissue and blood vessels.[2] Most of the immune system cellular components occur in the substantia propria. The stroma contains lymphocytes, lymphoid follicles, neutrophils, plasma cells, and mast cells, all of which proliferate extensively in conjunctival inflammatory disease. This proliferation leads to the formation of papillae and follicles.[4–6]

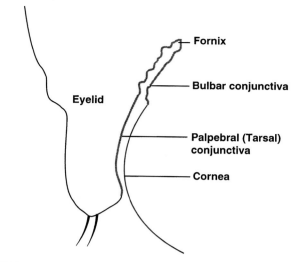

FIGURE 26.1   **Anatomic division of the conjunctiva.**

Fornix Conjunctiva

The conjunctival fornix extends over the globe beginning and ending at the medially located plica semilunaris and caruncle.[3] The fornix adheres loosely to the underlying stroma. A small fold in the fornix conjunctiva permits free motion during eye movements. The lower fornix contains an abundance of lymphoid follicles and inflammatory cells. The accessory lacrimal gland of Krause is located in the superior fornix with few accessory lacrimal glands situated in the lower fornix.[7]

Bulbar Conjunctiva

The conjunctiva proceeds onto the globe from the fornix to form the bulbar conjunctiva, which overlies Tenon's capsule and merges with the limbal cornea. Loosely attached to the capsule over the entire globe, the bulbar conjunctiva forms a homogeneous layer of stratified squamous epithelium at the limbus and contains many goblet cells near the fornix.[7] The goblet cells secrete mucopolysaccharides that form the mucin layer of the tear film.[8] Loss of goblet cells may result in various forms of ocular surface disease ranging from dry eye syndrome to cicatricial disorders. The limbal conjunctival substantia propria has many sensitive unmyelinated nerve fibers and free nerve endings as well as a complex network of perilimbal vessels and vascular arcades. Medially, the bulbar conjunctiva is bordered by the caruncle which forms a mucocutaneous junction between the bulbar conjunctiva and the epidermis of the skin. Accessory lacrimal glands may occasionally be located in the caruncle.[7]

A substantial concentration of Langerhans' cells occurs at the limbus. These cells, known as monocytes within the blood and macrophages when deposited in tissues, derive from bone marrow and have a dendritic morphologic shape. They occur within all epithelial surfaces and mucous membranes. Langerhans cells initiate the ocular immune response by functioning as antigen-presenting cells. Foreign antigens displayed on their surfaces are recognized by T lymphocytes in a complex interaction.[9-11]

Inflammation of the Conjunctiva

The clinical signs exhibited by the conjunctival inflammatory response usually depend on the nature of the causative agent. Conjunctival tissue may be exposed to antigens or pathogens through airborne transmission; direct contact (hand to eye, person to person, or from contaminated instruments or surfaces); and sexual transmission. Acute or chronic conjunctivitis may present with any of five clinical manifestations of conjunctival inflammation. These are chemosis, hyperemia, discharge or exudate, follicles, and papillae (Table 26.1).

All immune system inflammatory cells may be elicited in extraordinary numbers in conjunctival tissues. Lymphocytes, neutrophils, mast cells, and plasma cells are present from birth and increase in quantity with age and antigenic exposure. Lymphoid tissue, however, is not present at birth but develops within the first few months.[12] Increased vascular permeability resulting from the ocular immune response to antigens, infectious agents, toxins, or other environmental stimuli, such as smoke or wind, often results in hyperemia, chemosis, or exudative discharge. The severity of the clinical presentation depends on both the causative agent and type of immune response. The exudative discharge may be serous, mucoid, purulent, fibrinous, or hemorrhagic.[13,14]

In the presence of exudates consisting of fibrin cellular debris, true or pseudomembranes may form on the conjunctiva. These membranes indicate a severe inflammatory response. A true membrane exists when the exudate attaches firmly to the underlying epithelium. True membranes leave raw, bleeding surfaces following removal, due to the defacement of the epithelium during the procedure. Pseudomembranes are loosely attached to the conjunctiva and easily removed with forceps.[14]

Papillary hypertrophy represents a nonspecific inflammatory response of the conjunctiva seen most commonly in allergic or bacterial conjunctivitis. It results from cellular infiltration of the substantia propria by inflammatory cellular material such as eosinophils, lymphocytes, mast cells, and polymorphonuclear leukocytes. Papillary hypertrophy results in elevations of the conjunctival epithelium and stroma termed *papillae,* which have a delineating margin with a small central vascular tuft. The central vessel is the source of

TABLE 26.1
Clinical Manifestations of Conjunctival Inflammation

Clinical Entity	Physical Appearance	Etiology
Chemosis	Edematous, swollen tissue	Increased vascular permeability
Hyperemia	Pale to bright red engorged vessels	Pathophysiologic response to injury
Exudates		
Serous	Clear, watery discharge	Increased vascular permeability
Mucoid	Clear to yellowish tinged, translucent sticky or stringy discharge	Increased mucus from goblet cell irritation
Mucopurulent	Yellowish white, less translucent, sticky discharge	Increased mucus combined with inflammatory cells, such as eosinophils and macrophages
Purulent	Yellowish white to yellowish-green tinged, opaque, thick discharge	High concentration of inflammatory cells, such polymorphonuclear leukocytes and macrophages
Fibrinous	White, opaque, flat appearing discharge that follows contour of conjuctiva and may be attached to the underlying tissue	High degree of fibrin mixed with inflammatory cells, such as polymorphonuclear leukocytes and macrophages
Hemorrhagic	Red streaked discharge which may also have any of the above characteristics	Red blood cells in discharge from increased vascular permeability or trauma
Papillary Hypertrophy	Elevations of conjunctival epithelium and stroma with a delineating margin and small central vascular tuft; when papillae are small, conjunctiva has velvety appearance	Cellular infiltration of the substantia propria by inflammatory cellular material such as eosinophils, lymphocytes, mast cells, and polymorphonuclear leukocytes
Follicles	Elevated, avascular, rounded lesions, translucent to whitish-gray, usually located in fornices; small vessel may surround the follicle; no central vascular tuft is present	Germinal cells (immature lymphocytes) and macrophages comprise central portion with mature cells forming the periphery

the cellular infiltration. When the papillae are small, the conjunctiva has a smooth, velvety appearance.[13,15,16]

Follicles result from focal lymphoid hyperplasia usually in response to chlamydial, viral, or toxic agents. Clinically, follicles appear as elevated, avascular, rounded lesions that are translucent to whitish-gray in color and usually located in the conjunctival fornices. Small external vessels may envelop the follicle, but it has no central vascular tuft. Germinal cells (immature lymphocytes) and macrophages comprise the central portion with mature cells forming the periphery. Follicles located in the fornices are usually nonspecific; however, follicles located on the superior tarsus or at the limbus frequently represent chlamydial disease.[13,15,17]

Microbiology of the Conjunctiva

Normal Flora

The normal conjunctiva, as with other mucous membranes, sustains a permanent flora of indigenous bacteria. These organisms constitute a protective host defense mechanism that helps prevent pathogens from multiplying efficiently. Normal flora may become pathogens in immunocompro-

mised or debilitated patients. Viruses and parasites, while often present in asymptomatic individuals, are not considered part of the normal flora. Several studies[18–20] have documented that the normal flora of the conjunctiva resembles that of the upper respiratory tract and eyelid skin. The primary microbial organisms retrieved are *Staphylococcus epidermidis, Staphylococcus aureus,* and *Corynebacterium* species (diphtheroids). *Staphylococcus epidermidis* is the most common organism. The distribution of organisms in the normal flora is relatively equal among patients of all ages except for a slightly higher yield of diphtheroids in individuals over age 20 years. At least one of these organisms could be isolated from 61% of the specimens from 92 healthy eyes during repetitive cultures of the conjunctiva.[21] Other organisms found on a transient basis include *Streptococcus pneumoniae,* the viridans group of streptococci, *Haemophilus influenzae,* and *Pseudomonas aeruginosa.* Occasionally, even enteric Gram-negative rods such as *Escherichia coli* occur. Obligate gram-positive rod anaerobes are isolated in 50% of the eyes cultured. *Propionibacterium acnes,* commonly isolated from the skin, is the most frequently isolated anaerobe.[22] Factors such as the presence of blepharitis, dry eye syndrome, meibomian gland dysfunction, and contact lens use may influence the composition of the normal flora or cause its disruption, which can lead to a disease state in

TABLE 26.2
Causes of Infectious Conjunctivitis

Bacterial		Viral	Chlamydial	Fungal
Gram Positive	Gram Negative			
Staphylococcus aureus	Haemophilus influenzae	Adenoviruses	Chlamydia trachomatis	Candida albicans
Staphylococcus epidermidis	Neisseria gonorrhoeae	Herpes simplex		Aspergillus species
Streptococcus pneumoniae	Escherichia coli	Varicella zoster virus		
Streptococcus pyogenes	Pseudomonas aeruginosa	Molluscum contagiosum		
Corynebacterium diphtheriae	Proteus mirabilis	Enterovirus 70		
	Moraxella lacunata	Epstein-Barr		
	Moraxella catarrhalis			

any given patient. Although immunocompromised individuals may harbor *Candida albicans,* fungi are considered opportunistic pathogens.[23] Little evidence supports the existence of any indigenous fungi in the normal conjunctival flora.[24]

Common Microbial Pathogens

Almost any microbial organism can cause infectious conjunctivitis. The infectious organisms include bacteria, chlamydia, fungi, and viruses. In immunocompetent persons, the primary causes of conjunctivitis are bacteria and viruses in children younger than 12 years of age, and viruses in adults and children older than 12 years of age. The primary bacterial pathogens are *Staphylococcus aureus, Haemophilus influenzae,* and *Streptococcus pneumoniae.* Adenovirus and herpes simplex are the most common viral causes. The frequency of infection by one of these organisms varies depending on the particular region's climate and other environmental factors. Table 26.2 summarizes the most significant ocular infectious agents.

Mechanism of Infection

The conjunctiva has several nonimmune defense barriers that protect it from infection. These include the intact mucous membrane surface, constant epithelial cell replacement, cool temperature due to tear evaporation, mechanical action of the eyelids, and the flushing action of the tears. The normal bacterial flora and tear film constituents, such as lactoferrin, beta-lysine, and lysozyme, have antibacterial action and supplement the anatomic barriers.[25] The prominently vascularized conjunctiva has highly active immunologic barriers. All cellular components of the immune system, except basophils and eosinophils, are typically found in the conjunctival substantia propria. These barriers work in conjunction with one another to provide protection against infection. Conjunctivitis may result from a disruption in any of the barriers, leading to invasion by a pathogen or overgrowth of one of the normal flora organisms. Irregular eyelid margins, irregular blinking, or poor tear film may compromise the epithelial surface. When an inoculum of sufficient quantity invades the conjunctiva, overcolonization by the infectious organism results either from a disruption in the normal flora or from exceeding the antibacterial capabilities of the tear constituents. For example, tear lysozyme is not effective against *Staphylococcus aureus.*[26] Once an infectious conjunctivitis becomes established, the severity of the infection depends on several factors, including the organism's virulence, invasiveness, level of toxin production, environmental elements such as temperature and pH, and the quality of the active nonimmune and immune barriers.

Laboratory Diagnosis of Conjunctivitis

Indications for Laboratory Analysis

Although all infectious conjunctivitis ideally should be cultured or have ocular smears performed to determine the exact etiology, the experienced practitioner does not find this approach necessary in the majority of cases. Conjunctivitis usually can be diagnosed accurately and treated by assessing the clinical history, signs, and symptoms. Some forms of conjunctivitis, due to the disease severity or increased risks for ocular tissue damage, must have laboratory diagnosis as part of the workup and management plan. In other cases, laboratory diagnosis is suggested but not mandatory. Conjunctival pathology requiring mandatory laboratory analysis includes severe chronic conjunctivitis, hyperacute conjunctivitis, membranous conjunctivitis, ophthalmia neonatorum, Parinaud's oculoglandular syndrome, and postoperative infections. Laboratory diagnosis is recommended for moderate chronic conjunctivitis, conjunctivitis secondary to canaliculitis or dacryocystitis, conjunctivitis secondary to infectious eczematous or ulcerative blepharitis, conjunctivitis unresponsive to therapy, and medicamentosa (Table 26.3). The inexperienced clinician may find laboratory evaluation helpful in confirming clinical judgments.[27]

Cultures

Whenever bacterial or fungal etiologies are suspected, ocular specimens for culture should be plated directly on agar plates containing enriched or selective bacteriologic media. Commercially available transport media are usually not sufficient for bacteria or fungi because most ocular specimens contain diminutive quantities of fastidious microorganisms. However, transport solutions for viruses and chlamydia can effectively maintain specimens for laboratory analysis. Innoculating agar plates directly enhances the practitioner's ability to isolate an offending organism successfully. Solid media plates also enable laboratory technicians to identify the organism's morphology more efficiently and thus shorten the waiting time for reports. Three types of solid media and one liquid medium are recommended for routine innoculation: blood agar, chocolate agar, Sabouraud's agar, and thioglycolate broth. The liquid medium provides for transport of any anaerobic microorganisms and permits the laboratory to innoculate additional media plates if necessary. Other selective media may be indicated when attempting to isolate specific microorganisms, such as the *Neisseria* species.

Blood agar is an all-purpose enriched medium appropriate for isolating most ocular aerobic or anaerobic pathogens except *Haemophilus, Neisseria,* and *Moraxella* species. When incubated under anaerobic conditions, blood agar is useful for isolating most anaerobes, including *Actinomyces.* This medium is trypticase-soy agar with 5% to 10% sterile, defibrinated sheep blood. Blood agar is the standard bacteriologic medium used for cultivating fastidious microorganisms and determining hemolytic reactions.[27]

Chocolate agar is a polypeptone or beef infusion agar enriched with 2% hemoglobin released from defibrinated, heated rabbit or sheep's blood. The blood hemolysis creates the chocolate color. Free hemin and nicotinamide adenine dinucleotide permit cultivation of *Haemophilus, Neisseria,* and *Moraxella* species. Since chocolate agar has a more limited usefulness, it cannot take the place of blood agar.[28]

Sabouraud's agar is a glucose-peptone agar combination with its pH adjusted to 6.7 to 7.1 to favor isolation of opportunistic fungi. The addition of antibiotics such as chloramphenicol or gentamicin prevents the growth of bacteria, thus enhancing the growth environment for fungal microorganisms. This medium should not contain cyclohexamide, which inhibits the majority of fungi causing ocular infection.[29,30]

Thioglycolate broth is an enriched trypticase peptone broth usually containing glucose, hemin, and vitamin K.

TABLE 26.3
Indications for Laboratory Diagnosis of Conjunctivitis

Mandatory	*Recommended*
Severe chronic conjunctivitis	Any chronic conjunctivitis
Hyperacute conjunctivitis	Conjunctivitis secondary to
Ophthalmia neonatorum	canalicultis or dacryocystitis
Membranous conjunctivitis	Conjunctivitis secondary to
Parinaud's oculoglandular	infectious eczematous or
syndrome	ulcerative blepharitis
Postoperative infections	Conjunctivitis unresponsive to
	therapy
	Medicamentosa

This medium is favorable for culturing a variety of fastidious aerobic or anaerobic microorganisms. Although it is superior to commercially available bacterial transport media systems for conveying specimens to the laboratory, thioglycolate broth should not be used as the sole medium. Solid media are still superior for isolating and quantifying microorganisms. In addition, extra care must be taken not to use a contaminated plate due to the relatively low numbers of microorganisms found in most ocular specimens. This care is important to minimize the risk for overgrowth of unwanted organisms when using a medium that will support multiple microbial species.[31,32]

Mannitol salt agar is a selective medium for the isolation of *Staphylococcus* species that ferment mannitol from non-mannitol fermenting species. The peptone-based agar contains mannitol with 7.5% sodium chloride and a phenol red indicator dye. The salt concentration inhibits most other bacteria.[29]

Thayer-Martin medium is a selective agar for isolating *Neisseria gonorrheae* or *Neisseria meningitidis* from specimens contaminated with bacteria and fungi. It consists of an enriched chocolate agar with vancomycin, colistin, trimethoprim, and nystatin added to inhibit the growth of other bacteria and fungi.[33] Chocolate agar should be inoculated in conjunction with Thayer-Martin medium because some strains of pathogenic *Neisseria* species are inhibited by the additives.

Several viral transport systems are available commercially or through medical laboratories. These transport solutions contain antibiotics to inhibit the growth of bacteria and are adequate for maintaining all types of viruses until the laboratory can culture them.

A dacron-tipped or calcium alginate swab is recommended for obtaining all conjunctival specimens for culture. The use of cotton-tipped swabs should be avoided since the fatty acids in the cotton material may inhibit the growth of many bacteria. Specimens should also be obtained without the use of topical anesthesia. All topical anesthetics have

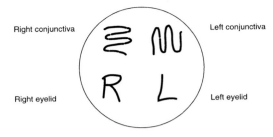

FIGURE 26.2   **Standard convention for streaking agar plates.**

some antimicrobial effects in addition to preservatives that may inhibit the recovery of some microorganisms.[34] The swab should be moistened with either thioglycolate broth or sterile saline and gently rolled through the full length of the conjunctival fornix. Specimens should be obtained from both eyes using one swab for each eye to innoculate all media. Avoid contacting the lid margins in order not to contaminate the conjunctival specimen. Innoculate the agar plates by streaking (lightly dragging) the swab across the surface of the plate. Gently roll the swab during the streaking process. After swabbing the conjunctiva, obtain specimens from the lid margins using a second moistened swab. The innoculums from both the conjunctiva and lid margins may be placed on the same plate using the standard convention shown in Figure 26.2. Following innoculation of the agar plates, plunge the swab into the thioglycolate broth, twirl the swab, and break or cut off the end that was handled,

allowing the lower portion to drop into the broth. The same procedure is followed for innoculating the viral or chlamydial transport media as with thioglycolate broth. However, dry swabs may be used to collect these samples. The practitioner is strongly advised to wear disposable latex gloves when obtaining ocular specimens with swabs or other ophthalmic instruments.

Until the laboratory sends results, empirical therapy is always started based on the clinical findings. The results of most aerobic bacterial cultures are usually known in 24 to 48 hours, anaerobic cultures in 3 to 7 days, and fungal cultures in 1 to 2 weeks.[35] Antibiotic sensitivity testing should be routinely ordered for all culture specimens. This testing allows for the proper management of the conjunctivitis following receipt of the laboratory report. Antibiotic sensitivity testing either confirms the appropriateness of the initial empirical therapy or indicates organism resistance, requiring the selection of another anti-infective agent (Table 26.4). Sensitivity testing is usually performed by a microbroth dilution method and should encompass all categories of antibiotics. The agents to be tested may vary based on availability of antibiotic disks, geographic prevalence rates of infection, or practitioner preference (Table 26.5).

Smears and Scrapings

Conjunctival smears and scrapings are used to investigate the exudative discharge or perform a cytological analysis of the conjunctival tissue. These techniques provide more immediate information regarding the disease process. A

TABLE 26.4
Efficacy of Commonly Used Topical Antibacterial Agents

Antimicrobial Agent	Bacterial Species Typically Susceptible
Bacitracin	*Staphylococcus, Streptococcus, Actinomyces, Corynebacterium, Neisseria*
Ciprofloxacin	*Staphylococcus, Streptococcus, Corynebacterium, Neisseria, Escherichia, Haemophilus, Moraxella, Proteus, Pseudomonas, Serratia, Chlamydia*
Erythromycin	*Staphylococcus, Streptococcus, Corynebacterium, Neisseria, Moraxella, Chlamydia*
Gentamicin	*Staphylococcus, Escherichia, Haemophilus, Proteus, Pseudomonas, Serratia*
Gramicidin	*Staphylococcus, Streptococcus, Actinomyces, Corynebacterium*
Neomycin	*Neisseria, Escherichia, Moraxella, Proteus, Serratia*
Norfloxacin	*Staphylococcus, Streptococcus, Neisseria, Escherichia, Haemophilus, Moraxella, Proteus, Pseudomonas, Serratia*
Ofloxacin	*Staphylococcus, Streptococcus, Neisseria, Escherichia, Haemophilus, Moraxella, Pseudomonas, Serratia*
Polymyxin B	*Echerichia, Haemophilus, Moraxella, Pseudomonas*
Sulfonamides	*Haemophilus, Moraxella, Chlamydia*
Tetracycline	*Actinomyces, Neisseria, Chlamydia*
Tobramycin	*Staphylococcus, Escherichia, Haemophilus, Proteus, Pseudomonas, Serratia*
Trimethoprim	*Staphylococcus, Streptococcus, Escherichia, Haemophilus, Moraxella, Proteus, Serratia, Chlamydia*

Adapted from Smolin G, Thoft RA. The cornea. 3 ed. Boston: Little, Brown and Co. 1994;5:135.

TABLE 26.5
Suggested Agents for Antibiotic Sensitivity Testing[a]

Ampicillin
Bacitracin
Carbenicillin
Cefazolin
Ciprofloxacin
Colistin (Polymyxin E)
Erythromycin
Gentamicin
Neomycin
Ofloxacin
Polymyxin B
Sulfisoxazole
Tetracycline
Tobramycin
Trimethoprim
Vancomycin

[a]If *Neisseria gonorrhoeae* is suspected, test ceftriaxone and penicillin G.

Kimura platinum spatula is the instrument of choice for obtaining conjunctival scraping specimens. After anesthetizing the conjunctiva with two drops of 0.5% proparacaine solution, the spatula is used to scrape the inferior palpebral conjunctival epithelial surface. Although some conjunctival blanching may occur, care should be taken to avoid any bleeding. The material is spread in a thin layer onto a clean glass microbiological slide, it is then either fixed with a commercial solution, methyl alcohol, or air dried. The smear is then stained to inspect for the presence of bacteria or inflammatory cells. The gram stain identifies bacteria as gram-positive (stains blue or purple) or gram-negative (stains pink). This information aids selecting the initial antibiotic for therapy until receiving the culture report. A conjunctival scraping often reveals a definitive inflammatory cell response indicating a particular disease process. Staining with Giesma solution is the most useful because Giesma stains inflammatory cells, epithelial cells, fungi, and chlamydial inclusion bodies present in the smear[36,37] (Table 26.6). Wright's solution or the Diff-Quik system stains conjunctival inflammatory cells, but chlamydial inclusion bodies will not be adequately stained. The Papanicolaou stain is superior for eliciting viral intranuclear inclusion bodies as well as cytological examinations for premalignancies or malignancies. The clinician should consult standard ocular microbiology and cytology texts for additional information on standard stain preparation techniques.[38]

Direct fluorescent antibody smears have become a more efficient method than Giesma stains or tissue cultures for identifying chlamydia. Commercially prepared kits make specimen collection convenient, and results are available in approximately 24 hours. Good results, however, depend on obtaining an adequate specimen. Fluorescein-labeled monoclonal antibodies in the staining reagent specific for *Chlamydia trachomatis* outer membrane proteins bind to the *Chlamydia trachomatis* in the smear. Studies[39–41] comparing direct fluorescein antibody techniques to tissue culture results have found acceptable sensitivity and specificity values. When using a commercial kit (e.g., MicroTrak), the specimen is collected with a dacron swab following topical anesthesia.[42] The superior and inferior palpebral conjunctiva should be swabbed. Direct fluorescent antibody testing can also be performed on conjunctival scrapings smeared on

TABLE 26.6
Ocular Smear Interpretation for Gram and Giesma Stains

Stain	Cells	Appearance
Gram	Gram positive	Violet to blue-black color
	Gram negative	Pinkish-red color
Giesma	Basophil	Dark blue nucleus, blue cytoplasm with dark blue-black granules
	Eosinophil	Blue nucleus, light blue cytoplasm with red to pink granules
	Epithelial	Blue nucleus, light blue cytoplasm
	Lymphocyte	Dark purple nucleus, light blue cytoplasm that may contain reddish granules
	Monocyte (macrophage)	Light purple nucleus, light gray to blue cytoplasm
	Mast	Dark blue-purple nucleus, blue cytoplasm with dark blue-black granules
	Neutrophil	Dark purple nucleus, light pink cytoplasm containing small light pink to blue-black granules
	Plasma cell	Dark purple, eccentric nucleus, light to dark blue cytoplasm, distinct perinuclear halo

Adapted from Haesaert CT. Clinical manual of ocular microbiology and cytology. St. Louis: Mosby-Year Book. 1993;4:80–84.

glass slides. Dacron swabs, however, are less traumatic and safer for infants.[43]

Enzyme-linked immunosorbent assay (ELISA) tests can identify *Chlamydia trachomatis,* herpes simplex types 1 and 2, and adenoviruses through the detection of microbial antigens. In the direct ELISA, an enzyme is covalently linked to an antigen specific monoclonal or polyclonal antibody. The antigen is then mixed with serial dilutions of the enzyme-labeled antibody. A chromogenic substrate mixed with the conjugated enzyme yields a water-soluble product whose absorbance can be measured by a spectrophotometer.[44] Recent technology has led to the development of rapid tests that do not require intact cells, live organisms, or cell cultures. ELISAs using monoclonal antibody techniques for the rapid detection of herpes simplex viruses, adenoviruses, and *Chlamydia trachomatis* have high sensitivity and specificity.[40,45,46]

Principles of Therapy

Whenever possible, therapy for infectious conjunctivitis should be specific for the offending microbial organism. In many cases, however, treatment is based on the clinical history, signs, and symptoms rather than on laboratory results from ocular cultures or smears. Although a broad-spectrum topical antibiotic is preferred when providing empirical treatment for bacterial infection, initial therapy should be based on the known antibiotic sensitivity characteristics of the various microorganisms (see Table 26.4).

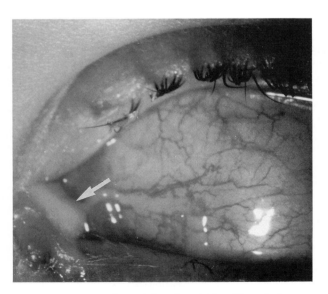

FIGURE 26.3 **Acute bacterial conjunctivitis with typical mucopurulent discharge (arrow).**

Severe disease such as gonococcal conjunctivitis may require systemic therapy. If the definitive cause is known, then antimicrobial selection should be specific for the offending organism. Treatment of viral infections is often directed at relieving patient symptomatology, since specific antiviral agents often do not exist. Chlamydial disease requires systemic therapy frequently combined with adjunctive topical therapy. The following sections will discuss specific protocols for the various categories of conjunctivitis.

Papillary Conjunctivitis

Acute Bacterial Conjunctivitis

ETIOLOGY

Both gram positive and negative organisms can cause acute bacterial conjunctivitis. In general, gram negative bacterial conjunctivitis is more severe than conjunctivitis induced by gram-positive organisms. *Staphylococcus aureus, Streptococcus pneumoniae,* and *Haemophilus influenzae* most frequently precipitate acute bacterial conjunctivitis.[47] *Staphylococcus aureus* is the most common infectious agent in patients of all ages. Less common causative organisms include *Staphylococcus epidermidis, Moraxella lacunata, Corynebacterium diphtheriae, Serratia marcescens,* and *Pseudomonas aeruginosa. Streptococcus pneumoniae* and *Haemophilus influenzae* occur more commonly in pediatric patients.[48,49]

DIAGNOSIS

Acute bacterial conjunctivitis usually begins suddenly in one eye with hyperemia and a mild to moderate mucopurulent or purulent discharge (Fig. 26.3). Associated mild to moderate lid edema and erythema may give the appearance of pseudoptosis. No preauricular lymph node swelling or tenderness occurs. The hyperemia may be either diffuse or localized to a particular sector, often nasally due to the higher accumulation of organisms from the natural tear circulation pattern. The hyperemia tends to be more intense toward the fornix and lessens at the limbus. This pattern results from the increased concentration of bacterial organisms and toxins in the fornices. Complaints of unilateral tearing and vague irritation are usually the first symptoms. Exudative material may accumulate on the eyelashes, resulting in complaints of the eyelids sticking together upon awakening. The fellow eye may become involved two to three days after the first eye. In some cases, a diffuse superficial punctate keratitis may be present, caused by microbial exotoxins damaging the corneal epithelium. Pseudomembrane or membrane formations may occur when *Streptococcus pyogenes* or *Corynebacterium diphtheria* causes the conjunctivitis. Conjunctival cultures and smears assist in the diagnosis and treatment of moderately severe or severe acute bacterial conjunctivitis.

Acute *Staphylococcus aureus* conjunctivitis occurs less commonly than chronic staphylococcal conjunctivitis. It is usually characterized by inferior palpebral conjunctival hyperemia with a mucopurulent discharge. In many cases, the bulbar conjunctiva covered by the eyelid is more hyperemic than the exposed bulbar tissue. Due to the release of staphylococcal exotoxins, superficial punctate keratitis and marginal corneal infiltrates frequently accompany the conjunctivitis.

Streptococcus pneumoniae is a frequent cause of acute bacterial conjunctivitis in children[48,49] (Fig. 26.4). Concurrent upper respiratory tract infections and otitis media, especially in children less than 4 years of age, are common.[50] In moderate climates, *S. pneumoniae* is often the etiology of epidemics of acute bacterial conjunctivitis. It is usually characterized by diffusely scattered petechial hemorrhages especially on the superior bulbar conjunctiva, and in the fornix, a mucopurulent discharge, and marginal corneal infiltrates with a somewhat transient course. Occasionally pseudomembranes form.

Haemophilus influenzae also frequently causes acute bacterial conjunctivitis in children and may concurrently cause upper respiratory infections and otitis media.[48,49,51] Conjunctivitis caused by *Haemophilus* species tends to occur more frequently in warmer climates and last longer than *Streptococcus pneumoniae* infections. The clinical appearance consists of bulbar and palpebral hyperemia with occasional petechial hemorrhages, mucopurulent discharge, and marginal corneal infiltrates. *Haemophilus influenzae biogroup aegyptius* causes a severe conjunctivitis that may precede the life-threatening pediatric disease Brazilian purpuric fever.[52] Young children with severe or improperly treated *Haemophilus* infections may present with periorbital bluish discoloration and edema suggestive of preseptal cellulitis or incipient orbital cellulitis.[53,54]

MANAGEMENT

Many cases of mild bacterial conjunctivitis are self-limiting and resolve without treatment. However, intervention with antibiotic therapy often lessens the patient's anxiety and ocular symptomatology, shortens the duration of the disease, and prevents recurrence or spread to the fellow eye.[55] The initial treatment is almost always a topical broad-spectrum antibiotic such as trimethoprim-polymyxin B, gentamicin, or tobramycin solution applied one drop 4 times per day for 5 to 7 days.[56–59] Bacitracin-polymyxin B, erythromycin, gentamicin, or tobramycin ointment may be used at bedtime as supplemental therapy or 4 times per day in children or other patients who are not comfortable with eyedrops. Moderate conjunctivitis may require a more frequent initial dosage, such as 6 to 8 times per day tapering to 4 times per day over 7 to 10 days. In moderate to severe bacterial conjunctivitis,

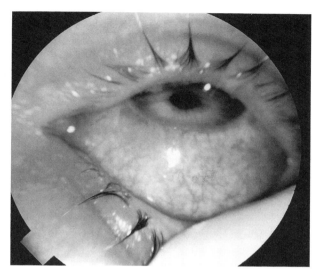

FIGURE 26.4   *Streptococcus pneumoniae* **conjunctivitis with petechial hemorrhages.**

conjunctivitis with pseudomembrane or membrane formation, or cases of drug resistance, one of the fluoroquinolones may be the initial drug of choice. These antibiotics are often applied 6 to 8 times per day initially and then tapered as the condition responds to therapy. Moderate to severe conjunctivitis often requires antibiotic therapy for 7 to 14 days to achieve complete resolution. Severe acute bacterial conjunctivitis with risk of preseptal cellulitis or conjunctivitis associated with otitis media requires concurrent oral antibiotic therapy,[54] especially in children with severe *Haemophilus* infections.[60] Possible systemic agents include amoxicillin, cefaclor, or cefotaxime with dosages appropriate for the patient's age and body weight (see Chap. 24).

Topical steroids are not indicated for most patients with acute bacterial conjunctivitis. The exception is any case demonstrating severe inflammation or the presence of pseudomembranes or true membranes. Concurrent topical antibiotic-steroid therapy hastens resolution of the inflammatory response in these cases.

Sulfonamide, chloramphenicol, and tetracycline antibiotics are generally not drugs of choice for treating bacterial conjunctivitis. The sulfonamides have a broad spectrum of activity against gram positive and negative organisms, but they are bacteriostatic agents that require normal immune responses to eliminate the infection. Since *Staphylococcus aureus* is often resistant to these agents, sulfonamides may delay resolution of the infection or create a low grade chronic conjunctivitis. The anti-infective activity of the sulfonamides is also inhibited by para-aminobenzoic acid (PABA) found in purulent exudates. Topical 10% sodium sulfacetamide and 4% sulfisoxazole are effective in mild cases of acute bacterial conjunctivitis when little or no mucopurulent discharge is present. The sulfonamides are also contraindicated in patients with allergies to these drugs, which may lead to erythema multiforme. Although not common, erythema multiforme has reportedly followed topical application of 10% sodium sulfacetamide.[61]

Chloramphenicol has a broad spectrum of activity against *Streptococcus pneumoniae* and many gram negative organisms, but several other available anti-infective agents are more efficacious and have lower risks of adverse effects. Chloramphenicol has been linked to numerous cases of aplastic anemia. The reaction is not dose-related and occurs weeks or months following completion of therapy.[62]

Tetracycline is useful as adjunctive therapy for chlamydial infections but not for initial therapy of acute bacterial conjunctivitis. Numerous organisms are resistant to tetracycline therapy.

Trimethoprim is a bactericidal agent effective against most gram positive and negative organisms except for *Pseudomonas aeruginosa*. When combined with polymyxin B, which is effective against *Pseudomonas*, it provides broad spectrum antimicrobial activity for the initial therapy of acute bacterial conjunctivitis. The usual dosage for the solution is one drop 4 times per day. Studies[59,63–65] indicate that trimethoprim is a safe and effective agent for treating conjunctivitis caused by a variety of organisms in patients of all ages above 2 months. Trimethoprim-polymyxin B is as effective as neomycin-polymyxin B-gramicidin for treating acute bacterial conjunctivitis.[59] It is particularly useful for children because of its antimicrobial activity against *Streptococcus pneumoniae* and *Haemophilus influenzae*.[65]

Gentamicin and tobramycin are aminoglycosides that are bactericidal against most gram negative bacteria, especially *Pseudomonas aeruginosa*, and some gram positive bacteria, particularly *Staphylococcus aureus*. *Haemophilus influenzae* and *Neisseria* species have a variable susceptibility to the aminoglycosides. Anaerobes, *Streptococcus pneumoniae* and the alpha hemolytic streptococci are resistant to the aminoglycosides.[66,67] The usual dosage frequency for these agents is 4 times per day whether in solution or ointment. Potential adverse effects include a toxic epitheliopathy or superficial punctate keratitis, and hypersensitivity reactions. The risk of adverse reactions is greater when the drugs are applied more often than 6 times per day or are applied as ointments. Other rarely occurring adverse events reported with gentamicin are pupillary mydriasis, conjunctival paresthesia, and neuromuscular blocking activity. Aminoglycosides should be used cautiously in patients with myasthenia gravis. These patients are more susceptible to the potential neuromuscular blocking action, which may lead to respiratory failure.[68]

Neomycin is a widely used topical aminoglycoside agent for skin wounds and in otolaryngology. Its antibacterial activity resembles gentamicin and tobramycin except for *Pseudomonas aeruginosa*, *Streptococcus pneumoniae*, and the alpha hemolytic streptococci, which are resistant. Neomycin's usefulness for treating acute bacterial conjunctivitis is limited by the relatively high rate of hypersensitivity reactions. Allergic reactions occur in about 6% to 8% of patients treated and are often more severe than the original infection. For these reasons, most clinicians avoid neomycin for routine use in treating acute bacterial conjunctivitis.[69]

Bacitracin is bactericidal for most gram positive organisms, especially *Staphylococcus* and *Streptococcus* species. It is particularly useful when combined with polymyxin B in an ophthalmic ointment. Bacitracin-polymyxin B ointment provides broad spectrum antibacterial activity for patients who require nighttime therapy or who are not comfortable with eyedrops. Bacitracin-polymyxin B ointment is particularly effective in the pediatric population due to the high incidence of *Streptococcus* infection. The usual dosage frequency is 3 to 4 times per day. Although adverse events are rare, hypersensitivity reactions can occur.

Polymyxin B is bactericidal for most gram negative organisms, especially *Haemophilus* and *Pseudomonas* species. *Neisseria* and *Proteus* species, however, are resistant. Combining polymyxin B with bacitracin or trimethoprim achieves broad spectrum antibacterial activity for treating acute bacterial conjunctivitis. Polymyxin B is primarily used for superficial infections since it is not absorbed through mucous membrane or skin tissue. Adverse reactions are rare.

Erythromycin is bactericidal for many gram positive organisms, such as *Staphylococcus aureus* and *Streptococcus pneumoniae*. Although erythromycin may have some bacteriostatic activity against *Haemophilus* and *Neisseria*, it is not a drug of choice for these organisms. Resistant strains of *Staphylococcus aureus* can be encountered. Because of its low incidence of adverse reactions, erythromycin is extremely well tolerated, particularly by children. Erythromycin is primarily used as adjunctive therapy at bedtime.

The fluoroquinolone antibiotics are potent agents with strong bactericidal activity for most gram positive and negative organisms.[70] Fluoroquinolones are usually indicated for moderate to severe acute bacterial conjunctivitis. The usual initial dosage is 6–8 times per day, tapering to 4 times per day over 5 to 7 days. Use of these agents for routine therapy or prophylactic purposes is controversial. Three fluoroquinolones are currently available: ciprofloxacin, norfloxacin, and ofloxacin.

Ciprofloxacin is effective against virtually all gram negative and most gram positive organisms including aminoglycoside-resistant *Pseudomonas*, methicillin-resistant *Staphylococcus*, *Neisseria* species and *Chlamydia trachomatis*.[71–74] However, *Streptococcus pneumoniae* infections tend to have a higher possibility for resistance and should be treated with more frequent dosing to achieve higher tissue concentrations and effect satisfactory resolution.[70] Despite ciprofloxacin's mechanism of action and strong clinical performance, reports indicate the existence of some resistant bacterial strains of *Pseudomonas* and

Staphylococcus.[75,76] Ciprofloxacin, however, does not exhibit any significant epithelial toxicity common with aminoglycosides, and the white drug precipitate seen in 16% of the patients receiving keratitis therapy does not generally occur when treating acute bacterial conjunctivitis.[71,77]

Norfloxacin has bactericidal activity similar to ciprofloxacin but is not as effective against *Pseudomonas aeruginosa, Streptococcus* species, and *Chlamydia trachomatis.*[73,78] The drug may not sufficiently inhibit *Streptococcus pneumoniae.*[70] Clinical studies[79–82] indicate that norfloxacin effectively eradicates most bacterial strains in acute bacterial conjunctivitis. Although norfloxacin has greater epithelial toxicity than does ciprofloxacin or ofloxacin, it is a safe and effective agent for treating bacterial conjunctivitis, with only 4.2% of the patients treated having adverse reactions.[77,83]

Ofloxacin has a bactericidal potency and spectrum closer to ciprofloxacin than to norfloxacin. It has strong antibacterial activity against a wide spectrum of gram negative and positive organisms including *Streptococcus pneumoniae,* but more frequent dosages should be used when infection with *Streptococcus* species is suspected.[70,84] Compared to gentamicin, ofloxacin had a greater clinical (98% to 92%) and microbiologic (78% to 67%) resolution in a study of 198 patients. Only 3.2% reported side effects for ofloxacin versus 7.1% for gentamicin.[85] Ofloxacin achieved better clinical resolution than tobramycin in a multicenter study on days three to five following initiation of treatment, but the efficacy of the two agents was relatively equal at day 11.[86] Ofloxacin also maintains tear concentration levels greater than its MIC_{90} values for 4 hours after administration.[87] Thus, ofloxacin appears to have prolonged contact time with infected tissues, making it an appropriate agent for more severe acute bacterial conjunctivitis. Additionally, when compared to ciprofloxacin and norfloxacin, ofloxacin has the highest level of corneal penetration and attained aqueous levels, 4 times greater than the other agents.[88]

Vancomycin is being more frequently used for topical therapy due to the increasing resistance of some *Staphylococcus* strains. Use of topical vancomycin at a concentration of 31 mg/ml has been successful in treating patients with chronic *Staphylococcus epidermidis* and methicillin-resistant *Staphylococcus aureus* infection. For most clinical situations, however, this therapy should be considered only after commercially formulated agents have failed to achieve resolution.[89]

Hyperacute Bacterial Conjunctivitis

ETIOLOGY

Hyperacute bacterial conjunctivitis most commonly results from *Neisseria gonorrhoeae* and less frequently from *Neisseria meningitidis.*[90] Other pathogens that can cause hyperacute conjunctivitis include *Staphylococcus aureus,*

Streptococcus species, *Haemophilus influenzae, Moraxella (Branhamella) catarrhalis, Escherichia coli,* and *Pseudomonas aeruginosa.*

DIAGNOSIS

Hyperacute bacterial conjunctivitis is characterized by a sudden, rapid onset of a purulent conjunctivitis with a copious discharge, chemosis, and severe hyperemia (Fig. 26.5). Complaints of ocular pain, tenderness of the globe, periorbital discomfort, and lid swelling commonly occur. Preauricular lymphadenopathy and preseptal cellulitis with associated fever are present concurrently in many cases. Typically, the purulent discharge quickly recurs when wiped away. Depending on the offending pathogen, if not managed properly hyperacute conjunctivitis can lead to subsequent conjunctival membrane or symblepharon formation, bacterial keratitis, peripheral corneal ulcers, and corneal perforation. Laboratory assessment is mandatory for hyperacute conjunctivitis, including both conjunctival cultures and smears prior to instilling any medications. Smears should be analyzed with gram stain at the time of the initial visit. Cultures should be performed using blood, chocolate, and Thayer-Martin agar media.

Neisseria gonorrhoeae hyperacute conjunctivitis, a disease primarily of the neonate and of sexually active adolescents or young adults, most likely results from direct contact with infected genitals or indirect contact by the hands.[90] Ocular involvement does not occur frequently. Only four cases of hyperacute conjunctivitis were reported among 800,000 cases of gonorrhea.[91] The patient's medical and

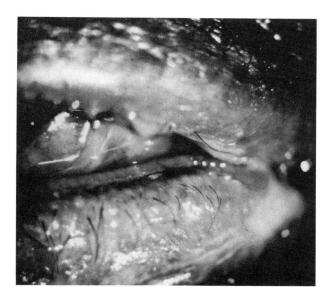

FIGURE 26.5 **Hyperacute bacterial conjunctivitis with copious purulent discharge.**

sexual history must be reviewed, since associated systemic findings such as urethritis or vaginitis frquently occur. Potential sexual abuse should be considered when a child develops gonococcal conjunctivitis.[92] Gonococcal conjunctivitis is usually unilateral and progresses rapidly, often with periocular involvement. Ocular pain with preauricular lymphadenopathy is common. The marked conjunctival inflammatory response includes chemosis and hyperemia with lid edema and a profuse, thick yellow-green purulent exudate. If not treated promptly, the conjunctivitis can lead to preseptal cellulitis, keratitis, corneal ulceration, dacryoadenitis, and potential septicemia. If left untreated, *Neisseria gonorrhoeae* can penetrate an intact cornea in 48 hours.[90,91,93]

Neisseria meningitidis hyperacute conjunctivitis usually occurs in children and causes a milder conjunctivitis similar to *Neisseria gonorrhoeae*. The disease is often bilateral and may occur in conjunction with meningococcemia, meningitis, and endogenous endophthalmitis. One report indicates that meningococcal conjunctivitis led to systemic meningococcal infection in 6 of 21 patients.[94] In a study[95] of 21 patients and literature review of another 63 patients with primary meningococcal conjunctivitis, 9 were neonates, 55 were children, and 20 were adults with a male to female ratio of 1.76 to 1.00. The most common ocular complication was corneal ulcer. Systemic disease developed in 17.8% of the patients and was significantly more frequent in patients receiving only topical therapy.

MANAGEMENT

Hyperacute bacterial conjunctivitis must be treated aggressively, since potentially blinding consequences may result. Topical and systemic antibiotics should start immediately following tissue specimen collection for laboratory analysis. Frequent irrigation of the conjunctiva with normal saline removes the purulent exudate, permitting better antibiotic access to the affected tissues. If *Neisseria gonorrhoeae* or *N. meningitidis* is suspected, the patient should receive full doses of systemic antibiotics.[96] A study of 13 patients indicated that a single 1-gram dose of intramuscular ceftriaxone is curative for gonococcal conjunctivitis. All patients cultured negative 6 hours and 12 hours following treatment.[97] However, the treatment can be repeated for five consecutive days if necessary. The historical drug of choice for therapy is penicillin G 100,000 U/kg/day administered in four divided doses or 4.8 million units intramuscularly divided into two doses and preceded by 1 g oral probenecid. Spectromycin 4 g intramuscularly given in two divided doses at one visit or 1.5 g oral tetracycline followed by 0.5 g 4 times per day for 4 days may be effective alternatives for adult patients sensitive to penicillin. Adjunctive topical therapy consists of bacitracin, gentamicin, or tetracycline ointments or penicillin G 100,000 U/ml every 2 hours.[93,96]

Due to their broad, potent bactericidal activity,[70–73,84,87,88] the fluoroquinolone antibiotics, specifically ciprofloxacin and ofloxacin, are also promising for topical therapy of hyperacute conjunctivitis. Topical ciprofloxacin or ofloxacin should be administered initially two drops every hour, concurrently with a systemic penicillin or cephalosporin for hyperacute bacterial conjunctivitis caused by organisms other than *Neisseria* species. Examples of adjunctive systemic therapy include ampicillin, amoxicillin, or cefaclor 250 mg 4 times per day depending on the patient's body weight and antibiotic sensitivities.

Chronic Bacterial Conjunctivitis

ETIOLOGY

Staphylococcus aureus or *Moraxella lacunata* most often cause chronic bacterial conjunctivitis. Other microorganisms commonly found in the normal flora may be implicated if an overgrowth occurs that disrupts the normal balance among the organisms. Frequently *Staphylococcus epidermidis* is the etiologic agent in chronic blepharitis, which may alter the normal tear film composition. *Proteus mirabilis*, *Escherichia coli*, *Klebsiella pneumoniae*, or *Serratia marcescens* may on occasion be the etiology of the chronic conjunctivitis. Environmental factors such as air pollution, allergies, and contact lens wear may also influence the nature of the offending bacterial agent and the subsequent immunologic response.[90,98,99]

DIAGNOSIS

Chronic bacterial conjunctivitis may present with various nonspecific symptoms and signs that are difficult to evaluate. Complaints of intermittent irritation, foreign body sensation, burning, tearing, redness, and sticky eyelids are common. Clinically, the conjunctiva may have a mild diffuse hyperemia, a thickened appearance, mucoid or mucopurulent discharge, and a papillary or follicular reaction. Patients with chronic bacterial conjunctivitis must undergo a thorough evaluation of the eyelids due to the high correlation of lid disease with chronic bacterial conjunctivitis. In the presence of chronic blepharitis or angular blepharoconjunctivitis, the lid margins often appear hyperemic and crusty with markedly reduced tear film quality and break-up time. The clinician should also carefully evaluate the lacrimal drainage system for signs of dacryocystitis or stagnant tear flow. Other clinical findings include bacterial exotoxin hypersensitivity reactions, marginal corneal infiltrates, and phlyctenules.[90,98,99] Conjunctival smears stained with Giesma and gram stains are extremely useful for evaluating the infectious versus inflammatory components of chronic bacterial conjunctivitis. Cultures on blood and chocolate agar media with drug sensitivities prove helpful in isolating the offending organism and determining the appropriate anti-infective agent.

MANAGEMENT

Adequate treatment almost always depends on good eyelid hygiene by the patient in conjunction with topical antibiotics. The bacterial pathogen often inhabits the lid margins or the base of the eyelashes even in asymptomatic patients. This concurrent blepharitis must be addressed with lid therapy consisting of a routine of warm compresses for 10 to 15 minutes, massaging of the lid margins, and lid scrubs 2–4 times per day. These procedures are crucial for a positive therapeutic outcome and must be performed by the patient on an ongoing basis. The lid scrubs may be accomplished with a warm washcloth, cotton-tipped applicator, or a commercially available cleansing agent (see Chap. 3). Since *Staphylococcus aureus* is often the etiology, treatment may also require topical erythromycin, bacitracin, or bacitracin-polymyxin B ointment applied 2 or 3 times per day. If gram negative bacteria are the offending organisms, bacitracin-polymyxin B or an aminoglycoside ointment is the drug of choice. In cases of primary meibomianitis, adjunctive oral treatment consisting of tetracycline 250 mg four times per day or doxycycline 50 mg twice per day for 10 to 21 days significantly improves the patient's symptoms. The chronic bacterial conjunctivitis is treated with topical antibiotics that have broad antibacterial activity, such as trimethoprim-polymyxin B or gentamicin solution applied four times per day. Antibiotic therapy should be limited to periods of disease exacerbation with the lid hygiene and scrubs providing the daily maintenance regimen. Occasionally topical erythromycin, bacitracin, or bacitracin-polymyxin B ointment applied at bedtime for several weeks proves beneficial as part of the therapeutic protocol. This type of therapy, however, always carries the risk of developing resistant organisms.[98,99]

If significant bacterial exotoxin hypersensitivity, marginal corneal infiltrates, or phlyctenules are present, treatment may require concurrent topical steroid therapy. When chronic dacryocystitis is involved, treatment should include irrigation of the lacrimal system with trimethoprim-polymyxin B or gentamicin. Adjunctive systemic antibiotic therapy may also be required (see Chap. 25).[98,99]

Follicular Conjunctivitis

The appearance of conjunctival follicles in the setting of acute or chronic conjunctivitis is a specific clinical finding that limits the differential diagnosis to clinical entities. Conjunctival follicles appear as avascular, translucent, amorphous lumps usually within the tarsal conjunctiva. Conjunctival follicles are lymphoid germinal centers. The conjunctival lymphatic system responds to antigen exposure with hyperplasia of the T-lymphocytes contained within the lymphoid germinal center of the follicle. This antigenic response can occur in viral and certain bacterial infections and in response to exposure to toxic agents.

Viral Agents

ADENOVIRAL CONJUNCTIVITIS

Etiology   Adenoviral infection is a common cause of acute follicular conjunctivitis. Over 45 immunologically distinct serotypes have been identified, 33 of which are pathogenic for humans.[100] Most adenoviral infections initially involve the upper respiratory tract and/or nasal mucosa. Epidemic outbreaks of adenoviral conjunctivitis have been recognized as distinct clinical entities including epidemic keratoconjunctivitis (EKC) and pharyngoconjunctival fever (PCF). In clinical practice, the exact etiologic agent is rarely identified, and different viral serotypes have been identified as the causative agent of both EKC and PCF. Viral transmission in epidemic outbreaks occurs through direct contact, contact with contaminated ophthalmic instruments and solutions, and in swimming pools.

Diagnosis.   Adenoviral conjunctivitis classically presents as an acute follicular conjunctivitis. The infection is usually unilateral at onset and often becomes bilateral after several days, although the second eye is frequently less involved than the first. Marked conjunctival injection is present, along with variable degrees of chemosis. In addition to conjunctival injection, moderate to marked eyelid and periorbital edema may also occur (Fig. 26.6). Occasionally petechial subconjunctival hemorrhages form and may coalesce, resulting in diffuse subconjunctival hemorrhage. Ipsilateral preauricular or submandibular lymphadenopathy, with or without tenderness, is a common and often distinguishing feature of adenoviral conjunctivitis (Fig. 26.7). Patients complain of moderate foreign body sensation as well as profuse tearing. They often also complain of eyelid crusting, particularly upon awakening. In severe cases, pseudomembranes or true conjunctival membranes may form on the lower or upper tarsal conjunctiva. These membranes represent the accumulation of mucus and inflammatory debris.[101] The membranes can cause significant discomfort and foreign body sensation. In rare instances, severe conjunctival membrane formation can result in conjunctival scarring and secondary cicatricial entropion.

When acute conjunctivitis is accompanied by mild fever and pharyngitis, the clinical triad is recognized as pharyngoconjunctival fever (PCF). An adenoviral infection seen most commonly in children, PCF is highly contagious and is often spread from contaminated swimming pools.

Corneal involvement, however, distinguishes EKC from other forms of adenoviral conjunctivitis. The first manifestation of corneal disease in EKC is the appearance of discrete diffuse punctate epitheliopathy. A focal epithelial keratitis (coarses epithelial erosions) follows. Ten to 14 days after the onset of infection, faint subepithelial opacities begin to form under the epithelial lesions (Fig. 26.8). The punctate epithelial lesions resolve, but the subepithelial infiltrates may

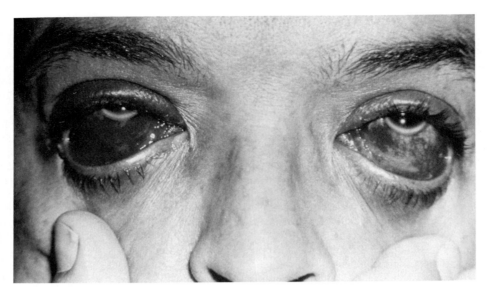

FIGURE 26.6 **Epidemic keratoconjunctivitis affecting right eye first, then left eye. Note more intense involvement of right eye. Marked conjunctival injection and chemosis, subconjunctival hemorrhages, and lid edema are present. (Courtesy William Wallace, O.D.)**

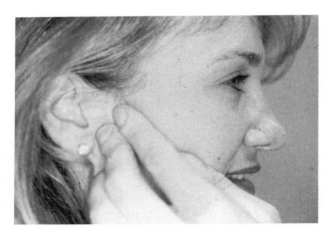

FIGURE 26.7 **Palpation of preauricular node in patient with adenoviral conjunctivitis.**

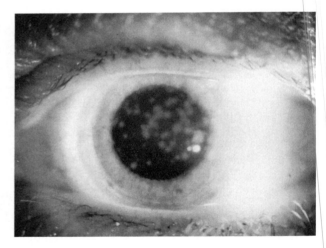

FIGURE 26.8 **Multiple subepithelial corneal opacities in epidemic keratoconjunctivitis.**

remain for an extended period, months or even years. When infiltrates or epithelial lesions occur on the visual axis, patients may experience decreased visual acuity. Besides loss of vision, the epithelial lesions and subepithelial opacities can cause bothersome glare, photophobia, and foreign body sensation.

Since microbiologic investigation is often not necessary in cases of nonspecific viral conjunctivitis, the clinician makes the diagnosis of adenoviral conjunctivitis based on clinical signs and symptoms. Other conditions that can have a similar clinical appearance include herpetic conjunctivitis, adult inclusion conjunctivitis, and hemorrhagic conjunctivitis. Severe membranous conjunctivitis can also occur in infections from beta *Streptococcus, Corynebacterium*

TABLE 26.7
Differentiation of Epidemic Keratonjunctivitis (EKC) from Pharyngoconjunctival Fever (PCF)

Condition	Age	Conjunctiva	Cornea	Associated Findings	Etiologic Agent
EKC	Any age	Follicles, hyperemia, membranes	Subepithelial infiltrates common	Tender, palpable preauricular node	Adenovirus type 8 and 19
PCF	Predominantly children	Follicles, hyperemia, membranes	Superficial punctate keratitis; subepithelial infiltrates not common	Fever, pharyngitis, nontender node	Adenovirus type 3 and 7

diphtheriae, or, uncommonly in Stevens-Johnson syndrome. The almost 50% occurrence of significant subepithelial infiltrates and their time course best differentiates EKC from these conditions. The conjunctivitis associated with EKC tends to be more severe than that caused by nonspecific adenoviral infection (Table 26.7).

Management. Adenoviral conjunctivitis is a self-limited infection. Most cases resolve spontaneously over approximately 14 to 21 days. In patients who develop keratitis and subepithelial infiltrates, corneal manifestations can last for many months. During the acute phase of adenoviral conjunctivitis, particularly in patients who are moderately symptomatic, supportive therapy including cold compresses, decongestants, or lubricants can help to relieve patients' symptoms. Topical antihistamines may be helpful if itching is significant. Topical antibiotics are generally not useful in the management of adenoviral infections. Although secondary bacterial infection is possible, the risk of hypersensitivity and toxic reactions to topical antibiotics must be weighed against the potential benefit of preventing secondary bacterial infection. Patients can experience a considerable degree of discomfort and reduced visual function when infiltrates are extensive. They should, therefore, receive assurance that symptoms often worsen from the time of initial presentation.

The role of steroids in the management of EKC remains controversial. The subepithelial infiltrates represent a cell-mediated immune response, most likely to viral protein.[102] Suppressing the immune response with steroids may interfere with clearing the viral antigen and ultimately prolong the course of the corneal disease. Patients who start steroids may develop a steroid dependence. Discontinuation of the steroid may result in recurrence of the subepithelial infiltrates.[103] The existence of an EKC-like variant of herpes simplex keratoconjunctivitis should further discourage the use of topical steroids.[104] Steroids should be reserved for patients who are highly symptomatic or functionally impaired due to their symptoms. Steroids are also indicated for patients who are significantly visually impaired due to subepithelial infiltrates on or near the visual axis. Clinicians should inform patients about the potential risks and benefits prior to instituting steroid treatment.

The use of antiviral agents in the management of adenoviral conjunctivitis has proved uniformly disappointing. Although inhibition of adenoviral replication *in vitro* has been demonstrated, Ward and associates[105] demonstrated no difference in the duration or outcome of EKC in patients treated with trifluridine, dexamethasone, or artificial tears.[106] Because of the relatively high degree of toxicity of antiviral agents, and due to the generally self-limited course of the infection, antivirals are generally not indicated.[107]

Educating patients regarding appropriate hygiene and following appropriate infection control procedures in the office are extremely important aspects of management. Adenoviral infections are contagious, and infected individuals continue to shed virus in tears and from the nasopharynx for approximately two weeks.[108] Patients should be appropriately educated with regard to transmission of the infection and should be carefully instructed to wash hands and to avoid sharing personal items such as linens and pillowcases. Direct hand-to-eye contact may result in the transmission of infection.

The practitioner's office should follow proper infection control procedures to prevent transmission of adenoviral conjunctivitis.[109] Staff should carefully disinfect equipment used in examining infected patients. Any tonometer tips used should be carefully disinfected. Adenovirus can persist on nonporous surfaces for up to 34 days.[110] Safe practice includes the use of barrier protection, such as gloves, while examining patients with adenoviral conjunctivitis. Careful handwashing before and after patient examination is mandatory.

HERPES SIMPLEX CONJUNCTIVITIS

Etiology. In the United States, 70% of the population has immunologic evidence of prior herpes simplex virus (HSV) infection by the age of 15 to 20 years and 97% by the age of 60.[111] Primary HSV infection is subclinical in 85% to 90% of cases.[112] Of the two types of herpes simplex virus, type 1 and type 2, type 1 predominates in approximately 85% of adult cases and is responsible for infection above the waist.[113]

Type 1 and type 2 ocular infections are clinically indistinguishable, although type 2 infections tend to be more severe.

Herpetic conjunctivitis is usually a manifestation of primary HSV infection. Primary HSV infection generally occurs in children between the ages of 6 months and 5 years. Most cases of herpetic ocular infection result from the nonvenereal form of the virus (HSV type 1). Ocular infection with HSV type 2 occurs in newborns and adults. Infection may result from contact with the virus in the infected birth canal or from auto-inoculation after sexual contact with an infected partner.

Diagnosis.   Careful examination of the lids and periorbital skin may reveal the typical vesicular eruptions characteristic of herpes simplex dermatitis (Fig. 26.9). These erythematous vesicular eruptions may have an appearance similar to ulcerative staphylococcal blepharitis (see Chap. 24). The dermatologic signs do not always occur, and acute follicular conjunctivitis may be the only manifestation of the primary infection. The acute onset of unilateral bulbar conjunctival injection and tearing in a young child should always bring to mind the possibility of primary herpetic infection. If the disease is bilateral, the second eye will most commonly become inflamed less than one week from the onset of infection in the fellow eye. Conjunctival follicles are a prominent feature, and pseudomembrane formation is not uncommon.[114] Many patients develop preauricular lymphadenopathy. Corneal involvement is not uncommon with the development of diffuse punctate epitheliopathy, subepithelial infiltrates, or the appearance of a typical dendritic or geographic corneal ulcer (see Chap. 27). Occasionally, dendritic or geographic bulbar conjunctival ulcerations occur.[245]

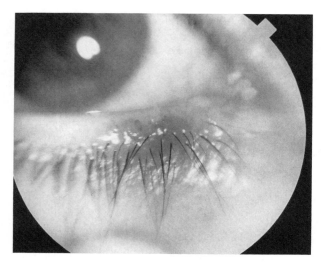

FIGURE 26.9   **Vesicular herpes simplex lesions of eyelid margin.**

Care must be taken to diagnose cases of herpetic conjunctivitis accurately. Herpetic conjunctivitis shares many of the clinical features of adenoviral conjunctivitis, and in the absence of recognizable corneal disease, the two entities cannot easily be distinguished. Differentiation is particularly important if the practitioner plans to use steroids as part of the contemplated management of adenoviral conjunctivitis—the use of topical steroids exacerbates herpetic infections.

Management.   Up to 50% of patients with herpetic eye disease experience a second episode of ocular involvement within 2 years of their initial episode.[115] Herpetic conjunctivitis without corneal involvement, however, is usually benign and self-limited.[116,117]

In patients with primary herpetic blepharoconjunctivitis, prophylactic treatment with antiviral agents to prevent corneal involvement is common practice. Trifluridine (Viroptic) is usually well tolerated and is effective against many strains of HSV. Topical dosage is one drop every 2 hours for a maximum of 9 drops daily. This dosage is reduced to one drop every 4 hours when clinical improvement occurs. Treatment continues for 3 to 5 days after clinical resolution of the infection. Vidarabine, available in a 3% ointment, can also be effective for cases resistant to trifluridine. Vidarabine is used 3 to 5 times daily until clinical resolution of the infection. Idoxuridine (IDU) as a 0.1% solution administered hourly during the day and every 2 hours at night is also effective against herpetic infection. Idoxuridine, however, is more toxic than either trifluridine or vidarabine and can cause toxic or hypersensitivity reactions. Chronic topical use of IDU may result in conjunctival cicatrization.[118] Lack of response to IDU in suspected HSV conjunctivitis should suggest resistance to the drug, and practitioners should place the patient on a different antiviral agent. Note that steroids are specifically contraindicated in the treatment of HSV conjunctivitis since steroids can increase virus replication. Topical antibiotics are also of limited value in treating herpes simplex virus. The risk of bacterial superinfection is low, and the potential toxic and hypersensitivity reactions associated with their use may obscure the clinical course of the underlying viral infection.

VARICELLA ZOSTER CONJUNCTIVITIS

Etiology.   Herpes zoster results from reactivation of the dormant varicella virus. This is the same virus generally acquired during childhood and manifested as "chicken pox." The incidence and severity of herpes zoster infection increases with age.[119] An increased incidence of herpes zoster is also associated with immune compromise. Peak incidence occurs between the age of 50 and 75 years. In young patients with no history of malignancy or immunosuppression, herpes zoster infection may be the presenting sign of AIDS-related complex (ARC) or AIDS.[120] Ocular lesions can occur in approximately 50% to 71% of the patients who develop active herpes zoster infection involving the first (ophthalmic) division of the trigeminal nerve.[121]

Diagnosis.   Acute follicular conjunctivitis is the most common ocular manifestation of herpes zoster infection. Patients typically present with vesicular eruptions localized to the dermatome innervated by the affected nerve ganglia. The vesicular eruptions respect the midline, revealing the neurologic nature of the infection. The vesicles may affect the skin of the eyelids and extend onto the side and tip of the nose (Hutchinson's sign) (Fig. 26.10), a result of spread along the nasociliary branch of the ophthalmic division of the trigeminal nerve. Ocular involvement most commonly includes the appearance of lid swelling, bulbar conjunctival injection, and chemosis. Regional lymphadenopathy may occasionally develop. Other ocular manifestations can include the development of keratitis (punctate, dendritic or disciform), anterior uveitis, and increased intraocular pressure. Cranial nerve palsies, optic neuritis, and retinitis can also rarely occur.[122]

Management.   The acute conjunctivitis can be treated with broad-spectrum topical antibiotics to help prevent secondary bacterial infection. The use of topical steroids may help the patient feel more comfortable and relieve some of the conjunctival inflammation. In contrast to herpes simplex infection, in which steroids are specifically contraindicated, topical steroids do not exacerbate herpes zoster infection. If steroids are used, the patient should be carefully monitored for the development of increased intraocular pressure. Oral acyclovir 800 mg five times daily for 7 days effects a rapid resolution of the signs and symptoms of acute herpes zoster ophthalmicus (HZO), particularly if treatment is initiated within 72 hours of the skin eruption.[123] Oral acyclovir also reduces the incidence of postherpetic neuralgia, which occurs in approximately 20% of patients.[124–126]

MOLLUSCUM CONTAGIOSUM

Etiology.   Molluscum contagiosum is a dermatologic lesion caused by a pox virus and is responsible for causing chronic or recurrent follicular conjunctivitis in patients who have lesions of the periorbital skin or eyelids.

Diagnosis.   The eyelid lesion is smooth with a central area of umbilication (Fig. 26.11). Some lesions may be difficult to detect, since they can be obscured by eyelashes. Clinical manifestations of conjunctivitis include the chronic and intermittent occurrence of conjunctival hyperemia, tearing and follicular hypertrophy of the lower tarsal conjunctiva. Symptoms often wax and wane, with patients often receiv-

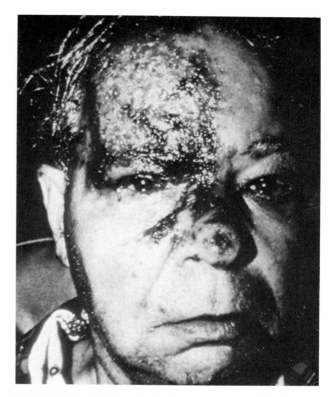

FIGURE 26.10   Hutchinson's sign in herpes zoster ophthalmicus. Note simultaneous involvement of the eye and the side and tip of the nose. (Courtesy William Wallace, O.D.)

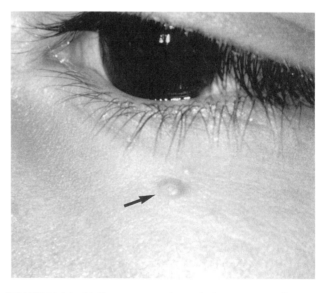

FIGURE 26.11   Molluscum contagiosum lesion (arrow) on lower eyelid of young child.

ing multiple antibiotics and steroids. The treatment causes the condition to improve; however, the untreated skin lesion continues to shed virus particles that cause a toxic reaction and chronic inflammation.

Management. The management of chronic follicular conjunctivitis associated with molluscum contagiosum involves removal of the dermatologic lesion to prevent further spread of virus particles into the eye.

ACUTE HEMORRHAGIC CONJUNCTIVITIS

Etiology. In 1970, Chatterjee and associates[127] described an unusual type of acute viral conjunctivitis. The enterovirus was recognized as causing acute hemorrhagic conjunctivitis (AHC). Coxsackievirus has also been implicated as a cause of AHC. Although serologically distinct from the enterovirus, the coxsackievirus causes disease with a similar clinical appearance. Over the past 25 years, many outbreaks of epidemic AHC have occurred worldwide.

Diagnosis. Bulbar conjunctival injection, tearing, and pain characterize the rapid onset of AHC. The conjunctiva develops moderate to severe hyperemia. Small petechial hemorrhages may subsequently form on the bulbar conjunctiva. Most patients develop follicles in the lower tarsal conjunctiva and demonstrate regional lymphadenopathy. The superior bulbar conjunctival petechial hemorrhages may increase and spread until there is diffuse and extensive subconjunctival hemorrhage. However, extensive subconjunctival hemorrhage is not a universal feature of the infection.[128] Ocular examination or lid eversion may bring on

hemorrhaging. The cornea often demonstrates a fine punctate epithelial keratitis. One or more subepithelial infiltrates may occur. The incubation period for AHC is frequently one day or less. This rapid onset contrasts with most cases of adenoviral conjunctivitis, which have a longer incubation period and duration. In addition to the acute conjunctivitis, several reports describe late neurologic complications, including asymmetric flaccid motor paralysis and cranial nerve palsies.[129]

Management. AHC is self-limited over a period of 10 to 14 days. Since antiviral agents are ineffective, the preferred treatment consists of topical application of cool compresses and astringents. Patient education should stress the severe communicability of this disorder. Topical steroids have not demonstrated any significant effect and may actually prolong the infection. Patients should also be reassured since the appearance of diffuse subconjunctival hemorrhage in the presence of pain and tearing can prove quite distressful.

NONSPECIFIC VIRAL CONJUNCTIVITIS

Acute conjunctivitis is a common feature of many other viral illnesses. The clinical manifestations are nonspecific, and knowledge of the systemic manifestations of these diseases leads to the appropriate diagnosis. Most cases result in mild, acute, transient, bilateral, follicular conjunctivitis. Treatment of the conjunctivitis in each case is generally supportive, with cold compresses, decongestants and lubricants used to ease the symptoms of acute conjunctivitis. Table 26.8 summarizes clinical features of the most common viral illnesses with associated conjunctivitis.

TABLE 26.8
Systemic Viral Diseases with Associated Conjunctivitis

Disease	Virus	Systemic Findings	Conjunctival Findings	Other
Infectious mononucleosis	Epstein-Barr virus	Malaise, headache, fever, sore throat, lymphadenopathy	Lid edema, hyperemia, follicles, membranes	Dacryoadenitis, episcleritis, epithelial and nummular keratitis
Newcastle's	Paramyxovirus	Mild upper respiratory symptoms, lympadenopathy	Unilateral follicular conjunctivitis	Associated with poultry exposure
Measles	Rubeola	Fever, cough, brownish pink maculopapular eruptions of skin	Hyperemia, chemosis commonly associated with prodrome	Koplik's spots
German measles	Rubella	Malaise, fever, rhinitis, fine pinkish macules	Mild hyperemia, follicles	Tender postauricular lymphadenopathy
Mumps	Paramyxovirus	Malaise, headache, anorexia, parotiditis	Hyperemia, follicles	Rare disciform keratitis
Influenza	Influenza	Cough, fever, malaise, headache	Hyperemia, follicles	Epidemic seasonal outbreaks

Nonviral Infectious Etiologies

Several other infectious agents can cause follicular conjunctivitis and should be included in the differential diagnosis of either acute or chronic follicular conjunctivitis.

MORAXELLA CONJUNCTIVITIS

Moraxella lacunata has been a recognized cause of conjunctivitis for many years. It causes at least two types of conjunctival infection: acute angular blepharoconjunctivitis and chronic follicular conjunctivitis. Conjunctival hyperemia, pain, and adherent eyelids upon awakening characterize *Moraxella* conjunctivitis.[130] Clinical signs often include chronic follicular conjunctivitis. Epidemic outbreaks can occur, and sharing eye makeup among school-age girls has been identified as a risk factor for infection.[131] Conjunctival scrapings demonstrate the characteristically large, square-shaped diplobacillus organism. Traditional treatment of *Moraxella* conjunctivitis has included topical zinc sulfate 0.25%. However, topical erythromycin 0.5% or topical tetracycline 1.0% is probably more effective and less toxic. Oral antibiotics (rifampin) may reduce the rate of recurrence and interrupt transmission of the infection.[131]

AXENFELD'S CHRONIC FOLLICULAR CONJUNCTIVITIS

Axenfeld's chronic follicular conjunctivitis is a mild asymptomatic follicular conjunctivitis involving mainly the upper palpebral conjunctiva.[132] This type of conjunctivitis occurs mostly in children in institutions. The clinical characteristics include mild superior follicular conjunctivitis without significant corneal involvement. This condition may represent a mild form of trachoma, similar to that seen in native Americans Indians in the southwest.[133] Treatment is similar to that for mild trachoma and consists of oral tetracycline or erythromycin.

LYME DISEASE

Lyme disease, caused by the spirochete *Borrelia burgdorferi,* has a variety of ocular manifestations, the most common of which is conjunctivitis. Although the characteristics of the conjunctivitis have not been clearly defined, several reports have described follicular conjunctivitis.[134,135] Increased antibody titers to *B. burgdorferi* indicate the presence of Lyme disease. A history of tick bite or erythema chronicum migrans should alert the clinician to consider Lyme disease in areas of the country where it is prevalent. Treatment of Lyme disease conjunctivitis should include topical tetracycline as an adjunct to oral doxycycline 100 mg daily for three weeks.[136]

PARINAUD'S OCULOGLANDULAR SYNDROME

Parinaud's oculoglandular syndrome constitutes a broad spectrum of conjunctival diseases caused by a variety of

TABLE 26.9
Causes of Parinaud's Oculoglandular Syndrome

Common
  Cat scratch disease
  Tularemia
  Sporotrichosis
Occasional
  Tuberculosis
  Syphilis
  Coccidioidomycosis
Rare
  Pasteurella septica
  Yersinia pseudotuberculosis
  Chancroid
  Lymphogranuloma vereneum
  Listerellosis
  Actinomycosis
  Blastomycosis
  Mumps

infectious agents. The manifestations of the condition vary and are nonspecific to the etiologic agent. Unilateral follicular conjunctivitis and conjunctival granulomas and ulcerations associated with regional lymphadenopathy are the primary clinical characteristics of the condition. The conjunctivitis and adenopathy usually resolve in 4 to 5 weeks. The specific clinical entity most commonly associated with Parinaud's is cat scratch disease. This disease is now believed to be caused by *Rochalimaea henselae,* a *Rickettsia*-like organism.[246] Table 26.9 lists the other agents responsible for Parinaud's oculoglandular syndrome.[137] Although cat scratch disease is usually benign and self-limited, prolonged morbidity and permanent complications can occur. Anecdotal reports indicate successful treatment of cat scratch disease with a variety of anti-infective drugs, including gentamicin, trimethoprim-sulfamethoxazole, ciprofloxacin, and rifampin.[246]

INCLUSION CONJUNCTIVITIS

Etiology. Chlamydia are obligate intracellular parasites that depend on the host cell to carry out metabolic biosynthesis. The genus has two major species: *Chlamydia trachomatis,* which causes disease in humans, and *Chlamydia psittaci,* which infects primarily nonhumans. The many different serotypes cause a wide spectrum of disease states, including inclusion conjunctivitis, trachoma, lymphogranuloma venereum, and venereal disease.

Chlamydial infections are the most common sexually transmitted disease in the United States, with 3 to 5 million new cases per year.[138] The disease can be relatively asymptomatic in terms of urogenital symptoms. However, nonspecific urethritis and chronic vaginal discharge are not uncommon. Ocu-

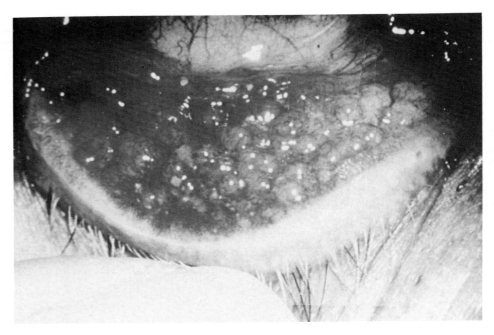

FIGURE 26.12   **Mixed follicular-papillary hypertrophy in adult inclusion conjunctivitis. (Courtesy William Wallace, O.D.)**

lar infection commonly occurs by autoinoculation in the infected individual. Chlamydial infections represent one of the most common causes of chronic conjunctivitis.[139]

Diagnosis.   Inclusion conjunctivitis presents in teens and adults as an acute follicular conjunctivitis often accompanied by a mucopurulent discharge. Upper respiratory symptoms and fever are generally lacking. The disease typically occurs in sexually active young adults who have acquired a new sexual partner in the past 1 to 2 months. After an incubation period of 5 to 12 days, an acute onset of conjunctival injection, mixed follicular-papillary hypertrophy and foreign body sensation develop (Fig. 26.12). The disease is usually unilateral with a small, preauricular node on the affected side. During the second week, epithelial keratitis may develop along with marginal or central infiltrates, superficial pannus and even EKC-like opacities. Patients often seek treatment for the acute phase of the disease, which practitioners frequently misdiagnose as a viral or routine bacterial conjunctivitis. Treatment with a variety of broad-spectrum antibiotics or topical steroids may initially help the patient's symptoms, but if left inadequately treated, the patient invariably returns with complaints of recurrent episodes of ocular redness and mucopurulent discharge. As in all cases of chronic conjunctivitis, only conjunctival cultures and scrapings should be performed to establish a definitive diagnosis. Several laboratory tests have been developed to establish a diagnosis of inclusion conjunctivitis.[140,141]

Management.   Topical therapy of adult inclusion conjunctivitis cannot effect a cure. Oral tetracycline 250 mg 4 times daily for 21 days has been the traditional treatment of choice. *Chlamydia* is quite sensitive to tetracyclines. Topical adjunctive therapy with tetracycline may also hasten resolution of the patient's symptoms. Semi-synthetic tetracyclines such as minocycline and doxycycline have been shown to be more active *in vitro* against *Chlamydia trachomatis*.[142] Doxycycline has several distinct advantages: a less frequent dosing schedule, better absorption following oral administration, and absorption that is less affected by dietary consumption. The usual dosage of doxycycline is 100 mg twice daily for 1 week followed by 100 mg daily for 2 additional weeks. Pregnant and lactating women, and children under the age of 8 years should avoid oral tectracycline therapy. In these patients, erythromycin 250 mg 4 times a day can be considered an alternative to doxycycline.

For patients with uncomplicated genital chlamydial infections, azithromycin 1 g for one day is equally effective as 100 mg of doxycycline twice a day for 7 days. This bolus dose of azithromycin should be considered particularly for patients in whom compliance may be a problem.[143,144] Topical tetracycline in suspension or ointment may be used as an adjunct.

Treating the genital infection requires systemic medication. This treatment should be done by a gynecologist or urologist. If left untreated, chlamydial vaginitis can result in severe pelvic inflammatory disease and infertility. Sexual partners of infected individuals should also receive systemic antibiotics even if no symptoms are present.

TRACHOMA

Etiology.   Although *Chlamydia trachomatis* is the infectious agent of both trachoma and adult inclusion conjunctivitis, the clinical presentations as well as the epidemiologic characteristics of the two diseases are quite different. Trachoma and its complications still represent a serious world health problem and today remain a major cause of preventable blindness. The incidence of trachoma is highest in unhealthy, dirty, crowded conditions typically associated with a low socioeconomic environment. Trachoma affects approximately one-seventh of the world population. In the United States, the disease is limited mostly to native American populations living in the southwest.[145]

Diagnosis.   In its early stages, trachoma presents as a chronic follicular conjunctivitis with a predilection for the superior tarsal and bulbar conjunctiva. As time passes, the conjunctival reaction becomes papillary in nature and with the inflammatory infiltration that occurs, the follicular character of the infection can become obscured. Patients begin to experience symptoms of photophobia, tearing, and mucoid or mucopurulent discharge. Limbal edema and superior bulbar conjunctival hyperemia also may occur. Conjunctival follicles that form at the limbus are characteristic of severe trachoma. Primary corneal involvement often includes superior epithelial keratitis and superficial superior pannus formation. A wide variety of corneal infiltrates (superior, diffuse, limbal) may occur, and marginal ulcerations are not uncommon. As the disease progresses, conjunctival subepithelial scarring begins to replace the acute inflammatory signs. Fine linear horizontal subepithelial scars that form on the upper tarsal conjunctiva are known as Arlt's lines (Fig. 26.13). The scarring can result in entropion and trichiasis which can, in turn, lead to corneal ulceration and scarring; these are the major blinding complications of trachoma. The involution of limbal follicles results in sharply demarcated limbal depressions known as Herbert's pits, which are considered pathognomonic for trachoma. Patients with severe conjunctival scarring can also develop many other secondary complications including severe dry eye syndrome and punctal stenosis.

The course of trachoma usually follows the MacCallen classification system, which is based solely on the conjunctival findings[146] (Table 26.10). Table 26.11 summarizes a simplified system for the assessment of trachoma and its complications.[147]

In areas endemic for trachoma, the presence of two of the

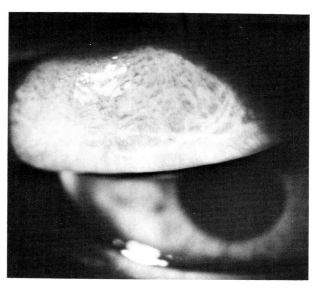

FIGURE 26.13   **Conjunctival scarring with Arlt's lines in stage IV trachoma.**

TABLE 26.10
MacCallen Classification of Trachoma

Stage	Conjunctival Signs
I	Soft immature follicles of upper tarsal conjunctiva
IIa	Mature follicles of upper tarsal conjunctiva with papillary response
IIb	Follicular reaction of upper tarsal plate obscured by papillary hypertrophy
III	Follicles on tarsal conjunctiva with conjunctival scarring
IV	No follicles but definite scarring

TABLE 26.11
Simplified Classification of Trachoma

Stage	Signs
Trachomatis inflammation (TF)	Five or more follicles of upper tarsal conjunctiva
Trachomatis intense (TI)	Pronounced inflammatory thickening obscuring more than one-half of the normal deep tarsal vessels
Trachomatis scarring (TS)	Scarring of upper tarsal conjunctiva
Trachomatis trichiasis (TT)	At least one eyelash rubs on globe
Corneal opacity (CO)	Easily visible corneal opacity

typical signs—upper tarsal follicles, pannus or limbal folli-cle—is sufficient for the diagnosis of trachoma. Laboratory studies may be useful in mild cases, either by isolating *Chlamydia* in tissue culture or by detecting chlamydial antibodies in serum or tears by means of immunofluorescent assay. In nonendemic populations, trachoma must be differ-entiated from other causes of chronic follicular conjunc-tivitis, such as *Moraxella,* adenoviral infection, herpetic infection, molluscum and chemical conjunctivitis. The prac-titioner should obtain a careful history, including whether the patient has traveled to any area with endemic trachoma. The predilection of trachoma to affect the upper tarsal con-junctiva as well as the superior cornea has great diagnostic value.

Management.   Trachoma usually responds to a 3-week course of oral tetracycline 250 mg 4 times a day or oral erythromycin 500 mg 4 times a day. The clinical response to treatment is relatively slow and may not appear significant for 3 to 4 months. Reinfection rates are high, especially in endemic areas. In pregnant patients and children under the age of 8 years, tetracycline is contraindicated because it can discolor the teeth and depress bone development. Topical treatment alone is generally considered ineffective for a complete cure, but topical tetracycline or erythromycin may be applied as adjunctive therapy. In patients with severe conjunctival cicatrization, surgical intervention may be re-quired to correct trichiasis and entropion and to prevent the possibility of corneal scarring. For patients who present with significant corneal scarring and decreased vision, penetrat-ing keratoplasty can be considered once the disease has been controlled.

Toxic Etiologies

Chronic exposure of the conjunctiva to chemicals and for-eign agents may result in a chronic follicular conjunctivitis. The conjunctivitis is limited to the eye in which the agent is instilled and resolves upon discontinuation of the offending agent.

Many agents including topical antibiotics, decongestants, preservatives, and other ophthalmic preparations cause toxic conjunctivitis. Chronic administration of almost any oph-thalmic drug can result in the characteristic findings of toxic conjunctivitis. Patients treated for glaucoma with miotic and epinephrine compounds frequently encounter toxic conjunc-tivitis. Over-treatment of infectious conjunctivitis with topi-cal antibiotics may produce conjunctival hyperemia and irritation, which can mask the clinical resolution of the original infection. The patient may then be subjected to a variety of additional treatments when the original treatment is "failing." The term *medicamentosa* describes this cycle of over-treatment.

A careful history, with particular attention to the patient's past medication history, establishes the diagnosis. The pa-tient should be questioned directly about the use of over-the-counter (OTC) eye preparations and contact lens solutions.

Treatment consists of removing the offending agent. In the patient who has chronic conjunctivitis and who has used numerous ophthalmic preparations without success, dis-continuing all topical medications except for unpreserved artificial tears for several days can prove rewarding. The conjunctivitis often begins to resolve spontaneously, al-though complete resolution may take weeks.

Ophthalmia Neonatorum

Ophthalmia neonatorum, or conjunctivitis of the neonate, deserves special consideration because of its relatively com-mon occurrence: Up to 12% of newborns have this condi-tion.[148] Because of the potentially devastating effects of neonatal infections resulting from *Neisseria gonorrhoeae, Pseudomonas, Chlamydia,* and herpes simplex, laboratory investigation is essential in attempting to establish an etiolo-gic diagnosis. Infants usually acquire infection from an infected birth canal. Premature membrane rupture and pro-longed delivery can also cause increased exposure to mater-nal pathogens and an increased risk of neonatal infection.

Neisseria Gonorrhoeae

In 1881 Credé first described the advantage of silver nitrate prophylaxis for the prevention of gonococcal infection.[149] Since that time, the incidence of infection from *Neisseria gonorrhoeae* has decreased from approximately 10% to less than 0.66%.[150] Gonococcal neonatal conjunctivitis is charac-terized by the development of a hyperacute conjunctivitis between two and five days postpartum. Conventional teach-ing holds that time of onset of conjunctivitis after birth provides useful diagnostic information in distinguishing the etiologic agent. Many factors, however, are now known either to delay or accelerate the development of conjunctivi-tis. Most cases of gonococcal conjunctivitis are bilateral; periorbital edema, chemosis, and purulent exudate are prom-inent (Fig. 26.14). Because of the ability of *N. gonorrhoeae* to penetrate intact epithelium, prompt and accurate diagno-sis is imperative to prevent corneal ulceration and perfora-tion. *N. gonorrhoeae* can also be associated with systemic infection. Specific dermatologic abnormalities are possible, and careful neurologic monitoring for evidence of central nervous system involvement is imperative. A lumbar punc-ture is mandatory if evidence of meningitis is present.

Presumptive diagnosis is based on the finding of intracel-lular gram negative diplococci on gram staining of conjunc-tival smears (Fig. 26.15). Conjunctival cultures should be

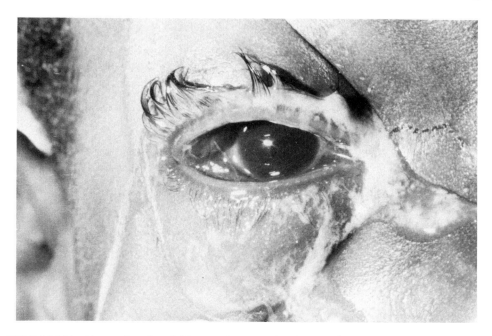

FIGURE 26.14   Neonatal conjunctivitis secondary to *Neisseria gonorrhoeae.* Note the copious purulent exudate and pronounced chemosis. (Courtesy William Wallace, O.D.)

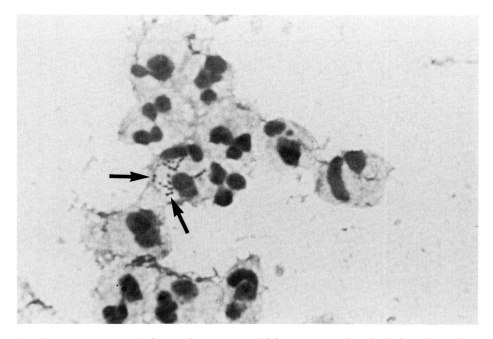

FIGURE 26.15   Gram-stained smear from neonate with hyperacute conjunctivitis shows intracellular *Neisseria gonorrhoeae* (arrows). (Courtesy William Wallace, O.D.)

obtained and incubated on Thayer-Martin or chocolate agar at 37°C under 2% to 10% CO_2. Antibiotic sensitivities are essential on all isolates due to the increasing incidence of penicillin-resistant strains of *N. gonorrhoeae*.[151]

Treatment of *N. gonorrhoeae* ophthalmia neonatorum includes mainly systemic agents. Patients should be hospitalized for observation of systemic infection, and the acute conjunctivitis should be treated with frequent saline lavage. Topical antibiotic agents are unnecessary if systemic treatment is administered.[153] Systemic treatment with ceftriaxone is curative and is the treatment now recommended by the Centers for Disease Control[152,153] The recommended regimen is ceftriazone 25 to 50 mg/kg intravenously or intramuscularly in a single dose, not to exceed 125 mg.[153] A single dose of cefotaxime intramuscularly is also effective.[154]

Chlamydia trachomatis

The leading infectious cause of ophthalmia neonatorum is *Chlamydia trachomatis*. It has been estimated to occur in 2% to 6% of all newborns.[155] The high incidence of this infection is due to the fact that up to 13% of women shed *Chlamydia* from the urogenital tract during the third trimester of pregnancy.[155] The high incidence of infection may also be related to the ineffectiveness of silver nitrate in preventing chlamydial infection.

Chlamydia ophthalmia neonatorum is characterized by the onset of a mild to moderate unilateral or bilateral mucopurulent conjunctivitis 5 to 14 days postpartum (Fig. 26.16). Lid edema, chemosis, and conjunctival membrane or pseudomembrane formation may also accompany this condition. Corneal findings occasionally include punctate opacities and micropannus formation. Ophthalmia neonatorum secondary to *Chlamydia* was once considered a benign and self-limited condition. However, systemic chlamydial infection, especially pneumonitis, is now well recognized in patients with chlamydial conjunctivitis.[156] Over 50% of infants who develop chlamydial pneumonitis may also have oppthalmia neonatorum.[157]

Diagnosis of *Chlamydia* ophthalmia neonatorum is established by conjunctival smears that reveal typical basophilic intracytoplasmic inclusions with Geimsa stain (Fig. 26.17). Direct immunofluorescent monoclonal antibody testing can also be helpful in confirming the diagnosis.

Optimal treatment of chlamydial ophthalmia neonatorum has not been determined. The Centers for Disease Control have recommended erythromycin 50 mg/kg/day in four divided doses for 10 to 14 days.[158] Because of its known side effects, systemic tetracycline therapy is contraindicated in infants. Another important aspect of treatment is concurrent therapy of the mother and her sexual partners.

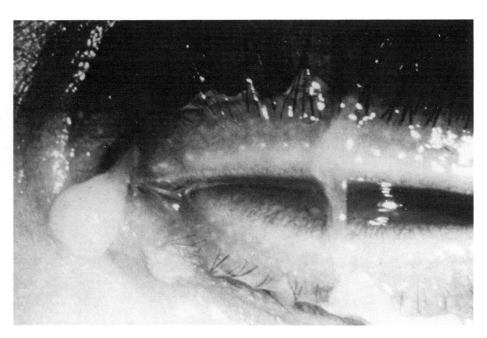

FIGURE 26.16   Neonatal inclusion conjunctivitis with prominent mucopurulent exudate. (Courtesy William Wallace, O.D.)

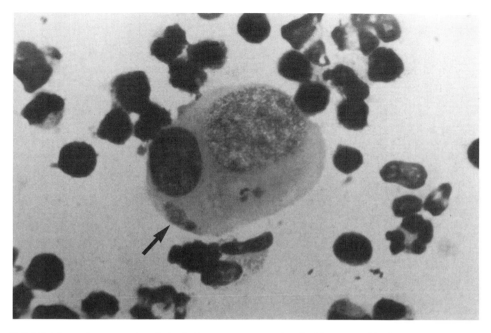

FIGURE 26.17   **Intracytoplasmic inclusions (arrow) associated with neonatal inclusion conjunctivitis. (Courtesy William Wallace, O.D.)**

Other Bacterial Etiologies

Many cases of ophthalmia neonatorum result from nongonococcal bacterial infections. *Staphylococcus aureus, Haemophilus* species, *Streptococcus viridans, E. coli,* and *Pseudomonas aeruginosa* have been implicated as causative agents in ophthalmia neonatorum.[158] The pathogen is most likely acquired as the newborn travels through the birth canal. All of these bacteria are part of the normal bacterial flora of the female genital tract.[159] Other sources are responsible as well, since 20% to 79% of the conjunctivas of infants delivered by cesarean section show bacterial growth.[160,161]

Clinical manifestations of bacterial ophthalmia neonatorum are nonspecific and similar to those caused by other pathogens already discussed. Infants experience the acute onset of hyperemia, chemosis, lid edema, and purulent or mucopurulent exudate 5 to 21 days postpartum. Care should be taken to rule out nasolacrimal duct obstruction, a finding that is relatively common in newborns and that can be associated with a secondary bacterial infection. Since the etiology of ophthalmia neonatorum cannot be distinguished on the basis of clinical examination alone, laboratory investigations (smears and cultures) are mandatory. Differentiation of bacterial infections, particularly *Pseudomonas,* is

important since these pseudomonal infections in premature infants can lead to septicemia and infant death if not aggressively and appropriately treated.[162]

Initial treatment of bacterial ophthalmia neonatorum should be directed by the results of conjunctival scrapings. Broad-spectrum antibiotics with low toxicity should be employed. Topical erythromycin or tetracycline ointment can be used 4 to 6 times daily for gram positive organisms, and gentamicin or tobramycin solution 4 to 6 times daily can be started if gram negative organisms are isolated. Trimethoprim-polymyxin B has broad-spectrum activity against a range of both gram-positive and gram-negative organisms, including *Pseudomonas* species.

Herpes Simplex Virus

Herpes simplex infection is an uncommon but important neonatal infection and can be associated with conjunctivitis in 5% to 10% of cases.[163] The clinical manifestations are nonspecific, with the occurrence of conjunctival hyperemia, chemosis, periorbital edema and mucous discharge. Corneal involvement is not uncommon and can include dendritic, geographic, or stromal keratitis. Herpetic ophthalmia neonatorum represents a primary herpetic infection. Central nervous system involvement, retinitis, optic neuritis, uveitis, choroiditis, and a fatal viremia can be important sequelae of primary herpetic infections.[164]

Diagnosis is often difficult, but laboratory testing can help in establishing a diagnosis. An absence of bacteria with conjunctival scrapings should alert the clinician to the possibility of viral infection. Papanicolaou stain may reveal intranuclear inclusions, and multinucleated giant cells can be seen on Giemsa staining. Maternal history of HSV infection and the characteristic corneal findings can also help establish the diagnosis. Viral cultures can be obtained, particularly in cases that are refractory to antibiotic treatment.

The prognosis for an infant with neonatal HSV infection is guarded. Treatment of the conjunctivitis should include topical trifluridine 1% every 2 hours until the infection begins to resolve, then tapered according to the clinical response. Systemic therapy with intravenous acyclovir is indicated in the presence of viremia and disseminated disease.[165]

Chemical Ophthalmia Neonatorum

Chemical conjunctivitis is the most common cause of ophthalmia neonatorum, occurring in up to 90% of infants administered silver nitrate. Mild transient conjunctival hyperemia and watery discharge occurring 1 to 2 days postpartum characterize chemical conjunctivitis. The conjunctivitis is self-limited over the course of 1 to 2 days. Most cases are the direct result of toxic reactions to silver nitrate used as prophylaxis for ophthalmia neonatorum. Silver nitrate can damage the corneal and conjunctival epithelium, disrupting the protective epithelial barrier and making the infant more susceptible to secondary bacterial infections. If the history confirms the use of silver nitrate, no treatment is necessary. If the condition does not improve after several days, other etiologic mechanisms must be considered (Table 26.12).

Prevention

In 1881, Credé first introduced the use of silver nitrate 1% for the prevention of gonococcal ophthalmia neonatorum.[149] Since that time the incidence of ophthalmia neonatorum has decreased dramatically. Silver nitrate prophylaxis, however, is not without limitations. This agent is toxic to the epithelium, since it acts by sloughing epithelial cells. It therefore usually induces chemical conjunctivitis. In addition, silver nitrate prophylaxis is not completely effective, failing to act against *Chlamydia,* a major cause of ophthalmia neonatorum. Various alternatives to silver nitrate prophylaxis have been advocated, including 0.5% erythromycin or 1% tetracycline ointment. When compared to silver nitrate, erythromycin ointment does not decrease the incidence of chlamydial ophthalmia neonatorum.[166–168] Despite its shortcomings, silver nitrate continues to provide effective prophylaxis for gonococcal ophthalmia neonatorum. Both erythromycin and tetracycline ointment are effective and less toxic alternatives.[153]

Oculodermatologic Disorders

Dermatologic disease and its related ocular complications are among the most common entities seen in general ophthalmic practice. Although numerous dermatologic conditions can affect the eye, this section deals only with the conditions most frequently encountered. These include acne rosacea, psoriasis, and atopic dermatitis.

Etiology

A disease of unknown etiology, acne rosacea typically occurs in the age group between the third and fifth decades and is significantly more frequent in women than men. Specific trigger factors may relate to the onset of the disease, includ-

TABLE 26.12
Causes of Ophthalmia Neonatorum

Etiologic Agent	Onset	Conjunctival Features	Cytology
Chemical	24 hours	Diffuse hyperemia, purulent exudate	Polymorphonuclear lymphocytes
Chlamydia	5–10 days	Diffuse hyperemia, purulent exudate	Basophilic cytoplasmic inclusion bodies
Other Bacterial	> 5 days	Diffuse hyperemia, mucopurulent discharge	Causative agent
Neisseria gonorrhoeae	3–5 days	Hyperacute conjunctivitis with mucopurulent discharge	Intraepithelial gram-negative diplococci
Herpetic	5–15 days	Diffuse hyperemia, watery discharge	Multinucleated giant cells

ing trauma and ethnic predisposition. Use of alcohol was once considered a factor, but it is now known that alcohol use is not associated with the onset of the disease.

Rosacea is a chronic skin disorder with characteristic clinical findings. These include an acneform papular-pustular eruption associated with erythema and hypertrophic sebaceous glands. Typically these changes appear on the cheeks, nose, and forehead, or the "facial flush" areas. Acne rosacea has no known relationship to any previous juvenile acne.[169]

Psoriasis vulgaris is a relatively chronic skin disease, of unknown etiology, that affects 1% to 4% of the population. Typically the disease presents with circumscribed, erythematous, plaque-like elevations with a coarse dry texture. As with other oculodermatologic conditions, it is typically more common in women, caucasians, and individuals below the age of 40 years. Most patients present with focal outbreaks of the disease usually on extensor surfaces such as the knee and elbow. It is also sometimes seen on the scalp. The majority of patients have a local or limited form of psoriasis, with approximately 1 in 7 progressing to a more severe generalized disease process.[170] The overall incidence of ocular involvement in patients with generalized psoriatic disease may be approximately 1 in 10, and the degree of clinical symptomatology is quite variable.

Atopic dermatitis is a unique form of hypersensitivity that presents with eczematous skin eruptions. Primarily it is a disease of childhood and early adolescence although it can develop in adults. Immunologic factors have been implicated in the onset of this entity. Other etiologic factors relate to potential genetically mediated defects in metabolism or biochemical response to exogenous substances. A decrease in cellular immunity and an abnormality in the IgE antibody response system have also been identified.[171]

Diagnosis

Acne rosacea can manifest itself in a wide spectrum of clinical presentations from extremely subtle, early telangiectatic changes to the more extreme pustular eruptive states noted in some patients. Ocular rosacea typically involves the eyelids, conjunctiva, and cornea in a variety of disease states. Ocular changes include meibomianitis, chalazion, hordeolum, and conjunctivitis. Corneal involvement includes superficial punctate keratitis, infiltration near the limbus with subsequent progression toward the apex, and neovascularization (Fig. 26.18). In severe disease the cornea can actually show thinning and subsequent perforation.[172]

Typical symptoms include foreign body sensation and hyperemia without significant bacterial findings. Because of the chronic nature of this disease, recurrent episodes are common, which should lead the practitioner to consider rosacea as a potential etiology.[173,174]

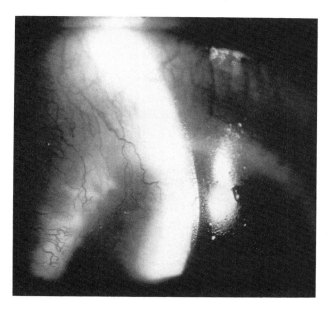

FIGURE 26.18   **Corneal neovascularization in patient with acne rosacea.**

An unusual clinical finding with rosacea in its more advanced state is the development of rhinophyma. This involves hypertrophy of the sebaceous glands of the skin of the nose and includes both the nasal folds and associated areas. The typical appearance is that of a bulbous, extremely disruptive epidermal surface with extensive hyperemia and telangiectatic changes that are pathognomonic of the disease (Fig. 26.19).

Psoriasis only infrequently affects the eye. When involvement is present, it is commonly noted as the typical epidermal plaque formations on the conjunctiva or eyelids (Fig. 26.20). Keratitis has been noted in some individuals, but this is primarily of a limbal nature and is thought to be related to the localized activity in the conjunctiva and lid margin area. There is also an increased frequency of uveitis, although it is not a significant component of this disease. Secondary involvement of the lids in the form of ectropion, entropion, and trichiasis usually relates to the lid lesions themselves and does not represent a primary component of the disease. Because of the diffuse nature of the psoriasis, it can occur in association with chronic juvenile arthritis as well as Reiter's syndrome.[175-177] Other investigators[177,178] have demonstrated a significant increase in prevalence in patients with HIV infection. The pathogenesis of this relationship is unclear, but an immune recognition event may occur related to the HLA-B27 antigen.

Atopic dermatitis is primarily characterized by a patchy excoriation of the skin, lability to heat and pressure stimulus,

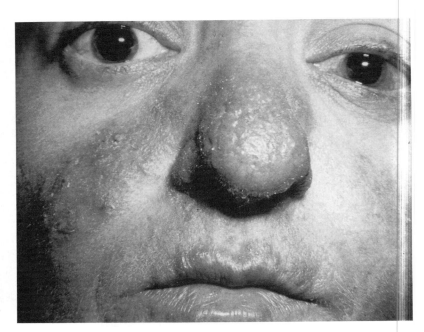

FIGURE 26.19   **Ocular rosacea with conjunctivitis, maculopustular involvement of skin, and rhinophyma. (Courtesy William Wallace, O.D.)**

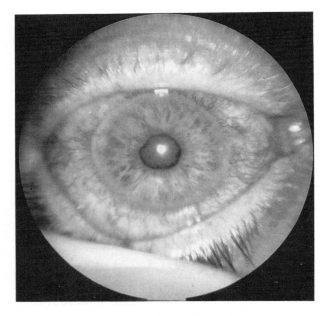

FIGURE 26.20   **Psoriatic blepharoconjunctivitis.**

and occurrence on all aspects of the body surface. Ocular involvement includes erythema, scaling of the eyelids and secondary staphylococcal blepharitis. The conjunctiva frequently presents with chemosis and hyperemia as well as a papillary response (Fig. 26.21). As the disease progresses, shrinkage of the fornices and subsequent scarring can take place. Corneal involvement can range from superficial punctate keratitis to cicatrization and vascularization (Fig. 26.22). There is more than a casual association between patients with an atopic history and keratoconus. A significant hereditary component to the ocular disease has been noted among patients with either a personal or family history of atopic dermatitis. Abnormalities in IgE production, leukocyte cyclic AMP response and abnormal methacholine inhalation testing have all been noted in association with the disease.[179–181]

Management

The treatment of acne rosacea has remained relatively constant over the last decade, and recent variations in management use longer-acting synthetic tetracyclines such as doxycycline. Standard dosage for tetracycline is 250 mg 4 times daily for approximately 4 to 6 weeks. The patient is then assessed, and the medication is tapered over a more extended period. Doxycycline is equally effective as tetracycline when used in a dosage of 100 mg daily over a 6-week period. As with tetracycline, this dose, if effective, is then tapered to 50 mg per day for approximately one month and then subsequently every other day for several weeks. When doxycycline is not effective, the recommended therapy is tetracycline 250 mg 4 times daily. In most instances, patients demonstrate significant improvement of clinical symptomatology and physical signs in the first 2 to 3 weeks. Many patients, however, require chronic therapy and demonstrate exacerbations of the disease during its course. Metronidazole (Metrogel) is a topical gel developed to treat the skin of the facial area in patients with chronic disease and thus reduce the reliance on oral antimicrobial agents. It is used twice daily but should not be used on the eyelids due to potential ocular toxicity.

Although topical antibiotics are frequently used in the management of ocular rosacea, no firm evidence demonstrates their efficacy as the sole therapeutic agent. Topical steroids, however, are effective for treatment of the inflammatory aspects and are frequently used 4 times daily in conjunction with antibiotics in combination products such as Tobradex, Pred-G, or Maxitrol. Because of potential steroid-induced side effects, chronic use of these agents should be avoided, and the patient should be placed on lid scrubs if any evidence of concurrent blepharitis appears. The primary concern of the ophthalmic practitioner is to prevent corneal involvement and the subsequent scarring and vascularization that occur secondary to inflammation.

The pharmacotherapeutic management of psoriasis has met with variable success. Therapy focuses primarily on altering the abnormal physiology of the epidermis. Topical agents such as anthralin have generally not been successful, and most individuals require oral therapy to show significant improvement in the more severe disease states. Currently, methotrexate is approved for systemic use in severe psoria-

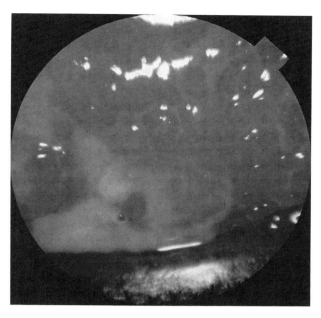

FIGURE 26.21   **Papillary response of upper tarsal conjunctiva in patient with atopic conjunctivitis.**

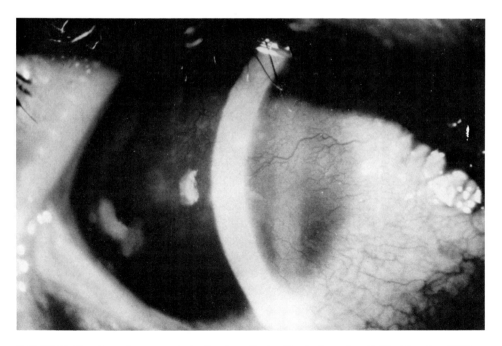

FIGURE 26.22   **Corneal neovascularization in patient with atopic conjunctivitis. (Courtesy William Wallace, O.D.)**

sis. The standard dosage is 2.5 to 5 mg 4 times daily 3 times per week. Other agents such as hydroxyurea, aminopterin, and retinoid etretinate have been shown to be effective.[182,183] Cyclosporine may be useful in the treatment of severe recalcitrant disease but has also been demonstrated to have significant side effects. The use of photochemotherapy in the form of PUVA is one of the most effective forms of treatment. It involves the use of an oral agent (psoralen) which sensitizes the epidermis to ultraviolet light. The patient is treated intensively over a 2- to 3-week period and subsequently placed on maintenance UV therapy for an extended time. Studies show that the effectiveness of this therapy in the acute period is up to 90% in remediating the disease, and in long-term therapy over 60% of patients have remained in remission at the 1-year period.[184] Risks associated with PUVA therapy include nonmelanoma skin cancers similar to those changes noted in any chronic solar exposure.

Ocular therapy includes management of the inflammatory component of the disease, which can manifest itself in the form of keratoconjunctivitis or uveitis. Appropriate steroid therapy should be implemented for those conditions. In cases of severe uveitis, the use of topical agents may be insufficient and patients may need oral steroids. Therapy of the skin involves the use of agents such as triamcinolone, hydrocortisone applied by either an occlusive dressing or other method to potentiate their effect. In less severe cases the use of topical solutions such as emollients, lubricants, oils, lotions, and creams can successfully keep the skin moist.

Therapy for the patient with atopic dermatitis can be divided into three distinct categories: topical therapy for the skin, systemic therapy, and ocular therapy. The predominant modality for topical therapy includes the use of fluorinated corticosteroids such as triamcinolone or betamethasone. As in other severe dermatologic disorders, coaltar derivatives can be used in cases where steroids are ineffective. Systemic management is primarily oriented toward the use of oral corticosteroids. In the acute phase, high-dose prednisone is the most effective agent, but patients can be managed chronically on low-dose therapy of 5 to 10 mg per day for prolonged periods. In patients with severe pruritus, oral antihistamines can minimize itching and provide symptomatic relief.[184]

Therapy for the eye-related complications of atopic dermatitis focuses on reducing inflammation. Appropriate agents include sodium cromolyn or other mast cell stabilizers as well as topical antihistamines or decongestants. These agents can be successfully used on a prolonged basis if necessary. In more severe cases, the use of topical corticosteroids can be initiated as a pulse dose of every 2 to 3 hours and subsequently tapered rapidly to 4 times daily and then more slowly until discontinued.

Surgical intervention in atopic dermatitis has been associated with a relatively high rate of complication. In particular, the incidence of retinal detachment is relatively high. The etiology is not clear, but one study noted breaks in the pars plicata of the ciliary body in four eyes of three patients with atopic dermatitis.[185]

Mucous Membrane Disorders

Etiology

Although several mucous membrane disorders have a generalized effect on the body, only benign mucous membrane pemphigoid (BMMP) and erythema multiforme commonly produce ocular complications. Both of these disorders are of unknown etiology and produce inflammatory changes of the mucosal tissue of the anterior segment with secondary complications.

BMMP is an uncommon inflammatory disease that is chronic in nature and has a typical onset late in life, usually during the sixth decade. Women are more commonly affected than men, and of the mucous membranes involved, the conjunctiva and buccal cavity are most often affected. Involvement of the nasal passages as well as occasional involvement of the genitalia and rectal mucosa occur. Although the disorder is relatively rare, 1 in 30,000, the incidence of significant visual loss is as high as 25% to 33% in patients with ocular involvement.[186]

Mucous membrane diseases are an immune-mediated reaction to antigens in the mucosal tissue's basement membrane. Studies indicate that ocular cicatricial pemphigoid is a unique clinical and immunopathologic entity separate from other subepithelial blistering diseases of the mucous membranes such as bullous pemphigoid and necrotizing epidermolysis.[187] Current research explores the role of mast cells and T cells as potential mediators in the development of the disease and the atypical response of fibroblasts in the cicatricial changes noted in this process.[188–190]

Unlike BMMP, erythema multiforme has an acute onset, occurs most commonly before the age of 30 years, and is more frequently seen in men than women. Although no specific etiology has been determined, factors such as drug administration and treatment of infectious disease such as *Mycoplasma* pneumonia and herpes simplex have been closely related to the development of erythema multiforme in younger patients.[191,192] Stevens-Johnson syndrome is the specific component of erythema multiforme that involves the ocular tissue and produces the classic signs of a catarrhal, pseudomembranous conjunctivitis.

Diagnosis

The most common initial sign of ocular cicatricial pemphigoid is a conjunctivitis associated with subepithelial fibrosis. The chronic inflammation accompanying the fibrotic

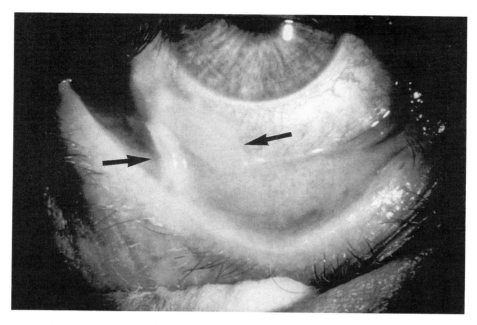

FIGURE 26.23   **Conjunctival shrinkage and symblepharon formation (arrows) in benign mucous membrane pemphigoid.**

changes produces progressive shrinkage of the ocular tissue with subsequent symblepharon formation (Fig. 26.23). In the more advanced stages of the disease, cicatrization begins to occur. The chronic contraction of conjunctival tissue can lead to entropion and subsequent trichiasis. In more advanced presentations, the cornea may demonstrate stromal thinning and develop an ulcerative process secondary to the architectural changes present and the chronic exposure of the eye to bacterial challenge. Keratinization of the conjunctiva and cornea can lead to profound vision loss (Fig. 26.24). A frequent finding is cicatricial closure of the puncta and lacrimal ducts. Cicatrization takes place in much the same way as the conjunctival adhesions and can produce marked epiphora or dry eye, depending on the degree of conjunctival scarring.[193–196]

Although BMMP presents primarily as an ocular manifestation, erythema multiforme initially occurs more frequently as a disseminated disease of epidermal tissue and usually does not involve the eye unless significant systemic manifestations are present. In individuals who develop ocular symptoms and signs, the most typical is that of a bacterial-like pseudomembranous conjunctivitis frequently associated with a discharge. It is typical for the conjunctiva to show vascular changes with necrosis and subsequent scarring. If the eyelids are involved in the cicatricial process, entropion and trichiasis are frequently noted, and in many individuals an ulcerative, bullous-type process develops

near or on the eyelid margin. The condition may demonstrate a wide spectrum of clinical manifestations from minimal punctal stenosis to severe corneal opacification and infiltration with scarring. More remarkable ocular involvement typically occurs only in individuals with extremely severe disease.[197–200]

The differential diagnosis relates to those conditions that produce similar cicatricial changes of the anterior segment, such as chemical trauma and radiation injury. Pseudomembranous changes are most typically associated with EKC and can also appear in other viral diseases such as herpes simplex. This type of change rarely occurs in a bacterial infection, although some organisms can mount this level of challenge to the ocular tissue and subsequently provoke the production of a pseudomembrane as part of the inflammatory process.

Management

Although the predominant clinical findings are ocular in BMMP, topical therapy alone generally proves insufficient. Historically, the most significant success follows the use of oral corticosteroids. Unfortunately, steroids act simply as a mechanism to suppress the response and are not curative. In most instances, patients are placed on initial high-dose steroids, show significant remission of symptoms, and can be

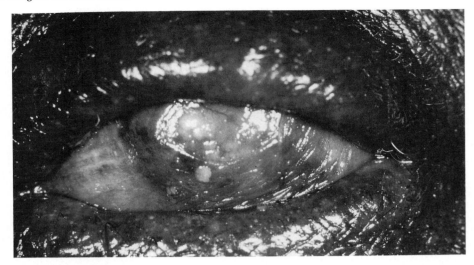

FIGURE 26.24   **Keratinization of conjunctiva and cornea in benign mucous membrane pemphigoid.**

tapered to a maintenance dosage level. Initial dosage is generally 40 to 60 mg prednisone daily. Maintenance therapy can be as little as 5 mg every other day. Unfortunately, approximately 25% of patients cannot continue long-term steroid therapy due to complications, and these patients eventually progress to severe visual impairment or blindness. Only one-third of patients on chronic immunosuppressive therapy can achieve long periods of remission off medication.[201]

Dapsone is effective in the treatment of the acute inflammatory stage of ocular pemphigoid. As with steroids, dapsone does not significantly impact the cicatricial component of the disease, but it does control the inflammatory aspect. In recent studies,[202,203] an initial dose of 100 mg a day was well tolerated with no toxicity. The use of 150 mg a day brought on significant side effects. Once an initial response was obtained usually in one to four weeks, a maintenance dose of 50 to 100 mg on alternate days could be used. Many patients experienced significant periods of remission, but in all instances therapy had to be reinstituted on a regular basis.

In patients with more advanced disease and in individuals who show rapid progression of disease or fail with either steroids or dapsone, immunosuppressive agents such as cyclophosphamide and azathioprine may produce sustained remission. The standard dose for cyclophosphamide is 1 to 2 mg/kg body weight/day combined with an equal amount of prednisone. Following a 1-month to 6-week initial treatment period, the effectiveness of therapy is assessed, and cyclophosphamide dosage may increase if the disease is still present or progressive. In most instances, steroids can be reduced at this point because of the obvious complications with long-term use. Cyclophosphamide therapy routinely continues for a period of 12 months or longer. In the treatment of acute severe ocular cicatricial pemphigoid, cyclophosphamide was successful in 96% of the patients when administered for 10 months or longer. Azathioprine was successful in 85% of the patients over the same period.[203]

Ocular therapy is directed toward management of the dry eye associated with BMMP. In this disease dry eye results from the damage to goblet cells in the conjunctiva and a decrease in surface mucin. Numerous agents are available for treatment, but chronic lubricant therapy should make use of non-preserved agents. Ointments are extremely effective in providing lubrication either overnight or, in the more advanced forms of the disease, during the daytime hours. The patient's symptoms determine dosage frequencies. Use of adjunctive therapy such as lid hygiene and the treatment of secondary infections should be implemented on an individual basis. However, the chronic use of antibiotics is contraindicated because of potential overgrowth of nonsusceptible organisms and antibiotic toxicity.

The goal of therapy is the maintenance of corneal integrity and patient comfort. Procedures such as eyelash epilation, lid scrubs, and antibiosis can help in the early phases of the disease process. In the more advanced disease states, surgical procedures have effectively improved outcomes. These include procedures for the correction of entropion and trichiasis as well as oculoplastic surgery for the resolution of symblepharon and conjunctival shrinkage. Buccal mucosal grafting shows promise in the rehabilitation of this disease, and investigators have evaluated nasal mucosal grafts as adjunctive therapy.[196,204,205] Surgical intervention should generally be withheld until the disease progresses unchecked by more conservative methods. Surgery itself can induce further inflammatory involvement. Unfortunately, keratoplasties and other corneal procedures are not particularly successful in the treatment of this disease.

Stevens-Johnson syndrome is treated in similar fashion to ocular cicatricial pemphigoid—use of systemic steroids and, in some instances of severe disease, immunosuppressive agents have been successful. Also included in systemic management is the use of oral agents such as tetracycline and ciprofloxacin to combat any secondary infections of the bullous regions of the epidermis. Fluid and electrolyte levels must be monitored to assess potential dehydration secondary to the skin lesions, and intravenous fluids shoud be administered as necessary. Ocular therapy is directed primarily at the prevention of infectious complications secondary to the colonization of organisms such as *Staphylococcus* species and other skin flora. This can be accomplished with antibiotics such as the aminoglycosides or other broad-spectrum drugs. Dosage frequencies are variable depending on the severity of the disease, but in most instances a dosage regimen of every 3 to 4 hours is recommended. The use of topical steroids has been advocated in the management of the inflammatory components of this disease. Prednisolone acetate 1% used every 2 to 3 hours initially and tapered after the inflammatory response begins to subside is a reasonable adjunct to antibiotic therapy. The use of lid scrubs, epilation in the case of trichiasis, sweeping of the fornices with a glass rod to prevent adhesions, and the use of cool compresses to provide symptomatic relief can prove extremely valuable in conjunction with topical pharmacotherapy.

The management of dry eye associated with Stevens-Johnson syndrome can be accomplished in an aggressive fashion with the use of nonpreserved lubricant solutions and bland ointments. Unfortunately, patients with Stevens-Johnson syndrome as well as BMMP frequently have chronic severe dry eye. The ophthalmic practitioner's challenge in managing this condition is to provide the best environment and visual performance possible in the face of rather severe compromise of the ocular surface. The best approach may entail using a variety of mechanisms to preserve lacrimal function, such as moisture chambers, lacrimal occlusion, and bandage lenses. These techniques should be considered on an individual basis when topical therapy alone is inadequate.

Although the majority of patients are successfully managed with topical therapy and adjunctive procedures, some require more extensive management in the form of surgical intervention. Tarsorrhaphy prevents excessive drying of the ocular surface. Other procedures to manage the sequelae of entropion or trichiasis, such as diathermy or cryosurgery, are effective for short-term resolution but frequently regress with time and must be repeated.[206]

Connective Tissue Disorders

The connective tissue disorders comprise a unique family of systemic diseases that have distinctive yet nonspecific systemic manifestations associated with organ involvement. Diseases such as rheumatoid arthritis, rheumatic fever, systemic lupus erythematosus (SLE), scleroderma, and periarteritis nodosa all demonstrate the typical histologic and clinical findings related to this category of diseases.

The histologic changes noted in these patients relate primarily to diffuse inflammatory damage to the connective tissue and vascular system. The nonspecific deposition of fibrin material in both the connective tissue and blood vessels typify this damage. This grouping of diseases is somewhat arbitrary, relating to the general acceptance of an autoimmune mechanism as an etiologic factor. While many of the diseases have common clinical findings, each also has unique and differentiating elements. Because recent evidence implicates Reiter's syndrome as belonging to this general category of autoimmune disease, it will also be considered in this discussion. Most of these diseases do not present with significant ocular manifestations. However, systemic lupus erythematosus, periarteritis nodosa, Reiter's syndrome, juvenile rheumatoid arthritis, and rheumatoid arthritis, in some instances, can be clinically identified through their overall ophthalmic presentations at an early stage in the disease.

Etiology

Connective tissue consists of a diverse group of physical elements that include collagen, elastin, proteoglycans, and other typical glycoproteins. The process by which these agents come together in any individual organ and the percentages of their distribution allow for the unique construction of each of the connective tissues within the body. Collagen and glycoproteins make up basement membranes and as such occur throughout the body as unique biologic and physical barriers. Little evidence exists that primary disease of these tissues is the pathologic agent. On the contrary, the connective tissue and vascular system are secondarily involved as the sites in which the inflammatory process develops. Hence, the traditional term *collagen-vascular disease* has been used to describe this broad category of disease, although it is no longer considered an acceptable term. Most of these conditions can produce diffuse involvement of the body's organs and tissues. The American College of Rheumatology has developed a series of diagnostic criteria that are used to identify each of these clinical entities.

Systemic lupus erythematosus (SLE) is a chronic inflammatory disease of unknown etiology that affects the skin, cardiovascular system, nervous system, mucous membranes, and kidneys. Prevalence of this disease is approximately 1 per 1,000. Although occurrence is slightly greater in blacks versus caucasians, the most notable epidemiologic factor is the remarkably high incidence among females, 5 to 10 times more frequent than in males.[207] The typical age of onset is in the third to fourth decade.[207] A variety of factors have been postulated as potential etiologic agents. These include endocrine, genetic, viruses, retroviruses, autoimmune mechanisms, and exogenous antigens. There have been cases of disease remission during pregnancy and exacerbation postpartum as well as correlations with use of anti-infective agents.[207,208]

Polyarteritis nodosa is a diffuse vasculitis that can produce necrotizing changes and predominantly involves the small and medium size arteries. The lesions in this disease are generally diffuse throughout the vascular system and asymmetric in presentation. The necrotizing inflammatory component is quite evident in the acute stage, and usually an accompanying infiltration of inflammatory cells occurs throughout the vessel walls and surrounding tissue. Vascular damage secondary to this inflammatory process usually relates to thrombosis and fibrosis with subsequent blockage of the blood flow to that area. Tissue infarction can occur. Unlike systemic lupus, polyarteritis nodosa more commonly occurs in males than females. Although patients of all ages can have the disease, the onset most typically occurs in the third to sixth decade.[207,211] Many etiologies have been postulated, including hypersensitivity reactions and response to

microorganisms such as *Streptococcus* species and viral entities.[209–212]

Reiter's syndrome has classically been associated with a triad of clinical presentations that include arthritis, conjunctivitis, and urethritis. These are associated with a relatively high incidence of positive HLA-B27 antigen as well as latex negative erosion. It has been implicated as a complication of such disease states as nonspecific urethritis, postgonococcal urethritis, or gastrointestinal disease involving organisms such as *Salmonella, Clostridium,* and *Yersinia.*[213,214] Although *Chlamydia* has been associated with Reiter's syndrome, recently researchers have identified *Chlamydia* as the most common pathogen associated with Reiter's syndrome. In addition, researchers have found that synovial biopsy tissue from most patients with Reiter's syndrome shows significant levels of apparently intact chlamydial RNA.[215–218] Although some investigators postulate an association between Reiter's syndrome and HIV infection, others indicate that Reiter's syndrome shows no significant relationship to HIV infection.[219,220]

Diagnosis

Systemic lupus can have ocular manifestations. Differential diagnosis of the disease is based on the presence of 4 of the 11 diagnostic criteria listed by the American College of Rheumatology. Ocular signs can include a variety of clinical manifestations, but the ocular disease most characteristically occurs as keratoconjunctivitis sicca. Other findings can include chemosis, recurrent episcleritis, conjunctival scarring and symblepharon (Fig. 26.25). Also noted is a relatively high incidence of anterior uveitis and in a small percentage of patients the presence of eyelid plaques.[221–223] Other common findings include corneal infiltration as well as marginal corneal ulcers.[224]

Although ocular manifestations may contribute to the diagnosis of SLE, it is important to evaluate the patient for systemic manifestations as well. These include fever, weight loss, arthralgia, nephritis, and the typical butterfly rash seen on the face. This particular presentation is evident in fewer than half the patients with systemic lupus. In many instances, more subtle signs may include a blush and swelling of the skin on the cheeks following exposure to the sun. These lesions frequently scale and are termed discoid when they present in this fashion. Subsequent episodes can produce either a hyper- or hypopigmented state and atrophy of the epidermal tissue. Raynaud's phenomenon is not uncommon, and many individuals develop ulcerative changes of the extremities in association with this aspect of the disease. Patients can show evidence of purpura and ecchymosis.[225] Antiphospholipid antibodies, or lupus anticoagulant, may play a role in retinal vaso-occlusive disease in the formation of either branch retinal or central retinal vein occlusion.[226]

As with SLE, polyarteritis nodosa has a wide range of

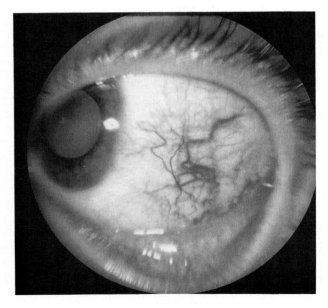

FIGURE 26.25 **Episcleritis in patient with systemic lupus erythematosus.**

clinical manifestations. These include fever, weight loss, severe abdominal and musculoskeletal pain, tachycardia, acute glomerulonephritis, polyneuritis, myocardial infarction, and pulmonary manifestations such as bronchial asthma. The frequency of this disease is approximately 8 per 1000, but the clinical diagnosis is considerably lower than postmortem studies indicate. Renal involvement is one of the most devastating aspects of the disease and can be manifested by simple hematuria or, in more severe cases, infarction and subsequent acute decompensation, resulting in pain in the lower back. Renal disease occurs in approximately 75% of patients, and hypertension occurs in over 50%.[227] Typical findings of the anterior segment include keratoconjunctivitis sicca with lacrimal gland atrophy, conjunctival hyperemia, subconjunctival hemorrhages, and chemosis. The cornea can demonstrate marginal ulceration or necrotizing sclerokeratitis. Retinal vaso-occlusive disease in the form of cotton wool spots, edema, hypertensive retinopathy, and hemorrhage are typical, and some instances of more extreme disease display nonrhegmatogenous retinal detachments (Fig. 26.26). Other, less common, findings include optic nerve involvement as well as extraocular muscle palsies. In severe cases nodular episcleritis or scleritis can progress to a necrotizing state. As with all connective tissue diseases, anterior uveitis can occur.

Ocular involvement relates primarily to the vascular inflammatory aspect of the disease. In the central nervous system, the disease manifests itself as neurologic deficits and in the retina as typical vaso-occlusive episodes.

Reiter's syndrome is a disease in which the systemic symptoms generally precede the ocular findings. Most commonly the patients experience genitourinary or gastrointestinal disturbances prior to the onset of ocular findings. In most instances, onset of the ocular disease follows these symptoms in a relatively short time, but in some patients the onset of ocular disease can be delayed for several months. The polyarthritis that is commonly associated with the disease is generally asymmetric and has a predilection for the joints of the lower extremities.[228,229] In most patients, remission occurs within several weeks to months following onset of the disease. Only a small number of individuals progress to the chronic or recurrent form of psoriatic arthritis. Less typical complications include cardiac and neurologic involvement, ankylosing spondylitis, amyloid disease, and aortic incompetence.[230–232] An unusual but clinically important finding is that of painful deformity of the feet in the form of keratoderma blenorrhagica (Fig. 26.27), which is primarily confined to the plantar surfaces of the foot. Although it occurs in a small percentage of patients (5% to 7%), when seen in conjunction with other findings, it can prove extremely helpful in the diagnosis. Nonspecific laboratory findings in patients with Reiter's syndrome include an increase in peripheral blood leucocytosis and elevated sedimentation rate. Radiographic abnormalities are typical of rheumatoid arthritis.

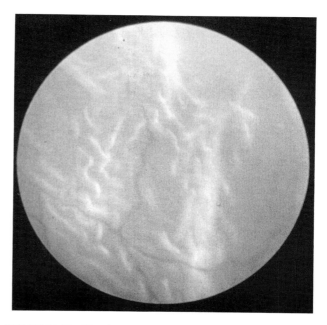

FIGURE 26.26   **Nonrhegmatogenous retinal detachment in polyarteritis nodosa.**

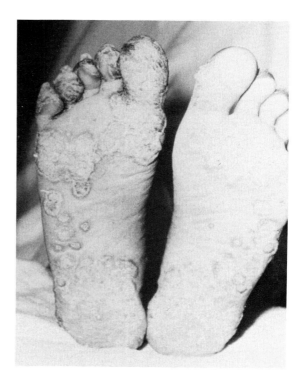

FIGURE 26.27   **Keratoderma blenorrhagica in Reiter's syndrome. (Courtesy William Wallace, O.D.)**

Unlike the other entities already discussed, the conjunctiva is one of the focal points of the ocular involvement in Reiter's syndrome. Changes in the conjunctiva include bilateral papillary hypertrophy with a mucopurulent discharge, although patients are frequently not extremely symptomatic. Associated chemosis, a follicular reaction, and variable hyperemia occur. In association with conjunctival changes, one frequently sees the presence of subepithelial opacities of the cornea as well as superficial punctate keratitis and edema. The concurrent presence of uveitis with the apparent bacterial disease is typical of Reiter's syndrome, and in conjunction with a positive systemic history of genitourinary complications, is pathognomonic for the disease. Other less typical ocular findings include the presence of optic nerve inflammation in the form of neuritis or disc edema. In some instances, the patient may present with macular edema, which is thought to be secondary to the inflammatory process. The anterior uveitis is typically severe and of relatively long duration. In patients with lumbar inflammatory disease, up to 50% develop recurrent uveitis, while only 10% of those who do not have lumbar involvement develop recurrent episodes.[233]

Management

Therapy of SLE is both complex and in many instances disappointing for both the patient and the practitioner. In general, management of the systemic signs and symptoms does little to improve the ocular manifestations of the disease. The most common therapy for the arthritic and cardiac complications is the use of nonsteroidal anti-inflammatory agents. Hydroxychloroquine and chloroquine are particularly effective in the treatment of the discoid rash associated with the disease. In some cases oral steroids are used. Immunosuppressive agents such as cyclophosphamide and azathioprine are used in individuals in whom the disease state is relatively severe and steroid therapy proves insufficient.

Ocular therapy for SLE is primarily directed at the treatment of the ocular surface disease complications. Maintenance of the tear film with adjunctive lubricant therapy is most common. Because of the chronic nature of the disease and the risk of development of preservative allergy, patients should be treated with nonpreserved artificial tears and ointments. Management of associated bacterial conjunctivitis should be undertaken with appropriate antibiotic therapy, but chronic antibiotic therapy can complicate the disease process and should be avoided. In some instances, clinicians have advocated the use of bandage lenses, punctal or canalicular occlusion, and other methods for enhancement of ocular surface quality, but these often have limited effectiveness in long-term management.

The underlying etiology of the disease determines the treatment of polyarteritis nodosa. The survival rate over 5 years for untreated patients with polyarteritis nodosa is approximately 10%.[234,235] Thus, the use of aggressive systemic management is of vital importance. Corticosteroid therapy has demonstrated improvement in the mortality rate and in some studies has increased the 5-year survival to over 50%.[234,235] Regimens for steroid therapy can be as high as 1 to 2 mg per kg body weight per day. This type of management requires following the patient carefully and tapering steroid therapy as rapidly as possible. Unfortunately, even with the use of steroids some patients are not successfully managed and require immunosuppressive therapy. As with SLE, cyclophosphamide and azathioprine are the two most commonly used agents. These are generally administered concurrently with steroids and in many instances allow significant reduction in steroid dosage while patient symptomatology is stabilized. Unfortunately, the morbidity associated with this disease is significant, and management of the complications related to systemic hypertension as well as organ failure can be extremely important in allowing the patient to maintain a more normal lifestyle. Because of the persistent presence of joint and muscle discomfort associated with the disease, the use of analgesic agents can be helpful in minimizing symptoms.

As with other connective tissue diseases, ocular therapy focuses on the disturbance of the ocular surface and makes use of topical nonpreserved lubricants. If uveitis is present concurrently, the use of topical steroids along with a cycloplegic agent is appropriate. The most effective means of controlling the ocular complications is to manage the systemic component of the disease aggressively. In some instances, patients are relatively asymptomatic systemically while being treated with steroids and immunosuppressive therapy but still demonstrate active disease. In these individuals the presence of continuing ocular inflammatory changes can be helpful in assessing the effectiveness of systemic therapy.

Therapy for Reiter's syndrome is best approached from both a systemic and ocular perspective. The current recommended ocular therapy involves the use of tetracycline 250 mg 4 times daily for a minimum of 3 to 4 weeks. The long-acting tetracyclines such as doxycycline can also be used. The use of erythromycin is recommended in individuals sensitive to tetracycline, in pregnant women, or in children. The normal adult dosage is 500 mg every 12 hours. While children can be managed in the primary care setting, comanaging the systemic aspects of the disease entails consulting the pediatrician. In instances of Reiter's syndrome that have been precipitated by enteric organisms, treatment with trimethoprim-sulfamethoxazole should be instituted.

Management of the ocular aspects of Reiter's syndrome is directed toward control of inflammation. The uveitis can be quite severe and resistant to therapy. In most instances the use of topical steroids such as prednisolone acetate 1% or dexamethasone 0.1% is recommended. Dosage is variable but in severe cases should be administered initially every 1 to 2 hours, accompanied by the use of cycloplegic agents such as homatropine 5% or scopolamine 0.25% 2 to 3 times daily. The sequelae that can occur relative to synechia and subsequent secondary glaucomas should be minimized. In patients who have severe uveitis associated with the disease, either subTenon's or oral steroids may be used in conjunction with topical management. The conjunctivitis associated with Reiter's syndrome usually responds quite well once the systemic condition has been identified and the patient is under appropriate oral antibiotic management. The use of a topical aminoglycoside, erythromycin or combination agent such as trimethoprim-polymyxin B is effective in minimizing ocular symptoms. However, the use of topical steroids to treat the conjunctivitis is not usually required since most ocular symptoms are dramatically diminished within the first few days of systemic and topical antibiotic therapy.

With any of the connective tissue diseases the potential for recurrence is relatively high, and in most instances the disease becomes chronic. Therefore, the practitioner must educate the patient to the potential for long-term involvement with the disease. Also, the patient should not be managed in isolation. The ophthalmic practitioner should consult with the patient's primary physician to optimize therapeutic management.

Localized Conjunctival Inflammation

Phlyctenulosis

ETIOLOGY

Phlyctenular conjunctivitis is an allergic hypersensitivity response of the conjunctiva and occasionally the cornea to antigens to which the patient is sensitive. Although the disease is world-wide in its distribution, the etiologic factors vary considerably depending on geographic location. In general, phlyctenular conjunctivitis occurs more commonly in areas of poor sanitation and health care. It is typically more common in women (60% to 70%) than men and occurs with greater frequency in children. The condition has numerous etiologic agents. In those populations in which poverty is endemic, tuberculosis is a common cause. In patient populations with access to health care and appropriate sanitation, the bacterial protein from the staphylococcal organism may be the causative agent. Other agents such as intestinal parasites are also potential sources of phlyctenular disease.

DIAGNOSIS

Although phlyctenular conjunctivitis can occur without obvious associated disease, patients with phlyctenules can have concurrent evidence of either dermatologic or systemic disease states, such as acne rosacea and seborrheic blepharo-

conjunctivitis. The symptoms associated with phlyctenulosis are similar to those of a mild to moderate conjunctivitis. The patient frequently has foreign body sensation as well as discomfort and injection. Although not common, mucopurulent discharge may occur concurrently with bacterial infection. In most instances, the patient complains of the mucus-like discharge seen in ocular allergy. Phlyctenules appear as small, raised, nodular lesions that are usually pinkish-white and surrounded by dilated blood vessels. The conjunctival lesions are self-limiting and rarely produce significant symptoms beyond those already mentioned. The more typical response occurs when the lesion develops at the limbal margin and encroaches onto the corneal surface. These junctional lesions can produce significant symptoms in the form of photophobia, ciliary spasm, and lacrimation. The limbus-based lesions resemble those of the conjunctiva, but they bridge the corneal limbus (see Fig. 27.24). Limbus-based lesions usually occur in the inferior aspect of the eye near the lid margin, while the conjunctival lesions develop within the interpalpebral aperture (Fig. 26.28). The diagnosis of phlyctenular conjunctivitis is based primarily on the typical appearance of the lesion, its location, and a thorough ocular examination and health history.

Differential diagnosis includes such entities as chlamydial conjunctivitis, pterygium, nodular episcleritis, and vernal conjunctivitis. Chlamydial infection presents with a much more chronic course and a follicular reaction typical of the disease. In its early phases, acne rosacea can appear subtle, but typical dermatologic changes allow easy differentation. Limbal vernal conjunctivitis, by producing similar allergic-like mucous discharge, can be difficult to diagnose in its early phase but has a seasonal component that helps to differentiate it from phlyctenulosis. Trantas' dots, associated with limbal vernal conjunctivitis, are also much smaller than phlyctenules.

MANAGEMENT

Therapy is directly dependent on etiologic factors. In individuals who are suspected of having tuberculosis, diagnosis should make use of a PPD skin test, chest x-ray, and sputum cultures if necessary. These individuals should be referred for comanagement to their primary physician or an infectious disease specialist. While antituberculin agents are systemically administered, the ocular lesions are appropriately treated with topical steroids. In most instances, patients respond to 1% prednisolone acetate every 3 to 4 hours for the first day and then subsequently tapered rapidly based on the patient's response.

When patients are suspected of having a staphylococcal infection, the clinician should manage both the inflammatory and bacterial components, which is best accomplished through the use of a steroid-antibiotic combination. Initial doses should be administered every 2 to 4 hours, depending on severity, for the first 24 to 48 hours. In most instances,

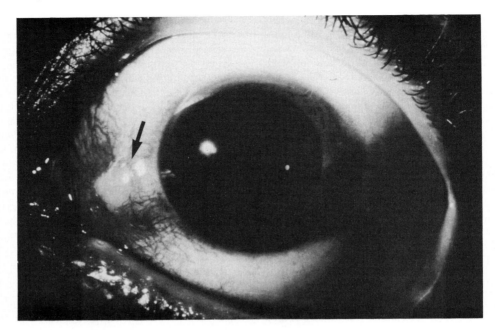

FIGURE 26.28   Conjunctival phlyctenule (arrow) in interpalpebral aperture. (Courtesy William Wallace, O.D.)

patients obtain dramatic relief of symptoms and can diminish use of the drug in 7 to 10 days. Because of the presumed etiology of *Staphylococcus*, these patients should receive lid therapy. Antibiotic ointments such as erythromycin, bacitracin, or bacitracin-polymyxin B can be used twice daily as a lid scrub. For recurrent cases, oral tetracycline is helpful.

Patients suspected of having oculodermatologic disease should be treated with oral antibiotics such as tetracycline or doxycycline. Tetracycline is given in a dosage of 250 mg 4 times daily for approximately 4 to 6 weeks, or doxycycline 100 mg twice daily for 4 to 6 weeks. When other etiologic agents such as intestinal parasites, *Chlamydia*, gonococcus, and herpes simplex are suspected, patients should receive appropriate systemic medications.

Superior Limbic Keratoconjunctivitis (SLK)

ETIOLOGY

This chronic inflammatory disease produces a papillary reaction of the upper tarsal conjunctiva and the bulbar conjunctival surface immediately superior to the limbal margin. The condition is usually bilateral although significant asymmetry can exist. For many patients the disease resolves within several weeks, while others experience no significant relief. One of the unusual aspects is its variable intensity from one eye to the other without significant remission

taking place in either eye. This finding frequently accompanies symptoms of fluctuating ocular pain.

Although there is no defined etiology for this disease, in Theodore's original study many patients had dry eye. Also, some patients may have thyroid dysfunction.[236]

DIAGNOSIS

The diagnosis of SLK is based on several unique factors. First is the chronicity of the patient's complaint. Second and more important is that patients are frequently more symptomatic than the clinical examination justifies. The clinical picture is that of a sectoral area of involvement at the limbal margin (10 to 2 o'clock position), demonstrating mild to moderate injection and in more advanced cases thickening of the limbal conjunctiva. Some individuals can also demonstrate filaments and a mild mucous discharge, but these findings may relate more directly to the reduction of aqueous tears and subsequent disproportionate level of mucin development. The classic clinical feature of this disease is the relatively intense punctate stain noted with rose bengal dye. This feature is typically much more severe than the conjunctival hyperemia or thickening would suggest and frequently correlates well with the patient's symptoms. The cornea, although it can demonstrate punctate staining, filament development, and occasionally pannus, is usually not as severely involved as the conjunctiva.

A variant of the classic form of SLK is that of soft contact lens-induced superior limbic keratoconjunctivitis. Although these individuals typically show findings very similar to those patients with SLK, they almost universally respond to discontinuing contact lenses and aggressive use of non-preserved artificial tears.

MANAGEMENT

Although SLK has no defined etiology, the most appealing hypothesis is that of a mechanical problem. For many years therapy has consisted of a wide variety of agents including steroids, antibiotics, ocular lubricants, and other more aggressive means of treatment. Unfortunately, topical pharmacotherapy has not been particularly successful. However, since some patients do respond, it is a prudent course of treatment prior to initiating more aggressive therapeutic intervention.[236]

Other topical therapy used with some success includes 10% to 20% acetylcystine applied every 4 hours, 4 times daily, and 4% sodium cromolyn used every 4 hours. Both of these agents have demonstrated modest success and should be considered prior to more aggressive intervention.[237] If these topical agents give no relief, the current recommended therapy is 0.25% to 0.5% silver nitrate solution followed by irrigation, selectively applied to the tarsal and bulbar conjunctival surfaces. Such therapy may not promote permanent resolution, but most patients achieve symptomatic relief for a period of time following the chemical cautery. Similar treatments include scraping of the tarsal conjunctiva, diathermy, cryotherapy, or laser. Other less invasive forms of therapy include the use of pressure patching of the affected eye, as well as bandage contact lenses. While none of these treatments has been universally successful, they have demonstrated some capacity to relieve symptoms in patients for finite periods of time.[238]

In individuals who do not respond to these therapeutic regimens, resection of the involved conjunctiva should be considered. This surgery involves the removal of a 5- to 6-mm section of conjunctiva in the affected area.[239]

Unfortunately, no one remedy has proved consistently successful, and the patient frequently demonstrates symptomatic relief followed by exacerbation. For this reason the clinician must provide adequate counselling to the patient regarding the potential chronicity of the disease. Any associated problems that develop during the course of therapy must also betreated, since they may produce an increase in symptoms. These include dry eye and bacterial conjunctivitis.

Pterygium

ETIOLOGY

Pterygia are a degeneration of the conjunctival stroma and are identical in cellular composition to pinguecula. The primary etiologic factors may relate to both heredity and environment. The incidence of pterygia is significantly higher in individuals who live in proximity to the equator. It also typically occurs in individuals who spend significant amounts of time outdoors and have high levels of ultraviolet exposure. Other agents that may contribute to the development of pterygium include external stimuli such as allergens, noxious chemicals, and irritants. Because of the marked similarity in cellular composition, pinguecula may in many instances be a precursor to pterygium. The term pterygium means "wing" and is descriptive of its typical appearance in most patients. Pterygia are primarily located in the interpalpebral area and more frequently occur in the nasal aspect of the bulbar conjunctiva. They appear as a wedge-like structure with its base towards the medial or lateral canthus and its apex towards the corneal surface (Fig. 26.29).

DIAGNOSIS

A thorough history and examination of the anterior segment can readily establish a diagnosis of pterygium. Typically the type of wedge-like elevated mass seen in pterygium is not characteristic of other lesions. On the other hand, when this occurs outside the palpebral aperture, one must consider the possibility of other etiologies such as phlyctenule or actinic keratosis. The clinical picture depends on the duration of the lesion's growth as well as the current level of inflammation. The mass is often relatively quiescent with little vascular involvement, but patients can present with significant inflammation and marked injection of the conjunctiva and associated tissue overlying the cornea. In advanced cases, pterygia can produce up to 4 to 6 diopters of curvature change. A more important and clinically significant finding is that of the associated dry area or dellen adjacent to the leading edge of the pterygium. This dry area may result from an inadequacy of the lid/corneal or lid/conjunctival contact on blinking and subsequent lack of mucin in that area. Patients with advanced pterygia complain often of changes in visual acuity related to the topographical changes in the cornea's surface. These changes are generally correctable to normal visual levels unless the pterygium has encroached upon the visual axis, in which case a rather marked reduction in visual acuity can occur. In some instances patients can have pterygia on both the nasal and temporal aspect of each eye and have a remarkable injection of the interpalpebral area with a relatively quiet conjunctiva beneath the upper and lower lids.

MANAGEMENT

The management of pterygia usually involves palliative therapy. Patients show significant relief of symptoms with the use of artificial tears and ointments. When these are insufficient, the use of mild steroids such as fluorometholone can be implemented 4 times daily to combat the inflammatory component. Chronic use of steroids, however, is not

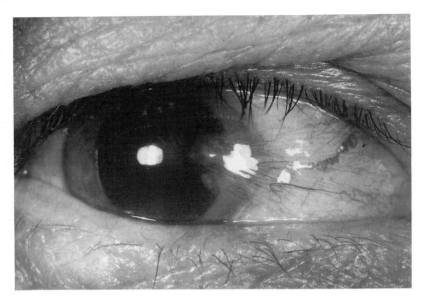

FIGURE 26.29   **Pterygium. Note base toward canthus and apex on corneal surface.**

recommended. An environmental history can indicate whether sources of stimulation can be modified or reduced through the use of protective eyewear or the reduction of exogenous irritants. If the predominant response is inflammatory in nature, antibiotic agents have little, if any, value and, in fact, can complicate the process because of allergic reactions or toxicity associated with the anti-infective agent. Surgical treatment of the disease is considered only for patients in whom cosmesis or visual compromise has produced a need for therapy beyond the use of topical agents.

Aside from the standard surgical techniques for removal, there have been numerous attempts to develop methods to limit the recurrence of pterygial growth. Currently, primary resection alone has a 40% to 50% recurrence rate.[240] The use of beta irradiation with strontium 90 has been recommended, and this is accomplished through the use of 1,000 to 1,500 rads in divided doses. Some clinicians advocate the use of Thiotepa.[241] This agent is applied topically in a concentration of 1:2000 for approximately 6 to 8 weeks. Success rates are significantly enhanced over controls, but complications have limited its use.[241]

Antimetabolites such as mitomycin C have demonstrated some success. By inhibiting fibroblast proliferation, mitomycin C may decrease the rate of pterygium recurrence after surgical excision. The drug has been applied intraoperatively by holding a sponge soaked in 0.02% to 4% mitomycin against the sclera for 3 to 5 minutes.[247,248] The medication has also been administered postoperatively with success.[249] Long-term complications include delayed epithelialization and degenerative calcification of conjunctiva.[249]

Conjunctival Trauma

Injuries to the conjunctiva result from many household, school, sport, or workplace activities. Children and young adults are particularly at risk. Monestam and Bjornstig[242] found that 40% of eye injuries resulted from foreign bodies on the conjunctiva or cornea. A disproportionate number of severe injuries occurred in children and young adults age 10 to 19 years. Clinical findings may include foreign bodies, chemical or thermal burns, and abrasions, lacerations, or contusions from blunt trauma. All conjunctival trauma should be considered an ocular urgency because of the risk of concurrent corneal injury or the possibility of penetration of the globe in high-speed impact foreign body situations.

Foreign Bodies

ETIOLOGY

Environmental foreign bodies consisting of dirt, dust, glass, metal, or other material may contact and adhere to the conjunctiva. Often the affected patient reports that something blew into the eye on a windy day. The workplace is also a frequent source of foreign body material, particularly for individuals not wearing protective eyewear.

DIAGNOSIS

A thorough history and biomicroscopic examination are crucial for all conjunctival injuries, both to assess the degree of conjunctival damage and to determine the extent of any corneal or scleral involvement. The case history needs to determine painstakingly the source and impact speed of the foreign material, since this information guides the clinician's examination and helps to determine the need for adjunctive testing such as radiologic studies. The eyelids must be everted to assess the palpebral conjunctiva carefully (Fig. 26.30). Occasionally a double lid eversion may be required. In some cases, topical anesthesia may be necessary to adequately evaluate the eye. The evaluation should also include a Seidel test using sodium fluorescein dye to rule out any aqueous or vitreous leakage from penetration of the globe. Most conjunctival foreign bodies are superficial and usually found on the superior palpebral conjunctiva (Fig. 26.30). Depending on the length of time the foreign body has been present, the wound site may have some surrounding hyperemia. When foreign bodies become embedded in the conjunctiva, a subconjunctival hemorrhage or conjunctival granuloma may envelop the impact site.

MANAGEMENT

Copious lavage of the conjunctiva with normal saline or extraocular irrigating solution may loosen and remove some foreign bodies. Swabbing the affected area with a moistened cotton-tipped applicator is often effective when the foreign body is partially adherent. When the foreign material is difficult to visualize, as with fiberglass particles, swabbing the fornices is often necessary to remove the foreign material. Any swabbing should be followed by a saline lavage. Embedded foreign bodies may be removed with a sterile needle or spud. A broad-spectrum topical antibiotic such as trimethoprim-polymyxin B solution or bacitracin-polymyxin B ointment should be applied to the eye after removal of the foreign body to prevent secondary infection. The antibiotic may be continued for 24 hours if necessary following the removal of embedded foreign bodies. Semipressure patching with cycloplegia and topical antibiotic may be indicated following removal of deeply embedded foreign bodies.

Burns

ETIOLOGY

Chemical burns of the conjunctiva usually result from inadvertent splashes of chemicals into the face or from hydrogen peroxide contact lens solutions. Occasionally patients may instill a chemical irritant directly into the eye, resulting in severe injury. Cigarettes, curling irons, or overexposure to ultraviolet radiation frequently cause thermal burns.

DIAGNOSIS

The diagnosis of conjunctival burns requires essentially all the procedures outlined for foreign bodies. For chemical

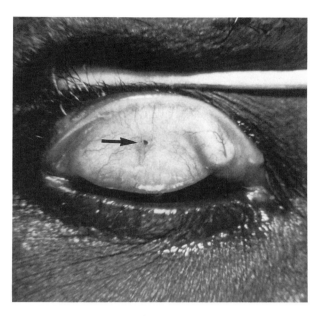

FIGURE 26.30 **Foreign body (arrow) on upper palpebral conjunctiva. (Courtesy Larry J. Alexander, O.D.)**

burns, the clinician must determine whether the offending chemical is acid or alkaline. If the chemical is not familiar to the clinician, the local poison control center can provide information. The conjunctival fornix and tear film can be tested with pH paper to determine whether an acid or base is present. The conjunctiva must then be carefully assessed to determine the depth of the burn. Most acid burns will cause superficial epithelial damage as indicated by punctate staining with sodium fluorescein. In severe cases, however, blanching of the conjunctiva is possible. Alkaline burns from chemicals such as lye or lime usually blanch the conjunctiva and cause more severe injury due to their collagenolytic capabilities. Thermal burns may cause either superficial or severe injury depending on contact time of the offending agent.

MANAGEMENT

For chemical burns, therapy begins with copious irrigation of the conjunctiva with normal saline or extraocular irrigating solution. The lavage should continue for at least 5 minutes for acid burns and 30 minutes for alkaline burns or until a neutral pH is obtained. Prophylactic topical trimethoprim-polymyxin B or aminoglycoside solution should be instilled 4 times per day for 3 to 5 days. The conjunctiva must then be carefully monitored for signs of fibroblast activity and scar formation for several days in acid burns or weeks for alkaline burns. A topical steroid 4 times per day may be necessary to prevent cicatricial tissue and subsequent development of symblepharon. Acetylcysteine 20% applied 4 times per day may inhibit collagenase activity.[243] Since secondary glaucoma may result from significant corneal involvement, intraocular pressure should be closely monitored in patients with alkaline burns. Most conjunctival thermal burns are treated similar to acid burns. Frequent instillation of nonpreserved artificial tears is also important for keeping the conjunctival tissue well lubricated in burn injuries.

Abrasions, Contusions, and Lacerations

ETIOLOGY

Direct trauma is the most frequent cause of conjunctival abrasions, contusions, or lacerations. The nature of the contact instrument usually determines what type of wound the patient suffers. For example, a thrown object may cause only a contusion, whereas a sharp pencil point can lacerate the conjunctiva.

DIAGNOSIS

The diagnosis of these conjunctival injuries is determined through the history and careful biomicroscopic examination. Symptoms usually consist of mild irritation or foreign body sensation. Clinical findings accompanying conjunctival abrasions include superficial epithelial cell loss, chemosis, or subconjunctival hemorrhage. Most conjunctival contusions result in subconjunctival hemorrhages. Lacerations are usually associated with hemorrhaging and frequently result in loose conjunctival tissue flaps if they are full-thickness tears. The white sclera may be visible, flanked by clumping of conjunctival tissue, chemosis, and subconjunctival hemorrhages. The sclera must be carefully evaluated to rule out perforation of the globe. A Seidel test should be performed.

MANAGEMENT

Conjunctival abrasions and lacerations should be irrigated with sterile normal saline or extraocular irrigating solution to remove any foreign material. Abrasions may be treated with topical trimethoprim-polymyxin B or aminoglycoside solution applied 4 times per day for several days or until healed. In pediatric cases, bacitracin-polymyxin B ointment may be substituted if necessary to improve patient comfort. Many conjunctival abrasions do not require patching. Lacerations may be managed with bacitracin-polymyxin B or aminoglycoside ointment applied 4 times per day for 5 to 7 days or until sufficient wound healing has occurred. Conjunctival lacerations will frequently require semipressure patching with cycloplegia and topical antibiotic ointment to achieve adequate resolution. Sutures are not needed for uncomplicated conjunctival lacerations.[244] Once healing has begun, frequent use of nonpreserved artificial tears often improves patient comfort. No specific therapy is required for conjunctival contusions since most involve only subconjunctival hemorrhages that are self-limiting. Nonpreserved artificial tears can improve patient comfort, and warm compresses used for 15 to 20 minutes several times daily may hasten resorption of blood.

References

1. National Center for Health Statistics. Ganley JP, Roberts J. Eye conditions and related need for medical care among persons 1–74 years of age—United States 1971–1972. Vital and Health Statistics. Series 11, No. 228. DHHS Pub(PHS) 83–1678. Public Health Service. Washington, DC. US Government Printing Office. March 1983.
2. Apple DJ, Rabb MF. Ocular pathology. Clinical applications and self assessment. St. Louis: Mosby-Year Book, 1991;10:454.
3. Wolff E. Anatomy of the eye and orbit. Philadelphia: WB Saunders Co, 1976;7:206.
4. Sachs EH, Wieczorek R, Jakobiec FA, et al. Lymphocytic subpopulations in the normal human conjunctiva: a monoclonal antibody study. Ophthalmology 1986;93:1276.
5. Spinak M. Cytological changes of the conjunctiva in immunoglobulin producing dyscrasias. Ophthalmology 1981;88:1207.
6. Allansmith MR, Greiner JV, Baird BS. Number of inflammatory cells in the normal conjunctiva. Am J Ophthalmol 1978;86:250.
7. Apple DJ, Rabb MF. Ocular pathology. Clinical applications and self assessment. St. Louis: Mosby-Year Book, 1991;10:456.
8. Greiner JV, Henriquez AS, Covington HI, et al. Goblet cells of the human conjunctiva. Arch Ophthalmol 1981;99:2190.
9. Bron AJ, Mengher LS, Davey CC. The normal conjunctiva and its response to inflammation. Trans Ophthalmol Soc UK 1985;104:424–435.
10. Gillette TE, Chandler JW, Greiner JV. Langerhans cells of the ocular surface. Ophthalmology 1982;89:700.
11. Friedlaender MH. Allergy and immunology of the eye. New York. Raven Press: 1993;1:9–10.
12. Friedlaender MH. Allergy and immunology of the eye. New York. Raven Press: 1993;3:54.
13. Friedlaender MH. Allergy and immunology of the eye. New York. Raven Press: 1993;3:55.
14. Yanoff M, Fine BS. Ocular pathology. Philadelphia: JB Lippincott Co, 1989;7:216–217.
15. Apple DJ, Rabb MF. Ocular pathology. Clinical applications and self assessment. St. Louis: Mosby-Year Book. 1991;10:460.
16. Yanoff M, Fine BS. Ocular pathology. Philadelphia: JB Lippincott Co, 1989;7:218–219.
17. Yanoff M, Fine BS. Ocular pathology. Philadelphia: JB Lippincott Co, 1989;7:219.
18. Khorazo D, Thompson R. The bacterial flora of the normal conjunctiva. Am J Ophthalmol 1935;18:1114.
19. Allansmith MR, Ostler HB, Butterworth M. Concomitance of bacteria in various areas of the eye. Arch Ophthalmol 1969;82:37.
20. Locatcher-Khorazo D, Seegal BC. Microbiology of the eye. St. Louis: CV Mosby Co, 1972;2:14–15.
21. McNutt J, Allen SD, Wilson LA, et al. Anaerobic flora of the normal human conjunctival sac. Arch Ophthalmol 1978;96:1448.

22. Perkins RE, Kundsin RB, Pratt MV, et al. Bacteriology of normal and infected conjunctiva. J Clin Microbiol 1975;1:145.

23. Friedberg DN, Stenson SM, Orenstein JM, et al. Microsporidial keratoconjunctivitis in acquired immunodeficiency syndrome. Arch Ophthalmol 1990;108:504.

24. Wilson L, Ahearn D, Jones D, Sexton R. Fungi from the normal outer eye. Am J Ophthalmol 1969;67:52.

25. Ostler HB. Diseases of the external eye and adnexa. Baltimore: Williams & Wilkins, 1993;8:361.

26. Friedlaender MH. Allergy and immunology of the eye. New York: Raven Press, 1993;3:53–55.

27. Washington JA. Laboratory procedures in clinical microbiology. New York: Springer-Verlag, 1985;App. B:771.

28. Washington JA. Laboratory procedures in clinical microbiology. New York: Springer-Verlag, 1985;App. B:776–777.

29. Baron EJ, Finegold SM. Diagnostic microbiology. St. Louis. CV Mosby. 1990;8:84.

30. Wilson LA, Sexton RR. Laboratory diagnosis in fungal keratitis. Am J Ophthalmol 1968;66:646.

31. Washington JA. Laboratory procedures in clinical microbiology. New York. Springer-Verlag. 1985;App. B:795.

32. Perry LD, Brinser JH, Kolodner H. Anaerobic corneal ulcers. Ophthalmology 1982;89:636.

33. Washington JA. Laboratory procedures in clinical microbiology. New York. Springer-Verlag. 1985;App. B:794.

34. Kleinfeld J, Ellis PP. Effects of topical anesthetics on the growth of microorganisms. Arch Ophthalmol 1966;76:712.

35. Perkins RE, Kundsin RB, Pratt MV, et al. Bacteriology of normal and infected conjunctiva. J Clin Microbiol 1975;1:147.

36. Jones BR. Laboratory tests for chlamydial infection. Br J Ophthalmol 1974;58:438.

37. Yoneda C, Dawson CR, Daghfous T, et al. Cytology as a guide to the presence of chlamydial inclusions in Giesma stained conjunctival smears in severe endemic trachoma. Br J Ophthalmol 1975; 59:116.

38. Washington JA. Laboratory procedures in clinical microbiology. New York. Springer-Verlag. 1985;Appendix B.

39. Bialasiewicz AA, Jahn GJ. Evaluation of diagnostic tools for adult chlamydial keratoconjunctivitis. Ophthalmology 1987;94:532.

40. Sheppard JD, Kowalski RP, Meyer MP, et al. Immunodiagnosis of adult chlamydial conjunctivitis. Ophthalmology 1988;95:434.

41. Roblin PM, Hammerschlag MR, Cummings C, et al. Comparison of two rapid microscopic methods and culture for detection of *Chlamydia trachomatis* in ocular and nasopharyngeal specimens from infants. J Clin Microbiol 1989;27:968.

42. MicroTrak Manual. Palo Alto, CA. Syva Co. 1987.

43. Rapoza PA, Johnson S, Taylor HR. Platinum spatula vs. dacron swab in the preparation of conjunctival smears. Am J Ophthalmol 1986;102:400.

44. Brinser JH, Weiss A. Laboratory diagnosis in ocular disease. In: Tasman W, Jaeger EA, eds. Duane's clinical ophthalmology. Philadelphia: JB Lippincott Co, 1993;vol 4;1:1–14.

45. Kowalski RP, Gordon YJ. Comparison of direct rapid tests for the detection of adenovirus antigen in routine conjunctival specimens. Ophthalmology 1989;96:1106.

46. Pavan-Langston DP, Dunkel EC. A rapid clinical diagnostic test for herpes simplex infectious keratitis. Am J Ophthalmol 1989; 107:675.

47. Limberg MB. A review of bacterial keratitis and bacterial conjunctivitis. Am J Ophthalmol 1991;112:2S.

48. Giglotti F, Williams WT, Hayden FG, et al. Etiology of acute conjunctivitis in children. J Pediatr 1981;98:531.

49. Weiss A, Brinser JH, Nazar-Stewart V. Acute conjunctivitis in childhood. J Pediatr 1993;122:10.

50. Ostler HB. Diseases of the external eye and adnexa. Baltimore: Williams & Wilkins, 1993;8:87.

51. Trotter S, Stenberg K, Von Rosen IA, Svanborg C. *Haemophilus influenzae* causing conjunctivitis in day-care children. Pediatr Infect Dis J 1991;10:578.

52. Erwin AL, Munford RS. Comparison of lipopolysaccharides from Brazilian purpuric fever isolates and conjunctivitis isolates of *Haemophilus influenzae biogroup aegyptius*. Brazilian Purpuric Fever Study Group. J Clin Microbiol 1989;27:762.

53. Londer L, Nelson DL. Orbital cellulitis due to *Haemophilus influenzae*. Arch Ophthalmol 1974;91:89.

54. Harrison CJ, Hedrick JA, Block SL, Gilchrist MJ. Relation of the outcome of conjunctivitis and the conjunctivitis-otitis syndrome to identifiable risk factors and oral microbial therapy. Pediatr Infect Dis J 1987;6:536.

55. Baum JL. Antibiotic use in ophthalmology. In: Tasman W, Jaeger EA, eds. Duane's clinical ophthalmology. Philadelphia: JB Lippincott, 1993;vol 4, 26:1–26.

56. Timewell RM, Rosenthal AL, Smith JP, et al. Safety and efficacy of tobramycin and gentamicin sulfate in the treatment of external ocular infection in children. J Pediatr Ophthalmol Strabismus 1983;20:22–26.

57. Gigliotti F, Hendley O, Morgan J, et al. Efficacy of topical antibiotic therapy for acute conjunctivitis in children. J Pediatr 1984;104:623–626.

58. Baum J. Therapy for ocular bacterial infection. Trans Ophthalmol Soc UK 1986;105:69–77.

59. Nozik RA, Smolin G, Knowlton G, Austin R. Trimethoprim-polymyxin B ophthalmic solution in treatment of surface ocular bacterial infections. Ann Ophthalmol 1985;17:746.

60. Bodor FF. Systemic antibiotics for treatment of the conjunctivitis-otitis media syndrome. Pediatr Infect Dis J 1989;8:287.

61. Genvert GI, Cohen EJ, Donnenfeld ED, et al. Erythema multiforme after use of topical sulfacetamide. Am J Ophthalmol 1985; 99:465.

62. Fraunfelder FT, Bagby GC, Kelly DJ. Fatal aplastic anemia following topical administration of ophthalmic chloramphenicol. Am J Ophthalmol 1982;93:356.

63. The Trimethoprim-polymyxin B Sulphate Ophthalmic Ointment Study Group. Trimethoprim-polymyxin B sulphate ophthalmic ointment versus chloramphenicol ophthalmic ointment in the treatment of bacterial conjunctivitis – a review of four clinical studies. J Antimicro Chemo 1989;23:261.

64. Behrens-Bauman W, Quentin CD, Gibson TR, et al. Trimethoprim-polymyxin B sulphate ophthalmic ointment in the treatment of bacterial conjunctivitis: a double blind study versus chloramphenicol ophthalmic ointment. Cur Med Res Opin 1988;11:227.

65. Lohr JA, Austin RD, Grossman M, et al. Comparison of three topical antimicrobials for acute bacterial conjunctivitis. Pediatr Infect Dis J 1988;7:626.

66. Annable WI. Therapy for ocular infections. Pediatr Clin N Am 1983;30:389–396.

67. Ashley KC. The anti-bacterial activity of topical anti-infective eye preparations. Med Lab Sci 1986;43:157–162.

68. Awan KJ. Mydriasis and conjunctival paraesthesia from local gentamicin. Am J Ophthalmol 1985;99:723–724.

69. McGill JI. Bacterial conjunctivitis. Trans Ophthalmol Soc UK 1986;105:37–40.

70. Neu HC. Microbiologic aspects of fluoroquinolones. Am J Ophthalmol 1991;112:15S–24S.

71. Leibowitz HM. Clinical evaluation of ciprofloxacin 0.3% ophthalmic solution for treatment of bacterial keratitis. Am J Ophthalmol 1991;112:34S–47S.

72. Insler MS, Fish LA, Silbernagel J, et al. Successful treatment of methicillin-resistant *Staphylococcus aureus* keratitis with topical ciprofloxacin. Ophthalmology 1991;98:1690.

73. Reidy JJ, Hobden JA, Hill JM, et al. The efficacy of topical ciprofloxacin and norfloxacin in the treatment of experimental *Pseudomonas* keratitis. Cornea 1991;10:25.

74. Leibowitz HM. Antibacterial effectiveness of ciprofloxacin 0.3% ophthalmic solution in the treatment of bacterial conjunctivitis. Am J Ophthalmol 1991;112:29S–33S.

75. Kaatz GW, Seo SM. Mechanism of ciprofloxacin resistance in *Pseudomonas aeruginosa.* J Infect Dis 1988;158:537.

76. Trucksis M, Hooper DC, Wolfson JS. Emerging resistance to fluoroquinolones in staphylococci: an alert (editorial). Ann Intern Med 1991;114:424.

77. Cutarelli PE, Lass JH, Lazarus HM, et al. Topical fluoroquinolones: antimicrobial activity and in vitro corneal epithelial toxicity. Curr Eye Res 1991;10:557.

78. Heessen FW, Muytjens HL. In vitro activities of ciprofloxacin, norfloxacin, pipemidic acid, cinoxacin, and nalidixic acid against *Chlamydia trachomatis.* Antimicrob Agents Chemother 1984;25:123.

79. Huber-Spitzy V, Arocker-Mettinger E, Baumgartner I. Efficacy of norfloxacin in bacterial conjunctivitis. Euro J Ophthalmol 1991;1:69.

80. Miller IM, Wittreich J, Vogel R, Cook TJ. The safety and efficacy of topical norfloxacin compared with chloramphenicol for the treatment of external ocular bacterial infections. The norfloxacin-chloramphenicol ophthalmic study group. Eye 1992;6(pt1):111.

81. Jacobson JA, Call NB, Kasworm EM, et al. Safety and efficacy of topical norfloxacin versus tobramycin in the treatment of external ocular infections. Antimicrob Agents Chemother 1988;32:1820.

82. Miller IM, Vogel R, Cook TJ, Wittreich J. Topically administered norfloxacin compared with topically administered gentamicin for the treatment of external ocular bacterial infections. The Worldwide Norfloxacin Ophthalmic Study Group. Am J Ophthalmol 1992;113:638.

83. Miller IM, Wittreich J, Vogel R, Cook TJ. The safety and efficacy of topical norfloxacin compared with placebo in the treatment of acute, bacterial conjunctivitis. The Norfloxacin-placebo Ocular Study Group. Euro J Ophthalmol 1992;2:58.

84. Osato MS, Jensen HG, Trousdale MD, et al. The comparative in vitro activity of ofloxacin and selected antimicrobial agents against ocular bacterial isolates. Am J Ophthalmol 1989;108:380–386.

85. Gwon A. Topical ofloxacin compared with gentamicin in the treatment of external ocular infection. Ofloxacin Study Group. Br J Ophthalmol 1992;76:714–718.

86. Gwon A. Ofloxacin vs. tobramycin for the treatment of external ocular infection. Ofloxacin Study Group II. Arch Ophthalmol 1992;110:1234–1237.

87. Borrmann L, Tang-Liu DD, Kann J, et al. Ofloxacin in human serum, urine, and tear film after topical application. Cornea 1992;11:226–230.

88. Donnenfeld ED, Schrier A, Perry HD, et al. Penetration of topically applied ciprofloxacin, norfloxacin, and ofloxacin into the anterior chamber. Ophthalmology 1994;101:902–905.

89. Ross J, Abate MA. Topical vancomycin for the treatment of *Staphylococcus epidermidis* and methicillin resistant *Staphylococcus aureus* conjunctivitis. DICP 1990;24:1050.

90. Limberg MB. A review of bacterial keratitis and bacterial conjunctivitis. Am J Ophthalmol 1991;112:2S–9S.

91. Wan WL, Farkas GC, May WN, et al. The clinical characteristics and course of adult gonococcal conjunctivitis. Am J Ophthalmol 1986;102:575–583.

92. Lewis LS, Glauser TA, Joffe MD. Gonococcal conjunctivitis in prepubertal children. Am J Dis Child 1990;144:546–548.

93. Ullman S, Roussel TJ, Forster RK. Gonococcal keratoconjunctivitis. Surv Ophthalmol 1987;32:199.

94. Moraga FA, Domingo P, Barquet N. et al. Invasive meningococcal conjunctivitis. JAMA 1990;264:333.

95. Barquet N, Gasser I, Domingo P, et al. Primary meningococcal conjunctivitis: report of 21 patients and review. J Infect Dis 1990;12:838–847.

96. Foulks GN. Bacterial infections of the conjunctiva and cornea. In: Albert DM, Jakobiec FA, eds. Principles and practice of ophthalmology. Philadelphia: Saunders, 1994;(1)7:164.

97. Haimovici R, Roussel TJ. Treatment of gonococcal conjunctivitis with single-dose intramuscular ceftriaxone. Am J Ophthalmol 1989;107:511–514.

98. Mannis MJ. Bacterial conjunctivitis. In: Tasman W, Jaeger EA, eds. Duane's clinical ophthalmology. Philadelphia: JB Lippincott, 1993;vol 4, 5:1–7.

99. Foulks GN. Bacterial infections of the conjunctiva and cornea. In: Albert DM, Jakobiec FA, eds. Principles and practice of ophthalmology. Philadelphia: Saunders, 1994;(1)7:165–166.

100. Fedukowitz HB, Stenson S. External infections of the eye. 3 ed. Norwalk CT: Appleton-Century-Crofts, 1985:150.

101. Kivela T, Tervo K, Ravila E, et al. Pseudomembranous and membranous conjunctivitis: Immunohistochemical features. Acta Ophthalmol 1992;70:534–542.

102. Knopf HL, Hierholzer JC. Clinical and immunologic responses in patients with viral keratoconjunctivitis. Am J Ophthalmol 1975;80:661–672.

103. Laibson PR, Dhiri S, Oncover J. Corneal infiltrates in epidemic keratoconjunctivits. Arch Ophthalmol 1970;84:36–40.

104. Darougar S, Hunter PA, Viwalingam M, et al. Acute follicular conjunctivitis due to herpes simplex virus in London. Br J Ophthalmol 1978;62:843–849.

105. Ward JB, Siojo LG, Waller SG. A prospective clinical trial of trifluridine, dexamethasone, and artificial tears in the treatment of epidemic keratoconjunctivitis. Cornea 1993;12:216–221.

106. Lennette DA, Eiferman RA. Inhibition of adenoviral replication in vitro by trifluridine. Arch Ophthalmol 1978;96:1662–1663.

107. Adams CP Jr, Cohen EJ, Albrecht J, Laibson PR. Interferon treatment of adenoviral conjunctivitis. Am J Ophthalmol 1984;98:429–432.

108. Dawson C, Hanna L, Wood TR, et al. Adenovirus type 8 keratoconjunctivitis in the United States. Epidemic, clinical and microbiologic features. Am J Ophthalmol 1970;69:473–480.

109. Primary Care and Ocular Disease Committee, American Optometric Association. Infection control guidelines for the optometric practice. J Am Optom Assoc 1993;64:853–861.

110. Gordon YC, Gordon RY, Romanowski EG, Araullo-Cruz T. Pro-

longed recoverability of desiccated adenoviral serotypes 5, 8, and 19 from plastic and metal surfaces in vitro. Ophthalmology 1993; 100:1835–1839.

111. Smith J, et al. Incidence of herpes virus H antibody in the population. J Hygiene 1967;65:365.

112. Darrell RW. Ocular infections caused by the herpes virus group. In: Locatcher-Khorato D, Seegal BC, eds. Microbiology of the eye. St. Louis: Mosby-Year Book, 1972:302–312.

113. Hanna L, Ostler HB, Keshishyan BA, et al. Observed relationship between herpetic lesions and antigenic type. Surv Ophthalmol 1976;21:110–114.

114. Arffa RC. Grayson's diseases of the cornea. 3 ed. St. Louis: Mosby-Year Book. 1991:242.

115. Nahias AJ, Starr SE. Infections caused by herpes simplex viruses. In: Hoeprich PD, ed. Infectious diseases. Hagerstown, MD: Harper & Row, 1977;2:727.

116. Simon JW, Longo F, Smith RS. Spontaneous resolution of herpes simplex blepharoconjunctivitis in children. Am J Ophthalmol 1986;102:598–600.

117. Ostler MB. Management of ocular herpes virus infection. Surv Ophthalmol 1976;21:136–140.

118. Lass JH, Thoft RA, Dohlman CH. Idoxuridine-induced conjunctival cicatrization. Arch Ophthalmol 1983;101:747–750.

119. Rogers RS, Tindal JP. Geriatric herpes zoster. J Am Geriat Soc 1971;19:495.

120. Sandor EV, Millman A, Croxson TS, et al. Herpes zoster ophthalmicus in patients at risk for the aquired immune deficiency syndrome (AIDS). Am J Ophthalmol 1986;101:153–155.

121. Strommen GL, Pucino F, Tight RR, et al. Human infection with herpes zoster: etiology, pathophysiology, diagnosis, clinical course, and treatment. Pharmacother 1988;8:52–68.

122. Marsh RJ, Dudley B, Kelly V. External ocular motor paresis in ophthalmic zoster: a review. Br J Ophthalmol 1977;61:677–682.

123. Cobo LM, Foulks GN, Liesegang T, et al. Oral acyclovir in the treatment of acute herpes zoster ophthalmicus. Ophthalmology 1986;93:763–770.

124. Hoang-Xuang T, Buchi ER, Herbort CP, et al. Oral acyclovir for herpes zoster ophthalmicus. Ophthalmology 1992;99:1062–1072.

125. Bowsher D. Acute herpes zoster and post-herpetic neuralgia: Effects of acyclovir and outcome of treatment with amitriptyline. Br J Gen Prac 1992;42:244–246.

126. Harding SP, Lipton JR, Wells JCD. Natural history of herpes zoster ophthalmicus: predictors of postherpetic neuralgia and ocular involvement. Br J Ophthalmol 1987;71:353–358.

127. Chatterjee S, Quarcoopome CO, Apenteng A. Unusual type of epidemic conjunctivitis in Ghana. Br J Ophthalmol 1970;54:628–630.

128. Babalol OE, Amoni SS, Samaila E, et al. An outbreak of acute haemorrhagic conjunctivitis in Kaduna, Nigeria. Br J Ophthalmol 1990;74:89–92.

129. Hung T. Central nervous system complications of enterovirus type 70 infections: Epidemiologic and clinical features. In: Uchida Y, Ishii K, et al, eds. Acute hemorrhagic conjunctivitis. Japan. University of Toyko Press. 1989;235–250.

130. Kowalski RP, Harwick JC. Incidence of *Moraxella* conjunctival infection. Am J Ophthalmol 1986;101:437–440.

131. Schwartz B, Harrison LH, Motter JS, et al. Investigation of an outbreak of *Moraxella* conjunctivitis at a native American boarding school. Am J Ophthalmol 1989;107:341–347.

132. Thygeson D, Dawson CR. Trachoma and follicular conjunctivitis in children. Arch Ophthalmol 1966;75:3–12.

133. Dawson CR, Sheppard JD. Follicular conjunctivitis. In: Tasman W, Jaeger EA, eds. Duane's clinical ophthalmology. Philadelphia: JB Lippincott 1993;vol 4;Chap. 7:20.

134. Flach AJ, Lavoie MD. Episcleritis, conjunctivitis and keratitis as ocular manifestations of Lyme disease. Ophthalmology 1990;97: 973–975.

135. Mombaerts IM, Maudgal PC, Knockaert DC. Bilateral follicular conjunctivitis as a manifestation of Lyme disease. Am J Ophthalmol 1991;98:96–97.

136. Cameron DJ. Treatment of early Lyme disease. Am J Med 1993; 94:553.

137. Chin GN, Hyndiuk RA. Parinaud's oculoglandular conjunctivitis. In: Tasman W, Jaeger EA, eds. Duane's clinical ophthalmology. Philadelphia. JB Lippincott Co, 1993;vol 4;4:1.

138. Judson FN. Assessing the number of genital chlamydial infections in the United States. J Reprod Med 1985;30:269.

139. Rapoza PA, et al. A systematic approach to the diagnosis and treatment of chronic conjunctivitis. Am J Ophthalmol 1990;109: 138–142.

140. Darougar S, et al. Rapid serologic test for the diagnosis of chlamydia ocular infections. Br J Ophthalmol 1978;62:503–508.

141. Sheppard JD, Kowalski RP, Meyer MP, et al. Immunodiagnosis of *Chlamydia* conjunctivitis. Ophthalmology 1988;95:434–442.

142. Viswalingam ND, Daroughar S, Yearsley P. Oral doxycyline in the treatment of adult chlamydial ophthalmia. Br J Ophthalmol 1986; 70:301–304.

143. Smolin G. The cornea. 3 ed. Boston: Little Brown & Co. 1994: 292.

144. Stamm WE. Azithromycin in the treatment of uncomplicated genital chlamydial infections. Am J Med 1991;91:19S–22S.

145. Fedukowitz HB, Stenson S. External infections of the eye. 3 ed. Norwalk, CT: Appleton-Century-Crofts. 1985:83.

146. MacCallan A. The epidemiology of trachoma. Br J Ophthalmol 1931;15:369.

147. Thylefors B, Dawson CR, Jones BR, et. al. A simple system for the assessment of trachoma and its complications. Bull World Health Organ 1987;65:477–483.

148. Sandstorm KI, Bell TA, Chandler JW, et al. Microbial causes of neonatal conjunctivitis. J Pediatr 1984;105:706–711.

149. Crede CSF. Die verhutung der augenentzundung der neugeborenen, Arch Gynak 1881;21:179.

150. Greenberg M, Vandow JE. Ophthalmia neonatorum: Evaluation of different methods of prophylaxis in New York City. Am J Pub Health 1961;51:836–845.

151. Lockie P, Leong LK, Louis A. Penicillinase-producing *Neisseria gonorrhoeae* as a cause of neonatal and adult ophthalmia. Aust NZ J Ophthalmol 1986;14:49–53.

152. Haimovici R, Rousell TJ. Treatment of gonococcal conjunctivitis with single dose intramuscular ceftriaxone. Am J Ophthalmol 1989;107:511–514.

153. Centers for Disease Control and Prevention. 1993 Sexually transmitted diseases treatment guidelines. MMWR 1993;42(RR14): 61–67.

154. Lepage P, et al. Single-dose cefotaxime intramuscularly cures gonococcal ophthalmia neonatorum Br J Ophthalmol 1988;72: 518–520.

155. Chandler JW, Alexander, ER, Pheiffer TA, et al. Ophthalmia

neonatorum associated with maternal *Chlamydia* infections. Ophthalmology 1977;83:302–308.

156. Beam MO, Saxon EM. Respiratory tract colonization and a distinctive pneumonia syndrome in infants infected with *Chlamydia trachomatis*. N Engl J Med 1977;296:306–310.

157. Harrison JR, Phil D, English MG, et al. *Chlamydia trachomatis* infant pneumonitis. N Engl J Med 1978;298:702–708.

158. Centers for Disease Control and Prevention. 1993 Sexually transmitted diseases treatment guidelines. MMWR 1993;42(RR14):54.

159. Brook I, Barrett C, Brinkman III C, et al. Aerobic and anaerobic bacterial flora of the maternal cervix and newborn gastric fluid and conjunctiva. Pediatr 1979;63:451–455.

160. Bezirtzoglou E, Romond C. Nosocomial infections of ocular conjunctiva in newborns delivered by cesarian section. Ophthalmic Res 1991;23:79–83.

161. Isenberg SJ, Apt L, Yoshimori R, et al. Source of the conjunctival bacterial flora at birth and implications for ophthalmia neonatorum prophylaxis. Am J Ophthalmol 1988;106:458–462.

162. Burns RP, Rhodes DH. *Pseudomonas* eye infection as a cause of death in premature infants. Arch Ophthalmol 1961;65:517–520.

163. Arffa RC. Grayson's diseases of the cornea. 3 ed. St. Louis: Mosby-Year Book, 1991:118.

164. Nahmias AJ, Visitine AM, Caldwell DR, et al. Eye infections with herpes simplex viruses in neonates. Surv Ophthalmol 1976;21:100–105.

165. Rotkis WM, Chandler JW. Neonatal conjunctivitis. In: Tasman W, Jaeger EA, eds. Duane's clinical ophthalmology. Philadelphia: JB Lippincott, 1993;(4)6:6.

166. Zanoni D, Isenberg SJ, Apt L. A comparison of silver nitrate with erythromycin for prophylaxis against ophthalmia neonatorum. Clin Pediatr 1992;31:295–298.

167. Hammerschlag MR, Cummings C, Roblin PM, et al. Efficacy of neonatal ocular prophylaxis for the prevention of chlamydial and gonococcal conjunctivitis. N Engl J Med 1989;320:769–772.

168. Black-Payne C, Bocchini JA, Cedotal C. Failure of erythromycin ointment for post-natal ocular prophylaxis of chlamydia conjunctivitis. Pediatr Infect Dis J 1989;8:491–495.

169. Jenkins MS, Brown SI, Lempert SL, Weinberg NJ. Ocular rosacea. Am J Ophthalmol 1979;97:622.

170. Huber-Spitzy V, Baumgartner I, Bohler-Sommeregger K, Grabner G. Blepharitis—a diagnostic and therapeutic challenge. A report on 407 consecutive cases. Graefe's Arch Clin Exp Ophthalmol 1991;229:224–227.

171. Friedlander MH. Allergy and immunology of the eye. Hagerstown, MD: Harper & Row, 1979;3:76–79.

172. Brown SI, Shahinian J, Jr. Diagnosis and treatment of ocular rosacea. Ophthalmology 1978;85:779–786.

173. Ersurum SA, Feder RS, Greenwald MJ. Acne rosacea with keratitis in childhood. Arch Ophthalmol 1993;111:228–230.

174. Patrinely JR, Font RL, Anderson RL. Granulomatous acne rosacea of the eyelids. Arch Ophthalmol 1990;108:561–563.

175. Koo E, Balogh Z, Gomor B. Juvenile psoriatic arthritis. Clin Rheumatol 1991;10:245–249.

176. Shupack JL, Stiller MJ, Haber RS. Psoriasis and Reiter's syndrome. Clin Dermatol 1991;9:53–58.

177. Brancato L, Itescu S, Skovron ML, et al. Aspects of the spectrum, prevalence and disease susceptibility determinants of Reiter's syndrome and related disorders associated with HIV infection. Rheumatol Internat 1989;9(3–5):137–141.

178. Reveille JD, Conant MA, Duvic M. Human immunodeficiency

179. Tuft SJ, Ramkrishnan M, Seal DV, et al. Role of *Staphylococcus aureus* in chronic allergic conjunctivitis. Ophthalmology 1992;99:180–184.

180. Hanifin JM. Recognizing and managing clinical problems in atopic dermatitis. Allergy Proceed 1989;10:397–402.

181. Frucht-Pery J, Chayet AS, Feldman ST, et al. The effect of doxycycline on ocular rosacea. Am J Ophthalmol 1989;107:434–435.

182. Halioua B, Saurat JH. Risk: benefit ratio in the treatment of psoriasis with systemic retinoids. Br J Dermatol 1990;122(suppl 36):135–150.

183. Belz J, Breneman DL, Nordlund JJ, Solinger A. Successful treatment of a patient with Reiter's syndrome and acquired immunodeficiency syndrome using etretinate. J Am Acad Dermatol 1989;20(5 Pt 2):898–903.

184. Wolff K. Side effects of psoralen photochemotherapy. Br J Dermatol 1990;122(suppl 36):117–125.

185. Iijima Y, Wagai K, Matsuura Y, et al. Retinal detachment with breaks in the pars plicata of the ciliary body. Am J Ophthalmol 1989;108:349–355.

186. Mondino BJ, Brown SI, Lempert S, Jenkins MS. Acute manifestations of ocular cicatricial pemphigoid: diagnosis and treatment. Ophthalmology 1979;89:543–552.

187. Chan LS, Yancev KB, Hammerberg C et al. Immune-mediated subepithelial blistering diseases of mucous membranes. Arch Dermatol 1993;129:448–455.

188. Hoang-Xuan T, Foster CS, Raizman MB, Greenwood B. Mast cells in conjunctiva affected by cicatricial pemphigoid. Ophthalmology 1989;96:1110–1114.

189. Sacks EH, Jakobiec FA, Wieczorek R, et al. Immunophenotypic analysis of the inflammatory infiltrate in ocular cicatricial pemphigoid. Further evidence for a T cell-mediated disease. Ophthalmology 1989;96:236–243.

190. Roat MI, Sossi G, Lo CY, Thoft RA. Hyperproliferation of conjunctival fibroblasts from patients with cicatricial pemphigoid. Arch Ophthalmol 1989;107:1064–1067.

191. Mondino BJ. Cicatricial pemphigoid and erythema multiforme. Ophthalmology 1990;97:939–952.

192. Brook U, Singer L, Fried D. Development of severe Stevens-Johnson syndrome after administration of slow-release theophylline. Pediatr Dermatol 1989;6:126–129.

193. Wolfley DE. Trichiasis preceding conjunctival changes in cicatricial pemphigoid. Cornea 1992;11:272–273.

194. Vandeveer MR. Ocular cicatricial pemphigoid. J Am Optom Assoc 1991;62:166–169.

195. Francis IC, McCluskey PJ, Walls RS, et al. Ocular cicatricial pemphigoid. Aust NZ J Ophthalmol 1990;18:43–50.

196. Mondino BJ. Cicatricial pemphigoid and erythema multiforme. Ophthalmology 1990;97:939–952.

197. Wilkins J, Morrison L, White CR Jr. Oculocutaneous manifestations of the erythema multiforme/Stevens-Johnson syndrome/toxic epidermal necrolysis spectrum. Dermatol Clin 1992;10:571–582.

198. Kivela T, Tervo K, Ravilla E, et al. Pseudomembranes and membranous conjunctivitis. Acta Ophthalmol 1992;70:534–542.

199. Belfort R Jr, de Smet M, Whitcup SM, et al. Ocular complications

of Stevens-Johnson syndrome and toxic epidermal necrolysis in patients with AIDS. Cornea 1991;10:536–538.

200. Auran JD, Hornblass A, Gross ND. Stevens-Johnson syndrome with associated nasolacrimal duct obstruction treated with dacryocystorhinostomy and Crawford silicone tube insertion. J Ophthalmic Plast Reconstruc Surg 1990;6:60–63.

201. Foster CS, Neumann R, Tauber J. Long-term results of systemic chemotherapy for ocular cicatricial pemphigoid. Doc Ophthalmol 1992;82:223–229.

202. Fern AI, Jay JL, Young H, et al. Dapsone therapy for the acute inflammatory phase of ocular pemphigoid. Br J Ophthalmol 1992; 76:332–335.

203. Tauber J, Sainz de la Maza M, Foster CS. Systemic chemotherapy for cicatricial pemphigoid. Cornea 1991;10:185–195.

204. Shore JW, Foster CS, Westfall CT, Rubin PA. Results of buccal mucosal grafting for patients with medically controlled ocular cicatricial pemphigoid. Ophthalmology 1992;99:383–395.

205. Bialasiewicz AA. Nasal mucosa grafting in ocular pemphigoid. Ophthalmology 1991;98:273.

206. Jones LT, Wolig JL. Surgery of the eyelids and lacrimal system. Birmingham, AL: Aesculapus, 1976;123–131.

207. Dubois EL, Tuffanelli DL. The natural history of systemic lupus erythematosus by prospective analysis. Medicine 1971;50:85.

208. Harvey AM, Shulman LE, Tumulty A, et al. Systemic lupus erythematosus: Review of the literature and clinical analysis of 138 cases. Medicine 1954;33:291.

209. Churg J, Strauss L. Allergic granulomatosis, allergic angiitis, and periarteritis nodosa. Am J Pathol 1951;27:277.

210. Fink CW. Polyarteritis and other diseases with necrotizing vasculitis in children. Arth Rheumatol 1977;20(suppl):378.

211. Rose GA. The natural history of polyarteritis. Br Med J 1957;2: 1148.

212. Barnett EV, et al. Nuclear antigens and antinuclear antibodies in mink sera. Arth Rheumatol 1968;11:92.

213. Keat A, Rowe I. Reiter's syndrome and associated arthritides. Rheumatic Dis Clin N Am 1991;19:25–42.

214. Cope A, Anderson J, Wilkins E. *Clostridium* difficile toxin-induced arthritis in a patient with chronic Reiter's syndrome. Euro J Clin Microbiol Infect Dis 1992;11:40–43.

215. Rahman MU, Husdon AP, Schumacher HR Jr. *Chlamydia* and Reiter's syndrome. Rheumatic Dis Clin N Am 1992;18:67–79.

216. Smith RJ. Evidence for *Chlamydia trachomatis* and *Ureaplasma urealyticum* in a patient with Reiter's disease. J Adoles Health Care 1989;10:155–159.

217. Rahman MU, Cantwell R, Johnson CC, et al. Inapparent genital infection with *Chlamydia trachomatis* and its potential role in the genesis of Reiter's syndrome. DNA Cell Biol 1992;11:215–219.

218. Hermann Em Mayet WJ, Thomssen H, Sieper J, et al. HLA-DP restricted *Chlamydia trachomatis* specific synovial fluid T cell clones in *Chlamydia* induced Reiter's disease. J Rheumatol 1992; 19:1243–1246.

219. Fuente C, Velez A, Martin N, et al. Reiter's syndrome and human immunodeficiency virus infection: case report and review of the literature. Cutis 1991;47:181–185.

220. Brancato L, Itescu S, Skovron ML, et al. Aspects of the spectrum, prevalence and disease susceptibility determinants of Reiter's syndrome and related disorders associated with HIV infection. Rheumatol Internat 1989;9:137–141.

221. Clark MR, Solinger AM, Hochberg MC. Human immunodeficiency virus infection is not associated with Reiter's syndrome.

222. Lealhey AB, Connor TB, Gottsch JD. Chemosis as a presenting sign of systemic lupus erythematosus. Arch Ophthalmol 1992; 110:609–610.

223. Frith P, Burge SM, Millard PR, et al. External ocular findings in lupus erythematosus:a clinical and immunopathological study. Br J Ophthalmol 1990;74:163–167.

224. Drosis AA, Petris CA, Petroutsos GM, Moutsopoulos HM. Unusual eye manifestations in systemic lupus erythematosus patients. Clin Rheumatol 1989;8:49–53.

225. Rafus PE, Canny CL. Initial identification of antinuclear-antibody negative systemic lupus erythematosus on ophthalmic examination: a case report, with a discussion of the ocular significance of anticardiolipin (antiphospholipid) antibodies. Can J Ophthalmol 1992;27:189–193.

226. Fitzpatrick EP, Chesen N, Rahn EK. The lupus anticoagulant and retinal vaso-occlusive disease. Ann Ophthalmol 1990;22:148–152.

227. Frohnert PP, Sheps SG. Long term follow-up study of polyarteritis nodosa. Am J Med 1967;43:8–14.

228. Mielants H, Veys EM. Clinical and radiographic features of Reiter's syndrome and inflammatory bowel disease related to arthritis. Curr Opin Rheumatol 1990;2:570–576.

229. Sharp JT. Reiter's syndrome. In: Hollander JL, McCarty DJ Jr. Arthritis and allied conditions. 8 ed. Philadelphia: Lea & Feiger, 1972.

230. Anderson CJ, Gregory MC, Groggel GC, Clegg DO. Amyloidosis and Reiter's syndrome:report of a case and review of the literature. Am J Kidney Dis 1989;14:319–323.

231. Misukiewicz P, Carlson RW, Rowan L, et al. Acute aortic insufficiency in a patient with presumed Reiter's syndrome. Ann Rheumatic Dis 1992;51:686–687.

232. Schwimmbeck PL, Oldstone MB. *Klebsiella* pneumoniae and HLA B27–associated diseases of Reiter's syndrome and anklyosing spondylitis. Curr Topics Microbiol Immunol 1989;145:45–56.

233. Calin A. Reiter's syndrome. Med Clin Am 1977;61:365–376.

234. Lieb ES, Restivo C, Paulus HE. Immunosuppressive and corticosteroid therapy of polyarteritis nodosa. Am J Med 1979;67:941–947.

235. Schien PS, Winokur SH. Immunosuppressive and cytotoxic chemotherapy long term complications. Ann Intern Med 1975;82: 84–95.

236. Wright P. Superior limbic keratoconjunctivitis. Trans Ophthalmol Soc UK 1972;92:555–560.

237. Confino J, Brown SI. Treatment of superior limbic keratoconjunctivitis with topical sodium cromolyn. Ann Ophthalmol 1987;19: 124–131.

238. Mondino BJ. Use of pressure patching and soft contact lenses in superior limbic keratoconjunctivitis. Arch Ophthalmol 1982;100: 1932–1934.

239. Donshik PC, et al. Conjunctival resection treatment and ultrastructural histopathology of superior limbic keratoconjunctivitis. Am J Ophthalmol 1978;85:101–110.

240. Bahrassa F, Datta R. Post-operative beta radiation treatment of pterygium. Int J Rad Oncol Bio Phys 1983;9:679–684.

241. Kleis W, Guillermo P. Thio-peta therapy to prevent post-operative pterygium occurrence and neovascularization. Am J Ophthalmol 1973;76:371–373.

242. Monestam E, Bjornstig U. Eye injuries in northern Sweden. Acta Ophthalmol 1991;69:1–5.

243. Ostler HB. Diseases of the external eye and adnexa. Baltimore: Williams & Wilkins, 1993;4:194.

244. Casser-Locke L. Conjunctival abrasions and lacerations. J Am Optom Assoc 1987;58:488.

245. Yao Y, Inoue Y, Shimomura Y, et al. Primary herpes simplex virus infection with geographic conjunctival ulceration. Am J Ophthalmol 1994;118:670–671.

246. Golnik KC, Marotto ME, Fanous MM, et al. Ophthalmic manifestations of *Rochalimaea* species. Am J Ophthalmol 1994;118:145–151.

247. Frucht-Pery J, Ilsar M, Hemo I. Single dosage of mitomycin C for prevention of recurrent pterygium: preliminary report. Cornea 1994;13:411–413.

248. Mastropasqua L, Carpineto P, Ciancaglini M, et al. Effectiveness of intraoperative mitomycin C in the treatment of recurrent pterygium. Ophthalmologica 1994;208:247–249.

249. Frucht-Pery J, Ilsar M. The use of low-dose mitomycin C for prevention of recurrent pterygium. Ophthalmology 1994;101:759–762.

CHAPTER 27

Diseases of the Cornea

Linda Casser
Nada J. Lingel

As the transparent, richly innervated convexity forming the anterior-most surface of the globe, the cornea is the eye's primary refracting surface.[1] As a result of these characteristics, diseases and disorders of the cornea can result in symptomatology that generally prompts the patient to seek care: loss of vision, pain, and photophobia.[2] Both the prevalence and potential severity of corneal conditions motivate the eye care provider to be fully versed in the diagnosis, treatment and management of corneal diseases and disorders.

This chapter provides practical information regarding common corneal conditions that require therapeutic treatment and management. By nature of its anatomic proximity to and integration with other ocular and adnexal structures, corneal abnormalities may result from diseases primary to the eyelids, conjunctiva, lacrimal system, episclera, and other tissues, such as sclera. These secondary corneal accompaniments are not emphasized in this chapter, and the reader should refer to other appropriate chapters for this information.

Clinical Anatomy and Physiology

The Normal Corneal State

Histologic cross section of the cornea reveals five identifiable layers: the epithelium, Bowman's membrane or layer, the stroma, Descemet's membrane, and the endothelium.[2] Fluid surrounds the cornea in the forms of the tear film in front and the aqueous behind. The various corneal layers combine to form a structure that is approximately 0.65 mm thick at the periphery and 0.52 mm thick centrally.[3]

The epithelium is stratified, being composed of five layers of interconnected squamous cells of various sizes and shapes. The deepest layer of cells, known as the basal cell layer, adheres to a basement membrane and serves as the germinal layer for new cells that are gradually pushed into the more superficial layers. An intact corneal epithelium helps to protect the cornea from most potential pathogenic organisms.[4]

Bowman's membrane or layer (anterior limiting membrane) is a thin homogeneous sheet of acellular, irregularly arrayed, fine caliber collagen fibers lying between the epithelial basement membrane and the stroma.[5] Bowman's membrane is a relatively tough layer of the cornea that provides substantial resistance to injury or infection. Since it cannot regenerate, unlike other corneal layers, scarring results when it is disrupted.

The stroma is a modified connective tissue comprising approximately 60 alternating fibrous lamellae, the planes of which are parallel to the corneal surface.[6] Adjacent lamellae are oriented at right angles to each other, and each is composed of very fine transparent fibers. It is the regularity of the stromal tissue array that contributes to corneal transparency, in contrast to the opaque and less regularly arranged fibers of the sclera. Occasionally, cells are noted histologically in the stroma. These cells include keratocytes, which are involved in collagen synthesis in wound healing, polymorphonuclear leukocytes, plasma cells, and histiocytes.[3,7] Disruption of the stromal layer results in scar formation.

Descemet's membrane (posterior limiting membrane) is easily differentiated from the corneal stroma. It is a strong homogeneous and very resistant membrane consisting of very fine collagen fibers in a regular array.[5] Descemet's membrane will regenerate if damaged. The endothelium consists of a single layer of interlocking epithelial-like cells. The abundance of cellular organelles occurring within the endothelial cells is consistent with the high level of metabolic activity provided by these cells as they actively transport aqueous fluid out of the cornea. Maintenance of relative corneal dehydration also is achieved by the barrier functions of the epithelium and endothelium against the influx of tears and aqueous, respectively.[8]

The transition of the cornea to its surrounding structures occurs at the limbus, defined as a "border" between two tissue types.[9] Here the corneal epithelium is continuous with the conjunctival epithelium. Bowman's membrane ends abruptly at the limbus, and the fibers of the corneal stroma are continuous with the fibers of the sclera. Descemet's membrane terminates at Schwalbe's ring. The corneal endothelium is continuous around the anterior chamber angle, then joins with cells on the front of the iris. The limbal area contains several melanin cells that may be highly pigmented in certain patients. A palisade cellular appearance at the limbus is common (palisades of Vogt).[3]

The cornea is normally avascular, with conjunctival vascular loops ending in the limbal area.[6] Nourishment to the cornea is provided by lymphatic permeation through the inter-lamellae spaces from the limbal vessels, as well as nutrients from the aqueous and tears.[2] The flow and diffusion of substances across the "physiologic" limbus is important to the normal physiology and pathophysiology of the eye and cornea.[10] The anterior ciliary nerves, branches of the fifth cranial nerve, pierce the sclera a short distance behind the limbus, combine to form pericorneal plexuses, and enter the cornea as 60 to 80 radially oriented myelinated trunks. After transversing the cornea for approximately 2 mm to 4 mm, the nerves lose their myelin sheaths and divide into anterior and posterior groups. The anterior group forms a plexus in Bowman's membrane and an intraepithelial plexus, terminating in the epithelium without a specific end organ, which would reduce corneal transparency. The posterior nerve group passes through the posterior cornea, although there are no nerves in Descemet's membrane or the endothelium.[3]

Using a parallelepiped with the slit-lamp biomicroscope, the anterior surface of the cornea is normally very smooth and covered by the precorneal tear layer. It is difficult to distinguish clinically between the epithelial layer and Bowman's membrane. The stroma comprises about 90% of the depth of the cornea and appears as a milky, finely reticular structure.[11] Although it is not possible to distinguish clinically between Descemet's membrane and the endothelium, specular reflection illumination will reveal the mosaic appearance of the endothelium. The posterior surface of the cornea contrasts sharply with the start of the optically empty anterior chamber.[12]

Response of the Cornea to Insult

The various types of potential insult to the cornea (traumatic, inflammatory, infectious, etc.) result in a variety of tissue responses. Significant disruption to the regularity of the corneal surface or corneal transparency may result in reduced visual acuity.[13] Stimulation of the numerous corneal nerve endings through tissue disruption can result in pain, which can be severe even with small lesions. The exception to this is the relative hypoesthesia in conditions such as recurrent herpes simplex keratitis. The symptoms of pain and photophobia related to corneal lesions also are exacerbated by discomfort from iris and ciliary body spasm.[2] Corneal insult results in the intraocular release of prostaglandins and other chemical mediators. Prostaglandin-mediated miosis, breakdown of the blood-aqueous barrier, and vasodilation contribute to the development of anterior uveitis associated with corneal lesions.[14] Unusually severe traumatic anterior uveitis resulting from corneal trauma has occurred in association with occult ankylosing spondylitis.[15] The development of corneal edema can be relatively focal due to epithelial disruption, or it can be diffuse as a result of interference with the endothelial pump mechanism. Opaque infiltrates may appear as inflammatory cells enter the cornea from the limbal vasculature or the pre-corneal tear film in response to antigens, toxins or other irritants.[16]

The term *superficial punctate keratitis* (SPK) is commonly used to refer generally to superficial punctate corneal epithelial disruptions of multiple etiologies, despite the specific condition described by Thygeson (see page 712). Recently, authors have introduced the terms *punctate epithelial erosions* (PEE) and *punctate epithelial keratopathy* (PEK).[17] PEEs refer to fine corneal epithelial lesions, usually slightly depressed, that stain prominently with fluorescein sodium or rose bengal and are found in many primary and secondary corneal conditions. PEKs describe accumulations of epithelial cells that are surrounded by a focal inflammatory cell infiltrate, as often accompanies viral keratoconjunctivitis. Disruption of the corneal epithelium in any form increases the risk of corneal invasion by pathogens, with potentially devastating outcomes. As a result, when using prophylactic topical antibiotics to protect the healing cornea from secondary infection, broad-spectrum agents are selected with efficacy against both gram-positive and gram-negative organisms.

Depending on the nature and extent of corneal insult, healing may proceed uneventfully with no scar development, as in the case of purely epithelial lesions, or the healing process may result in significant disruption of the corneal regularity and transparency.[13] Individual corneal epithelial cells have an average life span of approximately one week.[18] Davanger and Evensen[19] believe that the corneal limbal palisade cells, coupled with the normal cell renewal activity of the basal layer of the epithelium, serve as generative tissue for corneal epithelial cells. Moreover, limbal basal epithelial cells likely serve as regenerative stem cells for corneal epithelial cell proliferation.[20] A high molecular weight plasma and extracellular matrix glycoprotein, fibronectin, is deposited following epithelial cell loss and serves as a transient matrix for attachment and migration of epithelial cells.[21,22] Clinical observations support the theory of centripetal movement of epithelial resurfacing from the corneal periphery, visualized as three to six convex leading fronts of centrally migrating epithelial sheets that eventually fuse.[23–26] In contrast, the healing of stromal lesions involves the formation of collagen fibrils as well as changes in the synthesis of corneal proteoglycans that lack the regular organization of normal stroma and are therefore less transparent.[27,28] Following inflammation or injury, blood vessels and cell-lined lymphatic vessels may invade the corneal tissue.[29] The mechanisms involved in corneal healing remain under continuous and intense study.[30–33]

Examination Considerations

Examination of the cornea is best performed using the slit-lamp biomicroscope. It is helpful to begin examination of the cornea using a 1-mm-wide parallelepiped illumination beam at moderate magnification (16×).[34] The parallelepiped technique results in a three-dimensional view of various corneal segments (Fig. 27.1). This initial view helps to avoid "passing over" often subtle corneal findings, particularly when small fixational shifts occur by the patient. It also is important to maintain a 60-degree angle between the slit-lamp illumination source and the eyepieces, so that the corneal parallelepiped is sufficiently separated optically from the reflection of the beam from the iris surface.

If a corneal lesion is detected using the parallelepiped, or if the clinician suspects variation from normal corneal thickness, then the beam should be narrowed to a two-dimensional optic section.[34] This procedure illuminates a "slice" through the cornea, which the examiner views laterally to examine the various corneal layers to localize the depth of an identified lesion or to assess relative corneal thickness. It is helpful to increase the slit-lamp magnification (25–40×) to assess effectively the optic section corneal view (Fig. 27.2).

The examiner incorporates specialty slit-lamp illumination techniques, as needed, to assess corneal abnormalities or normal variations.[35] By using the corneal endothelium as a convex reflecting surface, specular reflection illumination allows assessment of the regularity of the endothelium. Indirect illumination is particularly helpful in assessing refractile, non-opaque lesions. Retroillumination "back-lights" corneal lesions using light reflected off the iris when the pupil is undilated, or using the "red reflex" of light reflected from the retina when the pupil is dilated. The

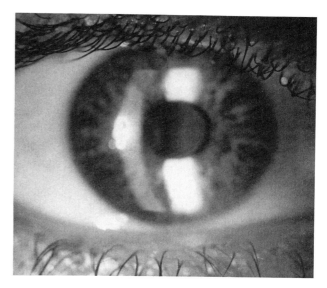

FIGURE 27.1 **The parallelepiped illumination technique results in a three-dimensional view of the cornea that is effective for detecting corneal lesions.**

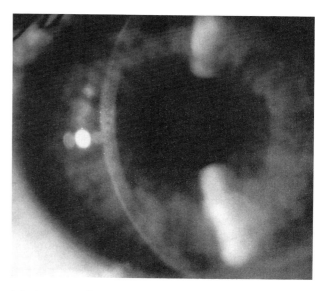

FIGURE 27.2 **The two-dimensional optic section view of the cornea allows examination of the various corneal layers, localization of the depth of an identified lesion, or assessment of relative corneal thickness.**

sclerotic scatter technique allows for gross assessment of corneal transparency.

The use of topical vital dye staining provides valuable diagnostic information in the assessment of the cornea (see

Chap. 17).[36] Areas of corneal epithelial loss, whether induced by mechanical, inflammatory, chemical, or other causes, will exhibit fluorescein sodium or fluorexon dye uptake ("positive" staining). Delineation of the size, shape and distribution of corneal epithelial disruption helps the examiner to diagnose its etiology. Conversely, areas of intact corneal epithelial elevation cause focal thinning in the precorneal tear film that, when stained with fluorescein sodium, produces black areas in the tear film fluorescence ("negative" staining). Corneal epithelial cells that are intact but lacking adequate protection from the tear film will take up rose bengal dye.

It is helpful to conduct a brief corneal evaluation following pupillary dilation using a 1-mm-wide parallelepiped beam. Full pupillary dilation provides a black background against which to view the three-dimensional corneal parallelepiped without the confounding iris structure that is present without dilation. With this enhanced view, the examiner has the opportunity to detect many subtle corneal lesions that might otherwise go undetected.[37]

Mechanical/Traumatic Conditions

Corneal Abrasion

ETIOLOGY

Corneal abrasions result from superficial traumatic "rub off" of the corneal epithelium. Corneal abrasions are common and are caused by a wide variety of etiologic agents—any object that may strike the patient's eye or facial area has the potential for causing a corneal abrasion. Some of the common causes include injuries from fingernails, tree branches, contact lens overwear or mishandling, mascara wands, and non-retained foreign bodies.[38] A recently reported cause of corneal and periorbital abrasions is the accident-activated automobile airbag.[39]

DIAGNOSIS

A patient with a corneal abrasion typically will report a history of a recent traumatic event, such as being struck by something flying into the eye or by a finger striking the eye. Patients with moderate- to large-sized corneal abrasions usually seek treatment within 24 hours of the injury because of the significance of their symptoms.

The severity of patient symptomatology associated with corneal abrasion tends to be proportional to the extent of the abrasion. Patients with very small corneal abrasions may experience only a mild "scratchiness" or foreign body sensation; patients with larger abrasions usually exhibit significant discomfort, including pain, reflex tearing and photophobia. Since the cornea is so richly innervated, even small corneal abrasions can cause significant pain, which

also is influenced by pain tolerance levels of the individual patient. Some lag time in the onset of pain associated with corneal abrasion is often encountered clinically, with the pain becoming most pronounced 4 to 6 hours following the traumatic event. In contrast, patients with reduced corneal sensitivity, such as may be associated with pre-existing corneal disease, long-term contact lens wear, or prior ocular surgery, may have minimal pain associated with even large abrasions. Thus, the timing of in-office patient presentation related to corneal abrasion can vary considerably.

During examination with the slit lamp, the size, shape, and location of corneal abrasions will vary widely based on the nature of the traumatic event. The use of fluorescein sodium staining will help to more fully delineate the area of corneal epithelial loss. Lesions may range from superficial foreign body tracking due to non-retained debris, to large areas of epithelial loss. Abrasions resulting from fingernail injuries or tree branches are often linear in shape (Fig. 27.3). If the lesion has been present for 24 hours or longer, the onset of corneal healing may affect the shape of the abrasion. During the examination and when considering the history of the traumatic episode, it is important to rule out possible corneal laceration or perforation, retained foreign bodies, or other ocular traumatic sequelae.[40] "Clean" corneal abrasions should not exhibit opaque infiltration suggestive of bacterial or fungal keratitis. Often patient symptomatology and pain-induced blepharospasm are severe enough to require instillation of a topical anesthetic to allow adequate examination.

Moderate to severe corneal abrasions usually are accompanied by several other ocular signs. Diffuse or focal conjunctival injection will be present, depending upon the size and location of the abrasion. Lid edema is common when profuse reflex lacrimation occurs. If the lesion has been present for at least 12 to 24 hours, a secondary traumatic anterior uveitis may result as indicated by an anterior chamber reaction (cells and flare), ciliary flush, and miosis (see Chap. 30).

MANAGEMENT

If particulate debris was a factor in the cause of the corneal abrasion, it is important to evert the lids and remove or irrigate debris from the eye. If a "flap" of displaced epithelium is present, it is helpful to debride this tissue to provide a "clean" leading edge for the start of corneal healing (Fig. 27.4).[41]

Small corneal abrasions with minimal associated symptomatology tend to heal quickly (24–36 hours). Topical prophylactic antibiotic therapy protects the disrupted corneal epithelium from secondary infection as the tissue heals. Broad-spectrum ophthalmic antibiotic drops may be prescribed during the day, such as 0.3% tobramycin or polymyxin B-trimethoprim instilled 3 to 4 times a day, along with a broad-spectrum antibiotic ointment instilled into the

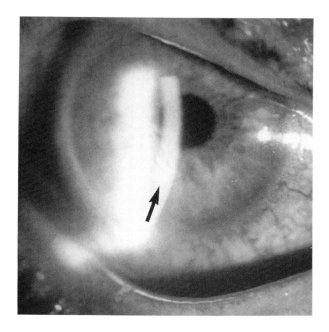

A

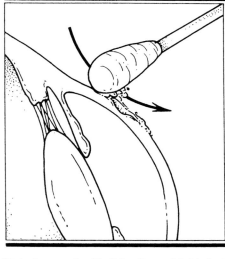

FIGURE 27.4   **Loosened epithelial cells are debrided using a cotton-tipped applicator. (Reprinted with permission from Fingeret M, Casser L, Woodcome HT. Corneal debridement. In: Atlas of primary eyecare procedures. Norwalk, CT: Appleton & Lange, 1990:160–161.)**

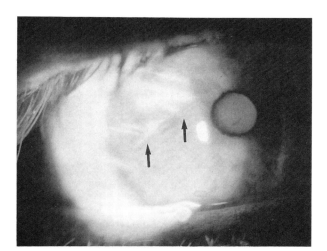

B

FIGURE 27.3   *(A)* **Example of a corneal abrasion (arrow) (Courtesy James L. Dixon, O.D.).** *(B)* **Multiple linear corneal abrasions (arrows) are shown stained with fluorescein sodium following injury from flying wood chips (courtesy William L. Jones, O.D.).**

conjunctival sac at bedtime, such as 0.3% tobramycin or polymyxin B-bacitracin. Discontinue prophylactic topical antibiotic therapy once the corneal epithelium is healed.

Moderate– to large–sized corneal abrasions are usually managed with pressure patching. The patch helps to control pain and promote epithelial healing by immobilizing the upper eyelid and applying mild pressure to the eye for 24 hours.

Prior to applying the pressure patch, the eye is dilated and cyclopleged to help control pain by reducing ciliary spasm and to help minimize a secondary anterior uveitis. Although epithelial loss due to the abrasion helps to enhance corneal penetration of the cycloplegic agent, the often pronounced ciliary spasm and inflammatory reaction may reduce the therapeutic effect of the cycloplegic. Clinical experience suggests that dilating the abraded eye with the traditional diagnostic agents of 0.5% to 1% tropicamide and 2.5% phenylephrine followed by instillation of a long-acting cycloplegic after 15 to 20 minutes results in pupillary dilation of quicker onset and one that tends to last for the duration of the pressure patch. Thus, once the pupil is fully dilated with the short-acting agents, add one to two drops 5% homatropine or 0.25% scopolamine prior to pressure patching. In patients with lightly pigmented irides and whose lesions are likely to heal in 24 hours, 5% homatropine is the agent of choice. In patients with darkly pigmented irides, who exhibit a significant anterior chamber reaction at the time of presentation, or whose abrasion may require several days to heal, 0.25% scopolamine may more effectively produce mydriasis and cycloplegia of longer duration. Since the mydriatic and cycloplegic agents cause some burning upon instillation, it is helpful to instill a topical anesthetic beforehand. Once the pupil is fully dilated, it is prudent to perform a dilated fundus

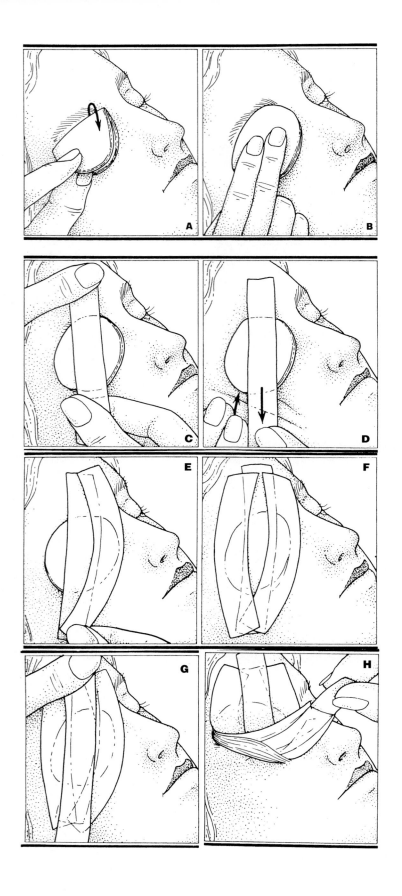

examination, particularly if a degree of contusion accompanied the abrasion or if a penetrating wound is suspected.

A pressure patch is applied following instillation into the conjunctival sac of a broad spectrum antibiotic ointment such as polymyxin B-bacitracin or 0.3% tobramycin (Fig. 27.5). The pressure of the patch should be sufficient to maintain lid closure but not so excessive as to cause discomfort. During the ensuing 24 hours when the patch is in place, patient comfort levels will be enhanced by reducing activity levels, using sunglasses, and taking over-the-counter analgesic agents, as required. In cases of extreme pain, opioid analgesics may be necessary (see Chap. 7). If it is anticipated that the lesion will heal substantially in 24 hours, the patient may be advised to remove the patch just prior to the follow-up appointment. In the instance of a large abrasion, however, the patch should be removed in-office.

At the 24-hour follow-up examination, the cornea is assessed with the slit lamp to determine the degree of healing. Patients may vary in their relative healing rates—younger patients tend to exhibit faster healing, older or diabetic patients tend to exhibit slower healing. With a moderate– to large–sized abrasion, particularly if the patch is removed in-office, the signs of corneal healing can be rather pronounced. Conjunctival injection is common and can be related to hypoxia induced by the patch. Several corneal changes that may accompany the healing abrasion are the formation of epithelial fusion lines that exhibit positive or negative staining, possibly including a pseudodendrite appearance; vortex-type changes of positive and negative staining as the sheets of resurfacing epithelium come together; filaments; epithelial (anterior) mosaic pattern, a cobblestone-shaped configuration of pressure lines in the epithelium related to the patch; edema, producing a "ground glass" appearance in the area of the resolving abrasion; transient pseudoguttata; and folds in Descemet's membrane related to edema, relative globe hypotony from any accompanying anterior uveitis, or mechanical pressure resulting from the patch (Table 27.1).[11,17,26,42] The development of corneal edema may be related to hypoxia or globe hypotony produced by tight pressure patches.[43]

The degree of corneal healing and anterior uveitis observed at the first follow-up visit will determine subsequent management.[40] Lesions that are not healed substantially should be treated the same as the initial abrasion—pupil dilation and cycloplegia, pressure patching, and follow-up in another 24 hours. If healing has progressed substantially and the patient is comfortable without the patch, discontinue the patch and use prophylactic topical antibiotics until the tissue

TABLE 27.1
Corneal Findings That May Accompany Healing Abrasions

Epithelial fusion lines
Pseudodendrites
Vortex changes
Filaments
Epithelial (anterior) mosaic
Edema
Pseudoguttata
Descemet folds

is completely healed. Pupil dilation and cycloplegia can be maintained to control the anterior chamber reaction, since resolution of the uveitis usually occurs in conjunction with the healing of the cornea. If significant corneal edema is present, supplement the prophylactic antibiotic therapy with hyperosmotic agents, such as 5% sodium chloride drops during the day and 5% sodium chloride ointment at bedtime. To enhance patient compliance, it is helpful to advise the patient that the hyperosmotic agents will cause some burning, particularly if the epithelium is still disrupted. The use of an antibiotic and/or hyperosmotic ointment instilled into the conjunctival sac at bedtime is particularly helpful to prevent re-irritation of the cornea upon awakening when the lids are opened. "Cut-like" abrasions that disrupt the epithelial basement membrane, such as caused by a fingernail, paper cut, etc., have a higher risk of resulting in recurrent corneal erosions.[44] Following resolution of the initial abrasion in these instances, the subtle signs of corneal healing should be monitored and the patient treated for at least 8 weeks with bland ophthalmic lubricating or hyperosmotic ointment instilled in the conjunctival sac at bedtime to prevent recurrent corneal erosion (see page 693).

Although the 24-hour pressure patch using eyepads and tape has been a widely used, clinically successful, and very acceptable technique for treating corneal abrasion, other treatment modalities are available and are becoming more commonly utilized. These include the Presspatch, collagen shields, and bandage contact lenses. The Presspatch (Precision Therapeutics) is a commercially available product with a plastic outer shell and a foam patch back that can be used for pressure patching.[38] The Presspatch is held in place with elastic bands secured with Velcro tabs. Use of the Presspatch can be helpful in instances when ointment re-instillation is needed, when the patient's facial hair precludes tape adhesion, or if the patient is allergic to the pressure patching tape. Abrasions caused by artificial fingernails may be contaminated by *Pseudomonas* from beneath the nail or in the nail fold, which may give a green to blue-gray discoloration of the nails (*Pseudomonas chromonychia*).[45] It has been suggested that abrasions caused by

FIGURE 27.5 **Traditional pressure patching procedures: *(A, B)* placement of eyepads; *(C–G)* positioning of tape; *(H)* removal of pressure patch. (Reprinted with permission from Fingeret M, Casser L, Woodcome HT. Pressure patching. In: Atlas of primary eyecare procedures. Norwalk, CT: Appleton & Lange, 1990:156–159.)**

artifical fingernails be treated similar to contact lens-induced abrasions and that traditional pressure patching be avoided (see page 725).[45]

Some investigators have questioned the value of a pressure patch for treatment of corneal abrasions in otherwise normal eyes. Anderson and associates[46] used tarsorrhaphy to simulate pressure patching in rabbits with abrasions 4 mm in size and found no statistically significant differences in corneal healing rates in occluded versus unoccluded eyes. Kirkpatrick and associates[47] found a significantly improved healing rate of corneal abrasions in patients treated with antibiotic ointment and mydriatic alone, as compared to patients treated with pressure patching. No significant difference in discomfort was noted between the two groups. In studying ocular effects produced by pressure patching in normal volunteers, Frucht-Pery and associates[48] found that pressure patching may contribute to the development of signs and symptoms such as conjunctival injection, pain or discomfort, and reduced visual acuity, generally attributed to other causes related to corneal healing. Collagen shields and bandage contact lenses are available to protect the cornea while avoiding use of the pressure patch. The porcine scleral collagen shield has been shown to result in accelerated corneal epithelial wound closure.[49,50] Wedge and Rootman[51] found that the collagen shield was as effective as a pressure patch after 24 hours, was significantly more comfortable than a pressure patch, but did not accelerate healing rates. They suggest that the collagen shield is an effective, yet more expensive, choice for patients who cannot tolerate a pressure patch or for patients with contact lens-induced abrasions that require frequent antibiotic instillation.

Archeson and associates[52] successfully used high-water content soft contact lenses as primary treatment for corneal abrasions, with the resultant advantages of retained visual function and binocularity during healing of the lesion. The use of cycloplegics and prophylactic antibiotics is continued with the lens in place; the patient is re-examined after 24 hours and at appropriate intervals thereafter. The contact lens is removed when healing is complete.[38] Careful monitoring is needed due to the potential risk of bacterial keratitis associated with soft contact lens wear.[52]

The nature of corneal healing remains under intense study.[53] Investigations currently are underway regarding the role of epidermal growth factor (EGF), a polypeptide hormone initially isolated from the mouse submaxillary gland, in promoting corneal healing.[54] EGF has a known potent stimulating effect on epidermal and epithelial cell proliferation; these mitogenic effects of EGF produce hyperplasia in the regenerating epithelium which grows over denuded and damaged stroma.[55] In a randomized clinical trial involving 104 patients treated with an ophthalmic EGF solution or placebo, Pastor and Calonge[56] found that mean epithelial healing time of traumatic corneal abrasions greater than 5 mm² in size and less than 6 hours in duration was signifi-

cantly enhanced in the EGF-treated group. The EGF was given 5 times daily along with 1% gentamicin drops and was well tolerated. It is reasonable to expect that EGF therapy has the potential to play an important future role in the treatment of corneal abrasion.

Diclofenac sodium 0.1% solution, a nonsteroidal anti-inflammatory drug (NSAID), effectively controls pain following photorefractive keratectomy (PRK).[57,58] In the future, this and other topical NSAIDs may play an important role in controlling pain caused by corneal abrasions and other traumatic or mechanical corneal lesions. The instillation of diclofenac and antibiotic drops following the application of a disposable soft contact lens can provide significant pain relief while the abrasion heals.[357] This approach also permits binocular vision in lieu of pressure patching.

Since most corneal abrasions involve loss of only the superficial epithelial cells, they generally heal without scar formation. As the healing cornea is monitored during follow-up care, it is important to determine that the signs and symptoms are consistent with the healing of a "clean" abrasion, and that bacterial or fungal keratitis does not develop, particularly in abrasions caused by vegetative matter.[59,60] Once the acute care aspects associated with the abrasion are resolved, it is helpful to discuss with the patient the appropriateness of protective eyewear, particularly if the patient is monocular. Protective eyewear may be needed in occupational, domestic, or recreational settings.[61]

Foreign Bodies

ETIOLOGY

Any foreign material debris that may strike the eye has the potential of becoming a corneal foreign body. Among the most common corneal foreign bodies diagnosed clinically are superficial metallic foreign bodies, as may result when a patient is doing body work on a car and metallic particulate debris flies or drops into the patient's eye(s) (Fig. 27.6). Other types of corneal foreign bodies include glass, plastic, insect parts, plant debris, wood splinters, and paint chips (Fig. 27.7).[62] Although most corneal foreign bodies tend to be superficial and lodge at Bowman's membrane, corneal perforation may occur from a high speed projectile foreign body or sharp objects such as spines from a plant.[63] History-taking is crucial for patients with corneal foreign bodies, since it is very important to determine, to the extent possible, the mechanism resulting in the foreign body.[64] If an etiology associated with high speed is present or suspected, such as a nylon cord weed trimmer, a grinding wheel, or hammer pounding on a nail, the likelihood of corneal perforation is greater.[65] A vegetative foreign body may result in a secondary fungal keratitis.[59] One study[66] indicated that most corneal foreign bodies are work-related and occur in men.

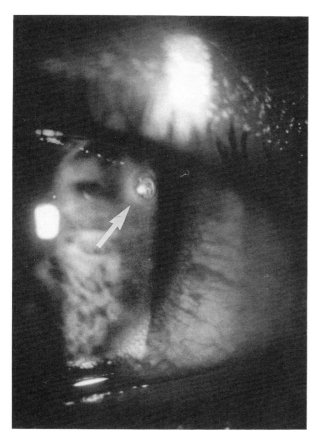

FIGURE 27.6   **Example of a metallic corneal foreign body (arrow).**

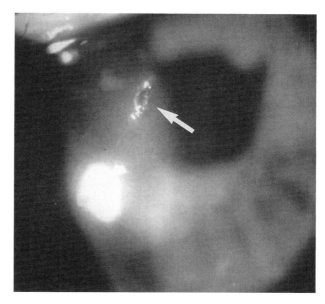

FIGURE 27.7   **Patient accidentally struck her cornea with a mascara wand, which resulted in this foreign body (arrow).**

DIAGNOSIS

Patient symptomatology related to a corneal foreign body may vary widely. Occasionally, an asymptomatic patient who presents for a routine examination may incidentally exhibit a small epithelial foreign body. More commonly, patients with corneal foreign bodies present acutely with symptoms similar to corneal abrasion—pain, photophobia, and reflex tearing. The patient may not be able to identify or recall the inciting event, and symptoms may have been present for a few days before their persistence or worsening prompted the patient to seek care.

Slit-lamp examination will reveal the presence of the foreign body. The appearance of the foreign body will often reveal its etiology, e.g., a metallic foreign body may exhibit oxidative rusting. A ring of edema and white blood cell infiltration may surround the foreign body. Other ocular signs that often accompany the corneal findings include conjunctival hyperemia and lid edema if profuse tearing is present. If the foreign body and resultant inflammation have

been present for 24 hours or longer, an anterior uveitis will often be present, manifested as an anterior chamber reaction (cells and flare) and miosis.

Careful slit-lamp technique is necessary to determine specifically the depth of the corneal foreign body. A thin optic section is used to determine the degree of corneal penetration. If it is determined that corneal penetration by the foreign body is sufficiently deep so that removal may risk corneal perforation, then a consultation for surgical removal is appropriate. Lid eversion is helpful to rule out the presence of an accompanying foreign body on the palpebral conjunctiva. A thorough dilated fundus examination assists in ruling out an accompanying intraocular foreign body. It is especially important to conduct a thorough dilated fundus examination if the etiologic mechanism of the corneal foreign body has the potential for corneal perforation.

Some clinicians advocate the use of orbital x-rays to rule out the possibility of a metallic intraocular foreign body when a metallic corneal foreign body is discovered. Although this practice is not universal and perhaps is not a practical use of health care resources, if clinical signs suggest the possibility of a metallic intraocular foreign body, then orbital x-rays or CT scanning is indicated.[65]

MANAGEMENT

Of the several effective techniques available for removal of a corneal foreign body, the one chosen often depends on the embeddedness of the foreign body, the cooperation of the

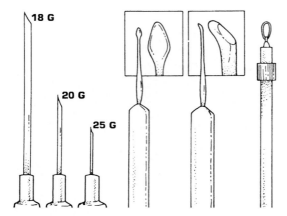

FIGURE 27.8   **From left to right, sterile needles, spuds or a loop may be used to remove a corneal foreign body. (Reprinted with permission from Fingeret M, Casser L, Woodcome HT. Corneal foreign body removal. In: Atlas of primary eyecare procedures. Norwalk, CT: Appleton & Lange, 1990:146–151.)**

patient, and personal preference of the clinician (Fig. 27.8). Instillation of a topical anesthetic precedes removal of the foreign body. Instillation of anesthetic drops in both eyes helps to control the patient's blink reflex during removal.

If the foreign body is very superficial, if patient cooperation is poor (e.g., a small child), or if particulate debris in the conjunctival sac accompanies the corneal foreign body, re-

moval can be attempted by irrigation with sterile irrigating solution. It is helpful to direct the stream of solution from the bottle toward the foreign body in an attempt to dislodge it.

The commonly used techniques for removing corneal foreign bodies include the use of a sterile 25-gauge needle or spud in conjunction with the slit lamp. The tip of the needle or edge of the spud is directed tangentially to the corneal surface to lift the edge of the foreign body and dislodge it (Fig. 27.9). Once the foreign body is dislodged, it is helpful to irrigate the conjunctival sac to remove residual particulate debris from the surface of the globe. The advantage of the spud over the needle technique is that a broader edge is available with which to contact the foreign body, and small movements of the patient's eye or the examiner's hand may be less likely to induce superficial corneal epithelial irritation. Other procedures used to remove corneal foreign bodies include an ophthalmic loop and magnetized forceps. Since many corneal foreign bodies are ferromagnetic, Arnold and Erie[67] report that attaching a small magnet to a sterile jeweler's forceps allows easier dislodging of the foreign body, followed by magnetically lifting or grasping it from the ocular surface.

Rust ring development is common when a metallic corneal foreign body has been present for 24 hours or longer (Fig. 27.10). When the foreign body is removed by irrigation, a needle, or spud, a "bed" of rust or a surrounding rust ring may remain. Although some of this residual rust will tend to slough as the cornea heals, it is preferable to remove the rust ring at the time of foreign body removal.[68] The rust

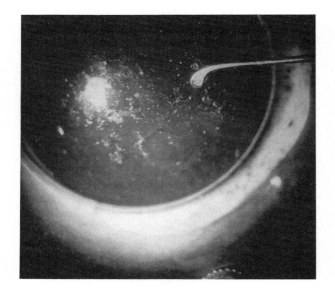

A

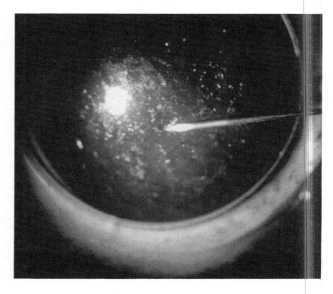

B

FIGURE 27.9   **Using a mounted bovine eye, the techniques of corneal foreign body removal are illustrated. (A) Spud is directed tangentially to the cornea, and the edge is used to lift the foreign body. (B) The tip of a sterile 25G needle is used to lift the foreign body. Note that the bevel of the needle is positioned away from the cornea.**

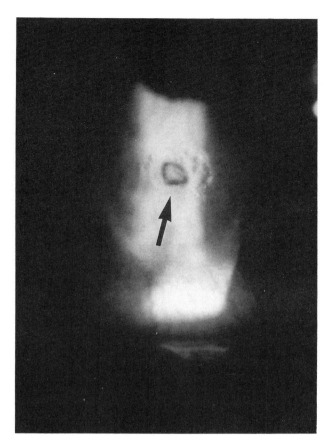

FIGURE 27.10 **Rust ring (arrow) noted following removal of a metallic corneal foreign body.**

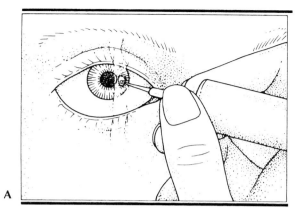

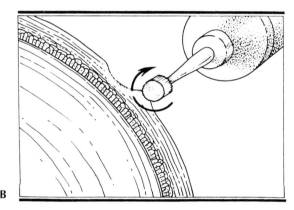

FIGURE 27.11 **Corneal rust ring removal. Introduced tangentially to the cornea (A), the Alger brush is used to remove rust-containing epithelial cells gently (B). (From Fingeret M, Casser L, Woodcome HT. Corneal rust ring removal. In: Atlas of primary eyecare procedures. Norwalk, CT: Appleton & Lange, 1990:152–155.)**

can be removed effectively using the edge of a spud or needle to "scrape" it away, or an Alger brush can be used to "burr" it away (Fig. 27.11).[69] Sigurdsson and associates[70] concluded that use of an electric drill was a quicker method of rust ring removal compared to a needle. Since rust ring removal tends to generate some debris, irrigation following this technique is helpful.

Following removal of a corneal foreign body and any accompanying rust ring, a small "crater-like" depression will result. Once the foreign body is removed, the therapeutic management aspects are similar to treating a corneal abrasion.[64] If the corneal disruption is minimal and accompanying symptoms are not significant, then broad-spectrum antibiotics, such as 0.3% tobramycin or polymyxin B-trimethoprim drops during the day and polymyxin B-bacitracin ointment at bedtime, are used until the corneal tissue heals. Hulbert[71] found that with small epithelial defects (1–2 mm) following corneal foreign body removal, patient comfort was enhanced and healing rates unaffected if antibiotic prophylaxis was used alone without a pressure patch (Fig. 27.12).

With more severe involvements, cycloplegic agents are instilled and a pressure patch is used along with a broad-spectrum antibiotic ointment, such as polymyxin B-bacitracin. A follow-up examination is performed 24 hours later. During follow-up examinations, it is important to monitor for signs of secondary bacterial keratitis, secondary fungal keratitis, or an intraocular foreign body that may have been overlooked initially.

If the foreign body disrupted Bowman's membrane and the anterior stroma, a small, usually circular, corneal opacity will result following the healing process. Even when located on the visual axis, these small opacities tend not to affect visual acuity and often are noted during routine eye examinations. If a metallic foreign body and rust ring had been present, often a light brown "tinge" to the resultant opacity persists. It also is not uncommon to note a Coat's white ring during routine slit-lamp examination in an asymptomatic

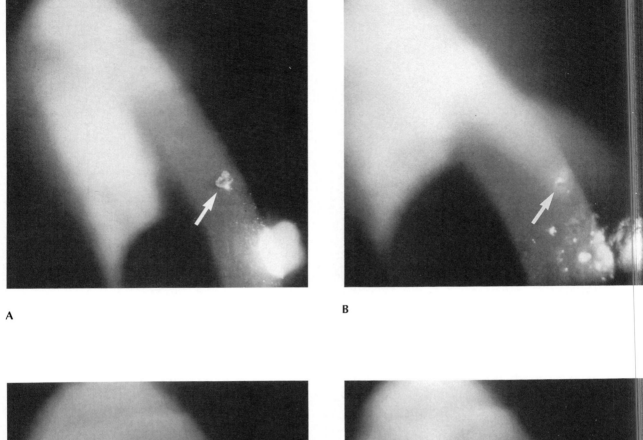

A   B

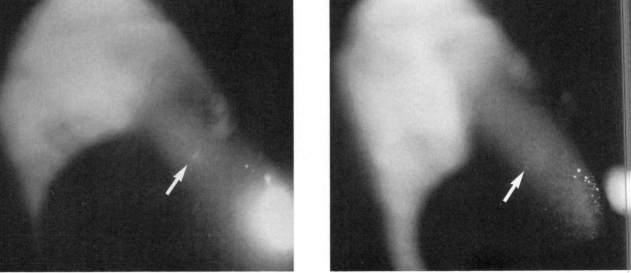

C   D

FIGURE 27.12   **Corneal foreign body removal with subsequent healing.** *(A)* Small metallic corneal foreign body (arrow) is noted in superior cornea. *(B)* Following removal with a spud, a small "crater-like" depression remains which stains with fluorescein sodium (arrow). *(C)* The following day, the epithelium is virtually healed, but a small focal area of edema and leukocyte infiltration remains (arrow). *(D)* Five days later the epithelium has healed completely, and a small diffuse spot of edema is noted (arrow), which ultimately resolved.

patient. This granular white ring opacity is thought to represent residual iron deposits at the site of a prior corneal foreign body (Fig. 27.13).[11]

Once the acute episode related to a corneal foreign body has resolved, it is important to provide patient education about the value of protective eyewear to help prevent future corneal foreign bodies. This primary care aspect of patient education is especially important if the patient is monocular, exhibits multiple corneal opacities from past foreign bodies, or is engaged in an occupation in which the likelihood of debris striking the eyes is great.

Lacerations and Perforations

ETIOLOGY

Any sharp object, such as glass, wire, or pins, that enters the eye with sufficient force may result in a corneal laceration in which the stroma is penetrated to any depth.[72,73] If the sharp object or foreign body passes completely through the cornea, then corneal perforation has occurred. Patients who have undergone radial keratotomy may be susceptible to corneal perforation at an incision site, as well as corneal rupture following blunt trauma.[74,75] Penetrating injuries caused by metal wire are not infrequently associated with intraocular cilia, which may be difficult to detect.[76]

One obvious concern in the event of deep stromal corneal laceration or corneal perforation is the resultant insult to the regularity and clarity of the corneal surface and the potential impact on visual acuity. This issue will also impact the method chosen for repair of the corneal laceration or perforation. In the case of corneal perforation, there also is concern about the impact on globe contents, including potential damage to intraocular structures and the risk of endophthalmitis.

DIAGNOSIS

A careful patient history will help to elucidate the etiology of the traumatic event, although the possibility of corneal laceration or perforation may not be determined definitively from the history alone. If patient history or initial examination indicates that deep laceration or penetration is present, care must be taken to avoid undue pressure on the globe during the examination.[77] The use of topical or regional anesthesia will help to minimize blepharospasm as a cause of pressure on the globe.

Patient symptomatology associated with corneal laceration or perforation may vary widely. In the event of a small corneal perforation that has self-sealed, associated symptomatology may be relatively minor.[65] More extensive involvement will produce symptoms of pain, photophobia, tearing, and blepharospasm.

In the event of a large object impaled into the eye, such as a fishhook, the etiology of the corneal wound will be obvious.[78] Otherwise, careful slit-lamp examination is needed to

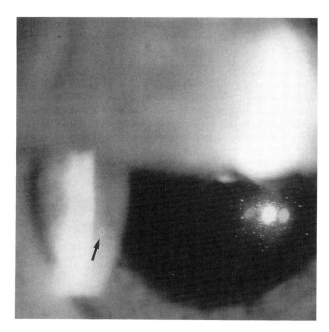

FIGURE 27.13 **Small Coat's white ring (arrow) noted during routine examination of an asymptomatic patient.**

determine the extent of the injury. An optic section at the site of the wound should be evaluated under high magnification to determine the depth of the laceration.[63] A full thickness corneal "track" suggests that perforation has occurred.

Evaluating for Seidel's sign at the site of the wound also will help to determine whether corneal perforation has occurred (see Chap. 31).[79] It is possible, however, that small lacerations or puncture wounds may self-seal so that Seidel's sign is negative even when perforation has occurred. An anterior chamber reaction (cells and flare), shallowing of the anterior chamber, and dramatic lowering of intraocular pressure (IOP) in the involved eye may be indicative of corneal perforation. Herniation of intraocular contents may occur through large corneal or corneoscleral defects, along with the presence of a flattened anterior chamber. It is important to examine thoroughly for retained foreign material that entered the eye through the cornea. When indicated, orbital x-rays and CT scanning should be ordered. MRI scanning is contraindicated when a metallic intraocular foreign body is suspected because of potential interaction between the magnetic field and the metallic foreign object, which may exacerbate globe damage.[65]

MANAGEMENT

Small, non-perforating corneal lacerations may be treated as corneal abrasions (Fig. 27.14). Small, self-sealing corneal perforations with no sign of active aqueous loss may be

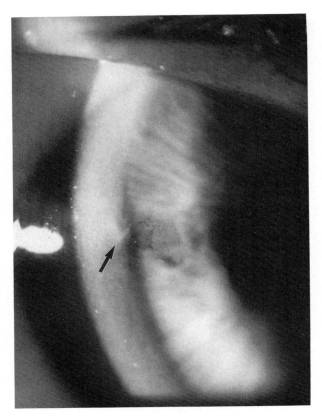

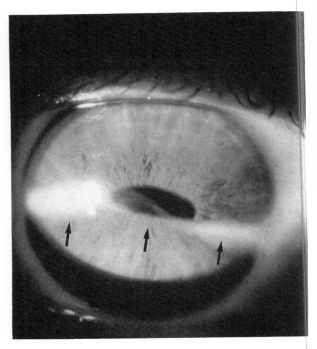

FIGURE 27.15   **Horizontal scar with anterior synechiae is noted following repair of a large corneoscleral laceration. (Courtesy William L. Jones, O.D.)**

FIGURE 27.14   **During routine examination a small full-thickness corneal scar was noted from prior corneal perforation (arrow). Patient also exhibits an iris sphincter tear and small rosette cataract but denies a prior traumatic ocular event.**

treated conservatively with topical antibiotic prophylaxis, systemic antibiotic prophylaxis to prevent endophthalmitis, and pupillary dilation and cycloplegia. Larger lacerations with tissue loss and obvious corneal perforations require aggressive treatment by a subspecialist (Fig. 27.15).[77] Taping a metal Fox shield over the eye to prevent further injury is appropriate while the patient is transported (Fig. 27.16).[38] Once examined, corneal suturing, corneal grafting, keratoplasty, adhesives, or conjunctival flaps may be utilized by the subspecialist.[80,81]

Alternative therapies have been proposed for the repair of corneal perforations. Bandage contact lenses in conjunction with topical and systemic prophylactic antibiotics have been used for small perforations exhibiting good apposition of wound edges.[82] Medical grade isobutyl cyanoacrylate tissue adhesive has been used to seal corneal perforations.[83] Erdey and associates[84] described a modified technique in which cyanoacrylate adhesive is applied along with a small collagen disk. A bandage contact lens can be added after the collagen disk dissolves in 24 hours if patient discomfort develops.

After surgical repair of a corneal laceration, visual rehabilitation may be obtained with the fitting of a contact lens, even with prominent central scarring and sutures intact.[85] This is especially necessary to help retain binocularity and prevent amblyopia in pediatric patients who have undergone corneal laceration repair.[86] A positive visual outcome with a contact lens may preclude the need for penetrating keratoplasty in these patients.[85]

Penetrating keratoplasty may restore functional vision when post-traumatic corneal scars are dense and centrally located.[87] Although emergency penetrating keratoplasty may be needed in the event of a large traumatic corneal perforation, Nobe and associates[88] determined that the chances of a clear graft post-penetrating keratoplasty improve if the procedure is delayed for at least three months.

A late onset complication of penetrating corneal wounds, particularly in children, is the development of a traumatic intracorneal cyst, probably due to epithelial cells forced into the stroma which subsequently proliferate.[89] Patient education regarding the use of protective eyewear may help to prevent corneal laceration and perforation injuries.[87] This is particularly important to protect the remaining normal eye in a patient who is monocular. Tetanus immunization is recommended following corneal perforating injuries.[90]

Recurrent Corneal Erosion

ETIOLOGY

Recurrent corneal erosions (RCE) are episodes of spontaneous breakdown or sloughing of the epithelial layer of the cornea. They are caused by poor adhesion between the epithelial basement membrane and Bowman's layer, and may be due to abnormalities of the basement membrane alone or in conjunction with an absence of hemidesmosomes.[91,92] They occur most frequently after sudden, sharp trauma to the cornea. Brown and Bron[93] reported that 60% of all RCEs were preceded by a fingernail scratch or paper cut to the eye. They are seldom associated with projectile foreign body trauma.[94]

When they occur bilaterally the most likely cause is a corneal dystrophy. Many corneal dystrophies, including Fuchs' and lattice, have been associated with RCEs, but the most frequent one is anterior basement membrane dystrophy (see page 720). It has been estimated that half of all patients with RCEs have anterior basement membrane dystrophy,[95] as compared to 2% to 15% of the general population.[93,96]

There are many other causes of RCE, but they occur much less frequently. They include chemical or thermal burns, damage from herpes simplex keratitis, neuroparalytic keratitis, bullous keratopathy, severe dry eyes, nocturnal lagophthalmos, and diabetes mellitus due to basement membrane abnormalities.

To understand the development of RCEs, the mechanism by which a corneal abrasion heals also must be understood. The corneal epithelium is 5 to 6 cell layers thick and rests on its basement membrane. Firm attachments called *hemidesmosomes* connect the cells to the underlying membrane. When the epithelium is damaged, surrounding cells liberate fibronectin, a polypeptide hormone that loosens cellular attachments to the basement membrane to allow the cells to slide and cover the damaged area.[21,22] After the area is covered, the cells begin to duplicate, but it takes 7 days for the regenerating epithelium to form firm attachments to undamaged basement membrane. If the anterior basement membrane is destroyed, it may take as long as 8 weeks for the attachments to reform.[97]

In RCE the original epithelial abrasion heals rapidly, usually with no visible sequelae. At some later time the symptoms suddenly recur. The mean time to recurrence in one study of 80 patients was 18 months. Although 63% occurred within the first four months, the range of time from initial injury to recurrence was reported to be as short as two days and as long as 16 years.[93] Because some RCEs occur without a positive history for injury, it is possible that patients with longer intervals are actually experiencing a spontaneous erosion. Although RCEs can start at any age, early adulthood to middle age is commonly observed.

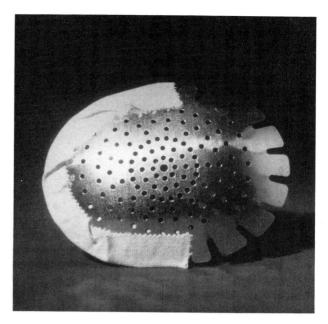

FIGURE 27.16   **If a patient is referred for consultation due to a suspected corneal perforation, it is appropriate to tape a metal Fox shield over the eye to protect from further trauma during transportation. Tape is placed over the edge of the Fox shield to enhance patient comfort (here shown partially completed).**

DIAGNOSIS

The most common symptom of RCE is acute pain. Of 80 patients in one study, 93% experienced sharp eye pain; most of these patients reported that the attacks of RCE occurred upon awakening, and symptoms improved during the day.[93] Other common symptoms include photophobia, tearing, blurred vision, redness, burning, blepharospasm, and foreign body sensation. These symptoms can resolve quickly as the epithelium is repositioned on the cornea, but they usually last hours to days. The symptoms tend to recur in cycles of days, weeks, or months.

Slit-lamp examination of patients with acute symptoms will show lesions varying from an area of localized roughening of the epithelium to a true corneal abrasion. This area often is just below the pupil in the approximate location of most Hudson-Stahli lines (Fig. 27.17).[93,98] Investigators believe that RCEs occur in this location because epithelial stem cells come from the limbus, and healing of central corneal lesions is accomplished by movement of peripheral epithelial cells toward the center.[99]

It also is possible to see microcysts, bullae, white cystic spaces, and loose sheets of epithelium in acute cases of RCE. If the epithelium is loose but still in position, it may appear as a slightly wavy or irregular area with surrounding edema.

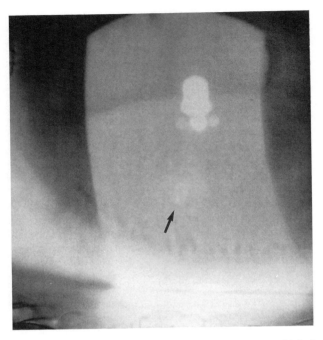

FIGURE 27.17   **Recurrent corneal erosion in the inferior third of the cornea (arrow) exhibits positive fluorescein sodium staining centrally. Note the surrounding punctate positive and negative stains.**

Stromal edema can cause a rusty hue in the area of epithelial detachment.[100] The area will stain irregularly with fluorescein sodium, and the tear break-up time will be very rapid. Perilimbal injection, upper lid edema, and blepharospasm are possible in severe cases.

Between episodes the most common signs of RCE are epithelial microcysts, surface irregularities and subepithelial scarring. A pseudodendrite appearance is possible due to apposition of the loose and well-attached epithelium.

MANAGEMENT

Treatment generally focuses on decreasing symptoms and encouraging regrowth and re-anchoring of the epithelium by keeping the eye moist. It is important to warn the patient of the recurrent nature of the condition, and to continue all treatment for some time after the eye appears to be healed.

During acute episodes a cycloplegic agent, such as 5% homatropine, should be instilled to decrease ciliary spasm and pain. A broad-spectrum topical prophylactic antibiotic ointment, such as 0.3% tobramycin, and pressure patch should also be applied. Oral analgesics can be prescribed as needed for pain (see Chap. 7). The eye should be examined every 24 hours while patched and the therapy continued until the epithelial defect is healed. During corneal healing it

is important to monitor for any signs of intraocular inflammation such as anterior uveitis.

If the epithelium is not healing or if the patient presents with grossly loose and elevated epithelium, the area should be debrided. Apply a topical anesthetic to anesthetize the cornea and to loosen the epithelium. A dry cellulose ophthalmic sponge or a wet sterile cotton-tipped applicator can be used to gently remove the epithelium (see Fig. 27.4).[101] It is important to avoid scraping too hard, since this could damage the basement membrane and increase healing time. Debridement should be followed by the usual therapy of cycloplegics, antibiotics, and pressure patching. Debridement speeds up the healing process but does not affect the incidence of recurrences.[93]

Once the epithelial defect is healed, artificial tears should be used 4 to 8 times each day, and nonpreserved 5% sodium chloride ointment should be instilled into the conjunctival sac each night. This lubrication decreases lid adhesion and also may create an osmotic gradient that draws fluid from the epithelium, keeping it close to Bowman's membrane and thereby promoting adherence.

Although some clinicians believe bland ointment may be just as effective, Trobe[102] showed that artificial tears, steroids and boric acid were not as effective as hyperosmotic ointment for controlling recurrences. It has been reported that 80% to 90% of patients with symptomatic recurrent corneal erosions experience some improvement in symptoms with the use of hyperosmotic ointment.[93,100] Patients who are concerned about blurred vision due to the ointment may irrigate the eye with artificial tears each morning.

Although it is generally believed that 6 to 8 weeks are needed to repair the epithelium, minor recurrent episodes can prolong the healing process. For this reason, patients should continue using hyperosmotics for at least 2 to 3 months after the last episode, since there is a tendency for recurrence of the erosion if the hyperosmotic therapy is withdrawn prematurely.[93] Clinical anecdotal information suggests that patients may benefit from increasing the frequency of hyperosmotic ointment use to four or five times a day for a brief period after a recurrence.

If the patient experiences persistent recurrences more frequently than once a month, an extended wear therapeutic or disposable soft contact lens may be helpful, especially if a diffuse area is involved. A thin, medium water content lens should be fit to allow minimal movement. These lenses are fitted in an attempt to protect the epithelium from lid trauma during blinking, and from adhering to the tarsal conjunctiva. The lenses tend to increase patient comfort and decrease the severity and frequency of recurrences, but they do not always prevent recurrences. Besides erosions occurring underneath the contact lens, other problems associated with contact lens wear may develop, including contact lens loss, discomfort, deposits, vascularization, stromal infiltrates, and infection. To monitor for these complications, it is suggested that the patient be examined 24 hours after contact lens dispensing.

1 week later, and each month after that.[97] If the patient is tolerating the lens well, it should be left in place for 2 months following healing of the erosion. This typically results in 3 to 6 months of wearing time. When lenses are discontinued, instruct the patient to instill 5% sodium chloride ointment into the conjunctival sac at bedtime for several months.

Anterior stromal puncture is an alternative to hydrophilic lens wear for the treatment of RCE. It was once reserved only for cases that did not respond to other therapy but is now considered earlier in the course of treatment, especially if the area of erosion is well defined.[103] The process of stromal puncture disrupts the epithelium and Bowman's membrane, allowing normal healing which secures the epithelium and basement membrane to the anterior stroma. The resultant scarring from anterior stromal puncture appears to be minimal enough to cause no apparent effect on visual acuity even if it is performed on the visual axis.[94,104]

Anterior stromal puncture involves the use of a standardized LOOK, Inc. needle or, if unavailable, a bent-tipped 23- to 25-gauge needle to make punctures through loose epithelium and Bowman's layer into the anterior stroma.[96] Enough pressure should be applied to indent the cornea 1/4 to 1/3 the depth of the anterior chamber, which should cause about 50% stromal thickness penetration. The bent tip prevents accidental perforation and controls the penetration depth. These punctures are placed approximately 0.5 mm apart over the entire area of loose epithelium, and about 1 mm outside the area delineated by fluorescein.[104]

After the procedure, instill a cycloplegic agent and a topical ophthalmic antibiotic such as 0.3% tobramycin ointment. The eye is pressure patched and examined each day until the epithelium is healed. After the pressure patch is no longer needed, a broad-spectrum antibiotic solution, such as 0.3% tobramycin or polymyxin B-trimethoprim, should be instilled four times a day for one week.[94] Patients should instill hyperosmotic ointment into the conjunctival sac at bedtime for several months and should be examined at one-week and two-month intervals after the epithelium is healed.

Some authors have suggested use of the Nd:YAG laser instead of a needle to decrease scarring and increase repeatability of penetration.[105] However, one major disadvantage of the laser procedure is the need, in some cases, to debride the corneal epithelium before the treatment is administered. This makes the procedure more painful for the patient, and recovery time is prolonged. There is controversy as to which method of anterior stromal puncture is more reasonable when comparing cost, discomfort, and repeatability.[103,105]

Surgical interventions usually are reserved for severe cases. These include superficial epithelial keratectomy with a variable speed diamond burr;[101,106] corneal basement membranectomy, which may be the best treatment for recurrent corneal erosion caused by anterior basement membrane dystrophy;[105] microdiathermy; and surface cautery or diathermy, used primarily for symptom relief if there is no visual potential.

Exposure Keratopathy

ETIOLOGY

Numerous local ocular or systemic factors may result in chronic corneal drying due to infrequent or incomplete blinking, or inadequate eyelid closure (lagophthalmos).[2] The resultant irritation to the corneal tissue is known as *exposure keratopathy*.

Ectropion (see Fig. 24.18) is an example of a local eyelid abnormality that may result in exposure keratopathy. Bell's palsy usually includes disrupted innervation to the orbicularis oculi muscle. The resultant retraction of the lower eyelid together with reduced blink capability of the upper lid may result in exposure keratopathy. Graves' disease is an example of a systemic condition that can produce exophthalmos (see Fig. 33.5) and accompanying exposure keratopathy. Nocturnal lagophthalmos, in which the eyelids do not close fully during sleep, is a relatively common cause of exposure keratopathy.

DIAGNOSIS

Patients with exposure keratopathy typically present with symptoms of foreign body sensation, irritation, and redness. The symptomatology may be more pronounced in the morning following a night of corneal desiccation, particularly in the case of nocturnal lagophthalmos. In the less frequent event of secondary corneal ulceration or infection, the symptoms will be more pronounced and consistent with these conditions.

Depending on the patient's lid configuration, slit-lamp examination will reveal punctate epithelial erosions in the interpalpebral area of the cornea or the inferior cornea.[107] These lesions will stain prominently with fluorescein sodium and often rose bengal (Fig. 27.18). Corresponding conjunctival injection is common. In more severe, long-standing cases, inferior micropannus, scarring or corneal thinning may be noted.

A thorough patient history along with other observed ocular, facial or systemic findings will assist in determining the etiology of exposure keratitis. The potential for lagophthalmos can be assessed by asking the patient to close his or her eyes and grossly inspecting for incomplete lid closure and exposure of the globe.[108] In patients with lagophthalmos a portion of the globe will be visible through the incompletely closed fissure (see Fig. 24.17). If the patient has a normal Bell's reflex, the bulbar conjunctival/scleral portion of the globe will be visible; if the patient has a poor Bell's reflex, the cornea will be visible through the incompletely closed fissure and exposure keratopathy will result. Friends or family members can observe the patient's eyelids during sleep to help determine if nocturnal lagophthalmos is present.

MANAGEMENT

If exposure keratopathy is the result of an ocular or systemic abnormality, the underlying condition should be addressed

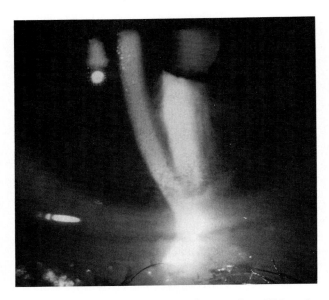

FIGURE 27.18 **Patient with exposure keratopathy exhibits staining inferiorly with rose bengal.**

as fully as possible. Patients with exposure keratopathy resulting from Bell's palsy or Grave's disease often are co-managed by a physician caring for the systemic problem together with the optometrist or ophthalmologist managing ocular complications.

Therapeutic measures for the management of exposure keratopathy are directed toward reinstating lubrication to the globe and cornea as long as the lagophthalmos is present. These measures typically include ocular lubricating drops during the day and bland ophthalmic lubricating ointment instilled into the conjunctival sac at bedtime. If ointment lubrication is not sufficient, and often as an interim measure, the eyelids may be taped closed with hypoallergenic tape to prevent corneal exposure during sleep. Moreover, several types of plastic shields are available commercially to reduce tear evaporation and resultant corneal desiccation.[108] Low-water content bandage or disposable soft contact lenses also may be used, but patients using these therapeutic measures should be monitored closely since they are at risk for secondary infection.[107]

If an underlying lid abnormality such as ectropion is the cause of the exposure keratitis, then consultation for a lid surgical procedure is appropriate. In extreme cases of exposure, a tarsorrhaphy may be performed to preserve corneal health. In the event that exposure keratitis has become complicated by secondary infection, appropriate treatment must be initiated.

Mild Acid Burns

ETIOLOGY

Any chemical solution that is splashed or thrown into the face has the potential to cause a chemical burn to the cornea, conjunctiva, and eyelids. One such type of injury are burns related to acid solutions. The most common solutions implicated in these types of corneal burns include sulfuric acid (a commonly used industrial acid, also used in car batteries), sulfurous acid, acetic acid, hydrochloric acid, hydrofluoric acid, nitric acid, and chromic acid.[80,109] Although burns caused by acids in high concentration may result in serious corneal and ocular injury, most acid burns result in local, superficial effects. Acid injury results in a barrier of precipitated tissue that tends to limit further ocular damage.[110]

DIAGNOSIS

A patient with a mild corneal or ocular acid burn typically reports a history of the offending solution splashing into the eye(s) or face. The patient generally presents soon after the injury or will seek care if ocular irritation persists after a day or two. The degree of symptomatology tends to be consistent with the extent of the ocular burn. Symptoms range from mild irritation and focal redness to significant irritation, burning, redness, tearing, and photophobia. During history-taking, the patient, a friend, or family member should identify the offending solution as accurately as possible. Resources are available to help identify the potential ocular effects of an identified chemical agent, such as a poison control "hotline" or Grant's *Toxicology of the Eye*.[111,112]

Since the ocular tissue exposed in the palpebral fissure is most likely to be involved in a splash chemical injury, the clinical signs tend to be most prominent in that area. Bulbar conjunctival injection will be most pronounced within the palpebral fissure. Punctate epithelial erosions will be noted at the areas of acid solution contact with the cornea. Fluorescein staining of the bulbar conjunctiva and corresponding inferior palpebral conjunctiva may be present. Depending on the extent of the injury, the skin of the eyelids and face also may exhibit acid burn involvement.

MANAGEMENT

When a history of recent acid solution injury is reported, institute copious ocular irrigation immediately. If a patient telephones with this complaint, instruct the patient, a friend, or family member to begin irrigation immediately before traveling for care. Copious ocular irrigation will help to neutralize the offending solution and will serve to wash away any accompanying particulate debris from the eye. Sterile saline or eyewash solution is preferred for irrigation, but on-site irrigation with clean water is satisfactory. Immediate ocular irrigation with saline or water for 20 to 30 minutes has been recommended.[80,109] The patient should be instructed to present for in-office care following thorough irrigation.

If the patient presents as an office ocular urgency, reporting a recent acid burn injury, immediate ocular irrigation should be instituted even before implementing other aspects of patient check-in and ocular examination. Instilling a drop of topical anesthetic into each eye will enhance patient cooperation during the irrigation. The globe should be thoroughly irrigated using sterile saline or extraocular irrigating solution (see Figs. 3.28 and 3.29).[111] The solution stream should also be directed toward the fornices. A 20 to 30-minute irrigation has been recommended, and litmus paper may be used to determine the effectiveness of irrigation in neutralizing the acid solution (endpoint of 7.3–7.7).[110] If particulate debris also is present in the eye, it should be removed using appropriate techniques. If patient cooperation is poor for ocular irrigation, use of a lid speculum may be helpful (Fig. 27.19).[113]

Following thorough irrigation and examination, additional therapeutic measures are instituted, as needed. Antibiotic prophylaxis using broad-spectrum topical agents, such as 0.3% tobramycin or polymyxin B-trimethoprim drops 4 times a day and 0.3% tobramycin or polymyxin B-bacitracin ointment in the conjunctival sac at bedtime, will protect the tissue from secondary infection during healing. Concurrent use of a low-potency topical steroid such as 0.12% prednisolone or 0.1% fluorometholone alcohol 4 times a day will help reduce the inflammatory response. More extensive acid burns may require pupillary dilation and cycloplegia with a long-acting agent such as 5% homatropine, along with a pressure patch using a broad-spectrum antibiotic ointment such as polymyxin B-bacitracin. Consultation with a corneal specialist may be indicated for severe acid burns involving more than superficial tissue injury.

Patient education about the use of protective eyewear in circumstances when chemical injury may occur is very important and may help to prevent future injury.

Mild Alkali Burns

ETIOLOGY

Alkali injuries to the eye represent true medical emergencies since the impact on ocular tissue, including the cornea, may be devastating. Common alkali agents that may cause ocular burns include ammonia, a common cleaning agent; sodium hydroxide, in lye, drain cleaners, or caustic soda; calcium hydroxide in lime, plaster, cement, mortar and whitewash; potassium hydroxide in caustic potash; and magnesium hydroxide, a component of flares and fireworks.[109] The alkaline substance may be in liquid form, or as in the case of lime-containing mortar, may involve solid contaminants. The

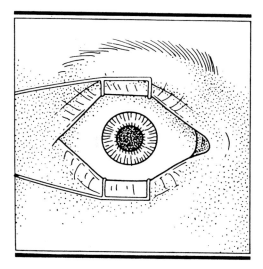

FIGURE 27.19 **Spring-type Barraquer lid speculum is shown in place. (Reprinted with permission from Fingeret M, Casser L, Woodcome HT. Speculum insertion. In: Atlas of primary eyecare procedures. Norwalk, CT: Appleton & Lange, 1990:90–91).**

form of the alkali impacts ocular contact time and the degree of resultant ocular damage. Mild alkali corneal burns may result from accidents involving household products; severe alkali burns occur from industrial accidents or deliberate assaults.[38,109]

The chemical composition of alkaline substances promotes rapid penetration through all corneal layers without being neutralized.[80] Corneal tissue damage is pronounced and includes epithelial denudation, cell membrane disruption and coagulation of keratocytes, and severe disruption of the mucopolysaccharide ground substance. Alkali agents coagulate blood vessels, resulting in ischemia and tissue necrosis.

DIAGNOSIS

A patient with a mild corneal or ocular alkali burn typically reports a history of having the offending solution or solid splashed into the eye(s) or face. The patient generally presents soon after the injury or will seek care if ocular irritation persists after a day or two. The degree of symptomatology tends to be consistent with the extent of the ocular burn. Symptoms range from mild irritation and focal redness, as may be seen from mild alkali burns from household products, to severe pain, burning, redness, tearing, and photophobia. During history-taking, the patient, a friend, or family member should identify the offending agent as accurately as possible. Resources are available to help predict potential damage to the eye caused by an identified chemical agent, such as a poison control "hotline" or Grant's *Toxicology of the Eye*.[111,112]

Since the ocular tissue exposed in the palpebral fissure is most likely to be involved in an alkali burn, the clinical signs tend to be most pronounced in that area. Severe alkali burns usually are associated with eyelid and facial skin involvement. In mild alkali burns, punctate epithelial corneal erosions will be noted at the point of alkali contact with the cornea. Fluorescein staining of the bulbar conjunctiva and corresponding inferior palpebral conjunctiva also may be present. Focal or diffuse conjunctival injection will be present.

In evaluating the severity of the alkali burn, it is very important to determine the degree of tissue involvement. Corneal haze and limbal or conjunctival ischemia indicate more severe involvement and a poorer visual and ocular prognosis. Areas of limbal or conjunctival ischemia or necrosis appear white and devoid of blood vessels.[109] A grading system has been described to determine the severity of an alkali ocular burn, which also impacts prognosis (Table 27.2). Severe alkali burns cause destruction of superficial ocular tissue to result in corneal scarring, symblepharon, entropion and keratitis sicca. Corneal penetration of the alkaline substance produces uveitis, cataract, and secondary glaucoma. Damage to ocular tissue may continue long after the initial injury occurred.[110]

MANAGEMENT

When a history of recent alkali injury is reported, institute copious ocular irrigation immediately. If a patient telephones with this complaint, instruct the patient, a friend, or family member to perform irrigation before traveling for care. Copious ocular irrigation is instituted in an effort to neutralize the offending agent and wash away any accompanying particulate debris from the eye. Sterile saline or eyewash solution is preferred for irrigation, but on-site irrigation with clean water is satisfactory. Immediate ocular irrigation with saline or water for 30 minutes is imperative.[80] The patient should then be instructed to present for in-office care following thorough irrigation. A patient with a severe alkali burn to the eyes and face should be transported immediately to an emergency medical facility following ocular irrigation, unless life-threatening issues take precedence.

If the patient presents as an office ocular emergency reporting a recent alkali burn injury, institute ocular irrigation immediately, even before performing other aspects of patient check-in and ocular examination. Instilling a drop of topical anesthetic into each eye will enhance patient cooperation during irrigation. Thoroughly irrigate the globe using sterile saline or extraocular irrigating solution (see Figs. 3.28 and 3.29).[111] The solution stream also should be directed toward the fornices. A 30-minute irrigation is needed, and litmus paper may be used to determine the effectiveness of irrigation in neutralizing the alkaline solution (endpoint of 7.3–7.7).[110] Remove all particulate debris using appropriate techniques. If patient cooperation is poor for ocular irrigation, use of a lid speculum may be helpful (see Fig. 27.19).[113]

The following additional therapeutic regimen applies to mild (grade 1) alkali burns, as needed. All other alkali burns should be treated and managed promptly by a subspecialist. Antibiotic prophylaxis using broad-spectrum agents, such as 0.3% tobramycin or polymyxin B-trimethoprim drops 4 times a day and polymyxin B-bacitracin ointment instilled into the conjunctival sac at bedtime, will protect the tissue from secondary infection during healing. Concurrent use of a low-potency topical steroid, such as 0.12% prednisolone or 0.1% fluorometholone alcohol, will help to reduce the inflammatory response. Pupillary dilation and cycloplegia with a long-acting agent, such as 5% homatropine, along with a pressure patch using a broad-spectrum antibiotic ointment, such as polymyxin B-bacitracin, may enhance patient comfort and healing. If healing of the mild alkali burn does not proceed as expected, it is possible that ischemia is present, necessitating re-evaluation of the treatment and management plans.

Investigators continue to study the corneal changes that result from alkali burns, not only as models of corneal healing, but also to identify effective therapeutic regimens to

TABLE 27.2
Hughes-Roper-Hall Classification of Alkali Burns

Grade	Corneal Findings	Limbal Ischemia	Prognosis
I	Epithelial damage	None	Good
II	Hazy but iris details visible	< 1/3	Good
III	Total epithelial loss	1/3–1/2	Guarded
	Stromal haze blurring iris details		
IV	Opaque; neither iris nor pupil visible	> 1/2	Poor

Modified from Arffa RC. Chemical injuries. In: Grayson's Diseases of the Cornea, 3rd ed. St. Louis: Mosby-Year Book, 1991:649–665.

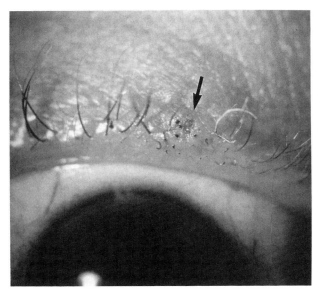

FIGURE 27.20 Focal area of singed lashes and lid erythema (arrow) in patient soon after a lighted matchhead flew into his eye.

counteract the potentially devastating outcomes of severe involvements.[114] For severe alkali burns, several agents have been studied or proposed to reduce stromal ulceration and stimulate epithelial regeneration and adhesion. These agents include collagenase inhibitors, ascorbic acid, therapeutic contact lenses, anti-inflammatory agents, fibronectin, epithelial growth factors, and topical citrate.[55,115-118] A multifaceted therapeutic approach to managing an eye with a severe alkali burn may enhance the integrity of the damaged eye and the potential for a positive outcome.[55,119]

Patient education about the use of protective eyewear in circumstances when alkali injury may occur is very important and may help to prevent future injury.

Mild Thermal Burns

ETIOLOGY

The cornea may be exposed to thermal burns from a variety of sources. The nature of the resultant injury will be determined by the form and temperature of the causative agent. Common causes of mild epithelial thermal burns include heated particles or objects—such as cinders, match heads, boiling fluids, firecracker particles, lit ends of cigars and cigarettes, and curling irons—that momentarily come into contact with the cornea.[120,121] Steam may cause corneal thermal burns, as has been reported following preparation of microwave popcorn.[122] Hot objects or liquid, such as molten metal or glass, that continue to radiate heat while in contact with the eye may cause severe corneal burns.[123] This is likely to involve the corneal stroma and result in permanent scarring. Very deep thermal burns may result in corneal perforation.[80] Lid and facial thermal burns may also accompany the ocular findings. In a study of 59 patients (66 eyes), Vajpayee and associates[121] found that 90% of corneal thermal burns were caused by domestic incidents and 10% by industrial accidents.

DIAGNOSIS

Typically, the patient will report the source of the thermal burn. Patient symptomatology may range from mild to severe, depending on the extent of the burn. Symptoms commonly include ocular pain, burning, redness, tearing, and photophobia.

External examination may reveal eyelid and facial skin thermal burn involvement, including lash and brow singeing, depending on the nature of the injury (Fig. 27.20). Slit-lamp examination will reveal varying degrees of bulbar conjunctival injection. A superficial epithelial corneal burn will appear as a focal, milky, gray-white coagulation of tissue which will tend to slough (eschar), often within the palpebral fissure (Fig. 27.21). Deeper, more severe corneal burns will reveal stromal involvement, which also may be

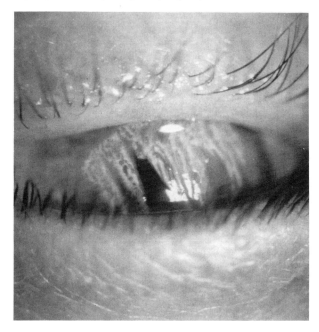

FIGURE 27.21 Corneal eschar in patient who sustained a thermal burn from a curling iron. Visual acuity was 20/100. (Courtesy James L. Dixon, O.D.)

due to an associated mechanical component to the injury.[121] Particulate debris from ashes or cinders may be evident in the globe and lid areas.

MANAGEMENT

Re-epithelialization of small areas of corneal eschar occurs readily, and is similar to the healing of a small corneal abrasion. In this instance, it is appropriate to use topical antibiotic prophylaxis therapy for a few days to protect the cornea from infection while it heals—for example, 0.3% tobramycin or polymyxin B-trimethoprim drops 4 times a day and polymyxin B-bacitracin ointment instilled into the con- junctival sac at bedtime. For larger corneal epithelial thermal burns, it is appropriate to debride the coagulated epithelium using a sterile cotton-tipped applicator (see Fig. 27.4). The lesion is then treated like a corneal abrasion, including pupil- lary dilation and cycloplegia with a long–acting agent, such as 5% homatropine, and pressure-patching for 24 hours with a broad-spectrum antibiotic ointment, such as polymyxin B- bacitracin. Continue supportive treatment of the epithelial thermal burn until healing is complete (Fig. 27.22).

Deep stromal thermal burns or burns causing corneal perforation require prompt intervention by a corneal special- ist. In the case of widespread thermal injury, eyelid and conjunctival damage may be extensive enough to result in

symblepharon, with the need for reconstructive surgical intervention. Severe facial burns also may require immedi- ate medical intervention.

The patient should be counseled as to the advisability of using protective eyewear when the risk of ocular thermal injury is high.

Ultraviolet Radiation Burns

ETIOLOGY

The most common type of radiation burn sustained by the cornea is that resulting from excessive exposure to ultravio- let (UV) light. The most common sources of excessive UV light exposure include sunburn, sunlamps, reflection of sun- light off snow without protective sunwear (''snow blind- ness''), and exposure to an electric welding arc without filter protection. An irritative keratoconjunctivitis may result, and the onset of ocular symptoms usually occurs approximately 6 to 12 hours after excessive UV light exposure.[110]

DIAGNOSIS

The patient with UV keratoconjunctivitis typically will report a recent history of excessive UV light exposure. When the cause is related to excessive sunlight or sunlamp exposure,

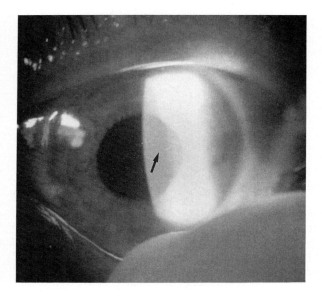

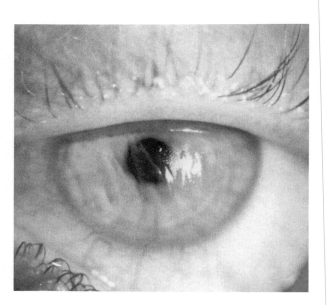

FIGURE 27.22 (A) Following debridement of the corneal eschar in the patient illustrated in Figure 27.21, the visual acuity improved to 20/25. Note the irregular corneal light reflex. Following instillation of 5% homatropine and gentamicin ointment, the patient was pressure patched. (B) Upon removal of the pressure patch 24 hours later, epithelial fusion lines are noted from the advancing sheets of healing epithelium (arrow). Resolution was complete in 48 hours. (Courtesy James L. Dixon, O.D.)

A   B

the patient generally will exhibit the dermatologic manifestations of sunburn on the face or other skin areas, including
erythema and blistering if severe. Ocular symptoms include
pain, photophobia, tearing, and blepharospasm.

External examination reveals erythema and swelling of
the affected skin areas. Slit-lamp examination reveals diffuse conjunctival injection and punctate epithelial erosions
of the cornea with corresponding fluorescein sodium staining. If the epithelial lesions are extensive and if lacrimation
is profuse, corneal edema also may be noted.

MANAGEMENT

As with any superficial keratitis, the corneal lesions related
to excessive UV radiation will generally resolve within a
few days. Supportive therapy for mild cases may include
topical lubricating agents only, including drops during the
day and ointment at bedtime. As with any sunburn, cold
compresses applied to the eyes 3 to 4 times daily also may
provide some symptomatic relief.

Broad-spectrum antibiotic drops, such as polymyxin
B-trimethoprim, may be instilled four times daily to prevent
secondary infection as the epithelium heals. A broad-
spectrum ophthalmic ointment, such as polymyxin
B-bacitracin, may be instilled into the conjunctival sac at
bedtime for prophylaxis. In more pronounced cases, pupillary
dilation and cycloplegia with a long-acting agent such as 5%
homatropine may help to relieve pain from associated ciliary
spasm.

Anecdotal clinical evidence suggests that some burning
pain associated with UV radiation keratitis may last for days
to weeks, even after complete resolution of the keratitis.
Patients should be advised of the value of protective
eyewear to prevent UV radiation keratoconjunctivitis, including appropriate filters for occupational/industrial use, as
well as appropriate sunwear for outdoor use that includes
UV light-blocking capability.

Bacterial and Bacterial-Related Keratitis

Superficial Punctate Keratitis

ETIOLOGY

Superficial punctate keratitis (SPK) with a bacterial origin
usually is associated with blepharitis, the most common
cause of which is an infection of the lid margins and glands
with *Staphylococcus*. Conjunctivitis from organisms such as
Streptococcus, *Moraxella*, and *Haemophilus* also may cause
superficial punctate keratitis.

DIAGNOSIS

Patients with SPK typically report a foreign body sensation,
photophobia, redness, and tearing of the eyes. Patients with
an associated blepharitis may also complain of debris on the
lids and redness of their lid margins. Usually, the patient will
report previous episodes, characterized by exacerbations and
remissions. If there is an associated conjunctivitis, the patient
typically will report an acute recent onset of discharge from
the eye and difficulty opening the lids in the morning.

Examination typically reveals diffuse superficial punctate
epithelial erosions (PEES), focal areas of epithelial disruption that stain well with fluorescein sodium.[124] Examination
also may reveal punctate epithelial keratopathy (PEK) that is
visible without dyes as small, grayish opacities in the epithelium.[17] PEKs stain poorly with fluorescein but stain well
with rose bengal.[124,125] The location and appearance of this
keratitis can be helpful in determining its cause. SPK from
blepharitis usually is more severe in the inferior one-third of
the cornea where it contacts the staphylococcal exotoxins
from infection of the lower lid. In cases of SPK caused by
bacterial conjunctivitis, the entire cornea may be involved.
Associated findings also help determine the cause. In
blepharitis the lid margins usually are thickened, red, and
scaly. Lashes also may be missing (madarosis). With conjunctivitis there is infection of the conjunctiva and a mucopurulent discharge.

MANAGEMENT

Treatment of SPK is directed toward the underlying infectious cause. Conjunctivitis should be treated with topical
antibiotics (see Chap. 26), and blepharitis should be treated
with lid hygiene and antibiotics (see Chap. 24). Additional
supportive treatment to reduce symptomatology caused by
SPK may include the use of artificial tears 4 to 6 times daily.

Marginal Infiltrative Keratitis

ETIOLOGY

Marginal infiltrative keratitis is known by many names,
including toxic keratitis, hypersensitivity keratitis, immune
keratitis, and marginal ulcers. *Marginal ulcer* is a commonly
used but less-preferred term because these infiltrates are not
due to corneal infection, but rather are caused by an antigen-
antibody reaction. Gram and Giemsa stains of corneal scrapings from these areas show neutrophils but no bacteria.
Although marginal infiltrative keratitis usually stems from
long-standing staphylococcal blepharoconjunctivitis, it also
occurs in acute conjunctivitis caused by beta-hemolytic
Streptococcus, *Haemophilus aegyptius*, and *Moraxella
lacunata*.[126] This condition also has been reported in association with chronic dacryocystitis.[127]

DIAGNOSIS

Patients with marginal infiltrative keratitis complain of pain,
tearing, foreign body sensation, and photophobia. When

asked, they typically report a history of staphylococcal lid disease. Marginal infiltrative keratitis is common in adults but is quite rare in children.[128]

Examination with the biomicroscope reveals single or multiple intraepithelial infiltrates separated from the limbus by a clear (lucid) interval (Fig. 27.23). This lucid area is about 2 mm wide and can be bridged by vessels. The infiltrates are usually between 0.5 mm and 1.5 mm in size and are most commonly found at the 2, 4, 8, and 10 o'clock positions where the lid margins cross the cornea.[128] Early in the process the infiltrate is elevated due to the accumulation of cells and debris. The infiltrate can become ulcerated and exhibit positive superficial staining in the center. Edema can develop around the infiltrates. Although this edema usually is limited to the epithelium, it also can be found in the anterior stroma. As the eye becomes more involved, the infiltrates can become more extensive. The spread of lesions usually is concentric with the limbus.[128] making it possible for the individual infiltrates to coalesce and form a ring-like infiltrate around the entire cornea.

Rarely, patients develop true "sterile ulcers" due to exotoxins causing tissue destruction and loss. Unlike marginal infiltrates, these appear as pale gray depressions with fuzzy edges. They are usually 1 mm to 2 mm in diameter and stain deeply with fluorescein because of the loss of stromal substance. Patients with true sterile ulcers also have intense symptoms and an anterior chamber reaction.

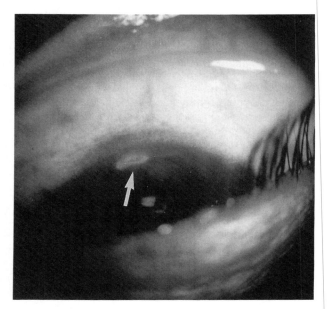

FIGURE 27.23 Marginal infiltrate (arrow). Note the lucid interval between the infiltrate and limbus.

MANAGEMENT

It is important to differentiate between true infection of the corneal tissue and marginal keratitis. The examiner must look for signs and symptoms of bacterial corneal ulcers and evaluate the patient's history for risk factors known to be associated with infectious keratitis. These risk factors include extended wear of contact lenses, contaminated ophthalmic solutions, poor personal hygiene, diabetes mellitus, recent or concurrent use of ocular steroids, a compromised immune system, recent ocular surgery, dry eyes, and epithelial damage.[120]

If marginal infiltrative keratitis is diagnosed and the patient has signs of blepharitis, treatment should be aimed at resolving the blepharitis. This includes warm compresses and lid scrubs 3 to 4 times a day, along with the application of a topical antibiotic ointment such as bacitracin or erythromycin (see Chap. 24). Antibiotic drops such as gentamicin may be administered 4 times a day, primarily for prophylaxis. Topical 1% prednisolone acetate also may be used 4 times a day to reduce inflammation and aid resolution of the infiltrates. For severe symptoms, administer a cycloplegic agent, such as 5% homatropine, 2 times a day. These patients should be re-examined in 2 to 3 days and should exhibit definite improvement in the signs and symptoms. The topical steroid should be tapered, with the goal of discontinuing the drug in about two weeks.

If there is true corneal ulceration and a definitive diagnosis between sterile ulcers and infectious keratitis cannot be made, obtain corneal cultures before starting any antibiotic or steroid therapy. If multiple risk factors are present, treat the ulcer as an infectious keratitis (see page 704). If there are no risk factors, Catania[120] suggests initiating treatment with a cycloplegic, such as 5% homatropine followed by 5 drops of 0.3% tobramycin in 5 minutes as a loading dose. The patient should then use three drops of 0.3% tobramycin every hour for the next 24 hours except during sleep, when three drops should be used every 2 hours.[120] The patient should be re-evaluated within 24 hours to assess any changes in corneal health.

Phlyctenulosis

ETIOLOGY

A phlyctenule is a round, focal nodule composed of leukocytes, and generally is the result of an allergic reaction to microbes or their toxins. For the allergic response to occur, the patient must have a history of previous exposure and sensitization to the causative organism or allergen. Reintroduction of the allergen causes development of the phlyctenule approximately 48 hours later.[129]

In the United States, the most common cause of phlyctenulosis is *Staphylococcus aureus. Staphylococcus aureus* is a prevalent microbe, and its cell wall antigens have been proven to cause phlyctenulosis in rabbits.[128,130,131]

Tuberculosis (TB) is another common cause of phlyctenulosis. This is especially true among recent immigrants to the United States and in patients with acquired immune deficiency syndrome (AIDS).[132] Patients in these demographic groups who exhibit phlyctenulosis also have a high rate of positive skin and radiology tests for TB. It also is common for patients with phlyctenulosis to relate a history of recent exposure to, or family members with, known TB.

Rarely, other organisms such as pneumococcus, Koch-Weeks, *Candida albicans, Chlamydia,* and round worm nematodes have been implicated in phlyctenulosis.[128,129,133] Malnutrition, vitamin deficiency, and poor public health conditions increase the incidence of phlyctenulosis.

DIAGNOSIS

The most common symptoms of phlyctenulosis include bilateral tearing, irritation or pain, mild to severe photophobia, and itching. Symptoms may include blepharospasm and usually are more severe if there is corneal involvement. The patient may report previous similar episodes.

Slit-lamp examination reveals single or multiple phlyctenules that appear as pinkish-white nodules on the cornea or conjunctiva, ranging in size from just visible to several millimeters in diameter (Fig. 27.24). They typically appear first at the limbus, and can easily be mistaken for catarrhal ulcers. Unlike catarrhal ulcers, phlyctenules are adjacent to the limbus, and the long axis of a phlyctenule is perpendicular to the limbus rather than parallel to it.

Along with the phlyctenule, examination often reveals conjunctival hyperemia, a scanty, often watery discharge, and diffuse corneal staining. If the phlyctenule is caused by *Staphylococcus,* an associated blepharitis is common. Phlyctenules typically last from 10 to 14 days and occur primarily in children,[128] with girls more frequently affected than boys.[129]

There are two major types of phlyctenules. Conjunctival phlyctenules appear on either the bulbar or palpebral conjunctiva in rows. They often are surrounded by hyperemia and are located near the free lid margin. Corneal phlyctenules typically start at the limbus accompanied by a leash of conjunctival vessels. These phlyctenules can progress toward the center of the cornea as the more peripheral margin heals and the central area remains active. The vessels associated with the phlyctenule also migrate toward the center of the cornea and produce focal neovascularization. Triangular corneal scars with their base at the limbus often form as phlyctenules heal. Scarring in the central cornea can decrease visual acuity if the phlyctenulosis is long-standing.[134]

MANAGEMENT

Thorough examination is important to determine the cause of phlyctenulosis. Inspect the lid margins for signs of staphylococcal blepharitis, and question the patient about any recent infections or TB exposure. If there is any reason to

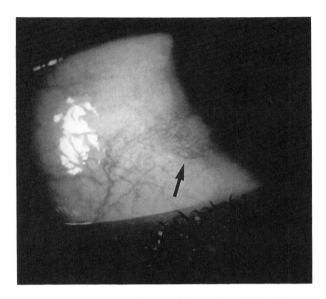

FIGURE 27.24   **Phlyctenule (arrow) in 13-year-old female.**

suspect TB, or if no other cause can be found, a tuberculin skin test may be indicated. If diarrhea or gastrointestinal distress is present, consider a stool examination for nematodes.

Although phlyctenules can resolve spontaneously, they usually ulcerate and scar prior to resolution. To prevent scarring, treatment should include 1% prednisolone acetate, one drop every 2 to 4 hours for 3 to 4 days. Also, instill prophylactic antibiotic ointment or drops, such as bacitracin, erythromycin, or gentamicin, into the conjunctival sac four times a day and continue as long as the steroid is used. The steroid should be tapered rapidly once improvement is noted—total antibiotic/steroid therapy generally lasts 10 to 14 days. If *Staphylococcus* is suspected, recommend warm compresses and lid scrubs 2 to 3 times a day followed by an application of antibiotic ointment, such as bacitracin, to the lid margins. Because many cases of staphylococcal blepharitis are chronic, lid scrubs with baby shampoo or commercial preparations may be necessary each day indefinitely. Vasoconstrictors or artificial tears can be used up to four times a day for comfort, and cycloplegic agents can be used to decrease photophobia or pain.[135] Culbertson and associates[136] studied the medical records of 17 patients aged 5 to 18 years with chronic or recurrent phlyctenular keratoconjunctivitis and noted long-lasting remission of this condition after a course of oral tetracycline or erythromycin.

Patients with phlyctenulosis should be re-evaluated in 3 to 4 days. Significant improvement in signs and symptoms should occur within 48 hours. If the tuberculin skin test is positive, chest x-rays and a medical consultation are indicated.

Bacterial Ulcers

ETIOLOGY

Bacterial ulcers are most often found in eyes made susceptible to infection by pre-existing conditions. There are many predisposing risk factors, and their incidence in patients with bacterial ulcers varies over time and from region to region in the United States. In a recent study[137] evaluating the incidence of ulcerative keratitis in Olmsted County, Minnesota, from 1950 through 1988, the most common predisposing factor was contact lens wear, which occurred in 40% of the patients. Trauma was the second most commonly associated factor, found in 18% of the patients. When evaluated by time periods, trauma was found to be a more common predisposing factor in the 1950s through the 1970s, with contact lens wear becoming the primary factor in the 1980s.[137] A 1983 study[138] performed in Michigan showed surgical and nonsurgical trauma to be the most common predisposing factor leading to bacterial keratitis, with 49% of the patients reporting a positive recent history of trauma. Contact lens wear was reported in only 11% of this study population.[138] Other reported predisposing factors include a history of herpes simplex virus, dry eye,[138] AIDS,[139] steroid use, and malnutrition. One study[140] found alcoholism as a risk factor in 72 of 227 patients with corneal ulcers. Any condition that causes epithelial damage, such as bullous keratopathy, recurrent corneal erosion, eyelid abnormalities, and neurotrophic keratitis, may increase the risk of infectious corneal ulcers. The use of prophylactic antibiotics can cause corneal ulcers due to an overgrowth of resistant bacteria.[141,142]

In one study[143] that evaluated risk factors in children, nonsurgical trauma was found in 44% of the cases, prior corneal surgery in 24%, and systemic illness in 14%. Males were more likely to have corneal ulceration than females.

Corneal ulcers seem to be bimodal in occurrence, with the highest incidence in patients in their twenties and those in their sixties to seventies.[137,138] This pattern probably is due to the increased incidence of trauma in the younger group, and pre-existing corneal damage in the older group.

The type of bacteria isolated from corneal ulcers is determined by several issues, including the presence of predisposing factors, the examiner's technique and media used for isolation and culture, patient age, and the patient's geographical location. *Pseudomonas aeruginosa* will penetrate an intact cornea and is isolated from 8% to 32% of corneal ulcers.[138,144–147] In contact lens wearers, however, the incidence of *Pseudomonas aeruginosa* isolate increases, accounting for as many as 62% to 64% of cases.[144,148,149] Asbell and Stenson[145] studied 677 cases over 30 years in New York and found an 8% incidence of *Pseudomonas aeruginosa*. Liesegang and Forster[146] studied 238 cases in Florida and found *Pseudomonas aeruginosa* in 31% of all infections, making it the most common cause of bacterial ulcers in their study.

Staphylococcus aureus also is a frequent isolate from bacterial corneal ulcers, ranging from 14% to 33% of all cases.[138,144,145,147,150] Bacterial corneal ulcers caused by *Staphylococcus aureus* typically occur in eyes that were previously compromised. Other common causes of bacterial corneal ulceration include *Moraxella*,[144,145] *Streptococcus pneumoniae*,[144,145,147] alpha-hemolytic *Streptococcus*,[147] *Staphylococcus epidermidis*,[144,145,147,150] *Klebsiella, Proteus* and *Serratia*.[146] The main isolates in children are *Pseudomonas* in 34%, *Staphylococcus aureus* in 20%, and fungi in 18%.[143]

Many organisms once considered to be normal flora are now being viewed as possible ocular pathogens. Some examples are *Staphylococcus epidermidis, Diphtheroids*[151] and *Mycobacterium* species.[152]

The clinical appearance of bacterial corneal ulcers is similar irrespective of the causative organism, and laboratory studies are needed to make a definitive diagnosis. It can be useful, however, to evaluate the clinical appearance of a corneal ulcer as an aid in choosing the initial antibiotic. In general, ulcers caused by gram-negative organisms are diffuse, gray-white, and have a "wet" or "soupy" appearance. The central cornea often is involved and the ulcer spreads rapidly. Gram-positive organisms cause more discrete, round, or oval ulcers. These are also gray-white but are "drier" in appearance. Some of the gram-positive organisms can cause a severe anterior chamber reaction.

Staphylococci are gram-positive cocci that tend to be cultured easily. An ulcer caused by Staphylococci tends to be centrally located, round or oval in shape, with a yellow-white, well demarcated infiltrate directly beneath it. Typically superficial at the start, the ulcer generally remains indolent with minimal anterior chamber reaction. If left untreated, stromal edema, multiple small satellite infiltrates, and perforation are possible. Response to treatment is rapid for *Staphylococcus epidermidis,* with improvement expected in the first 24 to 48 hours of treatment. *Staphylococcus aureus* is less rapid in its response to treatment and will often show no change in the first 48 hours.[153]

Streptococcus pneumoniae is a gram-positive, lancet-shaped organism that causes a rapidly progressing, gray-yellow, disc-shaped ulcer. It commonly spreads by "creeping" toward the center of the cornea, and the advancing edge usually has an over-hanging margin (serpiginous ulcer). Corneal perforation is common if left untreated, and a sterile hypopyon is characteristic of *Streptococcus pneumoniae.*

Alpha-hemolytic *Streptococcus* usually occurs in patients who are immunosuppressed, and typically produces a gray-white, well-circumscribed, "dry" looking epithelial defect. This ulcer is slow to progress, has a minimal to moderate anterior chamber reaction, and responds rapidly to antibiotics.

An unusual crystalline keratitis is reported to be caused by nutritional variant Streptococci. The keratitis presents as a branching pattern that looks like cracked glass, needles, snowflakes or ferns in the corneal stroma. It is covered by an intact epithelium and has minimal intraocular inflammation. With time, the crystalline infiltrate may coalesce into a homogeneous infiltrate. This unusual presentation is known as infectious crystalline keratopathy (ICK), and often is found after penetrating keratoplasty with topical steroid treatment. Although it progresses slowly, it responds poorly to treatment with antibiotics.[154]

Pseudomonas aeruginosa is common in the environment and may contaminate make-up or contact lens solutions. As previously noted, it is the most common cause of bacterial corneal ulcers in contact lens wearers.[148,149] It also is commonly found in patients with corneal injury or extensive body burns. Patients receiving respiratory assistance are prone to develop *Pseudomonas aeruginosa* corneal ulcers because the organism frequently colonizes humidifiers.[145]

Pseudomonas is cultured easily and appears as a gram-negative rod in smears. The corneal ulcer appears as a central, gray infiltrate with an overlying epithelial defect. It progresses very rapidly over a large area of the cornea and can cause corneal perforation within 24 to 48 hours.[155] The area adjacent to the ulcer usually has a hazy appearance due to edema, which causes a "soupy" appearance. Hypopyon is common, as is a yellow-green discharge that fluoresces in cobalt blue light. *Pseudomonas* corneal ulcers often are difficult to treat. Resistant strains are common, and even if treatment is effective, the ulcer often appears worse in the first 24 to 48 hours after the initiation of therapy.[144,153] This is in part due to toxins that continue to destroy stromal and epithelial tissue after live bacteria are no longer present.

Moraxella is more commonly found in hot, dry areas and can cause angular blepharitis and conjunctivitis. It is most commonly found as the cause of corneal ulcers in alcoholic, malnourished, or debilitated patients,[145,156,157] or in patients who are immunosuppressed. The prevalence of *Moraxella* infection seems to be decreasing in recent years.[145]

Moraxella is a gram-negative diplobacillus that can appear to be gram-positive and can be difficult to culture. One of the significant findings with this ulcer is that it is often painless.[156] It tends to start in the central or inferior areas of exposed corneas and appears as a gray-white, dense, anterior stromal abscess.[156] The epithelial defect is well delineated and deeply invades the cornea, commonly causing perforation or a descemetocele if left untreated.[157] Hypopyon and hyphema have been reported to occur.[156,157] *Moraxella* ulcers are slow to heal,[156] respond poorly to antibiotics, and are very slow to reepithelialize. It has been suggested that there may be two types of *Moraxella* ulcers—one indolent and shallow, and the other very severe.[157]

DIAGNOSIS

Patients with corneal ulcers present with the same basic symptoms regardless of the causative agent. These include photophobia, decreased visual acuity, redness, swelling of the lids, discharge, reports of a "white spot" on the eye, and

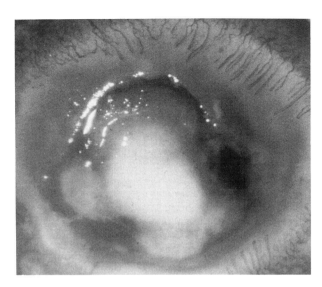

FIGURE 27.25   **Central bacterial corneal ulcer. (Courtesy Casey Eye Institute, Portland, OR)**

variable degrees of pain. Patients with ulcers caused by *Moraxella* are less likely to report pain, as are patients who have corneal hypoesthesia due to prior cataract extraction or penetrating keratoplasty. In one study,[141] 25% of the patients reported no pain, no discharge, and no visual loss with corneal ulcers that occurred after penetrating keratoplasty.

Slit-lamp examination typically reveals moderate to severe edema and inflammation of the lid and conjunctiva, a purulent discharge, and ulceration of the corneal epithelium (Fig. 27.25). As previously described, these ulcerations can take on many appearances, usually accompanied by surrounding corneal edema and stromal infiltration underneath the ulcer. A mild to severe anterior chamber reaction, which can cause hypopyon, cataracts, synechiae, and elevated intraocular pressure, also is frequently associated with corneal ulcers. Descemetoceles, perforation, and scarring have been reported.

A thorough history should be performed on all patients presenting with corneal ulcers to determine which risk factors, if any, are present. A detailed clinical examination should then be performed, including slit-lamp biomicroscopy, to evaluate the severity of the ulcer and to help determine the possible causative organism. Photodocumentation or detailed corneal diagramming of the ulcer helps to monitor resolution of the lesion.

Some authors argue that the high cost and low recovery rate of corneal cultures along with the successful treatment of most corneal ulcers with broad-spectrum antibiotics makes corneal cultures unnecessary.[158–160] Most authorities advise, however, that microbiology evaluation be performed prior to initiating treatment.[144,150,161,162] Microbiologic smear evaluation can immediately determine whether a bacterium is prevalent in the ocular tissues, and whether the organism is gram-positive or gram-negative. Cultures and sensitivity tests can later determine the actual pathogen and the antibiotics to which it is sensitive. This allows the selection of the most appropriate antibiotic and prevents overuse of ineffective antibiotics. Conservative management supports the use of corneal cultures prior to treatment, since it is very difficult to isolate organisms after initiating antibiotic therapy.

Microbiologic evaluation of a corneal ulcer is aimed at determining the causative organism and the appropriate specific treatment. Benson and Lanier[163] demonstrated that more positive cultures were obtained by using a calcium alginate swab instead of a platinum spatula and suggested the following method of obtaining corneal material for cultures. Obtain culture specimens of the conjunctiva and eyelid margins with a calcium alginate swab moistened with trypticase soy broth. Directly plate specimens onto solid blood and chocolate agar plates using an "R" and "L" pattern for the conjunctiva, and a horizontal line for the lids. Collect these specimens without anesthesia because the preservative in the anesthetic can inhibit bacterial growth. Rayon, dacron, and cotton swabs are not recommended since they also may inhibit the growth of some bacteria, although dacron has been reported to be acceptable.[164] Moistening the swab may increase the number of bacteria that are collected and released when plated.

For the second step, instill a topical anesthetic solution such as proparacaine 0.5% and use a sterile platinum spatula to obtain material from the corneal ulcer for gram and Giemsa staining. This material should be smeared onto clean glass slides, heat fixed with an alcohol lamp for gram staining and air dried for Giemsa staining, and then stained following each stain manufacturer's suggestions. gram stains are useful for determining if the most prevalent organism is gram-positive or gram-negative, but it is important to realize that the topical anesthetic can cause damage to the cell walls of gram-positive bacteria, causing them to stain more like gram-negative organisms.[161] Gram stains will correlate with culture results in approximately 65% to 77% of cases.[141,145,150] Giemsa stains are useful for determining the type of inflammatory cell present, and, more importantly in patients with corneal ulcers, can reveal fungal components.

The third step involves using a sterile platinum spatula to scrape the corneal ulcer and inoculating two blood agar plates, one chocolate agar plate and a Sabouraud's dextrose agar plate without cyclohexamide, with one row of "C's" each. Store one of the blood agar plates at 37°C. The other blood agar plate and the Sabouraud's agar are stored at 25°C to improve the chances of fungal growth. Aerobic and facultatively anaerobic bacteria, such as *Neisseria* and *Haemophilus,* are more likely to grow on the chocolate agar plate.

The next step is to rub the ulcer with a sterile calcium alginate swab moistened with trypticase soy broth and inoculate three rows of "C" on each of the blood, chocolate, and Sabouraud's plates. Place this swab in a tube of thioglycolate broth media to isolate anaerobes. A freshly moistened swab should then be rubbed across the corneal ulcer and used to reinoculate the same "C" streaks on the agar plates. This swab should then be placed in trypticase soy broth. If there are any indications that the corneal ulcer may be caused by *Acanthamoeba,* cultures also should be performed on nonnutrient agar with an *E. coli* overgrowth. Benson and Lanier[163] suggest the use of both the swab and the spatula because filamentous bacteria or fungi may be cultured more easily with the spatula.

Twenty-four to 48 hours are needed to obtain information from cultures. From 28% to 93% will be culture positive.[137,141,145,160] If a fungal ulcer is suspected, 2 to 6 weeks are necessary before the cultures should be declared negative. Some of the bacteria recently considered pathologic instead of normal flora also take longer to grow on cultures. These include *Diphtheroids,* which require one week to grow, and *Mycobacterium,* which may require as long as 8 weeks to grow on normal culture media.[151,152]

Once an organism has grown on culture, sensitivity testing can be performed to determine which antibiotics will be the most effective. The Kirby-Bauer diffusion disc system is the most commonly used method of performing sensitivity testing. This method usually takes 48 hours to perform and can be inaccurate because of the lower concentrations of antibiotic on the test discs compared to levels that can be achieved in the cornea through topical application. In addition, some topical ocular preparations are not available on discs for sensitivity testing.[161]

Other diagnostic laboratory tests are available, although they are used much less frequently. These include staining with acridine orange, which causes an orange fluorescence of bacteria, fungi, and *Acanthamoeba,* but stains human cells yellow-green. One of the major drawbacks to this staining technique is the need for a fluorescence microscope.[165]

Limulus lysate assay is available in kit form and indicates the presence of gram-negative organisms by testing for endotoxins. It is rapid, detecting even small amounts of endotoxins in 24 hours, but does not indicate which gram-negative organism is present. It is more sensitive than gram stains and may be useful when antibiotic treatment has already been started.[161]

MANAGEMENT

Treatment of bacterial corneal ulcers typically is started once laboratory testing has been performed but before the results are obtained. Initial treatment has traditionally included broad-spectrum antibiotics that were chosen based on the gram stain results, history, and clinical impression. If no organisms or multiple organisms are seen on the gram stain, or if there are risk factors that differ from the gram stain result, treatment may be initiated with cefazolin (50 mg/ml), one drop every 15 to 30 minutes, and gentamicin or tobramycin (13.6 mg/ml), one drop every 15 to 30 minutes.[144,149] If gram-positive cocci are seen, one drop of cefazolin (50 mg/ml) every 15 to 30 minutes is suggested.[144] Gram-positive rods should be treated with gentamicin (13.6 mg/ml) and penicillin (100,000 units/ml), one drop each every 15 to 30 minutes.[144] Ulcers caused by gram-negative cocci may be treated with ceftriaxone or ceftazidime, 50 mg/ml one drop every 15 to 30 minutes.[144] Gram-negative rods may be treated with gentamicin (13.6 mg/ml) or tobramycin (13.6 mg/ml), one drop every 15 to 30 minutes.[144] When initiating treatment, it is important to give a loading dose by instilling five drops of each of the suggested antibiotics, one minute apart.

Ciprofloxacin, a fluoroquinolone antibiotic, is available in an aqueous 0.3% ophthalmic solution and often is considered the drug of first choice for bacterial keratitis. It has a broad spectrum of action against mycobacteria, mycoplasmas, chlamydiae, gram-positive and gram-negative organisms.[147,166] Ciprofloxacin has been shown to be successful in treating a corneal ulcer caused by methicillin-resistant *Staphylococcus aureus,*[167] and is reported to be more effective against *Staphylococcus aureus* than are vancomycin and cefazolin.[168] It is effective against *Pseudomonas,* and one *in vitro* study has shown it to be more effective than tobramycin against this organism.[169]

Ciprofloxacin has many advantages over traditional treatment. It is available as commercially prepared 0.3% topical solution which does not need to be fortified to be effective. As a result, there is less chance of contamination and less epithelial toxicity compared to fortified drops. Ciprofloxacin's wide spectrum of activity allows the patient to use only one medication, which may increase patient compliance.

Leibowitz[147] reported that 91.9% of 148 corneal ulcers were treated successfully with ciprofloxacin compared to 88.3% with "standard treatment," which usually consisted of cefazolin (33 mg/ml) and gentamicin or tobramycin (14 mg/ml). The usual dosage of ciprofloxacin solution for the treatment of bacterial ulcers is two drops every 15 minutes for 6 hours, then two drops every 30 minutes for 18 hours, followed by two drops every hour for 24 hours. Ciprofloxacin is then used every 4 hours for the next 12 days.[147] Ciprofloxacin ointment also is effective in the treatment of bacterial keratitis.[169,170] It has the advantage of being applied every 1 to 2 hours in the first two days and then every 4 hours for the next 12 days.

When ciprofloxacin is used in either form, a white precipitate is deposited on the cornea in 16.6%[147] to 42% of patients treated with the drug.[166] This white precipitate, which is actually ciprofloxacin, usually occurs at the ulcer site from 1 to 7 days after initiating treatment. Its presence makes it more difficult to evaluate the corneal ulcer and may decrease the patient's visual acuity. Clinical anecdotal infor-

mation suggests that this decrease in visual acuity may be severe enough for alternative pharmacotherapy to be chosen in a monocular patient. Although the white precipitate resolves without adverse effect once ciprofloxacin therapy is discontinued, it may disappear spontaneously even with continued treatment. A metallic taste is noted by 5% to 36% of patients using topical ciprofloxacin,[147,166] and local burning and discomfort have also been reported.[155]

Although ciprofloxacin is a relatively new drug, some resistant organisms have already been found. These include some strains of *Staphylococcus epidermidis, Xanthomonas maltophila,*[162] anaerobic gram-positive cocci, *Clostridia, Bacteroids,* and *Streptococcus* to a variable degree.[144,166] Additional resistant bacterial strains may develop, and cultures and sensitivities are necessary to ensure that the causative organism is sensitive to ciprofloxacin. In instances in which ciprofloxacin is not effective against the causative bacterial organism, more traditional corneal ulcer therapy may be effective.[162]

A newer fluoroquinolone, ofloxacin 0.3%, has been shown to be effective in the treatment of corneal ulcers,[171] including those caused by *Pseudomonas.*[172] White corneal precipitates have not been reported in association with ofloxacin therapy.

In situations in which patient compliance is questionable, subconjunctival injections of traditional antibiotics such as cefazolin, gentamicin, and penicillin G may be necessary.[150] Some practitioners feel the risks of subconjunctival injections are outweighed by the benefit of constant and high corneal drug levels achieved by this method,[150] while others seldom use this method of drug delivery.[144] The use of corneal collagen shields as drug delivery devices can often achieve corneal antibiotic levels significantly higher than those obtained by subconjunctival injection (see Chap. 3).

Cycloplegic agents, such as homatropine 5% instilled three times a day or atropine 1% two times a day, may help decrease the anterior chamber reaction associated with bacterial corneal ulcer and decrease the patient's discomfort.

It is important to determine if hospitalization is necessary by evaluating the likelihood of corneal perforation as well as the patient's ability to comply with the frequency of drop instillation and the follow-up schedule. The patient must be examined at least daily to evaluate the size and depth of the ulcer, the degree of anterior chamber reaction, the development of satellite lesions, and the amount of pain the patient is experiencing. Ulcers caused by gram-negative organisms often appear worse in the first 24 hours following initiation of therapy, even if treatment is successfully decreasing the bacterial colony. In milder ulcers it is possible to see subtle signs of improvement after 18 to 24 hours of appropriate therapy. If the ulcer is no worse, continue the original antibiotics for at least 36 to 48 hours. If the ulcer appears worse, therapy should be changed based on the culture results, which usually are available after 48 hours. As the clinical findings and cornea are assessed, it is important to consider the potential for epithelial toxicity caused by the antibiotics.

The results from sensitivity testing can be used to alter the medication schedule, to discontinue the less effective drug if two are being administered, or to substitute equally effective medications if the patient is experiencing an adverse reaction to the original antibiotic(s).

If the ulcer appears to be responding to the antibiotic after 48 to 72 hours of treatment, the frequency of administration can be decreased to four times a day if ciprofloxacin is used, and to every 2 hours if fortified antibiotics are used. If the ulcer is not responding to treatment, the possibility of nonbacterial causes must be considered, and corneal scraping may need to be repeated. If possible, discontinue antimicrobial therapy for 24 to 48 hours prior to the scraping and culturing.

As the corneal ulcer responds to antibiotics, the frequency of instillation can be tapered slowly. Patients with ulcers caused by gram-negative rods must be tapered even more slowly. These patients may be on medications for as long as 2 to 4 weeks.[153] Patients should continue to use antibiotics for one week after resolution of the ulcer.

Prepared solutions of fortified tobramycin and cefazolin can be kept for at least four weeks. Although tobramycin can be either refrigerated or stored at room temperature, it is suggested that cefazolin be kept refrigerated. Cefazolin stored at room temperature causes an increased pH, which results in greater discomfort on instillation.[173]

The use of a collagen shield as a method for drug delivery may reduce the frequency of antibiotic instillation by maintaining a more uniform drug concentration in the eye over time. It also has been suggested that collagen shields may compete for the collagen-damaging enzymes released by *Pseudomonas*.[174] Unfortunately, collagen shields are uncomfortable and many patients do not tolerate them well.

The use of topical steroids for the treatment of bacterial corneal ulcers is controversial. Because some of the damage that occurs with bacterial corneal ulcers is inflammatory in nature, some authors believe topical steroids may be used if adequate antibacterial drugs are instilled concurrently. However, steroids should not be used until the infecting organism and the most effective antibiotic have been identified through microbiologic evaluation. Furthermore, steroids are not generally used until progressive improvement in the ulcer has been noted for 2 to 3 days. At that time prednisolone acetate 1% or dexamethasone 0.1% can be instilled 2 to 4 times a day if the infiltrate is compromising the visual axis. If steroids are used, the antibiotic must be instilled more frequently than the steroid.[144]

In a study of 40 patients, Carmichael and associates[175] reported no delay in healing of corneal ulcers with the use of dexamethasone 0.1% four times a day. Unfortunately, there also was no improvement reported in the final visual outcome. If topical steroids are used, it is important to monitor the patient very closely. Steroids will decrease the host response to bacteria, and, since sensitivity discs are not able to distinguish between bactericidal and bacteriostatic agents, it is possible for the bacteria to increase in number once steroids are started. Stern and Buttross[176] suggest that if the eye is improving without steroids, the benefits of instituting steroids may not outweigh the associated potential risks.

The use of steroids is contraindicated in eyes in which there is a threat of perforation, because the steroid will negatively affect collagen synthesis. When a penetrating keratoplasty is necessary, use steroids up to 24 hours prior to surgery to lessen postsurgical inflammation and improve the chances of success.

Ablative treatment with the excimer laser has been used successfully to treat infectious crystalline keratopathy.[177] It also was shown to be effective in rabbits infected with *Candida* 48 hours prior to treatment.[178] However, rabbit studies with keratitis from *Fusarium* or atypical mycobacterial infections have shown a high incidence of corneal perforation during this treatment, along with failure to eradicate the organism if allowed to incubate longer than 24 hours.[179]

Fungal Keratitis

Etiology

Although corneal infection can be caused by more than 100 fungal species, the primary pathogens come from two main groups. Septate filamentous organisms most commonly cause corneal ulcers and include *Fusarium*, *Aspergillus*, *Cephalosporium*, *Curvularia* and *Penicillium* species.[150] *Candida* species, another common corneal pathogen, is from the yeast group.[141]

The most common fungal isolates vary by geographic location. In the United States the septate filamentous organisms are the most common cause of fungal corneal ulcers in southern regions, while *Aspergillus* or *Candida* is most likely in northern regions.[180] Worldwide, *Aspergillus* and *Fusarium* are the leading fungal ocular pathogens.[181]

The incidence of fungal keratitis also varies by geographic location. In a nine-year study in Florida, 133/371 (35%) of culture-positive ulcers were found to be fungal in origin,[146] compared to 1% of 547 culture-positive cases in New York.[145] The incidence of fungal corneal ulcers appears to be increasing. This may be due to long-term topical steroid or antibiotic use, or to improvements in diagnosis.[141,176,182]

Patients who develop fungal keratitis frequently have a history of previous corneal trauma with vegetation such as sticks, branches, and wood. Liesegang and Forster[146] reported that 60% of 133 patients with fungal keratitis had such a history, and Clinch and associates[60] described three cases of fungal keratitis resulting from injuries associated with nylon line lawn trimmers. Extended wear of contact lenses is also a risk factor.[358] Other conditions associated with fungal keratitis, especially that caused by *Candida,* include diabetes and the chronic use of topical steroids or antibiotics.[141,183]

Diagnosis

Patients with fungal corneal ulcers present with the same basic symptoms as those with bacterial corneal ulcers. These include photophobia, decreased visual acuity, redness, swelling of the lids, discharge, and reports of a "white spot" on the eye. Pain typically is less than that expected from the clinical picture, and Harris and associates[141] reported that 59% of all cases without symptoms at presentation were caused by fungi.

Although there is no pathognomonic clinical picture of fungal ulcers, there are characteristics that aid in the correct diagnosis. The patient reports symptoms no sooner than five days after injury, and more often from 10 days to three weeks later.[184] The eye tends to react severely, even if the ulcer is superficial, including folds in Descemet's layer, ciliary flush, and an anterior chamber reaction with a large hypopyon. Filamentous fungal ulcers will appear as unifocal or multifocal infiltrates with fine feathery edges and relatively mild stromal inflammation (Fig. 27.26). Corneal yeast infections appear as unifocal or multifocal dense suppurative infiltrates.[144] The ulcer can be elevated above the corneal surface and can exhibit branching lines that radiate from the ulcer margin into the stroma. Satellite infiltrates often develop subsequent to, and in the same location as, these distinct branching lines. The formation of a dense, white, endothelial plaque and a white ring of polymorphonuclear cells in the midperiphery of the cornea are fairly common,[184] but corneal vascularization is rarely present.

Laboratory evaluation of suspected fungal ulcers should be performed in the same way as for suspected bacterial ulcers. Gram and Giemsa stains assist in the diagnosis of fungal infection by staining the fungal hyphae. Jones[150] found that gram stains positively identified fungi in 78% of ulcers that were positively cultured for fungi. Liesegang and Forster[146] found Giemsa staining to be more accurate than gram staining, correctly identifying 66% compared to 55% of positive fungal cultures, respectively.

Sabouraud's agar without cyclohexamide is one of the most reliable media for growing fungi, having 74.8% to 79% positive culture yields.[146,181] Although some fungi grow in Sabouraud's medium within 36 to 48 hours,[146,183] others can take as long as 2 to 3 weeks.[180] Thioglycolate broth is another useful medium for culturing fungi.[180]

Management

Treatment of fungal keratitis is a prolonged process, with therapy typically lasting at least 6 weeks. Due to this long-

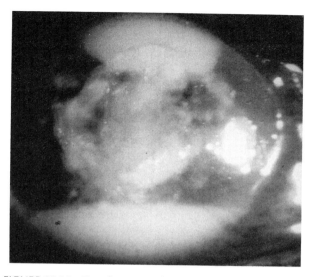

FIGURE 27.26 *Fusarium* **corneal ulcer showing dried, crusting edges. A hypopyon is present in the anterior chamber. (Courtesy J. James Rowsey, M.D.)**

term treatment and the known toxicity of antifungal drugs, treatment generally is not started unless there is microbiologic (culture or smear) support for a fungal infection.

If the smear shows a septate hyphal fragment suggestive of filamentous fungi, natamycin 5% is the drug of choice. It is generally administered topically every hour, including during sleeping hours, for several days; the dosage frequency is then gradually reduced. If natamycin is not available, amphotericin B 0.15% is the next drug of choice.[182]

Natamycin 5% is the only antifungal agent commercially available for ophthalmic use in the United States. It is a stable, relatively non-irritating suspension that must be shaken before administration. It is most effective against *Fusarium* and *Aspergillus* and much less effective against *Candida.* Its use can cause a punctate epithelial keratitis and low grade inflammation.[182]

If the smear shows the oval buds or pseudohyphae of yeast, treatment is initiated with amphotericin B 0.15% by administering one drop every 5 minutes for 1 hour, then one drop each hour.[144] Amphotericin B is insoluble in water, unstable to temperature and light, and will last one week when stored at 36°C. It must be reconstituted in an aseptic manner from powder and diluted to desired concentrations that may range from 0.05% to 1%. Higher concentrations are toxic to the cornea and cause chemosis, burning, epithelial clouding, and punctate epithelial erosions.[182] Amphotericin B is most effective against yeasts and works poorly against filamentous fungi, with the exception of *Aspergillus.* Mechanical debridement of the corneal epithelium is necessary when using either natamycin or amphotericin B because each penetrates the cornea very poorly.

If the ulcer fails to respond to amphotericin B, other anti-infective agents can be administered concurrently. Flucytosine, a drug that inhibits fungal growth, is given orally in divided doses of 150 mg/kg/day, or topically as a 1.0% solution every 15 to 30 minutes. Animal studies have shown that subconjunctival injection of rifampin, an antibiotic agent, will increase the efficacy of amphotericin B in treating *Candida albicans* keratitis.[185] In humans, successful treatment of *Candida* enophthalmitis has been reported using this combination of therapeutic agents.[186]

Topical steroids generally are contraindicated in the treatment of fungal ulcers because steroids allow the fungi to replicate more freely,[176] especially since antifungal agents are fungistatic and not fungicidal.[182]

Because fungal ulcers resolve very slowly and antifungal agents are toxic to the cornea, it can be difficult to determine clinically if the ulcer is improving. Improvement is suggested when the patient has decreased pain, the infiltrate is smaller, satellite lesions are disappearing, and the feathery margins of the ulcer are becoming more rounded. Continue therapy for at least 6 weeks, and modify treatment, if needed, primarily from the culture results.

Other antifungal agents are available for the treatment of corneal fungal ulcers but are seldom, if ever, used. Nystatin is not used because it is too toxic to the cornea and penetrates very poorly. Clotrimazole can be formulated for instillation into the eye, but it is not available in the United States. This drug has poor water solubility, is usually made with peanut oil, and is most effective against *Aspergillus* and *Candida albicans*.

Miconazole is available for intravenous use, but can be formulated for topical or subconjunctival administration. Mohan and associates[187] suggest that miconazole 1% be used every 2 hours for one week, then every 4 hours until the ulcer is healed. They report an overall treatment success rate of 64.7%. Topically applied miconazole can cause conjunctival injection and punctate epithelial erosions.[182]

Ketoconazole is a relatively new but promising antifungal drug for use against *Candida, Fusarium* and *Curvularia*. It is administered orally in doses of 300 mg/day, or topically in concentrations of 1% to 5%.[182]

Viral Keratitis

Epidemic Keratoconjunctivitis

ETIOLOGY

As its name implies, epidemic keratoconjunctivitis (EKC) is highly contagious and communicable. It is typically caused by adenoviruses, with types 8 and 19 most commonly re-

ported. Adenoviruses can cause severe epidemics and can be spread by finger-to-eye contact, medical instruments such as tonometers,[188,189] and possibly chairs, magazines, and other articles found in the practitioner's reception area. The contagious period may last as long as three weeks, and the virus is recoverable from all body secretions the first 10 days after ocular involvement occurs.[190]

It has been shown that adenovirus type 8 survives up to four days on a metal tonometer,[188] and type 19 has been recovered up to 8 days from paper and 35 days from dry plastic.[191] The incubation period from exposure to onset of symptoms is 4 to 18 days, with a mean of 10 days.[188,192,193]

DIAGNOSIS

Patients will usually present with complaints of acute onset of redness of the eye, foreign body sensation, burning, profuse tearing, lid swelling, photophobia, and lid matting, especially in the morning.[190,193] The symptoms typically are unilateral, with the second eye becoming involved over time. Due to systemic immune responses, the second eye usually is affected less severely than the first.[190]

History will often elicit an acquaintance, family member, or co-worker with similar signs or symptoms. These symptoms usually are more severe in adults.[188] Rarely, the patient will report a low-grade fever and respiratory symptoms.

Examination reveals an often marked conjunctivitis with a papillary and follicular response of the palpebral conjunctiva (Fig. 27.27). The follicles typically are worse in the inferior palpebral conjunctiva, with papillae more common in the superior.[194] Preauricular lymphadenopathy will be present in about 64% of patients at presentation[195] and lasts approximately one week.[196] Small subconjunctival hemorrhages are not an uncommon characteristic of the bulbar conjunctival reaction.

The conjunctivitis and symptoms last 7 to 16 days, with a mean between 8.6 and 10 days.[190,195] A diffuse superficial epithelial keratitis usually develops in the first week and may be caused by proliferation of live virus within the corneal epithelium. With time (approximately one week) this fine keratitis progresses to become deeper, positively staining, slightly elevated focal epithelial lesions. These epithelial lesions fade slowly, usually disappearing by 4 weeks.

Granular or fluffy subepithelial opacities typically develop under the focal epithelial lesions 11 to 15 days after the onset of symptoms (Fig. 27.28). These lesions likely represent antigen-antibody complexes that form in response to the viral antigen. Subepithelial infiltrates occur in 10% to 90% of cases depending on the serotype of the causative agent.[190,192] Severe subepithelial infiltrates may decrease the patient's visual acuity to 20/200 or worse. They may last from three months to two years, and focal permanent anterior stromal scars may result.

Additional findings in EKC can include pseudomembrane formation and corneal epithelial sloughing. Sym-

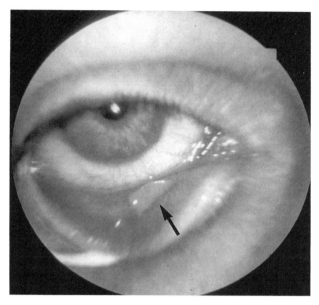

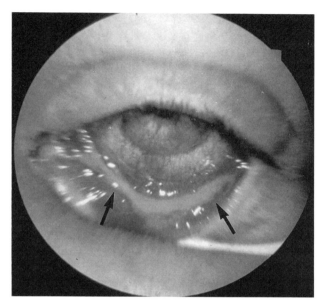

A

B

FIGURE 27.27   **Right** *(A)* **and left** *(B)* **eyes of patient with EKC. As is typically the case, the initially involved (left) eye shows a more dramatic presentation compared to the secondly involved eye. Pseudomembranes (arrows) are noted in both inferior palpebral conjunctivae.**

blepharon,[197] scleritis, and anterior uveitis rarely develop.[190] Nasolacrimal system obstruction due to inflammation or adhesion of opposing surfaces, as occurs in symblepharon formation, also is a rare complication.[194]

MANAGEMENT

Treatment of EKC is primarily supportive. It is very important to inform the patient of the expected course of the disease, including the likelihood that the symptoms will increase in severity for several days and then spontaneously resolve in 2 to 4 weeks. Artificial tears or lubricants, topical ophthalmic decongestants, and cold compresses may be used for symptomatic relief. Cleaning the lids and lashes of mucus and the use of analgesics and sunglasses also may increase patient comfort.

It is equally important to warn the patient of the contagious nature of EKC. Instruct the patient of the need to wash his or her hands frequently, to use separate towels and soap,[195] to dispose of facial tissues, and to avoid direct contact with others. It may be necessary to instruct the patient to remain at home for up to two weeks after the onset of symptoms. To avoid spreading EKC to other patients and staff members in the practitioner's office, it is important to minimize the number of return visits, isolate affected patients from others by using a single room for examining these patients when possible,[192] and cleansing or disinfecting one's hands and instruments carefully between each patient.

The use of topical ophthalmic steroids is not recommended by most authors as a general course, but may be necessary if central infiltrates are affecting visual acuity or if signs and symptoms are particularly severe. If steroids are used, the formation of subepithelial infiltrates may be suppressed, but they usually reappear when the steroids are discontinued.[198] When used, milder potency steroids generally are chosen and tapered slowly.

The use of topical ophthalmic antiviral agents, such as idoxuridine and adenine arabinoside, generally has been found ineffective in the treatment of EKC.[189,199–201] However, 1% trifluridine has been shown to decrease replication of adenovirus types 8, 13 and 19 *in vitro,* with types 13 and 19 being affected most.[202] Kana[203] reported seven cases of subepithelial infiltrates of greater than one year in duration that responded to the use of trifluridine, but no systematic controlled studies have been undertaken. Ward and associates[190] compared dexamethasone, trifluridine, and artificial tears, each administered five times a day until resolution of the signs and symptoms. Each of the drugs was tapered and discontinued within three weeks. No statistically significant differences were found in the duration or severity of the keratoconjunctivitis, but the outbreak studied was fairly mild with few subepithelial infiltrates.

Pharyngoconjunctival fever (PCF) and acute hemor-

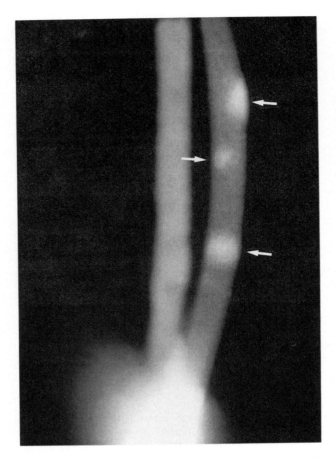

FIGURE 27.28   **Subepithelial infiltrates (arrows) in patient with EKC.**

rhagic conjunctivitis (AHC) are similar to EKC in presentation except for a recent history of upper respiratory problems and fever in PCF, and development of large subconjunctival hemorrhages in AHC. The cornea typically is less involved in each of these conditions, but they are treated in the same manner as EKC (see Chap. 26).

Thygeson's Superficial Punctate Keratitis

ETIOLOGY

Although the exact etiology of Thygeson's superficial punctate keratitis (Thygeson's SPK) is unknown, it is suggested that it may be due to chronic subclinical viral infection in the deep layers of the basal epithelium.[204] Support for this theory includes the protracted course of this condition, its tendency to recur, the lack of effect by antibiotics on its clinical course, and lack of bacterial isolation from eyes affected by

the condition. The clinical presentation of corneal mononuclear cell infiltrates,[205] the rapid resolution of these infiltrates with use of topical steroids, and their rapid reappearance if topical steroids are stopped too quickly support the possibility that the primary presentation is that of a typical immunologic response.[204] Lemp and associates[206] believe that the remissions and exacerbations characteristic of Thygeson's SPK suggest a latent type of infection.

Herpes zoster or a similar virus has been suggested as the most likely cause of this condition.[204,206] Attempts have been made to culture virus from corneas affected by Thygeson's SPK with variable results. Lemp and associates[206] isolated varicella zoster virus from a 10-year-old patient with Thygeson's by using a cotton-tipped swab without anesthetic. The swab was swirled in viral inoculating broth, which was directly inoculated to five cell lines. No growth was found on any of the cell lines, including human embryonic kidney, except Hep-2.

Braley and Alexander[207] obtained daily scrapings of the cornea from a patient with Thygeson's SPK. They cultured these scrapings and found virus only in the tissue culture from the second and fifth days. These cultures produced a clinical response similar to Thygeson's SPK when placed on abraded rabbit corneas. Braley and Alexander also checked the serum titer of the patient to the isolated virus and found that the serum titer was increased during remission. Inoculations with the attenuated virus in seven patients resulted in two developing an increased serum titer and decreased disease. Unfortunately, the virus was lost in a laboratory accident.[207] Braley and Alexander's case included superior conjunctival hyperemia, which Thygeson originally reported to be part of Thygeson's SPK but later felt represented mild cases of superior limbic keratoconjunctivitis.[208]

Tabbara and associates[205] were unable to isolate virus from any of 10 patients. Their methods included the use of anesthetic, freezing the medium before inoculation, and use of human embryonic kidney cells as the growth medium even though Lemp and associates' isolate had not grown on that medium.

As Lemp and associates[206] point out, herpes zoster virus is recoverable from skin lesions only for the first several days in varicella zoster, and spread of the virus from deeper ganglia is only a sporadic event. This decreases the chances of obtaining a positive culture. It also is important to note that a positive culture does not prove the etiology of the disease.

Hardten and associates[209] reported two cases of Thygeson's SPK that developed 9 months and 10 days, respectively, after being treated for follicular conjunctivitis secondary to *Chlamydia trachomatis*. Both patients were treated with oral medications effective against *Chlamydia*. These authors felt that in some patients the appearance of Thygeson's may be an immune response due to prior chlamydial infection in which the TRIC agent persisted in the epithelial cells.[209] Except for these cases, no associated systemic disease or allergy history has been reported.

Most authors have reported no gender or age predilection except van Bijsterveld and associates,[211] who reported a higher incidence in women than men. The age of onset ranges from 2.5 years to 70 years,[205] with a mean in the 20's.[205,211]

Examination of these patients reveals multiple gray-white, coarse, granular, intraepithelial lesions (Fig. 27.29).[208] Subepithelial opacities, which may be caused by edema, also may be seen, and patients with a history of idoxuridine use often will have more obvious infiltrates.[205] The intraepithelial lesions are of variable size and may number between 12 and 20.[205,214] They are more numerous in the pupillary zone and appear as stellate, round, or oval areas made up of smaller punctate opacities (Fig. 27.30).

The lesions stain variably with fluorescein sodium, but appear to be slightly raised (Fig. 27.31).[205,208,210,212] They come and go, and change locations quickly. The eye usually

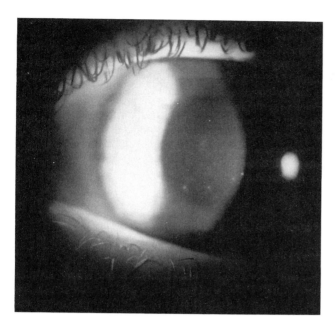

FIGURE 27.29 **Scattered central epithelial infiltrates in patient with Thygeson's superficial punctate keratitis.**

DIAGNOSIS

When Thygeson described this condition in 1961, he noted that the disease was chronic, bilateral, and had a long duration with exacerbations and remissions. Also noted was the typical punctate epithelial keratitis that showed no response to antibiotics or epithelial debridement, a rapid response to very low doses of steroids, and eventual healing without scars.[210] These features, with few variations, are still characteristic of the disease today. Although the disease is bilateral in 96% of patients, there are reports of unilateral cases.[205,211,212]

The duration of the disease is quite long, lasting weeks to years. Thygeson[213] initially reported a duration of 6 months to 4 years. In contrast, the average duration reported by van Bijsterveld and associates[211] was 2.5 years, with one patient still affected after 32 years. The average found by Tabbara and associates[205] was 3.5 years with a range of 1 month to 24 years. The possibility that the use of topical ophthalmic steroids may be increasing the duration of the disease has been suggested by several authors.[204,205,209]

Patients with Thygeson's SPK usually report an insidious onset of symptoms such as foreign body sensation, tearing, photophobia, slightly decreased vision, burning, and itching. These symptoms are primarily the result of epithelial disruption, with decreased vision occurring due to infiltrates on the visual axis and irregularity of the corneal surface. Rafieetary and associates[212] reported a case without symptoms.

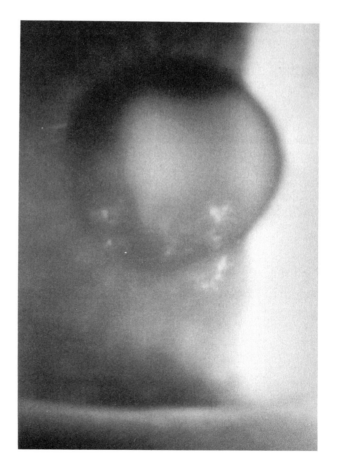

FIGURE 27.30 **Higher magnification view of epithelial infiltrates in Thygeson's SPK illustrates their granular nature.**

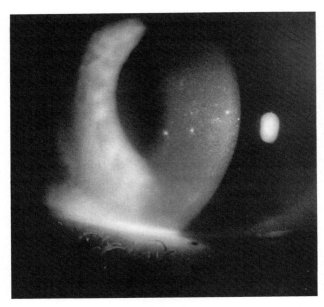

FIGURE 27.31 **Instillation of fluorescein sodium in the patient illustrated in Figure 27.29 illustrates the positive staining of these epithelial infiltrates.**

is white with little, if any, accompanying conjunctivitis.[210] Corneal sensitivity may be reduced[208,214] or normal.[205,210,211]

The differential diagnoses of Thygeson's SPK include viral, toxic, bacterial, chlamydial, exposure and dry eye causes of punctate epithelial keratopathy. Most of these will resolve in shorter time periods and will be found to have a more obvious conjunctivitis.

MANAGEMENT

Mild cases of Thygeson's SPK can be treated with artificial tears 4 to 8 times a day and lubricating ointment at bedtime for symptomatic relief. It is important to counsel the patient regarding the chronic nature of the disease.

Moderate to severe cases may require topical steroids for relief of symptoms. A mild steroid such as 0.12% prednisolone or 0.1% fluorometholone should be used four times a day for one week and then tapered slowly. The use of steroids has been found to control exacerbations in about 50% of cases.[205]

Although idoxuridine has been shown to cause long-lasting subepithelial opacities in patients with Thygeson's,[205,208,211,213] 1% trifluridine solution used 8 to 10 times per day for 14 days and then tapered, decreased symptoms in 5 of 6 treated eyes with long-standing disease.[204] Nesburn and associates[204] noted that trifluridine did not produce as rapid or dramatic a resolution of Thygeson's

SPK as steroids, but the symptoms disappeared in 2 to 3 weeks and the lesions in 2 to 3 months.

Soft contact lenses may also be used to increase comfort, but they can be responsible for inducing exacerbations.[205,211,215–217] Contact lenses generally improve symptoms by covering nerves and exposed epithelium and by improving the optical characteristics of the eye. The lenses need to be worn every day, and patients wearing them should be monitored closely for contact lens-induced problems.

Patients experiencing exacerbations of Thygeson's SPK may be followed weekly while undergoing therapy. Patients in remission may be followed every 3 to 12 months.

Herpes Simplex Keratitis

ETIOLOGY

Humans are the only natural host to the herpes simplex viruses (HSV),[218] and more than 80% of the population carries systemic antibodies to them.[219] The primary, or initial, HSV infection usually occurs by the age of five years[220] and often goes unnoticed or is too mild for the parent to seek medical attention for the child. After the primary infection, the virus settles into the central nervous system and localizes in the nerve ganglia. From there it can be reactivated by many factors, including UV exposure, trauma, stress, extreme temperatures, steroid use, and menstruation. When activated, the virus travels along the sensory nerve to the peripheral tissue to cause recurrent HSV infection.

Herpes simplex infections are caused by two strains of virus. Typically, but not universally, HSV type 1 infects tissue above the waist and includes the oral and ocular area. It is transmitted by kissing or other close contact with individuals who are shedding the virus in active lesions. The virus remains latent in the trigeminal nerve, may remain in the cornea,[221,222,223] and has been reported in tears.[224]

HSV type 2 usually infects the genital areas and is transmitted sexually, but it can be the cause of ocular infection if transmitted to the eye via infected genital secretions. This most commonly occurs in neonates who are exposed to the virus in the birth canal. In neonates, herpes simplex can cause a fatal systemic infection.

An estimated 300,000 to 500,000 cases of primary and recurrent HSV infections develop each year.[224] Herpes simplex keratitis (HSK) is one of the most common infectious causes of blindness, second only to trauma as a cause of corneal blindness in the United States. Recurrent HSK occurs through HSV reactivation by mechanical, chemical, or photochemical injuries or stimulation, and by immunosuppressive therapy. It has been reported in patients who have had penetrating keratoplasty, radial keratotomy, or have been treated with excimer lasers.[218,225]

Most herpes simplex keratitis in adults is caused by HSV type 1, but there is one reported case of simultaneous ocular infection with both type 1 and type 2 in a patient with AIDS.[226]

DIAGNOSIS

Pain, photophobia, and decreased vision are symptoms reported by patients with either primary or secondary infection,[226] but primary HSV ocular infection usually has very mild symptoms. The patient with primary infection often has signs and symptoms similar to an upper respiratory infection, including mild rhinitis, pharyngitis, fever, and malaise with a generalized skin rash.[227] A vesicular blepharitis, especially on the lower lid (see Chap. 24),[228] or an acute follicular conjunctivitis occurs in approximately 54% of patients with primary HSV infection.[229] Although the preauricular lymph node often is swollen, the patient frequently reports no tenderness.[228]

Corneal involvement in primary HSV infection can occur in the form of epithelial keratitis or dendrites, but these tend to be small, late in onset, and very transitory. These superficial corneal changes occur in approximately 63% of the patients with primary HSV infection and tend to last only 1 to 3 days.[229] Stromal disciform keratitis, which presents as a round area of stromal edema with an overlying intact epithelium, is much less frequent in patients with primary HSV infection, occurring in about 6% of patients.

Unrecognized primary HSV keratoconjunctivitis is most commonly misdiagnosed as epidemic keratoconjunctivitis due to the follicular conjunctivitis and corneal changes.[230] One clinical feature helpful in making the diagnosis is the tendency for primary herpes simplex keratitis to be unilateral and epidemic keratoconjunctivitis to be bilateral.

Recurrent herpes simplex keratitis occurs from reactivation of the latent virus. After the first episode there is approximately a 10% risk of recurrence within the first year and a 23% risk within the second year. Half the patients who have experienced one episode of recurrent herpes simplex keratitis will have a second episode within 10 years. The risk of recurrence increases with each episode.[229] The patient usually is most symptomatic during the first episode of recurrent HSK. Symptoms tend to decrease with each subsequent episode because of reduced corneal sensitivity (corneal hypoesthesia), which is a classic but not pathognomonic sign of herpes simplex keratitis.[228]

Recurrent HSK will have accompanying lid and conjunctival involvement in about 31% of cases.[229] This involvement typically appears as unilateral follicular conjunctivitis with moderate to severe diffuse conjunctival hyperemia. Involvement of the superficial epithelium occurs in approximately 78% of patients with recurrent herpes simplex keratitis.[229] Although dendritic or ameboid keratitis is the most common manifestation,[224] a diffuse punctate keratitis often develops first. This keratitis is caused by a plaque-like swelling of the epithelial cells from intracellular replication of herpes simplex virus.[231] Initially, this swelling will cause

fluorescein to pool around the cells,[228] but within 24 hours the cells die and a coarse punctate or stellate keratitis develops. As these areas of punctate keratitis coalesce, they develop into the typical branching dendritic or ameboid herpes simplex keratitis (Fig. 27.32).[220]

Dendritic ulcers from herpes simplex stain brightly with fluorescein sodium and have dichotomous branching, terminal end bulbs and a delicate pattern (see Fig. 27.32). The edges of these lesions are formed by swollen, opaque cells that stain well with rose bengal. Although these lesions are typical of herpes simplex keratitis and will often suggest the diagnosis, it is important to rule out other causes of dendritiform lesions. These include pseudodendrites caused by contact lens wear, herpes zoster ophthalmicus, healing epithelial defects, Epstein-Barr, medicamentosa primarily from antivirals, corneal dystrophy, *Acanthamoeba* keratitis, systemic tyrosinemia type II, and Thygeson's superficial punctate keratitis.[232] Herpes simplex dendritic lesions can enlarge to form an ameboid (geographic) shape. Stromal edema and subepithelial infiltrates can develop under the dendrite in just a few days. These infiltrates can leave faint scars in the superficial stroma, which can be useful for diagnosing previous episodes of HSK (Fig. 27.33).

Noninfectious, indolent epithelial ulcers also can occur in herpes simplex keratitis. These ulcers, formerly referred to as *metaherpetic* lesions, tend to be round with smooth, rolled edges. Generally 2 mm to 8 mm in size, they may be caused by damage to the epithelial basement membrane due to

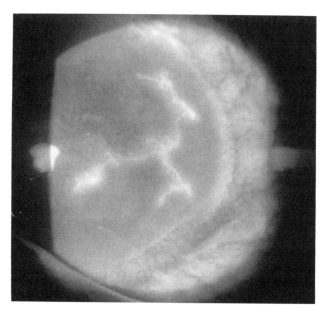

FIGURE 27.32 **Recurrent epithelial herpes simplex keratitis stained with fluorescein sodium. (Courtesy William L. Jones, O.D.)**

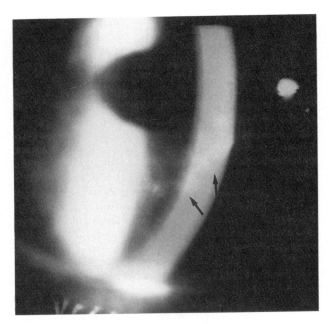

FIGURE 27.33 **Central anterior stromal corneal scarring (arrows) following recurrent herpes simplex keratitis.**

inflammation, tear film problems, neurotrophic problems, and toxicity from the antiviral medications. These ulcers may be long lasting, resulting in neovascularization and scarring.

Disciform keratitis may develop beneath the dendrite in recurrent herpes simplex keratitis,[228] or can occur months after the initial episode.[220] It will appear as a 5 mm to 7 mm, disc-shaped area of edema in the corneal stroma, which can cause folds in Descemet's membrane (Fig. 27.34). Disciform keratitis is probably a cell-mediated immune response to antigens and occurs in approximately 17% of patients with recurrent HSK.[229] The development of disciform keratitis may be a function of the strain of herpes simplex or may be due to some patient-specific response factor.[224]

Epithelial bullae can be found in some cases of disciform keratitis,[224] as can a Wessley ring, which is composed of immune cells surrounding the discoid edema. A mild to moderate uveitis with keratic precipitates usually is present, although it may not be visible due to the corneal edema.[224,228] Secondary glaucoma also can develop, primarily due to the intraocular inflammation.

The diagnosis of herpes simplex disciform keratitis usually is based on clinical appearance. If ghost scars, a history of previous episodes, or decreased corneal sensation is found, herpes simplex is the likely cause. It is important to rule out other causes of disciform keratitis, such as herpes zoster, varicella, vaccinia, mumps, and syphilis.

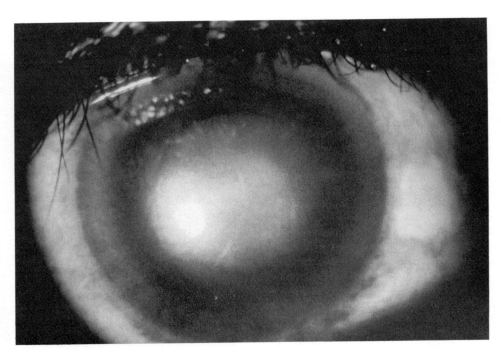

FIGURE 27.34   **Herpes simplex disciform keratitis with disc-shaped central stromal edema and folds in Descemet's membrane.**

Necrotizing interstitial keratitis may occur after multiple attacks. It is characterized by a white, dense, cottage cheese-like infiltrate of the stroma with epithelial ulceration. Anterior uveitis, secondary glaucoma, vascularization, scarring, corneal thinning, and perforation can occur with necrotizing interstitial keratitis.

Laboratory tests are available to help diagnose herpes simplex keratitis in cases that are clinically uncertain. One of the most reliable and fastest tests is the Herpchek, which is an enzyme immunoassay test that yields results in one day.[233] Viral culture microbiologic studies also can be performed.[234]

MANAGEMENT

Treatment of HSK is primarily based on whether the corneal condition is caused by active virus, as is found in epithelial dendritic keratitis, or by an immune response, as is typical of disciform keratitis. No treatment has been proven to remove the virus from the ganglia or to prevent recurrences in humans, although studies in mice suggest that oral acyclovir may be useful when administered prophylactically to patients exposed to a known inciting factor.[235]

Corneal epithelial disease should be treated with trifluridine 1% ophthalmic drops 5 to 8 times a day. Trifluridine is the drug of choice because it is the most potent antiviral currently available.[220] Vidarabine 3% ophthalmic ointment can be used at bedtime to increase corneal contact time while the patient is sleeping. If there is no improvement after one week or an adverse reaction occurs, use a different antiviral. Vidarabine ointment five times a day is the most common alternative choice because idoxuridine is more toxic to the epithelium.[224]

If the corneal lesions are superficial, the patient is an adult, and no topical steroids have been used, corneal debridement can be performed as an adjunct to the use of antivirals. Debridement is performed by instilling topical anesthetic drops such as proparacaine and using a sterile cotton-tipped applicator to remove the lesions (see Fig. 27.4).

If there is an anterior chamber reaction or if debridement has been performed, a cycloplegic agent such as homatropine 5% or scopolamine 0.25% should be used 2 to 3 times a day. Topical steroids should be tapered in any patient using them, since they are contraindicated in the presence of active HSV corneal epithelial disease. Animal studies have shown that topical steroids increase the resistance of certain genomes of herpes simplex virus to antiviral medications.[236] Antibiotics have no proven use in the treatment of herpes simplex epithelial disease.

HSV drug resistance is rare, and 97% of the cases resolve within two weeks of using trifluridine 1% solution.[224] Since antivirals are toxic to the corneal epithelium and may delay healing, their frequency of use should be decreased after the first week and tapered once the lesion is resolved. A suggested tapering schedule is four times a day for the second week, three times a day for the third week, and two times a day for the fourth week.[120] Tapering also allows time for the dormant virus to be shed.

Indolent ulcers can be very difficult to treat. Any topical medications should be discontinued, since antivirals and the preservatives in other medications can contribute to the problem. A prophylactic antibiotic such as polymyxin B-bacitracin ointment should be instilled followed by pressure patching, or instilled 2 to 4 times a day without a pressure patch. A cycloplegic agent such as homatropine 5% should be used 2 to 3 times a day. These patients must be monitored to make sure a secondary infection does not occur. If the ulcer deepens, a new infiltrate forms, or there is an increase in the anterior chamber reaction while the patient is being treated, cultures should be performed to rule out bacterial or fungal infection. If healing does not occur with this regimen, conjunctival flap surgery or tarsorrhaphy may be required.[237]

Treatment of disciform keratitis should be directed toward decreasing inflammation. If the disciform keratitis is very mild, treat it with cycloplegics such as homatropine 5% three times a day to decrease pain and to prevent the formation of synechiae.[228] If the disciform keratitis is affecting vision because of its severity or location, topical steroids are used. Disciform keratitis responds rapidly to steroids but will tend to recur if the therapy is not continued for an appropriate length of time or is tapered too quickly.[359] Topical antivirals should always be administered concurrently and in equal dosage frequency as the topical steroid.[224] Prednisolone acetate 1% or dexamethasone 0.1% four to five times a day for 1 week along with trifluridine five times a day is a suggested therapy, but it is prudent to use the lowest dose of topical steroid that will resolve the inflammation.

Improvement occurs quickly in disciform keratitis, but the topical steroid must be tapered very slowly. It is common for the patient to instill a drop of prednisolone acetate 1% every day or every other day after three months of treatment. It is not uncommon to have the patient use lower concentrations of topical steroids, such as prednisolone 0.12%, every other day for more than a year.[228] The antiviral agents can be discontinued when the steroids are being used no more than once a day. If the steroid is tapered too quickly and the disciform keratitis recurs, the topical steroid and antiviral agent should both be reinstituted at a higher frequency of instillation. Disciform keratitis generally leaves a scar after resolution of the acute inflammation, and a penetrating keratoplasty may be necessary for the patient to regain useful vision.

There is some evidence to suggest that oral acyclovir may be helpful in treating HSV epithelial keratitis or uveitis, but its use is still experimental in the United States. Investigative treatment currently includes 200 mg to 400 mg of acyclovir by mouth five times a day for 14 to 21 days.[238,239] Although there seems to be some benefit to the use of oral acyclovir, a case of acyclovir-resistant herpes simplex keratitis has been reported already.[240] For patients with stromal keratitis without concomitant epithelial keratitis, the use of oral acyclovir appears to offer no benefit when used with topical steroids and trifluridine.[360]

Generally, necrotizing interstitial keratitis should be treated in the same manner as disciform keratitis, but necrotizing keratitis is much less responsive to steroids. As with disciform keratitis, the steroid must be tapered very slowly, often over a period of months or years. Conjunctival flaps may be necessary as may permanent or temporary tarsorrhaphy.

Herpes Zoster Ophthalmicus

ETIOLOGY

First exposure to the varicella-zoster virus causes chickenpox, after which the virus remains latent in the nerve ganglia.[221] Herpes zoster is caused by reactivation of the latent varicella-zoster virus and most often occurs in patients who are immunocompromised. Factors such as physical and emotional trauma, immunosuppressive medications, irradiation, cancer, tuberculosis, malaria, and syphilis are known to reactivate the virus. Herpes zoster ophthalmicus also can be an early presenting sign in patients with AIDS.[241]

Herpes zoster is found world-wide and affects both sexes equally. It is more common in individuals over the age of 40 and rarely occurs in children. Approximately 90% of all adults in the United States have blood antibodies to herpes zoster, and about 20% will experience a reactivation of the virus.

When reactivation occurs, the virus passes along the sensory nerve and erupts on the tissue innervated by that nerve (dermatome). The ophthalmic division of the trigeminal nerve is involved in 8% to 56% of the cases of herpes zoster, a condition known as herpes zoster ophthalmicus (HZO).[242] Ocular complications occur in 50% to 75% of patients with involvement of the ophthalmic division of the trigeminal nerve.[243,244]

The nasociliary branch of the trigeminal nerve supplies the conjunctiva, cornea, iris, ciliary body, anterior choroid, and the skin of both lids and the tip of the nose. Herpes zoster involvement of the nasociliary branch is indicated by cutaneous vesicles on the tip of the nose. Vesicles in this location are often referred to as *Hutchinson's sign,* and their presence increases the chances of serious corneal involvement.

DIAGNOSIS

Patients with HZO typically report a history of headache, malaise, fever, and chills for 2 to 3 days. At the same time they may notice pain, tingling, burning, itching, erythema and edema of the skin over the affected nerve. Some patients also have ocular symptoms of pain, tearing, and foreign body sensation.[245] A few days later patients develop flushing of the skin and an eruption of vesicles along the distribution of the nerve. These vesicles become pustular and hemorrhagic in 3 to 4 days, developing crusts in 7 to 10 days.[246] Severe pain is common both while the vesicles are present, due to inflammation of the neurons, and after the vesicles are healed because of scarring in and around the nerves. Permanent scarring of the skin also is quite common unless aggressive therapeutic measures are taken with systemic antiviral therapy before the vesicles erupt. It is possible, but rare, to have herpes zoster without skin lesions. Involvement of the ophthalmic branch of the trigeminal nerve usually causes lymphadenopathy.[242]

Ocular involvement can develop as soon as several days, to as long as years, after the formation of vesicles.[242,247] Ocular involvement may include lid edema, follicular conjunctivitis, corneal changes, anterior uveitis, glaucoma, episcleritis, scleritis, Horner's syndrome, extraocular muscle palsy, chorioretinitis, optic neuritis, and scarring of the lids and lacrimal canalicular system.

Corneal changes can occur within the first week of the disease, or months later. These changes include punctate epithelial keratitis and pseudodendritic keratitis, and occur in approximately 74% of patients with HZO.[245] The punctate epithelial keratitis is coarse in appearance, with blotchy, swollen epithelial cells. The lesions are numerous and located peripherally in the cornea. In one study,[245] these lesions coalesced to form pseudodendrites in about 55% of the patients.

The dendritic corneal lesions of HZO are more superficial, smaller, finer, and have blunter ends than do the dendrites caused by herpes simplex (Table 27.3). They usually occur 4 to 6 days after the skin vesicles erupt and stain moderately well with rose bengal and fluorescein (Fig. 27.35).[245]

Anterior stromal infiltrates can develop under the dendritic HZO lesions. These stromal infiltrates appear as hazy, granular, nummular subepithelial opacities.[248] They can be self-limiting or chronic. They are most likely caused by an antigen-antibody reaction to viral particles and respond to topical steroids.[249] Serpiginous ulceration, which is another corneal change likely to be caused by an immune response, occurs in approximately 7% of patients. In this condition, a crescent-shaped peripheral ulcer develops with acute stromal and cellular infiltration. This ulcer appears to have smooth edges and is associated with decreased corneal sensation and uveitis. With time the ulcer results in thinning and vascularization of the cornea in the majority, and perforation in a minority of cases. These ulcers respond to steroids and should not be confused with neurotrophic ulceration.

Mucous plaque keratitis can occur almost anytime in the course of the disease.[242] These plaques appear as elevated, sharply demarcated, opaque, gray-white lesions. They are variable in size and shape. They stain well with rose bengal but poorly with fluorescein. A poor tear film and neuro-

TABLE 27.3
Differential Diagnosis of Herpes Simplex and Herpes Zoster

	Herpes Simplex	*Herpes Zoster*
Dermatomal distribution	Limited	More complete
Pain	Mild to moderate	Severe
Dendrite appearance	Larger, more branching, discrete, delicate pattern, more central	Smaller, less branching, coarse, blunted pattern, usually peripheral
Epithelium	Ulcerated	Plaque-like dendrite with slightly raised edges
NaFl staining	Prominent	Dull and irregular
Endbulbs	Present	Absent
Scarring of skin	Rare	Common
Postherpetic neuralgia	Rare	Common
Iris atrophy	Rare	Common
Recurrence	Common	Rare

Modified from Nichols B, ed. Basic and Clinical Science Course. External Disease and the Cornea, Section 7. American Academy of Ophthalmology, 1990–1991.

trophic corneal changes are common in these cases. Viral cultures are negative, and the lesions appear to be mucous deposits on abnormal epithelial cells, which can migrate or disappear with time (Fig. 27.36).[245]

Deep corneal edema with folds in Descemet's membrane, in the presence of an intact epithelium, can develop from 3 to 4 months after acute HZO.[242] This disciform keratitis involves the full thickness of the cornea and often occurs in areas of previous infiltrate. It also is considered to be an immune response to viral antigens and responds quickly to topical steroid use. Unfortunately, it is common to have recurrences when steroids are tapered or discontinued.

Exposure keratitis in HZO usually is the result of lid changes from scarring. Scarring prevents complete blinking and causes a punctate keratitis. Neurotrophic keratitis often is associated with exposure keratitis and occurs in approximately 25% of patients with HZO.[245] It can be easily overlooked in the early stages, because the decreased corneal sensitivity often is localized to a small area of the cornea.[242] The loss of corneal sensation causes a breakdown of the corneal epithelium, often in a horizontally oval pattern.

Many of these corneal conditions associated with HZO can cause stromal scarring. Liesegang[245] found scars that affected visual acuity in approximately 15% of patients.

MANAGEMENT

Systemic acyclovir promotes resolution of HZO skin lesions and reduces the incidence and severity of dendriform keratopathy, uveitis, and stromal keratitis by decreasing the rate of virus replication. Acyclovir usually is administered orally in dosages of 600 mg to 800 mg five times per day for 10 days. Recently, however, Hoang-Xuan and associates[250] found that 800 mg of oral acyclovir and topical 3% acyclovir ointment, each administered five times a day for only 7 days,

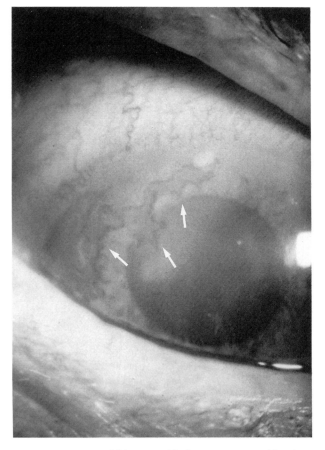

FIGURE 27.35   **Dendritic corneal lesion (arrows) resulting from herpes zoster ophthalmicus, shown stained with rose bengal and fluorescein sodium.**

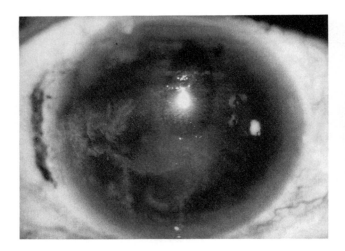

A

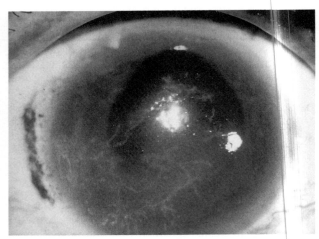

B

FIGURE 27.36   **Corneal mucous plaque keratitis associated with herpes zoster. *(A)* Initial presentation. *(B)* Note migratory nature of lesions three weeks later. (Courtesy Marc A. Michelson, M.D.)**

was as effective as 14 days of oral acyclovir treatment in decreasing subjective symptoms, skin lesions, and ocular complication. This shorter treatment should be considered due to the expense of oral acyclovir and the increased risk of side effects with longer treatment. For acyclovir to have the maximum effect, treatment must be started within 72 hours of the vesicular eruptions.[251] Unlike acyclovir, the antiviral agents cytosine arabinoside, idoxuridine, and adenosine arabinoside have not been proven to be helpful in decreasing the severity or incidence of ocular manifestations of HZO.[242]

The early corneal changes of superficial punctate keratitis and pseudodendrites usually are self-limiting, lasting weeks to months, and require no treatment. In a study of nine patients, Piebenga and Laibson[252] found that dendritic lesions resolved in an average of 30 days. Artificial tears and cool compresses may be helpful for symptomatic relief.[247]

Use of topical steroids usually is not necessary if there is only mild inflammation and good vision. Prednisolone acetate 1% can be used four times a day for corneal changes caused by inflammation such as stromal infiltrates, serpiginous ulceration, and disciform keratitis. Some authors suggest using prophylactic antibiotics along with the steroid.[248,252] If there is any possibility that herpes simplex is present, a topical ophthalmic antiviral agent should be used concurrently with the steroid. To avoid recurrences of inflammation, steroids must be tapered very slowly. A cycloplegic agent such as homatropine 5% used two to three times a day can decrease pain and help prevent or control uveitis and synechiae.

Mucous plaque keratitis can be treated with 10% acetylcysteine, but also will resolve without treatment. Keeping

the eye moist with artificial tears may be helpful. Exposure keratitis and neurotrophic keratitis are best treated with artificial tears, lid taping at bedtime and, if necessary, tarsorrhaphy. Bandage contact lenses should not be used due to the risk of developing infectious ulcers in an eye with decreased sensitivity.[247]

Corneal scarring that affects vision is best treated with penetrating keratoplasty. Penetrating keratoplasty generally is considered to have a poor outcome after herpes zoster ophthalmicus because of recurrent or chronic inflammation, vascularization, glaucoma, and poor tear film. The chances of success seem to improve, however, if the corneal surface is protected after surgery by lubricants, bandage lenses or tarsorrhaphy, or if there has been a long interval since the previous occurrence.[244,253]

Degenerations and Dystrophies

Anterior Basement Membrane Dystrophy

ETIOLOGY

Abnormal corneal epithelial regeneration and maturation, along with an abnormal basement membrane, are the primary features found in anterior basement membrane dystrophy (ABMD). The prevalence of anterior basement membrane dystrophy has been reported to be as low as 2%[254] and as high as 42% of all patients.[255] In patients over the age of 70, the estimates are as high as 76%.[255] Although anterior basement membrane dystrophy often is considered the most

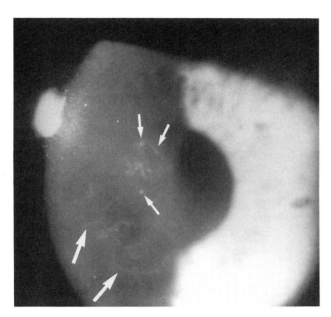

FIGURE 27.37 Using diffuse illumination, maps (large arrows) and dots (small arrows) are noted in patient with ABMD.

A very careful slit-lamp examination is needed to diagnose the condition. The most common findings in ABMD are gray, chalky patches; intraepithelial microcysts; and fine lines, or a combination of these seen in the central two-thirds of the cornea. These findings are known as *maps, dots,* and *fingerprints.* All of the corneal changes in anterior basement membrane dystrophy may vary in appearance at each examination.

Maps appear as diffuse gray patches with sharp margins, and thick irregular lines that may be surrounded by a haze. Maps often are separated by clear zones and may contain lacunae or white microcysts within their borders (Figs. 27.37 and 27.38). They are seen most easily with tangential illumination.[100] The tears over map areas breakup rapidly, and fluorescein sodium helps outline areas of mapping due to negative staining (Fig. 27.39). Maps are caused by thickening of the basement membrane due to a proliferation of collagen material.[258]

Dots contain degenerated epithelial cells that are trapped in intraepithelial extensions of the basement membrane. This prevents the normal migration of these cells toward the epithelial surface. Dots develop two different appearances.[259,260] Some will appear gray-white and have distinct edges. They often form clusters and vary in size from barely visible to 1 mm (Fig. 27.40). These dots are seen easily on direct illumination and stain only when they break through to the corneal surface. If the dots are very prominent, the condition is known as Cogan's microcystic

common corneal dystrophy, it may be an age-related degeneration. Werblin and associates[255] evaluated 215 patients from the general population and 93 relatives of 19 patients known to have ABMD but were unable to prove either the existence or lack of dominant inheritance. The large number of patients with the condition, its increasing prevalence with increasing age, and its late onset support classifying ABMD as a degeneration instead of a dystrophy.[255,256]

DIAGNOSIS

Not all patients with this condition are symptomatic. The estimates of symptomatic ABMD patients range from lows of 10% to 20%[254] to highs of 69%.[100] The most common symptom is a mild foreign body sensation that usually is worse in dry weather, wind, and air conditioning.[100] Blurred vision from irregular astigmatism or a rapid tear break-up time may occur, especially in patients over the age of 45.[257] Pain, when reported, usually is caused by recurrent corneal erosion, which is estimated to occur in 10% of patients with ABMD.[95]

It is easy to overlook ABMD during a clinical examination. This may be the reason for such wide variations in reported prevalence. The condition typically is bilateral but often asymmetric. Females are affected more often than males. It often is first diagnosed between the ages of 40 and 70 years, but it has been reported in patients as young as five years of age.[95]

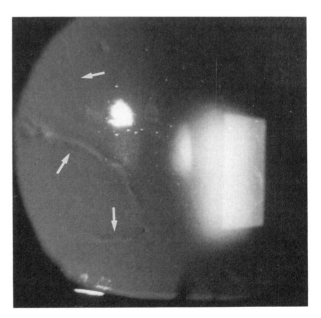

FIGURE 27.38 ABMD mapping is seen in retroillumination (arrows). The irregular corneal surface caused by this condition may result in reduced visual acuity.

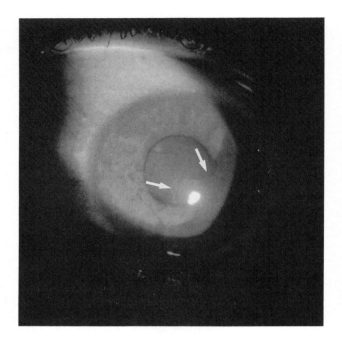

FIGURE 27.39   **Negative staining (arrows) following instillation of fluorescein sodium helps to outline ABMD mapping.**

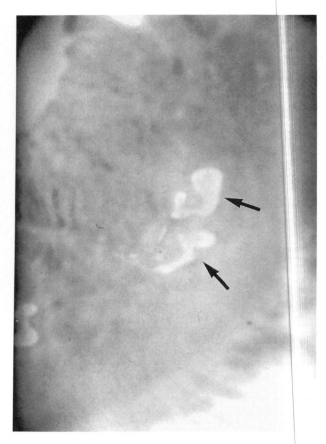

FIGURE 27.40   **Large dots in ABMD (arrows).**

dystrophy. Blebs, the second type of dots, are fine, clear, closely clustered refractile opacities that are seen only on retroillumination. They have no effect on tear breakup time and do not enhance the likelihood of recurrent corneal erosions. Blebs are formed by the accumulation of fibrogranular material between the basement membrane and Bowman's layer.[261]

Fingerprint lines are thin, relucent, hair-like lines often arranged parallel to each other, giving the appearance of fingerprints. They are caused by a thickened and reduplicated basement membrane that extends into the epithelial layers.[258] Retroillumination or indirect illumination are the best methods for seeing these lines, but a rapid tear breakup time over the areas also helps distinguish them (Fig. 27.41). Lines similar to fingerprint lines also can develop in association with herpes simplex keratitis and bullous keratopathy.[262,263]

A scalloped line of tear film thinning in patients with anterior basement membrane dystrophy was reported by Shahinian.[264] It occurred in the superior one-third of the cornea as a fine blue line of negative staining with pooling along its margins. Shahinian called this condition *corneal valance* and reported that it was visible with a photokeratoscope.

MANAGEMENT

Treatment is directed toward preventing recurrent corneal erosions and most commonly consists of the use of 5% sodium chloride ointment instilled into the conjunctival sac at bedtime. This is especially indicated for patients who notice blurring of their vision upon awakening in the morning due to associated edema. If epithelial edema consistently contributes to a reduction is visual acuity, then 5% sodium chloride drops may be added during the day. Nonhypertonic lubricating solutions may enhance patient comfort and visual acuity. The use of punctal plugs may be helpful to improve lubrication.[265]

If a recurrent corneal erosion develops acutely as a result of ABMD, appropriate treatment should be instituted (see page 693). If ABMD is severe enough to cause significant visual loss, then debridement or superficial keratectomy may be considered.

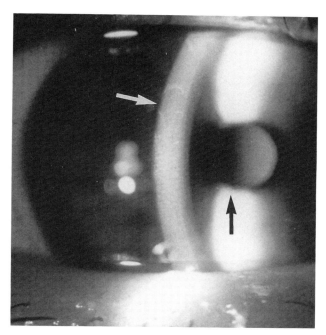

FIGURE 27.41   Subtle fingerprint lines (black arrow) are noted in indirect illumination. This patient with ABMD also exhibits mapping in direct parallelepiped illumination (white arrow).

Guttata and Fuchs' Dystrophy

ETIOLOGY

The development of corneal guttata is a common form of endothelial anomaly. Guttata are wart-like prominences on Descemet's membrane and result from abnormal corneal endothelial secretions. Histologic studies indicate that guttata are accompanied by thinning of the overlying endothelial cells along with thickening of Descemet's membrane.[11] Guttata generally are located in the central cornea, except in the case of Fuchs' endothelial dystrophy, when the peripheral endothelium also becomes involved. When these lesions are noted in the peripheral corneal endothelium only, they are termed Hassall-Henle bodies. Guttata usually are first noticed clinically in patients in their 30's and 40's or older, although the density of the guttata may vary significantly from patient to patient.[120] Mild guttata commonly appear as occasional scattered lesions in the central cornea. Moderate guttata appear as a relatively dense collection of lesions in the central cornea. Pigment is commonly associated with guttata and may be entrapped in the irregular endothelial surface. Moderate guttata may take on a plaque-like appear-

ance in the central cornea, which somewhat obscures the typical guttata detail due to clinically significant thickening of Descemet's membrane. In the presence of mild to moderate guttata, the overlying stroma and epithelium remain clear, and these conditions tend to remain stationary for years.[266] Guttata have also been reported in association with keratoconus.[267]

Fuchs' (endothelial) dystrophy has a component of guttata, but the involvement is such that corneal physiology is affected adversely. Fuchs' dystrophy occurs bilaterally, most commonly affects women in the fourth or fifth decade of life, and probably is transmitted dominantly. Prominent guttata initially occur centrally, then become extensive enough to involve the peripheral cornea. In Fuchs' dystrophy, the endothelial cells become sufficiently compromised to interfere with their metabolic "pump" ability, thus permitting aqueous fluid to enter the corneal tissue. As a result, and over a course lasting several decades, stromal edema, epithelial edema, and bullous keratopathy will ensue. Histologic studies suggest an initial increase in the pump site activity in early Fuchs', followed by a gradual deterioration toward end-stage Fuchs'.[268] Secondary abnormalities in the basement membrane and Bowman's layer also develop.[11]

Transient secondary guttata may develop in association with degenerative corneal disease, trauma, or inflammation.[13] Transient guttata associated with corneal edema have been termed *pseudoguttata*.[16]

DIAGNOSIS

The diagnosis of corneal guttata is made using the slit-lamp biomicroscope. In direct illumination, particularly with a parallelepiped, guttata will appear as small refractile "drops" on the corneal endothelium. Closer inspection using specular reflection illumination reveals orange peel-like "dimpling" of the endothelium caused by the guttata, appearing as dark spots in the reflected light (Fig. 27.42). This clinical presentation may be accentuated by evaluating the cornea following pupillary dilation. The pigmentation and plaque-like haze of moderate guttata will be quite apparent.

Established Fuchs' dystrophy consists of dense guttata, most pronounced centrally but involving the entire corneal endothelium. The endothelium may take on a bronzed, beaten metal-like appearance. Accompanying stromal edema appears as a central, whitish haze (Fig. 27.43). Epithelial edema may appear as corneal bedewing, best seen in indirect illumination, and frank bullae may be present. Long-standing corneal edema may result in corneal scarring, and advanced cases may exhibit subepithelial fibrosis and vascularization.[8]

Patient symptomatology varies with the extent of the guttata. Mild corneal guttata have no effect on visual func-

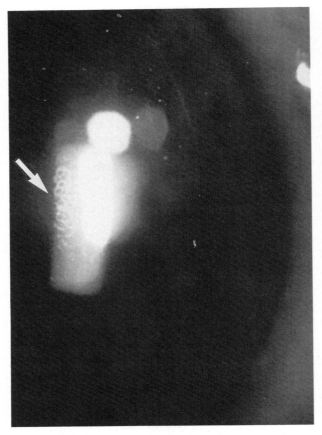

FIGURE 27.42   **Specular reflection illumination reveals the orange peel-like "dimpling" of the endothelium caused by guttata (arrow).**

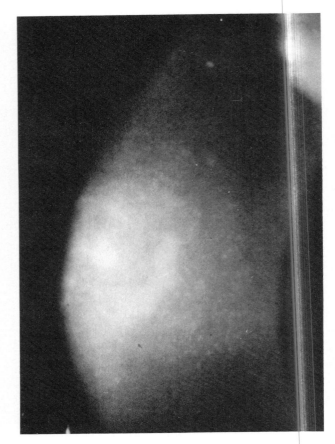

FIGURE 27.43   **High magnification view of central stromal haze of Fuchs' dystrophy.**

tion. Moderate corneal guttata, with its central and rather dense distribution, may affect visual function, including light scatter and reduced visual acuity to approximately 20/25 to 20/30. Decreased visual acuity due to corneal edema may be noticed upon awakening. This condition may improve during the course of the day as the corneal fluid evaporates. The visual impact of moderate guttata will be most noticeable under conditions of pupillary constriction. Overlying corneal edema in association with moderate guttata is not generally visible using a biomicroscope; however, clinical anecdotal evidence suggests that patients with this condition may report blurring of vision upon awakening in the morning, which may represent an exacerbation of corneal edema resulting from closure of the lids overnight.[269]

The edema and other corneal changes associated with Fuchs' dystrophy will adversely affect visual acuity. Symptoms will be worse when corneal edema is more pronounced, particularly upon awakening. Rupture of associated bullae will produce symptoms of foreign body sensation, pain, and redness.

MANAGEMENT

The use of topical ophthalmic hypertonic agents may reduce epithelial edema related to Fuchs' dystrophy; however, these agents will not reduce stromal edema. The use of topical 5% sodium chloride drops 6 to 8 times daily, along with 5% sodium chloride ointment instilled into the conjunctival sac at bedtime, may be instituted to determine the effect on symptoms and visual acuity. Although epithelial edema is not an obvious factor in moderate corneal guttata, 5% sodium chloride ointment instilled into the conjunctival sac at bedtime may relieve the symptoms of those patients who experience accentuated blurring of vision upon awakening.

To help relieve patient discomfort due to the rupture of epithelial bullae, a bandage soft contact lens may be tried (see page 733). Effective restoration of patient comfort and visual function for well-established Fuchs' dystrophy, however, may be best achieved through penetrating keratoplasty. Growth factors are under study as a potential method for regenerating damaged endothelial cells.[270]

Corneal Hydrops Secondary to Keratoconus

ETIOLOGY

Keratoconus is an ectatic corneal dystrophy that tends to be bilateral, but may be asymmetric, and generally manifests in the second or third decade of life. The familiar slit-lamp manifestations include central corneal thinning, Fleischer's ring, scarring at the level of Bowman's layer or anterior stroma, and vertical endothelial striae (Vogt's lines).[271] The keratoconic cornea exhibits an accentuated outward bowing of the lower lid in downgaze, known as *Munson's sign.* Common refractive or topographic effects include irregular astigmatism and poor best-corrected visual acuity with spectacles. Visual acuity typically is maximized following correction with rigid gas permeable contact lenses. Characteristic conic steepening patterns will be noted on corneal surface topography evaluation.

Keratoconus tends to progress over 7 to 8 years, then stabilizes.[271] The severity of keratoconus varies among patients and often is asymmetric when comparing the two eyes. In some keratoconic patients, the progressive corneal thinning proceeds to such an extent that Descemet's membrane ruptures. In this event, a sudden influx of aqueous into the cornea occurs, known as acute *hydrops.*

DIAGNOSIS

Patients presenting with acute corneal hydrops typically will be aware of the pre-existing diagnosis of keratoconus. Symptoms of hydrops include a sudden decrease in best corrected visual acuity, redness, and a foreign body sensation or pain in the involved eye.[271]

Slit-lamp examination of acute hydrops reveals prominent central or inferior corneal edema and clouding along with conjunctival hyperemia (Fig. 27.44). The contralateral eye will generally exhibit findings of keratoconus but without hydrops.

MANAGEMENT

Acute hydrops secondary to keratoconus tends to be self-limiting in approximately 8 to 10 weeks when the corneal endothelial cells regenerate across the rupture in Descemet's membrane, re-establishing stromal deturgescence.[11] Conservative therapeutic measures typically are instituted during this resolution period, including the use of topical 5% sodium chloride drops during the day and 5% sodium chloride ointment instilled into the conjunctival sac at bedtime.[271] Broad-spectrum topical ophthalmic antibiotics may be instituted to protect the inflamed eye from secondary bacterial infection.

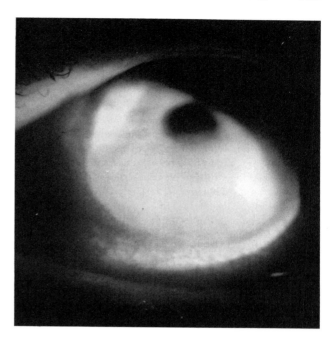

FIGURE 27.44   **Acute corneal hydrops secondary to keratoconus. (Courtesy William L. Jones, O.D.)**

It is common for corneal scarring to remain once the edema related to acute hydrops resolves. Topical ophthalmic steroid drops may be used in an effort to minimize resultant scar formation.

Penetrating keratoplasty currently is the most common surgical management for keratoconus. This intervention is considered when contact lens intolerance occurs or if the visual acuity can no longer be corrected adequately using a contact lens. Acute hydrops may result in chronic corneal edema or central corneal scarring that adversely impacts best corrected visual acuity. Both of these conditions also may be indications for surgical intervention. It is possible, however, that the corneal edema due to hydrops will leave a sufficiently small scar that contact lens wear can be resumed without the need for penetrating keratoplasty.[8]

Contact Lens-Related Corneal Complications

Contact Lens-Induced Abrasions

ETIOLOGY

Contact lenses are a very specific and not uncommon source of corneal abrasion. The cause of the abrasion may involve many factors, including physiologic, toxic, and mechanical.[272] Contact lens–induced corneal abrasions may be related to overwear, difficulties with insertion or removal, problems with the lens-cornea relationship, a damaged lens, or a foreign body trapped under the lens.[273,274] Abrasions related to contact lens wear can occur from the use of rigid or soft materials, daily or extended wear, but are more common in rigid contact lens wearers.[275]

DIAGNOSIS

The clinical signs and symptoms of contact lens-induced corneal abrasion are comparable to those described from other causes (Fig. 27.45). The pain and redness associated with the abrasion will typically cause the patient to discontinue lens wear, although soft lenses may exert a bandage effect.[272]

A careful patient history is important to establish parameters associated with development of the abrasion. Questions should be asked about the type of lens worn, wearing time immediately prior to development of the abrasion, usual wearing time, age of the current lenses, duration of contact lens wear, cleaning regimen, unusual events just prior to the development of symptoms such as unusual difficulty with removal, etc.[272]

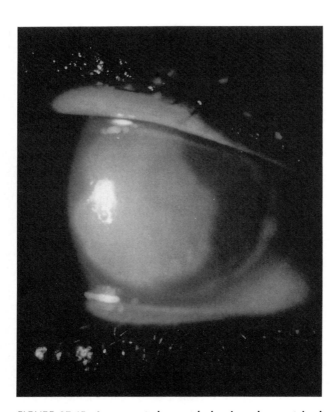

FIGURE 27.45   **Large central corneal abrasion, shown stained with fluorescein sodium, resulting from overwear of a rigid gas permeable contact lens.**

Careful slit-lamp examination is needed to determine whether the lesion is an abrasion related to contact lens wear versus a contact lens-induced infiltrate or ulcerative keratitis. The "clean" abrasion should not exhibit corneal infiltration, severe corneal edema, a severe anterior chamber reaction, or mucopurulent discharge. Careful examination and close monitoring are needed, however, since atypical bacterial keratitis has been reported in contact lens wearers that presented as an epithelial defect without apparent signs of infiltration.[276] In addition, contact lens-induced abrasions exhibit definite traumatic epithelial loss rather than diffuse areas of edema and extensive epithelial erosion, referred to as the *soft lens-associated corneal hypoxia (SLACH) syndrome*.[277] The SLACH syndrome worsens with pressure patching due to a further reduction in oxygen levels to the cornea.

MANAGEMENT

The treatment of corneal abrasions in contact lens wearers poses a management challenge because of the altered normal flora and the risk of potentially devastating secondary infection by gram-negative organisms, especially in extended wear patients.[59] Epithelial defects associated with contact lenses may predispose the patient to ulcerative keratitis, particularly in the patient using extended-wear lenses.[278] Cases have been reported of *Pseudomonas* ulcers that developed following a single application of topical ophthalmic antibiotic ointment and pressure patching.[279]

To avoid the development of a secondary bacterial keratitis during treatment with a traditional pressure patch, several options are available. First, patching may be avoided altogether and prophylactic topical antibiotic therapy instituted to protect the cornea from infection while it heals. Cycloplegia is utilized, just as it is in the non–contact lens abrasion, using long-acting agents. Broad-spectrum antibiotics are used, such as 0.3% tobramycin drops every 2 to 4 hours during the day and ointment at bedtime.[272] Ciprofloxacin 0.3% solution used at the same dosage is an excellent alternative to tobramycin. Oral analgesics (see Chap. 7) will be needed along with sunglasses to reduce photophobia. The patient should be examined every 24 to 48 hours while the tissue heals.

Alternatively, the Presspatch may be used to treat this condition. The Presspatch offers the benefits of patching, such as enhanced comfort and protection from lid blinking, but will allow for reinstillation of broad-spectrum ophthalmic ointment such as 0.3% tobramycin every 2 to 4 hours.

Finally, collagen shields or bandage soft contact lenses may be used along with topical antibiotic prophylaxis while the corneal abrasion re-epithelializes.[51] In the event of a soft contact lens–related abrasion, it is important to use a fresh bandage or disposable soft contact lens rather than the patient's own lens. Broad-spectrum antibiotic agents are

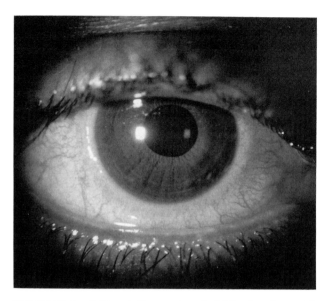

FIGURE 27.46 **Diffuse bulbar conjunctival injection along with perilimbal injection and chemosis in patient with acute red eye reaction syndrome. The patient was wearing two-year-old daily wear soft contact lenses and had not had follow-up care in two years. Scattered small focal infiltrates were noted in the inferior nasal quadrant of the cornea (not shown).**

instilled while the bandage lens or collagen shield is in place.

Once the abrasion has healed, careful reinstitution of contact lens wear may proceed. As contact lens wear is resumed, it is important to monitor for subtle signs of persistent corneal healing, such as epithelial basement membrane disruption. It also is important to address with the patient, in an appropriate manner, issues that led to the abrasion, such as poor handling technique, damaged lenses, poor cleaning regimen, so that a future similar episode may be avoided. If signs of bacterial keratitis develop, the appropriate treatment regimen must be instituted (see page 704).

Acute Red Eye Reaction (Infiltrative Keratitis)

ETIOLOGY

The acute red eye reaction syndrome, which tends to be associated with extended-wear soft contact lenses, also has been called *tight lens syndrome, lens intolerance,* and *idiopathic red eye.*[280–282] The average yearly reported incidence of this condition ranges from 2.5% to as high as 56%.[281,283] The development of corneal infiltrates also has been reported with the use of daily-wear soft contact lenses.[275]

Several etiologies have been suggested as contributing to the development of this condition, including contact lens

solution hypersensitivity, especially to preservatives; tight-fitting lenses providing insufficient tear exchange and resulting in a build-up of irritants behind the lens; mechanical compression on the limbus by the lens; entrapment of leukocytes from the tear film and conjunctival vessels between the eye and the contact lens; contact lens deposits; bacterial endotoxins; anoxia; decreased tear pH; and hypersensitivity to the contact lens itself.[16,282,284–290] Corneal hypoxia related to a tight-fitting lens commonly is viewed as a cause of this problem.[291]

DIAGNOSIS

Patients experiencing the acute red eye reaction tend to have a common set of signs and symptoms. The onset of symptoms typically is acute and may be noticed upon awakening, or the patient may be awakened in the middle of the night with the problem. Symptoms of unilateral ocular discomfort or pain, redness, tearing, and photophobia are reported. A detailed patient history should be taken to determine the nature of the onset of symptoms as well as any unusual circumstances leading to the episode, such as failure to clean the lenses, excessive wearing time, etc.

Slit-lamp examination reveals moderate bulbar conjunctival injection, particularly in the perilimbal area (Fig. 27.46). The cornea may exhibit a varying degree of infiltration, ranging from a diffuse band of small, hazy, grayish opacities that give the cornea a dull, grainy appearance, to single or multiple focal opaque lesions (Fig. 27.47).[16] The infiltrates tend to be located in the anterior stroma and may be periph-

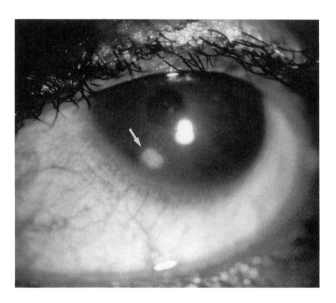

FIGURE 27.47 **Corneal infiltrate (arrow) in patient with acute red eye reaction syndrome. The patient was wearing extended-wear soft contact lenses on a daily wear basis for 16 hours a day.**

eral or central.[361] A mild anterior chamber reaction is common. Instillation of fluorescein sodium tends not to reveal significant epithelial involvement, although small foci of positive staining may be noticed overlying areas of limbal chemosis and corneal infiltration.[16] Negative staining overlying the corneal infiltrates also is common.[16]

The definitive diagnosis of acute red eye reaction can pose a clinical challenge with respect to ruling out other conditions that cause an acute red eye with corneal infiltration. Epidemic keratoconjunctivis (EKC), chlamydial keratoconjunctivitis, marginal infiltrates, *Acanthamoeba* keratitis, and bacterial keratitis are among the most prominent differential diagnoses. To rule out other possible diagnoses, other signs and symptoms need to be assessed thoroughly. Such signs and symptoms include the presence or absence of conjunctival follicles, lymphadenopathy, mucopurulent or purulent discharge, and bilateral involvement.[273,288] Clinical anecdotal experience suggests that prominent perilimbal injection and chemosis is an important feature of the acute red eye reaction syndrome.

One critical distinction to make is whether a focal corneal infiltrate is infected with bacteria or is a sterile, immunologic response. Many clinicians advocate routine scraping for smears and cultures of corneal infiltrates associated with soft contact lens wear to determine definitively whether active bacterial keratitis is present. In a prospective study, Stein and associates[292] compared the clinical characteristics of infected versus sterile corneal infiltrates in contact lens wearers. These investigators found that sterile infiltrates usually were smaller (less than 1 mm), multiple or arcuate, and lacked significant pain, epithelial staining or anterior chamber reaction. Conversely, infected ulcers were associated with increased pain, a larger size (over 2 mm), more extensive epithelial staining, a discharge, and a more prominent anterior chamber reaction. When in doubt, it is best to assume that a lesion is infected and initiate appropriate laboratory analysis and aggressive therapeutic intervention.

MANAGEMENT

The acute red eye reaction syndrome necessitates discontinuation of contact lens wear. With significant corneal involvement and an anterior chamber reaction, cycloplegia with a long-acting agent such as 5% homatropine will enhance patient comfort and help to relieve iris congestion.

Once contact lens wear is discontinued, the acute red eye reaction syndrome will be self-limiting over a few days to a week. The infiltrates take longer to resolve than does the conjunctival hyperemia. Epithelial microcysts may develop in the acute red eye reaction syndrome, which may prolong resolution time (see page 729).[16]

Topical prophylactic antibiotic therapy is appropriate to protect the inflamed eye from infection as it heals.[292] With the potential for gram-negative pathogens in a soft contact lens wearer, especially extended wear, choose broad-spectrum agents such as 0.3% tobramycin drops four times a

day or 0.3% ciprofloxacin drops four times a day, and 0.3% tobramycin ointment at bedtime. If bacterial keratitis is suspected or while waiting for culture results, more aggressive dosage intervals may be initiated (see page 704).

Some clinicians advise against the use of topical steroid therapy in this condition.[291] However, the addition of a topical steroid, such as 0.12% or 1% prednisolone four times a day, will accelerate resolution of the stromal infiltrates and the accompanying inflammatory response of the eye.[293] The use of 1% prednisolone or 0.25% fluorometholone is appropriate if an anterior chamber reaction is present. The addition of topical steroids should be judicious pending the definitive diagnosis issues discussed previously. Clinical anecdotal reports have supported the use of aggressive topical antibiotic therapy for the first 24 hours with the addition of the topical steroid once the clinical picture becomes clearer. Drug therapy usually is needed for 5 to 7 days. The patient should be monitored closely for the development of new signs or symptoms that alter the initial diagnosis of acute red eye reaction syndrome.

The acute red eye reaction syndrome may recur if contact lens wear is reinstituted too soon and the eye has not been given adequate time to heal. Ideally, contact lens wear should not be resumed until all infiltrates, epithelial defects (including microcysts and subtle negative staining), and signs of inflammation have resolved, which may take up to several weeks.[291,293] It is not uncommon, however, for prominent anterior stromal infiltrates to leave a persistent opacity (Fig. 27.48) that does not preclude resumption of contact

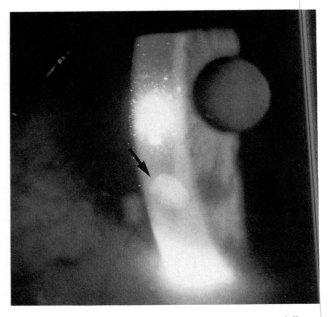

FIGURE 27.48 **An anterior stromal scar remains (arrow) following resolution of the acute red eye reaction syndrome and corneal infiltrate.**

lens wear following complete resolution of the acute signs and symptoms.

Once contact lens wear is resumed, it is important to evaluate the lens fit, wearing time, and cleaning regimen in an effort to avoid recurrences of the acute red eye reaction syndrome. Contact lens replacement, a temporary or ongoing switch from extended to daily wear, refitting to a flatter lens, changing to disposable lenses, or refitting with rigid gas permeable lenses may be needed, singly or in combination.[291] It also is important to remind the patient of appropriate contact lens follow-up care intervals in an effort to minimize the development of acute problems.

Epithelial Microcysts

ETIOLOGY

The term *epithelial microcysts* refers to an abnormal corneal response at the cellular level to chronic hypoxia from contact lens wear. When present, they tend to be observed in soft contact lens wearers, particularly those wearing extended-wear soft contact lenses.[275] An hypoxic state can result in the development of microcysts due to such causes as excessive wearing time and reduced corneal oxygen levels from aging lens material, a tight fitting lens, or excessive coating and depositing on the lenses.

Epithelial microcysts likely represent small pockets of cellular debris and disorganized cell growth arising from the basement membrane and basal layers of the cornea.[293] The inciting event to microcyst development may be the accumulation of fluid in the intracellular spaces of the epithelium.[273] Microcysts appear as tiny, refractile spheroidal dots in the central and paracentral corneal epithelium.[291] Due to normal cell turnover, the microcysts tend to migrate through the corneal epithelium where they may rupture and erode onto the epithelial surface.[294] Although an occasional epithelial microcyst may be noted in an asymptomatic extended-wear soft contact lens patient, a patient who develops large numbers of densely aggregated microcysts eventually will develop symptomatology. It is the latter patient who will require therapeutic intervention.

DIAGNOSIS

The soft contact lens patient who becomes symptomatic from epithelial microcysts tends to develop symptoms rather suddenly following uneventful contact lens wear. It is not uncommon for the patient with microcysts to have been remiss in timely follow-up care, when the formation of microcysts may have been detected before symptoms developed. Symptoms associated with this condition include burning, foreign body sensation, tearing, and photophobia, all likely related to the disrupted epithelium. Decreased visual acuity will result, even with the best spectacle correction in place, because of the now irregular anterior corneal surface.

Mild to moderate conjunctival injection occurs and may be enhanced in the perilimbal area. Careful slit-lamp examina-

tion reveals a dense collection of tiny, clear epithelial cysts in the central cornea. This appearance is best viewed using indirect illumination and retroillumination techniques (Fig. 27.49).[293] Instillation of fluorescein sodium reveals an irregular central epithelial surface with almost a discoid collection of punctate "positive" and "negative" stains. Positive stains occur when the microcysts have emptied onto the epithelial surface and caused microerosions; negative stains occur over the tiny "bumps" in the epithelium where the microcysts have invaded the epithelium but not yet eroded it.

MANAGEMENT

Treatment requires discontinuation of contact lens wear until the epithelial microcysts resolve. Therapeutic measures primarily are supportive in nature while the tissue heals and returns to a normal state. Patients who are acutely symptomatic may benefit from cycloplegia, using long-acting agents such as 5% homatropine for several days. Prophylactic topical antibiotic therapy, such as polymyxin B-trimethoprim or 0.3% tobramycin drops instilled four times daily, will protect the cornea from secondary infection. A topical ophthalmic ointment, such as polymyxin B-bacitracin or 0.3% tobramycin instilled into the conjunctival sac at bedtime, will provide a cushioning layer between the lid and the irritated epithelium. Additionally, the instillation of a mild topical steroid drop, such as 0.12% prednisolone or 0.1% fluorometholone four times a day, will enhance patient comfort.

Epithelial microcysts may take weeks to months to resolve, although the therapy described above is generally needed only for the first 1 or 2 weeks after acute presentation. Once the patient becomes asymptomatic, it can be a challenging management issue to convince the patient that contact lens wear should be discontinued until the corneal tissue is observed to be healed. While corneal healing is being monitored, it is important to observe closely for subtle positive and negative staining, which are indicative of persistent epithelial disruption.

Once the microcysts resolve completely, contact lens wear may be reinstituted carefully. If age of the lens material, deposited lenses, tight fitting lenses, or low water content was related to the development of the microcysts, then pursue contact lens refitting. Patient education must be addressed regarding the need for proper lens hygiene, wearing time and follow-up care. Once contact lens wear is resumed, careful periodic corneal examination is needed to monitor for recurrence of epithelial microcysts.

Acanthamoeba Keratitis

ETIOLOGY

Acanthamoeba is a free-living, nonparasitic protozoan found in soil, fresh water, salt water, distilled water, and saliva.[295] Twenty-two species of *Acanthamoeba* have been identified,

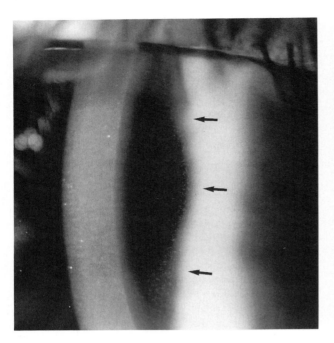

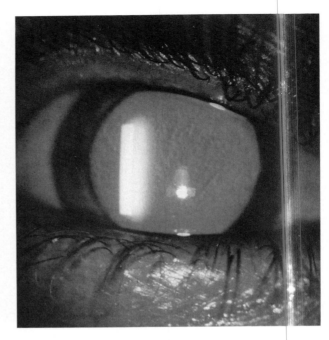

A

B

FIGURE 27.49   **Epithelial microcysts (arrows) observed in indirect illumination *(A)* and retroillumination *(B)*. The patient was wearing daily-wear soft contact lenses and last had a follow-up examination 11 months earlier. Due to the irregular corneal surface, best corrected visual acuity was reduced to 20/50.**

five of which may cause keratitis.[296] The exact mechanism of corneal infection by this organism is uncertain but seems to involve many factors, including epithelial trauma, a large inoculum of organism, and compromised host defense mechanisms.[297]

Acanthamoeba ocular infection was first described in 1973.[296] The majority of *Acanthamoeba* keratitis cases described in the mid-1980s involved daily-wear soft contact lens wearers who were using saline made from distilled water and salt tablets. Cases have also been described in extended-wear soft contact lens wearers and rigid contact lens wearers. In a survey of corneal specialists, Stehr-Green and associates[298] found that 85% of the reported cases were in contact lens patients using primarily daily-wear or extended-wear soft lenses.

Acanthamoeba keratitis can occur in patients other than contact lens wearers. This condition may result following corneal contamination or injury from water or vegetative matter.[299] *Acanthamoeba* keratitis has been reported following penetrating keratoplasty in a patient with no identifiable risk factors for this condition.[297] Parrish and associates[297] theorize that the post-keratoplasty development of this condition may have been the result of surgically induced epithelial trauma and alteration of the eye's normal flora following postoperative use of topical steroids, although they do not discount the possibility of transmission of the organism through the donor corneal tissue. Fungal, viral, chlamydial, and bacterial infections, including crystalline keratopathy caused by the viridans group of streptococci, have been reported concurrent with *Acanthamoeba* keratitis.[300,301] It is theorized that these organisms, along with damaged host cells, may potentiate *Acanthamoeba* infection by serving as an initial source of nutrition for the protozoan.[300]

DIAGNOSIS

The patient with *Acanthamoeba* keratitis typically presents with symptoms of redness, irritation, pain, photophobia, and reduced visual acuity.[302] A history of corneal contamination with water, saliva, or vegetative matter may be elicited with careful questioning. The duration of symptoms may vary from days to weeks, with waxing and waning of signs and symptoms common. Not infrequently, the condition has been present for weeks or months, and treatment with multiple agents for viral or bacterial keratitis had been attempted without result.[303]

Clinical signs of *Acanthamoeba* keratitis include lid edema, conjunctival injection and usually a mild anterior chamber reaction. Early in the disease course a dendritiform keratitis,[304,305] central or paracentral infiltration, or elevated epithelial lines[306] may be evident. Late in the course a prominent complete or partial stromal ring-shaped infiltrate with recurrent epithelial breakdown is highly suggestive of this condition (Fig. 27.50).[307] Subepithelial infiltrates, similar to those seen in viral or chlamydial corneal infections, have been noted late in the disease course away from the site of original infection and with minimal to no accompanying inflammatory signs.[308] Holland and associates[308] theorize that an immunologic mechanism may be responsible for these late-onset, steroid-responsive infiltrates.

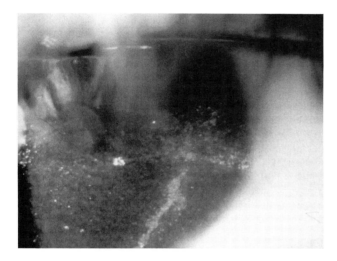

A

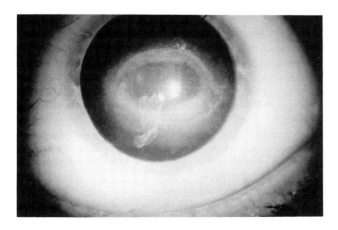

B

FIGURE 27.50 *Acanthamoeba* keratitis. *(A)* Dendritiform. *(B)* Ring-infiltrative pattern of late-stage infection. (Courtesy J. James Rowsey, M.D.)

Acanthamoeba keratitis should be suspected in at-risk patients who exhibit a deteriorating corneal condition unresponsive to multiple therapy regimens. Definitive diagnostic information is obtained through laboratory analysis.[309] Keratoplasty biopsy has been used to identify encysted organisms as well as trophozoites, the stage when the amoebas emerge from dormant cysts to become actively feeding cells.[310] Specular microscopy has been used as a noninvasive "photographic biopsy" to identify *Acanthamoeba* cysts within the corneal stroma.[311] Alternative microbiologic techniques have been evaluated to diagnose *Acanthamoeba* keratitis.[312] More recently, routine microbiologic techniques have been used to identify *Acanthamoeba* keratitis. The cysts may be identified using gram and Giemsa stains, and *Acanthamoeba* may be isolated from a corneal scraping plated onto a nutrient agar enriched with *E. coli.*[299,300]

MANAGEMENT

Acanthamoeba keratitis is an extremely challenging clinical management problem with the potential for treatment failure and should be treated by a provider experienced in its management. Aggressive medical therapy is initiated using multiple antibacterial, antifungal, and antiamoebic agents. Therapeutic agents that have been reported to be successful, used either alone or in combination, include propamidine isethionate, neomycin, paromomycin, miconazole, clotrimazole, ketoconazole (systemic), and itraconazole (systemic).[313,314] Polyhexamethylene biguanide, a newer antiparasitic agent first reported in 1991 as a successful pharmacotherapeutic agent for *Acanthamoeba* keratitis, has been used successfully in combination with propamidine and neomycin by Varga and associates[315] to treat five patients. The antiamoebic treatment regimen may be continued for 3 to 6 months following resolution of the clinical signs.[316] Topical steroids may be added to control symptoms and reduce late-onset infiltrates, although withdrawal of the steroid may prove to be difficult.[308,317]

In many instances, patient symptoms of pain and photophobia are proportionately higher than the clinical signs may predict.[295] Sulindac, a systemic nonsteroidal anti-inflammatory agent, has been reported to control severe pain associated with this condition when other nonopioid and opioid analgesic agents failed.[318]

Bacon and associates[316] reported that patients who are diagnosed and treated appropriately for *Acanthamoeba* keratitis within one month of initial symptoms have a much higher cure rate with good visual outcomes compared with those for whom antiamoebic therapy was started later in the disease course. Clinical signs common in early *Acanthamoeba* keratitis include limbitis; epitheliopathy in a disc, ring, or dendritiform distribution; perineural infiltrates; and a low-grade anterior uveitis.[316] The successful response of early *Acanthamoeba* keratitis to pharmacotherapy may reflect concentration of the organism in the corneal epithelium before stromal penetration has occurred.

Penetrating keratoplasty may be needed after pharmacotherapy if a visually debilitating corneal scar remains. The use of keratoplasty as a therapy for *Acanthamoeba* keratitis that is not responding to medical therapy is a subject of debate. It is preferable to perform the surgery when active inflammation is not present, and recurrence appears to be common if it is performed too soon; however, the success rate is higher before the organism has disseminated throughout the cornea and caused excessive tissue damage.[300,319] Continued efforts toward successful medical therapies may increasingly preclude the need for penetrating keratoplasty.

Prevention of *Acanthamoeba* keratitis is its best treatment.[295] Contact lens–wearing patients must be educated carefully as to the proper use and care of their lenses. Homemade saline is no longer an approved or accepted contact lens solution.[320] It is advisable not to wear contact lenses while swimming or in hot tubs, although nonprescription swimming goggles may provide some protection from water exposure. Prescription swimming goggles may be preferable for correction of high refractive errors in this setting. Rigid contact lens wearers should be advised not to contaminate their lenses with saliva. Water contamination of contact lenses, including the case, should be avoided. It also is important that eye care providers remain alert to the possibility of this diagnosis so that the signs and symptoms of *Acanthamoeba* keratitis might be recognized as early in the disease course as possible, which may enhance the success of medical treatment.

Miscellaneous Corneal Conditions

Dellen

ETIOLOGY

Dellen are small areas of corneal thinning typically located at the limbus. They are caused by localized drying of the cornea usually due to poor spreading of the tear film. The tear film disruption is often due to a local surface elevation of the conjunctiva in the adjacent paralimbal area. Pterygium, pinguecula, conjunctival chemosis, scarring from cataract or muscle surgery, filtering blebs for the treatment of glaucoma, nerve palsies, scleritis, and episcleritis are common causes of dellen, but any mass that prevents close apposition of the lids to the cornea can be responsible for their formation. The use of systemic medications with anticholinergic side effects, such as antihistamines, may precipitate or exacerbate the clinical signs or symptoms.[321]

DIAGNOSIS

Patients with dellen usually present with a foreign body sensation or slight discomfort. They often have a history of irritated eyes which have recently become worse. They commonly report redness of their eyes, and focal conjunctival injection usually is visible on slit-lamp examination.

Slit-lamp examination reveals a small, oval, saucer-like excavation usually less than 2.0 mm in size located on the corneal side of the limbus. Although the lesion has clearly defined borders, its base appears hazy and dry. The wall of the excavation will be steeper on the corneal side and more sloping on the limbal side.[322] Fluorescein sodium will pool in the excavation, and actual staining of the lesion may vary from minimal to prominent (Fig. 27.51).

Early in the development of a delle, the stroma is intact but thinned due to loss of fluid (Fig. 27.52). Stromal degeneration can occur, and true scarring with or without vascularization develops if the delle is allowed to persist. The formation of a descemetocele in a long–standing delle that required a corneoscleral patch graft has been reported.[323]

MANAGEMENT

Treatment for dellen is directed toward rehydrating the cornea and removing the cause, if possible. Artificial tears administered every 2 hours and lubricating ointment instilled into the conjunctival sac at bedtime usually will allow resolution within 48 hours. If the delle is diagnosed early in its development and treated aggressively, it can resolve within 24 hours.[322] Very severe dellen may require pressure patching with prophylactic topical antibiotics such as polymyxin B-bacitracin or erythromycin ointment, for 24 hours. If the delle has formed due to an inflammation such as scleritis or episcleritis, appropriate therapy with topical ste-

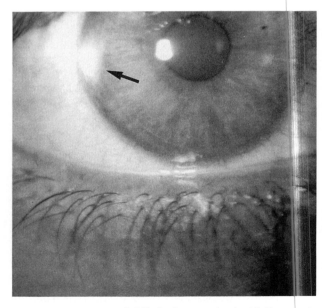

FIGURE 27.51   **Corneal delle is shown stained with fluorescein sodium (arrow).**

roids should be initiated. Patients should be asked to return for evaluation in 1 to 7 days after instituting therapy depending on the severity of the lesion.

Bullous Keratopathy

ETIOLOGY

If fluid enters the cornea at a rate faster than it is removed by the pump mechanism of the endothelial cells, edema will result. Fluid accumulates in the epithelium as well as the stroma and causes the epithelium to separate from Bowman's layer. Clinically, these areas of separation between Bowman's layer and the epithelium are called *bullae,* which appear like small blisters on the front surface of the cornea. With time and the normal growth of epithelial cells, these bullae will be pushed anteriorly in the cornea and erupt at its surface.

In recent years, most bullous keratopathy has developed after cataract surgery and intraocular lens (IOL) implantation. In 1983, Taylor and associates[324] showed that pseudophakic bullous keratopathy was found more often with intracapsular cataract extraction and anterior chamber IOLs (4.3%) when compared to extracapsular cataract extraction and posterior chamber IOLs (0.3%). When it occurs, the average length of time from cataract surgery to the development of bullous keratopathy is 18 to 24 months.[324,325] The occurrence of bullous keratopathy after cataract surgery is thought to be due primarily to trauma to the endothelium from contact with the intraocular lens implant or surgical instruments. Other authors argue that corneal decompensation results from the release of inflammatory mediators due to continuous trauma to the eye by the intraocular lens implant[326] or by shock waves from pseudophakodonesis.[324]

Although cataract surgery is a potential precursor to bullous keratopathy, there are many other causes. Fuchs' endothelial dystrophy, infection, trauma, retained foreign body, posterior polymorphous dystrophy, chronic uveitis, chronically elevated intraocular pressure, and vitreous touch are all known causes of bullous keratopathy.

DIAGNOSIS

Subjectively, the patient with bullous keratopathy will report tearing, a foreign body sensation, and pain. The pain is caused by either the exposure of nerves with the eruption of the bullae, or the stretching of nerves as they pass through swollen, edematous epithelium. Another common symptom is decreased vision due to edema and distortion of the anterior corneal surface.

Evaluation of the cornea reveals an edematous, thickened, usually hazy cornea with bullae (Fig. 27.53). Some areas of the cornea will stain with fluorescein sodium due to ruptures of the bullae. Focal involvement of the cornea is possible, especially if there has been local trauma such as birth trauma or foreign body injury.

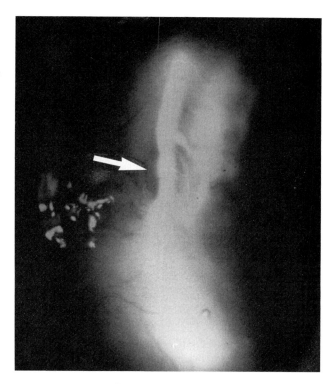

FIGURE 27.52 **Focal stromal thinning at the site of a corneal delle (arrow). (Courtesy William L. Jones, O.D.)**

MANAGEMENT

A thorough examination should be performed to determine the cause of bullous keratopathy. The specific treatment plan depends on both the cause as well as the severity of the keratopathy. Examination of the endothelium, internal structures, and fundus can be enhanced by the use of topical ophthalmic glycerin to decrease the epithelial edema.[327] Because glycerin will sting when applied to the cornea, its use should be preceded by instillation of a topical anesthetic. Internal examination is essential to determine if there is corneal touch by the intraocular lens or vitreous face, and to rule out cystoid macular edema or intraocular inflammation.

Although corneal edema can affect the measurement of IOP, it is nevertheless important to perform tonometry. The incidence of open angle glaucoma in patients with Fuchs' dystrophy and its potential bullous keratopathy is estimated to be 10% to 15%,[327] and angle-closure glaucoma can cause corneal edema similar to that seen with bullous keratopathy.

If there is a known treatable cause, its management is necessary for resolution of the edema. If, however, the corneal edema appears to be due to changes in endothelial function, hyperosmotic therapy with 5% sodium chloride solution 4 to 8 times a day and 5% sodium chloride ointment

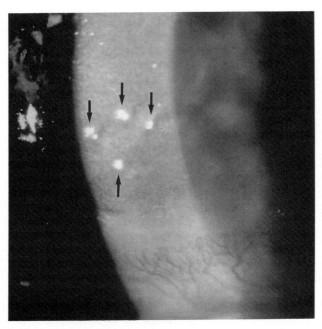

FIGURE 27.53   **Bullous keratopathy (arrows) in patient with end-stage neovascular glaucoma. Intraocular pressure was 56 mm Hg.**

in the conjunctival sac at bedtime is the most appropriate treatment. Treatment with hypertonic agents is limited by stinging on instillation and by the difficulty caused by frequent applications.

Hair dryers, used on a low setting and directed toward the eyes at arm's length, may also prove useful. The evaporation of tears changes their tonicity which, in turn, draws fluid from the epithelium and stroma to decrease corneal edema.

If patients are experiencing pain or poor vision, a hydrophilic bandage lens often is applied. Aquavella[328] reported 13 out of 20 patients experienced complete relief of pain with the continuous wear of hydrophilic contact lenses. An additional 5 patients reported partial relief. The relief of pain from soft contact lenses probably is due to protection of the nerves exposed by ruptured bullae.

In the same study, Aquavella[328] reported an improvement in visual acuity for 69% of patients with bullous keratopathy when wearing contact lenses. The most likely explanation is the covering of an irregular cornea with the regular surface of a soft contact lens. The usefulness of hydrophilic contact lenses for pain relief and vision improvement is well supported.[329–332] Maximum relief of symptoms is obtained when soft contact lenses are used on an extended-wear basis, but daily-wear use also has been successful. Although Aquavella also reported improvement in the slit-lamp appearance of the corneas when contact lenses were used, others have found no evidence of this benefit.[332]

Patients with bullous keratopathy wearing soft contact lenses should be monitored closely. The corneal breaks caused by bullous keratopathy, along with decreased endothelial function, may make these patients more susceptible to complications from contact lens wear such as infection, ulceration, neovascularization, increased edema, and inflammation. Andrew and Woodward[329] found that 13% of their bullous keratopathy patients developed suppurative keratitis after one year of contact lens wear. Leibowitz and Rosenthal[332] suggest monthly evaluations for patients using contact lenses on an extended-wear basis for bullous keratopathy.

Some practitioners prefer not to recommend the use of soft contact lenses during episodes of bullae eruption. When a patient presents with corneal epithelial defects due to ruptured bullae, a prophylactic antibiotic ointment such as erythromycin or tobramycin can be administered, along with a cycloplegic agent and pressure patching for 24 to 48 hours. As with all cases that involve pressure patching, patients should be seen within 24 hours after applying the patch.

Although there is concern about the uptake of medications or their preservatives by hydrophilic contact lenses, some authors support the concurrent use of bandage soft contact lenses and medications such as prophylactic antibiotics and hypertonics.[328–332] Many of these authors, however, used nonpreserved formulations.

Because even normal IOP can force fluid into the cornea if the endothelium is not functioning properly, many authors suggest the use of topical or oral medications to decrease the IOP in patients with bullous keratopathy.[327,333–335] It is important, however, to avoid epinephrine derivatives if the patient is aphakic or pseudophakic due to the potential development of cystoid macular edema.

As bullous keratopathy becomes more severe, surgical intervention may be considered. Pseudophakic bullous keratopathy has recently become the most common indication for penetrating keratoplasty in the United States.[326,336] Results indicate that grafts remain clear in a large percentage of patients who have penetrating keratoplasty.[337]

If the patient has limited visual potential due to factors such as age-related macular degeneration, cystoid macular edema, or end-stage glaucoma, surgery for bullous keratopathy is designed to make the patient more comfortable. A Gunderson conjunctival flap procedure, in which the superior bulbar conjunctiva is drawn over the cornea, is one of the most common types of surgical intervention in these patients. Electrocautery of Bowman's layer also has been reported as a successful method of pain control.[333]

Follow-up for patients with bullous keratopathy varies depending on contact lens wear and the severity of the disease. Most patients should be monitored every 1 to 6 months.

Toxic Keratitis

ETIOLOGY

A wide range of substances toxic to the cornea may produce epithelial insult known as toxic keratitis. This terminology generally is reserved for mild, superficial corneal irritation not related to a specific clinical entity such as chemical burns, discussed elsewhere in this chapter. Contact with solutions that are foreign to the eye are common causes of toxic keratitis. These may include such common entities as shampoos, lotions used in the periocular area, and chlorinated pool water. Toxic corneal reactions have been reported from tonometer tips contaminated with 70% isopropyl alcohol or hydrogen peroxide that was not fully removed after disinfection of the probe.[338–340] Irreversible corneal scarring has resulted from inadvertent ocular contamination with chlorhexidine gluconate, a skin cleanser used preoperatively.[341] A number of topical ophthalmic preparations are known to cause toxic keratitis, including antivirals, fortified antibiotics, antifungals, aminoglycosides, anesthetics, and contact lens solutions.[275,342,343] The causative agents may be the active ingredients of these preparations or the preservatives used in formulating them.[343,344] The mistaken use of nonophthalmic products for eyedrops may result in toxic keratitis or even corneal trauma.[345,346]

The term *medicamentosa* is used to refer to a type of toxic keratitis related to topical ophthalmic medication use. It frequently manifests as a collection of punctate epithelial erosions in the inferior third of the cornea following ophthalmic drop or ointment use.[17] Its location in the inferior third of the cornea is likely related to the accumulation of medication in this area, resulting in toxic epithelial insult. An accompanying mechanical component from instillation of the medication in this part of the globe seems reasonable. Following routine use of topical ophthalmic anesthetic and mydriatic or cycloplegic agents, it is common to observe a toxic keratitis that can be fairly prominent in the inferior one-third to one-half of the cornea. The resulting punctate epithelial keratopathy appears as a grayish, irregular "softening" of the epithelium.

DIAGNOSIS

The patient with toxic keratitis or medicamentosa will generally report recent exposure to the offending substance, or the use of an ophthalmic preparation on a short- or long-term basis. In the case of mild toxic keratitis, the patient may have few or no symptoms. More involved cases may produce very definite symptoms of redness, irritation, burning, and tearing.

Clinical signs are also of variable severity. Mild medicamentosa may manifest as scattered punctate epithelial erosions in the inferior third of the cornea in a patient who is being treated for an anterior segment condition such as bacterial conjunctivitis. More pronounced toxic keratitis may present as diffuse punctate epithelial erosions and punctate epithelial keratopathy in the exposed interpalpebral corneal area or over the entire cornea (Fig. 27.54). Conjunctival involvement may range from none, to mild inferior bulbar injection, to prominent diffuse injection and chemosis.[347] Accompanying dermatitis of the lids

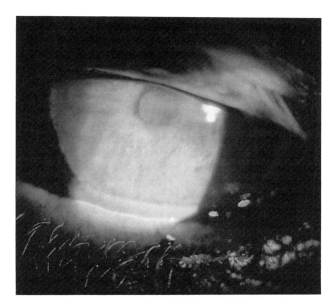

FIGURE 27.54 **Diffuse punctate epithelial erosions in patient with toxic keratitis.**

suggests an allergic hypersensitivity reaction rather than a toxic keratitis.

MANAGEMENT

Discontinuation or avoidance of the offending agent usually brings resolution of the toxic keratitis. The risk/benefit ratio of treating this condition should be assessed, since adding topical ophthalmic medications may exacerbate the condition. In general, mild medicamentosa can be tolerated easily without treatment, both from the patient and examiner standpoints, until the condition prompting initial treatment is resolved and the medication is discontinued. If toxic keratitis results in intolerance of a certain contact lens solution or a needed therapeutic agent, alternative therapy should be chosen.

In the case of mild, transient toxic keratitis, patient comfort may be enhanced with the use of topical nonpreserved lubricating agents while the condition resolves within a few days. In the case of more pronounced toxic keratitis, particularly involving conjunctival injection, topical decongestant agents may be used, such as 0.1% naphazoline drops instilled four times daily until resolution occurs.

More severe forms of toxic keratitis may require prophylactic topical antibiotic therapy to protect the inflamed globe while it heals. The use of aminoglycosides should be avoided, however, since they tend to be associated with this condition. In addition, the use of a mild topical steroid, such as 0.12% prednisolone drops four times a day, will aid the resolution of more severe toxic keratitis. Any allergic component involving the lids or conjunctiva should be treated appropriately.

Calcific Band Keratopathy

ETIOLOGY

The deposition of calcium carbonate salts in the epithelium, subepithelial tissue, stroma, and particularly in Bowman's layer commonly is called *band keratopathy* because of its characteristic band-like appearance. Chronic ocular inflammation is one of the most common causes and includes conditions such as anterior uveitis, severe superficial keratitis, interstitial keratitis, trachoma, and prolonged glaucoma. The chronic anterior uveitis of juvenile rheumatoid arthritis (JRA) is frequently associated with band keratopathy, one study reporting its development in 30% of patients with JRA.[348]

Topical and intraocular medications have been reported as common causes of band keratopathy. Exposure to silicone oil used for surgery to treat trauma and retinal detachments can result in the rapid development of band keratopathy,[349,350] as does the original formulation of sodium chondroitin sulfate (Viscoat) when used with BSS-Plus during cataract surgery.[351,352] Viscoat had a high phosphate level which may have bound to the calcium in the BSS-Plus at the time of these reports, but has since been formulated with less phosphate.[353] Chronic exposure to topical medications with phenylmercuric preservatives also has been reported as a cause of band keratopathy.

Alterations in systemic calcium-phosphorus ratios is a known cause of band keratopathy formation. This includes hypercalcemia caused by conditions such as hyperparathyroidism, sarcoidosis, and vitamin D intoxification, as well as the elevated serum phosphorus commonly found with kidney failure.

Gout is another known cause of band keratopathy. There are many reported cases of idiopathic band keratopathy, some of which seem to have an hereditary component.

DIAGNOSIS

The patient with band keratopathy reports decreased visual acuity, visual halos, or a white spot on the eye. If an epithelial erosion develops, the patient also may report a foreign body sensation, photophobia and lacrimation. A patient who develops band keratopathy in a non-seeing eye may be asymptomatic for this condition.

Examination will show a dusting of gray white deposits in Bowman's layer or a slight hazing of the cornea early in the course of the disease. It typically starts at 3 and 9 o'clock and progresses slowly toward the center, usually taking several months to years to coalesce and form a complete band across the cornea in the interpalpebral opening (Fig. 27.55). A clear zone between the limbus and the deposit and multiple clear areas within the plaque are characteristics that confirm the diagnosis.

There are reports of development of less characteristic band keratopathies. Patients with severely dry eyes seem to develop band keratopathy much more quickly. Freddo and Leibowitz[354] reported a case that developed within 24 hours, and Lemp and Ralph[355] reported its development in 2 to 3 weeks, all in patients with dry eyes. Band keratopathy due to gout appears more brown in color instead of gray-white. Band keratopathy due to phenylmercuric nitrate preservatives has been reported, in which the bands tend to start centrally and progress toward the periphery.[349]

MANAGEMENT

A careful history along with slit-lamp examination for signs of chronic anterior segment inflammation, end-stage glaucoma, or other underlying conditions should be performed to determine the cause of band keratopathy. If no cause can be detected, laboratory tests can be performed to evaluate kidney function, including BUN, serum albumin, magnesium, creatinine, and phosphorus levels. Serum calcium should be evaluated to rule out hyperparathyroidism, and uric acid level should be ascertained if there is a possibility of gout.

Treatment of band keratopathy should be directed toward any underlying cause. If the patient's symptoms are mild, artificial tears 4 to 6 times a day with lubricating ointment at bedtime may be all that is necessary. Patients with only mild symptoms may be monitored every 3 to 12 months.

If the symptoms are severe or vision is poor, the calcium band should be removed. This is performed at the slit-lamp with a mixture of 2% to 3% EDTA. After instillation of a topical anesthetic, the corneal epithelium over the band keratopathy is debrided with a sterile scalpel. The calcium band is wiped with a cotton swab or ophthalmic cellulose sponge saturated with the 3% EDTA solution for 5 to 30 minutes until the calcium clears. Scraping of the calcium is discouraged since it can cause damage to Bowman's layer.

Because this procedure can cause anterior uveitis, a cycloplegic agent such as 5% homatropine should be administered. A prophylactic antibiotic ointment such as tobramycin or polymyxin B-bacitracin should be instilled into the conjunctival sac, and a pressure patch applied. The patient should return in 24 hours for evaluation, and pressure patching should be repeated until the epithelium is healed. Oral analgesics (see Chap. 7) will make the patient more comfortable.

Recently, phototherapeutic keratectomy with a 193 nm excimer laser was reported to be effective for the treatment of band keratopathy.[356]

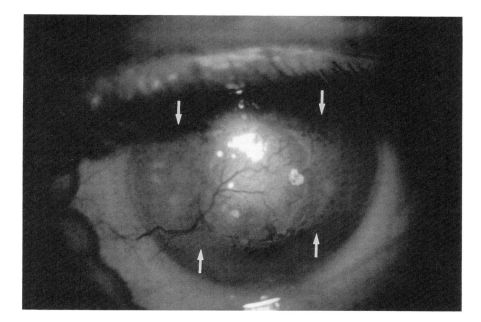

A

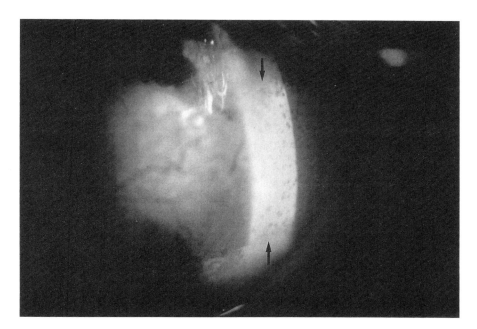

B

FIGURE 27.55   *(A)* Band keratopathy (arrows) in patient with a phthisical eye secondary to multiple failed retinal detachment surgeries. *(B)* Parallelepiped view shows the typical "Swiss cheese" appearance of calcific band keratopathy (arrows).

References

1. Last RJ. The eyeball. In: Eugene Wolff's Anatomy of the eye and orbit, 6th ed. Philadelphia: WB Saunders Company, 1973:30–181.
2. Vaughn D. Cornea. In: Vaughan D, Asbury T, Tabbara KF, eds. General ophthalmology, 12th ed. Norwalk, CT: Appleton & Lange, 1989:104–125.
3. Arffa RC. Anatomy. In: Grayson's Diseases of the cornea, 3rd ed. St. Louis: Mosby Year Book, 1991:1–24.
4. Arffa RC. Infectious ulcerative keratitis: bacterial. In: Grayson's Diseases of the cornea, 3rd ed. St. Louis: Mosby Year Book, 1991: 163–198.
5. Klyce SD, Beuerman RW. Structure and function of the cornea. In: Kaufman HE, Barron BA, McDonald MB, Waltman SR, eds. The cornea. New York: Churchill Livingstone, 1988:3–54.
6. Waltman SR, Hart WM, Jr. The cornea. In: Moses RA, Hart WM, Jr., eds. Adler's Physiology of the eye. Clinical application. St. Louis: CV Mosby Company, 1987:36–59.
7. Katakami C, Fujisawa K, Sahori A, et al. Localization of collagen (I) and collagenase mRNA by *in situ* hybridization during wound healing after epikeratophakia or alkali burn. Jpn J Ophthalmol 1991;36:10–22.
8. Doughman DJ. Corneal edema. In: Tasman W, Jaeger EA, eds. Duane's Clinical ophthalmology, Vol. 4, revised edition. Philadelphia: JB Lippincott Company, 1991;16A:1–17.
9. Van Buskirk EM. The anatomy of the limbus. Eye 1989;3:101–108.
10. McCulley JP. The circulation of fluid at the limbus (flow and diffusion at the limbus). Eye 1989;3:114–120.
11. Kenyon KR, Fogle JA, Grayson M. Dysgeneses, dystrophies and degenerations of the cornea. In: Tasman W, Jaeger EA, eds. Duane's Clinical ophthalmology, Vol. 4, revised edition. Philadelphia: JB Lippincott Company, 1991;16:1–56.
12. Last RJ. Slit-lamp appearance. In: Wolff's Anatomy of the eye and orbit, 6th ed. Philadelphia: WB Saunders Company, 1973:241–250.
13. Kenyon KR. Morphology and pathologic responses of the cornea to disease. In: Smolin G, Thoft RA, eds. The cornea. Scientific foundations and clinical practice, 2nd ed. Boston: Little, Brown and Company, 1987:63–98.
14. Bonomi L, Perfetti S, Bellucci R, et al. Prevention of surgically induced miosis by diclofenac eye drops. Ann Ophthalmol 1987; 19:142–145.
15. Seymour R, Ramsey MS. Unusually severe traumatic uveitis associated with occult ankylosing spondylitis. Can J Ophthalmol 1991;26:156–158.
16. Zantos SC. Management of corneal infiltrates in extended-wear contact lens patients. Int Contact Lens Clin 1984;10:604–610.
17. Coster DJ. Superficial keratopathy. In: Tasman W, Jaeger EA, eds. Duane's Clinical ophthalmology, Vol. 4, revised edition. Philadelphia: JB Lippincott Company, 1991;17:1–13.
18. Dohlman CH. The function of the corneal epithelium in health and disease. Invest Ophthalmol 1971;10:383–407.
19. Davanger M, Evensen A. Role of the pericorneal papillary structure in renewal of corneal epithelium. Nature 1971;229:560–561.
20. Tseng SC. Concept and application of limbal stem cells. Eye 1989;3:141–157.
21. Murakami J, Nishida T, Otori T. Coordinated appearance of beta 1 integrins and fibronectin during corneal wound healing. J Lab Clin Med 1992;120:86–93.
22. Phan TM, Foster CS, Wasson PJ, et al. Role of fibronectin and fibrinogen in healing of corneal epithelial scrape wounds. Invest Ophthalmol Vis Sci 1989;30:377–385.
23. Bron AJ. Vortex patterns of the corneal epithelium. Trans Ophthalmol Soc UK 1973;93:455–472.
24. Dua HS, Forrester JV. Clinical patterns of corneal epithelial wound healing. Am J Ophthalmol 1987;104:481–489.
25. Thoft RA, Wiley LA, Sundarraj N. The multipotential cells of the limbus. Eye 1989;3:109–113.
26. Locke LC, Blesch K. Vortex keratopathy. Clin Eye Vis Care 1989; 1:143–156.
27. Sakai J, Hung J, Zhu G, et al. Collagen metabolism during healing of lacerated rabbit corneas. Exp Eye Res 1991;52:237–244.
28. Funderburgh JL, Chandler JW. Proteoglycans of rabbit corneas with nonperforating wounds. Invest Ophthalmol Vis Sci 1989;30: 435–442.
29. Junghans BM, Collin HB. Limbal lymphangiogenesis after corneal injury: an autoradiographic study. Curr Eye Res 1989;8:91–100.
30. Ormerod LD, Garsd A, Reddy CV, et al. Dynamics of corneal epithelial healing after an alkali burn. A statistical analysis. Invest Ophthalmol Vis Sci 1989;30:1784–1793.
31. Hurst JS, Balazy M, Bazan HE, et al. The epithelium, endothelium and stroma of the rabbit corneal generate (12S)-hydroxyeicosatetranoic acid as the main lipoxygenase metabolite in response to injury. J Biol Chem 1991;266:6726–6730.
32. SunderRaj N, Rizzo JD, Anderson SC, et al. Expression of vimentin by rabbit corneal epithelial cells during wound repair. Cell Tissue Res 1992;267:347–356.
33. Tervo T, Tervo K, van Setten GB, et al. Plasminogen activator and its inhibitor in the experimental corneal wound. Exp Eye Res 1989;48:445–449.
34. Fingeret M, Casser L, Woodcome HT. Overview biomicroscopic examination. In: Atlas of primary eyecare procedures. Norwalk, CT: Appleton & Lange, 1990:20–25.
35. Fingeret M, Casser L, Woodcome HT. Corneal evaluation. In: Atlas of primary eyecare procedures. Norwalk, CT: Appleton & Lange, 1990:30–35.
36. Fingeret M, Casser L, Woodcome HT. Vital dye staining. In: Atlas of primary eyecare procedures. Norwalk, CT: Appleton & Lange, 1990:46–49.
37. Locke LC, Hill S. Polymorphic amyloid degeneration of the cornea. Clin Eye Vis Care 1992;4:3–12.
38. Messner SS. Corneal trauma. In: Onofrey BE, ed. Clinical optometric pharmacology and therapeutics. Philadelphia: JB Lippincott Company, 1992;27:1–18.
39. Larkin GL. Airbag-mediated corneal injury. Am J Emerg Med 1991;9:444–446.
40. Melton NR, Maino JH, Thomas RK. Management of corneal abrasions. Optom Clin 1991;1(4):119–126.
41. Fingeret M, Casser L, Woodcome HT. Corneal debridement. In: Atlas of primary eyecare procedures. Norwalk, CT: Appleton & Lange, 1990:160–161.
42. Kowalik BM, Rakes JA. Filamentary keratitis: the clinical challenge. J Am Optom Assoc 1991;62:200–204.
43. Levy B, Nguyen N, Abbott RL, et al. Hypotony and corneal edema secondary to patching in normal eyes. Optom Vis Sci 1992;69:72–75.
44. Arffa RC. Epithelial diseases. In: Grayson's Diseases of the cornea, 3rd ed. St. Louis: Mosby Year Book, 1991:324–332.

45. Parker AV, Cohen EJ, Arentsen JJ. *Pseudomonas* corneal ulcers after artificial fingernail injuries. Am J Ophthalmol 1989;107: 548–549.

46. Anderson C, Moretti S, Greser RG. The effect of tarsorrhaphy on normal healing of corneal epithelial defects in a rabbit model. Cornea 1991;10:478–482.

47. Kirkpatrick JNP, Hoh HB, Cook SD. No eye pad for corneal abrasion. Eye 1993;7:468–471.

48. Frucht-Pery J, Stiebel H, Hemo I, et al. Effect of eye patching on ocular surface. Am J Ophthalmol 1993;115:629–633.

49. Shaker GJ, Ueda S, LoCascio JA, et al. Effect of a collagen shield on cat corneal epithelial wound healing. Invest Ophthalmol Vis Sci 1989;30:1565–1568.

50. Frantz JM, Dupery BM, Kaufman HE, et al. The effect of collagen shields on epithelial wound healing in rabbits. Am J Ophthalmol 1989;108:524–528.

51. Wedge CI, Rootman DS. Collagen shields: efficacy, safety and comfort in the treatment of human traumatic corneal abrasion and effect on vision in healthy eyes. Can J Ophthalmol 1992;27:295–298.

52. Archeson JF, Joseph J, Spalton DJ. Use of soft contact lenses in an eye casualty department for the primary treatment of traumatic corneal abrasions. Br J Ophthalmol 1987;71:285–289.

53. Essepian JP, Wei F, Hildesheim J, et al. Comparison of corneal epithelial wound healing rates in scrape vs lamellar keratectomy injury. Cornea 1990;9:294–298.

54. Gonul B, Koz M, Ersoz G, et al. Effect of EGF on the corneal wound healing of alloxan diabetic mice. Exp Eye Res 1992;54: 519–524.

55. Singh G, Foster CS. Growth factors in treatment of nonhealing corneal ulcers and recurrent erosions. Cornea 1989;8:45–53.

56. Pastor JC, Calonge M. Epidermal growth factor and corneal wound healing. A multicenter study. Cornea 1992;11:311–314.

57. Herschel MK, McDonald MB, Ahmed S, et al. Voltaren for treatment of discomfort after excimer ablation. Invest Ophthalmol Vis Sci 1993;34(Suppl):893.

58. Sher NA, Frantz JM, Talley A, et al. Ocular pain control after excimer laser PRK. Invest Ophthalmol Vis Sci 1993; 34(Suppl):893.

59. Smolin G, Tabbara K, Whitcher J. The cornea. In: Infectious diseases of the eye. Baltimore: Williams & Wilkins, 1984:81–131.

60. Clinch TE, Robinson MJ, Barron BA, et al. Fungal keratitis from nylon line lawn trimmers. Am J Ophthalmol 1992;114:437–440.

61. Wellington DP, Johnstone MA, Hopkins RJ. Bull's-eye corneal lesion resulting from war game injury. Arch Ophthalmol 1989; 107:1727.

62. Augeri PA. Corneal foreign body removal and treatment. Optom Clin 1991;1(4):59–70.

63. Miller KB. Attack of the sand brier. Ann Emerg Med 1991;20: 418–420.

64. Melton R, Thomas RK. Conjunctival and corneal foreign-body removal. In: Onofrey BE, ed. Clinical optometric pharmacology and therapeutics. Philadelphia: JB Lippincott Company, 1992;55: 1–10.

65. Migneco MK, Simpson DE. Penetrating injury from hammering with subtle ocular damage. J Am Optom Assoc 1992;63:634–637.

66. Alexander MM, MacLeod JDA, Hall NF, et al. More than meets the eye: a study of time lost from work by patients who incurred injuries from corneal foreign bodies. Br J Ophthalmol 1991;75: 740–742.

67. Arnold RW, Erie JC. Magnetized forceps for metallic corneal foreign bodies. Arch Ophthalmol 1988;106:1502.

68. Zuckerman BD, Lieberman TW. Corneal rust ring. Arch Ophthalmol 1960;63:254–264.

69. Fingeret M, Casser L, Woodcome HT. Corneal rust ring removal. In: Atlas of primary eyecare procedures. Norwalk, CT: Appleton & Lange, 1990;152–155.

70. Sigurdsson H, Hanna I, Lockwood AJ, et al. Removal of rust ring, comparing electric drill and hypodermic needle. Eye 1987;1:430–432.

71. Hulbert MFG. Efficacy of eyepad in corneal healing after corneal foreign body removal. Lancet 1991;337:643.

72. Keenan JM, Raines MF. Ocular injury from external rear view mirrors. Eye 1990;4:649–650.

73. Wilson SE, Bannan RA, McDonald MB, et al. Corneal trauma and infection caused by manipulation of the eyelashes after application of mascara. Cornea 1990;9:181–182.

74. Nolan BT. Perforation by a foreign body through a pre-existing radial keratotomy wound. Milit Med 1991;156:151–154.

75. McDermott ML, Wilkinson WS, Tukel DB, et al. Corneoscleral rupture ten years after radial keratotomy. Am J Ophthalmol 1990; 110:575–577.

76. Metrikin DC, Fante RG, Hodes BI. Intraocular cilia after penetrating eye injury. Arch Ophthalmol 1992;110:921.

77. Hamill MB, Thompson WS. The evaluation and management of corneal lacerations. Retina 1990;10:S1–S7.

78. Aiello LP, Iwamoto M, Taylor HR. Perforating ocular fishhook injury. Arch Ophthalmol 1992;110:1316–1317.

79. Fingeret M, Casser L, Woodcome HT. Seidel test. In: Atlas of primary eyecare procedures. Norwalk, CT: Appleton & Lange, 1990:290–291.

80. McMahon TT, Robin JB. Corneal trauma: I-classification and management. J Am Optom Assoc 1991;62:170–178.

81. Lam S, Rapuano CJ, Krachmer JH, et al. Lamellar corneal autograft for corneal perforation. Ophthalmic Surg 1991;22:716–717.

82. Hugkulstone CE. Uses of a bandage contact lens in perforating injuries of the cornea. J R Soc Med 1992;85:322–323.

83. Hirst LW, Smiddy WE, Stark WJ. Corneal perforations: changing methods of treatment, 1960–1980. Ophthalmology 1982;89:630–635.

84. Erdey PA, Lindahl KJ, Temnycky GO, et al. Techniques for application of tissue adhesive for corneal perforations. Ophthalmic Surg 1991;22:352–354.

85. Smiddy WE, Hamburg TR, Kracher GP, et al. Contact lenses for visual rehabilitation after corneal laceration repair. Ophthalmology 1989;96:293–298.

86. LaRoche GR. Children benefit from contact lens fitting after corneal laceration repair. Ophthalmology 1989;96:1679.

87. Doren GS, Cohen EJ, Brady SE, et al. Penetrating keratoplasty after ocular trauma. Am J Ophthalmol 1990;110:408–411.

88. Nobe JR, Moura BT, Robin JB, et al. Results of penetrating keratoplasty for the treatment of corneal perforations. Arch Ophthalmol 1990;108:939–941.

89. Chan MY, Liao HR, Cheng FJ. Traumatic intracorneal cyst. Ann Ophthalmol 1989;21:303–305.

90. Parrish CM, Chandler JW. Corneal trauma. In: Kaufman HE, Barron BA, McDonald MB, Waltman SK, eds. The cornea. New York: Churchill Livingstone, 1988:599–646.

91. Goldman JN, Dohlman CH, Kravitt BA. The basement membrane

of the human cornea in recurrent epithelial erosion syndrome. Trans Am Ophthalmol Soc 1969;73:471–481.

92. Tripathi RC, Bron AJ. Ultrastructural study of non-traumatic recurrent corneal erosion. Br J Ophthalmol 1972;46:73–85.

93. Brown N, Bron A. Recurrent erosion of the cornea. Br J Ophthalmol 1976;60:84–96.

94. McLean EN, MacRae SM, Rich LF. Recurrent erosion. Treatment by anterior stromal puncture. Ophthalmology 1986;93:784–787.

95. Waring GO III, Rodrigues MM, Laibson PR. Corneal dystrophies. I. Dystrophies of the epithelium, Bowman's layer and stroma. Surv Ophthalmol 1978;23:71–122.

96. Waltman SR. Recurrent corneal erosion. Arch Ophthalmol 1989; 107:1436.

97. Kenyon KR. Recurrent corneal erosion: pathogenesis and therapy. Int Ophthalmol Clin 1979;19:169–195.

98. Wood TO. Recurrent erosion. Trans Am Ophthalmol Soc 1984; 82:850–898.

99. Huang AJW, Tseng SCG. Corneal epithelial wound healing in the absence of limbal epithelium. Invest Ophthalmol Vis Sci 1991;32: 96–105.

100. Trobe JD, Laibson PR. Dystrophic changes in the anterior cornea. Arch Ophthalmol 1972;87:378–382.

101. Kell HM, Prouty RE. Recurrent corneal epithelial erosions: advanced approaches to management. South J Optom 1991;9:28–33.

102. Trobe JD. Recurrent corneal erosion. Int Ophthalmol Clin 1973; 13:155–165.

103. Rubinfeld RS, MacRae SM, Laibson PR. Successful treatment of recurrent corneal erosion with Nd: YAG anterior stromal puncture. Am J Ophthalmol 1991;111:252–255.

104. Rubinfeld RS, Laibson PR, Cohen EJ, et al. Anterior stromal puncture for recurrent erosion: further experience and new instrumentation. Ophthalmic Surg 1990;21:318–326.

105. Katz HR, Snyder ME, Green WR, et al. Nd:YAG laser photo-induced adhesion of the corneal epithelium. Am J Ophthalmol 1994;118:612–622.

106. Buxton JN, Fox ML. Superficial epithelial keratectomy in the treatment of epithelial basement membrane dystrophy. Arch Ophthalmol 1983;101:392–395.

107. Bass LJ. Exposure keratitis. In: Onofrey BE, ed. Clinical optometric pharmacology and therapeutics. Philadelphia: JB Lippincott Company, 1992;59:1–4.

108. Arffa RC. Tear film abnormalities. In: Grayson's Diseases of the cornea, 3rd ed. St. Louis: Mosby Year Book, 1991:310–323.

109. Arffa RC. Chemical injuries. In: Grayson's Diseases of the cornea, 3rd ed. St. Louis: Mosby Year Book, 1991:649–665.

110. Asbury T, Tabbara KF. Trauma. In: Vaughan D, Asbury T, Tabbara KF, eds. General ophthalmology, 12th ed. Norwalk, CT: Appleton & Lange, 1989:343–349.

111. Fingeret M, Casser L, Woodcome HT. Conjunctival/ocular irrigation. In: Atlas of primary eyecare procedures. Norwalk, CT: Appleton & Lange, 1990:130–131.

112. Grant WM. Toxicology of the eye, 3rd ed. Springfield, IL: CC Thomas, 1986.

113. Fingeret M, Casser L, Woodcome HT. Speculum insertion. In: Atlas of primary eyecare procedures. Norwalk, CT: Appleton & Lange, 1990:90–91.

114. Haseba T, Nakazawa M, Kao CW, et al. Isolation of wound-specific cDNA clones from a cDNA library prepared with mRNA's of alkali-burned rabbit corneas. Cornea 1991;10:322–329.

115. Schultz GS, Strelow S, Stern GA, et al. Treatment of alkali-injured rabbit corneas with a synthetic inhibitor of matrix metalloproteinases. Invest Ophthalmol Vis Sci 1992;33:3325–3331.

116. Chung JH, Fagerholm P, Lindstom B. Hyaluronate in healing of corneal alkali wound in the rabbit. Exp Eye Res 1989;48:569–576.

117. Fagerholm P, Fitzsimmons T, Harfstrand A, et al. Reactive formation of hyaluronic acid in the rabbit corneal alkali burn. Acta Ophthalmol 1992;202:67–72.

118. Haddox JL, Pfister RR, Yuille-Barr D. The efficacy of topical citrate after alkali injury is dependent on the period of time it is administered. Invest Ophthalmol Vis Sci 1989;30:1062–1068.

119. Burns FR, Stack MS, Gray RD, et al. Inhibition of purified collagenase from alkali-burned rabbit corneas. Invest Ophthalmol Vis Sci 1989;30:1569–1575.

120. Catania LJ. Diseases of the cornea. In: Primary care of the anterior segment, Norwalk, CT: Appleton & Lange, 1988:83–181.

121. Vajpayee RB, Gupta NK, Angra SK, et al. Contact thermal burns of the cornea. Can J Ophthalmol 1991;26:215–218.

122. DeRespinis PA, Frohman LP. Microwave popcorn-ocular injury caused by steam. New Engl J Med 1990;323:1212.

123. Terry JE. Diseases of the cornea. In: Bartlett JD, Jaanus SD, eds. Clinical ocular pharmacology, 2nd ed. Boston: Butterworths, 1989;567–611.

124. Jones BR. Differential diagnosis of punctate keratitis. Trans Ophthalmol Soc UK 1960;80:664–675.

125. Petit TH, Meyer KT. The differential diagnosis of superficial punctate keratitis. Int Ophthalmol Clin 1984;24:79–92.

126. Taylor PB, Tabbara KF. Peripheral corneal infections. Int Ophthalmol Clin 1986;26:29–48.

127. Cohn H, Mondino BJ, Brown SI, et al. Marginal corneal ulcers with acute beta streptococcal conjunctivitis and chronic dacryocystitis. Am J Ophthalmol 1979;87:541–543.

128. Mondino BJ. Inflammatory diseases of the peripheral cornea. Ophthalmology 1988;95:463–472.

129. McCulloch D, Alexander A. Phlyctenular keratoconjunctivitis. J Am Optom Assoc 1983;54:435–439.

130. Mondino BJ, Adamu SA, Pitchekian-Halabi H. Antibody studies in a rabbit model of corneal phlyctenulosis and catarrhal infiltrates related to *Staphylococcus aureus*. Invest Ophthalmol Vis Sci 1991;32:1854–1863.

131. Mondino BJ, Dethlefs B. Occurrence of phlyctenules after immunization with ribitol teichoic acid of *Staphylococcus aureus*. Arch Ophthalmol 1984;102:461–463.

132. Farson C. Phlyctenular keratoconjunctivitis at Point Barrow, Alaska. Am J Ophthalmol 1961;51:585–588.

133. Jeffery MP. Ocular diseases caused by nematodes. Am J Ophthalmol 1955;40:41–53.

134. Thygeson P. The etiology and treatment of phlyctenular keratoconjunctivitis. Am J Ophthalmol 1951;34:1217–1236.

135. Jones WL. Phlyctenular keratoconjunctivitis. Rev Optom 1981; 118:74–76.

136. Culbertson WW, Huang AJW, Mandelbaum SH, et al. Effective treatment of phlyctenular keratoconjunctivitis with oral tetracycline. Ophthalmology 1993;100:1358–1366.

137. Erie JC, Nevitt MP, Hodge DO, et al. Incidence of ulcerative keratitis in a defined population from 1950 through 1988. Arch Ophthalmol 1993;111:1665–1671.

138. Musch DC, Sugar A, Meyer RF. Demographic and predisposing factors in corneal ulceration. Arch Ophthalmol 1983;101:1545–1548.

139. Hemady RK, Griffin N, Aristimuno B. Recurrent corneal infections in a patient with the acquired immunodeficiency syndrome. Cornea 1993;12:266–269.

140. Ormerod LD, Gomez DS, Schanzlin DJ, et al. Chronic alcoholism and microbial keratitis. Br J Ophthalmol 1988;72:155–159.

141. Harris DJ, Stulting RD, Waring GO, et al. Late bacterial and fungal keratitis after corneal transplantation. Spectrum of pathogens, graft survival and visual prognosis. Ophthalmology 1988; 95:1450–1457.

142. Kent HD, Cohen EJ, Laibson PR, et al. Microbial keratitis and corneal ulceration associated with therapeutic soft contact lenses. CLAO J 1990;16:49–52.

143. Cruz OA, Sabir SM, Capo H, et al. Microbial keratitis in childhood. Ophthalmology 1993;100:192–196.

144. Matoba AY. Infectious keratitis. Focal points. Clinical Modules for Ophthalmologists 1992;X(8):1–12.

145. Asbell P, Stenson S. Ulcerative keratitis. Survey of 30 years' laboratory experience. Arch Ophthalmol 1982;100:77–80.

146. Liesegang TJ, Forster RK. Spectrum of microbial keratitis in south Florida. Am J Ophthalmol 1980;90:38–47.

147. Leibowitz HM. Clinical evaluation of ciprofloxacin 0.3% ophthalmic solution for treatment of bacterial keratitis. Am J Ophthalmol 1991;112:34S–47S.

148. Alfonso E, Mandelbaum S, Fox MJ, et al. Ulcerative keratitis associated with contact lens wear. Am J Ophthalmol 1986;101: 429–433.

149. Derick RJ, Kelley CG, Gersman M. Contact lens related corneal ulcers at the Ohio State University Hospitals 1983–1987. CLAO J 1989;15:268–270.

150. Jones DB. Decision-making in the management of microbial keratitis. Ophthalmology 1981;88:814–820.

151. Rubinfeld RS, Cohen EJ, Arentsen JJ, et al. Diphtheroids as ocular pathogens. Am J Ophthalmol 1989;108:251–254.

152. Bullington RH, Lanier JD, Font RL. Nontuberculous mycobacterial keratitis. Arch Ophthalmol 1992;110:519–524.

153. Shovlin J. Contact lens troubleshooter. What to expect "the morning after." Optom Manag 1992;27(5):73.

154. Ormerod LD, Ruoff KL, Meisler DM, et al. Infectious crystalline keratopathy. Role of nutritionally variant *Streptococci* and other bacterial factors. Ophthalmology 1991;98:159–169.

155. Scott A. Ciloxan for the management of corneal ulcers. J Ophthal Nurs Tech 1991;10:207–210.

156. Parker P. *Moraxella* corneal ulcer. J Ophthal Nurs Tech 1988;7: 87–89.

157. Marioneaux SJ, Cohen EJ, Arentsen JJ, et al. *Moraxella* keratitis. Cornea 1991;10:21–24.

158. Pepose JS, Wilhelmus KR. Divergent approaches to the management of corneal ulcers. Am J Ophthalmol 1992;114:630–632.

159. McDonnell PJ, Nobe J, Gauderman WJ, et al. Community care of corneal ulcers. Am J Ophthalmol 1992;114:531–538.

160. Kowal VO, Mead MD. Community acquired corneal ulcers: the impact of cultures on management. Invest Ophthalmol Vis Sci 1992;33(suppl):1210.

161. Perrigin J. Laboratory workup of microbial keratitis. J Am Optom Assoc 1992;63:243–248.

162. Snyder ME, Katz HR. Ciprofloxacin-resistant bacterial keratitis. Am J Ophthalmol 1992;114:336–338.

163. Benson WH, Lanier JD. Comparison of techniques for culturing corneal ulcers. Ophthalmology 1992;99:800–804.

164. Varga JH, Wolf TC, Jensen HG. Swab culture of corneal ulcers. Ophthalmology 1992;99:1346.

165. Gomez JT, Robinson NM, Osato MS, et al. Comparison of acridine orange and gram stains in bacterial keratitis. Am J Ophthalmol 1988;106:735–737.

166. Parks DJ, Abrams DA, Sarfarazi FA, et al. Comparison of topical ciprofloxacin to conventional antibiotic therapy in the treatment of ulcerative keratitis. Am J Ophthalmol 1993;115:471–477.

167. Insler MS, Fish LA, Silbernagel J, et al. Successful treatment of methicillin-resistant *Staphylococcus aureus* keratitis with topical ciprofloxacin. Ophthalmology 1991;98:1690–1692.

168. Callegan MC, Hobden JA, Hill JM, et al. Topical antibiotic therapy for the treatment of experimental *Staphylococcus aureus* keratitis. Invest Ophthalmol Vis Sci 1992;33:3017–3023.

169. Hobden JA, O'Callaghan RJ, Insler MS, et al. Ciprofloxacin ointment versus ciprofloxacin drops for therapy of experimental *Pseudomonas* keratitis. Cornea 1993;12:138–141.

170. Wilhelmus KR, Hyndiuk RA, Caldwell DR, et al. 0.3% Ciprofloxacin ophthalmic ointment in the treatment of bacterial keratitis. Arch Ophthalmol 1993;111:1210–1218.

171. Lambert JN, Gritz GC, McDonnell PJ, et al. The potential of ofloxacin as a topical treatment for bacterial ulcers. Invest Ophthalmol Vis Sci 1991;32(suppl):1184.

172. Gritz DC, McDonnell PJ, Lee TY, et al. Topical ofloxacin in the treatment of *Pseudomonas* keratitis in a rabbit model. Cornea 1992;11:143–147.

173. Bowe BE, Levartovsky S, Eiferman RA. Neurotrophic corneal ulcers in congenital sensory neuropathy. Am J Ophthalmol 1989;107:303–304.

174. Clinch TE, Hobden JA, Hill JM, et al. Collagen shields containing tobramycin for sustained therapy (24 hours) of experimental *Pseudomonas* keratitis. CLAO J 1992;18:245–247.

175. Carmichael TR, Gelfand Y, Welsh NH. Topical steroids in the treatment of central and paracentral corneal ulcers. Br J Ophthalmol 1990;74:528–531.

176. Stern GA, Buttross M. Use of corticosteroids in combination with antimicrobial drugs in the treatment of infectious corneal disease. Ophthalmology 1991;98:847–853.

177. Eiferman RA, Forgey DR, Cook YD. Excimer laser ablation of infectious crystalline keratopathy. Arch Ophthalmol 1991;110:18.

178. Serdarevic O, Darrell RW, Krueger RR, et al. Excimer laser therapy for experimental *Candida* keratitis. Am J Ophthalmol 1985;99:534–538.

179. Gottsch JD, Gilbert ML, Goodman DR, et al. Excimer laser ablative treatment of microbial keratitis. Ophthalmology 1991;98: 146–149.

180. O'Day DM. Selection of appropriate antifungal therapy. Cornea 1987;6:238–245.

181. Vajpayee RB, Surendra KA, Sandramouli S, et al. Laboratory diagnosis of keratomycosis: comparative evaluation of direct microscopy and culture results. Ann Ophthalmol 1993;24:68–71.

182. Johns KJ, O'Day DM. Pharmacologic management of keratomycoses. Surv Ophthalmol 1988;33:178–188.

183. Forster RK, Rebell G. The diagnosis and management of keratomycoses. Arch Ophthalmol 1975;93:975–978.

184. Kaufman HE, Wood RM. Mycotic keratitis. Am J Ophthalmol 1965;59:993–1000.

185. Stern GA, Okumoto M, Smolin G. Combined amphotericin B and rifampin treatment of experimental *Candida albicans* keratitis. Arch Ophthalmol 1979;97:721–722.

186. Lou P, Kazdan J, Bannatyne RM, et al. Successful treatment of *Candida* endophthalmitis with synergistic combination of amphotericin B and rifampin. Am J Ophthalmol 1977;83:12–13.

187. Mohan M, Panda A, Gupta SK. Management of human keratomycosis with miconazole. Aust NZ J Ophthalmol 1989;17:295–297.

188. Wegman DH, Guinee VF, Millian SJ. Epidemic keratoconjunctivitis. Am J Public Health 1970;60:1230–1237.

189. Hecht SD, Hanna L, Sery TW, et al. Treatment of epidemic keratoconjunctivitis with idoxuridine (IUDR). Arch Ophthalmol 1965;73:49–54.

190. Ward JB, Siojo LG, Waller SG. A prospective, masked clinical trial of trifluridine, dexamethasone, and artificial tears in the treatment of epidemic keratoconjunctivitis. Cornea 1993;12:216–221.

191. Nauheim RC, Romanowski EG, Araullo-Cruz T, et al. Prolonged recoverability of desiccated adenovirus type 19 from various surfaces. Ophthalmology 1990;97:1450–1453.

192. Colon LE. Keratoconjunctivitis due to adenovirus type 8: report on a large outbreak. Ann Ophthalmol 1991;23:63–65.

193. Murrah WF. Epidemic keratoconjunctivitis. Ann Ophthalmol 1988;20:36–38.

194. Hyde KJ, Berger ST. Epidemic keratoconjunctivitis and lacrimal excretory system obstruction. Ophthalmology 1988;95:1447–1449.

195. Paparello SF, Rickman LS, Mesbahi HN. Epidemic keratoconjunctivitis at a U.S. Military Base: Republic of the Philippines. Milit Med 1991;156:256–259.

196. Reed K. Epidemic viral keratoconjunctivitis diagnosis and management. J Am Optom Assoc 1983;54:141–144.

197. Hammer LH, Perry HD, Donnenfeld ED, et al. Symblepharon formation in epidemic keratoconjunctivitis. Cornea 1990;9:338–340.

198. Laibson PR, Dhiri S. Oconer J, et al. Corneal infiltrates in epidemic keratoconjunctivitis. Response to double-blind corticosteroid therapy. Arch Ophthalmol 1970;84:36–40.

199. Dudgeon J, Bhargava SK, Roxx CAC. Treatment of adenovirus infection of the eye with 5-iodo-2′-deoxyuridine. A double-blind trial. Br J Ophthalmol 1969;53:530–533.

200. Pavan-Langston D, Dohlman CH. A double blind clinical study of adenine arabinoside therapy of viral keratoconjunctivitis. Am J Ophthalmol 1972;74:81–88.

201. Waring GO III, Laibson PR, Satz JE, et al. Use of vidarabine in epidemic keratoconjunctivitis due to adenovirus types 3, 7, 8, and 19. Am J Ophthalmol 1976;82:781–785.

202. Lennette DA, Eiferman RA. Inhibition of adenovirus replication in vitro by trifluridine. Arch Ophthalmol 1978;96:1662–1663.

203. Kana JS. Delayed trifluridine treatment of subepithelial corneal infiltrates. Am J Ophthalmol 1992;113:212–214.

204. Nesburn AB, Lowe GH, Lepoff NJ, et al. Effect of topical trifluridine on Thygeson's superficial punctate keratitis. Ophthalmology 1984;91:1188–1192.

205. Tabbara KF, Ostler HB, Dawson C, et al. Thygeson's superficial punctate keratitis. Ophthalmology 1981;88:75–77.

206. Lemp MA, Chambers RW, Lundy J. Viral isolate in superficial punctate keratitis. Arch Ophthalmol 1974;91:8–10.

207. Braley AE, Alexander RC. Superficial punctate keratitis. Isolation of a virus. Arch Ophthalmol 1953;50:147–154.

208. Thygeson P. Superficial punctate keratitis. JAMA 1950;144:1544–1549.

209. Hardten DR, Doughman DJ, Holland EJ, et al. Persistent superficial punctate keratitis after resolution of chlamydial follicular conjunctivitis. Cornea 1992;11:360–363.

210. Thygeson P. Further observations on superficial punctate keratitis. Arch Ophthalmol 1961;66:158–162.

211. van Bijsterveld OP, Mansour KH, Dubois FJ. Thygeson's superficial punctate keratitis. Ann Ophthalmol 1985;17:150–153.

212. Rafieetary MR, Sharpe JS, Heavener PH. Thygeson's superficial punctate keratitis. Clin Eye Vis Care 1991;3:183–186.

213. Thygeson P. Clinical and laboratory observations on superficial punctate keratitis. Am J Ophthalmol 1966;61:1344–1349.

214. Tantum LA. Superficial punctate keratitis of Thygeson. J Am Optom Assoc 1992;53:985–986.

215. Forstot SL, Binder PS. Treatment of Thygeson's superficial punctate keratopathy with soft contact lenses. Am J Ophthalmol 1979;88:186–189.

216. Goldberg DB, Schanzlin DJ, Brown SI. Management of Thygeson's superficial punctate keratitis. Am J Ophthalmol 1980;89:22–24.

217. Ramsay WK, Brown LA. Thygeson's superficial punctate keratitis: a case report. South J Optom 1988;6:43–44.

218. Pepose JS, Laycock KA, Kelvin J, et al. Reactivation of latent herpes simplex virus by excimer laser photokeratectomy. Am J Ophthalmol 1992;114:45–50.

219. Cook SD. Herpes simplex virus in the eye. Br J Ophthalmol 1992;76:365–366.

220. Kaufman HE. Synopsis: diseases of the cornea. Herpetic dendritic ulcer. Clin Sci Ophthalmol 1982;V(5).

221. Liesegang TJ. Biology and molecular aspects of herpes simplex and varicella-zoster virus infections. Ophthalmology 1992;99:781–799.

222. Cantin E, Chen J, Willey DE, et al. Persistence of herpes simplex virus DNA in rabbit corneal cells. Invest Ophthalmol Vis Sci 1992;33:2470–2475.

223. Pepose JS. Herpes simplex keratitis: role of viral infection versus immune response. Surv Ophthalmol 1991;35:345–352.

224. Kaufman HE. Herpetic keratitis: Proctor Lecture. Invest Ophthalmol Vis Sci 1978;17:941–957.

225. Vrabec MP, Durrie DS, Chase DS. Recurrence of herpes simplex after excimer laser keratectomy. Am J Ophthalmol 1992;114:96–97.

226. Rosenwasser GOD, Greene WH. Simultaneous herpes simplex types 1 and 2 keratitis in acquired immunodeficiency syndrome. Am J Ophthalmol 1992;113:102–103.

227. Vila-Coro AA, del Cotero JF, Bonafonte S. Pediatric herpes simplex masquerading as varicella-zoster. Ann Ophthalmol 1992;21:47–48.

228. Laibson PR. Current therapy of herpes simplex virus infection of the cornea. Int Ophthalmol Clin 1973;13(4):39–52.

229. Liesegang TJ. A community study of ocular herpes simplex. Curr Eye Res 1991;10:111–115.

230. Deutsch FH. Concurrent adenoviral and herpetic ocular infections. Ann Ophthalmol 1989;21:432–438.

231. Holbach LM, Font RL, Wilhelmus KR. Recurrent herpes simplex keratitis with concurrent epithelial and stromal involvement. Immunohistochemical and ultra structural observations. Arch Ophthalmol 1991;109:692–695.

232. Shovlin JP. Dendriform lesions of the cornea: an important differential diagnosis in contact lens wearers. Int Contact Lens Clin 1991;18:165–166.

233. Pavan-Langston D, Dunkel EC. A rapid clinical diagnostic test for

herpes simplex infectious keratitis. Am J Ophthalmol 1989;107: 675–677.

234. Kowalski RP, Gordon YJ, Romanowski EG, et al. A comparison of enzyme immunoassay and polymerase chain reaction with the clinical examination for diagnosing ocular herpetic disease. Ophthalmology 1993;100:530–533.

235. Blatt AN, Laycock KA, Brady RH, et al. Prophylactic acyclovir effectively reduces herpes simplex virus type 1 reactivation after exposure of latently infected mice to ultraviolet B. Invest Ophthalmol Vis Sci 1993;34:3459–3465.

236. Kaufman HE, Varnell ED, Centifanto YM, et al. Effect of the herpes simplex genome on the response of infection to corticosteroids. Am J Ophthalmol 1985;100:114–118.

237. Brown DD, McCulley JP, Bowman RW, et al. The use of conjunctival flaps in the treatment of herpes keratouveitis. Cornea 1992; 11:44–46.

238. Schwab IR. Oral acyclovir in the management of herpes simplex ocular infections. Ophthalmology 1988;95:423–430.

239. Teich SA, Cheung TW, Friedman AH. Systemic antiviral drugs used in ophthalmology. Surv Ophthalmol 1992;37:19–53.

240. Sonkin PL, Baratz KH, Frothingham R, et al. Acyclovir-resistant herpes simplex virus keratouveitis after penetrating keratoplasty. Ophthalmology 1992;99:1805–1808.

241. Sandor EV, Millman A, Croxson TS, et al. Herpes zoster ophthalmicus in patients at risk for the acquired immune deficiency syndrome (AIDS). Am J Ophthalmol 1986;101:153–155.

242. Karbassi M, Raizman MB, Schuman JS. Herpes zoster ophthalmicus. Surv Ophthalmol 1992;36:395–410.

243. Pavan-Langston D, McCulley JP. Herpes zoster dendritic keratitis. Arch Ophthalmol 1973;89:25–29.

244. Reed JW, Joyner SJ, Knauer WJ. Penetrating keratoplasty for herpes zoster keratopathy. Am J Ophthalmol 1989;107:257–261.

245. Liesegang TJ. Corneal complications from herpes zoster ophthalmicus. Ophthalmology 1985;92:316–324.

246. Liesegang TJ. Diagnosis and therapy of herpes zoster ophthalmicus. Ophthalmology 1991;98:1216–1229.

247. Marsh RJ. Current management of ophthalmic zoster. Aust NZ J Ophthalmol 1990;18:273–279.

248. Jones WL. Herpes zoster dendritic keratitis. J Am Optom Assoc 1982;53:813–814.

249. Womack LW, Liesegang TJ. Complications of herpes zoster ophthalmicus. Arch Ophthalmol 1983;101:42–45.

250. Hoang-Xuan T, Buchi ER, Herbort CP, et al. Oral acyclovir for herpes zoster ophthalmicus. Ophthalmology 1992;99:1062–1070.

251. Cobo LM, Foulks GN, Liesegang T, et al. Oral acyclovir in the therapy of acute herpes zoster ophthalmicus. Ophthalmology 1985;92:1574–1583.

252. Piebenga LW, Laibson PR. Dendritic lesions in herpes zoster ophthalmicus. Arch Ophthalmol 1973;90:268–270.

253. Soong HK, Schwartz AE, Meyer RF, et al. Penetrating keratoplasty for corneal scarring due to herpes zoster ophthalmicus. Br J Ophthalmol 1989;73:19–21.

254. Findley HM. Recurrent corneal erosions. J Am Optom Assoc 1986;57:392–396.

255. Werblin TP, Hirst LW, Stark WJ, et al. Prevalence of map-dot-fingerprint changes in the cornea. Br J Ophthalmol 1981;65:401–409.

256. Ehlers N, Moller HU. Dot-map-fingerprint dystrophy—Cogan's microcystic dystrophy—normal reactions of the corneal epithelium? Acta Ophthalmol 1987;65:62–66.

257. Payant JA, Eggenberger LR, Wood TO. Electron microscopic findings in corneal epithelial basement membrane degeneration. Cornea 1991;10:390–394.

258. Rodrigues MM, Fine BS, Laibson PR, et al. Disorders of the corneal epithelium. Arch Ophthalmol 1974;92:475–482.

259. Cogan DG, Kuwabara T, Donaldson DD, et al. Microcystic dystrophy of the cornea. A partial explanation for its pathogenesis. Arch Ophthalmol 1974;92:470–474.

260. Bron AJ, Brown NA. Some superficial corneal disorders. Trans Ophthalmol Soc UK 1971;91:13–29.

261. Dark AJ. Bleb dystrophy of the cornea: histochemistry and ultrastructure. Br J Ophthalmol 1977;61:65–69.

262. Brodrick JD, Dark AJ, Peace GW. Fingerprint striae of the cornea following herpes simplex keratitis. Ann Ophthalmol 1976;8:481–484.

263. DeVoe AG. Certain abnormalities of Bowman's membrane with particular reference to fingerprint lines in the cornea. Trans Am Ophthalmol Soc 1962;60:195–201.

264. Shahinian L, Jr. Corneal valance: a tear film pattern in map-dot-fingerprint corneal dystrophy. Ann Ophthalmol 1984;16:567–571.

265. Gurwood AS, Kern BC. Punctal plugs help manage corneal dystrophy. Rev Optom 1991;128:77–79.

266. Arffa RC. Disorders of the cornea. In: Grayson's Diseases of the cornea, 3rd ed. St. Louis: Mosby Year Book, 1991:417–438.

267. Orlin SE, Raber IM, Eagle RC, et al. Keratoconus associated with corneal endothelial dystrophy. Cornea 1990;9:299–304.

268. McCartney MD, Wood TO, McLaughlin BJ. Moderate Fuchs' endothelial dystrophy ATPase pump site density. Invest Ophthalmol Vis Sci 1989;30:1560–1564.

269. Bass SJ. Corneal dystrophies. Optom Clin 1991;1(4):31–44.

270. Brogdon JD, McLaughlin SA, Brightman AH, et al. Effect of epidermal growth factor in healing of corneal endothelial cells in cats. Am J Vet Res 1989;50:1237–1243.

271. Arffa RC. Dystrophies of the epithelium, Bowman's layer, and stroma. In: Grayson's Diseases of the cornea, 3rd ed. St. Louis: Mosby Year Book, 1991:364–416.

272. Catania LJ. Management of corneal abrasions in an extended-wear patient population. Optom Clin 1991;1(3):123–133.

273. Larke JR. Contact lens wear and the epithelium. In: The eye and contact lens wear. London: Butterworths, 1985:94–101.

274. Dougal J. Abrasions secondary to contact lens wear. In: Tomlinson A, ed. Complications of contact lens wear. St. Louis: Mosby-Year Book, 1992:123–156.

275. Stapleton F, Dart J, Minassian D. Nonulcerative complications of contact lens wear: relative risks for different lens types. Arch Ophthalmol 1992;110:1601–1606.

276. Nauheim RC, Nauheim JS. Contact lens-related *Streptococcus viridans* keratitis presenting as an epithelial defect. Arch Ophthalmol 1991;109:1354.

277. Wallace W. The SLACH syndrome. Int Eye Care 1985;1:220.

278. Lin ST, Mandell RB. Corneal trauma from overnight wear of rigid or soft contact lenses. J Am Optom Assoc 1991;62:224–227.

279. Udell IJ, Ormerod LD, Boniuk V, et al. Treatment of contact lens-associated corneal erosions. Am J Ophthalmol 1987;104:306–307.

280. Binder PS. Complications associated with extended wear of soft contact lenses. Ophthalmology 1979;86:1093–1101.

281. Nilsson SE, Persson G. Low complication rate in extended wear of contact lenses. Acta Ophthalmol 1986;64:88–92.

282. Kenyon E, Polse KA, Seger RG. Influence of wearing schedule on extended-wear complications. Ophthalmology 1986;93:231–236.

283. Kotow M, Grant T, Holden BA. Avoiding ocular complications during hydrogel extended wear. Int Contact Lens Clin 1987;14: 95–99.

284. Josephson JE, Caffery BE. Proposed hypothesis for corneal infiltrates, microabrasions, and red eye associated with extended wear. Optom Vis Sci 1989;66:192.

285. Gordon A, Kracher GP. Corneal infiltrates and extended-wear contact lenses. J Am Optom Assoc 1985;56:198–201.

286. Phillips AJ, Badenoch PR, Grutzmacher R, et al. Microbial contamination of extended-wear contact lenses: an investigation of endotoxin as a cause of acute ocular inflammation reaction. Int Eyecare 1986;2:469–475.

287. Holden BA. The Glenn A. Fry Award Lecture 1988:The ocular response to contact lens wear. Optom Vis Sci 1989;66:717–733.

288. Josephson JE, Caffery BE. Infiltrative keratitis in hydrogel lens wearers. Int Contact Lens Clin 1979;6:223–239.

289. Vikoren Mertz PH, Bouchard CS, Mathers WD, et al. Corneal infiltrates associated with disposable extended wear soft contact lenses: a report of nine cases. CLAO J 1990;16:269–272.

290. Mondino BJ, Groden LR. Conjunctival hyperemia and corneal infiltrates with chemically disinfected soft contact lenses. Arch Ophthalmol 1980;98:1767–1770.

291. Silbert JA. Complications of extended wear. Optom Clin 1991; 1(3):95–121.

292. Stein RM, Clinch TE, Cohen EJ, et al. Infected vs sterile corneal infiltrates in contact lens wearers. Am J Ophthalmol 1988;105: 632–636.

293. Josephson JE, Zantos S, Caffery B, et al. Differentiation of corneal complications observed in contact lens wearers. J Am Optom Assoc 1988;59:679–685.

294. Weissman BA, Mondino BJ. Complications of extended-wear contact lenses. Int Eye Care 1985;1:230–240.

295. Dornic DI. *Acanthamoeba.* In: Onofrey BE, ed. Clinical optometric pharmacology and therapeutics. Philadelphia: JB Lippincott Company, 1992;41:1–9.

296. Jones DB. Acanthamoeba—the ultimate opportunist. Am J Ophthalmol 1986;102:527–530.

297. Parrish CM, Head WS, O'Day DM, et al. *Acanthamoeba* keratitis without other identifiable risk factors. Arch Ophthalmol 1991; 109:471.

298. Stehr-Green JK, Bailey TM, Visvesvara GS. The epidemiology of *Acanthamoeba* keratitis in the United States. Am J Ophthalmol 1989;107:331–336.

299. Sharma S, Srinivasan M, George C. *Acanthamoeba* keratitis in non-contact lens wearers. Arch Ophthalmol 1990;108:676–678.

300. Reddy VM, Pepose JS, Lubniewski AJ, et al. Concurrent chlamydial and *Acanthamoeba* keratoconjunctivitis. Am J Ophthalmol 1991;112:466–468.

301. Davis RM, Schroeder RP, Rowsey JJ, et al. *Acanthamoeba* keratitis and infectious crystalline keratopathy. Arch Ophthalmol 1989; 105:1524–1527.

302. Cohen EJ, Parlato CJ, Arentsen JJ, et al. Medical and surgical treatment of *Acanthamoeba* keratitis. Am J Ophthalmol 1987;103: 615–625.

303. Cohen EJ, Buchanan HW, Laughrea PA, et al. Diagnosis and management of *Acanthamoeba* keratitis. Am J Ophthalmol 1985; 100:389–395.

304. Lindquist TD, Neal AS, Doughman DJ. Clinical signs and medical therapy of early *Acanthamoeba* keratitis. Arch Ophthalmol 1988;106:73–77.

305. Hsieh WC, Dornic DI. *Acanthamoeba* dendriform keratitis. J Am Optom Assoc 1989;60:32–34.

306. Florakis GJ, Folberg R, Krachmer JH, et al. Elevated corneal epithelial lines in *Acanthamoeba* keratitis. Arch Ophthalmol 1988;106:1202–1206.

307. Berger ST, Mondino BJ, Hoft RH, et al. Successful medical management of *Acanthamoeba* keratitis. Am J Ophthalmol 1990; 110:395–403.

308. Holland EJ, Alul IH, Meisler DM, et al. Subepithelial infiltrates in *Acanthamoeba* keratitis. Am J Ophthalmol 1991;112:414–418.

309. Mathers W, Stevens G, Rodrigues M, et al. Immunopathology and electron microscopy of *Acanthamoeba* keratitis. Am J Ophthalmol 1987;103:626–635.

310. Silvany RE, Luckenbach MW, Moore MB. The rapid detection of *Acanthamoeba* in paraffin-embedded sections of corneal tissue with calcofluor white. Arch Ophthalmol 1987;105:1366–1367.

311. Wilhelmus KR, McCulloch RR, Osato MS. Photomicrography of *Acanthamoeba* cysts in human cornea. Am J Ophthalmol 1988; 106:628–629.

312. Robin JB, Chan R, Andersen BR. Rapid visualization of *Acanthamoeba* using fluorescein-conjugated lectins. Arch Ophthalmol 1988;106:1273–1276.

313. Larkin DFP, Kilvington S, Dart JKG. Treatment of *Acanthamoeba* keratitis with polyhexamethylene biguanide. Ophthalmology 1992;99:185–191.

314. Driebe WT, Stern GA, Epstein RJ, et al. *Acanthamoeba* keratitis, potential role for topical clotrimazole in combination chemotherapy. Arch Ophthalmol 1998;106:1196–1201.

315. Varga JH, Wolf TC, Jensen HG, et al. Combined treatment of *Acanthamoeba* keratitis with propamidine, neomycin, and polyhexamethylene biguanide. Am J Ophthalmol 1993;115:466–470.

316. Bacon AS, Dart JKG, Ficker LA, et al. *Acanthamoeba* keratitis, the value of early diagnosis. Ophthalmology 1993;100:1238–1243.

317. Horsburgh B, Hirst LW, Carey T, et al. Steroid sensitive *Acanthamoeba* keratitis. Aust NZ J Ophthalmol 1991;19:349–350.

318. Solomon JM, Koenig SB, Hyndiuk RA. Medical and surgical treatment of *Acanthamoeba* keratitis. Am J Ophthalmol 1987;104: 309–310.

319. Moore MB, McCulley JP, Luckenbach M, et al. *Acanthamoeba* keratitis associated with soft contact lenses. Am J Ophthalmol 1985;100:396–403.

320. FDA Safety Alert: Homemade saline solutions for contact lenses (HFZ-460). Public Health Service, Food and Drug Administration, Rockville, MD, January 24, 1989.

321. Bartlett JD. Medications and contact-lens wear. In: Silbert JA, ed. Anterior segment complications of contact lens wear. New York: Churchill Livingstone, 1994:473–485.

322. Baum JL, Mishima S, Boruchoff A. On the nature of dellen. Arch Ophthalmol 1968;79:657–662.

323. Insler MS, Tauber S, Packer A. Descemetocele formation in a patient with postoperative corneal dellen. Cornea 1989;8:129–130.

324. Taylor DM, Atlas BF, Romanchuk KG, et al. Pseudophakic bullous keratopathy. Ophthalmology 1983;90:19–24.

325. Cohen EJ, Brady SE, Leavitt K, et al. Pseudophakic bullous keratopathy. Am J Ophthalmol 1988;106:264–269.

326. Lindquist TD, McGlothan JS, Rotkis WM, et al. Indications for penetrating keratoplasty: 1980–1988. Cornea 1991;10:210–216.

327. Boruchoff SA. Clinical causes of corneal edema. Int Ophthalmol Clin 1968;8:581–600.

328. Aquavella JV. Chronic corneal edema. Am J Ophthalmol 1973;76:201–207.

329. Andrew NC, Woodward EG. The bandage lens in bullous keratopathy. Ophthalmic Physiol Opt 1989;9:66–68.

330. Gasset AR, Kaufman HE. Therapeutic uses of hydrophilic contact lenses. Am J Ophthalmol 1970;69:252–259.

331. Lerman S, Sapp G. The hydrophilic (hydron) corneoscleral lens in the treatment of bullous keratopathy. Ann Ophthalmol 1970;2:142.

332. Leibowitz HM, Rosenthal P. Hydrophilic contact lenses in corneal disease. II. Bullous keratopathy. Arch Ophthalmol 1971;85:283–285.

333. DeVoe AG. Electrocautery of Bowman's membrane. Arch Ophthalmol 1966;76:768–771.

334. Brown SI. Peripheral corneal edema after cataract extraction. Am J Ophthalmol 1970;70:326–328.

335. Kornmehl EW, Steinert RF, Odrich MG, et al. Penetrating keratoplasty for pseudophakic bullous keratopathy associated with closed-loop anterior chamber intraocular lenses. Ophthalmology 1990;97:407–412.

336. Brady SE, Rapuano CJ, Arentsen JJ, et al. Clinical indications for and procedures associated with penetrating keratoplasty, 1983–1988. Am J Ophthalmol 1989;108:118–122.

337. Zaidman GW. Penetrating keratoplasty for pseudophakic bullous keratopathy associated with closed-loop anterior chamber intraocular lenses. Ophthalmology 1990;97:413–414.

338. Soukiasian SH, Asdourian GK, Weiss JS, et al. A complication from alcohol swabbed tonometer tips. Am J Ophthalmol 1988;105:424–425.

339. Pogrebniak AE, Sugar A. Corneal toxicity from hydrogen peroxide-soaked tonometer tips. Arch Ophthalmol 1988;106:1505.

340. Levenson JE. Corneal damage from improperly cleaned tonometer tips. Arch Ophthalmol 1989;107:1117.

341. Tabor E, Bostwick DC, Evans CC. Corneal damage due to eye contact with chlorhexidine gluconate. JAMA 1989;261:557–558.

342. Morgan JF. Complications associated with contact lens solutions. Ophthalmology 1979;86:1107–1119.

343. Arffa RC. Toxic and allergic reactions to topical opthalmic medications. In: Grayson's Diseases of the cornea, 3rd ed. St. Louis: Mosby Year Book, 1991:632–648.

344. Rietschel RL, Wilson LA. Ocular inflammation in patients using soft contact lenses. Arch Dermatol 1982;118:147–149.

345. Gray PJ. Aerosals causing ocular trauma. BMJ 1991;302:238.

346. Lyons C, Stevens J, Bloom J. Superglue inadvertently used as eyedrops. BMJ 1990;300:328.

347. Stenson S. Ocular surface disease complicating hydrophilic lens wear. CLAO J 1986;12:158–164.

348. Wolf MD, Lichter PR, Ragsdale CG. Prognostic factors in the uveitis of juvenile rheumatoid arthritis. Ophthalmology 1987;94:1242–1248.

349. Brazier DJ, Hitchings RA. Atypical band keratopathy following long term pilocarpine treatment. Br J Ophthalmol 1989;73:294–296.

350. Beekhuis WH, van Rij G, Zivojnovic R. Silicone oil keratopathy: indications for keratoplasty. Br J Ophthalmol 1985;69:247–253.

351. Binder JS, Deg JK, Kohl S. Calcific band keratopathy after intraocular chondroitin sulfate. Arch Ophthalmol 1987;105:1243–1247.

352. Coffman MR, Mann PM. Corneal subepithelial deposits after use of sodium chondroitin. Am J Ophthalmol 1986;102:279–280.

353. Nevyas AS, Raber IM, Eagle RC, et al. Acute band keratopathy following intracameral Viscoat. Arch Ophthalmol 1987;105:958–964.

354. Freddo TF, Leibowitz HM. Bilateral acute corneal calcification. Ophthalmology 1985;92:537–542.

355. Lemp MA, Ralph RA. Rapid development of band keratopathy in dry eyes. Am J Ophthalmol 1977;83:657–659.

356. Campos M, Nielsen S, Szerenyi K, et al. Clinical follow-up of phototherapeutic keratectomy for treatment of corneal opacities. Am J Ophthalmol 1993;115:433–440.

357. Salz JJ, Reader AL, Schwartz LJ, et al. Treatment of corneal abrasions with soft contact lens and topical diclofenac. J Refract Corneal Surg 1994;10:640–646.

358. Rosa RH, Miller D, Alfonso EC. The changing spectrum of fungal keratitis in South Florida. Ophthalmology 1994;101:1005–1013.

359. Wilhelmus KR, Gee L, Hauck WW, et al. Herpetic eye disease study. A controlled trial of topical corticosteroids for herpes simplex stromal keratitis. Ophthalmology 1994;101:1883–1896.

360. Barron BA, Gee L, Hauck WW, et al. Herpetic eye disease study. A controlled trial of oral acyclovir for herpes simplex stromal keratitis. Ophthalmology 1994;101:1871–1882.

361. Snyder C. Infiltrative keratitis with contact lens wear—a review. J Am Optom Assoc 1995;66:160–177.

Allergic Eye Disease

John H. Nishimoto

Ocular tissues frequently are compromised by allergens. Because of the bothersome symptoms or disfiguring signs induced by ocular allergy, the clinician must understand the pathophysiology, clinical presentations, and therapeutic management of allergic conditions. This chapter considers allergic disorders of the eyelids and conjunctiva, the most common sites of allergic involvement encountered in primary eyecare.

General Immunopathology

The eye resists exogenous agents through the body's established defense mechanisms, and is capable of withstanding most with little change in ocular structure or function.[1] The eye's natural resistance depends heavily on the anatomy and physiology of external ocular structures such as the lids, tears, conjunctiva, and cornea.[2,3] Immunologic responses to antigens can be important causes of inflammation and are termed hypersensitivity reactions. Although four types of hypersensitivity reactions occur, the most common associated with ocular tissues are Type I, *immediate* or *anaphylactic reaction,* and Type IV, the *cell-mediated* or *delayed reaction.*[4] Type I reactions are triggered when an allergen (e.g., dust, pollens, animal danders, drugs, preservatives) attaches to adjacent IgE molecules that are bound to the surface of the mast cell or basophil. The cell membrane undergoes physical changes initiating the release of various mediators, including histamine (see Fig. 13.1). Examples of allergies involving Type I hypersensitivity are allergic conjunctivitis, vernal conjunctivitis, urticaria, and angioedema. Type IV reactions are the

result of interactions between T-lymphocytes and the antigen itself. Usually within 24 to 48 hours of exposure to the antigen, the patient develops erythema and other signs of inflammation. Examples of Type IV[5] hypersensitivity reactions include allergic contact dermatitis and phlyctenular keratoconjunctivitis. Ocular allergies can be a combination of two or more types of hypersensitivity reactions. The distinction between the two major types of allergies becomes important when developing a strategy for pharmacotherapeutic management.

Eyelid Disease

The eyelid is one of the most common sites of ocular allergy. Since the palpebral conjunctiva and eyelid margins adjoin, allergic involvement of each may occur simultaneously. In addition, the eyelid skin is extremely thin, making this area vulnerable to allergic involvement.[6] Since the skin of the lids possesses the same microbial properties as skin elsewhere in the body, allergic ocular reactions may also involve other areas of the body. Table 28.1 summarizes the important allergic eyelid disorders.

Allergic Edema and Angioedema

Allergic edema, also known as *hives* or *urticaria,* refers to localized patches of edema, usually involving the superficial layers of skin. In comparison, angioedema is a condition involving the deeper subcutaneous tissues.[7]

TABLE 28.1
Allergic Eyelid Diseases

Condition	Etiology	Signs	Symptoms	Treatment/Management
Allergic edema	Insect bites/stings, ingestion of food/drugs, use of topical drugs	Circular plaques of edema, erythematous margin and blanched center, (+) intradermal skin test	Mild, moderate discomfort, itching	Oral antihistamines q 4–6 hrs. Cold compresses 10 min. 4 times/day, alternate with warm compresses; topical steroids for severe cases
Angioedema	Insect bites/stings, ingestion of foods, use of topical drugs	Generalized local edema, normal appearing epidermis	Itching, discomfort	Oral antihistamines q 4–6 hrs. Cold compresses 10 min. 4 times/day, alternate with warm compresses; topical steroids
Allergic contact dermatitis	Cosmetics, medications, jewelry, preservatives in contact lens solutions	Erythema, vesiculation, oozing, crusting, scaling, spreads to periorbital skin and conjunctiva (chemosis and papillae), (+) skin patch test	Itching	Avoid offending agent. Cool compresses with Burow's solution (1:15–20), Domeboro powder with water, 0.5%–1.0% hydrocortisone for dry, chronic conditions
Irritant contact dermatitis	Cosmetics, medications, jewelry, preservatives in contact lens solutions	Localized scaling, slight edema, erythema	Irritation, slight itching	Avoid offending agent. Cool compresses with Burow's solution (1:15–20), Domeboro powder with water, oral antihistamine

ETIOLOGY

Most cases of allergic edema and angioedema are thought to represent Type I hypersensitivity reactions.[8,9] Among the many causes are insect stings or bites, or ingestion of a food or drug to which the patient is sensitive. The prevalence of this condition in the general population is estimated to be between 10% and 25%. No specific cause can be found in 70% of patients with chronic urticaria.[10] In others, psychogenic, allergic, and physical factors may play a role. In general, the urticarias are classified as immunologic and non-immunologic. Immunologic causes include hypersensitivity responses to infections, foods, and drugs. These responses may be mediated by any one of the four types of hypersensitivity reactions. Drugs commonly associated with urticaria include aspirin, tetracycline, acetazolamide and other sulfonamide derivatives, penicillin, neomycin, and opium alkaloids such as morphine, codeine, and meperedine. Berries, shellfish, nuts, and eggs are some of the common dietary causes of urticaria. Infections with parasites, viruses, and bacteria have also been implicated in urticaria. Pollens and contact sensitizers are known to produce urticaria and can be evaluated easily for allergenic potential. Non-immunologic causes of urticaria include physical and emotional factors, and cholinergic stimuli. Psychogenic factors may play a role in approximately 25% of cases, but the associated pathophysiology is completely

unknown. Urticaria may be observed during the course of certain systemic diseases including collagen vascular disease (particularly systemic lupus erythematosus), Hodgkins disease, other lymphomas, carcinoma, and amyloidosis.[1]

Urticaria can also be produced by certain physical agents including light, heat, cold, and trauma.[11] Light-induced urticaria occurs on areas of the skin that have been exposed to sunlight. Heat-induced urticaria may be produced by emotional stress, physical exertion, or exogenous heat. It may be related to an increase in body temperature and excitation of the autonomic nervous system. Cold-induced urticaria is one of the most common physical allergies. It may be due to an antibody mechanism since in some cases the sensitivity to cold can be transferred passively by serum to normal skin. The nature of the antigen, however, is unknown. Skin trauma or pressure on the skin are physical factors that are also capable of inducing urticaria in susceptible individuals.

DIAGNOSIS

The history and clinical findings usually provide an immediate diagnosis. Patients often complain of itching and discomfort. The allergic reaction may occur within seconds or minutes following allergen exposure and reveals itself independently in the eyelid or in concert with acute allergic reactions elsewhere in the body.

Both urticaria and angioedema may present with similar

symptoms, but physical appearances differ. Circular plaques of edema with blanched centers are characteristic of urticaria. This differs from angioedema, in which only generalized edema occurs in the dermis, while the overlying epidermis remains essentially normal (Fig. 28.1).

The intradermal skin test, used to confirm the diagnosis, actually promotes an allergic reaction. This test consists of applying a small amount of the suspected allergen to a superficial epidermal scratch or injecting the allergen intradermally. Within seconds or minutes, a round wheal (elevation of skin that is white in the center and red in the periphery), redness, and itching indicate a positive response.[7] As an alternative, instill a small amount of the substance topically into the conjunctival sac—the nearly immediate onset of eyelid swelling, chemosis, conjunctival hyperemia, and itching indicates a positive response. It must be emphasized, however, that these skin and conjunctival tests can cause anaphylaxis in highly susceptible individuals.[7] Thus, when performing the conjunctival test, it is prudent to use relatively low drug concentrations or to instill relatively small amounts. Unfortunately, a negative skin or conjunctival test does not ensure that the drug can be administered safely. Severe, even fatal, reactions have been reported following negative skin testing.[8]

MANAGEMENT

Although urticaria and angioedema may appear debilitating, they rarely lead to complications. Thus, management usually includes reassurance. The use of oral antihistamines, such as chlorpheniramine 4 mg every 4 to 6 hours, is more effective than topical antihistamines for Type I reactions. Cold compresses for 10 to 15 minutes 4 times a day for 24 to 48 hours, followed with warm compresses can provide relief of itching and discomfort.[7,8] If the condition is severe, immediate therapy may include the subcutaneous administration of 0.3 to 0.5 ml epinephrine 1:1000.[12] Systemically or topically administered steroids can be employed for general discomfort and itching, but due to their potential complications they should be used only when the condition is severe or debilitating. Orally administered aspirin can be a valuable antipruitic agent in some cases.[12]

It is important to determine the cause of the reaction since reexposure will often lead to recurrence of the problem. In cases in which continued exposure cannot be prevented, it may be necessary to refer the patient to an allergist for desensitization to the offending allergen.

Contact Dermatitis

ETIOLOGY

Contact dermatitis is an inflammation of the skin evidenced by itching, redness, and various skin lesions that are caused by an offending agent. The condition is classified as either nonallergic (irritant) or allergic (Table 28.2).[13] Nonallergic contact dermatitis occurs when an offending irritant such as acids, alkalis, resins, or chemicals comes in contact with the skin and ocular tissues. Allergy or hypersensitivity plays a role in irritant contact dermatitis. Nonallergic dermatitis is provoked by substances with primary irritant properties, or by frequent defatting of the skin caused by excessive moisture. With continued defatting of the skin or repeated irritant exposure, edema, erythema, vesiculation, and scaling of the skin develop. The damaged or inflamed eczematous skin has

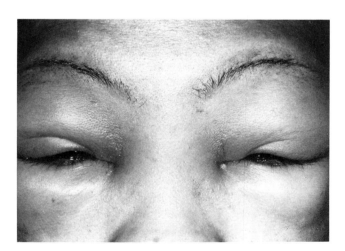

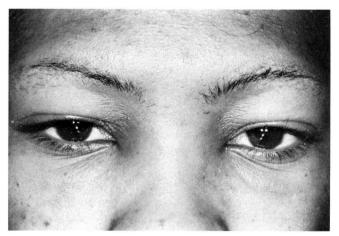

A   B

FIGURE 28.1 *(A)* **Angioedema secondary to hair dressing solution.** *(B)* **Complete resolution after 3 days of oral antihistamines and application of warm compresses.**

TABLE 28.2
Characteristics of Contact Dermatitis

Characteristic	Primary Irritant Dermatitis	Allergic Contact Dermatitis
Incidence	Common	Uncommon
Occurrence	Occurs upon first exposure	Occurs with previous sensitizing exposure
Onset	1–24 hours	12–72 hours
Immunity	None	Cell-mediated
Clinical appearance	Flat, dry, scaly	Papular, vesicular
Exposure required	Concentration dependent	Minimal exposure

Modified from Rich LF, Hanifin JM. Ocular complications of atopic dermatitis and other eczemas. Int Ophthalmol Clin 1985;25:61–76.

a high risk of developing a true allergic contact dermatitis. Removal of the irritant causing skin inflammation will allow the irritant dermatitis to resolve. On the other hand, allergic contact dermatitis is a cell-mediated, delayed (Type IV) hypersensitivity that usually involves the eyelid skin and conjunctiva.[7] In allergic contact dermatitis, an individual becomes sensitized to a given substance and upon reexposure to the same chemical or related congeners, an erythematous, delayed skin reaction is elicited.[1]

In allergic contact dermatitis, the sensitizing substances generally are haptens of small molecular weight that bind to dermal proteins, forming complete antigens. The haptens do not cause significant changes to configuration of these carrier proteins. Upon initial application of a contact sensitizer, most of the applied chemical is removed rapidly by the blood stream. Initial exposure results in the production of sensitized T-lymphocytes capable of responding to the antigen when reexposure occurs. A second application of the sensitizing substance, therefore, leads to an inflammatory response or an accumulation of mononuclear cells and other inflammatory cells characteristic of cell-mediated responses.

Many substances can cause allergic contact dermatitis. Although virtually any medication or substance has the potential to cause allergic contact dermatitis, several are especially potent sensitizers (Table 28.3).[14–19] Facial creams and cosmetics are particularly common causes of allergic contact dermatitis in women.[20] Sensitization usually requires at least 5 to 10 days for strongly sensitizing allergens, but can require months or even years when less potent sensitizers are involved.[21] After the patient has been sensitized, the time interval between subsequent exposure to the allergen and appearance of the reaction is usually 12 to 72 hours.

Allergic contact dermatitis from topically administered ocular medications usually occurs following contact conjunctivitis. On the other hand, allergic contact dermatitis without conjunctivitis is usually caused by a drug or substance coming in contact with the eyelids without having been instilled into the conjunctival sac.[22]

DIAGNOSIS

Due to many possible irritants and allergens, diagnosis can be difficult. A careful history and physical examination are necessary for proper diagnosis and management.

The primary signs of irritant contact dermatitis are mild eyelid edema, erythema, and scaly eruptions.[13] Irritant contact dermatitis is often localized to the skin of the eyelid, whereas allergic contact dermatitis can spread to involve periorbital skin. Signs of allergic contact dermatitis include erythema, vesiculation, oozing, crusting, scaling, or thickening (Fig. 28.2). The predominant symptom is itching. Conjunctival involvement is similar to that of acute allergic conjunctivitis and may include hyperemia, chemosis, watery discharge, or papillary hypertrophy.

Sensitization from the offending allergen can cause allergic reactions to occur in other ocular tissues. Besides the

TABLE 28.3
Drugs or Substances Known to Cause Allergic Contact Dermatitis or Dermatoconjunctivitis

- Cosmetics (including nail polish)
- Local anesthetics
- Neomycin
- Tobramycin
- Gentamicin
- Bacitracin
- Benzalkonium chloride
- Thimerosal
- Parabens
- Atropine
- Timolol
- Phenylephrine
- Lanolin
- Rubber or nickel (eyelash curler)
- EDTA

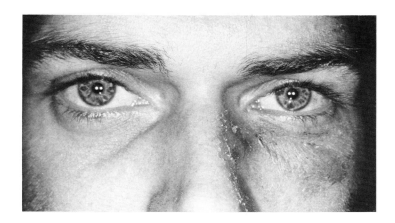

FIGURE 28.2 **Eczematoid reaction of left lower lid, cheek, and nose characteristic of allergic contact dermatitis.**

skin lesions of contact dermatitis, contact sensitizers may produce a conjunctivitis characterized most often by a papillary response, pronounced vasodilation, chemosis, and watery discharge. An erythematous blepharitis may occur, and in very severe cases a keratitis may develop that is typified by yellow necrotic opacities just inside the limbus. The fine epithelial punctate keratitis can be attributed to chronic use of gentamicin, topical anesthetics, echothiophate, or phenylephrine.

Rubbing the eyes after handling soaps, detergents, or chemicals may provoke a contact dermatitis. Allergic reactions to cosmetics affect primarily the eyebrows and upper lid because of the method of application. Mascara, eyebrow pencil, and facial creams can act as allergens, and nail polish can cause sensitization around the eye by accidental touching of the area. Lip gloss and eye gloss cosmetics contain lanolin fractions that may also act as sensitizers.[1]

Parabens, used as preservatives in many lotions, creams, and cosmetics, are one of the primary causes of contact dermatitis. Nickel sulfate is a common sensitizer found in jewelry and undergarments. Other common offenders are chromates, which are used in costume jewelry, leather products, bleaches, and automobile products.[1]

Confirmation of the offending allergen can be made by using the skin patch test. Apply the drug or substance to be tested to a relatively hairless area of the skin, usually the back, leg, or forearm. Cover the substance with a Band-Aid or cotton ball that is sealed with tape or plastic wrap to prevent contamination. The adhesive eye patches that are used for amblyopia therapy may be used. Application should last for 48 hours, and the skin should be observed 24 to 48 hours after removal of the dressing to allow the pressure-induced effects to subside (Fig. 28.3). It is possible for false-negative results to occur because the skin to which the substance has been applied is relatively resistant to the development of allergic contact dermatitis. Similarly, false-positive results may occur from the application of a sub-

stance that is too concentrated and therefore produces an eczematous reaction by irritation rather than by immunologic hypersensitivity.[7] Since asymptomatic individuals can demonstrate positive skin patch tests, a positive result does not necessarily indicate the specific cause of the dermatitis. Thus, a careful history is probably more important than skin patch-testing in delineating the specific cause.

Another important test for positive diagnosis of allergic contact dermatitis is simply to instruct the patient to use the suspected allergen (such as a cosmetic). By employing such a usage test either alone or in combination with skin patch-testing, the accuracy of diagnosis increases significantly.[13,20]

MANAGEMENT

The most effective treatment for contact dermatitis is to eliminate the offending substance. This may be the only treatment necessary, but persistent or severe cases may require more aggressive treatment. For symptomatic relief, the patient can apply cool compresses, Burow's solution (aluminum acetate and water, 1:15–20), or Domeboro powder or tablets (aluminum sulfate and calcium acetate) dissolved in water. This is especially effective for the acute, weeping, oozing stages of the disorder and often causes drying of the dermatitis within a few days.[7,12] For dry, subacute, or chronic conditions, applications of steroid cream or ointment such as 0.5% or 1.0% hydrocortisone can be effective. The steroid can be applied to the eyelids several times daily, but must be monitored closely due to potential complications (infection, elevated intraocular pressure) from steroid use.[23] Oral antihistamines can provide relief from the associated itching, but topically applied antihistamines have no effect on this Type IV hypersensitivity and may even be sensitizing.[7] Desensitization to offending substances has largely been ineffective.[24]

If contact with the offending substance continues, allergic contact dermatitis may continue or worsen even with the use

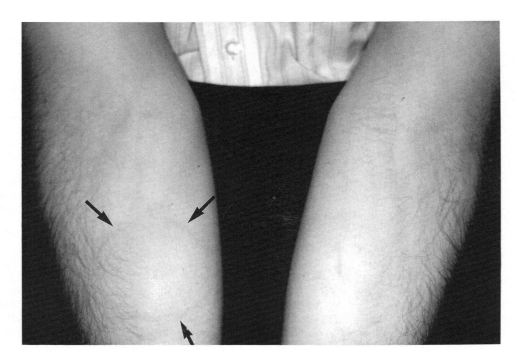

FIGURE 28.3   **Results of positive occlusive patch test performed for 48 hours by taping a cotton pad soaked in thimerosal-preserved saline to the inner surface of the right forearm. The left arm serves as a control by taping a nonmedicated cotton pad to its inner surface. Arrows indicate the well-circumscribed area of redness reflecting thimerosal sensitivity. (Courtesy Joseph F. Molinari, O.D.)**

of steroid therapy. Thus, the use of combination preparations such as neomycin-hydrocortisone can exacerbate the dermatitis, especially if neomycin is the offending agent causing the hypersensitivity. Moreover, topically applied fluorinated steroids can cause persistent periocular dermatitis.[25] If treatment does not appear to improve the condition after 7 days, withdrawal of the preparation is necessary to eliminate persistent dermatitis and possible sensitization. Subsequent treatment with topical 0.5 to 1.0% hydrocortisone along with oral tetracycline (250 mg 4 times daily) can prove successful. The only form of contact dermatitis that may require a systemic steroid is widespread, severe poison ivy dermatitis.[26] A 10- to 14-day course of oral prednisone or its equivalent may be used since it can lessen the intensity of the disease, and decrease the amount of time lost from work or school.

Conjunctival Disease

Allergic conditions that involve the conjunctiva may be caused by airborne allergens, contact allergens, and reactions to allergens associated with various microbial agents.

The pathophysiology of allergic conjunctivitis is clearly linked to the cascade of events triggered by mast cell degranulation. Human conjunctiva has a mast cell density of approximately 5,000 cells/mm^3 with the limbus having the highest concentration.[27,28] The high concentration of mast cells in the conjunctiva is especially important because these cells play a major role in ocular allergy. Each mast cell contains hundreds of granules filled with preformed chemical medicators, such as histamine, as well as precursors of biologically potent prostaglandins, thromboxanes, and leukotrienes.[29] Release of these mediators is associated with subsequent signs and symptoms of itching, tearing, hyperemia, and swelling. Table 28.4 summarizes the important allergic conjunctival disorders.

Allergic Conjunctivitis

ETIOLOGY

Allergic conjunctivitis occurs most often in persons aged 20 to 30 years. These patients may have a history of atopic conditions such as hay fever. Determination of an etiology often is difficult because multiple allergens are common.

TABLE 28.4
Allergic Conjunctival Diseases

Condition	Etiology	Signs	Symptoms	Treatment/Management

Allergic conjunctivitis	History of hay fever, airborne dust & pollens, topical drug use, cosmetics, soaps, animal hair & dander	Eosinophils, papillary hypertrophy, chemosis, diffuse hyperemia	Itching, ropy discharge	Avoid offending agent
				Mild cases: Nonpreserved artificial tears qid
				  Cool compresses qid
				  Decongestants qid
				Moderate: Decongestant-antihistamine combination qid
				  Ketorolac tromethamine 0.5%
				  Levocabastine 0.05% qid
				Severe: Topical steroids q 1–2 h × 24–48 h, then bid-qid until symptoms minimized or relieved

Giant papillary conjunctivitis	Contact lens wear, ocular prosthesis, exposed sutures	Conjunctival papillae > 0.3 mm diameter on upper tarsal conjunctiva	Itching, decreased lens tolerance, mucous production	Decrease/discontinue lens wear Frequent lens replacements and improved cleaning Cromolyn sodium 4% qid 1–2% N-acetyl-L-cysteine 4–6× day Suprofen 1.0% qid

Vernal keratoconjunctivitis	Seasonal, occurring in warm months and warm climate	Eosinophils, giant "cobblestone" papillae, superior punctate epithelial keratitis, corneal shield ulcer, limbal papillae	Intense itching, ropy discharge, possible photophobia	Mild cases: Cold compresses qid
				  Cromolyn sodium 4% qid
				Topical antihistamine-decongestant qid
				  Lodoxamide 0.1% qid
				Severe: "Pulse" of topical prednisolone acetate 1% q 1–2h × 48 hrs
				Lodoxamide 0.1% qid

Most hypersensitivity reactions of the conjunctiva are one of two types based on the time between antigen exposure and appearance of the immune response. Immediate, or Type I, hypersensitivity is mediated by serum immunoglobulins (antibodies) and produces a predominantly eosinophilic cellular response. Delayed, or Type IV, hypersensitivity is mediated by cells (T-lymphocytes) sensitized to antigen and produces a predominantly mononuclear cellular response.

The immediate, antibody-mediated response develops within minutes after exposure to the offending antigen and is characterized by conjunctival hyperemia and chemosis secondary to vascular dilatation and serous exudation. Histopathologically, there is a pattern of eosinophil infiltration, goblet cell discharge, and epithelial damage similar to that produced by histamine alone. Conjunctival itching is a prominent symptom in most patients, and micropapillary reaction of the palpebral conjunctiva is often seen in more chronic antigen exposure states. Seasonal allergic (hay fe-

ver) conjunctivitis is the prototype Type I allergic eye disease.

The delayed, cell-mediated response develops within hours or days after introduction of the antigen. This response is characterized by the same general conjunctival signs of chemosis and hyperemia as in the immediate reaction, but in many cases a mild follicular reaction may be superimposed. Type IV, or cell-mediated, hypersensitivity often plays a major role in many forms of allergic conjunctivitis, especially in those associated with hypersensitivity to topical antibiotics and preservatives.

One study of 5,000 children[30] undergoing treatment for allergy found ocular involvement in 3.5%. In those children exhibiting eye signs, 94% demonstrated anterior segment signs, with 80% of those having conjunctivitis. Respiratory or dermatologic involvement was present in 66% of patients, while 32% showed ocular involvement as the only sign of the allergic disorder. Conjunctival allergy to airborne dust and pollen is common in the spring and summer, while allergic states secondary to topical drug use and cosmetics show no seasonal variation.

Airborne pollens, dust, and other environmental contaminants may constitute the largest single group of agents responsible for allergic conjunctivitis. The allergens responsible mainly are graminaceae pollen, along with house dust, animal hair, and yeasts. Cosmetics, perfumes, soaps, detergents, aftershave lotions, and hair dressings are also frequent causes. Ophthalmic drugs such as neomycin, sulfonamide preparations, proparacaine, and atropine are commonly encountered etiologic agents along with cyclopentolate, timolol, thimerosal, epinephrine and its prodrug, dipivefrin.[19,31]

DIAGNOSIS

A careful history is important to determine the responsible agent. In addition, patients with allergic conjunctivitis often demonstrate eosinophils in Giemsa (Diff-Quik) stains of conjunctival scrapings. Tada and associates[32] reported that of 175 patients with atopic asthma, allergic rhinitis, and dermatitis, 61% exhibited conjunctival signs. Of those, 52% demonstrated a positive skin test for house dust, 35% for *Candida* species, and 12% for pollen. This illustrates the value of antigen testing in assessing the cause of recalcitrant cases of allergic conjunctivitis.

Signs of acute allergic conjunctivitis include conjunctival and lid edema, dilation of conjunctival vessels, and papillae. Symptoms include itching, tearing, burning, and, occasionally, a "pressure" sensation behind the eyes. A stringy discharge may be present. Chronic allergic conjunctivitis presents with a relatively quiet conjunctiva, mild chemosis, and prominent papillae (Fig. 28.4). A watery or mucopurulent discharge may be present. The itching and tearing symptoms are often more prominent than signs of chemosis and hyperemia.[33,34] The use of sodium fluorescein helps to enhance the presence of papillae by pooling between the papillae, thereby creating a fluorescein "cobblestone" appearance (Fig. 28.5).

Performing a conjunctival provocation test by applying a suspected allergen to the conjunctiva occasionally may lead to tissue inflammation and accumulation of neutrophils, eosinophils, and lymphocytes. This fact has proven useful in diagnosing a specific allergen-induced itching and redness.[35–39]

Eliciting appropriate information from the patient is essential to successful management. For example, bilateral involvement is expected with most environmental allergies, and there is often a family history of hay fever.[40] Although there are no pathognomonic symptoms of allergic conjunctivitis, the diagnosis often can be suggested by an almost normal appearing eye, mild to moderate symptoms of itching and tearing, and the absence of specific signs.[41,42]

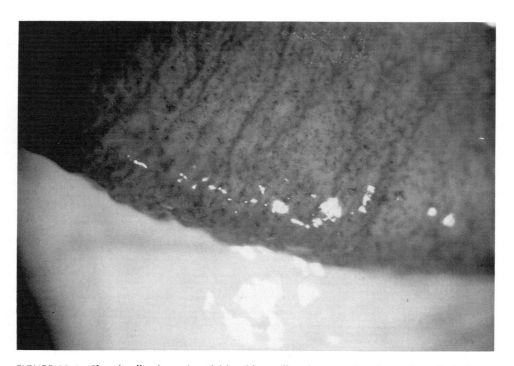

FIGURE 28.4 **Chronic allergic conjunctivitis with papillary hypertrophy of superior palpebral conjunctiva.**

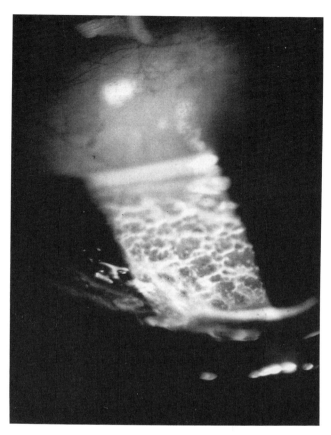

FIGURE 28.5 Pooling of sodium fluorescein among papillae in allergic conjunctivitis.

Evidence of eosinophilis in scrapings from the inner surface of the upper and lower lid is helpful in determining the diagnosis. Eosinophils are not found in conjunctival scrapings from nonallergic persons. The presence of even one eosinophil or eosinophilic granule on Giemsa stain would support the diagnosis of allergic conjunctivitis.[43] However, since the prevalence of eosinophils may vary (20–80%), the absence of eosinophils should not preclude the diagnosis.[44,45] In severe cases a scratch or prick test may be needed to establish a hypersensitivity to specific allergens.

Differential diagnosis includes blepharitis and infectious conjunctivitis. Most cases of allergic conjunctivitis are seasonal, and patients have a history of allergy. The clinician should consider symptoms and signs in relation to environmental stimuli. For example, if symptoms correlate with the pollen season or the acquisition of a new pet, this may provide supportive evidence for a diagnosis of allergy. Blepharitis and other infectious types of conjunctivitis usually are not seasonal. Signs and symptoms are often worse upon awakening. In addition, itching, a prominent feature in allergy, often is absent in infectious conjunctivitis. In contrast, burning, stinging, and matting of the eyelids are common features of blepharitis.[46] Tear levels of IgE are elevated in most patients with allergic rhinoconjunctivitis but are normal in patients with blepharitis. Cultures are helpful in the diagnosis of infectious conjunctivitis. Contact allergy often affects the skin of the lower lids, and withdrawal of the suspected contact allergen is often the best way to confirm the diagnosis.

MANAGEMENT

The general approach to the management of allergic conjunctivitis includes avoiding the offending agent, promoting the judicious use of pharmacologic agents, and desensitization. Avoiding the offending allergen may be impossible, as in the case of dust allergy, or impractical, as in the case of hay fever. However, management by avoiding allergens is quite successful in cases of allergic conjunctivitis secondary to ophthalmic drug preparations and facial cosmetics. Desensitization may be of value in cases associated with pollen or other airborne allergens. Tada and associates[32] desensitized 120 children to graminaceae pollen, alone or in combination with dust. The results were encouraging since 47% were cured and 24% demonstrated considerable improvement. Most of the failures involved children with multiple allergies, including vernal conjunctivitis.

Pharmacotherapy depends on the severity of signs and symptoms. It is prudent to consider using the mildest therapy needed to control annoying symptoms.[33] Mild allergic conjunctivitis can be treated with an over-the-counter preparation such as a decongestant or artificial tear. Topical decongestants containing naphazoline, phenylephrine, or oxymetazoline can be effective. When used in the typical dosage of 4 to 6 times daily, the vasoconstrictive action of these drugs reduces congestion and edema and can greatly relieve the patient's symptoms. However, long-term or indiscriminant use of phenylephrine or combinations containing phenylephrine may be accompanied by rebound hyperemia.

The release of histamine and other vasoactive substances from tissue is largely responsible for the hyperemia, tearing, and itching that accompany acute allergic conjunctivitis. Drugs that inhibit the actions of histamine usually are effective in the relief of allergic signs and symptoms. Topical decongestant-antihistamine combinations, such as naphazoline-pheniramine (Naphcon-A) and naphazoline-antazoline (Vasocon-A) used 4 times a day, can provide relief of symptoms associated with allergic conjunctivitis.[47,48] The usual dosage is one drop every 3 to 4 hours as required to relieve symptoms, but these preparations are well tolerated and may be instilled initially as often as every 1 to 2 hours for severe cases. Levocabastine 0.05%, a second generation H_1 antihistamine, is also effective when used 4 times daily.[49–51]

Cromolyn sodium 4% (Crolom) inhibits mast cell degranulation and is particularly effective for hay fever conjunctivitis and giant papillary conjunctivitis. Cromolyn is also useful in conjunction with other medications used to control various types of ocular allergies. In the event of unavailability of ophthalmic cromolyn sodium, cromolyn used for allergic rhinitis (Nasalcrom) has been suggested as an alternative. It has been recommended that Nasalcrom be prepared for ophthalmic use by filtering through a 0.22 μm filter into a sterile dropper bottle under aseptic conditions. No adverse effects have been reported with this solution, and patient acceptance has been good.[52]

Ketorolac tromethamine 0.5% (Acular), a nonsteroidal anti-inflammatory agent that inhibits prostaglandin synthetase, is also effective in relieving signs and symptoms of acute allergic conjunctivitis.[53,54] In severe cases, ophthalmic steroids may play a vital role in providing palliative therapy. A typical dose is one drop every 1 to 2 hours for the first 24 to 48 hours, then 2 to 4 times a day until symptoms are relieved or minimized. The most common topical steroids used are prednisolone acetate 1.0%, prednisolone sodium phosphate 1.0%, dexamethasone 1%, fluorometholone 0.1%, and medrysone 1.0%. Since elevated intraocular pressure and secondary infection can occur, tonometry and careful anterior segment evaluations should be performed.[53,54]

Giant Papillary Conjunctivitis

ETIOLOGY

Giant papillary conjunctivitis (GPC) is a specific conjunctival inflammatory reaction to soft and rigid contact lens wear and can also occur in patients wearing prosthetic eyes.[33,55,56] It is characterized by papillary hypertrophy primarily affecting the superior tarsal conjunctiva. Eosinophils and basophils, as well as mast cells, characterize the cellular infiltrate. Analysis of soft contact lenses from individuals with contact lens-associated GPC has not shown differences in the types of lens surface deposits in those patients compared with asymptomatic patients. In addition, studies of bacterial attachments to soft contact lens in patients with GPC and asymptomatic soft contact lens wearers have also failed to show any significant differences between the two groups. These results solidify the fact that the development of GPC is a reflection of individual immunologic response rather than individual differences in lens deposits or bacterial contamination.[57] Recent reports, however, have established an association between GPC and stimuli that are inert and therefore unlikely to stimulate an immune response. These include exposed sutures, extruded scleral buckle, cyanoacrylate adhesive, and an epithelialized foreign body.[58]

Tear levels of lactoferrin are reduced considerably in patients with GPC.[59] The reduced levels return to normal as the GPC subsides. Lactoferrin, an iron-complexing protein found in normal tears, has both bacteriostatic and bactericidal properties that make it an important component of the defense system of the external eye. Lactoferrin also has a strong inhibitory effect on the complement system by blocking the formation of C3 convertase. Thus, the reduced levels of tear lactoferrin observed in patients with GPC, the cause of which is unknown, could further contribute to the inflammation and tissue damage observed in this disorder.[59]

Soni and Hathcoct[60] reported an increase in the incidence of GPC and associated conjunctival inflammatory response during the month of March. This suggests that seasonal allergy may explain, at least in part, some of the clinical manifestations of this disorder.

Several studies[61,62] suggest a strong correlation between the severity of GPC and the severity of meibomian gland dysfunction. Since GPC occurs most often in soft contact lens wearers, the degree of mucin adherence to lens materials has been suggested as a contributing factor. Other investigators implicate contact lens polymers, deposits on the contact lens surface, and chemicals in lens solutions. According to one theory,[63] the external eye becomes sensitive to the antigen coating on the contact lens. The ensuing immunologic response results in release of vasoactive amines from mast cells and basophils that are responsible not only for allergic symptoms, but also for the collagen fibrovascular changes that become manifest as longer papillae. Lens-induced trauma to the tarsal conjunctiva with release of neutrophilic chemotactic factor and other inflammatory mediators is a possible immunologic etiology for GPC.[64] It is likely that both irritative and immunologic factors contribute to the pathogenesis. The more intimate association between the contact lens and the upper palpebral conjunctiva probably explains the location of the giant papillary hypertrophy.

DIAGNOSIS

GPC is defined by the presence of papillae greater than 0.3 mm in diameter on the upper tarsal conjunctiva.[33,65,66] Therefore, the upper lids of patients wearing contact lenses, especially soft lenses, should be everted for careful inspection of the upper tarsal conjunctiva (Fig. 28.6). Symptoms include itching, contact lens intolerance, increased mucous production and conjunctival injection. The clinical findings are similar to those of vernal conjunctivitis, and it is thought that similar immunologic mechanisms may be involved in both diseases. Other symptoms include loose lenses and fluctuating vision. Symptoms usually diminish when the lenses are removed.

In the early stages of GPC, patients frequently complain of mild itching on removal of the lens, mucus in the nasal corners of the eye, and slight blurring of vision. Patients also report an increased awareness of the contact lens. The blurred vision may be the result of accumulation of mucus or coating on the lens.[33] Such symptoms may not be reported to

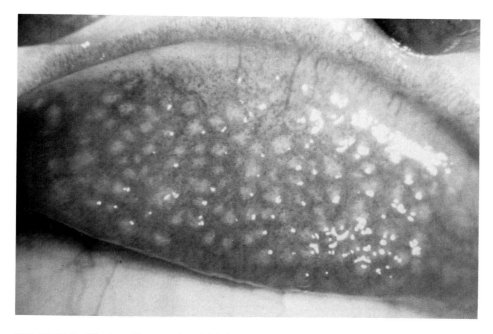

FIGURE 28.6   **Giant papillary conjunctivitis in a 27-year-old soft contact lens wearer.**

the clinician because of their mildness or a belief that they are unavoidable effects of contact lens wear.

Clinical signs usually follow the onset of symptoms. Early signs include mild hyperemia and the presence of small strands of mucus. Careful examination may reveal abnormal thickening of the conjunctiva.

Progression of GPC is marked by opacification of the tarsal conjunctiva, a result of infiltration by eosinophils and other inflammatory cells. Large conjunctival papillae (>0.3 mm in diameter) begin to grow and push aside normal papillae. These large papillae can persist for months and even years. Infrequently, limbal and corneal lesions may accompany the conjunctival papillae.[67] Mucous production increases and symptoms become more bothersome; there is an increase in itching and greater awareness of the lens. The symptoms intensify in proportion to the size of newly forming papillae. When GPC reaches the final stage, the upper tarsal plate shows a cobblestone arrangement of giant papillae as in vernal keratoconjunctivitis. At this stage there may be complete contact lens intolerance, intense itching, and copious mucous production. Lenses can become clouded by mucus shortly after insertion.[67] Other symptoms include pain and foreign body sensation.

MANAGEMENT

When found in the early stages, GPC will resolve if lens wear is discontinued. However, most patients want to con-

tinue wearing contact lenses. In more advanced cases, topical antihistamine-decongestant preparations can provide symptomatic relief. Increased mucous production may be a prominent component of GPC. Mucolytic agents such as N-acetyl-L-cysteine (Mucomyst) applied topically in 1% to 2% solution in artificial tears 4 to 6 times daily can reduce this problem. Once the patient becomes asymptomatic, it may be possible to reinstitute contact lens wear. Since most patients want to continue wearing contact lenses, the management of GPC may include lens replacement, improved lens care using a more vigorous schedule of enzymatic and daily cleaning, the use of nonpreserved saline, changing the lens design and polymer, and the use of disposable[78] or frequent replacement lenses.

Cromolyn sodium 4% is useful for treatment of GPC. Donshik and associates[68] found that by using cromolyn sodium in combination with frequent contact lens replacement, 82% of the patients with GPC were able to continue wearing lenses. Artificial tears used 4 times daily, or irrigating the conjunctiva with nonpreserved saline 2 to 3 times daily, may provide some relief, possibly by diluting the antigenic stimulus.[69] Suprofen 1.0% used 4 times daily also reduces signs and symptoms, such as papillae and mucous strands.[70]

Following the diagnosis of active GPC, contact lens wear should be discontinued for at least 4 weeks. If inflammation is mild, increased topical lubrication may be the only required therapy. If severe inflammation occurs, cromolyn sodium or suprofen may be needed 4 times daily. Although topical steroids generally are ineffective in the treatment of GPC, loteprednol has been shown to reduce the papillary hypertrophy in many patients with GPC.[69]

Vernal Conjunctivitis

ETIOLOGY

Vernal conjunctivitis or keratoconjunctivitis (VKC) is a bilateral inflammation affecting primarily the upper palpebral conjunctiva. It is a rare form of allergic ocular disease that affects males more than females. The allergy begins in prepubescent years, with a peak incidence between ages 11 and 13. The condition usually resolves during the late teens or early twenties[71] It is more common in dry, warm climates. Patients usually have a history of atopy, with seasonal allergies, asthma, atopic dermatitis, and a family history of allergies. Although the disease is self-limited, signs and symptoms are often severe and difficult to control. The highest incidence occurs between April and August, although many patients have virtually continual disease. Histologically, patients with VKC demonstrate basophils, eosinophils, and mast cells in the conjunctival epithelium. In normal patients, few if any mast cells occur in the upper palpebral conjunctiva, whereas in patients with VKC the density of mast cells in this area can exceed 15,000/mm3.[72] Tear histamine levels are significantly higher than in healthy eyes.

DIAGNOSIS

Most patients complain of extreme itching, with occasional foreign body sensation, photophobia, blurred vision and blepharospasm. Giant papillae, commonly termed "cobblestone" papillae, typically occur on the upper palpebral conjunctiva (Fig. 28.7). These represent new blood vessel formation with surrounding accumulations of inflammatory cells, especially eosinophils and plasma cells. The papillae are polygonal, flat-topped, and at least one millimeter in size. Mucous strands, which can sometimes be pulled from the eyes, may be present between the papillae. Conjunctival scrapings show many eosinophils as well as eosinophilic granules on Giemsa staining. Limbal papillae may have a gelatinous or fleshy appearance and can occur throughout the limbal circumference, although they are often located in the superior region. Trantas' dots (Fig. 28.8), located within the limbal papillae, are whitish-chalky calcifications of eosinophils. Although patients may complain of a thick, ropy discharge, the lids typically do not stick together.

The cornea may undergo significant, although rare, findings. Corneal involvement is an index of disease severity and can include punctate epithelial keratitis, epithelial

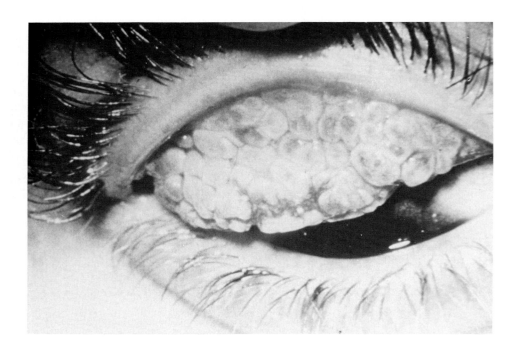

FIGURE 28.7   **Vernal conjunctivitis with cobblestone papillae on upper palpebral conjunctiva.**

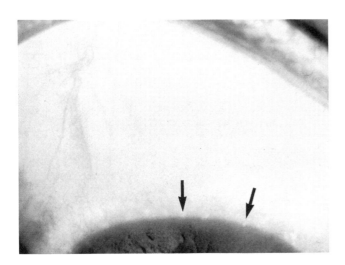

FIGURE 28.8   **Trantas' dots (arrows) in limbal vernal conjunctivitis.**

macroerosion, plaques, and subepithelial scarring. Fine punctate keratopathy may progress to erosion or to a characteristic "shield-ulcer" (Fig. 28.9), which can lead to superficial stromal scarring upon resolution.[33]

MANAGEMENT

Management of patients with vernal conjunctivitis involves relief of ocular symptoms and control of ocular signs. In mild forms of the disease, cold compresses, in combination with topical antihistamines or decongestants, are effective for symptomatic control. The use of 4% cromolyn sodium 4 times daily has proven effective in many patients through its stabilizing effect on mast cells. Patients appear to tolerate this medication and report few adverse effects. The use of oral antihistamines is also helpful in relieving symptoms. When used 4 times daily, 0.1% Iodoxamide, a mast cell stabilizer, appears to be significantly more effective than 4% cromolyn sodium in relieving the signs and symptoms of VKC, including its corneal complications (see Chap. 13).

Topical steroids can provide symptomatic relief from VKC, especially in severe cases. A "pulse" of topical steroids may reduce the symptoms to a level where other treatment modalities can be used. Since long-term use of steroids increases the risk of glaucoma, infection, and cataract, it is important to reduce or discontinue the steroid as soon as symptoms are reduced. A typical regimen consists of topical 1.0% prednisolone acetate (Pred Forte) every 1 to 2 hours (while awake) for 48 hours and then tapered over a 1- to 2-week period. Pulses of steroids several times a year may be helpful in severe cases. It is important to educate the patient not to become dependent on steroids for any mild recurrence. Since the disease tends to run a chronic course, steroids with low IOP-elevating potential should be used

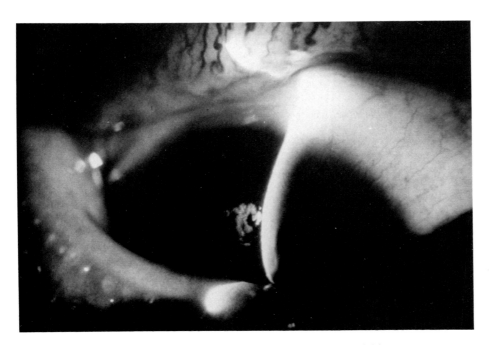

FIGURE 28.9   **Shield corneal ulcer associated with vernal keratoconjunctivitis.**

when possible. These include fluorometholone, rimexolone, or loteprednol.

There is some clinical evidence[72,73] that aspirin given orally (0.5 to 1.5 g per day) may provide symptomatic relief in some individuals whose symptoms are not controlled by cromolyn or steroids. Although the efficacy of this approach varies widely, a therapeutic trial may be warranted in severe cases. Recommended dosage is 650 mg 3 times daily, with careful attention to the potential side effects of aspirin.[72] Aspirin prevents the formation of prostaglandin D_2, a secondary mast cell mediator that may play a key role in allergic conditions.

Dramatic clinical improvement in some patients with severe chronic vernal conjunctivitis has been described after topical treatment with a 2% solution of cyclosporine,[74–77] an immunomodulating agent. The therapeutic effect of cyclosporine may result from a direct stabilizing effect on conjunctival mast cells or the drug's inhibitory effect on both the release of interleukins and the clonal expansion of T helper-inducer lymphocytes.[77] Although the drug was well-tolerated, most patients in these studies demonstrated recurrence of disease after discontinuing the cyclosporine.

As a last resort, desensitization may be used, but this management approach does not appear to be as effective in VKC patients as it is in patients suffering from hay fever conjunctivitis. Although not generally practical, moving to a cooler climate often reduces symptoms. This is probably the result of the lower concentration of pollens in the air and the vasoconstrictive effect of the cool air itself.

References

1. Friedlaender MH. Allergy and immunology of the eye. New York: Raven Press, 1993.
2. Friedlaender MH. Ocular allergy and immunology. J Allergy Clin Immunol 1970;104:463.
3. Friedlaender MH, Allansmith MR. Ocular allergy. Ann Ophthalmol 1975;7:1171.
4. Gell PG, Coombs RRA. Clinical aspects of immunology. Philadelphia, PA: FA Davis, 1964.
5. Allansmith MR. Immunology of the external ocular tissues. J Am Optom Assoc 1990;61(6)(suppl):16–22.
6. Friedlaender MH. Ocular allergy. J Allergy Clin Immunol 1985;76:645–657.
7. Wilson FM. Adverse external ocular effects of topical ophthalmic medications. Surv Ophthalmol 1979;24:57–88.
8. Zimmerman MC. The prophylaxis and treatment of penicillin reactions with penicillinase. Clin Med 1958;5:305–311.
9. Bloomfield SE. Clinical allergy and immunology of the external eye. In: Tasman W, Jaeger EA, eds. Duane's Clinical ophthalmology. Philadelphia: J B Lippincott Co, 1993;Vol.4,Chap. 2.
10. Green GR, Koelsche GA, Kerland RR. Etiology and pathogenesis of chronic urticaria. Ann Allergy 1965;23:30.
11. Schaeffer AC. Urticaria and angioedema. Pediatr Clin North Am 1975;22:193.
12. Ellis PP. Ocular therapeutics and pharmacology. St. Louis: C. V. Mosby Co, 1985;7:105–120.
13. Rich LF, Hanifin JM. Ocular complications of atopic dermatitis and other eczemas. Int Ophthalmol Clin 1985;25:61–76.
14. Hatinen A, Terasvirta M, Fraki JE. Contact allergy to components in topical ophthalmologic preparations. Acta Ophthalmol 1985;63:424–426.
15. Richmond PP, Allansmith MR. Allergic disorders of the anterior segment. Int Ophthalmol Clin 1983;23:43–61.
16. Romaguera C, Grimolt F, Vilaplana J. Contact dermatitis by timolol. Contact Derm 1986;14:248.
17. Ducombs G, de Casammayor J, Verin P, Whaleville J. Allergic contact dermatitis to phenylephrine. Contact Derm 1986;15:107–108.
18. Jennings B. Mechanisms, diagnosis and management of common ocular allergies. J Am Optom Assoc 1990;61(6)(suppl):32–41.
19. Fernandez-Vozmediano JM, Blasi NA, Romero-Cabera MA, et al. Allergic contact dermatitis to timolol. Contact Derm 1986;14:252.
20. Sher MA. Contact dermatitis of the eyelids. S Afr Med J 1979;55:511–513.
21. de Weck AL. Contact eczematous dermatitis. In: Fitzpatrick TB, Arndt VA, Clark WH, et al, eds. Dermatology in general medicine. New York: McGraw-Hill, 1971:669–679.
22. Theodore FH, Schlossman A. Ocular allergy. Baltimore: Williams and Wilkins, 1958:64–77.
23. Eisenlohr JE. Glaucoma following the prolonged use of topical steroid medication to the eyelids. J Am Acad Dermatol 1983;8:878–881.
24. Fisher AA. Contact dermatitis. Philadelphia: Lea and Febiger, 1973;2:39–70.
25. Fisher AA. Periocular dermatitis akin to the periorbital variety. J Am Acad Dermatol 1986;15:642–644.
26. Freedman SO, Gold P. Clinical Immunology, ed. 2. Hagerstown, MD: Harper and Row, 1976.
27. Baum JL. Antibiotic use in ophthalmology. In: Tasman W, Jaeger EA, eds. Duane's Clinical ophthalmology. Philadelphia: J B Lippincott Co, 1993, Vol. 4;Chap. 26:1–20.
28. Bergmanson JPG. Clinical anatomy of the external eye. J Am Optom Assoc 1990;61(6)(suppl):7–11.
29. Allansmith MR, Ross RN. Ocular allergy and mast cell stabilizers. Surv Ophthalmol 1986;30:229–244.
30. Marrache F, Brunet D, Frandeboeuf J, et al. The role of ocular manifestation in childhood allergy syndromes. Rev Fr Allerg/Immuno Clin 1978;18:151–155.
31. Fisher AA. Allergic reactions to contact lens solutions. Cutis 1985;36:209–211.
32. Tada R, Yuasa T, Shimomura Y. Response of the conjunctiva in atopic disease. Acta Soc Ophthalmol Jpn 1979;83–921.
33. Friedlaender MH. Conjunctivitis of allergic origin: Clinical presentation and differential diagnosis. Surv Ophthalmol 1993;38(suppl):105–114.
34. McMonnies CW, Chapman-Davies A. Assessment of conjunctival hyperemia in contact lens wearers–Part 1. Am J Optom Physiol Opt 1987;64:246–250.
35. Bonini S, Bonini S, Berruto A, et al. Conjunctival provocation test as a model for the study of allergy and inflammation in humans. Int Arch Allergy Appl Immunol 1989;88(1–2):144–148.
36. Schoeneich M, Pecoud AR. Effect of cetirizine in a conjunctival provocation test with allergens. Clin Exp Allergy 1990;20(2):171–174.

37. Pastorello EA, Codecasa LR, Provettoni V, et al. Clinical reliability of diagnostic tests. In: Allergic rhinoconjunctivitis. Boli-1st-Sieroter-Milan 1988;67(5–6):377–385.

38. Garcia-Ortega P, Costa B, Richart C. Evaluation of the conjunctival provocation test in allergy diagnosis. Clin Exp Allergy 1989; 19(5):529–532.

39. Friedlaender MH, Sweet J. Conjunctival provocation tests and naturally occurring allergic conjunctivitis in clinical trials. Int Ophthalmol Clin 1988;28(4):338–339.

40. Sikes CV Jr. How to manage allergic conjunctivitis. Optom Manage 1991;27(5):41.

41. Allansmith MR, Ross RN. Ocular allergy. Clin Allergy 1988;18:1–13.

42. Donshik PC. Allergic conjunctivitis. Int Ophthalmol Clin 1988;28: 294–302.

43. Friedlaender MH, Chisari FV, Baer H. The role of the inflammatory response of skin and lymph nodes in the induction of sensitization to simple chemicals. J Immunol 1973;111:164–170.

44. Abelson MB, Madiwale N, Weston JH. Conjunctival eosinophils in allergic ocular disease. Arch Ophthalmol 1983;101:555–556.

45. Friedlaender MH, Ohashi Y, Kelley J. Diagnosis of allergic conjunctivitis. Arch Ophthalmol 1984;102:1198–1199.

46. Smolin G, Okumoto M. Staphylococcal blepharitis. Arch Ophthalmol 1977;95:812–816.

47. Duzman E, Warman A, Warman R. Efficacy and safety of topical oxymetazoline in treating allergy and management of conjunctivitis. Ann Ophthalmol 1986;18:28–31.

48. Abelson MB, Paradis A, George MA, et al. Effects of Vasocon-A in the allergen challenge model of acute allergic conjunctivitis. Arch Ophthalmol 1990;108(4):520–524.

49. Awouters F, Niemegeers CJ, Jansen T, Megens AA, Janssen PA. Levocabastine: Pharmacological profile of a highly effective inhibitor of allergic reactions. Agents-Actions 1992;35(1–2):12–18.

50. Dechant KL, Goa KL. Levocabastine: A review of its pharmacological properties and therapeutic potential as a topical antihistamine in allergic rhinitis. Drugs 1991;41(2):202–224.

51. Janssens MM. Levocabastine: A new topical approach for the treatment of pediatric allergic rhinoconjunctivitis. Rhino 1992;13: 39–49.

52. Fiscella RG, Siegel FP, Weisbecker C. Alternative solution for Opticrom. Am J Hosp Pharm 1992;49:70.

53. Abelson MB, Schaeffer K. Conjunctivitis of allergic origin: Immunologic mechanisms and current approaches to therapy. Surv Ophthalmol 1993;38(suppl):115–140.

54. Ballas Z, Blumenthal MD, Tinkelman MD, et al. Clinical evaluation of ketorolac tromethamine 0.5% ophthalmic solution for the treatment of seasonal allergic conjunctivitis. Surv Ophthalmol 1993;38(suppl):141–148.

55. Srinivasan RD, Jakobick FA, Iwamoto T, et al. Giant papillary conjunctivitis with ocular prostheses. Arch Ophthalmol 1979;97: 892.

56. Douglas JP, Lowder CY, Lasorik R, et al. Giant papillary conjunctivitis associated with rigid gas permeable contact lenses. CLAO J 1988;14(3):143–147.

57. Fowler SA, Greiner JV, Allansmith MR. Soft contact lenses from patients with giant papillary conjunctivitis. Am J Ophthalmol 1979; 88:1056.

58. Friedlaender MH. Some unusual non-allergic causes of giant papillary conjunctivitis. Trans Am Ophthalmol Soc 1990;88:343–349.

59. Ballow M, Donshik PC, Rapaca P, et al. Tear lactoferrin levels in patients with external inflammatory ocular disease. Invest Ophthalmol Vis Sci 1987;28:543–545.

60. Soni PS, Hathcoct G. Complications reported with hydrogel extended wear contact lenses. Am J Optom Physiol Opt 1988; 65(7):545–551.

61. Martin NF, Rubinfeld RS, Malley JD, et al. Giant papillary conjunctivitis and meibomian gland dysfunction blepharitis. CLAO J 1992;18:165–169.

62. Mathes WD, Billborough M. Meibomian gland dysfunction and giant papillary conjunctivitis. Am J Ophthalmol 1991;114(2):188–192.

63. Richard NR, Anderson JA, Tasevska ZG, Binder PS. Evaluation of tear protein deposits on contact lenses from patients with and without giant papillary conjunctivitis. CLAO J 1992;18(3):143–147.

64. Elgebaly SA, Donshik PC, Rahhal F, et al. Neutrophil chemotactic factors in the tears of giant papillary conjunctivitis patients. Invest Ophthalmol Vis Sci 1991;32:208–213.

65. Lustine T, Bouchard CS, Cavanaugh HD. Continued contact lens wear in patients with giant papillary conjunctivitis. CLAO J 1991; 17(2):104–107.

66. Kruger CJ, Ehlers WH, Luistro AE, et al. Treatment of giant papillary conjunctivitis with cromolyn sodium. CLAO J 1991; 18(1):46–48.

67. Allansmith MR, Ross RN. Giant papillary conjunctivitis. Int Ophthalmol Clin 1988;28:309–316.

68. Donshik PC, Ballow M, Luistro A, et al. Treatment of contact lens associated giant papillary conjunctivitis. Arch Ophthalmol 1979: 97–473.

69. Bartlett JD, Howes JF, Ghormley NR, et al. Safety and efficacy of loteprednol etabonate for treatment of papillae in contact lens-associated giant papillary conjunctivitis. Curr Eye Res 1993;12: 313–321.

70. Wood TS, Stewart RH, Bowman RW, et al. Suprofen treatment of contact lens-associated giant papillary conjunctivitis. Ophthalmology 1988;95:822–826.

71. Friedlaender MH. Ocular allergy. In: Middleton E, Jr., Reed CE, Ellis EF, et al, eds. Allergy: Principles and practice, ed. 3. St. Louis: C. V. Mosby, 1988:1469–1480

72. Abelson MB, Butrus SI, Weston JH. Aspirin therapy in vernal conjunctivitis. Am J Ophthalmol 1983;95:502–505.

73. Chaudhary KP. Evaluation of combined systemic aspirin and cromolyn sodium in intractable vernal catarrh. Ann Ophthalmol 1990;22(8):314–318.

74. Secchi AG, Tognan MS, Leonardi A. Topical use of cyclosporine in the treatment of vernal keratoconjunctivitis. Am J Ophthalmol 1990;110(6):641–645.

75. Ben Ezra D, Matamoros N, Cohen E. Treatment of severe vernal keratoconjunctivitis with cyclosporine eyedrops. Transplant Proc 1988;20(2)(suppl 2):644–649.

76. Bleik JH, Jabbara KF. Topical cyclosporine in vernal keratoconjunctivitis. Ophthalmology 1991;98(11):1679–1684.

77. Ben Ezra D, Pe'er J, Brodsky M, et al. Cyclosporine eyedrops for the treatment of severe vernal keratoconjunctivitis. Am J Ophthalmol 1986;101:278–282.

78. Bucci FA, Lopatynsky MD, Jenkins PL, et al. Comparison of the clinical performance of the Acuvue disposable contact lens and CSI lens in patients with giant papillary conjunctivitis. Am J Ophthalmol 1993;115:454–459.

CHAPTER 29

Diseases of the Sclera

William L. Jones

The sclera is the outer protective coat of the eye and, along with the cornea, is primarily responsible for maintaining the shape of the eye. Composed chiefly of collagen and ground substances, the sclera also contains a scant vascular and nervous system. Diseases of the collagen and vascular tissues can manifest themselves in the sclera. This chapter discusses three forms of scleral disease: episcleritis, scleritis, and scleromalacia perforans.

Episcleritis

Episcleritis is usually a benign inflammation that occurs most often in young adults. It is relatively common and seems to occur spontaneously. Involvement is unilateral in approximately two-thirds of cases.[1] There may be recurrences at the same location or in a different area of the same eye, and it may reappear in the fellow eye. Episcleritis is found twice as often in females and has a peak incidence in the fourth decade of life.

Clinical Anatomy of the Episclera

The episclera is a thin vascular fibroelastic tissue covering the sclera. It acts as a synovial membrane for smooth movements of the globe and, along with the check ligaments, limits excessive eye movement.

The episclera consists of the outer parietal and the inner visceral layer, both of which are attached loosely to one another by connecting fibers. Each layer is supplied with a vascular network derived from the anterior and posterior ciliary arteries. These vessel complexes anastomose at the limbus with the conjunctival vessels. The visible vessels are usually veins derived from the superficial and deep intrascleral veins that drain the anterior region of the ciliary body and Schlemm's canal. Conjunctival, episcleral, and scleral vessels constitute the three vessel networks visible in the anterior segment of the eye. The topical instillation of 10% phenylephrine or 1:1000 epinephrine will blanch the superficial vessels but has little effect on the deep scleral vessels. This is an important clinical tool used to differentiate superficial from deep inflammation. Another way to distinguish superficial from deep inflammation is to mechanically move the conjunctival vessels by applying pressure through the lids onto the sclera. The episcleral vessels remain stationary, while the loose conjunctiva moves freely.

Etiology

Approximately 30% of patients with episcleritis have a known associated systemic condition, but the majority of cases are of unknown etiology.[2,100] Of those patients with known causes reported by Watson,[2] 5% were associated with collagen disease, 7% with herpes zoster, 3% with gout, and 3% with syphilis. The remainder were associated with such conditions as Schönlein-Henoch purpura, penicillin sensitivity, erythema nodosum, and contact with industrial solvents, all of which are believed to be antigen-antibody reactions. Rheumatoid arthritis has also been associated with episodes of episcleritis.[3] Many of these patients had a strong family history of atopy, but they uniformly did not test positive themselves. Episcleritis is the most common ocular finding in relapsing polychrondritis, and it is also seen in Wegener's granulomatosis.[4,5] Systemic diseases such as tuberculosis, gonorrhea, staphylococcal infection, coccidioidomycosis, and Lyme disease have been implicated as sources for delayed types of bacterial allergies.[6–9] Other known causes are episcleral foreign bodies, surgical trauma, and skin diseases such as psoriasis, lichen planus, and erythema elevantum diutinum.[10] Attacks often are related to stress caused by family or work problems.[11] It also has been found in patients with familial Mediterranean fever.[12]

Light and electron microscopic studies have failed to elucidate the underlying causes of episcleritis. The involved area is packed with lymphocytes, but there are no mast cells, plasma cells, or eosinophils.[2]

Diagnosis

Episcleritis is often acute in onset (as short as half an hour), is usually unilateral, and tends to recur. The redness is often seen in a sectorial configuration within the interpalpebral fissure (Fig. 29.1), but it can encompass the entire anterior portion of the globe. The vessels are usually tortuous, and it is not uncommon to observe saccular dilatations (Fig. 29.2). The patient may complain of a sensation of heat, prickling, photophobia, and mild discomfort. The eye is rarely tender to the touch.[2,3] Ocular pain may be absent but on occasion can be severe. The pain is usually localized to the eye, but it may radiate to the forehead. Although tearing is common, there is no ocular discharge. In rare instances, the lids may become edematous, and if photophobia is present, an associated keratitis should be suspected. Visual acuity is usually

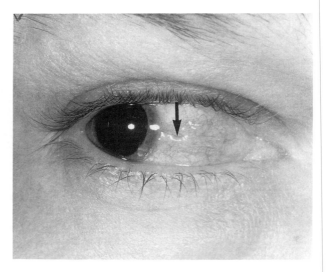

FIGURE 29.1   **Nodular episcleritis in sectorial configuration. Arrow points to elevated, edematous nodule.**

not affected, and intraocular structures are usually not involved. Pathologically, episcleritis is characterized by widespread hyperemia, edema, and lymphocytic infiltration. The lesions heal without leaving a scar.[13]

Episcleritis can be classified as either simple or nodular.

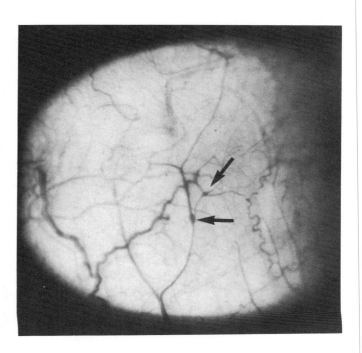

FIGURE 29.2   **Diffuse episcleritis demonstrating vessel injection, tortuosity, and saccular dilatations (arrows).**

Each form differs in its clinical course and appearance. Both forms, however, have areas of edema and infiltration that are localized to the episclera. Although most of the congestion is in the superficial episcleral vessels, some congestion is observed in the conjunctival and deep episcleral vessels.

The vessel injection in simple episcleritis can vary from a mild red flush to an intense fiery red. However, it does not have the bluish tinge that is so characteristic of scleritis. The congested vessels tend to retain their normal radial configuration. The edema is distributed diffusely, and there may be grayish infiltrates present that appear yellow in red-free light.

Nodular episcleritis is localized to discrete areas, each of which consists of an elevated edematous nodule associated with surrounding congestion. The nodule is mobile over the underlying sclera.[14] These nodules may be single or multiple. After many attacks of nodular episcleritis in the same location, the superficial scleral lamellae may show alterations and become slightly transparent.[2] Since the edema is isolated to the episclera, the slit beam from the biomicroscope will not show any upward deviation of the underlying sclera.

Management

The course of simple episcleritis is usually 10 to 21 days. It periodically reappears, but the recurrences become less frequent with time until the disease no longer recurs. Most episodes of nodular episcleritis last 5 to 10 days, but durations vary considerably. Some cases may last up to 2 months. Over half the patients have intermittent attacks for 3 to 6 years, and some patients have had intermittent attacks for as long as 30 years.[15] As with simple episcleritis, recurrences of nodular episcleritis become less frequent until the disease no longer recurs.

A simple episcleritis may recur in a nodular form, or vice versa. Although episcleritis does not develop into a scleritis, scleritis will produce an overlying episcleritis. Complications of episcleritis include an occasional minor reduction in visual acuity, mild uveitis, and, in some patients with nodular episcleritis, mild changes of the pars plana.[2]

Since it is a self-limiting disease with little or no permanent damage to the eye, episcleritis generally does not require treatment.[2,15] However, many patients desire symptomatic relief from the redness and associated ocular discomfort. Treatment depends on the severity of the disease, and mild cases can be treated satisfactorily with topical decongestants or corticosteroids several times a day. With appropriate treatment, the condition generally resolves within a few days. For patients who suffer recurrent attacks, steroid treatment should be continued for several days after the condition has subsided. In severe cases of episcleritis, systemic steroids may be necessary along with the use of topical steroids. Since episcleritis is sometimes seen in association with systemic disorders, such as collagen diseases, resolution of the disease will depend on the severity of the systemic condition. In cases of persistent or recurrent attacks of episcleritis, an internist should assist in evaluating the patient for systemic disease[100].

Treatment of mild episodes of episcleritis can consist of cold compresses and decongestants such as phenylephrine 0.12%. These offer symptomatic relief without greatly affecting the inflammatory process. Orally administered aspirin and other nonsteroidal anti-inflammatory drugs (NSAIDs) have also been used.[16] Antihistamines and histamine desensitization have been attempted, but the response has not been nearly as effective as the response to local steroid therapy.[16] Desensitization has been known to precipitate an attack.[15] If an allergy is suspected, the definitive treatment entails elimination of the offending allergen.

Treatment of simple episcleritis usually consists of local steroids, such as prednisolone 1% or dexamethasone 0.1%, which can be administered every 1 or 2 hours until the redness disappears, and then 3 or 4 times a day for 4 to 5 days. Continuation of the topical steroid after the redness has dissipated prevents a rebound recurrence, but topical steroid treatment should not continue for more than a month due to the possibility of steroid-induced glaucoma. However, simple episcleritis frequently will improve by 50% in the first week and completely resolve within 3 weeks without treatment. Steroid therapy serves only to hasten its resolution.[2,15,17]

Since nodular episcleritis tends to resolve much more slowly than does simple episcleritis, local treatment is more advantageous. Topical steroid therapy is generally used, but in more severe cases systemic therapy is sometimes necessary. All patients undergoing steroid therapy should have periodic evaluations of intraocular pressure to detect possible steroid-induced glaucoma. NSAIDs such as oxyphenbutazone and indomethacin are generally preferred over systemic steroids because of their effectiveness and less rebound phenomenon. Patients who do not respond to one of the two aforementioned drugs will often respond to the other. The recommended oral dosage of oxyphenbutazone is 100 mg 3 or 4 times daily. When used in a 10% ointment, oxyphenbutazone has been of some value in the treatment of recurrent episcleritis.[16] The recommended oral dosage of indomethacin is 25 mg daily for 2 days, 50 mg daily for 2 days, then 75 mg daily until the condition is controlled.[15]

Scleritis

Unlike the more commonly encountered episcleritis, inflammation of the sclera is relatively rare. Women are affected more frequently, and scleritis is usually seen in the fourth to sixth decades of life. Scleritis is bilateral in 52% of patients. In half of the bilateral cases, it occurs simultaneously in both eyes, and the remainder become bilateral in 5 or more years.[2]

Clinical Anatomy of the Sclera

The sclera is composed of collagen and elastic tissue that allow it to be resilient enough for variation in intraocular pressure, yet strong enough to prevent distortion of the globe by either the extraocular muscles or external forces. The collagen fibers are irregular in size and are spaced in a parallel and interlacing crisscross fashion, which produces a white opaque structure. The sclera is approximately 1 mm thick, except at the insertions of the recti muscles, where it is about 0.3 mm thick. It is continuous with the cornea anteriorly and with the dura sheath of the optic nerve posteriorly. A few strands of scleral tissue transgress the optic nerve, creating a structure known as the lamina cribrosa.

The posterior portion of the sclera is penetrated by the long and short posterior ciliary nerves and arteries; the equatorial region is penetrated by the vortex veins; and the anterior region is penetrated by the anterior ciliary arteries, veins, and nerves. Thus, the neural innervation to the sclera is through the long and short posterior ciliary nerves and the anterior ciliary nerves. Inflammation and scleral distention result in pain mediated by each of these nervous networks. Nourishment to the sclera is provided by the many branches of the long and short posterior ciliary arteries, the anterior ciliary arteries, the underlying choroid, and the overlying episclera. These vascular channels can transport various substances capable of producing inflammation within the sclera.

Etiology

A causative factor is more often found in scleritis than in episcleritis. Systemic and ocular conditions known to cause scleritis are listed in Table 29.1. In a series reported by Watson,[2] 40% of the patients with necrotizing scleritis had evidence of collagen disease, while only 20% of the patients with diffuse anterior or nodular scleritis had associated collagen disease. Of the patients with diffuse anterior and nodular scleritis, 12% had ankylosing spondylitis, and 15% occurred in patients following an attack of herpes zoster ophthalmicus. Other studies have found scleritis associated with connective tissue disease in 15% to 89% of cases.[18-20] Rheumatoid arthritis is a connective tissue disease most commonly associated with scleral disease, and scleritis is seen in 0.5% to 0.7% of patients with this disease.[21,22] Watson and Hazelman[23] found an 8% incidence of scleritis in patients with systemic lupus erythematosus. A number of other conditions such as Reiter's disease, tuberculosis, gout, IgA nephropathy,[24] erythema nodosum,[25] and syphilis have been implicated as etiologic factors.

Since approximately 50% of patients with scleral inflammation have an underlying systemic disease,[26,100] it is incumbent upon the clinician to rule out infections such as tuberculosis and venereal diseases, skeletal and collagen diseases such as rheumatoid arthritis and Wegener's granulomatosis,[28-31] and skin diseases such as psoriasis and erythema nodosum. AIDS-related opportunistic infections have also been cited as causing scleritis.[27]

TABLE 29.1
Systemic and Ocular Conditions Known to Cause Scleritis

Collagen Diseases	Metabolic Diseases	Granulomatous Diseases	Infectious Diseases	Ocular Conditions
Rheumatoid arthritis[a]	Thyrotoxicosis	Syphilis	Herpes zoster	Penetrating injuries
Ankylosing spondylitis	Gout	Leprosy	Herpes simplex	Thermal burns
Systemic lupus erythematosus		Tuberculosis	Onchocerciasis	Alkali and acid burns
Polyarteritis nodosa		Sarcoidosis[d]	*Pseudomonas*	Irradiation
Relapsing polychondritis[b]			*Acanthamoeba*[e]	
Wegener's granulomatosis[c]			Toxoplasmosis[f]	
Ulcerative colitis			*Sporothrix schenskii*[g]	
Crohn's disease				
Behçet's syndrome				
Dermatomyositis				
Sjögren syndrome (complete)				
Psoriatic arthritis				
Erythema nodosum				

[a]Barr CC, Davis H, Culbertson WW. Rheumatoid scleritis. Ophthalmology 1981;88:1269–1273.
[b]Isaak BL, Liesegang TJ, Michet CJ Jr. Ocular and systemic findings in relapsing polychondritis. Ophthalmology 1986;93:681–689.
[c]Bullen CL, Liesegang TJ, McDonald TJ, et al. Ocular complications of Wegener's granulomatosis. Ophthalmology 1983;90:279–290.
[d]Henkind P. Sarcoidosis: An expanding ophthalmic horizon. J R Soc Med 1982;75:153–159.
[e]Dougherty PJ, Binder PS, Mondino BJ, et al. *Acanthamoeba* sclerokeratitis. Am J Ophthalmol 1994;117:475–479.
[f]Schuman JS, Weinberg RS, Ferry AP, et al. Toxoplasmic scleritis. Ophthalmology 1988;95:1399–1403.
[g]Brunette I, Stulting RD. *Sporothrix schenskii* scleritis. Am J Ophthalmol 1992;114:370–371.

Experimentally, pathologic and clinical data seem to support an immunologic basis as the cause of many attacks of scleritis.[17,32–34] Circulating antigen-antibody complexes that involve the complement system cause inflammation at the sites where the complexes concentrate. This does not mean that the sclera is necessarily liberating the antigen, since the focus of antigen production may be at a distant tissue location. Circulating immune complexes have a predilection for the basement membranes of blood vessels, and it is there that they activate the complement system, initiate inflammation, and produce tissue damage.[35,36] Immunologic injury may lead to a chronic granulomatous response (Type IV hypersensitivity) mediated by macrophages, epithelioid cells, multinucleated giant cells, and lymphocytes.[33,34] It has been proposed that since the posterior segment of the eye has fewer blood vessels, posterior scleral inflammation is less severe than inflammation of the anterior sclera.[15,35] Examples of immune complex diseases that can have an associated scleritis include rheumatoid arthritis, systemic lupus erythematosis, and polyarteritis nodosa. Scleritis has been found following uneventful cataract surgery with or without intraocular lens implantation.[37–39]

Histopathologic studies from nodular scleritis have shown areas adjacent to the necrotic tissue as swollen, excavated, and ulcerated with a thin overlying layer of fibrous tissue. What appears clinically as inflammation and edema in scleritis is histopathologically a granulomatous lesion of the sclera consisting largely of plasma cells, lymphocytes, and mast cells.[2] Adjacent areas show activation of fibrocytes that release proteoglycans, causing the collagen fibrils of the sclera to unravel.[40] The vessels in the involved areas show mild necrosis and perivascular cuffing with lymphocytes, vascular occlusion, and aneurysmal formation in the center of the lesions.[41]

Diagnosis

Scleritis can be an extremely destructive disease leading to loss of vision, severe pain, perforation of the globe, and loss of the eye. Therefore, early diagnosis and treatment are crucial. Although episcleritis rarely involves the sclera, scleritis always produces a concurrent episcleritis.[2,42,43]

The onset of scleritis is slow, and symptoms increase over many days. Tearing and photophobia are common complaints in scleritis, with or without a concurrent keratitis. One of the hallmark symptoms of scleritis is severe pain, often boring in nature, which prompts the patient to seek eyecare. The pain may be localized to the eye, but in many instances it is much more diffuse and may be described as radiating to the jaw, sinuses, and temple.[2] It is not uncommon for the pain to awaken the patient in the night or to prevent the patient from falling asleep during an attack, and it is only temporarily relieved by analgesics. The eye can become exquisitely tender to the touch, and the slightest digital pressure through the lids can cause the patient to recoil from the examiner. The pain experienced by such patients seems much greater than can be explained by the ocular findings. This is particularly true in posterior scleritis, since the inflammation is not visible to the clinician. The sclera varies in thickness from 0.3 to 1.0 mm, but in scleritis it can become as thick as 6 mm.[45] The pain is secondary to distension of the sensory nerve endings as they become edematous, and an even more severe pain can result from actual destruction of the nerves in necrotizing scleritis. In some cases intractable pain may be relieved only by the use of retrobulbar alcohol injections.[44]

Inflammation is a prominent feature in anterior scleritis, and it produces a bluish red (violaceous) color instead of the bright red injection observed in episcleritis (Fig. 29.3). Since the violaceous color is seen more easily in the daylight and is often overlooked in tungsten fluorescent light, the clinician may want to examine the patient next to a window or outside the office. Red-free (green) light can be used to enhance blood vessels and may allow the clinician to observe any avascular areas within the lesion. The episcleral congestion can be differentiated from that of the sclera by instilling phenylephrine 10% or epinephrine 1:1000, which will blanch the episcleral vessels but have little effect on the deeper scleral vessels.

Another test that can be used is instillation of a topical anesthetic followed by application of a cotton swab to the inflamed site. If this elicits a pain response, then scleritis or episcleritis should be suspected. The absence of pain suggests a diagnosis of conjunctivitis or anterior uveitis. The degree of inflammation depends on the amount of episcleral tissue. Thus, younger patients have more inflammation and older patients with rheumatoid arthritis have the least.[2]

Laboratory tests should include hemoglobin, WBC with differential, erythrocyte sedimentation rate, rheumatoid factor, antinuclear and anti-DNA antibodies, circulating immune complexes (polyethylene glycol method preferred), LE cells search, C-reactive protein, serum uric acid, full serologic tests for syphilis, and radiologic films of the sacroiliac joints and other joints, as deemed necessary.[34] The practitioner should be careful to exclude intraocular causes of scleral inflammation. Yeo and associates[45] have reported intraocular metastatic carcinoma that masqueraded as scleritis. Also, ophthalmoscopy should be performed to distinguish an exudative retinal detachment from a granulomatous disease with posterior involvement.

ANTERIOR SCLERITIS

Anterior scleritis can be classified into three types: diffuse, nodular, and necrotizing. Patients with necrotizing scleritis can be subdivided into those with and those without scleromalacia perforans. In a study by Tuft and Watson,[46] scleritis had a recurrence of 35.9%. Of 290 patients, only 12 progressed from diffuse to nodular, and 10 with nodular scleritis

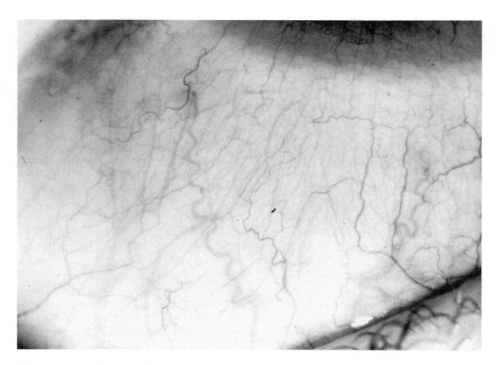

FIGURE 29.3   **Diffuse scleritis with deep vessel injection and associated episcleritis.**

developed necrosis. Women with rheumatoid arthritis had the greatest tendency to progress to necrotizing scleritis.

Diffuse scleritis is more common than the other forms, and involves inflammation that occurs over a small area or encompasses the entire anterior segment. The vessels of the superficial and deep layers become engorged and tortuous, losing their normal radial pattern, and they may become beaded in appearance. The term "brawny scleritis" is used when there is severe inflammation of the superficial tissues. Fluorescein angiography shows a relatively benign scleritis with rapid transit time, as is seen in episcleritis. There can be mild anomalous changes in the blood vessels that may persist even following successful treatment. This form of scleritis has a 9% incidence of visual loss.[46]

Nodular scleritis consists of one to many immovable nodules of scleral tissue. The adjacent episclera usually is edematous and lightly affixed to the underlying sclera. The sclera may become transparent beneath the nodule. Fortunately, the sclera does not become necrotic, and the scleral inflammation does not extend beyond the nodule. About half of affected patients have a bilateral occurrence. Fluorescein angiography has findings similar to the diffuse form of the disease, exhibiting deep scleral staining. Nodular scleritis can on occasion resemble a scleral buckle.[47] This type of scleritis has a 26% incidence of visual loss, and it is typically seen in older patients who have an associated systemic disease.[46]

Necrotizing scleritis is relatively rare but is the most serious form of scleritis and has the highest complication rate.[100] Over 60% of patients develop complications other than scleral thinning, and 40% to 74% have loss of visual acuity.[1,46] The mortality rate for patients with necrotizing scleritis secondary to rheumatoid arthritis is 45% in 5 to 10 years of follow-up.[48,49] The scleritis begins in a localized area with acute congestion of the vessels, which become greatly distorted or occluded. The usual presentation is that of gradual onset of a painful, injected eye; the pain can become severe enough to require enucleation. The underlying sclera becomes transparent, and the choroid may be observed when viewed in daylight. If the inflammation remains uncontrolled, it may spread to newly formed areas of scleritis in adjoining locations. The progression can occur rapidly (within 2 to 4 weeks) and leave the area behind the advancing edge very thin or perforated.[50] The entire anterior segment can become involved if efforts are not made to control the inflammation. Serious complications generally do not occur until the necrotizing process is almost circumferential. Staphylomas are uncommon unless the intraocular pressure is above 40 mm Hg.[2,18] With successful treatment, necrotic areas may disappear or may leave a thin film of conjunctiva or episclera covering the uvea. In other cases there may be actual uveal exposure. Small defects are usually covered by new collagen, but large defects may require a scleral graft. Necrotizing scleritis may indicate a potential lethal underlying systemic vasculitis.[49]

Fluorescein angiography is useful in diagnosing necrotizing scleritis and shows hypoperfusion of deeper vessels that are occluded or partially occluded during the early dye transit phase, and deep leakage on the late phase due to newly formed vessels within the granuloma. These angiographic findings are helpful in differentiating early necrotizing scleritis from diffuse and nodular scleritis.[50,51]

Necrotizing anterior scleritis without accompanying inflammation is known as scleromalacia perforans. It most commonly affects women between 50 and 75 years of age who suffer from chronic polyarticular rheumatism. It is characterized by a melting of episcleral and scleral tissue with almost a total lack of symptoms. The underlying uvea may be covered by conjunctiva or be totally exposed (Fig. 29.4). Fluorescein angiography is not very helpful and may show only areas of vascular occlusion.

POSTERIOR SCLERITIS

Posterior scleritis is usually unilateral and is more difficult to diagnose, since it is hidden from direct view. The underestimation of posterior scleritis is rather high as suggested by studies in which 43% to 62% of enucleated eyes had a posterior scleritis or posterior extension of anterior disease.[43,52] When the patient experiences considerably more ocular pain and discomfort than can be justified by the examination, posterior scleritis should be suspected. Scleral depression can localize an area of posterior scleritis by eliciting intense pain when applied to the involved inflammatory site. Exudative retinal and choroidal detachment, optic disc edema, macular edema, retinal hemorrhages, proptosis, ophthalmoplegia and, rarely, angle-closure glaucoma may develop in posterior scleritis.[1,2,53–57] The proptosis and ophthalmoplegia result from the outward extension of inflammation to involve the extraocular muscles. Lower lid retraction can occur, thought to be the result of inflammation of the muscle cone and tendons.[18] Angle-closure glaucoma results from an anterior ciliochoroidal effusion that displaces the iris forward.[58] Posterior scleritis can develop as a posterior extension of anterior scleritis, and posterior scleritis can extend forward to cause anterior disease.

The diagnosis of posterior scleritis may be facilitated by ultrasonography, which shows thickened sclera and a possible clear zone immediately posterior to the globe (Fig. 29.5). This clear zone consists of transudates produced by the adjacent scleritis.[59,60] Computed tomography (CT) can also reveal the inflammation as a thickening of the sclera and a separation between the sclera and Tenon's capsule.[61,62] The

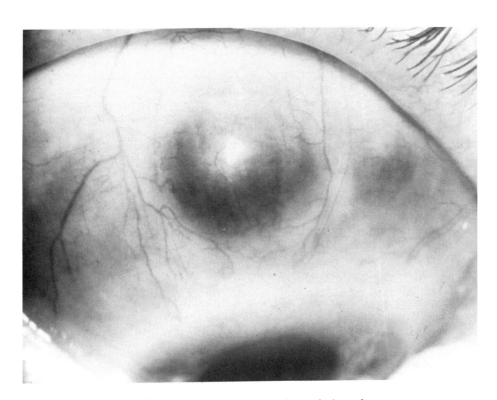

FIGURE 29.4 **Rheumatoid nodules seen in a case of scleromalacia perforans.**

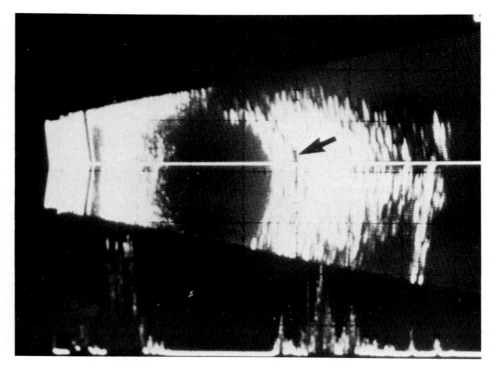

FIGURE 29.5   **B-scan ultrasonogram of posterior scleritis demonstrating the edematous zone (arrow) produced by the posterior scleritis.**

thickening of the sclera is made obvious by comparing it to the fellow globe on the CT scan. Magnetic resonance imaging (MRI) is advantageous for detecting soft tissue masses within or next to the sclera. It is not uncommon for an eye to be removed because of a suspected intraocular tumor,[53,54,63] only to be discovered later by the pathologist that the lesion in question was an area of posterior scleritis.

In a study by Tuft and Watson,[46] 12% of 290 patients with scleral inflammation had posterior scleritis, and 84% of those patients suffered visual loss. Patients with posterior scleritis have the highest incidence of visual loss, which is mainly due to retinal edema and optic nerve involvement. The progress of posterior scleritis approximates that of nodular scleritis. Posterior scleritis can mimic a subretinal mass such as choroidal melanoma or hemangioma, metastatic carcinoma, or uveal lymphoid hyperplasia.[57,63–65] Clinical signs and symptoms that distinguish posterior scleritis from a neoplasm are ocular redness, periorbital pain, and choroidal folds.

Management

Aggressive treatment of scleritis is important to prevent complications that occur in the later stages of the disease and vary according to the degree of inflammation. They include uveitis, glaucoma,[3,18,66] keratitis, corneal ulceration, scleral thinning, proptosis, diplopia, cataract, macular edema, optic disc edema, exudative retinal detachment, annular choroidal detachment, lid edema, chemosis, hyperemia of the conjunctiva, paresis of extraocular muscles, and myopia.[2,3,66–68] Many of these complications can result in reduced vision.

In a series reported by Watson,[2] 27% of the patients lost a significant amount of vision within a year of onset of the condition despite aggressive treatment, and this was usually caused by cataracts and keratitis. However, only 4% of the patients over a 15-year period had permanent loss of vision. Early and intensive treatment was very successful in preserving the eye; over a 6-year period in which 343 eyes were treated, only 4 were enucleated for intractable pain. All 4 patients had severe necrotizing scleritis and maintained reasonable visual acuity until the entire anterior segment became involved.

Treatment of scleritis is determined primarily by its etiology and severity of the inflammation. Associated ocular and systemic diseases are more commonly found in patients with scleritis than in those with episcleritis. A known bacterial infection or other known condition should be treated with a specific therapeutic regimen.[69–72]

Scleritis secondary to infections has been found in 6% to 18% of patients with scleritis.[18,72,73] Infectious scleritis is difficult to treat, probably due to the poor penetration of antibiotics into the nearly avascular sclera, and due to the ability of microbial organisms to persist within the avascular intrascleral lamellae for long periods without inciting an immune response.[21] Often, when the sclera develops an infectious inflammation, medical treatment alone is usually not effective. Approximately 60% of eyes with infectious keratoscleritis undergo evisceration or enucleation or are left blind.[74] Modes of treatment include intensive antibiotic eyedrops, subconjunctival injections, and parenteral antibiotics.

Scleritis associated with brucellosis should be treated with 500 to 700 mg of tetracycline 4 times a day, or 1g to 2 g of streptomycin per day for 3 to 4 weeks. Scleritis associated with syphilis should be treated with penicillin in a total dose varying from 5 to 10 million units. Scleritis associated with tuberculosis should be treated with streptomycin, 1g to 2 g daily; rifampin, 600 mg daily; or ethambutol, 15 mg/kg body weight daily. This can be administered in combination with isoniazid, 5 to 10 mg/kg body weight in 2 to 3 daily doses.[75,76] Gouty scleritis can be treated with colchicine, 0.6 mg every 2 hours until the symptoms are relieved or gastrointestinal disturbances appear, but in mild cases only 0.6 mg daily may be sufficient. Phenylbutazone is used in acute cases of gout, and the initial dosage is 200 to 400 mg orally, then 200 mg every 6 hours for 4 days, followed by 100 mg 3 times a day until symptoms dissipate. Because of the risk of severe and sometimes fatal toxic reactions, therapy should not exceed 7 to 10 days. Indomethacin has been found to be effective in gout; the dosage is 50 mg 3 times daily in the acute phase and 25 mg twice daily in the quiescent phase.[16]

Scleritis secondary to leprosy should be treated with sulfone drugs, such as dapsone, in oral doses of 25 mg twice weekly and then increased by 25 mg twice weekly until a maintenance weekly dosage of 300 mg is achieved after 4 to 6 months of therapy. Sulfoxone sodium may be given for leprosy in an oral dosage of 330 mg twice weekly for the first 2 weeks and gradually increasing to 330 mg daily after 1 month of therapy. In all the systemic diseases mentioned above, the use of topical steroids can relieve pain and dramatically reduce the scleral inflammation. They may be used to treat the associated scleritis as long as the underlying systemic disease is controlled adequately.[16,21,77] Cryotherapy may be useful in the treatment of infectious scleritis,[21,78] and this may be due to the mechanical destruction of the microorganisms by the extracellular ice, or it may enhance antibiotic absorption through damage to bacterial cell walls or disrupted scleral tissue.[79]

If no local or systemic disease process can be identified or if a collagen disease is discovered, then systemic anti-inflammatory or immunosuppressive agents should be administered. Scleritis is most often associated with the rheumatoid group of diseases, and the associated scleritis usually varies with the severity of the systemic condition.[19,80] The scleritis may develop while the patient is receiving salicylate or steroid therapy for the arthritis.[16]

Many parameters can be used to assess the effectiveness of treatment, including episcleral and deep scleral injection, tenderness, pain, and corneal and intraocular involvement. Pain is especially useful in determining the response of scleritis to treatment, and it is often used as an indicator to modify the treatment regimen. If the pain disappears, the steroid dosage can often be reduced with confidence.

Scleritis is usually treated with topical steroid drops or ointment. Prednisolone 1% or dexamethasone 0.1% can be used 4 times daily to once every hour, depending on the severity of the inflammation. Such local steroids are used when the inflammation is mild and the pain is slight. They can be used to maintain the patient in a state of remission or may be used between severe attacks. Topical steroids can decrease symptoms and shorten the period of inflammation. However, topical steroid therapy is usually not adequate by itself to treat scleritis, and the preferred treatment plan is systemic anti-inflammatory or immunosuppressive agents. High doses of systemic anti-inflammatory drugs are necessary to achieve a therapeutic level in the poorly vascularized scleral tissue.[2]

Nonsteroidal anti-inflammatory drugs (NSAIDs) should be the initial treatment for diffuse and nodular scleritis, and high dosages of NSAIDs can often be useful in controlling the inflammation of necrotizing scleritis.[80,81] Dosages commonly employed include indomethacin 75 mg bid, naproxen 375–500 mg bid, ibuprofen 400 to 600 mg qid, piroxicam 20 mg qd, diflunisal 500 mg bid, or sulindac 200 mg bid. If one NSAID fails, then another should be attempted before changing to steroids or immunosuppressive drugs.[20] Watson[2] prefers flurbiprofen or indomethacin as the initial therapy. Flurbiprofen is given in doses of 100 mg tid for one week, and the scleritis pain usually disappears in 48 hours. Indomethacin is administered if the response to flurbiprofen is poor and is given as a 25 mg dose tid.

If NSAID treatment fails to control the inflammation, second-line therapy is steroids. These should be tapered as soon as possible and remission maintained with NSAIDs. A useful systemic steroid dosage is prednisone 60 to 120 mg per day for one week, tapered to 20 mg daily within 2 to 3 weeks by lowering the dosage in 2.5 mg steps.[20] The required dosage may be as high as 120 mg daily in severe cases, and as high as 300 mg if lower dosages fail to control the inflammation.[82] Sometimes, a pulse method is used to treat diffuse and nodular scleritis, accomplished by an intravenouus injection of methylprednisolone.[83] In some cases where neither steroid nor NSAID controls non-necrotizing scleritis, satisfactory control may be achieved by combining oral prednisone and indomethacin.[84] In patients with diffuse or nodular scleritis, over 90% will have control of the inflammation with an NSAID as the first drug of choice. The addition of steroids or immunosuppressive drugs will bring the scleral inflammation under control in most of the remaining cases.[20]

Immunosuppressive drugs may be necessary in cases of necrotizing scleritis when high doses of steroids and NSAIDs have failed. The immunosuppressive drug cyclosporine is commonly used in treating scleritis, and it has shown efficacy in the management of ocular inflammation and in immunologically mediated eye diseases.[85–90] The dosage is 2 to 5 mg/kg/day for 1 to 2 weeks.[20] Side effects involve the neurologic, gastrointestinal, cardiovascular, and dermatologic systems, resulting in tremors, nausea, diarrhea, and hypertrichosis.[91,92] Since NSAIDs can potentiate renal disease in patients on cyclosporine, patients should be removed from NSAIDs when placed on this drug.[93] The risk of nephrotoxicity is reduced with lower cyclosporine doses, but it is important to monitor blood levels of the drug to minimize renal toxicity. Immunosuppressives as the first drug of choice were successful in controlling inflammation in 74% of patients with necrotizing scleritis.[20] Tuft and Watson[46] reported that only 29% of patients with necrotizing scleritis responded sufficiently to systemic steroid treatment, whereas 67% required the addition or substitution of immunosuppressive agents. Foster and associates[49] reported that patients with necrotizing scleritis secondary to rheumatoid arthritis showed no destructive progression when placed on immunosuppressive drugs, whereas those on systemic steroids or NSAIDs demonstrated progression.

Retrobulbar injections of adrenocorticotropic hormone (ACTH) have been attempted, primarily for patients who cannot tolerate systemic steroids.[57] Subconjunctival or sub-Tenon's steroid injections should be avoided, since the involved sclera is thin and easily perforated.[16,18] Such injections can also lead to scleral perforation due to lysis of collagen, and this may be due to the particulate matter in the suspension exacerbating the granulomatous reaction. Thus, it appears that periocular injections have little if any beneficial effect.[94] Watson[2] has reported that the removal of a subconjunctival deposit of steroid resulted in the resolution of a progressive necrotizing scleritis. Recently, however, there has been some success in the treatment of non-necrotizing scleritis with the use of orbital floor injection of 40 mg methylprednisolone acetate.[95] This treatment helps avoid many of the side effects of systemic steroids used for extended periods.

Treatment of scleromalacia perforans consists of topical steroids, such as prednisolone 0.12% 3 times daily, to limit the accompanying anterior uveitis. Active cases require 40 to 80 mg of oral prednisolone daily combined with 200 mg of phenylbutazone. This approach may prevent progression of the destructive process.[15]

Surgery is rarely necessary for scleral defects because of scleral tissue's regenerative capabilities. Grafting is generally reserved for eyes in which there is an imminent danger of perforation. New collagen is produced readily in the base of small scleral defects when there is adequate medical treatment. Large defects, however, may require a scleral graft, which is usually successful when properly covered by conjunctiva. In addition to sclera, other grafting materials have included fascia lata and aortic tissue.[96–98] Unfortunately, the successful graft may become involved in the necrotizing process if the scleral disease is out of control.[99] Scleral grafts do not survive in patients with active vasculitis without systemic immunosuppression.[48]

Since scleritis may be the presenting sign of an underlying systemic disease, the patient must be treated in conjunction with a rheumatologist or internist. The required evaluation can be extensive.

References

1. Yanoff M, Fine FS. Ocular pathology—A text and atlas. Hagerstown, MD:Harper & Row, 1982:383–388.
2. Watson P. Diseases of the sclera and episclera. In: Tasman W, Jaeger E, eds. Duane's Clinical ophthalmology. Philadelphia: JB Lippincott, 1993;4:1–43.
3. McGavin DDM, Williamson J, Forester JV, et al. Episcleritis and scleritis: A study of their clinical manifestations and associations with rheumatoid arthritis. Br J Ophthalmol 1976;60:192–226.
4. Bullen CL, Liesegang TJ, McDonald TJ, et al. Ocular complications of Wegener's granulomatosis. Ophthalmology 1983;90:279–290.
5. Haynes BF, Fishman ML, Fauci AS, et al. The ocular manifestations of Wegener's granulomatosis. Am J Med 1977;63:131–141.
6. Scheie HG, Albert DM. Aldler's textbook of ophthalmology. Philadelphia: WB Saunders Co, 1969:15.
7. Vaughn D, Asbury T. General ophthalmology. Los Altos, CA: Lange, 1977:102–105.
8. Hogan MJ, Zimmerman LE. Ophthalmic pathology. An atlas and textbook. Philadelphia: WB Saunders Co, 1962:337.
9. Flach AJ, Lavoie PE. Episcleritis, conjunctivitis, and keratitis as ocular manifestations of Lyme disease. Ophthalmology 1990;67:973–975.
10. Roy FH. Ocular differential diagnosis. Philadelphia: Lea & Febiger, 1975;2:206–207.
11. Curtis EM. Recurrent episcleritis and emotional stress. Arch Ophthalmol 1984;102:821–824.
12. Scharf J, Meyer E, Zonis S. Episcleritis associated with familial Mediterranean fever. Am J Ophthalmol 1985;100:337–339.
13. Sexton RR. Diseases of the sclera. In: Dunlap ED, ed. Gordon's medical management of ocular disease. Hagerstown, MD: Harper & Row, 1976:171–175.
14. Gold GH. Ocular manifestations of connective tissue disease. In: Duane TD, ed. Clinical ophthalmology. Hagerstown, MD: Harper & Row, 1987;5:1–30.
15. Fraunfelder FT, Roy FH. Current ocular therapy. Philadelphia: WB Saunders Co, 1990:689–693.
16. Ellis PP. Ocular therapeutics and pharmacology. St. Louis: C.V. Mosby Co, 1981:136–138.
17. Sainz de la Maza M, Foster CS. Necrotizing scleritis after ocular surgery. Ophthalmology 1991;98:1720–1726.
18. Watson P, Hayreh SS. Scleritis and episcleritis. Br J Ophthalmol 1976;60:163–191.

19. Lyne AJ, Pitkeathly DA. Episcleritis and scleritis: Association with connective tissue disease. Arch Ophthalmol 1968;80:171–176.

20. Sainz de la Maza M, Jabbur NS, Foster CS. An analysis of therapeutic decision for scleritis. Ophthalmology 1993;100:1372–1376.

21. Reynolds MG, Alfonso E. Treatment of infectious scleritis and keratoscleritis. Am J Ophthalmol 1991;112:543–547.

22. Williamson J. The rheumatic eye. Practitioner 1982;226:863–874.

23. Watson PG, Hazelman BL. The sclera and systemic disorders. London: WB Saunders, 1976:236–246.

24. Morrison JC, Van Buskirk M. Anterior collateral circulation in the primate eye. Ophthalmology 1983;90:707–710.

25. Schuettenberg SP. Nodular scleritis, episcleritis and anterior uveitis as ocular complications of Crohn's disease. J Am Optom Assoc 1991;62:377–381.

26. Wilhelmus KR, Yokoyama CM. Syphilitic episcleritis and scleritis. Am J Ophthalmol 1987;104:595–597.

27. Mohit N, Pflugfelder SC, Holland G. Fulminant pseudomonal keratitis and scleritis in human immunodeficiency virus-infected patients. Arch Ophthalmol 1991;109:503–505.

28. Wirtschafter J. Wegener's granulomatosis presenting sclerokeratitis diagnosed by antineutrophil cytoplasmic autoantibodies (ANCA). Surv Ophthalmol 1993;37:373–376.

29. Soukiasian S, Foster S, Niles JL, Raizman MB. Diagnostic value of antineutrophil cytoplasmic antibodies in scleritis associated with Wegener's granulomatosis. Ophthalmology 1992;99:125–132.

30. Sacks RD, Stock EL, Crawford SE, Greenwald MJ, O'Grady RB. Scleritis and Wegener's granulomatosis in children. Am J Ophthalmol 1991;111:430–433.

31. Sullivan RL, Austin JK, Jones WL. Wegener's granulomatosis: Case report and review. Clin Eye Vision Care 1991;3:114–122.

32. Rahi AHS, Garner A. Immunopathology of the eye. Oxford: Blackwell Scientific, 1976:282.

33. Nomoto Y, Sakai H, Enhdoh M, et al. Scleritis and IgA nephropathy. Arch Intern Med 1980;140:783–785.

34. Fong LP, Sainz de la Maza M, Rice BA, Kupferman AM, Foster CS. Immunopathology of scleritis. Ophthalmology 1991;98:472–479.

35. Jabs DA, Prendergast RA. Autoimmune ocular disease. Invest Ophthalmol Vis Sci 1991;32:2718–2722.

36. Bloomfield SE. Clinical allergy and immunology of the external eye. In: Tasman W, Jaeger E, eds. Duane's Clinical ophthalmology. Philadelphia: J B Lippincott, 1993;4:1–25.

37. Salamon SM, Bartly JM, Zaidman GW. Peripheral corneal ulcers, conjunctival ulcers, and scleritis after cataract surgery. Am J Ophthalmol 1982;93:334–337.

38. Soong HK, Kenyon KR. Adverse reactions to virgin silk sutures in cataract surgery. Ophthalmology 1984;91:479–483.

39. Glasser DB, Bellor J. Necrotizing scleritis of scleral flaps after transscleral suture fixation of an intraocular lens. Am J Ophthalmol 1992;113:529–532.

40. Watson PG, Young RD. Changes at the periphery of a lesion in necrotising scleritis: Anterior segment fluorescein angiography correlated with electron microscopy. Br J Ophthalmol 1985;69:656–660.

41. Watson PG. The nature and treatment of scleral inflammation. Trans Ophthalmol Soc UK 1982;102:257.

42. Watson PG. The diagnosis and management of scleritis. Ophthalmology 1980;87:716–720.

43. Clerey PE, Watson PG, McGill JI, et al. Visual loss due to posterior segment disease in scleritis. Trans Ophthalmol Soc UK 1975;95:297–300.

44. Michels PG. Ocular manifestation in arthritis. In: Ryan SJ Jr, Smith RE, eds. Selected topics on the eye in systemic disease. New York: Grune and Stratton, 1974:365.

45. Yeo JH, Jakobiec F, Iwamoto T, et al. Metastatic carcinoma masquerading as scleritis. Ophthalmology 1983;90:184–194.

46. Tuft SJ, Watson PG. Progression of scleral disease. Ophthalmology 1991;96:467–471.

47. Bidwell AE, Jampol LM, O'Grady R. Scleritis resembling a scleral buckle. Arch Ophthalmol 1993;111:865.

48. Sainz de la Maza M, Tauber J, Foster CS. Scleral grafting for necrotizing scleritis. Ophthalmology 1989;96:306–310.

49. Foster CS, Forstot SL, Wilson LA. Mortality rate in rheumatoid arthritis patients developing necrotizing scleritis or peripheral ulcerative keratitis. Effects of systemic immuno-suppressing. Ophthalmology 1984;91:1253–1263.

50. Meyer P, Watson PG. Low dose fluorescein angiography of the conjunctiva and episclera. Br J Ophthalmol 1987;92:1.

51. Watson PG, Bovey E. Anterior segment fluorescein angiography in the diagnosis of scleral inflammation. Ophthalmology 1985;92:1.

52. Fraunfelder FT, Watson PG. Evaluation of eyes enucleated for scleritis. Br J Ophthalmol 1976;60:227–230.

53. Hurd ER, Snyder WB, Ziff M. Choroidal nodules and retinal detachments in rheumatoid arthritis. Am J Med 1970;48:273–278.

54. Sevel D. Rheumatoid nodule of the sclera. Trans Ophthalmol Soc UK 1965;357–366.

55. Wolter JR, Bentley MD. Scleromalacia perforans and massive granuloma of the sclera. Am J Ophthalmol 1961;51:71–80.

56. Manschot WA. The eye in collagen diseases. Adv Ophthalmol 1961;51:71–80.

57. Benson WE. Posterior scleritis. Surv Ophthalmol 1988;32:297–316.

58. Quilan MP, Hitchings RA. Angle closure glaucoma secondary to posterior scleritis. Br J Ophthalmol 1978;62:330–335.

59. Coleman DJ, Lizzie FL, Jack RL. Ultrasonography of the eye and orbit. Philadelphia: Lea & Febiger, 1977:306.

60. Marushak D. Uveal effusion attending scleritis posterior. A case report with A-scan and B-scan echograms. Acta Ophthalmol 1982;60:773–778.

61. Trokel SL. Computed tomographic scanning of orbital inflammations. Int Ophthalmol Clin 1982;22:81–98.

62. Litwak AB. Posterior scleritis with secondary ciliochoroidal effusion. J Am Optom Assoc 1989;60:300–306.

63. Feldon SE, Segelman J, Albert DM, et al. Clinical manifestations of brawny scleritis. Am J Ophthalmol 1978;85:781–787.

64. Brod RD, Saul RF. Nodular posterior scleritis. Arch Ophthalmol 1990;108:1170–1171.

65. Shields J. Differential diagnosis of posterior uveal melanomas. In: Diagnosis and management of intraocular tumors. St Louis: C.V. Mosby Co, 1983:185.

66. Wilhelmus KR, Grierson I, Watson PG. Histopathologic and clinical associations of scleritis and glaucoma. Am J Ophthalmol 1981;91:697–705.

67. Manshot WA. Progressive scleroperikeratitis. Arch Ophthalmol 1954;52:375–384.

68. Benson WE, Shields JA, Tasman W, et al. Posterior scleritis. A cause of diagnostic confusion. Arch Ophthalmol 1981;91:697–705.

69. Alfonso E, Kenyon KR, Ormerod LD, et al. *Pseudomonas* corneoscleritis. Am J Ophthalmol 1987;103:90–98.

70. Stenson S, Brookenr A, Rosenthal S. Bilateral endogenous necrotizing scleritis due to *Aspergillus oryzase*. Ann Ophthalmol 1982;14:67–72.

71. Callwell DR, Kastle P, Ottman D. A fungal infection as an intrascleral abscess. Ann Ophthalmol 1981;13:841–842.

72. Hemady R, Sainz de la Maza M, Raizman MB, et al. Six cases of scleritis associated with systemic infection. Am J Ophthalmol 1992;114:55–62.

73. Rao NA, Marak GE, Hidayat AA. Necrotizing scleritis. A clinicopathologic study of 41 cases. Ophthalmology 1985;92:1542–1549.

74. Raber IM, Laibson PR, Kruz GH, et al. *Pseudomonas* corneoscleral ulcers. Am J Ophthalmol 1981;92:353–355.

75. Bloomfield SE, Mondino B, Gray GF. Scleral tuberculosis. Arch Ophthalmol 1976;94:954–957.

76. Nanda M, Pflugfelder SC, Holland S. Mycobacterium tuberculosis scleritis. Am J Ophthalmol 1976;108:736–737.

77. Harbin T. Recurrence of a corneal *Pseudomonas* infection. Am J Ophthalmol 1964;58:670–675.

78. Alpren TVP, Hyndiuk RA, Davis SD, et al. Cryotherapy for experimental *Pseudomonas* keratitis. Arch Ophthalmol 1979;97:711–713.

79. Eiferman RA. Cryotherapy of *Pseudomonas* keratitis and scleritis. Arch Ophthalmol 1979;97:1637–1640.

80. Jayson MI, Jones DEP. Scleritis and rheumatoid arthritis. Ann Rheum Dis 1971;30:343–347.

81. Meyer PAR, Watson PG, Frands WK, Dubord P. "Pulse" immunosuppressive therapy in the treatment of immunologically induced corneal and scleral disease. Eye 1987;1:487–495.

82. Tessler H. Uveitis. In: Peyman GA, Sanders DR, Goldberg MF, eds. Principles and practices of ophthalmology. Philadelphia: W.B. Saunders, 1980:1567–1570.

83. McCluskey P, Wakefield D. Intravenous pulse methylprednisolone in scleritis. Arch Ophthalmol 1987;105:793–797.

84. Mondino BJ, Phinney RB. Treatment of scleritis with combined oral prednisone and indomethacin therapy. Am J Ophthalmol 1988;106:473–479.

85. McCarthy JM, Dubord PJ, Chalmers A, et al. Cyclosporine A for the treatment of necrotizing scleritis and corneal melting in patients with rheumatoid arthritis. J Rheumatol 1992;19:1358–1361.

86. Hill JC, Potter P. Treatment of Mooren's ulcer with cyclosporin A: A report of three cases. Br J Ophthalmol 1987;71:11–15.

87. Wakefield D, McKluskey P, Penny R. Intravenous pulse methylprednisolone therapy in severe inflammatory eye disease. Arch Ophthalmol 1986;104:847.

88. Wakefield D, Robinson L. Cyclosporine therapy in Mooren's ulcer. Br J Ophthalmol 1987;71:415–417.

89. Wakefield D, McKluskey P. Cyclosporin therapy for severe scleritis. Br J Ophthalmol 1989;73:743–746.

90. Hakin KN, Lightman SL. Use of cyclosporin in the management of steroid dependent non-necrotising scleritis. Br J Ophthalmol 1991;75:340–341.

91. Foster CS. Immunosuppressive therapy for external ocular inflammatory disease. Ophthalmology 1980;87:140–150.

92. Hemady R, Tauber J, Foster CS. Immunosuppressive drugs in immune and inflammatory ocular disease. Surv Ophthalmol 1991;35:369–385.

93. Keown PA. Emerging indications for the use of cyclosporin in organ transplantation and autoimmunity. Drugs 1990;40:315–325.

94. Jakobiec FA, Jones IS. Orbital inflammations. In: Tasman W, Jaeger E, eds. Duane's Clinical ophthalmology. Philadelphia: J B Lippincott, 1993;2:1–75.

95. Hakin KN, Ham J, Lightman SL. Use of orbital floor steroids in management of patients with uniocular non-necrotising scleritis. Br J Ophthalmol 1991;67:337–339.

96. Bick MW. Surgical treatment of scleromalacia perforans. Arch Ophthalmol 1959;61:907–917.

97. Torchia RT, Dunn RE, Pease PJ. Fascia lata grafting in scleromalacia perforans. Am J Ophthalmol 1959;61:907–917.

98. Merz EH. Scleral reinforcement with aortic tissue. Am J Ophthalmol 1964;57:766–790.

99. Jayson MI, Easty DL. Ulceration of the cornea in rheumatoid arthritis. Ann Rheum Dis 1977;36:428–432.

100. Sainz de la Maza M, Jabbur NS, Foster CS. Severity of scleritis and episcleritis. Ophthalmology 1994;101:389–396.

CHAPTER 30

Uveitis

Murray Fingeret
Felicia A. Fodera

The iris, ciliary body, and choroid compose the uvea, a highly vascularized structure that can be affected by numerous disease processes leading to infection or inflammation. Pharmacologically, a variety of drugs may be used in the treatment of uveal inflammation. This chapter considers how these drugs can be used to modify the natural course of uveitis to prevent serious complications from the disease.

Definition and Classification

Uveitis is usually defined as an inflammation of the iris, ciliary body, or choroid of the eye. The inflammation can be limited to the anterior, intermediate, or posterior structures, and clinical features will depend on the site of involvement. The etiology of many cases of uveitis is often unknown or presumed,[1] and treatment is often nonspecific, aimed at reducing inflammation and preventing ocular complications.

A variety of methods are used to classify uveitis.[2,3] One method is based on the anatomic site of inflammation. For example, uveitis that involves the iris only is termed *iritis*. Another, more contemporary method is to classify the uveal inflammation based on whether it affects the anterior, intermediate, or posterior structures of the eye. A third way is to classify the inflammation as either granulomatous or nongranulomatous. A granulomatous uveal inflammation may present acutely or, more likely, be chronic and insidious in onset. It may involve either the anterior or the posterior uvea, and often presents with a white eye.[4] Such inflammation may be due to an infectious agent, can involve the choroid or the retina, and may produce large, greasy keratic

precipitates that can be observed along with epithelioid cells and macrophages in the anterior chamber. In contrast, a nongranulomatous uveal inflammation usually involves the anterior segment of the eye and has an acute onset accompanied by a cellular reaction in the anterior chamber that represents smaller cell types (lymphocytes) than those in granulomatous inflammation. There is considerable overlap in any clinical classification system, but these classifications provide some opportunity to differentiate various presentations and predict the natural course of the inflammation.

New immunologic developments are on the forefront of a better understanding of the etiology and course of uveitis.[2] In many cases of uveitis, there is limited response to antimicrobial therapy, and the cause of the inflammation is discovered only occasionally.[5] Concepts in immunology, including human leukocyte antigen (HLA) typing, may add much to our knowledge of uveal inflammation. Certain types of uveitis are associated with specific HLAs, indicating that a specific subset of the population might be at greater risk for certain types of uveal inflammation.[6]

Epidemiology

Anterior uveitis is more common than posterior uveitis, accounting for approximately 12 cases per 100,000 population, whereas posterior uveitis accounts for approximately 3 cases per 100,000 population. Thus, anterior uveitis is approximately 4 times as common as posterior uveitis.[7]

The peak prevalence for cases of uveitis is in persons age

20 to 50 years.[8] This age group also parallels the peak activity of T-lymphocytes.

Uveitis may have a sexual predilection depending on the specific condition.[9,10] Reiter's syndrome and ankylosing spondylitis, for example, are more common in males, whereas sarcoid and juvenile rheumatoid arthritis are more common in females. Race can also be a factor. Ocular toxoplasmosis and histoplasmosis are more frequently observed in caucasians, while ocular sarcoidosis occurs more often in blacks. In addition, there may be a geographic predisposition for certain uveal inflammations.[9,10] Ocular histoplasmosis is observed in persons from the midwestern United States, Behçet's disease is more typically observed in persons from Mediterranean countries and Japan, and sarcoid is seen in whites from Scandinavia.

Etiology

At one time an infectious agent was thought to cause most uveitis. Currently, however, uveitis is thought to be an immune-complex disorder with some type of T-cell antigen dysfunction playing a major role. A previous infection may alter the patient's immunologic condition, or a primary immunologic condition can underly the presenting uveitis.[11] HLA studies are being undertaken to identify persons who might be predisposed to recurrent episodes of uveitis or whose uveitis might be associated with specific immunologic conditions. HLA systems are the antigenic complexes involved with histocompatibility, including graft rejection. Of the four groups of HLA antigens (A, B, C, and D), types A and B are observed most frequently.[11] They are present on the surface membranes of leukocytes and are regulated by the gene loci on chromosome 6. The HLA system is a genetic marker for cell surface antigens and can be used to identify the subgroup that may be at risk for a certain condition. Certain HLA phenotypes are at a greater risk for specific inflammatory conditions.

About 35% of patients with ankylosing spondylitis will have uveitis at some point in the natural course of the disease.[2] Of patients with ankylosing spondylitis, about 90% will have HLA-B27.[12,13] HLA-B27 has also been found in Reiter's syndrome and persons with acute anterior uveitis of unknown etiology.[5] HLA-B27 has been observed in 50% to 70% of patients with acute anterior uveitis compared with a control group manifesting 4% to 8% HLA-B27.[12] However, an individual with HLA-B27 has only a 1% chance of developing uveitis, which suggests that other factors exist in the etiology of uveal inflammation.[5] Such risk factors remain unknown. An individual may not have an HLA-B27 marker and incur ankylosing spondylitis, but the chance of acquiring uveitis is only 7%, compared with 35% if the gene is present.[5]

Diagnosis

The symptoms and signs of uveitis depend on the anatomic site of inflammation. Acute anterior uveitis is usually characterized by a painful, often photophobic, red eye. The redness, known as ciliary flush, occurs in a circumcorneal fashion. The pupil may be miotic, the intraocular pressure may be reduced, and there can be slit-lamp findings of posterior synechiae (Fig. 30.1) or of keratic precipitates on the corneal endothelium (Fig. 30.2). Such keratic precipitates can vary in size and appearance from small and pinpoint to large and waxy.

The hallmark anterior segment reaction that is virtually pathognomonic of anterior uveitis is the appearance of cells and flare in the anterior chamber (Fig. 30.3). Cells appear as small individual white particles floating in the anterior chamber. They represent the passage of lymphocytes through the dilated spaces of the iris blood vessels into the anterior chamber, as the blood-aqueous barrier has broken down. Flare represents transudation of protein into the aqueous and appears as a haziness or milkiness in the anterior chamber. Cells and flare are best detected by using the biomicroscope and carefully observing the aqueous in the anterior chamber using the dilated pupil as the background. This procedure works best when performed in a dark room, after allowing time for the examiner to dark-adapt. A bright, short optic section under moderate to high magnification (10X– 20X) is oscillated back and forth and up and down in the anterior chamber while searching for the cells and flare to come into focus. A typical grading system for cells and

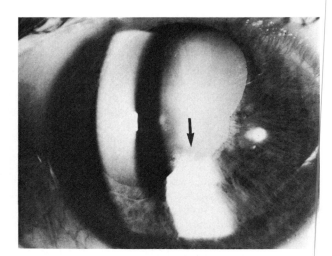

FIGURE 30.1   **Posterior synechia (arrow) associated with anterior uveitis. (Courtesy Scott Richter, O.D.)**

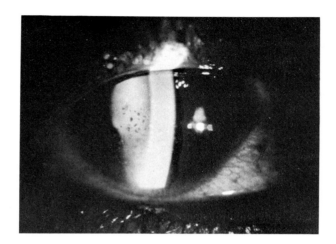 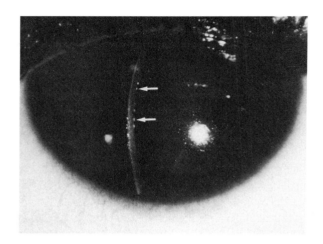

A   B

FIGURE 30.2   **Large keratic precipitates associated with anterior uveitis.** *(A)* **As seen with wide slit-lamp beam.** *(B)* **Viewed with thin optic section. (Courtesy Scott Richter, O.D.)**

flare is shown in Table 30.1. Laser flare-cell photometry is now available to quantify the anterior chamber reaction. This procedure, however, is used primarily for research purposes.[60]

Patients with anterior uveitis often present with symptoms of ocular pain, photophobia, and blurred vision. Pain is usually acute in onset, isolated deep in the eye, and dull or pulsating. Photophobia is a constant symptom in many cases and may present as the first sign of the condition. Photophobia can be reduced with cycloplegia, which places the iris and ciliary body muscles at rest. Blurred vision results from lacrimation or the accumulation of cells and flare in the anterior chamber.

Cases of anterior uveitis that are bilateral, recurrent, refractory to treatment, or occuring in a child necessitate a more extensive diagnostic evaluation. Such anterior uveitis often results from an endogenous condition, with the more common etiologies including tuberculosis, syphilis, arthritic and rheumatologic conditions, herpetic disease, and sarcoidosis.

Posterior uveitis is characterized by a white eye with little or no pain. Although there may be some cell and flare reaction in the anterior chamber, if present it is most remarkable in the vitreous. Histoplasmosis is an example of a posterior uveitis without cells or flare. Blurred vision is present if the macula is involved or if the vitreous is sufficiently hazy to diminish vision. In addition, there may be flare in the posterior chamber, which can be noted with a conical beam or optic section from the slit lamp. When viewed with the binocular indirect ophthalmoscope, flare in the posterior chamber can appear as a green-tinted haze.

The most frequently encountered cases of posterior uveitis are from endogenous causes that include toxoplasmosis, histoplasmosis, and toxocariasis.[13] The immune system may be altered by the suspected endogenous cause, or it may respond to an underlying systemic disease that predisposes the person to other immunologic diseases.[14] Only occasion-

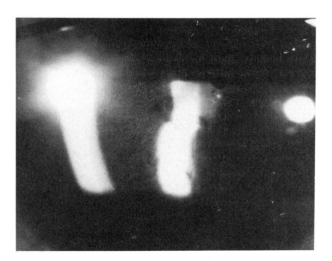

FIGURE 30.3   **Anterior chamber cells and flare associated with anterior uveitis.**

TABLE 30.1
Grading Scale for Anterior Chamber Cells and Flare

Anterior Chamber Sign	Grade				
	Trace	*+*	*++*	*+++*	*++++*
Cells	1–3 cells noted in beam	4–8 cells	9–15 cells	Too many cells to count	Appearance of snowstorm
Flare	None to questionable	Faint haze just detectable	Moderate haze; iris detail clear	Marked haze; iris detail fuzzy	Plastic iritis; fibrin clot

ally can an infectious agent be identified in the ocular tissues. Instead, the uveitis may represent the immunologic focus of an endogenous condition. Many of the endogenous causes can be identified or suspected based on laboratory testing.

Selecting and Interpreting Laboratory Tests

Determining the etiology for a particular case of uveitis requires a systematic approach, using laboratory testing along with ocular examination, history, and medical examination to help corroborate a suspected clinical disease (Table 30.2). Laboratory testing should be tailored for each individual case rather than ordering the same battery of tests for every patient.[15] The examination process begins with a thorough history and ocular examination, which can provide initial direction for specific laboratory testing.[16] The history should include questions about the present attack, such as the nature of the symptoms and onset (acute vs. insidious). The patient should be questioned about past episodes, including their duration and treatment. Ocular, medical, and social histories must be reviewed. Family ocular, medical, and geographic histories also need to be pursued. Finally, a review of systems is needed that should include a survey of dermatologic, rheumatologic, respiratory, gastrointestinal, genitourinary, and neurologic systems (Table 30.3). A medical examination in selected cases may also be useful in investigating specific etiologies.

Laboratory testing is required in cases of bilateral or recurrent uveitis, atraumatic pediatric uveitis, granulomatous anterior uveitis, episodes unresponsive to treatment, or nonspecific cases of posterior uveitis.[17] Laboratory evaluation is not required for traumatic uveitis, one-time, uncomplicated adult cases, or cases of uveitis with a definite clinical diagnosis such as Fuchs' heterochromic iridocyclitis or lens-induced uveitis.[18] Approximately half the patients with anterior uveitis have an associated systemic component.[15]

Serologic laboratory tests may be part of the battery used to confirm the diagnosis of a particular disease. These tests identify specific antibodies that are found in the patient's blood, indicating previous exposure to the antigen associated with a specific disease. The serum is diluted progressively with an innocuous solution, to as low as one part serum to more than one thousand parts of diluent (e.g., 1:1064). The result is described as a titer, with the highest titer representing the weakest solution in which antibodies

TABLE 30.2
Laboratory Tests in the Etiologic Diagnosis of Uveitis

Suspected Etiology	Laboratory Test
Ankylosing spondylitis	Sacroiliac joint x-ray film HLA testing
Histoplasmosis	Chest x-ray film
Tuberculosis	Purified protein derivative (PPD) skin test Chest x-ray film
Sarcoidosis	Serum angiotensin converting enzyme (ACE) Serum lysozyme Limited gallium scan Biopsy of suspected lesion (skin, conjunctiva, lacrimal gland) Chest x-ray film
Syphilis	Fluorescent treponemal antibody absorption (FTA-ABS) test Venereal Disease Research Laboratory (VDRL) test
Rheumatoid conditions	Rheumatoid factor Sedimentation rate HLA testing
Toxocara	Enzyme-linked immunosorbent assay (ELISA)
Toxoplasmosis	Fluorescent antibody test ELISA test
Juvenile rheumatoid arthritis	Antinuclear antibody (ANA) Sedimentation rate
Reiter's syndrome	HLA testing Sacroiliac joint x-ray film
Behçet's disease	HLA testing

TABLE 30.3
Characteristics of Uveitic Syndromes

Associated Systemic Disease	Etiology	Age (yr), Race, Sex	Signs, Symptoms	Laboratory Tests	Systemic Disease Treatment	Sequelae
Ankylosing Spondylitis	Unknown	20–30, white, male	Lower back pain, limited movement of lower back, late stage cardiac failure and pulmonary fibrosis	Sacroiliac joint x-ray (men), shoulder x-ray (women) HLA-B27	Steroids, NSAIDs, physical therapy, rheumatology consult	Cardiac and pulmonary complications, limited movement of lower back
Reiter's Syndrome	Unknown	20–30, white, male	Arthritis, conjunctivitis, urethritis	HLA-B27, S-I x-ray, ESR	Steroids, oral antibiotics, NSAIDs	Arthritis
Inflammatory Bowel Disease	Unknown	15–30, M = F	Abdominal pain, bloody diarrhea, fever, arthritis	G-I series, joint x-ray, HLA-B27	Diet, steroids	G-I
Syphilis	Treponema pallidum	Any age, M = F	Chancre (primary), flu (secondary), cardiac, neuro (tertiary)	FTA-ABS, VDRL, MHA-TP	Penicillin	Tertiary stage
Lyme Disease	Borrelia burgdorferi	Any age, M = F	Rash, flu (primary), arthritis, cardiac (secondary), neurologic (tertiary)	ELISA, joint x-ray	Systemic antibiotics	Systemic problems in tertiary stage
Sarcoidosis	Unknown	20–40, black, female	Pulmonary, skin lesions, arthritis, CNS, liver, spleen	Chest x-ray, ACE, biopsy, gallium scan	Steroids	May affect any organ system, with devastating results
Tuberculosis	Tubercle bacilli	35–44, M = F	Weight loss, fever, cough	PPD, chest x-ray	INH	Pulmonary
Behçet's Disease	Unknown immune disorder	15–40, Eastern European, Mediterranean male	Oral, genital, or skin ulcers	HLA-B5	Cytotoxic medications	Rheumatology consult
Juvenile Rheumatoid Arthritis	Unknown	age < 15, F > M (early onset), M > F (late onset)	Arthritis of medium to large joints	ANA (+), ESR, joint x-rays, RF (–), HLA-B27	Steroids, NSAIDs	Rheumatology consult

are found.[19] A titer over 1:64 may be needed to confirm the presence of active disease.[19]

For cases in which the history and examination do not reduce the list of suspected clinical entities, a chest x-ray and FTA-ABS (fluorescent treponemal antibody-absorption test) often are useful. These results will confirm or rule out sarcoidosis or syphilis, respectively, two diseases that can be asymptomatic aside from their ocular manifestations. The presence of bilateral hilar adenopathy, seen on chest x-ray, without any other symptoms, is diagnostic of sarcoidosis. It is important to order a chest x-ray at the onset of ocular inflammation because the hilar adenopathy may resolve eventually despite persistent ocular inflammation.[16] An elevated angiotensin-converting enzyme (ACE), a positive gallium scan, and a positive biopsy of the lacrimal gland or a conjunctival granuloma will help to confirm the diagnosis of sarcoidosis. The FTA-ABS test or MHA-TP (microhemagglutination) test have very high levels of sensitivity and specificity and should be the test of first choice in ruling out syphilis. The VDRL (Venereal Disease Research Laboratory) and the RPR (rapid plasma reagin) screening tests are less sensitive tests for syphilis.[20] Combinations of these tests can be ordered to determine the state of syphilitic activity:

(−)FTA-ABS with (+)VDRL → False Positive

(+)FTA-ABS with (−)VDRL → Inactive Disease, Past Exposure

(+)FTA-ABS with (+)VDRL → Active Disease

A purified protein derivative (PPD) test is used to rule out tuberculosis, but its limited specificity and uncertain sensitivity reduces its role as a routine screening test. The high false-positive rate associated with the PPD suggests that its role be limited to confirming the diagnosis of tuberculosis. The CBC (complete blood count) with differential provides diagnostic information for hemoglobinopathies, bacterial and viral infections, and some rheumatologic disorders.[21] An ESR (erythrocyte sedimentation rate) can be elevated in a number of different situations including infection, inflammation, malignancy, rheumatoid disease, pregnancy, obesity, and tissue necrosis. Due to its nonspecific nature, an ESR should not be used for routine screening evaluation. It is helpful in monitoring therapeutic efficacy and disease activity as well as in the differential diagnosis of temporal arteritis.

The ANA (antinuclear antibody) titer, an invaluable test for establishing the diagnosis of systemic lupus erythematosus (SLE), is another test with a high false-positive rate. Therefore, it should be reserved for patients with uveitis and other signs of SLE such as rash, arthritis, nephritis, or pleuropericarditis. It is also helpful in the diagnosis of juvenile rheumatoid arthritis (JRA), a condition more commonly associated with uveitis than is SLE.

Rheumatoid factor (RF) testing is not helpful in the screening of uveitis patients for systemic disease. Patients with JRA, the form of rheumatoid arthritis most commonly associated with uveitis, will have a negative RF. HLA-B27 typing will be positive in up to 70% of patients with acute, unilateral, anterior uveitis. These patients have a high likelihood of ankylosing spondylitis.[22,23] The prevalence of Lyme disease and associated uveitis varies geographically. Current Lyme serologic testing has a high false-positive rate and should be reserved for uveitic patients with other symptoms or signs of Lyme disease, such as arthritis, rash, carditis, or neurologic disease.

Management

Anterior Uveitis

The objectives in the treatment of anterior uveitis are to: (1) reduce the severity of the attack(s) or exacerbations, (2) prevent posterior synechiae, (3) prevent damage to the iris blood vessels and blood-aqueous barrier, (4) reduce the frequency of attacks, (5) prevent the development of secondary cataracts, and (6) prevent phthisis bulbi.

Posterior synechiae can often be prevented with use of cycloplegics. Cycloplegia places the ciliary body and iris at rest and reduces many of the associated symptoms. Table 30.4 lists the spectrum of drugs that can be used for therapeutic cycloplegia. At one end of the spectrum is tropicamide 1%, which has a cycloplegic effect lasting up to 6 hours. Cyclopentolate 1% is a more effective cycloplegic and is useful when administered 2 or 3 times daily in mild to moderate cases of anterior uveitis. Homatropine 5% is an intermediate-strength cycloplegic usually employed 3 to 4 times daily or, in more severe cases, up to every 2 hours. Atropine 1% is the strongest cycloplegic. Although atropine cycloplegia can last up to 2 weeks in a healthy eye, the drug must be instilled twice daily to induce cycloplegia in the inflamed eye. If atropine is contraindicated because of hypersensitivity, scopolamine 0.25%, another strong cycloplegic, can be used. Patients with uveitis with an excessive protein (flare) component are at great risk for posterior synechiae and must be managed aggressively with cyclople-

TABLE 30.4
Drugs for Therapeutic Cycloplegia

Drug	Indication
Tropicamide 1%	Mild to moderate anterior uveitis
Homatropine 2%	
Cyclopentolate 1%	
Homatropine 5%	Moderate anterior uveitis
Atropine 1%	Moderate to severe anterior uveitis
Scopolamine 0.25%	

gics. The cycloplegia should be reduced as the inflammation begins to subside.

It is helpful to use a cycloplegic that will provide some iris movement, keeping the pupil somewhat mobile.[24] This will prevent posterior synechiae. A drug that will keep the pupil dilated and fixed in an 8 mm state may promote synechia formation just as a fixed 3 mm pupil would. Because of this, atropine is often avoided in favor of homatropine 5%, which will permit some movement of the pupil. In cases of suspected noncompliance, however, it is better to use a longer-acting cycloplegic such as atropine. When in doubt, it is better to use a stronger rather than weaker cycloplegic.

It is necessary to measure the intraocular pressure in uveitis. Inflammation of the ciliary body often reduces aqueous production, and intraocular pressure will be low. An increased intraocular pressure may be measured if the trabeculum becomes inflamed and does not allow the aqueous to filter properly, or if inflammatory cells block the meshwork. In addition, a high intraocular pressure may occur if there is formation of posterior synechiae with iris bombé, or if anterior synechiae form and block aqueous outflow. The treatment of uveitic glaucoma is discussed in Chapter 35.

Steroid therapy can be delivered to the eye by several routes. Topical steroid administration is the most common method for treatment of anterior uveitis. In more severe cases, however, periocular injections or oral steroids may be indicated. For posterior uveitis, topical steroids have little effect, and periocular and oral steroids are the methods of choice.

Historically, the most effective steroid administered topically has been 1% prednisolone acetate, because it can effectively penetrate the intact epithelium of the cornea to gain access to the anterior chamber (Table 30.5).[25] Since they are suspensions, prednisolone acetate preparations should be shaken vigorously to resuspend the steroid particles before the medication is instilled. Other steroids, such as rimexolone and loteprednol, may also have anti-inflammatory effects comparable to prednisolone acetate. Dosage frequency may be as often as hourly for severe inflammations, and every 2 to 3 hours for moderate involvements. Use of weaker preparations or less frequent instillation will depend on the severity of the inflammation. Frequently administered, high-concentration steroids should be tapered to prevent a rebound phenomenon. The tapering is done over 1 to 2 weeks to try to preserve the remission. Patients should be monitored at 1- to 2-week intervals during the active phase of the uveitis until all signs of inflammation have disappeared.

Any uveal inflammation must be managed aggressively to minimize damage to the iris blood vessels and the blood-aqueous barrier, which, if affected, can allow an acute presentation to become chronic and difficult to manage. Once the active inflammation has subsided, the steroid dosage should be tapered to preserve the remission. If the patient has been receiving the steroid more than 4 times daily, the medication should be reduced to 4 times daily for 4 days, 3 times daily for 3 days, 2 times daily for 2 days, once for 1 day, and then discontinued. Further modification may be needed depending on circumstances, since too sudden withdrawal can reactivate the uveitis.

Occasionally, a case of chronic anterior uveitis requires continual low-dose topical steroids to maintain the quiet eye. The risks of once to twice daily topical steroid used indefinitely must be weighed against the potential damage due to further exacerbations of the uveitis.

Many side effects of systemic steroid use can be avoided by using periocular injections. In particular, periocular steroids are useful in the treatment of posterior uveitis. They can be administered by injection in the anterior subconjunctiva, posterior sub-Tenon's capsule, or in a retrobulbar fashion. Periocular steroids can be injected so that they are placed close to the site of inflammation.

Oral steroids may reach all parts of the body with reduced concentration in the eye. They are administered easily but can lead to significant systemic side effects. An alternate-day dosage can be used when the condition is stabilized because the anti-inflammatory effect is comparable to daily dosage, and the depressive effects on immunity and the adrenal glands are much less intense.[24]

Pulse dosages of intravenous methylprednisolone have been shown to be effective for severe or recalcitrant forms of uveitis while minimizing the side effects associated with more conventional routes of steroid administration.[26]

TABLE 30.5
Anti-Inflammatory Effectiveness of Topical Steroids with Intact Corneal Epithelium

Minimal Effectiveness	Moderate Effectiveness	Maximal Effectiveness
Dexamethasone sodium phosphate 0.05% (ointment)	Prednisolone sodium phosphate 1.0%	Dexamethasone alcohol 0.1%
		Fluorometholone acetate 0.1%
		Rimexolone 1.0%
Dexamethasone sodium phosphate 0.1%	Fluorometholone alcohol 0.1%	Prednisolone acetate 1.0%

Modified from Leibowitz HM, Kupferman A. Anti-inflammatory medications. Int Ophthalmol Clin 1980;20:117–134.

Oral nonsteroidal anti-inflammatory drugs (NSAIDs) (e.g., indomethacin, aspirin, ibuprofen) have held great promise but up to now have been a clinical disappointment. They do not appear to be potent enough for use during an attack of uveitis. Flurbiprofen (Ocufen), a topical NSAID, is used to prevent miosis due to the release of prostaglandins during cataract surgery. Flurbiprofen inhibits the synthesis of prostaglandins, decreasing miosis and presumably the inflammatory component mediated by prostaglandins (see Chap. 12). If topical NSAIDs can be shown to decrease inflammation associated with endogenous uveitis, their potential is great, since they do not elevate intraocular pressure or cause cataracts, side effects associated with steroid use.

Immunosuppressive therapy can be used in severe cases where steroids may not be effective and the eye is worsening. Chlorambucil, for example, has been effective in Behçet's disease and other types of uveitis, including juvenile rheumatoid arthritis and sympathetic ophthalmia.[24] However, immunosuppressive agents have many serious side effects and require immunologic consultation (see Chap. 12).[27]

Cyclosporine is a second-generation immunosuppressive drug that attempts to modify the immune response without destroying cells from the immune system. An 11-amino acid cyclic peptide, it has been used extensively in the field of organ transplantation with dramatic results.[28] However, at the dosage levels used to prevent organ rejection, nephrotoxicity almost always occurs. This is acceptable for the liver or heart patient near death but is unacceptable for patients with uveitis. The dosage levels of cyclosporine have been reduced by using it with other medications such as systemic steroids or bromocriptine.[28]

Patients receiving cyclosporine have chronic autoimmune conditions and will require treatment for a long time, further increasing the risk of side effects. Thus, cyclosporine is now viewed as a second-line medication for Behçet's disease and other sight-threatening uveitic conditions not responding to topical, periocular, or systemic steroids.

Posterior Uveitis

Management of the patient with posterior uveitis is quite different from management of a patient with anterior uveitis. The objectives of treating and managing posterior uveitis include: (1) protecting the macula, (2) protecting the optic nerve, (3) protecting the vitreous, (4) preventing loss of ciliary body or retinal function, and (5) preventing cataract formation.

Uveitis posterior to the iris and lens has little chance of creating posterior synechiae, so cycloplegia is not necessary. Because of the posterior inflammatory site, topical steroids are not effective in therapeutic doses, and systemic or periocular administration is necessary. Systemic and periocular steroids have greater risks and must be used carefully. It is important that steroid-treated uveitis, if of an infectious origin, be covered concurrently with the appropriate antimicrobial agent(s). Periocular steroids should not be used in an infectious condition because of the risks of reactivation to an uncontrollable level. If periocular steroids are used, a sub-Tenon's injection of a repository form may be given up to every 2 weeks. Systemic steroids are usually started with a full dose divided into 4 parts per 24 hours. When the condition stabilizes, the medication can be given every other morning to reduce the amount of immune system suppression. If used for less than 2 weeks, the dose of systemic steroid may be reduced quickly, but in most cases a slower withdrawal of steroid will preserve the remission.

Each encounter with uveitis, either anterior or posterior, must be considered individually. The decision to treat with cycloplegics, steroids, or immunosuppressive agents should be made carefully. Patients with uveitis that is bilateral, recurrent, or refractory to treatment should undergo more extensive evaluation for underlying systemic disease.

Specific Uveitic Syndromes

Trauma

Trauma to the eye can result in anterior uveitis. Contusion injury can create a mild to severe inflammation, with moderate cases requiring only cycloplegia for a short time. Severe inflammation will require more aggressive therapy, including the use of topical steroids. In addition to uveitis, trauma may cause other ocular problems, including perforating injury, angle recession glaucoma, and retinal breaks with or without retinal detachment.

A traumatic corneal abrasion can cause anterior uveitis from vasodilation and increased permeability of the iris blood vessels in response to the primary insult. As the corneal abrasion resolves with treatment that might include antibiotics and patching, the uveitis also will resolve. Some patients may require cycloplegia to reduce ocular pain associated with the anterior segment inflammation.

Trauma can lead to bleeding in the anterior chamber—a few red blood cells to frank hemorrhage. Such hemorrhage, or hyphema, usually fills less than one-third of the anterior chamber[29] (Fig. 30.4). So-called microscopic hyphemas may be observable only with the slit lamp and consist of a few red blood cells in the anterior chamber. This may be difficult to differentiate from the cells seen in anterior uveitis, but use of the green filter may enable differentiation. Red cells will not be apparent with the green filter, but the white cells of uveitis can be observed.

The clinician should also investigate for associated conditions, including blow-out fractures of the orbit, corneal edema, subluxated lens, retinal breaks, or retinal detachment. Gonioscopy, to rule out the possibility of angle reces-

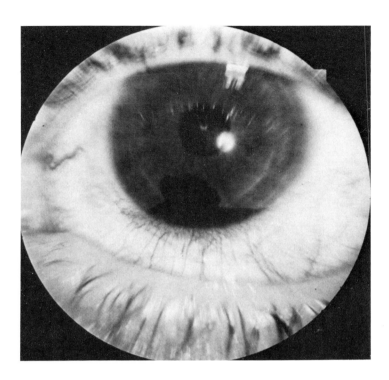

FIGURE 30.4 **Traumatic hyphema filling less than one-third of anterior chamber.**

sion, should be delayed until the hyphema has cleared enough to permit adequate visualization of ocular structures without reinjury to any tissue.

The majority of hyphemas last about 5 days, and from 2% to 38% rebleed. This 5-day period represents the period of greatest risk for a rebleed.[29] If no rebleed has occurred after 5 days, the chances of rebleed decrease significantly. Conversely, with each episode of rebleed, the chances of good visual recovery diminish.

The initial height of the hyphema tends to correlate with the chance for rebleeding. A significantly higher rate of secondary hemorrhage is found among patients with larger initial hyphemas, but the severity of the injury cannot be determined from the height of the hyphema at initial presentation.

Treatment of hyphema is controversial. Miotics have been used to increase the area of absorption on the iris. However, because most of the resorption of hyphema probably takes place in the angle rather than in the iris, cycloplegics and mydriatics are now advocated.[30] Cycloplegics may improve comfort associated with anterior uveitis, and mydriatics may reduce the likelihood of secondary synechiae. Some authors, however, contend that any manipulation of the iris, even with medication, increases the potential for rebleed.[29] Topical steroid therapy may be implemented in protracted cases,[29] and topical β blockers or carbonic anhydrase inhibitors can be used in cases where the intraocular pressure is elevated.

Oral antifibrinolytic agents have been advocated for use in the medical management of hyphemas.[30–32] Aminocaproic acid (Amicar) has lowered the rate of rebleeding from approximately 30% to 3%.[33] The full dose is 100 mg/kg body weight every 4 hours, up to a maximal dose of 30 g daily. The drug is expensive and causes numerous side effects including dizziness, hypotension, syncope, nausea, and vomiting. In one study[33] the dose was reduced by half while maintaining the impressive low rate of rebleeding and causing fewer side effects, except for nausea and vomiting.

Aminocaproic acid has been shown to be ineffective for traumatic hyphemas in children,[34] but another antifibrinolytic agent, tranexamic acid (Cyklokapron), has been shown to reduce the incidence of secondary hemorrhage significantly in the pediatric population. Because of the cost of therapy and its side effects and medicolegal issues regarding the labelling of tranexamic acid,[61] some investigators question the value of systemic treatment with antifibrinolytic agents.

There is general agreement that patients with hyphema should be at rest, but there is controversy over the methods to be implemented. Some practitioners place patients in the hospital with complete bedrest, bilateral patches, and sedation. Evidence, however, suggests that there is no difference in prognosis if the patient is not hospitalized.[35] As a general rule, any child with hyphema or an adult with a rebleed should be hospitalized. If the patient is not hospitalized, the eye should be protected with a shield at bedtime, and the patient should have periodic bedrest with the head elevated at a 30° to 45° angle.[29] The angle of the head helps settle the hyphema in the inferior anterior chamber angle.

Cataract Surgery

Immediately following cataract extraction, with or without the implantation of an intraocular lens, prophylactic antibiotic and steroid eyedrops are used. Antibiotics are generally discontinued within the first 3 weeks, and steroids are used for 3 to 6 weeks. Antibiotics are usually discontinued abruptly, whereas topical steroids must be tapered gradually. In general, 1 fewer daily drop is used each week once tapering of topical steroids has begun. As an example, during weeks 1 through 3 the steroid dosage frequency might be 4 times daily, and during week 4 it would be 3 times daily. Then, during week 5 the frequency would be twice daily, and for week 6 it would be 1 drop daily. During the first 3 weeks the cells and flare should diminish, and by the sixth week no anterior chamber reaction should be observed. Postoperative management of the cataract patient is discussed in detail in Chapter 31.

Retinal Tears

A patient presenting with anterior uveitis, especially one resistant to treatment, requires a careful dilated fundus examination with the binocular indirect ophthalmoscope. Small, peripheral, hitherto asymptomatic retinal tears, with or without accompanying retinal detachment, may be the causative agent. Repair of the retinal disorder usually causes the anterior uveitis to resolve.

Arthritis

Although the relationship is not fully understood, uveitis and arthritis are related. Uveitis occurs more frequently in patients with arthritis than in the general population.[36] An immunologic basis has been implicated, and data from HLA testing have substantiated such a relationship.[36]

In children, especially girls, a higher prevalence of anterior uveitis is associated with juvenile rheumatoid arthritis.[37] Children affected with uveitis have limited debilitation from the systemic condition. In juvenile rheumatoid arthritis, the onset of uveitis is insidious, and affected children may have cells, flare, and synechiae without ocular symptoms. Because the eye may not be injected and there may be no symptoms, the uveitis, which is generally bilateral, may be an elusive diagnosis. Such uveitis is typically chronic, with the child developing a secondary cataract or band keratopathy before the diagnosis is established.[38] In fact, loss of vision from either band keratopathy or secondary cataract

may be the reason for the child's eye examination. The treatment for uveitis in children with rheumatoid arthritis requires cycloplegia and careful use of topical or systemic steroids. Because steroids do not always control the inflammation adequately, immunosuppressive drugs may be required in some cases.[39]

Ankylosing spondylitis (Marie-Strümpell disease) is a chronic form of arthritis involving the sacroiliac joint, spine, and soft surrounding tissue (Fig. 30.5). The condition is found most frequently in young men as an acute anterior, episodic, nongranulomatous inflammation. It is uncommon for this nongranulomatous anterior segment inflammation to become chronic, and the patient may have the uveitis many years before having back pain. About one-third of patients will have anterior uveitis at some point in the course of this systemic disease.[11]

Adult males who have recurrent episodes of bilateral, acute nongranulomatous anterior uveitis should have x-ray studies of the sacroiliac joints. HLA-B27 has been observed

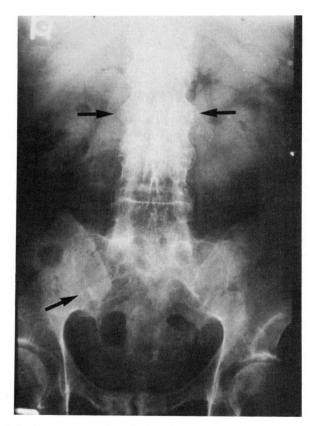

FIGURE 30.5   **X-ray film of spine of patient with ankylosing spondylitis. The sacroiliac joint margin (lower arrow) is blurred and poorly defined. This anteroposterior view also reveals the appearance of a bamboo spine (upper arrows), diagnostic of ankylosing spondylitis.**

in 80% to 90% of patients with anterior uveitis in ankylosing spondylitis.[6] Treatment, as in other forms of nongranulomatous anterior uveitis, is aimed at decreasing inflammation and preventing complications. Topical steroids and cycloplegics can be used to accomplish these therapeutic goals.

Inflammatory Bowel Disease (Crohn's Disease and Ulcerative Colitis)

Patients with manifest ulcerative colitis have an increased frequency of acute, bilateral, nongranulomatous anterior uveitis—0.5% to 12% level.[11] This anterior uveitis occurs between the second and fourth decades of life. In patients with both ulcerative colitis and sacroiliitis, the frequency of anterior uveitis is about 50%.[11,40] Although topical and systemic steroids have been the mainstay of therapy for the anterior uveitis, Soukiasian and associates[62] have found that most patients with HLA-B27-positive anterior uveitis are refractory to steroid therapy. These patients often respond favorable to systemic immunosuppressive therapy.

Reiter's Syndrome

Reiter's syndrome is a triad of nongonococcal urethritis, polyarthritis, and acute conjunctivitis. It has been observed most often in young men, with 8% to 40% having an acute anterior uveitis. The arthritis is usually oligoarticular and asymmetric, affecting the large, weight-bearing joints of the lower extremities. Inflammation of the axial skeleton presenting as a sacroiliitis may be seen. The etiology of Reiter's syndrome is obscure, but an infectious cause has been suggested. A history of dysenteric or venereal disease can often be elicited.[9] The conjunctivitis is often bilateral and mucopurulent and may be accompanied by keratoderma blennorrhagica and a circinate balanitis. In addition, HLA-B27 is seen in 63% to 96% of patients with Reiter's syndrome compared with 4% to 8% in a control population.[6] Systemic antibiotics can be used to treat the urethritis, felt to be due to *Chlamydia trachomatis, Ureaplasma urealyticum, Salmonella, Shigella,* or *Yersinia.* Unfortunately, exposure to any of these organisms, even when treated successfully, triggers changes in the immune system leading to anterior uveitis.[2] For the anterior uveitis, topical steroids and cycloplegics are indicated to limit the inflammation.

Behçet's Disease

Behçet's disease is a condition consisting of major findings that include nongranulomatous, bilateral, hypopyon uveitis; aphthous ulcers of the tongue and mouth; genital ulcers; and nonulcerative skin lesions. Minor findings include arthritis, thrombophlebitis, cardiovascular disease, gastrointestinal disease, and central nervous system (CNS) disorders. The ocular components account for a great deal of the morbidity, but the so-called minor findings can be extremely serious. A vasculitis appears to be the underlying pathology.

Behçet's disease occurs in persons of Mediterranean and Japanese ancestry.[9,41] The etiology is unknown, but some evidence suggests a viral, immunologic, and hereditary condition. HLA-B51 has been demonstrated in several ethnic groups with the disease.[42] Ocular lesions occur in 75% of cases.[43] Complications include occlusive retinal vasculitis, cataract formation, and glaucoma. Almost half the cases with retinal involvement will lead to blindness in 4 to 8 years if untreated.[43] Steroids have not proved effective, but the use of immunosuppressive agents, such as chlorambucil or cyclosporine, for at least 1 year after the inflammation has subsided, may reduce the morbidity in most cases.[9]

Cyclosporine, because of reduced toxicity, has become the immunosuppressive agent of choice for patients with Behçet's disease with ocular or CNS involvement.[28] Topical and systemic steroids are often used concurrently, with cyclosporine, and such combination therapy may be less toxic than treatment with cyclosporine alone.[63]

Sarcoidosis

Sarcoid disease is a granulomatous condition of unknown etiology. It can affect any organ, and 25% to 50% of patients with the condition will have ocular problems, usually uveitis.[11] Sarcoid disease occurs more often in females[11] and is more common among black Americans than in black Africans. It also occurs in white Scandinavians.

The most frequent ocular presentation of sarcoid disease is an acute, granulomatous anterior uveitis. With chronic sarcoidosis, mutton-fat keratic precipitates, synechiae, and cataracts may form. A retinochoroiditis may develop with retinal lesions characterized by "candle-wax drippings" beginning in the peripheral retina around the equator. In addition, a vitritis may be present, and retinal periphlebitis can occur, leading to macular edema.

The primary method to establish the diagnosis of sarcoid disease is the chest x-ray film. The classic picture is one of bilateral hilar adenopathy (Fig. 30.6). When findings are questionable, a conjunctival biopsy may prove useful. Even if there is no ocular disease, a conjunctival biopsy will be positive in about one-third of patients with sarcoid disease.[11] If the x-ray studies and conjunctival biopsy are equivocal, a biopsy of the liver or mediastinum can be performed. Noninvasive tests useful in determining the diagnosis include angiotensin-I-converting enzyme (ACE), gallium scan, and serum lysozyme levels.[9,44,45]

Topical and periocular steroids along with cycloplegics remain the therapy of choice for the anterior uveitis, but many patients require the long-term use of systemic steroids to control the inflammation. Because uveitis in sarcoid disease is chronic, drug therapy for each patient must be individualized.

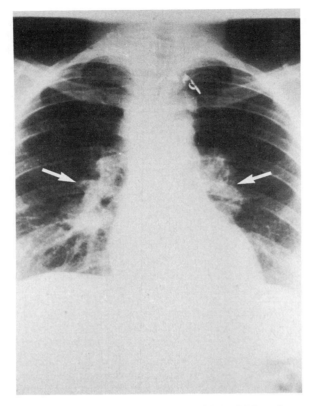

FIGURE 30.6 **Chest x-ray film showing bilateral hilar adenopathy (arrows) in patient with sarcoidosis.**

Fuchs' Heterochromic Iridocyclitis

Fuchs' heterochromic iridocyclitis is a mild, unilateral anterior uveitis with onset in early adulthood. The involved iris is heterochromic, usually lighter, and appears moth-eaten. The heterochromia, often the first sign of the disease, occurs because the iris stroma is atrophic. Multiple iris nodules may assist in the identification of Fuchs' uveitis, especially in black patients.[64] The eye is usually white with some cells and little flare. Clear or white clumps of lymphocytes, which do not accumulate pigment, are seen on the corneal endothelium. Synechia formation is uncommon in Fuchs' heterochromic iridocyclitis, but complications can include posterior subcapsular cataract formation and glaucoma.

The associated cataract can be removed surgically since synechiae formation is rare. The secondary glaucoma can occur from two causes. A trabeculitis may lead to decreased aqueous outflow. The trabeculitis can be controlled with topical or periocular steroids. Iris neovascularization may also occur, leading to neovascular glaucoma. In these cases, vessels grow from the iris root to the trabecular meshwork,

closing the angle. Laser photocoagulation can be used to control the glaucoma.

Since Fuchs' heterochromic iridocyclitis occurs in young persons, patients will require a lifetime of follow-up including periodic angle evaluation to rule out neovascular growth. Many cases of Fuchs' heterochromic iridocyclitis are difficult to diagnose in the early stages because the eye is white, and the condition is rare enough to escape initial recognition. Since the iridocyclitis does not respond well to steroids, these agents are indicated only if the inflammation becomes symptomatic or if trabeculitis occurs. Finally, cycloplegia is not usually required because there is little risk of synechia formation.

Herpes Simplex

Anterior uveitis associated with herpes simplex virus (HSV) is generally of two types. First, anterior uveitis can result from corneal epithelial dendritic formation, which causes an axonal reflex with vasodilation of the blood vessels of the iris and ciliary body. This produces the characteristic cells and flare. Second, and more severe, is anterior uveitis resulting from corneal stromal involvement from HSV. Although the virus is probably not the direct cause, it alters the immune system, leading to inflammation. This severe uveitis is unilateral and quite painful. In addition, there may be hemorrhage or red blood cells in the anterior chamber. This severe form of anterior uveitis may last for months, whereas the epithelial herpetic uveitis is limited to the duration of the epitheliopathy. Synechiae, keratic precipitates, and occasionally trabeculitis with resulting glaucoma can result from anterior uveitis associated with stromal HSV.

The most appropriate therapy for anterior uveitis associated with epithelial HSV is topical antiviral agents and cycloplegia. As the epithelium heals, the anterior uveitis resolves. In contrast, stromal herpetic keratitis can cause an anterior uveitis that may be quite difficult to manage. Because such uveitis can readily cause synechia formation, cycloplegia is imperative. In addition, high dosages of topical steroids may be required to control the anterior segment inflammation, with topical antiviral agents administered concomitantly to combat the steroid-induced viral replication. Trabeculitis may precipitate a secondary glaucoma that should be managed with oral carbonic anhydrase inhibitors such as acetazolamide, or topical β blockers. Miotics should be avoided, since they can exacerbate the uveitis.

Herpes Zoster

Like HSV, herpes zoster can present with two different forms of anterior uveitis. Anterior uveitis can occur from a corneal axonal reflex as in HSV uveitis. The second form, seen in older persons with herpes zoster, consists of an immunologic uveitis characterized by an intense anterior uveitis. This second form of uveitis eventually leads to patchy necrosis of the iris and secondary segmental iris atrophy that will transilluminate. This characteristic wedge defect in the iris can be helpful in confirming the clinical diagnosis of herpes zoster uveitis. The chronic form of herpes zoster uveitis is felt to be an immune reaction[9] and is therefore quite difficult to control with steroids.

Treatment is aimed at reducing the local hypersensitivity to the zoster virus and includes the use of oral acyclovir, topical cycloplegics, and topical or oral steroids.

Intermediate Uveitis

Intermediate uveitis is a recent term.[3] It describes a collection of conditions having inflammatory cells in the vitreous (Fig. 30.7), little, if any, anterior segment reaction, no synechia, and mild periphlebitis.[46] Fundus lesions are not present, but macular and optic disc edema are part of the presentation. Symptoms, which may be absent, can include blurred vision or floaters. Pain or redness of the eye is rarely seen.

Subclassifications of intermediate uveitis include pars planitis, chronic cyclitis, and senile vitritis. Several systemic conditions may present with intermediate uveitis. These include multiple sclerosis, reticulum cell sarcoma, sarcoidosis, or Whipple's disease. A retinal detachment may appear with cells or pigment in the anterior vitreous and mimic the appearance of intermediate uveitis.

Pars planitis is a condition of unknown etiology, usually occurring in teenagers or young adults. The signs and symptoms are typical of those of intermediate uveitis, but also include a cellular exudation or cyclitic membrane forming over the inferior pars plana.[47] Binocular indirect ophthal-moscopy with scleral depression is required to see these "snowbanks" in the periphery (Fig. 30.8). Cystoid macular edema is often the cause of decreased vision in patients with pars planitis. Pars plana snowbanks are not necessary for the diagnosis of intermediate uveitis, but the presence of snowbanks is associated with a more severe vitreal disease and an increased incidence of cystoid macular edema.[48]

Many cases of intermediate uveitis do not require therapy. If cystoid macular edema is present but mild (visual acuity better than 20/40), the condition may be monitored.[47] However, if the vision drops below 20/40 or the patient is extremely symptomatic, then treatment should be instituted using oral or periocular steroids. Since intermediate uveitis often persists for 10 to 20 years with periods of exacerbations and remissions, the risks of long-term systemic steroid use must be weighed against the potential benefits. In patients with refractory pars planitis and snowbanking, cryopexy of the vitreous base may decrease the peripheral exudation.[65]

Multiple Sclerosis

Multiple sclerosis (MS) is a chronic disease associated with demyelination of the central nervous system. The condition usually affects young adults from 20 to 40 years old, which is similar to the age range associated with most forms of uveitis. Recent theories have proposed that the demyelination process is of an autoimmune nature, similar to the etiology of many forms of uveitis. The ocular findings associated with MS include optic neuritis, motility disturbances, periphlebitis, intermediate uveitis, and granulomatous anterior uveitis.[49] The granulomatous anterior uveitic presentation includes mutton-fat keratic precipitates. Individuals presenting with a granulomatous anterior uveitis of

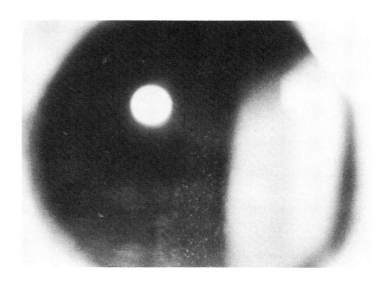

FIGURE 30.7 **Cells in vitreous associated with pars planitis. (Courtesy Scott Richter, O.D.)**

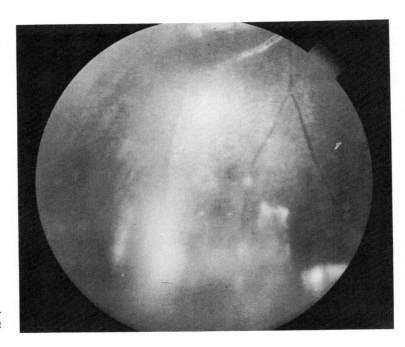

FIGURE 30.8 **Inferior peripheral exudates (snow-banks) associated with pars planitis. (Courtesy Scott Richter, O.D.)**

unknown etiology should have a careful medical history, including neurologic symptoms that may be associated with MS. A neurologic examination is indicated when multiple sclerosis is suspected.

Treatment is similar to other forms of anterior uveitis, with topical steroids and cycloplegics the mainstay of therapy. The dosage of each medication is based on the intensity of the inflammatory response.

Tuberculosis

Both anterior and posterior uveitis have been associated with tuberculosis and have been observed in 3% of the population of a clinic specializing in uveitis.[9] Two types of uveitis are related to tuberculosis. The first is due to perforated tuberculosis lesions with direct infection of the uveal tissues. Second, tuberculosis may alter the immune status in an infected individual. Such alteration of the immune system may lead to a granulomatous uveitis. The diagnosis of tuberculosis is often presumptive and is based on a positive purified protein derivative (PPD) skin test and positive chest x-ray films,[50] but without obtaining cultures of the organism. Anterior uveitis can vary from an acute onset of a painful red eye to a smoldering, chronic, low-grade inflammation. The latter manifestation leads to formation of cataract, glaucoma, and phthisis and responds very poorly to therapy. Finally, a fulminating reaction may occur leading to corneal perforations. In addition to the anterior uveitis with its attendant synechiae and mutton-fat keratic precipitates, a posterior uveitis may occur that is characterized by diffuse chorioretinitis.

Because it penetrates the eye so well, isoniazid (INH) is the drug of choice for therapy of uveitis in tuberculosis. However, INH can cause hepatitis or peripheral neuropathy, and many patients may develop tolerance to the medication. For some patients, ethambutol can be used in combination with INH, and in those patients who develop tolerance to INH, rifampin can be used. INH is used for 1 year, and ethambutol is used for at least 2 months while the patient is monitored monthly for liver toxicity. If peripheral neuropathy occurs during therapy, pyridoxine (vitamin B_6) can be used for prevention. Steroids have been used on occasion, but only with extreme caution, since they can aggravate or precipitate a local or systemic tuberculosis reaction.

Syphilis

Either congenital or acquired syphilis can cause uveitis. Because of transplacental transfer in the congenital form, an acute anterior uveitis can be seen in the newborn with congenital syphilis. However, the acute anterior uveitis is usually observed at about 6 months. The uveitis is generally bilateral, and the diagnosis is established by obtaining a positive fluorescent treponemal antibody absorption (FTA-ABS) test from both child and mother. The therapy for syphilis is penicillin, but despite therapy the patient may develop interstitial keratitis, a bilateral immunologic corneal reaction usually seen between 6 and 12 years. A secondary anterior uveitis may occur in patients with interstitial keratitis.

The most common ocular finding in congenital syphilis is chorioretinitis, which occurs in about half the cases.[51] The chorioretinitis represents an inflammation of the retinal pigment epithelium, with the pigment migrating in a perivascular pattern, revealing a bone spicule or "salt and pepper" appearance similar to that seen in retinitis pigmentosa. This fundus picture and the occurrence of associated deafness in congenital syphilis can lead the clinician to suspect a diagnosis of Usher's syndrome. However, normal acuities, laboratory testing, and full visual fields help provide the diagnosis.

In the secondary stages of acquired syphilis there may be a chorioretinitis and an anterior uveitis. The condition may be unilateral and be associated with excellent visual acuities and full visual fields.

In any recurrent or bilateral anterior uveitis not responding to therapy, Venereal Disease Research Laboratory (VDRL) and FTA-ABS tests should be considered. If the tests are positive for syphilis, penicillin therapy should be instituted to eradicate potential treponemes and prevent the onset of tertiary syphilis and its associated neurosyphilis. Since penicillin will not diminish the inflammation, steroids and cycloplegics are necessary to treat the anterior uveitis.

Phacoantigenic Uveitis

Phacoantigenic uveitis can be seen in traumatic conditions where the capsule of the lens has been ruptured, or in mature cataract that leaks protein into the anterior chamber. The severe anterior uveitis that results is due to the antigenic nature of the lens proteins, which stimulate an inflammatory reaction. Although such a uveitis is quite severe, it is rare. Generally, the history is most useful in the diagnosis. The patient usually reports a traumatic incident or is elderly and has a history of poor vision with one eye for years. The anterior chamber is filled with flare so pronounced that it is often difficult to visualize the lens. Until the lens is removed surgically, the patient can receive topical cycloplegics and steroids to reduce the inflammation, but the best treatment is removal of the lens. If there is severe inflammation, macrophages laden with lens material may clog the trabeculum and lead to phakolytic glaucoma. Although there is no clear understanding of the etiology, immunology may play an important role in the pathogenesis of phacoantigenic uveitis.

Sympathetic Ophthalmia

Sympathetic ophthalmia is a bilateral, granulomatous uveitis that may occur after ocular trauma or surgery, with the inflammation usually occurring from 2 to 8 weeks after the antecedent event. It has been reported to occur as early as 9 days to as late as 50 years after the initial insult.[2] Because of the autoimmune processes involved in sympathetic ophthalmia, the pathogenesis has been studied extensively. The inflammation of sympathetic ophthalmia is a delayed hypersensitivity reaction that causes a panuveitis of insidious onset in the uninvolved eye. There is evidence to suggest that retinal S antigens from the retinal photoreceptors may be the cause of the delayed hypersensitivity reaction.[52,53] Affected patients become sensitized to their retinal rod outer segments, a type of cell-mediated hypersentivity occurs, and uveitis that affects the entire uvea ensues.[53]

Treatment of sympathetic ophthalmia involves reducing the body's immune response. Early, high dosages of steroids should be employed, but in cases where steroid therapy is unsuccessful or contraindicated, immunosuppressive therapy may be used with some success.[9,54] Methotrexate, chlorambucil, cyclophosphamide, and cyclosporine have been used,[54] but they are extremely toxic. Cycloplegia is needed to prevent synechiae, and steroids may be required topically, subconjunctivally, or orally. Because sympathetic ophthalmia occurs only rarely, and because it may not occur until many years after the initial insult, prophylactic steroid therapy is controversial.[9] The uveal inflammation of sympathetic ophthalmia occurs in only 0.1% of patients with significant ocular trauma,[55] but because it affects the uninvolved eye, it causes great concern. Often the fellow eye may be so damaged from the panuveitis that the traumatized eye may have better resulting vision. Occasionally a perforated, painful eye must be enucleated because of the threat of sympathetic ophthalmia, but each case should be considered on its own merits, since sympathetic ophthalmia is rare. If enucleation is indicated, it must be done within 2 weeks of the injury. If panuveitis has begun in the sympathizing eye, removal of the injured eye will not alter the course.

Histoplasmosis

Histoplasmosis is an infection that occurs both systemically and ocularly, and is caused by the fungus *Histoplasma capsulatum*. Both the systemic and the ocular diseases are encountered most frequently in the Ohio and Mississippi river valleys in the United States. The systemic disease occurs in all races and age groups, with an acute pulmonary reaction being the most frequently observed manifestation of the disease.

Ocular histoplasmosis consists of a triad of peripapillary chorioretinal atrophy, peripheral atrophic scars, and macular scarring noted in young adults (Fig. 30.9). The fundus scars predispose the patient to active macular disease, best noted by the fluid and hemorrhage surrounding the old scars. Interestingly, ocular histoplasmosis is uncommon in blacks.[56] The choroiditis occurs in both eyes, and there is no anterior uveitis or vitritis. Most cases are called presumed

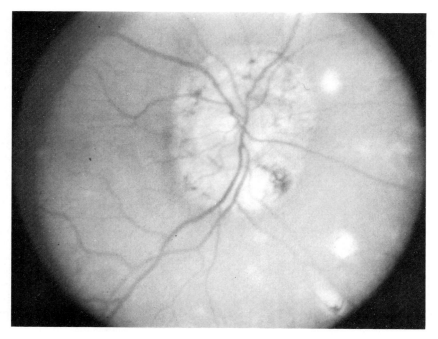

FIGURE 30.9. **Peripapillary chorioretinal atrophy and peripheral atrophic scars in presumed ocular histoplasmosis syndrome.**

ocular histoplasmosis syndrome (POHS), because it is rare for the fungus to be isolated from affected choroidal tissue. The diagnosis is based on the ophthalmoscopic findings. Although characteristic lung lesions are usually noted on the chest x-ray film, it is rarely needed for diagnostic purposes. Skin tests are not recommended because they may reactivate the ocular lesions and lead to vision loss.

The systemic condition is treated with amphotericin B, which is extremely toxic and has no effect on the eye.[57] For ocular histoplasmosis, the major concern is the potential for loss of vision from both atrophic and hemorrhagic lesions at the maculae. Because the atrophic lesions can provide an environment where subretinal neovascularization can occur, resulting in hemorrhagic maculopathy, therapy for the ocular manifestations of histoplasmosis is aimed at preserving macular function. High dosages of systemic steroids are sometimes used, and argon laser photocoagulation is implemented to control the subretinal neovascularization. No therapy is indicated for inactive scars.

There may be an altered immune mechanism in histoplasmosis, and HLA-DRW-2 and HLA-B7 have been observed in cases of ocular histoplasmosis.[56,58] In addition, there may be a trigger mechanism in some cases, since both emotional and physical stress have been known to reactivate ocular histoplasmosis.[59]

References

1. Hendly DE, Genetler AJ, Smith RE, Rao NA. Changing patterns of uveitis. Am J Ophthalmol 1987;103:131–136.
2. Nussenblatt RB, Palestine AG. Uveitis fundamentals and clinical practice. Chicago: Yearbook Medical Publishers, 1989;59–77.
3. Bloch-Michel E, Nussenblatt RB. International uveitis study group recommendations for evaluations of intraocular inflammatory disease. Am J Ophthalmol 1987;103:234–235.
4. Tessler HH. Classification and symptoms and signs of uveitis. In: Tasman W, Jaeger EA, eds. Duane's Clinical ophthalmology. Philadelphia: J B Lippincott, 1992:4:Chap. 32, pp. 1–10.
5. Godfrey WA. Acute anterior uveitis. In: Tasman W, Jaeger EA, eds. Duane's Clinical ophthalmology. Philadelphia: J B Lippincott, 1992;4:Chap. 40.
6. Scharf Y, Zonis S. Histocompatibility antigens (HLA) and uveitis. Surv Ophthalmol 1980;24:220–228.
7. Darrell RW, Kurland L, Wagenerti P. Epidemiology of uveitis. Incidence and prevalence in a small community. Arch Ophthalmol 1962;68:4.
8. Sheppard JD, Nozik RA. Practical diagnostic approach to uveitis. In: Tasman W, Jaeger EA, eds. Duane's Clinical ophthalmology. Philadelphia: J B Lippincott, 1992;4:Chap. 33.
9. Schlaegel TF. Perspectives in uveitis. Ann Ophthalmol 1981;13: 799–806.
10. Rothova MD, van Veenendall WG, Linssen A, et al. Clinical features of anterior uveitis. Am J Ophthalmol 1987;103:137–145.

11. Friedlander MH. Allergy and immunology of the eye, ed. 2. New York, NY: Raven, 1992.

12. Brewerton DA, Caffrey M, Nicholls A, et al. Acute anterior uveitis and HLA-27. Lancet 1973;2:994–996.

13. Rothova A, Buitenhuis HJ, Meenken C, et al. Uveitis and systemic disease. Br J Ophthalmol 1992;76:137–141.

14. Nussenblatt RB, Palestine AG. Uveitis fundamentals and clinical practice. Chicago: Yearbook Medical Publishers, 1989;21–23.

15. Nussenblatt RL, Palestine AG. Uveitis fundamentals and clinical practice. Chicago: Yearbook Medical Publishers, 1989;80–93.

16. Rosenbaum JT, Wernick R. Selection and interpretation of laboratory tests for patients with uveitis. Int Ophthalmol Clin 1990;30: 238–243.

17. Parker JA, Nozik RA. Laboratory tests in diagnosis of uveitis. In: Karcioglu ZA, ed. Laboratory diagnosis in ophthalmology. New York: Macmillian, 1987;185–205.

18. Friedberg MA, Rapuano CJ. Uveitis. In: Office and emergency room diagnosis and treatment of eye disease. Philadelphia: J B Lippincott, 1990:331–365.

19. Pickney C, Pinckney ER. The patient's guide to medical tests. New York: Facts on File Publications, 1986;8–12.

20. Tamesis RR, Foster S. Ocular syphilis. Ophthalmology 1990;97: 1281–1287.

21. Talley DK. Clinical laboratory testing for the diagnosis of systemic disease associated with anterior uveitis. Optom Clin 1992;2:105–123.

22. Rosenbaum JT. Characterization of uveitis associated with spondyloarthritis. J Rheumatol 1989;16:792–796.

23. Wakefield D, Montanaro A, McCluskey P. Acute anterior uveitis and HLA-B27. Surv Ophthalmol 1991;36:223–232.

24. Nussenblatt RL, Palestine AG. Uveitis fundamentals and clinical practice. Chicago: Yearbook Medical Publishers, 1989;104–144.

25. Leibowitz HM, Kupferman A. Anti-inflammatory medications. Int Ophthalmol Clin 1980;20:117–134.

26. Wakefield D. Methylprednisolone pulse therapy in severe anterior uveitis. Aust NZ J Ophthalmol 1985;13:411–415.

27. Lightman S. Uveitis: management. Lancet 1991;338:1501–1504.

28. Nussenblatt RB, Palestine AG. Cyclosporine: Immunology, pharmacology and therapeutic uses. Surv Ophthalmol 1986;31:159–169.

29. Crouch ER, Read JE. Trauma: Ruptures and bleeding. In: Tasman W, Jaeger EA, eds. Duane's Clinical ophthalmology. Philadelphia: J B Lippincott, 1992;4:Chap. 61, pp 6–18.

30. Kutner B, Fourman S, Brein K, et al. Aminocaproic acid reduces the risk of secondary hemorrhage in patients with traumatic hyphema. Arch Ophthalmol 1987;105:206–208.

31. Crouch ER Jr, Frenkel M. Aminocaproic acid in the treatment of traumatic hyphema. Am J Ophthalmol 1976;81:355–360.

32. McGetrick JJ, Jampol LM, Goldberg MF, et al. Aminocaproic acid decreases secondary hemorrhage after traumatic hyphema. Arch Ophthalmol 1983;101:1031–1033.

33. Palmer DJ, Goldberg MF, Frenkel M, et al. A comparison of two dose regimens of epsilon aminocaproic acid in the prevention and management of secondary traumatic hyphemas. Ophthalmology 1986;93:102–108.

34. Kraft SP, Christianson MD, Crawford JS, et al. Traumatic hyphema in children. Treatment with epsilon-aminocaproic acid. Ophthalmology 1987;94:1232–1237.

35. Read JE, Goldberg MF. Traumatic hyphema: Comparison of medi-

cal treatment. Trans Am Acad Ophthalmol Otolaryngol 1974;78: 799.

36. Rothova A, van Veenendaal WG, Linssen A, et al. Clinical features of acute anterior uveitis. Am J Ophthalmol 1987;103:137–145.

37. Nussenblatt RB, Palestine AG. Uveitis fundamentals and clinical practice. Chicago: Yearbook Medical Publishers, 1989;Chap. 9.

38. Wolf MD, Licter PR, Ragsdale CR. Prognostic factors in the uveitis of juvenile rheumatoid arthritis. Ophthalmology 1987;94:1242–1248.

39. Mehra R, Moore T, Catalano JD, et al. Chlorambucil in the treatment of iridocyclitis in juvenile rheumatoid arthritis. J Rheumatol 1981;8:141–144.

40. Salmon JF, Wright JP, Murray ADN. Ocular inflammation in Chron's disease. Ophthalmology 1991;98:480–484.

41. Mamo JG, Azzam SA. Treatment of Behçet's disease with chlorambucil. Arch Ophthalmol 1970;84:446.

42. Mizuki N, Inoko H, Ando H, et al. Behçet's disease associated with one of the HLA-B51 subantigens, HLA-B5101. Am J Ophthalmol 1993;116:406–409.

43. Chajek T, Fainru M. Behçet's disease. Report of 41 cases and a review of the literature. Medicine 1975;54:179–196.

44. Baarsma GS, Lahey E, Glasuis E, et al. The predictive value of serum converting enzyme and lysozyme levels in the diagnosis of ocular sarcoidosis. Am J Ophthalmol 1987;104:211–217.

45. Weinreb RN, Tessler H. Laboratory diagnosis of ophthalmic sarcoidosis. Surv Ophthalmol 1984;26:653–664.

46. Tessler H. The uvea—what is intermediate uveitis. In: Ernest JT, ed. The yearbook of ophthalmology 1985. Chicago: Yearbook Publishers, 1985:155–156.

47. Henderly DE, Genstler AJ, Smith RE, Rao NA. Pars planitis. Trans Ophthalmol Soc UK 1986;105:227.

48. Smith RE, Nozik RA. Uveitis: A clinical approach to diagnosis and management, ed. 2. Baltimore: Williams and Wilkins, 1988.

49. Lim JI, Tessler H, Goodwin JA. Anterior granulomatous uveitis in patients with multiple sclerosis. Ophthalmology 1991;98:142–145.

50. Abrams J, Schlaegel TF. The tuberculin skin test in the diagnosis of tuberculosis uveitis. Am J Ophthalmol 1983;96:295–298.

51. Weinberg R. Syphilis. In: Tasman W, Jaeger EA, eds. Duane's Clinical ophthalmology. Philadelphia: J B Lippincott, 1992; 4:Chap. 50.

52. Wacker WB, Rao NB, Marak GE. Experimental sympathetic ophthalmia. In: Silverstein AM, O'Connor GR, eds. Immunology and immunopathology of the eye. New York: Masson, 1979;121–126.

53. Wacker WB. Experimental allergic uvitis. J Immunol 1977;199: 1949–1950.

54. Corwin JM, Weiter JJ. Immunology of chorioretinal disease. Surv Ophthalmol 1981;25:287–305.

55. Aronson SB, Elliot JH. Ocular inflammation. St. Louis: C.V. Mosby Co, 1972.

56. Meridith TA, Smith RE, Duguesnoy RJ. Association of HLA-DRW2 antigen with presumed ocular histoplasmosis. Am J Ophthalmol 1980;89:70–76.

57. Schlaegel TF. Ocular histoplasmosis. New York: Grune & Stratton, 1977.

58. Meridith TA, Smith RE, Braley RE, et al. The prevalence of HLA-B7 in presumed ocular histoplasmosis in patients with peripheral atrophic scars. Am J Ophthalmol 1978;86:325–328.

59. Becker N, Tessler HH. Ocular histoplasmosis syndrome. In: Tas-

man W, Jaeger EA, eds. Duane's Clinical ophthalmology. Philadelphia: J B Lippincott, 1992;4:Chap. 48.

60. Guex-Crosier Y, Pittet N, Herbort CP. Evaluation of laser flare-cell photometry in the appraisal and management of intraocular inflammation in uveitis. Ophthalmology 1994;101:728–735.

61. Mindel JS. Problems in the use of tranexamic acid by ophthalmologists. Arch Ophthalmol 1989;107:486–487.

62. Soukiasian SH, Foster CS, Raizman MB. Treatment strategies for scleritis and uveitis associated with inflammatory bowel disease. Am J Ophthalmol 1994;118:601–611.

63. Whitcup SM, Salvo EC, Nussenblatt RB. Combined cyclosporine and corticosteroid therapy for sight-threatening uveitis in Behçet's disease. Am J Ophthalmol 1994;118:39–45.

64. Rothova A, La Hey E, Baarsma GS, et al. Iris nodules in Fuch's heterochromic uveitis. Am J Ophthalmol 1994;118:338–342.

65. Josephberg RG, Kanter ED, Jaffee RM. A fluorescein angiographic study of patients with pars planitis and peripheral exudation (snowbanking) before and after cryopexy. Ophthalmology 1994;101:1262–1266.

operative eyes were treated with either 0.1% dexamethasone phosphate or saline, 3 times daily. Topical atropine or scopolamine was administered twice daily. The patients who received steroid once daily failed to demonstrate a statistically significant anti-inflammatory effect. However, eyes treated 3 times daily showed a somewhat greater, although minimal, anti-inflammatory effect.

The first study to demonstrate substantial therapeutic efficacy of steroids following cataract extraction was reported in 1976 by Corboy.[27] A multicenter, double-masked, randomized clinical trial was conducted in which topical betamethasone phosphate 0.1% or placebo was used 5 times daily for two weeks following uncomplicated ICCE. Each of the 107 patients had moderate to severe postoperative inflammation on the first postoperative day. In terms of the rate of clinical improvement, the difference between the betamethasone-treated groups was significant, beginning at postoperative day 4 to the final visit. There were no ocular complications attributable to steroid treatment, and Corboy[27] concluded that frequent application of topical betamethasone following uncomplicated ICCE is effective in reducing inflammatory signs and symptoms.

Clobetasone butyrate has been compared with prednisolone phosphate and placebo for treatment of inflammatory signs and symptoms following uncomplicated ICCE.[28] Both clobetasone and prednisolone were found to be significantly more effective in reducing postoperative inflammatory signs than was placebo, and the two steroids were judged to be clinically equivalent as anti-inflammatory agents.

Periocular steroids have also been studied for their usefulness as anti-inflammatory agents following cataract extraction. Buxton and associates[29] studied 200 consecutive patients undergoing cataract extraction who were given subconjunctival steroids at the time of cataract surgery. Postoperative flat or shallow anterior chambers, iris prolapse, surgical wound dehiscence, uveitis, infection, and glaucoma were observed less frequently when steroids were used. Although these authors did not advocate the routine use of subconjunctival steroids following cataract extraction, this route of steroid administration appears to be useful in complicated cases, especially in eyes with previous keratoplasties or those with active or inactive uveitis. Patients with pre-existing uveitis often respond to surgical procedures better during extended periods of remission. They may also be treated prophylactically with either topical or subconjunctival steroids prior to surgery. Postoperatively, they may require an enhanced anti-inflammatory regimen, as compared with routine cases.

More recently a randomized, double-masked study of 1% rimexolone (Vexol) and the rimexolone vehicle (placebo) was conducted in 197 patients who had undergone cataract extraction by either extracapsular methods or phacoemulsification with implantation of a posterior chamber IOL.[30] These investigators concluded that rimexolone is significantly more effective in reducing postoperative inflamma-

tory signs and symptoms than is placebo. This is consistent with the positive results reported previously[26,27] where multiple daily doses of topical steroids were used. The rate of clinical improvement with rimexolone was comparable to that reported for betamethasone.[27] The difference between rimexolone and placebo-treated eyes was statistically significant beginning at postoperative day 3, while Corboy[27] found statistically significant differences for betamethasone beginning at day 4. Moreover, neither rimexolone nor placebo induced any clinically significant adverse events, including elevated IOP, infection, wound dehiscence, or shallow or flat anterior chamber. Thus, rimexolone appears to be effective for treatment of inflammatory signs and symptoms following cataract extraction with implantation of posterior chamber IOLs, but without inducing adverse side effects characteristic of many other steroidal compounds.

The typical postoperative anti-inflammatory regimen includes the use of a topical steroid separate from or in combination with an antibiotic. Commonly used steroids are listed in Table 31.1.[31] Patients who experience an abnormal elevation in IOP due to steroid therapy may experience a delayed or diminished pressure rise with fluorometholone acetate 0.1% (Flarex) versus the other agents, and still have the desired anti-inflammatory effect.[32]

Steroids are typically administered using a regimen of one drop 4 times daily for the first postoperative week, then tapered to 3 times daily for the second week, 2 times daily for the third week, once daily for the fourth week, then discontinued.[31] The dosage may be more frequent and the tapering more prolonged if there is significantly increased postoperative inflammation.

To enhance convenience and reduce cost, antibiotic/steroid combinations are often used instead of prescribing the individual drugs separately. Commonly used combinations are listed in Table 31.1. The primary disadvantage in using a combination is that the practitioner is less able to prescribe in a way that uses the individual components to their maximum effectiveness. The frequency and duration of administration are driven by the desired anti-inflammatory effect of the steroid component, rather than by the anti-infective effect of the antibiotic component. In general, however, the advantages of using antibiotic/steroid combinations usually outweigh the disadvantages.

Nonsteroidal Anti-Inflammatory Drugs

Corticosteroids are the mainstay for treatment of inflammation following routine cataract extraction. Their usefulness, however, can be limited by side effects. For this reason, efforts have been made to develop compounds with fewer adverse reactions. The demonstration by Vane[33] that aspirin inhibits prostaglandin synthesis, along with the well-known observations that aspirin can have prominent anti-inflammatory actions, has resulted in development of other compounds in the same therapeutic class. All are thought to act in some way on prostaglandin or leukotriene biosynthetic mechanisms.[34–38] Table 31.2 lists the commercially available nonsteroidal anti-inflammatory drugs (NSAIDs) employed in cataract surgery.

The fact that prostaglandin release during cataract surgery can induce miosis and thus contribute to surgical complications, has provided a basis for the use of NSAIDs prophylactically to inhibit such intraoperative miosis.[39–41] A number of clinical trials[42–45] have shown that topically applied NSAIDs have a statistically significant effect on pupil size, compared to placebo, when administered preoperatively with topically applied mydriatic agents. These data, however, suggest that the pharmacologic effect on the pupil is small,[45,46] and that the slight inhibition of intraoperative miosis appears to vary according to the surgical technique employed. Nevertheless, flurbiprofen 0.03% (Ocufen) and suprofen 1.0% (Profenal) are approved for use as inhibitors of intraoperative miosis. Although the published studies document statistically significant inhibitory effects on the pupil following preoperative use of these topically applied NSAIDs, it is unclear whether these effects are always clinically significant. As a result, many surgeons remain unconvinced and therefore do not routinely use topical NSAIDs preoperatively.[13,47]

Numerous investigators[21,48–50] have reported clinical effectiveness of topical indomethacin in reducing postoperative anterior segment inflammatory signs following cataract extraction. Most of these studies, however, allowed the routine concomitant use of topical steroids. Thus, the study designs do not allow definitive conclusions regarding the clinical efficacy of topical indomethacin alone. Rather, the results of these studies seem to reflect a degree of synergism or additivity between topical indomethacin and steroids. Sawa[17] conducted one of the few studies of topical indomethacin without concurrent steroid use and found that topically applied 0.5% indomethacin was effective in suppressing the postoperative increase in aqueous flare but had little effect on the cellular reaction in the anterior chamber.

TABLE 31.2
Topical Ophthalmic NSAIDs Used in Cataract Surgery

Generic Name	Trade Name	Indication
Flurbiprofen	Ocufen (Allergan)	Inhibition of intraoperative miosis
Suprofen	Profenal (Alcon)	Inhibition of intraoperative miosis
Diclofenac	Voltaren (Ciba Vision Ophthalmics)	Treatment of postoperative inflammation

The clinical efficacy of orally administered ibuprofen in reducing postoperative inflammation following ICCE was reported by Sabiston.[51] This study showed that orally administered ibuprofen, 1600 mg daily, produced greater improvement in inflammatory signs in the lids, conjunctiva, cornea, and anterior chamber than in subjects receiving no ibuprofen. Furthermore, suppression of the inflammatory response was delayed in the cornea and anterior chamber, achieving more immediate results in the lids and conjunctiva.

Several studies have been conducted to explore the anti-inflammatory efficacy of flurbiprofen,[42, 51–54] ketorolac,[15,55] and diclofenac.[56,57] Flach and associates[15] studied the efficacy of 0.5% ketorolac solution compared to placebo following ECCE without implantation of an IOL. Treatment with ketorolac significantly decreased inflammatory signs of lid edema, conjunctival vasodilation, and ciliary flush on postoperative days 2, 12, and 19, and was significantly more effective than placebo in decreasing anterior chamber cells on day 12. A similar study by Flach and associates[55] compared the anti-inflammatory effects of ketorolac 0.5% solution or placebo on postoperative inflammation in 129 patients undergoing ECCE with implantation of a posterior chamber IOL. A statistically significant postoperative anti-inflammatory effect was observed in patients treated with ketorolac compared with placebo-treated patients.

Investigators have studied the anti-inflammatory effects of flurbiprofen following topical[42,51,52] or oral[53,54] administration. Sabiston and associates[52] reported reduced postoperative inflammation following ICCE without implantation of an IOL in 72 patients who used topical 0.03% flurbiprofen, compared with placebo. Although the conjunctival hyperemia, as well as anterior chamber cells and flare, were greater in the placebo-treated group on postoperative days 3, 7, and 14, the differences between the treatment and placebo groups did not reach statistical significance until day 14. Other studies have likewise suggested the relative ineffectiveness of topically applied flurbiprofen as an anti-inflammatory agent following cataract surgery. Tsuchisaka and Takase[42] used topical flurbiprofen 0.1% or placebo preoperatively and 3 times daily following ECCE. These investigators found that nearly all the inflammatory signs evaluated were not suppressed by flurbiprofen, compared with the control group. Sabiston[51] conducted a double-masked trial with 40 subjects, 20 of whom received topical flurbiprofen 0.03%, and 20 received placebo. There was no significant difference in the inflammatory responses in patients receiving flurbiprofen compared with those receiving placebo.

The results reported with orally administered flurbiprofen have been varied. Hillman and associates[53] administered flurbiprofen 100mg or placebo 3 times daily for 8 days, beginning 24 hours before cataract surgery. The only statistically significant clinical effect was improvement in corneal inflammation at the sixth postoperative day. These results are in contrast to those reported by Sabiston and Robinson,[54] who reported significantly less postoperative inflammation in patients receiving flurbiprofen 100mg twice daily in addition to routine postoperative therapy. These authors suggest that flurbiprofen does reduce postoperative inflammatory responses following ICCE without implantation of an IOL.

Two reports[56,57] describe the effects of topically applied or orally administered diclofenac following cataract surgery. Ronen and associates[56] conducted a study of 100 patients undergoing ICCE. All patients were treated with dexamethasone phosphate 0.1% twice daily, and atropine 1.0% twice daily, for 28 days. Patients were randomized to either diclofenac 50mg or placebo 3 times daily, beginning 24 hours before surgery and continuing for 4 weeks. Compared with placebo-treated subjects, patients receiving oral diclofenac had a significant reduction in pain, conjunctival hyperemia, chemosis, and cells and flare in the anterior chamber.

The anti-inflammatory efficacy of topically applied diclofenac 0.1% ophthalmic solution was evaluated in a study of 309 patients recovering from cataract extraction and implantation of an IOL.[57] This study found that topically administered diclofenac was significantly more effective than placebo in reducing postoperative anterior chamber cells and flare, as well as conjunctival and ciliary inflammatory responses.

These studies suggest, therefore, that several of the currently available NSAIDs are effective, compared with placebo, in reducing anterior segment inflammation following ICCE or ECCE, both with or without implantation of an IOL, and both with or without concurrent steroid administration.

Maintaining Desired Intraocular Pressure

Prior to cataract extraction, it is desirable to lower IOP to prevent loss of vitreous, intraocular hemorrhage, and associated complications. This is especially critical in patients with pre-existing glaucoma. Mechanical, medical, and surgical techniques are used to reduce preoperative IOP. Mechanical pressure from digital massage, Honan balloon, or "Super Pinkie" rubber ball can be applied either before or after retrobulbar anesthesia to create a "soft eye." Hyperosmotics such as oral 50% glycerin (Osmoglyn), oral or intravenous acetazolamide, or intravenous 20% mannitol are also effective in lowering IOP. If neither mechanical nor medical techniques are effective, a posterior sclerotomy is used occasionally to reduce IOP prior to creating the incision for cataract extraction.[58]

The careful monitoring of IOP with applanation tonometry at each follow-up visit is an important aspect of postoperative management. Pressures that are either elevated or depressed outside the expected range for a particular patient are considered to be a postoperative complication and should be managed accordingly (see Managing Complications).

Controlling Pain

The three basic methods of controlling intraoperative pain during cataract extraction are general, retrobulbar, or periocular (peribulbar) anesthesia. General anesthesia was the primary method used prior to the development of long-acting local and regional anesthetics. Of these newer agents, retrobulbar anesthesia became the mode of choice because systemic complications, such as cardiac or pulmonary arrest, are much less frequent than with general anesthesia. In addition, improvements in surgical techniques significantly reduced surgical time, thus decreasing the need for general anesthesia.[59] Agents commonly used for retrobulbar anesthesia include 2% lidocaine with epinephrine, 0.75% bupivacaine, and hyaluronidase. Bicarbonate may be added to adjust the pH and decrease the onset time of the anesthesia.[60,61]

With most cataract extractions being performed in outpatient surgical centers where anesthesiologists or nurse anesthetists are not always available, some surgeons advocate periocular (peribulbar) over retrobulbar anesthesia. The same agents are used in periocular as in retrobulbar anesthesia. Although it is less effective in producing extraocular muscle akinesia compared with retrobulbar techniques, periocular administration is thought to produce fewer complications such as retrobulbar hemorrhage, central retinal artery occlusion, globe perforation, or injection into the subarachnoid space or optic nerve sheath. Moreover, it is often tolerated better by the patient.[59,62,63] Since the early 1990s, some surgeons have performed cataract surgery using only topical anesthesia. This procedure can be successful in cooperative patients with uncomplicated cataract extractions.

Sometimes premedication agents are used in addition to anesthesia. These agents help to relieve anxiety, produce sedation, and, in some cases, produce short-term anterograde amnesia. Oral or intravenous diazepam (Valium) or intravenous midazolam (Versed) are commonly used for preoperative sedation.[64]

Cataract patients, in general, have relatively little immediate postoperative pain. This is at least in part due to the long duration of action (up to 12 hours) of bupivacaine used in retrobulbar anesthesia.[60] Some practitioners recommend the use of oral analgesics, such as acetaminophen or ibuprofen, as needed, if the patient experiences minor discomfort in the immediate postsurgical period (see Chap. 7). Significant or persistent postoperative pain is considered to be abnormal and may be a symptom of such complications as corneal abrasion, bullous keratopathy, high IOP, or endophthalmitis.[65]

Optimizing Vision

The three methods of correcting distance vision after cataract extraction are aphakic spectacles, contact lenses, and

IOL implantation. The latter method is now used almost exclusively. The power of the IOL is determined by preoperative measurements of axial length and corneal curvature.

Although it is relatively easy to bring the spherical component of the refractive error close to emmetropia with an IOL, a residual astigmatic component may remain. Astigmatism may also be iatrogenically induced by incision and suturing techniques. With limbal incisions, a moderate amount of with-the-rule postoperative astigmatism (2 to 4 D) that decreases as the wound heals is considered to be normal.[31]

Several procedures, including using small incisions, modifying incision placement, and judiciously placing or removing sutures can be used to help control postoperative astigmatism surgically. The appropriate time to cut a suture for astigmatism control depends on the surgeon's technique. Continuous sutures, for example, should not be cut for at least 6 weeks after surgery. Single interrupted sutures placed specifically for astigmatism control, on the other hand, may be cut as early as one week after surgery.[65] Note that with continuing advances in surgical techniques, including the ''one-stitch'' and ''no stitch'' procedures, the need for suture removal to control astigmatism has diminished significantly.

To remove a suture, the eye must first be anesthetized topically with an agent such as 0.5% proparacaine. The eye also may be treated prophylactically with an antibiotic drop, such as 0.3% gentamicin or 0.3% tobramycin. Once the eye is anesthetized, a small beaver blade or 22 gauge needle is slipped under the suture to cut it near the inferior insertion. Forceps are then used to grasp the free end of the suture and pull it downward. Care should be taken to minimize the amount of exposed, contaminated suture that is pulled back through the cornea.[65] The wound integrity should be evaluated using the Seidel test (Fig. 31.1). This involves painting the wound site with topical sodium fluorescein and then examining it closely with a slit lamp under cobalt-filtered illumination. If aqueous is leaking from the wound (positive Seidel test), it will cause the fluorescein to glow bright green and stream downward.[66] If the Seidel test is negative, the patient should be prescribed a prophylatic topical antibiotic and followed as necessary. A similar technique may be used to remove symptomatic, protruding suture barbs in the late postoperative period.[67]

Topical steroids may control postoperative astigmatism pharmacologically. Increasing the dosage or duration of steroids can delay wound healing, which may reduce with-the-rule astigmatism.[31]

In the absence of other pathology, the patient's vision should be fully correctable within a few weeks after cataract surgery. Vision that is initially clear after cataract extraction, but then deteriorates, is suggestive of a postoperative complication such as capsular opacification, bullous keratopathy, cystoid macular edema, or retinal detachment.[65]

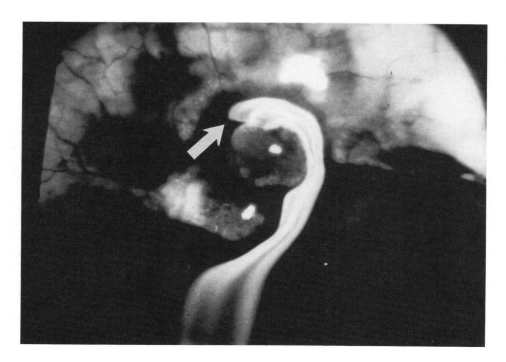

FIGURE 31.1   Positive Seidel test. Arrow points to site of wound leak highlighted by stream of sodium fluorescein. (Courtesy Oli Traustason, M.D.)

Managing Complications

Cataract extraction is considered to be a "safe" surgical procedure with relatively few postoperative complications.[135] Use of the newer small incision and "no stitch" techniques in preference to the larger incision techniques has reduced the rate of most complications even further. The most common complications noted in the early postopera-tive period include lid edema, subconjunctival hemorrhage, conjunctival injection, corneal edema, and anterior chamber reaction. Although serious complications are uncommon, the practitioner who is providing postoperative care must be able to diagnose and manage these conditions if they arise. Table 31.3 is a suggested guide to patient care following cataract extraction.[3] Note, however, that each surgeon has a preferred postoperative regimen and follow-up schedule.

TABLE 31.3
Postoperative Management of the Aphakic/Pseudophakic Patient

Examination Schedule	Medications	Examination	Patient Instructions
Immediately postoperative	• Topical antibiotic ointment or • Topical antibiotic-steroid ointment		• Eye shield, to be removed by practitioner • Return in 1 day • Acetaminophen or ibuprofen p.r.n.
Day 1	• Topical antibiotic and steroid drops q.i.d. • If IOP elevated, topical antiglaucoma therapy	• History • Visual acuity (pinhole) • Slit-lamp examination • Tonometry	• Use medications as prescribed • Acetaminophen or ibuprofen p.r.n. • Eye shield at bedtime • Wear glasses/sunglasses during day • Limit lifting or straining • Avoid rubbing eye • Return in 1 week
1 Week	• Taper antibiotic and steroid drops	• History • Visual acuity (pinhole) • Slit-lamp examination • Keratometry (optional) • Refraction (optional) • Tonometry • Dilated fundus examination if vision less than 20/50	• Same as day 1 instructions • Return in approximately 1 month
3–5 Weeks	• Discontinue medications	• History • Visual acuity (pinhole) • Slit-lamp examination • Keratometry • Refraction • Tonometry • Dilated fundus examination if vision less than 20/50 • If high astigmatism, cut suture, if appropriate • Check clarity of posterior capsule	• Discontinue eye shield • Prescribe spectacles or contact lens if refraction stable • Resume normal activity • Return in approximately 1 month
6–8 Weeks		• Similar to 3–5 week examination	• Return in approximately 4 months
6 Months		• History • Visual acuity (best-corrected) • Slit-lamp examination • Tonometry • Dilated fundus examination • Check clarity of lens capsule	

Complications of the Lids and Conjunctiva

Eyelid bruising and ptosis are caused by trauma from the lid speculum or local anesthesia. Bruising resolves spontaneously, as does ptosis, but the latter may persist and, if severe, require surgical correction.[65]

Subconjunctival hemorrhage is usually caused by damage to the episcleral vessels at the incision site and may appear to be enlarging as gravity pulls it downward. Subconjunctival hemorrhages typically resolve spontaneously within 2 to 3 weeks.[68]

Both the lids and conjunctiva may become red and edematous following surgery. A small amount of redness and edema during the first postoperative week is usually considered to be normal. These signs may be due to an allergic reaction to one of the topical postoperative medications or may be an indication of endophthalmitis. Allergic reactions can be managed by removing the sensitizing agent, while endophthalmitis requires more aggressive treatment.[69]

Endophthalmitis

As mentioned previously, mild to moderate inflammation is normal in the early postoperative period. However, severe inflammation or endophthalmitis is one of the most catastrophic postoperative complications. It can be classified as either infectious or sterile (aseptic).[10,69] *Staphylococcus epidermidis, S. aureus, Streptococcus, Proteus,* and *Pseudomonas* are the most common organisms that have been isolated in postoperative eyes with infectious endophthalmitis.[70] *Bacillus* species and *Propionibacterium acnes* are less common causes, and in rare cases fungal species are the infectious agent.[7,71] Acute endophthalmitis usually becomes manifest between 1 and 4 days following cataract surgery. Bacterial endophthalmitis is characterized by vitritis and a marked anterior chamber reaction with or without hypopyon (Fig. 31.2). It is often accompanied by severe reduction of visual acuity, pain, elevated IOP, proptosis, chemosis, and swollen eyelids.[69] The exception is endophthalmitis caused by *Propionibacterium acnes,* which has a delayed onset and indolent course similar to that seen with fungal infection.[71] If a bacterial or fungal infection is suspected, an anterior chamber or vitreous sample should be taken, and the fluid should be investigated aggressively using standard culture and smear techniques.[72]

Sterile endophthalmitis has many causes. It may be a phacoanaphylactic response to released crystalline lens material; a reaction to chemicals, drugs or foreign bodies introduced during surgery; or may rarely be a response to the IOL material. Sterile endophthalmitis typically begins 1 to 14 days following surgery. The inflammation is usually not as severe as in infectious endophthalmitis and is accompanied by little or no lid swelling or pain.[70]

Treatment of infectious endophthalmitis entails adminis-tration of broad-spectrum antibiotics into the vitreous in combination with systemic, periocular, and topical antibiotic therapy. Agents used include gentamicin, vancomycin, and cefazolin. Once the infectious organism has been identified and the patient has been on appropriate antibiotic therapy for at least 24 hours, steroids may be administered orally, subconjunctivally, and topically to reduce inflammation.[72,73] In advanced cases vitrectomy may be indicated.[74] The success of endophthalmitis treatment depends on both the virulence of the organism and the speed with which therapy is initiated.[74] Fortunately, endophthalmitis is an extremely rare complication of contemporary cataract surgery.[136]

Decreased Intraocular Pressure (Hypotony)

Decreased IOP, or hypotony, is caused by insufficient aqueous production or excessive aqueous drainage. Trauma to the ciliary body, or ciliochoroidal detachment due to cataract surgery, can result in low IOP and a shallow anterior chamber. The Seidel test will be negative. In most cases, ciliary body function and normal IOP will return spontaneously.[75]

Another cause of low IOP is wound leak. This is usually evident at the first postoperative visit and can be confirmed with a positive Seidel test. Wound leaks are managed initially by instilling a cycloplegic agent, such as 5% homatropine or 1% cyclopentolate, and patching the eye. A bandage contact lens may be used instead of an eye patch.[75] Topical or oral broad-spectrum antibiotics are administered to prevent infection, and topical steriods may be discontinued to promote wound healing. An alternate method is to introduce an air bubble into the anterior chamber through a limbal stab wound, then patch the eye. The air bubble serves to seal the leak and allows the aqueous to reform the anterior chamber.

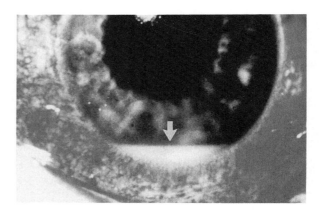

FIGURE 31.2 **Endophthalmitis with hypopyon (arrow). (Courtesy of Jeff Miller, O.D.)**

If neither of these methods is effective, surgical repair of the wound is necessary.[75]

A third potential cause of hypotony is the formation of a cyclodialysis cleft, which allows aqueous to leak under the conjunctiva into the suprachoroidal space. In such cases, the anterior chamber is shallow and the Seidel test is negative. Surgical repair or laser photocoagulation is used to treat this condition.[68,75]

Elevated Intraocular Pressure (Ocular Hypertension)

There are many causes of elevated IOP following cataract surgery, but most are related to impairment of aqueous outflow. Postoperative inflammation can cause changes in the blood/aqueous barrier with release of white blood cells and other inflammatory debris that block the trabecular meshwork. Other endogenous materials that can clog the trabecular meshwork include particles of retained lens nucleus or cortex, pigment, red blood cells, and vitreous.[76–78] In addition, the ingrowth of fibrous connective tissue or downgrowth of corneal epithelium introduced into the eye during surgery can cover the trabecular meshwork and block outflow.[79]

Certain exogenous materials may also impair aqueous outflow. Included in this group are the viscoelastic substances that are used to maintain the anterior chamber, expand the capsule, and protect the corneal endothelium during surgery[80] (see Table 19.3) Several studies[81–83] have shown that sodium hyaluronate, if not completely aspirated following IOL implantation, may cause an IOP rise, but this has been refuted in a study by Stamper and associates.[84] Burke and associates[85] found that retained 1% sodium hyaluronate was more likely to cause a longer duration of IOP elevation than a 3% sodium hyaluronate: 1% chondroitin sulfate combination (Viscoat).

Other exogenous agents include alpha-chymotrypsin, a chemical used for lysing zonules in ICCE procedures. It may elevate IOP during the first postoperative week.[86] Topical steroids, including those found in antibiotic/steroid combinations used routinely to control postoperative inflammation, can also cause ocular hypertension in susceptible patients.[87,88]

The location and placement of IOL implants may be responsible for IOP elevations in certain cases. Inflammation and damage caused by IOLs with haptics placed in the ciliary sulcus can cause the formation of peripheral anterior synechiae which, in turn, block aqueous outflow.[89] The positioning of the optic portion of certain lens designs, particularly anterior chamber IOLs, can prevent aqueous from passing through the pupil into the anterior chamber. This pupillary block causes iris bombé, narrowing of the anterior chamber, and elevated IOP.[68]

Another cause of postoperative ocular hypertension is a water-tight wound closure. This is more likely to occur with the newer, small incision, sutureless techniques than with the older, large incision procedures.[90]

Postoperative elevated IOP is treated according to the underlying etiology if it can be determined. For example, topical steroid therapy can be modified or discontinued if the patient is a steroid responder.[87] Nonspecific pressure rise is usually managed with apraclonidine, one drop 3 times daily, or a topical β blocker administered using a regimen of one drop twice daily. Carbonic anhydrase inhibitors may be added if a further decrease in aqueous production is necessary.[77,78] The need for these drugs often diminishes as the underlying condition causing impaired aqueous outflow resolves.

Pupillary block with an anterior chamber IOL can be prevented or treated with a surgical iridectomy or laser iridotomy.[68] In the case of a water-tight wound closure, sliding a 25-gauge needle into the wound site and allowing a small amount of aqueous to escape will immediately reduce IOP. Topical antiglaucoma medications are then used short-term to maintain IOP in the normal range.[91]

Corneal Edema

A certain amount of corneal edema is a normal finding immediately following cataract extraction. At the one-day postoperative visit, moderate to severe edema may cause visual acuity to be dramatically reduced; epithelial microcysts, bullae, and folds in Descemet's layer are often evident on slit lamp examination. This edema typically resolves over the next 1 to 2 weeks.[68,92]

Persistent microcystic edema may be associated with high IOP. Topical hyperosmotic agents, such as 5% sodium chloride or glycerin, may temporarily reduce the edema (see Chap. 15), but treatment of the underlying IOP elevation with antiglaucoma agents is necessary for long-term resolution of the problem.[92,93]

Bullous keratopathy is usually caused by damage to the corneal endothelium from prolonged use of intraocular irrigating solutions, trauma during surgery, or adherence of the vitreous, iris, or lens capsule to the corneal endothelium.[92,93] It is more likely to occur after phacoemulsification than following other extraction procedures, and occurs more often in patients with pre-existing corneal disease, such as Fuchs' dystrophy.[94,95] Minimizing the amount of phacoemulsification time and using viscoelastic substances help to protect the endothelium and reduce the incidence of bullous keratopathy.[68,95]

Bullous keratopathy affects all layers of the cornea (Fig. 31.3). Stromal and epithelial edema causes blurred vision, and erupting bullae can be quite painful. Prolonged edema can result in stromal vascularization and permanent vision loss.[96]

Initial treatment of bullous keratopathy involves reducing epithelial edema with topical hyperosmotic drops and/or

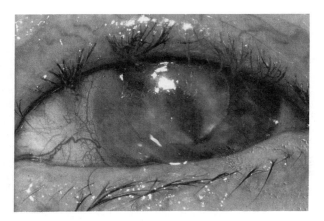

FIGURE 31.3   **Bullous keratopathy secondary to cataract extraction and anterior chamber IOL implantation.**

ointments. Warm air blown across the cornea using a hair dryer held at arm's length may also be helpful. Bandage contact lenses can reduce the pain of erupting bullae. Moderate to severe stromal edema may be reduced with an aggressive steroid regimen. In advanced cases where no response is seen following extensive topical steroid therapy and corneal decompensation is evident, penetrating keratoplasty may be the treatment of choice.[96,97]

Pupil Distortion

Pupil distortion can be caused by many factors. If a wound leak is present, a wick of vitreous or prolapsed iris may become incarcerated in the wound, causing a distorted or "peaked" pupil. The peak of the pupil often points toward the incarcerated area.[65]

Surgical trauma can also cause irregularly shaped pupils. In intracapsular procedures, inadvertent touching of the cryoextraction probe to the iris can cause permanent damage. In planned extracapsular procedures, the iris may become damaged if the surgeon attempts to remove the nucleus through an insufficiently dilated pupil. In phacoemulsification procedures, the iris can be traumatized by accidently touching it with the phacoemulsifier tip.[68,76] Occasionally the iris is damaged intentionally during cataract extraction. Patients whose pupils dilate poorly due to long-term miotic therapy may require a surgical sphincterotomy.[98]

Other causes of pupil distortion are related to the type and location of IOL implants. Some of the early iris-fixated and iris-plane lenses often caused square pupils, and some of the early anterior chamber IOLs, such as the Choyce lens, caused the pupil to be stretched ovally. The older lenses were also more likely to irritate the iris and anterior chamber

angle, causing chronic low-grade iritis. This, in turn, resulted in iris atrophy and synechiae formation.[99,100] These lenses have been replaced by newer designs that are less likely to cause pupil distortion and chronic inflammation. Although patients with iris-fixated IOLs are now encountered only rarely, it is important to remember that routine pupil dilation is contraindicated with these lenses. Inadvertent dilation can cause these lenses to become dislocated and create permanent damage by touching the retina or corneal endothelium.[100] Occasionally, the pupil will become distorted if the iris is captured by the edge of the IOL optic or if the lens becomes displaced (see Fig. 21.19.). Superior displacement of an IOL is called "sunrise syndrome," while inferior displacement is termed "sunset syndrome."[100,101]

Surgical or laser intervention is usually necessary to treat irregular pupils caused by iris or vitreous prolapse or by malpositioned IOLs.[98–100] If detected early, pupil distortion caused by IOL capture can occasionally be treated by dilating the pupil with mydriatic or mydriatic/cycloplegic agents, and applying gentle pressure to the sclera. Once synechiae have formed, however, surgical or laser procedures are usually needed to relieve the captured iris.[101] In general, the earlier the intervention, the more successful the pupil repair procedure.

Hyphema

Hyphema following cataract surgery may vary in appearance from a few red blood cells floating in the aqueous (microhyphema) to a distinct layer or clot of blood in the anterior chamber. Early in the postoperative period, a hyphema is usually caused by surgical trauma to the vessels of the sclera or iris.[76] It is more commonly associated with phacoemulsification through a scleral incision, but is occasionally seen with ECCE procedures.[31] It is also more likely to occur in patients with blood dyscrasias or those taking anticoagulants, such as Coumadin.[65]

In the late postoperative period, hyphemas may be caused by neovascularization and subsequent bleeding at the limbal wound, or by the IOL's chafing a vessel.[65] The UGH syndrome, a combination of chronic uveitis, glaucoma, and hyphema, is associated primarily with use of some of the early anterior chamber IOLs, but it can still occur with posterior chamber lenses if they become dislocated.[99,102]

Small hyphemas noted in the early postoperative period usually resolve spontaneously and require no treatment. The usual postoperative precautions of wearing a shield at bedtime and avoiding excessive lifting should be emphasized with these patients.[68] Significant hyphema (blood filling ≥50% of the anterior chamber) is more serious because it can cause elevated IOP and permanent blood staining of the cornea (Fig. 31.4). An anterior chamber washout procedure may be indicated with these patients and antiglaucoma therapy added, if necessary.[68,76]

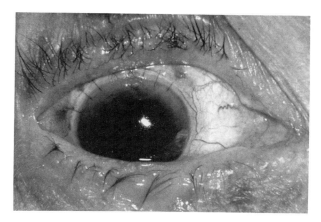

FIGURE 31.4   **Large "eight-ball" hyphema.**

Late hyphemas from neovascularization of the limbal wound can be prevented by laser photocoagulation.[68] Chronic UGH syndrome may be treated with topical steroids and cycloplegics to control inflammation, and ocular hypotensive medications to control glaucoma. Miotics, such as 1% pilocarpine, may also be used to fix the pupil and prevent iris chafing. The treatment of choice, however, is often surgical removal or replacement of the IOL.[102]

Capsular Opacification

Capsular opacification is one of the most common complications following otherwise uncomplicated planned extracapsular and phacoemulsification/aspiration procedures. The incidence may be as high as 50% in elderly patients and even higher in younger patients.[103,104]

Capsular opacification is caused by the proliferation of anterior lens epithelial cells that have migrated to the posterior capsule. These cells may form Elschnig pearls, thought to be an aberrant attempt at generating new lens fibers. Occasionally, capsular opacification is caused by fibrous metaplasia secondary to inflammation or a remnant of a posterior subcapsular cataract.[104]

Capsular opacification manifests clinically as a cloudy, wrinkled, or granular appearance of the posterior capsule and is visible with the slit lamp biomicroscope. The patient experiences reduced vision compared with the earlier postoperative acuity, and increased glare sensitivity. This typically becomes apparent several weeks to months after surgery.[65]

Posterior capsulotomy, a procedure in which an opening is made in the opacified capsule along the visual axis, was performed initially with a surgical knife or needle.[76] Most practitioners now use the noninvasive Nd:YAG laser tech-

nique, which creates a clear opening in the capsule via photodisruption of the involved tissues (Fig. 31.5).[105,106]

The Nd:YAG capsulotomy procedure, however, is not without complications. One of the most common complications is IOP elevation, which usually occurs within 4 hours after the procedure.[107] This can often be prevented by treating the eye with apraclonidine (Iopidine). The recommended dosage is one drop applied topically 1 hour prior to the capsulotomy, and one drop immediately after the procedure.[108,109] Topical β blockers and oral carbonic anhydrase inhibitors also can prevent or control post-capsulotomy pressure spikes.[106]

Another common complication associated with laser capsulotomy is anterior segment inflammation, which typically manifests as flare in the anterior chamber.[106,110] This can be prevented or treated with topical steroids. A suggested regimen is one drop of 1% prednisolone acetate administered 4 times daily for 4 to 7 days following the procedure.[9]

Other complications of Nd:YAG capsulotomy, though uncommon, are numerous. These include damage to the IOL, corneal endothelial cell loss and edema, iris hemorrhage, rupture of the anterior hyaloid face, cystoid macular edema, macular holes, and retinal detachment.[106,110]

Cystoid Macular Edema

Cystoid macular edema (CME) has long been recognized as a troublesome complication of cataract surgery. The syndrome, first described by Irvine,[111] is characterized by gradual reduction of visual acuity occurring several weeks or months following an uneventful cataract extraction. Although ophthalmoscopic and biomicroscopic retinal examinations may be normal, fluorescein angiography reveals

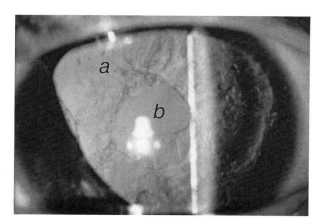

FIGURE 31.5   **Posterior capsule opacification (a) with clear central area (b) following Nd:YAG laser capsulotomy.**

cystic spaces of edema within the sensory retina in the macular area (see Fig. 32.1).[112,113] This condition usually resolves spontaneously,[114] but 1 to 2% of cases can become chronic and result in permanently reduced visual acuity.[115]

The pathophysiology of aphakic and pseudophakic CME is poorly understood. One theory is that vitreous fibers trapped in the wound cause traction on the macula. This, in turn, causes the perifoveal capillaries to leak and form cystoid macular edema. The use of posterior chamber IOLs and advances in surgical techniques have reduced the incidence of vitreous entrapment in the wound.[115]

Other investigators maintain that inflammation plays the major role in the development of postoperative CME.[111,112,116,117] An inflammatory process would help to explain many of the clinical signs and symptoms, the increased capillary permeability, and the retinal cellular infiltration.[117,118] An extremely important finding has been the association between prostaglandins and the inflammatory process seen in CME.[119,120] Prostaglandins are known to be released following the trauma of ocular surgery[121] or postoperative anterior uveal irritation,[115] and they are associated with disruption of the blood-aqueous barrier.[116,122] A transvitreal pathway from the anterior segment of the eye to the retina has been identified.[123] The ocular effects produced by prostaglandins are consistent with many of the anatomic changes seen in CME, such as capillary dilatation and increased capillary leakage, as well as disruption of the blood-aqueous barrier.[124] Prostaglandins also can induce miosis,[125] which can lead to vitreous loss and lysis of zonules supporting the lens.[126]

Chronic CME secondary to vitreous or iris incarceration in the wound may respond to Nd:YAG laser vitreolysis or anterior or posterior surgical vitrectomy. These procedures may be performed subsequent to, or concurrently with, pharmacologic therapy.[68,115] However, pharmacologic therapy is often ineffective in cases of chronic CME, where an abnormal anterior uveovitreal relationship exists.

Chronic CME that appears to be primarily inflammatory in nature has been treated with a variety of anti-inflammatory agents. Steroids have been used with variable success.[127] Systemic or peribulbar steroids may be more effective than topical administration, because the topical agents penetrate poorly to the posterior segment. The efficacy of steroids in the treatment of CME is unclear, because most of the studies to date have been uncontrolled patient series rather than double-masked randomized clinical trials.[115]

Nonsteroidal anti-inflammatory agents, which reduce or prevent the production of prostaglandins, have been used to prevent or treat CME associated with cataract surgery.[13] Neither topical fenoprofen[128] nor oral indomethacin[129] was shown to be effective; however, Flach and associates[130,131] showed some improvement in visual acuity after treatment of CME with topical ketorolac.

A third drug class that has been used to treat CME is the carbonic anhydrase inhibitors such as acetazolamide. They are thought to work by enhancing the fluid pumping action of the retinal pigment epithelium. This treatment appears to be effective in only a small percentage of patients with CME. In addition, the common systemic side effects of oral carbonic anhydrase inhibitors prevent them from being the treatment of choice in most cases.[132,133]

Retinal Detachment

Another serious complication of cataract surgery is retinal detachment. Kraff and Sanders,[134] in a series of 4,329 eyes, found the overall incidence of retinal detachment to be 1.4% in eyes that had had cataract extraction with posterior chamber IOL implantation. These investigators found the incidence in cases with an intact posterior capsule to be 0.8%, while the incidence in cases with an opened capsule increased to 1.9%. They also found that high axial myopes had a greater risk of retinal detachment following surgery, and a combination of axial myopia and open capsule increased the risk 10-fold.

It is important for the primary eye care provider to be aware of the increased risk of postoperative retinal detachment when counseling patients with high myopia or lattice degeneration about the risks and benefits of cataract surgery. The practitioner should perform a dilated fundus examination (see Chap. 21) as part of routine preoperative and postoperative care, so that retinal tears and detachments can be detected and treated in a timely fashion.[67]

References

1. Stark WJ, Leske MC, Worthen DM, et al. Trends in cataract surgery and intraocular lenses in the United States. Am J Ophthalmol 1983;96:304–310.
2. Stark WJ, Whitney CE, Chandler JW, et al. Trends in intraocular lens implantation in the United States. Arch Ophthalmol 1986; 104:1769–1770.
3. Cataract Management Guideline Panel. Management of functional impairment due to cataract in adults. Guideline Report, number 4. Rockville, MD. U.S. Department of Health and Human Services, Public Health Service, Agency for Health Care Policy and Research. AHCPR Pub. No. 93–0541. August 1993.
4. Percival SPB, ed. Color atlas of lens implantation. St. Louis: Mosby-Yearbook, 1991.
5. Ajamian PC. Pre- and postoperative care of the cataract patient. Boston: Butterworth-Heinemann 1993:51–58.
6. Bezan D, Halverson K, Schaffer K, Thomas P. Optometric guide to surgical co-management. Boston: Butterworth-Heinemann 1992:v.
7. Peyman GA, Daun M. Prophylaxis of endophthalmitis. Ophthalmic Surg 1994;25:671–674.
8. Hall GW. Operative profile. Ocular Surg News 1993;11:98.
9. Weinstein GW. Cataract surgery. In: Tasman W, Jaeger EA, eds.

Duane's clinical ophthalmology. Philadelphia: J.B. Lippincott, 1990;5(7):35.

10. Allen HF, Grove AS. Early acute aseptic iritis after cataract extraction. Trans Am Acad Ophthalmol Otolaryngol 1976;81: 145–150.

11. Jaffe NS, Jaffe MS, Jaffe GE. Cataract surgery and its complications. St. Louis: C.V. Mosby Co, 1993:543–559.

12. Yourston D, Whicher J, Chambers R, et al. The acute phase response in acute anterior uveitis. Trans Ophthalmol Soc UK 1985;104:166–170.

13. Flach AJ. Cyclo-oxygenase inhibitors in ophthalmology. Surv Ophthalmol 1992;36:259–284.

14. Fearnley IR, Spalton DJ, Smith SE. Anterior segment fluorophotometry in acute anterior uveitis. Arch Ophthalmol 1987;105: 1550–1555.

15. Flach AJ, Graham J, Kruger L, et al. Quantitative assessment of postsurgical breakdown of the blood aqueous barrier following administration of ketorolac tromethamine solution: A double-masked, paired comparison with vehicle-placebo solution study. Arch Ophthalmol 1988;106:344–347.

16. Mishima S, Tanishima T, Masuda K. Pathophysiology and pharmacology of intraocular surgery. Aust NZ J Ophthalmol 1985;13: 147–158.

17. Sawa M. Clinical application of laser flare-cell meter. Jpn J Ophthalmol 1990;34:346–363.

18. Hogan MJ, Kimura SJ, Thygeson P. Signs and symptoms of uveitis. Am J Ophthalmol 1959;47:155–170.

19. Komuro Y, Matsumoto S, Shirato S, et al. A new apparatus for automatic counting of aqueous floaters. Acta Soc Ophthalmol Jpn 1985;89:556–561.

20. Sawa M, Tsurimaki Y, Tsuru T, et al. New quantitative method to determine protein and cells in aqueous in vivo. Jpn J Ophthalmol 1988;32:132–142.

21. Sanders DR, Kraff MC. Steroidal and nonsteroidal anti-inflammatory agents. Effects on postsurgical inflammation and blood-aqueous barrier breakdown. Arch Ophthalmol 1984;102:1453–1456.

22. Flach AJ, Stegman RC, Graham J. Prophylaxis of aphakic cystoid macular edema without corticosteroids. Ophthalmology 1990;97: 1253–1258.

23. Duke-Elder S. The clinical value of cortisone and ACTH in ocular disease. Br J Ophthalmol 1951;35:637.

24. Knope MM. A double-blind study of fluorometholone. Am J Ophthalmol 1970;69:739–740.

25. Burde RM, Waltman SR. Topical corticosteroids after cataract surgery. Ann Ophthalmol 1972;4:290.

26. Mustakallio A, Kaufman HE, Johnston G, et al. Corticosteroid efficacy in postoperative uveitis. Ann Ophthalmol 1973;5:719–730.

27. Corboy JM. Corticosteroid therapy for the reduction of postoperative inflammation after cataract extraction. Am J Ophthalmol 1976;82:923–927.

28. Ramsell TG, Bartholomew RS, Walker SR. Clinical evaluation of clobetasone butyrate: A comparative study of its effects in postoperative inflammation and on intraocular pressure. Br J Ophthalmol 1980;64:43–45.

29. Buxton JN, Smith DE, Brownstein S. Cataract extraction and subconjunctival repository corticosteroids. Ann Ophthalmol 1971;3:1376–1379.

30. Lehmann R, Assil K, Stewart R, et al. Comparison of rimexolone

1% ophthalmic suspension to placebo in control of postcataract surgery inflammation. Invest Ophthalmol Vis Sci 1995;36(suppl): S793.

31. Ajamian PC. Pre- and postoperative care of the cataract patient. Boston: Butterworth-Heinemann, 1993:72–82.

32. Stewart RH, Smith JP, Rosenthal AL. Ocular pressure response to fluorometholone acetate and dexamethasone sodium phosphate. Curr Eye Res 1984;3:835–839.

33. Vane JR. Inhibition of prostaglandin synthesis as a mechanism of action of aspirin-like drugs. Nature 1971;231:232–235.

34. Jaanus SD. Anti-inflammatory drugs. In: Bartlett JD, Jaanus SD, eds. Clinical ocular pharmacology, ed. 2. Boston: Butterworth-Heinemann, 1989:163–197.

35. Flower RJ, Moncada S, Vane JR. Analgesic-antipyretics and anti-inflammatory agents. Drugs employed in the treatment of gout. In Gilman AG, Goodman LS, Rall TW, et al, eds. The pharmacological basis of therapeutics. New York: McMillan Co, 1985:674–715.

36. Waitzman MB. Possible new concepts relating prostaglandins to various ocular functions. Surv Ophthalmol 1970;14:301–326.

37. Podos SM. Prostaglandins, nonsteroidal anti-inflammatory agents and eye disease. Trans Am Ophthalmol Soc 1976;74:637–660.

38. Kulkarni PS, Srinivasan BD. Nonsteroidal anti-inflammatory drugs in ocular inflammatory conditions. In: Lews AS, Furst DE, eds. Nonsteroidal anti-inflammatory drugs. New York: Marcel Dekker, 1987:Chap. 7.

39. Kramer SG, Oyakawa RT, Drake M. Enhancement of pupillary dilation during intraocular surgery by prostaglandin inhibition. Invest Ophthalmol Vis Sci 1976;15:63.

40. Bito LZ. Species differences in the responses of the eye to irritation and trauma, an hypothesis of divergence in ocular defense mechanisms, and the choice of experimental animals for eye research. Exp Eye Res 1984;39:807–829.

41. Mishima S, Masuda K. Clinical complications of prostaglandins and synthesis inhibitors. In: Leopold RH, Burns RP, eds. Symposium on ocular therapy, vol 10. New York: John Wiley, 1977:1–19.

42. Tsuchisaka H, Takase M. Topical flurbiprofen in intraocular surgery on diabetic and nondiabetic patients. Ann Ophthalmol 1985; 17:577–581.

43. Keulen-DeVos HC, VanRij JCG, deLavalette J, et al. Effect of indomethacin in preventing surgically induced miosis. Br J Ophthalmol 1983;67:94–96.

44. Keates RH, McGowan KA. The effect of topical indomethacin in maintaining mydriasis during cataract surgery. Ann Ophthalmol 1984;16:1116–1121.

45. Keates RH, McGowan KA. Clinical trial of flurbiprofen to maintain pupillary dilation during cataract surgery. Ann Ophthalmol 1984;16:919–921.

46. Stark WJ, Fagadu WR, Stewart RH. Reduction of pupillary constriction during cataract surgery using suprofen. Arch Ophthalmol 1986;104:364–366.

47. Bito LZ. Surgical miosis: Have we been misled by a bunch of rabbits? Ophthalmology 1990;97:1–2.

48. Mochizuki M, Sawa M, Masuda K. Topical indomethacin in intracapsular extraction of senile cataract. Jpn J Ophthalmol 1977; 21:215–226.

49. Sanders DR, Kraff MC, Lieberman HL, et al. Breakdown and reestablishment of the blood aqueous barrier following implant surgery. Arch Ophthalmol 1982;100:588–590.

50. Arie M, Sawa M, Takase M. Effect of topical indomethacin on the

blood aqueous barrier after intracapsular extraction of senile cataract—a fluorophotometric study. Jpn J Ophthalmol 1981;25:237–247.

51. Sabiston DW. Non-steroidal anti-inflammatory agents for post-cataract patients. Trans Ophthalmol Soc NZ 1983;35:98–100.

52. Sabiston D, Tessler H, Sumers K, et al. Reduction of inflammation following cataract surgery by the nonsteroidal anti-inflammatory drug, flurbiprofen. Ophthalmic Surg 1987;18:873–877.

53. Hillman JS, Frank GJ, Kheskani MB. Flurbiprofen and human intraocular inflammation. In: Samuelsson B, Ramwell PW, Paoletti R, eds. Advances in prostaglandin and thromboxane research. New York: Raven Press,1980:1723–1725.

54. Sabiston DW, Robinson IG. An evaluation of the anti-inflammatory effect of flurbiprofen after cataract extraction. Br J Ophthalmol 1987;71:418–421.

55. Flach AJ, Lavelle CJ, Olander KW, et al. The effect of ketorolac tromethamine solution 0.5% in reducing postoperative inflammation after cataract extraction and intraocular lens implantation. Ophthalmology 1988;95:1279–1284.

56. Ronen S, Rozenman Y, Zylbermann R, Berson D. Treatment of ocular inflammation with diclofenac sodium: Double-blind trial following cataract surgery. Ann Ophthalmol 1985;17:577–581.

57. Vickers FF, McGuigan LJB, Ford C, et al. The effect of diclofenac sodium ophthalmic on the treatment of postoperative inflammation. Invest Ophthalmol Vis Sci 1991;32(suppl):793.

58. Jaffe NS, Jaffe MS, Jaffe GE. Cataract surgery and its complications. St. Louis: C.V. Mosby Co, 1993:341–358.

59. Aquavella JV. Comment (Limbal anesthesia for cataract surgery). Ophthalmic Surg 1990;21:26.

60. Wilson RP. Local anesthesia in ophthalmology. In: Tasman W, ed. Duane's clinical ophthalmology. Philadelphia: JB Lippincott Co, 1991;5:1–20.

61. Zahl K, Jordan A, McGroaty J, et al. Peribulbar anesthesia. Effect of bicarbonate on mixtures of lidocaine, bupivacaine and hyaluronidase with or without epinephrine. Ophthalmology 1991;98:239–242.

62. Furata M, Toriumi T, Kashiwagi K et al. Limbal anesthesia for cataract surgery. Ophthalmic Surg 1990;21:22–25.

63. Redmond RM, Dallas NL. Extracapsular cataract extraction under local anesthesia without retrobulbar injection. Br J Ophthalmol 1990;74:203–204.

64. Jaffe NS, Jaffe MS, Jaffe GE. Cataract surgery and its complications. St. Louis: C.V. Mosby Co, 1993:34–35.

65. Bezan D, Halverson K, Schaffer K, Thomas P. Optometric guide to surgical co-management. Boston: Butterworth-Heinemann, 1992:16–47.

66. Drake S. There must be more to Seidel test. Rev Optom 1992; Jun:28.

67. Dornic D. How to treat suture barbs. Rev Optom 1987:67–68.

68. Ajamian PC. Pre- and postoperative care of the cataract patient. Boston: Butterworth-Heinemann, 1993:83–110.

69. Wilson FM, Wilson FM II. Postoperative uveitis. In: Tasman W, ed. Duane's clinical ophthalmology. Philadelphia: JB Lippincott Co. 1990;4:1–18.

70. Driebe WT, Mandelbaum S, Forster RK, et al. Pseudophakic endophthalmitis: Diagnosis and management. Ophthalmology 1986;93:442–448.

71. Sawusch MR, Michels RG, Stark WJ, et al. Endophthalmitis due to *Propionibacterium acnes* sequestered between IOL optic and posterior capsule. Ophthalmic Surg 1989;20:90–92.

72. Allen HF. Bacterial endophthalmitis after cataract extraction. In: Bellows JG, ed. Cataract and abnormalities of the lens. New York: Grune & Stratton, 1975:421–428.

73. Stonecipher KG, Parmley VC, Jensen H, et al. Infectious endophthalmitis following sutureless cataract surgery. Arch Ophthalmol 1991;109:1562–1563.

74. Mandelbaum S, Forster RK. Bacterial endophthalmitis. In: Fraunfelder FT, Roy FH. Current ocular therapy, ed. 3. Philadelphia: WB Saunders Co, 1990:533–535.

75. Jaffe NS, Jaffe MS, Jaffe GE. Cataract surgery and its complications. St. Louis: C.V. Mosby Co, 1993:366–375.

76. Goodman DF, Stark WJ, Gottsch JD. Complications of cataract extraction with intraocular lens implantation. Ophthalmic Surg 1989;20:132–140.

77. Kooner KS, Cooksey JC, Perry P, et al. Intraocular pressure following ECCE, phacoemulsification and PC-IOL implantation. Ophthalmic Surg 1988;19:570–575.

78. Rowes JR. Postoperative IOP in cataract surgery. Ophthalmic Surg 1989;20:145–146.

79. Loane M, Weinreb R. Glaucoma secondary to epithelial downgrowth and 5–fluorouracil. Ophthalmic Surg 1990;21:704–706.

80. Liesegang TJ. Viscoelastic substances in ophthalmology. Surv Ophthalmol 1990;34:268–293.

81. Passo MS, Ernest JT, Goldstick TK. Hyaluronate (Healon) increases intraocular pressure when used in cataract extraction. Br J Ophthalmol 1985;69:572–575.

82. Glasser DB, Matsuda M, Edelhauser HF. A comparison of the efficacy and toxicity of and intraocular pressure response to viscous solutions in the anterior chamber. Arch Ophthalmol 1986; 104:1819–1824.

83. McRae SM, Edelhauser HF, Hyndiuk RA. The effects of Healon, chondroitin sulfate and methylcellulose on the corneal endothelium and intraocular pressure. Am J Ophthalmol 1983;95:333–341.

84. Stamper RL, Diloreto D, Schacknow P. Effect of intraocular aspiriation of sodium hyaluronate on postoperative intraocular pressure. Ophthalmic Surg 1990;21:486–491.

85. Burke S, Sugar J, Farber MD. Comparison of the effects of two viscoelastic agents, Healon and Viscoat, on postoperative intraocular pressure after penetrating keratoplasty. Ophthalmic Surg 1990;21:821–826.

86. Jaffe NS, Jaffe MS, Jaffe GE. Cataract surgery and its complications. St. Louis: C.V. Mosby Co, 1993:400–402.

87. Mindel JS, Tavitian HO, Smith H, Walker EC. Comparative ocular pressure elevations by medrysone, fluorometholone, and dexamethasone phosphate. Arch Ophthalmol 1980;98:1577–1578.

88. Bartlett JD, Woolley TW, Adams CM. Identification of high intraocular pressure responders to topical ophthalmic corticosteroids. J Ocular Pharmacol 1993;9:35–45.

89. Evans RB. Peripheral anterior synechia overlying the haptics of posterior chamber lenses: Occurrence and natural history. Ophthalmology 1990;94:415–423.

90. Ernest PH, Grabow HB, McFarland MS. Advantages and disadvantages of sutureless surgery. In: Gills JP, Martin RG, Sanders DR, eds. Sutureless cataract surgery. Thorofare, NJ: Slack, Inc., 1992:50.

91. Stewart RH, Kimbrough RL, Davidovski F. Office management of excessive postoperative intraocular pressure. Ophthalmic Surg 1989;20:824.

92. Jaffe NS, Jaffe MS, Jaffe GE. Cataract surgery and its complications. St. Louis: C.V. Mosby Co, 1993:412–433.

93. Koch DD. The dilemma of pseudophakic bullous keratopathy. Ophthalmic Surg 1989;20:463–464.

94. Lugo M, Cohen EJ, Eagle RC, et al. The incidence of preoperative endothelial dystrophy in pseudophakic bullous keratopathy. Ophthalmic Surg 1988;19:16–19.

95. Ajamian PC. Pre- and postoperative care of the cataract patient. Boston: Butterworth-Heinemann, 1993:88–99.

96. Sugar J. Corneal edema. In: Fraunfelder FT, Roy FH. Current ocular therapy, 3rd ed., Philadelphia: WB Saunders Co. 1990:442.

97. Kornmehl EW, Steinert RF, Odich MG. Penetrating keratoplasty for pseudophakic bullous keratopathy associated with closed loop anterior chamber intraocular lenses. Ophthalmology 1990;97:407–414.

98. Jaffe NS, Jaffe MS, Jaffe GE. Cataract surgery and its complications. St. Louis: C.V. Mosby Co,1993:68.

99. Findley HM, Dilorio RC. A review of intraocular lenses. J Am Optom Assoc 1984;55:811–817.

100. Ajamian PC. Pre- and postoperative care of the cataract patient. Boston: Butterworth-Heinemann 1993:104–110.

101. Lindstrom RL, Herman WK. Pupil capture: Prevention and management. Am Intra-ocular Implant Soc J 1983;9:201–204.

102. Percival SPB. UGH syndrome after posterior chamber lens implantation. Am Intraocular Implant Soc J 1983;9:200.

103. Moisseieve J, Bartov E, Schochat A, et al. Long-term study of the prevalence of capsular opacification following extracapsular cataract extraction. Ophthalmic Surg 1989;20:321–324.

104. Maltzman BA, Haupt E, Notic C. Relationship between age at time of cataract extraction and time interval before capsulotomy for opacification. Ophthalmic Surg 1989;20:321–324.

105. Mainster MA, Ho PC, Mainster KJ. Nd:YAG laser photodisrupters. Ophthalmology 1983;90:45–47.

106. Aron-Rosa D, Abitbol Y. Laser capsulotomy. Ophthalmol Clin N Am 1989;2:549–554.

107. Richter CU, Arzeno G, Pappas HR, et al. Intraocular pressure elevation following Nd:YAG laser posterior capsulotomy. Ophthalmology 1985;92:636–640.

108. Pollack IP, Brown RH, Crandall AS, et al. Prevention of the rise in intraocular pressure following neodymium YAG posterior capsulotomy using topical 1% apraclonidine. Arch Ophthalmol 1988;106:754–757.

109. Robin AL. Medical management of acute postoperative intraocular pressure rises associated with anterior segment ophthalmic laser surgery. In Ophthalmol Clin 1990;30:102–110.

110. Flohr MJ, Robin AL, Kelley JS. Early complications of Q-switched neodymium:YAG posterior capsulotomy. Ophthalmology 1985;92:360–363.

111. Irvine SR. A newly defined vitreous syndrome following cataract surgery: Interpreted according to recent concepts of the structure of the vitreous. Am J Ophthalmol 1953;36:699–719.

112. Gass JDM, Norton EWD. Cystoid macular edema and papilledema following cataract extraction. Arch Ophthalmol 1966;76:646–661.

113. Jampol LM, Sanders DR, Draff MC. Prophylaxis and therapy of aphakic cystoid macular edema. Surv Ophthalmol 1984;28(suppl):535–539.

114. Jacobson DR, Dellaporta A. Natural history of cystoid macular edema after cataract extraction. Am J Ophthalmol 1974;77:445–447.

115. Spaide RF, Yannuzzi LA. Post-cataract surgery cystoid macular edema. Clin Signs Ophthalmol 1992;8:2–15.

116. Cunha-Vaz JG, Travassos A. Breakdown of the blood-retinal barriers and cystoid macular edema. Surv Ophthalmol 1984;28(suppl):485–492.

117. Martin WF, Green WR, Martin LW. Retinal phlebitis in the Irvine-Gass syndrome. Am J Ophthalmol 1977;83:377–386.

118. Sears ML. Aphakic cystoid macular edema. The pharmacology of ocular trauma. Surv Ophthalmol 1984;28(suppl):525–534.

119. Kremer M, Bailkoff G, Charbonnel B. The release of prostaglandins in human aqueous after intraocular surgery; effect of indomethacin. Prostaglandins 1982;23:695–702.

120. Miyake K. Prostaglandins as a causative factor of the cystoid macular edema after lens extraction. Acta Soc Ophthalmol Jpn 1977;81:1449–1464.

121. Eakins KE. Prostaglandin and non-prostaglandin mediated breakdown of the blood-aqueous barrier. Exp Eye Res 1977;80(suppl):483–498.

122. Bonnet M, Bievelez B. Iris fluorescein angiography and Irvine-Gass syndrome. Albrecht vonGraefes Arch klin Exp Ophthalmol 1980;213:187–194.

123. Peyman GA, Spitznas M, Straatsma BR. Chorioretinal diffusion of peroxidase before and after photocoagulation. Invest Ophthalmol 1971;10:489–495.

124. Gass JDM, Norton EWD. Follow-up of aphakic cystoid macular edema. Trans Am Acad Ophthalmol Otolaryngol 1969;73:665–682.

125. Camras CB, Miranda OC. The putative role of prostaglandins in surgical miosis. In: Bito LZ, Stjernschantz J, eds. The ocular effects of prostaglandins and other eicosanoids. New York: Alan R Liss, 1989.

126. Guzek JP, Holm M, Cotter JB, et al. Risk factors for intraoperative complications in 1000 extracapsular cataract cases. Ophthalmology 1987;94:461–466.

127. McDonnell PJ, Ryan SJ, Walonker AF, et al. Prediction of visual acuity recovery in cystoid macular edema. Ophthalmic Surg 1992;23:354–358.

128. Burnett J, Tessler M, Isenberg S, et al. Double masked trial of fenoprofen sodium treatment of chronic aphakic cystoid macular edema. Ophthalmic Surg 1983;14:150–152.

129. Yannuzzi LA, Klein RM, Watlyn RH, et al. Ineffectiveness of indomethacin in the treatment of chronic cystoid macular edema. Am J Ophthalmol 1977;84:517–519.

130. Flach AJ, Dolan BJ, Irvine AR. Effectiveness of ketorolac 0.5% solution for chronic aphakic and pseudophakic cystoid macular edema. Am J Ophthalmol 1987;103:479–486.

131. Flach AJ, Jampol LM, Weinberg D, et al. Improvement in visual acuity in chronic aphakic and pseudophakic cystoid macular edema after treatment with topical ketorolac tromethamine. Am J Ophthalmol 1991;112:514–519.

132. Cox SN, Hay E, Bird AC. Treatment of chronic macular edema with acetazolamide. Arch Ophthalmol 1988;106:1190–1195.

133. Tripathi RC, Fekrat S, Tripathi BJ, et al. A direct correlation of the

resolution of pseudophakic cystoid macular edema with acetazolamide therapy. Ann Ophthalmol 1991;23:121–124.

134. Kraff MC, Sanders DR. Incidence of retinal detachment following posterior chamber intraocular lens surgery. J Cataract Refract Surg 1990;16:477–480.

135. Powe NR, Schein OD, Gieser SC, et al. Synthesis of the literature on visual acuity and complications following cataract extraction with intraocular lens implantation. Arch Ophthalmol 1994;112: 239–252.

136. Javitt JC, Street DA, Tielsch JM, et al. National outcomes of cataract extraction. Retinal detachment and endophthalmitis after outpatient cataract surgery. Ophthalmology 1994;101:100–106.

Diseases of the Retina

Larry J. Alexander

Although diseases of the retina, specifically of the macular area, represent a serious threat to vision, pharmacologic management of these conditions has been disappointing. This chapter considers only retinal conditions in which pharmacologic intervention has a major role in diagnosis or therapy.

Fluorescein Angiography

Fluorescein angiography and oral fluorography are gaining importance as diagnostic tools now that new developments are being made in laser treatment of retinal vascular disease. Laser modifications and a better understanding of ocular vasculopathy allow for earlier therapeutic intervention, treatment closer to the foveal avascular zone (FAZ), and better visual results.

Fluorescein has been used in vision care for over 100 years.[1] Oral administration fluorescein to study the retinal vasculature was attempted in 1910.[2] The first use of intravenous fluorescein was reported in 1930,[3] and several other reports followed over the next 30 years. In 1961, photographs were used to document fluorescein studies, allowing for a more detailed and logical approach to understanding fluorescein angiography.[4] The first comprehensive text on fluorescein studies was published in 1977[5] and was soon followed by other works.[6]

The concept of oral fluorography was reintroduced in 1979 to allow fluorescein studies without potential systemic side effects.[7] Further studies in oral fluorography established the technique as an effective viable alternative in the diagnosis of retinal vascular diseases.[8,9] The Oral Fluorescein Study Group was formed in 1984 to further evaluate the orally administered fluorescein technique. The Group's report, published in 1985, concluded that oral fluorography was not a substitute for the diagnostic capabilities of intravenous fluorescein angiography but was a significant diagnostic tool, especially for fundus disorders that demonstrated fluorescein leakage. That report also established the fact that minimal side effects occur with oral fluorescein administration.[10]

Fluorescein angiography is especially useful in detecting subclinical retinal changes in diabetic patients. Yamana and associates[11] reported that of 272 eyes of 166 patients with no ophthalmoscopically visible vascular changes, fluorescein angiography demonstrated diabetic vascular changes in 66.5%. Other studies have found angiographic changes in diabetic children that were not observed by ophthalmoscopy alone.[12,13] Fluorescein studies also have demonstrated significant vascular changes in the mid-periphery that were overlooked previously.[14] Prudent clinical judgment dictates that fluorescein studies be performed in diabetic patients with any unexplained reduction in macular function, with encroachment of diabetic retinopathy into the macular area, with any sign of proliferative retinopathy, with the appearance of intraretinal microvascular abnormalities (IRMA), and with the appearance of 3 or more signs of preproliferative diabetic retinopathy.

New technology demonstrates that infrared scanning laser fluorescein angiography, using both fluorescein and indocyanine green, can facilitate the early detection of choroidal and retinal vascular anomalies.[15–19] Experimental work with calcein dye, which remains in the circulatory system longer, also may improve imaging characteristics.[20] New work in targeted dye delivery, utilizing lipid-enveloped fluorescein, promises to improve visualization by eliminating cluttering of the image caused by background fluorescence, as found in current studies.[21] In addition, digitization of images is improving our ability to differentially diagnose both retinal and choroidal conditions.[22-23] Table 32.1 lists some ocular disease processes that indicate the need for fluorescein angiography to assist in the differential diagnosis and management.

Technique

Fluorescein studies may be performed with or without an appropriate fundus camera. If performed with a binocular indirect ophthalmoscope, the technique is known as fluorescein angioscopy. To perform fluorescein angioscopy successfully, the binocular indirect ophthalmoscope must be equipped with a high-intensity light source and appropriate filters.

If fluorescein photographic studies are desired, it is necessary to use a fundus camera equipped with a high-intensity flash system, a rapid recycle time, and appropriate blue excitation and yellow-green barrier filters. The excitation filter should be the Baird Atomic B4 470 or Kodak

TABLE 32.1
Ocular Diseases Indicating the Need for Fluorescein Angiography

Acute posterior multifocal placoid pigment epitheliopathy (APMPPE)
Angiomatosis retinae
Anterior ischemic optic neuropathy
Behçet's disease
Branch retinal vein occlusion
Cavernous hemangioma of the retina
Choroidal rupture (when developing choroidal neovascularization)
Coats' disease (Retinal Telangiectasia)
Cystoid maculopathy (Irvine-Gass syndrome)
Diabetic retinopathy
Eale's disease
Fuchs' spot (degenerative myopia)
Hemicentral retinal vein occlusion
Idiopathic central serous choroidopathy
Iris neovascularization
Maculopathy of angioid streaks
Malignant choroidal melanoma
Preretinal macular fibrosis
Presumed ocular histoplasmosis (macular changes)
Proliferative peripheral retinal disease
Retinal capillary hemangioma
Retinal macroaneurysm
Retinal pigment epithelial dystrophies (central)
Retinal pigment epithelial detachment
Retinal tumors
Sensory retinal detachments
Tumors of the iris and ciliary body

Wratten 47 to create wavelengths to stimulate fluorescence. The barrier filter should be a Kodak Wratten B, Ilford 109 Delta Chromatic 3, or Kodak Wratten G15 to block the exciting light from the film plane, allowing only visualization of the fluorescing blood.[24] Note that both barrier and excitation filters lose specificity (fade) with age and should be replaced according to manufacturer's guidelines. It is also advisable to fit the camera back with a power winder, since the early phases of fluorescein studies necessitate rapid-fire photography.

Several films and developing processes are available to enhance study results. Although any high-speed 200 to 400 ASA black-and-white film can be used, it is difficult to advise on processing. It is best to contact a local film processing laboratory or an experienced angiographer regarding optimal processing and film use. Some practitioners advocate using color film to eliminate autofluorescence,[25] but adoption of this technique has met with resistance. Using Kodak T-Max P3200 (3200 ASA) film for fluorescein angiography allows the photographer to reduce the flash intensity and thus perform the study more effectively on patients known to be severely photophobic.[26]

Although other dyes have been used,[27] sodium fluorescein is still the accepted standard. Sodium fluorescein for intravenous injection is available in 10% and 25% concentrations. Generic brands are available at considerably reduced cost and may be used without fear. One study does, however, report the presence of a toxic substance, dimethyl formamide, an industrial solvent, in commercially prepared sodium fluorescein for injection.[28] Moreover, outdated fluorescein carries the potential for side effects, such as an increase in the incidence of nausea. It is advised that some form of documentation of informed consent be obtained from the patient prior to performing fluorescein angiography.[29]

Sodium fluorescein is considered pharmacologically inert and fluoresces when stimulated by an excited light source. Fluorescein is injected into a suitable vein in the antecubital space or on the hand. It reaches ocular circulation bound to serum albumin and in a free, unbound state. This then fluoresces, allowing for easy visualization of vascular alterations and leakage from altered vessels. Factors affecting the quality of the results include clarity of the ocular media, maximal dilation of the pupil, and especially the concentration of fluorescein reaching the retinal-choroidal vascular system.[30] Improper injection is the most significant factor contributing to decreased retinal-choroidal concentration. The injection must be into the vein and performed within 10 to 15 seconds.

A crash cart (cardiopulmonary resuscitation unit) must be available on site to accommodate any potential side effects. Before the procedure the practitioner must ensure the following: (1) an informed consent form has been read and signed by the patient (see Chap. 5), (2) the patient is aware of what is about to happen, (3) the patient's pupils are maximally dilated, (4) color photographs of the fundus have been taken, (5) red-free photographs of the fundus have been taken on the black-and-white angiographic film, (6) the fundus camera and patient are adjusted to a comfortable height, (7) the filters are placed in the camera, (8) the proper flash settings are made, and (9) an appropriate intravenous line has been established and maintained with heparinized saline. Next, 5 ml of 10% sodium fluorescein should be ready in a syringe to replace the heparinized saline. The patient should be situated in the camera and the syringe of fluorescein should be attached. When the appropriate area of the fundus is in focus and the filters are moved into place, the bolus of fluorescein should be injected rapidly. The photography usually begins within approximately 15 seconds, which is the choroidal flush phase. Rapid sequence photographs are taken within the first few minutes, then intermittently for the next 10 to 20 minutes. Late phase photographs will detect leakage problems such as sensory retinal detachments associated with choroidal neovascular nets. Particular timing sequences depend on the suspected disease being investigated.

Complications

Complications are inherent in any procedure such as fluorescein angiography. Fortunately, the more common complications can be managed easily without aborting the diagnostic procedure. One study[31] reported adverse reactions in 4.82% of 5000 procedures. Of these, nausea was most frequent (2.24%), followed by vomiting (1.78%) and urticaria and pruritus (0.34%). No higher rate of side effects was found when 25% sodium fluorescein was used than when 10% sodium fluorescein was employed.[31] The itching and hives are thought to be associated with a change in the plasma complement associated with a rise in the histamine level.[32] In another study[33] of 2631 procedures, it was found that males and young patients experienced side effects at a higher rate. In this study, only one life-threatening event, acute pulmonary edema, was reported.[33]

Although some clinicians[34] discount the beneficial effect of prophylaxis against the side effects of fluorescein, a double-blind study reported that 20 mg of intravenous metoclopramide hydrochloride significantly decreased the incidence of nausea and vomiting.[35] The primary side effect of nausea or warm flush usually occurs within the first 30 seconds after injection and is transient. If the patient is advised of this potential side effect in advance, the procedure usually can be completed without difficulty. It is also wise to advise the patient that the skin and urine will be discolored for several days following the procedure.

A severe anaphylactic reaction has been reported after the use of indocyanine green as an angiographic dye.[36] Note also that fluorescein angiography performed during pregnancy does not appear to create a higher rate of birth anomalies or complications.[37]

Oral Fluorography

Oral fluorography can offer results similar to those obtained with intravenous fluorescein angiography but without the potential side effects. Oral fluorography is especially useful in cases where late dye leakage is expected. Oral fluorography can be performed using either USP bulk powder sodium fluorescein, 500 mg capsules, or commercially available 5-ml vials of 10% injectable sodium fluorescein. The powdered form is difficult to obtain, but 2 to 3 of the 5-ml vials of 10% fluorescein is usually sufficient to obtain good results. The fluorescein is mixed with a citrus drink and allowed to cool in crushed ice. The patient is asked to fast for about 8 hours before the test. The patient then is instructed to remove any dentures, since the solution will discolor these prosthetic devices. Before the procedure the practitioner must ensure the following (1) an informed consent form has been read and signed by the patient (see Chap. 5), (2) the patient is aware of what is about to happen, (3) the patient's pupils are maximally dilated, (4) color photographs of the fundus have been taken, (5) red-free photographs have been taken, (6) the fundus camera has been adjusted, and (7) the proper film has been loaded, filters put in place, and flash settings set. The patient is then instructed to drink the solution rapidly through a straw to prevent staining the lips.

Photography begins at the first sign of retinal circulation (15 to 30 minutes), with the late phase showing in approximately 1 hour. As with intravenous studies, the skin and urine will be slightly discolored for several days.

Reported complications of oral fluorography are few and minor.[38–41] It has been suggested that it would require ingestion of 90 g of fluorescein by a 100-pound person to produce a toxic effect.[39]

The oral fluorescein technique can be beneficial in aphakic children,[42] in patients with vaso-occlusive diseases of the retina,[43] and in patients with many other retinal diseases that manifest late-stage leakage such as idiopathic central serous choroidopathy (ICSC) and cystoid macular edema (CME) (Fig. 32.1).[44]

Interpretation

A fundamental understanding of retinal-choroidal anatomy and vasculature is crucial in interpreting fluorescein angiography. Some basic features of the retinal and choroidal system create the diagnostic capabilities of fluorescein angiography. These features are as follows: (1) healthy retinal vessels do not leak fluorescein because the vessel walls are not fenestrated; (2) healthy choriocapillaris vessels are fenestrated and leak freely, creating a sponge-like tissue; (3) in

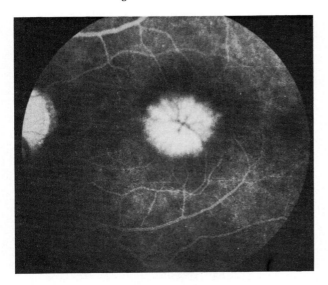

FIGURE 32.1 **Characteristic "rose petal" configuration of fluorescein staining in cystoid macular edema (CME) following administration of oral fluorescein sodium. (Courtesy James Hunter, O.D.)**

a healthy retina the fluid in the choriocapillaris is kept away from the sensory retina by an intact retinal pigment epithelium (RPE)/Bruch's membrane barrier. The RPE also serves as a filter to allow only part of the choroidal glow to show through. If the RPE is absent, more glow (hyperfluorescence) will be visible, and if there is an excess of RPE, less glow (hypofluorescence) will be visible. Dense RPE and xanthophyl mask the choroidal flush in a healthy macula.

In addition to the basic anatomic characteristics, the time-related stages of the angiogram are also important. The stages are classically described as the choroidal flush (prearterial phase), the arterial-venous phase, and the late phase. The choroidal flush occurs within seconds after injection. The posterior ciliary arteries supply the choroidal system in a patchy pattern, which is quickly masked by the fluorescein leaking into the choroidal swamp through fenestrated vasculature. This fluorescein will stay within the swamp if the RPE/Bruch's membrane barrier is healthy. Observation of the choroidal flush stage is especially useful in detecting diseases of the choroidal vasculature or the RPE/Bruch's membrane barrier, such as choroidal neovascularization in age-related maculopathy.

Within a few more seconds the retinal arteries start to fill in a laminar flow pattern. The central core of the artery glows first, followed by filling to the limits of the walls. The capillaries then fill, followed by the laminar filling of the veins. With the veins, the area of the blood column near the walls glows first, followed by filling to the center. The walls

of the arteries, capillaries, and veins in the healthy retina are not fenestrated and, therefore, should not leak. Any condition that creates breakdown of vessel walls with subsequent leakage or neovascularization would be most apparent in this stage. An example is leaking microaneurysms in diabetic retinopathy.

The late stages of fluorescein angiography usually occur approximately 10 minutes after injection. During this stage the arteries and veins have almost emptied of fluorescein, and the underlying choroidal flush is minimized. The optic nerve remains hyperfluorescent because the dye adheres to the nerve tissue. Leakage of choroidal and retinal vessels becomes more apparent by the diffusely spreading staining pattern overlying the vascular lesion. Late staining also occurs in sensory retinal detachments and RPE detachments due to choriocapillaris leakage.

Application of the time-stages of fluorescein angiography and the basic retinal-choroidal anatomy will allow for effective interpretation of fluorescein angiograms. The practitioner must realize that 2 basic situations occur in diseased conditions: (1) hypofluorescence, or a blockage of the glow, where one would normally expect it; and (2) hyperfluorescence, or an excessive glow, where one would not normally expect it. Table 32.2 outlines conditions that create hypofluorescence and hyperfluorescence, and Figure 32.2 illustrates some of the conditions best interpreted with fluorescein angiography.

Retinal Vascular Occlusive Disease

Retinal vascular occlusive disease is important from the standpoint of both vision loss and associated systemic disease. The retinal process invariably compromises some vision and reflects an underlying systemic disease condition. Although there is an intimate relationship among all retinal vaso-occlusive diseases, they are often divided into 5 categories: (1) branch vein occlusion (BVO), (2) central vein occlusion (CVO), (3) hemicentral vein occlusion (HCVO), (4) branch artery occlusion (BAO), and (5) central artery occlusion (CAO). The vein occlusion categories are then subdivided into ischemic and nonischemic categories depending on the degree of retinal hypoxia present.

Central Vein Occlusion

CVO is a visually debilitating condition with a strong association with systemic cardiovascular disease. CVO has a strong male predominance, with peak occurrences in the fifth to sixth decades.

TABLE 32.2

Common Ocular Conditions Creating Hypofluorescence or Hyperfluorescence During Fluorescein Angiography

	Hypofluorescence	*Hyperfluorescence*
RPE/Bruch's membrane	APMPPE (early) Congenital hypertrophy of RPE RPE hyperplasia	Age-related maculopathy (dry) Angioid streaks APMPPE (late) Choroidal folds Chorioretinal scars Drusen ICSC (cystoid maculopathy) Retinal hole RPE detachment RPE window defects Serous sensory retinal detachment
Choroid	Benign choroidal melanoma with no overlying serous detachment	Choroidal neovascularization Malignant choroidal melanoma
Retina	BAO CAO Cotton wool spots Preretinal hemorrhages Retinal exudates Subretinal hemorrhages	Angiomatosis retinae Capillary hemangioma Cavernous hemangioma (stasis) Leaking compromised veins Macroaneurysms Microaneurysms Neovascularization (retinal) Periphlebitis Telangiectasia
Optic nerve		Anterior ischemic optic neuropathy Neovascularization (disc) Papilledema

RPE, retinal pigment epithelium: APMPPE, acute posterior multifocal placoid pigment epitheliopathy; ICSE, idiopathic central serous choroidopathy; BAO, branch artery occlusion; CAO, central artery occlusion.

ETIOLOGY

CVO presents as a sudden, variable loss of vision. The etiology is complex and is age-dependent. Table 32.3 categorizes systemic factors as related to age. Several causes for CVO have been reported[45]: antithrombin deficiency,[46] associated with spontaneous carotid-cavernous fistula,[47] secondary to hemodialysis,[48] increase in platelet aggregability,[49,50] elevation of thrombocyte aggregation,[51] hypercholesterolemia, hypertriglyceridemia, hyperlipidemia,[52] hyperhomocysteinemia,[53] and HIV infection.[54]

Predisposing factors for CVO include glaucoma, papilledema, subdural hematoma, hemorrhage within the optic nerve, drusen of the optic nerve, hypertension, cardiovascular and cerebrovascular disease, diabetes, leukemia, thrombocytopenia, mitral valve prolapse, sclerodermatous vascular disease, Reye's syndrome, systemic lupus erythematosus, and trauma.[55–63] CVO often occurs in young adults with no apparent association to systemic disease and is referred to as papillophlebitis.[64,65]

DIAGNOSIS

From an ophthalmoscopic standpoint, CVO can present as 2 distinct clinical entities. These are not always easily differentiated, however, since the conditions exist as part of a continuum. The recognized types are nonischemic retinopathy and ischemic retinopathy. The primary difference is determined by the presence of significant retinal ischemia.[66] The most effective method to differentiate ischemic from nonischemic CVO is the observation of capillary obliteration present with fluorescein angiography. The relative afferent pupillary defect is also more obvious in the ischemic form.[67]

The CVO in either case can present with the prodromal symptom of transient obscurations (brief blurring of vision

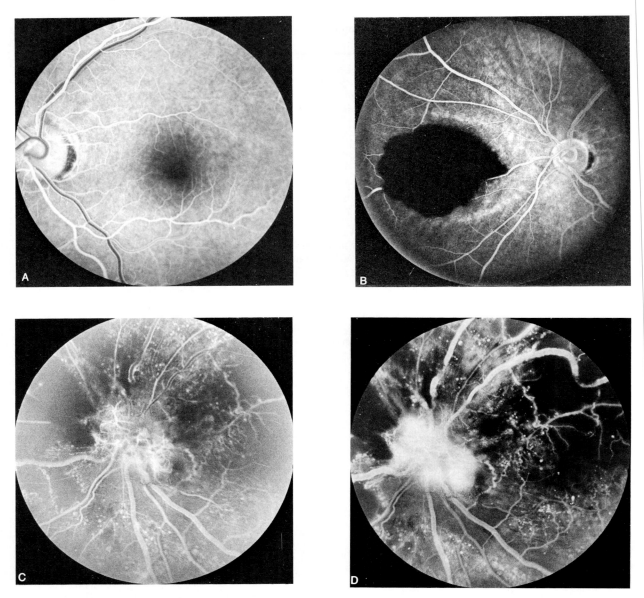

FIGURE 32.2   **Examples of fluorescein angiography.** *(A)* Choroidal-arterial phase showing laminar flow in the veins. *(B)* Blockage of background choroidal fluorescence as well as arteries and veins by a preretinal hemorrhage. *(C)* Early-phase angiogram of disc neovascularization. *(D)* Later-phase angiogram of disc neovascularization demonstrating leakage into the vitreous. *(E)* Microaneurysms surrounding the macula. *(F)* Demonstration of the intraretinal edema caused by leaking microaneurysms. *(G)* Subretinal pigment epithelial neovascularization, early phase. *(H)* Subretinal pigment epithelial neovascularization, early phase. *(I)* Subretinal pigment epithelial neovascularization, late phase, demonstrating fluid accumulation in overlying sensory retinal detachment.

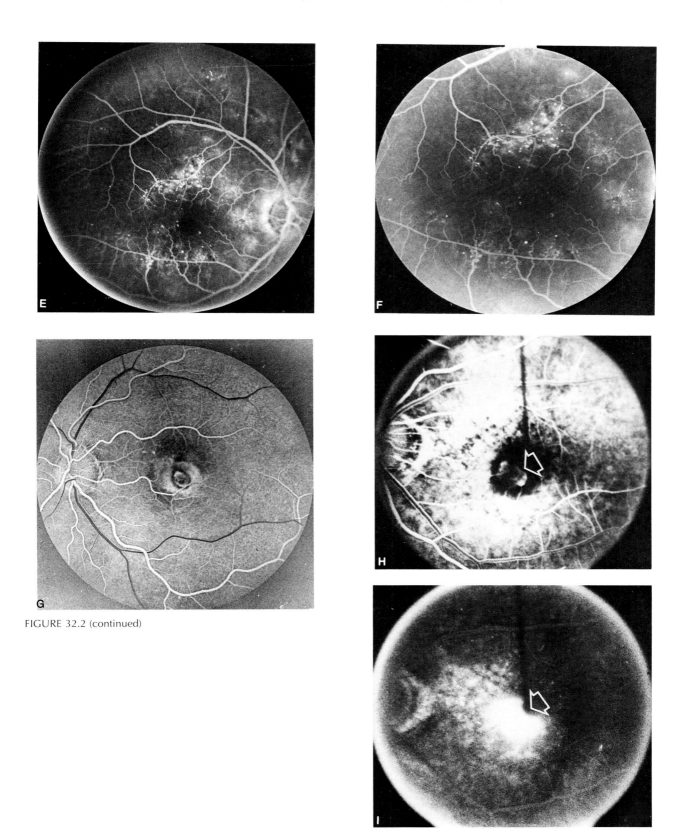

FIGURE 32.2 (continued)

TABLE 32.3
Systemic Factors in Central Vein Occlusion as Related to Age

Age (yr)	Causes
Under 50	Head injuries
	Hyperlipidemia
	Estrogen-containing preparations
	Hyperviscosity syndromes
	Cryofibrinogenemia
Over 50	Hypertension
	Abnormal GTT
	Hyperlipidemia
	Chronic lung disease
	Elevated serum IgA
	Hyperviscosity syndromes
	Cryofibrinogenemia

GTT, glucose tolerance test.
Adapted from McGrath MA, Wechsler F, Hunyor AB, et al. Systemic factors contributory to retinal vein occlusion. Arch Intern Med 1978;138:216–220.

associated with postural changes) and the prodromal sign of a yellowish hue in the posterior pole when comparing one eye with the other. The prodromata may last months, with the active phase being heralded by dot and blot hemorrhages and intraretinal edema. The hemorrhages extend from the posterior pole to the retinal periphery. Evidence of capillary dilation may occur near the optic disc or temporal vascular arcade as seen by fluorescein angiography. Vision loss is relatively sudden, since the macular area is very susceptible to intraretinal edema.

The two major types of CVO have specific characteristics, prognosis, and management procedures. Nonischemic CVO is characterized by dot and blot hemorrhages, intraretinal edema, and various degrees of macular edema (Fig. 32.3). The ischemic CVO presents as dot and blot hemorrhages, superficial flame-shaped hemorrhages, cotton wool spots, silver wire or sheathed arteries, very dense intraretinal and macular edema, and at least 10 disc diameters of retinal capillary non-perfusion. (Fig. 32.4). Another clinical finding that accompanies the acute stage of the occlusion is lowered intraocular pressure. There is a greater initial reduction of pressure in ischemic CVO than in nonischemic CVO, and both have a greater reduction than does BVO.[68,69] Two cases of transient angle-closure glaucoma have been reported in patients with CVO.[70] It has also been reported that there is a difference in relative afferent pupillary defects between ischemic and nonischemic CVO.[71]

Fluorescein angiographic findings in CVO will vary considerably depending on the type of occlusion as well as the elapsed time after onset. Initially there will be blockage of background choroidal fluorescence by the intraretinal and flame-shaped hemorrhage. The retina will be stained with fluorescein because of intraretinal leakage, and the macula will demonstrate varying degrees of edema. Neovascularization may develop along with its classic fluorescein angiographic picture.

MANAGEMENT

An attempt must be made to ascertain the underlying systemic or local cause in all cases of CVO. The visual prognosis of CVO is guarded, but one can expect a more favorable outcome in nonischemic CVO than in ischemic CVO.[72–74] Although recovery of visual acuity is variable, neovascular glaucoma is

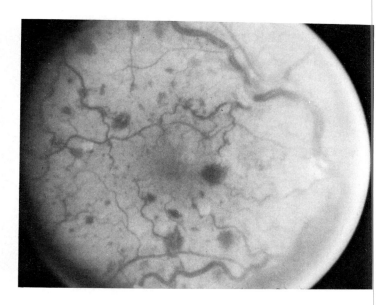

FIGURE 32.3 **Nonischemic central vein occlusion (CVO). Note tortuosity and dilation of veins and deep retinal hemorrhages.**

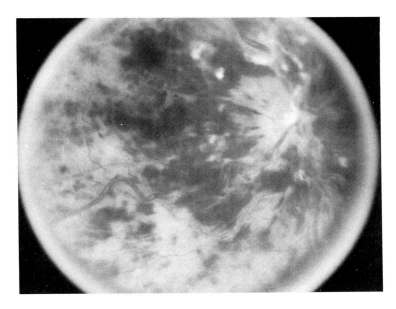

FIGURE 32.4   **Ischemic CVO. Note cotton wool spots and nerve fiber layer hemorrhages.**

an identified complication in 14% to 20% of all CVO cases.[75] The risk of neovascular glaucoma is even higher (60%) in ischemic CVO.[76,77] The incidence of primary open-angle glaucoma in patients with CVO is 5.7% to 66%, and CVO occurs in 3.5% to 5% of patients with primary open-angle glaucoma and in 3% of patients with ocular hypertension.[78] Disc and retinal neovascularization do not represent as significant a threat in CVO as in BVO because of the retinal capillary endothelial death that occurs in the former.

Any drugs, such as oral contraceptives, suspected of precipitating the CVO should be discontinued. The use of IOP-lowering drugs that also may have the potential to improve vascular perfusion at the nerve head may relieve some of the pressure at the lamina, facilitating breakup of the thrombus. Anticoagulants do not actively dissolve a thrombus once it has formed, but they may prevent its propagation. Monitoring of anticoagulant levels is essential once therapy has been instituted. Heparin is often the drug of choice, but hospitalization is required because of the intravenous or intramuscular route of administration. The usual dosage of heparin is 100 mg followed by 50 mg every 4 to 6 hours to stabilize the anticoagulant level.

Coumarin drugs are then instituted because they may be given orally on an outpatient basis. Since this drug group specifically depresses prothrombin levels, these levels should be monitored. There should be a 24- to 48-hour overlap of heparin therapy to ensure establishment of coumarin activity.

Warfarin may be administered in an initial dosage of 20 to 25 mg, followed by 2 to 10 mg daily as a maintenance dosage. Oral prednisone therapy can be used to treat the inflammatory component.[79]

Anticoagulation therapy, although controversial, does seem to give slightly more favorable results than no therapy at all. Anticoagulation therapy may minimize the progression from nonischemic to ischemic CVO, actually reducing the incidence of development of neovascular glaucoma.[80,81] Monitoring of blood prothrombin times is a crucial aspect of any anticoagulation therapy.

Despite good results with retrobulbar injections of lidocaine and acetylcholine, coupled with systemic administration of low molecular weight dextran and papaverine hydrochloride, investigators suggest that this therapy is only moderately beneficial.[82]

Recent work has indicated that isovolemic hemodilution improves the visual outcome of patients with CVO and does offer some hope.[83] Improvement in visual acuity may occur with 150 mg bifemelane hydrochloride daily for up to 11 months as an adjunct to other therapies.[84]

One indisputable mode of therapy is the use of panretinal photocoagulation to prevent the development of neovascular glaucoma. Visual outcome is not necessarily improved by photocoagulation,[85] but the chance of development of neovascular glaucoma is minimized.[86-89] Panretinal photocoagulation has little effect in nonischemic CVO unless it is secondary to ipsilateral carotid artery occlusion,[90] but it is of significant benefit in ischemic CVO. Photocoagulation minimizes the vasoproliferative stimulus created by the hypoxic retina, which minimizes iris neovascularization.[91] Photocoagulation alters but does not eliminate all of the retinal ischemia leading to the development of retinal neovascularization.[92] It also appears that to be effective in the prevention of iris neovascularization, the panretinal photocoagulation must be performed within 90 days of the onset of the CVO.[93] In the event that the retina cannot be viewed for photocoagulation, cryotherapy may be of benefit.

If nonischemic retinopathy appears to be worsening and there is associated orbital pain, bypass surgery of the carotid system may produce beneficial results.[94,95] It is important to note that patients with neovascular glaucoma but without an obvious precipitating fundus condition should be suspected of having ipsilateral carotid artery disease until proven otherwise.[96,97]

Hemicentral Vein Occlusion

The basis of an HCVO lies in the fact that a 2-trunked central retinal vein exists in some patients.[98] This occurs when the vein bifurcates in the anterior portion of the optic nerve before piercing the lamina cribrosa. One of the 2 trunks may become occluded to produce the picture of an HCVO. Although the clinical findings may resemble a BVO, from a pathogenesis standpoint the condition is more related to CVO. This analysis, however, is controversial, since some clinicians believe that HCVO is actually simultaneous BVOs of different branches.[99] The HCVO may present in either a nonischemic or ischemic form and usually involves half the retina (Fig. 32.5). HCVO differs from CVO from the standpoint that a full half of the retina is nonperfused while the other half is viable. This lends more easily to the development of retinal and disc neovascularization.

Prognosis depends on macular involvement and the development of neovascularization. Neovascularization is not

expected in the nonischemic form but can develop in the ischemic variety within 6 months.[100]

Retinal Arterial Occlusion

Retinal arterial occlusions occur in two forms—CAO and BAO. Both conditions have similar origins and similar treatment modalities, although prognosis differs in the two conditions.

CENTRAL ARTERY OCCLUSION

Etiology.   Patients with increased vascular resistance, such as internal carotid artery obstruction, are highly susceptible to CAO.[101,102] Any condition contributing to this increased resistance may act as a causative factor. These include emboli from cardiac lesions,[103,104] mitral valve prolapse,[105] emboli from artificial cardiac valves,[106] emboli from bacterial endocarditis,[107] thrombi secondary to giant cell arteritis, syphilis, fungal infections of the ethmoid or sphenoid sinuses,[108] occlusion secondary to oral contraceptives,[109] and occlusion secondary to polyarteritis nodosa.[110] Both CAO and BAO may occur secondary to methylprednisolone acetate injections of the head and neck soft tissue.[111,112] Additional reports implicate cardiac catherization,[113] Sneddon's disease associated with antiphospholipid antibodies,[114] complications of rhinoplasty,[115] endarterectomy,[116] pregnancy,[117] and osteogenesis imperfecta.[118] Retinal artery occlusion has been reported in a diver suffering from a decompression disorder,[119] as well as in association with postherpetic cerebral vasculopathy.[120]

Diagnosis.   The typical clinical presentation of a CAO is a sudden, painless loss of vision in a nondiseased eye. The visual acuity loss is severe, and there is loss of the direct pupillary response. If there remains a patent cilioretinal artery (origin from the choroidal vascular supply), a variable central island of vision may be maintained.

The ophthalmoscopic appearance of the retina depends on time elapsed since the occlusion. Initially the retinal arteries appear narrowed in contrast to the veins, and there is a subtle haziness of the retinal tissue. The veins may become distended and may exhibit a box car segmentation. Within hours the inner retinal tissue becomes milky white (Fig. 32.6) and contrasts markedly with the red-appearing macula, which receives its nutrition from the choroid.

After weeks, the retina is replaced by glial tissue, the arterial tree assumes a more normal appearance except for irregular narrowing, and optic atrophy may ensue. Neovascular glaucoma is rare in CAO. The presence of neovascular glaucoma associated with arterial obstructive disease usually indicates the ocular ischemic syndrome, which includes aqueous flare, rubeosis iridis, mid-peripheral intraretinal hemorrhages, narrowed retinal arteries, cherry red spot,

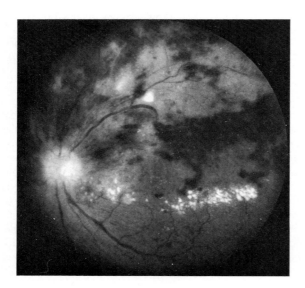

FIGURE 32.5   **Hemicentral vein occlusion (HCVO). The superior half of the retina is involved with hard exudates demarcating the retinal edema.**

neovascularization of the disc or retina, and ipsilateral or bilateral common carotid artery obstruction.[121]

Management. From a visual standpoint prognosis is grim unless therapy is begun within 1 to 2 hours after the occlusion. Management of the underlying systemic condition is also of immediate concern.

Management of CAO depends on the precipitating factor. If CAO is secondary to facial trauma resulting in retrobulbar hemorrhage, the treatment is surgical drainage of the hematoma.[122] If the CAO is due to sickle cell occlusion, exchange transfusions have offered some success.[123]

The most important aspect of the management of CAO is to ascertain the underlying source of the embolus. A complete cardiovascular and carotid system evaluation is in order. Blood tests should include a test for antiphospholipid antibodies in unexplained cases of CAO. Temporal arteritis must also be ruled out.[124]

Some general statements regarding therapy can be made. The occlusions caused by emboli may exhibit some recovery if therapy is instituted within 1 to 2 hours. Digital massage of the globe through the eyelid may dislodge the embolus. Massage coupled with inhalation of a mixture of 5% CO_2 (vasodilator) combined with 95% O_2 for 15 minutes, followed by breathing room air for 15 minutes over 6 to 12 hours may be of value. However, when considering the fact that CAO occurs at the lamina and that vasodilators will not affect this collagen-like structure, the use of vasodilators is illogical. Deutsch and associates[125] have concluded that attempts at vasodilation are of little benefit. Paracentesis of the anterior chamber will quickly lower the intraocular pressure and may facilitate dislodgement of the embolus. The intraocular pressure should be maintained low for several days by oral administration of acetazolamide, 250 mg every 6 hours.[108] Retrobulbar injections of acetylcholine, atropine, or tolazoline may be beneficial. Papaverine plus heparin through the infraorbital artery has been attempted.[126] If the CAO is proven to be secondary to temporal arteritis, intravenous methylprednisolone 15 to 30 mg/kg/day has been shown to stabilize vision function.[127] Microcatheter urokinase infusion or tissue plasminogen activator may also promote visual recovery in patients with CAO.[128]

Any attempt to restore circulation is worthwhile, since the prognosis is otherwise grim. Particular attention must be given to the patient's general health status, since CAO implies generalized cardiovascular compromise. Sheng and associates[129] concluded that over 50% of patients with CAO who undergo carotid angiography have an ipsilateral carotid lesion. This suggests that CAO is a significant marker for extracranial carotid disease.

BRANCH ARTERY OCCLUSION

Etiology. Etiology of BAO is similar to that of CAO, with the additional precipitating factors of self-injected emboli or

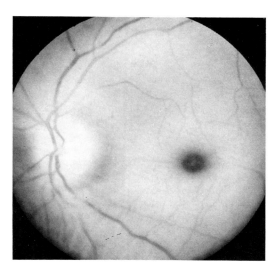

FIGURE 32.6   **Central artery occlusion (CAO). (Courtesy Hernan Benavides, O.D.)**

emboli secondary to diagnostic procedures.[130,131] In general, individuals with BAO secondary to generalized cardiovascular disease have lesions that are more amenable to surgical intervention than do individuals with CAO.[102] It has also been suggested that there is an idiopathic form of BAO that may be a variety of focal arteritis.[132] BAO can also be associated with pseudotumor cerebri and Lyme disease.[133,134]

Diagnosis. The most frequently affected region of the retina is the superior temporal area. Vision and visual fields are variable, but the ophthalmoscopic appearance is similar to that of CAO. The major difference in the evolution is the tendency toward development of arterial shunts in CAO. The vision remains compromised in the affected area, and segmental optic atrophy may be a complication.

Management. The likelihood for return of vision or visual field is minimal unless therapy is instituted within 1 to 2 hours. The visual field that remains is sharp-edged along the horizontals, representing termination of the inner retinal arterial supply at the horizontal raphé.

Management of BAO depends on the extent of visual loss. If vision is severely compromised, aggressive therapy should be used as in CAO.[135] If loss of visual field occurs without severe loss of vision, the procedure of greatest importance is an aggressive search for the cause of the BAO.

Some clinicians advocate pentoxifylline, 300 to 600 mg daily over a 3-month period, to prevent retinal or intravitreal neovascularization caused by retinal ischemia.[136] This method of management of retinal occlusive disease is still under investigation and has yet to be proved as a beneficial therapeutic procedure.

Hereditary Diseases

Hereditary Gyrate Atrophy of the Choroid and Retina with Hyperornithinemia

ETIOLOGY

This autosomal recessive and progressive dystrophy is associated with hyperornithinemia (plasma ornithine levels are typically 800 to 1300 μM) and deficient mitochondrial ornithine ketoacid aminotransferase activity. Serum lysine levels are typically lower than normal. A deficiency of creatinine or phosphocreatinine may also be involved in the pathogenesis.[137,138]

However, cases of gyrate atrophy can occur with normal plasma ornithine levels, and cases of hyperornithinemia occur without gyrate atrophy.[139]

DIAGNOSIS

The classic clinical presentation is myopia in the first decade, night blindness in the second decade, cataracts of such severity that extraction is needed in the third decade, and progressive visual impairment caused by macular changes in the fourth to fifth decades. However, there appear to be variations depending on serum ornithine levels.[140]

The fundus has a characteristic appearance with irregular, sharply defined areas of chorioretinal atrophy beginning in the periphery and progressing toward the posterior pole. The areas of atrophy tend to merge and take on scalloped borders. The fundus takes on a yellowish appearance, as does the disc, as pigment migrates and retinal vessels attenuate. The cataract that occurs in 40% of patients begins as a posterior subcapsular complicated variety, but anterior subcapsular cataract has also been associated with gyrate atrophy.[141] Abnormal electrodiagnostic signs are present, and seizure disorders may become a problem.[139,142]

MANAGEMENT

Visual acuity remains intact until macular encroachment occurs, but visual fields exhibit a concentric constriction with accompanying night vision problems. Color vision loss eventually ensues.

Since this is a hereditary disorder, genetic counseling and examination of siblings is crucial. Considerable work is ongoing regarding the molecular genetics associated with gyrate atrophy of the choroid and retina.[143–146] Management is directed at reducing serum ornithine levels. This can be achieved by restricting protein.[147,148] Arginine-deficient diets may reduce serum ornithine levels, especially in patients who

do not respond to oral pyridoxine therapy. Oral pyridoxine (vitamin B_6), 15 to 18 mg daily, may reduce serum ornithine, while massive doses (600 to 750 mg) may improve retinal function.[149,150] Orally administered α-aminoisobutyric acid aids the reduction in serum ornithine.[147]

If serum ornithine is maintained between 55 and 355 μM by any means, it appears that chorioretinal degeneration does not progress.[147] No direct evidence exists to firmly support any particular therapy, but any method that reduces serum ornithine levels will improve the prognosis of hereditary gyrate atrophy. Dietary restrictions are safe as long as amino acid requirements are met by supplements.

Acquired or Degenerative Diseases

Cystoid Macular Edema

ETIOLOGY

Cystoid macular edema (CME) occurs secondary to many ocular conditions. The most familiar form is associated with cataract surgery and is referred to as the Irvine-Gass syndrome. Other causes include BVO,[151] retinitis pigmentosa,[152] progressive pigmentary degeneration,[153] YAG laser capsulotomy,[154] pars planitis,[155] severe carotid artery obstruction,[156] corneal relaxing incision,[157,158] long-standing venous stasis retinopathy,[159] retinal surgery, ocular inflammation,[160] and ocular tumors. In general, any condition that can produce intraretinal fluid accumulation, including drug toxicities such as with epinephrine, can cause CME.

Cystoid maculopathy occurs when fluid seeps into Henle's fiber layer of the fovea. It is obvious that the leakage occurs as the result of venous stasis in vascular disease and inflammatory conditions, but the etiology in dystrophic conditions and toxic reactions is not identified as easily. Following cataract surgery with vitreous face complications, cystoid maculopathy may develop (Irvine-Gass syndrome). There is usually a delay in the onset of this condition postsurgically, with the peak incidence occurring at about the sixth postoperative week. By fluorescein studies, it has been shown that approximately 40% to 50% of aphakic eyes develop cystoid maculopathy, but only 2% to 3% present a significant problem.[161,162] The prognosis is reasonably good because approximately 50% of affected patients recover normal vision within about 6 months. Twenty percent have the condition for 1 to 3 years.[163]

DIAGNOSIS

As mentioned previously, it is well known that cystoid maculopathy may result from any number of ocular conditions. The majority of these conditions are related to systemic disease processes such as hypertension, atherosclerosis, hyperlipidemia, and hypercholesterolemia and their ocular manifestations. The clinical picture will be characteristic in these conditions. In the Irvine-Gass syndrome, the fundus may reveal only a loss of foveal reflex or, in more severe cases, a retinal elevation. Visual acuity will be reduced, there will be a prolonged macular photostress recovery time, and metamorphopsia will be revealed by the Amsler grid. The definitive clinical diagnosis can be made by fluorescein studies (see Fig. 32.1).

Differential diagnosis is best accomplished by fluorescein angiography, which assists in differentiating cystoid maculopathy from dystrophic or degenerative conditions as well as from subretinal pigment epithelial neovascularization.

MANAGEMENT

Management of CME is controversial because the disease is difficult to study. The condition appears to be quite prevalent by angiographic studies, but true clinical manifestations appear to be rare.[161-163] However, management of any condition that can precipitate CME is mandatory.

The controversy arises when CME occurs as the primary condition. Oral inhibitors of prostaglandin synthesis, such as indomethacin, have been advocated, but their efficacy is not proved. Topical steroids are inadequate, and oral steroids have numerous and sometimes serious side effects. Periocular steroid injections may be attempted in cases where there is an immediate, severe threat to vision. A sub-Tenon's injection of methylprednisolone, 40 to 80 mg, is placed in the superior temporal quadrant posterior to the equator after topical anesthesia is achieved with 4% lidocaine. One or two treatments may result in remission, but edema often returns after the therapeutic effect has resolved.[162] Caution should be exercised regarding the possibility of inducing a rise in intraocular pressure associated with the use of steroids.[163a]

Many studies have reported the benefits to aphakic CME of prostaglandin inhibitors, such as 1% topical indomethacin drops 4 times daily for 1 to 4 months. There appears to be a strong positive effect of topical indomethacin in chronic CME after cataract extraction, since there is a worsening of vision with cessation of the drops.[164] Actual prophylaxis against angiographically proved aphakic CME has also been achieved by topical indomethacin.[165-167] Some authors advocate combining topical 1% indomethacin with 1% prednisolone.[168-170] The question remains whether management of angiographically proved CME is necessary, since there may be no significant difference in visual outcome with or without pharmacologic intervention.[171] Other prostaglandin inhibitors, such as fenoprofen sodium, have produced similar, equivocal results.[172] Prostaglandin inhibitors are widely available and are used worldwide both as a method of inhibiting intraoperative miosis and as anti-inflammatory agents in the treatment of CME.[173] Flach and associates[174] used 0.5% topical ketorolac tromethamine solution and demonstrated that this nonsteroidal anti-inflammatory drug (NSAID) may reverse vision loss in some patients with long-standing aphakic and pseudophakic CME. Controlled studies have further substantiated the positive benefit of 0.5% ketorolac tromethamine used alone in the management of CME.[175-176]

Treatment with systemic acetazolamide may also result in visual improvement in cases of chronic CME. Both low dosages (125 mg) over a prolonged period, as well as higher dosages (500 mg timed-release), have been recommended. In either case, slow tapering of treatment is recommended to minimize reactivation.[177-181]

Pars plana vitrectomy may be considered if vitreous strands are apparent or in cases that are unresponsive to oral, sub-Tenon's and topical steroids.[182] Laser photocoagulation has been used in an attempt to drain the macular area, with some positive results attained with grid photocoagulation.[183-185] Hyperbaric oxygen therapy may be of benefit in the treatment of aphakic CME.[186,187] Lysing of vitreous strands with the neodymium:YAG laser to relieve potential vitreoretinal stress also helps in the treatment of some cases of CME.[188]

Inflammatory Diseases

Ocular Toxoplasmosis

ETIOLOGY

Toxoplasma gondii is an obligate intracellular protozoan parasite that is one of the most likely causes of posterior uveitis in the United States. *T. gondii* uveitis is rarely acquired but, rather, is thought to be congenital with a delayed ocular onset.[189] The factors that lead to reactivation as well as the occasional acquired infection involve a compromise of the patient's immune status.

The prevalence of toxoplasmosis varies considerably in different studies. In general, it is accepted that 70% to 80% of females are at risk during child-bearing years.[190] Congenital infection occurs as a consequence of primary maternal infection during pregnancy.[191] The rate of fetal infection increases throughout the pregnancy,[192,193] and the incidence of congenital infection is 0.01% of live births.[194] Toxoplasmosis can, however, be transmitted to the fetus only during maternal parasitemia.[195] When the parasite reaches the ocular circulatory system, it lodges in retinal vessels, often in the nerve fiber layer. When active parasites are present, a necrotizing retinitis ensues. It is thought that the live organism rather than the toxins is the cause of the retinochoroiditis,[195,196] and that the major disruption of the choroidoretinal interface is probably secondary to invasion by the parasite.[197] Humoral and cell-mediated immunity inhibit the active process that results in encystation of still viable *T. gondii*. It has been suggested that the body produces an antibody that protects the parasite.[198] The encysted *T. gondii* then await a future compromise of the immune system, which leads to successful reactivation.[199] This results in the typical toxoplasmosis scar with satellites of reactivated lesions. The compromised immune system in the patient with acquired immunodeficiency syndrome (AIDS) significantly increases the risk of reactivation of toxoplasmic encystations.

The anterior uveitis that accompanies the retinal lesion is believed to be a manifestation of hypersensitivity, since *T. gondii* have never been recovered from the anterior chamber.[198] There has been a reported association of ocular toxoplasmosis and Fuchs' heterochromic iridocyclitis, but the evidence is arguable.[200,201]

In the past, acquired *T. gondii* retinochoroiditis was considered to be rare. Fewer than 1% of patients with acquired systemic toxoplasmosis manifest retinal lesions.[194] However, more reports are surfacing that suggest an increase in the acquired form. Toxoplasmic retinochoroidal lesions in patients with AIDS are not often associated with a pre-existing scar, suggesting that the lesions are a manifestation of an acquired disease rather than reactivation of a congenital lesion.[202] There are even reports of miniepidemics of acquired toxoplasmosis that involve retinal lesions.[203–207] The incidence of acquired toxoplasmic retinochoroiditis will probably increase because of the increased use of immunosuppressive therapy.[204,208]

DIAGNOSIS

Reactivated congenital toxoplasmic retinochoroiditis typically occurs as an indistinct yellow-white lesion with an overlying vitritis (Fig. 32.7). The active lesion usually occurs at the margin of an old toxoplasmic scar, which suggests a rupture of an encysted toxoplasmic colony. There may be an associated posterior vitreous detachment with keratic precipitates on the vitreous face. The frequent association of retinal arteritis,[209,210] occlusive vasculitis,[211,212] iridocyclitis, optic neuritis (papillitis), and macular edema[213] reflects the inflammatory aspect of the disease.[214,215] The inflammatory response indicates the need to incorporate steroids into the treatment regimen. Subretinal pigment epithelial neovascularization can also occur in active toxoplasmic retinochoroidopathy.[207]

It has been suggested that reactivation of congenital toxoplasmosis can manifest itself neurologically. Robinson and Bauman[216] described a girl with focal encephalitis associated with a reactivation of ocular toxoplasmic retinochoroidopathy. The brain and eye share a similar vascular system, resulting in the following characteristics of congenital toxoplasmosis: (1) convulsions, (2) intracranial calcification, and (3) retinochoroiditis.

Active toxoplasmosis is common in the teen years but is rare over age 40 years. An active attack lasts 1 week to 2 years, with an average of 4.2 months.[194] Several laboratory tests are available to assist in the diagnosis of toxoplasmic retinochoroidopathy. The Sabin-Feldman methylene blue dye test (SFDT) is the diagnostic test used most often in toxoplasmosis.

Laboratory testing to differentiate the causes of uveitis is of variable effectiveness. HLA-B27 typing coupled with testing for the angiotensin converting enzyme (ACE) is of

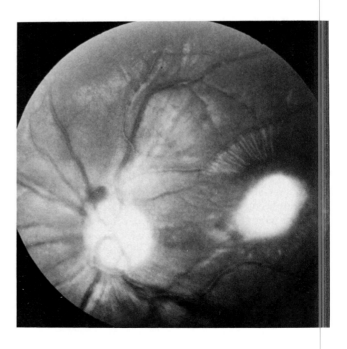

FIGURE 32.7   Active ocular toxoplasmosis involving the macula. (Courtesy John F. Amos, O.D.)

value for sarcoid uveitis. *Toxoplasma* serology is of value. Analysis of local intraocular antibody production with commercially available kits is becoming a valuable adjunct to assist in the differential diagnosis of all ocular granulomatous lesions.[217,218] It is recommended that in patients suspected of having toxoplasmic infection with negative immunofluorescent antibody toxoplasmic titers, that SFDT or ELISA titers be obtained as well.[219]

The SFDT is of limited usefulness in congenital toxoplasmosis, since the mother's antibodies cross the placenta whether or not the infection is transmitted. The SFDT does, however, measure antibodies that are detectable for decades.[220] The complement fixation test (CFT) measures antibodies of comparatively short duration after infection and, therefore, has value in indicating which children have been infected during the first 6 years of life.[221] The indirect fluorescent antibody test is a useful adjunct to the SFDT but has some limitations due to availability. The presence of an IgM antibody is significant because this antibody will not pass the placental barrier; therefore, its presence indicates infection.[222–226] The lymphocyte transformation test may also be of some benefit for detecting infection in the first year of life.[194]

Since many diseases may mimic toxoplasmic retinochoroidopathy, other laboratory tests should be routinely performed, including screening for AIDS. A PPD coupled with a chest x-ray film will rule out tuberculosis. FTA-ABS will assist in the differential diagnosis of syphilitic retinitis. Other conditions necessitate more sophisticated laboratory analyses.

MANAGEMENT

Visual prognosis in cases of ocular toxoplasmosis depends on the time elapsed between activation or reactivation of the retinitis and initiation of therapy. If the lesion progresses to necrosis (even 5 or 6 days), therapy will act only to limit the extent of damage. Indications for treatment of ocular toxoplasmosis are the following[227]: (1) active lesions near the macula or papillomacular bundle; (2) lesions threatening or involving the optic nerve; (3) lesions severe enough to cause significant vitreous traction or retinal detachment; (4) peripapillary lesions, especially those closer to the disc because of the associated sectorial visual field loss; and (5) visual acuity worse than 20/200.[228]

Accepted systemic therapy is the use of antitoxoplasmic agents with the addition of oral steroids when an inflammatory reaction exists. The synergistic use of triple sulfonamides with pyrimethamine is an effective antitoxoplasmic regimen because each works at a different point in the toxoplasmosis cycle.[229]

Pyrimethamine (Daraprim) is typically prescribed in an initial loading dose of 100 to 150 mg orally, followed by 25 to 50 mg daily for 4 to 6 weeks.[230,231] Pyrimethamine is a folate antagonist that can cause white blood cell and platelet depression as well as megaloblastic anemia. Should the platelet

count drop below 100,000/mm³, 10 mg of folinic acid (leucovorin) can be administered intramuscularly or orally (in orange or tomato juice) to reverse the effect without affecting the action of the pyrimethamine. Some authors advocate using 2 to 3 mg of leucovorin 3 times per week as a preventive measure.[232,233] One may also use 1 tablet of Brewer's yeast 3 times daily as a substitute for folinic acid.[234]

Chlortetracycline can be used as a substitute for pyrimethamine at a loading dose of 2 g, followed by 250 mg 4 times daily for 1 month. Spiramycin at 2 g daily can be used as a substitute in pregnant women because it does not cross the placental barrier.[191]

Triple sulfonamides (sulfadiazine-sulfamerazine-sulfamethazine) lessen the chance of renal calculus formation while being effective antitoxoplasmic agents. The loading dose is 2 to 4 g, followed by 1 g 4 times daily. Therapy should be continued for 4 to 6 weeks.[235]

Clindamycin (Cleocin) is an antitoxoplasmic drug with a high rate of ocular penetration. If oral clindamycin is given, the dosage is 300 mg 4 times daily for 4 weeks. The alternative to this dosage is 50 mg administered subconjunctivally on alternate days for 4 weeks.[236] The major concern with clindamycin is the side effect of severe colitis, which can prove fatal. Should bowel movement exceed 4 times daily beyond normal, the drug should be discontinued and the patient should notify the physician. Vancomycin, 500 mg every 6 hours for 10 days, can be effective in controlling the colitis.[237]

Steroids have some value in the management of ocular toxoplasmosis. However, it is likely that all toxoplasmic retinochoroiditis is infectious and that the steroid's immunosuppressive action is potentially dangerous. When used alone in injectable or oral form, steroids will cause a brief improvement in the inflammatory process, followed by a worsening.[230] However, when used in conjunction with antitoxoplasmic agents, steroids will improve some of the inflammatory responses and allow for less overall damage. The standard therapeutic dosage is 100 mg of oral prednisone daily for 7 to 10 days, followed by a tapering of dosage on alternate days.[235]

Tessler[235] proposed a variation on antitoxoplasmosis therapy that he contends minimizes the hematologic problems associated with pyrimethamine therapy. He calls this approach quadruple therapy:

Pyrimethamine	75 mg loading dose followed by 25 mg daily, discontinued in 1 to 2 weeks
Triple sulfonamides	2 g loading dose followed by 1 g 4 times daily, discontinued in 3 weeks
Clindamycin	300 mg 4 times daily, discontinued in 3 weeks
Oral prednisone	60 to 80 mg every other day at breakfast, tapering off in 3 to 4 weeks

If a toxoplasmosis lesion is threatening the macula or optic disc, or if vision is reduced to 20/70 or less due to vitreous opacification, quadruple therapy results in a response of over 50% in two weeks and over 80% in three weeks.[238] Treatment of patients with ocular toxoplasmosis threatening vision results in positive effects in approximately 50% of patients, while 20% of the lesions will reduce in size if left untreated. The recurrence of inflammation in both treated and untreated cases approaches 50% within a 3-year follow-up.[239] It has been reported that trimethoprim-sulfamethoxazole (Bactrim DS) may be an effective substitute for sulfadiazine, pyrimethamine, and folinic acid, with minimal side effects.[240]

Treatment of toxoplasmosis lesions in patients with AIDS is effective with pyrimethamine, clindomycin, and sulfadiazine, but systemic steroid treatment may be associated with the development of CMV retinitis. Treatment becomes effective within a median period of 6 weeks.[241] The relationship of toxoplasmosis in the ocular and neurological form is becoming more apparent in the patient with AIDS. AIDS patients with any type of retinitis or other ocular granulomatous signs should be suspected of having toxoplasmic infection along with CMV, progressive outer retinal necrosis, and syphilitic retinitis.[242,243] Inflammatory optic neuropathy in these patients also implies toxoplasmosis.[244]

One other aspect of ocular toxoplasmosis that must be managed is that of associated iridocyclitis. The degree of cells, flare, and keratic precipitates dictates the mode of therapy. Mydriatic-cycloplegic agents, such as cyclopentolate 1% or homatropine 5%, should be instilled 2 to 4 times daily in less severe cases. Atropine 1% should be instilled twice daily in severe cases. Topical steroids assist in alleviating the inflammatory process. Prednisolone acetate 0.5% to 1% has the best ocular penetration and may be used at intervals that correspond to the degree of inflammation.

When using pyrimethamine, it is important to obtain a CBC and platelet count on a weekly basis. Follow-up for treated ocular toxoplasmic lesions should be every 3 to 7 days depending on severity.

Ocular Toxocara canis

ETIOLOGY

Toxocara is a parasite that infects dogs, wolves, foxes, and other canids and is transferrable to humans through feces. The human infection is manifest in two forms, ocular larva migrans and visceral larva migrans. Affected patients are usually between 2 and 40 years, with an average age of 7.5 years.[245] The syndrome of visceral larva migrans is diagnosed most frequently in the southcentral and southeastern region of the United States.[246]

It has been shown that the major risk factor is exposure to dogs in the household or contact with puppies. Pica has been implicated, and this is conceivable, since 10% to 30% of soil

samples in public playgrounds and parks has been found contaminated with *Toxocara* eggs.[247] It is not known if larval invasion of the eye occurs immediately after ingestion of the eggs or after months or years.[248] It is believed, however, that the number of eggs ingested may determine whether the ocular, visceral, or oculovisceral form of *Toxocara* infection develops.[249]

DIAGNOSIS

Visceral larva migrans is rarely acute. The patient usually complains of a wheezy cough, chest pain, intermittent fever, loss of appetite, and sometimes right upper abdominal pain. In children, pruritic eruptions occasionally occur over the trunk and lower extremities, accompanied by transient tender nodules. There also may be some focal or generalized seizures. In the systemic condition, eosinophils and neutrophils are predominant in the peripheral blood smear.[250]

Ocular larva migrans can occur up to 3 years after the time of presumed infection. Ocular toxocariasis may vary from a low-grade iritis with peripheral anterior synechiae to posterior pole or peripheral retinal granulomas. Peripheral granulomas represent a minimal threat to vision and are the least common of the clinical presentations.[251] Toxocariasis has also been associated with scleritis.[252]

The posterior pole lesion may be characterized by decreased vision or strabismus, depending on the location of the lesion. The lesion is typically round, raised, and white and approximately 1 disc diameter in size (Fig. 32.8). There

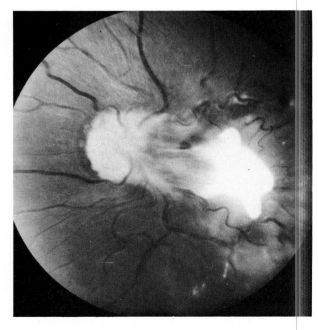

FIGURE 32.8 **Ocular toxocariasis involving the macular region. (Courtesy Randall Coshatt, O.D.)**

can be surrounding pigmentary migration. Fibrous bands may radiate from the lesion, and a crescentic dark area in the lesion is thought to be the larval position within the granuloma.[253]

Tables 32.4 and 32.5 summarize the differences between the ocular and the visceral larva migrans syndromes. It should be noted that it is rare to have concurrent ocular and visceral syndromes.

The clinical diagnosis is based on the enzyme-linked immunosorbent assay (ELISA). The ELISA gives a diagnostic sensitivity of 78% with a 92% specificity.[246] Although this degree of sensitivity and specificity may be overestimated, ELISA remains the laboratory test of choice for ocular *Toxocara canis*.[254] This test is performed in a communicable disease center on 10 ml of clotted blood.[255,256] The percentage of seropositive patients with visceral *Toxocara* decreases with age, while the percentage of seropositive patients with the ocular form increases with age.[257] In an instance where the differential diagnosis of a posterior pole lesion is uncertain and a nondiagnostic ELISA is performed on blood, it is suggested that an anterior chamber tap be performed, since the antibody level is higher in the aqueous than in the blood. This often can prevent an unnecessary enucleation.[258] It is also suggested that ultrasonography may be of some assistance in differential diagnosis.[259] When faced with a patient with an undiagnosed cause for leukocoria, ultrasound may be of benefit. The ultrasound characteristics of a *Toxocara* lesion include: (1) a solid, highly reflective mass; (2) a vitreous band extending from the mass; and (3) a traction retinal detachment extending from the mass.[260] When *Toxocara* is found in one family member, all other family members should be examined.[261]

MANAGEMENT

Management of ocular toxocariasis is controversial. The best management is elimination of the nematodes.

Diethylcarbamazine is the drug used most often in treatment of visceral larva migrans. The initial dosage is 0.5 mg/kg body weight according to tolerance. The dosage is then increased over 3 or 4 days to achieve a final dosage of 3 mg/kg, administered 3 times daily. This dosage level is maintained for 21 days.[262,263]

Steroid therapy, such as oral prednisone 40 mg daily for several weeks, may be of some value in managing the accompanying inflammatory response in the visceral form. The steroid must then be tapered. Although subconjunctival injections of steroids have been reported to aid improvement,[255,263] no proof exists.

Thiabendazole has been tried in systemic *Toxocara* infection with variable success. The usual dosage is 1.5 g twice daily for patients over 70 kg. The dosage is decreased proportionately for patients under 70 kg. This agent is thought to have more of an anti-inflammatory and analgesic effect than an anthelmintic effect.

Photocoagulation and cryopexy may be of some value in isolating the organism if the granuloma is out of the capillary-free zone of the macula. When the granuloma occurs in the macular area and these methods are employed, resultant visual acuity is usually less than 20/200 (6/60).[264]

Should a traction retinal detachment occur secondary to the inflammatory reaction to ocular larva migrans, vitreoretinal surgical intervention may be successful.[265]

Sarcoid Ophthalmopathy

ETIOLOGY

Sarcoidosis is a systemic disease of unknown etiology that is characterized by enhanced immune response at the sites of involvement.[266] It is probably an antigenic reaction of the reticuloendothelial system, but recent work also implicates genetically linked cofactors in the etiology of sarcoidosis.[267] Sarcoidosis is a granulomatous disease that affects many bodily functions. The process may be acute, which indicates

TABLE 32.4
Differences between Ocular and Visceral Toxocariasis

Characteristic	Ocular Larva Migrans	Visceral Larva Migrans
Average age of patient	7.5 years	2 years
White blood cell count	Normal	Elevated
Eosinophilia	Normal	Elevated (> 30%)
Hepatomegaly	None	Usually present
Splenomegaly	None	Usually present
Ocular findings	Posterior pole granuloma Endophthalmitis Peripheral granulomas	Very rare

From Schlaegel TF. Uveitis and miscellaneous parasites. Int Ophthalmol Clin 1977;17:177–194.

TABLE 32.5
The Relationship between Ocular and Visceral Larva Migrans Syndromes: A Hypothetical Model Based on Observations in Human and Experimentally Infected Animals

Toxocariasis	Infectious Dose	Incubation Period	ELISA Antibody Titer
Visceral	Moderate to high	Short (days to months)	High (> 1:16)
Ocular	Low	Long (months to years)	Low (< 1:512)
Visceral and ocular	Very high	Very short (days)	Very high (> 1:1024)

ELISA, enzyme-linked immunosorbent assay.
From Glickman LT, Shantz PM. Epidemiology and pathogenesis of zoonotic toxocariasis. Epidemiol Rev 1981;3:230–250.

a more favorable prognosis than does the chronic presentation. Onset usually occurs between the ages of 20 to 60 years, and approximately 27% to 50% of patients have ocular involvement.[268,269] The most common ocular manifestation is chronic granulomatous anterior uveitis, but the vitreous and retina may also be involved. Blacks are affected more often than are caucasians.[270]

DIAGNOSIS

Granulomatous anterior uveitis is often the first manifestation. While most causes of anterior granulomatous uveitis are often undetermined,[271] the most common systemic association is sarcoidosis.[272] Posterior ocular involvement occurs in about 25% to 37% of patients with ocular sarcoid. The vitreous may be involved, showing fluffy snowball infiltrates near whitish chorioretinal nodules in the inferior retinal periphery. These nodules can vary in size from a disc diameter to large masses.[273,274]

Periphlebitis is the most common fundus feature, and the equatorial retinal veins are most often involved. These changes range from marked, creamy-white perivascular exudation (candlewax drippings) to changes present only in a fluorescein angiogram.[275] Focal subretinal lesions that could be choroidal granulomas occur most commonly in the equatorial retina. Patients with extensive subretinal lesions have less severe periphlebitis. Conditions that may occur as components of ocular sarcoid are: optic disc edema, neovascularization, "snowball" or "string-of-pearls" vitreous opacities,[276] trabecular nodules and tent-like peripheral anterior synechiae as well as Busacca nodules on the iris surface and Koeppe nodules at the pupillary margin,[277] isolated choroidal masses with the possibility of overlying fluffy infiltrates,[278] orbital masses,[279] keratoconjunctivitis sicca secondary to lacrimal gland infiltration,[280] or angiomas.[281,282] Subretinal neovascularization also has been reported as a complication.[283]

The diagnosis of sarcoidosis can be elusive. Transbronchial lung biopsy is diagnostic in approximately 60% of patients presenting with suspected ocular sarcoidosis without extraocular signs.[276] Conjunctival lesions occur in 50% of patients with ocular sarcoid, and biopsy of these lesions may aid in the diagnosis.[284,285] Conjunctival biopsy, while effective, is less sensitive than lung biopsy.[286] Chest x-ray studies also assist in the diagnosis. The elevation of ACE and serum lysozyme levels in some patients with granulomatous uveitis is strongly suggestive of sarcoidosis.[287,288] Gallium-67 imaging is also of value in differential diagnosis,[289] usually presenting the lambda sign (Greek letter lambda in the intrathoracic lymph node)[290] or the panda sign (symmetrical lacrimal and parotid gland uptake) with the most common site of uptake in the lacrimal glands.[291]

The systemic implications of sarcoidosis are crucial because the disease can affect numerous systems. Neurologic[292,293] and cardiovascular[294,295] complications can be severe. Dermatologic signs, such as hypopigmented maculae or nodular lesions on the face or eyelids, may occur in patients with sarcoidosis.[296,297] When managing the patient with ocular manifestations of sarcoidosis, the practitioner must not ignore the potential systemic morbidity of the disease.

MANAGEMENT

The course of the disease is variable, characterized by frequent remissions in the first 3 years, but may become chronic and progressive.[298] As previously mentioned, an acute onset has a more favorable prognosis than does the chronic disease. Visual prognosis is reasonably good if neovascularization does not develop. A final visual acuity of 20/30 (6/9) can be expected if the intraocular inflammation can be controlled.[273]

Note that sarcoidosis is a disease of remissions and exacerbations. This characteristic also applies to the ocular involvement. If active fundus involvement becomes a part of the disease complex, oral steroid therapy should be initiated. Prednisone is started at 60 mg daily and tapered as the inflammatory response diminishes. If the disease is unresponsive to steroids, chlorambucil may be used. This is started at a single daily dose of 4 to 6 mg, increasing weekly by 2 mg if necessary to a maximal dose of 12 mg daily. White blood cell count and platelet activity must be monitored while the patient is taking chlorambucil.[298]

Other options include phenylbutazone or oxyphenbutazone, 600 mg daily in divided doses during the first few days followed by a reduction to 300 mg daily. Other drugs include chloroquine and potassium paraaminobenzoate.[299] With proper surveillance for ocular side effects, chloroquine may be used to control the calcium abnormalities of sarcoidosis.[300]

The most severe ocular complication of sarcoidosis is neovascularization. Whether this appears in the subretinal or supraretinal form, laser photocoagulation may avert potential loss of vision.

Management of the accompanying granulomatous anterior uveitis is achieved through use of topical steroids and mydriatic-cycloplegic agents. The cycloplegic of choice will vary according to severity of the inflammation, with 1% atropine reserved for the stubborn cases. If better mydriasis is needed, 2.5% phenylephrine may be used in conjunction with the cycloplegic. Topical steroids are used initially every 2 hours during the day and should be tapered slowly as the inflammation subsides. If improvement is not noted after a few days, subconjunctival or oral steroids should be used.

The patient with ocular manifestations of sarcoidosis who is placed on therapy must be followed within 2 to 7 days and therapy adjusted according to the response. Any associated keratoconjunctivitis sicca (KCS) must also be managed appropriately. This multisystem disorder requires a multidisciplinary approach for effective management.

Cytomegalovirus (CMV) Retinitis Associated with Acquired Immunodeficiency Syndrome (AIDS)

ETIOLOGY

By the mid-1990s, there were over 350,000 persons diagnosed with AIDS in the United States. It is estimated that there are over 1.5 million persons infected with the human immunovirus (HIV) in the United States and over 10 million persons infected worldwide. Of the total adults and adolescents, approximately 70% have been the result of homosexual and bisexual intercourse, about 20% in intravenous (IV) drug users, 4% the result of heterosexual intercourse, 3% from blood and blood product transfusions, and the remainder undetermined.[301]

The now-recognized cause of AIDS is a retrovirus of the human T-cell lymphotropic class (HTLV-III). The vi-

TABLE 32.6
Diseases Indicating Underlying Cellular Immunodeficiency

Protozoal and helminthic infections
  Cryptosporidiosis
  Strongyloidosis
  Toxoplasmosis
Fungal infections
  Pneumocystis carinii
  Candidiasis
  Cryptococcosis
Bacterial infections
  Mycobacterium avium
  Mycobacterium tuberculosis
Viral infections
  Herpes zoster
  Cytomegalovirus
  Herpes simplex
Cancer
  Kaposi's sarcoma
  Diffuse lymphoma (undifferentiated)
  Lymphoma
  Hodgkin's disease
Other opportunistic infections
  Histoplasmosis
  Isosporiasis

rus has been called the lymphadenopathy-associated virus (LAV) and has been referred to as HTLV-III/LAV by the Centers for Disease Control (CDC). It is now referred to as human immunovirus (HIV). It is believed that all HIV-positive individuals will develop AIDS. The CDC defines a case of AIDS as an illness characterized by: (1) the presence of one or more opportunistic diseases (Table 32.6) that are at least moderately indicative of immunodeficiency, (2) absence of all known underlying causes of immunodeficiency, and (3) absence of all other possible causes of reduced resistance ordinarily associated with the opportunistic diseases.[302]

A minority of individuals currently infected with HIV has AIDS. Up to 25% of individuals infected have lymphadenopathy syndrome: chronic generalized lymphadenopathy, fever, fatigue, malaise, night sweats, weight loss, thrush, or diarrhea. About 10% to 30% of these individuals progress to AIDS within 2 to 3 years.[302]

HIV has been isolated from blood, semen, saliva, bone marrow, lymph nodes, brain, peripheral nerves, cerebrospinal fluid, and conjunctival and corneal epithelium.[303] Fortunately, although the virus is omnipresent, it is also eliminated by several conventional sterilization methods. Transmission is by: (1) sexual contact with exchange of body secretions, (2) infusion of blood or blood products, or (3) infected mother to child.

DIAGNOSIS

It is estimated that patients with AIDS will have at least one ophthalmic or neuro-ophthalmic manifestation at some point in their illness.[304] Cotton wool spots are the most common retinal manifestation of AIDS, occurring in at least two-thirds of patients. These lesions occur as the result of capillary damage, creating localized ischemia. The cotton wool spots are transient, lasting 4 to 6 weeks. Cotton wool spots have no particular prognostic significance.

Flame, white-centered, or dot-blot hemorrhages may also occur as a manifestation of the retinal microvasculopathy. These are seen in 15% to 40% of patients. Ischemic maculopathy may be present in about 6% of patients and is characterized by macular edema and macular star formation.[305]

Cytomegalovirus retinitis (CMVR) is the most common severe ocular manifestation of AIDS, affecting 25% to 45% of patients.[304] Approximately 2% of patients with AIDS have CMVR as the first manifestation of AIDS, and less than 1% of HIV-infected persons will develop CMVR as the initial presentation of AIDS during the first 7 years after HIV infection.[306] CMVR occurs in approximately 16% of terminal AIDS patients.[307] Although most adults have been exposed to CMVR, the intact immune system keeps the infection at bay. CMVR is a necrotizing infection that leads to full-thickness retinal destruction. CMVR may be multifocal and bilateral in 50% of patients. Early CMVR lesions are white and granular with variable degrees of associated hemorrhage, and may appear in the posterior pole or peripheral retina. There may be an accompanying low grade anterior uveitis and vitritis.[308] Bilateral CMVR may serve as a marker of HIV encephalitis, possibly indicating a severely immunosuppressed state.[309] Disc neovascularization may develop in some cases of AIDS and CMVR.[310] The CMVR usually spreads in a "brushfire" fashion accompanied by hemorrhage. Once established, the CMVR may spread rapidly and destroy vision within 6 months (Fig. 32.9). Plaque-like intraretinal calcifications may occur in areas of healed CMVR,[311] as well as persistent stable white borders of opacification on the edge of the healed CMVR.[312]

Unfortunately, retinal detachment is a complication of CMVR.[313,314] Jabs and associates[315] estimated a prevalence of 26% in patients with CMVR, with a probability of 50% within 1 year after the diagnosis of CMVR. Retinal repair is usually anatomically successful, but only 20% of eyes achieve vision of 5/200 or better since there is a high incidence of proliferative vitreoretinopathy.[316] Because of the severity of CMVR, patients who are HIV-positive should have dilated fundus examinations every 3 to 6 months, and patients with AIDS should have dilated fundus examinations every 3 months. The longest reported survival after the diagnosis of CMVR is 30 months while the median survival time is 8.4 months.[317]

Frosted branch angiitis can also be associated with CMVR. This condition manifests as sheathing of retinal vessels. The perivascular infiltration is usually thick and white, affecting both veins and arteries near veins. Fluorescein angiography demonstrates leakage from both arteries and veins. Frosted branch angiitis is usually not directly associated with any particular disease process and occurs most frequently in young patients. Note that the treatment of frosted branch angiitis, when associated with CMVR and AIDS, may result in the potentiation of CMVR.[318-320]

The primary diagnostic test for AIDS is the Western blot test. The laboratory diagnosis of AIDS is made by ELISA for HIV. ELISA is a highly specific screening test for the presence of antibodies to the HIV virus. Positive results on the ELISA must then be confirmed by a Western blot test or immunofluorescent assay (IFA). A positive ELISA means only that antibodies to the HIV virus are present and does not imply that the patient will necessarily progress to the full-blown AIDS complex.

MANAGEMENT

Opportunistic infections must be managed separately, and often the infection reappears when treatment ceases. For toxoplasmic retinitis, pyrimethamine and sulfadiazine are effective against the active organism, but there is a high recurrence rate when treatment is discontinued.[321,322] The use of corticosteroids in patients with immunosuppression secondary to HIV may result in an increased incidence of CMV disease throughout the body.[323]

Clinical trials confirm that CMVR can be treated successfully with antiviral agents. Patients respond more rapidly to ganciclovir than foscarnet, but both modes of therapy appear to be effective. Ganciclovir therapy is associated with more delayed reactivation and fewer side effects than is foscarnet,[324-328] but foscarnet may prolong survival (12.6 months) of persons with AIDS and CMVR as compared to treatment with ganciclovir (8.5 months).[329-331] To be effective, both antiviral agents must be dosed intravenously and then followed with maintenance dosages. Oral ganciclovir can be given for the maintenance treatment of CMVR in patients for whom the risk of more rapid disease progression is balanced by the benefit associated with avoiding intravenous infusions. Increasing the maintenance dosages of intravenous foscarnet to 120 mg/kg/day from 90 mg/kg/day lengthens survival time and delays CMVR progression without associated increases in toxicity.[332] Ganciclovir demonstrates toxicity in the form of neutropenia when given intravenously and endophthalmitis when delivered intravitreally.[333] Since foscarnet may induce nephrotoxicity, serum creatinine levels should be monitored.[334,335] Intravitreal foscarnet given in two injections of 1200 μg weekly for 3 weeks, followed by a maintenance treatment regimen of one injection weekly, has been effective for the treatment of CMVR, while minimizing toxic reactions.[336,337]

Despite treatment with ganciclovir, progression of CMVR

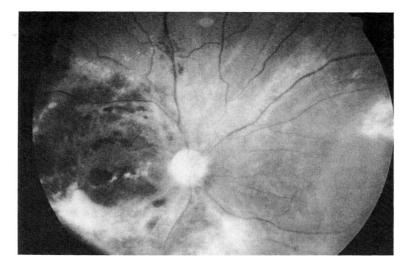

A

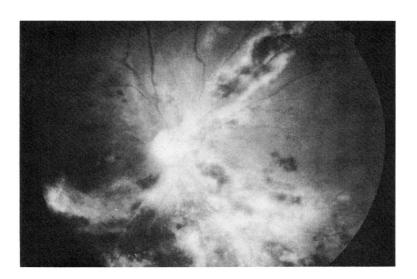

B

FIGURE 32.9   *(A)* CMV retinitis in a 27-year-old male with AIDS. *(B)* One month later, showing marked progression of retinitis. (Courtesy Brian P. Den Beste, O.D.)

may occur.[338,339] Clinically-resistant CMVR appears to be a manifestation of acquired CMV antiviral drug resistance, and the use of foscarnet combined with ganciclovir appears to be effective in halting progression in some patients.[340,341]

Although ganciclovir and foscarnet are the drugs of choice for CMVR, intravenous zidovudine combined with acyclovir may offer an effective alternative.[342,343]

In monitoring the patient treated for CMVR, fundus evaluation is crucial, but visual field testing offers another effective tool. Stabilization of the visual field defects occurring in many cases of CMVR indicates control of the destructive retinal process.[344]

Outer retinal necrosis, which is acute and rapidly progressive, is proposed to be the result of CMV. Ganciclovir appears to be effective in the treatment of this disorder, especially if used early in the disease process.[345]

Clearly the best possible management for AIDS is prevention through appropriate education and prophylaxis. The following is a summary of current recommendations to prevent transfer of HIV.[346–347]

1. Special care must be exercised regarding all sexual contacts.
2. Gloves should be worn when there is potential contact with body secretions or blood. Otherwise, routine examination followed by careful handwashing are sufficient.
3. Masks may be worn in the examination of patients suspected of having airborne opportunistic organisms.
4. Goggles or eye shields should be worn when infected fluids might be splashed into the eyes.
5. All needles and syringes should be disposed of properly in "sharps" containers.
6. Tonometer tips and all other instruments making contact with the eye should be disinfected after use. HIV is inactivated by 5 to 10 minute exposure to 3% hydrogen peroxide, a 1:10 dilution of household bleach, or 70% ethanol or isopropyl alcohol. Environmental surfaces may be disinfected in the same manner.
7. Rigid polymethylmethacrylate (PMMA) contact lenses and rigid gas-permeable lenses should be disinfected with commercially available hydrogen peroxide systems. Soft contact lenses may be heat-disinfected or disinfected with commercially available hydrogen peroxide systems.

Acute Retinal Necrosis Syndrome (ARNS)

ETIOLOGY

Acute retinal necrosis syndrome (ARNS) is a variation of an occlusive retinal vasculitis primarily affecting the arteries of the retina and choroid, and occurring usually in immunocompetent individuals.[365,366] There is a propensity for involvement of the peripheral retina. The end result in the majority of untreated cases is a rhegmatogenous retinal detachment that often occurs 2 to 3 months after the onset of the disease.[348] The strongest evidence implicates herpes viruses as the causative agent. Herpes simplex virus infections usually are associated with younger patients, while herpes zoster infections appear in the older patient population.[349] Chickenpox also has an association with ARNS.[350] ARNS occurs in patients aged 20 to 60 years, but there is considerable variability in the presentation. The condition is bilateral in approximately 33% of patients, with involvement of the second eye after several weeks. Males are affected slightly more often than females. There is thought to be a relationship to immunogenetic predisposition based on HLA antigen findings.[351] Immunocompromised patients are more prone to develop ARNS.

DIAGNOSIS

The patient with ARNS presents clinically with mild to moderate ocular or periorbital pain that may be enhanced by motion of the globe, a red eye, chemosis and lid edema, mild proptosis, subconjunctival hemorrhage, and a mild foreign body sensation. Mild to moderate anterior granulomatous uveitis is typical, with the possibility of an associated hypopyon. Intraocular pressure is often elevated in the affected eye. There may be hazy vision, floaters, and peripheral vision complaints, with loss of central vision possible late in the process secondary to optic neuritis or retinal detachment.[352]

The signs in the posterior segment include retinal and choroidal vasculitis, retinal necrosis, optic disc edema, and vitritis. The peripheral retina is usually involved first, followed by spreading toward the posterior pole. The larger arteries are narrowed and sheathed while periphlebitis is rare. Retinal hemorrhages may be present. Retinal necrosis presents as areas of confluent retinal whitening in the form of pseudopods that obscure underlying choroidal detail.[353–355] Vitreous cells are a feature of ARNS that help to differentiate the disease from CMVR.

The process is self-limiting in 6 to 12 weeks with subsequent atrophy of the inflamed areas. Retinal holes, retinal tears, and vitreous traction all contribute to the development of retinal detachment and proliferative vitreoretinopathy in up to 75% of patients with ARNS. Associated systemic viral findings are often present.[356,357]

MANAGEMENT

Diagnosis of ARNS is often by exclusion. Vitrectomy and retinal biopsy may produce a diagnostic culture,[353,358–360] and immunofluorescent studies of the aqueous may confirm herpes simplex or varicella virus.[361] Currently, standard diagnostic tests will not confirm the diagnosis of ARNS, but HIV testing is imperative prior to diagnosis and initiation of therapy. Fluorescein angiography demonstrates early blockage of the underlying choroidal fluorescence in areas of active retinitis with blockage of arterial flow.

Therapy is based on the assumption that ARNS is the result of herpes simplex virus (HSV) or varicella zoster virus (VZV) infection. Intravenous acyclovir, 1500 mg/m^2 per day in three doses for 5 to 10 days, is recommended. Progression of the retinitis often occurs over the first 48 hours of treatment, with regression within 4 days. After the intravenous treatment, oral acyclovir is given at 400 to 600 mg 5 times a day for 6 weeks, because of potential involvement of the second eye within 6 weeks of the first.[353,362] For immunocompromised patients, intravitreal injection of ganciclovir or foscarnet at initial diagnosis in conjunction with prolonged intravenous combination therapy with both drugs may prove beneficial.[363,365] Antiplatelet therapy in the form of aspirin 125 mg to 650 mg once or twice a day is indicated for the associated hyperactivity of the platelets in ARNS.

Systemic corticosteroids may suppress the inflammatory activity but also may exacerbate the viral infection.

Prophylactic laser photocoagulation applied to the areas of active retinitis appears to minimize the threat of subsequent retinal tears and detachment. Retinal detachment surgery with vitrectomy is necessary to treat complications of vitreous traction and rhegmatogenous detachment.[364]

References

1. Von Bayer A. Ber Deutsch Chemistrie. Ges 1871;4:555.
2. Burk A. Die Klinische, physiologische und pathologische bedeutung der fluoreazenz in augenach darreichung von uranin. Klin Monatsbl Augenheilkd 1910;48:454–455.
3. Kikai K. Ueber die vitalfarbung des hinteren bulbussabschnittes. Arch Augenheilkd 1930;103:541.
4. Novotny HR, Alvis DL. A method of photographing fluorescein in circulating blood in the human retina. Circulation 1961;24:82–86.
5. Patz A, Fine SL. Interpretation of the fluorescein angiogram. Boston: Little, Brown, 1977.
6. Schatz H. Interpretation of fundus fluorescein angiography. St. Louis: C.V. Mosby Co, 1978.
7. Kelley JS, Kincaid M. Retinal fluorography using oral fluorescein. Arch Ophthalmol 1979;97:2331–2332.
8. Hunter JE. Oral fluorography in retinal pigment epithelial detachment. Am J Optom Physiol Opt 1982;59:926–928.
9. Hunter JE. Oral fluorography in papilledema. Am J Optom Physiol Opt 1983;60:908–910.
10. The Oral Fluorescein Study Group. Oral fluorography. J Am Optom Assoc 1985;10:784–792.
11. Yamana Y, Ohnishi Y, Taniguchi Y, Ikeda M. Early signs of diabetic retinopathy by fluorescein angiography. Jpn J Ophthalmol 1983;27:218–227.
12. Starup K, Larsen HW, Enk B, Vestermark S. Fluorescein angiography in diabetic children. Acta Ophthalmol 1980;58:347–354.
13. Klemen UM, Freyler H, Schober E, Frisch H. Diagnosis of retinal vascular changes in diabetic children by means of fluorescein angiography. Monatsschr Kinderheilkd 1980;128:502–505.
14. Schimizu K, Kobayashi Y, Muraoka K. Midperipheral fundus involvement in diabetic retinopathy. Ophthalmology 1981;88:601–612.
15. Scheider A, Nasemann JE, Lund OE. Fluorescein and indocyanine green angiographies of central serous choroidopathy by scanning laser ophthalmoscopy. Am J Ophthalmol 1993;115:50–56.
16. Kuck H, Inhoffen W, Schneider U, et al. Diagnosis of occult subretinal neovascularization in age-related macular degeneration by infrared scanning laser videoangiography. Retina 1993;13:36–39.
17. Scheider A, Voeth A, Kaboth A, et al. Fluorescence characteristics of indocyanine green in the normal choroid and in subretinal neovascular membranes. Ger J Ophthalmol 1992;1:7–11.
18. Yannuzzi LA, Slakter JS, Sorenson JA, et al. Digitial indocyanine green videoangiography and choroidal neovascularization. Retina 1992;12:191–223.
19. Miki T, Kitashoji K, Kohno T. Intrachoroidal dye leakage in indocyanine green fundus angiography after experimental commotio retinae. Eur J Ophthalmol 1992;2:79–82.
20. Oncel M, Khoobehi B, Peyman GA. Calcein angiography: a preliminary report on an experimental dye. Int Ophthalmol 1990;14:245–250.
21. Zeimer RC, Guran T, Shahdi M, et al. Visualization of the retinal microvasculature by targeted dye delivery. Invest Ophthalmol Vis Sci 1990;31:1459–1465.
22. Spencer T, Phillips RP, Sharp PF, et al. Automated detection and quantification of microaneurysms in fluorescein angiograms. Graefe's Arch Clin Exp Ophthalmol 1992;230:36–41.
23. Phillips RP, Ross PG, Tyska M, et al. Detection and quantification of hyperfluorescent leakage by computer analysis of fundus flourescein angiograms. Graefe's Arch Clin Exp Ophthalmol 1991;229:329–335.
24. Terry J. Ophthalmic photography and fluorescein angiography. In: Terry J, ed. Ocular disease. Boston: Butterworths, 1984.
25. Bianchi C. Fluorescein angiography. Why not in color? J Fr Ophthalmol 1980;3:715–718.
26. Choromokos EA, Wilson CA, Raymond LA, et al. Fluorescein angiography using ultra-high speed film. Ann Ophthalmol 1990;22:299–301.
27. Hyvarinen L, Flower RW. Indocyanine green fluorescein angiography. Acta Ophthalmol 1980;58:528–538.
28. Jacob JS, Rosen ES, Young E. Report of the substance, dimethyl formamide, in sodium fluorescein used for fluorescein angiography. Br J Ophthalmol 1982;66:567–568.
29. Lee PP, Yang JC, Schachat AP. Is informed consent needed for fluorescein angiography? Arch Ophthalmol 1993;111:327–330.
30. Romanchuk KG. Fluorescein. Physiochemical factors affecting its fluorescence. Surv Ophthalmol 1982;26:269–283.
31. Butner RW, McPherson AR. Adverse reactions in intravenous fluorescein angiography. Ann Ophthalmol 1983;15:1084–1086.
32. Arroyave CM. Plasma complement and histamine changes after intravenous administration of sodium fluorescein. Am J Ophthalmol 1969;87:474–479.
33. Pacurariu RI. Low incidence of side effects following fluorescein angiography. Ann Ophthalmol 1982;14:32–36.
34. Ellis PP, Schoenberger M, Rendi MA. Antihistamines as prophylaxis against side reactions to intravenous fluorescein. Trans Am Ophthalmol Soc 1980;78:190–205.
35. Brown RE, Sabates R, Drew SJ. Metoclopramide as prophylaxis for nausea and vomiting induced by fluorescein. Arch Ophthalmol 1987;105:658–659.
36. Wolf S, Arend O, Schulte K, et al. Severe anaphylactic reaction after indocyanine green fluorescence angiography. Am J Ophthalmol 1992;114:638–639.
37. Olk RJ, Halperin LS, Soubrane G, et al. Fluorescein angiography—is it safe to use in a pregnant patient? Eur J Ophthalmol 1991;1:103–106.
38. Irwin R. Practical aspects of oral fluorography. J Ophthal Photog 1981;4:16–18.
39. Noble MJ, Cheng H, Jacobs PM. Oral fluorescein and cystoid macular edema: Detection in aphakic and pseudophakic eyes. Br J Ophthalmol 1984;68:221–224.
40. Emerson GA, Anderson HH. Toxicity of certain proposed antileprosy dyes: Fluorescein, eosin, erythrosin and others. Int J Leprosy 1934;2:257–263.
41. Kelley JS, Kincaid M, Hoover RE, McBeth C. Retinal fluorograms using oral fluorescein. Ophthalmology 1980;87:805–811.

42. Morgan KS, Franklin RM. Oral fluorescein angioscopy in aphakic children. J Pediatr Ophthalmol Strabismus 1984;21:33–36.

43. El-Mofty A, Barada A, Yaqoub M. Fundus fluorescein angioscopy in vaso-occlusive diseases of the retina. Bull Ophthalmol Soc Egypt 1982;75:237–241.

44. Balogh VJ. The use of oral fluorescein angiography in idiopathic central serous chorioretinopathy. J Am Optom Assoc 1986;57:909–913.

45. McGarth MA, Wechsler F, Hunyor AB, Penney R. Systemic factors contributory to retinal vein occlusion. Arch Intern Med 1978;2:216–220.

46. Ririe DG, Cosgriff TM, Martin B. Central retinal vein occlusion in a patient with familial antithrombin III deficiency: Case report. Ann Ophthalmol 1979;11:1841–1845.

47. Brunette I, Boghen D. Central retinal vein occlusion complicating spontaneous carotid cavernous fistula: Case report. Arch Ophthalmol 1987;105:464–465.

48. Barton CH, Viziri ND. Central retinal vein occlusion associated with hemodialysis. Am J Med Sci 1979;277:39–47.

49. Priluck IA. Impending central retinal vein occlusion associated with increased platelet aggregability. Ann Ophthalmol 1979;11:79–84.

50. Walsh PN, Goldberg RE, Tax RL, Magargal LE. Platelet coagulant activities and retinal vein thrombosis. Thromb Haemostas 1977;38:399–406.

51. Heidrich H, Hofner J, Wollensak J, Schneider D. Retinal vascular occlusion and thrombocyte aggregation. J Med 1980;11:127–131.

52. Dodson PM, Galton DJ, Hamilton AM, Black PK. Retinal vein occlusion and the prevalence of lipoprotein abnormalities. Br J Ophthalmol 1982;66:161–164.

53. Wenzler EM, Rademarkers AJ, Boers GH, et al. Hyperhomocysteinemia in retinal artery and retinal vein occlusion. Am J Ophthalmol 1993;115:162–167.

54. Roberts SP, Haefs TM. Central retinal vein occlusion in a middle-aged adult with HIV infection. J Optom Vis Sci 1992;69:567–569.

55. Hedges TR Jr, Giliberti OL, Magargal LE. Intravenous digital subtraction angiography and its role in ocular vascular disease. Arch Ophthalmol 1985;103:666–669.

56. Brown GC, Shah HG, Magargal LE, Savino PJ. Central retinal vein obstruction and carotid artery disease. Ophthalmology 1984;91:1627–1633.

57. Gonder JR, Magargal LE, Walsh PN, et al. Central retinal vein obstruction associated with mitral valve prolapse. Can J Ophthalmol 1983;18:220–222.

58. Green WR, Chan CC, Hutchins GM, Terry JM. Central retinal vein occlusion: A prospective histopathologic study of 29 eyes in 28 cases. Trans Am Ophthalmol Soc 1981;79:371–422.

59. Priluck IA, Robertson DM, Holenhorst RW. Long-term follow-up occlusion of the central retinal vein in young adults. Am J Ophthalmol 1980;2:190–202.

60. Littlejohn GO, Urowitz MB, Paulin CJ. Central retinal vein occlusion and scleroderma: Implications for sclerodermatous vascular disease. Ann Rheum Dis 1981;40:96–99.

61. Smith P, Green WR, Miller NR, Terry JM. Central retinal vein occlusion in Reye's syndrome. Arch Ophthalmol 1980;98:1256–1260.

62. Silverman M, Lubeck MJ, Briney WG. Central retinal vein occlusion complicating systemic lupus erythematosus. Arthritis Rheum 1978;21:839–843.

63. Kline LB, Kirkham TH, Belanger G, Remillard G. Traumatic central retinal vein occlusion. Ann Ophthalmol 1978;10:587–591.

64. Fong AC, Schatz H. Central retinal vein occlusion in young adults. Surv Ophthalmol 1993;37:393–417.

65. Fong AC, Schatz H, McDonald HR, et al. Central retinal vein occlusion in young adults (papillophlebitis). Retina 1992;12:3–11.

66. Hayreh SS, van Heuven WA, Hyareh MS. Experimental retinal vascular occlusion. Pathogenesis of central retinal vein occlusion. Arch Ophthalmol 1978;96:311–323.

67. Spires R. Central retinal vein occlusion. J Ophthalmic Nurs Tech 1993;12:57–63.

68. Frucht J, Shapiro A, Merin S. Intraocular pressure in retinal vein occlusion. Br J Ophthalmol 1984;68:26–28.

69. Hayreh SS, March W, Phelps CD. Ocular hypotony following retinal vein occlusion. Arch Ophthalmol 1978;96:827–833.

70. Bloome MA. Transient angle-closure glaucoma in central retinal vein occlusion. Ann Ophthalmol 1977;9:44–48.

71. Servais GE, Thompson HS, Hayreh SS. Relative afferent pupillary defect in central retinal vein occlusion. Ophthalmology 1986;93:301–303.

72. Zegarra H, Gutman FA, Conforto J. The natural course of central retinal vein occlusion. Ophthalmology 1979;86:1931–1942.

73. Frucht J, Hanko L, Norin S. Central retinal vein occlusions in young adults. Acta Ophthalmol 1984;62:780–786.

74. Zegarra H, Gutman FA, Zakov N, Carim M. Partial occlusion of the central retinal vein. Am J Ophthalmol 1983;96:330–357.

75. Little HL, Chan CC. Infrequency of retinal neovascularization following central retinal vein occlusion attributed to endothelial death. Mod Probl Ophthalmol 1979;20:121–126.

76. Magargal LE, Brown GC, Augsburger JJ, Parrish RK. Neovascular glaucoma following central retinal vein obstruction. Ophthalmology 1981;88:1095–1101.

77. Tasman W, Magargal LE, Augsburger JJ. Effects of argon laser photocoagulation on rubeosis iridis and angle neovascularization. Ophthalmology 1980;87:400–402.

78. Lunta MH, Schenker HI. Retinal vascular accidents in glaucoma and ocular hypertension. Surv Ophthalmol 1980;25:163–167.

79. Ellis PP. Retinal vein occlusion. In: Fraunfelder FT, Roy FH, eds. Current ocular therapy. Philadelphia: W.B. Saunders Co, 1980;561–562.

80. Minturn J, Brown GC. Progression of nonischemic central retinal vein obstruction to the ischemic variant. Ophthalmology 1986;93:1158–1162.

81. Jaeger EA. Venous obstructive disease of the retina. In: Duane TD, ed. Clinical ophthalmology. Philadelphia: Harper & Row, 1981;3:Chap. 15, pp. 12–13.

82. Gombos GM. Retinal vascular occlusions and their treatment with low molecular weight dextran and vasodilators: Report of six years' experience. Ann Ophthalmol 1978;10:579–583.

83. Hansen LL, Daniseyski P, Arntz HR, et al. A randomized prospective study on treatment of central retinal vein occlusion by isovolemic hemodilution and photocoagulation. Br J Ophthalmol 1985;69:108–116.

84. Hirayama Y, Matsunaga N, Tashiro J, et al. Bifemelane in the treatment of central retinal artery or vein obstruction. Clin Therapeutics 1990;12:230–235.

85. Laatikainen L. Photocoagulation in retinal venous occlusion. Acta Ophthalmol 1977;55:478–488.

86. Laatikainen L. Preliminary report on effect of panphotocoagula-

tion on rubeosis iridis and neovascular glaucoma. Br J Ophthalmol 1977;61:278–284.

87. Smith RJ. Rubeotic glaucoma. Br J Ophthalmol 1981;65:606–609.

88. Demeler U. Management of retinal venous occlusion. Ophthalmologica 1980;180:61–67.

89. May DR, Klein ML, Peyman GA, Raichand M. Xenon arc panretinal photocoagulation for central retinal vein occlusion: A randomized prospective study. Br J Ophthalmol 1979;63:725–734.

90. Carter JE. Panretinal photocoagulation for progressive ocular neovascularization secondary to occlusion of the common carotid artery. Ann Ophthalmol 1984;16:572–576.

91. Laatikainen L, Kohner EM, Khoury D, Black RK. Panretinal photocoagulation in central retinal vein occlusion: A randomized controlled clinical study. Br J Ophthalmol 1977;61:741–753.

92. Murdoch IE, Rosen PH, Shilling JS. Neovascular response in ischaemic central retinal vein occlusion after panretinal photocoagulation. Br J Ophthalmol 1991;75:459–461.

93. Hayreh SS, Klugman MR, Podhajsky P, et al. Argon laser panretinal photocoagulation in ischemic central retinal vein occlusion. A 10–year prospective study. Graefe's Arch Clin Exp Ophthalmol 1990;228:281–296.

94. Kerns TP, Siekert RG, Sandt TM. The ocular aspects of bypass surgery of the carotid artery. Mayo Clin Proc 1979;54:3–11.

95. Kerns TP, Younge BR, Piepgras DG. Resolution of venous stasis retinopathy after carotid bypass surgery. Mayo Clin Proc 1980;55:342–346.

96. Cowan CL Jr, Butler G. Ischemic oculopathy. Ann Ophthalmol 1983;15:1052–1057.

97. Brown GC, Magargal LE, Schachat A, Shah H. Neovascular glaucoma. Etiologic considerations. Ophthalmology 1984;91:315–320.

98. Chopdar A. Dual trunk central retinal vein incidence in clinical practice. Arch Ophthalmol 1984;102:85–87.

99. Sanborn GE, Magargal LE. Characteristics of the hemispheric retinal vein occlusion. Ophthalmology 1984;91:1616–1626.

100. Hayreh SS, Hayreh MS. Hemi-central retinal vein occlusion. Pathogeneses, clinical features, and natural history. Arch Ophthalmol 1980;98:1600–1609.

101. Sayegh F. Obstruction of the central retinal artery. Comparison of the ophthalmodynamometry measurements in relation to the time. Ophthalmologica 1979;179:322–329.

102. Wilson LA, Warlow CP, Russell RW. Cardiovascular disease in patients with retinal arterial occlusion. Lancet 1979;1:292–294.

103. Cullen JG, Korcusba K, Masser G, et al. Calcified left ventricular thrombus causing repeated retinal arterial emboli: Clinical, echocardiographic, and pathologic features. Chest 1981;79:708–710.

104. Brockmeier LB, Adolph RJ, Gustin BW, et al. Calcium emboli to the retinal artery in calcific aortic stenosis. Am Heart J 1981;101:32–37.

105. Baker RS, Tibbs PA, Millett AJ. Carotid-retinal embolism with coexistant mitral valve prolapse. Neurology 1981;31:1192–1193.

106. Rush JA, Kearns TP, Danielson GK. Cloth-particle retinal emboli from artificial cardiac valves. Am J Ophthalmol 1980;89:845–850.

107. Reese LT, Shafer D. Retinal embolization from endocarditis. Ann Ophthalmol 1978;10:1655–1657.

108. Appen RE. Central retinal artery occlusion. In: Fraunfelder FT, Roy FH, eds. Current ocular therapy. Philadelphia: W.B. Saunders Co, 1980;549–550.

109. Stowe GC III, Zakov ZN, Albert DM. Central retinal vascular occlusion associated with oral contraceptives. Am J Ophthalmol 1978;86:798–801.

110. Solomon SM, Solomon JH. Bilateral central retinal artery occlusions in polyarteritis nodosa. Ann Ophthalmol 1978;10:567–569.

111. Wilson RS, Havener WH, McGrew RN. Bilateral retinal artery and choriocapillaris occlusion following the injection of long-acting corticosteroid suspension in combination with other drugs. I. Clinical studies. Ophthalmology 1978;85:967–973.

112. Whiteman DW, Rosen DA, Pinkerton RM. Retinal and choroidal microvascular embolism after intranasal corticosteroid injection. Am J Ophthalmol 1980;89:851–853.

113. Hallerman D, Singh B. Iatrogenic central retinal artery embolization: A complication of cardiac catherization. Ann Ophthalmol 1984;16:1025–1027.

114. Jonas J, Kolbe K, Volcker HE, et al. Central retinal artery occlusion in Sneddon's disease associated with antiphospholipid antibodies. Am J Ophthalmol 1986;102:37–40.

115. Cheney ML, Blair PA. Blindness as a complication of rhinoplasty. Arch Otolaryngol Head Neck Surg 1987;113:768–769.

116. Etre JM, Magnus DE, Jones WL. Central retinal artery occlusion with an irido-embolus following carotid endarterectomy. J Am Optom Assoc 1987;58:419–422.

117. LaMonica CB, Foye GJ, Silberman L. A case of sudden retinal artery occlusion and blindness in pregnancy. Obstet Gynecol 1987;69:433–435.

118. Bradish CF, Flowers M. Central retinal artery occlusion in association with osteogenesis imperfecta. Spine 1987;12:193–194.

119. Hsu AA, Wong TM, How J, et al. Retinal artery occlusion in a diver. Singapore Med J 1992;33:299–301.

120. Wilson CA, Wander AH, Choromokos EA. Central retinal artery obstruction in herpes zoster ophthalmicus and cerebral vasculopathy. Ann Ophthalmol 1990;22:347–351.

121. Brown GC, Magargal LE, Simeone FA, et al. Arterial obstruction and ocular neovascularization. Ophthalmology 1982;89:139–146.

122. Hodes BL, Edelman D. Central retinal artery occlusion after facial trauma. Ophthalmic Surg 1979;10:21–23.

123. Weissman H, Nadel AJ, Dunn M. Simultaneous bilateral retinal arterial occlusions treated by exchange transfusions. Arch Ophthalmol 1979;97:2151–2153.

124. Wray SH. The management of acute visual failure. J Neurol Neurosurg Psych 1993;56:234–240.

125. Deutsch TA, Read JS, Ernest JT, et al. Effects of oxygen and carbon dioxide on the retinal vasculature in humans. Arch Ophthalmol 1983;101:1278–1280.

126. Henbink P, Chambers JK. Arterial occlusive disease of the retina. In: Duane TD, ed. Clinical ophthalmology. Philadelphia: Harper & Row, 1981;3;Chap. 14, p. 14.

127. Matzkin DC, Slamovits TL, Sachs R, et al. Visual recovery in two patients after intravenous methylprednisolone treatment of central retinal artery occlusion secondary to giant-cell arteritis. Ophthalmology 1992;99:68–71.

128. Schmidt D, Schumacher M, Wakhloo AK. Microcatheter urokinase infusion in central retinal artery occlusion. Am J Ophthalmol 1992;113:429–434.

129. Sheng FC, Quinones-Baldrich W, Machleder HI, et al. Relationship of extracranial carotid occlusive disease and central retinal artery occlusion. Am J Surg 1986;152:175–178.

130. Schatz H, Drake M. Self-injected retinal emboli. Ophthalmology 1979;86:468–483.

131. Nehen AM, Damgaard-Jensen L, Hansen PE. Foreign body embolism of retinal arteries as a complication of carotid angiography. Neuroradiology 1978;15:85–88.

132. Gass JD, Tiedeman J, Thomas MA. Idiopathic recurrent branch retinal arterial occlusion. Ophthalmology 1986;93:1148–1157.

133. Lam BL, Siatkowski RM, Fox GM, et al. Visual loss in pseudotumor cerebri from branch retinal artery occlusion. Am J Ophthalmol 1992;113:334–336.

134. Lightman DA, Brod RD. Branch retinal artery occlusion associated with Lyme disease. Arch Ophthalmol 1991;109:1198–1199.

135. Nielsen NV. Treatment of acute occlusion of the retinal arteries. Acta Ophthalmologica 1979;57:1078–1081.

136. Iwafune Y, Yoshimoto H. Clinical use of pentoxifylline in haemorrhagic disorders of the retina. Pharmatherapeutica 1980;2:429–438.

137. Sipila I. Inhibition of arginino-glycine aminotransferase by ornithine. A possible mechanism for the muscular and chorioretinal atrophies in gyrate atrophy of the choroid and retina with hyperornithinemia. Biochem Biophys Acta 1980;613:79–84.

138. Ramesh V, Gusella JF, Shih VE. Molecular pathology of gyrate atrophy of the choroid and retina due to ornithine aminotransferase deficiency. Mol Biol Med 1991;8:81–93.

139. Francois J. Gyrate atrophy of the choroid and retina. Ophthalmologica 1979;178:311–320.

140. Kaiser-Kupfer MI, Valle D, Bron AJ. Clinical and biochemical heterogeneity in gyrate atrophy. Am J Ophthalmol 1980;89:219–222.

141. Steel D, Wood CM, Richardson J, et al. Anterior subcapsular plaque cataract in hyperornithinaemia gyrate atrophy—a case report. Br J Ophthalmol 1992;76:762–763.

142. Potter MJ, Berson EL. Diagnosis and treatment of gyrate atrophy. Int Ophthalmol Clin 1993;33:229–236.

143. Park JK, O'Donnell JJ, Shih VE, et al. A 15–bp deletion in exon 5 of the ornithine aminotransferase (OAT) locus associated with gyrate atrophy. Human Mutation 1992;1:293–297.

144. Mashima Y, Weleber RG, Kennaway NG, et al. A single-base change at a splice acceptor site in the ornithine aminotransferase gene causes abnormal RNA splicing in gyrate atrophy. Human Gen 1992;90:305–307.

145. Akaki Y, Hotta Y, Mashima Y, et al. A deletion in the ornithine aminotransferase gene in gyrate atrophy. J Biol Chem 1992;267:12950–12954.

146. Reichel E, Berson EL. New techniques for evaluating pediatric retinal disease: molecular genetics. Int Ophthalmol Clin 1992;32:153–161.

147. Valle D, Walser M, Brusilow SW, Kaiser-Kupfer M. Gyrate atrophy of the choroid and retina. Amino acid metabolism and correction of hyperornithinemia with an arginine-deficient diet. J Clin Invest 1980;63:371–378.

148. Kaiser-Kupfer MI, Caruso RC, Valle D. Gyrate atrophy of the choroid and retina. Long-term reduction of ornithine slows retinal degeneration. Arch Ophthalmol 1991;109:1539–1548.

149. Vannus-Sulonen K, Sipila I, Vannus A, et al. Gyrate atrophy of the choroid and retina: A five-year follow-up of creatine supplementation. Ophthalmology 1985;92:1719–1727.

150. Kennaway NG, Weleber RG, Buist NRM. Gyrate atrophy of the choroid and retina with hyperornithinemia: Biochemical and histologic studies in response to vitamin B_6. Am J Hum Genet 1980;32:529–541.

151. Ogura Y, Takahashi M, Ueno S, Honda Y. Hyperboric oxygen treatment for chronic cystoid macular edema after branch retinal vein occlusion. Am J Ophthalmol 1987;104:301–302.

152. Heckenlively JR. Grid photocoagulation for macular edema in patients with retinitis pigmentosa (letter). Am J Ophthalmol 1987;104:94–95.

153. MacKay CJ, Shek MS, Carr RE, et al. Retinal degeneration with nanophthalmos, cystic macular degeneration, and angle closure glaucoma. A new recessive syndrome. Arch Ophthalmol 1987;105:366–371.

154. Lewis H, Singer TR, Hanscom TA, Straatsma BR. A prospective study of cystoid macular edema after neodymium:YAG laser posterior capsulotomy. Ophthalmology 1987;94:478–482.

155. Henderly DE, Hammond RS, Rao NA, Smith RE. The significance of the pars plana exudate in pars planitis. Am J Ophthalmol 1987;103:669–671.

156. Brown GC. Macular edema in association with severe carotid artery obstruction. Am J Ophthalmol 1986;102:442–448.

157. Dulaney DD. Cystoid macular edema and corneal-relaxing incisions (letter). Arch Ophthalmol 1987;105:742–743.

158. Carter J, Barron BA, McDonald MB. Cystoid macular edema following corneal-relaxing incisions. Arch Ophthalmol 1987;105:70–72.

159. Brough GH, Jones WL. Long-standing venous stasis retinopathy with resultant cystoid macular edema. J Am Optom Assoc 1987;58:423–425.

160. Nussenblatt RB. Macular alterations secondary to intraocular inflammatory disease. Ophthalmology 1986;93:984–988.

161. Irvine AR. Cystoid maculopathy. Surv Ophthalmol 1976;21:1–17.

162. Irvine AR. Cystoid maculopathy (cystoid macular edema, Irvine-Gass syndrome). In: Fraunfelder FT, Roy FH, eds. Current ocular therapy. Philadelphia: W.B. Saunders Co, 1980;517–519.

163. Watzke RC. Acquired macular disease. In: Duane TD, ed. Clinical ophthalmology. Philadelphia: Harper & Row, 1981;3:Chap. 23, pp. 22–24. 163a. Melberg NS, Olk RJ. Corticosteroid-induced ocular hypertension in the treatment of aphakic or pseudophakic cystoid macular edema. Ophthalmology 1993;100:164–167.

163a. Melberg NS, Olk RJ. Corticosteroid-induced ocular hypertension in the treatment of aphakic or pseudophakic cystoid macular edema. Ophthalmology 1993;100:164–167.

164. Peterson M, Yoshizumi MO, Hepler R. Et al. Topical indomethacin in the treatment of chronic cystoid macular edema. Graefe's Arch Clin Exp Ophthalmol 1992;230:401–405.

165. Yamaaki H, Hendrikse F, Deutman AF. Iris angiography after cataract extraction and the effect of indomethacin eyedrops. Ophthalmologica 1984;188:82–86.

166. Urner-Bloch U. Pravention des zystoiden Makuloedems nach Kataraktextraktion durch lokale Indomethacin Applikation. Klin Monatsbl Augenheikd 1983;183:479–484.

167. Miyake K. Indomethacin in the treatment of postoperative cystoid macular edema. Surv Ophthalmol 1984;28:554–568.

168. Yannuzzi LA. A perspective on the treatment of aphakic cystoid macular edema. Surv Ophthalmol 1984;28:540–553.

169. Sanders DR, Kraff M. Steroidal and nonsteroidal anti-inflammatory agents; effect on postsurgical inflammation and blood-aqueous humor barrier breakdown. Arch Ophthalmol 1984;102:1453–1456.

170. Jampol LM. Pharmologic therapy of aphakic and pseudophakic cystoid macular edema. Ophthalmology 1985;92:807–810.

171. Kraff MC, Sanders DR, Jampol LM, et al. Prophylaxis of

pseudophakic cystoid macular edema with indomethacin. Ophthalmology 1982;89:886–889.

172. Burnett J, Tessler H, Isenberg S, Tso MOM. Double-masked trial of fenoproxen sodium: Treatment of chronic aphakic cystoid macular edema. Ophthalmic Surg 1983;14:150–152.

173. Flach AJ. Cyclo-oxygenase inhibitors in ophthalmology. Surv Ophthalmol 1992;36:259–284.

174. Flach AJ, Dolan BJ, Irvine AR. Effectiveness of ketorolac tromethamine 0.5% ophthalmic solution for chronic aphakic and pseudophakic cystoid macular edema. Am J Ophthalmol 1987; 103:479–486.

175. Flach AJ, Jampol LM, Weinberg D, et al. Improvement in visual acuity in chronic aphakic and pseudophakic cystoid macular edema after treatment with topical 0.5% ketorolac tromethamine. Am J Ophthalmol 1991;112:514–519.

176. Flach AJ, Stegman RC, Graham J, et al. Prophylaxis of aphakic cystoid macular edema without corticosteroids. A paired-comparison, placebo-controlled double-masked study. Ophthalmology 1990;97:1253–1258.

177. Weene LE. Cystoid macular edema after scleral buckling responsive to acetazolamide. Ann Ophthalmol 1992;24:423–424.

178. Steinmetz RL, Fitzke FW, Bird AC. Treatment of cystoid macular edema with acetazolamide in a patient with serpiginous choroidopathy. Retina 1991;11:412–415.

179. Tripathi RC, Fekrat S, Tripathi BJ, et al. A direct correlation of the resolution of pseudophakic cystoid macular edema with acetazolamide therapy. Ann Ophthalmol 1991;23:127–129.

180. Gelisken O, Gelisken F, Ozceten H. Treatment of chronic macular oedema with low dosage acetazolamide. Bull De La Societe Belge D Ophtalmo 1990;238:153–160.

181. Chen JC, Fitzke FW, Bird AC. Long-term effect of acetazolamide in a patient with retinitis pigmentosa. Invest Ophthalmol Vis Sci 1990;31:1914–1918.

182. Dugel PU, Rao NA, Ozler S, et al. Pars plana vitrectomy for intraocular inflammation-related cystoid macular edema unresponsive to corticosteroids. A preliminary study. Ophthalmology 1992;99:1535–1541.

183. Watzke RC, Burton TC, Woolson RF. Direct and indirect laser photocoagulation of central serous choroidopathy. Am J Ophthalmol 1979;88:914–918.

184. Braustein RA, Gass JDM. Serous detachments of the retinal pigment epithelium in patients with senile macular disease. Am J Ophthalmol 1979;88:652–660.

185. Newsome DA, Blackarski PA. Grid photocoagulation for macular edema in patients with retinitis pigmentosa. Am J Ophthalmol 1987;103:161–166.

186. Ploff DS, Thom SR. Preliminary report on the effect of hyperbaric oxygen on cystoid macular edema. J Cataract Refract Surg 1987; 13:136–138.

187. Benner JD, Miao XP. Locally administered hyperoxic therapy for aphakic cystoid macular edema. Am J Ophthalmol 1992;113:104–105.

188. Tchah H, Lindstrom RL. Lysis of vitreous strands with neodymium:YAG laser. Korean J Ophthalmol 1990;4:34–39.

189. Perkins ES. Ocular toxoplasmosis. Br J Ophthalmol 1973;57: 1–17.

190. Feldman HA. Toxoplasmosis. N Engl J Med 1968;279:1431–1437.

191. Desmonts F, Couvreur J. Congenital toxoplasmosis. A prospective study of 378 pregnancies. N Engl J Med 1974;290:1110–1116.

192. Kimball AC, Kean BH, Fuchs F. Congenital toxoplasmosis. A prospective study of 4,048 obstetric patients. Am J Obstet Gynecol 1971;111:211–218.

193. Amos CS. Posterior segment involvement in selected pediatric infectious diseases. J Am Optom Assoc 1979;50:1211–1220.

194. Schlaegel TF. Toxoplasmosis. In: Duane TD, ed. Clinical ophthalmology. Philadelphia: Harper & Row, 1981;4 Chap. 51, pp. 1–17.

195. Carter AD, Frank JW. Congenital toxoplasmosis: Epidemiologic features and control. Can Med Assoc J 1986;135:618–623.

196. Corwin JM, Weiter JJ. Immunology of chorioretinal disorders. Surv Ophthalmol 1981;25:287–305.

197. Tabbara KF. Disruption of the choroidoretinal interface by toxoplasma. Eye 1990;4:366–373.

198. O'Conner GR. Protozoan diseases of the uvea. Int Ophthalmol Clin 1977;17:163–176.

199. Streilein JW, Kaplan HJ. Immunologic privilege in the anterior chamber. In: Silverman AM, O'Connor GR, eds. Immunology and immunopathology of the eye. New York: Masson, 1979;174–179.

200. LaHey E, Rothova A, Baarsma GS, et al. Fuchs' heterochromic iridocyclitis is not associated with ocular toxoplasmosis. Arch Ophthalmol 1992;110:806–811.

201. Schwab IR. The epidemiologic association of Fuchs' heterochromic iridocyclitis and ocular toxoplasmosis. Am J Ophthalmol 1991;111:356–362.

202. Gagliuso DJ, Teich SA, Friedman AH, Orellana J. Ocular toxoplasmosis in AIDS patients. Trans Am Ophthalmol Soc 1990;88: 63–86.

203. O'Connor GR. Manifestations and management of ocular toxoplasmosis. Bull NY Acad Med 1974;50:192–210.

204. Reese LT, Shafer DM, Zweifach P. Acute acquired toxoplasmosis. Ann Ophthalmol 1981;13:467–470.

205. Masur H, Lempert JA, Cherubini TD. Outbreak of toxoplasmosis in a family and documentation of acquired retinochoroiditis. Am J Med 1978;64:396–402.

206. Gump DW, Holden RA. Acquired chorioretinitis due to toxoplasmosis. Ann Intern Med 1979;90:58–60.

207. Willerson D, Aaberg TM, Reeser F, Meredith TA. Unusual ocular presentation of acute toxoplasmosis. Br J Ophthalmol 1971;61: 693–698.

208. Hoerni B, Vallat M, Durand M, Pesme D. Ocular toxoplasmosis and Hodgkin's disease. Arch Ophthalmol 1978;96:62–63.

209. Orzalesi N, Ricciardi L. Segmental retinal periarteritis. Am J Ophthalmol 1971;72:55–59.

210. Schwartz PL. Segmental retinal periarteritis as a complication of toxoplasmosis. Ann Ophthalmol 1977;9:157–162.

211. Nicholson D. Ocular toxoplasmosis in an adult receiving long-term corticosteroid therapy. Arch Ophthalmol 1976;94:248–254.

212. Braunstein RA, Gass JDM. Branch artery obstruction caused by acute toxoplasmosis. Arch Ophthalmol 1980;98:512–513.

213. Saari M. Toxoplasmic chorioretinitis affecting the macula. Acta Ophthalmologica 1977;55:539–547.

214. Moreno RJ, Weisman J, Waller S. Neuroretinitis: An unusual presentation of ocular toxoplasmosis. Ann Ophthalmol 1992;24: 68–70.

215. Rose GE. Papillitis, retinal neovascularisation and recurrent retinal vein occlusion in Toxoplasma retinochoroiditis: A case report with uncommon clinical signs. Aust NZ J Ophthalmol 1991;19: 155–157.

216. Robinson RO, Bauman RJ. Late cerebral relapse of congenital toxoplasmosis. Arch Dis Child 1980;55:231–232.

217. Phaik CS, Seah S, Guan OS, et al. Anti-toxoplasma serotitres in ocular toxoplasmosis. Eye 1991;5:636–639.

218. Kijlstra A. The value of laboratory testing in uveitis. Eye 1990;4: 732–736.

219. Weiss MJ, Velazquez N, Hofeldt AJ. Serologic tests in the diagnosis of presumed toxoplasmic retinochoroiditis. Am J Ophthalmol 1990;109:407–411.

220. Kean BH, Kimball AC. The complement-fixation test in the diagnosis of congenital toxoplasmosis. Am J Dis Child 1977;131: 21–28.

221. Sabin A. Complement fixation test in toxoplasmosis and persistence of the antibody in human beings. Pediatrics 1949;4:443–452.

222. Potasman I, Araujo FG, Remington JS. Toxoplasma antigens recognized by naturally occurring human antibodies. J Clin Microbiol 1986;24:1050–1054.

223. Lindenschmidt EG. Demonstration of immunoglobulin M class antibodies to toxoplasma gondii antigenic component p 35000 by enzyme-linked antigen immunoabsorbent assay. J Clin Microbiol 1986;24:1045–1049.

224. Tomasi JP, Schlit AF, Stadtsbaeder S. Rapid double-sandwich enzyme-linked immunoabsorbent assay for detection of human immunoglobulin M anti-*Toxoplasma gondii* antibodies. J Clin Microbiol 1986;249:849–850.

225. Lin TM, Chin-See MW, Halbert SP, Joseph JM. An enzyme immunoassay for immunoglobulin M antibodies to *Toxoplasma gondii* which is not affected by rheumatoid factor or immunoglobulin G antibodies. J Clin Microbiol 1986;23:77–82.

226. Holliman RE, Stevens PJ, Duffy KT, Johnson JD. Serological investigation of ocular toxoplasmosis. Br J Ophthalmol 1991;75: 353–355.

227. Martin WG, Grown GC, Parris RK, et al. Ocular toxoplasmosis and visual field defects. Am J Ophthalmol 1980;90:25–29.

228. Engstrom RE, Holland GN, Nussenblatt RB, Jabs DA. Current practices in the management of ocular toxoplasmosis. Am J Ophthalmol 1991;111:601–610.

229. Schlaegel TF. Perspectives in uveitis. Ann Ophthalmol 1981;13: 799–806.

230. Sabates R, Pruett RC, Brockhurst RJ. Fulminant ocular toxoplasmosis. Am J Ophthalmol 1981;92:497–503.

231. O'Connor GR. Toxoplasmosis (ocular toxoplasmosis, toxoplasmic retinochoroiditis). In: Fraunfelder FT, Roy FH, eds. Current ocular therapy. Philadelphia: W.B. Saunders Co, 1980;99–101.

232. Schlaegel TF. Essentials of uveitis. Boston: Little, Brown, 1969; 181–207.

233. Fenkel JK, Jacobs L. Ocular toxoplasmosis. Arch Ophthalmol 1958;59:260–279.

234. Sabates R, Pruett RC, Brockhurst RJ. Ocular toxoplasmosis treated with pyrimethamine (letter). Am J Ophthalmol 1982;93: 371–372.

235. Tessler HH. Ocular toxoplasmosis. Int Ophthalmol Clin 1981;21: 185–189.

236. Ferguson JG. Clindamycin therapy for toxoplasmosis. Ann Ophthalmol 1981;13:95–100.

237. Antibiotic colitis-new cause, new treatment. Med Lett Drugs Ther 1979;21:97.

238. Lam S, Tessler HH. Quadruple therapy for ocular toxoplasmosis. Can J Ophthalmol 1993;28:58–61.

239. Rothova A, Meenken C, Buitenhuis HJ, et al. Therapy for ocular toxoplasmosis. Am J Ophthalmol 1993;115:517–523.

240. Opremcak EM, Scales DK, Sharpe MR. Trimethoprim-sulfamethoxazole therapy for ocular toxoplasmosis. Ophthalmology 1992;99:920–925.

241. Cochereau-Massin I, LeHoang P, Lautier-Frau M, et al. Ocular toxoplasmosis in human immunodeficiency virus-infected patients. Am J Ophthalmol 1992;114:130–135.

242. Moorthy RS, Smith RE, Rao NA. Progressive ocular toxoplasmosis in patients with acquired immunodeficiency syndrome. Am J Ophthalmol 1993;115:742–747.

243. Berger BB, Egwuagu CE, Freeman WR, Wiley CA. Miliary toxoplasmic retinitis in acquired immunodeficiency syndrome. Arch Ophthalmol 1993;111:373–376.

244. Falcone PM, Notis C, Merhige K. Toxoplasmic papillitis as the initial manifestation of acquired immunodeficiency syndrome. Ann Ophthalmol 1993;25:56–57.

245. Brown DH. Ocular *Toxocara canis*. J Pediatr Ophthalmol 1970;7: 182–191.

246. Schantz PM, Glickman LT. Current concepts in parasitology. Toxocaral visceral larva migrans. N Engl J Med 1978;298:436–439.

247. Berrocal J. Prevalence of *Toxocara canis* in babies and in adults as determined by the ELISA test. Trans Am Ophthalmol Soc 1980; 78:376–413.

248. Shantz PM, Weis PE, Pollard ZF, White MC. Risk factors for toxocaral ocular larval migrans. A case-control study. Am J Public Health 1980;70:1269–1272.

249. Glickman LT, Shantz PM. Epidemiology and pathogenesis of zoonotic toxocariasis. Epidemiol Rev 1981;3:230–250.

250. Morris PD, Katerndahl DA. Human toxocariasis. Review with report of a probable cause. Postgrad Med 1987;81:263–267.

251. Dernouchamps JP, Verougstraete C, Demolder E. Ocular toxocariasis: a presumed case of peripheral granuloma. Int Ophthalmol 1990;14:383–388.

252. Hemady R, Sainz de la Maza M, Raizman MB, Foster CS. Six cases of scleritis associated with systemic infection. Am J Ophthalmol 1992;114:55–62.

253. Dugid IM. Features of ocular infestation by *Toxocara*. Br J Ophthalmol 1961;45:789–796.

254. Safar EH, Azab ME, Khalil HM, et al. Immunodiagnostics of *Toxocara canis* in suspected ocular and visceral manifestations. Folia Parasit 1990;37:249–254.

255. Schlaegel TF. Uveitis and miscellaneous parasites. Int Ophthalmol Clin 1977;17:177–194.

256. Pollard ZF, Jarrett WH, Hagler WS, et al. ELISA for diagnosis of ocular toxocariasis. Ophthalmology 1979;86:743–752.

257. Logar J, Kraut A, Likar M. Toxocara antibodies in patients with visceral or ocular disorder in Slovenia. Infection 1993;21:27–29.

258. Felberg NT, Shields JA, Federman JF. Antibody to *Toxocara canis* in the aqueous humor. Arch Ophthalmol 1981;99:1563–1564.

259. Kennedy JJ, Defeo E. Ocular toxocariasis demonstrated by ultrasound. Ann Ophthalmol 1981;13:1357–1358.

260. Wan WL, Cano MR, Pince KJ, Green RL. Echographic characteristics of ocular toxocariasis. Ophthalmology 1991;98:28–32.

261. Pollard ZF. Ocular *Toxocara* in siblings of two families. Diagnosis confirmed by ELISA test. Arch Ophthalmol 1979;97:2319–2320.

262. Woodruff AW. Toxocariasis (visceral larva migrans). In: Fraunfelder FT, Roy FH, eds. Current ocular therapy. Philadelphia: W.B. Saunders Co, 1980;98–99.

263. Nolan J. Chronic toxocaral endophthalmitis: Successful treatment

of a case with subconjunctival depot corticosteroids. Br J Ophthalmol 1976;60:365–370.

264. Crane TB, Christensen GR. Presumed subretinal nematode infestation with visual recovery. Ann Ophthalmol 1981;13:345–348.

265. Hagler WS, Pollard ZF, Jarrett WH, Donnelly EH. Results of surgery for ocular *Toxocara canis.* Ophthalmology 1981;88:1081–1086.

266. Angi MR, Forattini F, Chilosi M, et al. Immunopathology of ocular sarcoidosis. Int Ophthalmol 1990;14:1–11.

267. Nowack D, Goebel KM. Genetic aspects of sarcoidosis. Class II histocompatability antigens and a family study. Arch Intern Med 1987;147:481–483.

268. Bernardino VB, Naidoff MA. Retinal inflammatory disease. In: Duane TD, ed. Clinical ophthalmology. Philadelphia: Harper & Row, 1981;3:Chap. 10, p. 7.

269. Jabs DA, Johns CJ. Ocular involvement in chronic sarcoidosis. Am J Ophthalmol 1986;102:297–301.

270. Obenauf CD, Shaw HE, Sydnor CF, Klintworth GK. Sarcoidosis and its ophthalmic manifestations. Am J Ophthalmol 1978;86:648–655.

271. Simmons CA, Mathews D. Prevalence of uveitis: A retrospective study. J Am Optom Assoc 1993;64:386–389.

272. Rothova A, Buitenhuis HJ, Meenken C, et al. Uveitis and systemic disease. Br J Ophthalmol 1992;76:137–141.

273. Spalton DJ, Sanders MD. Fundus changes in histologically confirmed sarcoidosis. Br J Ophthalmol 1981;65:348–358.

274. Mizuno K, Takahashi J. Sarcoid cyclitis. Ophthalmology 1986;93:511–517.

275. O'Day J, Schilling JS, Ffytche TJ. Retinal vasculitis. Trans Ophthalmol Soc UK 1979;99:163–166.

276. Ohara K, Okubo A, Kamata K, et al. Transbronchial lung biopsy in the diagnosis of suspected ocular sarcoidosis. Arch Ophthalmol 1993;111:642–644.

277. Ohara K, Okubo A, Sasaki H, Kamata K. Intraocular manifestations of systemic sarcoidosis. Jpn J Ophthalmol 1992;36:452–457.

278. Tingey DP, Gonder JR. Ocular sarcoidosis presenting as a solitary choroidal mass. Can J Ophthalmol 1992;27:25–29.

279. Satorre J, Antle CM, O'Sullivan R, et al. Orbital lesions with granulomatous inflammation. Can J Ophthalmol 1991;26:174–195.

280. Koopmans PP, Bodeutsch C, de Wilde PC, Boerbooms AM. Primary Sjogren's syndrome presenting as a case of sarcoidosis and suspected pancreatic tumour. Ann Rheum Dis 1990;49:407–409.

281. Noble KG. Ocular sarcoidosis occuring as a unilateral optic disk vascular lesion. Am J Ophthalmol 1979;87:490–493.

282. Doxans MT, Kelley JS, Prout TE. Sarcoidosis with neovascularization of the optic nerve head. Am J Ophthalmol 1980;90:347–351.

283. Gragoudas ES, Regan CDJ. Peripapillary subretinal neovascularization in presumed sarcoidosis. Arch Ophthalmol 1981;99:1194–1197.

284. Merritt JC, Lipper SL, Peiffer RL, Hale LM. Conjunctival biopsy in sarcoidosis. J Natl Med Assoc 1980;72:347–349.

285. Nicols CW, Eagle RC, Yanoff M, Menocal NG. Conjunctival biopsy as an aid in the evaluation of the patient with suspected sarcoidosis. Ophthalmology 1980;87:287–289.

286. Spaide RF, Ward DL. Conjunctival biopsy in the diagnosis of sarcoidosis. Br J Ophthalmol 1990;74:469–471.

287. Weinreb RN, Kimura SJ. Uveitis associated with sarcoidosis and

288. Lieberman J, Sastree A. An angiotensin-converting enzyme (ACE) inhibitor in human serum. Increased sensitivity of the serum ACE assay for detecting active sarcoidosis. Chest 1986;90:869–875.

289. Nidiry JJ, Mines S, Hackney R, Nabhani H. Sarcoidosis: A unique presentation of dysphagia, myopathy, and photophobia. Am J Gastroenterol 1991;86:1679–1682.

290. Sulavik SB, Spencer RP, Weed DA, et al. Recognition of distinctive patterns of gallium-67 distribution in sarcoidosis. J Nucl Med 1990;31:1909–1914.

291. Sulavik SB, Palestro CJ, Spencer RP, et al. Extrapulmonary sites of radiogallium accumulation in sarcoidosis. Clin Nucl Med 1990;15:876–878.

292. Stern BJ, Griffin DE, Luke RA, et al. Neurosarcoidosis: Cerebrospinal fluid lymphocyte subpopulations. Neurology 1987;37:878–881.

293. Sethi KD, el Gammal T, Patel BR, Swift TR. Dural sarcoidosis presenting with transient neurologic symptoms. Arch Neurol 1986;43:595–597.

294. Valantine H, McKenna WJ, Nihoyannopoulas P, et al. Sarcoidosis: A pattern of clinical and morphological presentation. Br Heart J 1987;57:256–263.

295. Ohtahara A, Kotake H, Hisatome I. Mashiba H. Complete atrioventricular block with a 22 month history of ocular sarcoidosis: A case report. Heart Lung 1987;16:66–68.

296. Callen JP, Mahl CF. Oculocutaneous manifestations observed in multisystem disorders. Derm Clin 1992;10:709–716.

297. Brownstein S, Liszauer AD, Carey WD, Nicolle DA. Sarcoidosis of the eyelid skin. Can J Ophthalmol 1990;25:256–259.

298. Kataria YP. Chlorambucil in sarcoidosis. Chest 1980;78:36–43.

299. Letocha CE. Sarcoidosis. In: Fraunfelder FT, Roy FH, eds. Current ocular therapy. Philadelphia: W.B. Saunders Co, 1980;320–321.

300. O'Leary TJ, Jones G, Yip A, et al. The effects of chloroquine on serum 1, 25–dihydroxyvitamin D and calcium metabolism in sarcoidosis. N Engl J Med 1986;315:727–730.

301. Alexander LJ. Primary Care of the Posterior Segment. ed. 2. E Norwalk: Appleton & Lange, 1993.

302. Spira TJ. The acquired immunodeficiency syndrome. In: Inslor MS, ed. AIDS and other sexually transmitted diseases and the eye. Orlando, FL: Grune & Stratton, 1987;119–144.

303. Den Beste BP, Hummer J. AIDS: A review and guide for infection control. J Am Optom Assoc 1986;57:675–682.

304. Springer M. Ophthalmologists on the front line treating AIDS patients. Arch Ophthalmol 1987;105:325.

305. Holland GN. Ophthalmic disorders associated with the acquired immunodeficiency snydrome. In: Inslor MS, ed. AIDS and other sexually transmitted diseases and the eye. Orlando, FL: Grune & Stratton, 1987;145–172.

306. Sison RF, Holland GN, MacArthur LJ, et al. Cytomegalovirus retinopathy as the initial manifestation of the acquired immunodeficiency syndrome. Am J Ophthalmol 1991;112:243–249.

307. Morinelli EN, Dugel PU, Lee M, et al. Opportunistic intraocular infections in AIDS. Trans Am Ophthalmol Soc 1992;90:97–109.

308. Heinemann MH. Characteristics of cytomegalovirus retinitis in patients with acquired immunodeficiency syndrome. Am J Med 1992;92:12S–16S.

309. Faber DW, Wiley CA, Lynn GB, et al. Role of HIV and CMV in

angiotensin converting enzyme. Trans Am Ophthalmol Soc 1979;77:280–293.

the pathogenesis of retinitis and retinal vasculopathy in AIDS patients. Invest Ophthalmol Vis Sci 1992;33:2345–2353.

310. Lee S, Ai E. Disc neovascularization in patients with AIDS and cytomegalovirus. Retina 1991;11:305–308.

311. Faber DW, Crapotta JA, Wiley CA, Freeman WR. Retinal calcifications in cytomegalovirus retinitis. Retina 1993;13:46–49.

312. Keefe KS, Freeman WR, Peterson TJ, et al. Atypical healing of cytomegalovirus retinitis. Significance of persistent border opacification. Ophthalmology 1992;99:1377–1384.

313. Chuang EL, Davis JL. Management of retinal detachment associated with CMV retinitis in AIDS patients. Eye 1992;6:28–34.

314. Freeman WR, Quiceno JI, Crapotta JA, et al. Surgical repair of rhegmatogenous retinal detachment in immunosuppressed patients with cytomegalovirus retinitis. Ophthalmology 1992;99:466–474.

315. Jabs DA, Enger C, Haller J, de Bustros S. Retinal detachments in patients with cytomegalovirus retinitis. Arch Ophthalmol 1991;109:794–799.

316. Sidikaro Y, Silver L, Holland GN, Kreiger AE. Rhegmatogenous retinal detachments in patients with AIDS and necrotizing retinal infections. Ophthalmology 1991;98:129–135.

317. Geier SA, Klauss V, Matuschke, et al. 2.5 years survival with sequential ganciclovir/forcarnet treatment in a patient with acquired immune deficiency syndrome and cytomegalovirus retinitis. Ger J Ophthalmol 1992;1:110–113.

318. Spaide RF, Vitale AT, Toth IR, Oliver JM. Frosted branch angiitis associated with cytomegalovirus retinitis. Am J Ophthalmol 1992;113:522–528.

319. Secchi AG, Tognon MS, Turrini B, Carniel G. Acute frosted retinal periphlebitis associated with cytomegalovirus retinitis. Retina 1992;12:245–247.

320. Rabb MF, Jampol LM, Fish RH, et al. Retinal periphlebitis in patients with acquired immunodeficiency syndrome with cytomegalovirus retinitis mimics acute frosted retinal periphlebitis. Arch Ophthalmol 1992;110:1257–1260.

321. Meredith JT. Toxoplasmosis of the central nervous system. Am Fam Physician 1987;35:113–116.

322. Haverkos HW. Assessment of therapy for *Toxoplasma* encephalitis. The TE Study Group. Am J Med 1987;82:907–914.

323. Nelson MR, Erskine D, Hawkins DA, Gazzard BG. Treatment with corticosteroids—a risk factor for the development of clinical cytomegalovirus disease in AIDS. Aids 1993;7:375–378.

324. Moyle G, Harman C, Mitchell S, et al. Foscarnet and ganciclovir in the treatment of CMV retinitis in AIDS patients: A randomised comparison. J Infect 1992;25:21–27.

325. AIDS Clinical Trials Group (ACTG). Studies of ocular complications of AIDS Foscarnet-Ganciclovir Cytomegalovirus Retinitis Trial: 1. Rationale, design, and methods. Controlled Clin Trials 1992;13:22–39.

326. Drew WL. Cytomegalovirus infection in patients with AIDS. Clin Infect Dis 1992;14:608–615.

327. Polis MA. Design of a randomized controlled trial of foscarnet in patients with cytomegalovirus retinitis associated with acquired immunodeficiency syndrome. Am J Med 1992;92:22S–25S.

328. Palestine AG, Polis MA, DeSmet MD, et al. A randomized, controlled trial of foscarnet in the treatment of cytomegalovirus retinitis in patients with AIDS. Ann Intern Med 1991;115:665–673.

329. Polis, MA, DeSmet MD, Baird BF, et al. Increased survival of a cohort of patients with acquired immunodeficiency syndrome and cytomegalovirus retinitis who received sodium phosphonoformate (foscarnet). Am J Med 1993;94:175–180.

330. Reddy MM, Grieco MH, McKinley GF, et al. Effect of foscarnet therapy on human immunodeficiency virus p24 antigen levels in AIDS patients with cytomegalovirus retinitis. J Infect Dis 1992;166:607–611.

331. AIDS Clinical Trials Group (ACTG). Mortality in patients with the acquired immunodeficiency syndrome treated with either foscarnet or ganciclovir for cytomegalovirus retinitis. Studies of Ocular Complications of AIDS Research Group, in collaboration with the AIDS Clinical Trials Group. N Engl J Med 1992;326:213–220.

332. Jacobson MA, Causey D, Polsky B, et al. A dose-ranging study of daily maintenance intravenous foscarnet therapy for cytomegalovirus retinitis in AIDS. J Infect Dis 1993;168:444–448.

333. Young SH, Morlet N, Heery S, et al. High dose intravitreal ganciclovir in the treatment of cytomegalovirus retinitis. Med J Aust 1992;157:370–373.

334. Balfour HH, Drew WL, Hardy WD, et al. Therapeutic algorithm for treatment of cytomegalovirus retinitis in persons with AIDS. A roundtable summary. J Acquired Immune Deficiency Syndromes 1992;1:S37–S44.

335. Katlama C, Dohin E, Caumes E, et al. Foscarnet induction therapy for cytomegalovirus retinitis in AIDS: comparison of twice-daily and three-times-daily regimens. J Acquired Immune Deficiency Syndromes 1992;1:S18–S24.

336. Diaz-Llopis M, Chipont E, Sanchez S, et al. Intravitreal foscarnet for cytomegalovirus retinitis in a patient with acquired immunodeficiency syndrome. Am J Ophthalmol 1992;114:742–747.

337. Keijer WJ, Burger DM, Neuteboom GH, et al. Ocular complications of the acquired immunodeficiency syndrome. Focus on the treatment of cytomegalovirus retinitis with ganciclovir and foscarnet. Pharm World Sci 1993;15:56–67.

338. Bernauer W, Meyer P, Zimmerli W, et al. Failure to control AIDS-related CMV-retinitis with intravenous ganciclovir. Int Ophthalmol 1992;16:453–457.

339. Holland GN, Shuler JD. Progression rates of cytomegalovirus retinopathy in ganciclovir-treated and untreated patients. Arch Ophthalmol 1992;110:14335–14342.

340. Flores-Aguilar M, Kuppermann BD, Quiceno JI, et al. Pathophysiology and treatment of clinically resistant cytomegalovirus retinitis. Ophthalmology 1993;100:1022–1031.

341. Kuppermann BD, Flores-Aguilar M, Quiceno JI, et al. Combination ganciclovir and foscarnet in the treatment of clinically resistant cytomagelovirus retinitis in patients with acquired immunodeficiency syndrome. Arch Ophthalmol 1993;111:1359–1366.

342. Carter JE, Shuster AR. Zidovudine and cytomegalovirus retinitis. Ann Ophthalmol 1992;24:186–189.

343. Sha BE, Benson CA, Deutsch TA, et al. Suppression of cytomegalovirus retinitis in persons with AIDS with high-dose intravenous acyclovir. J Infect Dis 1991;164:777–780.

344. Bachman DM, Bruni LM, DiGioia RA, et al. Visual field testing in the management of cytomegalovirus retinitis. Ophthalmology 1992;99:1393–1399.

345. Laby DM, Nasrallah FP, Butrus SI, Whitmore PV. Treatment of outer retinal necrosis in AIDS patients. Graefe's Arch Clin Exp Ophthalmol 1993;231:271–273.

346. Centers for Disease Control. Recommendations for prevention of

HIV transmission in health-care settings. MMWR 1987;36(Suppl no. 25):3–18.

347. Centers for Disease Control. Recommendations for preventing possible transmission of human T-lymphotropic virus type III/ lymphadenopathy-associated virus from tears, MMWR 1985;34: 533–534.

348. Prasad P, Upadhyaya NS. Bilateral acute retinal necrosis—a case report. Ind J Ophthalmol 1992;40:96–98.

349. Rummelt V, Wenkel H, Rummelt C, et al. Detection of varicella zoster virus DNA and viral antigen in the late stage of bilateral acute retinal necrosis syndrome. Arch Ophthalmol 1992;110: 1132–1136.

350. Culbertson WW, Brod RD, Flynn HW, et al. Chickenpox-associated acute retinal necrosis syndrome. Ophthalmology 1991;98: 1641–1646.

351. Matsuo T, Matsuo N. HLA-DR9 associated with the severity of acute retinal necrosis syndrome. Ophthalmologica 1991;203:133–137.

352. Spires R. Acute retinal necrosis syndrome. J Ophthal Nurs Tech 1992;11:103–108.

353. Gerling J, Neumann-Haefelin D, Seuffert HM, et al. Diagnosis and management of the acute retinal necrosis syndrome. Ger J Ophthalmol 1992;1:388–393.

354. Duker JS, Blumenkranz MS. Diagnosis and management of the acute retinal necrosis (ARN) syndrome. Surv Ophthalmol 1991; 35:327–343.

355. Gartry DS, Spalton DJ, Tilzey A, Hykin PG. Acute retinal necrosis syndrome. Br J Ophthalmol 1991;75:292–297.

356. Cartwright MJ. Acute retinal necrosis: An unusual presentation. Ann Ophthalmol 1991;23:452–453.

357. Matsuo T, Morimoto K, Matsuo N. Factors associated with poor visual outcome in acute retinal necrosis. Br J Ophthalmol 1991; 75:450–454.

358. Hellinger WC, Bolling JP, Smith TF, Campbell RJ. Varicella-zoster virus retinitis in a patient with AIDS-related complex: Case report and brief review of the acute retinal necrosis syndrome. Clin Infect Dis 1993;16:208–212.

359. Nishi M, Hanashiro R, Mori S, et al. Polymerase chain reaction for the detection of the varicella-zoster genome in ocular samples from patients with acute retinal necrosis syndrome. Am J Ophthalmol 1992;114:603–609.

360. Foulds WS. The uses and limitations of intraocular biopsy. Eye 1992;6:11–27.

361. Pepose JS, Flowers B, Stewart JA, et al. Herpesvirus antibody levels in the etiologic diagnosis of the acute retinal necrosis syndrome. Am J Ophthalmol 1992;113:248–256.

362. Palay DA, Sternberg P, Davis, et al. Decrease in the risk of bilateral acute retinal necrosis by acyclovir therapy. Am J Ophthalmol 1991;112:250–255.

363. Laby DM, Nasrallah FP, Butrus SI, Whitmore PV. Treatment of outer retinal necrosis in AIDS patients. Graefe's Arch Clin Exp Ophthalmol 1993;231:271–273.

364. McDonald HR, Lewis H, Kreiger AE, et al. Surgical management of retinal detachment associated with the acute retinal necrosis syndrome. Br J Ophthalmol 1991;75:455–458.

365. Kuppermann BD, Quiceno JI, Wiley C, et al. Clinical and histopathologic study of varicella zoster virus retinitis in patients with the acquired immunodeficiency syndrome. Am J Ophthalmol 1994;118:589–600.

366. Holland GN, The Executive Committee of the American Uveitis Society. Standard diagnostic criteria for the acute retinal necrosis syndrome. Am J Ophthalmol 1994;117:663–666.

CHAPTER 33

Thyroid-Related Eye Disease

David P. Sendrowski
Eduardo Gaitan

Parry (1825), Graves (1835), and Von Basedow (1840) provided the first classic accounts of exophthalmic goiter.[1] However, Robert J. Graves,[2] an Irish physician, is usually credited with the first publication describing most accurately the suspected association between thyroid disease and the eye. The eponym "Graves' ophthalmopathy" has accordingly been proposed as the standard term describing the orbital disease that may result from or relate to abnormalities of the thyroid gland. Although approximately 75% of patients with Graves' disease have some degree of ocular involvement, only 15% of those patients ever develop serious functional impairment of vision.[3] Nevertheless, the diagnosis and management of thyroid-related eye disease are often a significant challenge to the eye care practitioner and endocrinologist. This chapter considers the diagnostic features of Graves' ophthalmopathy and discusses the management of this important clinical syndrome.

Epidemiology

Noninfiltrative (Class 1) thyroid-related eye disease, the mildest form of ocular involvement, is the most frequent ocular manifestation of hyperthyroidism. This occurs in up to 50% of patients with toxic diffuse goiter and can begin at any age.[4] The more severe infiltrative (Classes 2 through 6) forms of ocular involvement, however, usually do not occur before adulthood. The incidence of ocular changes is inversely proportional to the severity of the manifestation; that is, most patients with ocular changes have relatively mild disease, and very few patients develop the severe involve-

ment characterized by significant corneal and optic nerve changes. Noninfiltrative disease occurs predominantly in females in a ratio of 4 to 6:1, with the most common age of onset during the second to third decade of life. Infiltrative disease, in contrast, is equally prevalent in male and female, but usually occurs at a later age.

Graves' ophthalmopathy develops in more than 80% of the cases within 18 months of diagnosis of Graves' hyperthyroidism.[5,6] Thyroid-related ophthalmopathy is associated with Graves' hyperthyroidism in 90% of the cases and with autoimmune thyroiditis (Hashimoto's disease) in some 5%. No clinical evidence of thyroid disease is found in 5 to 10% of patients.[7] This situation is called euthyroid Graves' ophthalmopathy.

Etiopathogenesis

Although the precise etiopathogenesis of Graves' ophthalmopathy is not well understood, a basic knowledge of the pathology associated with the disease is essential for an understanding of the mechanisms of action of the various drugs and other therapeutic modalities used in managing this disorder. The ocular involvement associated with thyrotoxicosis is primarily an orbital disease, and pressure-volume relations within the orbit are critical in the pathogenesis of Graves' ophthalmopathy.[6] The most striking pathologic feature of thyroid-related ophthalmopathy is the marked enlargement of the extraocular muscles. This is accompanied by mononuclear cell (activated T-cells, B-cells, plasma cells, macrophages, and mast cells) infiltration and proliferation of orbital fibroblasts with increased production of collagen and glycosaminoglycans (GAG) into the interstitial space of extraocular muscle fibers, orbital fat and orbital connective tissue, resulting in increased edema of these tissues, and in degenerative changes within the muscle cells.[8,9] This diffuse orbital infiltration involves all the connective tissues and extraocular muscles and is responsible for the proptosis and many of the other signs of Graves' ophthalmopathy.[10] Cant and Wilson[10] hypothesized that almost all the secondary effects of thyroid-related orbital infiltration are circulatory, and that the visual field loss and color vision dysfunction are typical of optic nerve involvement either by direct compression or by interference with circulation.

The role of the immune system in the pathophysiology of Graves' disease is well established.[11–16] A considerable amount of information links the human major histocompatibility complex (HLA) with Graves' disease.[14,17] For instance, there is an increased frequency of HLA-B8 in whites with this disorder. This is also true for the HLA-Dw3 that confers an even greater relative risk for Graves' disease than HLA-B8. On the other hand, Graves' disease in the Japanese has been found to be associated with HLA-B35, while in patients of Chinese origin HLA-Bw46 confers a greater risk. Risk ratios indicating an increased probability for patients to develop Graves' hyperthyroidism have been in the range of 3 to 5 fold, which suggest a relatively weak association.[18]

In contrast to the systemic disorder, however, there is considerable disagreement regarding the association of HLA antigens and Graves' ophthalmopathy.[17] Although the immune system is clearly implicated, the immunologic basis and precise mechanism have not yet been defined to provide an explanation for the ocular disorder.[15,16,19,20] Graves' disease is an autoimmune disorder, but its precise relationship with thyroid ophthalmopathy is unclear.[9] Graves' hyperthyroidism results from overstimulation of thyroid cells by TSH-receptor autoantibodies (TSHR-Ab), but the role of TSHR-Ab or the target antigen in orbital tissue has not been established in thyroid-related ophthalmopathy. Furthermore, in general, TSHR-Ab titers do not correlate with the severity of Graves' ophthalmopathy.[21] Immunoglobulin G (IgG) circulating antibodies to eye muscle and orbital fibroblasts have been implicated in the pathogenesis of thyroid-related ophthalmopathy.[22] Antibodies against a periorbital muscle membrane protein 64kDa have been detected in patients with Graves' ophthalmopathy, but their pathogenic role has not been demonstrated.[7,23] The current view is that thyroid-related ophthalmopathy is a T-cell mediated autoimmune disease. Activated T-cells (CD8+>CD4+) releasing the cytokines interleukin-1 (IL-1), γ-interferon (Γ-IFN), and tumor necrosis factor (TNF) stimulate retroorbital fibroblast GAG production, with attendant edema, swelling of the muscles and an increase in retroorbital tissue, resulting in clinical manifestations of ophthalmopathy.[7,9] The mechanism responsible for initiation of the autoimmune response awaits further study.[7,9,24,25] Abnormal cell-mediated immunity appears to play an important role in the pathogenesis of Graves' ophthalmopathy.[14–16,26]

Diagnosis

The clinical diagnosis of Graves' ophthalmopathy can frequently be made without laboratory testing. Indeed, 5% of patients will present with the classic signs of Graves' ophthalmopathy but will be found to be chemically and clinically euthyroid. In the patient who has a present or previous history of hyperthyroidism, the diagnosis is usually immediate. However, in those patients without such history, evidence of lid retraction is virtually pathognomonic. Vertical diplopia is particularly common, and intraocular pressure elevated more than 4 mm Hg on attempted upgaze signifies fibrosis of the inferior rectus muscle, an important diagnostic sign. The use of rose bengal solution may reveal superior limbic keratoconjunctivitis, which has been shown to have a possible association with hyperthyroidism.[27] These and other clinical findings, to be described, may serve to secure the clinical diagnosis. In a series of 52 patients,[27] a diagnosis of Graves' ophthalmopathy based on the clinical findings alone was made in 42 of the patients with laboratory documentation of thyrotoxicosis.

Although Graves' disease and Hashimoto's thyroiditis account for the largest proportion of patients with bilateral proptosis, it can also be produced by neoplastic, vascular, and inflammatory processes as well as by infections, granulomatous processes, and other endocrine (Cushing's and acromegaly) diseases.[6,12,28] Thus, the diagnosis of Graves' ophthalmopathy can be made only by carefully excluding other possible causes of proptosis.[29,30,31]

Diagnosis of Thyrotoxicosis

In most cases the diagnosis of Graves' disease can be made on the basis of a careful clinical history and physical examination. Nervousness, palpitations, weight loss, hyperhydrosis, and heat intolerance are symptoms occurring in more than 80% of hyperthyroid patients, and tremor, hyperreflexia, tachycardia, skin changes, stare, and lid lag are observed in more than 60%. Goiter is present in more than 95% of Graves' disease patients.[32,33] In all cases, however, the laboratory confirmation of thyrotoxicosis is necessary to corroborate the diagnosis.

The American Thyroid Association (ATA) issued updated guidelines for the use of laboratory tests in thyroid disorders.[34–36] The emergence of highly sensitive thyrotropin (TSH) assays capable of clearly separating normal from subnormal serum TSH levels,[37] constitutes a practical, useful, and significant laboratory advance in clinical thyroidology. Measurement of serum TSH, complemented by an appropriate free-thyroxine (FT₄) estimate, represents the best and most efficient combination of blood tests for diagnosis of hyperthyroidism. The thyroid hormones thyroxine (T₄) and triiodothyronine (T₃) are present in blood both in the free form (FT₄ and FT₃) and bound to serum proteins, i.e., thyroid hormone binding globulin (TBG), thyroxine-binding prealbumin (TBPA) or transthyretin, and albumin. Only 0.04% of T₄ and 0.4% of T₃ are unbound in the free bioactive form in blood. FT₄ measured by equilibrium dialysis is largely free from artifactual error, and considered ideal, but it is laborious, time-consuming, and expensive. Other methods to estimate FT₄ are intrinsically susceptible to inaccuracies. A practical estimate of FT₄ is offered by the free thyroxine index (FT₄I). To calculate this index, total thyroxine (T₄) measured by radioimmunoassay (RIA) is multiplied by the radioactive triiodothyronine resin uptake (T₃U). The product is the FT₄I value, which correlates well in most instances with FT₄ concentrations. T₃U is an indirect but simple *in vitro* technique reflecting the concentration and affinity of thyroxine binding proteins. A subnormal serum TSH level with an elevated FT₄ estimate or FT₄I establish a diagnosis of hyperthyroidism. In patients with mild hyperthyroidism, the FT₄ by any method is less sensitive than the TSH. Therefore, when hyperthyroidism is suspected and FT₄ is normal, the measurement of total triiodothyronine (T₃) by RIA in serum is appropriate. Under these conditions a subnormal TSH level with an elevated T₃ will establish the diagnosis of T₃-toxicosis. Finally, the thyrotropin-releasing hormone (TRH) test, which involves intravenous administration of 200 μg of TRH and serum TSH measurements at the moment of injection and at 30 minutes thereafter, has been relegated to those rare situations of patients with subnormal serum TSH levels but normal concentrations of both FT₄ and T₃. A positive TSH response after TRH discards the diagnosis of "subclinical" hyperthyroidism.

Thyrotropin receptor antibodies (TSHR-Ab or TRAb) are found in over 90% of patients with hyperthyroidism of Graves' disease, occurring otherwise only in variants of this disorder, such as in some patients with euthyroid Graves' ophthalmopathy, Hashimoto's disease, and hypothyroid Graves' ophthalmopathy.[21,38–40] Only two assays for thyroid stimulating antibody (TSAb), a TSHR-Ab, are in common use today.[38,39] One uses human thyroid cells and the other functioning rat thyroid (FRTL-5) cells, in culture as the target preparation. An increase in cyclic AMP indicates the presence of TSAb. At present, there appears to be no justification for inclusion of TSAb measurements as part of the general diagnostic work-up of Graves' disease patients. This is in view of their cost, availability, and the adequacy of other routine laboratory tests such as TSH, FT₄, and T₃. Actually, measurement of the thyroid peroxidase (microsomal) antibody (TPOAb), which is less expensive and more readily available, has equivalent diagnostic significance to that of TRAb assays to establish the diagnosis of underlying

autoimmune thyroid disease.[38] Determination of TPOAb may be helpful in the diagnosis of euthyroid Graves' ophthalmopathy and in characterizing those patients with Hashimoto's thyroiditis and ophthalmopathy, in whom positive antibodies against thyroid peroxidase (TPOAb) and thyroglobulin (TgAb) are found in almost 100%, using the more sensitive immunoassays.[21,38–40] Finally, there is no available assay that reliably measures, in serum, Graves' disease specific antibodies to ocular antigens, i.e., extraocular muscle and retroorbital fibroblasts.[7,21–25]

Classification of Graves' Ophthalmopathy

In an attempt to achieve uniformity in terminology regarding the various ocular changes associated with thyroid disease, the American Thyroid Association adopted in 1968 an initial classification of the ocular changes of Graves' disease.[41] Various modifications to the original classification system have been proposed,[42,43] and one has been approved by the American Thyroid Association[42] (Tables 33.1 and 33.2). Each class usually, but not necessarily, includes the changes indicated in the preceding class. This classification, however, suffers from several flaws. There is a lack of natural progression from one class to the next. Also, the classification fails to distinguish between the active and inactive forms of the disease.[44,45] Finally, there seems to be a poor relationship between the class and the severity of the ophthalmopathy.[44,45] In the past several years, new classification systems have been attempted,[45] but the system that is still in wide use is the NO SPECS classification. The first letters of each definition form the mnemonic NO SPECS, the NO indicating the usually non-threatening prognosis of Classes 0 and 1, and SPECS indicating the relatively serious nature of Classes 2 through 6.

TABLE 33.1
Abridged Classification of the Eye Changes of Graves' Disease

Class[a]	Definition
0	No physical signs or symptoms
1	Only signs, no symptoms (e.g., upper eyelid retraction, stare, and eyelid lag)
2	Soft tissue involvement (symptoms and signs)
3	Proptosis
4	Extraocular muscle involvement
5	Corneal involvement
6	Sight loss (optic nerve involvement)

[a]Each class usually, but not necessarily, includes the involvements indicated in the preceding class.

From Werner SC. Modification of the classification of the eye changes of Graves' disease. Am J Ophthalmol 1977;83:725–727, and ETA, LATS, Japanese-AOTA, ATA. Classification of eye changes of Graves' disease. Thyroid 1992;2: 235–236.

TABLE 33.2
Detailed Classification of the Eye Changes of Graves' Disease

Class	Grade	Suggestions for Grading
0		No physical signs or symptoms
1		Only signs
2		Soft tissue involvement with symptoms and signs
	o	Absent
	a	Minimal
	b	Moderate
	c	Marked
3		Proptosis 3 mm or more in excess of upper normal limits, with or without symptoms
	o	Absent
	a	3–4 mm increase over upper normal
	b	5–7 mm increase
	c	8 or more mm increase
4		Extraocular muscle involvement; usually with diplopia, other symptoms, and other signs
	o	Absent
	a	Limitation of motion at extremes of gaze
	b	Evident restriction of motion
	c	Fixation of a globe or globes
5		Corneal involvement primarily caused by lagophthalmos
	o	Absent
	a	Stippling of cornea
	b	Ulceration
	c	Clouding, necrosis, perforation
6		Sight loss caused by optic nerve involvement
	o	Absent
	a	Disc pallor or choking, or visual field defect; acuity 6/6 (20/20)–6/18 (20/60)
	b	Same; acuity 6/22 (20/70)–6/60 (20/200)
	c	Blindness (failure to perceive light), acuity less than 6/60 (20/200)

From Werner SC. Modification of the classification of the eye changes of Graves' disease. Am J Ophthalmol 1977;83(5):725–727.

The American (ATA), European (ETA), Latin-American (LATS), Japanese and Asia-Oceania (AOTA) Thyroid Associations reexamined the content and applications of the NOSPECS classification, reaching consensus on the following points[46]: (1) The NOSPECS classification is an ingenious memory aid for clinical examination of the orbital changes of Graves' disease and has useful educational application, (2) NOSPECS and its numerical indices are less satisfactory for objective assessment of the orbital changes of Graves' disease and for reporting results of clinical studies. For these purposes specific and separate measurements relating to the status of eyelids, cornea, extraocular muscles, proptosis, and optic nerve function should be provided.

An assessment of the activity of Graves' ophthalmopathy is relevant to therapy. Disease activity at one time may be assessed by assigning 1 point to each of the following signs and symptoms: spontaneous retrobulbar pain, pain on eye movement, eyelid erythema, conjunctival injection, chemosis, swelling of the caruncle, and eyelid edema or fullness. The sum of these points defines the clinical activity score (range 0–7). Finally, an important element in evaluating the effects of treatment of Graves' ophthalmopathy is the patient self-assessment. Such assessments, described on scales of best to worst, should include appearance, visual acuity, eye discomfort, and diplopia.

CLASS 1 DISEASE

Class 1 disease, formerly termed *mild* or *noninfiltrative* disease, is characterized by upper lid retraction (Fig. 33.1) and occurs in over 90% of patients with hyperthyroidism.[10] This sign may initially occur unilaterally or bilaterally and is often asymmetric.[47] A helpful diagnostic sign often associated with lid retraction is the lid tug sign,[48] in which the retracted upper lid offers a sensation of increased resistance on attempted manual lid closure. The resistance to lid closure is noted by simply grasping the lashes of the upper lid and gently pulling down. The amount of resistance is compared with the contralateral lid in unilateral cases, or with a control normal lid in cases of bilateral lid retraction. This

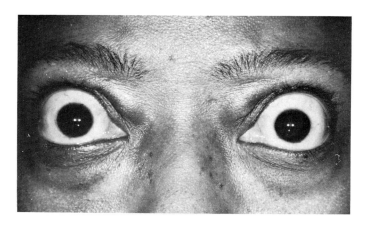

FIGURE 33.1 **Upper lid retraction characteristic of Class 1 Graves' ophthalmopathy.**

test is particularly helpful in cases of questionable bilateral retraction or ambiguous unilateral retraction versus contralateral ptosis.

Lid retraction can produce findings in several associated tests that may correlate with the onset of the ophthalmopathy. For example, measurement of the palpebral fissure width is helpful in the diagnosis of unilateral cases. Another potential finding is a reduction in the tear break-up time (TBUT) of one or both eyes. Lid retraction causes an increase in the ocular surface area that must be covered by the tear film, and there is an associated decrease in blink frequency in Graves' patients.[44] The combination of these two factors affects the stability of the tear film.

The most common cause of lid retraction is hyperthyroidism.[49] Thus, this sign is virtually pathognomonic of Graves' ophthalmopathy. There are three major hypotheses for the pathogenesis of thyroid-associated lid retraction[49–52]: (1) in the early stages there is excessive stimulation of Müeller's muscle in the upper lid associated with the sympathicotonia of Graves' disease, resulting from the marked inhibition of liver monoamine oxidase synthesis by high circulating thyroxine levels; (2) in long-standing Graves' disease, there may be overaction of the levator muscle, resulting from excessive stimulation of the superior rectus muscle acting against a fibrotic inferior rectus muscle[172]; and (3) mechanical restriction or infiltration of the levator muscle.

There is negligible lymphocytic infiltration, and the extracellular volume is not increased in the levator muscle. However, the muscle fibers become greatly enlarged, leading to hypertrophy of the levator muscle and upper eyelid retraction.[53] This is in contrast to the changes that occur in the extraocular muscles.[53]

Lid retraction can appear in the presence of chemical and clinical euthyroidism and is often unrelated to control of any existing thyroid dysfunction. Lid lag (Von Graefe's sign) often accompanies lid retraction (Fig. 33.2). Lid retraction

disappears spontaneously after 15 years in about 60% of patients.[4]

CLASS 2 DISEASE

Classes 2 through 6 disease, formerly termed *severe* or *infiltrative* disease, represent the more significant and vision-threatening changes associated with Graves' disease. The ocular manifestations of Class 2 disease include a variety of important clinical signs: swelling of the lids; prolapse of orbital fat, nasally in the upper lid and temporally in the lower lid; palpable lacrimal gland; injection of the conjunctival and episcleral vessels; and chemosis (Fig. 33.3). These changes result in symptoms relating to lacrimation, light sensitivity, and gritty or sandy foreign body sensation. Some patients may complain of sudden intolerance to contact lens wear. These symptoms are frequently worse in the morning on awakening. Inflammation and hypertrophy of the insertions of the extraocular muscles (Fig. 33.4) are common and are of diagnostic value in those patients without proptosis.[27]

CLASS 3 DISEASE

The incidence of proptosis in patients with hyperthyroidism is high, with estimates ranging from 40% to 75%.[54] Two-thirds of patients with Graves' ophthalmopathy develop proptosis of 21 mm or more.[4] Although computed tomography (CT) and ultrasound evaluations reveal extraocular muscle involvement, the degree of proptosis does not necessarily parallel the severity of the orbital inflammatory process.[55] One mechanism for proptosis associated with thyroid orbitopathy has been partially clarified. Increased orbital deposition of glycosaminoglycans (mucopolysaccharides) occurs as the result of both hormonal and immunologic mediators.[45] Approximately 50% of thyroid patients have an increase in orbital fat, and of these patients 10% show this

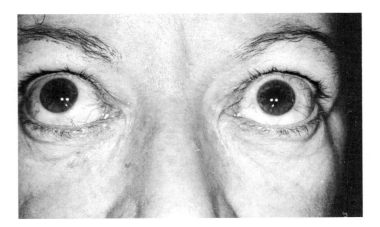

A

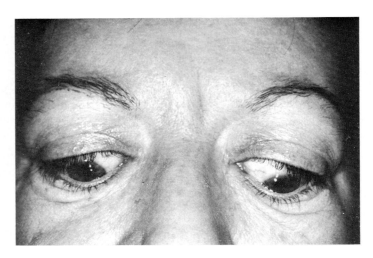

B

FIGURE 33.2   **Lid lag (Von Graefe's sign). Following extreme upgaze (A), the upper lids remain retracted and fail to assume their normal depressed position on downgaze (B).**

increase as the only sign on CT or MRI examination.[56] The proptosis may give rise to secondary lagophthalmos (Fig. 33.5).

Like lid retraction, proptosis can begin unilaterally and should therefore be differentiated from the apparent proptosis simulated by unilateral lid retraction. This can be accomplished clinically by measurement using the Luedde or Hertel exophthalmometer,[57] with which the upper limits of normal are approximately 18 mm for Orientals, 20 mm for whites, and 23 mm for blacks[42,58] (Table 33.3). A difference between eyes of 2 mm or more should be considered abnormal and justification for further study.[59] Another helpful test is palpable retropulsion. Having the patient close his or her

eyes and pushing on the globe will result in less detectable resistance in thyroid orbital disease as opposed to a greater resistance from an orbital tumor. Since hyperthyroidism is the most common cause of unilateral proptosis, the investigation of unilateral proptosis in patients without other signs of Graves' ophthalmopathy should include serum TSH, complemented by FT_4I or FT_4 estimate determinations.

CLASS 4 DISEASE

Approximately 14% of patients with thyrotoxicosis[60] and 33% of patients with Graves' ophthalmopathy[4] develop Class 4 involvement, in which the inflammatory changes

subtotal thyroidectomy or after radioactive iodine (RAI) therapy.[4] The onset is usually subacute, with one eye frequently being affected before its fellow. The natural history of the ocular disease from onset to spontaneous remission usually covers 6 months to 3 years (mean 2 years), after which the patient usually manifests a residual lid retraction, lid fullness, proptosis, and fibrotic changes of the extraocular muscles. Because of the tendency for Graves' ophthalmopathy to undergo spontaneous remission, medical or surgical treatment is intended to prevent permanent ocular damage rather than to arrest or retard progression of the disease process.

The clinical course of the ocular changes in hyperthyroidism seems to have two distinct phases,[77] rapid and plateau. The rapid phase lasts from several weeks to 6 months. During this time the ocular changes progress rapidly. During the plateau phase, the condition of the eyes either remains stationary or slowly moderates over several years before significant improvement occurs.

Management

Since the natural history of Graves' ophthalmopathy is to undergo spontaneous remission, the effectiveness of various forms of treatment is sometimes difficult to evaluate. However, with the knowledge that some eyes are lost solely due to failure to provide treatment, appropriate therapeutic measures may serve to reduce the risk to visual function and provide the patient with symptomatic relief. In general, management of the ocular involvement includes treatment of the underlying hyperthyroidism, if present, and the provision of local treatment to protect the ocular tissues and preserve visual functions. Surgical intervention should be withheld until the ocular and thyroid disorders are stable. The presence of active Class 2 through Class 6 disease calls for prompt and aggressive treatment as soon as the diagnosis is confirmed. Since the clinical manifestations of Class 2 through Class 6 disease are mostly caused by loss of critical pressure-volume relations within the orbit, therapy should be directed to restoring those relations toward normal.[6] Regardless of the stage of ocular involvement, the following general principles of management apply[78]:

- Since most patients with Graves' ophthalmopathy go through a period of initial worsening followed by a plateau of variable length, and finally spontaneous improvement, patients should be monitored more closely if in the worsening phase. If spontaneous improvement is occurring, more vigorous forms of treatment such as surgery or high-dose steroids should be withheld.
- Many patients, if relieved of the fear of losing vision, are willing to accept surprising degrees of cosmetic change and sometimes demanding treatment modalities. Several

studies have shown that patients with severe eye signs smoked significantly more tobacco than did those with less serious signs.[79] There are no data on the impact of smoking cessation on the degree of thyroid ophthalmopathy, but patients should be educated as to the potential relationship between smoking and ophthalmopathy.
- The patient should be advised of the marked variations in the course of the ocular disease and its relatively imprecise association with thyrotoxicosis; this will serve to reassure the patient and maintain rapport with the practitioner if the condition should worsen in its later stages.

A major problem in devising effective treatment has been an inadequate understanding of the factors that cause the ocular disease. Despite this, management of Graves' ophthalmopathy involves treating the thyroid dysfunction, relieving ocular pain and discomfort, restoring and protecting vision, and improving cosmetic appearance.[69] The following recommendations are representative of the most effective treatment modalities currently available.

Management of the Thyrotoxicosis

As part of the treatment of Graves' ophthalmopathy, adequate control of the hyperthyroid state, if it exists, is essential.[80,81] The antithyroid drugs propylthiouracil (PTU) and methimazole (MMI), radioactive iodine (^{131}I), and surgery are the three major modalities used in the treatment of hyperthyroidism. In addition, β-adrenergic blocking agents such as propranolol are useful for the rapid control of sympathetic nervous system manifestations. There is general agreement that the hyperthyroid state and the ocular disease run their own courses. Although control of hypermetabolism is necessary, this control does not ensure that the ophthalmopathy will improve concomitantly with treatment of the hyperthyroidism. However, it is essential in the treatment of the thyrotoxicosis to bring the patient gradually to euthyroidism by avoiding abrupt and exaggerated changes in the thyroid state. The ocular changes may be more likely to progress following systemic treatment that causes rapid alteration in thyroid function.[3]

Results of survey studies among thyroid specialists who treat Graves' hyperthyroidism in Europe, Japan, or the United States[82] have shown consensus only on the relative lack of a role of thyroidectomy, except for narrow indications. Graves' hyperthyroidism in the United States is treated in most adults (69%) with radioactive iodine (RAI-^{131}I), while the rest receive treatment with the antithyroid drugs, PTU or MMI. Conversely, antithyroid drugs are used in Europe (77%) and Japan (88%) in most Graves' disease patients, while the rest are treated with RAI.

Most patients with Graves' disease will respond adequately to an initial dose of PTU, 300 to 450 mg, or MMI, 30 to 45 mg, daily in divided doses. Doses should be adjusted subsequently by clinical response and thyroid hormone determinations. Several management options exist once the patient's hyperthyroidism has been controlled with antithyroid drugs.[83] Some physicians reduce the dose of medication while others, to maintain a euthyroid state, provide thyroid hormone replacement without modifying the amount of antithyroid drug. Radioactive iodine (RAI) treatment is generally reserved for patients over 30 years of age. Most patients with Graves' disease will respond adequately to doses between 5 and 10 mCi of [131]I. Subtotal thyroidectomy is used only in selected cases, but should not be performed until the patient is under adequate control with antithyroid drugs. Patients developing hypothyroidism due to treatment should receive L-thyroxine, 0.1 to 0.2 mg (1.6 µg per kg body weight) daily. These patients should be monitored at regular intervals by serum TSH and FT_4I or FT_4 estimate determinations.[84]

The frequency and types of toxic reactions to PTU and MMI are similar but appear to be related to the doses employed. In about 5% of patients there are mild side effects, ranging from gastrointestinal complaints to mild skin reactions and pruritis, that can usually be controlled adequately with antihistamines without discontinuing the drug. The most severe and worrisome complication, however, is agranulocytosis, which occurs in about 0.2% of patients treated with these drugs. It always responds to discontinuation of the medication, but, in a few instances, concomitant administration of steroids may be indicated. Since this complication can be lethal if not quickly recognized, the patient should be advised to report to the physician whenever infection, sore throat, or general malaise occurs, in which case a complete blood count (CBC) should be obtained.

Although Tallstedt and associates[85] suggest that RAI treatment for Graves' disease is associated with a higher incidence and worsening of ophthalmopathy than is treatment with either antithyroid drugs (MMI) or surgery, other studies have not established such a relationship. It is generally accepted that the outcome of Graves' ophthalmopathy after treatment of the hyperthyroidism with antithyroid drugs, radioactive iodine, or surgery is similar for the three groups.[86] There is also clinical evidence that the development of severe ophthalmopathy does not seem to be related to the degree of hypothyroidism or hyperthyroidism, but that the careful, gradual control of thyroid function is important in minimizing the danger to these patients' eyes.

Local Management of the Ophthalmopathy

A variety of local measures can be used to provide the patient with symptomatic relief while protecting ocular tissues and preserving visual functions. These are discussed for each disease classification.

CLASS 1 DISEASE (LID RETRACTION)

The patient with Class 1 disease may have lagophthalmos ranging from very mild to very severe. The lid retraction and lagophthalmos accelerate tear film evaporation, thus increasing tear film osmolarity and causing ocular surface damage.[87] Any associated exposure keratopathy should be managed with ocular lubricating solutions or ointments. The clinician should try several types of artificial tears. This allows the patient to choose the formulation that gives the greatest symptomatic relief. A variety of general measures may be helpful, such as the wearing of tinted lenses to shield the cosmetic appearance and to protect the eye from wind, dust, and other environmental factors. The eyelids can be taped shut at bedtime to protect the cornea. Likewise, a Saran Wrap shield can be constructed and taped over the eye, thus creating a moisture chamber during sleep. Moreover, certain sleep positions may increase the effects of the lagophthalmos. Many clinicians have observed patients who sleep in the prone position to have more ocular symptoms than do those who sleep supine.[67] For moderate to severe cases of corneal exposure, applying a topical broad-spectrum antibacterial ointment (e.g., gentamicin or bacitracin-polymyxin B) at bedtime or continuously during the day may prevent infection of the exposed corneal and conjunctival tissues.

In many instances, however, the patient's primary desire is to have an improved cosmetic appearance of the lid retraction. Since the relationship between the clinical signs of thyrotoxicosis and the effects of increased catecholamine activity has been apparent for many decades, various attempts have been made to control or alleviate the upper lid retraction by using adrenergic blocking agents such as guanethidine, reserpine, and thymoxamine. Because upper lid retraction may be mediated through sympathetic activity of Müeller's muscle, drugs with α-adrenergic blocking properties have been used topically and orally to manage this condition. However, these drugs do not affect the degree of proptosis, if present, because proptosis is associated with increased volume of the retrobulbar tissues and is not mediated through autonomic nervous system control. Topical bethanidine, an adrenergic blocking agent, has been used in 10% and 20% solutions to treat lid retraction.[88] When used in a dosage of 2 or 3 drops daily, it effectively induces a pharmacologic Horner's syndrome with associated ptosis and miosis. Three or more weeks may be required to reach a maximum ptotic effect. No serious adverse ocular or systemic side effects have been observed. Propranolol, a β-adrenergic blocking agent, has been used both orally[62] and topically[89] to relieve lid retraction. For acute cases of lid retraction, propranolol, 10 mg 4 times daily, may be helpful. The topical use of 1% propranolol solution has produced variable results.[89] In addition, topical timolol has been used by some practitioners for lid retraction, but with variable results.[90]

Dapiprazole HCL (REV-Eyes) is an α-adrenergic blocking agent introduced for the treatment of iatrogenically induced mydriasis. One of the side effects of this topical agent is ptosis (see Fig. 8.14). In theory, this effect could potentially be useful for early lid retraction of Graves' disease. Other side effects, however, include burning upon instillation, and moderate to severe conjunctival injection. There have been no published studies on the efficacy of dapiprazole to relieve lid retraction in Class 1 disease.

The most commonly employed drug for the relief of lid retraction is orally or topically administered guanethidine. Guanethidine depletes sympathetic storage sites, initially causing release of norepinephrine that may lead to mydriasis and lid retraction, but that eventually produces a chemical sympathectomy resembling postganglionic Horner's syndrome. Although guanethidine is somewhat unpredictable in

the management of lid retraction, it seems to offer the best results with the fewest toxic effects when used in lower concentrations. Orally administered guanethidine, 15 mg daily, has been shown to lower the eyelid in some patients,[90] but most clinicians prefer the topical route of administration. When employed topically in a 10% concentration, this agent substantially reduces lid retraction (Fig. 33.9) but is associated with significant superficial punctate keratitis in about 50% of patients.[91] The 5% solution is equally effective but without the attendant side effects.[91] Unlike the effect associated with thymoxamine, the maximum effect on lid retraction requires several days (Fig. 33.10). Cartlidge and associates[92] found that the ptosis produced by 5% topical guanethidine was approximately 1.5 mm. Systemic side effects have not been noted in most studies, but a report of two patients with severe abdominal pains and diarrhea re-

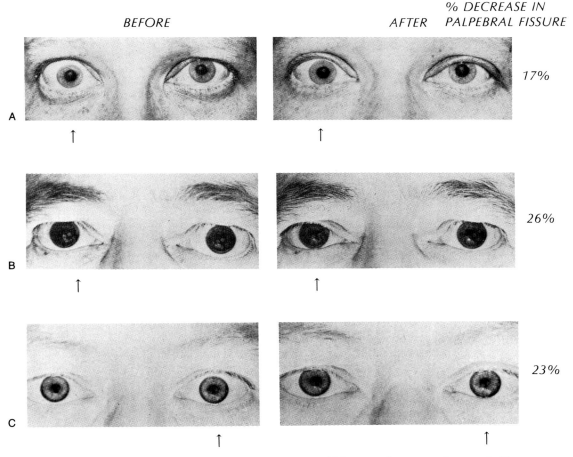

BEFORE

AFTER   % DECREASE IN PALPEBRAL FISSURE

A   17%

B   26%

C   23%

FIGURE 33.9   **Response of three patients to treatment with guanethidine 10% in one eye for 1 week. The average reduction in the palpebral fissure of the treated eye is about 1.5mm. (From Sneddon JM, Turner P. Adrenergic blockade and the eye signs of thyrotoxicosis. Lancet 1966;2:525–527, with permission of the authors and publisher.)**

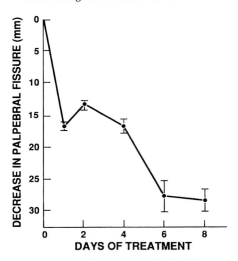

FIGURE 33.10 **The mean decrease in palpebral fissure of one eye compared with pretreatment values in 14 patients receiving guanethidine 10%, 2 drops twice daily. Each point represents the mean (± SEM). Measurements were obtained by projecting the clinical photographs to 8 times their original size. (From Sneddon JM, Turner P. Adrenergic blockade and the eye signs of thyrotoxicosis. Lancet 1966;2:525–527, with permission of the authors and the publisher.)**

quiring emergency hospital admission should call for caution in the use of this drug.[93] The clinician should initiate therapy with 5% guanethidine,[a] 1 drop 3 times daily, until maximum improvement in the lid position is obtained, and then reduce the frequency of administration to daily instillation if this is adequate and, if possible, further reduce the instillation to alternate days.

Several conditions may adversely affect the ability of guanethidine to lower the upper lid[51]: (1) if the patient is thyrotoxic, rather than euthyroid or hypothyroid[95]; (2) if the patient is concomitantly undergoing drug therapy with adrenergic agonists, either systemically or topically; and (3) if adhesions form between the levator and the superior rectus muscles in the later stages of the disease process.[90]

If conservative measures are insufficient to promote patient comfort or acceptance, botulinum A toxin can be injected directly into the affected levator muscle. Injection of 2.5 to 7.5 units of toxin may lower the affected lid by 2 to 3 mm, lasting 1 to 8 months.[174,175]

Surgery for Class 1 disease is usually not indicated because these patients are typically asymptomatic and because the lid retraction may resolve after treatment of the underlying thyrotoxicosis. Surgery, however, is a reasonable and necessary alternative for patients with severe lid retraction

---

[a] Not FDA-approved for topical use in the United States.

not responding to more conservative measures. The two most common reasons for surgical repair are cosmesis and relief of symptoms arising from ocular exposure. Many surgical procedures are available, including those affecting the levator muscle, Müeller's muscle, a combination of the two procedures, and tarsorrhaphy. In some patients with fibrosis of the inferior rectus muscle, recession of the tight muscle may reduce or eliminate upper lid retraction.[172] Eyelid retraction procedures seem to be most effective in patients with minimal to moderate proptosis (less than 25 mm).[67] In most cases, surgery for lid retraction should not be considered until the ocular condition has been stable for at least 6 months to 1 year. If proptosis is present and is severe enough to require orbital decompression, this procedure should be done first, since the decompression itself may reduce the lid retraction.[96] The decision to lower the lids should then be postponed for several months. However, in emergencies in which corneal integrity is threatened, lid surgery could be contemplated together with the orbital decompression.[49]

CLASS 2 DISEASE (SOFT TISSUE INVOLVEMENT)

Many patients with mild Class 2 disease can be managed adequately with ocular lubricants. Elevating the head of the bed on 6 inch blocks during sleep can minimize lid and periocular swelling on awakening.[3,4,62,93] Reduction of periorbital swelling may be measured by inserting a small, straight-edged ruler into the upper lid fold and allowing periorbital tissue to rest on it. The number of millimeters the periorbital tissue covers is a quantitative measure of the swelling. The use of tinted lenses will provide relief from light sensitivity. Tinted lenses not only guard against irritation and light sensitivity, but they also have the advantage of masking the cosmetic problem. Occasionally, the use of orally administered diuretics is indicated. If the patient has unquestioned glaucoma concomitantly with Class 2 Graves' ophthalmopathy, the diuretic of choice, conveniently, is acetazolamide.[62] For patients with moderate to severe Class 2 disease, the use of systemically administered corticosteroids may be of immense benefit (Fig. 33.11). There is no doubt that the use of steroids in adequate dosages can decrease the severity of ocular complications, although they have minimal, if any, influence on the duration of the thyrotoxicosis.[93] The use of systemic steroids seems to have the greatest benefit on patients with acute orbitopathy.[66] These patients are often without history of thyroid disease, and diagnostic imaging confirms the thyroid orbitopathy.

Locally administered steroids have been used with variable success. Although topically applied steroids are completely ineffective in alleviating the ocular signs or symptoms associated with Class 2 disease,[4] periocular steroids have been employed with some success.[4,62,78,93,97,98] Subconjunctival or retrobulbar injections of methylprednisolone are used, and sub-Tenon's injection of aqueous triamcinolone (Kenalog 40 mg/ml) can also be used.[62,93] The

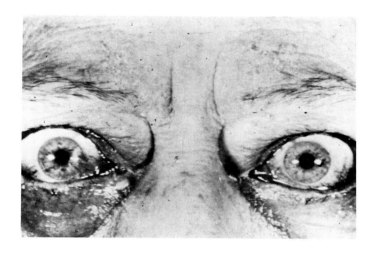

FIGURE 33.11   **Same patient as in Figure 33.3 following systemic steroid therapy. Note the marked improvement in lid swelling, conjunctival and episcleral injection, and chemosis.**

precise dosage of methylprednisolone must be guided by the individual patient, but 10 to 20 mg per injection (40 mg/ml) has been effective when repeated at varying intervals.[93] More concentrated preparations of methylprednisolone (Depo-Medrol 80 mg/ml) permit the injection of higher doses with smaller volumes,[93] which is particularly important when giving retrobulbar injections into an already tense orbit. Periocular injections may be repeated at monthly or longer intervals as required.

The results obtained from the use of periocular steroids can be quite dramatic. Most patients obtain relief from the symptoms of ocular discomfort after the first injection.[97] If periocular steroids are to be used, treatment should not be delayed until after the ocular disease becomes severe but, rather, should be employed at an early stage to prevent complications. The results of steroid use are most beneficial in the early years of the orbital disease. The anti-inflammatory and immunosuppressive actions are initially effective, but there is some doubt as to their effects as the extraocular muscles become fibrotic.

The duration of steroid therapy is controversial. Starting the patient on oral prednisone 80 mg daily for 10 days and then abruptly stopping the steroid has shown several interesting results. Approximately 30% of patients treated with this regimen appear to have a relatively permanent effect on their symptoms.[56] Continuation of the medication or slowly tapering the drug may give a higher response rate but can increase the likelihood of secondary complications.[99] Orbital radiation is indicated when the short course of high-dose steroid has no response, a partial response, or when a relapse occurs after steroid therapy has been discontinued.

CLASS 3 DISEASE (PROPTOSIS)

Since proptosis is a variable finding in Graves' ophthalmopathy, it is not a useful indication of the degree of orbital infiltration or of the response to treatment. Moreover, longstanding proptosis tends to be permanent, presumably because of the permanent changes in the tissues of the orbit, and is thus not often amenable to medical therapy.

As previously stated, Graves' ophthalmopathy may be more likely to progress following systemic treatment that causes rapid alteration in thyroid tissue and function.[3] Gwinup and associates,[100] however, have shown that proptosis progresses more slowly in patients treated with subtotal thyroidectomy and radioactive iodine in contrast to treatment with antithyroid drugs. The loss of thyroid tissue by these means may limit the progression of proptosis.

Proptosis as an isolated finding rarely requires treatment unless there is secondary exposure keratopathy or unless it represents a significant cosmetic problem.[52] Such patients may benefit from a trial of systemic or periocular corticosteroids. A significant decrease in the severity of proptosis may be observed in some patients. In general, if regression of the proptosis occurs after the institution of steroid therapy, it will begin soon after the onset of therapy and reach a maximum in 2 or 3 months.[101]

Adrenergic blocking agents, such as propranolol, have been used but are generally ineffective in relieving proptosis, since this condition is associated with increased volume of the retrobulbar tissues rather than with sympathetic autonomic nervous system control of the eye.[102]

CLASS 4 DISEASE (EXTRAOCULAR MUSCLE INVOLVEMENT)

Many patients, perhaps up to 50%, may experience return of normal eye movements following medical control of the thyrotoxicosis.[60] For patients who do not experience improvement, the only pharmacologic interventions that have been shown to be effective for the specific changes associated with Class 4 disease are systemic prednisone[4,101,103] and local injections of botulinum toxin.[104–106]

In the early stages of Class 4 involvement, treatment with small doses of prednisone may be initiated when control of the hyperthyroidism or adequate therapy of hypothyroidism has not arrested the ocular activity. Improvement in motility usually occurs within 4 to 12 weeks.[52] Many patients experience enough subsequent improvement in ocular motility that severe Class 4 disease may be considered a relative but not absolute indication for steroid therapy.[101,107] However, conservative therapy is prudent in many cases and may include exercising the eyes to lessen the tendency for muscle fibrosis;[62] the use of Fresnel prisms, which have a definite advantage in the management of unstable motility disorders; or simple monocular patching.

In patients with motility disorders with onset of less than 12 months, botulinum toxin can be injected directly into the affected muscle(s).[104,106] Following injection the toxin rapidly binds to the muscle, where it inhibits liberation of the neurotransmitter, acetylcholine, into the neuromuscular junction.[105] Such "chemodenervation" can effectively, although temporarily, decrease or eliminate symptoms of diplopia.[104] The use of botulinum, however, is usually limited to patients with diplopia of less than 6 months duration.

Many patients should be considered surgical candidates following the failure of steroid therapy or other, more conservative therapeutic measures. Marked improvement can often be obtained in elevation of the globe following appropriate recession of the fibrotic inferior rectus muscle.[108–110] The recession of other extraocular muscles to correct existing heterotropias and associated diplopia should also be considered.[108,111] In general, surgery should be postponed at least 6 to 12 months after stabilization of the metabolic and ocular conditions, since early surgical manipulation may acutely exacerbate the original disease process.[93,112] Significant complications from eye muscle surgery are rare but include an increase of the proptosis following release of the fibrotic ocular muscles.[113] For this reason, if the proptosis is more than 22 or 23 mm, serious consideration should be given to orbital decompression before muscle surgery even if there is no significant threat to vision.

CLASS 5 DISEASE (CORNEAL INVOLVEMENT)

Patients with Class 5 disease are at risk of serious ocular complications and loss of vision. In the milder forms of exposure keratopathy the administration of bland ocular lubricants at bedtime or continuously during the day may be of significant benefit in alleviating associated symptoms and preventing or delaying more serious ocular involvement. The topical application of broad-spectrum antibiotics (e.g., gentamicin) may be indicated for the prophylaxis of infection. Taping the lids shut at bedtime or employing a Saran Wrap shield may also prove beneficial. When frank corneal ulceration is imminent, systemic steroid therapy can prove useful.[114] In these cases high doses of steroid given for short periods (e.g., prednisone 120 to 140 mg daily for 7 days and

gradually tapered) may bring about desired results. The use of systemic steroids sometimes obviates the need for surgery (orbital decompression) but generally involves long-term therapy with the possibility of adverse effects. Steroids are also useful for patients who cannot undergo orbital decompression because of contraindication to general anesthesia. In addition, the use of diuretics may be beneficial in some patients.

Orbital decompression should be considered for patients with severe Class 5 disease for whom steroids and orbital radiation are ineffective or contraindicated, for patients whose compliance may be poor, or for whom follow-up may be difficult.

CLASS 6 DISEASE (OPTIC NERVE INVOLVEMENT)

Although as many as 70% of patients with optic neuropathy spontaneously improve without treatment,[115] the risk to vision is significant, and loss of vision may become permanent if the optic neuropathy is not quickly recognized and aggressively treated.[116] The most common presentation is a patient with a complaint of visual acuity loss or a visual field defect. Ultrasonography often demonstrates optic disc edema. Ideally, therapy should begin with correction of the thyroid imbalance.[83] Replacement thyroid hormone is mandatory for hypothyroid states. Some patients with optic neuropathy can be managed entirely by adjustment of the thyroid state, particularly if the clinician and patient are willing to wait several weeks for improvement to begin.

Systemic steroids have been used for severe Class 6 disease since they first became available, but the early results were not satisfactory, probably because of the relatively small doses that were employed. Brown and associates[101] in 1963 were the first to show the often dramatic effects of large doses of prednisone in patients with Graves' ophthalmopathy, including documented optic nerve disease.

A gratifying response to steroid therapy may be observed in many patients with optic neuropathy (Fig. 33.12). Trobe and associates[117] reported a 48% success rate defined as two Snellen lines of improvement in visual acuity within 2 months of steroid treatment. A beneficial effect was usually noted within 72 hours of beginning therapy, and no further improvement was noted after 6 to 8 weeks. Fifty-two percent of eyes failed to respond to oral steroid therapy despite doses from 50 to 100 mg daily maintained for 2 to 6 months.

When steroid therapy is not effective, cytotoxic or immunosuppressive agents have been attempted. Prummel and associates[118] performed a single-masked study of 36 patients randomized to either 7.5 mg/kg cyclosporine or 60 mg oral prednisone. The prednisone group had a greater effect but more immediate complications than did the cyclosporine group. Perros and co-workers[119] found poor results with the use of azathioprine for moderate ophthalmopathy.

Trobe and associates[117] offer the following guidelines for the management of patients with optic neuropathy:

- Patients with minimal optic nerve dysfunction (visual acuity of 20/30 [6/9] or better) may be managed by observation alone. However, the tendency for rapid progression demands serial examinations of visual acuity, visual fields, and pupillary testing.
- Patients with progressive vision loss (with or without disc swelling), or with disc swelling and no visual defect should be treated. Oral steroids in large doses remain the primary therapeutic modality, but if a response has not occurred within 3 or 4 weeks, continued high doses are not likely to succeed.
- Prolonged steroid maintenance without improvement in visual function is not justified.

With failure of systemic steroids to control the optic nerve disease, low-dosage orbital irradiation (1600 to 2000 rad) may be considered or may be employed initially for patients with contraindications to steroids. With the failure of both oral steroids and orbital irradiation, orbital decompression must be considered the final management option.

Systemic Management of the Ophthalmopathy

As mentioned, the hyperthyroid state must be controlled before use of other therapeutic measures,[78,93] including diuretics, steroids, plasmapheresis, and immunosuppressive agents. Systemic treatment with steroids, plasmapheresis and immunosuppressive agents, either alone or in combination, is based on the assumption that Graves' ophthalmopathy is the consequence of an autoimmune process. These treatments attempt to relieve inflammatory or congestive signs by shrinking tissues within the orbit, resulting in decreased intraorbital pressure.

Diuretics are used occasionally in the treatment of Graves' ophthalmopathy, particularly when there is pronounced periorbital edema. These agents are thought to mobilize salt and water deposits retained locally by hydrophilic mucopolysaccharides. Diuretics might also be used in conjunction with other forms of treatment such as systemic steroids. As previously mentioned, the use of acetazolamide is a logical and convenient choice for patients who also have unquestioned glaucoma.[62]

Systemic steroids and plasmapheresis are effective only in ophthalmopathy that is recent or acute (less than 6 months) or that is rapidly advancing. These forms of treatment are ineffective in stable and chronic ophthalmopathy.

STEROIDS

Systemic steroids often effectively control the optic neuropathy and other inflammatory changes of the ophthalmopathy. However, systemic steroids must be used in high dosages at the expense of their known complications and side effects, including osteoporosis, hyperglycemia, hypertension, infec-

tion, gastric ulceration, cataract, Cushingoid features, and psychosis.[78,93,101,120,121] However, rapid progression of proptosis, ophthalmoplegia, and optic nerve involvement warrant such treatment. Development of visual field defects or decreased visual acuity are absolute indications for the use of steroids. High-dose steroids as monotherapy are of use in ameliorating many of the inflammatory features of the orbitopathy. Patients who benefit will do so very early in the course of treatment. Subjective improvement might occur within the first 24 hours, and extraocular muscle function and visual acuity might improve in a few days or weeks.[121] Treatment should be initiated with large doses of prednisone (50 to 100 mg daily). When improvement is apparent, the dosage should be reduced gradually. Whenever exacerbation occurs, the dosage must be increased until improvement is restored. Subsequently, the steroid should be tapered more gradually. Werner[120] reported dramatic results with the use of very high doses of oral prednisone, 140 mg daily, in extreme emergencies such as severe corneal compromise or optic nerve involvement. The use of intravenous methylprednisolone has also been reported.[122] This form of therapy produced rapid improvement in the majority of treated patients. Soft tissue signs showed the greatest improvement, and, as with oral therapy, patients with disease of shorter duration manifested the greatest improvement.

In general, if optic neuropathy is responsive to steroids, exacerbations will occur if the drug is withdrawn within 2 to 4 weeks.[115,121] Therefore, steroids must be administered until the disease process undergoes spontaneous remission. Although this increases the potential risk of serious steroid-related complications, this risk is justified in many instances. Because of the risks inherent in systemic steroid therapy, the practitioner should educate the patient regarding the potential side effects of steroids and the need for regular and long-term medical supervision.

Combining steroids with cyclosporine or orbital irradiation appears to enhance the efficacy of individual therapy.[5,118,123–125] Use of steroids has also been recommended to prevent progression of Graves' ophthalmopathy following RAI treatment of hyperthyroidism.[126]

PLASMAPHERESIS

Plasmapheresis as a form of therapy for Graves' ophthalmopathy was first reported by Dandona and associates[127,128] in 1979. A more recent study by Glinoer and associates[129] confirmed the earlier results that plasmapheresis was ineffective in chronic nonprogressive forms of Graves' disease. It was, however, quite successful in more acute forms. The effects of this form of therapy were not permanent and were without associated immunosuppressive effect. Recurrences were observed in approximately 6 months in one-third of patients. However, its cost-effectiveness has been questioned[12,28,130]; the procedure consists of 3 or 4 sessions of plasmapheresis, each of which involves removal of 2 or 3

CENTRAL 30 - 2 THRESHOLD TEST

NAME

STIMULUS III, WHITE, BCKGND 31.5 ASB BLIND SPOT CHECK SIZE III

STRATEGY FULL THRESHOLD

FASTPAC

BIRTHDATE 01-11-22 DATE 03-26-93

FIXATION TARGET CENTRAL   ID 35023   TIME 11:42:22 AM

RX USED +3.75 DS   DCX   DEG   PUPIL DIAMETER   VA 20/25

LEFT

AGE   71

FIXATION LOSSES 0/19

FALSE POS ERRORS 1/12

FALSE NEG ERRORS 0/10

QUESTIONS ASKED 375

TEST TIME 00:11:02

HFA S/N

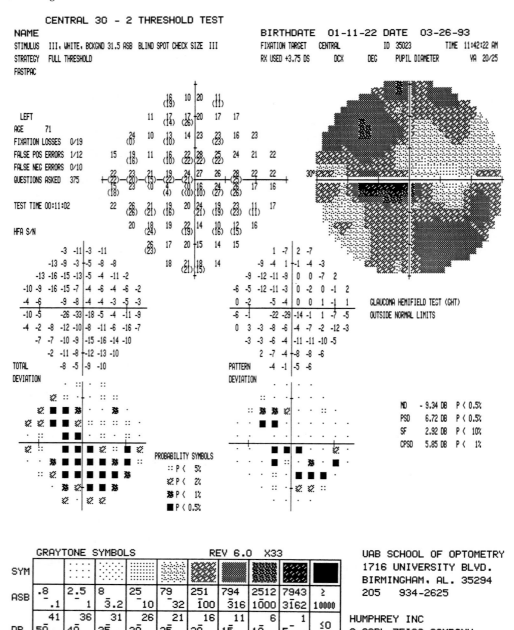

GLAUCOMA HEMIFIELD TEST (GHT)

OUTSIDE NORMAL LIMITS

TOTAL DEVIATION

PATTERN DEVIATION

MD	- 9.34 DB	P < 0.5%	
PSD	6.72 DB	P < 0.5%	
SF	2.92 DB	P < 10%	
CPSD	5.85 DB	P < 1%	

PROBABILITY SYMBOLS

:: P < 5%

⊠ P < 2%

▨ P < 1%

■ P < 0.5%

GRAYTONE SYMBOLS						REV 6.0 X33				
SYM										
ASB	.8 - .1	2.5 - 1	8 - 3.2	25 - 10	79 - 32	251 - 100	794 - 316	2512 - 1000	7943 - 3162	≥ 10000
DB	41 50	36 40	31 35	26 30	21 25	16 20	11 15	6 10	1 5	≤0

UAB SCHOOL OF OPTOMETRY

1716 UNIVERSITY BLVD.

BIRMINGHAM, AL. 35294

205   934-2625

HUMPHREY INC

A CARL ZEISS COMPANY

A

FIGURE 33.12   71-year-old female with acute Class 6 Graves' ophthalmopathy. *(A)* Central and paracentral defects in left visual field are associated with 20/60 (6/18) visual acuity. *(B)* Left visual field after 3-week course of oral prednisone, 60 mg daily, then tapered. Visual acuity improved to 20/40 (6/12).

CENTRAL 30 - 2 THRESHOLD TEST

NAME
STIMULUS   III, WHITE, BCKGND 31.5 ASB BLIND SPOT CHECK SIZE III
STRATEGY   FULL THRESHOLD
FASTPAC

BIRTHDATE   01-11-22 DATE   04-23-93
FIXATION TARGET   CENTRAL   ID   TIME 01:56:24 PM
RX USED +3.75 DS   DCX   DEG   PUPIL DIAMETER   VA

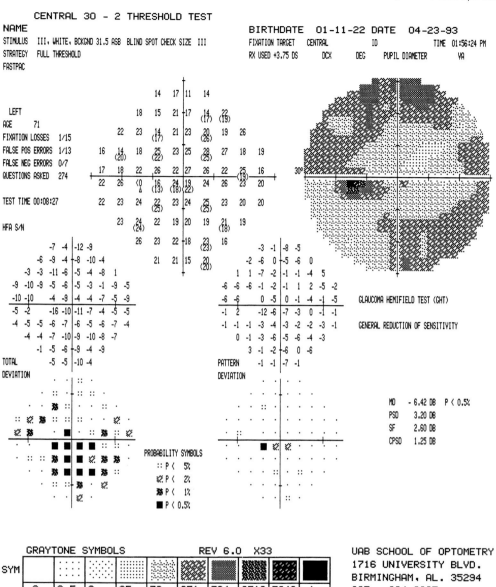

LEFT

AGE   71
FIXATION LOSSES   1/15
FALSE POS ERRORS 1/13
FALSE NEG ERRORS 0/7
QUESTIONS ASKED   274

TEST TIME 00:08:27

HFA S/N

GLAUCOMA HEMIFIELD TEST (GHT)

GENERAL REDUCTION OF SENSITIVITY

TOTAL
DEVIATION

PATTERN
DEVIATION

MD   - 6.42 DB   P < 0.5%
PSD   3.20 DB
SF   2.60 DB
CPSD   1.25 DB

PROBABILITY SYMBOLS
:: P < 5%
▧ P < 2%
▨ P < 1%
■ P < 0.5%

GRAYTONE SYMBOLS				REV 6.0	X33				
SYM									
ASB	.8 .1	2.5 1	8 3.2	25 10	79 32	251 100	794 316	2512 1000	7943 3162	≥ 10000
DB	41 50	36 40	31 35	26 30	21 25	16 20	11 15	6 10	1 5	≤0

UAB SCHOOL OF OPTOMETRY
1716 UNIVERSITY BLVD.
BIRMINGHAM, AL. 35294
205   934-2625

HUMPHREY INC
A CARL ZEISS COMPANY

B

FIGURE 33.12   **(Continued)**

liters of plasma. Lost plasma is replaced by human plasma or human albumin in 0.9% saline solution. Best results are obtained in patients with acute, recent, or rapidly advancing eye disease.[131] The treatment should be instituted concurrently with the administration of prednisone 80 mg for the first day, and then decreasing every second day to 60, 40, and 20 mg doses, which is then maintained for at least 3 weeks. Improvement in the ocular condition has been observed within 48 to 72 hours, even before steroids have been administered. The question still remains, however, whether the dramatic improvement in the ocular condition is due more to the administration of steroids than to the plasmapheresis itself. Dandona and associates[127,128] observed that the levels of TSAb markedly decrease after the procedure, but this does not necessarily correlate with the ocular response. However, if steroids are not concomitantly administered, there is rebound in the production of these antibodies to values higher than those before treatment, with potential aggravation of the hyperthyroid state.

IMMUNOSUPPRESSIVE AGENTS

There is convincing evidence that Graves' disease is related to a defective immune system.[11,132,133] TSAb, which are immunoglobulins (IgG) that bind the TSH receptor (TSHR-Ab), are present in the serum of patients with Graves' disease.[21,38,39] The long-acting thyroid stimulator (LATS) was the first immunoglobulin, class IgG, identified and the one that initiated the concept of the autoimmune origin of Graves' disease. Thyroid-related ophthalmopathy is also likely to be an autoimmune disorder in which activated T and B cells appear to play a key role.[7,9,24,25,125] On the basis of these findings, it seemed justifiable to attempt immunosuppressive therapy in an effort to control the ocular changes. However, several therapeutic attempts using immunosuppressive drugs, such as azathioprine and ciamexone, have generally been unsuccessful in improving the ocular involvement.[3,114,123,134,135] Burrow and associates[135] administered azathioprine to five patients with the active eye changes of Graves' disease and noted objective evidence of immune suppression in each patient; despite this, however, there was no significant improvement in the ophthalmopathy. Two possible explanations for the failure of immunosuppressive therapy are: (1) the orbital infiltration may occur and stabilize before therapy is begun, and (2) TSAb may not play a role in the etiology of the ocular changes; therefore suppression of TSAb production has no effect on the ocular disease.

Bigos and associates[134] administered cyclophosphamide in the management of advanced Graves' ophthalmopathy with proptosis and diplopia. Withdrawal of steroid therapy was permitted in one patient, symptoms of diplopia completely resolved in two patients and improved in a third patient coincident with administration of the drug, and deteriorating visual acuity resolved in one patient. Although chemosis improved in the two affected patients, proptosis remained unchanged in all three patients. Cyclophosphamide appears to have modest efficacy but has not been used in many patients.[6,123]

Cyclosporine A is a potent immunosuppressive agent with a high degree of specificity for T-cells.[137] Therapeutic results obtained with this drug have varied. Use of cyclosporine was unsuccessful in small groups of patients reported by Howlett and associates[138] and Brabant and associates.[139] Conversely, the drug improved ocular motility, visual acuity, proptosis, and muscle swelling in two patients reported by Weetman and associates[137] and in nine patients reported by Utech and associates.[140] Concomitantly, thyroid antibodies fell and T-cell abnormalities returned toward normal.[137] More recent controlled trials have demonstrated that the efficacy of cyclosporine is similar to that of steroids, and that patients who may not respond to either drug, when used alone, may respond when the two are combined.[6,118,123] However, the use of cyclosporine A in the treatment of Graves' ophthalmopathy appears to be limited by its potentially serious side effects, cost, and lack of superiority over steroids.

Several other immunomodulator agents are currently under investigation. Ciamexone inhibits the expressions of HLA-DR antigens. These antigens play a role in the antigen-recognition pathway. Several patients with ophthalmopathy have been treated with this drug, and the early results are encouraging.[136]

The use of bromocriptine has been shown to be effective in thyroid ophthalmopathy.[41,161] Bromocriptine binds to dopamine receptors, which in turn has several effects including decreasing prolactin levels, inhibiting thyroid stimulating hormones, and an anti-T-lymphocyte reaction. Many patients have been treated with this drug, and some have experienced improvement after failure of conventional therapy. Patients generally receive approximately 2.5 mg bromocriptine three times daily for several months.[141,161]

The Role of Other Forms of Management

ORBITAL IRRADIATION

Attempts at orbital irradiation were begun over 50 years ago but involved relatively low-dose, low-energy, or poorly collimated beams. The results were generally unsatisfactory. In 1968, Donaldson[142] began an experimental program of supervoltage orbital radiotherapy for Graves' ophthalmopathy. The design was to treat the orbit laterally, targeting the muscle cone only, and sparing the lens, cornea, pituitary, and hypothalamus. The results have been favorable, and this approach seems to offer a reasonable alternative to steroid therapy and surgical decompression in some patients. Prummel and associates[176] found orbital irradiation to be as effective as oral prednisone in patients with moderately severe disease but without optic neuropathy. The irradiation has several effects on the orbital tissues, which include the biochemical effect of correcting acidosis produced by the inflammatory response, and suppressing lymphocytes. The most antiphlogistic effect of irradiation is the suppression of fibroblast production by relatively small radiation doses.[56,143] Existing hyperthyroidism should be corrected, if possible, before irradiation. Supervoltage radiation therapy combined with corticosteroids is more effective than radiotherapy alone.[5,124] When systemic steroids are administered simultaneously, the dose should be kept constant during the period of irradiation and for several weeks thereafter.[115,144] Overall, approximately 60 to 70% of irradiated patients improve.[5,123]

In general, orbital irradiation produces the most impressive results in patients with active and progressive ophthalmopathy, rather than in patients with a more indolent disease course. The procedure is indicated for patients with the following[145,146]:

- Rapidly progressive severe ophthalmopathy
- Troublesome soft tissue signs and symptoms
- Contraindications to use of steroids
- Side effects from or lack of disease control with steroids

Therapy may result in improved proptosis, lid retraction, visual acuity, and soft tissue signs,[146–148] but motility disorders respond less satisfactorily.[146,150] If treatment is administered early (within 6 to 24 months[148,151]), a positive response usually occurs within 6 weeks.[147] Acute and long-term complications are negligible,[146] but radiation retinopathy can occur as a rare side effect.

ORBITAL DECOMPRESSION

When steroid therapy or orbital irradiation is unsatisfactory in improving the severe changes associated with Class 5 and

6 disease, surgical enlargement of the orbital volume should be considered. Dollinger[152] first reported orbital decompression for Graves' ophthalmopathy in 1911.[153–155,157,169,170,171] Since then, several surgical approaches for orbital decompression have been described (Fig. 33.13). In 1931, Naffziger introduced the concept of removal of the roof of the orbit by a neurosurgical transfrontal approach. Another approach, the Kronlein procedure, involves removing the lateral wall of the orbit with decompression into the temporal fossa. Both these procedures have the disadvantage of decompressing the orbit into an area of high tissue pressure. In addition, the Naffziger approach introduces the morbidity of an intracranial operation, and the Kronlein method is a lengthy procedure involving considerable bony resection. The most commonly used decompressive procedure for Graves' orbitopathy is the antralethmoidal method through either a transantral or translid approach.[156] In 1992, Antoszyk and associates[156] reported using a transorbital three-wall decompression through a modified blepharoplasty incision. This technique allowed a single incision with wide exposure, a low incidence of permanent strabismus, lateral orbital rim and canthal tendon preservation, and a large reduction in proptosis. Many ophthalmic surgeons still use modifications of Ogura's original procedure,[157] but regardless of the particular technique used, surgical experience is a major factor in success rate.[177,178]

Because of the inherent risks involved, orbital decompression should be considered only after more conservative therapeutic measures have been attempted. Most clinicians reserve the use of orbital decompression for patients with severe corneal compromise associated with progressive proptosis and corneal exposure, and for patients with optic neuropathy who have failed to respond to systemic steroids or for whom systemic steroids are contraindicated. In all cases, however, orbital decompression should not be considered until the thyroid state is stable.[113]

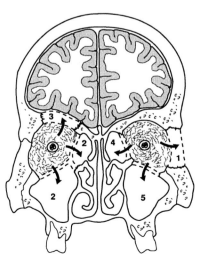

1 LATERAL (Kronlein)
2 TRANSANTRAL (Ogura)
3 TRANSFRONTAL (Naffziger)
4 ETHMOIDAL (Sewall)
5 MAXILLARY (Hirsch)

FIGURE 33.13 **Schematic diagram of approaches for orbital decompression. (Modified from Char DH. Thyroid eye disease, ed. 2. New York: Churchill Livingstone, 1990.)**

TABLE 33.4
**Medical and Surgical Management of Graves'
Ophthalmopathy**

Symptom/Sign	Management
Eye discomfort (e.g., dryness, "gritty sensation") and eyelid retraction	Ocular lubricants Eyelids closed with adhesive tape during sleep Dark spectacle lenses Adrenergic blocking agents (e.g., guanethidine) Eyelid surgery
Periorbital edema, chemosis, injection	Diuretics Sleep with head of bed elevated Corticosteroids Immunosuppressants Radiotherapy I.V. immunoglobulin Plasmapheresis Orbital decompression surgery
Diplopia	Patching or lens occlusion Prism eyeglasses Extraocular muscle surgery
Disfiguring proptosis	Orbital decompression Eyelid surgery
Decreased visual acuity (i.e., optic nerve compression)	Corticosteroids Immunosuppressants Radiotherapy Orbital decompression

Adapted from Garrity JA. Graves' ophthalmopathy: An ophthalmologist's perspective. Thyroid Today 1992; 15 (No. 1): 1–9 and Bahn RS, Garrity JA, Gorman CA. Diagnosis and management of Graves' ophthalmopathy. J. Clin. Endocrinol Metab 1990; 71:559–563.

Orbital decompression allows the volume of the orbit to be expanded by as much as two-fold,[158] often with significant improvement in visual acuity, visual field, disk edema, proptosis, lid closure, and corneal healing.[159] The degree of recession of proptosis can range from 2 to 12 mm.[160]

Although not without serious risks, this procedure, particularly the transantral approach, is remarkably free of significant complications in most patients. However, the major complication of the transantral approach is infraorbital nerve anesthesia, which may last up to 18 months.[160] Other complications have included blindness, accentuation of the appearance of upper lid retraction associated with inferior displacement of the globe, substantial blood loss, nasolacrimal duct obstruction, ascending infection from the sinuses, and meningitis associated with cerebrospinal fluid leakage.[54,159] Chronic sinusitis with polyps is the main contraindication to transantral decompression.[160]

Fortunately, Graves' ophthalmopathy severe enough to warrant high-dosage steroids, orbital radiotherapy, or orbital decompression is estimated to occur in not more than 3% of patients with Graves' disease.[134] In the vast majority of

cases, patients can be managed adequately with more conservative therapeutic measures. Table 33.4 summarizes the current therapeutic approaches to the patient with Graves' ophthalmopathy.

References

1. Medvei VC. A history of endocrinology. Boston: MTP Press Limited, 1982;159:259–266.
2. Graves RJ. Clinical lectures. Lond Med Surg J 1835;7:516.
3. Young LA. Dysthyroid ophthalmopathy: An update. J Natl Med Assoc 1979;71:855–860.
4. Werner SC, Fells P, Day RM, et al. Eye changes. In: Werner SC, Ingbar SH, eds. The thyroid: A fundamental and clinical text. Hagerstown, MD: Harper & Row, 1978;4:655–683.
5. Char DH. The ophthalmopathy of Graves' disease. Med Clin North Am 1991;75:97–119.
6. Gorman CA, Bahn RS, Garrity JA. Ophthalmopathy. In: Braverman LE, Utiger RD, eds. Werner and Ingbar's the thyroid: A fundamental and clinical text, ed. 6. Philadelphia, PA: J.B. Lippincott Co, 1991;657–676.

7. Weetman AP. Update: Thyroid-associated ophthalmopathy. Autoimmunity 1992;12:215–222.

8. Kroll AJ, Kuwabara T. Dysthroid ocular myopathy. Anatomy, histology, and electron microscopy. Arch Ophthalmol 1966;76:244–257.

9. Bahn RS, Heufelder AE. Pathogenesis of Graves' ophthalmopathy. N Engl J Med 1993;329:1468–1474.

10. Cant JS, Wilson TM. The ocular and orbital circulations in dysthyroid ophthalmopathy. Trans Ophthalmol Soc UK 1974;94:416–429.

11. Kidd A, Okita N, Row VV, et al. Immunologic aspects of Graves' and Hashimoto's diseases. Metabolism 1980;29:80–99.

12. DeGroot LJ, Larsen PR, Refetoff S, Stanbury JB, eds. The thyroid and its diseases, ed. 5. New York: John Wiley & Sons, 1984;458–496.

13. Weetman AP, McGregor AM. Autoimmune thyroid disease: Developments in our understanding. Endocr Rev 1984;5:309–355.

14. Walfish PG, Wall JR, Volpe R, eds. Autoiummunity and the thyroid. New York: Academic Press, 1985.

15. Wall JR, Koroki T. Immunologic factors in thyroid disease. In: Kaplan MM, Larsen PR, eds. Symposium on thyroid disease. Philadelphia: W. B. Saunders Co, 1985;59:913–936.

16. Gorman CA. Extrathyroid manifestations of Graves' disease. In: Ingbar SH, Braverman LE, eds. Werner's the thyroid: A fundamental and clinical text, ed. 5. Philadelphia: J. B. Lippincott Co, 1986;1015–1038.

17. Farid NR, Bear JC. The human major histocompatibility complex and endocrine disease. Endocr Rev 1981;2:50–85.

18. Davies F. New thinking on the immunology of Graves' disease. Thyroid Today 1992;15 (No. 4):1–11.

19. Riddick FA Jr. Immunologic aspects of thyroid disease. Ophthalmology 1981;88:471–475.

20. Sergott RC, Felberg NT, Savino PJ, et al. The clinical immunology of Graves ophthalmopathy. Ophthalmology 1981;88:484–487.

21. Rosenbaum D, Davies TF. The clinical use of thyroid autoantibodies. The Endocrinologist 1992;2:55–62.

22. Weightman D, Perros P, Sherif I, et al. Autoantibodies to eye muscle and orbital fibroblasts in the pathogenesis of thyroid associated ophthalmopathy. Exp Clin Endocrinol 1991;97:197–201.

23. Salvi M, Bernard N, Miller A, et al. Prevalence of antibodies reactive with a 64kDa eye muscle membrane antigen in thyroid-associated ophthalmopathy. Thyroid 1991;1:207–213.

24. Heufelder AE, Wenzel BE, Gorman CA, et al. Detection, cellular localization and modulation of heat shock proteins in cultured fibroblasts from patients with extrathyroidal manifestations of Graves' disease. J Clin Endocrinol Metab 1991;73:739–745.

25. Heufelder AE, Gorman CA, Bahn RS. Modulation of HLA-DR expression on retroocular fibroblasts from patients with active thyroid-related ophthalmopathy: In vitro effects of agents used in the management of hyperthyroidism and ophthalmopathy. Exp Clin Endocrinol 1991;97:206–211.

26. Wang PW, Hiromatsu Y, Laryea E, et al. Immunologically mediated cytotoxicity against human eye muscle cells in Graves' ophthalmopathy. J Clin Endocrinol Metab 1986;63:316–322.

27. Lawton NF. Dysthyroid eye disease: Medical investigations. Proc R Soc Med 1977;70:698–700.

28. Jacobson DH, Gorman CA. Diagnosis and management of endocrine ophthalmopathy. In: Kaplan MM, Larsen PR, eds. Symposium on thyroid disease. Philadelphia: W. B. Saunders Co, 1985;69:973–988.

29. Bullock JD, Bartley GB. Dynamic proptosis. Am J Ophthalmol 1986;102:104–110.

30. Hornblass A, Jakobiec FA, Reifler DM, et al. Orbital lymphoid tumors located predominantly within extraocular muscles. Ophthalmology 1987;94:688–697.

31. Garrity JA. Graves' ophthalmopathy: An ophthalmologist's perspective. Thyroid Today 1992;15(No. 1):1–9.

32. Volpe R. Graves' disease. In: Burrow GN, Oppenheimer JH, Volpe R, eds. Thyroid function and disease. Philadelphia, PA: W.B. Saunders Co, 1990;214–260.

33. Gaitan E. Toxic nodular goiter (Plummer's disease) and Graves' disease: Differential diagnosis, clinical features, and treatment. Thyroid Univ Case Reports 1980;2(No. 1):1–3.

34. Surks I, Chopra IJ, Mariash CN, Nicoloff JT, Solomon DH. American Thyroid Association guidelines for use of laboratory tests in thyroid disorders. JAMA 1990;263:1529–1532.

35. Hay ID, Bayer MF, Kaplan MM, Klee GG, Larsen PR, Spencer CA. American Thyroid Association assessment of current free thyroid hormone and thyrotropin measurements guidelines for future clinical assays. Clin Chem 1991;37(11):2002–2008.

36. Becker DV, Bigos ST, Gaitan E, et al. Public Health Committee ATA. Optimal use of blood tests for assessment of thyroid function. JAMA 1993;269:2736–2737.

37. Spencer CA, LoPresti JS, Patel A, Guttler RB, Eigen A, Shen D, Gray D, Nicoloff JT. Applications of a new chemiluminometric thyrotropin assay to subnormal measurement. J Clin Endocrinol Metab 1990;70:453–460.

38. McKenzie JM, Zakarija M. The clinical use of thyrotropin receptor antibody measurements. J Clin Endocrinol Metab 1989;69:1093–1096.

39. Pinchera A, Mariotti S, Vitti P, et al. Thyroid autoantigens and their relevance in the pathogenesis of thyroid autoimmunity. Biochimie 1989;71:237–245.

40. Kasagi K, Hidaka A, Nakamura H, et al. Thyrotropin receptor antibodies in hypothyroid Graves' disease. J Clin Endocrinol Metab 1993;75:504–508.

41. ETA, LATS, Japanese-AOTA, ATA. Classification of eye changes of Graves' disease. Thyroid 1992;2:235–236.

42. Werner SC. Modification of the classification of the eye changes of Graves' disease. Am J Ophthalmol 1977;83:725–727.

43. Van Dyk HJ. Orbital Graves' disease. A modification of the "NO-SPECS" classification. Ophthalmology 1981;88:479–483.

44. Mourits M, Koornneef L, Wiersinga WM, et al. Clinical criteria for the assessment of disease activity in Graves' ophthalmopathy: A novel approach. Br J Ophthalmol 1989;73:639–644.

45. Fells P. Thyroid-associated eye disease: Clinical management. Lancet 1991;338:29–32.

46. ETA, LATS, Japanese-AOTA, ATA. Classification of eye changes of Graves' disease. Thyroid 1992;2:235–236.

47. Uldry PA, Regli F, Scazziga BR, et al. Palpebral asymmetry and hyperthyroidism. Two cases in connection with Graves' disease. J Neurol 1986;233:126–127.

48. Laibovitz RA, Cain R. Lost lid signs in topical neuro-ophthalmic diagnosis. Tex Med 1977;73:68–69.

49. Meltzer MA. Surgery for lid retraction. Ann Ophthalmol 1978;10:102–106.

50. Dixon RS, Anderson RL, Hatt MU. The use of thymoxamine in eyelid retraction. Arch Ophthalmol 1979;97:2147–2150.

51. Gay AJ, Wolkstein MA. Topical guanethidine therapy for endocrine lid retraction. Arch Ophthalmol 1966;76:364–367.

52. Sergott RC, Glaser JS. Graves' ophthalmopathy. A clinical and immunologic review. Surv Ophthalmol 1981;26:1–21.

53. Weetman AP. Thyroid-associated eye disease: Pathophysiology. Lancet 1991;338:25–28.

54. Linberg JV, Anderson RL. Transorbital decompression. Indications and results. Arch Ophthalmol 1981;99:113–119.

55. Frueh BR, Musch DC, Garber FW. Exophthalmometer readings in patients with Graves' eye disease. Ophthalmic Surg 1986;17:37–40.

56. Char D. Advances in thyroid orbitopathy. Neuro-Ophthalmology 1992;25–39.

57. Greenberg DA. Basic evaluation of exophthalmos. J Am Optom Assoc 1977;48:1431–1433.

58. DeJuan E, Hurley DP, Sapira JD. Racial differences in normal values of proptosis. Arch Intern Med 1980;140:1230–1231.

59. Migliori ME, Gladstone GJ. Determination of the normal range of exophthalmometric values for black and white adults. Am J Ophthalmol 1984;98:438–442.

60. Schultz RO, Van Allen MW, Blodi FC. Endocrine ophthalmoplegia: with an electromyographic study of paretic extraocular muscles. Arch Ophthalmol 1960;63:217–225.

61. Shammus HJ, Minekier DS. Ultrasound in early thyroid orbitopathy. Arch Ophthalmol 1980;98:227–231.

62. Smith JL. Recent advances in therapy of thyroid eye disease. In: Smith JL, ed. Neuro-ophthalmology. St. Louis: C. V. Mosby Co, 1972;6:1–10.

63. Metz HS. Saccadic velocity studies in patients with endocrine ocular disease. Am J Ophthalmol 1977;84:695–699.

64. Jensen SF. Endocrine ophthalmoplegia. Is it due to myopathy or to mechanical immobilization? Acta Ophthalmol 1971;49:679–684.

65. Stetz CA, Roman SH, Podos S, et al. Prevalence and clinical associations of intraocular pressure changes in Graves' disease. J Clin Endocrinol Metab 1985;61:183–187.

66. Hallin ES, Felson SE. Graves' Ophthalmopathy II. Correlation of clinical signs with measures derived from computed tomography. Br J Ophthalmol 1988;72:678–682.

67. Char DH. Thyroid eye disease, ed. 2. New York: Churchill Livingstone, 1990;Chap. 4, pp. 35–85.

68. Gasser P, Flammer J. Optic neuropathy of Graves' disease. A report of a perimetric follow-up. Ophthalmologica 1986;192:22–27.

69. Bahn RS, Garrity JA, Gorman CA. Diagnosis and management of Graves' ophthalmopathy. J Clin Endocrinol Metab 1990;71:559–563.

70. Dallow RL. Ultrasonography of the orbit. Int Ophthalmol Clin 1986;26:51–76.

71. Leib MC. Computed tomography of the orbit. Int Ophthalmol Clin 1986;26:103–121.

72. Char DH, Normal D. The use of computed tomography and ultrasonography in the evaluation of orbital masses. Surv Ophthalmol 1982;27:49–63.

73. Holt JE, O'Connor PS, Douglas JP, et al. Extraocular muscle size comparison using standardized A-scan echography and computerized tomography scan measurements. Ophthalmology 1985;92:1351–1355.

74. Trokel SL. Computed tomographic scanning of orbital inflammations. Int Ophthalmol Clin 1982;22:81–98.

75. Gorman CA. Temporal relationship between onset of Graves' ophthalmopathy and diagnosis of thyrotoxicosis. Mayo Clin Proc 1983;58:515–519.

76. Gamblin GT, Harper DG, Galentine P, et al. Prevalence of increased intraocular pressure in Graves' disease—evidence of frequent subclinical ophthalmopathy. N Engl J Med 1983;308:420–424.

77. Ali AS, Akavaram NR. Neuromuscular disorders in thyrotoxicosis. Am Fam Physician 1980;22:97–102.

78. Gorman CA. Management of the patient with Graves' ophthalmopathy. Thyroid Today 1977;1:1–6.

79. Prummel MF, Wiersinga WM. Smoking and risk of Graves' disease. JAMA 1993;269:479.

80. Braverman LE. Thyrotoxicosis. Therapeutic considerations. Clin Endocrinol Metab 1978;7:221–240.

81. McClung MR, Greer MA. Treatment of hyperthyroidism. Ann Rev Med 1980;31:385–404.

82. Wartofsky L, Glinoer D, Solomon B, et al. Differences and similarities in the diagnosis and treatment of Graves' disease in Europe, Japan, and the United States. Thyroid 1991;129–135.

83. Knox DL. Optic nerve manifestations of systemic diseases. Trans Am Acad Ophthalmol Otolaryngol 1977;83:743–750.

84. Gaitan E, Cooper DS. Primary hypothyroidism. In: Bardin CW, ed. Current therapy in endocrinology and metabolism. Toronto, PA: BC Decker, Inc, 1991;75–78.

85. Tallstedt L, Lundell G, Torring O, et al. Occurrence of ophthalmopathy after treatment for Graves' hyperthyroidism. N Engl J Med 1992;326:1733–1738.

86. Riddick FA Jr. Update on thyroid diseases. Ophthalmology 1981;88:467–470.

87. Gilbard JP, Farris RL. Ocular surface drying and tear film osmolarity in thyroid eye disease. Acta Ophthalmol 1983;61:108–116.

88. Gay AJ, Salmon ML, Wolkstein MA. Topical sympatholytic therapy for pathologic lid retraction. Arch Ophthalmol 1967;77:341–344.

89. Sneddon JM, Turner P. Adrenergic blockade and the eye signs of thyrotoxicosis. Lancet 1966;2:525–527.

90. Hodes BL, Schoch DE. Thyroid ocular myopathy. Trans Am Ophthalmol Soc 1979;77:80–103.

91. Crombie AL, Lawson AAH. Long-term trial of local guanethidine in treatment of eye signs of thyroid dysfunction and idiopathic lid retraction. Br Med J 1967;4:592–595.

92. Cartlidge NE, Crombie A, Anderson J, Hall R. Critical study of 5 percent guanethidine in ocular manifestations of Graves' Disease. Br Med J 1969,4:645–647.

93. Kramar P. Management of eye changes of Graves' disease. Surv Ophthalmol 1974;18:369–382.

94. Cant JS, Lewis DRH, Harrison MT. Treatment of dysthyroid ophthalmopathy with local guanethidine. Br J Ophthalmol 1969;53:233–238.

95. Bowden AN, Rose FC. Dysthyroid eye disease. A trial of guanethidine eye drops. Br J Ophthalmol 1969;53:246–251.

96. Frueh BR, Musch DC, Garber FW. Lid retraction and levator aponeurosis defects in Graves' eye disease. Ophthalmic Surg 1986;17:216–220.

97. Garber MI. Methylprednisolone in the treatment of exophthalmos. Lancet 1966;1:958–960.

98. Gebertt S. Depot-methylprednisolone for subconjunctival and retrobulbar injections. Lancet 1961;2:344–345.

99. Brown J, Coburn JW, Wigod RA, Hiss JM Jr, Dowling JT.

Adrenal steroid therapy of severe infiltrative ophthalmopathy of Grave's Disease. Am J Med 1983;34:786–795.

100. Gwinup G, Elias AN, Ascher MS. Effect on exophthalmos of various methods of treatment of Graves' disease. JAMA 1982; 247:2135–2138.

101. Brown J, Coburn JW, Wigod RA, et al. Adrenal steroid therapy of severe infiltrative ophthalmopathy of Graves' disease. Am J Med 1963;34:786–795.

102. Grossman W, Robin NI, Johnson LW, et al. Effects of beta blockade on the peripheral manifestations of thyrotoxicosis. Ann Intern Med 1971;74:875–879.

103. Sisler HA, Jakobiec FA, Trokel SL. Ocular abnormalities and orbital changes of Graves' disease. In: Duane TD, Jaeger EA, eds. Clinical ophthalmology. Philadelphia: Harper & Row, 1987;2: 1–30.

104. Dunn WJ, Arnold AC, O'Connor PS. Botulinum toxin for the treatment of dysthyroid ocular myopathy. Ophthalmology 1986; 93:470–475.

105. Hoffman RO, Helveston EM. Botulinum in the treatment of adult motility disorders. Int Ophthalmol Clin 1986;26:241–250.

106. Fells P, McCarry B. Diplopia in thyroid eye disease. Trans Ophthalmol Soc UK 1986;105:413–423.

107. Frueh BR, Benger RS. Spontaneous reversal of vertical diplopia in Graves' eye disease. Trans Am Ophthalmol Soc 1985;83:387–396.

108. Schimek RA. Surgical management of ocular complications of Graves' disease. Arch Ophthalmol 1972;87:655–664.

109. Miller JE, van Heuven W, Ward R. Surgical correction of hypotropias associated with thyroid dysfunction. Arch Ophthalmol 1965;74:509–515.

110. Buckley EG, Meekins BB. Fadenoperation for the management of complicated incomitant vertical strabismus. Am J Ophthalmol 1988;105:304–312.

111. Long JC. Surgical management of the tropias of thyroid exophthalmos. Arch Ophthalmol 1966;75:634–638.

112. Apers RC, Bierlaagh JJM. Indications and results of eye muscle surgery in thyroid ophthalmopathy. Ophthalmologica 1976;173: 171–179.

113. Dyer JA. Ocular muscle surgery in Graves' disease. Trans Am Ophthalmol Soc 1978;76:125–139.

114. Sachdev Y, Chatterji JC, Sharma RC. Heterogeneity of failure of visual acuity in Graves' disease. Postgrad Med J 1979;55:241–247.

115. Ravin JG, Sisson JC, Knapp WT. Orbital radiation for the ocular changes of Graves' disease. Am J Ophthalmol 1975;79:285–288.

116. Trobe JD. Optic nerve involvement in dysthyroidism. Ophthalmology 1981;88:488–492.

117. Trobe JD, Glaser JS, Laflamme P. Dysthyroid optic neuropathy. Clinical profile and rationale for management. Arch Ophthalmol 1978;96:1199–1209.

118. Prummel MF, Mourits MP, Berghout A, et al. Prednisone and cyclosporine in the treatment of severe Graves' ophthalmopathy. N Engl J Med 1989;321:1353–1359.

119. Perros P, Weightman DR, Crombie AL, Kendall-Taylor P. Azathioprine in the treatment of thyroid associated ophthalmopathy. Acta Endocrinol 1990;122:8–12.

120. Werner SC. Management of the active severe eye changes of Graves' disease. Am Acad Ophthalmol Otolaryngol 1967;71: 631–637.

121. Day RM, Carroll FD. Corticosteroids in the treatment of optic nerve involvement associated with thyroid dysfunction. Trans Am Ophthalmol Soc 1967;65:41–51.

122. Kendall-Taylor P, Crombie AL, Stephson AM, Hardwick M, Hall K. Intravenous methylprednisolone in the treatment of Grave's ophthalmopathy. Br Med J 1988;297:1574–1578.

123. Wiersinga WM. Immunosuppressive treatment of Graves' ophthalmopathy. Thyroid 1992;2:229–233.

124. Saulter-Bihl ML, Heinze HG. Radiotherapy of Graves' ophthalmopathy. In: Pickardt CR, Boergen KP, eds. Graves' ophthalmopathy. Developments in diagnostic methods and therapeutic procedures. Dev Ophthalmol. Basel: Karger 1989;20:139–154.

125. Burman KD. Treatment of autoimmune ophthalmopathy. The Endocrinologist 1991;1:102–110.

126. Bartalena L, Marcocci C, Bogazzi F, et al. Use of corticosteroids to prevent progression of Graves' ophthalmopathy after radioiodine therapy for hyperthyroidism. N Engl J Med 1989;321:1349–1352.

127. Dandona P, Marshall NJ, Bidey SP, et al. Successful treatment of exophthalmos and pretibial myxoedema with plasmapheresis. Br Med J 1979;1:374–376.

128. Dandona P, Marshall NH, Bidey SP, et al. Treatment of acut malignant exophthalmos with plasma exchange. In: Stockigt JR, Nagataki S, eds. Thyroid research VIII. Canberra: Australian Academy of Science, 1980;583–586.

129. Glinoer D, Etienne-Decerf J, Schrooyen M et al. Beneficial effects of intensive plasma exchange followed by immunosuppressive therapy in severe Graves' ophthalmopathy. Acta Endocrinol 1986; 111:30.

130. McConahey WM. Ophthalmopathy. In: Van Middlesworth L, ed. The thyroid gland: A practical clinical treatise. Chicago: Year Book Medical Publishers, 1986:315–331.

131. Zeser W, Shubai J, Zutong Z. The effect of acupuncture in 40 cases of endocrine ophthalmology. J Trad Chinese Med 1985;5: 19–21.

132. UCLA Conference. Autoimmune thyroid diseases—Graves' and Hashimoto's. Ann Intern Med 1978;88:379–391.

133. McKenzie JM, Zakarija M, Sato A. Humoral immunity in Graves' disease. Clin Endocrinol Metab 1978;7:31–45.

134. Bigos ST, Nisula BC, Daniels GH, et al. Cyclophosphamide in the management of advanced Graves' ophthalmopathy. A preliminary report. Ann Intern Med 1979;90:921–923.

135. Burrow GN, Mitchell MS, Howard RO, et al. Immunosuppressive therapy for the eye changes of Graves' disease. J Clin Endocrinol Metab 1970;31:307–311.

136. Utech C, Wulle KG, Pfannenstiel P, Adaw W. Ciamexone—treatment in endocrine ophthalmopathy. Acta Endocrinol 1987; 281:342–343.

137. Weetman AP, Ludgate M, Mills PV, et al. Cyclosporin improves Graves' ophthalmopathy. Lancet 1983;2:486–489.

138. Howlett TA, Lawton NF, Fells P, et al. Deterioration of severe Graves' ophthalmopathy during cyclosporin treatment. Lancet 1984;2:1101.

139. Brabant G, Pater H, Becker H, et al. Cyclosporin infiltrative eye disease. Lancet 1984;1:515–516.

140. Utech C, Wulle KG, Bieler EU, et al. Treatment of severe Graves' ophthalmopathy with cyclosporin A. Acta Endocrinol 1985;110: 493–498.

141. Lopatynsky MO, Krohel GB. Bromocriptine therapy for thyroid ophthalmopathy. Am J Ophthalmol 1989;107:680–681.

142. Donaldson SS, Bagshaw MA, Kriss JP. Supervoltage orbital ra-

diotherapy for Graves' ophthalmopathy. J Clin Endocrinol Metab 1973;37:276–285.

143. Petersen IA, Kriss JP, McDougall IR, Donaldson SS. Prognostic factors in the radiotherapy of Grave's ophthalmopathy. Int J Radiation Oncol Biol Phys 1990;19:256–264.

144. Leone CR. The management of ophthalmic Graves' disease. Ophthalmology 1984;91:770–779.

145. Glaser JS. Graves' ophthalmopathy. Arch Ophthalmol 1984;102:1448–1449.

146. Olivotto IA, Ludgate CM, Allen LH, et al. Supervoltage radiotherapy for Graves' ophthalmopathy: CCABC technique and results. Int J Radiat Oncol Biol Phys 1985;11:2085–2090.

147. Pinchera A, Bartalena L, Chiovato L, et al. Radiotherapy of Graves' ophthalmopathy. In: Gorman CA, Waller RR, Dyer JA, eds. The eye and orbit in thyroid disease. New York: Raven Press, 1984;301–316.

148. Hurbli T, Char DH, Harris J, et al. Radiation therapy for thyroid eye disease. Am J Ophthalmol 1985;99:633–637.

150. Brennan MW, Leone CR, Janaki L. Radiation therapy for Graves' disease. Am J Ophthalmol 1983;96:633–637.

151. van Ouwerkerk BM, Wijingaarde R, Hennemann G, et al. Radiotherapy of severe ophthalmic Graves' disease. J Endocrinol Invest 1985;8:241–247.

152. Dollinger J. Die druchenllastung der augenhohle durch entfernung der ausseren orbitalwand bei hochgradigen exophthalmus und konsekotiver hornhauterkrantung. Dtsch Med Wochenschr 1911; 37:1888–1890.

153. Shorr N, Seiff SR. The four stages of surgical rehabilitation of the patient with dysthyroid ophthalmopathy. Ophthalmology 1986; 93:476–483.

154. Riley FC. Surgical management of ophthalmopathy in Graves' disease: Transfrontal orbital decompression. Mayo Clin Proc 1972;47:986–988.

155. Wirtschafter JD, Chu AE. Lateral orbitotomy without removal of the lateral orbital rim. Arch Ophthalmol 1988;106:1463–1468.

156. Antoszyk JH, Tucker N, Codere F. Orbital decompression for Graves' disease: Exposure through a modified blepharoplasty incision. Ophthalmic Surg 1992;23(8):516–521.

157. Ogura JH, Pratt LL. Transantral decompression for malignant exophthalmos. Otolaryngol Clin North Am 1971;4:193–203.

158. Anderson RL, Linberg JV. Transorbital approach to decompression in Graves' disease. Arch Ophthalmol 1981;99:120–124.

159. Ogura JH. Surgical results of orbital decompression for malignant exophthalmos. J Laryngol Otol 1978;92:181–195.

160. Fells P. Surgical management of dysthyroid eye disease: A review. Proc R Soc Med 1977;70:698–699.

161. Lopatynsky MO, Krokel GB. Bromocriptine therapy for thyroid ophthalmopathy. Am J Ophthalmol 1989;107:680.

162. Fledelius HC, Nielson H. Graves' orbitopathy clinical features and imaging results, by ultrasound and CT-scan. Orbit 1990; 9(4):235–240.

163. Sridama V, DeGroot LJ. Treatment of Graves' disease and the course of ophthalmopathy. Am J Med 1989;87:70–73.

164. Parker RG, Withers HR. Radiation Retinopathy. JAMA 1988;259: 43.

165. Miyakawa M, Tsushima T, Onoda N, Etoh M, Isozaki O, Arai M, Shizume K, Demura H. Thyroid ultrasonography related to clinical and laboratory findings in patients with silent thyroiditis. J Endocrinol Invest 1992;15(4):289–295.

166. Byrne SF, Gendron EK, Glaser JS, Fever W, Atta H. Diameter of normal extraocular recti muscles with echography. Am J Ophthalmol 1991;112:706–713.

167. Wilson WB, Manke WF. Orbital decompression in Graves' disease. Arch Ophthalmol 1991;109:343–345.

168. Guistina A, Buffoli MG, Bussi AR, Wehrenberg WB. Acute effects of clonidine and growth-hormone-releasing hormone on growth hormone secretion in patients with hyperthyroidism. Hormone Research 1991;36:192–195.

169. McCord CD. Current trends in orbital decompression. Ophthalmology 1985;92:21–33.

170. Taylor W. Transantral orbital decompression in dysthyroid eye disease. Trans Ophthalmol Soc NZ 1974;26:51–53.

171. Desanto LW. Surgical palliation of ophthalmopathy of Graves' disease: Transantral approach. Mayo Clin Proc 1972;47:989–992.

172. Hamed LM, Lessner AM. Fixation duress in the pathogenesis of upper eyelid retraction in thyroid orbitopathy. A prospective study. Ophthalmology 1994;101:1608–1613.

173. Ohnishi T, Noguchi S, Murakami N, et al. Extraocular muscles in Graves ophthalmopathy. Usefulness of T_2 relaxation time measurements. Radiology 1994;190:857–860.

174. Ebner R. Botulinum toxin type A in upper lid retraction of Graves' ophthalmopathy. J Clin Neuro-ophthalmol 1993;13:258–261.

175. Biglan AW. Control of eyelid retraction associated with Graves' disease with botulinum A toxin. Ophthalmic Surg 1994;25:186–188.

176. Prummel MF, Mourits MP, Blank L, et al. Randomized double-blind trial of prednisone versus radiotherapy in Graves' ophthalmopathy. Lancet 1993;342:949–950.

177. Weisman RA, Osguthorpe JD. Orbital decompression in Graves' disease. Arch Otolaryngol Head Neck Surg 1994;120:831–834.

178. Fatourechi V, Garrity JA, Bartley GB, et al. Graves' ophthalmopathy. Results of transantral orbital decompression performed primarily for cosmetic indications. Ophthalmology 1994;101:938–942.

CHAPTER 34

Pharmacologic Management of Strabismus

Paul L. Owens
David M. Amos

Management of strabismus includes amblyopia therapy, spectacle lenses, prisms, orthoptics, and eye muscle surgery. The goal is to produce equal vision, cosmetically straightened eyes, and functional binocularity, when possible. Pharmacologic agents have been used to aid in obtaining these goals. This chapter considers the clinical uses of anticholinesterase miotics for treatment of accommodative esotropia, and the use of botulinum toxin A (Botox) as an alternative and adjunct to conventional strabismus surgery.

Accommodative Esotropia

Etiology

Esodeviations are caused by innervational or mechanical factors, or a combination of both.[1] Accommodative esotropia is a convergent concomitant strabismus associated with increased convergence innervation, usually accommodative in origin, often occurring in hyperopes.[2] If the fusional divergence amplitude is sufficient to allow fusion, it is termed *accommodative esophoria*; however, if fusion is not maintained, it is termed *accommodative esotropia*. Accommodative esotropia has an acquired onset from as early as 3 or 4 months to as late as up to 7 years, averaging 2.5 years of age.[3] Accommodative esotropia is heritable, with siblings, parents, or relatives exhibiting the same disorder.[4] The esodeviation usually is intermittent at onset, becoming con-

stant when left untreated. For this reason, accommodative esotropia demands early and aggressive treatment to prevent suppression, amblyopia, and loss of binocularity.

Accommodative esodeviations have been classified into four basic types: (1) refractive accommodative esotropia (fully accommodative or high hyperopia) with the distance deviation equal to the near deviation—the AC/A ratio is normal; (2) nonrefractive accommodative esotropia (greater esodeviation at near fixation than at distance fixation—the AC/A ratio is high; (3) mixed mechanism esotropia—partially accommodative; and (4) decompensated accommodative esotropia, which is unresponsive to nonsurgical modalities of treatment.

Diagnosis

A cycloplegic refraction or retinoscopy should be performed on all children with suspected accommodative esotropia. It is essential to uncover the full hyperopic correction. Atropine usually is the drug of choice for retinoscopy of children up to age 4 years with suspected accommodative esotropia.[5-8] One preparation of choice is 1% atropine sulfate ophthalmic ointment. It can be administered once daily at bedtime, 3 nights before the refraction. The ointment is less irritating than atropine solution, is easier to instill, and there is much less risk of toxic reactions. In contrast, atropine solution passes much more rapidly into the systemic circulation by way of the nasolacrimal duct.

Children at least 5 years of age can receive an adequate cycloplegic refraction utilizing 1% or 2% cyclopentolate, which can be preceded by one drop of 0.5% proparacaine HCl to decrease the burning sensation and to increase absorption of the cycloplegic. The refraction should then be performed approximately 30 minutes later, provided the pupils are fully dilated and unresponsive to light.

It should be emphasized that both atropine and cyclopentolate can cause ocular and systemic reactions including contact blepharodermatitis,[9,10] angle-closure glaucoma,[11] hallucinations,[12] and severe anticholinergic effects[13] (see Chap. 9).

The degree of refractive error can be a distinguishing factor between types of accommodative esotropia. Refractive accommodative esotropia (normal AC/A) is characterized by high hyperopia in the range of +3.00 to +10.00, D with an average of +4.00 D. The esodeviation is the same at distance and near, with or without spectacles. Nonrefractive accommodative esotropia (high AC/A) is associated with a refractive error that is normal for the age, averaging +2.00 D, but may range from myopic to a high hyperopic correction. There is little or no deviation at distance fixation, but a moderate esotropia at near fixation of 20 to 30 prism diopters. In both refractive and nonrefractive accommodative esotropia, the angle may be variable, depending on the amount of accommodative effort expressed and the patient's attentiveness to the fixational target.

The clinical investigation of accommodative esotropia is not complete without an estimate of the AC/A ratio. Most clinicians employ the gradient method of measurement. The gradient method arrives at the AC/A ratio by measuring the change in near deviation in prism diopters divided by the change in lens power. To determine the AC/A ratio, the patient should wear the full cycloplegic refraction, or as much plus as the patient will accept for best distance vision. With this distance correction in place, the near deviation is measured at 13 inches (33 cm), first without, then with the addition of a +3.00 or -3.00 lens. Fixation is controlled with an accommodative target. The AC/A ratio is the change in the near deviation divided by 3.00. The normal AC/A ratio is between 3 and 5. Values above 5 denote a high or excessive accommodative convergence, and values under 3 a low or insufficient accommodative convergence.[14]

Divergent fusional reserve should also be estimated by

placing in the trial frame the least amount of hyperopic correction that permits fusion, and then performing the cover tests with increases in base-in prism. The divergent fusional amplitude range is usually between 12 and 20 prism diopters. Patients with intermittent esotropia usually have a much higher amount of divergent fusional reserve than will patients who develop constant esotropia.

Management

Accommodative esotropia should be diagnosed and treated as early as possible to avoid a permanent strabismus and other complications of delayed treatment. Complications of long-standing esodeviations such as amblyopia, eccentric fixation, suppression, and anomalous retinal correspondence greatly influence the choice of treatment and invariably require a more sophisticated treatment plan. Three possible methods of therapy can be used, either singularly or in combination, to produce alignment: (1) spectacles for hyperopia, (2) anticholinesterase miotics, and (3) vision therapy-orthoptics. All these methods may be used to relieve the accommodative stress. Spectacle therapy and vision therapy-orthoptics are not discussed in detail in this chapter.

SPECTACLE THERAPY

Spectacles provide the most conservative yet the most effective method of treatment for most patients with accommodative esotropia[15] (Table 34.1). Parks[4] recommends that the full correction determined by the cycloplegic refraction be prescribed for children under 4 years of age. If the full plus correction is not accepted by the patient, 1% atropine can be prescribed for a brief period to assist with the plus lens acceptance. The cycloplegic refraction should be repeated several times during the first year of treatment, since it is not uncommon to reveal even more hyperopia, especially in patients under 4 years of age.[6]

After the young patient with esotropia and hyperopia has worn the full plus correction for several weeks or months, reexamination will probably reveal one of the following conditions: (1) orthophoria with near and distance fixation, (2) reduced amount of esotropia with near and distance fixation, or (3) orthophoria with distance fixation but a significant esodeviation with near fixation. This near esodeviation is thought to be caused by a high AC/A ratio.[16] To alleviate the near esodeviation, a plus lens addition over the full distance hyperopic correction has proved quite successful. This bifocal addition is determined by adding +0.50 to +1.00 D increments to the patient's spectacles until the least power is found that reduces the angle of strabismus sufficiently to permit stable fixation and fusion. The bifocal addition is usually between +1.00 D and +3.50 D. A flat top, executive style bifocal bisecting the pupils with the eyes in primary position may be prescribed. However, some investi-

TABLE 34.1
Advantages of Glasses over Miotics

- No side effects
- Probably more effective for more patients
- Bifocals very effective for patients with high AC/A ratios
- More cosmetically acceptable to children now compared with years ago

gators[17,18] have shown that progressive-addition lenses are also effective in the management of accommodative esotropia.

MIOTIC THERAPY

Since some children will not wear or tolerate spectacles or bifocals for a variety of reasons, anticholinesterase miotics have been used therapeutically as a "substitute" for spectacles.

History.   Miotics have been used in the treatment of convergent strabismus for over 100 years. In 1896, Javal[19] specifically mentioned the use of pilocarpine and physostigmine as substitutes for spectacles in several cases of convergent strabismus. In 1949, Abraham[20,21] first reported the effective use of isoflurophate in accommodative esotropia. It offered a great advantage over pilocarpine or physostigmine because of its effectiveness when used only once a day, or less. In 1960, Miller[22] reported a similar effectiveness with the use of echothiophate iodide. Since then, many studies have been published concerning the effectiveness and safety of anticholinesterase miotics in the treatment of accommodative esotropia.

Pharmacology.   The contraction of the ciliary muscle for accommodation is effected through the parasympathetic outflow of the third cranial nerve. The efferent arc consists of the preganglionic fiber from the central nervous system (CNS) to the ciliary ganglion, and the postganglionic fiber from the ciliary ganglion to the effector cells in the ciliary muscle. Transmission of the nerve impulse is mediated by acetylcholine (ACh). Acetylcholine is hydrolyzed to choline and acetic acid by acetylcholinesterase. It is possible to simulate this cholinergic effect by using agents that mimic the actions of ACh, or by allowing ACh to accumulate on the effector cells. The latter action is accomplished by using anticholinesterase drugs to prevent Ach inactivation by acetylcholinesterase.[23]

The classic theory that is held to explain their success is that these anticholinesterase drugs increase the accommodative output (ciliary muscle contraction) without increasing the usually associated neuronal input into the ciliary muscle. As a result, there is no increase in convergence associated with the drug-induced ciliary muscle contraction. This theory explains to some extent why these drugs often reduce the AC/A ratio (Fig. 34.1 and 34.2). There are also indications of a more direct effect of cholinesterase inhibitors on the extraocular muscles. Bunke and Bito[24] demonstrated that with prolonged use of cholinesterase inhibitors in rabbit eyes, the extraocular muscles develop a hypersensitivity to the drugs, which causes direct stimulation of the muscle. This stimulation is relatively increased when the concentration of ACh surrounding the muscle is low. When the level of ACh is high, this stimulation becomes irrelevant, since there is increased stimulation at the

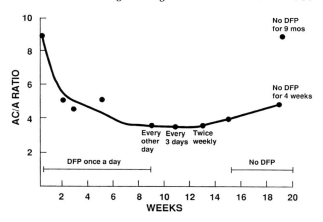

FIGURE 34.1   **Decrease in AC/A ratio during isoflurophate therapy and subsequent return to previous values. (Modified from Sloan LL, Sears ML, Jablonski MD. Convergence-accommodation relationships. Description of a simple clinical test and its application to the evaluation of isoflurophate (DFP) therapy. Arch Ophthalmol 1960; 63:283–306. Copyright 1960, American Medical Association)**

respective neuromuscular junction due to the presence of ACh. These factors help to explain why such drugs have more of a stimulative effect on the lateral rectus muscles, which are normally less active in accommodative esotropia than are the medial rectus muscles.

The anticholinesterase miotics most commonly used in the treatment of accommodative esotropia, isoflurophate and echothiophate, "irreversibly" inactivate cholinesterase, so that more enzyme must be regenerated. Thus, their effects last several days.

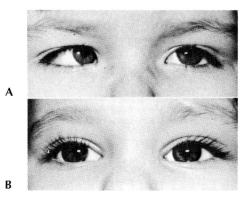

FIGURE 34.2   **Effect of miotic therapy on accommodative esotropia. (A) Before therapy. (B) During anticholinesterase therapy. (From von Noorden GK. Atlas of strabismus, ed. 4. St. Louis: C.V. Mosby Co, 1983, with permission of the author and publisher.)**

Indications.   As previously noted, anticholinesterase miotics can be useful in children with accommodative esotropia who will not wear glasses for a variety of reasons. These include the usual childhood problems with broken or poorly adjusted frames, undesirable cosmesis, peer pressure, and insignificant improvement in visual acuity. Other possible advantages of miotics are[25]: (1) to ensure a continuous therapeutic effect throughout the day; (2) to correct or diminish a near esotropia; (3) to replace glasses or bifocals, especially in accommodative esotropic patients with high AC/A ratios; and (4) to help wean older children (8 years and older) from their hyperopic glasses. Miotics do not seem to be effective when used in conjunction with glasses, since the patient tends to peer over the lenses.[4]

There has been considerable debate regarding the true effectiveness of miotics as a permanent replacement for spectacles in hyperopic patients with accommodative esotropia. Hill and Stromberg[26] reported that echothiophate may be an effective substitute for bifocals, especially in patients with high AC/A ratios. Wheeler and Moore[27] reported approximately the same findings with isoflurophate. Bedrossian and Krewson[28] found that glasses and miotics are equally effective in 42% of cases and that glasses were more effective in 48%. Hiatt and associates[29] found an equal reduction in esodeviation in 48% of cases treated with echothiophate for 2 months compared with treatment using full hyperopic correction. However, 48% had a larger reduction in the esodeviation with glasses than with echothiophate, while the miotic was more effective in only 4% of patients.

Goldstein[25] suggested the following guidelines for the use of miotics.

- Miotics should never be used unless some degree of binocularity can be achieved.
- Miotics tend to be less effective in the presence of amblyopia.
- Miotics are more useful in patients with high AC/A ratios.
- Miotics are more effective in reducing the near as compared to the distance deviation.

No studies have shown anticholinesterase miotics to be significantly *more* effective than glasses or bifocals in the treatment of accommodative esotropia.[30]

Dosage.   Since isoflurophate hydrolyzes in the presence of water, it has been dispensed in USP anhydrous peanut oil or as an ophthalmic ointment. Currently it is commercially available only as an ointment in 0.025% concentration (Table 34.2).[31] It should be instilled at bedtime to minimize blurring of vision.

In addition to its therapeutic use, isoflurophate may be employed as a diagnostic aid to determine if an accommodative component exists in very young children and in patients with relatively low hyperopic refractive errors. The ointment should be instilled nightly at bedtime for 2 weeks. An accommodative component is revealed if the esodeviation is reduced. This procedure is useful in supplementing standard evaluation techniques.

Echothiophate iodide is available in 0.03, 0.06, 0.125, and 0.25% solutions. The usual concentration for use in strabismus is 0.125%.[32] Echothiophate is relatively stable in water, but refrigeration improves its stability. Instillation is once a day, preferably at bedtime. A 0.06% solution is sometimes used in older children in an effort to remove the glasses by expanding the fusional divergence amplitude through increased accommodation.

As with isoflurophate, echothiopate may be used diagnostically to confirm the presence of an accommodative component. The 0.125% solution should be instilled at bedtime for 2 to 3 weeks. If the esotropia is accommodative, a reduction of the deviation will be revealed.

Side Effects.   The most significant ocular side effects of the anticholinesterase miotics are the formation of iris cysts (see Fig. 10.9) and the development of anterior subcapsular lens opacities (see Fig. 10.8). Other ocular complications include retinal detachment,[33] angle closure glaucoma,[34] iritis,[35] superficial punctate keratitis,[22] follicular conjunctivitis,[36] brow-ache, blurred distance vision, lid swelling, and fasciculation of eyelid muscles.[26]

TABLE 34.2
Anticholinesterase Miotics Used for Accommodative Esotropia

Generic Name	Trade Name	Dosage Form	Recommended Dosage
Diisopropylfluorophosphate (DFP, isoflurophate)	Floropryl	0.025% ointment	Instill at bedtime
Echothiophate iodide	Phospholine Iodide	0.03%–0.25% solution	Instill 0.125% solution at bedtime

The major systemic side effect of echothiophate is substantial reduction of plasma and erythrocyte cholinesterase, which can result in marked cholinergic overactivity.[37–47] Isoflurophate seems to depress cholinesterase levels less than does echothiophate, possibly due to rapid hydrolysis by plasma esterases. Serious systemic toxicity is rare in children using anticholinesterase miotics for strabismus.[47] Nausea, abdominal discomfort, and diarrhea are the most frequently reported symptoms, but these problems are usually mild and of no serious consequence. It should be noted, however, that children on long-term use of potent anticholinesterase drugs, such as echotiophate, may be at significant risk should they require emergency general anesthesia. Plasma and erythrocyte cholinesterase is needed for the hydrolysis of succinylcholine, a drug frequently used by anesthesiologists to facilitate intubation, and patients using anticholinesterase miotics may develop prolonged respiratory paralysis. For this reason, many clinicians use miotics only for short periods–for example, to replace glasses not being worn during summer months, when children engage in activities such as swimming. If serious systemic toxicity is noted, atropine and pralidoxime chloride (Protopam) are effective antidotes.

Use of Botulinum Toxin

Amblyopia therapy, spectacle lenses, prisms, and orthoptics are used in an effort to align strabismic eyes and achieve binocularity. When these modalities fail, eye muscle surgery is performed to correct the remaining strabismic angle or nonaccommodative component. Historically, the most common strabismic surgical procedures have been an extraocular muscle weakening (recession) and/or an extraocular muscle shortening (resection) or advancement. Of the two, weakening of the overacting extraocular muscle is the most effective.[48] However, its direct antagonist must be capable of contracting enough to change the position of the globe as a result of the weakening (recession) procedure. Until recently, this weakening procedure was performed intraoperatively with various surgical instruments. In 1973, Scott and associates[49] reported on several toxins which, when injected, would cause weakening of an overacting extraocular muscle without the use of the traditional incisional surgical recession. Agents evaluated in animal models included alcohol, cobra neurotoxin, botulinum neurotoxin type A, and diisopropylfluorophosphate (DFP). Scott found botulinum toxin (type A) in low doses to be most effective, without serious side effects.[49] Beginning in 1977, chemodenervational treatment of strabismus with botulinum toxin A was tried in human subjects under the auspices of the Food and Drug Administration (FDA).[50,51] The first clinical trials were limited to attempted correction of horizontal strabismic devi-

ations and the treatment of blepharospasm. Following successful clinical trials by over 290 investigators and 17,000 botulinum toxin A injections in over 8,000 patients, the FDA in 1989 approved the use of purified botulinum toxin A for the treatment of adult strabismus and blepharospasm. Allergan Pharmaceuticals currently distributes the drug under the name of Botox (formerly Oculinum).

Pharmacology

Botox, a highly purified, stable and crystalline form of botulinum toxin A, is manufactured easily in deep culture.[52,53] It is a derivative of one of eight exotoxins produced by *Clostridium botulinum.* The crystalline form of botulinum toxin A is a high-molecular-weight protein (900,000 daltons) consisting of two subunits that dissociate in solution. Each subunit can be broken down further into three peptide chains (one peptide chain is toxic and the other two are nontoxic peptides). One of the two nontoxic chains has hemagglutinating activity.[54]

When injected into muscle tissue, the neurotoxin acts at the level of the neuromuscular junction.[51,55] Botulinum A binds rapidly and firmly to receptor sites on the cholinergic nerve terminal and enters the intracellular compartment by way of a synaptic vesicle process.[51] At this point, the toxin prevents calcium exostosis and specifically blocks quantal ACh release.[56] Since the nerve terminals are not destroyed[57,58] and entry of calcium into the nerve terminal is not blocked,[59] paralysis is transient, with recovery of neuromuscular function usually complete within 6 to 9 months.[49,60] Scott,[61] however, states that upon recovery, the injected muscle may or may not resume its preinjection level of function.

The paralytic effect and duration of Botox is dose-related, with maximum effect occurring in 5 to 7 days.[53,62] This response is based on a satisfactory injection technique. Multiple injections have been given over time to the same patient without the toxin being recognized by the immune system.[63] An antitoxin is available, however, and can be used to counteract inadvertent overdoses, which are rare, as well as prevent spread of the toxin into adjacent muscles.[53,64] When injecting extraocular muscles and orbicularis muscles, the adjacent levator is most sensitive to diffusion and development of undesired, but transient, ptosis.

The amount of toxin injected for the treatment of strabismus, essential blepharospasm, and other human disorders is minute and not associated with any severe generalized toxicity.[52] Botox is supplied in vials containing 100 units of frozen, lyophilized toxin, which remains stable for up to 4 years. Each unit contains 0.25 nanograms, which is the lethal dose of 50% (LD_{50}) of mice.[64–66] Helveston[48] calculates that the human LD_{50} is approximately the full contents of 20 vials, making the drug safer than aspirin.

The freeze-dried Botox must be gently reconstituted without shaking, using nonpreserved saline. It must be used within 4 hours. In an adult, the initial dose for an extraocular muscle injection is usually 2.5 units (see Table 23.13). Subsequent doses may be increased until the desired effect is obtained.

Clinical Uses

The potential clinical uses for botulinum toxin A have expanded greatly since 1977 (Table 34.3).[51] In the management of strabismus, Botox injections have proven effective as an alternative to traditional (incisional) surgery. The toxin is injected into an extraocular muscle under topical anesthesia with the assistance of EMG equipment.[62] Botox injections work best in cases of: (1) acute third- and sixth-nerve paresis[67–69]; (2) other small to moderate angles of strabismus, especially in the presence of fusion[62]; (3) in some acute cases of thyroid myopathy; and (4) cases of complete sixth-nerve palsy, where total transposition of the superior rectus and inferior rectus to the insertion of the lateral rectus is accompanied by a Botox injection into the ipsilateral medial rectus. This technique reduces the risk of anterior segment ischemia.[70,71]

Botox injections are not effective as an alternative to conventional (incisional) surgery in treating large angles of strabismus or longstanding restrictive strabismus. In cases in which the patient has had a prior large eye muscle recession, injection is difficult using topical anesthesia and EMG equipment.[72,73] Owens[74,75] reported how these and other conditions might be aided by the use of botulinum toxin A as an adjunct to conventional (incisional) surgery. Botox is used at the time of traditional (incisional) surgery, under general

TABLE 34.3
Clinical Uses of Botox

1. Strabismus
   Horizontal nonparalytic, nonrestrictive strabismus less than 40 prism diopters
   Surgical undercorrection and overcorrection
   Sensory deviation
   Preoperative evaluation for intractable diplopia
   Vertical, nonparalytic, nonrestrictive strabismus
   Acute or chronic third- and sixth-nerve palsies
   Thyroid ophthalmopathy in the acute phase
   Strabismus after retinal detachment surgery
   Surgery contraindicated or refused
2. Acquired nystagmus
3. Essential blepharospasm
4. Hemifacial spasm
5. Aberrant regeneration of seventh nerve
6. Myokymia
7. Corneal exposure

anesthesia, with direct visualization of the injected muscle. No EMG equipment is needed. This approach has been successful in correcting a very large strabismic angle (100 prism diopters) in deeply amblyopic or blind eyes. In such cases, surgery had to be limited to the amblyopic or blind eye. Prior to the availability of Botox, a large 10mm lateral rectus recession and 10mm medial resection was performed. Postoperatively, a high percentage of undercorrections occurred in these eyes. Botox can now be used intraoperatively under direct visualization to enhance the effect of the 10mm lateral rectus recession.

At the time of surgery, the muscle to be recessed (weakened) is operated upon first. Prior to recessing the muscle, 5 to 10 units of purified botulinum toxin A in 0.1cc saline solution is injected through a 30-gauge hypodermic-infusion set needle directly into the rectus muscle. The injection is given slowly under direct visualization, approximately 10mm from the muscle insertion, while an assistant holds the muscle up and away from the globe with a muscle hook. The muscle body should be observed to swell. Upon completion of the injection, the area surrounding the muscle is blotted dry with a cotton-tipped applicator to limit unwanted diffusion of Botox. The muscle is then recessed and the ipsilateral direct antagonist is resected. With good technique, a significant esotropia should develop within 24 to 48 hours. This transient esotropia can last 8 to 12 weeks. During this period of transient paralysis, it is proposed that Botox induces additional lengthening of the lateral recti muscle fibers, resulting in a greater weakening of the recessed lateral rectus. While the lateral rectus is paretic, the resected medial rectus strongly contracts. This enhanced contracture acting in the presence of surgical inflammation and scars of healing results in a stronger resection than one might obtain without the use of Botox. Upon return of lateral rectus function, there is a significant reduction in the large preoperative strabismic angle (Fig. 34.3).

Another innovative use of Botox has been in the treatment of acquired neurologic nystagmus. Helveston[48] has injected 25 units of Botox into the retrobulbar space of several patients whose visual acuities were reduced to 20/100 or less, due to nystagmus from brainstem lesions. Following Botox retrobulbar injections, vision improved to as much as 20/30 in some patients. The effect from Botox lasted up to 3 months.

Patient Selection

Variation exists in the criteria used by strabismologists in choosing the patient population best suited for this alternative therapy. Some investigators believe the procedure has merit in children. Magoon and Scott[76] published the results of a series of 82 children, aged 13 years or younger, treated for horizontal strabismus by toxin injection. Improvement was achieved in 81 of the children, although reinjection was

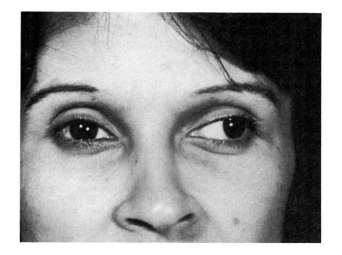

A

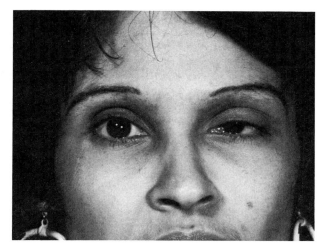

B

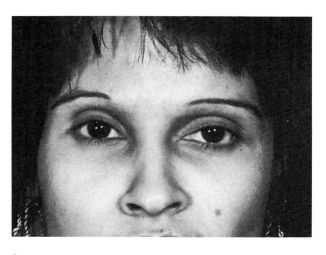

C

FIGURE 34.3   **Reduction of large angle left exotropia in a blind eye using combination of surgery and botulinum toxin injection.** *(A)* **Preoperative left exotropia measured 100Δ by Krimsky with 15Δ left hypotropia. At surgery the left lateral rectus was injected with 10 units of botulinum toxin, followed by 10mm recession of the left lateral rectus and 10mm resection of the medial rectus.** *(B)* **One week postoperatively, deviation in primary gaze was 30Δ left esotropia with no lateral rectus function. Note left ptosis.** *(C)* **Twelve weeks postoperatively, deviation was 3Δ left exotropia with 10Δ left hypotropia. Ptosis has resolved.**

necessary in 85% of the patients. The advantage of using a local anesthetic is lost in children, since in much of this population general anesthesia is required. Low dose ketamine anesthesia has typically been used in this age group.[77] However, the procedure can be carried out successfully in children younger than 1 year and older than 6 years of age using only topical drop anesthesia and no sedation.[76]

Most investigators, however, reserve the therapy primarily for teenage and adult patients, often those who have undergone prior surgical attempts at correction.[65] Some clinicians actually restrict botulinum toxin A injection to patients who represent a poor surgical risk for general anesthesia.

Complications

Pain, subconjunctival hemorrhage, expanded paralysis within the orbit, induced diplopia, and a prolonged period of ptosis have been reported.[65,77] Ptosis is a relatively common, but temporary, complication, occurring to some extent in up to 53% of cases[78] and to a significant degree in 17% to 21% of cases.[78,79] The ptosis generally resolves within 8 weeks (see Fig. 34.3). Diplopia is brought on when the altered, usually overcorrected gaze takes the treated eye into an area where suppression does not occur.[65] This temporary complication can be managed with a patch or prism.[79] In about 10% of cases, adjacent muscles will be affected by the toxin injection, with the levator being the most susceptible.[78] In some instances where the paralytic effect has expanded outside the injected muscle, surgical correction has been necessary.[79] The most serious complication associated with botulinum injection is inadvertent perforation of the globe. Five cases have been reported, with one patient suffering vitreous hemorrhage and subsequent decreased vision. Other rarely reported complications include retrobulbar hemorrhage, pupillary dilation, spatial disorientation, and rash.[65]

References

1. Von Noorden GK. Binocular vision and ocular motility, ed. 4. St. Louis: C.V. Mosby Co, 1990;285.

2. Duke-Elder S, Wybar K, eds. System of ophthalmology. St. Louis: C.V. Mosby Co, 1973;6:590–616.

3. Baker JD, Parks MM. Early onset accommodative esotropia. Am J Ophthalmol 1980;90:11–18.

4. Parks MM, Wheeler MB. Concomitant esodeviations. In: Tasman W, Jaeger EA, eds. Duane's Clinical ophthalmology. Philadelphia: J B Lippincott Co, 1992;Vol. 1, Chap. 12:1–14.

5. Chang FW. The pharmacology of cycloplegics. Am J Optom Physiol Opt 1978;55:219–222.

6. Amos DM. Cycloplegics for refraction. Am J Optom Physiol Opt 1978;55:223–226.

7. Bartlett JD. Administration of and adverse reactions to cycloplegic agents. Am J Optom Physiol Opt 1978;55:227–228.

8. Rosenbaum AL, Bateman JB, Bremer DL, et al. Cycloplegic refraction in esotropic children. Cyclopentolate versus atropine. Ophthalmology 1981;88:1031–1033.

9. Havener WH. Ocular pharmacology, ed. 5. St. Louis: C.V. Mosby Co, 1983;379–398.

10. Michaels DD. Visual optics and refraction: A clinical approach. St. Louis: C.V. Mosby Co, 1975:186–195.

11. Abraham SV. Mydriatic glaucoma—a statistical study. Arch Ophthalmol 1933;10:757–762.

12. Adcock EW. Cyclopentolate (Cyclogyl) toxicity in pediatric patients. J Pediatr 1971;79:127–129.

13. Gray LF. Avoiding adverse effects of cycloplegics in infants and children. J Am Optom Assoc 1979;50:465–470.

14. Sloan L, Sears ML, Jablonski MD. Convergence-accommodative relationships. Arch Ophthalmol 1960;63:283.

15. Wick B. Accommodative esotropia: Efficacy of therapy. J Am Optom Assoc 1987;58:562–566.

16. Von Noorden GK, Morris J, Edelman P. Efficacy of bifocals in the treatment of accommodative esotropia. Am J Ophthalmol 1978;85:830–834.

17. Jacob JL, Beaulieu Y, Brunet E. Progressive-addition lenses in the management of esotropia with a high accommodation-convergence ratio. Can J Ophthalmol 1980;15:166–169.

18. Smith JB. Progressive-addition lenses in the treatment of accommodative esotropia. Am J Ophthalmol 1985;99:56–62.

19. Javal E. Manuel du strabisme. Paris: Mason, 1896;45–87.

20. Abraham SV. The use of miotics in the treatment of convergent strabismus anisometropia: A preliminary report. Am J Ophthalmol 1949;32:233–240.

21. Abraham SV. The use of miotics in the treatment of non-paralytic convergent strabismus: A progress report. Am J Ophthalmol 1952;35:1191–1195.

22. Miller JE. A comparison of miotics in accommodative esotropia. Am J Ophthalmol 1960;49:1350–1355.

23. Taylor P. Anticholinesterase agents. In: Gilman AG, Rall TW, Nies AS, Taylor P, eds. Goodman and Gilman's The pharmacological basis of therapeutics, ed. 8. New York: Pergamon Press, 1990;131–149.

24. Bunke A, Bito LZ. Gradual increase in the sensitivity of extraocular muscles to acetylcholine during topical treatment of rabbit eyes with isoflurophate. Am J Ophthalmol 1981;92:259–267.

25. Goldstein JH. The role of miotics in strabismus. Surv Ophthalmol 1968;13:31–46.

26. Hill K, Stromberg AE. Echothiophate iodide in the management of esotropia. Am J Ophthalmol 1962;53:488–494.

27. Wheeler MC, Moore S. DFP in the handling of esotropia. Am Orthop J 1964;14:178–188.

28. Bedrossian EH, Krewson WE. Isoflurophate versus glasses in evaluating the accommodative element in esotropia. Arch Ophthalmol 1966;76:186–188.

29. Hiatt RL, Ringer C, Cope-Troupe C. Miotics vs glasses in esodeviation. J Pediatr Ophthalmol 1979;16:213–217.

30. Hiatt RL. Management of accommodative esotropia. J Pediatr Ophthalmol Strabismus 1983;20:199–201.

31. Bartlett JD, Ghormley NR, Jaanus, SD, et al. eds. Ophthalmic Drug Facts. St. Louis: Facts and Comparisons, 1995.

32. Moss HM. Strabismus: Current use of therapeutic drugs. In: Srinivasan BD, ed. Ocular therapeutics. New York: Masson, 1980; 114–124.

33. La Rocca V. Retinal detachment from diisopropyl fluorophosphate in an aphakic eye. NY State J Med 1952;52:1329–1330.

34. Butler WE. Acute glaucoma precipitated by DFP: Report of a case. Am J Ophthalmol 1952;35:1031–1033.

35. Becker B, Gage T. Demecarium bromide and echothiophate iodide in chronic glaucoma. Arch Ophthalmol 1960;63:102–107.

36. Knapp P. Use of miotics in esotropia. J Iowa State Med Soc 1956; 46:581–585.

37. De Roetth A, Dettbarn WD, Rosenberg P, et al. Effect of phopholine iodide on blood cholinesterase levels of normal and glaucoma subjects. Am J Ophthalmol 1965;59:586–592.

38. Humphreys JA, Holmes JH. Systemic effects produced by echothiophate iodide in the treatment of glaucoma. Arch Ophthalmol 1963;69:737–743.

39. Klendshoj NC, Olmstead EP. Observation of dangerous side-effects of phospholine iodide in glaucoma therapy. Am J Ophthalmol 1963;69:737–743.

40. McGavi DM. Depressed levels of serum pseudocholinesterase with echothiophate iodide eyedrops. Lancet 1965;2:272–250.

41. Ripps H. Miotics in the treatment of accommodative strabismus. Trans Ophthalmol Soc UK 1963;88:199–210.

42. Klendshoj NC, Feldstein M. Cholinesterase of blood in relation to organic phosphate insecticides. NY State J Med 1953;53:2667–2669.

43. Leopold IH, Comroe JH. Effect of diisopropyl fluorophosphate ("DFP") on the normal eye. Arch Ophthalmol 1946;36:17–32.

44. Leopold IH. Ocular cholinesterase and cholinesterase inhibitors. Am J Ophthalmol 1961;51:885–919.

45. Ellis PP, Esterdahl M. Echothiophate iodide therapy in children. Effect upon blood cholinesterase levels. Arch Ophthalmol 1967;77:598–601.

46. Sampson CR, Hermann JS. Isoflurophate in esotropic children: Effects on serum cholinesterase. J Pediatr Ophthalmol 1970;77:44–45.

47. Apt L. Toxicity of strong miotics in children. In: Leopold IH, ed. Symposium on ocular therapy V. St. Louis: C.V. Mosby Co, 1972;Chap. 2:30–35.

48. Helveston EM. Surgical management of strabismus, ed. 4. St. Louis: C.V. Mosby Co, 1993;14:345–354.

49. Scott AB, Rosenbaum A, Collins C. Pharmacological weakening of extra-ocular muscles. Invest Ophthalmol 1973;12:924–927.

50. Scott AB. Botulinum toxin: Role in ophthalmology, 1988 (unpublished).

51. Osako M, Keltner MD. Botulinum A toxin (Oculinum) in ophthalmology. Surv Ophthalmol 1991;36:28–46.

52. Scott AB, Suzuki D. Systemic toxicity of botulinum toxin by intramuscular injection in the monkey. Movement Disorders 1988; 3:333–335.

53. Scott AB. Botulinum toxin injection of eye muscles to correct strabismus. Trans Am Ophthalmol Soc 1981;79:735–770.

54. Das Gupta BR. The structure of botulinum neurotoxin. In: Simpson LL, ed. Botulinum neurotoxin and tetanus toxin. New York: Academic Press, 1989;53–67.

55. Kelly RB, Beutsch JW, Carlson SS, Wagner JA. Biochemistry of neurotransmitter release. Ann Rev Neurosci 1979;2:399–446.

56. Stanley EF, Drachman DB. Botulinum toxin blocks quantal but not non-quantal release of ACh at the neuromuscular junction. Brain Res 1983;261:172–175.

57. Dolly JO, Blach J, Williams RS, Melling J. Acceptors for botulinum neurotoxin reside on motor nerve terminals and mediate its internalization. Nature 1984;307:457–460.

58. Spencer RF, McNeer KW. Botulinum toxin paralysis of adult monkey extraocular muscle. Arch Ophthalmol 1987;105:1703–1711.

59. Melling J, Hambleton P, Shone CC. *Clostridium botulinum* toxins: Nature and preparation for clinical use. Eye 1988;2:16–23.

60. Gammon JA. Chemodenervation treatment of strabismus and blepharospasm with botulinum toxin. Ocular Therapy 1984;1:3–7.

61. Scott AB. Clostridium toxin as therapeutic agents. In: Simpson LL, ed. Botulinum neurotoxin and tetanus toxin. New York: Academic Press, 1989;399–412.

62. Magoon EH. Botulinum chemodenervation for strabismus and other disorders. Int Ophthalmol Clin 1985;25:149–159.

63. Scott AB. Botulinum toxin treatment of strabismus. American Academy of Ophthalmology Clinical Modules for Ophthalmologists, 1989;7:1.

64. Scott AB. Antitoxin reduced botulinum side effects. Eye 1988;2: 29–32.

65. Hoffman RO, Helveston EM. Botulinum in the treatment of adult motility disorders. Int Ophthalmol Clin 1986;26:241–250.

66. Scott AB, Kraft SP. Botulinum toxin injection in the management of lateral rectus paresis. Ophthalmology 1985;92:676–683.

67. Lee J, Harris S, Cohen J, et al. Results of a prospective randomized trial of botulinum toxin therapy in acute unilateral sixth nerve palsy. J Pediatr Ophthalmol Strabismus 1994;31:283–286.

68. Flynn JT, Bachynski B. Botulinum toxin therapy for strabismus and blepharospasm. Bascom Palmer Eye Institute experience. Trans New Orleans Acad Ophthalmol 1986;73–88.

69. Wagner RS, Frohman LP. Long-term results: Botulinum for sixth nerve palsy. J Pediatr Ophthalmol Strabismus 1989;26:106–108.

70. Fitzsimmons R, Lee JP, Elston J. Treatment of sixth nerve palsy in adults with combined botulinum toxin chemodenervation and surgery. Ophthalmology 1988;95:1535–1542.

71. Rosenbaum AL, Kushner BJ, Kirshchen D. Vertical rectus muscle transposition and botulinum (Oculinum) to medial rectus for abducens palsy. Arch Ophthalmol 1989;107:820–823.

72. Jampolsky A. Botulinum toxin injections in strabismus. Trans New Orleans Acad Ophthalmol 1986;522–536.

73. Scott AB. Botulinum toxin type A injection in the treatment of strabismus. Arch Ophthalmol 1991;109:1510.

74. Owens PL. Intraoperative uses of Oculinum. Pediatric ophthalmology and strabismus conference. Manhattan Eye, Ear and Throat Hospital: February 7, 1987.

75. Owens PL. New use of Oculinum: Adjunct to conventional surgical correction of large angle strabismus. American Association of Pediatric Ophthalmology and Strabismus: May 19–21, 1988.

76. Magoon E, Scott AB. Botulinum toxin chemodenervation in infants and children: An alternative to incisional strabismus surgery. J Pediatr 1987;110:719–722.

77. Metz HS. Botulinum injections for strabismus. J Pediatr Ophthalmol Strabismus 1984;21:199–201.

78. Burns CL, Gammon JA, Gemmill MC. Ptosis associated with botulinum toxin treatment of strabismus and blepharospasm. Ophthalmology 1986;93:1621–1627.

79. Elston JS. The use of botulinum toxin A in the treatment of strabismus. Trans Ophthalmol Soc UK 1985;104:208–210.

Medical Management of the Glaucomas

Jimmy D. Bartlett
Murray Fingeret

The term *glaukoma* was first used by Aristotle when referring to blue-eyed patients with "weakness of the eyes" in daylight.[1] It has been assumed that Aristotle was referring to blue-eyed patients with cataracts. Al-Tabari, an Arabian physician, is reported to be the first to associate the term *glaucoma* with an increased intraocular pressure (IOP).[2] In 1622, Banister, an English oculist, discussed the detection of glaucoma using finger palpation to evaluate hardness of the eyeball.[3] Over the years the term *glaucoma* came to be associated with an elevated IOP that produced damage to ocular structures. The emphasis in the theoretical considerations and in the clinical diagnosis was on elevated IOP.

Over the past several decades, however, the emphasis has shifted from elevated IOP to risk factors that might predict impaired visual function. An elevated IOP is a major risk factor for glaucoma, but the ability to predict the presence of impaired visual function from IOP alone is low. Glaucoma is a progressive optic neuropathy characterized by functional and structural impairment. This impairment is manifested by specific optic disc changes, nerve fiber layer defects, visual field losses, and other signs that are usually associated with a disturbance of aqueous drainage and a constant or intermittent unphysiologic IOP. This chapter emphasizes the pharmacotherapeutic management of the most common glaucomatous conditions.

Classification

The glaucomas can be divided into two broad etiologic classifications—primary and secondary. Primary glaucoma is associated with a direct disturbance of aqueous outflow, and, in general, with grossly normal ocular anatomy. Secondary glaucoma develops because of another recognizable disease mechanism. The glaucomas can be further classified anatomically by the degree of the anterior chamber angle, with 20° usually considered to be the magnitude dividing narrow angle (less than 20°) from open angle (greater than 20°). Although this classification can be made clinically, the work of Douglas and associates[4] and Horie and associates[5] suggest that the glaucomas may exist as a continuum from acute angle-closure, to subacute angle-closure, to chronic angle-closure, to open-angle glaucoma. These investigators found that patients with acute angle-closure glaucoma had normal visual fields and normal optic discs, but patients with chronic angle-closure glaucoma had visual field and optic disc changes similar to those in open-angle glaucoma. This suggests that, although there are specific differences, the basic etiopathogenesis of primary angle-closure glaucoma and primary open-angle glaucoma is similar.

Congenital (developmental) glaucoma is often classified

separately. This form of glaucoma occurs in the young as the result of fetal maldevelopment of the iridocorneal angle (goniodysgenesis).

A clinical classification of the glaucomas is shown in Table 35.1.

Epidemiology

Prevalence

Glaucoma is currently a leading cause of legal blindness in the United States, and the incidence does not appear to be decreasing.[6] Approximately 1.6 million persons aged 40 years or older in the United States have primary open-angle glaucoma.[7] Over 80,000 individuals are legally blind from glaucoma, and approximately 1 million have visual impairment. It is estimated that glaucoma is responsible for 15% of all cases of blindness worldwide, making it the third leading cause after cataract and trachoma.[436]

In a study of people over the age of 60 years in Sweden,[8] the prevalence of glaucoma was found to be 0.86% for open-angle glaucoma, 0.06% for angle-closure glaucoma, 0.05% for congenital glaucoma, and 0.27% for secondary glaucoma. This suggests that approximately 80% of glaucoma is primary and approximately 20% is secondary in Sweden.

The studies of Hollows and Graham[9] and of Bankes and associates[10] indicate that the prevalence of open-angle glaucoma in the population over 40 years of age is 0.43% to 1.02%. These investigators found the prevalence of angle-closure glaucoma to be 0.09% to 0.21%, suggesting that open-angle glaucoma is about 5 times more prevalent than angle-closure glaucoma. Klein and associates,[11] however, found angle-closure glaucoma to be extremely rare (2 cases out of 4926), and found the overall prevalence of open-angle glaucoma to be 2.1% of a rural white population.

Since open-angle glaucoma is an asymptomatic disease, and as many as half the patients with glaucomatous damage may be unaware of their condition,[12] the practitioner must be fully alert to the various factors that increase the risk of glaucoma.

Risk Factors

Several risk factors increase the probability of primary glaucoma in any given patient (Table 35.2). Appreciation of these factors is important for the diagnosis and management of primary glaucoma.

AGE

The prevalence of primary glaucoma increases with age. Colenbrander[13] reported that the prevalence of glaucoma is approximately 0.25% at age 20 years and that it nearly doubles every 10 years thereafter.

In white populations, the overall prevalence of open-angle glaucoma is approximately 2.0%. The prevalence increases with age from 0.9% in persons 43 to 54 years of age, to 4.7% in people 75 years of age or older.[11] An increasing prevalence with age has also been reported in African-Americans.[7] The age group most frequently affected with angle-closure glaucoma is between 50 and 60 years of age.[14]

TABLE 35.1
Clinical Classification of the Glaucomas

Congenital (developmental) glaucoma
Primary glaucoma
  Open angle
    Chronic open angle (High tension)
    Normal tension
  Angle closure
    With pupillary block
      Acute
      Subacute
      Chronic
    Without pupillary block
Secondary glaucoma
  Open angle
  Angle closure

TABLE 35.2
Risk Factors for Primary Glaucoma

General
  Age
  Family history of glaucoma
  Race

Ocular
  Ametropia
  Elevated IOP[a]
  Asymmetric IOP[a]
  Diffuse or focal narrowing of neuroretinal rim
  Asymmetry of cup-disc ratios
  Diffuse or focal dropout of nerve fiber layer

Non-Ocular
  Diabetes mellitus
  Hypothyroidism
  Systemic hypertension (?)
  Vasospasms

---

[a]IOP = intraocular pressure.
Modified from Lewis TL. Optometric clinical practice guideline. Care of the patient with open-angle glaucoma. Reference guide for clinicians. St. Louis: American Optometric Association, 1995.

FAMILY HISTORY

Substantial evidence indicates a genetic basis for primary glaucoma. Becker and associates[15] studied the close relatives (parents, siblings, children) of patients with primary open-angle glaucoma and found that the average values for intraocular pressure and outflow facility were significantly different from those for a normal population. They also found a 5.5% prevalence of primary open-angle glaucoma in close relatives. Shin and associates[16] found a family history of glaucoma in 50% of the patients with primary open-angle glaucoma. Perkins[17] studied the children and siblings of patients with glaucoma and found a prevalence of 5.3% with open-angle glaucoma and 6% with angle-closure glaucoma. Paterson[18] studied the relatives of patients with angle-closure glaucoma and also found a prevalence of primary angle-closure glaucoma of approximately 6%. These studies suggest that family history is an important risk factor for primary open-angle glaucoma. The Baltimore Eye Survey found that the age-adjusted associations of primary open-angle glaucoma with a history of glaucoma are higher in siblings than in parents or children.[437]

Although genetic factors are involved in primary glaucoma, the exact mode of inheritance is unclear. Studies have suggested that the inheritance patterns for angle-closure glaucoma could be multifactorial,[19] polygenic,[20] autosomal dominant,[21] and autosomal recessive.[22] Similarly, other studies suggest several modes of inheritance for open-angle glaucoma—multifactorial,[23] autosomal dominant with variable penetrance,[24] and autosomal recessive.[25]

Infantile glaucoma occurs in 1 in 10,000 births and is bilateral in 75% of the infants. It appears to have an autosomal recessive transmittance with incomplete penetrance.[26,27]

RACE

Several reports indicate that the prevalence of primary glaucoma varies among different racial groups. In their study of nearly 12,000 people, Packer and associates[28] found a prevalence of open-angle glaucoma of 1% in whites and 2.6% in blacks. In a comprehensive study of 15,000 patients by Turner,[29] the prevalence of open-angle glaucoma was 1% in whites and 3% in blacks. In the Baltimore Eye Survey,[7] the age-adjusted prevalence rates for primary open-angle glaucoma were 4 to 5 times higher in blacks compared to whites. Rates among blacks ranged from 1.23% in persons 40 to 49 years of age, to 11.26% in those 80 years of age or older. Rates for whites ranged from 0.92% to 2.16%, respectively.

Several investigators[7,30] have found that glaucoma occurs at a younger age in blacks than in whites. They also suggest that glaucoma is a more severe disease in blacks, since blacks appear to be less responsive to glaucoma therapy.[12,30] Martin and associates[31] found a higher incidence of open-angle glaucoma in blacks, and that the age of diagnosis was younger, the mean cup/disc ratio was higher, the IOP at the time of diagnosis was higher, and the visual field loss at the time of diagnosis was greater in blacks than in whites.

The prevalence of angle-closure glaucoma has also been reported to vary with race. Angle-closure glaucoma is 4 times more prevalent than open-angle glaucoma among the Singaporean Chinese,[32] and is the most prevalent form of glaucoma among adults in the Philippines.[34] Alper and Laubach[34] reported that acute angle-closure glaucoma, with its classic signs and symptoms, is rare in African-American blacks but that chronic angle-closure glaucoma occurs with significant frequency. However, Luntz[35] reported that the prevalence and clinical features of angle-closure glaucoma are similar for blacks and for whites in South Africa.

AMETROPIA

Angle-closure glaucoma occurs more frequently in hyperopic eyes.[36] The influence of myopia in glaucoma is not as significant, but Perkins and Phelps[37] found a high incidence of open-angle glaucoma in patients with myopia.

GENDER

There appears to be no difference in rates of primary open-angle glaucoma between men and women for either blacks or whites.[7,11] Several studies,[38,39] however, have suggested that angle-closure glaucoma is more common in females.

SYSTEMIC ILLNESS

Numerous systemic diseases such as diabetes, hypothyroidism, anemia, hypertension, and arteriosclerosis have been associated with glaucoma. The association of diabetes with primary open-angle glaucoma has been controversial and often confused by varying definitions of these two conditions. Recent population-based studies reached different conclusions. The Baltimore Eye Survey found no association between diabetes and primary open-angle glaucoma,[40] while the Beaver Dam Eye Study found an increased presence of open-angle glaucoma in individuals with older-onset diabetes.[41] Most clinic-based studies seem to support a positive association between diabetes and primary open-angle glaucoma.[40]

Smith and associates[42] demonstrated a significant association between hypothyroidism and primary open-angle glaucoma and suggested that treating the underlying thyroid disorder may be of benefit.

Studies examining the relationship between systemic blood pressure and primary open-angle glaucoma have been contradictory. Schulzer and Drance[43] have shown that, although systolic blood pressure does increase with age, there is no statistical association between systolic blood pressure and glaucoma. However, recent large population-based studies have demonstrated a positive association between systemic blood pressure, including hypertension, and primary open-angle glaucoma.[438,439] Lower perfusion pressure (blood pressure – intraocular pressure) is strongly associated with an increased prevalence of primary open-angle glaucoma.[439]

Treatment Rationale

The only interventional strategy that has consistently been shown to be of benefit in the treatment of glaucoma is reduction of IOP.[44–51] The goal of therapy is the maintenance or stabilization of existing optic nerve tissue and visual function. Many drugs are available to reduce IOP (see Table 10.1), and their ocular hypotensive mechanisms, clinical uses, side effects, and contraindications are discussed in Chapter 10. The following sections consider how these agents are used, either alone or in combination, for the control of specific glaucomatous conditions.

Congenital (Developmental) Glaucoma

Etiology

The etiology of congenital glaucoma varies with the specific iridocorneal angle abnormality. Some of the major causes and associated abnormalities are listed in Table 35.3. Congenital glaucoma is not due solely to genetic factors.[52,53] In most cases, the condition results from an interaction between genetic predisposition and a combination of environmental causes.[54] Glaucoma associated with congenital anomalies accounts for 46% of the patients, secondary infantile glaucoma is present in 32% of the patients, and primary congenital glaucoma occurs in about 22%.[55]

Diagnosis

Several conditions simulate congenital glaucoma and should be considered carefully in the differential diagnosis (Table 35.4). The diagnosis of congenital glaucoma is accomplished through careful patient history, family history, and examination.

PATIENT HISTORY

Some of the early indications of congenital glaucoma are lacrimation, epiphora, light sensitivity, and blepharospasm. Slight haziness or cloudiness of the cornea is also common. Buphthalmus may be present if the IOP has been elevated for some time. Infants should be observed closely for the presence of these signs. Another indication is the presence of any abnormality known to cause congenital glaucoma, such as aniridia, Reiger's anomaly, or Marfan's syndrome.

EXAMINATION

Using calipers for accuracy, the horizontal diameter of the cornea should be measured. Each corneal diameter should be approximately equal. The average in infants is 10.0 mm as compared with 11.9 mm in adults.[56] Corneal asymmetry exceeding 1.5 mm or a diameter over 12 mm in an infant suggests congenital glaucoma (Fig. 35.1)

Although the axial length is increased in congenital glaucoma, corneal diameter is a more sensitive and more reliable finding than axial length in the diagnosis of congenital glaucoma.[57] The use of A-scan ultrasonography, however, can be helpful in the long-term follow-up of patients being treated for congenital glaucoma.[58] Axial length changes can be used to evaluate the effectiveness of therapy.

Each cornea should be evaluated with a penlight, loupe,

TABLE 35.3
Congenital Glaucoma

Etiology	*Associated Congenital Abnormality*
Residual iris stump obstructing the trabecular meshwork	Aniridia
Anomalous attachment of iris tissue to the cornea, obstructing the trabecular meshwork	Anterior chamber cleavage syndrome
	Axenfeld's syndrome
	Reiger's anomaly
	Peters' anomaly
	Neurofibromatosis
Dislocated crystalline lens or microspherophakia, producing pupillary block	Marfan's syndrome
	Homocystinuria
	Marchesani's syndrome
Barkan's membrane (a thin translucent gelatinous-appearing membrane that covers the trabecular meshwork)	Infantile glaucoma
Improper development of the trabecular meshwork	Lowe's syndrome

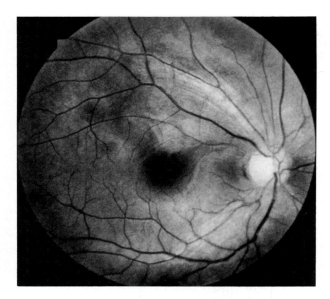

FIGURE 35.6   **Nerve fiber layer changes eminating from the optic disc and following the superior and inferior arcuate bundles.**

fundi increase visibility of the nerve fibers, which makes slight variations in the nerve fiber layer more apparent, resulting in detection of nerve fiber layer defects when none is actually present.[131] Defects are also more difficult to detect in patients with lightly pigmented fundi.[132] It is unfortunate that evaluation of the nerve fiber layer is more difficult in the elderly and blacks, because of the increased incidence of glaucoma in these populations.

Tuulonen and associates[133] have shown that many patients with normal appearing optic discs and normal routine visual fields, but with nerve fiber layer defects, may demonstrate subtle functional damage indicating early glaucoma. Nerve fiber layer examination, however, should not take precedence over optic disc evaluation, since the latter has greater diagnostic precision in correctly determining the presence or absence of structural damage in early glaucoma.[134] Quantitative grading of nerve fiber layer changes may improve the accuracy and reliability of this procedure.[135] Instrumentation to measure nerve fiber layer thickness by scanning laser polarimetry is now available.

VISUAL FIELDS

For many years, glaucoma was synonymous with visual field loss. In 1969, Armaly[136] suggested that a definitive diagnosis of glaucoma could not be made before the demonstration of a characteristic visual field loss. It is evident now that there is loss of optic nerve fibers and cupping of the optic disc before visual field loss can be detected. A histological study[137] of the optic nerve of patients with ocular

hypertension found a diffuse loss of 40% of the optic nerve fibers in a patient who had a medium sized, vertically oval cup and a normal visual field. Increases in cupping often precede the detection of visual field defects.[138] However, the testing of visual fields remains an essential part of the diagnostic evaluation of glaucoma and should be done on every patient suspected of having glaucoma. The results of visual field testing are also essential in determining the prognosis and effectiveness of medical and surgical therapy.

Although it is an essential part of the diagnostic evaluation for glaucoma, visual field testing is time-consuming, and the detection of glaucomatous visual field changes can be elusive. Sturmer[139] has shown that a relative scotoma, or early visual field loss, in glaucoma does not always consist of a sharply bordered area with a definite loss of sensitivity, but instead can be a region of increased scatter with poorly definable borders due to instability of the threshold. In other instances, diffuse rather than localized areas of sensitivity losses are seen.[140] These early threshold disturbances cannot be detected without static threshold perimetry, which has become the standard of care in visual field evaluation (Fig. 35.7).[141,142] Because of intratest variability, it is helpful to obtain at least two visual fields prior to initiating therapy in glaucoma suspects who have subtle optic disc findings with few, if any, additional risk factors.[143] Computerized algorithms are incorporated into these instruments that allow faster evaluations,[144] estimates of patient reliability,[141,142] and that compensate for extraneous variables such as cataract.[145] Short-wavelength testing, involving blue targets on yellow background, is now available and may dramatically increase the detection of early visual field losses before they would be seen on standard white-on-white perimetry.[146–148]

It is important to realize that visual field losses simulating glaucoma can occur with conditions such as cataract, pituitary tumor, drusen of the optic nerve head, sclerosis of the choroidal vessels, stenosis or sclerosis of the ciliary arteries, choroidal tumors, and ischemic optic neuropathy. If the optic disc topography does not correlate with the visual fields, the practitioner should search for other causes of the visual field loss.

Management

The availability of a wide variety of ocular hypotensive agents (see Chap. 10) often allows IOP to be controlled adequately, thereby minimizing further optic disc damage and visual field loss.[149] The successful management of POAG requires careful attention to the patient's optic discs, visual fields, IOPs and medication schedules. Failure of medical therapy to prevent further optic disc and visual field changes necessitates reevaluation and possibly laser or surgical intervention.[150] The planning of an appropriate treatment strategy may reduce the risk of treatment failure.

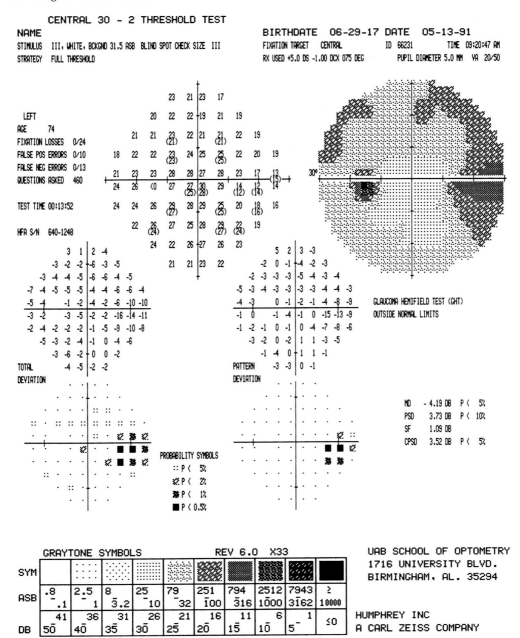

CENTRAL 30 - 2 THRESHOLD TEST

NAME

STIMULUS   III, WHITE, BCKGND 31.5 ASB BLIND SPOT CHECK SIZE III

STRATEGY   FULL THRESHOLD

BIRTHDATE   06-29-17 DATE   05-13-91

FIXATION TARGET   CENTRAL   ID 66231   TIME 09:20:47 AM

RX USED +5.0 DS -1.00 DCX 075 DEG   PUPIL DIAMETER 5.0 MM   VA 20/50

LEFT

AGE   74

FIXATION LOSSES   0/24

FALSE POS ERRORS   0/10

FALSE NEG ERRORS   0/13

QUESTIONS ASKED   460

TEST TIME 00:13:52

HFA S/N   640-1248

GLAUCOMA HEMIFIELD TEST (GHT)

OUTSIDE NORMAL LIMITS

TOTAL DEVIATION

PATTERN DEVIATION

MD   -4.19 DB   P < 5%

PSD   3.73 DB   P < 10%

SF   1.09 DB

CPSD   3.52 DB   P < 5%

PROBABILITY SYMBOLS

:: P < 5%

⊠ P < 2%

▩ P < 1%

■ P < 0.5%

GRAYTONE SYMBOLS					REV 6.0 X33				
SYM									
ASB	.8 .1	2.5 1	8 3.2	25 10	79 32	251 100	794 316	2512 1000	7943 3162	≥ 10000
DB	41 50	36 40	31 35	26 30	21 25	16 20	11 15	6 10	1 5	≤0

UAB SCHOOL OF OPTOMETRY

1716 UNIVERSITY BLVD.

BIRMINGHAM, AL. 35294

HUMPHREY INC

A CARL ZEISS COMPANY

A

FIGURE 35.7   **Examples of visual field results obtained with static threshold testing.** *(A)* **Inferior nasal step indicating early visual field loss.** *(B)* **Superior hemifield loss indicating more advanced glaucomatous damage.**

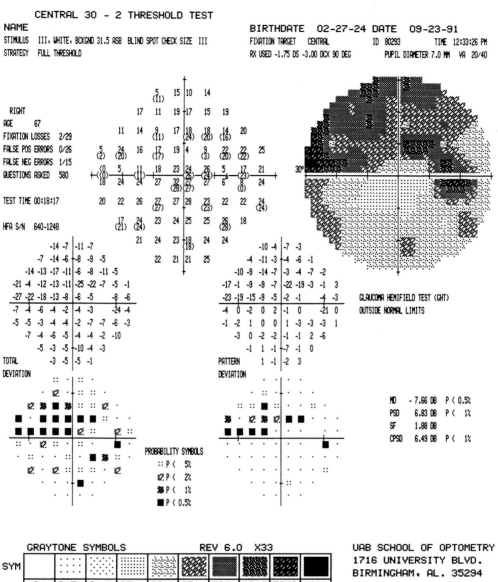

CENTRAL 30 - 2 THRESHOLD TEST

NAME

STIMULUS III, WHITE, BCKGND 31.5 ASB BLIND SPOT CHECK SIZE III
STRATEGY FULL THRESHOLD

BIRTHDATE 02-27-24 DATE 09-23-91
FIXATION TARGET CENTRAL   ID 80293   TIME 12:33:26 PM
RX USED -1.75 DS -3.00 DCX 90 DEG   PUPIL DIAMETER 7.0 MM   VA 20/40

RIGHT
AGE 67
FIXATION LOSSES 2/29
FALSE POS ERRORS 0/26
FALSE NEG ERRORS 1/15
QUESTIONS ASKED 580

TEST TIME 00:18:17

HFA S/N 640-1248

GLAUCOMA HEMIFIELD TEST (GHT)
OUTSIDE NORMAL LIMITS

TOTAL DEVIATION

PATTERN DEVIATION

PROBABILITY SYMBOLS
:: P < 5%
▨ P < 2%
▩ P < 1%
■ P < 0.5%

MD   - 7.66 DB   P < 0.5%
PSD   6.83 DB   P < 1%
SF   1.88 DB
CPSD   6.49 DB   P < 1%

	GRAYTONE SYMBOLS			REV 6.0	X33				
SYM									
ASB	.8 -.1	2.5 - 1	8 3.2	25 -10	79 -32	251 100	794 316	2512 1000	7943 3162	≥ 10000
DB	41 50	36 40	31 35	26 30	21 25	16 20	11 15	6 10	1 5	≤0

UAB SCHOOL OF OPTOMETRY
1716 UNIVERSITY BLVD.
BIRMINGHAM, AL. 35294

HUMPHREY INC
A CARL ZEISS COMPANY

B

FIGURE 35.7 (Continued)

INITIATING TREATMENT

Therapy for POAG is indicated when the IOP is above an arbitrary level (usually around 30 mm Hg), or at lower pressure levels when optic disc changes or visual field defects are noted. Individuals without definite nerve or field damage and whose IOP is over 21 mm Hg may be treated if additional risk factors accompany the presentation (see Table 35.2). Patients without risk factors may be followed closely, monitoring for any damage that may warrant therapy (see "Ocular Hypertension").

DETERMINING THE "TARGET PRESSURE"

The predominant objective in the treatment of POAG is to obtain a level of IOP that is compatible with preservation of optic nerve function and stability of the visual fields. In addition, the medical therapy must be compatible with the patient's lifestyle. Treatment that is inconvenient or that causes undesirable side effects encourages noncompliance, a significant factor in the failure of medical therapy. The most popular treatment strategies involve considering the initial status of the IOP, optic discs, and visual fields, and the use of uniocular therapeutic trials.

Initial Status of IOP, Optic Discs, and Visual Fields. The initial treatment strategy is based on evaluation of the initial IOPs as well as initial status of the optic discs and visual fields. From this information, a target pressure is determined that should prevent further damage to the visual system. By considering the initial pressure that presumably produced the observed optic disc and visual field changes, the clinician is able to estimate the level of IOP reduction that should prevent further visual field loss. Examples of such an approach are illustrated in Table 35.7. These exam-

TABLE 35.7
Examples of Choosing Level of Intraocular Pressure That Controls the Glaucoma

	Patient A	Patient B
Initial IOP before treatment (mm Hg)	36	29
Initial disc cupping (C/D ratio)	0.9	0.9
Initial visual field	Dense nasal step	Dense nasal step
"Target pressure"	Reduce IOP to mid to upper teens	Reduce IOP to low to mid teens

	Patient A	Patient B
Initial IOP before treatment (mm Hg)	36	29
Initial disc cupping (C/D ratio)	0.95	0.95
Initial visual field	Dense arcuate scotoma (hemifield loss)	Dense arcuate scotoma (hemifield loss)
"Target pressure"	Reduce IOP to low to mid teens	Reduce IOP to low teens

	Patient A	Patient B	Patient C
Initial IOP before treatment (mm Hg)	29	24	24
Initial disc cupping (C/D ratio)	0.7	0.7	0.7
Initial visual field	Dense arcuate scotoma (hemifield loss)	Dense arcuate scotoma (hemifield loss)	Complete loss of nasal field
"Target pressure"	Reduce IOP to high teens	Reduce IOP to mid teens	Reduce IOP to low teens

	Patient A	Patient B
Initial IOP before treatment (mm Hg)	26	34
Initial disc cupping (C/D ratio)	0.6	0.6
Initial visual field	No defect	No defect
"Target pressure"	(No treatment—ocular hypertension)	Reduce IOP to mid 20s

ples are intended merely to illustrate the process. They should not be interpreted as necessarily defining specific management procedures for individual patients with IOPs, optic discs, and visual fields described. An extremely important principle that guides medical therapy is to reduce IOP to a greater extent in eyes with more advanced glaucomatous damage. That is, the greater the initial damage, the greater the IOP should be reduced to obtain adequate control and prevent further damage.[151]

The findings in each eye are particularly useful in estimating the level of IOP at which control of the glaucoma should be obtained. Asymmetric findings, in particular, can be used to further define the decision to treat. This concept is illustrated in Table 35.8. Other factors may contribute to the decision regarding the level of IOP to be attained. Patients with central or branch vein occlusions may require lower IOP, as would those with low systemic blood pressure, cardiovascular disease, or diabetes.[152]

Since the changes in the optic discs and visual fields may have occurred at a pressure lower than that determined on the initial examination, the practitioner must not underestimate (i.e., select an IOP that is too high) the pressure level at which no further damage is likely to occur. Once the decision is made about the desired target IOP level that would be expected to control the glaucoma, the patient should be monitored carefully on treatment to determine the accuracy of this initial prediction. Serial examinations of IOPs, optic discs, and visual fields will verify the adequacy of the pressure reduction in controlling the glaucoma. Although these judgments are somewhat arbitrary in the beginning, the experienced clinician soon learns to predict such controlling IOP levels fairly accurately.

The Uniocular Therapeutic Trial. Uniocular therapeutic trials have been used to assess the therapeutic effective-

ness and potential side effects of a proposed drug regimen. They are based on the premise that the IOP of each eye varies synchronously, the difference in pressure between the two eyes remaining fairly constant for the full 24-hour period.[153] One eye is used as a control to evaluate the therapeutic efficacy of the intended drug regimen. Wilensky and associates,[94] however, demonstrated that erratic IOP curves without a diurnal rhythm are sometimes present in patients with ocular hypertension or POAG. Differences between the curves of an individual's two eyes are common, thus precluding use of one eye as a control for its fellow, treated eye. Moreover, topically applied β blockers often have a hypotensive effect on the fellow, untreated eye.[154] For these reasons, the uniocular therapeutic trial probably has limited practical usefulness. Despite these potential problems, however, some clinicians use this approach to help gauge the efficacy and safety of the initial therapeutic regimen before beginning treatment in both eyes.

TREATMENT GUIDELINES

Since POAG is a bilateral disease, treatment should generally be instituted in both eyes even if the glaucomatous damage is evident in only one eye. This often is not the case, however, in many of the secondary glaucomas such as those associated with trauma, in which unilateral treatment is justified.

In general, it is unnecessary to advise patients to reduce fluid intake (including coffee or other stimulants) or to withhold treatment with topical or systemic over-the-counter medications. Although the pharmaceutic labelling of many systemic drugs—anticholinergic agents or drugs with anticholinergic side effects, and other drugs such as vasodilators and corticosteroids—often states that these medications are contraindicated in glaucoma, this advice fails to recognize that glaucoma is a multifaceted disease rather than

TABLE 35.8
Example of Using Asymmetric Findings

	Normal Eye	Abnormal Eye	Maximal IOP Chosen for Control
Initial IOP before treatment (mm Hg)	18	26	18
Initial disc cupping (C/D ratio)	0.4	0.6	
Initial visual field	No defect	Nasal step	

	Normal Eye	Abnormal Eye	Maximal IOP Chosen for Control
Initial IOP before treatment (mm Hg)	27	33	
Initial disc cupping (C/D ratio)	0.6	0.6	High teens
Initial visual field	No defect	Nasal step	

TABLE 35.9
Estimate of Actual Risk Associated with Drugs "Contraindicated" in Glaucoma

Patient Group	High Risk (Avoid)	Slight Risk	Minimal Risk (in Usual Doses)
Patients with controlled open-angle glaucoma	None	Topical steroids 　Dexamethasone 　Prednisolone 　Bethamethasone Oral steroids	Topical and oral anticholinergics 　Antihistamines 　Tricyclic antidepressants 　Phenothiazines 　Benzodiazepines 　Transdermal scopolamine Vasodilators 　Nitrites 　Nitrates 　Tolazoline 　Hydralazine 　Nylidrin 　Nicotinic acid 　Cyclandelate 　Isoxuprine 　Papaverine
Patients predisposed to angle-closure glaucoma	Topical anticholinergics 　Atropine 　Homatropine 　Scopolamine 　Cyclopentolate 　Tropicamide Topical adrenergics 　Naphazoline 　Tetrahydrozoline 　Epinephrine 　Ephedrine 　Phenylephrine 　Hydroxyamphetamine	Oral anticholinergics 　Atropine 　Scopolamine 　Belladonna alkaloids Oral adrenergics 　Pseudoephedrine 　Phenylephrine 　Phenylpropanolamine 　Ephedrine 　Methoxphenamine Amphetamines Appetite suppressants Bronchodilators Central nervous system 　stimulants	Steroids Vasodilators Tricyclic antidepressants Phenothiazines Antihistamines

Modified from Durkee DP, Bryant BG. Drug therapy reviews: Drug therapy of glaucoma. Am J Hosp Pharm 1978;35:682–690; Maus TL, Larsson L, Brubaker RF. Ocular effects of scopolamine dermal patch in open-angle glaucoma. J Glaucoma 1994;3:190–194.

a single disease entity. In patients with medically controlled POAG, there is no definite contraindication to the use of most systemic medications because the concentration of drug reaching the eye is usually too low to be of any significant influence. Although there have been reports of aggravation of existing open-angle glaucoma with the use of systemic steroids, these drugs can generally be used safely in such patients if the IOP is monitored carefully.[155] The concomitant use of some topical and systemic medications is a greater risk in patients predisposed to angle-closure glaucoma (Table 35.9).[156]

In devising an effective treatment plan, the following guidelines listed (summarized in Table 35.10) should facilitate management of the patient by increasing the effectiveness of medical therapy, improving patient compliance, and reducing therapeutic failures[152,157]:

• Use the lowest concentration and dosage frequency compatible with acceptable control of IOP. This is determined by beginning with low drug concentrations and increasing as necessary until the desired IOP is attained. Low initial doses cause fewer side effects and often improve patient compliance with the prescribed therapy.

• Ideally, IOP should be determined just before a scheduled drug application to ensure that the desired effect is reasonably maintained from one dose to the next.

• Teach the patient how to administer a drop of medication. Considerable instruction regarding proper instillation technique may be required. If the patient has difficulty discerning when a drop of medication has been instilled properly, the drug can be refrigerated to improve the patient's sensitivity. In addition, the patient should be instructed to wait at least 5 minutes between drop instilla-

TABLE 35.10
Guidelines for the Medical Management of Primary Open-Angle Glaucoma

1. Start with low drug concentrations
2. If possible, measure IOP just before the next scheduled drug dosage
3. Teach proper eyedrop instillation technique, including nasolacrimal occlusion, *before* the patient begins therapy
4. Patient can refrigerate eyedrops to facilitate instillation awareness
5. Patient should wait at least 5 minutes between eyedrop instillations when more than one topical medication is used
6. Integrate therapy into patient's lifestyle
7. Keep continuing record of ophthalmic and systemic medications, primary physician, and pharmacist
8. Communicate with the patient, primary physician, and glaucoma subspecialist

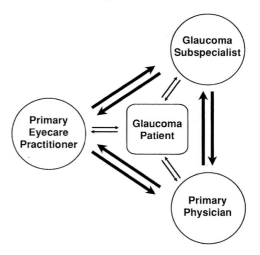

FIGURE 35.8 **"Communication triangle" in glaucoma management.**

tions when multiple topical medications have been prescribed. Washing one medication out with another is a frequent cause of failure to obtain expected additive drug effects when topical medications are used in combination.

• Every patient should be taught nasolacrimal occlusion (see Fig. 3.6). This procedure, or simple eyelid closure, for 3 to 5 minutes following eyedrop instillation may enhance drug efficacy and reduce the potential for systemic side effects.

• When initially devising a mediation schedule, the practitioner should attempt to integrate the therapy as smoothly as possible into the patient's daily routine. This is especially important in encouraging compliance with the use of every-6-hour medications (pilocarpine solutions). In such cases, the patient can be instructed to use the medication on arising, before lunch, before dinner, and before retiring. For some employed patients, the use of two bottles of medication, one for home and one for work, may be beneficial.

• The practitioner should have regard for the patient's safety by keeping a drug record that includes the name and address of the patient's primary physician as well as a complete list of all ophthalmic and systemic medications. In addition, the practitioner should remind the patient to inform his or her primary physician of the medications that have been prescribed for the glaucoma, or alternatively, the optometrist or ophthalmologist may communicate directly with the primary physician regarding the prescribed antiglaucoma regimen. This is especially important when the drug regimen includes a β blocker, anticholinesterase agent, epinephrine, or an oral carbonic anhydrase inhibitor. Ongoing communication among the primary eyecare practitioner, primary physician, and glaucoma subspecialist is critical if the needs of the glaucoma patient are to be fully met (Fig. 35.8).

DRUG SCHEMA

The general approach to the medical management of primary open-angle glaucoma is shown in Figure 35.9. When beginning treatment, the choice of drug should generally be a β blocker. This approach usually allows a significant reduction of IOP without the ocular side effects of miotics. In addition, dosage frequency is only once or twice daily, which reduces the opportunity for noncompliance when compared with the more frequent instillation required of pilocarpine solutions. Moreover, treatment with β-blockers, such as timolol, has been shown to preserve visual field better than does treatment with pilocarpine.[158,159] It must be stressed that the general recommendations given in Figure 35.9 must often be modified according to each patient's individual requirements. Some patients, for example, will have contraindications to specific drugs, and some medications will not be tolerated or will be ineffective. Some medications, such as dipivefrin or a β-blocker, may be tolerated well for many months or years, but then suddenly induce toxic or allergic effects.[160] Apraclonidine can cause allergic reactions in 14% to 48% of patients within several months after initiating treatment.[442,443] It is important to modify therapy promptly or discontinue any medications that are poorly tolerated or ineffective.

Once the patient has started initial drug therapy, 2 to 4 weeks is a useful follow-up time interval. This allows the patient to determine the ability to tolerate the medication and allows the practitioner to determine the clinical effectiveness of therapy. According to the results of this therapeutic trial, therapy can be increased, decreased, or otherwise modified to enhance the reduction of IOP while minimizing undesir-

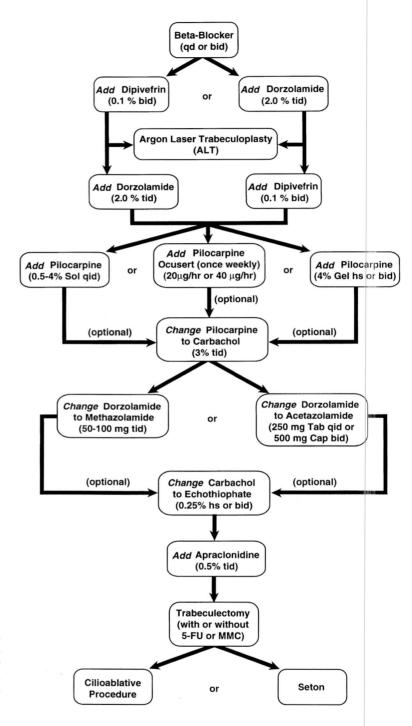

FIGURE 35.9 **Flowchart for the medical management of primary open-angle glaucoma. Nasolacrimal occlusion may allow dosage frequencies lower than indicated. Contraindications, drug intolerance, or other factors may alter the order of medications prescribed for individual patients.**

able side effects. After the medication has been titrated to achieve the desired "target pressure," the patient should be monitored every 3 to 6 months according to the severity of the glaucomatous damage and the susceptibility of the pa-

tient to further optic disc and visual field changes. Specific procedures and guidelines for the long-term management of patients with POAG are discussed below.

Although single-medication therapy is preferred, patients

often become tolerant to the initial drug or require additional medication as the glaucomatous damage progresses. In such cases, additional medication may be added to the drug regimen,[161] as shown in Figure 35.9. This step-wise approach reserves the more toxic medications, such as the oral carbonic anhydrase inhibitors, for patients with more advanced and resistant forms of glaucoma. Patients with early or moderate degrees of glaucomatous damage are unlikely to require these medications.

SPECIFIC MANAGEMENT PLANS

Although the drug schema illustrated in Figure 35.9 can be used to treat most patients with POAG, the specific management plan will vary according to the individual characteristics and requirements of each patient (Table 35.11). For example, miotic solutions may be used in elderly patients without cataracts, but the practitioner should be cautious in using oral carbonic anhydrase inhibitors because of drug-induced behavioral changes.

In patients with cataracts, miotic solutions are generally contraindicated because of their devastating effect on visual acuity and because of their acceleration of cataractous changes. A β blocker or dipivefrin is a reasonable drug of first choice for such patients, and, if needed, topical or oral carbonic anhydrase inhibitors may be added, followed finally by lower concentrations of pilocarpine.[152]

Miotic solutions should be avoided in young patients (under 40 years of age) because of drug-induced accommodative spasm and refractive changes. Instead, a β blocker or dipivefrin may be useful initial drugs that can be followed, if

necessary, by a topical carbonic anhydrase inhibitor. Pilocarpine in the form of Ocusert or gel may be beneficial. The anticholinesterase agents are generally not tolerated by these patients.

All strong miotics, including carbachol and echothiophate, should be avoided in patients with a history of retinal detachment or in patients with high myopia. Dipivefrin or a β blocker is preferred as the initial drug, followed, if necessary, by lower concentrations of pilocarpine or a topical or oral carbonic anhydrase inhibitor.

Epinephrine and dipivefrin should be avoided in aphakic or pseudophakic patients, since these drugs carry a risk of maculopathy. Instead, treatment should begin with low concentrations of pilocarpine or a β blocker and proceed, as needed, to a topical or oral carbonic anhydrase inhibitor.[152] Since the anticholinesterase agents have a greater risk of retinal detachment, they should be held in reserve until all other treatment modalities have been exhausted.

Patients with a history of kidney stones may be treated as shown in Figure 35.9. However, methazolamide should be the oral carbonic anhydrase inhibitor of choice because of its lower risk of kidney impairment.

PATIENT COMPLIANCE

The general factors contributing to noncompliance with medication schedules are discussed in Chapter 4. Primary open-angle glaucoma encompasses more of these factors than do most other ocular diseases because it is chronic, asymptomatic, sometimes requires complex therapeutic regimens often with associated side effects, and requires considerable time in patient education. It has been reported that patients take only about 75% of prescribed doses of pilocarpine drops, with 6% of patients taking less than one-fourth and 15% taking less than half of prescribed doses.[165] Unfortunately, there is no simple screening device that will help the practitioner identify the unreliable patient, or that will predict accurately at the time of initial diagnosis the potential for patient noncompliance.[166] In general, age, gender, education, visual ability, and ethnic background seem to have little influence on the potential for noncompliance.[167,168] The practitioner often assumes that the patient is complying properly with the prescribed treatment and interprets the progression of optic disc damage and visual field loss as indicating medication failure. This may be an inappropriate assumption, since the progression of glaucomatous damage may be related solely to patient failure to comply properly with the medical therapy.

Numerous factors contribute to noncompliance in patients with POAG (Table 35.12). The fact that POAG is a chronic disease that requires long-term management encourages at least occasional noncompliance with medication schedules. The asymptomatic nature of the disease, in which the beneficial effects of therapy are not readily appreciated or are associated with significant side effects, are other factors leading to noncompliance.

TABLE 35.11
Contraindicated Drugs or Drug Classes

Situation	Contraindicated Drug or Drug Class
Elderly patients	Oral carbonic anhydrase inhibitors
Cataract	Miotic solutions
Young patients (<40 years of age)	Miotic solutions
History of retinal detachment	Strong miotics (e.g., anticholinesterase agents)
High myopia	Strong miotics (e.g., anticholinesterase agents)
Aphakia or pseudophakia	Epinephrine and dipivefrin[a]
History of kidney disease	Acetazolamide
Chronic obstructive pulmonary disease	β blockers (β₁ blockers may be used with caution), acetazolamide
Congestive heart disease	β blockers
Pregnancy and lactation	Caution with all drugs[162,163]

[a]Relative rather than absolute contraindication.[164]

TABLE 35.12
Factors Contributing to Noncompliance in POAG

- Use of multiple medications requiring frequent daily administration
- Medication expense
- Medication side effects
- Patient's understanding of the disease
- Asymptomatic disease (no noticeable effects of therapy)
- Requires long-term medication (chronic disease)
- Patient's ability to understand treatment procedure and to comply with drop instillation or oral medication

Factors related to the therapeutic regimen itself may promote poor compliance. These include the use of multiple medications requiring frequent administration, and the frequency and severity of side effects. In general, the more a therapeutic regimen interferes with the patient's daily lifestyle, the less likely it is to be accepted and maintained.

Socioeconomic factors may contribute to noncompliance. Medication expense, cost of office visits, and transportation may limit use of medications in some patients despite the willingness of the patient to accept and comply with the prescribed therapy. Patients should be encouraged to compare prices of medications at different pharmacies to obtain the most economical dosage regimen, and the practitioner can help reduce overall cost of therapy by prescribing generic equivalent drugs, if available.[169]

Perhaps the most important factor is the patient's perception and understanding of the disease. Poor compliance occurs more frequently in patients who show little concern for their own health or well-being, who question the effectiveness of medical care or medications, or who do not understand the information or instructions provided by the practitioner or staff.[168]

Recognition of the patient's noncompliance is essential so that appropriate corrective measures can be instituted before further glaucomatous damage occurs. Noncompliance may be identified by instructing the patient to bring his or her medications to the office so that the amount used by the patient can be determined (Table 35.13). It is important to inspect the pupillary responses of patients taking miotics; normally reactive pupils that are not miotic are a strong indication of noncompliance. On the other hand, the practitioner should be alert to the occasional patient who instills the medication only on the day of examination. Despite acceptable IOPs, progression of glaucomatous damage to the optic disc and visual field is observed.[165] Once the clinician realizes the potential for such noncompliance, the assessment of visual fields and optic discs should take precedence over the measurement of IOP.

Methods for improving compliance are listed in Table 35.14.[170] Unfortunately, simple interventions rarely produce substantial, long-lasting improvement in compliance.[171] On the other hand, coercing or provoking fear may also be unsuccessful in improving compliance, because the patient may fear the consequences of the glaucoma so much that he or she does not use the required medications, which only reinforces a feeling of vulnerability to the disease.[171]

Perhaps the most effective method for improving compliance with medication schedules is by developing an attitude of concern and compassion and frequently communicating with the patient using understandable instructions for proper use of the medications. Brown and associates[172] found that 13% of glaucoma patients experienced in the use of topical eyedrops were unable to instill topical medications into both eyes successfully even after several attempts. In addition, counseling and education regarding the disease process and the importance of its treatment are vital.[173] This should be reinforced by the office assistant, technician, or nurse. On subsequent visits the practitioner or assistant should periodically reassess (by observation) the patient's ability to use the prescribed medication properly.[172,174] In addition, the patient should be asked to verbally recite the instructions for use of the medication. At each office visit the patient should be reminded about the importance of regular medication usage and should be reassured regarding minor medication side effects.

Another effective method for improving compliance is to devise an initial medication schedule that is easily integrated into the patient's daily lifestyle. This appears to be effective

TABLE 35.13
Approximate Longevity of Glaucoma Medications[a]

Medication	Bottle Size (ml)	Dosage Frequency		
		Once Daily	Twice Daily	Four Times Daily
β blocker, dipivefrin	10	100 days	50 days	
β blocker, pilocarpine, dipivefrin	15	150 days	75 days	38 days
Pilocarpine	30		150 days	75 days

[a]Assumes 20 drops/ml and good patient compliance for instillation into both eyes. Since drop sizes and bottle volumes vary, some medications may last longer.

TABLE 35.14
Effective Methods for Improving Compliance

- Improve doctor-patient communication and rapport
- Use understandable instructions
- Continually educate the patient about glaucoma and its treatment
- Periodically reassess eyedrop instillation technique
- Ascertain patient's understanding of drug regimen
- Continually remind patient about regular medication usage and side effects
- Devise medication schedule that is easily integrated into patient's lifestyle
- Use fewest medications consistent with achieving target pressure
- Use a medication timetable card
- Use C Cap Compliance Caps for pilocarpine, dipivefrin, or levobunolol
- Periodically substitute a "new," equally effective medication for older drug therapy

in reducing the number of missed doses and improving the regular dosage intervals. For example, the use of pilocarpine drops on awakening, before lunch, before dinner, and at bedtime avoids a rigid every-6-hour dosage schedule. On the other hand, patients who consistently administer their medication at unevenly spaced intervals may require such a rigid

dosage schedule. It may be helpful for these patients to change from a q.i.d. dosage interval to a q.6.h. schedule to reduce diurnal variations of IOP. Pilocarpine dosage can be reduced to b.i.d. if nasolacrimal occlusion is employed after the drops are instilled. The use of a β blocker, requiring only once- or twice-a-day dosage instead of 4 times a day, will interfere less with the patient's normal lifestyle and often improves compliance.[173,175] Recent studies,[176] however, have shown that, at least for timolol, instillation at bedtime is ineffective in reducing IOP during sleep. In this regard, a compromise may be required by both the practitioner and the patient. A realistic drug schedule with which the patient is likely to comply may be far superior to a medically ideal regimen that requires substantial changes in the patient's lifestyle. A medication timetable card similar to the one shown in Table 35.15 can be used to reinforce medication schedules.[177] Another measure that may improve compliance in some patients is the dispensing of pilocarpine, dipivefrin, or levobunolol with C Cap Compliance Caps (Allergan) (Fig. 35.10). This dosing formulation allows the patient to keep track of the daily doses of medication and may help to minimize dosing confusion when multiple medications are prescribed.[178]

Another method for improving compliance is to substitute a "new," equally effective medication for the older drug therapy. Novack and associates,[179] for example, have shown

TABLE 35.15
Glaucoma Medication Timetable Card

Medication	Bottle Cap or Pill Color	Eye		Time			
		R	L	AM	PM	PM	PM
Timoptic 0.25%, 0.5%							
Levobunolol 0.25%, 0.5%							
Betoptic-S 0.25%							
Betoptic 0.5%							
Optipranol 0.3%							
Ocupress 1.0%							
Iopidine 0.5%							
Propine 0.1%							
Pilocarpine 1%, 2%, 4%							
Carbachol 3%							
Phospholine Iodide 0.25%							
Trusopt 2%							
Neptazane tablets 25 mg, 50 mg							
Diamox tablets 250 mg							
Diamox capsules 500 mg							

Adapted from Kooner KS, Zimmerman TJ. A glaucoma medication timetable card. Ann Ophthalmol 1987;19:43–44.

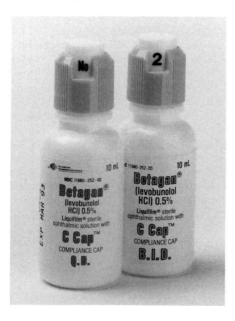

FIGURE 35.10 **Glaucoma medications with C Cap Compliance Caps (Allergan). When the medication cap is returned to the bottle after dispensing a drop of medication into the eye, the cap is turned to the next dosage indication. The number of instilled daily doses can thus be accounted for, and the device serves to remind the patient of the next indicated dosage. (Courtesy Allergan Pharmaceuticals, Inc.)**

TABLE 35.16
Color Identification of Antiglaucoma Medications[a]

Color	Medication
Topical	
Light Blue	Timoptic 0.25%
	Levobunolol 0.25%
	Betoptic-S 0.25%
Dark Blue	Betoptic 0.5%
Yellow	Timoptic 0.5%
	Levobunolol 0.5%
Purple	Propine 0.1%
Green	Pilocarpine 0.5–4.0%
	Carbachol 0.75–3.0%
White	Optipranolol 0.3%
	Ocupress 1.0%
	Iopidine 0.5%
Orange	Trusopt 2.0%
Oral	
White	Diamox
	Neptazane
Orange	Diamox Sequel

[a]Bottle cap color of topical medications; color of oral solid dosage form.

that patients may comply better with levobunolol as "new" therapy when they were previously uncontrolled with timolol. When two or more drugs are prescribed for use at different times, the patient must be able to identify the individual medications. He or she can be educated in this regard by identifying the pilocarpine as "the bottle with the green top" or the β blocker as "the bottle with the yellow top," and so on (Table 35.16). When a particular medication may be expected to cause unfamiliar or uncomfortable side effects, these should be explained to the patient before beginning therapy. In those instances in which the side effects will decrease or disappear, the patient should be advised of this in advance.

If the problem of noncompliance is not addressed properly, it usually leads to progressive glaucomatous damage. In these cases, laser therapy or filtering surgery become the only recourse.

LONG-TERM MANAGEMENT

The long-term management of patients with POAG requires careful attention to a variety of parameters that serve to indicate the effectiveness and safety of the glaucoma therapy (Table 35.17). The most important factors to be monitored

TABLE 35.17
Composition of Follow-up Examinations for Glaucoma Patients Under Treatment

Patient History
  Compliance
  Side effects of medication

Visual Acuity

Blood Pressure and Pulse[a]
Slit Lamp Examination
  Side effects of medications

Applanation Tonometry
  Diurnal stability

Gonioscopy
Stereoscopic Optic Disc Assessment
  Change over time
  Photographic documentation

Red-Free Nerve Fiber Layer Assessment
  Change over time
  Photographic documentation

Automated Perimetry
  Change over time

[a]Symptomatic patients using topical β-blocker.
Modified from Lewis TL. Optometric clinical practice guideline. Care of the patient with open-angle glaucoma. Reference guide for clinicians. St. Louis: American Optometric Association, 1995.

carefully are IOP, visual fields, and the optic discs. Depending on the extent of glaucomatous damage and rate of progression of the optic disc and visual field changes, it is useful to monitor patients every 3 to 6 months. IOP status should be determined at each visit, but visual fields and optic disc evaluations generally need to be performed only every 6 months. Table 35.18 suggests a long-term management plan for various kinds of glaucoma patients. Regardless of the time interval chosen for the monitoring schedule, it is essential that evaluations of visual fields and optic discs be performed during the same office visit, or within a few weeks of each other, so that the optic disc changes can be correlated accurately with changes of the visual fields.

The large amount and variety of information collected on individual patients necessitates use of a control sheet such as the one illustrated in Table 35.19. This control sheet facilitates the long-term monitoring of patients by consolidating the important diagnostic and therapeutic parameters into a single form that allows for rapid recognition of trends in the IOP or visual acuity.[180] A simple check mark may indicate that visual field or optic disc evaluations were performed. The patient's chart must then be consulted to determine the actual status of the visual fields or optic discs. For simplicity, therapeutic drug regimens can be documented using easily identifiable abbreviations (Table 35.20).

Use of Medications. As previously discussed, the patient's improper use of medication is one of the most important factors in failure to control the IOP. Therefore, it is vital to evaluate the patient's continued ability to use the prescribed medications properly. The practitioner should inquire about the frequency of medication use, the approximate percentage of missed doses, and convenience of the dosage schedule. Any medication side effects should be

TABLE 35.18
Frequency of Follow-up Examinations for POAG

Type of Patient	Frequency of Examination	Tonometry	Gonioscopy	Optic Nerve/NFL Assessment	Stereo Optic Nerve and NFL Photography	Automated Perimetry
New glaucoma patient or new glaucoma suspect	Weekly to bi-weekly to achieve target pressure	Yes: Multiple readings may be necessary to establish baseline	Yes: Standard classification and drawing at initial visit	Dilate: Optic nerve drawing at initial visit	Yes	Yes: Repeat to establish baseline
Glaucoma suspect	6–12 months depending on level of risk	Multiple readings may be necessary to establish baseline	Annual	Dilate at each visit	Every 2 years	Annual
Stable-mild stage	4–6 months	Every visit	Annual	Dilate every other visit	Annual	Annual
Stable-moderate stage	3–4 months	Every visit	Annual	Dilate every other visit	Annual	6 months
Stable-advanced stage	2–3 months	Every visit	6 months	Dilate every other visit	Annual	3–4 months
Unstable-IOP poorly controlled; ON and/or VF progressing	Weekly or bi-weekly until stability established	Every visit	Initial visit	Initial visit	Annual or each time ON or NFL changes	4–6 weeks or as needed to establish new baseline
Recently established stability	1–3 months	Every visit. Re-establish baseline	Depends on severity of the glaucoma	Dilate every other visit	Annual or each time ON or NFL changes	Depends on severity of the glaucoma

NFL = nerve fiber layer; IOP = intraocular pressure; ON = optic nerve; VF = visual field.
Modified from Lewis TL. Optometric clinical practice guideline. Care of the patient with open-angle glaucoma. Reference guide for clinicians. St. Louis: American Optometric Association, 1995.

TABLE 35.19
Glaucoma Control Sheet

NAME: *John A. Doe*
DOB: *6/17/27*
DIAGNOSIS: *POAG OU*
TARGET PRESSURE: *Below 21*

Primary Physician: *Dr. Jane Brown*
Systemic diseases: *Emphysema*
Systemic medication: *Albuterol*
Pharmacy: *Best Drugs*

| | IOP | | Visual | Optic Discs | | | Visual Acuity | | Blood | | Medication | |
Date	OD	OS	Fields	OD	OS	Gonio	OD	OS	Pressure	Pulse	Schedule	Comments
2/10/92	31	28	✓	✓	✓	✓	20/25	20/25	140/88	68	B-S OU BID	Emphysema
2/24/92	25	21					20/25	20/25	142/86	70	Add PP OU BID	
3/7/92	20	19					20/25	20/25	140/86	62		Good Compliance
7/8/92	19	18					20/30	20/25	140/88	72		
11/10/92	20	18	✓	✓	✓		20/25	20/30	136/86	68		
3/15/93	24	22					20/30	20/30	136/86	70		Missed last dosage
7/20/93	21	20	✓	✓	✓		20/30	20/30	140/88	64		
11/13/93	22	22					20/30	20/30	146/85	72		
3/11/94	25	24	✓	✓	✓	✓	20/30	20/30	145/88	74	Add P_1 OU QID	Patient refuses ALT
3/26/94	19	18					20/30	20/40	140/86	64		
8/3/94	21	21					20/40	20/30	142/84	66		
12/15/94	21	22	✓	✓	✓		20/40	20/40	138/90	66		
4/3/95	23	22					20/40	20/40	130/85	72	Δ P_1 to P_2 OU QID	
4/20/95	18	18					20/40	20/40	136/88	68		
8/18/95	25	24	✓	✓	✓	✓	20/40	20/40	140/92	66		Patient to consider ALT

elicited, particularly those that might limit use of the medication. Because IOP status directly reflects duration of action of the various medications, it is essential to record in the patient's chart the time of the most recent dose of each medication.

Visual Acuity. Stabilization of the IOP at a level that permits control of the glaucomatous optic disc changes should prevent any further loss of visual acuity. A gradual reduction in visual acuity may be associated with further visual field changes, indicating progression of optic disc damage. Corneal edema associated with corneal endothelial compromise may also reduce visual acuity. Other possible causes of visual acuity loss include retinal venous occlusive disease and retinal detachment. A gradual or sudden reduction of visual acuity should be an indication for pupillary dilation, repeat visual fields, and careful examination of the crystalline lens and retina.

Intraocular Pressure. The IOP should be correlated with the most recent dose of medication. An apparent increase in pressure may be related solely to the interval between the last medication dose and the time of IOP measurement, rather than to a true drug tolerance or exacerbation of the disease. Since diurnal variations have an important influence on IOP measurements, these influences should be taken into consideration when interpreting the IOP. The possibility of noncompliance should be considered when the IOPs are elevated only occasionally. Once the practitioner determines that a true, consistent elevation in IOP has occurred, the medication or dosage schedules should be adjusted accordingly. When a sudden decrease in IOP occurs, the possibility of uveitis or retinal detachment should be considered, as well as a possible change in systemic medications (e.g., antihypertensive).

Visual Fields. Assessment of visual fields provides a far more consistent measure of glaucoma progression than does IOP.[159] Thus, periodic reevaluation of the visual field is one of the most important factors in the patient's long-term management. In comparing the visual field from one visit to the next, it is important to look for consistent *trends* in visual field changes, rather than changing medical therapy solely on the basis of a single visual field evaluation. It is important, therefore, that the physical parameters of visual field testing—illumination, refractive correction, pupil size,[181] and procedure—be the same for each visual field assessment. Pupillary dilation with a combination of 2.5% phenylephrine and 0.5% to 1.0% tropicamide is usually satisfactory for these evaluations. It is important to realize that changes

TABLE 35.20
Commonly Used Abbreviations for Glaucoma Medications

Medication	Trade Name	Concentration (%)	Abbreviation
Timolol	Timoptic	0.25, 0.5	$T_{1/4}$, $T_{1/2}$
	Timoptic XE	0.25, 0.5	$TXE_{1/4}$, $TXE_{1/2}$
Levobunolol	Betagan	0.25, 0.5	$L_{1/4}$, $L_{1/2}$
Betaxolol	Betoptic	0.5	$B_{1/2}$
	Betoptic-S	0.25	B-S
Metipranolol	Optipranolol	0.3	Opti
Carteolol	Ocupress	1.0	Ocu
Dipivefrin	Propine	0.1	PP
Pilocarpine solution	Isoptocarpine	1.0, 2.0, 4.0	P_1, P_2, P_4
Pilocarpine gel	Pilopine H.S. Gel	4.0	P Gel
Carbachol	Isoptocarbachol	3.0	C_3
Apraclonidine	Iopidine	0.5, 1.0	$I_{1/2}$, I_1
Dorzolamide	Trusopt	2.0	Tru
Acetazolamide[a]	Diamox	250[a], 500[a]	D_{250}, D_{500}
Methazolamide[a]	Neptazane	25[a], 50[a]	N_{25}, N_{50}
Echothiophate	Phospholine Iodide	0.25	$PI_{1/4}$

[a]The concentration for these medications is in milligrams (mg).

in the visual field may be due not only to progressive glaucoma, but may also be caused by many other disorders such as retinal venous occlusive disease, retinal detachment, cataracts, diabetic retinopathy, or refractive error changes.[152]

Optic Discs.   It is crucial to dilate the pupil for careful stereoscopic evaluation of the optic discs. The optic discs must be reevaluated carefully for changes in cupping, pallor, or the presence of neuroretinal rim compromise, which may indicate inadequate control of IOP.[152]

Systemic Disease.   The patient's general health should be monitored. Patients who develop systemic hypertension or who have been given an increase of antihypertensive medication should be monitored more carefully for optic disc and visual field changes. In some cases it may be appropriate to adjust the patient's medication schedule to allow for some additional reduction in IOP so that an optimum perfusion-pressure gradient is maintained. In addition, the development of diabetes, with associated small-vessel disease, may indicate the need to further reduce IOP.

Although treatment with topical antiglaucoma medications does not lead to an increased risk of congestive heart disease or cardiac conduction disturbances in most patients who use them,[182] topical β-blockers may reduce plasma HDL cholesterol levels in some patients.[183] It is unknown if these changes in plasma lipids will increase the risk of coronary heart disease.

FAILURE OF MEDICAL THERAPY

A variety of factors contribute to the failure of medical therapy to adequately prevent further glaucomatous optic disc and visual field changes[152,184,185]:

- The IOP measurements may not completely reflect the pressure control because of diurnal variations of pressure.[186]
- The practitioner may inaccurately estimate the level of IOP that is expected to reduce the risk of further progression. Such underestimation (i.e., selecting an IOP that is too high) leads to further visual field loss even though lower pressures could have been obtained by adjusting the medical therapy.
- Drug tolerance may occur. This may lead to the use of maximum tolerated medical therapy. If tolerance develops to this drug regimen, laser or filtering surgery is required. In some cases, however, the practitioner may be able to change to a previously employed drug, with some occasional success in further reducing pressure.
- Medication side effects may necessitate discontinuation of certain drugs, leading in some cases to the need for laser or filtering surgery.
- The development and treatment of other diseases can contribute to progressive optic disc damage. Patients may unknowingly be given topical or systemic anticholinergic drugs or steroids by other practitioners. These medications may prevent adequate reduction of IOP. The presence of diabetes or treatment of systemic hypertension may accel-

erate glaucomatous changes of the optic disc despite maximum medical glaucoma therapy.

- Noncompliance can significantly affect the success of medical therapy.

LASER SURGERY

Since the late 1970s, argon laser trabeculoplasty (ALT) has been used to lower IOP in patients uncontrolled with maximum tolerated medical therapy.[187–194] The technique is performed at the slit lamp following topical anesthesia. After placement of a mirrored contact lens on the cornea, the operator places 50 to 100 "burns" evenly spaced on the anterior portion of the trabecular meshwork. Most clinicians initially treat only 180 of the angle, reserving the balance of the angle for later treatment, if indicated.[193,195] The procedure may produce an increase in aqueous outflow by opening the trabecular spaces due to the mechanical shrinkage of collagen at the burn sites.[195] Several investigators[196,197] have shown that laser trabeculoplasty induces mechanical, cellular, and biochemical changes within the trabecular meshwork, causing decreased outflow resistance.[198]

When first introduced into clinical practice, ALT was reserved for use only in patients who remained uncontrolled with maximum tolerated medical therapy. Now, however, some authors[172,190,199] advocate its use as primary therapy, even before attempting pharmacologic treatment. Although the indications for ALT are now more liberal than in the past, most clinicians favor using the procedure when patients cannot tolerate simple drug regimens or when noncompliance, drug tolerance, or advancing disease preclude the success of pharmacologic therapy[187,191,200] (Table 35.21). Contraindications to ALT are listed in Table 35.22.

Although the initial results of ALT can be impressive, the effectiveness of the procedure tends to decrease with time,[192,189,200] and most patients will continue to require medical therapy.[192,201] Pollack and associates[201] have shown that about 40% of eyes will require the prelaser medical regimen, while only about 20% can discontinue all prior medical therapy. Some patients, however, may be able to discontinue miotics or oral carbonic anhydrase inhibitors following ALT and can thus avoid annoying side effects from these medications. Although ALT can delay the need for filtering sur-

gery,[202] the probability of treatment success after 1 year is about 77%, at 5 years 50%, and 32% at 10 years.[203]

Several investigators[204–208] have studied the effectiveness of ALT used as primary therapy. Although the treatment protocols and definitions of success vary, the likelihood of a successful outcome at 4 years may be as high as 50%.[205] In the Glaucoma Laser Trial in the United States,[208] after 2 years of follow-up, 44% of "laser-first" eyes were controlled by ALT, 70% were controlled by ALT or ALT with timolol, and 89% were controlled within the specified medical regimen. In contrast, 30% of "medication-first" eyes remained controlled by timolol, and 66% were controlled within the specified medical regimen. There were no major differences between the two treatment approaches with respect to changes in visual acuity or visual field. Because of certain study design variables, however, these results have been controversial but do suggest the prospect of ALT as primary or early therapy in selected patients.

Table 35.23 lists the complications of ALT. Following the procedure, topical steroids are used routinely to control ocular inflammation, including anterior uveitis.[189,195] Although some patients do not need steroids, a regimen consisting of 1% prednisolone acetate 4 times daily for 5 to 7 days is effective in reducing both the incidence and severity of anterior uveal reactions. A more serious postlaser complication is acute elevation of IOP, which can lead to optic disc damage and further visual field loss in susceptible patients. Since the incidence of IOP elevations of 10 mm Hg or greater is 20% to 40% following ALT,[209] it is important to minimize these pressure responses to prevent iatrogenic glaucomatous damage. These IOP elevations can often be prevented or controlled by giving 4% pilocarpine postopera-

---

TABLE 35.21

Indications for Argon Laser Trabeculoplasty

- Medically uncontrolled POAG before filtering surgery
- Unacceptable side effects from medical therapy
- Poor compliance with medical therapy
- Patient inability to instill topical medications

Adapted from Goldberg I. Argon laser trabeculoplasty and the open-angle glaucomas. Aust NZ J Ophthalmol 1985;13:243–248.

TABLE 35.22

Contraindications to Argon Laser Trabeculoplasty

- Corneal opacities
- Extensive peripheral anterior synechiae
- Patient inability to cooperate at slit lamp

From Goldberg I. Argon laser trabeculoplasty and the open-angle glaucomas. Aust NZ J Ophthalmol 1985;13:243–248.

TABLE 35.23

Complications of Argon Laser Trabeculoplasty[209]

- Transient blurred vision
- Iritis
- Microhyphema
- Acute elevation of IOP
- Peripheral anterior synechiae
- Corneal burns
- Corneal edema

tively and monitoring IOP for 2 to 3 hours before dismissing the patient to regular postoperative care.[210] Currently, however, apraclonidine 1% (Iopidine), an α_2-adrenergic agonist, is commonly used 1 hour before laser treatment and immediately following ALT. This agent, which reduces IOP by inhibiting aqueous formation, is effective in reducing both the incidence and severity of acute postlaser IOP elevations.[211] The combined use of 4% pilocarpine and 1% apraclonidine can be even more effective than the use of either medication alone.[444]

FILTERING SURGERY AND OTHER TREATMENT MODALITIES

When ALT and maximum tolerated medical therapy fail to prevent further progression of optic disc damage and visual field loss, filtering surgery is indicated. Since the prognosis for retention of visual acuity and visual field is generally good following surgical intervention,[212] and since the risk of visual loss increases markedly in eyes with advanced glaucoma in which IOP exceeds 18 mm Hg, serious consideration should be given to a filtering procedure when the IOP is consistently over 22 mm Hg.[213]

Despite very definite risks, various filtering procedures may be used in an attempt to further reduce IOP. The most popular technique is trabeculectomy. This procedure involves providing a scleral filtration pathway to the subconjunctival space to allow the aqueous to escape. After a conjunctival flap is turned down over the cornea, a lamellar flap of sclera is created and the exposed corneo-trabecular block is excised. A peripheral iridectomy is performed, and the sclera and conjunctival flaps are replaced. This creates a filtering bleb at the site of aqueous drainage. (Fig. 35.11)

In recent years, arguments have been offered for earlier filtering surgery in patients with POAG.[214-217] There is evidence that earlier surgery may retain visual field better than the traditional medical approach,[215] and IOP may be significantly lower than in other treatment methods.[217] Successful surgery greatly reduces reliance on the patient for compliance with topical therapy. Although some studies[445] suggest that the preoperative use of topical antiglaucoma medication does not influence the outcome of surgery, prolonged medical therapy (>12 months) prior to filtering surgery may increase the risk of surgical failure.[218,446] This increased risk results from drug-induced inflammatory cells and fibroblasts that accelerate scarring and bleb failure following surgery.[219,220,447] Prolonged medical therapy may thus increase the need for antifibrotic agents, such as 5-fluorouracil or mitomycin,[216] which are themselves toxic (see Chap. 10). On the other hand, trabeculectomy can lead to serious surgical complications such as hypotony, endophthalmitis, and anesthesia-related morbidity.[214] It is clear that the specific therapy selected (i.e., medical vs. surgical) should be individualized for each patient after the risks and benefits of each approach are considered carefully. The most important consideration seems to be the level of IOP reduction

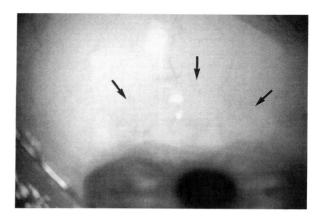

FIGURE 35.11　**Filtering bleb (arrows) at site of trabeculectomy.**

achieved by treatment. A similar reduction of IOP, whether achieved by medicine, laser, or surgery, would be expected to have the same ultimate effect on visual field preservation.[448]

Various procedures may be carried out to destroy ciliary body function, thereby decreasing aqueous production. These techniques, known as *cilioablative procedures*, are reserved for cases that are resistant to control by standard filtering operations. *Cyclocryotherapy* uses transcleral freezing of the ciliary body at multiple locations.[221,222] A modification of this procedure can be performed using the Nd:YAG laser rather than freezing.[223]

Setons, tubes placed in the anterior chamber to drain aqueous to the subconjunctival space, are also used in some patients with end-stage glaucoma or a high risk of trabeculectomy failure. Such drainage systems include the Baerveldt or Molteno implant (Fig. 35.12) and the anterior chamber tube shunt to encircling band procedure.[224,225]

Another approach currently receiving attention is strenuous aerobic exercise training. Passo and associates[226] have shown that after 3 months of exercise training, mean IOP decreased 4.6 mm Hg (20%). With cessation of exercise, however, IOP returned to preconditioning levels. Regular aerobic exercise may represent an effective nonpharmacologic intervention for patients with early glaucoma.[226,227]

Normal-Tension (Low-Tension) Glaucoma

Etiology

Traditionally, the term *low-tension glaucoma* has applied to the patient with typical glaucomatous optic disc damage, visual field losses, and open anterior chamber angles, but with statistically "normal" IOP ($\leq$ 21 mm Hg). Recent evidence, however, discounts the traditional distinction be-

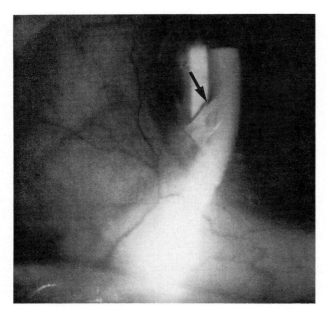

FIGURE 35.12   **Molteno drainage tube (arrow) in anterior chamber. (Courtesy Lyman Norden, O.D.)**

tween "low-tension" and "high-tension" glaucoma.[12] Adding to the apparent paradox of glaucomatous damage in the presence of "normal" IOP is the fact that some patients with normal IOP, disc damage, and visual field loss have stable visual acuity and visual fields even if left untreated, while others progress relentlessly despite aggressive lowering of IOP from its "normal" levels. Normal-tension glaucoma (NTG) remains an enigma, and many patients with NTG will have progressive deterioration of visual field despite our best efforts.

Investigators have been unable to develop a precise description of the pathogenesis of NTG. Aqueous dynamics appear to be similar to those in POAG.[228] Although visual field damage is almost always greater in the eye with the higher IOP,[229] other factors may also play a role in the development of visual field defects. Reduced optic nerve perfusion appears to be an important factor in some patients,[230] but generalized vascular disease of an atheromatous or hyperviscous nature has not been shown to play an important pathogenic role.[231] Instead, localized or vasospastic processes within the optic disc itself may produce local disc damage and associated visual field loss,[231,232] independent of IOP. Using magnetic resonance imaging, Stroman and associates[449] found diffuse cerebral small-vessel ischemic changes more often in patients with NTG than normal controls, providing indirect evidence of a vascular cause for the optic neuropathy. Humoral immune mechanisms may also play a role in the pathogenesis of this condition.[450]

Diagnosis

There are considerable racial differences in the prevalence of NTG. In Caucasians, the prevalence is approximately 15% of all patients with primary open-angle glaucoma.[233]

The differential diagnosis includes the disorders listed in Table 35.24. Many patients assumed to have NTG may actually have one of the following conditions:

- "Burned-out" open-angle glaucoma. These patients have had moderate POAG or pigmentary glaucoma for many years that produced the damage. When they are examined in later years, the damage is evident and they have normal or low IOP because of aqueous hyposecretion presumed to be due to ciliary body atrophy and advancing age. Even though the pressure is not high, damage may still be occurring. The appropriate treatment is usually filtering surgery if the damage is progressive.
- Patients with high diurnal variations. Some patients with visual field loss and optic disc changes will have IOPs of 17 to 19 mm Hg at certain times of the day and 28 to 30 mm Hg at other times. In other cases, patients' systemic medications (e.g., β-blockers for systemic hypertension) may mask high IOP. These patients may have POAG and should be treated as such.

TABLE 35.24
Differential Diagnosis of Normal-Tension Glaucoma

Nonprogressive	*Progressive*
Burned-out open-angle glaucoma	Internal carotid artery obstruction
Burned-out steroid glaucoma	Cavernous sinus fistula
Burned-out pigmentary glaucoma	Orbital varices
Burned-out uveitic glaucoma	Sturge-Weber syndrome
Hemodynamic shock	Optic atrophy
Resolved AION	Drug-induced optic neuropathy
Resolved elevated episcleral venous pressure (e.g., thyroid ophthalmopathy)	POAG with large diurnal variations of IOP
Optic nerve pit	Intermittent or chronic angle-closure glaucoma
Optic disc coloboma	Pituitary tumor
Tilted disc syndrome	Optic nerve tumor
Optic disc drusen (may be slowly progressive)	

AION = anterior ischemic optic neuropathy; POAG = primary open-angle glaucoma; IOP = intraocular pressure.

Modified from Cockburn DM, Gutteridge IF. Low-tension glaucoma. In: Lewis TL, Fingeret M. Primary care of the glaucomas. Norwalk, CT: Appleton & Lange, 1993:323–346.

- Patients with history of cardiovascular disease. Some patients with normal or low IOP, visual field loss, and optic disc changes may have histories of severe internal bleeding, low systemic blood pressure, myocardial infarction, or serious arrhythmia that produced a sudden and somewhat prolonged decrease in systemic blood pressure, resulting in ischemia of the optic nerve with glaucomatous disc changes and visual field losses.[234] This is more likely to occur in patients with myopia and preexisting large physiologic cupping. Generally no treatment is necessary if the cardiovascular problems have been treated properly. An increased prevalence of optic disc hemorrhages in patients with NTG[235] indicates the presence of a possible ischemic factor in the pathogenesis of this disorder.
- Patients with hereditary optic atrophy. These patients have low IOP, optic disc changes, and glaucoma-like visual field losses. A complete examination and thorough history, including a genetic evaluation, are necessary to determine the correct diagnosis. No medical or surgical treatment is effective.

Several investigators[236–240] have compared the optic discs in NTG and POAG and have concluded that the neuroretinal rim in NTG is significantly thinner than in POAG, especially in the inferior and inferotemporal areas. These differences, however, may be present even before visual field defects occur.[237] When analyzed by computerized imaging techniques, optic disc topography appears to be similar in patients with either POAG or NTG.[238] Cupping in NTG is often broadly sloping (shallow),[238] and the disc size is often larger than in POAG.[239] Focal notching of the neuroretinal rim appears to be more common in patients with NTG than with POAG,[241] but the degree of parapapillary halo or crescent appears to be the same in POAG and NTG.[242]

Although some investigators have shown the pattern of visual field defects in NTG to differ from those in POAG,[243–246] others have demonstrated that the visual field losses are similar.[238] The rate of visual field progression in NTG is generally greater than in patients with POAG.[244]

It is important to rule out intracranial and other neurologic causes of increased cupping in the presence of normal IOP. Several types of compressive lesions of the optic nerve or chiasm can induce cupping resembling that seen in NTG.[451] Neuroradiologic studies may be needed to distinguish glaucomatous cupping from compressive lesions.

Management

The significant risk factors that can contribute to NTG must be sought out and corrected, if possible. These conditions include incipient cardiac failure, paroxysmal arrhythmias, and therapy of systemic hypertension.[185] It is not necessary to treat the group of patients who have had a preceding hemodynamic crisis because the likelihood of further pro-

TABLE 35.25
Practical Evaluation of Patients with Suspected NTG

- Careful cardiovascular history
    Profound blood loss
    Shock
    Myocardial infarction
    Arrhythmia
    Stroke
- Signs or symptoms of temporal arteritis?[a]
    Temporal pain or headache
    Pain on chewing
    Elevated erythrocyte sedimentation rate (ESR)
- Blood pressure
- Pulse
- Evidence of carotid bruits?
    Carotid auscultation
- Evidence of optic disc drusen?
    Fundus biomicroscopy
    B-scan ultrasonography
- Evidence of "burned out" pigmentary or uveitic glaucoma?
    Slit lamp examination
    Gonioscopy
- Repeat IOP at different times of day

[a]In patients over age 60 years.

gression of the glaucomatous damage is remote. These patients can be considered to have a stable, nonprogressive optic neuropathy. It is reasonable to monitor without treatment all patients with suspected NTG for 6 to 12 months to ascertain progression of the optic discs and visual fields. When evidence of progression occurs, treatment can then be initiated.[233,247] A practical evaluation strategy, such as the one shown in Table 35.25, can be useful in selecting patients who may need earlier intervention.

Patients with progressive optic nerve damage and visual field loss should be treated aggressively. Marked IOP reduction can often be achieved and maintained on a long-term basis using a medical regimen consisting of a β blocker with or without pilocarpine.[248,249] Laser trabeculoplasty (ALT) is often employed.[248] Filtering surgery, however, not only effectively lowers IOP, but it has also been shown to slow further progression of visual field loss.[250]

Laser treatment or filtering surgery should be considered only after weighing the potential benefits and risks. Although not as effective in NTG as in patients with higher baseline IOPs,[251] ALT can further reduce the IOP to clinically acceptable levels that may slow the progression of optic disc damage and visual field loss.[252] Schwartz and associates[251] showed that ALT was clinically successful in 73% of patients with progressive NTG, and the procedure decreased the mean peak pressure during the diurnal curve, confirming the usefulness of laser therapy as an alternative to filtering surgery.

It is often difficult to determine the effectiveness of filtering surgery, since the natural course of visual field loss in NTG is less certain than in POAG. Thus, it may be less advisable to operate on the elderly patient with NTG who has a limited life expectancy than on the same patient with POAG. The spectrum of surgical results ranges from being completely ineffective to being occasionally successful.[253] In cases of NTG that are definitely progressive, surgery is likely to be more successful if the preoperative baseline IOP is in the upper normal range.[253] If filtering surgery is considered, it should be performed before visual field loss involves fixation. Abedin and associates[254] reported successful management of progressive NTG by performing filtering surgery to reduce the IOP to 10 mm Hg or less.

A recent strategy in treating NTG involves the use of oral Ca^{++} channel antagonists. In this novel approach, IOP control is essentially disregarded in favor of preventing or controlling local vasospastic processes within the optic nerve head. Although Lumme and associates[255] have shown no favorable influences on optic nerve progression using nifedipine, other investigators[256–258] have demonstrated either improvement or less progression of visual field or optic nerve changes. Kitazawa and associates[256] concluded that visual field is likely to improve with oral nifedipine in patients who are young, have less initial visual field loss, lower IOP, and have less reduction in diastolic blood pressure with nifedipine administration. In contrast to patients with NTG, patients with POAG seem to receive no benefit from Ca^{++} antagonists.[258] Calcium antagonist therapy may become an important part of the medical treatment of selected patients with NTG.

Ocular Hypertension

Definition

The term *ocular hypertension* is controversial. It was developed from a practical clinical perspective. Patients exhibiting high IOPs (greater than 21 mm Hg), open anterior chamber angles, healthy-appearing optic discs, and no visual field losses are said to have ocular hypertension. Other terms such as "glaucoma suspect" are sometimes used. Although some patients with IOPs greater than 21 mm Hg will develop glaucoma, most will not, so that any classifying term using the word *glaucoma* seems inappropriate. Furthermore, use of any term that includes "glaucoma" frightens the patient and may carry legal and employment consequences. Regardless of the terminology, since a large number of these patients does exist, it is essential for the practitioner to understand the condition and to develop a systematic approach to its management.

Epidemiology

The prevalence of ocular hypertension in patients over age 40 years is 3% to 8%.[259] Cockburn[260] evaluated 1000 consecutive adult patients in a private optometric practice and classified 5.4% as having ocular hypertension.

The incidence of glaucoma in patients with ocular hypertension who have been monitored for several years is very low.[259] Cockburn[260] reviewed 21 studies that reported long-term follow-up evaluations of ocular hypertensive patients. Although different criteria for ocular hypertension were used, different lengths of follow-up time were involved, and although there were considerable variations in the findings, the evaluation probably yields useful information. The 21 studies included 2178 ocular hypertensive patients, and 10.6% were found to have progressed to true glaucoma. Long-term follow-up has shown that, each year, visual field defects and/or optic disc damage develop in about 1% of ocular hypertensive patients.[261]

Diagnosis

The diagnosis of ocular hypertension is relatively straightforward. Those patients with open anterior chamber angles, healthy-appearing optic discs, and no visual field loss but with IOPs greater than 21 mm Hg on two or more occasions have ocular hypertension.

Management

The management of patients with ocular hypertension can be a challenging clinical problem. The problem is identifying the ocular hypertensive patients who will develop glaucomatous damage. Although definitive predictive information is not yet available, the evaluation of risk factors is very helpful.

Levene[262] has classified the most significant risk factors according to their importance in contributing to early optic disc damage and visual field loss (Table 35.26). The decision to treat ocular hypertension may be based solely on the more important factors, sometimes in combination with the less important factors, but the decision is rarely based solely on the less important factors.

Although color vision testing and evaluation of the pattern electroretinogram (PERG) have been advocated to identify patients who may be destined for glaucomatous damage,[263,264] it is generally agreed that it is not yet possible to predict, with precision, which individual patients with ocular hypertension will eventually develop glaucomatous visual field loss. A management decision for each ocular hypertensive patient must be made—to treat or to monitor without treatment. The prevailing management guideline is

TABLE 35.26
Risk Factors in Ocular Hypertension

More Important Factors	Less Important Factors
• Suspicious visual field	• Age and longevity
• Optic disc changes	• General vascular disease
• Retinal nerve fiber layer defects	• Unreliability in follow-up
• IOP elevation or asymmetry	• Poor cooperation in testing
• Useful vision in only 1 eye	• Psychological considerations
• Family history of glaucoma	• Myopia
• Idiopathic retinal vascular occlusion	

Modified from Levene RZ. Indications for medical treatment of ocular hypertension and the initial use of pilocarpine. Surv Ophthalmol 1980;25:183–187; Quigley HA, Enger C, Katz J, et al. Risk factors for the development of glaucomatous visual field loss in ocular hypertension. Arch Ophthalmol 1994;112:644–649; Jonas JB, Konigsreuther KA. Optic disk appearance in ocular hypertensive eyes. Am J Ophthalmol 1994;117:732–740.

to weigh carefully the benefits of "early" or "prophylactic" therapy against the risks of medication cost and side effects, noncompliance, and glaucomatous visual field loss. Despite the lack of convincing evidence for the effectiveness of "prophylactic" treatment, it is estimated that 1.5 million patients with ocular hypertension in the United States are being treated with ocular hypotensive medications.[259]

SELECTING PATIENTS FOR TREATMENT

There is no general agreement that reducing IOP in ocular hypertensive patients lowers the risk of developing glaucomatous damage.[259] Recent studies are almost equally divided on whether treatment does[265,266] or does not[261] prevent or delay the onset of visual field loss or optic disc changes. Despite medical therapy, some patients with ocular hypertension will develop glaucomatous damage. Moreover, medical therapy is often expensive and inconvenient, and it may produce adverse psychological effects. The side effects of medication can contribute to noncompliance in some patients. Thus, it is wise to carefully select patients for treatment based on the presence of substantial risk factors rather than to provide treatment for all patients with ocular hypertension.

The management decision should include an evaluation of systemic risk factors. Younger patients are likely to be treated more aggressively than are older patients because of their longer life expectancy.[267] Patients with one or more vascular diseases are more likely to be treated. These include diabetes, cerebrovascular disease, cardiac disease, and patients with systemic hypertension undergoing treatment. Levene,[262] however, believes that systemic vascular disease probably has only a weak association with glaucomatous

visual field loss. Elderly patients (over 70 years of age) with IOPs greater than 26 mm Hg who also have systemic vascular disease should probably be treated because of the increased risk of retinal vein occlusion.[268–270] However, if such patients have IOPs lower than 26 mm Hg, there is probably no advantage in prescribing treatment. In addition, patient lifestyle as well as attitude toward and understanding of the condition will help to determine patient reliability in complying with the proposed management plan.

The management decision may be based primarily on the elevated IOP. This decision is justified if reliable visual fields cannot be obtained because of poor patient cooperation. Patients who have normal visual fields and optic discs, and IOPs greater than 30 mm Hg, should receive treatment regardless of the presence or absence of other significant risk factors. Most practitioners consider the risk of impending visual field loss to be substantial when the IOP exceeds 30 mm Hg, regardless of the absence of other risk factors.

The practitioner may decide to treat based primarily on the optic disc changes. Progression of optic disc changes is an important indication for treatment even if visual field loss is not apparent or is unreliable. These patients likely have early POAG.

The management decision may be based primarily on visual field changes. If any consistent, reliable glaucomatous visual field change is present, it is essential that treatment be provided.

It has been reported that the use of medications in the treatment of ocular hypertension can improve compliance in patient follow-up by implying seriousness of the condition and by providing a daily reminder to the patient that an abnormal condition exists.[168] However, the institution of treatment for this reason alone cannot be advocated because of documented high noncompliance rates among the patients who are treated.[168] Instead, the decision to treat patients with ocular hypertension must be individualized by considering the major risk factors, with the potential for noncompliance being of secondary importance.

The existence of multiple risk factors increases the justification for medical therapy. Yablonski and associates[271] reported that patients with a mean IOP of 28 mm Hg or higher and a vertical C/D ratio of 0.6 or greater had a 100% incidence of glaucomatous visual field loss in 5 years. Under ideal situations it is probably more important to emphasize evaluation of the optic discs and visual fields rather than to rely on IOP, even though the only single risk factor that has been proved in prospective studies to be a valid predictor of glaucomatous visual field loss is the level of IOP.[268] However, when a dense cataract prevents adequate examination of the optic disc, or when the visual fields are unreliable, the IOP assumes greater importance. The evaluation of multiple risk factors in the decision to treat ocular hypertension is summarized in Table 35.27.[3262] This table illustrates seven specific clinical situations, with an approximate ranking of

TABLE 35.27
The Decision to Treat Ocular Hypertension Based on Six Risk Factors

	Visual Field	Optic Disc	Intraocular Pressure	Useful Vision in Only One Eye	Family History of Glaucoma	Retinal Vascular Occlusion
1	—	Abnormal	—	—	—	—
2	—	—	>30	—	—	—
3	Suspect	Suspect	—	—	—	—
4	—	Suspect	Progressive elevation or asymmetry	—	—	—
5	—	Suspect	—	+	—	—
6	—	Suspect	—	—	+	—
9	—	Suspect	—	—	—	+

Modified from Levene RZ. Indications for medical treatment of ocular hypertension and the initial use of pilocarpine. Surv Ophthalmol 1980;25:183–187.

the relative importance of six major risk factors from left to right. The importance of the optic disc is emphasized, since it is involved in six of the seven clinical situations. One risk factor alone is sufficient to justify treatment in two cases—a definitely abnormal optic disc or an IOP repeatedly over 30 mm Hg. A combination of two risk factors is sufficient to justify treatment in the remaining situations.

MEDICAL THERAPY

Most practitioners favor the use of β blockers for the initial medical therapy of patients with ocular hypertension. These drugs do not produce the miosis and accommodative spasm characteristic of pilocarpine, and their long-term effectiveness and side effects have been established. If the β blocker causes undesirable side effects or is contraindicated, dorzolamide, dipivefrin, or pilocarpine may be used.[272,273] Medications such as acetazolamide and echothiophate should be avoided because of their greater potentials for adverse effects. In addition, laser trabeculoplasty or filtering surgery is clearly without justification in patients with normal optic discs and visual fields, except in cases with extremely high IOP not controlled medically.

In the treatment of patients with ocular hypertension, it must be emphasized that medical therapy is elective, not imperative.[274] The practitioner should respect the wishes of the patient who prefers treatment despite the absence of significant risk factors.[272,273] In many instances it is acceptable to provide medical therapy as long as it does not cause severe drug-related side effects and the patient has been informed about[275]: (1) the individual risk factors present; (2) the insidious, painless nature of primary open-angle glaucoma; (3) the generally permanent nature of lost vision; (4) the treatable nature of primary open-angle glaucoma, especially in its early stages; (5) the low incidence of developing visual field changes; and (6) the economic aspects of life-long treatment.

MONITORING THE PATIENT WITHOUT TREATMENT

Although most patients with ocular hypertension can be managed without medical therapy, these patients must be monitored carefully so that treatment can be instituted before significant glaucomatous damage occurs. Patients who appear to be least likely to develop such changes are those having normal visual fields and optic discs, IOPs between 21 and 30 mm Hg, and no other significant risk factors. Unfortunately, ocular hypertensive patients not receiving medical therapy do not return for follow-up examinations as often as do ocular hypertensives who are receiving treatment. Bigger[168] found that over a 12- to 20-month period, 37% of ocular hypertensive patients were lost to follow-up evaluation. Noncompliance rates were highest in patients who were not prescribed medical therapy. The majority of noncompliant patients were lost to follow-up within 1 month following the initial diagnosis. Such high noncompliance rates can be decreased by careful patient education.

During the initial examination, complete baseline information should be obtained, including documentation of the appearance of the optic discs (preferably with stereophotography or computerized imaging techniques), visual fields, tonometry, gonioscopy, and evaluation of risk factors. According to the availability and reliability of the diagnostic information and clinical history, each patient's follow-up may be individualized according to the following general guidelines[274,276]: (1) reevaluate at yearly intervals if the IOP is 20 to 24 mm Hg, (2) reevaluate every 6 months if the IOP is 25 to 29 mm Hg, and (3) reevaluate every 3 or 4 months if the IOP is 30 mm Hg or higher if the decision is made to withhold treatment. Each follow-up visit should include evaluation of IOPs, visual fields, careful stereoscopic examination of the optic discs, and reevaluation of risk factors by assessing the ocular, medical, and family history. Since diurnal variations of IOP can make these general guidelines arbitrary, clinical judgment must always remain sovereign.

Primary Angle-Closure Glaucoma

Angle-closure glaucoma is caused by an anatomic obstruction of the anterior chamber angle, decreasing aqueous drainage from the eye. The reduced aqueous outflow increases the IOP. Tomlinson and Leighton[19] compared the ocular dimensions of patients with primary angle-closure glaucoma to those of matched normal control subjects and found that patients with primary angle-closure glaucoma have smaller corneal diameters and thicker crystalline lenses positioned more anteriorly than do normals. Thus, the anterior chamber depth is a useful diagnostic sign for identifying patients with primary angle-closure glaucoma and patients who are at risk for it.

Primary angle-closure glaucoma associated with pupillary block can be classified as acute, subacute, or chronic. There is a continuum from acute angle-closure glaucoma to chronic angle-closure glaucoma in symptoms and, to a lesser extent, in signs. Sudden, dramatic, severe, and persistent symptoms characterize acute angle closure, while episodic or recurrent symptoms indicate subacute angle closure. Chronic angle-closure glaucoma has few if any symptoms.

Acute Angle-Closure Glaucoma

DIAGNOSIS

This condition is a true ocular emergency. A sudden significant increase in IOP occurs with dilation of vessels at the limbus, steamy cornea, and mid-dilated pupil that is unreactive to light (Fig. 35.13), symptoms of blurred vision, colored rings around point sources of light, ocular pain and discomfort, nausea, and often vomiting. The "attack" follows sudden obstruction of the trabecular meshwork. If the patient is not treated, loss of vision can occur within 24 hours, and blindness may follow in 2 or 3 days.[277]

The clinical examination consists of history, biomicroscopy, gonioscopy, and tonometry. If corneal edema is significant, the use of topical glycerin (75% to 100%) following topical anesthesia will often reduce the edema so that gonioscopy can be performed. In some cases, use of glycerin as the gonioscopic bonding solution hastens the reduction of corneal edema by prolonging drug contact with the cornea.

Because of the discomfort and accompanying signs, the diagnosis of acute angle-closure glaucoma is usually

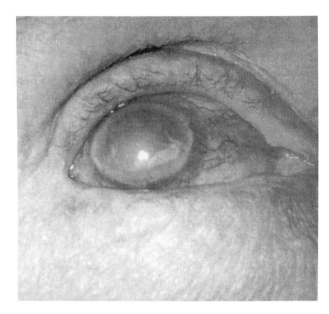

FIGURE 35.13 **Conjunctival hyperemia, corneal edema, and fixed, mid-dilated pupil in 72-year-old male with acute angle-closure glaucoma.**

straightforward. The patient is often an older, hyperopic individual with a small globe and a significantly narrow anterior chamber angle.[278,279] There is often a history of mild "attacks." In some instances, acute angle-closure glaucoma can be iatrogenically induced by routine pupillary dilation or by use of nebulized anticholinergic bronchodilators for treatment of chronic obstructive pulmonary disease.[280–282]

MANAGEMENT

Because the mechanism of acute angle closure almost always relates to pupillary block and subsequent iris bombé, the initial treatment involves use of mild miotics to break the pupillary block, pull the iris away from the angle, and reduce the IOP, followed by the use of laser iridotomy to eliminate the obstruction of aqueous flow from the posterior to the anterior chamber.[283]

Acute angle-closure glaucoma should be regarded as a true ocular emergency, and the immediate reduction of IOP is crucial to minimize vision loss. This reduction is usually achieved with the use of topically administered pilocarpine, β blocker, or apraclonidine,[284] along with orally administered isosorbide or glycerin, and parenteral or oral acetazolamide (Fig. 35.14). Although any of these medications, when used alone, may be sufficient to relieve the angle-closure attack, the combined use of several medications increases the chance of terminating the attack and shortening

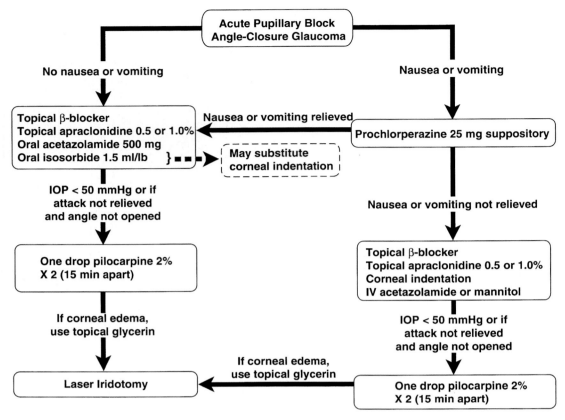

FIGURE 35.14   **Flowchart for the management of acute pupillary block angle-closure glaucoma.**

its duration.[285] Since the acute episode rarely resolves without medical treatment and may cause significant ocular damage, it is imperative to relieve the attack promptly. Following medical reduction of IOP, a laser iridotomy is indicated.

Pilocarpine concentrations exceeding 2% are contraindicated because these concentrations are no more effective than the 2% concentration. In addition, such strong miotics can cause further shallowing of the anterior chamber, leading to intensified pupillary block, permanent peripheral synechiae, and permanent angle closure.[285–287] For these reasons anticholinesterase agents such as echothiophate are contraindicated.

In the early stages of the attack, pilocarpine often is ineffective in producing miosis because of ischemia of the iris sphincter caused by IOP exceeding 50 to 55 mm Hg.[287] Once the IOP has been reduced by drugs that decrease aqueous formation or withdraw intraocular water (acetazolamide, a β blocker, apraclonidine, or isosorbide), normal blood flow is reinstated to the iris sphincter, which then responds to the pilocarpine.[287] Thus, the instillation of pilocarpine should often be delayed until the IOP has been reduced to levels that permit normal activity of the iris sphincter.[288] At that time, one drop of 2% pilocarpine can be instilled twice during a 15-minute interval. When this regimen is followed, excessive doses of pilocarpine become unnecessary.[286] This also eliminates the systemic side effects associated with the more traditional dosage recommendations, which administer approximately 40 to 80 mg of pilocarpine.[289] The symptoms of nausea, diaphoresis, and weakness frequently experienced by patients undergoing acute angle closure are often attributed to the glaucoma attacks themselves; however, these symptoms may also be associated with systemic pilocarpine toxicity.

In addition to the topical instillation of pilocarpine, apraclonidine, and a β blocker, the systemic administration of various drugs will hasten reduction of intraocular pressure. If the patient is not nauseated or vomiting, acetazolamide 500 mg and glycerin 1.5 g/kg body weight should be administered orally.[290] Glycerin is best tolerated if administered chilled, and the entire dose should be consumed within 5 minutes.[290] Isosorbide, however, is often the hyperosmotic of choice since this agent generally causes less nausea and does not induce hyperglycemia, making it safer for use in diabetic patients. If the patient is vomiting, oral drug administration is impossible, and the patient should be given the acetazolamide intravenously. Alternatively, the topical administration of apraclonidine and timolol or other β blocker may be substituted for acetazolamide. The use of topical 0.5% timolol, 2 drops within 1 hour, is effective in reducing the IOP to a level that permits pilocarpine to activate the iris sphincter and terminate the angle-closure attack.[291] Analgesics may be administered in cases of severe pain (see Chap. 7), and antiemetic agents, such as 25 mg prochlorperazine (Compazine) as a suppository, often relieve nausea or vomiting.

As an alternative to the use of oral hyperosmotics, a corneal indentation maneuver has been described by Anderson.[292] This procedure involves the use of a cotton-tipped applicator or Goldmann applanation prism to indent the cornea (Fig. 35.15), thereby deepening the anterior chamber and allowing aqueous to escape from the anterior chamber. This maneuver serves the same purpose as do hyperosmotic agents—the removal of intraocular fluid leading to reduced IOP and relief of iris sphincter ischemia. Thus, the procedure may be used in lieu of hyperosmotic agents. Following gonioscopy for the initial diagnostic evaluation, the cornea is indented for about 30 seconds followed by release of indentation for another 30 seconds. This process is continued for 15 to 20 minutes. The intermittent release of indentation reduces the risk of central retinal artery occlusion. The patient need not be positioned at the slit lamp, since the procedure can be performed with a hand-held device while the patient relaxes in the examination chair. It should be emphasized that this technique does not replace the need for pilocarpine, acetazolamide, or β-blockers because these agents help to prevent the immediate recurrence of angle closure during the interval before laser surgery. In addition, since this procedure is ineffective in eyes with total peripheral anterior synechiae and rubeosis, hyperosmotic agents and aqueous suppressants will be necessary in these eyes.[292]

The patient should be reevaluated periodically during the initial 2 or 3 hours of medical therapy. The desired response is a reduction of IOP, pupillary constriction, and deepening of the anterior chamber. After 2 or 3 hours of therapy, usually 1 of 3 responses is observed[283,290]: (1) The eye may become stable following termination of the attack, as evidenced by opening of the anterior chamber and reduction of IOP to normal levels. If the IOP has been reduced to normal levels and gonioscopy reveals entirely open angles, the condition is arrested temporarily, but it may recur even with the use of miotic therapy. Thus, the patient should proceed to laser surgery within 1 or 2 days, since it is impossible to predict which patients will have recurrence of the acute angle-closure episode. (2) The IOP may decrease to normal or subnormal levels, but gonioscopy may reveal much or all of the angle to have remained closed. In such cases the low pressure is the result of a reduction of aqueous formation caused by the acetazolamide, apraclonidine, or β blocker, or by the hyperosmotic effect of the isosorbide or glycerin

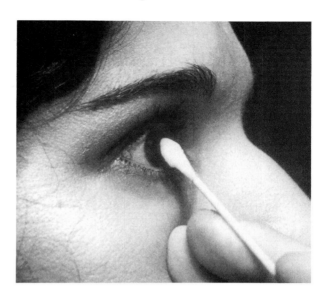

FIGURE 35.15 **Corneal indentation using cotton-tipped applicator.**

rather than a result of improvement in aqueous outflow. These patients should proceed to laser surgery within 2 to 4 hours. (3) The eye may be totally unresponsive to medical therapy, as evidenced by persistence of a considerably elevated IOP, a mid-dilated pupil, and a closed angle. Laser iridotomy or surgical peripheral iridectomy should be performed on such eyes within 2 to 4 hours.

Despite the success of pharmacologic therapy in lowering IOP and deepening the anterior chamber, surgical intervention is indicated to reduce the risk of a subsequent attack. Laser iridotomy is the treatment of choice.[293,294] Laser therapy has several advantages over surgical iridectomy, including simplicity, reduced cost, fewer complications, and the fact that it can be performed on an outpatient basis.[295,296] Although treatment with either argon or Nd:YAG laser can cause complications (Table 35.28), Nd:YAG laser iridotomy appears to be the preferred procedure in most patients because of its effectiveness and reduced complication rate.[293]

The laser iridotomy establishes a communication between the posterior and anterior chambers (Fig. 35.16), thus permitting aqueous to enter the anterior chamber. If the iridotomy remains patent, the laser procedure will generally protect the eye from further angle-closure attacks. For neglected cases of angle closure, in which the eye has been untreated for periods exceeding 48 hours and the IOP cannot be reduced with miotics or β blockers, iridotomy may succeed in completely normalizing the IOP.[297] In some cases of phacomorphic glaucoma, however, the angle closure will remain uncontrolled until cataract extraction is performed.[298,299] In other instances, miotic therapy[300] or argon

TABLE 35.28
Complications of Laser Iridotomy

- Iridotomy closure
- Corneal opacities/burns
- Microhyphema
- Reduced visual acuity
- Lenticular opacities
- Corectopia
- Hypopyon
- Transient elevation of IOP
- Posterior synechiae
- Anterior uveitis
- Retinal burns
- Malignant glaucoma (aqueous misdirection)
- Endophthalmitis

IOP = intraocular pressure.

laser iridoplasty[301,302] may be successful in treating angle-closure glaucoma unrelieved by laser iridotomy. Iridoplasty involves argon laser applications to the peripheral iris stroma to retract the iris and open the anterior chamber, a procedure especially helpful in cases of nonpupillary block angle closure.

Pilocarpine 2% can be instilled 20 or 30 minutes before laser treatment if a miotic has not been administered previously. This produces a stretched and thinned iris, allowing easier iridotomy. It also avoids motion of the pupil during the procedure.[303,304] Postoperatively, IOP increases in 25% to 40% of eyes undergoing laser iridotomy and has a peak incidence between 1 and 3 hours after the procedure.[303] Although these pressure spikes are transient, resolving within several days, it is important to protect against large pressure increases, particularly in patients with severe glaucomatous damage. To this end, many practitioners use topical β-blockers or oral carbonic anhydrase inhibitors postoperatively, as necessary.[295,303–305] Alternatively, topical apraclonidine 1% (Iopidine) can be administered 1 hour before laser surgery and immediately on completion of the procedure.[211,306,307] Topical steroids are also used postoperatively to reduce the inflammatory reaction and can be tapered from a dosage frequency of every 6 hours on the day of laser therapy to discontinuation after 4 or 5 days.

Angle-closure glaucoma eventually becomes bilateral in up to 70% of patients.[307] Thus, it is imperative that patients sustaining an acute angle-closure episode in one eye undergo prophylactic laser iridotomy in the fellow eye. The fact that optic nerve damage occurs within hours of the initial elevation in IOP emphasizes the need for routine prophylactic iridotomy in fellow eyes.[308,309] This can be performed at the same time that the initial eye receives treatment.[309]

Subacute and Chronic Angle-Closure Glaucoma

DIAGNOSIS

A subacute angle-closure attack requires prompt diagnosis and appropriate management, in part to avoid a possible acute attack in the future. The symptoms, although transient, are similar to those in acute angle-closure glaucoma (Table 35.29). These symptoms are present more often when the patient is tired, angry, worried, in a poorly lighted room, or during periods of inactivity or following emotional stress. These conditions are often associated with a mydriatic pupil.

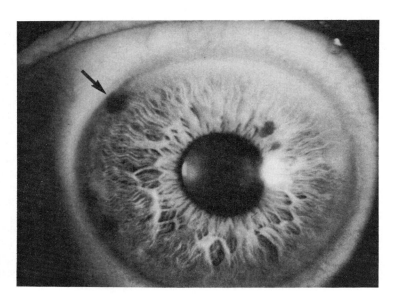

FIGURE 35.16   **Nd:YAG laser iridotomy (arrow). (From Catania LJ, Lewis TL, eds. Primary care of glaucoma. Dresher, PA: Primary Eyecare, 1986.)**

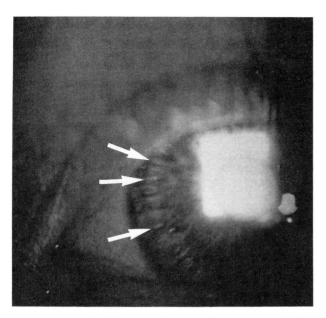

FIGURE 35.22   **Slit-like areas of iris transillumination typical of PDS. Arrows denote representative defects.**

belief that they reduce iridozonular contact and consequently decrease further pigment liberation. There is evidence to support such an approach (Fig. 35.23), but caution must be observed during miotic therapy because of the relatively high incidence of drug-induced retinal detachment.[342] Topical or oral carbonic anhydrase inhibitors may be employed according to the usual guidelines governing these drugs. They may be effective on a short-term basis during acute elevations of IOP. It has been speculated that dapiprazole or thymoxamine, α-adrenergic blocking agents, should be beneficial in these patients by constricting the pupil without affecting accommodation, thereby minimizing the iridozonular contact. This would tend to eliminate pigment release and accumulation in the trabecular meshwork.[337] Karickhoff,[350] however, has shown in a small number of patients that dapiprazole seems to increase, rather than decrease, iridozonular contact. Chronic drug-induced conjunctival hyperemia and variable miosis also argue against such an approach.

Many individuals with PDS or pigmentary glaucoma may have a shower of pigment into the angle following vigorous exercise. The immediate effect on IOP, however, appears to be negligible.[343,344] Patients with PDS or pigmentary glaucoma need not avoid exercise, and if marked exercise-induced pigment dispersion occurs, topical pilocarpine can be used before exercise to minimize the effect on pigment release.[344]

In some patients with pigmentary glaucoma, the pigment

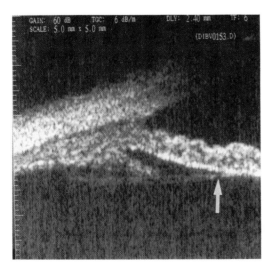

A

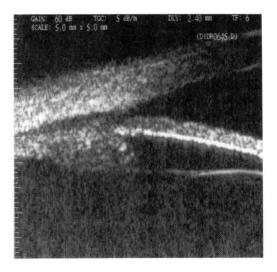

B

FIGURE 35.23   **Ultrasound biomicroscopy demonstrates effect of miotics on iridozonular contact.** *(A)* **Premiotic scan shows iris concavity and iridozonular touch (arrow).** *(B)* **Postmiotic scan shows convex iris configuration, deepening of posterior chamber, and resolution of iridozonular contact. (From Potash SD, Tello C, Liebmann J, Ritch R. Ultrasound biomicroscopy in pigment dispersion syndrome. Ophthalmology 1994;101:332–339.)**

decreases in the trabecular meshwork with time (years). Medical therapy can then be decreased or discontinued. Patients with glaucomatous damage may later be diagnosed erroneously as having normal-tension glaucoma.[341] Likewise, in pigmentary glaucoma associated with posterior chamber intraocular lenses (IOLs), the intensity of the glaucoma lessens with time as the pigment liberation from the localized area of IOL-iris contact decreases.[345,346] In the meantime, use of routine antiglaucoma medications is usually effective in controlling the pressure and preventing optic disc damage. Severe glaucoma not controlled medically may require repositioning of the IOL, laser trabeculoplasty, or trabeculectomy. Removal of the offending IOL is not generally advisable because of surgical complications.[345]

In patients for whom simple medical regimens do not allow adequate control of IOP, laser trabeculoplasty should be attempted.[338,340] This procedure seems to have a long-term efficacy similar to that in patients with POAG.[321] Although the initial effect on IOP may decline rapidly,[347] Ritch and associates[348] reported long-term success rates of 80% at 1 year, 62% at 2 years, and 45% at 6 years. Younger patients appear to have a more favorable prognosis with ALT than do older patients.

The surgical management of pigmentary glaucoma follows the same general guidelines as for POAG. If medical and laser therapy are not effective, filtration procedures are used and are usually successful.[338,349]

A new approach to treatment involves use of a laser peripheral iridotomy. Karickhoff[350] has introduced the concept of *reverse pupillary block* to explain the posterior bowing of the iris against the crystalline lens and zonules. Iridotomy equilizes pressure between the anterior and posterior chambers, bringing the iris forward and eliminating the mechanical rubbing of pigment from the iris epithelium (Fig. 35.24). Laser iridotomy for PDS or pigmentary glaucoma will require further study to support its usefulness for the prevention or treatment of these disorders.[351]

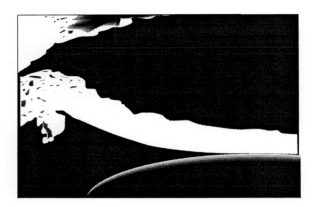

A

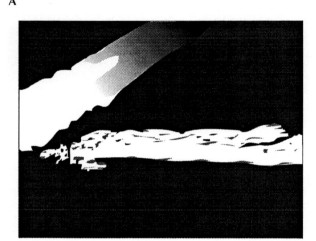

B

FIGURE 35.24 **Effect of laser iridotomy on posterior iris bowing.** *(A)* **Prelaser posterior bowing of iris.** *(B)* **Postlaser anterior movement of iris. (Computer simulation of ultrasound biomicroscopy)**

Exfoliation Glaucoma

ETIOLOGY

Exfoliation glaucoma is associated with the exfoliation syndrome. In 1917, Lindberg[352] first reported grayish flaky material at the pupillary margins, and Vogt[353] later associated the presence of the material with glaucoma resulting from decreased aqueous outflow due to exfoliated material in the trabecular meshwork. The flaky material was first considered to be desquamated debris from the crystalline lens capsule. Since further studies suggested that the material was not true exfoliation from the lens capsule, which is usually associated with exposure to an infrared-emitting heat source,[354] Dvorok-Theobald[355] proposed that the condition be called pseudoexfoliation syndrome. There is evidence, however, that the exfoliated material comes from multiple sources—lens epithelium, ciliary body epithelium, iris pigment epithelium, corneal endothelium, zonular fibrils, and endothelial cells in the trabecular meshwork[356,357]—so the term *exfoliation glaucoma* is generally accepted.

Initially, exfoliation syndrome was believed to be a degenerative ocular disorder involving the limiting basement membrane lining the anterior and posterior chambers.[358] Recent evidence, however, supports the concept of a generalized systemic disorder with ocular manifestations, since the exfoliative material has been identified in skin, heart, lung, liver, kidney, and cerebral meninges.[359,360] The material also occurs in extrabulbar tissues such as conjunctiva, extraocular muscles, and optic nerve sheath.[361] This evidence suggests that the exfoliation syndrome may actually be a systemic condition involving abnormal extracellular matrix synthesis, especially in connective tissues. Ocular hypoperfusion may also contribute to this process.[362]

The relationship between glaucoma and exfoliation syndrome is well established. The presence of exfoliation syndrome seems to increase the eye's vulnerability to develop glaucoma.[363] Most studies have shown the prevalence of glaucoma in patients with exfoliation syndrome to be about 30% to 40%.[364–366] Kozart and Yanoff[453] studied 100 patients with exfoliation syndrome and found that 7% had glaucoma. These investigators also reported that another 13% had ocular hypertension (IOP greater than 21 mm Hg) and that patients with bilateral exfoliation syndrome had a higher incidence of glaucoma. Other investigators have shown that the presence of exfoliation syndrome increases the risk of both ocular hypertension and glaucoma.[367,368]

Movement of the iris scrapes the exfoliation material off the anterior lens capsule, leaving a clear zone where the iris moves and depositing the material on the pupillary margins and on the lens surface in the pupillary area (Fig. 35.25). The flow of aqueous moves the debris to the iris, corneal endothelium, and trabecular meshwork, where it decreases aqueous outflow and produces a secondary glaucoma.

Exfoliation glaucoma develops slowly, and although it often occurs in only one eye, it becomes bilateral in many patients.[367] The incidence increases with age and is much more prevalent after age 70 years. The incidence appears to be higher in females, in people from Scandinavian countries,[364] and in Spanish Americans,[369] but much lower in people from central Europe and in African-Americans. Familial occurrence of the exfoliation syndrome suggests an autosomal dominant mode of inheritance.[370] It is found in patients with wide and with narrow anterior chamber angles, but the anterior chambers of affected patients are shallower than normal[371] and thus may predispose to a higher risk of angle-closure glaucoma.[372]

DIAGNOSIS

Exfoliation glaucoma is characterized by elevated IOP, optic disc or visual field changes, the presence of flaky, dandruff-like, white or light gray material on the pupillary margin, and a sugar-like frosting on the anterior lens capsule.[373] The material may be present on the iris and corneal endothelium, but it is difficult to see. There may be slight depigmentation of the pupillary margin and pigment on the corneal endothelium. There is generally heavy pigmentation of the trabecular meshwork, although less than that observed in pigmentary glaucoma. Since the diagnosis of exfoliation syndrome can be overlooked easily, the practitioner must not dismiss the subtle clinical signs that can reveal the disease (Table 35.30).

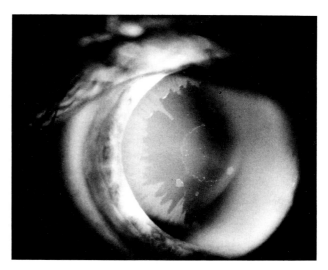

FIGURE 35.25 **Appearance of the crystalline lens in exfoliation syndrome.**

MANAGEMENT

The medical management of exfoliation glaucoma generally follows the same guidelines as for POAG.[374] However, medical therapy is usually not as satisfactory in exfoliation glaucoma as it is in POAG.[368,370,375] Pilocarpine can be used, but the stronger miotics, such as the anticholinesterase agents, should be avoided because of the possibility of drug-induced cataract. Because many of these patients have nuclear sclerotic or posterior subcapsular cataracts, it is advantageous to avoid miosis by employing adrenergic agents such as topical dipivefrin, β-blockers, or topical dorzolamide.

ALT appears to be a useful adjunct to medical therapy, especially for patients who remain uncontrolled with maximum-tolerated drug therapy.[374] Sherwood and Svedbergh[376] found a 70% success rate with use of ALT in patients with exfoliation glaucoma, and 40% of patients were able to

TABLE 35.30
Subtle Signs of Exfoliation Syndrome

- Pupillary ruff defects
- Iris sphincter transillumination
- Whorl-like particulate pigment deposition on iris sphincter
- Particulate pigment deposition on anterior iris surface and trabecular meshwork
- Exfoliation material on zonules and ciliary body

Adapted from Prince AM, Ritch R. Clinical signs of the pseudoexfoliation syndrome. Ophthalmology 1986;93:803–807.

reduce or discontinue their drug therapy. It should be noted, however, that the long-term efficacy of ALT in these patients may be less satisfactory than in patients with POAG.[377]

Filtering surgery is indicated in cases that are unresponsive to medical or laser therapy. Although lens extraction may be temporarily beneficial, deposition of exfoliation material can continue following cataract extraction.[378] Thus, it is probably unwise to depend solely on lens extraction as the primary therapeutic approach to lowering IOP in exfoliation glaucoma. Trabeculectomy appears to be an effective surgical procedure in most cases.[375] Tarkkanen[370] reported that 85% of patients with exfoliation glaucoma were well controlled without medication 5 years following trabeculectomy, and 92% were controlled with concomitant medical therapy.

Steroid-Induced Ocular Hypertension and Glaucoma

ETIOLOGY

Some patients receiving long-term topical steroid therapy, or in some cases systemic steroids, respond with a marked increase in IOP.[379] In these patients, the steroid decreases the efficiency of the aqueous outflow mechanism in the trabecular meshwork or endothelial vacuoles. Although the precise mechanisms are poorly understood, steroids may induce an overproduction of glycoproteins such as fibronectin that impede aqueous drainage.[380] In most instances of short-term steroid-induced ocular hypertension, there is an increase of IOP but no optic nerve damage or visual field loss. Prolonged IOP increases, however, can lead to true glaucomatous damage that is irreversible.

DIAGNOSIS

Before instituting steroid therapy—especially topical—baseline IOP should be recorded. During the course of therapy, close observation of the patient is mandatory, monitoring the IOP at least every 2 to 4 weeks, especially in patients known to be at risk for a steroid response. These include individuals with glaucoma, their first-degree offspring, and patients with a history of steroid response.[381] Although the risk of steroid-induced ocular hypertension is greatest during the first 4 to 6 weeks of therapy, the patient may develop an elevation of pressure at any time, sometimes after several months of treatment.

MANAGEMENT

Most cases of steroid-induced ocular hypertension respond promptly to tapering or discontinuation of the drug.[382] This is usually the only treatment required. In some cases of persistent elevation of IOP, treatment with ocular hypotensive medications may be necessary, following the principles outlined for treatment of POAG. Elevated IOP that is resistant to such medical management should be treated by laser trabeculoplasty or filtering procedures. However, it may be reasonable to monitor the patient carefully in cases in which there is no apparent optic nerve damage. Laser trabeculoplasty or filtering surgery should be reserved for patients with progressive optic nerve or visual field damage or for patients in whom such damage seems imminent.[382] Following filtering surgery, steroids can be used as necessary to control inflammation and scarring without the risk for drug-induced elevation of IOP.[382]

If anti-inflammatory therapy must be continued despite the presence of elevated IOP, use a lower steroid dosage frequency or drug concentration or continue therapy by changing to fluorometholone, loteprednol,[383] or rimexolone,[384] steroids with less propensity to elevate IOP. Substituting a topical nonsteroidal anti-inflammatory agent for the steroid can also be considered. If decreasing or changing steroid therapy does not reduce IOP, or if such changes are contraindicated, routine antiglaucoma therapy may be instituted.

Persistent elevation of IOP associated with the use of periocular steroids often responds to standard medical therapy. However, excision of the steroid material may be necessary if the pressure cannot be controlled medically.

Uveitic Glaucoma

ETIOLOGY

Anterior uveitis can produce several changes in the anterior chamber that decrease aqueous outflow and elevate IOP. Reduced aqueous outflow can result from a decrease in size of the pores in the trabecular meshwork, because the trabecular meshwork is swollen and edematous from the inflammation (trabeculitis). It also may be caused by blockage of some of the trabecular meshwork pores by inflammatory debris (white blood cells and macrophages) and by an increased viscosity of aqueous due to protein leakage from blood vessels in the iris and ciliary body. Elevated IOP associated with anterior uveitis may also result from the development of posterior or anterior synechiae, which compromise aqueous outflow.

DIAGNOSIS

There may be a significant and rapid elevation in IOP with ocular discomfort and corneal edema. A complete glaucoma workup should be performed, including gonioscopy to differentiate the condition from angle-closure glaucoma and to assess the extent of peripheral anterior synechiae.

MANAGEMENT

Management of glaucoma associated with active anterior uveitis is directed primarily toward the inflammation by employing cycloplegics, mydriatics, and steroids. Secondarily, management focuses on the elevated IOP by employing inhibitors of aqueous formation. If medical therapy fails to adequately control the IOP, surgical intervention may become necessary.

Posterior synechiae should be prevented or broken with the use of topical cycloplegic and mydriatic agents (Fig. 35.26). Use of a combination of 1% atropine or 5% homatropine 2 to 3 times daily, and 2.5% phenylephrine 4 times daily, often reduces patient discomfort associated with ciliary spasm, reduces intraocular inflammation associated with the uveitis, and prevents the development of posterior synechiae.

Topically applied steroids, along with the cycloplegic, will often control the anterior segment inflammation. Since the anti-inflammatory effect is related to the frequency of instillation, a useful dosage regimen is 1 drop of 1% prednisolone acetate every 1 or 2 hours during the acute state of inflammation. As the inflammatory process subsides, the dosage frequency may be decreased gradually. When persistent elevation of IOP is suspected to be associated with the steroid, changing the drug to fluorometholone, loteprednol,[383] or rimexolone[384] may be sufficient to reduce pressure while maintaining the steroid's desired anti-inflammatory effect. In some cases it is difficult to determine whether the elevated IOP is caused by the uveitis or the topical steroid.

If the anterior uveitis does not respond adequately to the use of topical steroids, subconjunctival or systemic steroids can be attempted. Subconjunctival steroid therapy is often effective with the use of dexamethasone phosphate 4 mg, prednisolone succinate 25 mg, triamcinolone acetonide 4

mg, or methylprednisolone acetate 20 mg.[385] The use of long-acting repository steroids should be avoided, since these may result in a sustained elevation of IOP. Systemic steroids become necessary when the topical or subconjunctival routes of administration have been ineffective. In such cases, prednisone, 80 to 100 mg daily, should be maintained until there is evidence of remission, at which time the daily dosage is decreased 5 mg every second or third day.[385]

Because the side effects of topical or systemic steroids are not insignificant, patients should be monitored carefully for the development of elevated IOP, posterior subcapsular cataracts, and other steroid-related effects. If the uveitis recurs after topical steroid therapy has been discontinued, the possibility of drug-induced rebound inflammation should be considered, and the steroid therapy should be reinstituted and then tapered more slowly.

In addition to control of the active anterior uveitis, treatment should be directed toward the elevated IOP by employing topical β blockers, dorzolamide, or dipivefrin. Miotics should be avoided since they can increase the inflammation and lead to the formation of posterior synechiae. When topical antiglaucoma therapy is unsuccessful in adequately controlling the elevated pressure, systemic carbonic anhydrase inhibitors such as methazolamide may be used. These agents are usually effective in treating glaucoma secondary to inflammatory diseases with obstruction of aqueous outflow.[385]

Elevated IOP that is unresponsive to medical therapy requires surgical intervention. Surgical results, however, are often disappointing in patients with active inflammation. Iridectomy is the procedure of choice if pupillary block is a

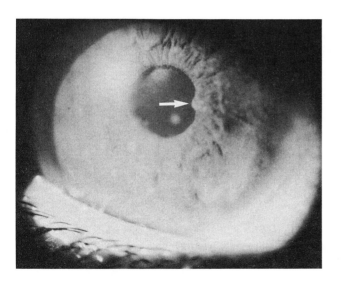

A

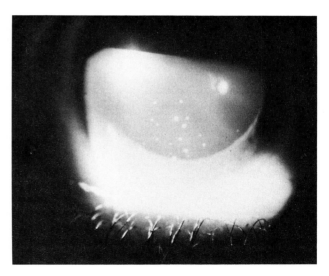

B

FIGURE 35.26 **Posterior synechiae. (A) Posterior synechiae (arrow) at the nasal pupillary margin before dilation. (B) The same eye after dilation. Small white spots are keratic precipitates on corneal endothelium.**

contributing factor.[385] ALT has been shown to be ineffective in cases of uveitic glaucoma and thus should not be attempted.[386] Trabeculectomy with antimetabolites can provide good results in patients with uveitic glaucoma, but setons may be more likely to control IOP in patients who are expected to have significant postoperative inflammation.[387]

Glaucoma Secondary to Cyclitis (Posner-Schlossman Syndrome)

DIAGNOSIS

Patients who have recurrent attacks of mild cyclitis can develop glaucoma, since cyclitis can produce an increase in IOP. The increase in IOP is usually rapid. This condition is called *glaucomatocyclitic crisis*, or the Posner-Schlossman syndrome.[388] It is generally unilateral and occurs in patients between the ages of 20 and 50 years, who report a history of recurrent attacks of unilateral blurred vision. There is usually only slight discomfort associated with the attack, and the attack may last from a few hours to several weeks. The patient may report that the eye with the blurred vision had a larger pupil during the attack, and the patient can even present with a larger pupil in the affected eye. These patients have open anterior chamber angles and do not have any posterior or anterior synechiae, ciliary injection, or numerous cells in the anterior chamber.[389] However, mild conjunctival injection is common. If the patient is not treated for the cyclitis, keratic precipitates can develop on the corneal endothelium, more cells can be present in the aqueous, and the visual acuity can be reduced. These patients generally have normal optic discs and no visual field loss. The increase in IOP is probably due to numerous mononuclear cells in the trabecular meshwork interspaces[390] and to increased aqueous formation.[390a]

MANAGEMENT

Since a glaucomatocyclitic crisis is self-limited, it usually subsides spontaneously within a few days regardless of treatment. Medical therapy, however, can be effective in controlling the acute elevations of IOP. The use of a topical β blocker, dipivefrin, or a systemic carbonic anhydrase inhibitor usually reduces the IOP to normal. Topical 1% apraclonidine has been shown to be especially beneficial in cases of glaucomatocyclitic crisis, reducing IOP approximately 50% in 4 hours.[391] Because of the inflammatory process, miotics should be avoided. In addition to this antiglaucoma regimen, topical steroids may be effective in controlling the inflammation, but the patient should be monitored carefully for the development of steroid-induced elevations of IOP.

Prolonged medical therapy with antiglaucoma agents and steroids should be avoided, since treatment does not prevent recurrences and is unnecessary between attacks. In addition, prolonged steroid therapy increases the risk of cataract, elevated IOP, and other undesirable steroid-related side effects.

Surgical procedures are generally ineffective in preventing recurrent attacks and, indeed, are contraindicated because of the risks they impose in this self-limited condition.[392] Varma and associates,[393] however, reported one patient who had no documented recurrent episodes of glaucomatocyclitis crisis during a 12-year period following a trabeculectomy for glaucomatous damage to the optic nerve.

Post-traumatic Glaucoma

Blunt trauma to the eye can result in damage to the anterior chamber angle, reduction in aqueous outflow, and secondary glaucoma. The most common abnormalities leading to elevated IOP include angle recession and hyphema.

ANGLE RECESSION

Etiology. The trauma can produce a tear in the ciliary muscle, usually between the circular and longitudinal muscles, creating a recession of the anterior chamber angle[394] (Fig. 35.27). Direct damage to the trabecular meshwork can also occur. In some patients, glaucoma can develop immediately following the trauma or may not occur until months or years later.[395]

The reported incidence of late-onset glaucoma following blunt trauma varies from 2% to 10%.[394,396] The incidence is higher if the angle recession involves 270° or more of the

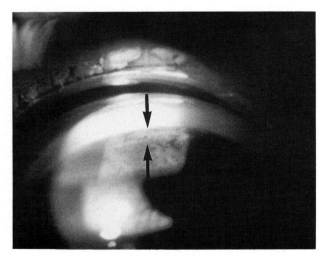

FIGURE 35.27 **Goniophotograph of angle recession. Note that the light beam on the iris exposes a wider than normal band of ciliary body (arrows).**

angle,[394] if the patient is older, and if there is familial predisposition for the development of POAG. The glaucoma is generally unilateral or asymmetric, with a tendency toward elevated IOP in the fellow eye.

The immediate elevation of IOP may be due to trabecular damage or to the presence of prostaglandins that are released in the anterior chamber. The elevated IOP often lasts for hours, days or weeks. It is usually self-limiting.

Some patients, months to years later, exhibit a gradual increase in IOP and develop glaucoma. These patients generally have a marked angle recession The elevation of pressure is due to a reduction of aqueous outflow believed to be caused by the resultant scarring of the trabecular meshwork or by the gradual growth of a membrane over the trabecular meshwork (Fig. 35.28)[397]

Diagnosis.   Patients who have sustained blunt trauma to the eye should be evaluated for possible angle-recession glaucoma by performing gonioscopy, tonometry, stereoscopic optic disc evaluation, and visual fields. Note that the recessed angle may scar closed and be difficult to detect on gonioscopy. The loss of iris processes may indicate previous ocular trauma with angle recession. Comparison of gonioscopic findings with the fellow eye can also be helpful in diagnosis. Slit-lamp examination may reveal patchy areas of *iridoschisis*, a local splitting of the iris into two layers, an indication of previous blunt ocular trauma.[398] In the absence of glaucoma, these patients should be monitored on an annual basis.[395]

Management.   Eyes with angle-recession glaucoma are treated following the same guidelines that apply to the

management of POAG. It should be realized, however, that miotics may be ineffective because of interruption of the normal ciliary muscle-scleral spur relationship induced by the initial traumatic episode. Rarely, a paradoxical elevation of IOP occurs in response to pilocarpine.[399] Paradoxically, the use of atropine in such cases may reduce the pressure and be of therapeutic value by forestalling the need for oral carbonic anhydrase inhibitors or surgical therapy.[399] Robin and Pollack[386] have shown poor responses to ALT in patients with angle-recession glaucoma. Nd:YAG laser trabeculopuncture (YLT) has been reported to have limited success but appears to be more effective than ALT.[400,401] For patients who are uncontrolled medically, trabeculectomy with adjunctive antimetabolite therapy offers the best chance of surgical success.[402,403]

HYPHEMA

Etiology.   Blunt, nonpenetrating trauma to the eye may cause hyphema. Blood in the anterior chamber (hyphema) can compromise aqueous outflow and produce glaucoma. Following a total hyphema where the entire anterior chamber is filled with blood ("8-ball" hyphema), the trabecular meshwork is overloaded with blood cells and blood clots, and aqueous outflow decreases, resulting in elevated IOP. On the other hand, hyphemas that occupy less than half the anterior chamber (Fig. 35.29) usually resolve spontaneously within 7 days without complications.[404] However, recession of the angle occurs in most eyes with hyphema, with the potential risk for acute or late-onset glaucoma.

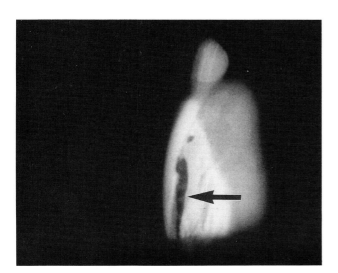

FIGURE 35.28   **Scarring of trabecular meshwork (arrow) in angle-recession glaucoma.**

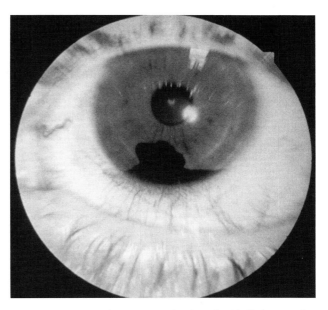

FIGURE 35.29   **Hyphema occupying less than half the anterior chamber.**

One of the most important developments in the patient with hyphema is secondary hemorrhage, or rebleeding. This occurs during the first 5 days in up to 25% of cases and has an even higher prevalence in patients with elevated IOP.[405,406] Rebleeding may be caused by lysis and retraction of the clot that occludes the traumatized iris or angle vessel.[407] Secondary hemorrhage is associated with a poorer visual prognosis because of the increased risk of corneal blood staining, development of peripheral anterior synechiae, and the need for surgical intervention.[407] Secondary hemorrhage is also associated with a higher incidence of elevated IOP than is the initial hyphema, the incidence of the former being about 50%.[408,409] Any hyphema, however, regardless of its size, can cause elevated IOP, but hyphemas filling at least half the anterior chamber are more likely to produce pressure increases.[410] About one-third of eyes with hyphema will develop an IOP exceeding 24 mm Hg during the acute episode.[405]

Management. The treatment of hyphema has been controversial[411] and has included miotics, cycloplegics, steroids, bed rest, unilateral or bilateral patching, hospitalization, and sedation. There is little difference in outcome, however, between patients treated with bilateral patching, bed rest, and sedation and those who remain ambulatory wearing a patch and shield over the injured eye.[405,412] As a practical matter, elevation of the head of the bed to 30° to 45° seems to facilitate the settling of blood in the anterior chamber, allowing more rapid improvement in vision and an earlier view of the fundus.[410] Since many patients have an associated anterior uveitis, treatment with cycloplegics and steroids improves comfort and places the iris at rest during the healing process. Hospitalization is not mandatory for small hyphemas, but it allows for daily monitoring of the resolution of the hyphema and of its effects on IOP.[410] However, hospitalization to ensure bed rest should be mandatory for children with hyphemas filling more than 50% of the anterior chamber.[411] Since patients with sickle cell trait are more susceptible to complications from hyphema,[413] black patients presenting with hyphema should be screened for hemoglobin abnormalities.

Although not effective in cases of total hyphema, topical β blockers can reduce elevated IOP. Miotics are generally contraindicated, since they increase vasodilatation and can aggravate any existing uveitis. In addition, one of the most effective drug groups for treatment of elevated IOP is the oral carbonic anhydrase inhibitors. One should be cautious, however, in using acetazolamide, since this drug can increase the ascorbate concentration of the aqueous and lower the pH, producing sickling of erythrocytes in the anterior chamber. This can possibly cause the hyphema to resolve more slowly and lead to additional complications. Methazolamide is a better choice, especially in patients with sickle cell disease.[412] If necessary, hyperosmotic agents (oral isosorbide or intravenous mannitol) can also be used.

Since the risk of complications increases with recurrent episodes, it is important to minimize the risk of secondary hemorrhage. Aminocaproic acid (Amicar), an antifibrinolytic agent, reduces the incidence of secondary hyphema in adults,[414-417] presumably by stabilizing the clot in the traumatized blood vessels[418] and allowing time for the integrity of the traumatized vessels to become reestablished.[407] Amicar is given in an oral dosage of 100 mg/kg body weight every 4 hours for 5 days. Side effects of nausea, vomiting, and systemic hypotension can often be minimized without diminishing efficacy by reducing the dosage to 50 mg/kg body weight.[416] This dosage has been shown to be equivalent to an oral dosage of 40 mg prednisone daily for reducing the risk of secondary hemorrhage.[418] Some patients, however, may be at risk for an early and significant increase in IOP following discontinuation of aminocaproic acid therapy due to rapid clot dissolution. Thus, patients with large residual clots should be monitored carefully during the first week after treatment is discontinued.[407] Moreover, aminocaproic acid should not be used for hyphemas larger than 75% because it may cause blood clotting in the anterior chamber.[410] The rate of secondary hemorrhage during aminocaproic acid use has been reported to be reduced from about 25% to 7%.[415-418]

Surgical intervention is necessary for cases of total hyphema that are unresponsive to medical therapy. Such treatment, however, should be delayed for at least 7 days, since early surgical intervention is often accompanied by rebleeding, and because a significant number of cases will resolve spontaneously during that time.[419] Surgical procedures include paracentesis, irrigation with balanced salt solution or fibrinolytic agents, aspiration with an emulsification or vitrectomy unit, or draining the anterior chamber through a trabeculectomy incision.[419] Sustained elevated IOP may require trabeculectomy.[454]

It should be noted that the ultimate visual outcome is determined more often by damage to the retina or optic nerve by the initial traumatic episode than by the elevation of IOP. In the future, spectrum analysis of high-frequency ultrasound data may be able to distinguish organized from recent hemorrhage, to evaluate the degree of absorption during follow-up, and to determine the degree of coagulation.[420] This might be helpful in planning or altering the course of medical or surgical management.

Secondary Angle-Closure Glaucoma: Neovascular Glaucoma

Etiology

Secondary angle-closure glaucoma develops as a consequence of another recognizable disease process that produces a marked narrowing of the anterior chamber angle either by pulling the iris forward or by pushing the iris into the angle. The typical glaucomatous signs of angle-closure glaucoma are usually present. Although secondary angle-closure glaucoma can result from a variety of diseases, only neovascular glaucoma is considered here. This disease is a highly complex condition that requires considerable care in establishing the etiologic diagnosis, and its management is often frustrating since the available treatment modalities are frequently unsuccessful.

Neovascular glaucoma results from growth of new vessels on the iris—*rubeosis iridis*.[421] Its incidence is highest in patients with diabetic retinopathy or central retinal vein occlusion. It also occurs in patients with other ocular disorders such as retinal arterial occlusion, chronic retinal detachment, Coats' disease, retinopathy of prematurity (ROP), ocular neoplastic disorders, sickle cell retinopathy,[422] and endophthalmitis. It has also developed following Nd:YAG laser posterior capsulotomy in diabetic patients.[423]

Diagnosis

The new vessels are generally observed first near the pupillary margin and in small isolated areas on the iris. The small vessels then extend in an irregular pattern to cover the iris and the posterior corneal surface near the angle[424] (Fig. 35.30). A fibrovascular membrane develops along the new vessels. Over time, it contracts and pulls the peripheral iris toward the cornea and physically restricts aqueous outflow, producing glaucoma. The glaucoma can occur weeks to years following neovascularization of the iris.

One of the earliest diagnostic signs of neovascularization is leakage of fluorescein from iris vessels into the anterior chamber. Another early sign is tiny dilated capillaries at the pupillary margin. These dilated capillaries can be mistaken for clumps of pigment. As the fibrovascular membrane develops in the pupillary area and contracts, it generally produces an ectropion uveae.

If angle-closure glaucoma does occur, there will be significant neovascularization, a markedly narrow or closed angle, corneal edema, and an extremely high IOP. Symptoms include ocular pain, conjunctival hyperemia, and blurred vision.

Management

Although neovascular glaucoma is one of the most difficult forms of glaucoma to manage successfully, recent advances have resulted in success rates up to 77%.[425] The most successful treatment occurs when the neovascular process is detected in its earliest phase, before the angle has become closed by peripheral anterior synechiae (PAS). Thus, it is imperative that all susceptible patients be evaluated periodically for the development of rubeosis at the pupillary margin and in the angle.[426] The use of anterior and posterior segment photocoagulation can maintain an open angle in up to 80% of eyes when they are treated before angle closure.[425] However, since progression from onset of neovascularization in the angle to a 360° closure of the angle may occur within weeks, treatment should be provided without delay. The underlying cause of neovascularization, such as diabetic retinopathy, must be sought out and managed aggressively.

It is practical to divide patients with neovascular glaucoma into those with and without useful vision (Fig. 35.31). Patients with useful vision may be treated with panretinal

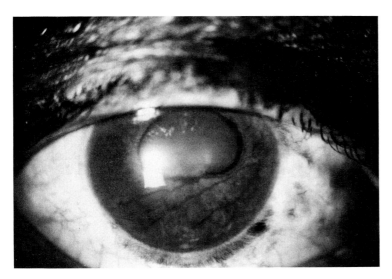

FIGURE 35.30 **Neovascularization of the inferior iris.**

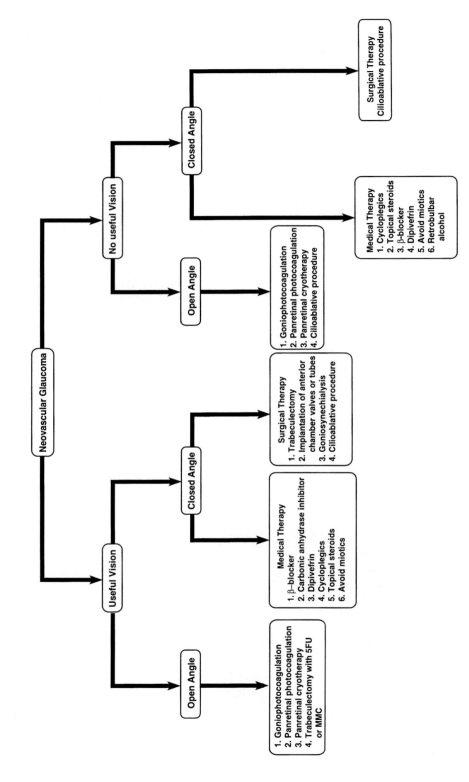

FIGURE 35.31 Flowchart for the management of neovascular glaucoma. (Modified from Weber PA. Neovascular glaucoma. Current management. Surv Ophthalmol 1981;26:149–153.)

photocoagulation (PRP), goniophotocoagulation (direct laser application to vessels in the angle), or both. PRP may result in regression of the anterior segment neovascularization,[427,428] while goniophotocoagulation may be successful in obliterating these vessels, thereby preventing angle closure. PRP generally requires several weeks to produce clinical regression of the neovascularization and can be effective in about 60% of cases.[429] Although not widely used, goniophotocoagulation usually causes immediate obliteration of the angle vessels.[425] In patients in whom media opacities preclude PRP, or in eyes that do not respond to photocoagulation therapy, panretinal cryotherapy may be effective.[430]

Once the angle has become completely closed by PAS, the prognosis diminishes considerably because laser therapy will be of no benefit in improving outflow facility. If the angle is closed 360° by PAS but there is potential for useful vision, a short clinical trial of medical therapy may be beneficial in some cases. A β blocker, dipivefrin, and topical or oral carbonic anhydrase inhibitor may be helpful in controlling the IOP.[425] Since the angle is closed, pilocarpine and other miotics are of no value. Cycloplegics and topical steroids, however, can often reduce discomfort in these inflamed eyes.[431] Although such medical therapy is justified on a short-term basis, most eyes will prove to be resistant, and various surgical approaches will be required (see Fig. 35.31). Trabeculectomy, goniosynechialysis, or cilioablative procedures (ciliary body destruction) can be attempted in an effort to control the IOP.[425,427,432] However, the presence of active neovascularization decreases the success of filtering surgery. Molteno tube implants, which drain aqueous from the anterior chamber to the subconjunctival space, reportedly have a success rate of 62% 1 year following surgery, but only about 10% at 5 years.[433] In severely compromised eyes, the primary advantage of these implants may be pain relief and delay of enucleation.[433–435]

If the angle is closed 360° by PAS and there is no potential for useful vision, the primary therapeutic goal is to provide comfort. This can be accomplished with the use of a β blocker, dorzolamide or dipivefrin.[425] Oral carbonic anhydrase inhibitors also may be employed, but they should generally be avoided because of potential systemic side effects. Pilocarpine also should be avoided because of its ineffectiveness in eyes with total PAS. In addition, pilocarpine causes increased vascular permeability, which leads to increased ocular inflammation and irritation. Additional comfort can be achieved in some eyes with the use of topical cycloplegics and steroids. When these efforts fail to provide an acceptable level of comfort, consideration may be given to cilioablative procedures, Molteno tube implantation, or retrobulbar alcohol injection.[425] Of these procedures, retrobulbar alcohol injection is the least expensive and the most convenient to use and offers immediate pain relief with a short convalescence.

References

1. Mailer CM. Glaucoma: An argument that began with Aristotle. Arch Ophthalmol 1966;76:623–636.
2. Duke-Elder S. System of ophthalmology. St. Louis: C.V. Mosby Co, 1969;3:381.
3. Banister R. A treatise of one hundred and thirteen diseases of the eyes and eye-liddes. London, 1622.
4. Douglas GR, Drance SM, Schulzer M. The visual field and nerve head in angle-closure glaucoma. Arch Ophthalmol 1975;93:409–411.
5. Horie T, Kitazawa Y, Nose H. Visual field changes in primary angle closure glaucoma. Jpn J Ophthalmol 1975;19:108–115.
6. Report of the Glaucoma Panel: Vision Research, a National Plan. Bethesda, MD: National Institutes of Health, 1983;vol. 2, part 4: 1–10.
7. Tielsch JM, Sommer A, Katz J, et al. Racial variations in the prevalence of primary open-angle glaucoma. The Baltimore Eye Survey. JAMA 1991;266:369–374.
8. Bengtsson B. The prevalence of glaucoma. Br J Ophthalmol 1981; 65:46–49.
9. Hollows FC, Graham PA. Intra-ocular pressure, glaucoma, and glaucoma suspects in a defined population. Br J Ophthalmol 1966; 50:570–586.
10. Bankes JLK, Perkins ES, Tsolakis S, et al. Bedford glaucoma survey. Br Med J 1968;1:791–796.
11. Klein BEK, Klein R, Sponsel WE, et al. Prevalence of glaucoma. The Beaver Dam Eye Study. Ophthalmology 1992;99:1499–1504.
12. Sommer A, Tielsch JM, Katz J, et al. Relationship between intraocular pressure and primary open-angle glaucoma among white and black Americans. The Baltimore Eye Survey. Arch Ophthalmol 1991;109:1090–1095.
13. Colenbrander MC. The early diagnosis of glaucoma. Ophthalmologica 1971;162:276–281.
14. David R, Tessler Z, Yassur Y. Epidemiology of acute angle-closure glaucoma: Incidence and seasonal variations. Ophthalmologica 1985;191:4–7.
15. Becker B, Kolker AE, Roth FD. Glaucoma family study. Am J Ophthalmol 1960;50:557–567.
16. Shin DH, Becker B, Kolker AE. Family history in primary open-angle glaucoma. Arch Ophthalmol 1977;95:598–600.
17. Perkins ES. Family studies in glaucoma. Br J Ophthalmol 1974; 58:529–535.
18. Paterson G. Studies on siblings of patients with both angle-closure and chronic simple glaucoma. Trans Ophthalmol Soc UK 1961; 81:561–576.
19. Tomlinson A, Leighton DA. Ocular dimensions in the heredity of angle-closure glaucoma. Br J Ophthalmol 1973;57:475–486.
20. Lowe RF. Aetiology of the anatomical basis for primary angle-closure glaucoma. Br J Ophthalmol 1970;54:161–169.
21. Lowe RF. Primary angle-closure glaucoma. Br J Ophthalmol 1964;48:191–195.
22. Biro I. Notes upon the question of hereditary glaucoma. Ophthalmologica 1951;122:228–238.
23. Armaly MF, Monstavicius BF, Sayegh RE. Ocular pressure and aqueous outflow facility in siblings. Arch Ophthalmol 1968;80: 354–360.

24. Francois J. Genetics and primary open-angle glaucoma. Am J Ophthalmol 1966;61:652–665.

25. Waardenburg PJ. Genetics and ophthalmology. Springfield, IL: Charles C Thomas, 1961.

26. Pollack IP. Diagnosis of the glaucomas. In: Symposium on glaucoma. St. Louis: C.V. Mosby Co, 1967;Chap. 2.

27. Luntz MH. Congenital, infantile, and juvenile glaucoma. Ophthalmology 1979;86:793–802.

28. Packer H, Deutsch AR, Lewis PM, et al. Study of the frequency and distribution of glaucoma. JAMA 1959;171:1090–1093.

29. Turner CC. Open-angle glaucoma—a survey of racial incidence. Am J Optom Physiol Opt 1967;44:56–57.

30. Wilensky JT, Gandhi N, Pan T. Racial influences in open-angle glaucoma. Ann Ophthalmol 1978;10:1398–1402.

31. Martin MJ, Sommer A, Gold EB, et al. Race and primary open-angle glaucoma. Am J Ophthalmol 1985;99:383–387.

32. Lim ASM. Primary angle-closure glaucoma in Singapore. Aust J Ophthalmol 1979;7:23–30.

33. Genio CA, Gavino BC. Glaucoma profile in the Phillipines General Hospital. Philipp J Ophthalmol 1983;15:1–2.

34. Alper MG, Laubach JL. Primary angle-closure glaucoma in the American Negro. Arch Ophthalmol 1963;79:663–668.

35. Luntz MH. Primary angle-closure glaucoma in urbanized South African caucasoid and negro communities. Br J Ophthalmol 1973;57:445–456.

36. Sugar HS. The mechanical factors in the etiology of acute glaucoma. Am J Ophthalmol 1941;24:851–873.

37. Perkins ES, Phelps CD. Open-angle glaucoma, ocular hypertension, low-tension glaucoma, and refraction. Arch Ophthalmol 1982;100:1464–1467.

38. Drance SM. Angle-closure glaucoma among Canadian Eskimos. Can J Ophthalmol 1973;8:252–260.

39. Alsbirk PH. Primary angle-closure glaucoma. Acta Ophthalmol 1976;Suppl 127:5–31.

40. Tielsch JM, Katz J, Quigley HA, et al. Diabetes, intraocular pressure, and primary open-angle glaucoma in the Baltimore Eye Survey. Ophthalmology 1995;102:48–53.

41. Klein BEK, Klein R, Jensen SC. Open-angle glaucoma and older-onset diabetes. The Beaver Dam eye study. Ophthalmology 1994;101:1173–1177.

42. Smith KD, Arthurs BP, Saheb N. An association between hypothyroidism and primary open-angle glaucoma. Ophthalmology 1993;100:1580–1584.

43. Schulzer M, Drance SM. Intraocular pressure, systemic blood pressure, and age: A correlational study. Br J Ophthalmol 1987;71:245–250.

44. Crick RP, Vogel R, Newson RB, et al. The visual field in chronic simple glaucoma and ocular hypertension; its character, progress, relationship to the level of intraocular pressure and response to treatment. Eye 1989;3:536–546.

45. Crick RP, Newson RB, Shipley MJ, et al. The progress of the visual field in chronic simple glaucoma and ocular hypertension treated topically with pilocarpine or with timolol. Eye 1990;4:563–571.

46. Chauhan BC, Drance SM. The relationship between intraocular pressure and visual field progression in glaucoma. Graefe's Arch Clin Exp Ophthalmol 1992;230:521–526.

47. Van Buskirk EM, Cioffi GA. Predicted outcome from hypotensive therapy for glaucomatous optic neuropathy. Am J Ophthalmol 1993;116:636–640.

48. Stewart WC, Chorak RP, Hunt HH, et al. Factors associated with visual loss in patients with advanced glaucomatous changes in the optic nervehead. Am J Ophthalmol 1993;116:176–181.

49. Mao LK, Stewart WC, Shields MB. Correlation between intraocular pressure control and progressive glaucomatous damage in primary open-angle glaucoma. Am J Ophthalmol 1991;111:51–55.

50. Rossetti L, Marchetti I, Orzalesi N, et al. Randomized clinical trials on medical treatment of glaucoma. Are they appropriate to guide clinical practice? Arch Ophthalmol 1993;111:96–103.

51. O'Brien C, Schwartz B, Takamoto T, Wu DC. Intraocular pressure and the rate of visual field loss in chronic open-angle glaucoma. Am J Ophthalmol 1991;111:491–500.

52. Mattox C, Walton DS. Hereditary primary childhood glaucomas. Int Ophthalmol Clin 1993;33:121–134.

53. Richards JE, Lichter PR, Boehnke M, et al. Mapping of a gene for autosomal dominant juvenile-onset open-angle glaucoma to chromosome 1q. Am J Hum Genet 1994;54:62–70.

54. Bardelli AM, Hadjistilianou T, Frezzotti R. Etiology of congenital glaucoma. Genetic and extragenetic factors. Ophthalmic Paediatr Genet 1985;6:265–270.

55. Barsoum-Homsy M, Chevrette L. Incidence and prognosis of childhood glaucoma. A study of 63 cases. Ophthalmology 1986;93:1323–1327.

56. Hetherington J. Congenital glaucoma. In: Duane TD, Jaeger EA, eds. Clinical ophthalmology. Philadelphia: Harper & Row, 1979;Chap. 51.

57. Kiskis AA, Markowitz SN, Morin JD. Corneal diameter and axial length in congenital glaucoma. Can J Ophthalmol 1985;20:93–97.

58. Krieglstein GK. Congenital glaucoma—diagnosis and management. Trans Ophthalmol Soc UK 1986;105:549–554.

59. Tucker SM, Enzenauer RW, Levin AV, et al. Corneal diameter, axial length, and intraocular pressure in premature infants. Ophthalmology 1992;99:1296–1300.

60. Duckman RH, Fitzgerald DE. Evaluation of intraocular pressure in a pediatric population. Optom Vis Sci 1992;69:705–709.

61. Richardson KT. Optic cup symmetry in normal newborn infants. Invest Ophthalmol 1968;7:137–140.

62. Shaffer RN. New concepts in infants glaucoma. Can J Ophthalmol 1967;2:243–248.

63. Morgan KS, Black B, Ellis FD, et al. Treatment of congenital glaucoma. Am J Ophthalmol 1981;92:799–803.

64. Feman SS, Reinecke RD, eds. Handbook of pediatric ophthalmology. New York: Grune & Stratton, 1978;85–86.

65. deLuise VP, Anderson DR. Primary infantile glaucoma (congenital glaucoma). Surv Ophthalmol 1983;28:1–19.

66. Boger WP. Timolol in childhood glaucoma. Surv Ophthalmol 1983;28:259–261.

67. Haskins HO, Hetherington J, Magee SD, et al. Clinical experience with timolol in childhood glaucoma. Arch Ophthalmol 1985;203:1163–1165.

68. Akimoto M, Tanihara H, Negi A, et al. Surgical results of trabeculotomy ab externo for developmental glaucoma. Arch Ophthalmol 1994;112:1540–1544.

69. Burke JP, Bowell R. Primary trabeculectomy in congenital glaucoma. Br J Ophthalmol 1989;75:186–190.

70. Haskins HD, Shaffer RN, Hetherington J. Goniotomy vs trabeculotomy. J Pediatr Ophthalmol Strabismus 1984;21:153–158.

71. Melamed S, Latina MA, Epstein DL. Neodymium: YAG laser

trabeculopuncture in juvenile open-angle glaucoma. Ophthalmology 1987;94:163–170.

72. Al Faran MF, Tomey KF, Al Mutlaq FA. Cyclocryotherapy in selected cases of congenital glaucoma. Ophthalmic Surg 1990;21:794–798.

73. Tomlinson A, Leighton DA. Ocular dimensions and the heredity of open-angle glaucoma. Br J Ophthalmol 1974;58:68–74.

74. Walker MW. Ocular hypertension. Trans Ophthalmol Soc UK 1974;94:525–534.

75. Weinstein BI, Munnangi P, Gordon GG, et al. Defects in cortisol-metabolizing enzymes in primary open-angle glaucoma. Invest Ophthalmol Vis Sci 1985;26:890–893.

76. Becker B, Unger HH, Coleman SL, et al. Plasma cells and gamma-globulin in trabecular meshwork of eyes with primary open-angle glaucoma. Arch Ophthalmol 1963;70:38–41.

77. Waltman SR, Yarian D. Antinuclear antibodies in open-angle glaucoma. Invest Ophthalmol 1974;13:695–697.

78. Segawa K. Ultrastructural changes of the trabecular tissue in primary open-angle glaucoma. Jpn J Ophthalmol 1975;19:317–338.

79. Rodrigues MM, Katz SI, Foidart JM, Spaeth GL. Collagen, factor VIII antigen, and immunoglobulins in the human aqueous drainage channels. Ophthalmology 1980;87:337–342.

80. Alvarado J, Murphy C, Juster R. Trabecular meshwork cellularity in primary open-angle glaucoma and nonglaucomatous normals. Ophthalmology 1984;91:564–579.

81. Johnson DH, Knepper PA. Microscale analysis of the glycosaminoglycans of human trabecular meshwork: A study in perfusion cultured eyes. J Glaucoma 1994;3:58–60.

82. Freddo TF. The Glenn A. Fry Award Lecture 1992:Aqueous humor proteins: A key for unlocking glaucoma? Optom Vis Sci 1993;70:263–270.

83. Johnson DH, Brubaker RF. Glaucoma: An overview. Mayo Clinic Proc 1986;61:59–67.

84. Brown RH, Zilis JD, Lynch MG, et al. The afferent pupillary defect in asymmetric glaucoma. Arch Ophthalmol 1987;105:1540–1543.

85. Kohn AN, Moss AP, Podos SM. Relative afferent pupillary defects in glaucoma without characteristic field loss. Arch Ophthalmol 1979;97:294–296.

86. Armaly MF. The visual field defect and ocular pressure level in open-angle glaucoma. Invest Ophthalmol 1969;8:105–124.

87. Cameron D, Finlay ET, Jackson CRS. Tonometry and tonography in the diagnosis of chronic simple glaucoma. Br J Ophthalmol 1971;55:738–741.

88. Spaeth GL. The effect of change in intraocular pressure on the natural history of glaucoma: Lowering intraocular pressure in glaucoma can result in improvement of visual fields. Trans Ophthalmol Soc UK 1985;104 (Pt. 3):256–264.

89. Ritch R, Reyes A. Moustache glaucoma. Arch Ophthalmol 1988;106:1503.

90. Klein BEK, Klein R, Linton KLP. Intraocular pressure in an American community. The Beaver Dam eye study. Invest Ophthalmol Vis Sci 1992;33:2224–2228.

91. David R, Zangwill LM, Tessler Z, et al. The correlation between intraocular pressure and refractive status. Arch Ophthalmol 1985;103:1812–1815.

92. Buguet A, Py P, Romanet JP. Twenty-four hour (nyctohemeral) and sleep-related variations of intraocular pressure in healthy white individuals. Am J Ophthalmol 1994;117:342–347.

93. Zeimer RC, Wilensky JT, Gieser DK. Presence and rapid decline of early morning intraocular pressure peaks in glaucoma patients. Ophthalmology 1990;97:547–550.

94. Wilensky JT, Gieser DK, Dietsche ML, et al. Individual variability in the diurnal intraocular pressure curve. Ophthalmology 1993;100:940–944.

95. Schappert-Kemmijser J. A five year follow-up of subjects with IOP of 22–30 mm Hg without anomalies of optic nerve and visual field typical for glaucoma at first investigation. Ophthalmologica 1971;162:289–295.

96. Pohjanpelto PEJ, Palva J. Ocular hypertension and glaucomatous optic nerve damage. Acta Ophthalmol 1974;52:194–200.

97. Bengtsson B. Some factors affecting the distribution of intraocular pressure in a population. Acta Ophthalmol 1972;50:33–46.

98. Kitazawa Y, Horie T. Diurnal variation of intraocular pressure and its significance in the medical treatment of primary open-angle glaucoma. In: Krieglstein GK, Leydhecker W, eds. Glaucoma update. New York: Springer-Verlag, 1979;169–176.

99. Carel RS, Korczyn AD, Rock M. Ocular tension: Comparison between the two eyes. Ophthalmologica 1985;190:98–101.

100. Varma R, Tielsch JM, Quigley HA, et al. Race-, age-, gender-, and refractive error-related differences in the normal optic disc. Arch Ophthalmol 1994;112:1068–1076.

101. Armaly MF. The optic cup in the normal eye. Am J Ophthalmol 1969;68:401–407.

102. Varma R, Steinmann WC, Scott IU. Expert agreement in evaluating the optic disc for glaucoma. Ophthalmology 1992;99:215–221.

103. Weisman RL, Asseff CF, Phelps CD, et al. Vertical elongation of the optic cup in glaucoma. Trans Am Acad Ophthalmol Otolaryngol 1973;77:157–161.

104. Caprioli J. Clinical evaluation of the optic nerve in glaucoma. Trans Am Ophthalmol Soc 1994;92:589–641.

105. Trobe JD, Glaser JS, Cassady J, et al. Non-glaucomatous excavation of the optic disc. Arch Ophthalmol 1980;98:1046–1050.

106. Quigley HA. The pathogenesis of optic nerve damage in glaucoma. Trans New Orleans Acad Ophthalmol. St. Louis: C.V. Mosby Co, 1985, 111–128.

107. Jonas JB, Fernandez MC, Sturmer J. Pattern of glaucomatous neuroretinal rim loss. Ophthalmology 1993;100:63–68.

108. Fishman RS. Optic disc asymmetry. Arch Ophthalmol 1970;84:590–594.

109. Armaly MJ. Genetic determination of cup/disc ratio of the optic nerve. Arch Ophthalmol 1967;78:35–43.

110. Odberg T, Riise D. Early diagnosis of glaucoma. The value of successive stereophotography of the optic disc. Acta Ophthalmol 1985;63:257–263.

111. Airaksinen PJ, Tuulonen A, Laanko HI. Rate and pattern of neuroretinal rim area decrease in ocular hypertension and glaucoma. Arch Ophthalmol 1992;110:206–210.

112. Rohrschneider K, Burk ROW, Kruse FE, et al. Reproducibility of the optic nerve head topography with a new laser tomographic scanning device. Ophthalmology 1994;101:1044–1049.

113. Weinreb RN, Lusky M, Bartsch DU, et al. Effect of repetitive imaging on topographic measurements of the optic nerve head. Arch Ophthalmol 1993;111:636–638.

114. Hoskins HD, Hetherington J, Glenday M, et al. Repeatability of the Glaucoma-Scope measurements of optic nerve head topography. J Glaucoma 1994;3:17–27.

115. Gloster J, Parry DG. Use of phonographs for measuring cupping in the optic disc. Br J Ophthalmol 1974;58:850–862.

116. Hoskins HD, Gelber EC. Optic disk topography and visual field defects in patients with increased intraocular pressure. Am J Ophthalmol 1975;80:284–290.

117. Hitchings RA, Spaeth GL. The optic disc in glaucoma. II. Correlation of the appearance of the optic disc with the visual field. Br J Ophthalmol 1977;61:107–113.

118. Motolko M, Drane SM. Features of the optic disc in preglaucomatous eyes. Arch Ophthalmol 1981;99:1992–1994.

119. Shihab ZM, Lee PF, Hay P. The significance of disc hemorrhage in open-angle glaucoma. Ophthalmology 1982;89:211–213.

120. Heijl A. Frequent disc photography and computerized perimetry in eyes with optic disc hemorrhage. A pilot study. Acta Ophthalmol 1986;64:274–281.

121. Poinoosawmy D, Gloster J, Nagasubramanian S, et al. Association between optic disc hemorrhages in glaucoma and abnormal glucose tolerance. Br J Ophthalmol 1986;70:599–602.

122. Cockburn DM. Clinical significance of hemorrhages in the optic disc. Am J Optom Physiol Opt 1987;64:450–457.

123. Bengtsson B, Holmin C, Krakau CET. Disc hemorrhage and glaucoma. Acta Ophthalmol 1981;59:1–14.

124. Jonas JB, Xu L. Optic disc hemorrhages in glaucoma. Am J Ophthalmol 1994;118;1–8.

125. Drance SM. Disc hemorrhages in the glaucomas. Surv Ophthalmol 1989;33:331–337.

126. Quigley HA, Miller NR, George T. Clinical evaluation of nerve fiber layer atrophy as an indicator of glaucomatous optic nerve damage. Arch Ophthalmol 1980;98:1564–1571.

127. Sommer A, Miller N, Quigley H, et al. Assessment of the nerve fiber layer as a predictor of glaucoma. Invest Ophthalmol Vis Sci 1985;26:122–128.

128. Airaksinen PJ, Drance SM, Douglas GR, et al. Diffuse and localized nerve fiber layer loss in glaucoma. Am J Ophthalmol 1984;98:566–571.

129. Fulk GW, Van Veen HG. How to photograph and evaluate the retinal nerve fiber layer. J Am Optom Assoc 1986;57:760–763.

130. Kini MM, Leibowitz HM, Colton T, et al. Prevalence of senile cataract, diabetic retinopathy, senile macular degeneration, and open-angle glaucoma in the Framingham Eye Study. Am J Ophthalmol 1978;85:28–34.

131. Pederson JE, Herschler JH. Reversal of glaucomatous cupping in adults. Arch Ophthalmol 1982;100:426–431.

132. Peli E, Hedges Tr, Schwartz B. Computerized enhancement of retinal nerve fiber layer. Acta Ophthalmol 1986;64:113–122.

133. Tuulonen A, Lehtola J, Airaksinen J. Nerve fiber layer defects with normal visual fields. Do normal optic discs and normal visual field indicate absence of glaucomatous abnormality? Ophthalmology 1993;100:587–598.

134. O'Connor DJ, Zeyen T, Caprioli J. Comparison of methods to detect glaucomatous optic nerve damage. Ophthalmology 1993;100:1498–1503.

135. Quigley HA, Reacher M, Katz J, et al. Quantitative grading of nerve fiber layer photographs. Ophthalmology 1993;100:1800–1807.

136. Armaly MF. Ocular pressure and visual fields. Arch Ophthalmol 1969;81:25–40.

137. Quigley HA, Addicks EN, Green WR. Optic nerve damage in human glaucoma. III. Quantitative correlation of nerve fiber loss and visual field defect in glaucoma, ischemic neuropathy, papilledema, toxic neuropathy. Arch Ophthalmol 1982;100:135–146.

138. Pederson JE, Anderson DR. The mode of progressive disc cupping in ocular hypertension and glaucoma. Arch Ophthalmol 1980;98:490–495.

139. Sturmer J. What do glaucomatous visual fields really look like in fine-grid computerized profile perimetry? Dev Ophthalmol 1985;12:1–47.

140. Drance SM. Diffuse visual field loss in open-angle glaucoma. Ophthalmology 1991;98:1533–1538.

141. Caprioli J. Automated perimetry in glaucoma. Am J Ophthalmol 1991;111:235–239.

142. Katz J, Tielsch JM, Quigley HA, et al. Automated perimetry detects visual field loss before manual Goldmann perimetry. Ophthalmology 1995;102:21–26.

143. Werner EB, Bishop KI, Koelle J, et al. A comparison of experienced clinical observers and statistical tests in detection of progressive visual field loss in glaucoma using automated perimetry. Arch Ophthalmol 1988;106:619–623.

144. Mills RP, Barnebey HS, Migliazzo CV, et al. Does saving time using FASTPAC or suprathreshold testing reduce quality of visual fields? Ophthalmology 1994;101:1596–1603.

145. Budenz DL, Feuer WJ, Anderson DR. The effect of simulated cataract on the glaucomatous visual field. Ophthalmology 1993;100:511–517.

146. Johnson CA, Brandt JD, Khong AM, et al. Short-wavelength automated perimetry in low-, medium-, and high-risk ocular hypertensive eyes. Initial baseline results. Arch Ophthalmol 1995;113:70–76.

147. Johnson CA, Adams AJ, Casson EJ, et al. Blue-on-yellow perimetry can predict the development of glaucomatous visual field loss. Arch Ophthalmol 1993;111:645–650.

148. Sample PA, Weinreb RN. Progressive color visual field loss in glaucoma. Invest Ophthalmol Vis Sci 1992;33:2068–2071.

149. Sears ML. Clinical and scientific basis for the management of open-angle glaucoma. Arch Ophthalmol 1986;104:191–195.

150. Quigley HA. A reevaluation of glaucoma management. Int Ophthalmol Clin 1984;24:1–11.

151. Grant WM, Burke JF. Why do some people go blind from glaucoma? Ophthalmology 1982;89:991–998.

152. Schwartz B. Primary open-angle glaucoma. In: Duane TD, Jaeger EA, eds. Clinical ophthalmology. Philadelphia: Harper & Row 1982;Chap. 52.

153. Kitazawa Y, Horie T. Diurnal variation of intraocular pressure in primary open-angle glaucoma. Am J Ophthalmol 1975;79:557–566.

154. Kwitko GM, Shin DH, Ahn BH, et al. Bilateral effects of long-term monocular timolol therapy. Am J Ophthalmol 1987;104:591–594.

155. Durkee DP, Bryant BG. Drug therapy reviews: Drug therapy of glaucoma. Am J Hosp Pharm 1978;35:682–690.

156. Soll DB, Saxon AM. Drugs and glaucoma. Am Fam Physician 1986;34:181–185.

157. Olander K, Zimmerman TJ. Practical aspects of controlling glaucoma medically or how to make your glaucoma medicines work for you. Ann Ophthalmol 1980;12:717–718.

158. Vogel R, Crick RP, Mills KB, et al. Effect of timolol versus pilocarpine on visual field progression in patients with primary open-angle glaucoma. Ophthalmology 1992;99:1505–1511.

159. Dallas NL, Sponsel WE, Hobley AJ. A comparative evaluation of

timolol maleate and pilocarpine in the treatment of chronic open-angle glaucoma. Eye 1988;2:243–249.

160. Gillies WE, Burdon JGW, Brooks AMV. The use of betaxolol in patients susceptible to nonselective beta-adrenergic blockers. Glaucoma 1993;15:181–184.

161. Parrow KA, Hong WJ, Shin DH, et al. Is it worthwhile to add dipivefrin HCl 0.1% to topical beta$_1$-, beta-$_2$ blocker therapy? Ophthalmology 1989;96:1338–1342.

162. Kooner K, Zimmerman TJ. Antiglaucoma therapy during pregnancy—Part I. Ann Ophthalmol 1988;20:166–169.

163. Kooner KS, Zimmerman TJ. Antiglaucoma therapy during pregnancy—Part II. Ann Ophthalmol 1988:20:208–211.

164. Borrmann L, Duzman E. Undetected cystoid macular edema in aphakic glaucoma patients treated with dipivefrin. J Toxicol-Cut Ocular Toxicol 1987;6:173–177.

165. Kass MA, Meltzer DW, Gordon M, et al. Compliance with topical pilocarpine treatment. Am J Ophthalmol 1986;101:515–523.

166. Kass MA, Gordon M, Meltzer DW. Can ophthalmologists correctly identify patients defaulting from pilocarpine therapy? Am J Ophthalmol 1986;101:524–530.

167. Granström P-A, Norell S. Visual ability and drug regimen—relation to compliance with glaucoma therapy. Acta Ophthalmol 1983;61:206–219.

168. Bigger JF. A comparison of patient compliance in treated vs untreated ocular hypertension. Trans Am Acad Ophthalmol Otolaryngol 1976;81:277–285.

169. Ball SF, Schneider E. Cost of β-adrenergic receptor blocking agent for ocular hypertension. Arch Ophthalmol 1992;110:654.

170. Zimmerman TJ, Zalta AH. Facilitating patient compliance in glaucoma therapy. Surv Ophthalmol 1983;28:252–257.

171. Ashburn FS, Goldberg I, Kass MA. Compliance with ocular therapy. Surv Ophthalmol 1980;24:237–248.

172. Brown MM, Brown GC, Spaeth GL. Improper topical self-administration of ocular medication among patients with glaucoma. Can J Ophthalmol 1984;19:2–5.

173. MacKean JM, Elkington AR. Compliance with treatment of patients with chronic open-angle glaucoma. Br J Ophthalmol 1983;67:46–49.

174. Zimmerman TJ, Ziegler LP. Successful topical medication: Methodology as well as diligence. Ann Ophthalmol 1984;16:109.

175. Kass MA, Gordon M, Morley RE, et al. Compliance with topical timolol treatment. Am J Ophthalmol 1987;103:188–193.

176. McCannel CA, Heinrich SR, Brubaker RF. Acetazolamide but not timolol lowers aqueous humor flow in sleeping humans. Graefe's Arch Clin Exp Ophthalmol 1992;230:518–520.

177. Kooner KS, Zimmerman TJ. A glaucoma medication timetable card. Ann Ophthalmol 1987;19:43–44.

178. Chang JS, Lee DA, Petursson G, et al. The effect of a glaucoma medication reminder cap on patient compliance and intraocular pressure. J Ocular Pharmacol 1991;7:117–124.

179. Novack GD, David R, Lee PF, et al. Effect of changing medication regimens in glaucoma patients. Ophthalmologica 1988;196:23.

180. Kowal DJ, Fingeret M. A glaucoma control chart. J Am Optom Assoc 1987;58:734–737.

181. Rebolleda G, Munoz FJ, Victorio JMF, et al. Effects of pupillary dilation on automated perimetry in glaucoma patients receiving pilocarpine. Ophthalmology 1992;99:418–423.

182. Monane M, Bohn RL, Gurwitz JH, et al. Topical glaucoma medications and cardiovascular risk in the elderly. Clin Pharmacol Ther 1994;55:76–83.

183. Freedman SF, Freedman SJ, Shields MB, et al. Effects of ocular carteolol and timolol on plasma high-density lipoprotein cholesterol level. Am J Ophthalmol 1993;116:600–611.

184. Sugar HS. Pitfalls in the medical treatment of simple glaucoma. Ann Ophthalmol 1979;11:1041–1050.

185. Drance SM. Medical control of open-angle glaucoma. Can J Ophthalmol 1978;13:123–127.

186. Wilensky JT, Gieser DK, Mori MT, et al. Self-tonometry to manage patients with glaucoma and apparently controlled intraocular pressure. Arch Ophthalmol 1987;105:1072–1075.

187. Remis LL, Epstein DL. Treatment of glaucoma. Ann Rev Med 1984;35:195–205.

188. Tuulonen A, Airaksinen PJ, Kuulasmaa K. Factors influencing the outcome of laser trabeculoplasty. Am J Ophthalmol 1985;99:388–391.

189. Grinich NP, Van Buskirk EM, Samples JR. Three-year efficacy of argon laser trabeculoplasty. Ophthalmology 1987;94:858–861.

190. Migdal C, Hitchings R. Primary therapy for chronic simple glaucoma. The role of argon laser trabeculoplasty. Trans Ophthalmol Soc UK 1984;104:62–66.

191. Watson PG, Allen ED, Graham CM, et al. Argon laser trabeculoplasty or trabeculectomy. A prospective randomised block study. Trans Ophthalmol Soc UK 1984;104:55–61.

192. Schwartz AL, Love DC, Schwartz MA. Long-term follow-up of argon laser trabeculoplasty for uncontrolled open-angle glaucoma. Arch Ophthalmol 1985;103:1482–1484.

193. Goldberg I. Argon laser trabeculoplasty and the open-angle glaucomas. Aust NZ J Ophthalmol 1985;13:243–248.

194. Krupin T, Patkin R, Kurata FK, et al. Argon laser trabeculoplasty in black and white patients with primary open-angle glaucoma. Ophthalmology 1986;93:811–816.

195. Thomas JV, Simmons RJ, Belcher CD, et al. Laser trabeculoplasty: Technique, indications, results, and complications. Int Ophthalmol Clin 1984;24:97–120.

196. Van Buskirk EM, Pond V, Rosenquist RC, et al. Argon laser trabeculoplasty. Studies of mechanism of action. Ophthalmology 1984;91:1005–1010.

197. Bylsma SS, Samples JR, Acott TS, et al. Trabecular cell division after argon laser trabeculoplasty. Arch Ophthalmol 1988;106:544–547.

198. Reiss GR, Wilensky JT, Higginbotham EJ. Laser trabeculoplasty. Surv Ophthalmol 1991;35:407–428.

199. Tuulonen A, Niva A-K, Alanko HI. A controlled five-year follow-up study of laser trabeculoplasty as primary therapy for open-angle glaucoma. Am J Ophthalmol 1987;104:334–338.

200. Fink AI, Jordan AJ, Lao PN, et al. Therapeutic limitations of argon laser trabeculoplasty. Br J Ophthalmol 1988;72:263–269.

201. Pollack IP, Robin AL, Sax H. The effect of argon laser trabeculoplasty on the medical control of primary open-angle glaucoma. Ophthalmology 1983;90:785–789.

202. Gilbert CM, Brown RH, Lynch MG. The effect of argon laser trabeculoplasty on the rate of filtering surgery. Ophthalmology 1986;93:362–365.

203. Shingleton BJ, Richter CU, Dharma SK, et al. Long-term efficacy of argon laser trabeculoplasty. A ten-year follow-up study. Ophthalmology 1993;100:1324–1329.

204. Bergea B, Svedbergh B. Primary argon laser trabeculoplasty versus pilocarpine. Short-term effects. Acta Ophthalmol 1992;70:454–460.

205. Elsas T, Johnsen H. Long-term efficacy of primary laser trabeculoplasty. Br J Ophthalmol 1991;75:34–37.

206. Searle AET, Rosenthal AR, Chaudhuri PR. Argon laser trabeculoplasty as primary therapy in open-angle glaucoma: a long-term follow-up. Glaucoma 1990;12:70–75.

207. Tuulonen A, Koponen J, Alanko HI, et al. Laser trabeculoplasty versus medication treatment as primary therapy for glaucoma. Acta Ophthalmol 1989;67:275–280.

208. The Glaucoma Laser Trial Research Group. The glaucoma laser trial (GLT). 2. Results of argon laser trabeculoplasty versus topical medicines. Ophthalmology 1990;97:1403–1413.

209. Hoskins HD, Hetherington J, Minckler DS, et al. Complications of laser trabeculoplasty. Ophthalmology 1983;90:796–799.

210. Ofner S, Samples JR, Van Buskirk EM. Pilocarpine and the increase in intraocular pressure after trabeculoplasty. Am J Ophthalmol 1984;97:647–649.

211. Brown RH, Stewart RH, Lynch MG, et al. ALO 2145 reduces the intraocular pressure elevation after anterior segment laser surgery. Ophthalmology 1988;95:378–384.

212. Lamping KA, Bellows AR, Hutchinson BT, et al. Long-term evaluation of initial filtration surgery. Ophthalmology 1986;93: 91–101.

213. Kolker AE. Visual prognosis in advanced glaucoma: A comparison of medical and surgical therapy for retention of vision in 101 eyes with advanced glaucoma. Trans Am Ophthalmol Soc 1977; 75:539–555.

214. Sherwood MB, Migdal CS, Sharir M, Zimmerman TJ, et al. Initial treatment of glaucoma: surgery or medications? Surv Ophthalmol 1993;37:293–305.

215. Jay JL, Allan D. The benefit of early trabeculectomy versus conventional management in primary open-angle glaucoma relative to severity of disease. Eye 1989;3:528–535.

216. Hitchings RA. Primary surgery for primary open-angle glaucoma—justified or not? Br J Ophthalmol 1993;77:445–448.

217. Sherwood MB, Migdal CS, Hitchings RA. Filtration surgery as the initial therapy for open-angle glaucoma. J Glaucoma 1993;2: 64–67.

218. Lavin MJ, Wormald RPL, Migdal CS, et al. The influence of prior therapy on the success of trabeculectomy. Arch Ophthalmol 1990; 108:1543–1548.

219. Sherwood MB, Grierson I, Millar L, et al. Long-term morphologic effects of antiglaucoma drugs on the conjunctiva and Tenon's capsule in glaucomatous patients. Ophthalmology 1989;96:327–335.

220. Baudouin C, Garcher C, Haouat N, et al. Expression of inflammatory membrane markers by conjunctival cells in chronically treated patients with glaucoma. Ophthalmology 1994;101:454–460.

221. Caprioli J, Strang SL, Spaeth GL, et al. Cyclocryotherapy in the treatment of advanced glaucoma. Ophthalmology 1985;92:947–954.

222. Brindler G, Shields MB. Value and limitations of cyclocryotherapy. Arch Clin Exp Ophthalmol 1986;224:545–548.

223. Marsh P, Wilson DJ, Samples JR, et al. A clinicopathologic correlative study of noncontact transscleral Nd:YAG cyclophotocoagulation. Am J Ophthalmol 1993;115:597–602.

224. Lloyd MAE, Baerveldt G, Heuer DK, et al. Initial clinical experience with the Baerveldt implant in complicated glaucomas. Ophthalmology 1994;101:640–650.

225. Smith MF, Sherwood MB, McGorray SP. Comparison of the double-plate Molteno drainage implant with the Schocket procedure. Arch Ophthalmol 1992;110:1246–1250.

226. Passo MS, Goldberg L, Elliot DL, et al. Exercise training reduces intraocular pressure among subjects suspected of having glaucoma. Arch Ophthalmol 1991;109:1096–1098.

227. Ashkenazi I, Melamed S, Blumenthal M. The effect of continuous strenuous exercise on intraocular pressure. Invest Ophthalmol Vis Sci 1992;33:2874–2877.

228. Larsson L-I, Rettig ES, Sheridan PT, et al. Aqueous humor dynamics in low-tension glaucoma. Am J Ophthalmol 1993;116: 590–593.

229. Crichton A, Drance SM, Douglas GR, et al. Unequal intraocular pressure and its relation to asymmetric visual field defects in low-tension glaucoma. Ophthalmology 1989;96:1312–1314.

230. Hamard P, Hamard H, Dufaux J, et al. Optic nerve head blood flow using a laser Doppler velocimeter and haemorheology in primary open angle glaucoma and normal pressure glaucoma. Br J Ophthalmol 1994;78:449–453.

231. Harris A, Sergott RC, Spaeth GL, et al. Color Doppler analysis of ocular vessel blood velocity in normal-tension glaucoma. Am J Ophthalmol 1994;118:642–649.

232. Gasser P, Flammer J, Guthauser U, et al. Do vasospasms provoke ocular disease? Angiology 1990;41:213–220.

233. Hitchings RA. Low-tension glaucoma—its place in modern glaucoma practice. Br J Ophthalmol 1992;76:494–496.

234. Demailly P, Cambien F, Plouin PF, et al. Do patients with low tension glaucoma have particular cardiovascular characteristics? Ophthalmologica 1984;188:65–75.

235. Kitazawa Y, Shirato S, Yamamoto T. Optic disc hemorrhages in low tension glaucoma. Ophthalmology 1986;93:853–857.

236. Caprioli J, Spaeth GL. Comparison of the optic nerve head in high- and low-tension glaucoma. Arch Ophthalmol 1985;103: 1145–1149.

237. Yamagami J, Araie M, Shirato S. A comparative study of optic nerve head in low-and high-tension glaucomas. Graefe's Arch Clin Exp Ophthalmol 1992;230:446–450.

238. Fazio P, Krupin T, Feitl ME, et al. Optic disc topography in patients with low-tension and primary open-angle glaucoma. Arch Ophthalmol 1990;108:705–708.

239. Tuulonen A, Airaksinen PJ. Optic disc size in exfoliative, primary open-angle and low-tension glaucoma. Arch Ophthalmol 1992; 110:211–213.

240. Nyman K, Tomita G, Raitta C, et al. Correlation of asymmetry of visual field loss with optic disc topography in normal-tension glaucoma. Arch Ophthalmol 1994;112–349–353.

241. Javitt JC, Spaeth GL, Katz LJ, et al. Acquired pits of the optic nerve. Increased prevalence in patients with low-tension glaucoma. Ophthalmology 1990;97:1038–1044.

242. Jonas JB, Xu L. Parapapillary chorioretinal atrophy in normal-pressure glaucoma. Am J Ophthalmol 1993;115:501–505.

243. Zeiter JH, Shin DH, Juzych MS, et al. Visual field defect in patients with normal-tension glaucoma and patients with high-tension glaucoma. Am J Ophthalmol 1992;114:758–763.

244. Gliklich RE, Steinmann WC, Spaeth GL. Visual field change in low-tension glaucoma over a five-year follow-up. Ophthalmology 1989;96:316–320.

245. Neureddin BN, Poinoosawmy D, Fietzke FW, et al. Regression analysis of visual field progression in low-tension glaucoma. Br J Ophthalmol 1991;75:493–495.

246. Araie M, Yamagami J, Suziki Y. Visual field defects in normal-

tension and high-tension glaucoma. Ophthalmology 1993;100: 1808–1814.

247. Rouhiainen HJ, Terasvirta ME. Hemodynamic variables in progressive and non-progressive low-tension glaucoma. Acta Ophthalmol 1990;68:34–36.

248. Schulzer M. The Normal Tension Glaucoma Study Group. Intraocular pressure reduction in normal-tension glaucoma patients. Ophthalmology 1992;99:1468–1470.

249. Nyman K. Intraocular pressure reduction with topically administered pilocarpine, timolol and betaxolol in normal-tension glaucoma. Acta Ophthalmol 1993;71:686–690.

250. deJong N, Greve EL, Hoyng PFJ. Results of a filtering procedure in low-tension glaucoma. Int Ophthalmol 1989;13:131–138.

251. Schwartz AL, Perman KI, Whitten M. Argon laser trabeculoplasty in progressive low-tension glaucoma. Ann Ophthalmol 1984;16: 560–566.

252. Sharpe ED, Simmons RJ. Argon laser trabeculoplasty as a means of decreasing intraocular pressure from "normal" levels in glaucomatous eyes. Am J Ophthalmol 1985;99:704–707.

253. Levene RZ. Low tension glaucoma: A critical review and new material. Surv Ophthalmol 1980;24:621–664.

254. Abedin S, Simmons RJ, Grant WM. Progressive low-tension glaucoma. Ophthalmology 1982;89:1–6.

255. Lumme P, Tuulonen A, Airaksinen PJ, et al. Neuroretinal rim area in low-tension glaucoma. Effect of nifedipine and acetazolamide compared to no treatment. Acta Ophthalmol 1991;69:293–298.

256. Kitazawa Y, Shirai H, Go FJ. The effect of Ca²⁺–antagonist on visual field in low-tension glaucoma. Graefe's Arch Clin Exp Ophthalmol 1989;227:408–412.

257. Gasser P. Ocular vasospasm: a risk factor in the pathogenesis of low-tension glaucoma. Int Ophthalmol 1989;13:281–290.

258. Netland PA, Chaturvedi N, Dryer EB. Calcium channel blockers in the management of low-tension and primary open-angle glaucoma. Am J Ophthalmol 1993;115:608–613.

259. Kass MA. The ocular hypertension treatment study. J Glaucoma 1994;3:97–100.

260. Cockburn DM. The prevalence of ocular hypertension in patients of an optometrist and the incidence of glaucoma occurring during long-term follow-up of ocular hypertensives. Am J Optom Physiol Opt 1982;59:330–337.

261. Schulzer M, Drance SM, Douglas GR. A comparison of treated and untreated glaucoma suspects. Ophthalmology 1991;98:301–307.

262. Levene R. Indications for medical treatment of ocular hypertension and the initial use of pilocarpine. Surv Ophthalmol 1980;25: 183–187.

263. Mantyjarvi M, Terasvirta M. Observations on color vision testing in ocular hypertension and glaucoma. Int Ophthalmol 1992;16: 417–422.

264. Pfeiffer N, Tillmon B, Bach M. Predictive value of the pattern electroretinogram in high-risk ocular hypertension. Invest Ophthalmol Vis Sci 1993;34:1710–1715.

265. Epstein DL, Krug JH, Hertzmark E, et al. A long-term clinical trial of timolol therapy versus no treatment in the management of glaucoma suspects. Ophthalmology 1989;96:1460–1467.

266. Kass MA, Gordon MO, Hoff MR, et al. Topical timolol administration reduces the incidence of glaucomatous damage in ocular hypertensive individuals. A randomized, double-masked, long-term clinical trial. Arch Ophthalmol 1989;107:1590–1598.

267. Caplan MB, Brown RH, Love LL. Pseudophakic pigmentary glaucoma. Am J Ophthalmol 1988;105:320–321.

268. David R, Livingston DG, Luntz MH. Ocular hypertension—a long-term follow-up of treated and untreated patients. Br J Ophthalmol 1977;61:668–674.

269. Luntz MH, Schenker HI. Retinal vascular accidents in glaucoma and ocular hypertension. Surv Ophthalmol 1980;25:163–167.

270. Allen PJ, Brooks AMV, Gillies WE. Hemicentral retinal vein occlusion associated with ocular hypertension and clotting abnormality. Ann Ophthalmol 1993;25:104–108.

271. Yablonski ME, Zimmerman TJ, Kass MA, et al. Prognostic significance of optic disc cupping in ocular hypertensive patients. Am J Ophthalmol 1980;89:585–592.

272. Shuster J, Kass MA. When to treat ocular hypertension. Ann Ophthalmol 1983;15:301–302.

273. Kass MA. When to treat ocular hypertension. Surv Ophthalmol 1983;28:229–232.

274. Phelps CD. The no treatment approach to ocular hypertension. Surv Ophthalmol 1980;25:175–182.

275. Johnson TD, Zimmerman TJ. Glaucoma? High-pressure decisions. Ann Ophthalmol 1986;18:207–209.

276. Phelps CD. Ocular hypertension: To treat or not to treat? Arch Ophthalmol 1977;95:588–589.

277. David R, Tessler Z, Yassur Y. Long-term outcome of primary acute angle-closure glaucoma. Br J Ophthalmol 1985;69:261–262.

278. Congdon N, Wang F, Tielsch JM. Issues in the epidemiology and the population-based screening of primary angle-closure glaucoma. Surv Ophthalmol 1992;36:411–423.

279. Panek WC, Christensen RE, Lee BA, et al. Biometric variables in patients with occludable anterior chamber angles. Am J Ophthalmol 1990;110:185–188.

280. Mulpeter KM, Walsh JB, O'Connor M, et al. Ocular hazards of nebulized bronchodilators. Postgrad Med J 1992;68:132–133.

281. Berdy GJ, Berdy SS, Odin LS, et al. Angle closure glaucoma precipitated by aerosolized atropine. Arch Intern Med 1991;151: 1658–1660.

282. Shah P, Bhurjon L, Metcalfe T, et al. Acute angle closure glaucoma associated with nebulised ipratropium bromide and salbutamol. BMJ 1992;304:40–41.

283. Chandler PA. Narrow-angle glaucoma. Arch Ophthalmol 1952; 47:695–716.

284. Krawitz PL, Podos SM. Use of apraclonidine in the treatment of acute angle closure glaucoma. Arch Ophthalmol 1990;108:1208–1209.

285. Kooner KS, Zimmerman TJ. Management of acute elevated intraocular pressure: Part II. Treatment. Ann Ophthalmol 1988;20:87–88.

286. Kramer P, Ritch R. The treatment of acute angle-closure glaucoma revisited. Ann Ophthalmol 1984;16:1101–1103.

287. Zimmerman TJ. Pilocarpine. Ophthalmology 1981;88:85–88.

288. Ganias F, Mapstone R. Miotics in closed-angle glaucoma. Br J Ophthalmol 1975;59:205–206.

289. Hillman JS, Marsters JB, Broad A. Pilocarpine delivery by hydrophilic lens in the management of acute glaucoma. Trans Ophthalmol Soc UK 1975;95:79–84.

290. Simons RJ, Dallow RL. Primary angle-closure glaucoma. In: Duane TD, Jaeger EA, eds. Clinical ophthalmology. Philadelphia: Harper & Row, 1982;Chap. 53.

291. Airaksinen PJ, Saari KM, Tiainen TJ, et al. Management of acute

closed-angle glaucoma with miotics and timolol. Br J Ophthalmol 1979;63:822–825.

292. Anderson DR. Corneal indentation to relieve acute angle-closure glaucoma. Am J Ophthalmol 1979;88:1091–1093.

293. Priore LVD, Robin AL, Pollack IP. Neodymium: YAG and argon laser iridotomy. Long-term follow-up in a prospective, randomized clinical trial. Ophthalmology 1988;95:1207–1211.

294. American Academy of Ophthalmology. Laser peripheral iridotomy for pupillary-block glaucoma. Ophthalmology 1994;101: 1749–1758.

295. Cashwell LF. Laser iridotomy for management of angle-closure glaucoma. South Med J 1985;78:288–291.

296. Cohen JS, Bibler L, Tucker D. Hypopyon following laser iridotomy. Ophthalmic Surg 1984;15:604–606.

297. Gieser DK, Wilensky JT. Laser iridectomy in the management of chronic angle-closure glaucoma. Am J Ophthalmol 1984;98:446–450.

298. Gunning FP, Greve EL. Uncontrolled primary angle closure glaucoma: results of early intercapsular cataract extraction and posterior chamber lens implantation. Int Ophthalmol 1991;15:237–247.

299. Tomey KF, Al-Rajhi AA. Neodymium:YAG laser iridotomy in the initial management of phacomorphic glaucoma. Ophthalmology 1992;99:660–665.

300. Lowenstein A, Geyer O, Goldstein M, et al. Argon laser gonioplasty in the treatment of angle-closure glaucoma (letter). Am J Ophthalmol 1993;115:399–400.

301. Weiss HS, Shingleton BJ, Goode SM, et al. Argon laser gonioplasty in the treatment of angle-closure glaucoma. Am J Ophthalmol 1992;114:14–18.

302. Lim ASM, Tan A, Chew P, et al. Laser iridoplasty in the treatment of severe acute angle closure glaucoma. Int Ophthalmol 1993;17: 33–36.

303. Drake MV. Neodymium: YAG laser iridotomy. Surv Ophthalmol 1987;32:171–177.

304. Haut J, Gaven I, Moulin F, et al. Study of the first hundred phakic eyes treated by peripheral iridotomy using the N.D.: YAG laser. Int Ophthalmol 1986;9:227–235.

305. Pollack IP. Current concepts in laser iridotomy. Int Ophthalmol Clin 1984;24:153–180.

306. Robin AL, Pollack IP, deFaller JM. Effects of topical ALO 2145 (p-aminoclonidine hydrochloride) on the acute intraocular pressure rise after argon laser iridotomy. Arch Ophthalmol 1987;105: 1208–1211.

307. Robin AL, Pollack IP, House B, Enger C. Effects of ALO 2145 on intraocular pressure following argon laser trabeculoplasty. Arch Ophthalmol 1987;105:646–650.

308. Hillman JS. Acute closed-angle glaucoma. An investigation into the effect of delay in treatment. Br J Ophthalmol 1979;63:817–821.

309. Ingram RM, Ennis JR. Acute glaucoma: Results of treatment by bilateral simultaneous iridectomy, now without admission to hospital. Br J Ophthalmol 1983;67:367–371.

310. Van Herick W, Shaffer RN, Schwartz A. Estimation of width of angle of anterior chamber. Am J Ophthalmol 1969;68:626–630.

311. Wilensky JT. Current concepts in primary angle-closure glaucoma. Ann Ophthalmol 1977;9:963–972.

312. Spaeth GL. Classification and management of patients with narrow or closed angles. Ophthalmic Surg 1978;9:39–44.

313. Forbes M. Gonioscopy with corneal indentation. A method for distinguishing between a positional closure and synechial closure. Arch Ophthalmol 1966;76:488–492.

314. Wishart PK. Can the pilocarpine phenylephrine provocative test be used to detect covert angle closure? Br J Ophthalmol 1991;75: 615–618.

315. Wishart PK. Does the pilocarpine phenylephrine provocative test help in the management of acute and subacute angle closure glaucoma? Br J Ophthalmol 1991;75:284–287.

316. Wilensky JT, Kaufman PL, Frohlichstein D, et al. Follow-up of angle-closure glaucoma suspects. Am J Ophthalmol 1993;115: 338–346.

317. Lewis RA, Phelps CD. A comparison of visual field loss in primary open-angle glaucoma and the secondary glaucomas. Ophthalmologica 1984;189:41–48.

318. Alvarado JA, Murphy CG. Outflow obstruction in pigmentary and primary open-angle glaucoma. Arch Ophthalmol 1992;110:1769–1778.

319. Murphy CG, Johnson M, Alvarado JA. Juxtacanalicular tissue in pigmentary and primary open-angle glaucoma. The hydrodynamic role of pigment and other constituents. Arch Ophthalmol 1992;110:1779–1785.

320. Ritch R, Steinberger D, Liebmann JM. Prevalence of pigment dispersion syndrome in a population undergoing glaucoma screening. Am J Ophthalmol 1993;115:707–710.

321. Farrar SM, Shields MB. Current concepts in pigmentary glaucoma. Surv Ophthalmol 1993;37:233–252.

322. Farrar SM, Shields MB, Miller KN, et al. Risk factors for the development and severity of glaucoma in the pigment dispersion syndrome. Am J Ophthalmol 1989;108:223–229.

323. Campbell DG. Pigmentary dispersion and glaucoma: A new theory. Arch Ophthalmol 1979;97:1667–1672.

324. Strasser G, Hauff W. Pigmentary dispersion syndrome. A biometric study. Acta Ophthalmol 1985;63:721–722.

325. Caprioli J, Spaeth GL, Wilson RP. Anterior chamber depth in open-angle glaucoma. Br J Ophthalmol 1986;70:831–836.

326. Ritch R, Alward WLM. Asymmetric pigmentary glaucoma caused by unilateral angle recession. Am J Ophthalmol 1993;115: 765–766.

327. Ritch R, Chaiwat T, Harbin TS. Asymmetric pigmentary glaucoma resulting from cataract formation. Am J Ophthalmol 1992; 114:484–488.

328. Semple HC, Ball SF. Pigmentary glaucoma in the black population. Am J Ophthalmol 1990;109:518–522.

329. Scheie HG, Cameron JD. Pigment dispersion syndrome; a clinical study. Br J Ophthalmol 1981;65:264–269.

330. Samples JR, Bellows AR, Rosenquist RC, et al. Pupillary block with posterior chamber intraocular lenses. Arch Ophthalmol 1987;105:335–337.

331. Smith JP. Pigmentary open-angle glaucoma secondary to posterior chamber intraocular lens implantation and erosion of the iris pigment epithelium. J Am Intraocul Implant Soc 1985;11:174–176.

332. Epstein DL, Freddo TF, Anderson PJ, et al. Experimental obstruction to aqueous outflow by pigment particles in living monkeys. Invest Ophthalmol Vis Sci 1986;27:387–395.

333. Migliazzo CV, Shaffer RN, Nykin R, et al. Long-term analysis of pigmentary dispersion syndrome and pigmentary glaucoma. Ophthalmology 1986;93:1528–1536.

334. Richter CU, Richardson TM, Grant WM. Pigmentary dispersion

syndrome and pigmentary glaucoma. A prospective study of the natural history. Arch Ophthalmol 1986;104:211–215.

335. Fine BS, Yanoff M, Scheie HG. Pigmentary glaucoma: A histological study. Trans Am Acad Ophthalmol Otolaryngol 1974;78: 314–325.

336. Epstein DL, Boger WP, Grant WM. Phenylephrine provocative testing in the pigmentary dispersion syndrome. Am J Ophthalmol 1978;85:43–50.

337. Richardson TM. Pigmentary glaucoma. In: Ritch R, Shields MB, eds. The secondary glaucomas. St Louis: C.V. Mosby Co, 1982; 84–98.

338. Sugar S. Pigmentary glaucoma and the glaucoma associated with the exfoliation-pseudoexfoliation syndrome: Update. Ophthalmology 1984;91:307–310.

339. Lehto I. Long-term prognosis of pigmentary glaucoma. Acta Ophthalmol 1991;69:437–443.

340. Ritch R. Pigmentary glaucoma: A self-limited entity? Ann Ophthalmol 1983;15:115–116.

341. Ritch R, Campbell DG, Camras C. Initial treatment of pigmentary glaucoma. J Glaucoma 1993;2:44–49.

342. Wesley P, Liebmann J, Walsh JB, Ritch R. Lattice degeneration of the retina and the pigmentary dispersion syndrome. Am J Ophthalmol 1992;114:539–543.

343. Smith DL, Kao SF, Rabbani R, et al. The effects of exercise on intraocular pressure in pigmentary glaucoma patients. Ophthalmic Surg 1989;20:561–567.

344. Haynes WL, Johnson AT, Alward WLM. Effects of jogging exercise on patients with the pigmentary dispersion syndrome and pigmentary glaucoma. Ophthalmology 1992;99:1096–1103.

345. Samples JR, Van Buskirk EM. Pigmentary glaucoma associated with posterior chamber intraocular lenses. Am J Ophthalmol 1985;100:385–388.

346. Woodhams JT, Lester JC. Pigmentary dispersion glaucoma secondary to posterior chamber intra-ocular lenses. Ann Ophthalmol 1984;16:852–854.

347. Lehto I. Long-term follow-up of argon laser trabeculoplasty in pigmentary glaucoma. Ophthalmic Surg 1992;23:614–617.

348. Ritch R, Liebmann J, Robin A, et al. Argon laser trabeculoplasty in pigmentary glaucoma. Ophthalmology 1993;100:909–913.

349. Gillies WE. Pigmentary glaucoma: A clinical review of anterior segment pigment dispersal syndrome. Aust NZ J Ophthalmol 1985;13:325–328.

350. Karickhoff JR. Pigmentary dispersion syndrome and pigmentary glaucoma: a new mechanism concept, a new treatment, and a new technique. Ophthalmic Surg 1992;23:269–277.

351. Karickhoff JR. Reverse pupillary block in pigmentary glaucoma: follow-up and new developments. Ophthalmic Surg 1993;24:562–563.

352. Lindberg JG. Klinska undersokningar over depigmentering av pupillarrandeh och genomlysbarket av aris. Helsingfors 1917.

353. Vogt A. Ein neues spaltlampenbild obschilferung der linsenvorderkapsel als wahrscheinliche ursache von seilem chronischen glaukom. Schweiz Med Wochenschr 1926;56:413–415.

354. Cashwell LF, Hollman IL, Weaver RG, et al. Idopathic true exfoliation of the lens capsule. Ophthalmology 1989;96:348–351.

355. Dvorak-Theobald G. Pseudoexfoliation of the lens capsule. Am J Ophthalmol 1954;37:1–12.

356. Schlotzer-Schrehardt UM, Dorfler S, Naumann GOH. Corneal endothelial involvement in pseudoexfoliation syndrome. Arch Ophthalmol 1993;111:666–674.

357. Chijiiwa T, Araki H, Ishibashi T, et al. Degeneration of zonular fibrils in a case of exfoliation glaucoma. Ophthalmologica 1989; 1623.

358. Sugar HS, Harding C, Barsky D. The exfoliation syndrome. Ann Ophthalmol 1976;8:1165–1181.

359. Schlotzer-Schrehardt UM, Koca MR, Naumann GOH, et al. Pseudoexfoliation syndrome. Ocular manifestation of a systemic disorder? Arch Ophthalmol 1992;110:1752–1756.

360. Streeten BW, Li ZY, Wallace RN, et al. Pseudoexfoliative fibrillopathy in visceral organs of a patient with pseudoexfoliation syndrome. Arch Ophthalmol 1992;110:1757–1762.

361. Schlotzer-Schrehardt U, Kuchle M, Naumann GOH. Electronmicroscopic identification of pseudoexfoliation material in extrabulbar tissue. Arch Ophthalmol 1991;109:565–570.

362. Repo LP, Terasvirta ME, Koivisto KJ. Generalized transluminance of the iris and the frequency of the pseudoexfoliation syndrome in the eyes of transient ischemic attack patients. Ophthalmology 1993;100:352–355.

363. Davanger M, Ringvold A, Blika S. Pseudo-exfoliation, IOP and glaucoma. Acta Ophthalmol 1991;69:569–573.

364. Ringvold A, Blika S, Elsas T, et al. The middle-Norway eye-screening study. II. Prevalence of simple and capsular glaucoma. Acta Ophthalmol 1991;69:273–280.

365. Ringvold A, Blika S, Elsas T, et al. The middle-Norway eye screening study. III. Prevalence of capsular glaucoma is influenced by blood-group antigens. Acta Ophthalmol 1992;70:207–213.

366. Lumme P, Laatikainen L. Exfoliation syndrome and cataract extraction. Am J Ophthalmol 1993;116:51–55.

367. Henry JC, Krupin T, Schmitt M, et al. Long-term follow-up of pseudoexfoliation and the development of elevated intraocular pressure. Ophthalmology 1987;94:545–552.

368. Brooks AMV, Gillies WE. The presentation and prognosis of glaucoma in pseudoexfoliation of the lens capsule. Ophthalmology 1988;95:271–276.

369. Jones W, White RE, Magnus DE. Increased occurrence of exfoliation in the male, Spanish American population of New Mexico. J Am Optom Assoc 1992;63:643–648.

370. Tarkkanen AH. Exfoliation syndrome. Trans Ophthalmol Soc UK 1986;105:233–236.

371. Gharagozloo NZ, Baker RH, Brubaker RF. Aqueous dynamics in exfoliation syndrome. Am J Ophthalmol 1992;114:473–478.

372. Gross FJ, Tingey D, Epstein DL. Increased prevalence of occludable angles and angle-closure glaucoma in patients with pseudoexfoliation. Am J Ophthalmol 1994;117:333–336.

373. Roth M, Epstein DL. Exfoliation syndrome. Am J Ophthalmol 1980;89:477–481.

374. Ritch R, Podos S. Laser trabeculoplasty in the exfoliation syndrome. Bull NY Acad Med 1983;59:339–344.

375. Konstas AGP, Jay JL, Marshall GE, et al. Prevalence, diagnostic features, and response to trabeculectomy in exfoliation glaucoma. Ophthalmology 1993;100:619–627.

376. Sherwood MB, Svedbergh B. Argon laser trabeculoplasty in exfoliation syndrome. Br J Ophthalmol 1985;69:886–890.

377. Higginbotham EJ, Richardson TM. Response of exfoliation glaucoma to laser trabeculoplasty. Br J Ophthalmol 1986;70:837–839.

378. Chen V, Blumenthal M. Exfoliation syndrome after cataract extraction. Ophthalmology 1992;99:445–447.

379. Goldmann H. Cortisone glaucoma. Arch Ophthalmol 1961;68: 621–626.

380. Steely HT, Browder SL, Julian MB, et al. The effects of dexamethasone on fibronectin expression in cultured human trabecular meshwork cells. Invest Ophthalmol Vis Sci 1992;33:2242–2250.

381. Bartlett JD, Woolley TW, Adams CM. Identification of high intraocular pressure responders to topical ophthalmic corticosteroids. J Ocular Pharmacol 1993;9:35–45.

382. Hodapp EA, Kass MA. Corticosteroid-induced glaucoma. In: Ritch R, Shields MB, eds. The secondary glaucomas. St Louis: C.V. Mosby Co, 1982;258–265.

383. Bartlett JD, Horwitz B, Laibovitz R, et al. Intraocular pressure response to loteprednol etabonate in known steroid responders. J Ocular Pharmacol 1993;9:157–165.

384. Leibowitz HM, Rich R, Crabb JL, et al. Intraocular pressure raising potential of rimexolone 1.0% in steroid responders. Invest Ophthalmol Vis Sci 1994;35(suppl):1508.

385. Krupin T. Glaucoma associated with uveitis. In: Ritch R, Shields MB, eds. The secondary glaucomas. St. Louis: C.V. Mosby Co, 1982;290–306.

386. Robin AL, Pollack IP. Argon laser trabeculoplasty in secondary forms of open-angle glaucoma. Arch Ophthalmol 1983;101:382–384.

387. Hill RA, Nguyen QH, Baerveldt G, et al. Trabeculectomy and Molteno implantation for glaucomas associated with uveitis. Ophthalmology 1993;100:903–908.

388. Posner A, Schlossman A. Syndrome of unilateral recurrent attacks of glaucoma with cyclitic symptoms. Arch Ophthalmol 1948;39:517–535.

389. Naveh-Floman N, Spierer A, Blumenthal M, et al. Protein glaucoma as a possible mechanism in a case of glaucomatocyclitic crisis and periphlebitis. Metab Pediatr Syst Ophthalmol 1983;7:85–88.

390. Harstad HK, Ringvold A. Glaucomatocyclic crises (Posner-Schlossman syndrome). A case report. Acta Ophthalmol 1986;64:146–151.

390a. Spivey BE, Armaly MF. Tonographic findings in glaucomatocyclitic crises. Am J Ophthalmol 1963;55:47–51.

391. Hong C, Song KY. Effect of apraclonidine hydrochloride on the attack of Posner-Schlossman syndrome. Korean J Ophthalmol 1993;7:28–33.

392. de Roetth A. Glaucomatocyclic crisis. Am J Ophthalmol 1970;69:370–371.

393. Varma R, Katz LJ, Spaeth GL. Surgical treatment of acute glaucomatocyclic crisis in a patient with primary open-angle glaucoma. Am J Ophthalmol 1988;105:99–100.

394. Herschler J. Trabecular damage due to blunt anterior segment injury and its relationship to traumatic glaucoma. Trans Am Acad Ophthalmol Otolaryngol 1977;83:239–248.

395. Pilger IS, Khwarg SG. Angle recession glaucoma: Review and two case reports. Ann Ophthalmol 1985;17:197–199.

396. Tonjum AM. Intraocular pressure and facility of outflow late after ocular contusion. Acta Ophthalmol 1968;46:886–908.

397. Kaufman JH, Tolpin DW. Glaucoma after traumatic angle recession: A ten year prospective study. Am J Ophthalmol 1974;78:648–654.

398. Salmon JF. The association of iridoschisis and angle-recession glaucoma. Am J Ophthalmol 1992;114:766–767.

399. Bleiman BS, Schwartz AL. Paradoxical intraocular pressure response to pilocarpine. A proposed mechanism and treatment. Arch Ophthalmol 1979;97:1305–1306.

400. Melamed S, Ashkenazi I, Gutman I, et al. Nd:YAG laser trabeculopuncture in angle-recession glaucoma. Ophthalmic Surg 1992;23:31–35.

401. Fukuchi T, Iwata K, Sawaguchi S, et al. Nd:YAG laser trabeculopuncture (YLT) for glaucoma with traumatic angle recession. Graefe's Arch Clin Exp Ophthalmol 1993;231:571–576.

402. Mermoud A, Salmon JF, Barron A, et al. Surgical management of posttraumatic angle recession glaucoma. Ophthalmology 1993;100:634–642.

403. Mermoud A, Salmon JF, Straker C, et al. Post-traumatic angle recession glaucoma: a risk factor for bleb failure after trabeculectomy. Br J Ophthalmol 1993;77:631–634.

404. Morin JD. Secondary glaucoma. In: Duane TD, Jaeger EA, eds. Clinical ophthalmology. Philadelphia: Harper & Row 1979;Chap. 54.

405. Read JE, Goldberg MF. Traumatic hyphema: Comparison of medical treatment. Trans Am Acad Ophthalmol Otolaryngol 1974;78:794–815.

406. Wilson TW, Nelson LB, Jeffers JB, et al. Outpatient management of traumatic microhyphemas. Ann Ophthalmol 1990;22:366–368.

407. Dieste MC, Hersh PS, Kylstra JA, et al. Intraocular pressure increase associated with episolon-aminocaproic acid therapy for traumatic hyphema. Am J Ophthalmol 1988;106:383–390.

408. Darr JL, Passmore JW. Management of traumatic hyphema: A review of 109 cases. Am J Ophthalmol 1967;63:134–136.

409. Thygeson P, Beard C. Observations of traumatic hyphema. Am J Ophthalmol 1952;35:977–985.

410. Jones WL. Posttraumatic glaucoma. J Am Optom Assoc 1987;58:708–715.

411. Little BC, Aylward GW. The medical management of traumatic hyphema. A survey of opinion among ophthalmologists in the U.K. J R Soc Med 1993;86:458.

412. Rakusin W. Traumatic hyphema. Am J Ophthalmol 1972;74:284–292.

413. Goldberg MF. Sickled erythrocytes, hyphema, and secondary glaucoma. Ophthalmic Surg 1979;10:17–31.

414. Crouch ER, Frenkel M. Aminocaproic acid in the treatment of traumatic hyphema. Am J Ophthalmol 1976;81:355–360.

415. McGetrick J, Jampol L, Goldberg MF, et al. Aminocaproic acid decreases secondary hemorrhage after traumatic hyphema. Arch Ophthalmol 1983;101:1031–1033.

416. Palmer DJ, Goldberg M, Frenkel M, et al. A comparison of two dose regimens of epsilon aminocaproic acid in the prevention and management of secondary traumatic hyphemas. Ophthalmology 1986;93:102–108.

417. Kutner B, Fourman S, Brien K, et al. Aminocaproic acid reduces the risk of secondary hemorrhage in patients with traumatic hyphema. Arch Ophthalmol 1987;105:206–208.

418. Farber MD, Fiscella R, Goldberg MF. Aminocaproic acid versus prednisone for the treatment of traumatic hyphema. A randomized clinical trial. Ophthalmology 1991;98:279–286.

419. Herschler J, Cobo M. Trauma and elevated intraocular pressure. In: Ritch R, Shields MB, eds. The secondary glaucomas. St Louis: C.V. Mosby Co, 1982;307–319.

420. Allemann N, Silverman RH, Reinstein DZ, Coleman DJ. High-frequency ultrasound imaging and spectral analysis in traumatic hyphema. Ophthalmology 1993;100:1351–1357.

421. Feibel RM, Bigger JF. Rubeosis iridis and neovascular glaucoma. Am J Ophthalmol 1972;74:862–867.

422. Bergren RL, Brown GC. Neovascular glaucoma secondary to sickle-cell retinopathy. Am J Ophthalmol 1992;113:718–719.

423. Weinreb RN, Wasserstrom JP, Parker W. Neovascular glaucoma following neodymium-YAG laser posterior capsulotomy. Arch Ophthalmol 1986;104:730–731.

424. Gartner S, Henkind P. Neovascularization of the iris (rubeosis iridis). Surv Ophthalmol 1978;22:291–312.

425. Weber PA. Neovascular glaucoma. Current management. Surv Ophthalmol 1981;26:149–153.

426. Rodgin SG. Neovascular glaucoma associated with uveitis. J Am Optom Assoc 1987;58:499–503.

427. Flanagan DW, Blach RK. Place of panretinal photocoagulation and trabeculectomy in the management of neovascular glaucoma. Br J Ophthalmol 1983;67:526–528.

428. Clearkin LG. Recent experience in the management of neovascular glaucoma by pan-retinal photocoagulation and trabeculectomy. Eye 1987;1:397–400.

429. Brooks AMV, Gillies WE. The development and management of neovascular glaucoma. Aust N Z J Ophthalmol 1990;18:179–185.

430. Sihota R, Sandramouli S, Sood NN. A prospective evaluation of anterior retinal cryoablation in neovascular glaucoma. Ophthalmic Surg 1991;22:256–259.

431. Pavan PR, Folk JC. Anterior neovascularization. Int Ophthalmol Clin 1984;24:61–70.

432. Shingleton BJ, Chang MA, Bellows AR, et al. Surgical goniosynechialysis for angle-closure glaucoma. Ophthalmology 1990;97:551–556.

433. Mermoud A, Salmon JF, Alexander P, et al. Molteno tube implantation for neovascular glaucoma. Long-term results and factors influencing the outcome. Ophthalmology 1993;100:897–902.

434. Lloyd MA, Heuer DK, Baerveldt G, et al. Combined Molteno implantation and pars plana vitrectomy for neovascular glaucomas. Ophthalmology 1991;98:1401–1405.

435. Molteno ACB. The dual chamber single plate implant—its use in neovascular glaucoma. Aust N Z J Ophthalmol 1990;18:431–436.

436. Thylefors B, Negrel A. The global impact of glaucoma. Bull World Health Org 1994;72:323–326.

437. Tielsch JM, Katz J, Sommer A, et al. Family history and risk of primary open angle glaucoma. The Baltimore Eye Survey. Arch Ophthalmol 1994;112:69–73.

438. Dielemans I, Vingerling JR, Algra D, et al. Primary open-angle glaucoma, intraocular pressure, and systemic blood pressure in the general elderly population. The Rotterdam Study. Ophthalmology 1995;102:54–60.

439. Tielsch JM, Katz J, Sommer A, et al. Hypertension, perfusion pressure, and primary open-angle glaucoma. A population-based assessment. Arch Ophthalmol 1995;113:216–221.

440. Fechtner RD, Weinreb RN. Mechanisms of optic nerve damage in primary open angle glaucoma. Surv Ophthalmol 1994;39:23–42.

441. Hendrickx KH, van der Enden A, Rasker MT, et al. Cumulative incidence of patients with disc hemorrhages in glaucoma and the effect of therapy. Ophthalmology 1994;101:1165–1172.

442. Butler P, Mannschreck M, Lin S, et al. Clinical experience with the long-term use of 1% apraclonidine. Incidence of allergic reactions. Arch Ophthalmol 1995;113:293–296.

443. Stewart WC, Ritch R, Shin DH, et al. The efficacy of apraclonidine as an adjunct to timolol therapy. Arch Ophthalmol 1995;113:287–292.

444. Dapling RB, Cunliffe IA, Longstaff S. Influence of apraclonidine and pilocarpine alone and in combination on postlaser trabeculoplasty pressure rise. Br J Ophthalmol 1994;78:30–32.

445. Johnson DH, Yoshikawa K, Brubaker RF, et al. The effect of long-term medical therapy on the outcome of filtration surgery. Am J Ophthalmol 1994;117:139–148.

446. Broadway DC, Grierson I, O'Brien C, et al. Adverse effects of topical antiglaucoma medication. II. The outcome of filtration surgery. Arch Ophthalmol 1994;112:1446–1454.

447. Broadway DC, Grierson I, O'Brien C, et al. Adverse effects of topical antiglaucoma medication. I. The conjunctival cell profile. Arch Ophthalmol 1994;112:1437–1445.

448. Migdal C, Gregory W, Hitchings R. Long-term functional outcome after early surgery compared with laser and medicine in open-angle glaucoma. Ophthalmology 1994;101:1651–1657.

449. Stroman GA, Stewart WC, Golnik KC, et al. Magnetic resonance imaging in patients with low-tension glaucoma. Arch Ophthalmol 1995;113:168–172.

450. Wax MB, Barrett DA, Pestronk A. Increased incidence of paraproteinemia and autoantibodies in patients with normal-pressure glaucoma. Am J Ophthalmol 1994;117:561–568.

451. Bianchi-Marzoli S, Rizzo JF, Brancato R, et al. Quantitative analysis of optic disc cupping in compressive optic neuropathy. Ophthalmology 1995;102:436–440.

452. Orgül S, Hendrickson P, Flammer J. Anterior chamber depth and pigment dispersion syndrome. Am J Ophthalmol 1994;117:575–577.

453. Kozart DM, Yanoff M. Intraocular pressure status in 100 consecutive patients with exfoliation syndrome. Ophthalmology 1982;89:214–218.

454. Graul TA, Ruttum MS, Lloyd MA, et al. Trabeculectomy for traumatic hyphema with increased intraocular pressure. Am J Ophthalmol 1994;117:155–159.

PART IV_____

Toxicology

The remedy often times proves worse than the disease.

—William Penn

CHAPTER 36

Drug Interactions

David S. Tatro

A drug interaction may be defined as a change in the effect of one drug, the *object drug,* by prior or concurrent administration of another drug, the *precipitant drug.*[1] For purposes of this chapter, the interaction effects of administering two drugs together should be greater than would be expected from additive effects of concomitant administration of the same drugs. An exception to this guideline is made for topically applied ophthalmic medications that interact with systemically administered drugs. Documentation is often insufficient to determine if the effects of these two routes of administration are additive or synergistic.[2] In addition, intravenous incompatibilities and clinically useful or intended interactions, such as the coadministration of probenecid with penicillin to delay penicillin elimination, are not discussed in this chapter. The focus of this chapter is drug interactions that can cause an increase, decrease, or loss of therapeutic effect of a medication, as well as increase in toxicity of the drug. Emphasis is placed on drug interactions that are substantiated by clinical data and that involve drugs most commonly administered systemically or topically for ophthalmic care. Note, however, that clinical documentation supporting drug interactions with topical ophthalmic medications is limited, frequently consisting of anecdotal case reports.[2]

A drug interaction may occur whenever a patient receives more than one medication. These drugs may be prescribed by a physician or self-administered for the treatment of conditions such as headaches, colds, or allergies. The medical literature is replete with case reports, clinical studies, and review articles about drug interactions, and books have been written on the subject.[3,4] Computer systems have been developed for the storage and retrieval of drug interaction information and for patient monitoring.

An estimated 6.5% of adverse drug reactions are due to drug interactions.[5] In a study involving 3028 patients in an outpatient setting, the incidence of potential drug interaction was 23%.[6] There was a dramatic increase in the frequency of potential interactions as the number of prescriptions received by a patient increased. Although patients may receive potentially interacting drugs, the frequency with which clinical consequences occur may be low. In a prospective study of 2422 patients, only 7 patients (0.03%) developed clinical evidence of a drug interaction.[7] Reports of drug interactions between systemic medications and topical ophthalmic agents are scarce. This may be due to under-reporting, since some physicians are not aware that administration of topical ophthalmic medications can result in serum concentrations that are great enough to interact with orally and parenterally administered drugs.[2] However, sufficient amounts of medications applied topically to the eye can be absorbed from the conjunctival, nasal, and oropharyngeal mucosa to interact systemically with other drugs.[2] For example, plasma concentrations following ophthalmic administration of timolol may approximate levels seen 6 to 8 hours after oral administration of timolol 10 mg. This level would be sufficient to cause some degree of systemic β-adrenergic blockade.[2,8]

Familiarity with the pharmacology and mechanisms of drug interactions can assist practitioners in preventing or minimizing the clinical consequences of drug interactions.

Drug Interaction Mechanisms

Drug interactions are of two general types, *pharmacokinetic* and *pharmacodynamic.* Pharmacokinetic interactions alter the disposition of a drug in the body, while pharmacodynamic interactions affect the pharmacologic activity of the interacting medications.

Pharmacokinetic Interactions

There are four mechanisms of pharmacokinetic interaction, each affecting the kinetics of the object drug. These mechanisms include alterations in gastrointestinal (GI) absorption, distribution, metabolism, and excretion. Pharmacokinetic interactions can affect the pharmacologic activity of drugs that have a concentration-dependent action.

ALTERATIONS IN GASTROINTESTINAL ABSORPTION

The precipitant drug can produce either an increase or decrease in absorption of the object drug. These changes in absorption are due to several factors, including modification in GI motility, stomach emptying time, pH, or the formation of drug complexes. Since interactions involving the GI tract often require both drugs to be in the stomach at the same time, separating the administration times by as much as possible will help minimize these interactions. Rarely, antibiotic therapy may affect absorption of a drug by altering the bacterial flora in the intestine. Examples of drugs that frequently alter GI absorption include antacids and cholestyramine.

DISPLACED PROTEIN BINDING

Plasma protein serves as a storage site for many drugs, and numerous drugs are reversibly bound to plasma protein. Protein-bound drugs are inactive pharmacologically and are not available for metabolism or excretion. An equilibrium exists between the quantity of free drug in the circulation and the amount bound to protein, and as metabolism and excretion of the drug occur, more drug is released from its protein-binding site. The affinity of a drug for a plasma protein binding site is based on the association constant of the drug and the binding site. Administration of more than one drug bound to the same plasma protein binding site can cause either drug to be displaced from its binding site, increasing the concentration of free drug in the circulation. The drug with the higher association constant for the protein binding site will displace the drug with the lower affinity. Once the object drug is displaced, more drug is free to act pharmacologically. Simultaneously, additional drug is available for redistribution to other tissues as well as for metabolism and excretion. To predict if a clinically important interaction will occur as the result of protein displacement, the net effect of these interrelated factors must be considered. Examples of drugs that are highly protein bound include phenytoin and warfarin.

ALTERATIONS IN METABOLISM

The effects of one drug on the metabolism of another are well documented. The precipitant drug may increase or decrease the rate of metabolism or change the first-pass metabolism of the object drug.

Increased metabolism involves an increase in synthesis of drug metabolizing enzymes by the precipitant drug. This mechanism has a slow onset, usually taking up to 3 weeks before the greatest effect is seen. As the number of enzymes increases, the plasma concentration of the object drug will decrease, reducing the pharmacologic effect and increasing the dosage requirement of the object drug. When the precipitant drug is discontinued, the process slowly reverses. Some drugs, such as carbamazepine, are capable of increasing their own metabolism. Examples of drugs that increase metabolism include barbiturates, carbamazepine, phenytoin, and rifampin.

Decreased metabolism frequently results from competition between the precipitant drug and the object drug for the same binding site on hepatic enzymes. Since direct competition for the binding site is involved, the onset of this interaction mechanism is faster than occurs with enzyme induction. When the precipitant drug inhibits the metabolism of the object drug, serum concentrations of the object drug are elevated, increasing both the pharmacologic and toxic effects of the object drug. Examples of drugs that inhibit metabolism include cimetidine, erythromycin, and oral contraceptives.

Following oral absorption, if the object drug is metabolized extensively by enzymes during its first-pass through the wall of the GI tract and liver, low concentrations will reach the systemic circulation. A drug that increases or decreases the first-pass metabolism of the object drug can have dramatic effects on the bioavailability of that drug. Compared to drugs taken orally, those administered by topical ophthalmic application attain higher levels relative to the amount administered.[2] This is because topically applied ophthalmic medications avoid first-pass metabolism by absorption from the conjunctival, nasal, and oropharyngeal mucosa.[2] Examples of drugs that are metabolized extensively by first-pass metabolism include propranolol and verapamil.

ALTERED RENAL EXCRETION

The primary means by which one drug increases or decreases the renal elimination of another drug involve competition for active tubular secretion and pH-dependent renal tubular transport. Drugs that are eliminated by active tubular secretion pass from the systemic circulation into the tubular lumen by combining with a protein. When a patient is receiving two drugs that are actively transported by this process, the drugs will compete for elimination. If the precipitant drug saturates the transport system, elimination of the object drug is decreased, producing increased serum concentrations of the object drug. Many drugs are eliminated from the renal tubules by passive diffusion. This process is dependent on the concentration and solubility of the drug on both sides of the cell membrane.[9] In an acidic urine, weakly acidic drugs will be reabsorbed, while more basic drugs will be eliminated. Conversely, in an alkaline urine, weakly basic drugs will be reabsorbed, while acidic drugs will be excreted.

Pharmacodynamic Interactions

Pharmacodynamic interactions relate to the pharmacologic activity of the interacting drugs. Thus, in a pharmacodynamic interaction, neither the pharmacokinetics nor serum concentration of the drugs is affected. Pharmacodynamic interactions can be antagonistic or synergistic, resulting in the two drugs interfering with or enhancing each other, respectively. Either or both medications may act as the precipitant or object drug, depending on the outcome of the interaction. Pharmacodynamic interactions also may occur at the receptor site. Thus, the precipitant drug may limit access of the object drug into a cell. The interaction between the thiazide diuretic hydrochlorothiazide and digoxin is an example of an indirect pharmacokinetic drug interaction. Hypokalemia induced by the diuretic increases the risk of occurrence of digitalis toxicity. Serum potassium should be monitored in patients receiving this combination, and supplemental potassium should be administered, if necessary.

Factors Predisposing Patients to Clinically Important Interactions

Therapeutic Index

If a medication has a narrow therapeutic index, the toxic dose may be only slightly greater than the therapeutic dose. Drugs with a narrow therapeutic index have the highest risk of being associated with clinically important drug interactions.[7,10,11] Examples of drugs with a narrow therapeutic index include digoxin, phenytoin, theophylline, and warfarin.

Severe Illness

The risk of clinically important interactions increases in severely ill patients.[10–12] These patients frequently are receiving multiple drug therapy and may have reduced hepatic or renal function, increasing the likelihood of a drug interaction.[10] In addition, patients with cardiac arrhythmias, epi-

lepsy, diabetes, asthma, or metabolic disorders may experience a severe exacerbation of their clinical condition if an interaction occurs.[10,13]

Individual Susceptibility

Due to individual variability and difficulty in correlating plasma drug concentrations to therapeutic outcome, it is difficult to predict the clinical importance of a drug interaction. Examples of factors that can affect variability in patient response include personal habits of the patient (including smoking or alcohol consumption), disease states (such as impaired hepatic or renal function), and genetics (e.g., acetylator phenotype).

Route of Administration

Since topically applied ophthalmic medications may be erroneously considered to be incapable of interacting with orally or parenterally administered drugs, they may be overlooked as contributing to a potential drug interaction. Adverse effects may continue for protracted periods of time without proper treatment if the symptoms are not recognized as resulting from a drug interaction.

Order of Administration

An interaction frequently will not occur if a patient's therapy with the precipitant drug is stabilized when the object drug is started. However, if the dose of the precipitant drug is changed significantly or the drug is stopped, it may be necessary to adjust the dose of the object drug to prevent an interaction.

Duration of Treatment

An interaction with a delayed onset, as occurs with hepatic enzyme induction, may not be seen if the precipitant drug is administered for an acute condition.

Dose

Many drug interactions are dose dependent. In these instances, the dose of the administered drugs must be sufficient to produce an interaction.

Approaches to Minimizing Clinically Important Drug Interactions

Awareness

Being aware that a drug interaction may occur whenever a patient receives more than one drug can help minimize the occurrence of a clinically important interaction. It is important to apply this same reasoning when considering topically administered ophthalmic agents. This awareness can lead to early recognition of a drug interaction and prevention of adverse clinical consequences.

Application Technique

If there is concern that a topically applied ophthalmic medication may interact systemically with other drugs, systemic absorption of the ophthalmic agent can be reduced by applying nasolacrimal occlusion procedures (see Fig. 3.6). Keeping the eyelid closed for 5 minutes after ophthalmic administration of a drug also decreases systemic absorption by inhibiting the nasolacrimal pump.[2,14,15]

Minimal Dose

Since many drug interactions are dose dependent, the occurrence of a drug interaction may be prevented or minimized by using the lowest possible dose necessary to achieve the desired clinical effect.

Number of Drugs

It is good practice to use the fewest number of drugs possible to achieve the necessary clinical effect.

Alternative Therapy

If there is a likelihood of a clinically important interaction, the practitioner should seriously consider using an alternative non-interacting drug. It may be necessary to choose a drug from a different chemical class that has the same or similar pharmacologic or therapeutic action. It may also be possible to select an alternative drug from the same chemical class if differences in absorption, distribution, metabolism, or excretion exist.

Order of Administration

Consider the consequences of starting, stopping, or altering the dose of one drug on the pharmacokinetics or pharmacodynamics of other drugs the patient is receiving. If the patient is taking the object drug chronically when the precipitant drug is started, dosage adjustments may be needed to prevent an interaction. However, if the precipitant drug has been taken chronically when the object drug is started, no interaction will occur if the dose of the object drug is titrated to the patient's clinical response. After the patient has been receiving both drugs chronically, it may be necessary to adjust the dose of the object drug if the dose of the precipitant drug is discontinued or altered significantly.

Route of Administration

Interactions that are route-dependent can be avoided by changing or avoiding the interacting route of administration. For example, an interaction resulting from interference with Gl absorption may be avoided by administering one of the drugs parenterally.

Therapeutic Monitoring

Monitoring therapy and adjusting treatment accordingly can help prevent serious drug interactions. Measuring plasma drug concentrations can help guide dosage adjustment if a drug interaction is suspected. However, plasma levels should not be the only criterion for making a clinical decision. The therapeutic status of the patient is a more reliable parameter on which to make a clinical evaluation of a possible drug interaction. Routine monitoring should always be performed in patients receiving drugs with a narrow therapeutic index.

Patient Education

Patients should be educated about the risks, signs, and symptoms of potential interactions of their current medications. This may help to prevent or minimize possible drug interactions. The potential for drug interactions should be communicated with the patient as well as the patient's other physicians when initiating treatment with a topically administered ophthalmic drug. Table 36.1 summarizes many of the drug interactions that may be encountered with agents that are most commonly administered systemically and topically for ophthalmic care. Drugs are listed alphabetically according to the precipitant drug. When neither drug is the precipitant, such as when synergistic interactions occur, the drugs are listed alphabetically.

Interacting Drugs	*References*

- Precipitant Drug: Erythromycin (e.g., EES), Troleandomycin (Tao)
- Object Drug: Astemizole (Hismanal) or terfenadine (e.g., Seldane)
- Summary: Increased astemizole or terfenadine concentrations may occur, producing life-threatening cardiac arrhythmias. This interaction is due to inhibition of the hepatic metabolism of astemizole or terfenadine. Torsades de pointes arrhythmias and other adverse cardiovascular drug interactions with erythromycin or troleandomycin do not appear to occur with loratadine (Claritin).
- Management: Concomitant administration of astemizole or terfenadine with either erythromycin or troleandomycin is contraindicated.

38, 60, 61, 112

- Precipitant Drug: Erythromycin (e.g., EES, E-Mycin)
- Object Drug: Carbamazepine (e.g., Tegretol)
- Summary: Erythromycin interferes with the metabolism of carbamazepine, producing increased levels of carbamazepine and possible toxicity, such as lethargy, ataxia, or neurotoxicity.
- Management: If it is not possible to avoid using these drugs concurrently, observe the patient for carbamazepine toxicity and adjust the dose as needed.

62–64

- Precipitant Drug: Erythromycin (e.g., EES, E-Mycin)
- Object Drug: Cyclosporine (Sandimmune)
- Summary: Elevated whole blood cyclosporine concentrations may occur, increasing the risk of renal toxicity.
- Management: Monitor serum creatinine and cyclosporine whole blood levels; observe the patient for toxicity. Adjust the dose of cyclosporine as needed.

65–67

- Precipitant Drug: Erythromycin (e.g., EES, E-Mycin)
- Object Drug: Digoxin (e.g., Lanoxin)
- Summary: Increased serum digoxin levels may occur in approximately 10% of patients taking oral digoxin and erythromycin. Digoxin toxicity may occur. The interaction is due to decreased metabolism of digoxin by GI bacteria in certain patients.
- Management: Observe the patient for digoxin toxicity and adjust the dose as needed. This interaction is less likely to occur with formulations of digoxin that have high bioavailability, such as digoxin capsules.

68–70

- Precipitant Drug: Erythromycin (e.g., EES, E-Mycin)
- Object Drug: Warfarin (e.g., Coumadin)
- Summary: Erythromycin may decrease the elimination of warfarin, thereby increasing the anticoagulant effect. Hemorrhage may occur.
- Management: Monitor anticoagulant function and adjust the dose of warfarin as needed.

71–74

- Precipitant Drug: Halothane
- Object Drug: Epinephrine (e.g., Propine)
- Summary: Ventricular fibrillation may occur during concurrent administration of epinephrine ophthalmic solution and halothane anesthesia. This effect has been attributed to halothane-induced increase in myocardial automaticity.
- Management: Alert anesthesiologist of the use of ophthalmic medications. Usual monitoring of cardiac function should be sufficient.

2

(continued)

Interacting Drugs	*References*

Indomethacin, see Nonsteroidal Anti-Inflammatory Drugs-Lithium
Indomethacin, see Nonsteroidal Anti-Inflammatory Drugs-Loop Diuretics
Insulin, see β-Blockers-Insulin

• Precipitant Drug: Iron Salts; e.g., ferrous sulfate	50, 75, 76
• Object Drug: Tetracyclines; e.g., doxycycline (e.g., Vibramycin), tetracycline (e.g., Achromycin V)	
• Summary: Iron salts can form insoluble chelates with tetracycline, decreasing absorption of the antibiotic. The anti-infective activity may be reduced.	
• Management: Separate the administration times of these agents by 3–4 hours.	

Isocarboxizide, see Monoamine Oxidase Inhibitors-Ephedrine
Isoflurophate, see Echothiophate-Succinylcholine
Itraconazole, see Azole Antifungal Agents-Astemizole
Ketoconazole, see Azole Antifungal Agents-Astemizole
Lithium, see Nonsteroidal Anti-Inflammatory Drugs-Lithium

• Precipitant Drug: Loop Diuretics; e.g., bumetanide (Bumex), ethacrynic acid (Edecrin), furosemide (e.g., Lasix)	77–79
• Object Drug: Aminoglycoside Antibiotics; e.g., gentamicin (e.g., Garamycin), Tobramycin (Nebcin)	
• Summary: Eighth nerve damage, resulting in irreversible hearing loss or damage may occur with concomitant use of loop diuretics and parenteral aminogycosides.	
• Management: Obtain a baseline hearing test and monitor hearing during concomitant use of these agents. Avoid use of large doses and prolonged therapy. Reduce the doses in patients with decreased renal function.	

Loop Diuretics, see Nonsteroidal Anti-Inflammatory Drugs-Loop Diuretics

• Precipitant Drug: Magnesium Salts; e.g., magnesium hydroxide (e.g., Milk of Magnesia)	50, 75, 80
• Object Drug: Tetracyclines; e.g., doxycycline (e.g., Vibramycin), tetracycline (e.g., Achromycin V)	
• Summary: Magnesium salts can form insoluble chelates with tetracycline, decreasing absorption of the antibiotic. The anti-infective activity may be reduced.	
• Management: Separate the administration times of these agents by 3–4 hours.	

Methazolamide, see Aspirin-Carbonic Anhydrase Inhibitors

Methotrexate, see Aspirin-Methotrexate

• Precipitant Drug: Methyldopa (Aldomet)	3, 81, 82
• Object Drug: Epinephrine (e.g., Adrenalin), Phenylephrine (e.g., Neo-Synephrine)	
• Summary: Hypertension may occur. Ophthalmic administration has not been studied.	
• Management: Monitor blood pressure. Discontinue the adrenergic agent if hypertension occurs.	

Methysergide, see β-Blockers-Ergot Alkaloids

• Precipitant Drug: Monoamine Oxidase Inhibitors (MAO-I); e.g., isocarboxizide (Marplan). Furazolidone (Furoxone), an antibacterial agent with MAO-I activity, is included in this interaction.	2, 3, 83
• Object Drug: Ephedrine	
• Summary: Hypertension may result from increased pressor effects due to release of large amounts of norepinephrine from nerve endings. This interaction has not been studied with ophthalmic administration.	
• Management: Closely monitor blood pressure.	

Neostigmine, see Prednisolone-Anticholinesterase

• Precipitant Drug: Nonsteroidal Anti-Inflammatory Drugs; e.g., ibuprofen (e.g., Motrin), indomethacin (e.g., Indocin)	3, 84, 85
• Object Drug: β-Blockers; e.g., betaxolol (Kerlone), timolol (Blocadren)	
• Summary: The antihypertensive effect of the β-blocker may be impaired due to inhibition of prostaglandin synthesis.	
• Management: This interaction has not been shown to affect the ocular hypotensive action of timolol (Timoptic). Monitor blood pressure when administering this combination. If possible, use alternative therapy.	

• Precipitant Drug: Nonsteroidal Anti-Inflammatory Drugs; e.g., ibuprofen (e.g., Motrin), indomethacin (e.g., Indocin)	3, 86–89

- Object Drug: Lithium (e.g., Eskalith)
- Summary: The pharmacologic and toxic effects of lithium may be increased due to increased plasma lithium concentrations.
- Management: When altering the dose of the nonsteroidal anti-inflammatory drugs, observe the patient for a change in clinical response to lithium. Adjust the dose as needed.

- Precipitant Drug: Nonsteroidal Anti-Inflammatory Drugs; e.g., ibuprofen (e.g., Motrin), indomethacin (e.g., Indocin)   90–93
- Object Drug: Loop Diuretics; e.g., bumetanide (Bumex), ethacrynic acid (Edecrin), furosemide (e.g., Lasix)
- Summary: The pharmacologic effects of loop diuretics may be reduced due to inhibition of prostaglandin synthesis and sodium retention.
- Management: Monitor the response of the patient to diuretic therapy. Adjust the dose of the loop diuretic or consider using aspirin.

Penicillins, see Tetracyclines-Penicillins
Phenylephrine, see β-Blockers-Epinephrine
Phenylephrine, see Chlorpromazine-Epinephrine
Phenylephrine, see Epinephrine-Guanethidine
Phenylephrine, see Methyldopa-Epinephrine
Phenylephrine, see Monoamine Oxidase Inhibitors-Epinephrine
Phenylephrine, see Reserpine-Epinephrine
Phenylephrine, see Tricyclic Antidepressants-Epinephrine
Phenothiazines, see Atropine-Phenothiazines

- Precipitant Drug: Phenytoin (e.g., Dilantin)   94–96
- Object Drug: Acetaminophen (e.g., Tylenol)
- Summary: The pharmacologic effects of acetaminophen may be reduced due to increased hepatic metabolism induced by phenytoin. However, more importantly, the potential for liver damage due to the presence of the hepatotoxic metabolite of acetaminophen may be increased.
- Management: This interaction is of greatest importance in patients who overdose with acetaminophen. Patients should avoid prolonged treatment with large doses of acetaminophen.

Prazosin, see β-Blockers-Prazosin

- Precipitant Drug: Prednisolone (e.g., Delta-Cortef)   3, 97
- Object Drug: Anticholinesterase, e.g., neostigmine (e.g., Prostigmin)
- Summary: In patients with myasthenia gravis, corticosteroids may antagonize the effects of anticholinesterase drugs, producing muscular weakness. Ophthalmic administration of corticosteroids has not been studied.
- Management: Monitor patients during combined therapy and have life support equipment available.

- Precipitant Drug: Probenecid (e.g., Benemid)   98, 99
- Object Drug: Zidovudine (Retrovir)
- Summary: Signs and symptoms of an interaction include cutaneous eruptions as well as fever, malaise, and myalgia. Probenecid may inhibit zidovudine metabolism.
- Management: Observe patients for a rash and systemic signs and symptoms. If necessary, reduce the dose of zidovudine.

Propranolol, see β-Blockers-Ergot Alkaloids
Propranolol, see β-Blockers-Epinephrine
Propranolol, see β-Blockers-Insulin
Propranolol, see β-Blockers-Prazosin
Quinidine, see β-Blockers-Quinidine

- Precipitant Drug: Reserpine (e.g., Serpasil)   3
- Object Drug: Epinephrine (e.g., Adrenalin), phenylephrine (e.g., Neo-Synephrine)
- Summary: Hypertension may occur. Ophthalmic administration has not been studied.
- Management: Monitor blood pressure, It may be necessary to decrease the dose of epinephrine or phenylephrine.

(continued)

| *Interacting Drugs* | *References* |

Scopolamine, see Atropine-Haloperidol
Scopolamine, see Atropine-Phenothiazines
Succinylcholine, see Echothiophate-Succinylcholine

- Precipitant Drug: Sulfinpyrazone (e.g., Anturane)   95, 100
- Object Drug: Acetaminophen (e.g., Tylenol)
- Summary: The pharmacologic effects of acetaminophen may be reduced due to increased hepatic metabolism induced by sulfinpyrazone. However, more importantly, the potential for liver damage due to the presence of the hepatotoxic metabolite of acetaminophen may be increased.
- Management: This interaction is of greatest importance in patients who overdose with acetaminophen. Patients should avoid prolonged treatment with large doses of acetaminophen.

Sulfonylurea Hypoglycemic Agents, see Aspirin-Sulfonylurea Hypoglycemic Agents
Terfenadine, see Azole Antifungal Agents-Astemizole
Terfenadine, see Erythromycin-Astemizole

- Precipitant Drug: Tetracyclines; e.g., tetracycline (e.g., Achromycin V)   70, 101
- Object Drug: Digoxin (e.g., Lanoxin)
- Summary: Increased serum digoxin levels may occur in approximately 10% of patients taking oral digoxin and tetracycline. Digoxin toxicity may occur. The interaction is due to decreased metabolism of digoxin by GI bacteria in certain patients.
- Management: Observe the patient for digoxin toxicity and adjust the dose as needed. This interaction is less likely to occur with formulations of digoxin that have high bioavailability, such as digoxin capsules.

- Precipitant Drug: Tetracyclines; tetracycline (e.g., Achromycin V)   3, 102
- Object Drug: Penicillins, cloxacillin (e.g., Tegopen), dicloxacillin (e.g., Dynapen), penicillin G
- Summary: The bactericidal effects of penicillin may be reduced by the bacteriostatic action of tetracycline.
- Management: Avoid concurrent administration when possible.

Tetracycline, see Aluminum Salts-Tetracyclines
Tetracycline, see Bismuth Salts-Tetracyclines
Tetracycline, see Calcium Salts-Tetracyclines
Tetracycline, see Iron Salts-Tetracyclines
Tetracycline, see Magnesium Salts-Tetracyclines
Tetracycline, see Zinc Salts-Tetracyclines
Theophylline, see β-Blockers-Aminophylline
Theophylline, see Erythromycin-Aminophylline
Timolol, see β-Blockers-Aminophylline
Timolol, see β-Blockers-Clonidine
Timolol, see β-Blockers-Digoxin
Timolol, see β-Blockers-Epinephrine
Timolol, see β Nonsteroidal Anti-Inflammatory Drugs–β-Blockers
Timolol, see β-Blockers-Quinidine
Timolol, see Verapamil–β-Blockers
Tobramycin, see Loop Diuretics-Aminoglycoside Antibiotics
Tolbutamide, see Aspirin-Sulfonylurea Hypoglycemic Agents

- Precipitant Drug: Tricyclic Antidepressants (TCAs); e.g., amitriptyline(e.g., Elavil)   2, 103, 104, 110
- Object Drug: Epinephrine (e.g., Adrenalin), phenylephrine (e.g., Neo-Synephrine)
- Summary: Hypertension may occur with concurrent administration of epinephrine or phenylephrine and TCAs.
- Management: Monitor blood pressure and adjust the dose of epinephrine or phenylephrine as needed.

Troleandomycin, see Erythromycin-Astemizole

Valproic Acid, see Aspirin-Valproic Acid

- Precipitant Drug: Verapamil (e.g., Calan)   105, 106
- Object Drug: β-Blockers; e.g., betaxolol (e.g., Betoptic, Kerlone), timolol (e.g., Blocadren, Timoptic)
- Summary: The antihypertensive effects of both drugs may be increased. In addition, adverse cardiovascular effects may occur. Sinus nodal dysfunction has been observed with systemic

absorption of timolol eye drops in patients receiving verapamil. This interaction is due to additive or synergistic effects.
- Management: Monitor cardiac function and adjust the dose of either drug as needed.

Warfarin, see Erythromycin-Warfarin
Warfarin, see Aspirin-Warfarin
Zidovudine, see Probenecid-Zidovudine

- Precipitant Drug: Zidovudine (Retrovir)   107, 108
- Object Drug: Ganciclovir (Cytovene)
- Summary: Life-threatening hematologic reactions have been reported, apparently due to combine toxicity.
- Management: Foscarnet (Foscavir) should be considered as an alternative to ganciclovir in treating CMV infections.

- Precipitant Drug: Zinc Salts; e.g., zinc sulfate (e.g., Orazinc)   50, 75, 109
- Object Drug: Tetracyclines; e.g., doxycycline (e.g., Vibramycin), tetracycline (e.g., Achromycin V)
- Summary: Zinc salts can form insoluble chelates with tetracycline, decreasing absorption of the antibiotic. The anti-infective activity may be reduced.
- Management: Separate the administration times of these agents by 3–4 hours.

References

1. Berkow R ed. The Merck manual of diagnosis and therapy, ed. 15. New Jersey: Merck Sharp & Dohme Research Laboratories, 1987.
2. Gerber SL, Cantor LB, Brater DC. Systemic drug interactions with topical glaucoma medications. Surv Ophthalmol 1990;35:205–218.
3. Tatro DS ed. Drug interaction facts. St. Louis: Facts and Comparisons, 1995.
4. Hansten PD, Horn JR. Drug interactions & updates. Vancouver: Applied Therapeutics, Inc, 1994.
5. Boston Collaborative Drug Surveillance Program: Adverse drug interactions. JAMA 1972;220:1238–1239.
6. Stanaszak WF, Franklin CE. Survey of potential drug interaction incidence in an outpatient clinic population. Hosp Pharm 1978;13:255–263.
7. Puckett WH, Visconti JA. An epidemiological study of the clinical significance of drug-drug interactions in a private community hospital. Am J Hosp Pharm 1971;28:247–253.
8. Munroe WP, Rindone JP, Kershner RM. Systemic side effects associated with the ophthalmic administration of timolol. Drug Intell Clin Pharm 1985;19:85–89.
9. Hansten PD, Horn JR. Interactions associated with modified drug excretion. Drug Interaction Newsletter 1989;9:497–503.
10. McInnes GT, Brodie MJ. Drug interactions that matter. A critical reappraisal. Drugs 1988;36:83–100.
11. Tatro DS. Drug interactions. In: Herfindal ET, Gourley DR, Hart LL, eds. Clinical pharmacy and therapeutics, ed. 5. Baltimore: Williams & Wilkins, 1992;37–46.
12. Hansten PD, Horn JR. Patients at increased risk for adverse drug interactions. Drug Interactions Newsletter 1990;10:589–595.
13. Tatro DS. Drugs interfering with control of the diabetic patient: Hypoglycemic drug-drug interactions. Rev Drug Interaction 1974;1:3–34.
14. Mort JR. Nightmare cessation following alteration of ophthalmic administration of a cholinergic and a beta-blocking agent. Ann Pharmacother 1992;26:914–916.
15. Zimmerman TJ, Sharir M, Nardin GF, et al. Therapeutic index of pilocarpine, carbachol, and timolol with nasolacrimal occlusion. Am J Ophthalmol 1992;114:1–7.
16. Boston Collaborative Drug Surveillance Program. Excess of ampicillin rashes associated with allopurinol or hyperuricemia. N Engl J Med 1972;286:505–507.
17. Jick H, Porter JB. Potentiation of ampicillin skin reactions by allopurinol or hyperuricemia. J Clin Pharmacol 1981;21:456–458.
18. Deppermann KM, Lode H, Hoffken G, et al. Influence of ranitidine, pirenzepine, and aluminum magnesium hydroxide on the bioavailability of various antibiotics, including amoxicillin, cephalexin, doxycycline, and amoxicillin-clavulanic acid. Antimicrob Agents Chemother 1989;33:1901–1907.
19. Nguyen VX, Nix DE, Gillikin S, et al. Effect of oral antacid administration on the pharmacokinetics of intravenous doxycycline. Antimicrob Agents Chemother 1989;33:434–436.
20. Schafer-Korting M, Kirch W, Axtheim T, et al. Atenolol interaction with aspirin, allopurinol, and ampicillin. Clin Pharmacol Ther 1983;33:283–288.
21. Sweeney KR, Chapron DJ, Antal EJ, et al. Differential effects of flurbiprofen and aspirin on acetazolamide disposition in humans. Br J Clin Pharmacol 1990;27:866–869.
22. Sweeney KR, Chapron DJ, Brandt L, et al. Toxic interaction between acetazolamide and salicylate: Case reports and a pharmacokinetic explanation. Clin Pharmacol Ther 1986;40:518–524.
23. Zucker MB, Peterson J. Effect of acetylsalicylic acid, other nonsteroidal anti-inflammatory agents, and dipyridamole of human blood products. J Lab Clin Med 1970;76:66–75.
24. Walker AM, Jick H. Predictors of bleeding during heparin therapy. JAMA 1980;244:1209–1212.
25. Mandel MA. The synergistic effect of salicylates on methotrexate toxicity. Plastic Reconstruct Surg 1976;57:733–737.
26. Taylor JR, Halprin KM. Effect of sodium salicylate and indometh-

acin on methotrexate-serum albumin binding. Arch Dermatol 1977;113:588–591.

27. Cattaneo AG, Caviezel F, Pozza G. Pharmacological interaction between tolbutamide and acetylsalicylic acid: Study on insulin secretion in man. Int J Clin Pharmacol Ther Toxicol 1990;28:229–234.

28. Farrell K, Orr JM, Abbott FS, et al. The effect of acetylsalicylic acid on serum free valproate concentrations and valproate clearance in children. J Pediatr 1982;101:142–144.

29. Abbott FS, Kassam J, Orr JM, et al. The effect of aspirin on valproic acid metabolism. Clin Pharmacol Ther 1986;40:94–100.

30. Goulden KJ, Dooley JM, Camfield PR, et al. Clinical valproate toxicity induced by acetylsalicylic acid. Neurology 1987;37:1392–1394.

31. Quick RM, Clesceri L. Influence of acetylsalicylic acid and salicylamide on the coagulation of blood. J Pharmacol Exp Ther 1960;128:95–98.

32. Singh MM, Kay SR. Therapeutic antagonism between anticholinergic antiparkinsonism agents and neuroleptics in schizophrenia. Neuropsychobiology 1979;5:74–86.

33. Singh MM, Smith JM. Reversal of some therapeutic effects of an antipsychotic agent by an antiparkinsonism drug. J Nerv Ment Dis 1973;157:50–58.

34. Rockland L, Cooper T, Schwartz F, et al. Effects of trihexyphenidyl on plasma chlorpromazine in young schizophrenics. Can J Psychiatry 1990;35:604–607.

35. Monahan BP, Ferguson CL, Killeavy ES, et al. Torsades de pointes occurring in association with terfenadine use. JAMA 1990;264:2788–2790.

36. Mathews DR, McNutt B, Okerholm R, et al. Torsades de pointes occurring in association with terfenadine use. JAMA 1991;266:2375–2376.

37. Honig PK, Wortham DC, Zamani K, et al. Terfenadine-ketoconazole Interaction: pharmacokinetic and electrocardiographic consequences. JAMA 1993;269:1513–1518.

38. Olin BR, ed. Drug facts and comparisons. St. Louis: Facts and Comparisons, 1995.

39. Bailey RR, Neale TJ. Rapid clonidine withdrawal with blood pressure overshoot exaggerated by beta-blockade. Br Med J 1976;1:942–943.

40. Vernon C, Sakula A. Fatal rebound hypertension after abrupt withdrawal of clonidine and propranolol. Br J Clin Pract 1979;33:112, 121.

41. Rynne MV. Timolol toxicity: Ophthalmic medication complicating systemic disease. J Maine Med Assoc 1980;71:82.

42. Gandy W. Severe epinephrine-propranolol interaction. Ann Emerg Med 1989;18:98–99.

43. Gandy W. Dihydroergotamine interaction with propranolol. Ann Emerg Med 1990;19:221.

44. Angelo-Nielsen K. Timolol topically and diabetes mellitus. JAMA 1980;244:2263.

45. Rubin P, Jackson G, Blaschke T. Studies on the clinical pharmacology of prazosin. II: The influence of indomethacin and of propranolol on the action and disposition of prazosin. Br J Clin Pharmacol 1980;10:33–39.

46. Dinai Y, Sharir M, Naveh N, et al. Bradycardia induced by interaction between quinidine and ophthalmic timolol. Ann Intern Med 1985;103:890–891.

47. Albert KS, Welch RD, DeSante KA, et al. Decreased tetracycline bioavailability caused by a bismuth subsalicylate antidiarrheal mixture. J Pharm Sci 1979;68:586–588.

48. Ericsson CD, Feldman S, Pickering LK, et al. Influence of subsalicylate bismuth on absorption of doxycycline JAMA 1982;247:2266–2267.

49. Poiger H, Schlatter CH. Compensation of dietary induced reduction of tetracycline absorption by simultaneous administration of EDTA. Eur J Clin Pharmacol 1978;14:129–131.

50. D'Arcy PF, McElnay JC. Drug-antacid interactions: assessment of clinical importance. Drug Intell Clin Pharm 1987;21:607–617.

51. Foster CA, O'Mullane EJ, Gaskell P, et al. Chlorpromazine: A study of its action on the circulation in man. Lancet 1954;2:614–617.

52. Pantuch EJ. Echothiophate eye drops and prolonged response to suxamethonium. Br J Anaesth 1966;38:406–407.

53. Gesztes T. Prolonged apnea after suxamethonium injection associated with eye drops containing an anticholinesterase agent. Br J Anaesth 1966;38:408–410.

54. Kinyon GE. Anticholinesterase eye drops—need for caution. N Engl J Med 1969;280:53.

55. Muelheims GH, Entrup RW, Paiewonsky D, et al. Increased sensitivity of the heart to catecholamine-induced arrhythmias following guanethidine. Clin Pharmacol Ther 1965;6:757–762.

56. Kozak PP, Cummins LH, Gillman SA. Administration of erythromycin to patients on theophylline. J Allergy Clin Immunol 1977;60:149–151.

57. Zarowitz BJM, Szefler SJ, Lasezkay GM. Effect of erythromycin base on theophylline kinetics. Clin Pharmacol Ther 1981;29:601–605.

58. Iliopoulou A, Aldhous ME, Johnston A, et al. Pharmacokinetic interaction between theophylline and erythromycin. Br J Clin Pharmacol 1982;14:495–499.

59. Ludden TM. Pharmacokinetic interaction of the macrolide antibiotics. Clin Pharmacokin 1985;10:63–79.

60. Woosley RL, Chen Y, Freiman JP, et al. Mechanism of the cardiotoxic actions of terfenadine. JAMA 1993;269:1532–1536.

61. Honig PK, Zamani K, Woosley RL, et al. Erythromycin changes terfenadine pharmacokinetics and electrocardiographic pharmacodynamics. Clin Pharmacol Ther 1992;51:156.

62. Macnab AJ, Robinson JL, Adderly RJ, et al. Heart block secondary to erythromycin-induced carbamazepine toxicity. Pediatrics 1987;80:951–953.

63. Barzaghi N, Gatti G, Crema F, et al. Inhibition by erythromycin of the conversion of carbamazepine to its active 10–,11–epoxide metabolite. Br J Clin Pharmacol 1987;24:836–838.

64. Miles MV, Tennison MB. Erythromycin effects on multiple-dose carbamazepine kinetics. Ther Drug Monit 1989;11:47–52.

65. Gupta SK, Bakran A, Johnson RWG, et al. Erythromycin enhances the absorption of cyclosporine. Br J Clin Pharmacol 1988;25:401–402.

66. Ben-Ari J, Eisenstein B, Davidovits M, et al. Effect of erythromycin on blood cyclosporine concentrations in kidney transplant patients. J Pediatr 1988;6:992–993.

67. Gupta SK, Bakran A, Johnson RWG, et al. Cyclosporine-erythromycin interaction in renal transplant patients. Br J Clin Pharmacol 1989;27:475–481.

68. Maxwell DL, Gilmour-White SK. Digoxin toxicity due to interaction of digoxin with erythromycin. Br Med J 1989;298:572.

69. Morton MR, Cooper JW. Erythromycin-induced digoxin toxicity. Drug Intell Clin Pharm 1989;23:668–670.

70. Lindenbaum J, Rund DG, Butler VP, et al. Inactivation of digoxin by the gut flora: reversal by antibiotic therapy. N Engl J Med 1981;305:789–794.

71. Schwartz JI, Bachmann KA. Erythromycin-warfarin interaction. Arch Intern Med 1984;144:2094.

72. Sato RI, Gray DR, Brown SE. Warfarin interaction with erythromycin. Arch Intern Med 1984;144:2413–2414.

73. Hassell D, Utt JK. Suspected interaction: warfarin and erythromycin. South Med J 1985;78:1015–1016.

74. Weibert RT, Lorentz SMC, Townsend RJ, et al. Effect of erythromycin in patients receiving long-term warfarin therapy. Clin Pharm 1989;8:210–214.

75. Neuvonen PJ. Interactions with the absorption of tetracyclines Drugs. 1976;11:45–54.

76. Neuvonen PJ, Penttila O. Effect of oral ferrous sulphate on the half-life of doxycycline in man. Eur J Clin Pharmacol 1974;7:361–363.

77. Quick CA. Hearing loss in patients with dialysis and renal transplants. Ann Otol Rhinol Laryngol 1976;85:776–790.

78. Kaka JS, Lyman C, Kilarski DJ. Tobramycin-furosemide interaction. Drug Intell Clin Pharm 1984;18:235–238.

79. Rybak LP. Furosemide ototoxicity: Clinical and experimental aspects. Laryngoscope 1985;95(Suppl 38):1–14.

80. Garty M, Hurwitz A. Effect of cimetidine and antacids on gastrointestinal absorption of tetracycline. Clin Pharmacol Ther 1980;28:203–207.

81. Dollery CT, Harington M, Hodge JV. Haemodynamic studies with methyldopa: Effect on cardiac output and response to pressor amines. Br Heart J 1963;25:670–676.

82. McLaren EH. Severe hypertension produced by interaction of phenylpropanolamine with methyldopa and oxprenolol. Br Med J 1976;2:283–284.

83. Harrrison WM, McGrath PJ, Stewart JW, et al. MAOIs and hypertensive crises: The role of OTC drugs. J Clin Psychiatry 1989;50:64–65.

84. Lichter M, Feldman F, Clark L, Cohen MM. Effect of indomethacin on the ocular hypotensive action of timolol maleate. Am J Ophthalmol 1984;98:79–81.

85. Mekki QA, Abrams SML, Petounis AD, et al. Indomethacin does not attenuate the ocular hypotensive effect of timolol. Br J Clin Pharmacol 1985;19:523–524.

86. Regheb M. The clinical significance of lithium-nonsteroidal anti-inflammatory drug interactions. J Clin Psychopharmacol 1990;10:350–354.

87. Khan IH. Lithium and non-steroidal anti-inflammatory drugs. Br Med J 1991;302:1537–1538.

88. Stein G, Robertson M, Nadarajah J. Toxic interactions between lithium and non-steroidal anti-inflammatory drugs. Psychol Med 1988;18:535–543.

89. Reimann IW, Frolich JC. Effects of diclofenac on lithium kinetics. Clin Pharmacol Ther 1981;30:348–352.

90. Patak RV, Mookerjee BK, Bentzel CJ, et al. Antagonism of the effects of furosemide by indomethacin in normal and hypertensive man. Prostaglandins 1975;10:649–659.

91. Brater DC. Analysis of the effect of indomethacin on the response to furosemide in man: Effect of dose of furosemide. J Pharmacol Exp Ther 1979;210:386–390.

92. Herchuelz A, Derenne F, Deger F, et al. Interaction between nonsteroidal anti-inflammatory drugs and loop diuretics: Modulation by sodium balance. J Pharmacol Exp Ther 1989;248:1175–1181.

93. Passmore AP, Copeland S, Johnston GD. The effects of ibuprofen and indomethacin on renal function in the presence and absence of furosemide in healthy volunteers on a restricted sodium diet. Br J Clin Pharmacol 1990;29:311–319.

94. Perucca E, Richens A. Paracetamol disposition in normal subjects and in patients treated with antiepileptic drugs. Br J Clin Pharmacol 1979;7:201–206.

95. Miners JO, Attwood J, Birkett DJ, et al. Determinants of acetaminophen metabolism: Effect of inducers and inhibitors of drug metabolism on acetaminophen's metabolic pathways. Clin Pharmacol Ther 1984;35:480–486.

96. Minton NA, Henry JA, Frankel RJ. Fatal paracetamol poisoning in an epileptic. Human Toxicol 1988;7:33–34.

97. Patten BM, Oliver KL, Engel W. Adverse interaction between steroid hormones and anticholinesterase drugs. Neurology 1974;24:442–449.

98. Kornhauser DM, Hendrix CW, Nerhood LJ, et al. Probenecid and zidovudine metabolism. Lancet 1989;2:473–475.

99. Petty BG, Kornhauser DM, Lietman PS. Zidovudine with probenecid: A warning. Lancet 1990;335(8696):1044–1045.

100. Abernethy DR, Greenblatt DJ, Ameer B, et al. Probenecid impairment of acetaminophen and lorazepam clearance: Direct inhibition of ether glucouronide formation. J Pharmacol Exp Ther 1985;234:345–349.

101. Lindenbaum J, Tse-Eng D, Butler VP, et al. Urinary excretion of reduced metabolites of digoxin. Am J Med 1981;71:67–74.

102. Lepper MH, Dowling HF. Treatment of pneumococcic meningitis with penicillin compared with penicillin plus aureomycin. Arch Intern Med 1951;88:489–494.

103. Svedmyr N. The influence of a tricyclic antidepressive agent (protriptyline) on some of the circulatory effects of noradrenaline and adrenaline in man. Life Sci 1968;7:77–84.

104. Boakes AJ, Laurence DR, Teoh PC, et al. Interactions between sympathomimetic amines and antidepressant agents in man. Br Med J 1973;1:311–315.

105. Sinclair NI, Benzie JL. Timolol eye drops and verapamil—a dangerous combination. Med J Aust 1983;1:548.

106. Pringle SD, et al. Severe bradycardia due to interaction of timolol eye drops and verapamil. Br Med J 1987;294:155–156.

107. Hochster H, Dietrerich D, Bozzette S, et al. Toxicity of combined ganciclovir and zidovudine for cytomegalovirus disease associated with AIDS. Ann Intern Med 1990;113:111–117.

108. Teich SA, Cheung TW, Friedman AH. Systemic antiviral drugs used in ophthalmology. Surv Ophthalmol 1992;37:19–53.

109. Anderson KE, Bratt L, Dencker H, et al. Inhibition of tetracycline absorption by zinc. Eur J Clin Pharmacol 1976;10:59–62.

110. Fraunfelder FT, Scafidi AF. Possible adverse effects from topical ocular 10% phenylephrine. Am J Ophthalmol 1978;85:447–453.

111. Brannan MD, Reidenberg P, Radwanski E, et al. Evaluation of pharmacokinetic and electrocardiographic parameters following 10 days of concomitant administration of loratadine with ketoconazole. J Clin Pharmacol 1994;34:1009–1033.

112. Brannan MD, Affrime MB, Reidenberg P, et al. Evaluation of the pharmacokinetics and electrocardiographic pharmacodynamics of loratadine with concomitant administration of erythromycin. Pharmacotherapy 1994;14:38.

CHAPTER 37

Ocular Effects of Systemic Drugs

Siret D. Jaanus
Jimmy D. Bartlett
Jeffrey A. Hiett

For the past several decades, the effects of systemic drug therapy on ocular function have received considerable attention.[1–8] Monographs and reviews have been devoted to this subject, and various mechanisms have been devised whereby clinical observations can be reported and possible causal connections between systemic drug use and ocular effects can be established.[3] Because of their unique position in the health care system, primary eye care practitioners are often the first to see adverse drug reactions (ADRs), and in particular, ocular adverse drug reactions (OADRs). The goal of early recognition and determination of how to best resolve the problem of OADRs can be complicated by numerous factors, such as multiple drug regimens, predisposing patient factors, and lack of conclusive evidence that the drug or drugs implicated are the cause of the observed reaction.[9] The aim of the practitioner should be to make careful observations, identify variables, and quantify the observations as much as possible.[10]

The eye, because of its rich blood supply and relatively small mass, exhibits an unusually high susceptibility to toxic substances. Drug molecules present in systemic circulation can reach the ocular structures by way of the uveal or retinal vasculature. Once in the eye, drugs and certain chemicals can be deposited in several anatomic sites acting as drug depots, such as the cornea, lens, and retina. In addition, many ocular functions, including pupil size, accommodation, intraocular pressure, and lid position, are controlled by what appears to be a delicate balance of interactions between the cholinergic and adrenergic nervous systems. Thus, many systemically ad-

ministered drugs can cause adverse ocular effects, and nearly all ocular structures are vulnerable.[5,6]

With our present state of knowledge, few ocular drug reactions are predictable or avoidable, since the patient's welfare usually depends on continued use of the drug. Nevertheless, OADRs can be reduced or prevented by understanding the major factors that lead to ocular side effects, and by knowing which systemic drugs cause adverse ocular effects.

Many cases of OADRs are individual case reports in which the administration of one or more drugs resulted in some unexpected sign or symptom. Seldom is the patient rechallenged with the implicated drug. Collectively, however, these isolated observations may represent significant findings.[10] This chapter considers primarily those drugs that have been frequently implicated in OADRs. Clinically important drug effects are related to the ocular structure or function involved, rather than to specific drug classes.

Determinants of Adverse Drug Reactions

Amount of Drug Administered

Nearly every drug, if administered in excessive dosage, may produce toxic effects. Toxic levels of drugs can result from high daily doses, following prolonged administration, or when drug detoxification or excretion mechanisms occur more slowly than normal.[5] The effect of excessive drug intake has been observed with several drugs and is particularly well documented with chloroquine.[9,11] When it is used as a malaria suppressant, ocular complications are rare. In control of rheumatoid arthritis and systemic lupus erythematosus, however, relatively larger dosages of chloroquine are administered and ocular complications involving the retina have been observed. Since the visual loss occurring with chloroquine is often irreversible,[12] regular ocular examinations of patients taking chloroquine or other quinoline derivatives are necessary.

Nature of Drug

The inherent pharmacologic properties of a drug determine its pharmacokinetic effects in the body, including its absorption, metabolism, and excretion. The ease with which a drug passes into the systemic circulation and its ability to penetrate the blood-brain, blood-aqueous, or blood-retinal barrier determine its ability to affect ocular tissue and function.

It has been suggested that the binding of drugs to melanin can lead to ocular toxicity.[6] The free, radical nature of melanin, present in ocular structures such as the uveal tract and retinal pigment epithelium, may contribute to the binding ability of certain drugs, including phenothiazines and chloroquine. Drugs can bind to ocular structures other than melanin. Digitalis has been observed to accumulate in the retina and ciliary body.[13] Other drugs may produce OADRs by their effects on the systemic circulation. For example, subconjunctival or retinal hemorrhages can be caused by use of anticoagulants, such as heparin or aspirin.[14]

Route of Administration

All routes of drug administration can affect ocular function. Most OADRs have been associated with oral or parenteral administration. However, topical application to the skin, particularly if abraded or burned, can result in sufficient systemic absorption to lead to ocular side effects. Dermatologic use of antibiotics has resulted in ocular hypersensitivity reactions.[1,2]

Pathophysiologic Variables

The presence of systemic disease can alter the way an individual detoxifies or excretes a drug. Liver and kidney disease, in particular, can markedly influence drug response by allowing the drug to accumulate to toxic levels. The rate of excretion of digoxin, for example, is reduced considerably in patients with renal impairment.[5] These patients could be more prone to ocular effects of this drug, such as the frequently observed alterations in color vision.

Sometimes the presence of systemic disease makes it difficult to determine whether the ocular effect is the result of the disease process itself or a toxic manifestation of the drug used in therapy. For example, ocular effects occurring in hypertensive patients could be associated with the disease process or be due to drugs used for control of blood pressure, such as clonidine, which has been implicated in macular depigmentation with reduced vision.[1]

Age and Gender

Adverse drug reactions are more likely to occur in the very young and the elderly. Deficiencies in liver and kidney function can result in marked delay of drug detoxification and elimination. Lower dosages of drugs are generally indicated at these two extremes of the human lifespan.

In general, more adverse systemic drug reactions are reported in women than in men. It is not clear whether this also applies to OADRs. A possible sex hormone-linked response to certain drugs may exist in humans.[5]

Multiple Drug Therapy

In general, the incidence of ADRs increases with the number of drugs administered. Interactions can occur when a drug is added to, or withdrawn from, a therapeutic regimen.

Many different sites or mechanisms can be involved. For example, one drug can alter the absorption, distribution, metabolism, or excretion of other drugs. In addition, a drug may alter the sensitivity of certain tissues to other drugs, or act at the same cellular site, or on the same physiologic system. Other factors, such as chemical incompatibility between drugs, can lead to inactivation and loss of pharmacologic activity.[5] Drug interactions of importance to the ophthalmic practitioner are discussed in Chapter 36.

History of Allergy to Drugs

Adverse reactions to drugs are more likely to occur in patients with a history of previous reactions. For a drug to cause an allergic reaction, it must combine with an endogenous protein and form an antigenic complex. Subsequent exposure of the patient to the drug or an agent similar to it results in an antigen-antibody interaction that provokes the allergic response. Such reactions are not usually dose related, and relatively small quantities of drugs that act as allergens can provoke a reaction.[5]

Allergic reactions are not infrequent and, more often than not, are unpredictable and sometimes difficult to manage. The skin is most commonly involved. Reactions can range from a mild rash to exfoliative dermatitis and erythema multiforme. Ocular structures most commonly affected are the eyelids and the conjunctiva.

Numerous systemic drugs have been implicated, including the penicillins and sulfonamides, which can cause swelling of the lids and conjunctiva as part of a generalized urticaria or localized angioneurotic edema. Other drugs implicated in ocular allergic reactions are antidepressants, antipsychotics, antihypertensives, antirheumatics, sedatives, and hypnotics.[1]

Individual Idiosyncrasy

Idiosyncrasy refers to an unexpected reaction that can occur in some patients following administration of ordinary doses of a drug. These qualitatively abnormal responses have been attributed to heritable characteristics that result in altered handling of, or abnormal tissue responsiveness to, drugs.[5,15]

In ocular therapeutics, the autosomal dominant inheritance of a glaucomatous response to topical ocular steroid therapy has been well documented. One-third of the general population responds to a 4- to 6-week challenge of topical ocular dexamethasone or betamethasone with a significant rise in intraocular pressure.[16,17] Patients with open-angle glaucoma, diabetes mellitus, or myopia greater than 5 D also have a greater incidence of increased intraocular pressure response to steroids. Genetic influences have also been implicated in the development of posterior subcapsular cataracts in patients receiving high-dose systemic steroid therapy.[18] Currently, the role of genetics in toxic drug reactions remains an enigma.

Alterations in enzymatic mechanisms could be responsible for some observed toxicities. Thus, the drug itself or metabolites formed in the liver or other organs of the body could enter the eye. It is also likely that metabolites can be formed locally in the eye, since a number of enzymes capable of metabolizing drugs have been isolated from various ocular tissues such as the corneal epithelium, iris, ciliary body, and retinal pigment epithelium.[6]

Diagnosis of Adverse Reactions

An effective approach to the diagnosis of OADRs is a detailed drug history that includes over-the-counter (OTC) drugs as well as prescription agents. A temporal relationship between drug use and ocular signs or symptoms is an important clue. Another, equally important factor is the practitioner's familiarity with the possible ocular effects of any drugs the patient is taking. This will allow prompt recognition and management.

Ocular Manifestations of Systemic Drug Therapy

When used in normal dosage amounts, most drugs have a relatively low incidence of drug-induced ocular complica-

tions.[19] Many drugs, however, may cause side effects, and others can affect ocular tissues or visual functions when taken in excessive quantities or when abused. The following sections consider the most important drugs that have the potential to affect the eye.

Drugs Affecting the Cornea and Lens

Sporadic reports implicate many drugs and other substances in adverse corneal and lenticular effects.[1,2,7,20] Several reports suggest an association between chronic allopurinol ingestion and cataract formation.[21] Other investigators, however, have found no evidence to confirm that allopurinol users were at higher risk of acquiring lens opacities.[22,23] Controlling for age, sex, hypertension, and diabetes, Clair and associates[23] reported no strong association between allopurinol and cataracts, based on either a blinded review of medical records or by prospective ophthalmic examination. There has been concern about whether lovastatin causes lens opacities. Laties and associates[24] reported no obvious effect on the lenses of over 8,000 patients who received either a placebo or lovastatin twice daily for 48 weeks. Analysis of the distribution of cortical, nuclear, and posterior subcapsular opacities showed no significant differences between the placebo and lovastatin groups. Chylack and associates[439] also observed no cataractogenic effect of lovastatin in a double-masked, randomized study of patients taking either 40 mg/day lovastatin or placebo for 2 years.

Other drugs that have been associated with lens opacities include phenytoin, diuretics, and, more recently, heavy alcohol consumption. [25–28,440] However, aside from isolated case reports, a variety of ocular toxicities are well recognized, and the drugs responsible for these side effects are listed in Tables 37.1 and 37.2.

TABLE 37.1
Drugs That Can Affect the Cornea

Drug	Side Effect
Chloroquine and hydroxychloroquine	Whorl-like epithelial opacities
Chlorpromazine	Pigmentation of endothelium and Descemet's membrane
Indomethacin	Stromal opacities or whorl-like epithelial opacities
Gold salts	Minute stromal gold deposits
Amiodarone	Whorl-like epithelial opacities
Isotretinoin	Corneal opacities, neo-vascularization
Crack cocaine	Ulceration, epithelial defects

TABLE 37.2
Drugs That Can Affect the Lens

Drug	Side Effect
Chlorpromazine	Anterior subcapsular stellate-shaped cataract
8-Methoxypsoralen	Cataract
Gold salts	Anterior capsular or subcapsular gold deposits
Corticosteroids	Posterior subcapsular cataract
Amiodarone	Anterior subcapsular opacities

Chloroquine and Hydroxychloroquine

Chloroquine and hydroxychloroquine are usually reserved for the treatment of rheumatoid arthritis, discoid and systemic lupus erythematosus, and other collagen diseases.[29,30] These quinoline drugs have been used for such purposes since the early 1950s. In 1958, Hobbs and Calnan[31] first reported corneal changes associated with these drugs.

CLINICAL SIGNS AND SYMPTOMS

The pattern of chloroquine keratopathy can be divided into three stages[11]: (1) in the early stages, diffuse punctate deposits appear in the corneal epithelium; (2) later the deposits aggregate into curved lines that converge and coalesce just below the central cornea; (3) finally, green-yellow pigmented lines appear in the center of the cornea as a whorl-like opacity.

Less than half of patients affected with corneal changes have visual symptoms,[32] but the most common complaints relate to halos around lights, glare, and photophobia. Visual acuity usually remains unchanged.[32,33] On discontinuation of drug therapy, both subjective symptoms and objective corneal signs disappear.[34–36]

Keratopathy occurs in 30% to 75% of patients treated with either chloroquine or hydroxychloroquine,[32,33,37] but the corneal changes are found much less frequently in patients treated with hydroxychloroquine.[32,33,35] Although Calkins[38] related the corneal findings to total (cumulative) drug dosage or duration of therapy, most recent studies[37,39] have found no correlation between the severity of keratopathy and the dosage or duration of drug therapy. Corneal deposits can be observed as early as 2 to 6 weeks after beginning therapy,[32,38] and there is no relationship between the development of corneal deposits and the occurrence of retinopathy.[39] About half of patients treated with chloroquine exhibit decreased or absent corneal sensitivity unrelated to the development of corneal opacities.[33]

Because of fewer side effects, hydroxychloroquine has become the preferred quinoline drug for the treatment of collagen diseases, and its ocular toxicity is considerably less than that of chloroquine.[36,40–42] Tobin and associates[40] monitored 99 patients treated with hydroxychloroquine during a 7-year period. All patients received the drug for at least 1 year, and most patients received a daily dosage of 400 mg. No keratopathy was observed in any patient. At higher dosage levels, however, a higher incidence of keratopathy has been reported.[41] In a group of patients receiving an average daily dosage of 800 mg of hydroxychloroquine, 6% developed keratopathy within 6 months of therapy, and the incidence increased to 32% during the second 6 months. Corneal changes were present in all patients after 4 years of hydroxychloroquine therapy. Shearer and Dubois[41] reported a rapid rise in the incidence of keratopathy when the total drug dosage exceeds 150 g. On reducing or discontinuing drug dosage, the corneal opacities decreased or disappeared during an average of 8 months.

ETIOLOGY

The origin of the corneal opacities is somewhat obscure but appears to represent reversible binding of the drug to intracellular nucleoproteins.[33] The changes are limited to the corneal epithelium, which the drug may reach by deposition in the tear film or by the limbal vasculature.[43]

Individual susceptibility probably plays an important role in the development of chloroquine keratopathy, since at lower dosages (e.g., 250 mg of chloroquine or 200 mg of hydroxychloroquine daily) there appears to be no relationship between the occurrence of keratopathy and total dosage or duration of therapy.[37] Patients receiving chloroquine doses exceeding 750 mg daily, or hydroxychloroquine doses exceeding 800 mg daily, appear to develop keratopathy earlier in the course of treatment.[38,41]

MANAGEMENT

Patients taking chloroquine or hydroxychloroquine should receive careful baseline and periodic slit-lamp examinations, with pupils dilated. Early identification of the corneal changes is facilitated by using retroillumination.[38] The practitioner should be careful to distinguish early chloroquine keratopathy from the normal development of Hudson-Stahli lines, which it can resemble. Fabry's keratopathy is another important condition in the differential diagnosis. The verticillate corneal findings are quite similar to those induced by chloroquine, but the systemic implications in Fabry's disease warrant consultation with an internist.

Since the condition is relatively benign and only rarely results in debilitating visual symptoms, the development of chloroquine keratopathy does not contraindicate continued use of the medication.[32,35] If, however, symptoms of glare, halos, or reduced vision bother the patient, drug therapy can be decreased or changed. This, however, must be done only in consultation with the prescribing physician.

Chlorpromazine

Chlorpromazine is a phenothiazine derivative used in the treatment of various psychiatric disorders.[44] Often high, prolonged dosages are required, and these have led to well-documented changes in the cornea and lens. In 1964, Greiner and Berry[45] reported the first cases of chlorpromazine-induced corneal and lens changes, and it is now generally accepted that chlorpromazine is the only phenothiazine to cause such ocular changes.[32]

CLINICAL SIGNS AND SYMPTOMS

Both corneal and lens changes are associated with chlorpromazine therapy.[46–51] Thaler and associates[46] describe lenticular pigmentation as occurring in 5 stages, and have assigned a grade (I–V) to each stage. The earliest sign of lenticular toxicity (grade I) is fine, dot-like opacities on the anterior lens surface. At this stage, the pigmentary deposits are small and tend to assume a disciform distribution within the pupillary area. Grade II lenticular changes consist of dot-like opacities that are more opaque and denser than in grade I. The pigmentary granules may begin to assume a stellate pattern. As the condition progresses, grade III changes are characterized by larger granules of pigment with an anterior subcapsular stellate pattern that is easily recognized. At this stage, the opacity can range from white, to yellow, to tan. The stellate pattern has a dense central area with radiating branches (Fig. 37.1). A readily visible stellate pattern with 3 to 9 star points characterizes grade IV lenticular pigmentation. The lens changes at this stage can be recognized with a penlight, and diagnosis does not necessarily require slit-lamp examination. Grade V lenticular changes are characterized by a central, lightly pigmented, pearl-like, opaque mass surrounded by smaller clumps of pigment.

Corneal pigmentary changes almost invariably occur only in patients who have concomitant lens opacities in the higher grades.[46,47,49] There is often little or no corneal involvement with lens grades I and II, but grades III and higher have detectable corneal pigmentation ranging from light to heavy.[46] The pigmentation is white, yellow-white, brown, or black and occurs at the level of the endothelium and Descemet's membrane, primarily in the interpalpebral fissure area (Fig. 37.2). In severe cases it can affect the deep stroma.[47]

The most prevalent ocular side effect associated with chlorpromazine therapy is anterior capsular and subcapsular lens pigmentation, followed by corneal endothelial pigmentary changes. Alexander and associates[44] found 67% of a group of patients to have the former, while 45% exhibited the latter. Both conditions, however, rarely reduce visual acuity, and patients may occasionally report glare, halos around lights, or hazy vision.

Usually, the corneal and lenticular pigmentary changes progress to a point beyond which no further changes are

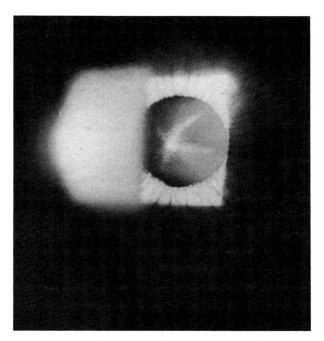

FIGURE 37.1 **Stellate pattern of anterior subcapsular cataract associated with chlorpromazine administration. (Courtesy Jerome Thaler, O.D.)**

observed.[50] On reduction or discontinuation of drug therapy, the pigmentary deposits are generally irreversible.[47,49,50] This is not surprising because the deposits associated with chlorpromazine therapy are located in avascular tissues. In rare instances the lenticular pigmentation can begin after chlorpromazine therapy is discontinued.[48]

The ocular changes associated with chlorpromazine are dose related. Lenticular pigmentation is rarely evident when the total dosage is less than 500 g, and the prevalence of pigmentary changes increases with total dosages between 1000 and 2000 g, until 90% of patients demonstrate pigmentation when the total dosage exceeds 2500 g.[44,46] Since some psychiatric conditions may require daily dosages exceeding 800 mg, lenticular pigmentation can appear in as early as 14 to 20 months of therapy.[46] Dosages consisting of 2000 mg daily have caused lenticular changes in as early as 6 months of therapy.[49]

Epidemiologic studies suggest an association between cataracts and a history of phenothiazine use.[52] Controlling for such suspect risk factors as diabetes and steroid use, a matched cohort study from a large health center indicated that use of phenothiazines increases the risk of cataract extraction by approximately 3.5 times in current users and in those exposed to the medications 2 to 5 years prior to the extraction.[52]

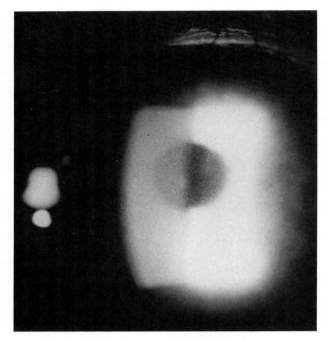

FIGURE 37.2   **Heavy pigment deposits on corneal endothelium, caused by chlorpromazine administration. (Courtesy Jerome Thaler, O.D.)**

Corneal toxicity has been reported to occur within 6 months of therapy in 12% of patients receiving 2000 mg of chlorpromazine daily, but in only 1% of patients receiving 300 mg of chlorpromazine daily.[49]

ETIOLOGY

The precise nature of the pigmentary granules in the cornea and lens is unknown. A popular hypothesis, however, is that the pigmentary changes are a result of drug interaction with ultraviolet light as it passes through the cornea and lens, causing exposed proteins to denature, opacify, and accumulate in the anterior subcapsular region of the lens as well as in corneal stroma.[53] This would explain why the keratopathy is localized to the interpalpebral fissure area.

MANAGEMENT

Patients receiving high-dosage or long-term, low-dosage chlorpromazine therapy should be monitored annually by careful slit-lamp examination. Since lens pigmentation is the most frequent ocular change observed, slit-lamp examination of the lens with the pupil dilated is the most direct method for detecting early chlorpromazine toxicity. Other tests, such as the Vistech gratings and Farnsworth Panel D-

15 tests, have been shown to be less reliable screening tests for ocular tissue changes.[54]

It may be possible to delay ocular pigmentary changes by avoiding long-term, high-dosage therapy or by employing intervals of treatment with nonphenothiazine drugs, such as haloperidol (Haldol).[47,49] The use of spectacle lenses, presumably to reduce the amount of ultraviolet light entering the eye, has been unsuccessful in reducing the prevalence of ocular toxicity.[44]

If corneal and lens changes occur but visual acuity is not affected and the patient is asymptomatic, the drug dosage can be continued without modification. If the patient becomes symptomatic, however, the dosage should be reduced or therapy should be changed to a different drug. The use of d-penicillamine has been unsuccessful in reversing the ocular pigmentary changes associated with long-term chlorpromazine therapy.[47]

Nonsteroidal Anti-Inflammatory Drugs

Nonsteroidal anti-inflammatory drugs (NSAIDs) are commonly used for their analgesic, anti-inflammatory, and antipyretic actions in the treatment of arthritis, musculoskeletal disorders, dysmenorrhea, and acute gout. Although these drugs are widely used and are often employed for prolonged periods, ocular side effects occur very rarely.[55]

CLINICAL SIGNS AND SYMPTOMS

The prevalence of corneal toxicity associated with indomethacin therapy has been reported to be 11% to 16%.[56,57] The corneal lesions appear either as fine stromal, speckled opacities or have a whorl-like distribution resembling that seen in chloroquine keratopathy. These corneal changes diminish or disappear within 6 months of discontinuing indomethacin therapy.[56,57] No definite relationship has been established between dosage of drug and corneal changes.[57] Palimeris and associates,[56] however, found corneal opacities in patients who had taken indomethacin for 12 to 18 months, with the daily dosage ranging from 75 to 200 mg and the total dosage ranging from 20 to 70 g.

Symptoms associated with the corneal opacities can include mild light sensitivity or even frank photophobia. Corneal sensitivity, however, is normal.[58]

Szmyd and Perry[58] observed whorl-like corneal opacities in a 76-year-old woman who had used naproxen for 2 months. There was complete regression of the corneal changes when the medication was discontinued.

ETIOLOGY

Carefully controlled epidemiologic studies are needed to further establish and clarify the association between NSAIDs and corneal opacities. The mechanism of these ocular changes is unknown.

MANAGEMENT

Since the corneal opacities associated with NSAIDs are benign and represent no significant threat to vision, patients taking these drugs can be monitored annually for evidence of corneal changes. Patients who develop evidence of keratotoxicity should be reassured regarding the benign nature of these changes, and the prescribing physician should be notified. The appearance of the corneal opacities does not necessitate reduction or discontinuation of drug therapy, except when severe corneal toxicity causes visual symptoms that are annoying or incapacitating.

Photosensitizing Drugs

Photosensitizing drugs are compounds that absorb optical radiation (ultraviolet [UV] and visible) and undergo a photochemical reaction, resulting in chemical modifications in nearby molecules of the tissue.[59] The psoralen compounds are photosensitizing drugs and are widely used by dermatologists to treat psoriasis and vitiligo. Commonly referred to as PUVA therapy, this treatment involves the administration of 8-methoxypsoralen (8-MOP) or related compounds, followed by exposure to UV radiation (320 to 400 nm) for short periods.[59] The most common photosensitizing reactions involve the skin and eye. Cataract formation is now well documented in patients undergoing PUVA therapy, but visual acuity usually does not deteriorate[59,60,441]

ETIOLOGY

The eye and the skin are the only tissues of the body that are particularly susceptible to damage from non-ionizing wavelengths of optical radiation (280 to 1400 nm).[59] The crystalline lens can absorb varying amounts of UV radiation and photobind susceptible drugs present in that tissue. Most ocular damage from photosensitizing drugs occurs on exposure to UV radiation.[59] Because the adult crystalline lens effectively filters most UV radiation, there is minimal risk of photobinding susceptible drugs in the retina. UV radiation, however, can penetrate to the retina in aphakic and some pseudophakic individuals and in young eyes, causing potential photosensitizing damage to the retina.[59]

MANAGEMENT

If the eye is protected from UV radiation during PUVA therapy, free 8-MOP can be found in the lens for only 24 hours.[59] Thus, to prevent permanent photobinding of this drug, dermatologists usually provide UV-filtering lenses to patients undergoing PUVA therapy. The patient should wear the lenses for at least 24 hours beginning when the drug is first taken.[60] These filters must be worn both indoors and outdoors, since there is sufficient UV radiation in ordinary fluorescent lighting to photobind the 8-MOP.[59] These measures are generally effective in preventing cataracts associated with PUVA therapy.

Gold Salts

Both parenteral and oral gold salts are used in the treatment of rheumatoid arthritis. After prolonged administration, gold can be deposited in various tissues of the body, a condition known as *chrysiasis*. Ocular chrysiasis was reported as early as 1937 by Bonnet[61] and can involve the conjunctiva, cornea, and lens. In 1987, Weidle[62] first reported ocular chrysiasis in a patient using oral gold.

CLINICAL SIGNS AND SYMPTOMS

Corneal chrysiasis consists of numerous, minute gold particles appearing as yellowish-brown to violet or red particles distributed irregularly in the stroma.[63–65] The deposition of gold generally spares the peripheral 1 to 3 mm as well as superior one-fourth to one-half of cornea,[63] and the deposits tend to localize to the posterior one-third of the stroma.[63,66] There is typically no involvement of the epithelium, Descemet's membrane, or endothelium.[63] Figure 37.3 shows the general distribution of gold deposits in a typical case of corneal chrysiasis.

Corneal chrysiasis is a common finding in patients receiving long-term maintenance gold therapy for rheumatoid arthritis. McCormick and associates[63] found gold deposits in 97% of patients receiving continuous gold therapy consisting of a cumulative dosage of at least 1000 mg. Gottlieb and Major[64] reported corneal chrysiasis in 45% of patients who had received a mean cumulative dosage greater than 7 g during a mean 6-year period. Although no correlation exists between the density of corneal deposits and the cumulative dosage, there is a positive correlation between the duration of gold therapy and the density of corneal deposits.[63]

Lenticular chrysiasis appears as fine, dust-like, yellowish, glistening deposits in the anterior capsule or in the anterior

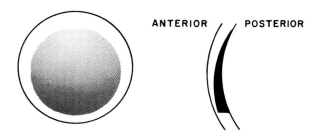

FIGURE 37.3 **General distribution of gold deposits in corneal chrysiasis. The deposits spare the peripheral and superior cornea and are more dense inferiorly. (Modified from McCormick SA, DiBartolomeo AG, Raju VK, et al. Ocular chrysiasis. Ophthalmology 1985;92:1432–1435.)**

suture lines.[64] Oral auranofin is deposited in the anterior subcapsular region[62] (Fig. 37.4).

Various studies[63,64] have established the prevalence of lenticular chrysiasis from parenteral gold to be from 36% to 55%. Although there is no correlation between the dosage of gold and the presence of lenticular deposits,[64] the deposition of gold deposits in the lens generally requires at least 3 years of parenteral chrysotherapy.[63] The lowest cumulative dosage to produce such lenticular deposits is about 2500 mg.[63] Weidle[62] reported lenticular chrysiasis in a 72-year-old woman who had received 960 mg of oral auranofin during a 5-month period.

There is no significant correlation between corneal chrysiasis and lenticular chrysiasis, and there is no evidence that gold therapy leads to cataract formation.[64] Deposits of gold in the cornea or lens do not cause visual disturbances or other symptoms.[63,64]

ETIOLOGY

The available evidence suggests that gold is deposited in the cornea and lens by circulation in the aqueous fluid in the anterior chamber.[63]

MANAGEMENT

Since ocular chrysiasis does not lead to visual impairment, inflammation, or corneal endothelial changes, gold therapy does not need to be reduced or discontinued.[62,63] This benign process requires only routine follow-up. The deposits often disappear within 3 to 6 months following cessation of therapy; occasionally, they are found years after chrysotherapy has been discontinued.

Corticosteroids

Because of the potential for systemic side effects, use of steroids is limited to conditions for which less conservative

therapy is inadequate. Steroids are sometimes used in the treatment of collagen diseases, such as rheumatoid arthritis and systemic lupus, and they are used in the treatment of sarcoidosis. The association between steroid use and cataracts has been well known for several decades. However, direct interpretation of published reports of patients with steroid-induced cataracts is often subject to error because of variations in duration of treatment and in the steroid dosages employed.

In 1960, Black and associates[67] first suggested that systemic steroid therapy could lead to posterior subcapsular (PSC) cataracts. They had observed PSC cataracts in 39% of a group of patients with rheumatoid arthritis who had undergone prolonged systemic steroid therapy. Although several authors subsequently refuted the relationship between systemic steroids and PSC cataracts,[68–70] it is now widely accepted that, under certain circumstances, systemic steroid therapy can induce cataract formation.

CLINICAL SIGNS AND SYMPTOMS

The use of systemic, topical ophthalmic, topical dermatologic, and nasal aerosol or inhalation steroids has been implicated to cause PSC cataracts that are clinically indistinguishable from complicated cataract and cataracts caused by exposure to ionizing radiation.[67,71–75] They often cannot be distinguished from age-related PSC cataracts, except that the latter frequently have other associated findings such as anterior capsular or subcapsular vacuoles, cortical opacities, or nuclear sclerosis. Even if the steroid dosage is reduced or discontinued, the cataract usually remains unchanged and will neither progress in size nor become smaller or less dense.[76,77] On rare occasions, however, the size of the opacity may decrease following reduction of steroid therapy. It has been suggested that spontaneous regression of steroid-induced PSC cataract might occur in cases associated with relatively low doses of steroid or when the duration of treatment is less than 2 years.[76] In other cases, progressive changes occasionally occur when the steroid dosage is reduced or discontinued.[76]

Several early studies of the relationship between systemic steroids and cataracts suggested that the dosage or duration of treatment was significantly correlated with the development of cataract.[77–79] Furst and associates,[77] however, proposed that it is possible for patients to develop steroid-induced cataract even when taking very low doses of steroid. In 1961, Oglesby and associates[78] provided data to suggest that no patient taking steroids for less than 1 year would develop PSC cataracts, whereas 48% of patients treated for 1 year or longer would develop lens opacities. Patients receiving less than 10 mg of prednisone daily, regardless of duration, or patients treated for less than 1 year, regardless of steroid dosage, would be unlikely to develop PSC cataracts. On the other hand, patients who receive at least 15 mg of prednisone daily for more than 1 year were very likely to

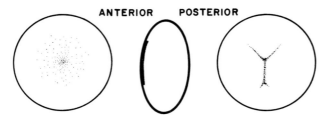

ANTERIOR   POSTERIOR

FIGURE 37.4 **Lenticular chrysiasis. Gold deposits can diffusely involve the anterior capsule and concentrate within the axial region, or can involve the anterior suture line. (Modified from McCormick SA, DiBartolomeo AG, Raju VK, et al. Ocular chrysiasis. Ophthalmology 1985;92:1432–1435.)**

develop PSC cataracts.[78] The relationship of dosage and duration of therapy was further defined by Crews,[80] who suggested that steroids could cause cataracts with short-term therapy only if the dosage was extremely high.

Allen and associates[73] reported three asthmatic patients, ages 40 to 57 years, who had been treated with inhaled beclomethasone dipropionate and small doses of systemic steroid for several years and who developed PSC cataracts. Subsequent, reports also implicated nasal aerosol or inhalation of steroids, both with and without additional systemic steroid use, with PSC cataracts[74,75] Conversely, Toogood and associates,[81] in a study of the associations between cataract occurrence and use of inhaled and oral steroid therapy in an adult population, found that neither the particular inhaled steroid used, its daily or cumulative dose, nor additional nonsteroidal risk factors present in some of the patients contributed significantly to the risk of developing PSC cataracts. Although the risk appears small in the general asthmatic population, inhaled steroid therapy might lead to cataracts if an individual has an exceptionally high inherent susceptibility.

The relationship between PSC cataract and daily dosage or duration of prednisone therapy has been called into question.[82,83] Because of considerable variation in the numbers of patients studied, dosage and duration of treatment, criteria for diagnosis, route of drug administration, and the underlying disease process itself, attention has focused on the possibility that PSC cataract formation may be related more to factors of individual susceptibility than to drug-related factors of dosage or duration of therapy.[18,84,85,442] Skalka and Prchal[85] found no statistically significant correlation between PSC opacities and total steroid dosage, weekly dosage, duration of therapy, or patient age. There may also be special susceptibility among various ethnic groups. Hispanics appear to be more predisposed to steroid-induced PSC cataracts than are either whites or blacks.[86,87]

It has been suggested that children are more susceptible than adults to develop steroid-induced cataracts,[76] developing them at a lower dosage and in a shorter time.[76,77] This can be attributed to the relatively massive doses of steroids in relation to body weight sometimes prescribed in children.[18]

A cause-and-effect relationship has been observed between PSC cataract formation and systemic steroid administration in children and adult bone marrow and renal transplant patients.[88-91] These patients generally receive significantly higher doses of steroids for immunosuppression than those used for patients with arthritis or other inflammatory disease. Although a relationship between total steroid dose, duration of therapy, and cataract formation has been reported,[91,443] other investigators[88-90] have found no significant correlation between cataract formation and the total dose of steroid administered. Moreover, cataracts have occurred in transplant patients receiving low steroid dosages.[88] These observations also suggest that an individual's susceptibility may be an important factor in cataract formation.

Visual impairment is rare in patients with steroid-induced PSC cataracts.[18,76,79] Astle and Ellis[82] reported that 88% of a group of patients with steroid-induced cataracts had visual acuity of 20/40 or better in each eye. Although severe visual reduction is uncommon, patients may report light sensitivity, photophobia, reading difficulty, or glare.

ETIOLOGY

Although the precise mechanism whereby steroids lead to cataract formation is unknown, Urban and Cotlier[18] proposed that steroids gain entry to the fiber cells of the crystalline lens and then react with specific amino groups of the lens crystallins. This alteration frees protein sulfhydral groups to form disulfide bonds, which subsequently lead to protein aggregation and, ultimately, to complexes that refract light. Other mechanisms have also been proposed.[92-94]

MANAGEMENT

Patients taking systemic steroids should have careful slit-lamp examinations performed through a dilated pupil every 6 months. Since it is possible for patients to develop cataracts even when taking very low doses of steroid,[95] every patient, regardless of dosage or duration of treatment, should be evaluated carefully for the presence of drug-induced cataract. When drug-induced cataracts are discovered, the prescribing practitioner should be notified so that the dosage can be reduced, if possible, to the minimum that will control the disease process. Other options include alternate-day therapy[85] or selecting an NSAID. Episodes of renal transplant rejection can often be controlled as effectively by lower doses of steroid, and these reduced dosages may help to prevent cataracts following transplantation.[83] If cataract extraction becomes necessary, the procedure generally carries an excellent prognosis.

Amiodarone

Amiodarone, a benzofurane derivative, has been used for several decades to treat a variety of cardiac abnormalities.[96,97] The drug is highly effective in the treatment of both atrial and ventricular arrhythmias and Wolff-Parkinson-White syndrome.[98] Amiodarone has been observed to cause keratopathy and anterior subcapsular lens opacities early in the course of treatment.[7,20]

CLINICAL SIGNS AND SYMPTOMS

Onset of keratopathy may be as early as 6 days following initiation of drug therapy,[99] but it more commonly appears after 1 to 3 months of treatment.[100] Virtually all patients will demonstrate corneal changes after 3 months of therapy.[99,101] The corneal deposits are bilateral but are often asymmetric,

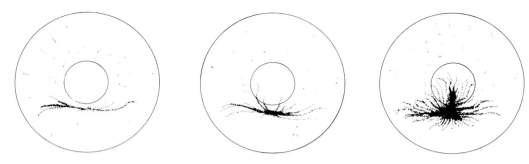

FIGURE 37.5   **Stages of amiodarone keratopathy. Left, grade I; Center, grade II; Right, grade III. (Modified from Klingele TG, Alves LE, Rose EP. Amiodarone keratopathy. Ann Ophthalmol 1984;16:1172–1176.)**

and they are observed easily with the slit lamp. The development of keratopathy can be divided into four stages.[99,100,102]

Grade 1. A faint horizontal line, similar to a Hudson-Stahli line, appears in the interpalpebral fissure at the junction of the middle and lower third of the cornea. It consists of golden-brown microdeposits in the epithelium just anterior to Bowman's layer.

Grade 2. Transition to grade II occurs by 6 months, during which the deposits become aligned in a more linear pattern and extend toward the limbus. The grade II pattern does not necessarily proceed to grade III.

Grade 3. The deposits increase in number and density, and the lines extend superiorly to produce a whorl-like pattern into the visual axis.

Grade 4. Irregular, round clumps of deposits characterize grade IV keratopathy. The development of each stage of keratopathy is shown in Figure 37.5, and a clinical representation of amiodarone keratopathy is shown in Figure 37.6.

The keratopathy gradually resolves within 6 to 18 months, after discontinuation of drug therapy.[100]

The severity of the keratopathy appears to be significantly correlated with total drug dosage as well as duration of treatment.[99,102,103] It is possible, however, for patients taking lower doses of amiodarone to demonstrate marked keratopathy while other patients taking high doses of drug show only mild corneal changes.[102] In general, patients taking low dosages of drug (100 to 200 mg daily) retain clear corneas or demonstrate only mild keratopathy regardless of duration of treatment or cumulative dosage. Patients taking higher dosages (400 to 1400 mg daily) demonstrate more advanced keratopathy depending on the duration of treatment.[97] Once the keratopathy becomes fully developed, it remains relatively stationary until the drug dosage is reduced or discontinued.[102]

Amiodarone-induced lens opacities have also been reported.[100,102,104] Fine anterior subscapular lens deposits occur in about 50% of patients taking amiodarone in moderate to high doses (600 to 800 mg daily)[104] after 6 to 18 months of treatment. The deposits first appear as small, golden-brown or white-yellow punctate opacities located just below the anterior lens capsule. They are packed loosely and cover an area greater than 2 mm within the pupillary aperture.[104] Unlike the lenticular deposits associated with chlorpromazine therapy, which develop before corneal changes, the lens opacities associated with amiodarone develop in the presence of marked keratopathy.

Amiodarone-induced lens deposits can be differentiated from the axial punctate opacities (epicapsular stars) found physiologically in about 10% of individuals over 40 years of age. The latter have a brown or metallic pigmentation and often penetrate several millimeters into the anterior cortex from their anterior subcapsular location.[100] The lenticular opacities related to amiodarone, however, are less darkly

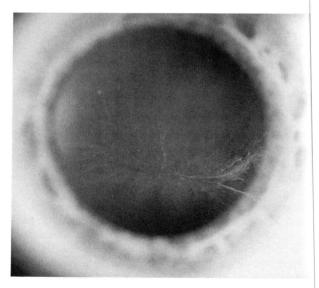

FIGURE 37.6   **Clinical photograph of grade III amiodarone keratopathy. (Courtesy Jerry Pederson, O.D.)**

pigmented and are limited to the superficial anterior subcapsular area. Once drug therapy is discontinued, it is unknown whether the lens opacities resolve.

Symptoms associated with amiodarone-induced corneal and lens changes are minimal or absent.[100–102] Lenticular opacities generally cause no visual symptoms, but moderate to severe keratopathy can lead to complaints of blurred vision, glare, halos around lights, or light sensitivity. Visual acuity usually is normal but may be slightly decreased if the keratopathy is severe.

ETIOLOGY

Amiodarone belongs to a group of drugs having the physical and chemical properties of cationic amphiphilia.[105] Amphiphilic drugs bind to polar lipids and accumulate within lysosomes. Several investigators[98,102,106,107] performed electron microscopy on ocular tissues of patients who had taken amiodarone, and these studies consistently revealed intracytoplasmic membrane-bound lamellar bodies similar to myelin. These changes have been noted not only in the corneal epithelium, the conjunctiva, and the lens, but have also been found in the corneal endothelium, the iris, ciliary body, choroid, and retina.[98,102] The presence of such complex lipid deposits within these tissues has led recent investigators to conclude that amiodarone keratopathy is probably a drug-induced lipid storage disease.[98,102,106] The whorl-like pattern of the keratopathy may result from an effect at the limbus on the epithelial cells that are migrating centripetally.[107a]

MANAGEMENT

Because the corneal and lenticular changes associated with amiodarone therapy are benign, special follow-up of affected patients is not required unless the opacities have induced visual symptoms. In the rare cases in which visual symptoms are annoying or incapacitating, reduction or discontinuation of drug dosage usually resolves the corneal findings. It is unusual for ocular side effects to necessitate discontinuation of drug therapy.[100] Occasionally, however, treatment must be discontinued because of drug intolerance or other side effects such as diarrhea, vomiting, pulmonary fibrosis, or liver damage.[102]

Light exposure may be a factor in the corneal and lenticular changes, since amiodarone is a photosensitizing agent and the observed lens changes are primarily localized to the pupillary aperture.[108] The use of UV-filtering lenses may provide a preventative measure.

Since the early stages of amiodarone keratopathy can mimic a Hudson-Stahli line, a drug history relative to amiodarone use should be elicited carefully. More advanced stages of amiodarone keratopathy may resemble the corneal changes of Fabry's disease or chloroquine toxicity. Because of the systemic implications of Fabry's disease, patients with no history of amiodarone or chloroquine use should be evaluated by an internist.

Donor corneas affected by amiodarone can be used safely in penetrating keratoplasty without removing the affected epithelium. The keratopathy has been reported to resolve quickly following the operation.[109]

Oral Contraceptives

CLINICAL SIGNS AND SYMPTOMS

Although ocular side effects have been widely reported with oral contraceptive use, most of these effects have been based primarily on isolated, anecdotal case reports. Animal studies as well as prospective clinical trials in humans have failed to document any significant relationship between use of oral contraceptives and ocular side effects.[110] Although various authors have speculated that oral contraceptives may influence contact lens wear, sometimes leading to contact lens intolerance, there is no evidence to suggest that such a relationship exists.[111,112]

ETIOLOGY

Anderson and Martin,[113] in an uncontrolled study, found that a significant number of women taking oral contraceptives experienced steepening of corneal curvature. The etiology of contact lens intolerance during use of oral contraceptives could potentially include changes in corneal curvature, corneal edema due to hypoxia,[114] or changes in the quality of the precorneal tear film, such as excessive mucus formation or a reduction of the aqueous component of the tears.[112] None of these changes, however, has been definitely implicated.

MANAGEMENT

The practitioner is cautioned to investigate other potential causes for any observed objective signs or subjective symptoms. The contact lens parameters, solutions, lens hygiene, wearing schedules, and other factors should be taken into consideration before recommendations are made regarding oral contraceptive use.

Although small anterior and posterior subcapsular opacities have been reported in patients using oral contraceptives,[115] most authorities believe there is no relationship between oral contraceptive use and cataract formation.[110] Interestingly, a recent survey of age-related eye disease in the Beaver Dam Eye Study suggests that estrogen may actually provide a modest protective effect on the crystalline lenses of women.[116]

Isotretinoin

An analog of vitamin A, isotretinoin (Accutane), or 13-*cis*-retinoic acid, is used for control of severe recalcitrant cystic acne and other keratinizing dermatoses.[117] Oral administration of 1 or 2 mg/kg body weight daily temporarily suppresses sebaceous gland activity, changes surface lipid composition of the skin, and inhibits keratinization. The therapeutic effect is resolution of lesions and, in most patients, prolonged remission of the disease.

Both systemic and ocular side effects have been reported with use of this drug. Dryness of the face and mucous membranes occurs frequently. Other systemic effects include hair loss, colitis, and skeletal hyperostosis.[117]

CLINICAL SIGNS AND SYMPTOMS

Adverse ocular effects can include keratitis, corneal opacities and corneal neovascularization.[118-121] Epithelial keratitis has been reported in patients treated with an average dose of 2 mg/kg for various dermatologic diseases.[122] Subepithelial corneal opacities may occur in both the peripheral and central cornea, and if the visual axis is involved, vision may be impaired.[119] Neovascularization can be exacerbated in patients being treated for acne with isotretinoin.[120]

ETIOLOGY

Since the meibomian glands anatomically are modified sebaceous glands, suppression of sebaceous gland activity can also cause deficiency of the normal lipid layer of the preocular tear film. This can lead to evaporation of the aqueous layer and subsequent drying of the ocular surface, followed by epithelial and subepithelial defects.

MANAGEMENT

Decreasing the dosage usually alleviates the side effects in some patients, but several months may be required before obtaining significant clinical improvement.[118]

Crack Cocaine

The use of cocaine, particularly the alkaline smoke from the crack form, can be associated with severe ocular problems, including corneal complications.[123,124]

CLINICAL SIGNS AND SYMPTOMS

Two possible patterns of clinical presentation have been observed.[124] One involves a painless loss of vision, redness, and purulent discharge in one or both eyes, usually associated with infectious corneal ulceration. The second pattern is characterized by painful loss of vision, redness, photophobia, tearing, and appears to be associated with vigorous eye rubbing and sterile epithelial defects.

ETIOLOGY

Several pathophysiologic mechanisms have been proposed.[124] A direct toxic effect may disrupt the structural and functional properties of the corneal epithelium. Other possibilities include decreased corneal sensation, neurotrophic changes, mechanical causes due to eye rubbing, and subclinical alkali burn due to the alkaline properties of crack cocaine. Each of these mechanisms alone, or in combination, could lead to chronic ocular surface disease and predispose to epithelial defects and subsequent corneal infection.

Although intranasal cocaine has not been detected in tears using high-performance liquid chromatography, the observed decrease in corneal sensitivity can be an indication that cocaine may travel retrograde through the nasolacrimal duct to reach the ocular tissues.[125]

MANAGEMENT

Therapy should be consistent with the clinical signs and symptoms present. Since patient compliance may be poor, aggressive initial therapy is recommended to prevent subsequent, more serious complications.[123,125]

Drugs Affecting the Conjunctiva and Lids

Drug effects on the conjunctiva and lids can be irritative, allergic, or involve pigmentary inclusions (Table 37.3)

Isotretinoin

The mucous membranes, including the conjunctiva, are sites that are associated most frequently with adverse effects of isotretinoin therapy.[118] Therefore, it is not surprising that blepharoconjunctivitis is the most common ocular adverse drug reaction associated with oral isotretinoin use, occurring in 20 to 50% of patients, usually within 2 months of therapy.[119,122]

CLINICAL SIGNS AND SYMPTOMS

Symptoms can vary from slight irritation associated with dry eyes, to severe discomfort and discharge. Examination of the

TABLE 37.3
Drugs That Can Affect the Conjunctiva and Lids

Drug	Side Effect
Isotretinoin	Blepharoconjunctivitis, dry eye, contact lens intolerance
Chlorpromazine	Slate-blue discoloration of conjunctiva and dermis of lids
Niacin	Lid edema
Sulfonamides	Lid edema, conjunctivitis, chemosis
Gold salts	Gold deposits in conjunctiva
Tetracycline	Pigmented conjunctival inclusion cysts

eyes may reveal scaly, crusty eyelids, dilated vessels at the lid margins, conjunctival injection, and punctate keratitis. Schirmer test and tear breakup time are usually decreased.[118,119,122]

In 1979, Blackman and associates[122] first reported blepharoconjunctivitis in association with isotretinoin therapy. Milson and associates[126] later observed a dose-dependent relationship between isotretinoin therapy and blepharoconjunctivitis. Isotretinoin dosages of 2 mg/kg body weight daily resulted in blepharoconjunctivitis in 43% of patients, whereas dosages of 1 mg/kg body weight daily showed a 20% incidence of blepharoconjunctivitis.

ETIOLOGY

Mathers and associates[127] have shown that isotretinoin treatment alters meibomian gland function. The glands appeared atrophic, and expressable excreta increased in thickness and decreased in volume.

MANAGEMENT

Since as many as half the patients who develop blepharoconjunctivitis have symptoms before the start of therapy, the drug may aggravate preexisting conditions.[122] Decreasing the dosage or discontinuing the drug usually alleviates the side effect, although a few months may be required before some patients obtain significant relief.

Chlorpromazine

Discoloration of the conjunctiva, sclera, and exposed skin have been reported with administration of phenothiazine derivatives.[51,128–131] The skin of the face and lids can be equally pigmented, while the palpebral folds contain an area of nonpigmented skin deep within the creases.[128] The discoloration usually is slate-blue. Melanin-like granules have been observed in the superficial dermis of the skin.[128,129] The oculo-skin syndrome is usually associated with pigmentary deposits in the exposed interpalpebral area of the bulbar conjunctiva, especially near the limbus.[128–131] The palpebral conjunctiva does not appear to be involved. Patients exposed to dosages of chlorpromazine ranging from 500 to 3000 mg daily for 1 to 6 years may develop discoloration of the exposed skin, lids, and bulbar conjunctiva.[130,131]

There have been sporadic reports of allergic conjunctivitis and edema of the lids associated with phenothiazine use.[132]

Sulfonamides

Ocular complications are rare with systemic use of this class of anti-infective drugs. Lid edema, conjunctivitis, chemosis, anterior uveitis, and scleral reactions have been reported with high-dose administration of sulfanilamide.[133,134] The

observed reactions appear to be analogous to systemic hypersensitivity reactions, such as urticaria and edema seen in some patients who are allergic to sulfonamides.

Gold Compounds

Chrysiasis, or gold deposition in various tissues of the body, can occur in the conjunctiva following gold injection for rheumatoid arthritis.

CLINICAL SIGNS AND SYMPTOMS

In 1956, Roberts and Wolter[66] observed via biomicroscopic examination the presence of irregular, brownish deposits in the cornea and superficial layers of the conjunctiva. On biopsy of the conjunctiva, the particles proved to be metallic gold. No deposits were found in the skin of the lid. Inflammation or foreign body reaction was not present. The patient had received a total of 4555 mg of sodium thiomalate (Myochrysine) and 2188 mg of aurothioglucose (Solganal) over a 9-year period.

One study of 34 patients with rheumatoid arthritis, who had received intramuscular injections of either Myochrysine or Solganal, failed to show deposits in the conjunctiva under slit-lamp examination although deposits were present in the cornea and lens (see above). The total dosage range of gold administered was 2250 to 10,410 mg. No tissue biopsies were performed on these patients.

MANAGEMENT

Conjunctival changes associated with gold treatment are generally benign. Discontinuation of therapy usually eliminates these effects.[63]

Tetracyclines

Tetracycline and its derivative, minocycline, are used for control of acne vulgaris. Conjunctival deposits similar to those seen in epinephrine-treated glaucoma patients have been observed in patients treated orally with these compounds.[135,136] Dosages ranged from 250 to 1500 mg daily of tetracycline and at least 100 mg daily of minocycline.

The deposits appear as dark-brown to black granules in the palpebral conjunctiva, located nasally and temporally in the upper tarsus and temporally in the lower tarsus.[135,137] The granules vary in size and are located in conjunctival cysts, surrounded by minute, gray-white, noncrystalline soft spots. Under UV light microscopy, the brown pigment concentrations give a yellow fluorescence characteristic of tetracycline.[136]

Along with pigment, calcium is also present in the cysts. It has been hypothesized that either tetracycline or its metabolites form an insoluble chelation complex that results in the pigmentation.[136] Considering the large number of patients who have received these drugs for prolonged periods for acne, it is interesting that conjunctival pigmentation has not been reported more frequently.

Amiodarone

Although chronic administration of this antiarrhythmic agent has produced no visible biomicroscopic changes in the conjunctiva, electron microscopic studies of human autopsy material have indicated that some ultrastructural changes may occur during therapy.[102,138] Intracytoplasmic membrane-bound deposits similar to myelin have been demonstrated in the cytoplasm of nearly all ocular structures, including the conjunctival epithelium.[138] It has been suggested that these findings represent a drug-induced lipidosis.[102,138] Amiodarone has also been reported to concentrate within a chalazion that developed in a patient who had been taking the drug for 2 years for ventricular arrhythmias.[139]

Miscellaneous Drugs

A variety of other systemic drugs can cause irritative or allergic reactions in the conjunctiva or lids.[2,11,132] Barbiturates rarely cause conjunctival hyperemia and chemosis. Dermatitis, lid swelling, and ptosis have also been related to chronic barbiturate use. The reaction can persist for months after the drug is discontinued.[140] Patients taking niacin for hyperlipidemia have shown a higher incidence of lid edema than a similar group not taking niacin.[444]

Salicylates may cause allergic conjunctivitis, which may be associated with urticaria of the lids.[132] Chloroquine has been reported to cause ptosis, and phenytoin may cause chronic conjunctivitis.[11] Drugs of abuse, such as marijuana, may lead to conjunctival injection, sometimes with eyelid edema.[1,2] Cocaine abuse during pregnancy can result in a prolonged and vision-threatening eyelid edema in infants.[141]

High-dose therapy with certain chemotherapeutic agents, including cytosine arabinoside, cyclophosphamide, methotrexate, and 5-fluorouracil, has been implicated to cause conjunctivitis.[8] However, it appears that low-dose therapy with the anti-cancer agent tamoxifen is infrequently associated with anterior segment toxicity.[142,143]

Subconjunctival hemorrhage has been reported in association with high-dosage use of aspirin and oral anticoagulant therapy with warfarin.[144]

Drugs Affecting the Lacrimal System

Human lacrimal fluid consists of a combination of secretions from the lacrimal gland, meibomian glands, and the goblet cells of the conjunctiva. Aqueous tear secretion from the lacrimal gland is controlled by the autonomic nervous system. The lacrimal gland is innervated by cholinergic fibers from the seventh cranial nerve as well as by adrenergic fibers from the pericarotid plexus.[145] Chemically, the tears are 98.2% water and 1.8% solids. Thus, drugs that directly or indirectly affect the autonomic nervous system may cause hypersecretion or, more commonly, dry eye.

Several classes of drugs can affect aqueous tear secretion, influence tear constituents, or appear in the tears following systemic administration.[146] Patients complaining of watery or dry eyes, eye infections, or uncomfortable contact lens wear could be exhibiting symptoms relating to actions on the tears from a variety of prescription as well as OTC drugs.[147]

Drugs reported to affect aqueous tear secretion are listed in Table 37.4. Among the agents that frequently reduce tear secretion are the anticholinergics and antihistamines. These classes of drugs are also present in numerous OTC products such as sedatives, sleep aids, cold preparations, antidiarrheals, and nasal decongestants.

TABLE 37.4
Drugs That Can Affect Aqueous Tear Secretion

Drug Class	Example
Agents decreasing aqueous tears	
Anticholinergics	Atropine Scopolamine
Antihistamines	Chlorpheniramine Diphenhydramine
Vitamin A analogs	Isotretinoin
Vitamins	Niacin
β-adrenergic blockers	Practolol Propranolol Timolol
Phenothiazines	Chlorpromazine Thioridazine
Antianxiety agents	Chlordiazepoxide Diazepam
Tricyclic antidepressants	Amitriptyline Doxepin
Agents increasing aqueous tears	
Adrenergic agonists	Ephedrine
Antihypertensives	Reserpine Hydralazine
Cholinergic agonists	Neostigmine Pilocarpine

Drugs That Decrease Aqueous Tears and Tear Film Constituents

ANTICHOLINERGICS

Dryness of mucous membranes is a common side effect of anticholinergic drug use, since atropine and related drugs inhibit glandular secretion in a dose-dependent manner.

In one study,[148] oral administration of atropine caused tear secretion to fall from 15 μl/min to 3 μl/min. A similar dose of atropine given subcutaneously gave a nearly 50% reduction in lacrimal secretion.[149] Scopolamine, 1 to 2 mg orally, reduced tear secretion from 5 μl/min to 0.8 μl/min.[148] One reported case study suggested that atropine combined with diphenoxylate (Lomotil) can cause severe keratoconjunctivitis sicca in susceptible individuals.[150]

ANTIHISTAMINES

This class of drugs consists of agents that block two types of histamine receptors, H_1 or H_2. Agents blocking H_1 receptor types are commonly used for symptoms associated with colds, hay fever and other allergies, to prevent motion sickness, and for control of Parkinson's disease. The H_2 receptor antagonists are clinically useful for gastric ulcer therapy.

In addition to their receptor-blocking effects, H_1 antihistamines have varying degrees of atropine-like actions, including the ability to alter tear film integrity.[147,149,151] Both aqueous and mucin production have been reported to decrease with antihistamine use.[148] Koeffler and Lemp[152] administered 4 mg daily of chlorpheniramine maleate to a group of young volunteers. Tear secretion was measured by use of the standard Schirmer's test. A significant reduction in tear flow was observed on the days when chlorpheniramine was taken. The difference between the mean values of Schirmer strip wetting for days on which antihistamines were taken and nondrug days was highly significant.

Systemic use of antihistamines can aggravate an existing condition of keratitis sicca.[153] Use of 200 mg daily of diphenhydramine (Benadryl) has resulted in recurrence of filamentary keratitis in a female arthritic patient. When the medication was discontinued, the symptoms disappeared. This suggests that patients with a compromised tear film may aggravate this condition by use of antihistamines or other agents that can affect ocular surface wetting.

ISOTRETINOIN

Dry eye symptoms frequently occur in patients taking isotretinoin.[154] The associated symptoms may, or may not, be accompanied by blepharoconjunctivitis.[118]

Isotretinoin has been observed to decrease tear breakup time.[154] It is possible that lipid secretion by the meibomian glands may be decreased, reducing the lipid layer and thereby increasing the evaporation rate of the aqueous tear film.[154]

Analysis of lacrimal gland fluid of rabbits and human tears from subjects treated with isotretinoin has shown the presence of this vitamin derivative in tears.[155,156] Thus, the actual presence of isotretinoin in tear fluid could decrease stability of the lipid layer of the tear film, which would enhance the formation of dry spots. This effect could be responsible, in turn, for the dry eye symptoms, contact lens intolerance, and conjunctival irritation accompanying isotretinoin therapy.[156] Use of artificial tear preparations may help to alleviate the associated discomfort.

BETA-ADRENERGIC BLOCKING AGENTS

Drugs classified as β-adrenergic blocking agents have become the mainstay in the treatment of systemic hypertension, ischemic heart disease, cardiac arrhythmias, and migraine headache. Use of these drugs is not without systemic and ocular side effects (see Chapter 10).

Reduced tear secretion is a reported side effect of oral β-blocking drugs. Although most of the reported cases deal with practolol,[157] other β blockers, such as propranolol and timolol, have also been implicated in dry eye syndrome.[158,159] Ocular side effects of practolol have been described as an oculomucocutaneous syndrome in which patients suffer from symptomatic lesions of the outer eye.[157] A reduction of lysozyme and an absence of IgA may also occur.[159] Because the ocular side effects of practolol can be so serious, this drug is no longer marketed for clinical use.

Atenolol, metoprolol, oxyprenolol, and pindolol have been implicated in patients with dry eye symptoms and in reduction of tear lysozyme.[159,160]

ORAL CONTRACEPTIVES

Although oral contraceptives have been implicated to cause reduced tear production and problems associated with contact lens wear, the literature is generally devoid of well-documented studies showing a definite cause-and-effect relationship.[161-163] Brennan and Efron[164] have shown, however, that oral contraceptive use in patients who also wear hydroxyethyl methacrylate (HEMA) contact lenses is more likely to result in symptoms of dryness and iritation than in non-users of these medications.[164] The symptom of dryness was reported more frequently by patients whose lenses were older than 6 months or who were wearing toric lenses.

MISCELLANEOUS AGENTS

Other drugs with possible anticholinergic actions, such as phenothiazines, antianxiety agents, tricyclic antidepressants, and niacin, have been associated with dry eye syndromes.[1,444] Diuretics such as hydrochlorothiazide and chemotherapeutic agents such as carmustine and mitomycin can also cause both qualitative and quantitative changes in the tear film.[165,445]

Drugs That Increase Aqueous Tears and Tear Film Constituents

Several studies indicate that systemic administration of certain cholinergic, adrenergic, and antihypertensive agents stimulates lacrimation (see Table 37.4). Subcutaneous pilocarpine can increase tear production in normal eyes.[148] Neostigmine, given subcutaneously or intramuscularly, also induces lacrimation.[166] Among the adrenergic agonists, ephedrine has been reported to increase tear production.[1,2] Several antihypertensive agents can increase tear production. Reserpine, hydralazine, and diazoxide at therapeutic dosages can induce lacrimation in humans.[2] Chronic use of marijuana has been reported to increase tear secretion.[167] Tear samples have shown the presence of small amounts of Δ^9-tetrahydrocannabinol. Other authors,[168] however, report a reduction in tear secretion following marijuana use, along with a subjective feeling of dryness.

Several investigators have studied the effects of systemic agents on tear protein and other constituents.[149,159] Atropine increases tear protein and lysozyme, but since tear secretion is reduced, production of protein and lysozyme per unit time remains unchanged.[149] In the same study, the adrenergic agonist, ephedrine, increased tear lysozyme production threefold per unit time.

Among the β-adrenergic antagonists, timolol and propranolol increase tear lysozyme, whereas practolol decreases its concentration, particularly in patients with the oculomucocutaneous syndrome of decreased tear secretion, conjunctival keratinization, scarring, and shrinkage.[159]

Drug penetration into tears has been reported with certain antimicrobial agents and aspirin. Sulfonamides, tetracyclines, erythromycin, and rifampin have been assayed in tears of human subjects.[169] Ampicillin and penicillin penetrate into the tears very poorly and most likely do not result in important bioactive concentrations.[169] In contrast, erythromycin levels in tears have been found to be higher than the serum concentration, implying active transport of this antibiotic into tears following systemic administration.[169] Following its oral administration, 36% to 88% of the daily erythromycin dosage is present in tears. Aspirin and isotretinoin also appear to penetrate into human tears following high-dose oral administration.[154,156]

An observation worth noting is that the tears can become discolored after the use of systemic rifampin.[170] The tears usually become orange, but may be light pink or red. Soft contact lenses may also stain; therefore, patients who secrete this drug into tears may need to discontinue lens wear during rifampin therapy.[171]

Drugs Affecting the Pupil

Pupil size and function can be affected by peripheral autonomic action and by centrally initiated impulses. The iris is an excellent indicator of autonomic activity because of the delicate balance between adrenergic and cholinergic innervation to the iris dilator and iris sphincter muscles, respectively. By acting directly on these muscles, both adrenergic and cholinergic agents can influence pupil size and activity.

Drugs Causing Mydriasis

Anticholinergics, central nervous system stimulants and depressants, antihistamines, and phenothiazines can all cause mydriasis (Table 37.5).

ANTICHOLINERGICS

Drugs with anticholinergic effects, such as atropine or related compounds, can cause significant mydriasis. Systemic administration of 2 mg or more of atropine can result in pupillary dilation and cycloplegia.[172]

Scopolamine, a semisynthetic derivative of atropine, is marketed as a transdermal delivery system (Transderm Scōp) to prevent motion sickness. The device, which is placed behind the ear, consists of a 2.5 cm² disk containing 1.5 mg of scopolamine in a polymeric gel. Approximately 0.5 mg of drug is released into systemic circulation over a 3-day period.[173] Both mydriasis and reduced pupillary light response can occur when this device is used for 3 or more days.[174] Direct contamination by rubbing the eye with fingers following application of the patch to the skin, or during wear, can cause the observed pupillary dilation.[173]

TABLE 37.5
Drugs That Can Cause Mydriasis or Miosis

Mydriasis	Miosis
Anticholinergics	Opiates
CNS stimulants	Heroin
Amphetamines	Codeine
Methylphenidate	Morphine
Cocaine	Anticholinesterases
CNS depressants	Neostigmine
Barbiturates	
Antianxiety agents	
Antihistamines	
Phenothiazines	

the dosage is reduced, and accommodation completely returns to pretreatment levels after drug therapy is discontinued.[212,216]

Drugs Affecting Intraocular Pressure

Several different classes of drugs may alter intraocular pressure (IOP) by influencing either aqueous humor production or outflow (Table 37.8).

Anticholinergics

Some systemic agents may possess sufficient anticholinergic activity to produce mydriasis and a weak cycloplegic effect. These medications include antimuscarinic drugs, antihistamines, phenothiazines, and tricyclic antidepressants (Table 37.9).[220]

CLINICAL SIGNS AND SYMPTOMS

Systemic antimuscarinic agents, including atropine and scopolamine, can be administered in doses that could produce mild dilation of the pupil and accommodative paresis. The degree of mydriasis and pupillary reactivity to light stimulation provide a clinical measure of antimuscarinic activity. Other commonly used systemic medications with antimuscarinic activity are the H_1-receptor antagonists. Of the systemic antihistamines, the ethanolamines, including diphenhydramine (Benadryl), have significant antimuscarinic activity. In addition, the antipsychotic agents, particularly the phenothiazines such as thioridazine (Mellaril), have well documented anticholinergic properties. Therapeutic doses of tricyclic antidepressants, like amitriptyline (Elavil) and imipramine (Tofranil), produce significant anticholinergic actions and thus have the potential for ocular side effects.[220,221]

TABLE 37.8
Drugs That Alter Intraocular Pressure

Increased IOP	Antimuscarinic agents
	Antihistamines
	Phenothiazines
	Tricyclic antidepressants
	Corticosteroids
Decreased IOP	β-blockers
	Cannabinoids
	Cardiac glycosides
	Ethyl alcohol

IOP = intraocular pressure.

TABLE 37.9
Systemic Drugs with Anticholinergic Actions

Agent	Dose Associated with Antimuscarinic Side Effects (mg)
Atropine	≥ 0.5
H_1-receptor antagonists	
Ethanolamines	
Diphenhydramine	25–50
Dimenhydrinate	50–100
Tricyclic antidepressants	
Amitriptyline	10–25
Doxepin	10–25
Imipramine	10–25
Antipsychotic agents	
Phenothiazines	
Chlorpromazine	200–800
Thioridazine	150–600

ETIOLOGY

Systemic agents with anticholinergic effects may produce sufficient mydriasis to produce pupillary block and precipitate acute or subacute angle-closure glaucoma in patients with narrow anterior chamber angles.[211,446] In addition, the weak cycloplegic effect may be sufficient to increase IOP in some open-angle glaucoma patients. Relaxation of the ciliary muscle may decrease traction on the trabecular meshwork and increase resistance to aqueous outflow, especially when relatively high doses of medication are used.[222] In contrast, Hiatt and associates[223] have shown that the risk is small of elevating IOP with systemically administered anticholinergic agents in normal doses, even in patients with narrow anterior chamber angles.

MANAGEMENT

If symptoms or signs suggestive of acute or subacute angle-closure glaucoma develop, patients with narrow anterior chamber angles should undergo a prophylactic laser iridotomy to prevent pupillary block and subsequent angle-closure glaucoma. If acute angle-closure glaucoma occurs, the patient should be managed according to the guidelines described in Chapter 35. The offending drug should be withdrawn if medically possible. Accommodative paresis (cycloplegia) can be managed with reading lenses, as necessary, depending on the expected duration of treatment with the anticholinergic medication.

TABLE 37.10
Commercially Available Oral β-Blockers

Generic Name	Trade Name	Dosage Range	Clinical Uses
Nonselective			
Carteolol	Cartrol	2.5–10 mg/day	Hypertension
Labetalol	Normodyne, Trandate	200–800 mg/day	Hypertension
Nadolol	Corgard	40–320 mg/day	Hypertension, angina pectoris
Penbutolol	Levatol	10–20 mg/day	Hypertension
Pindolol	Visken	10–60 mg/day	Hypertension
Propranolol	Inderal	80–640 mg/day	Hypertension, angina pectoris, arrhythmias, myocardial infarction, migraine, essential tremor, hypertrophic subaortic stenosis
Sotalol	Betapace	160–320 mg/day	Ventricular arrhythmias
Timolol	Blocadren	20–40 mg/day	Hypertension, myocardial infarction, migraine
β₁-selective			
Acebutolol	Sectral	200–1200 mg/day	Hypertension, ventricular arrhythmias
Atenolol	Tenormin	50–100 mg/day	Hypertension, angina pectoris
Betaxolol	Kerlone	5–10 mg/day	Hypertension
Bisoprolol	Zebeta	2.5–20.0 mg/day	Hypertension
Metoprolol succinate	Toprol XL	50–400 mg/day	Hypertension, angina pectoris
Metoprolol tartrate	Lopressor	100–450 mg/day	Hypertension, angina pectoris, myocardial infarction

Modified from Hiett JA, Carlson DM. Ocular adrenergic agents. In: Onofrey BE, ed. Clinical optometric pharmacology and therapeutics. Philadelphia: JB Lippincott Co, 1991;9:19.

β-Blockers

CLINICAL SIGNS AND SYMPTOMS

Systemic β-blockers are used extensively for the treatment of hypertension and other cardiovascular disorders. Of the available oral β-blockers (Table 37.10), atenolol,[224–227] metoprolol,[228,229] nadolol,[230–234] pindolol,[235] propranolol,[225,236–241] and timolol[242,243] have been documented to produce a dose-dependent reduction in IOP. Although specific studies have not been conducted with most of the remaining systemic β-blockers, these agents might also be expected to reduce IOP at clinically useful doses.

Atenolol.   A single oral 50-mg dose of atenolol has been shown to decrease IOP in patients with ocular hypertension, open-angle glaucoma, and chronic angle-closure glaucoma.[224–227] A significant ocular hypotensive effect may occur for about 7 hours.[224] The average maximum reduction occurs 5 hours after ingestion, and the degree of reduction is about 35% of the initial IOP.[224] In patients with open-angle and chronic angle-closure glaucoma, a single oral 50-mg dose of atenolol produced a significantly greater reduction in IOP than a single dose of either propranolol (40 mg)[225] or acetazolamide (500 mg).[226] Oral doses of atenolol (50 mg twice daily) have also been reported to reduce IOP in non-glaucomatous eyes.[227] In this latter study, the initial pressure reduction was maintained throughout the 8 days of administration.

Metoprolol.   The dose-response relationship of metoprolol's ocular hypotensive action was studied by Alm and Wickstrom,[228] who found that single 25-, 50-, or 100-mg doses of metoprolol reduced IOP in healthy men and women. A maximum effect was noted 2 to 5 hours after oral administration of all doses. The duration and magnitude of the pressure reduction increased with increasing doses, but a significant ocular hypotensive effect that lasted the duration of the study (8 hours) was found only with the 100-mg dose. This dose had a maximum effect 4 hours after administration and produced a 32% relative decrease in IOP from pretreatment levels. In a short-term study involving patients with previously untreated open-angle glaucoma, 50 mg of metoprolol, given every 8 hours for 24 hours, reduced IOP in the glaucomatous eyes from a mean pressure of 30.1 mm Hg to 20.6 mm Hg.[229]

Nadolol.   Oral nadolol produces a dose-dependent ocular hypotensive response in humans with both normal and elevated IOP.[230–234] In a study of patients with open-angle glaucoma, the ocular hypotensive effect of orally administered nadolol (20 or 40 mg once daily) was equivalent to that of 0.25% and 0.5% timolol eyedrops.[233] The ocular hypotensive effects of long-term nadolol were well maintained for the duration of the 2-year study. The investigators concluded that a 20- or 40-mg nadolol tablet, taken once daily, will control IOP in many patients with open-angle glaucoma.[233]

Pindolol.   Limited information is available regarding the effects of systemic pindolol on IOP. Smith and associates[235] administered intravenous pindolol to young healthy volunteers and found that IOP decreased to maximal levels within 1 hour. This study is of interest because these investigators compared the ocular hypotensive response and plasma concentrations of an intravenous dose of pindolol (1.13 mg) to an equivalent dose (2 drops of 1%) of pindolol applied topically to the eye. Both routes of administration produced equivalent pressure reductions of about 3 mm Hg. After topical application to the eye, pindolol 1% produced a bilateral reduction of IOP, although the untreated eyes exhibited a hypotensive response that was less than that of the treated eyes. Systemic absorption of topically applied pindolol was postulated to account for the reduction of IOP in the untreated eye. To support this contention, plasma pindolol concentrations were determined after topical ocular and intravenous administration of equivalent doses (2 drops of 1% and 1.13 mg, respectively). The plasma levels attained were much less after ocular instillation than following intravenous administration (6.8 μmol/l and 34.2 μmol/l, respectively).

Propranolol.   Systemic propranolol decreases IOP in both healthy and glaucomatous eyes.[225,236–241] Since the ocular hypotensive effect of propranolol is dose-dependent, a greater pressure reduction is observed when higher doses are given.[238] In 7 of 19 glaucomatous patients in one study, oral propranolol, in doses of 20 to 40 mg administered 3 to 4 times daily, reduced IOP to an acceptable level ($\leq$ 22 mm Hg) for up to 42 months.[239] Oral propranolol, 40 mg taken twice daily, reduces IOP to about the same level as does acetazolamide 250 mg taken twice daily.[240]

Timolol.   In nonglaucomatous eyes, the ocular hypotensive effect of oral timolol changes very little at doses above 5 mg daily, although higher doses would be expected to produce a more complete blockade of β receptors.[242] The dose-response relationship of oral timolol's ocular hypotensive effect has not been established for eyes with glaucoma. However, timolol, 20 mg twice daily, reduces IOP significantly in patients with open-angle glaucoma.[243] At these doses, an additional reduction in IOP does not occur following concomitant use of topical timolol.[243] At low doses

(5 mg) of oral timolol, the addition of topical epinephrine produces further reduction of IOP. Higher doses (20 mg) of oral timolol, however, antagonize the ocular hypotensive action of epinephrine.[244] This antagonistic interaction has also been reported following use of topical timolol.[245–247] Since timolol produces a dose-dependent competitive blockade of receptors, the higher doses of timolol appear to antagonize the β-receptor-mediated increase in facility of outflow produced by epinephrine.[242]

ETIOLOGY

Like topical β-blockers,[248–255] systemic β-blockers may decrease aqueous formation via an action linked to receptors (predominantly β_2 receptors) on the nonpigmented ciliary epithelium. Numerous studies[233,243] indicate that the ocular hypotensive effect of systemic β-blockers can be equivalent to that of topical β-blockers. The reduction of IOP produced by systemic β-blockers is linked with both the β-receptor selectivity and the drug's dose. Nonselective oral β-blockers have been particularly effective ocular hypotensive agents. The degree of β-receptor blockade in the ciliary body from oral nonselective β-blocker therapy appears to be nearly complete, since topical β-blockers often produce little additional IOP reduction with concomitant administration.[256]

MANAGEMENT

The reduction in IOP associated with systemic β-blocker therapy may confuse the diagnosis of open-angle glaucoma. Thus, patients exhibiting glaucomatous optic neuropathy may be diagnosed incorrectly as having normal tension glaucoma. If β-blocker therapy is subsequently discontinued, these patients may develop substantially higher IOP. In addition, glaucoma patients taking systemic nonselective β-blockers may not show any additional ocular hypotensive effect upon administering a topical nonselective β-blocker.[256] However, patients receiving a β_1-selective oral agent may show a further decrease in IOP with the concurrent use of a topical nonselective β-blocker.[256] To minimize ineffective topical therapy in these patients, a uniocular trial with a topical β-blocker may be useful to determine its ocular hypotensive effect. As with topical β-blockers, nonselective oral β-blockers inhibit the β_2-receptor mediated increase in outflow facility produced by epinephrine.[244] Thus, glaucoma patients on oral β-blockers may show only a slight long-term reduction in IOP with the addition of an epinephrine derivative. As a useful alternative, miotic therapy should be strongly considered since it offers the most effective means of lowering IOP in patients on systemic nonselective β-blocker therapy.[257] Although many patients currently use oral β-blockers for a variety of conditions, these agents are not approved for use as ocular hypotensive agents. Nevertheless, the ocular hypotensive activity of these agents may have a beneficial effect on IOP.

Cannabinoids

Derivatives of the marijuana plant, *Cannabis sativa*, make up a group of compounds known as *cannabinoids*. Various cannabinoids have been administered orally, topically, and by inhalation as a means of reducing IOP. Smoking and ingesting marijuana significantly reduces IOP. After smoking a single marijuana cigarette, patients with primary open-angle or secondary glaucomas exhibited a significant reduction in IOP.[258] The maximal ocular hypotensive response occurs 60 to 90 minutes after inhalation and lasts about 4 hours. These patients, however, have many systemic side effects including postural hypotension, tachycardia, anxiety, drowsiness, euphoria, and hunger.[258] Thus, systemic administration of presently available cannabinoids is an unacceptable route of administration for treatment of glaucoma, but the practitioner may encounter patients using marijuana and should be familiar with its ocular actions.

Cardiac Glycosides

CLINICAL SIGNS AND SYMPTOMS

When administered systemically, cardiac glycosides reduce IOP in humans. Systemic digoxin therapy has been shown to reduce IOP by 14% in the glaucomatous human eye,[259] and aqueous humor formation can be reduced by as much as 45% after several days of digoxin therapy.[260] Patients with uncontrolled IOP, however, despite maximum medical therapy, have been shown to remain uncontrolled after digitalization.[261]

ETIOLOGY

The effect on IOP of the cardiac glycosides, primarily digitalis derivatives and ouabain, has been of interest for many years. The physiologic effects of these agents are produced by their ability to inhibit Na^+-K^+ATPase, and a ouabain-sensitive Na^+-K^+ATPase has been demonstrated in the ciliary epithelium.[262] In the ciliary nonpigmented epithelium, like other types of secretory epithelium, Na^+-K^+ATPase is thought to be responsible for the active transport of sodium, a process necessary for aqueous secretion to occur.

MANAGEMENT

Systemic administration of cardiac glycosides may reduce IOP to some degree in glaucomatous and nonglaucomatous eyes, but it is unlikely to produce adequate control of IOP when maximal medical therapy has failed to achieve this goal. In addition, cardiac glycosides have a low margin of safety and are frequently associated with toxicity. Gastrointestinal disturbances, fatigue, and visual complaints are among the most common side effects encountered with cardiac glycosides.[263] Although all types of arrhythmias have been associated with cardiac glycoside toxicity, ventricular arrhythmias are of particular concern, since they may be life-threatening due to decreased cardiac output. For this reason, systemic cardiac glycosides currently have no place in the therapy of glaucoma.

Corticosteroids

CLINICAL SIGNS AND SYMPTOMS

Systemically administered glucocorticoids, by oral, nasal, or inhalation routes, can elevate IOP.[264–266,447] Oral steroids, such as prednisone, are less likely to increase IOP compared to topical ophthalmic steroids. This difference is probably due to a lower anterior chamber concentration of the steroid following systemic administration.[264,265] Nevertheless, systemic steroids have the potential to increase IOP to a level sufficient to produce glaucomatous optic neuropathy with associated visual field loss.[266]

Usually, long-term administration of systemic steroids causes only a slight increase in IOP.[78,267] The IOP returns to pretreatment levels as the steroid is tapered or discontinued. In one study,[268] 34% of patients receiving systemic steroids had IOP of 20 mm Hg or higher, while only 6% of the nontreated group had a similar IOP level. As with topically applied steroids, the degree of IOP response to systemic steroids is not related to dosage or duration of treatment but is due, rather, to factors of individual susceptibility or responsiveness to the effects of steroids.[268–271] In patients who respond to steroid use, IOP elevations with systemic steroids average about 60% of those produced by topically applied steroids.[272] Thus, one would expect patients with open-angle glaucoma to be particularly sensitive to the pressure-elevating effects of systemic steroids.

ETIOLOGY

As with topically applied steroids, systemic steroid administration may reduce aqueous outflow in susceptible patients.[272] There is also substantial evidence that systemically administered steroids may increase aqueous humor formation, thereby contributing to elevated IOP.[70,268,269,272,273] Diotallevi and Bocci[273] have shown that systemic steroids can increase aqueous production without elevating IOP, implying a concomitant increase in aqueous outflow. Compared to topical steroids, systemic steroids may evoke different changes in the ocular fluid dynamics because of the distinctly different route of administration.[268] Patients receiving long-term systemic steroids may accumulate excessive amounts of mucopolysaccharide in the trabecular meshwork, obstructing aqueous outflow by hydrating the trabeculum.[274]

TABLE 37.11
Drugs That Can Affect Retinal Function

Drug	*Side Effect*
Chloroquine and hydroxychloroquine	Retinal pigmentary changes, visual field defects, color vision loss
Thioridazine	Retinal pigmentary changes, disturbances of dark adaptation, color vision loss, visual field defects
Quinine	Impairment of dark adaptation, visual field defects, vascular attenuation
Talc	Intra-arteriolar talc particles, retinal nonperfusion, neovascularization
Cardiac glycosides	Color vision disturbances, entopic phenomena
Nonsteroidal anti-inflammatory agents	
Salicylates	Retinal hemorrhage
Indomethacin	Pigmentary changes, color vision loss, visual field defects
Antineoplastic agents	
Tamoxifen	Refractile opacities in posterior pole
Carmustine	Retinal vascular disease
Isotretinoin	Impairment of dark adaptation
Niacin	Cystoid macular edema

MANAGEMENT

Ocular hypertension or steroid-induced glaucoma should be managed according to guidelines given in Chapter 35. Reducing steroid dosage, if possible, almost always reduces the IOP. If continuation of systemic steroid therapy is necessary, the ocular pressure can often be controlled with topical antiglaucoma medications.[264]

Ethyl Alcohol

Ethyl alcohol, taken orally, may reduce IOP by increasing serum osmolarity and functioning as a short-acting hyperosmotic agent.[275,276] When consumed as alcohol-containing beverages, ethyl alcohol can reduce IOP in both normal and glaucomatous eyes. The maximal ocular hypotensive effect occurs 1 to 2 hours after consumption.[276] Therefore, the practitioner must consider the actions of ethyl alcohol if consumption by the patient has occurred prior to measuring IOP.

Drugs Affecting the Retina

Numerous drugs have been associated with retinal toxicity (Table 37.11). These include medications obtained by prescription as well as drugs available over the counter. For example, phenylpropanolamine, an adrenergic agonist available over the counter and used as an anorectic, has been reported to cause central retinal vein occlusion associated with systemic hypertension.[277] This emphasizes the importance of a careful drug history.

Several mechanisms can result in drugs becoming retinotoxic (Table 37.12). Depending on the specific drug, its dosage, and duration of treatment, these retinotoxic effects are often reversible if recognized early.[278]

The following sections discuss the systemic drugs that are well known to be toxic to the retina.

Chloroquine and Hydroxychloroquine

Practitioners have used chloroquine and hydroxychloroquine to treat rheumatoid arthritis, discoid and systemic

TABLE 37.12
Mechanisms of Retinal Drug Toxicity

- Overdosage
- Idiosyncrasy
- Side effects
- Secondary
- Hypersensitivity
- Photosensitization

Modified from Crews SJ. Some aspects of retinal drug toxicity. Ophthalmologica 1969;158:232–244.

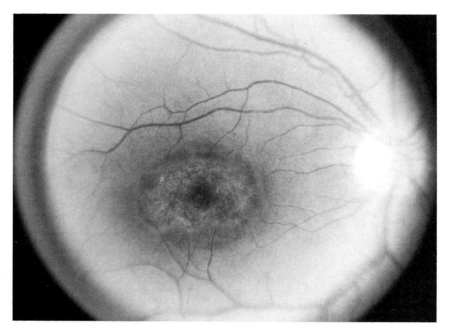

FIGURE 37.8   **Characteristic bull's eye maculopathy associated with chloroquine toxicity.**

lupus erythematosus, and other collagen diseases since the early 1950s. Currently, hydroxychloroquine (Plaquenil) is used almost exclusively as the quinoline agent of choice for the treatment of rheumatic diseases.[279,280] Cambiaggi[281] first described chloroquine retinopathy, although he believed the lesions to be associated with the patient's systemic lupus. In 1959, Hobbs and associates[282] confirmed these findings and correctly related them to the chloroquine treatment. Since that time, numerous cases of chloroquine-related retinopathy have been reported, and the mechanism underlying these drug-induced changes has been largely confirmed.[283]

CLINICAL SIGNS AND SYMPTOMS

The first visible evidence of chloroquine retinopathy is a fine pigmentary mottling within the macular area, with or without loss of the foveal reflex.[284,285] Even before visible ophthalmoscopic changes are detectable, however, a "premaculopathy" state can exist in which the drug interferes with metabolism of the macular tissues, causing subtle relative visual field defects in patients with ophthalmoscopically normal maculas.[213,214] As the macular pigmentary changes progress, a classic pattern develops consisting of a granular hyperpigmentation surrounded by a zone of depigmentation. The zone of depigmentation is, in turn, surrounded by another ring of pigment. Although this clinical picture can vary in intensity, it is pathognomonic of chloro-

quine retinopathy and is referred to as a "bull's eye" lesion[33,284–289] (Fig. 37.8).

Variations of retinal pigment epithelial (RPE) disturbances can occur, but most often appear as a well-circumscribed area of RPE atrophy in the macular area, which resembles a macular hole[33,284] (Fig. 37.9). In moderate to advanced cases of retinal toxicity, the arterioles may become attenuated, and the optic disc can become pale.[33,286,287] Occasionally, there may be signs of macular edema.[33,287] A high degree of bilateral symmetry between eyes usually occurs, but, occasionally, the toxicity can affect one eye more than the other.

Fluorescein angiography demonstrates dramatic fluorescence of the macular area in patients with chloroquine maculopathy. RPE atrophy allows the underlying choroidal fluorescence to become visible during the early, pre-arterial phase of the angiogram.[33,290]

Some patients with chloroquine retinopathy may have retinal changes resembling retinitis pigmentosa.[33,288,291–294] Chloroquine retinopathy does exhibit peripheral RPE hyperplasia, but, in contrast to retinitis pigmentosa, the pigment does not tend to accumulate around the retinal veins.[294] The peripheral lesions can occur with or without simultaneous macular involvement[33](Fig. 37.10). Other changes include attenuated retinal vessels, optic atrophy, peripheral visual field loss, and a subnormal electroretinogram (ERG). The fact that the dark-adaptation threshold is normal, or only

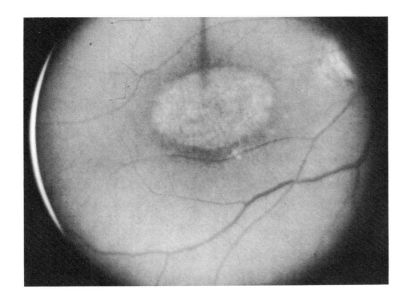

FIGURE 37.9 **Retinal pigment epithelial atrophy in macular area as a consequence of chloroquine therapy.**

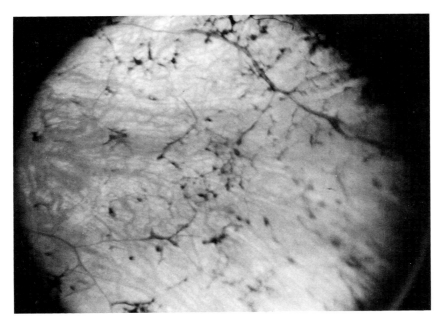

FIGURE 37.10 **Peripheral retinal pigment epithelial hyperplasia characteristic of pseudoretinitis pigmentosa in 42-year-old male with chloroquine toxicity.**

minimally abnormal, further differentiates this condition from retinitis pigmentosa.[292]

Although the visual fields may be normal even in the presence of definite macular pigmentary changes,[39] visual field loss generally correlates well with the degree of retinal damage. The typical visual field defects in chloroquine retinopathy consist of central, paracentral, or pericentral scotomas.[34,294–296] The paracentral scotomas may become confluent and form a complete ring scotoma.

In the early stages of retinopathy, electrodiagnostic studies tend to be of little value in detecting early chloroquine toxicity.[33,285] Both the ERG and electro-oculogram (EOG) can be normal or abnormal.[297] Advanced cases of chloroquine retinopathy, however, usually exhibit markedly abnormal, or even extinguished, ERGs.[292,294,298] This is especially true in cases involving the retinal periphery.

Although it is possible for patients with chloroquine maculopathy to be asymptomatic,[39] extensive macular damage often leads to symptoms of decreased visual acuity, metamorphopsia, and visual field disturbances.[33,213,286] Pericentral ring scotomas can cause reading difficulty.[299] Although color vision is normal in the early stages of chloroquine toxicity, more extensive macular damage can lead to severe impairment of color vision. Dark adaptation is typically normal, an important feature distinguishing the peripheral retinal changes from those seen in retinitis pigmentosa.[33]

Risk factors for the development of chloroquine retinopathy include daily dosage, duration of treatment, serum drug levels, and patient age. The incidence of retinopathy increases with patient age, and in older patients retinal toxicity appears to be correlated with total drug dosage.[39,300,301] Ehrenfeld and associates[300] contend that daily dosage is the most critical risk factor. Most cases of chloroquine retinopathy occur in patients taking 500 mg daily,[a] but dosages of 250 mg daily, or less, can also be retinotoxic.[32,33,288,302] Retinopathy can develop when the total cumulative dosage is as little as 100 g (the equivalent of 250 mg daily for 1 year), but the risk increases significantly when the total dosage exceeds 300 g.[32] Marks and Power[39] found retinopathy in 10% of patients receiving a total dosage of less than 200 g, while 50% of patients receiving more than 600 g developed retinopathy. The duration of therapy required to produce chloroquine retinopathy can be as little as 6 months, but most patients require 2 to 4 years of therapy before retinal changes develop.[32,286,303]

Chloroquine retinopathy tends to remain stable once therapy is discontinued.[288] Some patients, however, may demonstrate regression of macular changes if the retinal involvement is mild and if visual acuity is normal.[285,288] Although some patients with the classic "bull's eye" maculopathy may have reversible macular changes,[39] patients with moderately advanced retinopathy may show progression after discontinuing drug therapy.[288] Progressive impairment of visual acuity can occur for up to 5 years following discontinuation of chloroquine therapy.[304]

Occasionally, retinopathy does not develop until chloroquine therapy is discontinued. Such delayed-onset chloroquine retinopathy can occur from 1 to 10 years following discontinuation of drug therapy.[287,299,300]

The risk of retinopathy associated with hydroxychloro-

quine appears to be considerably less than that associated with chloroquine.[305,306] Tobin and associates[40] reported retinal toxicity in only 4 of 99 patients receiving hydroxychloroquine in a daily dosage of 400 mg for at least 1 year. No patient, however, sustained significant vision loss, and the abnormalities were reversible after the medication was discontinued. In some cases the macular changes may be reversible without recurrence even if the medication is reinstituted.[279] As little as 73 g of hydroxychloroquine taken over 6 months has been reported to cause retinopathy,[279] and the incidence of retinopathy may be as high as 29% if the cumulative dosage exceeds 800 g.[289] Several investigators,[40,307] however, have discounted the role of cumulative dosage and believe that the risk of maculopathy associated with hydroxychloroquine therapy is more closely related to daily dosage. Johnson and Vine[307] found no evidence of retinopathy in 9 patients treated with massive total dosages of hydroxychloroquine ranging from 1054 to 3923 g. Recent data seem to indicate that the risk of retinal toxicity is minimal if the daily dose of hydroxychloroquine is less than 6.5 mg/kg body weight, the duration of treatment is less than 10 years, and retinal function is normal.[305,306]

ETIOLOGY

Although the precise mechanism by which chloroquine and hydroxychloroquine cause retinal toxicity is unknown, it is widely recognized that these drugs bind tenaciously to melanin within the eye.[308,309] Moreover, histopathologic analysis has revealed that the pigmented tissues of the eye will continue to hold the drug for prolonged periods after drug therapy is discontinued.[308] This can lead to degenerative changes of the RPE. Rosenthal and associates,[308] however, have shown that chloroquine also accumulates in the retina itself, suggesting that the neurosensory retina may bind the drug. Investigations in monkeys have shown that chloroquine initially causes degenerative effects in the ganglion cells, followed by disruption of the photoreceptors, and finally the RPE and choroid.[308] Ramsay and Fine[310] confirmed in humans that the initial pathologic change occurs in the ganglion cells and that the changes within the RPE and photoreceptors occur late in the disease process. The destructive process within the RPE leads to migration of pigment-laden cells from the RPE to the outer nuclear and outer plexiform layers.[33,311] The foveal cones often are spared, which explains the ophthalmoscopic appearance seen in cases of bull's eye maculopathy.[309] Attenuation of the retinal arterioles is thought to be secondary to the extensive retinal damage.[309]

Vitreous fluorophotometry has shown that the blood-retinal barrier (BRB) breaks down in chloroquine retinopathy.[312] However, in asymptomatic patients who receive varying amounts of chloroquine or hydroxychloroquine, the BRB appears to remain intact.

---

[a]For comparison purposes, 500 mg of chloroquine phosphate is equivalent to 400 mg of hydroxychloroquine sulfate.

MANAGEMENT

Since early retinopathy often is reversible if drug dosage is reduced or discontinued, patients taking chloroquine or hydroxychloroquine should be monitored very carefully. Patients should receive baseline examinations before starting therapy and should be examined periodically for evidence of retinal changes. Baseline examinations of the fundus are especially important, since chloroquine and hydroxychloroquine maculopathy can resemble age-related macular disease. Once treatment has started, it is prudent to monitor patients every 6 months,[40,279,306,313] especially if the patient is over 65 years of age.[300,314] Practitioners should monitor elderly patients particularly carefully, because chloroquine and hydroxychloroquine are detoxified and eliminated by the liver and kidney, respectively, and these organs might be impaired in the elderly.[36]

Fundus and visual field evaluations are among the most important clinical procedures to be performed. Careful ophthalmoscopic examination of the fundus, including retinal periphery, is one of the most sensitive procedures used to detect early maculopathy.[289,315] Subtle macular changes can often be detected using slit lamp biomicroscopy. Visual field assessment using static threshold techniques can help to detect the early stages of visual field loss associated with chloroquine retinopathy.[295]

Testing of contrast sensitivity function is an additional screening procedure to detect early macular dysfunction, particularly in patients under 40 years of age.[297] In addition, patients should be encouraged to evaluate their condition themselves by using the Amsler charts every 2 weeks.[302,305,306]

The questionable nature of the ERG and EOG in cases of early maculopathy preclude their use in the detection of early chloroquine retinopathy. Similarly, fluorescein angiography is not as sensitive as routine ophthalmoscopy or color photography in the detection of early chloroquine retinopathy.[284] Thus, fluorescein angiography is not required to establish the diagnosis in most cases. However, in patients with preexisting macular disease, fluorescein angiography may help differentiate underlying macular disease from that induced by drug toxicity.

Since the clinical signs and symptoms of toxic retinopathy may not appear until after drug therapy is discontinued, it is important to monitor patients for several years after drug therapy has been stopped. This is more important for patients who have received at least 300 g of chloroquine, or the equivalent of hydroxychloroquine.[299,300]

Thioridazine

Chlorpromazine and thioridazine, both phenothiazine derivatives, are used for their antipsychotic effects. Pigmentary changes of the retina have been reported occasionally in association with chlorpromazine therapy,[217] Currently, however, it is recognized that only thioridazine produces retinal toxicity. Pigmentary retinopathy associated with thioridazine therapy was first reported in 1959 by Kinross-Wright.[316]

CLINICAL SIGNS AND SYMPTOMS

Blurred vision associated with thioridazine therapy is often due to the anticholinergic effects of the medication. More important, however, thioridazine can cause significant retinal toxicity, leading to reduced visual acuity, changes in color vision, and disturbances of dark adaptation. These symptoms typically occur 30 to 90 days after initiating treatment.[216,317] Visual field changes consist of concentric contraction or irregular paracentral or ring scotomas.[317] The fundus often appears normal during the early stages of symptoms, but within several weeks or months a pigmentary retinopathy develops characterized by fine clumps of pigment developing first in the periphery and progressing toward the posterior pole (Fig. 37.11).[216,318] In milder cases the pigment remains fine and peppery, but in more severe cases the pigment can form plaque-like lesions with multiple confluent areas of hypopigmentation and choroidal atrophy.[317] Retinal edema can also occur,[216] but the optic disc and retinal vasculature are usually normal.[318]

The ERG and EOG are often normal during the early stages of toxicity, but as the RPE becomes diffusely abnormal, the EOG becomes attenuated.[319] The amplitude of the oscillatory potential of the ERG decreases in proportion to the daily dosage of thioridazine, but the a- and b-waves and the latencies are normal.[320] In addition, the ERG response to red light will diminish in the early stages of thioridazine toxicity.[321] Cessation of therapy appears to increase the amplitude, at least in some patients.

It is now recognized that the primary clinical factor associated with thioridazine retinopathy is the daily drug dosage.[318] Before becoming aware of the dose-related retinal toxicity, practitioners commonly prescribed dosages exceeding 1600 mg daily.[317] Few cases of pigmentary retinopathy have been reported, however, with daily dosages of less than 800 mg.[322] Thus, it appears that thioridazine therapy will not induce retinal toxicity as long as patients receive daily dosages of less than 800 mg.[48,318,323]

Although it is possible for thioridazine retinopathy to resolve despite continued drug therapy, this usually occurs only in patients taking low dosages.[216] In general, for significant resolution to occur, drug therapy must be reduced or discontinued. Depending on the severity of toxicity, retinal function can return to normal, but the pigmentary changes are often permanent. Severe cases may result in permanent impairment of visual acuity, visual field, and dark adaptation.[48,318] The pigmentary retinopathy may even progress after the drug therapy has been discontinued, and some cases of progressive retinopathy can have a late onset, occurring from 4 to 10 years following discontinuation of thioridazine.[318,319,324]

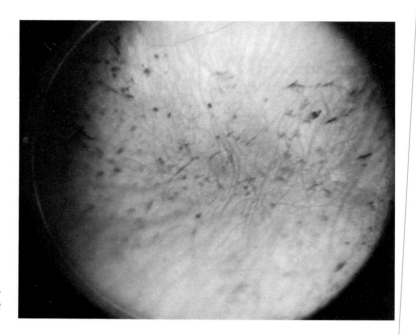

FIGURE 37.11   **Retinal pigment epithelial hyperplasia and atrophy in 33-year-old man with thioridazine retinopathy.**

ETIOLOGY

Thioridazine and other phenothiazines bind to melanin in the uveal tract, especially the choroid.[318,325] Drug uptake by the choroid occurs even in patients whose serum levels of thioridazine are in the nontoxic range.[326] Such drug binding may be retinotoxic by damaging the choriocapillaris, thus leading to changes in the RPE.[317,318] It is also possible that thioridazine may alter retinal enzyme kinetics, inhibiting the oxidation of retinol. Alterations in the enzyme systems of Mueller cells and photoreceptors may lead to atrophy and disorganization of the rods and cones as one of the initial degenerative changes, followed later by loss of the RPE and choriocapillaris.[317,324]

MANAGEMENT

Since the danger of retinal toxicity from thioridazine is significantly correlated with daily dosage, patients should be placed on dosages of less than 800 mg daily.[317,318] Patients should receive careful fundus examinations during the first 2 to 4 months of therapy and every 6 months thereafter.[318] Electrodiagnostic tests such as ERG and EOG are generally of no value in detecting early retinopathy.[327] If symptoms or objective signs of retinal toxicity are observed, promptly discontinue the medication to improve the chances of resolution. This must be done only in consultation with the patient's physician. Since the pigmentary retinopathy may be progressive even after thioridazine has been discontinued, patients should receive follow-up examinations on an annual basis.

Quinine

Historically, quinine has been employed for the treatment of malaria, but it is now used primarily for the management of leg cramps, myotonia congenita, and eyelid myokymia.[328] Quinine toxicity has been recognized for 150 years, and overdosage of quinine is still encountered in patients who attempt abortion or suicide. Accidental ingestion of quinine can lead to serious side effects. Among the various features of quinine toxicity, acute vision loss is one of the most significant and dangerous.

CLINICAL SIGNS AND SYMPTOMS

Mild toxic reactions are characterized by slight reduction of visual acuity, "flickering" of vision, tinnitus, weakness, or confusion. In more severe cases, symptoms consist of sudden complete loss of vision, dizziness, and even deafness. Coma with circulatory collapse characterize the most severe form of quinine toxicity.[328] Patients presenting with acute quinine overdose frequently have no light perception in both eyes, and pupils are often dilated and nonreactive to light.[329-331] Patients may complain of impairment of night vision, but color vision is usually normal.[331] The visual fields usually demonstrate concentric contraction, and improvement of the visual fields following the acute episode may require days or months, but the field loss may show no recovery and become permanent.[328,329]

Ophthalmoscopic examination of the fundus soon after acute quinine overdose may reveal a normal fundus,[331,332] but also may reveal constriction of the arterioles, optic disc pallor, venous dilatation, or retinal edema. Several authors[328,333] reported normal ERG findings in the early stages of quinine toxicity, but as visual acuity improves, the ERG becomes distinctly abnormal. Yospaiboon and associate[329] have shown, in contrast, an initially abnormal ERG that gradually improves as visual function recovers. Similarly, studies of EOG results have shown initial abnormality followed by improvement as visual function returned.[328,333]

The visual prognosis for patients with acute quinine toxicity is guarded. Visual acuity can improve from no light perception to 20/20 within days[331] to several weeks.[328,332] Sometimes vision does not improve to normal for several months.[329] As vision recovers, there is progressive constriction of the retinal vessels, and the optic disc becomes pale.[328,331] Although central vision often returns to normal levels, the visual fields can remain constricted.[328,330,332] Any impairment of night vision and color vision can be permanent.[328,330]

In general, the maximum daily dosage of quinine should not exceed 2 g; quinine toxicity is common in dosages over 4 g. The lethal oral dose in adults is approximately 8 g.[331] Toxic reactions to relatively small doses of quinine are probably idiosyncratic in nature, but can result in a clinical picture similar to that caused by higher doses.

ETIOLOGY

Our current understanding of the pathogenesis of quinine retinal toxicity is derived primarily from various electrodiagnostic studies that have demonstrated that quinine probably has a direct toxic effect on the photoreceptors and ganglion cells.[329,331,332,334] Moreover, fluorescein angiographic studies have shown no significant circulatory disturbances.[329] Damage to the RPE is indicated by the abnormal EOG, the increased visibility of the choroid in the late stages of toxicity, and the increased background fluorescence seen on angiography.[331,333] Visual evoked potential (VEP) findings confirm the conduction abnormality in the nerve fiber layer associated with the secondary optic atrophy.[328]

MANAGEMENT

Several decades ago, when the concept of vascular spasm was accepted as the cause of retinal damage in quinine toxicity, attempts at retinal vasodilatation were made to improve retinal circulation. Stellate ganglion block was commonly used for this purpose.[335–337] Efforts were also made to accelerate removal of quinine from the body with techniques such as hemodialysis, peritoneal dialysis, plasmapheresis, and forced diuresis.[338,339] More recent investigations, however, have shown that these procedures have no rational basis and are without proven benefit.[331,332,334] Since central vision tends to recover spontaneously even without treatment,[331] patients with acute quinine toxicity should be managed by immediate gastric emptying, administration of activated charcoal, and other supportive measures. It is important to emphasize preventive measures such as patient education and dispensing of quinine in child-resistant containers, and efforts should be made to reformulate quinine tablets to enhance their bitter taste.

Following the acute episode, patients should be carefully monitored for improvement in visual acuity, visual fields, and fundus appearance.

Talc

Tablets of medication intended for oral use contain inert filler materials such as talc (magnesium silicate), corn starch, cotton fibers, and other refractile and nonrefractile substances.[340] Chronic drug abusers are known to prepare a suspension of medication for injection by dissolving the crushed tablet of cocaine, heroin, methylphenidate, or other narcotic in water. They then boil the solution and filter it through a crude cigarette or cotton filter before injecting the solution intravenously, subcutaneously, or intramuscularly.[341,342] The talc particles eventually embolize to the retinal circulation and produce a characteristic form of retinopathy.[343] Talc retinopathy was first reported in 1972 by AtLee,[344] and since then numerous cases have been described.

CLINICAL SIGNS AND SYMPTOMS

Fundus examination reveals multiple, tiny, yellow-white, glistening particles scattered throughout the posterior pole, but they are more numerous in the capillary bed and small arterioles of the perimacular area[344–346] (Fig. 37.12). In addition to these characteristic lesions, some patients can have macular edema, venous engorgement, punctate and flame-shaped hemorrhages, and arterial occlusion.[344,347] Foreign body granulomas of the retina have also been described.[340]

Retinal neovascularization as a consequence of talc injection was first reported in 1979 by Kresca and associates.[348] These lesions appear in the retinal periphery as neovascular tufts in the shape of seafans at the junction of the perfused and nonperfused retina. This is a potentially serious complication of talc injection because it can lead to retinal detachment, massive vitreal hemorrhage, and optic disc neovascularization.[341,349]

Most patients have no significant visual symptoms, and visual acuity is normal.[349] Some patients, however, report blurring of vision, blind spots in the visual fields, and occasionally can have severe reduction of visual acuity.[341,347,349] Neither the extent of drug abuse nor the degree of filtration of the prepared suspension appears to be correlated with visual symptoms.[341]

The extent and concentration of talc particles observed in the posterior pole appear to correlate with the duration of drug abuse as well as with the cumulative number of tablets

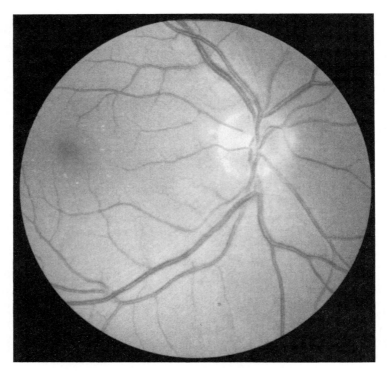

FIGURE 37.12 **Talc retinopathy characterized by numerous yellow-white intra-arteriolar particles scattered throughout perimacular area.**

injected.[341,344] Often the drug abuser injects from 10 to 40 tablets daily, and some abusers inject as many as 100 tablets daily for several years.[344,350] Talc retinopathy is usually not found in drug abusers who have injected less than 9000 tablets, but it is consistently found in most patients who have injected more than 12,000 tablets.[350,351]

ETIOLOGY

As the talc, corn starch, and other insoluble tablet fillers embolize to the lungs, they become trapped within the pulmonary tissues and eventually cause pulmonary hypertension. This leads to the development of collateral vessels that allow part of the venous return to bypass the lungs and enter the left side of the heart, where the particles are further embolized to the eye and other organs of the body.[341,345] The presence of talc particles in the eye indicates that substantial foreign body damage has occurred in the lungs.[344]

The talc particles are more numerous in the perimacular region than in other areas of the retina, probably because of the rich blood supply and greater blood flow in that area.[352] The particles lodge in the walls of the precapillary arterioles and capillaries, producing focal occlusion of these vessels in the retina and choroid.[353] The occlusions are caused primarily by the cellular reaction to the emboli.[354]

The neovascular lesions of talc retinopathy are thought to be associated with peripheral arteriolar nonperfusion, which leads to retinal ischemia and secondary neovascularization. Such a pathogenesis is quite similar to that seen in sickle cell retinopathy and is confirmed by the predominantly superotemporal location of the neovascular proliferation.[341,348,349]

MANAGEMENT

Because of the implications involved in the diagnosis, the practitioner must rule out other conditions that may have a similar clinical appearance. The differential diagnosis includes Gunn's dots, multiple cholesterol emboli, drusen, and Stargardt's disease.

Once the diagnosis has been established, appropriate drug abuse counseling should be given to prevent further risk of severe pulmonary or ocular complications. Consideration should also be given to pulmonary consultation, since patients with eye findings usually have acute or chronic impairment of pulmonary function.[350] The patient should be monitored carefully for the development of progressive ocular lesions, especially of the neovascular type. Proliferative retinopathy can be treated with the use of argon laser photocoagulation, and vitreal hemorrhage may require vitrectomy.[341]

Cardiac Glycosides

Digitoxin and digoxin, both digitalis derivatives, have been widely used in the treatment of congestive heart disease and certain cardiac arrhythmias. Visual symptoms associated with digitalis have been recognized since 1785, when Withering[355] recorded the effects from large doses of foxglove. Since that time, many patients have incurred symptoms of dimness of vision, flickering or flashing scotomas, and significant disturbances of color vision.

CLINICAL SIGNS AND SYMPTOMS

The most common symptoms reported by patients are changes in color vision and impaired vision.[356] These symptoms can take many forms and include the visual phenomena listed in Table 37.13. They often precede cardiac abnormalities as the earliest symptoms of digitoxin intoxication.[357] A common symptom is snowy vision (objects appear to be covered with frost or snow), and this observation is intensified in brightly illuminated environments.[356,358] Elevated dark-adaptation thresholds have been reported, which gradually return to normal within 2 to 3 weeks after digitalis is discontinued.[359] There is also evidence that digoxin may contribute to rhegmatogenous retinal detachment by decreasing the normal adhesion of the retina to the retinal pigment epithelium.[360]

Complaints of color vision disturbances are common with both digoxin and digitoxin, but color vision impairment can often be detected even in patients without symptoms.[361] Both the incidence and severity of color vision impairment tend to correlate with the plasma glycoside level.[361,362] Figure 37.13 shows the results of color vision testing in patients receiving therapeutic doses and toxic serum levels of digoxin. About 80% of patients with digoxin intoxication demonstrate generalized color vision deficiencies,[361] but detectable color vision impairment occurs even at therapeutic drug levels (Fig. 37.14). In contrast, patients treated with digitoxin in therapeutic concentrations usually show no significant color vision abnormality.[362] Haustein and associates[362] showed that, at toxic plasma concentrations, nearly all digoxin-treated patients, but only about half of digitoxin-treated patients, will demonstrate impaired color vision. Thus, at therapeutic concentrations digoxin tends to impair color vision more than does digitoxin. This difference may be related to plasma protein binding or to different distributions in the retina.[362] Digoxin can also interact with quinidine, raising the digoxin level approximately twofold.[358]

The prevalence of digitalis intoxication is from 16% to 20%,[363] and the incidence of visual complaints among intoxicated patients may be as high as 10% to 25%.[356] Color vision disturbances are especially common and may occur before, simultaneously with, or after the onset of cardiac toxicity.[361] However, although color vision disturbances are

TABLE 37.13
Visual Symptoms in Digitalis Intoxication[356,358]

- Dyschromatopsia
- Flickering or flashes of light
- Colored spots surrounded by coronas
- Snowy, hazy, or blurred vision
- Dimming of vision
- Glare sensitivity

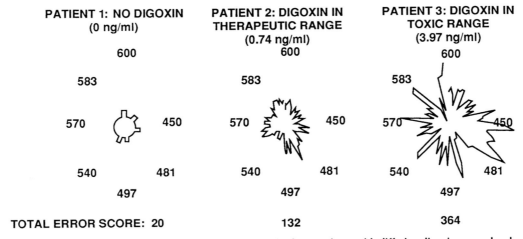

FIGURE 37.13   Farnsworth Munsell 100-hue test results in three patients with differing digoxin serum levels (0.0, 0.74, 3.97 ng/ml, respectively). Total error scores were 20, 132, and 364, respectively. (Modified from Rietbrock N, Alken RG. Color vision deficiencies: A common sign of intoxication in chronically digoxin-treated patients. J Cardiovasc Pharmacol 1980;2:93–99.)

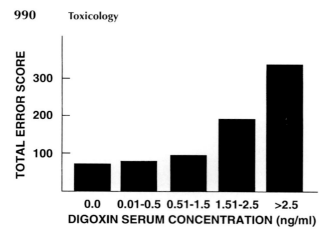

FIGURE 37.14   **Mean total error scores on Farnsworth Munsell 100-hue test according to digoxin serum concentration ranges. (Modified from Rietbrock N, Alken RG. Color vision deficiencies: A common sign of intoxication in chronically digoxin-treated patients. J Cardiovasc Pharmacol 1980;2:93–99.)**

associated with cardiac glycoside toxicity, decreased visual acuity without the accompanying classic symptom of xanthopsia is also common.[364]

Visual symptoms may occur as soon as 1 day following drug administration, but often occur within 2 weeks of initial therapy. Occasionally, ocular toxicity does not appear until after several years of treatment.[356] Once the serum level is decreased or digitalis therapy is discontinued, however, visual symptoms quickly subside, usually within several weeks.[364]

ETIOLOGY

Early reports suggested that the cause of the visual symptoms in patients with digitalis toxicity was retrobulbar neuritis or disturbances in the visual cortex.[365] Gibson and associates,[366] however, were among the first investigators to propose that the retina, rather than the optic nerve, was the site of digitalis toxicity. Binnion and Frazer[367] demonstrated in dogs that the highest concentrations of digoxin are found in the choroid and retina. In addition, ERG studies, as well as dark adaptometry, have confirmed cone dysfunction in patients with digitalis intoxication.[358,359,448,449]

The precise mechanism whereby digoxin produces a toxic effect may involve inhibition of Na^+-K^+-activated ATPase, an enzyme that plays a vital role in maintaining normal cone receptor function. This would explain the drug-induced interference with both dark adaptation and color vision.[358,359,449]

MANAGEMENT

Patients taking cardiac glycosides should be monitored carefully for visual symptoms, including color vision changes,

flashing or flickering lights, and other entoptic phenomena. Color vision evaluation, especially during the first several weeks of therapy, can be especially helpful in detecting signs of early intoxication. Although the Panel D-15 test can be useful for this purpose, the Farnsworth Munsell 100-hue test has been shown to be particularly sensitive for detecting digitalis-induced color vision deficiencies.[361,363] Periodic color vision testing should be performed as long as the patient continues taking the medication, and detectable changes in color vision should warrant consultation with the prescribing physician with regard to potential digitalis intoxication.

Nonsteroidal Anti-Inflammatory Agents

NSAIDs are commonly used for their analgesic, anti-inflammatory, and antipyretic actions in the treatment of arthritis, musculoskeletal disorders, dysmenorrhea, and acute gout. Although these drugs are widely used and are often employed for prolonged periods, retinal toxicity is rare.[55]

CLINICAL SIGNS AND SYMPTOMS

Salicylates are well known to have anticoagulant properties, and in high dosages or prolonged use these drugs can cause retinal hemorrhage.[368]

Most of the reported cases of retinopathy associated with NSAIDs have involved indomethacin therapy. Although there have been no epidemiologic studies investigating the relationship between indomethacin and retinopathy, there is evidence that the drug can induce pigmentary changes of the macula and other areas of the retina.[55–57,369,370] The lesions usually consist of discrete pigment scattering of the RPE perifoveally, as well as fine areas of depigmentation around the macula. In some cases, the pigmentary changes can be more marked in the periphery of the retina.[55] Depending on the amount of retinal involvement, the ERG and EOG can be normal or abnormal.[55–57] Likewise, the amount of retinopathy will dictate whether changes occur in visual acuity, dark adaptation, and visual fields. Acquired color vision deficiencies of the blue-yellow type have been reported.[56,369]

No definite relationship has been established between the dosage of indomethacin and retinal toxicity. When drug therapy is discontinued, however, most of the functional disturbances associated with the retinopathy usually improve, although the pigmentary changes of the retina are generally irreversible.[55–57,369] Significant improvement of color vision, visual acuity, dark adaptation, and visual fields may require at least 6 to 12 months following discontinuation of drug therapy.

ETIOLOGY

Most investigators have speculated that indomethacin may have a direct or indirect effect on the retinal pigment epithelium, but the precise mechanism has not been clarified.[55–57] The localization of the retinotoxic effect to the RPE is supported by changes observed in the ERG and EOG in patients with indomethacin retinopathy.[55]

MANAGEMENT

Patients taking high or prolonged doses of salicylates or indomethacin should be monitored carefully for evidence of retinal hemorrhage or pigmentary changes, especially in the macular area. Evaluation of color vision may be helpful in identifying patients with early retinotoxic effects associated with indomethacin.[369] Consideration should also be given to other functional disturbances, and these can be monitored by performing serial visual acuity, visual fields, and studies of dark adaptation. Once retinal toxicity is documented, the prognosis for improved retinal function is good provided indomethacin therapy is decreased or discontinued. Drug therapy, however, should be changed only on the advice of the prescribing physician.

Antineoplastic Agents

TAMOXIFEN

Tamoxifen citrate (Nolvadex), an orally administered non-steroidal antiestrogen, is one of the most effective antitumor agents for the palliative treatment of metastatic breast carci-noma in postmenopausal women.[371] This drug has been in clinical use since 1970 without serious side effects in most patients. It is used both alone and in combination with other agents, and the recommended oral dosage is 10 mg twice daily, increasing to 20 mg twice daily if no response is obtained within 1 month.[372]

Clinical Signs and Symptoms.   Tamoxifen retinopathy has been documented in many patients, and the retinal findings include white or yellow refractile opacities in the macular and perimacular area, with or without macular edema (Fig. 37.15).[373–377,450] Although the lesions are usually more numerous in the macular area, they can also extend to the ora serrata.[374] The lesions occur at all levels of the sensory retina, and many appear superficial to the retinal vessels. The patient may experience reduced visual acuity associated with the macular lesions, and the visual fields can show abnormalities.

Although tamoxifen is less likely to induce ocular toxic-ity, at the normal dosage level of 20 mg daily, clinical observations indicate that retinopathy does occur.[372,376–379] With high dosages (e.g., 90 to 120 mg twice daily), toxic effects can be observed within 17 to 27 months, as the total cumulative dosage exceeds 90 g.[371,373,374]

Once tamoxifen therapy is discontinued, the number and size of retinal lesions generally remain unchanged, and the degenerative changes are irreversible.[371,376,379]

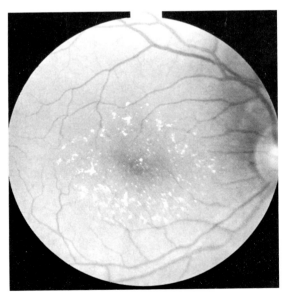
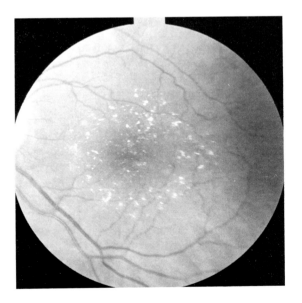

A

B

FIGURE 37.15   **Macular edema with yellow-white crystalline deposition in 66-year-old woman administered 120 mg of tamoxifen twice daily for 2 years.** *(A)* Right eye, visual acuity 20/180 (6/54). *(B)* Left eye, visual acuity 20/60 (6/18).

Etiology. Kaiser-Kupfer and associates[371] provided the first clinicopathologic correlation of tamoxifen retinopathy. These investigators have shown that high-dosage tamoxifen therapy causes widespread axonal degeneration, primarily in the paramacular area. The yellow-white lesions seen on fundus examination appear to represent products of the axonal degeneration. They are 3 to 10 μm in diameter in the macular area, from 30 to 35 μm in diameter in the paramacular area, and are confined to the nerve fiber and inner plexiform layers.

Management. Since tamoxifen retinopathy can occur at relatively low total doses of drug, it is important to obtain a baseline examination before therapy is begun. This should include best-corrected visual acuity, visual fields, Amsler grid evaluation, and fundus photography. It is important to monitor symptomatic patients carefully during therapy, since macular compromise can result in irreversible loss of vision. Annual examinations are sufficient if normal drug dosages are administered. However, patients receiving higher than normal doses, ranging from 80 mg once daily to 120 mg twice daily, should be monitored every 6 months.[375,377,450] The prevalence of ocular toxicity from low-dose tamoxifen therapy (10 mg twice daily) appears to be low.[450]

CARMUSTINE

Carmustine (BCNU) is a commonly used chemotherapeutic agent for the treatment of various malignant neoplasms, including metastatic malignant melanoma, malignant gliomas of the central nervous system, metastatic breast cancer, and leukemia.[380–382] It has been administered by infusion into the internal carotid artery as a method of increasing bioavailability of the drug to brain tumors within the supply of this vessel. This has led to ocular toxicity in some patients.[383]

Clinical Signs and Symptoms. Retinal toxicity usually begins within 2 to 14 weeks following intra-arterial infusion of BCNU.[380,382] Approximately 65% of patients develop retinal complications (Table 37.14).[384] It is common to have loss of vision from the retinopathy, and visual acuity can be reduced to 20/60, to light perception, or even no light perception.[380,384] A definite relationship between dosage of

TABLE 37.14
Retinal Complications of Carmustine

- Retinal infarction
- Retinal periarteritis
- Retinal periphlebitis
- Changes of retinal pigment epithelium
- Branch retinal artery occlusion
- Nerve fiber layer hemorrhages
- Macular edema

BCNU and retinopathy has not been established, but retinal complications can be avoided using intracarotid administration by passing the infusion catheter beyond the origin of the ophthalmic artery.[381,385]

Etiology. The retinal toxicity resulting from intracarotid BCNU is probably related to the increased flow of drug into the ophthalmic artery. The precise mechanism whereby BCNU causes retinal toxicity is unknown, but several investigators have suggested that the drug may be toxic to the retinal and choroidal vasculature, causing segmental intraretinal vasculitis with or without vascular obstruction. This process would lead to nerve fiber layer infarcts and retinal hemorrhage.[380,384]

Management. As previously mentioned, the retinotoxic effects of intracarotid BCNU can be largely minimized or avoided by employing an infusion catheter that is advanced beyond the origin of the ophthalmic artery.[385] If retinal complications develop, the risk/benefit ratio must be considered regarding the advisability of continued therapy.

MISCELLANEOUS AGENTS

Various other systemic chemotherapeutic agents have been associated with retinotoxic effects.[8,384,386] Use of alpha interferon, for example, has resulted in various retinal effects, including cotton-wool spot formation, capillary nonperfusion, arteriolar occlusion, and hemorrhage.[386]

Oral Contraceptives

Since the early 1960s, when oral contraceptives became a popular means of birth control, there have been numerous reports of ocular as well as systemic side effects associated with this medication. Although the relationship between the use of oral contraceptives and systemic thromboembolic disease is well established,[110,387] the evidence linking oral contraceptives with ocular side effects has been based solely on isolated case reports and uncontrolled retrospective studies. Most case reports of ocular side effects involve drug therapy from 48 hours to several years, and complications have been observed for up to 5 months following discontinuation of oral contraceptive use.[110] Controlled studies, however, have consistently failed to document any significant relationship between use of oral contraceptives and ocular side effects.[110,388–391] Nevertheless, there is circumstantial evidence that retinal vascular disease may be associated with oral contraceptives, because patients have been reported with retinal lesions that disappeared when the drug was discontinued, promptly reappeared when the drug was resumed, and then regressed when treatment was again discontinued.[392,393] Furthermore, the retinal vascular disturbances occur at an unusually young age when vascular damage associated with arteriosclerosis is quite rare. Thus, the practitioner should be aware of the most common retinal vascular lesions that have been linked with oral contraceptive therapy.

CLINICAL SIGNS AND SYMPTOMS

The most common retinal findings reportedly associated with oral contraceptive use are retinal vascular occlusions. These may present as typical branch or central retinal vein occlusion,[394] branch or central retinal artery occlusion,[395] or they may involve atypical presentations such as tortuosity of the perimacular venules[396] or combined central retinal artery and vein occlusion.[397]

Acquired color vision deficiencies have also been reported. Marre and associates[398] found acquired tritanomaly in 28% of women using oral contraceptives when tested with the Panel D-15 test.

Other retinotoxic effects reportedly associated with oral contraceptives are listed in Table 37.15.

ETIOLOGY

The mechanism underlying retinal vascular complications associated with oral contraceptives is unknown. Schenker and associates[399] showed that oral contraceptives may cause changes in the retinal microvasculature. Fluorescein angiography was used to demonstrate narrowing of the capillary arterioles and postcapillary venules. Women who complained of headache while taking oral contraceptives demonstrated dilatation of perimacular vessels several weeks after the drug was discontinued. Retinal vascular occlusive episodes might also occur as a consequence of marked intimal proliferation, or as a result of contraceptive-enhanced platelet adhesiveness. Fibrinogen and clotting factors may also be increased.[110,397]

MANAGEMENT

In general, the risk of retinal vascular disease associated with oral contraceptive use in women of child-bearing age is considered to be minimal. However, certain predisposing factors may increase the risk of retinal vascular episodes. Women with any of the conditions listed in Table 37.16 may be at increased risk for vascular complications associated with oral contraceptives.[110,114,392,400,401] These patients should therefore be monitored more carefully for evidence of retinal disease. If the patient develops retinal vascular complications that are suspected to be associated with the oral contraceptive, consideration can be given to changing the mode of contraception. This should be done only in consultation with the patient's primary physician.

Isotretinoin

Isotretinoin, or 13-*cis*-retinoic acid, is widely used for the treatment of cystic acne. Although this drug more commonly affects the external tissues of the eye, there is evidence to suggest that this agent may have a retinotoxic effect.

CLINICAL SIGNS AND SYMPTOMS

Impairment of dark adaptation with or without excessive glare sensitivity has been reported with isotretinoin therapy in dosages of 1 mg/kg body weight daily.[402] These complaints may be associated with an abnormal ERG or abnormal EOG. Once therapy is discontinued, both the abnormal dark adaptation and abnormal ERG usually resolve within several months.

ETIOLOGY

Although the precise mechanism explaining isotretinoin's effect on dark adaptation is unclear, it has been suggested that the drug could become incorporated into the rod photoreceptor elements during the process of outer disc shedding and renewal.[59] Weleber and associates[402] hypothesized that isotretinoin may compete for normal retinol binding sites on cell surfaces or transport molecules, accounting for the reduced retinal sensitivity.

TABLE 37.15
Reported Retinotoxic Effects of Oral Contraceptives[114,392]

- Central retinal vein occlusion
- Branch retinal vein occlusion
- Central retinal artery occlusion
- Branch retinal artery occlusion
- Perivasculitis
- Impending occlusion of central retinal vein
- Attenuation of retinal arteries
- Macular hemorrhage
- Retinal edema

TABLE 37.16
Risk Factors for Vascular Complications Associated with Oral Contraceptives

- Migraine headache
- Phlebitis
- Inclination to varicosity
- Systemic hypertension
- Hyperlipidemia or hypercholesterolemia
- Diabetes
- Cigarette Smoking
- Obesity

Patients taking isotretinoin should be monitored for changes in night vision. A history of night vision impairment should suggest more definitive evaluation procedures such as visual fields, dark adaptometry, and electroretinography. If retinal function is documented to be abnormal, the drug should be withdrawn in consultation with the patient's physician. Once drug therapy has been discontinued, retinal function should be monitored for improvement.

Drugs Affecting the Optic Nerve

Drug toxicity must always be considered in the differential diagnosis of optic neuropathy.[451] A careful history should attempt to uncover any prescribed or self-administered drugs that may have been taken in the past or present. There has been speculation that maternal drug use during pregnancy may lead to optic nerve hypoplasia. Drugs reported to cause this condition include phenytoin,[403] quinine,[404] alcohol and cocaine.[141,405] Other drugs known or reported to cause significant optic nerve disease are listed in Table 37.17. Two of those drugs, ethambutol and chloramphenicol, are addressed in some detail in the following sections.

Ethambutol

Introduced in 1961 for the treatment of tuberculosis, ethambutol supplanted paraaminosalicyclic acid for the initial and retreatment of tuberculosis.[406] Severe toxic side effects were reported initially, but these were linked to use of the racemic mixture of the drug. Consequently, the dextro isomer was selected as the most therapeutically useful and has been found to have a lower incidence of ocular toxicity than the racemic form.[407] Ocular side effects usually occur in the form of retrobulbar neuritis.

Ethambutol is well recognized to cause ocular symptoms of reduced visual acuity, changes in color vision, and visual field loss.[408,409] Signs of ocular toxicity can appear as early as several weeks following initial therapy, but the onset of ocular complications usually occurs several months after therapy is begun.[410–412] Although various forms of optic neuritis have been described,[413] the primary ocular manifestation of ethambutol toxicity is retrobulbar neuritis. This can occur in several forms (Table 37.18).[411,414–416] The most common form involves loss of visual acuity associated with a central or paracentral scotoma, along with color vision disturbances, and is caused by compromise of the central optic nerve fibers. Less commonly, ethambutol can affect the peripheral optic nerve fibers, causing defects in the peripheral visual field. Finally, in rare cases, ethambutol can cause visible retinal manifestations, including hyperemia and swelling of the optic disc, flame-shaped hemorrhages on the optic disc and in the retina, and macular edema. After several weeks, these signs can be followed by primary optic atrophy.[413,417]

Color vision deficiencies are probably the most sensitive indicator of early ethambutol optic neuropathy.[286,418] When the patient is examined with sensitive tests such as the Farnsworth Munsell 100-hue or desaturated Panel D-15, both red-green and blue-yellow defects may be observed in early stages of toxicity.[369,418] These changes in color vision can occur even before visual acuity and visual fields are affected.

Sometimes contrast sensitivity function can also be affected before visual acuity or color vision becomes impaired.[419] Salmon and associates[419] have suggested that testing with Arden contrast sensitivity plates may be effective in detecting subclinical toxic optic neuropathy associated with ethambutol.

Once changes have occurred in visual acuity, visual field, or color vision, these functional changes may continue to deteriorate even after ethambutol has been discontinued.[417]

TABLE 37.17
Drugs That Can Affect the Optic Nerve

Drug	Side Effect
Ethambutol	Retrobulbar neuritis
Chloramphenicol	Optic neuritis, retrobulbar neuritis
Isoniazid	Optic neuritis
Nonsteroidal anti-inflammatory drugs	Optic neuritis, papillitis
Oral contraceptives	Pseudotumor cerebri, optic neuritis
Tamoxifen	Optic neuritis
Corticosteroids	Pseudotumor cerebri
Tetracycline	Pseudotumor cerebri
Amiodarone	Papillitis

TABLE 37.18
Characteristics of Ethambutol Optic Neuropathy

	Central (Axial)	Peripheral
Toxic dosage	Low	High
Visual acuity	Reduced	Normal
Visual field	Central scotoma	Peripheral contraction
Color vision	Red-green deficiency	Normal

Modified from Garrett CR. Optic neuritis in a patient on ethambutol and isoniazid evaluated by visual evoked potentials: Case report. Military Med 1985;150:43–46.

More often, however, there is recovery of pretreatment visual acuity and visual field several months or years following discontinuation of the drug.[408,412] The degree of recovery depends largely on the extent to which ethambutol has compromised optic nerve function. If the ocular toxicity is not recognized early, the drug can cause permanent loss of vision.[417,420]

Considerable evidence indicates that ocular toxicity associated with ethambutol therapy is dose-related.[407,420] It is now recognized that ethambutol rarely induces ocular changes at a dosage of 15 to 20 mg/kg body weight daily,[412] and this has led to the current recommendation that ethambutol dosages should not generally exceed 15 mg/kg body weight daily. Some practitioners employ the drug in dosages of 25 mg/kg daily for a period not exceeding 2 months, followed by a maintenance dose of 15 mg/kg daily, and this has been shown to cause virtually no ocular complications.[410,415]

ETIOLOGY

Although the mechanism by which ethambutol causes retrobulbar neuritis is largely unknown, van Dijk and Spekreijse[421] suggested that ethambutol may affect the amacrine and bipolar cells of the retina, since color vision can be affected without altering visual acuity. This concept deserves further study before definitive conclusions can be reached.[422]

MANAGEMENT

It is important for patients beginning treatment with ethambutol to have baseline examination and frequent monitoring of visual acuity, visual fields, color vision, and fundus appearance. Since it is rare for ocular toxicity to occur with dosages as low as 15 mg/kg daily, patients taking such doses can be monitored every 3 to 6 months.[418] Patients with renal insufficiency, however, have impaired ability to excrete the drug and therefore may be at greater risk for developing ocular changes.[413,417] These patients should be monitored monthly.[423,424] Since there is some evidence that patients with lower plasma zinc levels have a higher incidence of

optic neuropathy, these patients should also be examined more frequently.[425]

Evaluations of color vision and visual fields are usually more sensitive indicators of early optic neuropathy than is visual acuity testing.[417,425] The desaturated Panel D-15 test or the Farnsworth Munsell 100-hue test can detect subtle color vision changes associated with early ethambutol toxicity.[412,418] Visual field studies using static threshold techniques will aid in detecting early visual field abnormalities.[426] Several authors have recommended use of VEPs for the routine monitoring of patients taking ethambutol.[414,420,427] This procedure has been effective in detecting subclinical optic nerve disease that can precede changes in visual acuity and color vision.

Nair and associates[406] suggested that symptoms of peripheral neuropathy may indicate early ethambutol toxicity and should serve as a warning sign of impending optic neuropathy. Thus, the ethambutol dosage in patients encountering peripheral neuropathy should be reduced to prevent the development of ocular toxicity. Ethambutol therapy must be discontinued in patients who develop reduced visual acuity, color vision deficiency, or visual field defects characteristic of optic neuropathy.[411,416,427] If discontinuation of drug therapy alone does not result in improvement of visual function, consideration can be given to treatment with hydroxycobalamin. Guerra and Casu[428] reported recovery of visual acuity in four patients treated with hydroxycobalamin several months after the discontinuation of ethambutol had failed to improve the visual acuity. Although the mechanism of action of hydroxycobalamin in the treatment of ethambutol-induced optic neuropathy is elusive, this vitamin may act by neutralizing the chelating action of ethambutol on the optic nerve. Further clinical trials are needed to clarify the role of hydroxycobalamin.

Chloramphenicol

Chloramphenicol is used for the treatment of typhoid fever, bacterial meningitis, and certain anaerobic infections. However, because of the risk of serious systemic toxicity, including blood dyscrasias and death, use of the drug is generally limited to conditions for which other, less toxic, agents are ineffective. Optic neuropathy as a consequence of chloramphenicol therapy is well known, especially when the drug is used to treat cystic fibrosis in children.

CLINICAL SIGNS AND SYMPTOMS

Chloramphenicol causes both optic neuritis and retrobulbar neuritis.[429] Characteristic of most cases is severe, bilateral reduction of visual acuity accompanied by dense central scotomas.[429–431] Visual acuity can range from 20/100 to 5/400.[432] Although there may be no fundus changes, the optic discs are usually edematous and hyperemic, the retinal veins are engorged and tortuous, and hemorrhages are often seen in the parapapillary area.[265,432] Optic atrophy is a late sign.[307] Peripheral neuritis characterized by numbness and cramps of the feet often precedes the visual complaints by 1 to 2 weeks, and may therefore serve as an early warning sign of impending ocular toxicity.[429]

Visual impairment associated with chloramphenicol therapy usually recovers after the drug is discontinued, but pretreatment visual acuity is often not regained and visual field defects may persist.[265,429,433] Some patients may tolerate further prolonged treatment with chloramphenicol without recurrent optic neuritis, and, occasionally, patients can demonstrate improvement of visual function despite continued therapy.[265]

Most cases of optic neuritis associated with chloramphenicol therapy have occurred in children with cystic fibrosis who were treated with large daily dosages of drug, 1 to 6 g daily. Although visual symptoms can occur as early as 10 days after beginning therapy, ocular toxicity commonly occurs after several months or years of treatment.[430,434] Harley and associates[430] reported a dosage-dependent relationship between chloramphenicol therapy and optic neuritis. The incidence of optic neuritis varied from 5% of patients treated with a daily dosage of 10 to 25 mg/kg body weight, to 38% of patients treated with a daily dosage exceeding 50 mg/kg body weight. There was no vision loss among patients treated for less than 3 months, but the incidence of optic neuritis increased to 16% in patients treated longer than 12 months.

ETIOLOGY

The precise mechanism by which chloramphenicol produces optic neuritis is unknown, but VEP abnormalities have confirmed optic nerve involvement in patients taking chloramphenicol.[435] Although not substantiated, several authors have proposed that chloramphenicol may induce optic neuropathy by causing a vitamin deficiency.[436] Genetic factors may be involved, and it has also been hypothesized that chloramphenicol may be metabolized to degradation products that are potentially toxic to the optic nerve.[265]

Histopathologic studies have found bilateral optic atrophy with primary involvement of the papillomacular bundle, loss of the retinal ganglion cells, and gliosis of the nerve fiber layer.[430] The presence of peripheral visual field defects in some patients is evidence that there is also involvement of the peripheral portion of the visual pathway.[431]

MANAGEMENT

Patients who are to receive long-term chloramphenicol therapy should receive a comprehensive baseline examination consisting of visual acuity, visual fields, color vision, and fundus examination. The risk of optic neuropathy is minimized if the daily dosage of drug is limited to 25 mg/kg body weight, or less, for a period not exceeding 3 months.[430] Patients or their parents should be encouraged to be alert to the development of peripheral neuritis, which might indicate impending loss of vision. Once signs or symptoms of optic neuropathy are detected, promptly discontinue drug therapy in consultation with the prescribing physician. Because the outcome of vitamin therapy is uncertain, the case for megadose vitamins is not compelling.[429]

Prevention of Adverse Reactions

Health care practitioners must protect their patients' well-being by detecting signs and symptoms of drug toxicities so that appropriate action can be taken to prevent or minimize serious ocular consequences. The detection process begins with the initial patient interview, during which a detailed drug history may reveal use of medications with potential ocular side effects.[437] A careful history is especially important in elderly patients, who typically use more medications than do younger individuals.[438] Although most patients over age 60 years regularly take several medications, many patients are unable to identify the drugs they take.[437] This emphasizes the importance of patient education regarding prescribed and self-administered medications.

The practitioner should record on the patient's chart both prescribed and self-administered medications, including drug dosage, duration of therapy, and any adverse reactions noted by the patient. If documented ocular side effects are discovered in the examination, it is wise to advise the prescribing practitioner so that appropriate remedial action can be taken. If no side effects are found, but the patient is using high-risk medications such as steroids, the patient should be monitored closely so that any significant adverse reaction can be detected before serious consequences develop.

References

1. Fraunfelder FT. Drug induced ocular side effects and drug interactions, ed. 2. Philadelphia: Lea & Febiger, 1989.

2. Grant WM. Toxicology of the eye. Springfield, IL: Charles C Thomas, 1994.

3. Fraunfelder FT, Meyer SM. The national registry of drug-induced ocular side effects. J Toxicol Cut Ocular Toxicol 1982;1:65–70.

4. Chiou GCY. Ophthalmic toxicology. New York: Raven Press, 1992.

5. McQueen EG. Pharmacological basis of adverse drug reactions. In: Avery GS, ed. Drug treatment. New York: Adis Press, 1980; Chap. 7.

6. Koneru PB, Lien EJ, Koda RT. Oculotoxicities of systemically administered drugs. J Ocul Pharmacol 1986;2:385–404.

7. Bartlett JD. Ophthalmic toxicity by systemic drugs. In: Chiou GCY, ed. Ophthalmic toxicology. New York: Raven Press, Ltd, 1992;Chap. 6.

8. Imperia PS, Lazarus HM, Lass JH. Ocular complications of systemic cancer chemotherapy. Surv Ophthalmol 1989;34:209–230.

9. Fincham JE. Monitoring and managing adverse drug reactions. Am Pharm 1992;32:74–82.

10. Green K. History of ophthalmic toxicology. In: Chiou GYC, ed. Ophthalmic toxicology. New York: Raven Press, Ltd, 1992; Chap. 1.

11. Hobbs HE, Eadie SP, Somerville F. Ocular lesions after treatment with chloroquine. Br J Ophthalmol 1961;45:284–298.

12. Leopold IH. Ocular complications of drugs. JAMA 1968;205:285–287.

13. Lufkin MW, Harrison CE, Henderson JW, et al. Ocular distribution of digoxin-H³ in the cat. Am J Ophthalmol 1967;64:1134–1140.

14. Yamamoto GK. Ocular drug toxicity. In: Langston-Pavan D. Manual of ocular diagnosis and therapy. Boston: Little, Brown, 1980; Chap. 15.

15. Abel A, Leopold IH. Ocular diseases. In: Avery GS, ed. Drug treatment. New York: Adis Press, 1980; Chap. 12.

16. Armaly MF. Statistical attributes of the steroid hypertensive response in the clinically normal eye. I. The demonstration of three levels of response. Invest Ophthalmol 1965;4:187–197.

17. Becker B. Intraocular response to topical corticosteroids. Invest Ophthalmol 1965;4:198–205.

18. Urban RC, Cotlier E. Corticosteroid-induced cataracts. Surv Ophthalmol 1986;31:102–110.

19. Davidson SI. Reports of ocular adverse reactions. Trans Ophthalmol Soc UK 1973;93:495–510.

20. Jaanus SD. Drug-related cataract. Optom Clin 1991;1(2):143–157.

21. Fraunfelder FT, Hanna C, Dreis MW, Cosgrove KW. Cataracts associated with allopurinol therapy. Am J Ophthalmol 1982;94:137–140.

22. Jick H, Brandt DE. Allopurinol and cataract. Am J Ophthalmol 1984;98:355–358.

23. Clair WK, Chylack LT, Cook EF. Allopurinol use and the risk of cataract formation. Br J Ophthalmol 1989;73:173–176.

24. Laties AM, Keates EU, Taylor HR, et al. The human lens after 48 weeks of treatment with lovastatin. N Eng J Med 1990;323:683–684.

25. Mathers W, Kattan H, Earll J, Lemp M. Development of presenile cataracts in association with high serum levels of phenytoin. Ann Ophthalmol 1987;19:291–292.

26. Sponsel WE, Rapoza PA. Posterior subcapsular cataracts associated with indapamide therapy. Arch Ophthalmol 1992;110:454–455.

27. Munoz B, Tajchman U, Bochow T, West S. Alcohol use and risk of posterior subcapsular opacities. Arch Ophthalmol 1993;111:110–112.

28. Ritter LK, Klein BEK, Klein R, Mares-Perlman J. Alcohol use and lens opacities in the Beaver Dam Eye Study. Arch Ophthalmol 1993;111:113–117.

29. Lozier JR, Friedlaender MH. Complications of antimalarial therapy. Int Ophthalmol Clin 1989;29:172–178.

30. Mazzuca SA, Yung R, Brandt KD, et al. Current practices for monitoring ocular toxicity related to hydroxychloroquine (Plaquenil) therapy. J Rheumatol 1994;21:59–63.

31. Hobbs HE, Calnan CD. The ocular complications of chloroquine therapy. Lancet 1958;1:1207–1209.

32. Bernstein NH. Some iatrogenic ocular diseases from systemically administered drugs. Int Ophthalmol Clin 1970;10:553–619.

33. Bernstein HN. Chloroquine ocular toxicity. Surv Ophthalmol 1967;12:415–447.

34. Goldhammer Y, Smith JL. Bitemporal hemianopia in chloroquine retinopathy. Neurology 1974;24:1135–1138.

35. Petrohelos MA. Chloroquine-induced ocular toxicity. Ann Ophthalmol 1974;6:615–618.

36. Mantyjarvi M. Hydroxychloroquine treatment and the eye. Scand J Rheumatol 1985;14:171–174.

37. Cullen AP, Chou BR. Keratopathy with low dose chloroquine therapy. J Am Optom Assoc 1986;57:368–372.

38. Calkins LL. Corneal epithelial changes occurring during chloroquine (Aralen) therapy. Arch Ophthalmol 1958;60:981–988.

39. Marks JS, Power BJ. Is chloroquine obsolete in treatment of rheumatic disease? Lancet 1979;1:371–373.

40. Tobin DR, Krohel GB, Rynes RI. Hydroxychloroquine. Seven-year experience. Arch Ophthalmol 1982;100:81–83.

41. Shearer RV, Dubois EL. Ocular changes induced by long-term hydroxychloroquine (Plaquenil) therapy. Am J Ophthalmol 1967;64:245–252.

42. Easterbrook M. Ocular effects and safety of antimalarial agents. Am J Med 1988;85:23–29.

43. Beebe WE, Abbott RL, Fung WE. Hydroxychloroquine crystals in the tear film of a patient with rheumatoid arthritis. Am J Ophthalmol 1986;101:377–378.

44. Alexander LJ, Bowerman L, Thompson LR. The prevalence of the ocular side effects of chlorpromazine in the Tuscaloosa Veterans Administration patient population. J Am Optom Assoc 1985;56:872–876.

45. Greiner AC, Berry K. Skin pigmentation and corneal and lens opacities with prolonged chlorpromazine therapy. Can Med Assoc J 1964;90:663–665.

46. Thaler JS, Curinga R, Kiracofe G. Relation of graded ocular anterior chamber pigmentation to phenothiazine intake in schizophrenics—quantification procedures. Am J Optom Physiol Opt 1985;62:600–604.

47. Mathalone MBR. Ocular effects of phenothiazine derivatives and reversibility. Dis Nerv Syst 1968;29:29–35.

48. Siddall JR. Ocular complications related to phenothiazines. Dis Nerv Syst 1968;29:10–13.

49. Prien RF, DeLong SL, Cole JO, et al. Ocular changes occurring with prolonged high dose chlorpromazine therapy. Arch Gen Psychiat 1970;23:464–468.

50. Rasmussen K, Kirk L, Faurbye A. Deposits in the lens and cornea

of the eye during long-term chlorpromazine medication. Acta Psychiat Scand 1976;53:1–6.

51. Brooks JG, Matoba AY. Chlorpromazine-induced anterior segment changes. Arch Ophthalmol 1992;110:126–127.

52. Isaac NE, Walker AM, Jick H, Gorman M. Exposure to phenothiazine drugs and risk of cataract. Arch Ophthalmol 1991;109:256–260.

53. Deluise VP, Flynn JT. Asymmetric anterior segment changes induced by chlorpromazine. Ann Ophthalmol 1981;13:953–955.

54. Scott R, Cunningham GT, Puddle JM, et al. Ocular side effects of phenothiazines. Clin Exp Optom 1991;74:11–14.

55. Henkes HE, van Lith GHM, Canta LR. Indomethacin retinopathy. Am J Ophthalmol 1972;73:846–856.

56. Palimeris G, Koliopoulos J, Velissaropoulos P. Ocular side effects of indomethacin. Ophthalmologica 1972;164:339–353.

57. Burns CA. Indomethacin, reduced retinal sensitivity, and corneal deposits. Am J Ophthalmol 1968;66:825–835.

58. Szmyd L, Perry HD. Keratopathy associated with the use of naproxen. Am J Ophthalmol 1985;99:598.

59. Lerman S. Photosensitizing drugs and their possible role in enhancing ocular toxicity. Ophthalmology 1986;93:304–313.

60. Cox NH, Jones SK, Downey DJ, et al. Cutaneous and ocular side effects of oral photochemotherapy: Result of an 8–year follow-up study. Br J Ophthalmol 1987;116:145–152.

61. Bonnet P. Sur une forme particuliere de granulations miliaires de l'iris. Bull Soc Ophthalmol Paris 1937;49:413–416.

62. Weidle EG. Lenticular chrysiasis in oral chrysotherapy. Am J Ophthalmol 1987;103:240–241.

63. McCormick SA, DiBartolomeo G, Raju VK, et al. Ocular chrysiasis. Ophthalmology 1985;92:1432–1435.

64. Gottlieb NL, Major JC. Ocular chrysiasis correlated with gold concentrations in the crystalline lens during chrysotherapy. Arth Rheumat 1978;21:704–708.

65. Tierney DW. Ocular chrysiasis. J Am Optom Assoc 1988;59:960–962.

66. Roberts WH, Wolter JR. Ocular chrysiasis. Arch Ophthalmol 1956;56:48–52.

67. Black RL, Oglesby RB, von Sallmann L, et al. Posterior subcapsular cataracts induced by corticosteroids in patients with rheumatoid arthritis. JAMA 1960;174:166–171.

68. Toogood JH, Dyson C, Thompson CA, et al. Posterior subcapsular cataracts as a complication of adrenocortical steroid therapy. Can Med Assoc J 1962;86:52–56.

69. Havre DC. Cataracts in children on long-term corticosteroid therapy. Arch Ophthalmol 1965;78:818–821.

70. Lindholm B, Linnér E, Tengroth B. Effects of long-term systemic steroids on cataract formation and on aqueous humour dynamics. Acta Ophthalmol 1965;43:120–127.

71. Becker B. Cataracts and topical corticosteroids. Am J Ophthalmol 1964;58:872–873.

72. Costagliola C, Cati-Giovannelli B, Piccirillo A. Cataracts associated with long-term steroids. Br J Dermatol 1989;120:472–479.

73. Allen MB, Ray SG, Leitch AG, et al. Steroid aerosols and cataract formation. Br Med J 1989;299:432–433.

74. Fraunfelder FT, Meyer SM. Posterior subcapsular cataracts associated with nasal or inhalation corticosteroids. Am J Ophthalmol 1990;109:489–490.

75. Karim AKA, Jacob TCS, Thompson GM. The human lens epithelium; morphological and ultrastructural changes associated with steroid therapy. Exp Eye Res 1989;48:215–224.

76. Kobayashi Y, Akaishi K, Nishio T, et al. Posterior subcapsular cataract in nephrotic children receiving steroid therapy. Am J Dis Child 1974;128:671–673.

77. Fürst C, Smiley WK, Ansell BM. Steroid cataract. Ann Rheum Dis 1966;25:364–368.

78. Oglesby RB, Black RL, von Sallmann L, et al. Cataracts in patients with rheumatic diseases treated with corticosteroids. Further observations. Arch Ophthalmol 1961;66:625–630.

79. Giles CL, Mason GL, Duff IF, et al. The association of cataract formation and systemic corticosteroid therapy. JAMA 1962;182:719–722.

80. Crews SJ. Posterior subcapsular lens opacities in patients on long-term corticosteroid therapy. Br Med J 1963;1:1644–1647.

81. Toogood JH, Markov AE, Baskervill J, Dyson C. Association of ocular cataracts with inhaled and oral steroid therapy during long-term treatment of asthma. J Allergy Clin Immunol 1993;91:571–579.

82. Astle JN, Ellis PP. Ocular complications in renal transplant patients. Ann Ophthalmol 1974;6:1269–1274.

83. Pavlin CR, de Veber GA, Cook GT, et al. Ocular complications in renal transplant recipients. Can Med Assoc J 1977;117:360–362.

84. Kristensen P. Posterior subcapsular cataract (PSC) and systemic steroid therapy. Acta Ophthalmol 1968;46:1025–1032.

85. Skalka HW, Prchal JT. Effect of corticosteroids on cataract formation. Arch Ophthalmol 1980;98:1773–1777.

86. Loredo A, Rodriguez RS, Murillo L. Cataracts after short-term corticosteroid treatment. N Engl J Med 1972;286:160.

87. Rooklin AR, Lampert SI, Jaeger EA, et al. Posterior subcapsular cataracts in steroid-requiring asthmatic children. J Allergy Clin Immunol 1979;63:383–386.

88. Debnath SC, Abomelha MS, Jawdat M, et al. Ocular side effects of systemic steroid therapy in renal transplant patients. Ann Ophthalmol 1987;19:435–437.

89. Adhikary HP, Sells RA, Basu PK. Ocular complications of systemic steroids after renal transplantation and their association with HLA. Br J Ophthalmol 1982;66:290–291.

90. Limaye SR, Pillai S, Tina LU. Relationship of steroid dose to degree of posterior subcapsular cataracts in nephrotic syndrome. Ann Ophthalmol 1988;20:225–227.

91. Dunn JP, Jabs DA, Wingard J, et al. Bone marrow transplantation and cataract development. Arch Ophthalmol 1993;111:1367–1373.

92. Harris JE, Gruber L. The electrolyte and water balance of the lens. Exp Eye Res 1962;1:372–384.

93. Mayman CI, Miller D, Tijerina ML. In vitro production of steroid cataract in bovine lens: II. Measurement of sodium-potassium adenosine triphosphatase activity. Acta Ophthalmol 1979;57:1107–1116.

94. Bucala R, Fishman J, Cerami A. Formation of covalent adducts between cortisol and 16 α-hydroxyestrone and protein: Possible role in the pathogenesis of cortisol toxicity and systemic lupus erythematosus. Proc Natl Acad Sci USA 1982;79:3320–3324.

95. Bluming AZ, Zeegen P. Cataracts induced by intermittent Decadron used as an antiemetic. J Clin Oncol 1986;4:221–223.

96. Ward DE, Butrous G, Camm J. Clinical uses of amiodarone—a potent antiarrhythmic drug. Intern Med Special 1985;6:44–55.

97. Kaplan LJ, Cappaert WE. Amiodarone keratopathy. Correlation to dosage and duration. Arch Ophthalmol 1982;100:601–602.

98. Chew E, Ghosh M, McCulloch C. Amiodarone-induced cornea verticillata. Can J Ophthalmol 1982;17:96–99.

99. Orlando RG, Dangel ME, Schaal SF. Clinical experience and grading of amiodarone keratopathy. Ophthalmology 1984;91: 1184–1187.

100. Dolan BJ, Flach AJ, Peterson JS. Amiodarone keratopathy and lens opacities. J Am Optom Assoc 1985;56:468–470.

101. Ingram DV, Jaggarao NSV, Chamberlain DA. Ocular changes resulting from therapy with amiodarone. Br J Ophthalmol 1982; 66:676–679.

102. Ghosh M, McCulloch C. Amiodarone-induced ultrastructural changes in human eyes. Can J Ophthalmol 1984;19:178–186.

103. Nielsen CE, Andreasen F, Bjerregaard P. Amiodarone-induced cornea verticillata. Acta Ophthalmol 1983;61:474–480.

104. Flach AJ, Dolan BJ, Sudduth B, et al. Amiodarone-induced lens opacities. Arch Ophthalmol 1983;101:1554–1556.

105. Gittinger JW, Asdourian GK. Papillopathy caused by amiodarone. Arch Ophthalmol 1987;105:349–351.

106. D'Amico DJ, Kenyon KR, Ruskin JN. Amiodarone keratopathy. Drug-induced lipid storage disease. Arch Ophthalmol 1981;99: 257–261.

107. Haug SJ, Friedman AH. Identification of amiodarone in corneal deposits. Am J Ophthalmol 1991;111:516–520.

107a. Bron AJ. Vortex patterns of the corneal epithelium. Trans Ophthalmol Soc UK 1973;43:455–472.

108. Flach AJ, Dolan BJ. Amiodarone-induced lens opacities: An 8-year follow-up study. Arch Ophthalmol 1990;108:1668–1669.

109. Garrett SN, Waterhouse WJ, Parmley VC. Amiodarone keratopathy in the donor cornea. Am J Ophthalmol 1988;105:425–427.

110. Wood JR. Ocular complications of oral contraceptives. Ophthal Sem 1977;2:371–402.

111. Koetting RA. The influence of oral contraceptives on contact lens wear. Am J Optom Arch Am Acad Optom 1966;43:268–274.

112. Ruben M. Contact lenses and oral contraceptives. Br Med J 1966; 1:1110.

113. Anderson RD, Martin PL. Oral contraceptives and eye changes. Pac Coast Oto-Ophthalmol Soc 1969;50:137–146.

114. Radnot M, Follmann P. Ocular side effects of oral contraceptives. Ann Clin Res 1973;5:197–204.

115. Varga M. Recent experiences on the ophthalmologic complications of oral contraceptives. Ann Ophthalmol 1976;8:925–934.

116. Klein BEK, Klein R, Ritter LL. Is there evidence of an estrogen effect on age-related lens opacities? The Beaver Dam Eye Study. Arch Ophthalmol 1994;112:85–91.

117. Dickens CH. Retinoids. A review. J Am Acad Dermatol 1984;11: 541–552.

118. Gold SA, Shupack JL, Nemec MA. Ocular side effects of the retinoids. Int J Dermatol 1989;28:218–225.

119. Fraunfelder FT, LaBraico JM, Meyer SM. Adverse ocular reactions possibly associated with isotretinoin. Am J Ophthalmol 1985;100:534–537.

120. Weiss J, Degnan M, Leupold R, et al. Bilateral corneal opacities: Occurrence in a patient treated with oral isotretinoin. Arch Dermatol 1981;117:182–183.

121. Hazen PG, Carney JM, Langston RH, et al. Corneal effects of isotretinoin: Possible exacerbation of corneal neovascularization in a patient with keratitis, ichthyosis deafness ("KID") syndrome. J Am Acad Dermatol 1986;14:141–142.

122. Blackman MJ, Peck GL, Olsen TG, et al. Blepharoconjunctivitis: A side effect of 13-cis-retinoic acid therapy for dermatologic disease. Ophthalmology 1979;86:753–758.

123. McHenry JG, Zeiter JH, Madion MP, Cowden JW. Corneal epithe-

124. Sachs R, Zagelbaum BM, Hersh PS. Corneal complications associated with the use of crack cocaine. Ophthalmology 1993;100: 187–191.

125. Strominger MB, Sachs R, Hersh PS. Microbial keratitis with crack cocaine. Arch Ophthalmol 1990;108:1672.

126. Milson J, Jones DH, King K. Ophthalmological effects of 13-cis-retinoic acid therapy for acne vulgaris. Br J Dermatol 1982;107: 491–495.

127. Mathers WD, Shields WJ, Sachdev MS, et al. Meibomian gland morphology and tear osmolarity: Changes with Accutane therapy. Cornea 1991;10:286–290.

128. Hays GB, Lyle CB, Wheeler CE. Slate gray color in patients receiving chlorpromazine. Arch Dermatol 1964;90:471–476.

129. Cairns RH, Capoore HS, Gregory JDR. Oculocutaneous changes after years of high doses of chlorpromazine. Lancet 1965;1:239–241.

130. Siddal JR. The ocular toxic findings with prolonged and high dosage chlorpromazine intake. Arch Opthalmol 1965;74:460–464.

131. McClanahan WS, Harris JE, Knobloch WH, et al. Ocular manifestations of chronic phenothiazine derivative administration. Arch Ophthalmol 1966;75:319–325.

132. Editorial. Iatrogenic symptoms in opthalmology. Br Med J 1969; 2:199–200.

133. Alvaro ME. Effects other than antiinfections of sulfonamide compounds on eye. Arch Ophthalmol 1943;29:615–632.

134. Tilden ME, Rosenbaum JT, Fraunfelder FT. Systemic sulfonamides as a cause of bilateral, anterior uveitis. Arch Ophthalmol 1991;109:67–69.

135. Brothers DM, Hidayat AA. Conjunctival pigmentation associated with tetracycline medication. Ophthalmology 1981;88:1212–1215.

136. Messmer E, Font RL, Sheldon G, et al. Pigmented conjunctival cysts following tetracycline/minocycline therapy. Ophthalmology 1983;90:1462–1468.

137. Westin EJ, Holdeman N, Perrigin D. Bulbar conjunctival pigmentation secondary to oral tetracycline therapy. Clin Eye Vis Care 1992;4:19–21.

138. D'Amico DS, Kenyon RR. Drug-induced lipidoses in the cornea and conjunctiva. Int Ophthalmol 1981;4:67–76.

139. Reifler DM, Verdier DD, Davy CL, et al. Multiple chalazia and rosacea in a patient treated with amiodarone. Am J Ophthalmol 1987;103:594–595.

140. Ruth JH. Luminal poisoning with conjunctival residue. Am J Ophthalmol 1926;9:533–534.

141. Good WV, Ferriero DM, Golabi M, Kobori JA. Abnormalities of the visual system in infants exposed to cocaine. Ophthalmology 1992;99:341–346.

142. Longstaff S, Sigurdsson H, O'Keefe M, et al. A controlled study of ocular effects of tamoxifen in conventional dosage in the treatment of breast carcinoma. Eur J Cancer Clin Oncol 1989;25: 1805–1808.

143. Vinding T, Vestinielsen N. Retinopathy caused by treatment with tamoxifen in low dosage. Acta Ophthalmol 1983;61:45–50.

144. Groomer AE, Terry JE, Westblom TU. Subconjunctival and external hemorrhage secondary to oral anticoagulation. J Am Optom Assoc 1990;61:770–775.

145. Fraunfelder FT, Meyer MS. Ocular toxicology. In: Duane TD,

lial defects after smoking crack cocaine. Am J Ophthalmol 1989; 108:732.

Jaeger EA, eds. Clinical opthalmology. Hagerstown, MD: Harper & Row, 1987; Vol. 5, Chap. 37.

146. Crandall DC, Leopold IH. The influence of systemic drugs on tear constituents. Ophthalmology 1979;86:115–125.

147. Farber AS. Ocular side effect of antihistamine-decongestant combinations. Am J Ophthalmol 1982;94:565.

148. Balik J. Effect of atropine and pilocarpine on the secretion of chloride ion into the tears. Cesk Oftalmol 1958;14:28–33.

149. Erickson OF. Drug influences on lacrimal lysozyme production. Stanford Med Bull 1960;18:34–39.

150. Mader TH, Stulting RD. Keratoconjunctivitis sicca caused by diphenoxylate hydrochloride with atropine sulfate (Lomotil). Am J Ophthalmol 1991;111:377–378.

151. Miller D. Role of the tear film in contact lens wear. Int Ophthalmol Clin 1973;13:247–262.

152. Koeffler BH, Lemp MA. The effect of an antihistamine (chlorpheniramine maleate) on tear production in humans. Am J Ophthalmol 1980;12:217–219.

153. Seedor JA, Lamberts D, Bermann RB, et al. Filamentary keratitis associated with diphenhydramine hydrochloride (Benadryl). Am J Ophthalmol 1986;101:376–377.

154. Ensink BW, Van Voorst Vader PC. Ophthalmological side effects of 13-cis-retinoic therapy. Br J Dermatol 1983;108:637–641.

155. Rismondo V, Ubels JL. Isotretinoin in lacrimal gland fluid and tears. Arch Ophthalmol 1987;105:416–420.

156. Ubels JL, MacRae SM. Vitamin A is present as retinol in tears of humans and rabbits. Curr Eye Res 1984;3:815–817.

157. Felix FH, Ive FA, Dahl MGC. Cutaneous and ocular reactions with practolol administration. Oculomucocutaneous syndrome. Br Med J 1975;1:595–598.

158. Scott D. Another beta blocker causing eye problems. Br Med J 1977;2:1221.

159. Mackie IA, Seal DV, Pescod JM. Beta-adrenergic receptor blocking drugs: Tear lysozyme and immunological screening for adverse reactions. Br J Ophthalmol 1977;61:354–359.

160. Almog Y, Monselise M, Almog CH, et al. The effect of oral treatment with beta blockers on tear secretion. Metab Ped Syst Ophthalmol 1983;6:343–345.

161. Chizek DJ, Franceschetti AT. Oral contraceptives: Their side effects and ophthalmological manifestations. Surv Ophthalmol 1969;14:90–101.

162. Verbeck B. Augenbefunde und stoffwechselverhalten bei einnahme von ovulation-schemmern. Klin Monatsbl Augenheilkd 1973;162:612–615.

163. Frankel SH, Ellis PP. Effect of oral contraceptives on tear production. Ann Ophthalmol 1978;10:1585–1588.

164. Brennan NA, Efron N. Symptomatology of HEMA contact lens wear. Optom Vis Sci 1989;66:834–838.

165. Berman MT, Newman BL, Johnson NC. The effect of a diuretic (hydrochlorothiazide) on tear production in humans. Am J Ophthalmol 1985;99:473–475.

166. De Haas EBH. Lacrimal gland response to parasympathomimetics after parasympathetic denervation. Arch Ophthalmol 1960;64:34–43.

167. Dawson WW, Jimenez-Antillon CF, Perez JM, et al. Marijuana and vision—after 10 years use in Costa Rica. Invest Ophthalmol Vis Sci 1977;16:689–699.

168. Shapiro D. The ocular manifestations of cannabinols. Ophthalmologia 1974;168:366–369.

169. Melon J, Reginster M. Passage into normal salivary, lacrimal and nasal secretions of ampicillin and erythromycin administered intramuscularly. Acta Otorhinolaryngol Belg 1976;30:643–651.

170. Fraunfelder FT. Orange tears. Am J Ophthalmol 1980;89:752.

171. Lyons RW. Orange contact-lenses from rifampin. N Engl J Med 1979;300:372.

172. Leopold IH, Comroe JH. Effect of intramuscular administration of morphine, atropine, scopolamine and neostigmine on the human eye. Arch Ophthalmol 1948;40:285–290.

173. Verdier DD, Kennerdell JS. Fixed dilated pupil resulting from transdermal scopolamine. Am J Ophthalmol 1982;93:803–804.

174. McCrary JA, Webb NR. Anisocoria from scopolamine patches. JAMA 1982;248:353–355.

175. Burns RP, Steele AS. Ocular change in drug abusers. In: Leopold IH. Symposium on ocular therapy. St Louis: C.V. Mosby Co, 1973; Vol. 6;6–10.

176. Goldey JA, Dick DA, Porter WL. Cornpicker's pupil: A clinical note regarding mydriasis from jimson weed dust (*Stramonium*). Ohio State Med J 1966;62:921.

177. Upholt JP, Qunby GE, Batchelor GS, et al. Visual effects accompanying TEPP induced miosis. Arch Ophthalmol 1956;56:128–134.

178. Lee HK, Wang SC. Mechanism of morphine induced miosis in the dog. Am J Ophthalmol 1982;14:436–438.

179. Crews SJ. Toxic effects on the eye and visual apparatus resulting from the systemic absorption of recently induced chemical agents. Trans Ophthalmol Soc UK 1962;82:387–406.

180. Rengstorff RH. Accidental exposure to sarin: Vision effects. Arch Toxicol 1985;56:201–203.

181. Leebeck MJ. Effect of drugs on ocular muscles. Int Ophthalmol Clin 1971;11:35–62.

182. Rosenberg ML. Reversible downbeat nystagmus secondary to excessive alcohol intake. J Clin Neuro-Ophthalmol 1987;7:23–25.

183. Chrousos GA, Cowdry R, Schuelein M, et al. Two cases of downbeat nystagmus and oscillopsia associated with carbamazepine. Am J Ophthalmol 1987;103:221–224.

184. Wilkinson IMS, Kime R, Purnell M. Alcohol and human eye movement. Brain 1974;97:785–792.

185. Bittencourt P, Wade P, Richens A, et al. Blood alcohol and eye movements. Lancet 1980;16:981.

186. Wilson G, Mitchell R. The effect of alcohol on the visual and ocular motor systems. Aust J Ophthalmol 1983;11:315–319.

187. Halperin E, Yolton RL. Is the driver drunk? Oculomotor sobriety testing. J Am Optom Assoc 1986;57:654–657.

188. Tiffany DV. Optometric expert testimony. Foundation for the horizontal gaze nystagmus test. J Am Optom Assoc 1986;57:705–708.

189. Coppetto JR, Montrieo ML, Lessel S, et al. Downbeat nystagmus. Long-term therapy with moderate-dose lithium carbonate. Arch Neurol 1983;40:754.

190. Halmagyi GM, Gresty MA, Rudge P, Sanders MD. Downbeating nystagmus. A review of 62 cases. Arch Neurol 1983;40:777.

191. Williams DP, Troost BT, Rogers J. Lithium-induced downbeat nystagmus. Arch Neurol 1988;45:1022–1023.

192. Halmagyi GM, Lessell I, Curthoys IS, et al. Lithium-induced downbeat nystagmus. Am J Ophthalmol 1989;107:664–670.

193. Bourgeois JA. Ocular side effects of lithium—a review. J Am Optom Assoc 1991;62:548–551.

194. Fraunfelder FT, Fraunfelder FW, Jefferson JW. The effects of lithium on the human visual system. J Toxicol—Cut Ocular Toxicol 1992;11:97–169.

195. Maddalena MA. Transient myopia associated with acute glaucoma and retinal edema. Arch Ophthalmol 1968;80:186–188.

196. Palestine AG. Transient acute myopia resulting from isotretinoin (Accutane) therapy. Ann Ophthalmol 1984;16:660–662.

197. Hook SR, Holladay JT, Prager TC, et al. Transient myopia induced by sulfonamides. Am J Ophthalmol 1986;101:495–496.

198. Chirls IA, Norris JW. Transient myopia associated with vaginal sulfanilamide suppositories. Am J Ophthalmol 1984;98:120–121.

199. Mattsson R. Transient myopia following the use of sulphonamides. Acta Ophthalmol 1952;30:385–398.

200. Beasley FJ. Transient myopia and retinal edema during hydrochlorothiazide (Hydrodiuril) therapy. Arch Ophthalmol 1961;65: 212–213.

201. Beasley FJ. Transient myopia and retinal edema during ethoxzolamide (Cardrase) therapy. Arch Ophthalmol 1962;68:490–491.

202. Galin MA, Baras I, Zweifach P. Diamox-induced myopia. Am J Ophthalmol 1962;54:237–240.

203. Michaelson JJ. Transient myopia due to Hygroton. Am J Ophthalmol 1962;54:1146–1147.

204. Muirhead JF, Scheie HG. Transient myopia after acetazolamide. Arch Ophthalmol 1960;63:315–318.

205. Yasuna E. Acute myopia associated with prochlorperazine (Compazine) therapy. Am J Ophthalmol 1962;54:793–796.

206. Sandford-Smith JH. Transient myopia after aspirin. Br J Ophthalmol 1974;58:698–700.

207. Bovino JA, Marcus DF. The mechanism of transient myopia induced by sulfonamide therapy. Am J Ophthalmol 1982;94:99.

208. Grinbaum A, Ashkenazi I, Gutman I, Blumenthal M. Suggested mechanism for acute transient myopia after sulfonamide treatment. Ann Ophthalmol 1993;25:224–226.

209. Fan JT, Johnson DH, Buck RR. Transient myopia, angle-closure glaucoma, and choroidal detachment after oral acetazolamide. Am J Ophthalmol 1993;115:813–814.

210. Laval J. Paresis of accommodation following sulfadiazine therapy. Am J Ophthalmol 1943;26:303.

211. Frucht J, Freimann I, Merin S. Ocular side effects of disopyramide. Br J Ophthalmol 1984;68:890–891.

212. Rubin ML, Thomas WC. Diplopia and loss of accommodation due to chloroquine. Arth Rheumat 1970;13:75–82.

213. Percival SPB, Behrman J. Ophthalmological safety of chloroquine. Br J Ophthalmol 1969;53:101–109.

214. Percival SPB, Meanock I. Chloroquine: Opthalmological safety, and clinical assessment in rheumatoid arthritis. Br Med J 1968;3: 579–584.

215. Howell R. Treatment of discoid lupus erythematosus. St John's Hosp Dermat Soc 1957;39:48.

216. Kjaer GCD. Retinopathy associated with phenothiazine administration. Dis Nerv Syst 1968;29:316–319.

217. Alkemade PPH. Phenothiazine-retinopathy. Ophthalmologica 1968;155:70–76.

218. Thaler JS. The effect of multiple psychotropic drugs on the accommodation of prepresbyopes. Am J Optom Physiol Opt 1979;56:259–261.

219. Thaler JS. Effects of benztropine mesylate (Cogentin) on accommodation in normal volunteers. Am J Optom Physiol Opt 1982; 59:918–919.

220. Ahronheim JC. Handbook of prescribing medications for geriatric patients. Boston: Little, Brown and Company, 1992;76,99,109, 136,385.

221. Ritch R, Krupin T, Henry C, Kurata F. Oral imipramine and acute angle closure glaucoma. Arch Ophthalmol 1994;112:67–68.

222. Layenby GW, Reed JW, Grant WM. Anticholinergic medication in open-angle glaucoma. Arch Ophthalmol 1970;84:719–723

223. Hiatt RL, Fuller IB, Smith L, et al. Systemically administered anticholinergic drugs and intraocular pressure. Arch Ophthalmol 1970;84:735–740.

224. Elliot MJ, Cullen PM, Phillips CI. Ocular hypotensive effect of atenolol. Br J Ophthalmol 1975;59:296–300.

225. Macdonald MJ, Cullen PM, Phillips CI. Atenolol versus propranolol. Br J Ophthalmol 1976;60:789–791.

226. Macdonald MJ, Gore SM, Cullen PM, Phillips CI. Comparison of ocular hypotensive effects of acetazolamide and atenolol. Br J Ophthalmol 1977;61:345–348.

227. Wettrell K, Pandolfi M. Effect of oral administration of various beta-blocking agents on the intraocular pressure in healthy volunteers. Exp Eye Res 1975;21:451–456.

228. Alm A, Wickstrom CP. Effects of systemic and topical administration of metoprolol on intraocular pressure in healthy subjects. Acta Ophthalmol 1980;58:740–747.

229. Alm A, Wickstrom CP, Ekstrom C, Ohman L. The effect of metoprolol on intraocular pressure in glaucoma. Acta Ophthalmol 1979;57:236–242.

230. Duff GR. The effect of twice daily nadolol on intraocular pressure. Am J Ophthalmol 1987;104:343–345.

231. Rennie IG, Smerdon DL. The effect of a once-daily oral dose of nadolol on intraocular pressure in normal volunteers. Am J Ophthalmol 1985;100:445–447.

232. Williamson J, Atta HR, Kennedy PA, Muir JG. Effect of orally administered nadolol on the intraocular pressure in normal volunteers. Br J Ophthalmol 1985;69:38–40.

233. Williamson J, Young JD, Atta H, et al. Comparative efficacy of orally and topically administered β blockers for chronic simple glaucoma. Br J Ophthalmol 1985;69:41–45.

234. Duff GR, Watt AH, Graham PA. A comparison of the effects of oral nadolol and topical timolol on intraocular pressure, blood pressure, and heart rate. Br J Ophthalmol 1987;71:698–700.

235. Smith SE, Smith SA, Reynolds R, Whitmarsh VB. Ocular and cardiovascular effects of local and systemic pindolol. Br J Ophthalmol 1979;63:63–66.

236. Phillips CI, Howitt G, Rowlands DJ. Propranolol as ocular hypotensive agents. Br J Ophthalmol 1967;51:222–226.

237. Pandolfi M, Ohrstrom A. Treatment of ocular hypertension with oral beta-adrenergic blocking agents. Acta Ophthalmol 1974;54: 464–467.

238. Wettrell K, Pandolfi M. Early dose response analysis of ocular hypotensive effects of propranolol in patients with ocular hypertension. Br J Ophthalmol 1976;60:680–683.

239. Ohrstrom A, Pandolfi M. Long-term treatment of glaucoma with systemic propranolol. Am J Ophthalmol 1978;86:340–344.

240. Wettrell K, Pandolfi M. Propranolol vs acetazolamide. Arch Ophthalmol 1979;97:280–283.

241. Borthne A. The treatment of glaucoma with propranolol (Inderal): A clinical trial. Acta Ophthalmol 1976;54:291–300.

242. Ohrstrom A. Dose response of oral timolol combined with adrenaline. Br J Ophthalmol 1982;66:242–246.

243. Batchelor ED, O'Day DM, Shand DG, Wood AJ. Interaction of topical and oral timolol in glaucoma. Ophthalmology 1979;86: 60–65.

244. Ohrstrom A. Dose-related interaction between timolol and adrenaline. Arch Klin Exp Ophthalmol 1981;216:55–59.

245. Thomas JV, Epstein DL. Study of additive effect of timolol and epinephrine in lowering intraocular pressure. Br J Ophthalmol 1981;65:596–602.

246. Ohrstrom A, Pandolfi M. Regulation of IOP and pupil size by beta-blockers and epinephrine. Arch Ophthalmol 1980;98:2182–2184.

247. Goldberg I, Ashburn FS Jr, Palmberg PF, et al. Timolol and epinephrine: A clinical study of ocular interactions. Arch Ophthalmol 1980;98:484–486.

248. Neufeld AH. Experimental studies on the mechanism of action of timolol. Surv Ophthalmol 1979;23:363–370.

249. Yablonski ME, Zimmerman TJ, Waltman SR, Becker B. A fluorophotometric study of the effect of topical timolol on aqueous humor dynamics. Exp Eye Res 1978;27:135–142.

250. Coakes RL, Brubaker RF. The mechanism of timolol in lowering intraocular pressure in the normal eye. Arch Ophthalmol 1978;96:2045–2048.

251. Zimmerman TJ, Harbin R, Pett M, Kaufman HE. Timolol and facility of outflow. Invest Ophthalmol Vis Sci 1977;16:623–624.

252. Sonntag JR, Brindley GO, Shields MB, et al. Timolol and epinephrine. Comparison of efficacy and side effects. Arch Ophthalmol 1979;97:273–277.

253. Schenker HI, Yablonski ME, Podos SM, Linder L. Fluorophotometric study of epinephrine and timolol in human subjects. Arch Ophthalmol 1981;99:1212–1216.

254. Vareilles P, Lotti VJ. Effect of timolol on aqueous humor dynamics in the rabbit. Ophthalmic Res 1981;13:72–79.

255. Reiss GR, Brubaker RF. The mechanism of betaxolol, a new ocular hypotensive agent. Ophthalmology 1983;90:1369–1372.

256. Gross FJ, Schuman JS. Reduced ocular hypotensive effect of topical β-blockers in glaucoma patients receiving oral β-blockers. J Glaucoma 1992;1:174–177.

257. Kass MA. Efficacy of combining timolol with other antiglaucoma medications. Surv Ophthalmol 1983;28:274–283.

258. Merritt JC, Crawford WJ, Alexander PC, et al. Effect of marihuana on intraocular and blood pressure in glaucoma. Ophthalmology 1980;87:222–228.

259. Simon KA, Bonting SL, Hawkins NM. Studies on sodium-potassium-activated adenosine triphosphatase. II. Formation of aqueous humour. Exp Eye Res 1962;1:253–261.

260. Simon K, Bonting SL. Possible usefulness of cardiac glycosides in the treatment of glaucoma. Arch Ophthalmol 1962;68:227–234.

261. Peczon JD. Clinical evaluation of digitalization in glaucoma. Arch Ophthalmol 1964;71:500–504.

262. Riley MV. The sodium-potassium-stimulated adenosine triphosphate of rabbit ciliary epithelium. Exp Eye Res 1964;3:76–84.

263. Lely AH, van Enter CHJ. Large scale digitoxin intoxication. Br Med J 1970;3:737–740.

264. Wilson DM, Martin JHS, Niall JF. Raised intraocular tension in renal transplant recipients. Med J Aust 1973:482–484.

265. Lieberman TW. Ocular effects of prolonged systemic drug administration (corticosteroids, chloramphenicol, and anovulatory agents). Dis Nerv Syst 1968;29:44–50.

266. Covell LL. Glaucoma induced by systemic steroid therapy. Am J Ophthalmol 1958;45:108–109.

267. Bernstein HN, Schwartz B. Effects of long-term systemic steroids on ocular pressure and tonographic values. Arch Ophthalmol 1962;68:742–743.

268. Godel V, Feiler-Ofry V, Stein R. Systemic steroids and ocular fluid dynamics. I. Analysis of the sample as a whole. Influence of dosage and duration of therapy. Acta Ophthalmol 1972;50:655–663.

269. Godel V, Feiler-Ofry V, Stein R. Systemic steroids and ocular fluid dynamics. II. Systemic versus topical steroids. Acta Ophthalmol 1972;50:664–676.

270. Godel V, Feiler-Ofry V, Stein R. The genetic nature of the hypertensive ocular response to long-term systemic steroids. Ann Ophthalmol 1970;1:462–467.

271. Schwartz B. The response of ocular pressure to corticosteroids. Int Ophthalmol Clin 1966;6:929–989.

272. Feiler-Ofry V, Godel V, Stein R. Systemic steroids and ocular fluid dynamics. III. The genetic nature of the ocular response and its different levels. Acta Ophthalmol 1972;50:699–706.

273. Diotallevi M, Bocci N. Effect of systemically administered corticosteroids on intraocular pressure and fluid dynamics. Acta Ophthalmol 1965;43:524–527.

274. Spaeth GL, Rodrigues MM, Weinreb S. Steroid-induced glaucoma. A. Persistent elevation of intraocular pressure. B. Histopathological aspects. Trans Am Ophthalmol Soc 1977;75:353–381.

275. Peczon JD, Grant WM. Glaucoma, alcohol, and intraocular pressure. Arch Ophthalmol 1965;73:495–501.

276. Krupin T, Kolker AE, Becker B. Alcohol and intraocular pressure. Invest Ophthalmol 1967;6:559–560.

277. Gilmer G, Swartz M, Teske M, et al. Over-the-counter phenylpropanolamine: A possible cause of central retinal vein occlusion. Arch Ophthalmol 1986;104:642.

278. Cerasoli JR. Effects of drugs on the retina. Int Ophthalmol Clin 1971;42:121–135.

279. Rynes RI, Krohel G, Falbo A, et al. Ophthalmologic safety of long-term hydroxychloroquine treatment. Arth Rheumat 1979;22:832–836.

280. Bernstein HN. Ocular safety by hydroxychloroquine sulfate (Plaquenil). So Med J 1992;85:274–279.

281. Cambiaggi A. Unusual ocular lesions in a case of systemic lupus erythematosus. AMA Arch Ophthalmol 1957;57:451–453.

282. Hobbs HE, Sorsby A, Freedman A. Retinopathy following chloroquine therapy. Lancet 1959;2:478–480.

283. Aylward JM. Hydroxychloroquine and chloroquine: Assessing the risk of retinal toxicity. J Am Optom Assoc 1993;64:787–797.

284. Cruess AF, Schachat AP, Nicholl J, et al. Chloroquine retinopathy. Is fluorescein angiography necessary? Ophthalmology 1985;92:1127–1129.

285. Henkind P, Carr RE, Siegel IM. Early chloroquine retinopathy: Clinical and functional findings. Arch Ophthalmol 1964;71:157–165.

286. Carlberg O. Three cases of chloroquine retinopathy. A follow-up investigation. Acta Ophthalmol 1966;44:367–374.

287. Martin LJ, Bergen RL, Dobrow HR. Delayed onset chloroquine retinopathy: Case report. Ann Ophthalmol 1978;10:723–726.

288. Brinkley JR, Dubois EL, Ryan SJ. Long-term course of chloroquine retinopathy after cessation of medication. Am J Ophthalmol 1979;88:1–11.

289. Mills PV, Beck M, Power BJ. Assessment of the retinal toxicity of hydroxychloroquine. Trans Ophthalmol Soc UK 1981;101:109–113.

290. Kearns TP, Hollenhorst RW. Chloroquine retinopathy: Evaluation

by fluorescein fundus angiography. Trans Am Ophthalmol Soc 1966;64:217–231.

291. Lowes M. Peripheral visual field restriction in chloroquine retinopathy. Report of a case. Acta Ophthalmol 1976;54:819–826.

292. Krill AE, Potts AM, Johanson CE. Chloroquine retinopathy. Investigation of discrepancy between dark adaptation and electroretinographic findings in advanced stages. Am J Ophthalmol 1971; 71:530–543.

293. Kolb H. Electro-oculogram findings in patients treated with antimalarial drugs. Br J Ophthalmol 1965;49:573–589.

294. Nylander U. Ocular damage in chloroquine therapy. Acta Ophthalmol 1966;44:335–348.

295. Hart WM, Burde RM, Johnston GP, et al. Static perimetry in chloroquine retinopathy. Perifoveal patterns of visual field depression. Arch Ophthalmol 1984;102:377–380.

296. Weiner A, Sandberg HA, Gaudio AR, et al. Hydroxychloroquine retinopathy. Am J Ophthalmol 1991;112:528–534.

297. Bishara SA, Matamoros N. Evaluation of several tests in screening for chloroquine maculopathy. Eye 1989;3:777–782.

298. Banks CN. Melanin: Blackguard or red herring? Another look at chloroquine retinopathy. Aust NZ J Ophthalmol 1987;15:365–370.

299. Burns RP. Delayed onset of chloroquine retinopathy. N Engl J Med 1966;275:693–696.

300. Ehrenfeld M, Nesher R, Merin S. Delayed-onset chloroquine retinopathy. Br J Ophthalmol 1986;70:281–283.

301. Finbloom DS, Silver K, Newsome DA, et al. Comparison of hydroxychloroquine and chloroquine use and the development of retinal toxicity. J Rheumatol 1985;12:692–694.

302. Easterbrook M. Dose relationships in patients with early chloroquine retinopathy. J Rheumatol 1987;14:472–475.

303. Voipio H. Incidence of chloroquine retinopathy. Acta Ophthalmol 1966;44:349–354.

304. Ogawa S, Kurumatani N, Shibaike N, et al. Progression of retinopathy long after cessation of chloroquine therapy. Lancet 1979; 1:1408.

305. Bernstein HN. Ocular safety of hydroxychloroquine. Ann Ophthalmol 1991;23:292–296.

306. Easterbrook M. The ocular safety of hydroxychloroquine. Sem Arthritis Rheumatol 1993;23:62–66.

307. Johnson MW, Vine AK. Hydroxychloroquine therapy in massive total doses without retinal toxicity. Am J Ophthalmol 1987;104: 139–144.

308. Rosenthal AR, Kolb H, Bergsma D, et al. Chloroquine retinopathy in the Rhesus monkey. Invest Ophthalmol Vis Sci 1978;17:1158–1175.

309. Bernstein HN, Ginsberg J. The pathology of chloroquine retinopathy. Arch Ophthalmol 1964;71:238–245.

310. Ramsey MS, Fine BS. Chloroquine toxicity in the human eye. Histopathologic observations by electron microscopy. Am J Ophthalmol 1972;73:229–235.

311. Wetterholm DH, Winter FC. Histopathology of chloroquine retinal toxicity. Arch Ophthalmol 1964;71:116–121.

312. Raines MF, Bhargava SK, Rosen ES. The blood-retinal barrier in chloroquine retinopathy. Invest Ophthalmol Vis Sci 1989;30: 1726–1730.

313. Easterbrook M. Is corneal deposition of anti-malarial any indication of retinal toxicity? Can J Ophthalmol 1990;25:249–251.

314. Falcone PM, Paolini L, Lou PL. Hydroxychloroquine toxicity despite normal dose therapy. Ann Ophthalmol 1993;25:385–388.

315. Fleck BW, Bell AL, Mitchell JD, et al. Screening for antimalarial maculopathy in rheumatology clinics. Br Med J 1985;291:782–784.

316. Kinross-Wright VJ. Newer phenothiazine drugs in treatment of nervous disorders. JAMA 1959;170:1283–1288.

317. Miller FS, Bunt-Milam AH, Kalina RE. Clinical-ultrastructural study of thioridazine retinopathy. Ophthalmology 1982;89:1478–1488.

318. Davidorf FH. Thioridazine pigmentary retinopathy. Arch Ophthalmol 1973;90:251–255.

319. Meredith TA, Aaberg TM, Willerson D. Progressive chorioretinopathy after receiving thioridazine. Arch Ophthalmol 1978;96: 1172–1176.

320. Miyata M, Imai H, Ishikawa S, et al. Change in human electroretinography associated with thioridazine administration. Ophthalmologica 1980;181:175–180.

321. Godel V, Loewenstein A, Lazar M. Spectral electroretinography in thioridazine toxicity. Ann Ophthalmol 1990;22:293–296.

322. Neves MS, Jordan K, Dragt H, et al. Extensive chorioretinopathy associated with very low dose thioridazine. Eye 1990;4:767–770.

323. Cameron ME, Lawrence JM, Olrich JG. Thioridazine (Melleril) retinopathy. Br J Ophthalmol 1972;56:131–134.

324. Marmor MF. Is thioridazine retinopathy progressive? Relationship of pigmentary changes to visual function. Br J Ophthalmol 1990;74:739–742.

325. Potts AM. The concentration of phenothiazines in the eye of experimental animals. Invest Ophthalmol Vis Sci 1962;1:522–530.

326. Kimbrough BO, Campbell RJ. Thioridazine levels in the human eye. Arch Ophthalmol 1981;99:2188–2189.

327. Henkes HE. Electro-oculography as a diagnostic aid in phenothiazin retinopathy. Trans Ophthalmol Soc UK 1967;87:285–287.

328. Gangitano JL, Keltner JL. Abnormalities of the pupil and visual-evoked potential in quinine amblyopia. Am J Ophthalmol 1980; 89:425–430.

329. Yospaiboon Y, Lawtiantong T, Chotibutr S. Clinical observations of ocular quinine intoxication. Jpn J Ophthalmol 1984;28:409–415.

330. Dickinson P, Sabto J, West RH. Management of quinine toxicity. Aust J Ophthalmol 1983;11:265–269.

331. Brinton GS, Norton EWD, Zahn JR, et al. Ocular quinine toxicity. Am J Ophthalmol 1980;90:403–410.

332. Dyson EH, Proudfoot AT, Bateman DN. Quinine amblyopia: Is current management appropriate? Clin Toxicol 1985–86;23:571–578.

333. Behrman J, Mushin A. Electrodiagnostic findings in quinine amblyopia. Br J Ophthalmol 1968;52:925–928.

334. Bacon P, Spalton DJ, Smith SE. Blindness from quinine toxicity. Br J Ophthalmol 1988;72:219–224.

335. Stuart P. Quinine blindness: The value of stellate ganglion block. Br J Anaesth 1963;35:728–730.

336. Bankes JLK, Hayward JA, Jones MBS. Quinine amblyopia treated with stellate ganglion block. Br Med J 1972;4:85–86.

337. Vainio-Mattila B, Zewi M. Quinine amblyopia and the electroretinogram (ERG). Acta Ophthalmol 1954;32:451–461.

338. Sabto J, Pierce RM, West RH, et al. Hemodialysis, peritoneal dialysis, plasmapheresis, and forced diuresis for the treatment of quinine overdose. Clin Nephrol 1981;16:264–268.

339. Floyd M, Hill AVL, Ormston BJ, et al. Quinine amblyopia treated by hemodialysis. Clin Nephrol 1974;2:44–46.

340. Michelson JB, Whitcher JP, Wilson S, et al. Possible foreign body granuloma of the retina associated with intravenous cocaine addiction. Am J Ophthalmol 1979;87:278–280.

341. Tse DT, Ober RR. Talc retinopathy. Am J Ophthalmol 1980;90:624–640.

342. Mclane NS, Carrol DM. Ocular manifestations of drug abuse. Surv Ophthalmol 1986;30:298–313.

343. O'Brien RJ, Schroedl BL. Talc retinopathy. Optom Vis Sci 1991;68:54–57.

344. AtLee WE. Talc and cornstarch emboli in eyes of drug abusers. JAMA 1972;219:49–51.

345. Lederer CM, Sabates FN. Ocular findings in the intravenous drug abuser. Ann Ophthalmol 1982;14:436–438.

346. Carman CR. Talc retinopathy. J Am Optom Assoc 1985;56:129–130.

347. Lee J, Sapira JD. Retinal and cerebral microembolization of talc in a drug abuser. Am J Med Sci 1973;265:75–77.

348. Kresca LJ, Goldberg MF, Jampol LM. Talc emboli and retinal neovascularization in a drug abuser. Am J Ophthalmol 1979;87:334–339.

349. Bluth LL, Hanscom TA. Retinal detachment and vitreous hemorrhage due to talc emboli. JAMA 1981;246:980–981.

350. Paré JAP, Fraser RG, Hogg JC, et al. Pulmonary "mainline" granulomatosis: Talcosis of intravenous methadone abuse. Medicine 1979;58:229–239.

351. Murphy SB, Jackson B, Paré JAP. Talc retinopathy. Can J Ophthalmol 1978;13:152–156.

352. Jampol LM, Setogawa T, Rednam KRV, et al. Talc retinopathy in primates. A model of ischemic retinopathy. I. Clinical studies. Arch Ophthalmol 1981;99:1273–1280.

353. Kaga N, Tso MOM, Jampol LM, et al. Talc retinopathy in primates: A model of ischemic retinopathy. II. A histopathologic study. Arch Ophthalmol 1982;100:1644–1648.

354. Kaga N, Tso MOM, Jampol LM. Talc retinopathy in primates: A model of ischemic retinopathy. III. An electron microscopic study. Arch Ophthalmol 1982;100:1649–1657.

355. Withering W. An account of the foxglove and some of its medical uses: With practical remarks on dropsy and other diseases. London: Broomsleigh Press, 1785.

356. Robertson DM, Hollenhorst RW, Callahan JA. Ocular manifestations of digitalis toxicity. Discussion and report of three cases of central scotomas. Arch Ophthalmol 1966;76:640–645.

357. Sykowski P. Digitoxin intoxication. Resulting in retrobulbar optic neuritis. Am J Ophthalmol 1949;32:572–574.

358. Weleber RG, Shults WT. Digoxin retinal toxicity. Clinical and electrophysiologic evaluation of a cone dysfunction syndrome. Arch Ophthalmol 1981;99:1568–1572.

359. Robertson DM, Hollenhorst RW, Callahan JA. Receptor function in digitalis therapy. Arch Ophthalmol 1966;76:852–857.

360. Frambach DA, Matthews JD, Weiter JJ, et al. Digoxin in the subretinal spaces of humans with rhegmatogenous retinal detachments. Am J Ophthalmol 1985;100:490–491.

361. Rietbrock N, Alken RG. Color vision deficiencies: A common sign of intoxication in chronically digoxin-treated patients. J Cardiovasc Pharmacol 1980;2:93–99.

362. Haustein K-O, Oltmanns G, Rietbrock N, et al. Differences in color vision impairment caused by digoxin, digitoxin, or pengitoxin. J Cardiovasc Pharmacol 1982;4:536–541.

363. Chuman MA, LeSage J. Color vision deficiencies in two cases of digoxin toxicity. Am J Ophthalmol 1985;100:682–685.

364. Piltz JR, Wertenbaker C, Lance SE, et al. Digoxin toxicity. J Clin Neuro-ophthalmol 1993;13:275–280.

365. Wagener HP, Smith HL, Nickeson RW. Retrobulbar neuritis and complete heart block caused by digitalis poisioning. Report of a case. Arch Ophthalmol 1946;36:478–483.

366. Gibson HC, Smith DM, Alpern M. II₅ specificity in digitoxin toxicity. A case report. Arch Ophthalmol 1965;74:154–158.

367. Binnion Pf, Frazer G. ³H digoxin in the optic tract in digoxin intoxication. J Cardiovasc Pharmacol 1980;2:699–706.

368. Mortada A, Abboud I. Retinal hemorrhages after prolonged use of salicylates. Br J Ophthalmol 1973;57:199–200.

369. Koliopoulos J, Palimeris G. On acquired colour vision disturbances during treatment with ethambutol and indomethacin. Mod Probl Ophthalmol 1972;11:178–184.

370. Graham CM, Blach RK. Indomethacin retinopathy: case report and review. Br J Ophthalmol 1988;72:434–438.

371. Kaiser-Kupfer MI, Kupfer C, Rodriques MM. Tamoxifen retinopathy. A clinicopathologic report. Ophthalmology 1981;88:89–93.

372. Beck M, Mills PV. Ocular assessment of patients treated with tamoxifen. Cancer Treat Rep 1979;63:1833–1834.

373. Kaiser-Kupfer MI, Lippman ME. Tamoxifen retinopathy. Cancer Treat Rep 1978;62:315–320.

374. McKeown CA, Swartz M, Blom J, et al. Tamoxifen retinopathy. Br J Ophthalmol 1981;65:177–179.

375. Gerner EW. Ocular toxicity of tamoxifen. Ann Ophthalmol 1989;21:420–423.

376. Pavlidis NA, Petris C, Briassoulis E, et al. Clear evidence that long-term, low-dose tamoxifen treatment can induce ocular toxicity. Cancer 1992;69:2961–2964.

377. Chern S, Danis RP. Retinopathy associated with low-dose tamoxifen. Am J Ophthalmol 1993;116:372–373.

378. Griffiths MFP. Tamoxifen retinopathy at low dosage. Am J Ophthalmol 1987;104:185–186.

379. Ashford AR, Donev I, Tiwari RP, Garrett TJ. Reversible ocular toxicity related to tamoxifen therapy. Cancer 1988;6:33–35.

380. Shingleton BJ, Bienfang DC, Albert DM, et al. Ocular toxicity associated with high-dose carmustine. Arch Ophthalmol 1982;100:1766–1772.

381. Kupersmith MJ, Frohman LP, Choi IS, et al. Visual system toxicity following intra-arterial chemotherapy. Neurology 1988;38:284–289.

382. Defer G, Fauchon F, Schiason M, et al. Visual toxicity following intra-arterial chemotherapy with hydroxyethyl-CNU in patients with malignant gliomas. Neuro-Radiol 1991;33:432–437.

383. Grimson BS, Mahaley MS, Dubey HD, et al. Ophthalmic and central nervous system complications following intracarotid BCNU (carmustine). J Clin Neuro-Ophthalmol 1981;1:261–264.

384. Miller DF, Bay JW, Lederman RJ, et al. Ocular and orbital toxicity following intracarotid injection of BCNU (carmustine) and cis-platinum for malignant gliomas. Ophthalmology 1985;92:402–406.

385. Chrousos GA, Oldfield EH, Doppman JL, et al. Prevention of ocular toxicity of carmustine (BCNU) with supraophthalmic intra-carotid infusion. Ophthalmology 1986;93:1471–1475.

386. Guyer D, Tiedeman J, Yannuzzi LA, et al. Interferon-associated retinopathy. Arch Ophthalmol 1993;111:350–356.

387. Kaplan NM. Clinical complications of oral contraceptives. Adv Intern Med 1975;20:197.

problems as hypoglycemia, analgesic overdose, stroke, and cardiopulmonary arrest.

The awake patient who suddenly develops crushing chest tightness associated with a presyncope feeling presents a special situation. The patient may well be suffering from ventricular tachycardia or ventricular fibrillation. In some of these patients, blood pressure, and thus consciousness, can be maintained for a short time by initiating a cough that increases peripheral vascular tone. Repeated coughing maintained cerebral perfusion until definitive therapy could be instituted in a small number of hospitalized patients. In addition, 10% of patients with ventricular dysrhythmia will cardiovert to a normal sinus with a vigorous cough. Thus, patients presenting chest tightness associated with a near syncope feeling should be directed to cough. This may prevent a full cardiopulmonary arrest.[14–16]

Although the following discussion outlines the current approach to basic cardiopulmonary resuscitation, it must be understood that proficiency in the techniques requires training that incorporates "hands-on" experience (with mannequins) and periodic recertification to maintain skills.

Once patient unresponsiveness is established, the first measure is to open the airway, "A." The patient should be positioned supine on a hard flat surface so that the airway can be opened and cardiopulmonary resuscitation performed, if indicated. In the unconscious patient, relaxation of the pharyngeal muscles may allow the tongue to fall back into the airway, resulting in mechanical obstruction. Simple maneuvers such as the head-tilt-neck-lift, head-tilt-chin-lift, or jaw thrust will relieve the obstruction. In some cases, restoration of airway patency may be all that is required to prevent deterioration of the patient's condition to complete cardiopulmonary arrest. Breathing, "B," can be ascertained by placing a hand or ear next to the patient's nose to detect air movement. If there is no air movement, breathing is inadequate. Four quick breaths should be delivered, and the chest wall should be observed for movement with each breath to reevaluate "A." Patients who have potential cervical spine injuries, although not likely to be encountered in the practitioner's office setting, pose a special problem. Maneuvers that depend on hyperextension of the neck in these patients should be avoided in favor of jaw thrust, which maintains the neck in the neutral position. The rescuer thereby minimizes the likelihood of a potential devastating spinal cord injury in the patient with a neck injury. The possibility of airway obstruction by vomitus, denture, or other foreign bodies must be kept in mind, and appropriate maneuvers should be undertaken to clear the airway. The lack of movement of the chest wall during rescue breathing means the airway has not been established. Prompt reevaluation and institution of additional maneuvers to restore patency must be performed before proceeding.

Breathing, "B," must be instituted immediately if the patient is not breathing once appropriate measures to open the airway have been performed. Mouth-to-mouth breathing using exhaled air is the technique of choice. Concentrations of oxygen approaching 18% to 20% can be delivered by this method.[17] Pocket masks (Fig. 38.1), available with a one-way valve preventing the regurgitation of stomach contents or air into the rescuer's mouth, are inexpensive and useful adjuncts to ventilation that can be used to overcome both aesthetic and health objections. These should be readily available to prevent delay in instituting CPR. A good seal over the face can be established, and with a simple oxygen delivery system it is possible to substantially increase the concentration of oxygen delivered to the patient. Observing movement of the chest wall confirms a patent airway and effective breathing, which together deliver oxygen to the alveolar capillary membrane for exchange.

The carotid pulse should be checked to assess circulation, "C," following the four quick breaths. The rescuer should attempt to palpate a spontaneous carotid pulse (femoral pulse is an acceptable alternative in the infant). If there is no palpable carotid pulse, a single firm precordial thump should be delivered. The thump will generate approximately 25 joules of energy and successfully cardiovert up to 25% of patients with ventricular fibrillation to a rhythm-producing cardiac output and thus a palpable carotid pulse. External cardiac compression should be initiated when no spontaneous pulse is present following the precordial thump. The heart serves as a passive conduit with blood flow resulting from the intrathoracic pressure changes produced during external chest compressions. When applied properly, external cardiac compressions can generate a cardiac output approaching 30% of normal.[17–19] When applied promptly and efficiently, external cardiac compressions support perfusion and oxygenation to vital organs until spontaneous circulation is reestablished.

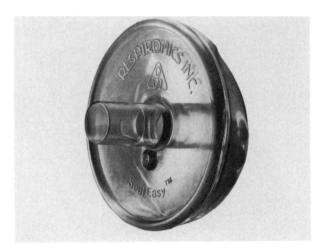

FIGURE 38.1 **Pocket mask, which aids ventilation procedures in CPR. (Courtesy Respironics, Inc., Monroeville, PA.)**

TABLE 38.1
Basic Emergency Equipment and Drugs

Item	Description
Airway	Oral, resuscitation mask, Ambu bag
Oxygen	With appropriate delivery tubing
Blood pressure cuff	
Drugs	Epinephrine 1:1000 injectable
	Diphenhydramine injectable
	Isoproterenol or metaproterenol inhaler

The time-critical nature of CPR must be recognized. Irreversible brain death occurs within 4 to 6 minutes from the cessation of cerebral perfusion. Variables such as body age, body temperature, certain drugs, and coexistent disease may modify tolerance of the brain to ischemia. However, the overriding consideration for the practitioner confronted with the unresponsive patient remains the prompt institution of measures for the support of breathing and circulation.

Adjunctive measures, including mechanical devices and drugs (Table 38.1), are used in keeping with statutory limitations imposed on the practitioner, availability of EMS resources, and the interest and commitment of the practitioner.[17,20,21] Commercially available kits (Fig. 38.2)

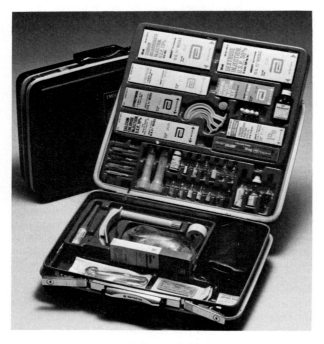

FIGURE 38.2 **Commercially available emergency drug kit. (Courtesy Banyan International Corporation, Abilene, TX)**

can be useful in an office setting where immediate access to equipment is essential. It must be reemphasized, however, that the critical element in the overall approach is the trained rescuer, and that basic CPR requires essentially no adjunctive equipment. Nevertheless, current concerns for disease transmission dictate the availability of a one-way valved pocket mask to prevent delays in instituting CPR.[22]

The institution of basic cardiopulmonary resuscitation is designed as an emergency measure before EMS personnel have arrived. What, then, is the responsibility of the practitioner in health care settings where cardiopulmonary arrest might reasonably be expected to occur on an infrequent basis? He or she should: (1) obtain cardiopulmonary certification, (2) provide cardiopulmonary resuscitation training for all office personnel, (3) maintain proficiency in the recognition and treatment of cardiopulmonary arrest by periodic retraining, and (4) educate office personnel about available EMS resources and how to activate these resources in an emergency.

References

1. Austen KF. Systemic anaphylaxis in the human being. N Engl J Med 1974;291:661–664.
2. Bristow MR, Ginsburg R, Harrison DC. Histamine and the human heart: The other receptor system. Am J Cardiol 1982;49:249–251.
3. Criep LH, Woehler TR. The heart in human anaphylaxis. Ann Allergy 1971;29:399–408.
4. Elenbaas RM. Anaphylactic shock. Crit Care 1980;2:77–84.
5. Hanashiro PK, Weil MH. Anaphylactic shock in man: Report of two cases with detailed hemodynamic and metabolic studies. Arch Intern Med 1967;119:129–139.
6. Lucke WC, Thomas H. Anaphylaxis: Pathophysiology, clinical presentations and treatment. J Emerg Med 1983;1:83–95.
7. Lockey RF, Bukantz SC. Allergic emergencies. Med Clin North Am 1974;58:147–156.
8. Ricker JG, Cacace LG. Double blind comparison of metaproterenol and isoetharine-phenylephrine solutions in intermittent positive pressure: Breathing in bronchospastic conditions. Chest 1980;78:723–725.
9. Kaliner M. Four immunologic mechanisms for release of chemical mediators of anaphylaxis from human lung tissue. Can Med Assoc J 1974;110:431–435.
10. American Heart Association. Heart attack: Signals and actions for survival. Dallas: 1976.
11. Feinleib M, Simon AB, Gillum RF, et al. Prodromal symptoms and signs of sudden death. Circulation 1975;52(suppl 3):155–159.
12. Simon RP. Coma. In: Ho MT, Saunders CE, eds. Current emergency diagnosis and treatment. Norwalk, CT: Appleton and Lange, 1990;77–92.
13. Baker, FJ II, Stauss R, Walter JJ. Cardiac arrest. In: Rosen P, Baker FJ II, et al, eds. Emergency medicine: Concepts and clinical practice. St. Louis: C.V. Mosby Co, 1988;83–141.
14. Caldwell G, Millar G, Quinn E, et al. Simple mechanical methods for cardioversion: Defense of the precordial thump and cough version. Br Med J 1985;291:627–630.

15. Criley JM, Neimann JT, Rosborough JP, et al. The heart is a conduit in CPR. Crit Care Med 1981;9:373–374.

16. Criley JM, Ung S, Neimann JT. What is the role of newer methods of cardiopulmonary resuscitation? Cardiovasc Clin 1983;13:297–307.

17. American Heart Association. Standards and guidelines for cardiopulmonary resuscitation (CPR) and emergency cardiac care (ECC). JAMA 1986;255:2905–2984.

18. Taylor GJ, Rubin R, Ticker M, et al. External cardiac compression. A randomized comparison of mechanical and manual techniques. JAMA 1978;240:644–646.

19. McDonald J. Systolic and mean arterial pressures during manual and mechanical CPR in humans. Ann Emerg Med 1982;11:292–295.

20. Goldberg A. Current concepts, cardiopulmonary arrest. N Engl J Med 1974;290:5.

21. Harris LC, Kirimli B, Safar P. Augmentation of artificial circulation during cardiopulmonary resuscitation. Anesthesiology 1967;28:730–734.

22. Centers for Disease Control. Recommendations for preventing transmission of infection with HIV during invasive procedures. MMWR 1986;35:221–223.

23. Dahlöf C, Mellstrand T, Svedmyr N. Systemic absorption of adrenaline after aerosol, eye-drop and subcutaneous administration to healthy volunteers. Allergy 1987;42:215–221.

Index

Note: Page numbers in italics indicate figures; page numbers followed by t indicate tables. Single drugs are listed under their generic names; trade names appear in small capitals and refer the reader to the generic name for the drug. Drug combinations are listed under their trade names.